Physical Rehabilitation

Physical Rehabilitation

FIFTH EDITION

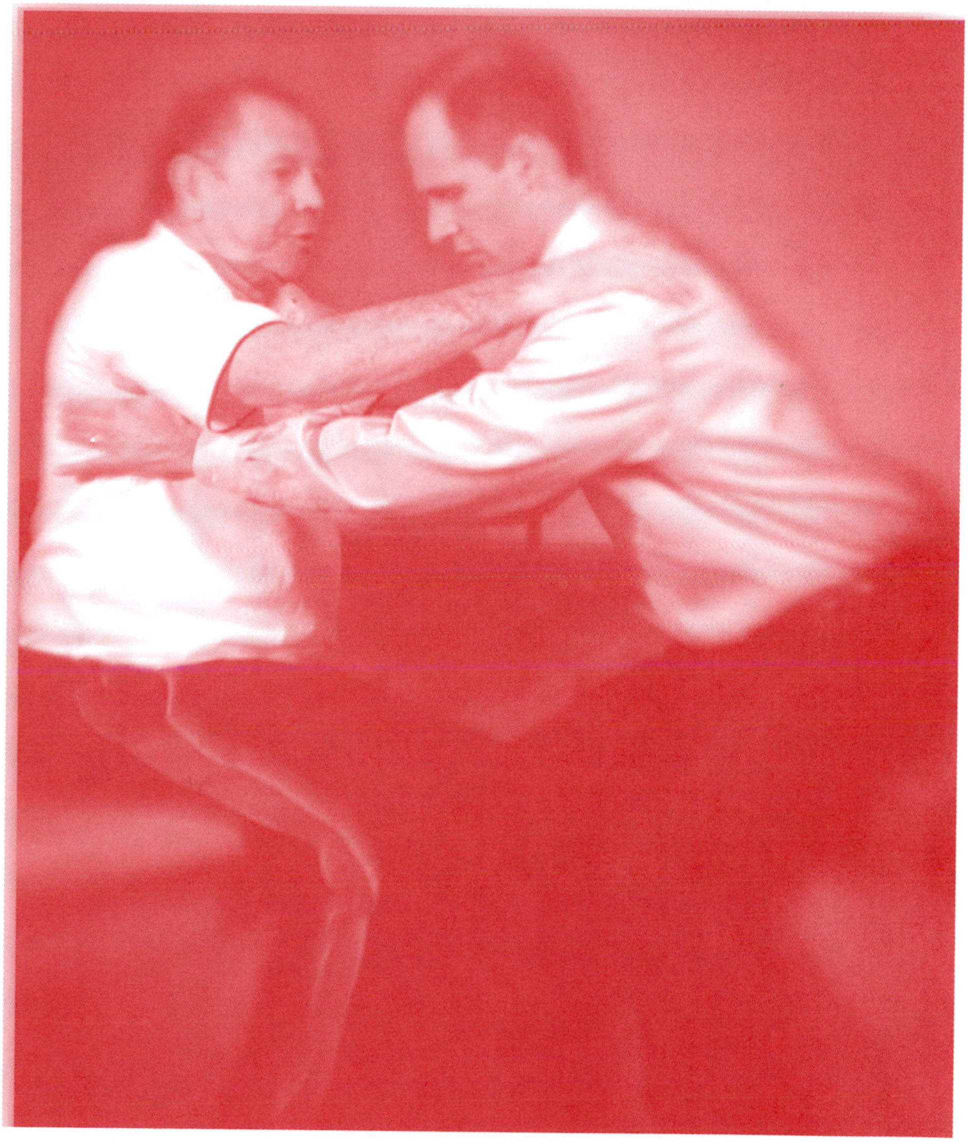

Susan B. O'Sullivan, PT, EdD
Professor and Chair
Department of Physical Therapy
School of Health and Environment
University of Massachusetts Lowell
Lowell, Massachusetts

Thomas J. Schmitz, PT, PhD
Professor
Division of Physical Therapy
School of Health Professions
Long Island University
Brooklyn Campus
Brooklyn, New York

F. A. DAVIS COMPANY • Philadelphia

F.A. Davis Company
1915 Arch Street
Philadelphia, PA 19103
www.fadavis.com

Printed in the United States of America

Last digit indicates print number: 10 9 8 7 6 5

Acquisitions Editor: Margaret Biblis
Manager, Content Development: Deborah Thorp
Developmental Editor: Jennifer Pine
Design Manager: Carolyn O'Brien
Photographer: Jaime Eric Eisman, ASMP
Models: Frank J. Ciuba, DPT, MS; Clifford Weller

Library of Congress Cataloging-in-Publication Data

Physical rehabilitation/[edited by] Susan B. O'Sullivan, Thomas J. Schmitz.—5th ed.
p. ; cm.
Includes bibliographical references and index.
ISBN-13: 978-0-8036-1247-1
ISBN-10: 0-8036-1247-8
1. Physical therapy. I. O'Sullivan, Susan B. II. Schmitz, Thomas J.
[DNLM: 1. Physical Therapy Modalities. 2. Disability Evaluation. WB 460 P57763 2007]
RM700.O88 2007
615.8′2—dc22
2006019334

Preface

With the fifth edition of *Physical Rehabilitation*, we continue a tradition of striving for excellence that began more than 20 years ago. We are gratified by the continuing wide acceptance of *Physical Rehabilitation* by both faculty and students.

The text is designed to provide a comprehensive approach to the rehabilitation management of adult patients. As such, it is intended to serve as a primary textbook for professional-level physical therapy students, and as an important resource for practicing therapists as well as for other rehabilitation professionals. This fifth edition recognizes the continuing growth of the profession and integrates basic and applied clinical research to guide and inform evidence-based clinical practice. It also integrates terminology, practice patterns, specific tests and measures, and interventions presented in the American Physical Therapy Association's *Guide to Physical Therapist Practice*.

Physical Rehabilitation is organized into four sections. Section One (Chapters 1–3) provides an introduction to patient care and includes chapters on clinical decision making, psychosocial factors, and values. Section Two (Chapters 4–12) focuses on examination of the sensory, motor, and cardiovascular systems as well as examination of functional status and the environment. Section Three (Chapters 13–30) addresses the common diseases, disorders, or conditions seen in the rehabilitation setting. Appropriate examination and intervention strategies are discussed for related impairments, functional limitations, and disabilities. Emphasis is placed also on parameters of learning critical to ensuring the patient/client can achieve an independent and active lifestyle. The final section, Section Four (Chapters 31–33) includes orthotics, prosthetics, and the prescriptive wheelchair.

A central element of the text is a strong pedagogical format designed to facilitate and reinforce the learning of key concepts. Each chapter of *Physical Rehabilitation* includes an initial content outline, learning objectives, an introduction and summary, study questions for self-assessment, and extensive references. Additional supplemental readings and recommended resources are also provided. Key terms are bolded throughout each chapter indicating their inclusion in a master glossary toward the end of the text. Application of important concepts is promoted through case study examples and problem-oriented guiding questions. New to the fifth edition, many chapters contain *Evidence Summary Boxes* that summarize and critically appraise research focused on a particular topic or intervention relevant to the chapter content. Our hope is that the boxes may provide a model for readers to continue to critically examine clinical practice using validated clinical methodologies. We also hope it will inspire enthusiasm about the importance of continuous, lifelong self-directed learning, without which practice may become rapidly and dangerously out-of-date.

The visual illustrations have been substantially enhanced with the addition of many new line drawings and photographs. Changes in design and the introduction of a two-color format provide a more reader-friendly environment as well as augment understanding of content.

Without question, our greatest asset in preparing the 5th edition of *Physical Rehabilitation* has been an outstanding group of contributing authors. We are most fortunate to have this group of talented individuals whose breadth and scope of professional knowledge and experience seems unparalleled. These individuals are recognized experts from a variety of specialty areas who have graciously shared their knowledge and clinical practice expertise by providing relevant, up-to-date, and practical information within their respective content areas.

The fifth edition has also benefited from the input of numerous individuals engaged in both academic and clinical practice settings who have used and reviewed the content. We are grateful for their constructive feedback and have instituted many of their suggestions and changes. As always, we welcome suggestions for improvements from our colleagues and students.

As physical therapists continue to take on more and greater professional responsibilities and challenges, the very nature of this text makes it a perpetual "work in progress." We are grateful for the opportunity to contribute to the academic literature in physical therapy as well as to the professional development of those preparing to enter a career devoted to improving the quality of life of those we serve.

We acknowledge the very important contributions that physical therapists make in the lives of their patients. This book is dedicated to those therapists—past, present, and future—who guide and challenge their patients to lead a successful and independent life.

Susan B. O'Sullivan
Thomas J. Schmitz

Acknowledgments

The on-going development of *Physical Rehabilitation* has been in all aspects a collaborative venture. Its fruition made possible only through the expertise and gracious contributions of many talented individuals. Our appreciation is considerable.

Heartfelt thanks are extended to our contributing authors. Each has brought a unique body of knowledge as well as distinct clinical practice expertise to their respective chapters. Their commitment to physical therapist education is collectively displayed in content presentations that carefully reflect the scope of knowledge and skills required of a dynamic, evolving physical therapy practice environment. We are extremely grateful to each of our contributors as well as heartened by the excellence they bring to the fifth edition.

Our gratitude is also extended to our guest editors and reviewers. Their collective expertise provided critical input during various phases of project development. We are particularly indebted to them for their content suggestions, pedagogical insights, and unconditional positive regard for the academic pursuits of physical therapy students.

We thank those individuals and companies who contributed new photographs to the individual chapters and to those patients/clients who allowed their photographs to be used throughout the text.

Our appreciation goes to the dedicated professionals at F.A. Davis Company, Philadelphia, PA: Margaret M. Biblis, Publisher, Jennifer A. Pine, Developmental Editor, Bob Butler, Production Manager, and Ron Moser, Marketing Manager. These individuals are recognized for their continued support, encouragement, and unwavering commitment to excellence. We would also like to thank Jean-Francois Vilain, Former Publisher, FA Davis, for his support throughout previous editions of this text. Thanks also are extended to Berta Steiner, Director of Production, Bermedica Production Ltd, and to Deborah Lynam for her considerable talents in preparing many of the new line illustrations.

We wish to thank the numerous students, faculty, and clinicians who over the years have used *Physical Rehabilitation* and provided us with meaningful and constructive comments that have greatly enhanced this edition. It is our sincere hope that this feedback will continue with the fifth edition.

Our thanks go also to the following individuals who provided assistance during different phases of the project: Diana Agoston, Elizabeth Blas, Ryanne Glasper, Ellen Godwin, Kim Harris, Cristiana Kahl Collins, Katherine Li, Mary Maloney, Eileen McAulay, Michele Mills, Evangelos Pappas, Alexander Rosado, Alexis Sams, and Gideon F. Shapiro. A particular note of thanks is extended to Stephen A. Caronia who contributed several Evidence Summary Boxes as well as considerable editorial assistance; to Alisa Yalan-Murphy, Faculty Liaison, Faculty Media Resource Center, Long Island University, for her great patience in creating many high quality photographs; and to Ivaldo Costa whose support has truly been immeasurable.

Finally, we are grateful for the continuing strong and productive working relationship that we maintain that has allowed us to complete a project of this scope through five editions.

Susan B. O'Sullivan
Thomas J. Schmitz

Guest Editors

Sharon A. Gutman, PhD, OTR
Associate Professor
Columbia University
Programs in Occupational Therapy
New York, New York

Raymond Marx, CPO, FAAOP
President
Ortho-Bionics Laboratory, Inc.
South Ozone Park, New York

Anne Hiller Scott, PhD, OTR, FAOTA
Associate Professor
Division of Occupational Therapy
School of Health Professions
Long Island University
Brooklyn Campus
Brooklyn, New York

Contributing Authors

Andrea L. Behrman, PT, PhD
Associate Professor
Department of Physical Therapy
University of Florida
Gainesville, Florida

Research Health Scientist
VA Brain Rehabilitation Research Center
Malcom Randall VA Medical Center
Gainesville, Florida

Adrienne Falk Bergen, PT, ATP
Seating Specialist
Delray Beach, Florida

Lisa Janice Cohen, PT, MS, OCS
The Body Mind Integration Center
Watertown, Massachusetts

Vanina Dal Bello-Haas, BScPT, PhD
Associate Professor
School of Physical Therapy
University of Saskatchewan
Saskatoon, Saskatchewan
Canada

Carol M. Davis, PT, EdD, MS, FAPTA
Professor and Assistant Chair
Department of Physical Therapy
University of Miami Miller School of Medicine
Coral Gables, Florida

John L. Echternach, PT, EdD, ECS, FAPTA
Professor and Eminent Scholar
School of Physical Therapy
Old Dominion University
Norfolk, Virginia

Joan E. Edelstein, PT, MA, FISPO
Special Lecturer
Program in Physical Therapy
Columbia University
New York, New York

George D. Fulk, PT, PhD
Assistant Professor
Department of Physical Therapy
Clarkson University
Potsdam, New York

Kate Grimes, DPT, MS, CCS
Clinical Assistant Professor
Graduate Programs in Physical Therapy
MGH Institute of Health Professions
Boston, Massachusetts

Andrew A. Guccione, DPT, PhD, FAPTA
Senior Vice President
Practice and Research Division
American Physical Therapy Association
Alexandria, Virginia

Deborah Graffis Kelly, PT, MSEd
Associate Professor
Division of Physical Therapy
University of Kentucky
Lexington, Kentucky

Bella J. May, PT, EdD, FAPTA
Professor Emerita
Medical College of Georgia
Augusta, Georgia

President, BJM Enterprises
Dublin, California

Marian A. Minor, PT, PhD
Professor and Chair
Department of Physical Therapy
School of Health Professions
University of Missouri
Columbia, Missouri

Cynthia C. Norkin, PT, EdD
Former Director and Associate Professor
School of Physical Therapy
Ohio University
Athens, Ohio

Sandra J. Olney, BSc (P & OT), MEd, PhD
Professor and Director
School of Rehabilitation Therapy
Queen's University
Kingston, Ontario
Canada

Susan B. O'Sullivan, PT, EdD
Professor and Chair
Department of Physical Therapy
School of Health and Environment
University of Massachusetts Lowell
Lowell, Massachusetts

Leslie G. Portney, DPT, PhD, FAPTA
Professor and Director
Graduate Programs in Physical Therapy
MGH Institute of Health Professions
Boston, Massachusetts

Pat Precin, OTR/L, MS, ABD
Assistant Professor
Department of Occupational Therapy
New York Institute of Technology
Old Westbury, New York

Executive Director
The Fostering Connection, Inc.
Brooklyn, New York

Consultant
Pathways to Housing, Inc.
New York, New York

Reginald L. Richard, PT, MS
Burn Clinical Specialist
Physical Therapy Department
Miami Valley Hospital Regional Burn Center
Dayton, Ohio

Serge H. Roy, PT, ScD
Research Professor
NeuroMuscular Research Center
Boston University
Boston, Massachusetts

Martha Taylor Sarno, MA, MD (hon)
Professor of Rehabilitation Medicine
School of Medicine
New York University
New York, New York

Director
Speech-Language Pathology Department
Rusk Institute of Rehabilitation Medicine
New York University Medical Center
New York, New York

David A. Scalzitti, PT, MS, OCS
Associate Director
Research Services
American Physical Therapy Association
Alexandria, Virginia

Thomas J. Schmitz, PT, PhD
Professor
Division of Physical Therapy
School of Health Professions
Long Island University
Brooklyn Campus
Brooklyn, New York

Michael C. Schubert, PT, PhD
Assistant Professor
The Department of Otolaryngology Head and Neck Surgery
Johns Hopkins University School of Medicine
Baltimore, Maryland

Julie Ann Starr, PT, MS, CCS
Clinical Associate Professor
Department of Physical Therapy and Athletic Training
Sargent College of Health and Rehabilitation Sciences
Boston University
Boston, Massachusetts

Carolyn A. Unsworth, OTR, PhD
Associate Professor
School of Occupational Therapy
La Trobe University
Bundoora, Victoria
Australia

R. Scott Ward, PT, PhD
Professor and Chair
Division of Physical Therapy
University of Utah
Salt Lake City, Utah

D. Joyce White, PT, DSc
Associate Professor
Department of Physical Therapy
School of Health and Environment
University of Massachusetts Lowell
Lowell, Massachusetts

Reviewers

Candy Bahner, PT, MS
Director and Assistant Professor
Physical Therapist Assistant Program
Washburn University
Topeka, Kansas

Marja Beaufait, PT, MA
Associate Professor
Physical Therapist Assistant Program
St. Petersburg College
St. Petersburg, Florida

Wendy Bircher, PT, EdD
Director
Physical Therapist Assistant Program
San Juan College
Farmington, New Mexico

Jill W. Bloss, PT, MPH
Former Associate Professor
Physical Therapy Program
Nazareth College
Rochester, New York

Kathy Brewer PT, MEd, GCS
Adjunct Faculty
Department of Physical Therapy
Arizona School of Health Sciences
A.T. Still University
Mesa, Arizona

Suzanne Robben Brown, PT, MPH
Director and Associate Professor
Department of Physical Therapy
Arizona School of Health Sciences
A.T. Still University
Mesa, Arizona

Alice F. Cain, PT
Clinical Coordinator
Physical Therapist Assistant Technology
Stark State College
North Canton, Ohio

Susan D. Calise, PT, MA
Brookdale Department of Geriatrics and Adult Development
Mount Sinai School of Medicine
New York, New York

Sean M. Collins, PT, ScD, CCS
Associate Professor
Department of Physical Therapy
School of Health and Environment
University of Massachusetts Lowell
Lowell, Massachusetts

Sam M. Coppoletti, MPT, BS, CSCS
Director and Assistant Professor
Physical Therapist Assistant Program
Shawnee State University
Portsmouth, Ohio

Linda Denney, PT, M.Appl.Sci. (Manip)
Adjunct Assistant Professor
Department of Physical Therapy
Arizona School of Health Sciences
A.T. Still University
Mesa, Arizona

George D. Fulk, PT, PhD
Assistant Professor
Department of Physical Therapy
Clarkson University
Potsdam, New York

Christine Kowalski, PTA, EdD
Director
Physical Therapist Assistant Program
Great Falls College of Technology
Montana State University
Great Falls, Montana

Steven G. Lesh, PT, PhD, MPA, SCS, ATC
Chair and Associate Professor
Department of Physical Therapy
Southwest Baptist University
Bolivar, Missouri

Marilyn Maxwell, PhD
Instructor, English Department
Hewlett High School
Hewlett, New York

Kathy Mercuris, PT, MGS
Former Associate Professor
Division of Physical Therapy
Des Moines University-Osteopathic Medical Center
Des Moines, Iowa

Robert J. Nelson, PT, MS, MPhil
H & D Physical Therapy
New York, New York

Susan Roehrig, PT, PhD
Associate Professor
Program in Physical Therapy
Arkansas State University
Jonesboro, Arkansas

Lynda L. Spangler, PT, MS, ACCE
Assistant Professor
Department of Physical Therapy
The College of St. Scholastica
Duluth, Minnesota

Doreen Stiskal, PT, PhD
Assistant Chair
Graduate Programs in Health Sciences
Seton Hall University
South Orange, New Jersey

Kristin von Nieda, DPT, MEd
Associate Professor
Director, Transitional DPT Program
Department of Physical Therapy
Temple University
Philadelphia, Pennsylvania

Denise Wise, PT, PhD
Chair and Assistant Professor
Department of Physical Therapy
The College of St. Scholastica
Duluth, Minnesota

Peter Zawicki, PT, MS
Director
Physical Therapist Assistant Program
Gateway Community College
Phoenix, Arizona

Table of Contents

Section Three: Intervention Strategies for Rehabilitation 469

S E C T I O N   O N E

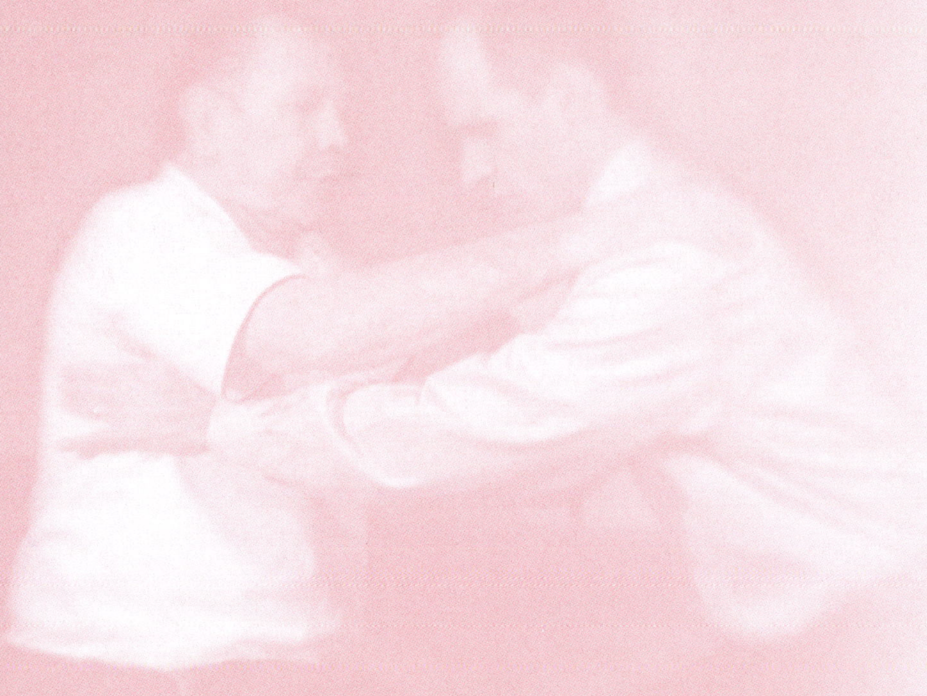

Introduction to Patient Care: Decision Making, Psychosocial Factors, and Values

CHAPTER

1

Clinical Decision Making

Susan B. O'Sullivan, PT, EdD

LEARNING OBJECTIVES

1. Define clinical reasoning. What factors impact on clinical decision making?
2. Describe the key steps in the patient/client management process.
3. Define the major responsibilities of the physical therapist in planning effective treatments.
4. Identify potential problems that could adversely affect the physical therapist's clinical reasoning.
5. Discuss strategies to ensure patient participation in the plan of care.
6. Discuss the importance of evidence-based practice in developing the plan of care.
7. Identify key elements of physical therapy documentation.
8. Differentiate between expert versus novice therapist clinical decision making.
9. Analyze and interpret patient/client data, formulate realistic goals and outcomes, and develop a plan of care when presented with a clinical case study.

OUTLINE

Clinical Reasoning/Clinical Decision Making

Clinical reasoning is a multidimensional process that involves a wide range of cognitive skills physical therapists use to process information, reach decisions, and determine actions. Reasoning can be viewed as an internal dialogue that one continuously employs while meeting the challenges of daily life; clinical reasoning forms the basis of patient/client management. A number of factors influence the clinical reasoning process. The clinician's goals, values and beliefs, psychosocial skills, knowledge base and expertise, problem-solving strategies, and procedural skills all impact on clinical reasoning. Many of these factors are the focus of discussion in later chapters in this text. Clinical reasoning is also influenced by patient/client characteristics (goals, values and beliefs, physical, psychosocial, educational, and cultural factors) as well as environmental factors (clinical practice environment, overall resources, time, level of financial support, level of social support). Experienced or expert clinicians tend to utilize a *forward reasoning process* in which the clinician is able to recognize cues and patterns as similar to previously identified cases. Decisions are formulated based on intuition. Hypothesis testing is not typically verbalized. Thus, actions are based on pattern recognition and experiential clinical knowledge. In contrast, a *backwards reasoning process* (also termed hypothetico-deductive process) is likely to be utilized by the novice or inexperienced clinician. This involves identifying cues, proposing a hypothesis, gathering supporting data and evaluating the hypothesis, and determining appropriate actions. Experts may use hypothesis-testing methods when routine problem recognition fails or they are practicing out of their area of expertise.[1]

Rothstein and Echternach developed a Hypothesis-Oriented Algorithm for Clinicians (HOAC) in 1986[2] and revised it in 2003 as the Hypothesis-Oriented Algorithm for Clinicians II (HOAC II).[3] An algorithm is a step-by-step guide designed to assist clinicians in decision making. It is based on specific clinical problems and identifies the decision steps and possible choices for remediation of a problem. A series of questions are posed, typically in yes/no format, addressing whether the measurements met testing criteria, the hypotheses generated were viable, goals were met, strategies were appropriate, and tactics were implemented correctly. Hypotheses are defined as the underlying reasons for the patient's problems, representing the therapist's conjecture as to the cause. Problems are defined in terms of functional limitations. A "no" response to any of the questions posed in an algorithm is an indication for reevaluation of the viability of the hypotheses generated and reconsideration of the decisions made. In using HOAC II as a model for clinical decision making, the therapist also distinguishes between existing problems and anticipated problems, defined as deficits that are likely to occur if an intervention is not used for prevention. The value of an algorithm is that it guides the therapist's decisions and provides an outline of the decisions made. See Chapter 20, Figures 20.8 to 20.10, for examples of problem-centered algorithms.

Clinical decisions are the outcomes of the clinical reasoning process. Physical therapists today practice in complex environments and are called upon to reach increasingly complex decisions under significant practice constraints. For example, the therapist may be required to determine a plan of care for the complicated patient with multiple comorbidities within 72 hours of admission to a rehabilitation facility. Reduced levels of treatment authorization with shorter and shorter stays in rehabilitation also complicate the decision making process. Novice practitioners can easily become overwhelmed. This chapter introduces a framework for patient/client management that can assist in organizing and prioritizing data and in planning effective treatments compatible with the needs and goals of the patient/client and members of the health care team. The disablement model has been widely incorporated into physical therapy practice and into the Guide to Physical Therapist Practice.[4] It provides an important framework for decision making. Evidence-based practice is another important element of decision making that allows the clinician to utilize research findings to inform and validate decision choices. Later chapters focus on interpreting and integrating the knowledge base with the framework for decision making needed to manage specific clinical problems and disabilities.

Steps in Patient/Client Management

Steps in patient/client management include: (1) examination of the patient; (2) evaluation of the data and identification of problems; (3) determination of the diagnosis; (4) determination of the prognosis and plan of care (POC); (5) implementation of the POC; and (6) reexamination of the patient and evaluation of treatment outcomes (Fig. 1.1).

Step 1. Examination

Examination involves identifying and defining the patient's problem(s) and the resources available to determine appropriate intervention. It consists of three components: the patient history, a review of relevant systems, and tests and measures. Examination begins with patient referral or initial entry, and continues as an ongoing process throughout the course of rehabilitation. Reexamination allows the therapist to evaluate progress and modify interventions as appropriate.[4]

History

Information about the patient's past history and current health status is obtained from review of the medical record and interviews. The medical record provides detailed reports from members of the health care team; processing these reports requires an understanding of disease and injury, medical terminology, differential diagnosis, laboratory and other diagnostic tests, and medical management. The use of resource material or professional consultation can assist the novice clinician. The types of data that may be generated from a patient history are presented in Figure 1.2.

The interview is an important tool used to obtain information directly from the patient, family, significant others, caregivers, and other interested persons. The therapist asks the patient to provide general information including past and present medical conditions/complications, mechanism of injury, prior diagnostic imaging/testing, medications, and prior surgical and therapy history. The patient is asked to describe his or her current condition/problem(s) and primary complaint (reason for referral to physical therapy). Typically the patient will describe his or her difficulties in terms of functional limitations or disabilities. The patient is then asked a series of questions designed to delineate the nature and history of the current condition/primary complaint. The therapist also needs to determine the patient's age, gender, ethnicity, primary language, cultural background, customs or religious beliefs that might affect care, educational level, social/health habits (e.g., smoking history, alcohol use, exercise likes and dislikes, frequency and intensity of regular activity), and family history. Sample interview questions are included in Box 1.1.

Pertinent information can also be obtained from the patient's family or caregiver. For example, patients with central nervous system deficit and severe cognitive and/or communication deficits or pediatric patients will be unable to accurately communicate their existing problems. The family member/caregiver then assumes the primary role of assisting the therapist in identifying problems and providing relevant aspects of the history.

The therapist should be sensitive to differences in culture and ethnicity that may influence how the patient or family member responds during the interview or examination process. Different beliefs and attitudes toward health care may influence how cooperative the patient will be. During the interview, the therapist should listen carefully to what the patient says. The patient should be observed for

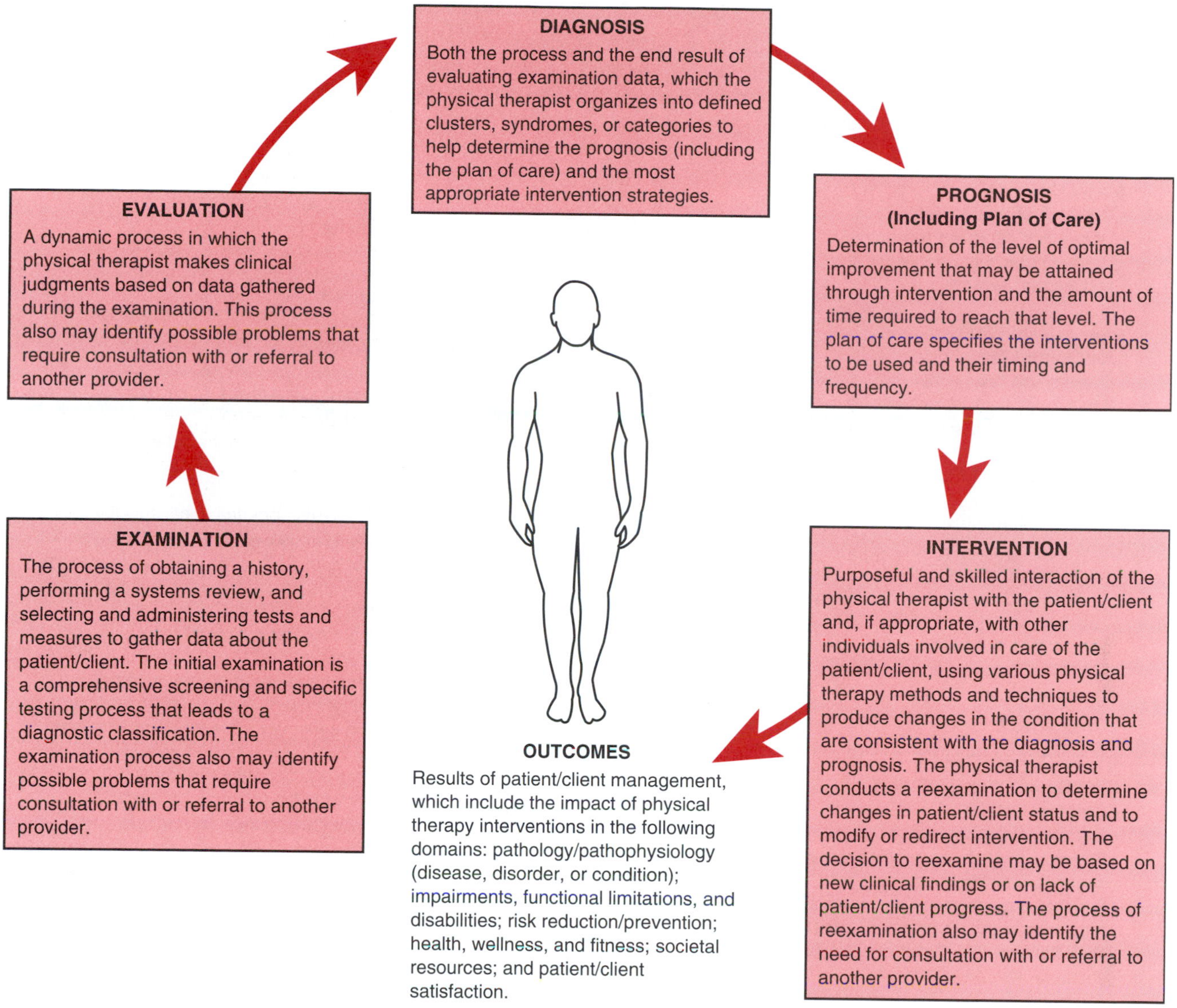
DIAGNOSIS
Both the process and the end result of evaluating examination data, which the physical therapist organizes into defined clusters, syndromes, or categories to help determine the prognosis (including the plan of care) and the most appropriate intervention strategies.
EVALUATION
A dynamic process in which the physical therapist makes clinical judgments based on data gathered during the examination. This process also may identify possible problems that require consultation with or referral to another provider.
PROGNOSIS
(Including Plan of Care)
Determination of the level of optimal improvement that may be attained through intervention and the amount of time required to reach that level. The plan of care specifies the interventions to be used and their timing and frequency.
EXAMINATION
The process of obtaining a history, performing a systems review, and selecting and administering tests and measures to gather data about the patient/client. The initial examination is a comprehensive screening and specific testing process that leads to a diagnostic classification. The examination process also may identify possible problems that require consultation with or referral to another provider.
INTERVENTION
Purposeful and skilled interaction of the physical therapist with the patient/client and, if appropriate, with other individuals involved in care of the patient/client, using various physical therapy methods and techniques to produce changes in the condition that are consistent with the diagnosis and prognosis. The physical therapist conducts a reexamination to determine changes in patient/client status and to modify or redirect intervention. The decision to reexamine may be based on new clinical findings or on lack of patient/client progress. The process of reexamination also may identify the need for consultation with or referral to another provider.
OUTCOMES
Results of patient/client management, which include the impact of physical therapy interventions in the following domains: pathology/pathophysiology (disease, disorder, or condition); impairments, functional limitations, and disabilities; risk reduction/prevention; health, wellness, and fitness; societal resources; and patient/client satisfaction.

Figure 1.1 Elements of patient management leading to optimal outcomes. (From APTA Guide for Physical Therapist Practice,[4, p. 35] with permission.)

any physical manifestations that reveal emotional context, such as slumped body posture, grimacing facial expression, poor eye contact, and so forth. Finally, the interview should be used to establish rapport, effective communication, and mutual trust. Patient cooperation serves to make the therapist's observations more valid and becomes crucial to the success of any rehabilitation plan of care.

Systems Review

The use of a brief **screening examination** allows the therapist to quickly scan the body systems and determine areas of intact function and dysfunction: cardiopulmonary, integumentary, musculoskeletal, and neuromuscular. Information is also obtained about communication, affect, cognition, and learning style. Areas of deficit confirm the need for further detailed examination by a physical therapist or referral to another health professional. Consultation with another physical therapist is appropriate if the needs of the patient/client are outside the scope of the expertise of the therapist assigned to the case. If the deficit is outside the scope of physical therapy, then referral to another health care provider is indicated.

Screening exams are also used for healthy populations. For example, the physical therapist can screen individuals to identify risk factors for disease such as decreased activity levels, stress, and obesity. Screening is also conducted in the case of pediatric clients (e.g., scoliosis screening), geriatric clients (e.g., to identify fall risk factors), athletes

General Demographics
- Age
- Sex
- Race/ethnicity
- Primary language
- Education

Social History
- Cultural beliefs and behaviors
- Family and caregiver resources
- Social interactions, social activities, and support system

Employment/Work (Job/School/Play)
- Current and prior work (job/school/play), community, and leisure actions, tasks, or activities

Growth and Development
- Developmental history
- Hand dominance

Living Environment
- Devices and equipment (eg, assistive, adaptive, orthotic, protective, supportive, prosthetic)
- Living environment and community characteristics
- Projected discharge destinations

General Health Status (Self-Report, Family Report, Caregiver Report)
- General health perception
- Physical function (eg, mobility, sleep patterns, restricted bed days)
- Psychological function (eg, memory, reasoning ability, depression, anxiety)
- Role function (eg, community, leisure, social, work)
- Social function (eg, social activity, social interaction, social support)

Social/health Habits (Past and Current)
- General health perception
- Physical function (eg, mobility, sleep patterns, restricted bed days)
- Psychological function (eg, memory, reasoning ability, depression, anxiety)
- Role function (eg, community, leisure, social, work)
- Social function (eg, social activity, social interaction, social support)

Family History
- Familial health risks

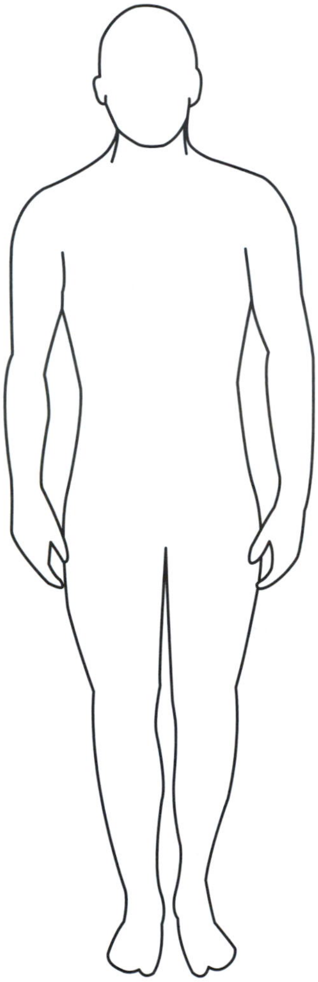

Medical/Surgical History
- Cardiovascular
- Endocrine/metabolic
- Gastrointestinal
- Genitourinary
- Gynecological
- Integumentary
- Musculoskeletal
- Neuromuscular
- Obstetrical
- Prior hospitalizations, surgeries, and preexisting medical and other health related conditions
- Psychological
- Pulmonary

Current Condtion(s)/ Chief Complaint(s)
- Concerns that led the patient/client to seek the services of a physical therapist
- Concerns or needs of patient/client who requires the services of a physical therapist
- Current therapeutic interventions
- Mechanisms of injury or disease, including date of onset and course of events
- Onset and patterns of symptoms
- Patient/client, family, significant other, and caregiver expectations and goals for the therapeutic intervention
- Previous occurence of chief complaint(s)
- Prior therapeutic interventions

Functional Status and Activity Level
- Current and prior functional status in self-care and home management, including activities of daily living (ADL) and instrumental activities of daily living (IADL)
- Current and prior functional status in work (job/school/play), community, and leisure actions, tasks, or activities

Medications
- Medications for current condition
- Medications previously taken for current condition
- Medications for other conditions

Other Clinical Tests
- Laboratory and diagnostic tests
- Review of available records (eg, medical, education, surgical)
- Review of other clinical findings (eg, nutrition and hydration)

Figure 1.2 Types of data that may be generated from patient history. (From APTA Guide for Physical Therapist Practice,[4, p 36] with permission.)

Box 1.1 Sample Interview Questions

I. Interview questions designed to identify the nature and history of the current problem(s):
   - What problems bring you to therapy?
   - When did the problem(s) begin?
   - What happened to precipitate the problem(s)?
   - How long has the problem(s) existed?
   - How are you taking care of the problem(s)?
   - What makes the problem(s) better?
   - What makes the problem(s) worse?
   - What are your goals and expectations for physical therapy?
   - Are you seeing anyone else for the problem(s)?

II. Interview questions designed to identify desired outcomes in terms of essential functional activities include:
   - What activities do you normally do at home/work/school?
   - What activities are you unable to do?
   - What activities are done differently and how are they different (i.e., extra time, extra effort, different strategy)?
   - What activities do you need help to perform that you would rather do yourself?
   - What leisure activities are important to you?
   - How can I help you be more independent?

III. Interview questions designed to identify environmental conditions in which patient activities typically occur include:
   - Describe your home/school/work environment.
   - How do you move around/access areas in the home (i.e., bathroom, bedroom, entering and exiting the home)? How safe do you feel?
   - How do you move around/access areas in the community (i.e., workplace, school, grocery store, shopping center, community center, stairs, curbs, ramps)? How safe do you feel?

IV. Interview questions designed to identify available social supports include:
   - Who lives with you?
   - Who assists in your care (i.e., Basic Activities of Daily Living [BADLs], Instrumental Activities of Daily Living [IADLs])?
   - Who helps you with the activities you want to do (i.e., walking, stairs, transfers)?
   - Are there activities you have difficulty with that would benefit from additional assistance?

V. Interview questions designed to identify the patient's knowledge of potential disablement risk factors include:
   - What problems might be anticipated in the future?
   - What can you do to eliminate or reduce the likelihood of that happening?

Sources: Section I: from the Documentation Template for Physical Therapist Patient/Client Management in the *Guide to Physical Therapist Practice*[4, pp 707–712]; Section II–IV adapted from Randall.[5, p 1200]

(e.g., pre-performance exams), and working adults (e.g., to identify the risk of musculoskeletal injuries in the workplace). These screens can involve any of the above steps: observation, chart review, oral history, and/or a brief examination. Additional screening exams may be mandated by institutional settings. For example, in a long-term care facility the therapist may be asked to review the chart for indications of changes in functional status or need for physical therapy, based on a review of the discharge notes from the prior acute care setting. The therapist makes a determination of the need for further physical therapy services based on an evaluation of the information obtained from the screening exam.[6]

Tests and Measures

More definitive tests and measures are used to provide objective data to accurately determine the degree of specific function and dysfunction (e.g., manual muscle test [MMT], range-of-motion [ROM] test, oxygen consumption, and so forth). Adequate training and skill in performing specific tests and measures are crucial in ensuring both validity and reliability of the tests. Failure to correctly perform an examination procedure can lead to the gathering of inaccurate data and the formation of an inappropriate plan of care. Later chapters focus on specific tests and measures and discuss issues of validity and reliability. The use of disability-specific standardized instruments (e.g., for individuals with stroke, the Fugl-Meyer Assessment of Physical Performance) can facilitate the examination process but may not always be appropriate for each individual patient. The therapist needs to carefully review the unique problems of the patient to determine the appropriateness and sensitivity of an instrument. Therapists should resist the tendency to gather excessive and extraneous data in the mistaken belief that more information is better. Unnecessary data will only confuse the picture, rendering clinical decision making more difficult and unnecessarily raising the cost of care. If problems arise that are not initially identified in the history or systems review, or if the data obtained are inconsistent, additional tests or measures may be indicated. Consultation with an experienced therapist can provide an important means to clarify inconsistencies and determine the appropriateness of specific tests and measures. Box 1.2 presents the categories for tests and measures identified in the Guide to Physical Therapist Practice.[4]

Step 2. Evaluation

Data gathered from the initial examination must then be analyzed and organized. Physical therapists must consider a number of factors when evaluating data, including the level of impairments, the degree of functional loss and disability, the patient's overall health and activity level, availability of social support systems, living environment, and potential discharge destination. Multisystem involvement,

Box 1.2 Categories for Tests and Measures

Aerobic Capacity/Endurance
Anthropometric Characteristics
Arousal, Attention, and Cognition
Assistive and Adaptive Devices
Circulation (Arterial, Venous, Lymphatic)
Cranial and Peripheral Nerve Integrity
Environmental, Home, and Work (Job/School/Play) Barriers
Ergonomics and Body Mechanics
Gait, Locomotion, and Balance
Integumentary Integrity
Joint Integrity and Mobility
Motor Function (Motor Control and Motor Learning)
Muscle Performance (Including Strength, Power, and Endurance)
Neuromotor Development and Sensory Integration
Orthotic, Protective, and Supportive Devices
Pain
Posture
Prosthetic Requirements
Range of Motion (Including Muscle Length)
Reflex Integrity
Self-Care and Home Management (Including Activities of Daily Living and Instrumental Activities of Daily Living)
Sensory Integrity
Ventilation and Respiration/Gas Exchange
Work (Job/School/Play), Community, and Leisure Integration or Reintegration (Including Instrumental Activities of Daily Living)

Adapted from APTA Guide for Physical Therapist Practice.[4]

severe impairment and functional loss, extended time of involvement (chronicity), comorbid conditions, and medical stability of the patient are important parameters that increase the difficulty and shape the decision making process.[4]

Disablement Terminology

Nagi used the terms pathology/pathophysiology, impairment, functional limitation, and disability to describe health status.[7–9] These terms can be used to categorize clinical observations systematically. **Disease** is "a pathological condition of the body or abnormal entity with a characteristic group of signs and symptoms that affect the body"[4, p 686] Etiology can be known or unknown. **Signs** are directly observable or measurable evidence of physical abnormality while **symptoms** are the more subjective reactions to the physical abnormality. **Impairments** (*direct*) are the result of pathology or disease states and include any loss or abnormality of physiologic, anatomic, or psychologic structure or function.[4] For a patient with stroke, examples of impairments that are the direct result of pathology might include sensory loss, paresis, dyspraxia, and hemianopsia. Impairments may or may not be permanent. **Secondary impairments** (*indirect*) are the sequelae or complications that originate from other systems.[4] They can result from preexisting impairments or the expanding multisystem dysfunction that occurs with prolonged inactivity, lack of adherence to suggested strategies/interventions, an ineffective plan of care, or lack of rehabilitation intervention. Examples of indirect impairments include decreased vital capacity, disuse atrophy and weakness, contractures, decubitus ulcers, deep venous thrombosis, renal calculi, urinary tract infections, pneumonia, and depression.

Functional limitation is defined as "the restriction of the ability to perform, at the level of the whole person, a physical action, task, or activity, in an efficient, typically expected, or competent manner."[4, p 687] Common functional limitations that might affect a person with stroke include limitations in the performance of locomotor tasks (gait), other basic mobility tasks (transfers), **basic activities of daily living** (BADLs: dressing, feeding, bathing), or **instrumental activities of daily living** (IADLs: housecleaning, preparing meals, shopping, telephoning, managing finances, and so forth). Thus functional limitations occur as a result of the inability to perform actions, tasks, and activities that constitute the "usual activities" for a given individual.

The term **disability** refers to societal rather than individual functioning. It is defined as an "inability to perform or a limitation in the performance of actions, tasks, and activities usually expected in specific social roles that are customary for the individual or expected for the person's status or role in a specific sociocultural context and physical environment. Categories of required roles included are self-care, home management, work (job/school/play), and community/leisure."[4,p 686] Thus the individual is unable to assume societal roles such as working, parenting, going to school, attending church or other group activities, or participating in leisure activities (sports, recreation, trips, and so forth).

The American Physical Therapy Association (APTA), in the *Guide to Physical Therapist Practice*,[4] as well as other professional bodies (National Advisory Board on Medical Rehabilitation Research[8]), have adopted Nagi's terminology framework. The World Health Organization has published a revised classification of its terminology, the International Classification of Impairments, Disabilities, and Handicaps (ICIDH-2).[9] Box 1.3 presents a guide to Disablement Terminology and is a compilation of these two sources. Clinical examples and applications of this terminology for decision making of patients with orthopedic and neurological dysfunction are evident in the physical therapy literature.[10–14]

Data obtained from functional examinations allow the therapist to determine functional limitations and disabilities. The level of performance is typically rated from complete independence to modified dependence to complete dependence. Figure 1.3 presents the Functional Independence Measure (FIM) levels of function and scoring rubric.[15] This instrument is used in the majority of rehabilitation

Box 1.3 Disablement Terminology

Activity: the nature and extent of functioning at the level of the person. Activities may be limited in nature, duration, and quality.[9]

Context: includes the features, aspects, attributes of, or objects, structures, human-made organization, service provision, and agencies in, the physical, social, and attitudinal environment in which people live and conduct their lives.[9]

Disability: inability to perform or a limitation in the performance of actions, tasks, and activities usually expected in specific social roles that are customary for the individual or expected for the person's status or role in a specific sociocultural context and physical environment. Categories of required roles are self-care, home management, work (job/school/play), and community/leisure.[4]

Disablement: an interaction/complex relationship between the health condition and the contextual factors (i.e., environmental and personal factors).[9]

Disease: a pathological condition of the body or abnormal entity with a characteristic group of signs and symptoms affecting the body and with known or unknown etiology.[4]

Function: those activities identified by an individual as essential to support physical, social, and psychological well-being and to create a personal sense of meaningful living.[4]

Functional limitation: the restriction of the ability to perform, at the level of the whole person, a physical action, task, or activity, in an efficient, typically expected, or competent manner.[4]

Health: state of complete physical, mental, and social well-being, and not merely the absence of disease and infirmity.

Health-related quality of life (HRQOL): the total effect of individual and environmental factors on function and health status; includes three major dimensions: physical function (BADLs, IADLs), psychological function, and social function.

Illness: forms of personal behavior that emerge as the reality of having a disease is internalized and experienced by an individual.

Impairment (direct): any loss or abnormality of anatomical, physiological, or psychological structure or function; the natural consequence of pathology or disease.[4]

Quality of life: the sense of total well-being that encompasses both the physical and psychosocial aspects of the patient's life.

Participation: the extent of a person's involvement in life situations in relation to impairments, activities, health condition, and contextual factors. Participation may be restricted in nature, duration and quality.[9]

Secondary impairment (indirect): sequelae or complications that originate from other systems, the result of preexisting impairments or expanding multisystem dysfunction.

Signs: directly observable or measurable changes in an individual's organs or systems as a result of pathology or disease.[4]

Symptoms: subjective evidence of physical abnormality the reactions to the changes experienced by an individual as a result of pathology or disease.[4]

Some terms from: (1) Guide to Physical Therapist Practice;[4] and (2) the International Classification of Impairments, Disabilities, and Handicaps (ICIDH-2).[9]

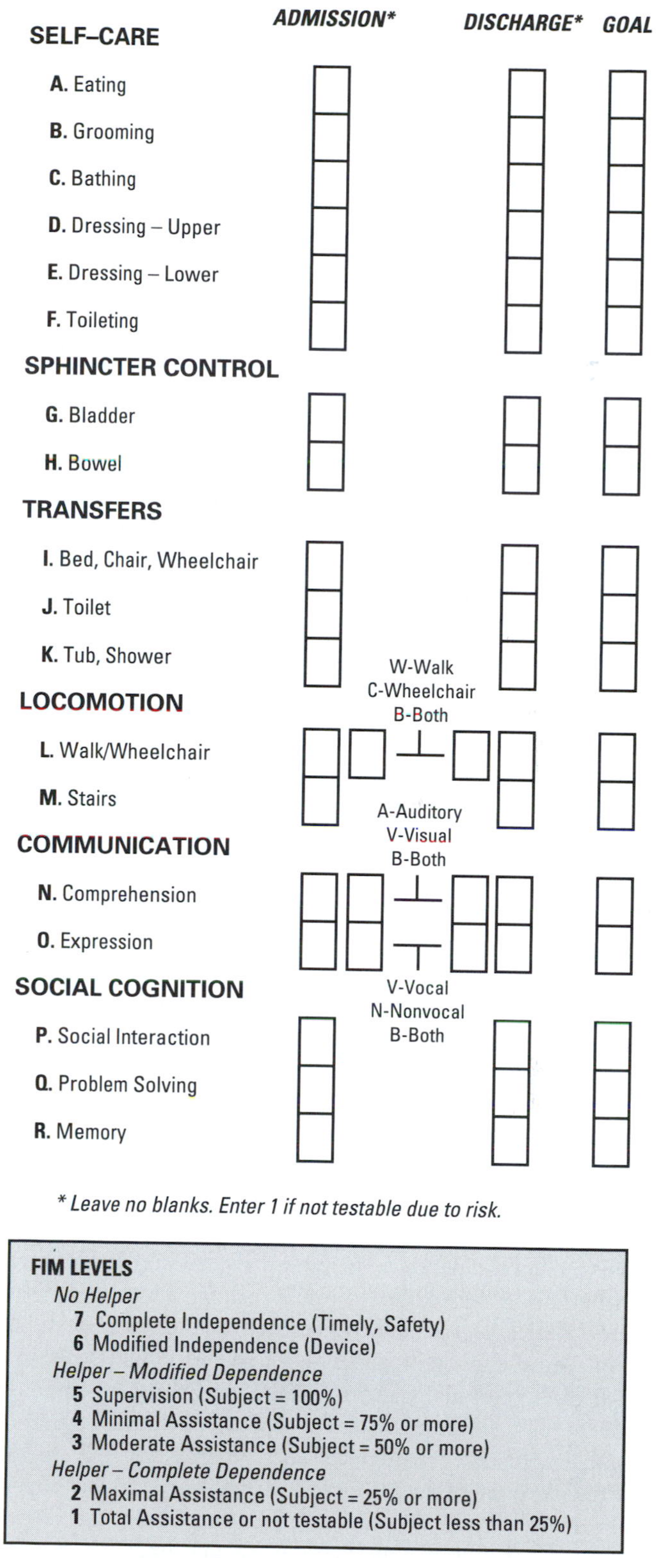

Figure 1.3 UDSmr[SM] FIM[SM] instrument. (Reprinted with permission of the Uniform Data System for Medical Rehabilitation, a division of U B Foundation Activities, Inc. [UDSmr[SM]]. Copyright 1996. Guide for the Uniform Data Set for Medical Rehabilitation [including the FIM[SM] instrument], Version 5.0. Buffalo, NY: State University of New York at Buffalo, 1996.)

facilities in the United States and is discussed more fully in Chapter 11.

Jette[14] suggests disablement risk factors and buffers should be evaluated. He defines **disablement risk factors** as behaviors, attributes, or environmental influences that increase the chances of developing impairments, functional limitations, or disability when an individual demonstrates an active pathology. For example, an individual may demonstrate predisposing characteristics (negative affect, psychosocial instability), demographics (limited financial/health resources, limited education), social and lifestyle factors (inadequate family support, disengaged life-style), or restrictive environment (numerous architectural barriers). **Buffers**, on the other hand, are defined as the actions or interventions on the part of the individual to resist the development of impairments, functional limitations, or disability. For example, an individual may adopt behaviors (positive attitudes, prayer, meditation) or helping strategies (use of adaptive equipment, peer support groups). Sometimes the strategies adopted are ineffective, leading to increased disablement (e.g., increased alcohol use).

Impairments, functional limitations, and disabilities must be analyzed to identify causal relationships. For example, shoulder pain in the patient with hemiplegia may be due to several factors, including hypotonicity and immobility, which are direct impairments, or soft tissue damage/trauma, which is an indirect impairment. Determining which of these factors is the primary cause of the problem is a difficult yet critical step in determining appropriate treatment interventions and resolving the patient's pain. An impairment may not be a major contributor to a patient's functional limitations and disability. Thus a plan of care that focuses on remediating the impairment is not likely to achieve successful clinical outcomes. Rather, the major focus of treatment should be on producing meaningful changes at the personal/social level by reducing functional limitations and disability. Achieving independence in ambulation or daily activities, return to work, or participation in recreational activities is far more important to the patient in terms of improving **quality of life (QOL)**.[16] QOL can be defined as the sense of total well-being that encompasses both physical and psychosocial aspects of the patient's life. Finally, not all impairments can be remediated by physical therapy. Some impairments are permanent and progressive, the direct result of unrelenting pathology such as amyotrophic lateral sclerosis (ALS). Therapists need to recognize the scope of physical therapy intervention. In this example, a primary emphasis on reducing the number and severity of indirect impairments and functional limitations is far more appropriate.

The generation of an **asset list** is also an important part of the clinical decision making process. The therapist analyzes the data and determines patient strengths, abilities, and buffers. These areas can be reinforced and emphasized during therapy, providing the patient with the opportunity for positive reinforcement and success. For example, the patient with stroke may at the same time have intact communication skills, cognitive skills, and good function of the uninvolved extremities. Assets can also include supportive and knowledgeable family members/caregivers, and an appropriate living environment. Improved motivation and compliance are the natural outcomes of reinforcement of patient assets.

Step 3. Diagnosis

A *medical diagnosis* refers to the identification of a disease, disorder, or condition (pathology/pathophysiology) by evaluating the presenting signs, symptoms, history, laboratory test results, and procedures. It is identified primarily at the cellular level. Physical therapists use the term **diagnosis** to "identify the impact of a condition on function at the level of the system (especially the movement system) and at the level of the whole person."[4, p 45] Thus the term takes on a different meaning and is used to clarify the body of knowledge in physical therapy and the role of physical therapists in health care. For example:

Medical diagnosis: cerebrovascular accident (CVA)
Physical therapy diagnosis: impaired motor function and sensory integrity associated with nonregressive disorders of the central nervous system—acquired in adolescence or adulthood[4, p 365]
Medical diagnosis: spinal cord injury (SCI)
Physical therapy diagnosis: impaired motor function, peripheral nerve integrity, and sensory integrity associated with nonregressive disorders of the spinal cord[4, p 437]

The use of diagnostic categories specific to physical therapy facilitates successful reimbursement when linked to functional outcomes and enhances direct access of physical therapy services.[16–21]

The diagnostic process includes integrating and evaluating the data obtained during the examination to describe the patient/client condition in terms that will guide the prognosis, the plan of care, and intervention strategies. The *Guide to Physical Therapist Practice* organizes diagnostic categories by **Preferred Practice Patterns**.[4] There are four main categories of conditions: Musculoskeletal, Neuromuscular, Cardiovascular/Pulmonary, and Integumentary with preferred practice patterns identified in each (Appendix A). The patterns are described fully according to the five elements of patient/client management. Each pattern also includes reexamination to evaluate progress, global outcomes, and criteria for termination of physical therapy services. Inclusion and exclusion criteria for the practice pattern and criteria for multiple-pattern classification are also presented. The patterns represent the collaborative effort of experienced physical therapists who detailed the broad categories of problems commonly seen by physical therapists within the scope of their knowledge, experience, and expertise. Expert consensus was thus used to develop and define the preferred practice patterns. The primary focus of preferred practice patterns is at the level of impairments and functional limitations. This is a far more appropriate level for clinical decision making by physical therapists than the medical diagnosis. Therapists unable to determine an identifiable practice pattern when referring to the *Guide to Physical Therapist Practice*[4] will need to plan interventions based on the specific deficits identified.

Therapists also need to identify the ICD-9-CM codes related to the preferred practice pattern, also listed in the *Guide to Physical Therapist Practice.*[4] The coding is from the World Health Organization's International Classification of Diseases. These codes are needed for billing purposes for some payers, including Medicare.

Step 4. Prognosis and Plan of Care

The term **prognosis** refers to "the predicted optimal level of improvement in function and amount of time needed to reach that level."[4, p 46] An accurate prognosis may be determined at the onset of treatment for some patients. For other, more complicated patients with extensive disability and multisystem involvement such as the patient with severe traumatic brain injury, a prognosis or prediction of level of improvement can be determined only at various increments during the course of rehabilitation. Knowledge of recovery patterns (stage of disorder) is sometimes useful to guide decision making. The amount of time needed to reach optimal recovery is an important determination, one that is required by Medicare and other insurance providers. Predicting optimal levels of recovery and time frames can be a challenging process for the inexperienced therapist. Use of experienced, expert staff as resources and mentors can facilitate this step in the decision making process. For each preferred practice pattern, the *Guide to Physical Therapist Practice*[4] includes a broad range of expected number of visits per episode of care.

The **plan of care (POC)** outlines anticipated patient management. The therapist must integrate data obtained from the patient history and examination to determine the diagnosis, prognosis, and appropriate interventions. This process requires skills in both interpretation and integration of data, as well as clinical reasoning. Essential components of the POC include (1) goals and outcomes; (2) specific interventions to be used; (3) duration and frequency of the interventions; and (4) criteria for discharge.

Anticipated Goals and Expected Outcomes

An important first step in the development of the POC is the determination of **anticipated goals** and **expected outcomes**. Goal and outcome statements address predicted changes in impairments, functional limitations, and disabilities. They can also address predicted changes in overall health, risk reduction and prevention, wellness and fitness, and optimization of patient/client satisfaction. All delineate the intended results of patient/client management. The difference is in terms of time frame. Outcomes define the patient's expected level at the conclusion of the episode of care or rehabilitation stay while goals define the interim steps that are necessary to achieve expected outcomes.[4]

Goal and outcome statements should be objective, measurable, and time limited. There are four essential elements:

1. ***Individual:*** Who will perform the specific behavior or aspect of care? Goals and outcomes are focused on the *patient* (individuals who receive direct care physical therapy services), or the *client* (individuals who benefit from consultation and advice, or services focused on promoting, health, wellness, and fitness). Goals can also be focused on family members or caregivers, for example, the parent of a child with a developmental disability.
2. ***Behavior/Activity:*** What is the specific behavior or activity the person will demonstrate? Goals and outcomes include changes in impairments (e.g., ROM, strength, balance) and changes in functional limitations or disability (e.g., transfers, ambulation, activities of daily living [ADLs]).
3. ***Condition:*** What are the conditions under which the patient's behavior is measured? The goal or outcome statement specifies the specific conditions or measures required for successful achievement, for example, distance achieved, required time to perform the activity, the specific number of successful attempts out of a specific number of trials. Statements focused on functional changes should include a description of the conditions required for acceptable performance (e.g., amount of supervision, verbal cues, assistance, use of assistive devices). The functional levels of performance used in the Functional Independence Measure (FIM) are defined in Figure 1.3. The type of environment required for a successful outcome of the behavior should also be specified: clinic/ home (e.g., one flight of eight stairs, carpeted surfaces), and community (e.g., uneven grassy surfaces, curbs, ramps).
4. ***Time:*** How long will it take to achieve the stated goal or outcome? Goals can be expressed as **short-term** (generally considered to be 2 to 3 weeks) and **long-term** (longer than 3 weeks). Outcomes describe the expected level of functional performance attained at the end of the episode of care or rehabilitation stay. In instances of severe disability and incomplete recovery, for example, the patient with traumatic brain injury, the therapist and team members may have difficulty determining the expected outcomes at the beginning of rehabilitation. Long-term goals can be used that focus on the expectations for a specific stage of recovery (e.g., minimally conscious states, confusional states). Goals

and outcomes can also be rewritten following a significant change in patient status. The level of patient participation in the activities is an important component of the goal or outcome statement.

Each POC has multiple goals and outcomes. Goals may be linked to the successful attainment of more than one outcome. For example, attaining ROM in dorsiflexion is critical to the functional outcome of independence in transfers and ambulation. The successful attainment of an outcome is also dependent on achieving a number of different goals. For example, independent ambulation (the outcome) is dependent on increasing strength, ROM, and balance skills. In formulating a POC, the therapist needs to accurately identify the relationship between goals and outcomes and to sequence them appropriately. Box 1.4 presents examples of outcome and goal statements.

The POC should also include a statement regarding the patient's overall **rehabilitation potential**. This is typically a one-word statement: excellent, good, fair, or poor. The therapist will need to consider multiple factors when determining rehabilitation potential such as the patient's condition and onset date, comorbidity, mechanism of injury, and baseline data.[22]

Interventions

The next step is to determine the specific interventions to achieve the goals and outcomes. Components of physical therapy interventions include (1) coordination, communication, and documentation; (2) patient/client-related instruction; and (3) procedural interventions (Fig. 1.4).[4]

Coordination and Communication

Case management requires that therapists be able to communicate effectively with all members of the rehabilitation team, directly or indirectly. For example, the therapist communicates with other professionals at case conferences, team meetings, or rounds or through documentation in the medical record. Effective communication enhances collaboration and understanding.

Therapists are also responsible for coordinating care at many different levels. The therapist delegates appropriate aspects of treatment to physical therapy assistants or aides. The therapist coordinates care with other professionals or family regarding a specific treatment approach or intervention. For example, for early transfer training to be effective, consistency in how everyone transfers the patient is important. The therapist also coordinates discharge planning with the patient and family and other interested persons. Therapists may be involved in providing POC

Box 1.4 Examples of Outcome and Goal Statements

The following are examples of expected outcomes, all to be achieved within the anticipated rehab stay:

The patient will be independent and safe in ambulation using an ankle-foot orthosis and a quad cane on level surfaces for unlimited community distances and for all daily activities within 8 weeks.

The patient will demonstrate modified dependence with close supervision in wheelchair propulsion for limited household distances (up to 50 feet) within 8 weeks.

The patient will demonstrate modified dependence with minimum assistance of one person for all transfer activities in the home environment within 6 weeks.

The patient will demonstrate independence in basic activities of daily living (BADLs) with minimal set up and equipment (use of a reacher) within 6 weeks.

The patient and family will demonstrate enhanced decision making skills regarding the health of the patient and use of health care resources within 6 weeks.

The following are examples of anticipated goals with variable time frames:

Short-Term Goals

The patient will increase strength in shoulder depressor muscles and elbow extensor muscles in both upper extremities from good to normal within 3 weeks.

The patient will increase ROM 10 degrees in knee extension bilaterally to within normal limits within 3 weeks.

The patient will be independent in the application of lower extremity orthoses within 1 week.

The patient and family will recognize personal and environmental factors associated with falls during ambulation within 2 weeks.

The patient will attend to task for 5 min out of a 30 min treatment session within 3 weeks.

Long-Term Goals

The patient will independently perform transfers from wheelchair to car within 4 weeks.

The patient will ambulate with bilateral KAFOs and crutches using a swing-through gait and close supervision for 50 feet within 5 weeks.

The patient will maintain static balance in sitting with centered, symmetrical weight-bearing and no upper extremity support or loss of balance for up to 5 minutes within 4 weeks.

The patient will sequence a three- to five-step routine task with minimum assistance within 5 weeks.

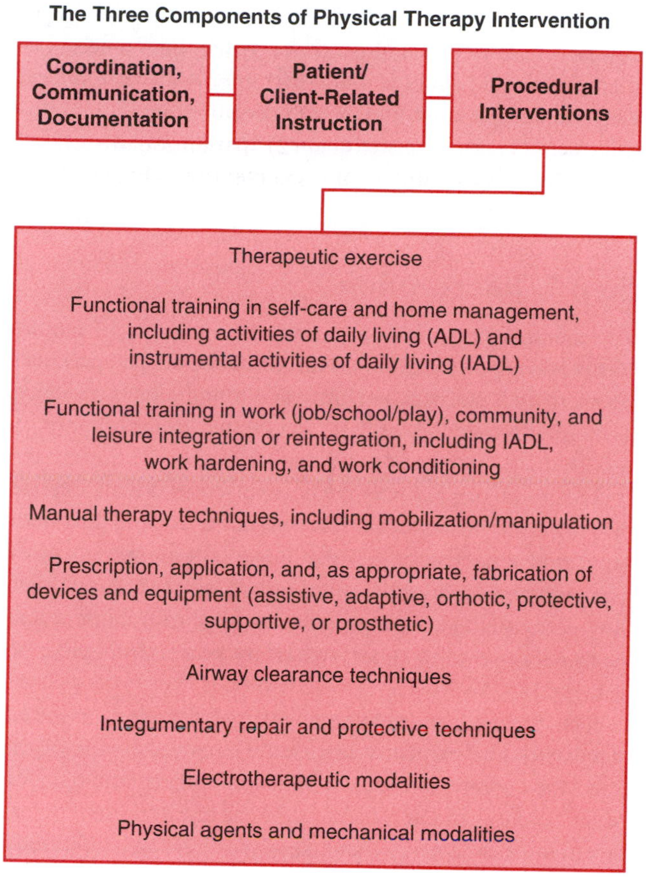

The Three Components of Physical Therapy Intervention
Coordination, Communication, Documentation
Patient/ Client-Related Instruction
Procedural Interventions
Therapeutic exercise
Functional training in self-care and home management, including activities of daily living (ADL) and instrumental activities of daily living (IADL)
Functional training in work (job/school/play), community, and leisure integration or reintegration, including IADL, work hardening, and work conditioning
Manual therapy techniques, including mobilization/manipulation
Prescription, application, and, as appropriate, fabrication of devices and equipment (assistive, adaptive, orthotic, protective, supportive, or prosthetic)
Airway clearance techniques
Integumentary repair and protective techniques
Electrotherapeutic modalities
Physical agents and mechanical modalities

Figure 1.4 The three components of physical therapy intervention. (From APTA Guide for Physical Therapist Practice,[4, p 98], with permission.)

recommendations to other facilities such as restorative nursing facilities.

Patient/Client-Related Instruction

Patient/client-related instruction is an important component of the POC. In an era of managed care and shorter durations of skilled physical therapy, effective patient-related instruction is critical in ensuring optimal care and successful rehabilitation. Communication needs to be modified based on age, cultural backgrounds, language and educational levels, and for individuals with impairments in communication or cognition. Therapists can provide direct one-on-one instruction to a variety of individuals, including patients, clients, families, caregivers, and other interested persons. Additional strategies can include group discussions or classes, or instruction through printed or audiovisual materials. Educational interventions are directed toward ensuring an understanding of the patient's condition, training in specific activities and exercises, the relevance of the interventions to improving function, and expected course in rehabilitation. In addition, educational interventions are directed toward ensuring a successful transition in returning home (training in home exercise programs [HEP]), returning to work (ergonomic training), or resuming social activities in the community. It is important to document what was taught, who was trained, and when the training occurred.[22]

Procedural Interventions

Skilled physical therapy includes a wide variety of procedural interventions, which can be broadly classified into three main groups. **Restorative interventions** are directed toward remediating or improving the patient's status in terms of impairments, functional limitations, and recovery of function. The involved segments are targeted for intervention. For example, the patient with incomplete spinal cord injury undergoes locomotor training using body weight support and a treadmill (BWSTT) to improve gait. Patients with chronic progressive pathology (e.g., the patient with Parkinson's disease) may not respond to restorative interventions aimed at resolving direct impairments; interventions aimed at restoring or optimizing function and modifying indirect impairments can, however, have a positive outcome. **Compensatory interventions** are directed toward promoting optimal function using residual abilities. The activity or task is adapted in order to achieve function and the uninvolved segments are targeted for intervention. For example, the patient with left hemiplegia learns to dress using the right upper extremity; the patient with complete T1 paraplegia learns to roll using upper extremities and momentum. Environmental adaptations are also used to facilitate relearning of functional skills and optimal performance. For example, the patient with traumatic brain injury is able to dress by selecting clothing from color-coded drawers. Compensatory interventions can be used in conjunction with restorative interventions to maximize function or when restorative interventions are unrealistic or unsuccessful. **Preventative interventions** are directed toward minimizing potential impairments, functional limitations, and disabilities and maintaining health. For example, early resumption of upright standing using a tilt table minimizes the risk of pneumonia, bone loss, and renal calculi in the patient with spinal cord injury.

Interventions are chosen on the basis of the data obtained, the diagnosis, prognosis, and anticipated goals and expected outcomes. It is important to identify all possible interventions early in the process, to carefully weigh those alternatives, and then to decide on the interventions that have the best probability of success. Narrowly adhering to one treatment approach reduces the available options and may limit or preclude successful outcomes. Use of a protocol (e.g., predetermined exercises for the patient with hip fracture) standardizes some aspects of care but may not meet the individual needs of the patient. Henry[23] points out that protocols foster a separation of evaluation findings from the selection of treatments.

Watts suggests that clinical judgment "is clearly an elegant mixture of art and science.[24, p 8] Professional consultation with expert clinicians is an effective means of helping the inexperienced therapist sort through the complex issues involved in decision making, especially when complicating factors intervene. For example, a consultation would be beneficial for the inexperienced therapist with a patient who is chronically ill, has multiple comorbidities or complications, impaired cognition, inadequate social supports, and/or severe functional limitations or disability.

A general outline of the POC is constructed. Schema can assist the therapist in organizing essential elements of the plan. One such commonly used schema is the **FITT equation (frequency-intensity-time-type)**. This includes an estimate of:

Frequency: how often the patient will receive skilled care; this is typically defined in terms of the number of times per week treatment will be given (e.g., three times per week), or the number of visits before a specific date.
Intensity: what are the prescribed number of repetitions of exercises or activities (e.g., 10 quad sets).
Time (duration): how long the patient will receive skilled care; this is typically defined in terms of days or weeks (e.g., three times per week for 7 weeks). The duration of an anticipated individual treatment session should also be defined (e.g., 30-minute sessions).
Type of intervention: what are the specific treatment strategies or procedural interventions used (e.g., neuromuscular electrical stimulation [NMES] to right dorsiflexors to increase dorsiflexor contraction).

Another example of a schema developed by Sullivan and Markos[25] identifies the specific components of a therapeutic exercise intervention. The components can be delineated by:

Posture and activity: a description of the specific posture and activity the patient must perform (e.g., sitting, weight shifting or standing, modified plantigrade, reaching).
Technique used: mode of therapist action or intervention used (guided, active-assisted, or resisted movement), or specific technique (e.g., rhythmic stabilization, slow reversals, and so forth).
Required elements: those components necessary to assist the patient in the exercise or activity (e.g., verbal commands, manual contacts, or equipment such as elastic band resistance, therapy ball, and so forth).

An example of this schema for the patient with stroke with poor dynamic sitting balance is: sitting, weight-shifting (position/activity), active-assisted reaching (mode of intervention), with verbal cueing and assisted stabilization of the affected upper extremity (required elements).

The therapist should ideally choose interventions that accomplish more than one goal and are linked to the expected outcomes. The interventions should be effectively sequenced to address key problems first and to achieve optimum motivational effects, interspacing the more difficult or uncomfortable procedures with easier ones. The therapist should include tasks that ensure success during the treatment session and, whenever possible, should end each session on a positive note. This helps the patient retain a positive feeling of success and look forward to the next treatment.

Step 5. Intervention

The therapist must take into account a number of factors in structuring an effective treatment session. The patient's comfort and optimal performance should be a priority. The environment should be structured appropriately to reduce distractions and focus the patient's attention on the task. Patient privacy should be respected, with adequate draping and positioning. The therapist should consider good body mechanics, effective use of gravity and position, and correct application of techniques and modalities. Any equipment should be gathered prior to treatment and be in good working order. All safety precautions must be observed.

The patient's pretreatment level of function or initial state should be carefully assessed. General state organization of the central nervous system and homeostatic balance of the somatic and autonomic systems are important determinants of how a patient may respond to treatment. Stockmeyer[26] points out that a wide range of influences, from emotional to cognitive to organic, may affect how a patient reacts to a particular treatment. Patients with altered homeostatic mechanisms (e.g., the patient with traumatic brain injury with either high or low arousal) can be expected to react to treatment in unpredictable ways. Responses to treatment should be carefully monitored throughout the course of rehabilitation, and treatment modifications implemented as soon as needed to ensure successful performance. Therapists develop the "art of clinical practice" by learning to adjust their input (e.g., verbal commands, manual contacts, and so forth) in response to the patient. Treatment thus becomes a dynamic and interactive process between patient and therapist. Shaping of behavior can be further enhanced by careful orientation to the purpose of the tasks and how they meet the patient's needs, thereby ensuring optimal cooperation and motivation.

Step 6. Outcomes

This last step is ongoing and involves continuous reexamination of the patient and a determination of the efficacy of treatment. The progress report summarizes reexamination findings, and evaluation of the patient's abilities in terms of the anticipated goals and expected outcomes set forth in the POC. A determination is made as to whether the goals and outcomes are reasonable given the patient's diagnosis and progress made. If the patient attains the desired level of competence for the stated goals, revisions in the POC are indicated. If the patient attains the desired level of competence for the expected outcomes, discharge is considered. If the patient fails to achieve the stated goals or outcomes, the therapist must determine why. Were the goals and outcomes realistic given the database? Were the interventions selected at an appropriate level to challenge the patient, or were they too easy or too difficult? Was the patient sufficiently motivated? Were intervening and constraining factors (disablement risk factors) identified? If the interventions were not appropriate, additional information is sought, goals modified, and different treatment interventions selected. Revision in the POC is also indicated if the patient progresses more rapidly or slowly than expected. Each modification must be evaluated in terms of its overall effect on the POC. Thus the plan becomes a fluid statement of how the patient is progressing and where he or she is going. Its overall success depends on the therapist's ongoing clinical decision making skills and on engaging the patient's cooperation and motivation. Patient adherence to the POC should be documented.

Discharge planning is initiated early in the rehabilitation process during the data collection phase and intensifies as goals and expected outcomes are close to being reached. Discharge planning may also be initiated if the patient refuses further treatment, or becomes medically or psychologically unstable. If the patient is discharged before outcomes are reached, the reasons for discontinuation of services must be carefully documented. Components of an effective **discharge plan** include (1) patient, family, or caregiver education; (2) plans for appropriate follow-up care or referral to another agency; (3) instruction in a home exercise plan (HEP); and (4) evaluation and modification of the home environment to assist the patient returning home. Essential equipment should be ordered before the discharge date in order to ensure any training in use and maintenance is completed. The therapist should also include the **discharge prognosis**, typically a one-word response such as excellent, good, fair, or poor. It reflects the therapist's judgment of the patient's ability to maintain the level of function achieved at the end of rehabilitation without continued skilled intervention.[24]

Patient Participation in Planning

Involving the patient and family in the planning process and evaluation of outcomes is essential in ensuring adherence to the POC and overall satisfaction. Noncompliance and dissatisfaction are frequently the result of failure to fully involve patient and family in the planning process or from miscommunication. Many rehabilitation plans have failed miserably simply because the patient did not see the relevance of the professionals' goals or outcomes (e.g., independent wheelchair mobility for the patient with complete transection of the cervical spinal cord). That same patient may have established a very different set of personal goals and expectations (e.g., return to walking). For many patients for whom complete recovery is not expected, the overall "goal of any rehabilitation program must be to increase the ability of individuals to manage their lives in the context of ongoing disability, to the greatest extent possible."[27, p 7] This cannot be effectively done if the therapist assumes the role of expert and sole planner, establishing the rules, regulations, and instructions for rehabilitation. Rather, it is important to empower individuals to assume a key role in planning and ensure the plan fits their life-style for life-long self-management. The patient's ability and motivation to participate in planning does vary. The more ill the patient, the less likely he or she will want to be actively involved in planning. As the illness resolves and the patient begins to feel better, the more likely he or she will want to be engaged in planning the treatment. Also the more difficult the problems encountered, the more likely patients are to put their trust in "the experts" and the less likely they are to trust their own abilities to reach effective decisions. The therapist needs to guard against promoting dependence on the expert and the patient's feelings of perceived helplessness in order to assist in developing the patient's own decision making abilities.

Ozer et al[27] address these issues in an excellent reference entitled *Treatment Planning for Rehabilitation—A Patient-Centered Approach*. The authors suggest asking the patient a series of *probing questions* to engage patients in the treatment planning process (Box 1.5).

The level of participation in this process may start out limited but can be expected to expand as the collaborative process is continued. A *Levels of Participation Scale* can be used to evaluate and document patient participation in the planning process (Box 1.6). In determining what level

Box 1.5 Questions Designed to Engage the Patient in the Treatment Planning Process

1. What are your concerns?
2. What is your greatest concern?
3. What would you like to see happen? What would make you feel that you are making progress in dealing with your chief concern? What are your goals?
4. What is your specific goal?
5. What results have you achieved?
6. What problems do you have? What questions do you have?
7. What would you like to see accomplished that would make you feel that you are making some progress in dealing with your greatest concern?

From Ozer M, Payton O, Nelson C. Treatment Planning for Rehabilitation: A Patient-Centered Approach. McGraw-Hill, New York, 2000, pp 37 and 60, with permission.

Box 1.6 Levels of Participation Scale

A = FREE CHOICE: The therapist asks an open-ended question. The patient explores and selects the answer (what) and further specifies where? and to what degree?
B = MULTIPLE CHOICE: The therapist asks questions, provides suggestions (three options). The patient selects one choice from the alternatives presented.
C = CONFIRMED CHOICE: The therapist asks questions, provides a recommendation (one choice) and asks for agreement. The patient puts into own words what has been selected.
D = FORCED CHOICE: The therapist asks questions, provides a recommendation (one option): the patient agrees (or disagrees) with what has been selected.
E = NO CHOICE: The therapist prescribes, does not ask; the patient is compliant (or noncompliant).

From Ozer M, Payton O, Nelson C. Treatment Planning for Rehabilitation: A Patient-Centered Approach. McGraw-Hill, New York, 2000, p 44, with permission.

the patient is functioning at, the therapist starts at the upper end of the scale (free choice) and moves down the scale as necessary. The lowest level of participation is recorded. For most patients, the lowest level of participation is optimally Level B Multiple Choice. Patients with significant cognitive or communication deficits (e.g., the patient with traumatic brain injury) typically will require lower levels of participation. The goal, however, as the patient recovers and progresses in rehabilitation, is to increasingly involve the patient in the planning process, to whatever extent possible. In these situations, the therapist can document improving levels of participation as evidence of recovery.

Evidence-Based Practice

The analysis of research evidence paired with the physical therapist's experience and expertise provides a powerful tool to guide clinical decision making. There are numerous areas of practice in physical therapy that lack rigorous examination and evidence. Therapists use some interventions all the time simply because they are in widespread use. Wolf[28] cautions against empiricism, that is, continuing to use a treatment simply because it has worked in the past. Therapists may also elect to use interventions because they are new and different or because they are the focus of "anecdotal testimonials" in continuing education courses. For example, nonstandard therapies have been described that are based on theories incongruent with anatomic or physiological function or have been proposed for a broad range of diagnoses without adequate scientific evidence in peer-reviewed journals (e.g., myofascial release, craniosacral mobilization). Harris points out that "the responsibility to deliver evidence-based treatment techniques rests with *all* physical therapists."[29, p 176] To that end, the American Physical Therapy Association (APTA) has developed a "clinical research agenda designed to support, explain, and enhance physical therapy clinical practice by facilitating research that is primarily useful to clinicians."[30, p 499] The APTA's *Hooked on Evidence* project provides links to *Evidence in Practice* (http://www.ptjournal.org) and provides training workshops to assist individuals in this process.

Evidence-based medicine (EBM) has been defined by Sackett et al as "the integration of best research evidence with clinical expertise and patient values."[31, p 1] This term has been expanded into **evidence-based practice** (EBP) to encompass a broader range of health professions.

The essential steps of EBP[31] are:

Step 1: A clinical problem is identified and an answerable question is formulated.
Step 2: A systematic literature review is conducted and evidence collected.
Step 3: The research evidence is critically analyzed for its validity, impact, and applicability.
Step 4: The critical appraisal is synthesized and integrated with the clinician's expertise and the patient's unique characteristics and values.
Step 5: The effectiveness and efficiency of the steps in the evidence-based process are evaluated.

A well built *research question* contains three elements: (1) a specific patient/client group or population, (2) the specific interventions or exposures to be studied, and (3) the outcomes achieved. For example, a published study[36] examined interventions commonly applied for low back pain (therapeutic exercise, TENS, thermotherapy, ultrasound, massage, E-stim, traction) using outcomes identified as important to the patient (pain, function, patient global assessment, quality of life, and return to work).

Systematic review (SR) is a comprehensive examination of the literature. The researcher determines key resources to provide the evidence. These include (1) peer-reviewed and evidence-based journals, (2) online services (e.g., Cochrane Reviews, Database of Abstracts of Reviews of Effectiveness or DARE, Physiotherapy-Evidence Database or Pedro), and (3) search engines (e.g., PubMed, Sum Search). Box 1.7 provides a brief list of EBP Internet resources. Specific criteria are developed for the inclusion and exclusion of the research studies selected for review. Studies employing different designs may be analyzed individually or compared qualitatively; studies of similar design may be combined quantitatively (e.g., meta-analysis).[31,32]

Critical analysis of research findings involves detailed examination of the methodology, results, and conclusions. The clinician should be able to answer the following questions: (1) What is the level of evidence?; (2) Is the evi-

Box 1.7 Evidence-Based Practice: Internet Resources

http://www.ncbi.nlm.nih.gov/PubMed	NLM free public access search engine
http://www.nhscrd.york.ac.uk/darehp.htm	database: abstracts of rehabilitation effectiveness
http://www.update-software.com/cochrane/	Cochrane Library
http://hiru.mcmaster.ca/cochrane/centers/Canadian	Canadian Cochrane Center
http://sumsearch.uthscsa.edu/searchform45.htm	Meta-search engine: Medline, DARE
http://ptwww.cchs.usyd.edu.au/pedro/	physiotherapy database
http://www.shef.ac.uk/~scharr/ir/core.html	links to all aspect of EBP
http://cebm.jr2.ox.ac.uk/cats/allcats.html	critical appraisal tools (CATS)
http://cebm.jr2.ox.ac.uk/docs/levels.html	UK-based Centre for EBM
http://cebm.utoronto.ca/	Sackett's EBM book, physiotherapy cases
http://consort-statement.org	guidelines for conducting good RCTs
http://ericae.net/faqs/meta-analysis/meta-analysis.htm	ERIC resource on meta-analysis

dence valid?; and (3) Are the results important and clinically relevant? Thus interpretation and synthesis of the evidence must be considered within the context of the specific patient/client problem. Examination begins with the purpose of the study, which should be clearly stated, and the review of literature, which should be relevant in terms of the specific question asked. The methods/design should be closely examined. Design types vary greatly and can be evaluated in terms of levels of evidence with grades of recommendation in order of most to least rigorous.[31,32]

Level 1 studies include large randomized controlled trials (RCTs) using meta-analyses of data. The essential feature of the studies included involves randomization into two or more groups including an experimental group(s) and a control group.

Level 2 studies include those with a cohort design and low-quality, smaller RCTs. In a cohort design, subjects are identified and followed over time (a prospective study) for changes/outcomes following exposure to an intervention. They may or may not have a control group (a comparison group). Since there is no randomization, it is difficult to know if the groups are truly similar. Confounding variables may account for some of the outcomes.

Level 3 studies include case-control studies (case-comparison) and studies with a single case-control design. In a case-control design, subjects are identified on the basis of a defining characteristic (e.g., cancer) and compared to another similar group without the defining characteristic to determine if a variable (e.g., smoking) is associated with the condition. The studies are retrospective in that they examine outcomes to a previous exposure/intervention or causal factor. Single-case design involves one subject evaluated over time. Varying designs (A B A, or A B A B) allow comparison of the intervention period (B) to a baseline period of no intervention (A).

Level 4 studies include case-series and poor quality cohort and case-control studies. These studies are largely descriptive. Subjects with a condition of interest are examined over time (e.g., stroke) and information about clinical outcomes is provided. No control or comparison group is used.

Level 5 studies include research based on expert opinion without explicit critical appraisal. While RCT provides the most rigorous design, there are times when the other designs are indicated. For example, there may be ethical issues involving control groups that receive no treatment when treatment is clearly beneficial. Or when outcomes are not clearly understood or defined (e.g., quality of life issues), designs such as singe-case studies may be indicated. See Table 1.1 for EBP: Levels of Evidence and Grades of Recommendation.

Critical Appraisal Tools (CATs) are available to assist the inexperienced clinician in the evaluation of research (e.g., in Law's *Evidence-Based Rehabilitation,* Appendix C/D[32]; and Helewa and Walker's *Critical Evaluation of Research in Physical Rehabilitation,* Appendix II[33]). Clinicians also need to utilize effective strategies to organize and store the data and to update data on a regular basis. Reference management systems such as Endnote and Reference Manager (ISI ResearchSoft, 800 Jones Street, Berkeley, CA 94710) are available to assist the therapist.

Evidence-based clinical practice guidelines (EBCPGs) are defined by the Institute of Medicine as systematically developed statements to assist practitioner and patient decisions about appropriate health care for specific clinical circumstances.[34] They are developed through a combination of (1) expert consensus (e.g., the Guide to Physical Therapist Practice[4]); (2) systematic reviews and meta-analysis; and (3) analysis of patient preferences combined with outcome-based guidelines. The *Philadelphia Panel* is a multidisciplinary, international panel of rehabilitation experts comprised of a group of Clinical Specialty Experts from the United States and the Ottawa Methods Group from Canada. The panel developed a structured and rigorous methodology to formulate evidence-based practice guidelines.[34,35] For example, the panel analyzed the evidence following a structured and rigorous review of selected interventions for low back pain.[36] The evidence was

Table 1.1 Evidence Based Practice: Levels of Evidence and Grades of Recommendation

Level of Evidence	Etiology, Intervention/ Prevention Studies	Grades of Recommendation
1	a: SR of multiple RCTs (with homogenicity, large *N*) b: Individual RCT with narrow confidence interval	A
2	a: SR (with homogeneity) of cohort studies b: Individual cohort study or low quality RCT (small *N*) c: Outcomes research	B
3	a: SR (with homogeneity) of case-control studies b: Individual case-control study	B
4	Case-series and poor quality cohort and case-control studies	C
5	Expert opinion without explicit critical appraisal, or based on physiology, bench research or first principles	D

SR = Systematic review (including meta-analysis); a review in which the primary studies are summarized, critically appraised, and statistically combined; usually quantitative in nature with specific inclusion/exclusion criteria.

RCT = Randomized controlled trial: an experimental study in which participants are randomly assigned to either an experimental or control group to receive different interventions or a placebo.

Cohort study = A prospective (forward-in-time) study; a group of participants (cohort) with a similar condition is followed for a defined period of time; comparison is made to a matched group that does not have the condition.

Homogeneity = SR free of variations (heterogeneity) in the directions and degree of results between individual studies.

N = Number of subjects.

Case control study = A retrospective (backward-in-time) study; a group of individuals with a similar condition (disease) is compared with a group that does not have the condition to determine factors that may have played a role in the condition.

Case report (study) = Type of descriptive research in which only one individual is studied in depth, often retrospectively.

Adapted from Centre for Evidence-based Medicine, Oxford-Centre for Evidence Based Medicine (http://www.cebm.net/levels of evidence.asp)

then translated into EBCPGs by reviewing key outcomes and deciding whether the intervention had clinical benefit. Categories of absolute and relative benefit were used. The panel established a clinical improvement of 15 percent or more relative to the control as an acceptable level of evidence. Recommendations were graded based on levels (methodological quality) of the studies. Grade A or B recommendations were required to demonstrate clinically important changes and statistical significance. The panel's positive recommendations were then sent to 324 clinical practitioners for their feedback. The panel reviewed practitioners' feedback and revised their recommendations accordingly. In the low back pain study, the panel recommended the following EBCPGs: (1) the use of therapeutic exercises for chronic, subacute, and post-surgery low back pain and (2) continuation of normal activities for acute low back pain. The panel found lack of evidence regarding efficacy for the use of other interventions (e.g., thermotherapy, therapeutic ultrasound, massage, electrical stimulation). A similar process was used to develop EBCPGs for rehabilitation of patients with knee pain[37] and shoulder pain.[38] According to Rothstein, these studies are clinically important in that they "are not telling us what is known and what is not known, but what is supported by evidence and what is not supported by evidence."[39, p 1620] The guidelines provide us with a summation of best possible evidence for use in clinical practice.

Documentation

Documentation is an essential requirement for timely reimbursement of services and communication among the rehabilitation team members. Written documentation is formally done at the time of admission and discharge, and at periodic intervals during the course of rehabilitation (interim or progress notes). The format and timing of notes will vary according to the regulatory requirements specified by institutional policy and third-party payers. Data included in the medical record should be meaningful (important, not just nice to have), complete and accurate (valid and reliable), timely (recorded promptly), and systematic (regularly recorded). All handwritten entries

Box 1.8 Documentation Guidelines from the APTA's Guide to Physical Therapist Practice[4]

Documentation should include:

1. Appropriate identification of the patient's full name and identification number, if applicable.
2. The date and the provider's full name and designation (i.e., PT or PTA). Services provided by students should include those designations (i.e., SPT or SPTA) and should be co-signed by a licensed physical therapist.
3. The manner in which physical therapy services are initiated (i.e., referral, direct access) should be indicated.
4. The results of the history, systems review, and administration of appropriate tests and measures. The results from a review of communication, affect, cognition, language, and learning style is also included.
5. The evaluation, diagnosis, and prognosis. This includes the identification of Preferred Practice Patterns and ICD-9-CM codes,[4, pp 725–735] as appropriate.
6. The POC including anticipated goals, expected outcomes, and interventions. This also includes patient/client and family/caregiver educational goals and appropriate collaboration and coordination of care with other professionals/services.
7. Results of interventions or services provided, including changes in patient status, i.e., progress, or regression. Documentation of individual visits should include: patient/client self-report, specific interventions provided (frequency, intensity, duration as appropriate), equipment provided, adverse reactions to the intervention. Also included are any factors that might modify the interventions and progress toward intended goals (i.e., patient adherence to instructions) and communication/consultation with patient/client, family members/caregivers, or other providers.
8. Results of reexamination and reevaluation. Documentation should include an updating of the patient's/client's status; interpretation of findings; and any revisions in the goals, outcomes, or POC.
9. Summation at the conclusion of the episode of care (discharge note). Documentation should include the criteria for discharge: (1) anticipated goals and outcomes have been achieved; (2) patient/client, caregiver or guardian declines to continue intervention; (3) patient/client unable to continue due to medical or psychosocial problems; or (4) patient/client will no longer benefit from physical therapy services. Also included are a determination of the patient's current physical and functional status, the degree to which the goals and outcomes have been achieved, and the reasons why the goals and outcomes were not achieved. The discharge note must also include the discharge plan related to the patient/client's continuing care needs, for example, referrals for home program, additional services, follow-up physical therapy service, continuing family and caregiver training, and a statement of any equipment provided.
10. Only acceptable medical terminology should be used in the medical record. Confusing abbreviations should be avoided. Generally, a facility will have an approved list of abbreviations. Physical therapists should ensure that notes are understandable to all who read and use the medical record.

The reader is referred to the Guidelines for Physical Therapy Documentation[4, pp 703–705] and the Documentation Templates for Physical Therapist Patient/Client Management.[4, pp 707–719]

should be in ink, legible, and signed with a legal signature. Charting errors should be corrected by a single line through the error with initialing and dating directly above the error. Errors should not be erased or covered with correction fluid. Electronic entries should comply with appropriate provisions for security and confidentiality. See Box 1.8 for documentation guidelines.

Problem-Oriented Medical Record

The *problem-oriented medical record* (POMR), originally developed by Weed and Zimny, has been adopted by many institutions.[40] The patient treatment process is divided into four phases:

Phase 1: The formation of a database, including history, physical examination, and laboratory and other test results.
Phase 2: Identification of a specific problem list from the interpretation of the database, including specific impairment of function (physical, psychological, social, and vocational) resulting from the disease process or from secondary impairments.
Phase 3: Identification of a specific POC that includes interventions for each of the problems described; evaluative and progress notes are included for each problem.
Phase 4: Determination of the effectiveness of the POC and subsequent changes as a result of patient progress.

The POMR thus highlights the relationship of the database to the POC and allows the specific patient problems to become the central focus of planning. Computerization of the POMR is available to store vast amounts of data and relates the information to a range of possible diagnoses and available management options.

Documentation Using SOAP Format

Progress notes are written in the subjective, objective, assessment, plan (**SOAP**) format. *Subjective findings* (S) are what the patient and his or her family tell the therapist about the current conditions/chief complaints, functional status/activity level, social history, living environment, social/health habits, family health history, and employment status. The patient's goals and prior response to treatment interventions are also included. Quoting the patient directly using direct quotes may be the most meaningful way to convey some information (e.g., "I don't need PT, there's nothing wrong with me"). Medical information obtained from the patient's chart can also be included under assessment because the therapist has not directly observed these findings.

Objective findings (O) are what the therapist observes, tests, or measures. The information is typically organized by specific headings based on (1) body systems, (e.g. musculoskeletal, neuromuscular, cardiopulmonary, integumentary); (2) types of specific tests and measurements performed (e.g., balance tests, gait tests, ROM tests, strength); and (3) areas of the body and functional skills (e.g., ADLs, upper extremities [UEs], lower extremities [LEs], trunk). Objective information must be stated in measurable terms.

Assessment (A) includes professional judgments about the subjective and/or objective findings. A prioritized problem list is generated with impairments linked to functional limitations. The physical therapy diagnosis is determined using the Preferred Practice Patterns (see Appendix A).

Plan (P) includes anticipated goals and expected outcomes and outlines the planned interventions to be used. Information should be provided concerning the frequency, specific interventions, treatment progression, equipment required and how it will be used, and education strategies. The plan also documents referrals to other professionals and recommendations for future interventions or follow-up care.[41]

Clinical Decision Making: Expert versus Novice

Jensen et al provide an excellent overview of the evidence accumulating on expertise in physical therapy practice.[42] The authors suggest that the knowledge, skills, and decision-making abilities used by expert clinicians can be identified, nurtured, and taught. Embrey et al[43] suggest that novices may benefit from a period of active mentoring by expert clinicians early in clinical practice. This information has important implications for novice therapists and for educators involved in teaching clinical decision making.

Knowledge Base and Experience

Decision making is influenced by knowledge and experience. Experts have more knowledge and experience and are able to organize, integrate, and shape information into a usable format. Their knowledge base is multidimensional and patient-centered. Their clinical reasoning is reflective, and focused. Expert clinicians collaborate effectively with patients and colleagues. The novice therapist, on the other hand, may collect similar data, but is unable to organize and categorize the information. Simple memorization of data and use of book-learned, declarative knowledge does not allow the novice to recognize meaningful relationships and generate accurate hypotheses within a realistic time frame. Organization of knowledge is specific and highly dependent on the mastery of a particular content area.[43–44] Content domains in physical therapy take the form of the specialty areas (orthopedic, neurological, pediatric, and so forth). As expertise increases, master clinicians increase their abilities to categorize information, improving in both mastery of depth and complexity of content. Jensen et al[42] found that master clinicians demonstrated increased confidence in evaluating patients and problem-solving. Novice therapists collected data but did not always recognize important data. They also tended to be rigidly governed by rules for decision making. For example, they adhered to standardized frameworks (protocols) whereas the expert group easily adapted and refocused their approach if a different direction was indicated. Experts also demonstrate improved procedural skills (practical knowledge) that are well integrated with their mastery of knowledge and clinical reasoning. Improved skills and expertise are developed through intense, focused, and deliberate practice. Jensen et al point out that experts are highly motivated and are constantly striving to improve their skills.[45] The APTA recognizes expertise in their board-certification process for clinical specialists.

Cognitive Processing Styles

The individual who utilizes a *receptive data-gathering style* generally suspends judgment until all possible data are gathered. The data are analyzed individually and collectively before a final determination is made of how to organize and use them. These same individuals are likely to adopt a systematic processing style, in which a methodical step-by-step approach is used, completing one step before progressing to the next. Contrasting styles are perceptive and intuitive. The individual who utilizes a *perceptive data-gathering style* will seek and respond to ongoing cues and patterns, defining and organizing problems early. Information processing is largely intuitive. Thus these clinicians are able to respond to a large number of stimuli as they occur and consider initiation of early treatment options.[42] Research suggests that styles may differ by expert group. May and Dennis[44] and Jensen et al[45] found that clinicians with expertise in orthopedics tended to utilize a receptive/systematic style, generating hypotheses only after a methodical and ordered search of data. Embrey et al[43] found that pediatric expert clinicians tended to utilize a perceptive data-gathering style and process information intuitively. Thus they responded rapidly to cues and patterns (movement scripts) and changes that occurred within the treatment session. Psychosocial sensitivity was a key factor in directing experienced pediatric clinicians during the physical therapy sessions. Novice therapists were less responsive to the psychosocial needs of the children and kept their attention focused on procedural matters. May and Dennis[44] reported that practitioners experienced in cardiopulmonary and neurological physical therapy also tended to respond more favorably to the perceptive/intuitive style. Thus the differences noted in terms of the types of cognitive strategies reported appear to be evoked by specific problem structure and domain.

Self-Monitoring Strategies

Important differences exist between expert versus novice clinicians in the area of self-monitoring. Expert clinicians were found to frequently and effectively utilize self-assessment to modify and redefine their clinical decisions. This reflective aspect of practice resulted in improved improvisational performance, the actions that occur when therapists are actually treating patients. They were better able to control the treatment situation (i.e., constant interruptions, the demands of many scheduled patients, multiple tasks, and so forth), and the time allotted. Conversely, novice therapists demonstrated self-monitoring, but were less able to utilize the information effectively to control the situation. They reacted more to external stimuli and the confusion of competing demands and were less able to offer alternate intervention strategies. Self-monitoring was viewed as a positive experience by the experts twice as often as by novice therapists, an indication that the inexperienced therapists were sensitive to their limitations. The experts were also more willing to take risks and to admit when they did not know something.[42]

Communication and Teaching Skills

Expert clinicians were able to maintain focus on the patient as evidenced in their verbal and nonverbal communications. They were able to provide hands-on examination and treatment while interacting socially with their patients. Their smooth interplay was responsive to the needs of each individual patient and demonstrated commitment and caring about the patient. Conversely, novice therapists were more structured by the demands of completing evaluations or interventions. Their focus was more on the mechanics of treatment rather than on the psychosocial needs of the patient.[43,47] Pediatric expert clinicians were able to consistently end each therapy session with a positive activity, frequently chosen by the children. Strong emotional bonding was evident. Novice pediatric therapists were less consistent in attention to the psychosocial needs of their patients. Expert clinicians affirmed the importance of teaching in assisting patients to assume control over their own health care. In an era of cost containment and limited services, this is an important value and one that is essential for ensuring successful long-term outcomes. Novice therapists, on the other hand, demonstrated greater interest in mastering hands-on skills and in ensuring the success of their treatments.[45]

Summary

An organized process of clinical decision making allows the therapist to systematically plan effective treatments. The steps identified in the patient/client management process are: (1) examine the patient, and collect data through history, systems review, and tests and measures; (2) evaluate the data and identify problems; (3) determine the diagnosis; (4) determine the prognosis and plan of care; (5) implement the plan of care; and (6) reexamine the patient and evaluate treatment outcomes.

Patient participation in planning is essential in ensuring successful outcomes. Evidence-based practice allows the therapist to select interventions that can provide meaningful change in patient's lives. Inherent to the therapist's success in this process are an appropriate knowledge base and experience, cognitive processing strategies, self-monitoring strategies, and communication and teaching skills. Documentation is an essential requirement for effective communication among the rehabilitation team members and for timely reimbursement of services.

Questions for Review

1. Describe the key steps in patient/client management.
2. Differentiate between impairments, functional limitations, and disability. Define and give an example of each.
3. What are the essential elements of goal and outcome statements? Write two examples of each.
4. In evaluating treatment outcomes, why might a patient fail to reach the stated outcome? What are possible risk factors for disablement? What are the possible buffers?
5. Select a research study and critically review it in terms of the essential steps of evidence-based practice.
6. What are the four components of the SOAP format of written documentation?

Case Study

PRESENT HISTORY

The patient is a 78-year-old woman who tripped and fell at home ascending the stairs outside the front door. She was admitted to the hospital after sustaining a transcervical, intracapsular fracture of the right femur. The patient had an open reduction internal fixation (ORIF) procedure of the RLE to reduce and pin the fracture.

PAST MEDICAL HISTORY

Patient is a very thin woman (98 pounds) with long-standing problems with osteoporosis (on medication for 8 years). She has a history of falls, three in the last year alone. Approximately 3 years ago she had a myocardial infarction, and presented with third-degree heart block, requiring implantation of a permanent pacemaker. She underwent cataract surgery with implantation 2 years ago; the left eye is scheduled for similar surgery.

MEDICAL DIAGNOSES

Coronary artery disease (CAD), hypertension (HTN), mitral valve prolapse, s/p permanent heart pacer, s/p right cataract with implant, osteoporosis (moderate to severe in the spine, hips, and pelvis), osteoarthritis with mild pain in right knee, s/p left elbow fracture (1 year ago), left ankle fracture (2 years ago), urinary stress incontinence.

MEDICATIONS

Fosamax 70 mg weekly
Atenolol 24 mg po qd
MVI with Fe tab po qd
Metamucil tbs prn po qd, Colace 100 mg po bid
Tylenol no. 3 tab prn/mild pain

SOCIAL SUPPORT/ENVIRONMENT

The patient is a retired schoolteacher who was recently widowed from her husband of 48 years. She has two sons and one daughter and four grandchildren, all of whom live within an hour's driving distance away. One of her children visits every weekend. She has a rambunctious black Labrador puppy that is 8 months old and was given to her "for company" at the time her husband died. She was walking the dog at the time of the accident. She is an active participant in a garden club, which meets twice a month and in weekly events at the local senior center. Previously she was driving her car for all community activities.

She lives alone in a large old New England farmhouse. Her home has an entry with four stairs and no rail. Inside she has 14 rooms on 2 floors. The downstairs living area has a step down into the family room with no rail. There are 14 stairs to the second floor with rails on either side. The upstairs sleeping area is cluttered with large, heavy furniture. The second floor bathroom is small, with a high old tub and pedestal feet and a lip. There is no added equipment.

PHYSICAL THERAPY EXAMINATION

1. Mental Status

Alert and oriented × 3
Pleasant, cooperative, articulate
No apparent memory deficits
Good problem solving and safety awareness about hip precautions

2. Cardiopulmonary Status

Pulse 74; BP 110/75
Endurance: good; min SOB with 20 min of activity

3. Sensation

Vision: wears glasses
Hearing: WFL
Depth perception impaired
Sensation BLEs intact

4. Skin

Incision is healed and well approximated
Wears bilateral TEDs q am × 6 wks

5. ROM

LLE, BUEs: WFL
Affected RLE:
- Flex 0 to 85°
- Ext NT
- Abd 0 to 20°
- Add NT
- IR, ER NT
- Right knee and ankle WFL

6. Strength

LLE, BUEs: WFL
Affected RLE:
- Hip flex NT (not tested)
- Hip ext NT
- Hip abd NT
- Knee ext 4/5
- Ankle DF 4/5, PF 4/5

7. Posture

Flexed, stooped posture: moderate kyphosis, flexed hips and knees
$^1/_2$-inch leg length shortening on RLE; uses wedge when sitting
Mild resting head tremor

8. Balance

Sitting balance: WFL

Standing balance:
Eyes open: good; leans slightly to left side
Eyes closed: unsteady, begins to fall
Arises from chair without help, some initial unsteadiness; sitting down: safe, smooth motion
Uses 2-inch foam cushions to elevate seat of kitchen chair and living room chair

9. Functional Mobility

Patient was completely independent (I) before her fall.
Results of functional assessment:
I bed mobility
I transfers; unable to do tub transfers at present
I ambulation with standard walker × 200 feet on level surfaces, partial weight-bearing RLE
Increased flexion of knees and dorsal spine
I one flight of stairs with rail and SBQC

10. ADLs

I dressing; requires minimal assist (MinA) of home health aide for sponge baths
Requires moderate assistance (ModA) of home health aide for homemaker activities

11. Patient Is Highly Motivated

"I want to get my life back together, get my dog home again so I can take care of him."

PRIMARY INSURANCE

Medicare

GUIDING QUESTIONS

1. Identify and categorize the patient's impairments into direct or indirect.
2. Identify her functional limitations, disabilities, and assets.
3. What are your concerns regarding potential disablement risk factors?
4. What is her rehabilitation prognosis?
5. Write two expected outcome and two goal statements to direct her POC.
6. Identify two treatment interventions you might include in her POC. What precautions should you observe?
7. What tests and measures will you use to determine successful attainment of outcomes?
8. What precautions are important to observe?

References

1. Jensen, G, Gwyer, J, Hack, L, et al: Expertise in Physical Therapy Practice. Butterworth Heinemann, Boston, 1999.
2. Rothstein, JM, and Echternach, JL: Hypothesis-oriented algorithm for clinicians: A method for evaluation and treatment planning. Phys Ther 66:1388, 1986.
3. Rothstein, JM, Echternach, JL, and Riddle, DL: The hypothesis-oriented algorithm for clinicians II (HOAC II): A guide for patient management. Phys Ther 83:455, 2003.
4. American Physical Therapy Association: Guide to Physical Therapist Practice, ed 2. Phys Ther 81:1, 2001.
5. Randall, KE, and McEwen, IR: Writing patient-centered functional goals. Phys Ther 80:1197, 2000.
6. Cohen, L: The screening process. PT Magazine Jan: 20–22, 2002.
7. Nagi, S: Disability and Rehabilitation. Ohio State Univ. Pr., Columbus, 1969.
8. National Advisory Board on Medical Rehabilitation Research: Draft V: Report and Plan for Medicare Rehabilitation Research. National Institutes of Health, Bethesda, MD, 1992.
9. The International Classification of Impairments, Disabilities, and Handicaps (ICIDH-2). World Health Organization, Geneva, 1999.
10. Schenkman, M, and Butler, R: A model for multisystem evaluation, interpretation, and treatment of individuals with neurologic dysfunction. Phys Ther 69:538, 1989.
11. Harris, B, and Dyrek, D: A model of orthopaedic dysfunction for clinical decision making in physical therapy practice. Phys Ther 69:548, 1989.
12. Wagstaff, S: The use of the International Classification of Impairments, Disabilities and Handicaps in Rehabilitation. Physiotherapy 68:233, 1982.
13. Guccione, A: Physical therapy diagnosis and the relationship between impairments and function. Phys Ther 71:499, 1991.
14. Jette, A: Physical disablement concepts for physical therapy research and practice. Phys Ther 74:380, 1994.
15. Guide for the Uniform Data Set for Medical Rehabilitation (including the FIM instrument), Version 5.0. State University of New York, Buffalo, 1996.
16. Rothstein, J: Disability and our identity. Phys Ther 74:375, 1994.
17. Sahrmann, S: Diagnosis by the physical therapists prerequisite for treatment. Phys Ther 68:1703, 1988.
18. Rose, S: Diagnosis: Defining the term. Phys Ther 69:162, 1989.
19. Jette, A: Diagnosis and classification by physical therapists: A special communication. Phys Ther 69:967, 1989.
20. Behr, D, et al: Diagnosis enhances, not impedes boundaries of physical therapy practice. J Orthop Sports Phys Ther 13:218, 1991.
21. Dekker, J, et al: Diagnosis and treatment in physical therapy: An investigation of their relationship. Phys Ther 73:568, 1993.
22. Baeten, A, Moran, M, Phillippi, L, et al: Documenting Physical Therapy—The Reviewer Perspective. Butterworth Heinemann, Boston, 1999.
23. Henry, J: Identifying problems in clinical problem solving. Phys Ther 65:1071, 1985.
24. Watts, N: Decision analysis: A tool for improving physical therapy education. In Wolf, S (ed): Clinical Decision Making in Physical Therapy. FA Davis, Philadelphia, 1985, p 8.
25. Sullivan, P, and Markos, P: Clinical Decision Making in Therapeutic Exercise. Appleton & Lange, East Norwalk,CT, 1995.
26. Stockmeyer, S: Clinical decision making based on homeostatic concepts. In Wolf, S (ed): Clinical Decision Making in Physical Therapy. FA Davis, Philadelphia, 1985, p 79.
27. Ozer, M, Payton, O, Nelson, C: Treatment Planning for Rehabilitation—A Patient-Centered Approach. McGraw-Hill, New York, 2000.
28. Wolf, S: Clinical Decision Making in Physical Therapy. FA Davis, Philadelphia, 1985.
29. Harris, S: How should treatments be critiqued for scientific merit? Phys Ther 76:175–181, 1996.
30. Guccione A, Goldstein, M, Elliott, S: Clinical research agenda for physical therapy. Phys Ther 80:499–513, 2000.
31. Sackett, D, and Haynes, B. Evidence-Based Medicine: How to Practice and Teach EBM, ed 2. Churchill-Livingstone, New York, 2000.
32. Law, M (ed): Evidence-Based Rehabilitation. Slack, Thorofare, NJ, 2002.

33. Helewa, A, and Walker, J: Critical Evaluation of Research in Physical Rehabilitation—Towards Evidence-Based Practice. WB Saunders, Philadelphia, 2000.
34. Scalzitti, D: Evidence-based guidelines: Application to clinical practice. Phys Ther 81:1622, 2001.
35. Philadelphia Panel: Evidence-based clinical practice guidelines on selected rehabilitation interventions: Overview and methodology. Phys Ther 81:1629, 2001.
36. Philadelphia Panel: Evidence-based clinical practice guidelines on selected rehabilitation interventions for low back pain. Phys Ther 81:1641, 2001.
37. Philadelphia Panel: Evidence-based clinical practice guidelines on selected rehabilitation interventions for knee pain. Phys Ther 81:1675, 2001.
38. Philadelphia Panel: Evidence-based clinical practice guidelines on selected rehabilitation interventions for shoulder pain. Phys Ther 81:1719, 2001.
39. Rothstein, J: Autonomous practice or autonomous ignorance? Phys Ther 81:1620, 2001.
40. Weed, LL, and Zimny, NJ: The problem-oriented system, problem-knowledge coupling, and clinical decision making. Phys Ther 69:656, 1989.
41. Kettenbach, G: Writing S.O.A.P. Notes, ed 3. FA Davis, Philadelphia, 2004.
42. Jensen, G, Gwyer, J, Hack, L, et al: Expertise in Physical Therapy Practice. Butterworth Heinemann, Boston, 1999.
43. Embrey, DG, et al: Clinical decision making by experienced and inexperienced pediatric physical therapists for children with diplegic cerebral palsy. Phys Ther 76:20, 1996.
44. May, BJ, and Dennis, JK: Expert decision making in physical therapy: A survey of practitioners. Phys Ther 71:190, 1991.
45. Jensen, GM, et al: Attribute dimensions that distinguish master and novice physical therapy clinicians in orthopedic settings. Phys Ther 72:711, 1992.
46. Riolo, L: Skill differences in novice and expert clinicians in neurologic physical therapy. Neurology Report 20:60, 1996.
47. Payton, O: Clinical reasoning process in physical therapy. Phys Ther 65:924, 1985.

Appendix A: Preferred Practice Patterns: APTA Guide to Physical Therapist Practice[4]

MUSCULOSKELETAL

Pattern A: Primary Prevention/Risk Reduction for Skeletal Demineralization

Pattern B: Impaired Posture

Pattern C: Impaired Muscle Performance

Pattern D: Impaired Joint Mobility, Motor Function, Muscle Performance, and Range of Motion Associated with Connective Tissue Dysfunction

Pattern E: Impaired Joint Mobility, Motor Function, Muscle Performance, and Range of Motion Associated with Localized Inflammation

Pattern F: Impaired Joint Mobility, Motor Function, Muscle Performance, Range of Motion and Reflex Integrity Associated with Spinal Disorders

Pattern G: Impaired Joint Mobility, Motor Function, Muscle Performance, Range of Motion Associated with Fracture

Pattern H: Impaired Joint Mobility, Motor Function, Muscle Performance, Range of Motion Associated with Joint Arthroplasty

Pattern I: Impaired Joint Mobility, Motor Function, Muscle Performance, Range of Motion Associated with Bony or Soft Tissue Surgery

Pattern J: Impaired Motor Function, Muscle Performance, Range of Motion, Gait, Locomotion, and Balance Associated with Amputation

NEUROMUSCULAR

Pattern A: Primary Prevention/Risk Reduction for Loss of Balance and Falling

Pattern B: Impaired Neuromotor Development

Pattern C: Impaired Motor Function and Sensory Integrity Associated with Nonprogressive Disorders of the Central Nervous System—Congenital Origin or Acquired in Infancy or Childhood

Pattern D: Impaired Motor Function and Sensory Integrity Associated with Nonprogressive Disorders of the Central Nervous System—Acquired in Adolescence or Adulthood

Pattern E: Impaired Motor Function and Sensory Integrity Associated with Progressive Disorders of the Central Nervous System

Pattern F: Impaired Peripheral Nerve Integrity and Muscle Performance Associated with Peripheral Nerve Injury

Pattern G: Impaired Motor Function and Sensory Integrity Associated with Acute or Chronic Polyneuropathies

Pattern H: Impaired Motor Function, Peripheral Nerve Integrity, and Sensory Integrity Associated with Nonprogressive Disorders of the Spinal Cord

Pattern I: Impaired Arousal, Range of Motion, and Motor Control Associated with Coma, Near Coma, or Vegetative State

CARDIOVASCULAR/PULMONARY

Pattern A: Primary Prevention/Risk Reduction for Cardiovascular/Pulmonary Disorders

Pattern B: Impaired Aerobic Capacity/Endurance Associated with Deconditioning

Pattern C: Impaired Ventilation, Respiration/Gas Exchange, and Aerobic Capacity/Endurance Associated with Airway Clearance Dysfunction

Pattern D: Impaired Aerobic Capacity/Endurance Associated with Cardiovascular Pump Dysfunction or Failure

Pattern E: Impaired Ventilation, Respiration/Gas Exchange Associated with Ventilatory Pump Dysfunction or Failure

Pattern F: Impaired Ventilation, Respiration/Gas Exchange Associated with Respiratory Failure

Pattern G: Impaired Ventilation, Respiration/Gas Exchange, and Aerobic Capacity/Endurance Associated with Respiratory Failure in the Neonate

Pattern H: Impaired Circulation and Anthropometric Dimensions Associated with Lymphatic System Disorders

INTEGUMENTARY

Pattern A: Primary Prevention/Risk Reduction for Integumentary Disorders

Pattern B: Impaired Integumentary Integrity Associated with Superficial Skin Involvement

Pattern C: Impaired Integumentary Integrity Associated with Partial-Thickness Skin Involvement and Scar Formation

Pattern D: Impaired Integumentary Integrity Associated with Full-Thickness Skin Involvement and Scar Formation

Pattern E: Impaired Integumentary Integrity Associated with Skin

CHAPTER

2

Influence of Psychosocial Factors on Rehabilitation

Pat Precin, OTR/L, MS, ABD

LEARNING OBJECTIVES

1. Recognize the psychosocial factors that influence rehabilitation.
2. Recognize the impact of psychological functioning and social interaction on health, disease, accident proneness, and adjustment to illness and physical trauma.
3. Recognize the psychological impact of disability on the patient.
4. Be aware of different professionals (and their roles) to which physical therapists can refer patients with psychosocial issues.
5. Be aware of the interventions used to handle challenging behavior—how to deescalate an agitated patient, manage violent patients, and identify signs of hypersexuality.
6. Identify the stages of psychosocial adaptation to loss and disability.
7. Understand the difference between psychosocial adaptation and psychosocial adjustment.
8. Understand different coping strategies that have been found to be important in psychosocial adaptation and adjustment to chronic disability and illness.
9. Understand the common defensive reactions to disability.
10. Understand how body image may be affected by disability and what a physical therapist can do to address body image issues.
11. Recognize the warning signs of possible posttraumatic stress disorder.
12. Describe the general adaptation syndrome, its aims, uses, and potential dangerous outcomes.
13. Identify crisis points in the rehabilitation process.
14. Understand the psychosocial techniques to facilitate client-centered therapy.
15. List strategies and resources for prevention, wellness, and psychosocial education.

OUTLINE

Psychosocial factors pertain to the psychological development of an individual in relation to his or her social environment.[1] Psychosocial factors are numerous, as a person's psyche is affected by countless events in the internal and external environments. This chapter focuses on the psychosocial factors that influence the direction of physical therapy intervention. Some psychosocial factors include premorbid mental illnesses, personality styles, coping strategies, defense mechanisms, and emotional reactions to disability. Others include spirituality, values, environment, adjustment, cognitive abilities, motivation, family, social supports, life roles, and educational level. All of these factors can affect patients and treatment outcomes.

This chapter (1) identifies and describes how psychosocial factors can influence rehabilitation; (2) demonstrates how to address such factors during physical therapy intervention; and (3) provides indications for referral to psychosocial rehabilitation specialists. Psychosocial factors profoundly affect a patient's ability to recover. Patients who are emotionally upset will have difficulty concentrating on physical therapy goals until emotional issues are addressed. If a patient is motivated to participate in rehabilitation, but his or her family members do not support the patient's rehabilitation goals, the patient will be unlikely to progress upon returning home. Mental health status has been shown to be one of the most important predictors of physical health.[2] Wickramasekera et al found that more than 50 percent of all visits to primary care doctors involved somatic complaints resulting from psychosocial problems.[3] Patients with physical disabilities may fail to respond to treatment if a prominent psychosocial issue is affecting them as well.

Patients' perceptions of their rehabilitation role influences treatment outcomes. Patients who believe that they possess control regarding their treatment and feel respected by staff tend to experience better health outcomes.[4,5] Empowerment, education, inclusion in goal setting, and a high level of engagement are important factors that positively influence recovery.

The mind and the body are highly connected.[6] Because of their reciprocal influence, psychosocial and physical issues should be addressed simultaneously to best facilitate recovery. A slow recovery may cause or prolong depression, which may in turn further delay the rehabilitation period. Watts believes that mental health interventions should be provided to all rehabilitation patients, as health outcomes tend to be poor and prolonged when psychosocial problems remain unaddressed.[7]

Physical therapists regularly encounter patients who have psychiatric illnesses. Psychiatric conditions occur with some frequency in the general population (Table 2.1), but occur at an even higher rate in rehabilitation settings.[8] For instance, panic disorder occurs in 10 to 30 percent of patients treated in cardiovascular, respiratory, and neurological rehabilitation units, and 60 percent of those treated in cardiology clinics (compared to 1 to 2 percent in the general population).[9] **Conversion disorder** has been reported to occur at a rate of up to 14 percent in general medical or surgical inpatient units (compared to .5 percent in the general population).[10] Friedland and McColl found the prevalence of depression and substance abuse to be significantly higher among people with disabilities than in the general population, as did Turner and Beiser, who documented the rate to be three times higher regardless of gender and age.[11,12] A *Healthy People 2010* survey reported that 28 percent of people with disabilities had sad feelings that interfered with daily activities.[13] Twenty-seven percent of patients with stroke were found to be depressed—a finding that correlated with poorer rehabilitation outcomes.[14] Patients with traumatic brain injury, spinal cord injury, and Parkinson's disease also reported higher levels of depression compared to the general public.[15,16]

Table 2.1 Lifetime World Prevalence of the Most Common Psychiatric and Personality Disorders[9]

Major Psychiatric or Personality Disorder	Lifetime World Prevalence (%)
Alzheimer's (85+ years old)	16–25
Alcohol abuse or dependence	15
Major depression	10
Marijuana abuse or dependence	5
Schizotypal personality disorder	3
Dependent personality disorder	3
Obsessive–compulsive disorder	2.5
Histrionic personality disorder	2.3
Borderline personality disorder	2
Antisocial personality disorder	2
Panic disorder	1–2
Schizophrenia	1

If a patient does not have a preexisting psychosocial illness, he or she is more likely to develop one after the onset of physical illness. Anxiety disorders can result from endocrine (e.g., hyper- and hypothyroidism, pheochromocytoma, hypoglycemia, and hyperadrenocorticism), cardiovascular (e.g., congestive heart failure, pulmonary embolism, and arrhythmia), respiratory (e.g., chronic obstructive pulmonary disease, pneumonia, and hyperventilation), metabolic (e.g., vitamin B_{12} deficiency and porphyria), and neurologic conditions (e.g., vestibular dysfunctions, encephalitis, and neoplasm).[9] The onset of depression has also been linked to the presence of an existing physical disability.[11,12] There is evidence for the converse as well; the longer one possesses some form of mental health concern, the greater the risk for developing a physical illness. Depression is a risk factor for heart disease and post-stroke mortality.[17,18] Heinemann et al found alcohol-related automobile accidents responsible for a significant number of spinal cord injuries, and Zegans reported that psychological problems can be exacerbated by physical illness or injuries.[19,20] Anxiety can also increase the risk of cardiovascular disease and hypertension.[21]

Although the co-occurrence of physical disabilities and mental illness is high, the rate of treatment for mental illness among people with disabilities is low. In 1997, only 23 percent of adults with depression, 38 percent with anxiety disorders, and 47 percent with serious mental illness received treatment.[13]

A thorough examination of the patient's psychological and social functioning can contribute significantly to a better understanding of needs, fears, anxieties, and capabilities, as well as furnish essential information about the patient's emotional adjustment to disability, assets and liabilities, personality structure, and cognitive functioning.

Box 2.1 Major Areas of Consideration in a Mental Health Examination

- Present and premorbid intellectual, emotional, and coping functioning
- Present and premorbid psychopathologies and personality structure and diagnosis of levels of depression, anxiety, and other mental disabilities
- Determination of suicidal tendencies, decompensation, and other risks
- Degree of organicity and cognitive disability and its relationship to the patient's rehabilitative capacity
- Symbolic meaning of the disability and loss, and the compensatory reserves that can be elicited
- Frustration tolerance, motivation, and secondary gain interference
- Levels of pain, stress, and tolerance
- Determination of vocational interests and background, and present functioning capacity
- Sexual attitudes and dysfunction
- Determination of present and pre-morbid family structure and interaction, social and economic status, and the natural support network (environmental support systems)

These can then be used to better understand the patient's emotional barriers and behavioral difficulties that can impede recovery. Although not inclusive, Box 2.1 highlights the major areas of consideration in a mental health examination.

Whether physical therapists should address psychosocial issues during treatment or refer psychologically impaired patients to other professionals depends on several variables: (1) the severity of the patient's psychosocial issue; (2) the level of comfort with which the physical therapist can address psychosocial problems; and (3) the patient's ability to progress in rehabilitation if existing psychosocial issues are not addressed. Professionals to whom referrals may be made for additional psychosocial intervention include but are not limited to psychiatrists, psychologists, psychiatric nurses, occupational therapists, social workers, creative arts therapists, vocational counselors, rehabilitation counselors, substance abuse professionals, and pastoral counselors.

Psychosocial Adaptation

The combination of intense psychological stress, uncertain prognosis, prolonged treatment, and interference with daily activities can greatly impact the rehabilitation of patients with disabilities and chronic illnesses. *Disability* is loss of or diminished ability to perform specific social roles normally expected of the patient. *Psychosocial adaptation* to disability and chronic illness is an ongoing, dynamic, evolving process through which a patient strives to attain an optimal state of function within his or her environment.[22] Successful psychosocial adaptation may be characterized by a sense of (1) personal mastery; (2) participation in social, recreational, or vocational pursuits; (3) successful negotiation of the environment; and (4) a realistic awareness of one's current strengths, deficits, and functional capacities.[23] Adjustment is the final phase in adaptation and includes striving to achieve life goals, feeling self-confident and having positive self-esteem, possessing a positive attitude toward one's disability, forming emotional connections to others, and establishing a community member role.[24]

The processes of adaptation and adjustment are influenced by whether or not a chronic illness or disability is congenital or adventitious, of sudden onset or gradually progressive, and stable or unstable. Patients born with a physical disability and those who acquire them as a result of accident or disease later in life have substantial psychological differences.[25] Children born with a physical disability have only experienced life with their impairment; the development of their self-identity commonly mirrors that of children without disabilities.

In contrast, patients with adventitious disabilities often experience acute loss and grief. Patients with gradually progressive diseases or disabilities of sudden onset often experience anxiety and shock when first becoming aware of their condition. Such anxiety and shock is often followed by anger and depression, as patients realize the magnitude and consequences of their diagnosis.[22] Disabilities of sudden onset (e.g., injuries or accidents) are usually experienced as crises that will change the lives of patients and their families for all time.

Grief, Mourning, and Sorrow

Grief is a psychological state of distress resulting from a significant loss. In reaction to a disability, grief may emerge from lost function, broken relationships, the loss of one's familiar self-identity, and disrupted roles. Grief is characterized by preoccupation with loss and feelings of worthlessness or helplessness. Specific symptoms include feelings of tightness of the throat, muscular weakness, emptiness in the abdomen, anxiety that is described as painful, shortness of breath and choking, and periodic waves of physical distress lasting up to an hour. Other symptoms may include forgetfulness, poor concentration, dissociation, insomnia, loss of appetite, compulsive behavior, decreased organization, social withdrawal, guilt, decreased ability to make decisions, excessive speech, and hostility.[26] Severe, prolonged cases of grief can compromise the immune system.[27] The grief–mourning period is unpredictable, lasting anywhere from 6 months to 2 or more years. According to Donatelle and Davis, the grieving process consists of 10 stages: (1) frozen feelings;

(2) emotional release; (3) loneliness; (4) physical symptoms; (5) guilt; (6) panic; (7) hostility; (8) selective memory; (9) struggle for a new life pattern; and (10) a sense that life is okay.[26] It is important to note that such stages do not always occur in a progressive linear fashion, and some stages may occur simultaneously.

Grief is a natural experience necessary to regain or adapt to one's losses and construct a new self-concept. New coping skills are learned as patients adjust to unfamiliar challenges. There may be a difference between people grieving over loss from a disability and those grieving over other types of losses. When grief occurs as a result of disability, it may become prolonged, as the patient must continuously strive to accept the disability and his or her altered self. Burke et al described the grief of people with disabilities as "chronic sorrow," or a grief regarding the loss of normality.[28] Lindgren et al defined chronic sorrow as (1) progressive sadness that often increases after the initial loss; (2) prolonged periods of sorrow with no predictable end; and (3) recurrent or cyclic in nature as the sadness is continuously triggered by internal or external events that reawaken loss.[29] Patients with chronic sorrow can eventually experience adaptation to their losses if they are highly motivated to rebuild their lives and find meaning in their experience. Conversely, patients with pathological grief often experience prolonged feelings of guilt, anger, and sadness that inhibit function and adaptation.

It is important to recognize that grief can be an all-encompassing experience that takes time and energy away from rehabilitation, but rehabilitation may not progress without it. Physical therapists must understand grieving, mourning, and sorrow so that a patient's lack of progress or motivation is not misinterpreted as malingering.

Phase Models of Psychosocial Adaptation

The literature regarding psychosocial adaptation to chronic disability and illness falls into two opposing theories of adaptation—one in which adaptation occurs as a set of nonsequential and independent patterns of behavior, and the other in which adaptation occurs progressively through a series of phases.

Phase models suggest that a patient's reaction to chronic disability or illness follows a stable sequence of phases, or stages, that are hierarchically and temporally ordered. This progression is gradual, linear, and involves the psychological assimilation of changes to one's body image and self-concept. The most frequently identified phases in the adaptation to chronic disability and disease are shock, anxiety, denial, depression, internalized anger, externalized hostility, acknowledgment, and final adjustment.[22]

Shock

Shock usually occurs as the initial reaction to a psychological trauma or severe and sudden physical injury. It results from an overwhelming experience and may include the inability to move or speak, psychic numbness, decreased cognitive skills, disorganization, and depersonalization.

During a traumatic event, an individual will respond primarily at the physiological level; emotional reactions are commonly delayed until the event is over and the individual is medically stable. Likewise, the medical emergency team will first implement immediate lifesaving attempts before addressing accompanying psychological issues.

During a perceived or real catastrophic event, an organism would most likely respond with what Selye termed the *general adaptation syndrome* (GAS).[30] Selye described GAS as an organism's defensive adaptation attempt, which expresses itself through physiological and emotional responses aimed at dealing with such emergencies. During GAS, there is a physiochemical chain reaction, whereby a peptide called corticotropin-releasing factor (CRF) is secreted to stimulate the release of adrenocorticotropic hormone (ACTH). ACTH sets into motion an increase of specific physiological activity designed to maximize the body's defense capacity while minimizing the utilization of nonessential physiological activities. Although an increase in CRF serves the person's self-defensive strategies, its inhibitory effect on other body functions—such as the production of insulin and calcium—is undesirable in the long run.

Studies have shown that injection of a CRF antagonist reduces anxiety in stressful situations.[31] When the inhibitory effects of CRF are prolonged, however, the additional undesirable effects of hypertension, digestive problems, and interference with the immune system result. Selye documented the devastating effect that a prolonged GAS response has on human mental and physical functioning. Theorell et al documented the occurrence of resultant illnesses long after the stress-producing event had ended.[32]

Anxiety

Once the magnitude of the traumatic event is comprehended, anxiety in the form of a panic-stricken reaction commonly occurs and is marked by compulsive activity, confusion, elevated pulse rate, difficulty breathing, and cognitive flooding. Situations that activate the sympathetic nervous system through repeated alarm or chronic stress may alter synaptic transmission and lead to depression and malfunction of normal body systems.

It should be noted that the physiological and psychological reaction to stress are not limited to catastrophic conditions. An extensive body of research shows stress reactions to be present in individuals under conditions that may not be traumatic but nevertheless persistent and disruptive. Everyday life frustrations, internal and external conflicts, and changes in life conditions are major causes of the stress reaction that, over time, have a deleterious effect on a person's function and health. Physical therapists should be cognizant that even though a patient's emergency situation is over, a stress reaction may continue to be present.

Denial

Denial is often used as a defense mechanism to alleviate the anxiety and pain associated with a disability or illness. Denial occurs as a specific phase early in the adaptation process and protects the person from having to confront the overwhelming implications of illness or injury at once. Instead, denial allows a gradual assimilation of one's altered reality. Breznitz identified seven types of denial[33]:

1. Denial of threatening information (using selective inattention and partial awareness)
2. Denial of vulnerability (exerting control and maximizing personal strengths)
3. Denial of urgency (using methods to see the situation as less pressing than it is)
4. Denial of affect (reduction of emotional impact)
5. Denial of affect relevance (diverting attention to other issues and believing that an emotion is coming from an unrelated cause)
6. Denial of personal relevance (attributing difficulties to a benign cause and blaming others when involvement was one's own)
7. Denial of all information (creating a barrier between external reality and one's psyche resulting in total disbelief of having an illness or disability)

Patients in the stage of denial may selectively attend to the environment, choose facts that support their beliefs about themselves and their condition, and ignore facts that remind them of their new challenges. They may have unrealistic and wishful goals for recovery and may be seen as indifferent and aloof.

Depression

The phase of depression occurs as denial lessens, allowing a greater awareness of one's losses. *Depression* is a reactive response of bereavement for impending death, suffering, or the loss of body function. Neurochemical and biological changes resulting from disability or disease, premorbid personality and family history, and reactions to stress have all been identified as risk factors for depression.[34,35]

Internalized Anger

Anger occurs in reaction to anxiety, misperception, threats of abandonment, feelings of helplessness, or fear of losing control. Characteristics of anger include hostility, resentment, or hatred. *Anger,* is a response to loss and if not expressed is termed *internalized anger*. Internalized anger is associated with self-blame and is a manifestation of self-directed bitterness and resentment. Signs of internalized anger include manipulation, sabotage, and passive–aggressive behavior. Sometimes anger emerges when a patient attributes his or her own behaviors to the onset of disability or disease. In such cases, internalized anger can result in depression, suicidal tendencies, or psychosomatic complaints—particularly in people who have a chronic condition.[36]

There are many reasons why patients may not express anger: fear of losing loved ones or social isolation, cultural restraints, lack of awareness, fear of losing control, or belief that expressing anger is inappropriate or dangerous. Repressed anger not only affects a patient's psychological well-being, but may also slow rehabilitation. It is important for physical therapists to encourage expression of angry feelings by providing a safe environment for patients to verbalize their anger in appropriate ways. Therapists might state that anger is a normal emotion—especially under the patient's circumstances—offer reasons why it is important to express anger, and provide anger management techniques. It is equally important for therapists to understand that while a patient's anger may be directed at the therapist, such anger more often reflects the patient's own projected feelings regarding his or her disability.

Externalized Hostility

Externalized hostility is anger directed toward other people or objects in the environment and is an attempt to retaliate against functional limitations. Challenges encountered during rehabilitation may trigger externalized hostility. As time from the onset of the disability passes, externalized hostility tends to become more apparent.[37] Signs include passive–aggressive behaviors that obstruct rehabilitation, aggressive acts, hypercriticism, demanding or antagonistic behaviors, falsely blaming others, and abusive accusations. Patients who express anger aggressively through physical or verbal abuse, sarcasm, or controlling behaviors need the help of the entire team to redirect their anger into productive therapeutic activities that further their rehabilitation goals.

Acknowledgment

Acknowledgment is the first sign that the patient has accepted or recognized the permanency of the condition and its future implications. The patient begins to integrate functional limitations into his or her self-concept. During this phase, the patient accepts him- or herself as a person with a disability, develops a new self-concept, reassesses values, and searches for new goals and meaning.

Adjustment

Adjustment is the final phase in adaptation and involves the development of new ways of interacting successfully with others and one's environment. The person is now adjusted to the outside world after having fully assimilated his or her functional limitations from disability into a new, cohesive self. In this phase, the person regains self-worth, understands that new potentials are possible, pursues vocational and social goals, and overcomes obstacles that arise in the attainment of goals.

There is evidence that the phase model of adjustment to chronic disability or illness is nonlinear, multidimensional, and progressive. Phase models tend to have 10 common assumptions[22]:

1. People may skip one or more phases or may regress to an earlier phase, but adaptation is not irreversible.
2. The pace and structure of adaptation can be influenced by external events or interventions (e.g., environmental changes or counseling) yet are mainly determined by internal processes.
3. Not everyone achieves adjustment; some fixate at earlier phases.
4. Adaptation is an unfolding, dynamic process that gradually shifts from initial experiences of distress to assimilation of loss and reconciliation.
5. The adaptation process is initiated by significant and permanent changes in the body's functional capacities and appearance, which are usually followed by alteration of self-concept and body image.
6. The amount of time spent in each phase varies and may be determined by a combination of the following factors: social support, financial and human resources, past exposure to crises, age at onset, severity, nature of the disability or illness, and premorbid personality.
7. Psychological maturity and growth occur as the patient progresses through the phases.
8. Psychological reequilibrium occurs through gradual adaptation and reintegration to the perceived misfortune.
9. Human variability and uniqueness have a strong influence on the temporal ordering of phases—the sequence of phases is not universal.
10. Occasionally, phases may overlap, be nondiscrete, or fluctuate, causing patients to experience more than one reaction at a time.

Chronic Illness and Disability: Differences in Adaptation

There are marked differences in the way that people adapt psychosocially to a disability associated with a traumatic event—such as traumatic brain injury—versus a chronic illness—such as multiple sclerosis. The onset of disability in a traumatic event is sudden, and medical stability may be achieved shortly after. The onset of a chronic illness is usually insidious and gradual; its course is often uncertain and marked by states of remission and deterioration.[38] In chronic illness each onset of symptoms can be experienced as a new illness.

Shock may not be experienced by people with gradually deteriorating medical conditions (e.g., Parkinson's disease, rheumatoid arthritis, or diabetes mellitus), but is usually experienced following a trauma (e.g., traumatic brain injury, myocardial infarction, amputation, or spinal cord injury). Shock may be present but not as strong in people with life-threatening or end-stage diseases (e.g., AIDS, cancer, or amyotrophic lateral sclerosis). The phases of anxiety and depression relate more to the past, such as grieving over the loss of premorbid functioning. In a chronic illness, anxiety and depression relate more to the future (e.g., fear of death, feelings of hopelessness, and fear of the unknown).[39] The acknowledgment and adjustment phases may be more difficult to achieve in chronic, life-threatening conditions that require the internalization of and acceptance that the condition may worsen and result in death.

Posttraumatic Rehabilitation

The posttraumatic period may include phases of anxiety, depression, denial, internalized anger, and externalized hostility mentioned earlier, and is usually the time during which much, if not most, of the rehabilitative intervention takes place. It is also the period during which the psychological effects of the traumatic experience are more strongly felt by the patient. It seems as if the psychological defenses and reactions that became secondary during the initial traumatic period (shock phase) begin emerging as the physical injury is dealt with. These repressed reactions seem to interact with a growing awareness of the effects of the disability creating fears, anxieties, and behaviors that the rehabilitation team must address.

Regardless of which phase the patient is in, physical therapists need to be aware of each patient's psychological needs. During the initial phases of adaptation, patients may experience an awareness of their injuries that facilitates panic and fear of total dependence. Patients may also experience anxiety as a result of anticipating painful medical treatment. Some patients react to these feelings by desperately seeking control over their rehabilitation. Others experience shock regarding their losses and become overly dependent. Patients may idealize the past and have unrealistic expectations about the duration of their recovery.

During these early stages, physical therapists should praise small gains and work with caregivers so they can offer hope and support to the patient. Therapists should be supportive but careful not to make unrealistic predictions about the expected degree of recovery, as this may lead to disappointment, resentment, and depression.[40] One of the first approaches physical therapists can use to help patients regain self-control is *diaphragmatic breathing*, which may decrease pain and anxiety through the relaxation response.[41]

During the middle stages, physical therapists may need to educate patients about medical precautions, contraindicated activities, how the patient's body has adapted to disability, and how to reformulate expectations. Psychosocial instruction should be integrated with direction about activities of daily living, mobility, strengthening, and endurance. The transition from the patient role to an independent adult member of society is a difficult adjustment and can result in anxiety, depression, and poor social integration.[22,42] Physical therapists should help patients prepare psychologically for discharge and reintegration into society. Some of the issues that patients may fear include negative reactions to their disability, feelings of inadequacy, having to identify new social supports, receiving help in the home environment, and adjusting to a new body image.

Body image includes judgment about one's appearance, an awareness of boundaries and personal space, judgment about one's bodily responses, perception of one's body parts and their movement, and an awareness of physical pleasure and pain. Body image is intimately related to self-concept and self-esteem. It affects not only a person's functional abilities, cognition, perceptions, attitudes, and emotions, but also the reactions of others to oneself. Because body image changes throughout life, it is thought to be both dynamic and developmentally based. Difficulties brought on by a disability—such as functional limitations and pain and disfigurement—alter body image and threaten its stability. Patients must then reconstruct their body image and self-perception to adapt to this physical change.[22]

Fisher has identified the following patterns in patients who experienced shifts in body image after disability: (1) denying the existence of one's body; (2) fantasizing about a lost or damaged body part being magically replaced or healthy; (3) concentrating solely on noninjured body parts in order to deny impairment of the affected area; and (4) experiencing a period of defensiveness followed by gradual acceptance and assimilation of their altered body.[43] The physical therapist's comfort level with the patient's physical disability and the therapist's attention to the affected body part may help the patient feel less ashamed about body changes.

Personality and Coping Styles

The more a patient has evolved socially and psychologically, the better he or she will be at using adaptive methods to deal with crises. Hence, a patient with a healthy premorbid personality but a severe physical disability may do better in rehabilitation than one with a less severe disability and a pathological premorbid personality.[44] When aware of their patients' personality styles, physical therapists will be more adept at developing treatment plans, strategizing interventions, and motivating and guiding patients through rehabilitation.

Personality Types

Although each personality is unique, personalities have been categorized into different types, such as type A, perfectionistic, authoritative, and passive–aggressive. These personality types are nonpathological and develop in response to one's environment when young.

Individuals with *type A personalities* have a compulsive need to be achievers in all aspects of life. They are extremely independent and productive. These qualities also serve as defenses against low self-esteem and interpersonal conflicts. These people usually derive satisfaction from being strong individuals who can help others. If they can no longer participate in this role, they may become depressed because of a perceived inability to confirm their worth through altruistic activities. Physical therapists can use these qualities in patients with type A personalities to motivate their interest in rehabilitation. Because they are often self-starters and take initiative for their own learning, they can usually be depended upon to independently practice home exercise programs.

Individuals with *perfectionistic personalities* uphold high standards in order to maintain self-esteem. These individuals judge themselves by inflexible and possibly unachievable criteria and may not be able to tolerate slow progress during rehabilitation. Physical therapists may aid these patients by helping them derive pleasure from simple things, such as a meal, a sunset, a new shirt, or interesting information. Helping them discover value in these things offers them sources of self-esteem other than meeting impossibly high standards.

Individuals with *authoritative personalities* need to be in control and need things to be done in a particular way because of rigid perceptions regarding values, rules, and the manner in which others should behave. They are often concerned with status, tend to be judgmental, and have difficulty empathizing with others. During rehabilitation, these patients may try to dictate their treatment and engage in a power struggle with their physical therapists. Patients with authoritative personalities have difficulty adapting to disability, which often requires acceptance and compromise. They may require alternative strategies to solve what may have been perceived as an unsolvable problem. Physical therapists should engage patients in problem solving to generate strategies to meet their goals.

Individuals with *passive–aggressive personalities* express hostility by using passive techniques such as procrastination, resistance, stubbornness, and intentional inefficiency. These personalities react to authority negatively and have difficulty working with others. Physical therapists may work more efficiently with passive–aggressive patients by placing the responsibility for progress onto them. Patients can be instructed to make decisions about their treatment whenever possible and then summarize their progress after each session. This deemphasizes the physical therapist's role as an authority figure, and therefore the need for a passive–aggressive response.

Personality Disorders

When an individual's personality style deviates from cultural norms over a long period of time, is inflexible or pervasive, causes distress to oneself and others, and leads to functional impairment, that personality style is considered to be dysfunctional.[9] Personality disorders have been thoroughly classified. They include paranoid, antisocial (also referred to as sociopath or psychopath), borderline, histrionic, narcissistic, avoidant, dependent, obsessive–compulsive, schizoid, and schizotypal personalities. Freidman et al state that disability exacerbates preexisting pathology, meaning that the stress of dealing with a physical illness can make personality disorders even more pronounced.[45]

Patients with *paranoid personality disorder* interpret the motives of others as malevolent when they may not be. This results from a pattern of suspiciousness and distrust. These patients believe that others are trying to exploit, deceive, or harm them. Because of such mistrust, they may discharge themselves from treatment. Physical therapists should look for behaviors that indicate paranoid thoughts such as hostile reactions, guardedness, argumentation, and stubbornness, and encourage patients to express their thoughts at that moment. If the patient seems paranoid, the physical therapist should help him or her to better understand the reality of a specific situation. For instance, if the patient complains about being forced to participate in an elaborate intervention so that, in his or her view, the therapist can make more money, the therapist should review the pros and cons of various treatments and discuss the clinical reasoning involved. Literature can be very convincing since it does not come directly from the therapist.

Patients with *antisocial personality* frequently engage in deceit and manipulation. In rehabilitation, they may use an alias, lie to the staff, or malinger. They are irresponsible and often fail to comply with self-care procedures such as hygiene and home maintenance. They seek out and take advantage of weaker staff members, often using wit and charm. When they do not receive what they want, they commonly become irritable and violent, especially when staff members attempt to impose restrictions. They frequently cause disruption to others in rehabilitation. These patients require a cohesive team approach with immediate and strong intercommunication to minimize disruptive behaviors and refocus on rehabilitation goals.

Patients with *borderline personality disorder* have instability in emotions, relationships, and self-image; are impulsive; use primitive defense mechanisms such as *splitting* and devaluation; and tend to engage in self-destructive behaviors such as abusing drugs or self-mutilation. On the surface, they may appear critical of others but these are signs of deep vulnerability and should be treated as such. Therapists should respond with understanding and empathy instead of anger, and should emphasize strengths and strategies for ongoing work. Self-mutilating behaviors, such as repetitive cutting with razor blades, pin pricking, or cigarette burning, should be immediately reported to a doctor and referral made to a psychiatrist.

Patients with *histrionic personality disorder* seek attention via excessive emotionality. Since these patients respond well to audiences, therapists should provide situations in which patients can gain positive attention from doing well in rehabilitation. Physical therapists should set boundaries to help patients achieve a balance between their need to express themselves and their need to focus on therapeutic interventions. A calm and logical approach to rehabilitation helps settle intense emotions. Referrals can be made to dance, music, art, or drama therapists to meet ongoing needs for attention and self-expression.

Patients with *narcissistic personality disorder* are condescending and have a need for admiration and feelings of superiority. If an illness causes a reduction in this image, they will require help from their physical therapists to identify strengths and feel acceptable.

Patients with *schizoid personality disorder* have a flat affect, or limited range of emotional expression, and are detached from social interactions. The therapist should attend to the patient's rehabilitation without trying to engage him or her in a great deal of social interaction. If the disorder has been long-standing, the patient will likely feel uncomfortable socializing.

Patients with *schizotypal personality disorder* have eccentric behavior, perceptual or cognitive distortions, and marked distress in social relationships. The social intimacy and physical restriction of a rehabilitation environment may cause anxiety. Slow, unforced integration into the therapeutic setting may be required. Asking patients whether their views of reality are accurate may help them remain focused on achieving rehabilitation goals.

Patients with *avoidant personality disorder* suffer from social inhibition, feelings of inadequacy, and hypersensitivity to criticism. Physical therapists should reassure these patients that they are doing well and emphasize their strengths.

Patients with *dependent personality disorder* exhibit clinging behavior, need others to care for them, and are submissive. They may fail to function independently in their life roles even after physical functioning has returned, continuing the pattern of dependency. They fear abandonment and require constant reassurances that staff members understand their condition and care about them. Some respond to clear explanations and feedback about their progress and treatment plans. The therapist should reinforce independent behavior through attention and positive feedback while extinguishing dependent behavior by ignoring or redirecting it.

Patients with *obsessive–compulsive personality disorder* have a long-standing preoccupation with control and order and are often perfectionists. If these patients perceive a loss of control, their self-esteem may suffer, and they may react by becoming more obstinate, demanding, and inflexible. Those who publicly express their anger may become ashamed. These patients require greater predictability in treatment than usual, dislike change, and do well when given an established routine to follow. The therapist should provide rehabilitative activities that promote a sense of control and predictability, and consider allowing patients to set treatment goals, then monitor their daily progress.

Coping Styles

Coping styles are ways that people deal with stress and include behavioral, emotional, and cognitive efforts to cope with internal and external challenges that strain ordinary resources.[46] Theories of coping suggest that it is not what happens to people that is important, but rather how they react.[47] Various coping strategies have been identified in the literature and summarized by Livneh and Antonak.[22] They include planning, problem solving, wishful thinking, avoiding, minimizing, seeking social support, searching for meaning, emoting feelings, blaming, accepting, negotiating, disengaging, and turning to religion. These and others can be categorized into three different types of coping: (1) seeking versus avoiding control and information; (2) expressing versus repressing emotional reactions; and (3) seeking versus withdrawing from social interactions and networks.

Coping strategies have been found to be of great importance in rehabilitation. Patients with higher level coping skills can more easily identify and report symptoms, make treatment decisions, comply with intervention, and accept support. Patients with good problem solving skills and positive attitudes have been found to make more positive adjustments to their disabilities than patients with low self-esteem and poor self-concept.[48] Coping styles often determine whether or not patients seek medical help and follow advice.[46]

Social influences, psychological characteristics, and health beliefs have been shown to modify the impact of disability and disease on an individual. Social activism, positive self-acceptance, and information seeking have predicted better ability to cope with a disability.[49] Krause and Rohe studied the relationship between adjustment and personality post-spinal cord injury to find that positive values, emotions, actions, and warmth correlated with superior outcomes.[50] Adaptive coping styles that result in positive outcomes for people with disabilities utilize positive, direct, and active problem solving, social support seeking, and information seeking. Maladaptive coping styles that lead to unfavorable adaptation outcomes include self-blame; nondirect, passive, and escape/avoidance modes of coping; and substance abuse.

Locus of control is a belief about one's ability to control life conditions and events.[51] Patients with an external locus of control believe that other people or outside factors determine outcomes. Patients with an internal locus of control take responsibility for change because they believe they can affect their own circumstances. The latter leads to goal-directed activity and active coping.

The ability to intentionally change the relative importance of events that occur in one's life requires constant practice.[52] It has been shown that patients with external loci of control experience stress and anxiety in rehabilitation, while patients with internal loci of control have quicker recoveries, better motivation, more hope, and more energy.

Coping styles can be examined through interviews, observations, self-report surveys, checklists, and information from the family. Treatment based on these findings should include emphasis on previous ways of successfully coping and expanding the range of coping strategies—such as maintaining a journal to increase self-expression. Taking care of a pet or using animal assistance can lend help, comfort, and companionship, as well as increase motivation. Group treatment can also be used to increase social networks.[53,54]

Many people with disabilities who have risk factors for emotional problems, such as lower education, less income, and social isolation, still do well in life because of a certain *resilience* defined as successful adaptation to stressful situations or events.[55] Researchers of resilience identify protective factors that safeguard people from adverse consequences. Protective factors can arise from the individual, family, and society and are concerned with how strengths and supports provide security, safety, and positive opportunities.

Turning points are important experiences and realizations that enable people to find new direction, purpose, or meaning in life. King et al reported four protective factors: determination, perseverance, spiritual beliefs, and social support.[56] Seven protective processes were also identified: transcending, self-understanding, accommodating, receiving a diagnosis that helps explain a patient's experiences, believing in oneself, using anger as motivation, and setting goals. These protective factors and processes help people with disabilities during turning points in their lives. Analysis of turning points revealed three major ways that patients maintained meaning in their lives: through doing, belonging, and understanding themselves in relationship to the world. Doing involves participating in activities that are fulfilling and facilitate competency. Belonging involves perceived acceptance by others or membership in a valued group. Understanding oneself in relationship to the larger world provides a sense of identity and sometimes purpose.

Common Defense Reactions to Disability

Defense mechanisms are coping styles that people use to defend against internal and external stressors. They happen automatically and unconsciously. Some individuals use many different defense mechanisms throughout their lives, but most tend to utilize only one or two. The goal is not to change or modify these defense mechanisms, but to identify them in order to understand the patient's psychological processes that underlie certain behaviors and resistance. Understanding these behaviors can help physical therapists to motivate or redirect patients during difficult times in their rehabilitation. The defense mechanisms described in Box 2.2 are common reactions to disability and can be

Box 2.2 Common Defense Mechanisms

Acting Out
Instead of expressing feelings verbally, the patient uses actions to release stress. For example, a patient is angry with the insurance company for not funding an athletic wheelchair, so refuses to use the standard wheelchair. Acting out occurs because certain feelings such as anger and hurt are too difficult to express verbally. Unexpressed feelings build anxiety until they are released through action.

The therapist should identify the feeling behind the acting out behavior by asking the patient why he or she behaved in that way. For instance, the therapist would ask the first patient above about using the wheelchair. The patient's responses will eventually trace back to the original unexpressed feeling. Through questioning, the therapist brings to the patient's awareness the link between the feeling and the action. The patient can now verbalize and discuss the feeling. In the case above, the patient may be more willing to use the wheelchair. A patient who does not have difficulty verbalizing feelings tends not to act out.

Altruism
The patient becomes dedicated to helping others in order to manage his or her own stress. An altruistic patient may stop treatment to help everyone else in the treatment room, including the therapist. Such a patient receives gratification through these actions, and hence decreases his or her stress.

Autistic Fantasy
The patient engages in excessive daydreaming instead of pursuing human relationships in order to decrease stress. The patient may have difficulty following directions, may appear to be in another world, but happily so, and may become emotional and tense when returned to reality. If asked what he or she is thinking about, the patient may describe his or her fantasies, which can be a rich source of wishes and desires that can be used by the therapist to motivate the patient to work on short-term goals. For instance, a male patient relates a fantasy of dating his favorite teen idol. However, in order to engage in dating, he must first develop interpersonal skills and practice them in simulated and real-life settings.

Denial
Denial protects the ego from being overwhelmed by pain through an unrelenting process of disbelief. In the case of disability, denial may be used to protect the patient from reminders of an altered external reality and the resultant sense of loss. Therefore, the patient may refuse to acknowledge an emotionally painful condition or situation that is apparent to others. The patient often denies the severity of a new disability, believing he or she can return to previous jobs or roles, despite reality testing from the therapist. The patient may refuse rehabilitation, claiming that he or she just wants to leave the hospital in order to care for his or her children.

It is important to help the patient work through denial slowly in order to avoid depression, which may occur if the patient becomes aware of his or her reality before psychologically ready to accept it. If the patient's denial is so great that treatment cannot proceed, he or she should be referred to a psychologist to explore what disability means to his or her future life.

Devaluation
The patient is overly critical of others and of him or herself and may insult therapists and other personnel. The therapist should not take such insults personally, but should offer empathy and kindness, which usually decrease devaluation and build rapport. Once a patient trusts the therapist, he or she may discuss insecurities and fears instead of defending against them through criticism. If the therapist becomes angry with the patient, the insults usually become worse and a power struggle may ensue.

Displacement
The patient transfers a response to, or feeling about, one object onto a less threatening object to minimize stress. For example, a patient may be angry with a spouse for driving the car recklessly and having an accident but takes the anger out on the physical therapist. In this situation, it may not be safe or helpful for the patient to express anger directly to the spouse, who may be the patient's only emotional support.

The therapist should help the patient transfer the misplaced feeling back to the object for which it was originally intended. The therapist might accomplish this by asking the patient a series of questions concerning the origin of the anger.

Dissociation
The patient deals with stress through a breakdown in memory, perception, consciousness, or sensorimotor behavior. The patient becomes detached from what is happening in the moment because it is too painful. The patient may stop speaking or participating in therapy and stare blankly into space for up to several minutes without responding to the environment. Afterward, the patient may not be aware of his or her dissociated state, or if he or she is, the patient may state that he or she "just spaced out." The patient who uses dissociation usually relies on it often; a physical therapist may note its occurrence several times during a session. It is important to notice what happened just before the dissociation to identify the painful thoughts, feelings, or actions that upset the patient.

Help-Rejecting
The patient deals with the stress of having covert hostile feelings toward caregivers by frequently asking for help and then rejecting every suggestion. Working with a patient who uses help-rejecting as a defense mechanism can be very frustrating. Such patients seem to sincerely seek help but reject all advice as ineffectual. In these cases, it may be helpful to point out to the patient that efforts to help have been thwarted. The patient is usually not aware that he or she has rejected all solutions and may then come up with a solution or be more open to one that has already been proposed.

Humor
Humor can be used to minimize stress by highlighting the ironic or amusing aspects of a stressful situation. For instance,

Box 2.2 (continued)

a patient states that he is going to open up a hardware store since he has so much hardware (meaning surgically placed pins and plates) in his leg. A patient who uses humor as a defense mechanism usually feels better if the physical therapist laughs at his or her jokes and participates in joking behavior. It is a safe way for the patient to recognize the difficulty of his or her situation.

Idealization

A patient endows another individual with overly positive attributes to enhance an otherwise negative situation. This other individual may be the therapist, in which case the therapeutic relationship is often strengthened. Or, it could be a spouse, in which case problems could arise if he or she is not such a positive support to the patient. It is important to uncover the reality of the situation so necessary treatment and discharge plans can be made.

Intellectualization

A patient uses intellectual reasoning rather than expressing emotions in order to avoid painful feelings. For example, the patient describes neurotransmitters and synapses when asked about a head injury. Therapists can relate to such patients by intellectualizing with them. In the preceding case, the therapist may speak about the patient's head injury in terms of science and facts instead of emotions.

Isolation of Affect

A patient separates feelings from ideas when thinking about and discussing an upsetting event to minimize negative feelings associated with it. He or she speaks of the details regarding the recent accident that caused a disability without mentioning any feelings associated with the event to avoid reexperiencing them. Therapists should help the patient integrate feelings about an event into his or her memory of it. This can be achieved by asking the patient how he or she feels about certain aspects of the event while talking about it.

Omnipotence

A patient feels or acts as if he or she is better than others to guard against feelings of inadequacy. For instance, a patient looks down on other patients with disabilities because he does not want to see himself as disabled. A therapist might observe criticism and devaluation of external objects, bragging about accomplishments or skills, conceit, and grandiosity. The therapist could use this defense mechanism to motivate the patient to get better in order to avoid feeling inferior.

Projection

A patient transfers his or her own unacceptable feelings, thoughts, and beliefs onto another person and becomes certain that the other person really feels, thinks, and believes that way. A patient cannot tolerate the idea of having unacceptable feelings such as anger, but expresses them by projecting them onto another person, remaining relatively guilt free. For example, a patient says that his therapist is annoyed with him when in fact the patient is annoyed with his therapist.

Rationalization

A patient uses elaborate explanations to reassure him that his actions are driven by sound motives, when he may truly be unsure. A family member caring for a relative with congestive heart failure asks for a do not resuscitate (DNR) status, citing extensive research studies. The family member states that the relative will die soon anyway, thereby concealing her real and less acceptable reason for seeking the DNR status—to relieve herself from caregiving responsibilities.

Repression

A patient unconsciously erases negative experiences, wishes, or thoughts from consciousness in order to decrease stress. For example, a patient finds an endearing letter to a spouse from a student and forgets to mention it because the possibility of the spouse having an affair is painful. Repressed material can be dangerous because it remains in the unconscious. Encouraging the patient to express his or her feelings, both good and bad, helps free him or her of these feelings and any possible negative urges to act upon them.

Splitting

A patient views a person or event through a positive or negative lens at any given point in time. Later, the patient may flip his or her feelings to the opposite end of the spectrum regarding the same person or situation, acting in this manner because he or she has difficulty integrating ambivalent feelings. Some patients will often attempt to split staff, identifying one staff member with unrealistic positive attributes, while identifying another staff member with unrealistic negative qualities. The staff member who has been identified as negative has usually denied some desire the patient requested. The patient may approach the positively identified therapist and complain that the first therapist is insensitive and doesn't understand her needs. The patient may express that only the positively identified therapist understands her problems. However, when the positively identified therapist also denies the patient's request, the patient then vilifies that therapist as well. The therapist may help the patient to integrate the opposite poles of his or her emotions by bringing both positive and negative emotions into consciousness. The patient then may be able to see the reality of his or her situation.

Sublimation

Sublimation occurs when patients transform unacceptable emotions or desires into socially acceptable actions. For example, a patient who is angry about his recent divorce may be unable to consciously express those feelings for fear of losing

(*continued*)

Box 2.2 Common Defense Mechanisms (continued)

the affection of his children. Instead of expressing his anger he may sublimate those emotions into a more socially acceptable action, such as working out in the gym and eventually training for marathons. By participating in an activity that is valued and admired in the society, he gains the positive support of others.

Suppression

A patient intentionally avoids thoughts of disturbing feelings, situations, experiences, or problems in order to reduce stress. When refusing to talk to his or her therapist about the accident that brought him to rehabilitation, the patient suppresses disturbing thoughts. Therapists can refer patients to creative arts therapists (e.g., dance, music, art, drama, or poetry therapists) to facilitate the expression of disturbing thoughts, as such emotions accrue over time if not expressed.

Undoing

A patient uses behavior or words to negate unacceptable actions, thoughts, or feelings. For example, one who is frequently bullied by another patient during rehabilitation feels rage against his aggressor, but invites him to lunch.

In both undoing and suppression, disturbing feelings are intentionally avoided. In suppression, the feelings are avoided and nothing else happens. Feelings are avoided and concealed through opposing words or actions. Both undoing and suppression differ from repression in that repression is an unconscious act.

further explored in the *Diagnostic and Statistical Manual of Mental Disorders*.[9]

Anxiety

The experience of *anxiety* varies in different patients. When someone is nervous (indicating a moderate level of anxiety) he or she may experience an upset stomach or headache. When someone is experiencing a panic attack (indicating a high level of anxiety), he or she may feel impending doom and terror. A symptom of anxiety in one patient may be heart palpitations, while in another it may be shortness of breath. What is anxiety-producing to one patient may cause little to no anxiety in another. Given these variables, the following definitions may facilitate physical therapists' understanding of their patients' conditions.

Anxiety is the apprehensive anticipation of future danger or misfortune accompanied by feelings of tension and agitation. The anticipated danger may be real or imagined, but is experienced both psychologically and physiologically.[57] A *panic attack* is a sudden onset of intense, overwhelmimg fear that may include feelings of imminent danger or impending doom. These attacks are marked by symptoms of palpitations, chest pain, smothering or choking sensations, shortness of breath, and fear of losing control, dying, or going crazy. Panic attacks may be unexpected (occurring without an internal or external trigger) or situational. It is unclear what kind of physiological change in the brain may trigger such a severe response. A *phobia* is an anxiety disorder characterized by intense anxiety resulting from thoughts of, or exposure to, a specific feared situation or object (such as heights, spiders, or exams) leading to avoidance of that object or situation. *Generalized anxiety disorder* is defined as excessive worry and anxiety without an apparent source persisting for at least 6 months.[9]

Causes of Anxiety

Twenty to 30 million Americans suffer from anxiety.[26] Some signs and symptoms of anxiety are listed in Table 2.2, and behaviors that may result from anxiety are listed in Table 2.3. Much of the literature on stress and coping has identified major life events as stressors. Life events refer to major changes in lifestyle, status, role, or situation. This view is consistent with the notion that stress, though individually mediated, is to some degree environmentally based and/or exacerbated by environmental and social conditions. Various life event measures have been developed and are used in examining potential environmental stress. One of the better known and used instruments is the *Holmes-Rahe Social Readjustment Rating Scale* (see Appendix A), which quantifies the effects of life changes on stress and health.[58] Such measures of life events assume a relatively global impact, and take into account only those items listed. Although there is justified validity in such an approach, there exist potentially more sensitive and valid measures, one of which is the Hassles Scale.

The *Hassles Scale* (Appendix B), developed by Kanner et al[59] requires subjects to identify the irritating and frustrating demands of everyday transactions with the environment. This approach takes into account the individual's perception of events believed to pose a threat. It is consistent with the theoretical assumption that chronic struggle may tax coping abilities and lead to greater difficulty in the management of daily life events. Considering the enormous changes in a person's function when disability occurs, patients are more likely to expect an increase in daily hassles and stressors. Dealing with life becomes more taxing when disabling circumstances block one's coping style, causing a gap between the person and his or her fit within the world. Repeat occurrences of stress and the continual need to adjust to new situations can result in repetition of the fight-or-flight response, which can, over time, result in high blood pressure leading to heart attack or stroke.[21]

Table 2.2 Signs and Symptoms Associated with Low, Moderate, and High Levels of Anxiety

Low-Level Anxiety	Moderate-Level Anxiety	High Level Anxiety
Agitation	Abdominal distress	Chest pains
Apprehension	Aches	Depersonalization
Distress	Chills	De-realization (feeling unreal)
Irritability	Decreased concentration	Difficulty sleeping
Motor restlessness	Diarrhea	Dizziness
Muscle tension	Fear	Dread
Nervousness	Feeling light-headed, unsteady or faint	Helplessness
Worry	Fever	Horror
	Heart palpitations	Hyper-vigilance
	Hot flashes	Increased sensitivity to pain
	Increased heart rate	Nausea
	Misperception	Paresthesia
	Shaking or trembling	
	Shortness of breath	
	Sweating	

Anxiety and Rehabilitation

Different levels of anxiety have different effects on patients. If anxiety is completely absent, patients may not be motivated to achieve treatment goals. Mild anxiety can be motivating if directed toward rehabilitation. Severe anxiety can escalate quickly and impair all aspects of the patient's life, including rehabilitation outcomes, by intensifying the perception of pain, inhibiting immunosuppression, and prolonging recovery time.[60,61] Patients who had difficulty managing anxiety prior to physical illness will probably have more difficulty managing stress brought on by disability.

Table 2.3 Behaviors Associated with Low, Moderate, and High Levels of Anxiety

Low-Level Anxiety	Moderate-Level Anxiety	High-Level Anxiety
Avoiding stressful situations	Going to the bathroom frequently	Holding hand over heart
Biting lips	Incessant talking	Reacting to irrelevant cues
Drumming fingers on a table top	Mumbling	Throwing up
Fidgeting	Overactivity	
Nail biting	Staring blankly	
Pacing	Verbalizing somatic preoccupations	
Pulling or twirling hair		
Rubbing an object such as worry beads		
Shaking legs		
Sighing heavily		
Tapping feet		

When a patient is anxious, thought and energy often become focused on the anxiety instead of physical therapy, resulting in decreased concentration. Decreased learning may be observed when a patient is unable to concentrate on the therapist's instructions. The patient may be unable to perform motor tasks that require multiple-step directions. Poor concentration can also result in safety risks as the patient's attention may be alternating between the anxiety and the demands of rehabilitation. To appear functional, the patient may try to perform a task having heard only part of the therapist's instructions. Such a patient may fail to understand directions given by the therapist and may not realize that he or she missed important information. Steps may be skipped and a patient may jump ahead too quickly, resulting in injuries to the patient or others.

If patients become fearful because of anxiety, they may avoid certain behaviors in an attempt to decrease their fear. Fearful, anxious patients are reluctant to try new things. They may refuse treatment, remain in their rooms, request a bedpan when they are capable of using the commode, or be reluctant to progress to the next step in therapy. Such patients will commonly make statements such as, "I can't. I don't feel well. I'm too tired. Leave me alone. Not now, I'll do it later. I'm afraid. You can't help me. You don't look strong enough. I'm going to fall."

Patients who express anxiety through overactivity may attempt to progress too quickly through rehabilitation. They often want to achieve everything at once and appear impatient. They tend to rush through each session without mastering each step. Such patients frequently talk of discharge before it is an option. They may make rash decisions regarding major life changes, such as purchasing new cars or planning vacations when neither would be in their best interest. Such behaviors may provide immediate relief from anxiety for both patients and their families yet cause more distress in the long run.

When anxiety causes misperception, patients may perceive their level of dysfunction and improvement differently than do their therapists. They often leave therapy sessions with an unrealistic opinion concerning any progress or gains made. Such patients may believe they performed at a higher level than they actually did.

Watching a patient experience a panic attack for the first time can be frightening. It may not be immediately evident to either the patient or physical therapist if the patient has never experienced one before. Patients experiencing a panic attack usually report fear of immediate death. They may start to hyperventilate, then suffer shortness of breath. Sometimes they believe they are having a heart attack as a result of chest pain, heart palpitations, and increased heart rate. Terror and panic ensue, and the therapist may call a code or, if in a clinic, rush the patient to the hospital.

How to Address Anxiety

Physical therapists need to help patients control anxiety so they can proceed with treatment. Some patients may find it beneficial to discuss their fears and concerns with their physical therapists. In such cases the therapist should initiate a dialogue with the patient, asking, "How are you feeling?" "What is your greatest concern?" "What is the worst thing you believe may happen?" and so forth. Physical therapists can work with patients to help defuse anxiety by using *cognitive restructuring*—or the reshaping of the patient's thoughts and beliefs regarding the feared event. For example, a therapist might help the patient to engage in reality testing by assisting the patient to understand that the occurrence of the feared event is unlikely.

Patients with real and imminent crises may benefit from assistance with problem solving, should their worst-case scenario occur. Such problem solving can help patients to believe that they can survive and live meaningful lives despite the occurrence of feared events. After patients have expressed their feelings, therapists can help them segue into treatment and transform their emotion into physical activity. It should be noted that patients who are verbose and cannot stop talking about their fears should not be encouraged to dwell upon them during physical therapy sessions. Encouraging patients to verbalize their anxieties is also contraindicated with patients whose psychosomatic complaints are fueled by conversation regarding their anxieties.

For patients who are very anxious, it may help to conduct treatment in a setting that is familiar, calm, and comfortable. An unfamiliar setting, too much stimulation in the environment, too many people, or too much noise can increase anxiety levels. It may be helpful to reorient patients to the therapy room and to treatment expectations—each session—to allow them to feel a greater sense of control.

Physical therapists should choose a purposeful activity with the patient's anxiety in mind. Some anxious patients have been known to respond to activities that consist of one repetitive motor action, as rhythmic motion helps to calm them.[62] Gross motor movements help decrease the physical symptoms of anxiety such as muscle aches, agitation, and restlessness. Therapists should begin by involving patients in a therapeutic activity that is easily performed and then increase the complexity of the task once the patient has gained confidence.

Anxious patients who may interrupt the physical therapist while he or she is with other patients may be reassured that they will be seen on a certain date and time. Physical therapists should ignore, without anger, all subsequent intrusions. Setting limits in this fashion helps patients improve their frustration tolerance. Very anxious people often welcome clear boundaries set by therapists because they have difficulty setting limits for themselves.

Stress management techniques are useful before and after a session. Techniques such as meditation, imagery, relaxation, stretching, stress management diaries, identifying stressors, biofeedback, nutrition, prioritizing, problem solving, decision making, anger management, Reiki, music therapy, therapeutic massage, and prayer have been shown to improve both the physical and emotional aspects of patients.[63–65] Some of these techniques work more effectively for some patients than others. Choosing one depends on the amount of time available, materials required, and the patient's preference.

Relaxation Response

Whichever stress management technique is selected, the overall goal is to teach patients how to experience the *relaxation response* and replicate it independently during stressful situations.[66] After studying the relaxation response for 20 years, Dr. Herbert Benson identified two essential components that elicit the response: (1) repetition of a sound, word, phrase, prayer, or muscular activity; and (2) disregarding distracting thoughts and returning to the repetition. Benson gives the following techniques for patients to use[21]:

1. Choose a phrase, word, or prayer that is part of your belief system.
2. Sit comfortably and quietly.
3. Close your eyes.
4. Relax your muscles beginning with your feet and working your way up your body.
5. Breathe naturally and slowly. Say your phrase, word, or prayer silently as you exhale.
6. Rid yourself of all distracting thoughts by letting them flow in and out of your mind like waves on the ocean, always returning to your phrase, word, or prayer.
7. Continue for up to 20 minutes.
8. Sit quietly for a minute, allowing your thoughts to return before opening your eyes. Sit for another minute before standing.
9. Practice this technique daily on an empty stomach if possible.

The relaxation response has proven to be effective in treating headaches, hypertension, anxiety, cardiac rhythm irregularities, mild and moderate depression, and premenstrual syndrome. The relaxation response works by decreasing heart rate, rate of breathing, metabolism rate, oxygen consumption and carbon dioxide elimination, and returning the body to a healthier balance.[21,66,67] When within-subject comparisons were made between blood pressure before and after meditation using the nine aforementioned steps above for several weeks, the average systolic blood pressure for the 36 subjects dropped from 146 to 137 mm Hg, while diastolic pressure dropped from 93.5 to 88.9; both are statistically significant changes.[21] The relaxation response seems to decrease blood pressure through counteracting the activity of the sympathetic nervous system—the same mechanism underlying the action of antihypertensive drugs. Lower blood pressure leads to lower risk for atherosclerosis and related diseases.

Guided Imagery

Another intervention is *guided imagery*, frequently used as a standard of care in multiple institutions to improve rehabilitation through relaxation. Guided imagery is said to work by decreasing the levels of cortisol that can inhibit the immune system and slow tissue repair.[68] As in eliciting the relaxation response, the patient should be guided to a state in which the mind is silent and calm. Through use of a tape, video, or therapy guide, the patient is asked to imagine a special place (e.g., the ocean, a forest, a sunset) and focus on vivid details using the five senses. By focusing on this location for increasing lengths of time, patients learn to gain relief from constant worry by releasing concerns for a period of time and returning to a place of relaxation and peace. Guided imagery enhances the mind–body–spirit connection through the induction of an altered state in which the mind communicates more effectively with the body.[60]

The use of guided imagery has achieved improved outcomes of care through significant reductions in pain, blood pressure, stress, side effects of treatments, headaches, uncertainty, depression, insomnia, blood glucose levels, and histamine response to allergies. Significant enhancement of the immune system and wound and bone healing has also been noted.[69] Because music may trigger emotional responses by influencing the limbic system when used with imagery, music used with guided imagery has been shown to decrease pain through increasing endorphin release.[70,71] Guided imagery with music has also been found to reduce the need for large doses of medication and reduce recovery time.[60]

Desensitization

One out of every eight American adults reports having phobias severe enough to interfere with daily functioning.[26] Patients suffering from phobias that interfere with treatment may require *desensitization techniques*, also called *situational exposure exercises*. For example, wheelchair-bound patients with a fear of elevators who always used stairs prior to injury now require help in coping with their fears. In a comfortable, calm treatment environment far from an elevator, the physical therapist can have the patient begin to talk about benign aspects of elevators (e.g., what they look like, where they are located, and how many floors are in the building). While the patient is answering these questions, the physical therapist should determine the patient's level of anxiety. What specific issue regarding the elevator is the patient discussing when his or her anxiety increases? If the patient has not as yet become too anxious, the therapist may ask more anxiety-producing questions, such as, "How high is the elevator's ceiling?" "Is there an emergency phone?" "Are you more fearful of taking an elevator by yourself or with a crowd of people and why?" "Have you ever taken an elevator before and if so, what happened?" The therapist should continue to examine the patient's level of anxiety during questioning, stopping just before the patient's anxiety reaches a point at which the patient cannot easily be calmed.

This process, called desensitization, allows the patient to discuss his or her fear in a safe environment where he or she does not feel overwhelmingly anxious. The physical therapist slowly increases the level of anxiety by asking more difficult questions, but only to a tolerable degree. The patient is then asked to visually imagine that he or she is in an elevator, while practicing relaxation techniques. The patient continues to practice this visualization, over time, until he or she can do so without experiencing fear. When the patient can visualize him- or herself in an elevator without experiencing fear, therapy progresses to the real-life experience of riding in an elevator with the therapist. Relaxation techniques continue to be used during such real-life practice. The activity of riding in an elevator with the therapist using relaxation techniques continues until the patient can do so without fear. The final step would be for the patient to practice riding in an elevator by him- or herself while using self-induced relaxation techniques. Desensitization therapy has a high rate of effectiveness in the treatment of phobias.

Cognitive–Behavioral Therapy

Cognitive-behavioral therapy (or cognitive restructuring) can help decrease anxiety by changing maladaptive thought patterns and modifying unhealthy behaviors.[72] Before unhealthy behaviors can be modified, they must first be identified and classified. Because many patients are not conscious of their anxiety, an initial step when using cognitive–behavioral therapy is to help patients recognize anxiety. Determine what the patient's first signs of stress tend to be. Many will reply that they react severely to stress, stating "I throw up," or "I cannot breathe." In these cases, therapists should ask about the existence of less severe signs, such as nail biting or leg shaking.

Next, patients should count how many times a day they experience stress, recording these in a journal. Physical therapists should help patients look for patterns in their anxiety. Are patients more anxious in the morning or evening, when they attend therapy, or when family members visit? The more patients can identify patterns of anxiety, the more they can anticipate it and prepare for anxiety before it occurs. Therapists should encourage patients to use stress management techniques as soon as they experience the first sign of stress so that their anxiety does not escalate. Keeping a stress management journal can give patients insight into how their thoughts affect their behavior. Research has shown that cognitive–behavioral therapy can be as effective as medication.[73–77] Evidence Summary Box 2.3 presents a summary of research data examining the effects of cognitive therapy versus use of antidepressants for depression.

Treatment for Panic Attacks

If the therapist knows that a patient has a history of panic attacks, the following techniques can be helpful. Have the patient describe the first signs of discomfort during the attack. Immediately help him or her to breathe long, deep, and slow breaths. This may require the use of a brown paper bag held by the patient over the mouth while breathing into it to slow the inhalation rate. It is beneficial to acknowledge that a panic attack is occurring and that the patient will be all right if he or she continues to focus on breathing slowly and deeply. The panic attack can become severe within minutes and pass just as quickly. The patient most likely will be seated or lying down throughout the panic attack, as it may render him or her incapable of doing anything else.

Patients are usually embarrassed after an attack and may avoid all situations in which they believe one may occur. They may sit on the end of the aisle while watching a movie, may avoid crowds, or, in extreme cases, stop leaving their homes entirely (referred to as agoraphobia). Therapists can help patients who experience panic attacks to achieve a more productive life by teaching them techniques to control the attacks before they become severe. Families and patients should be educated to understand that panic attacks involve a real physiological reaction, tend to last only several minutes, and often recur without further intervention. Patients with severe, continuous panic attacks should be referred to a psychiatrist for possible medication management.

When to Make a Referral for Anxiety

In many cases, medication does not fully alleviate patients' anxiety. However, it may decrease it sufficiently enough for patients to begin expressing their fears and implementing strategies to decrease stress. Becoming familiar with antianxiety medications may help physical therapists identify patients suffering from anxiety, especially if a diagnosis of anxiety is not documented in a patient's chart. Frequently prescribed antianxiety medications are listed in Box 2.4.

Multiple referrals may be necessary. Patients who have panic attacks should be referred to a psychiatrist for medication. Generalized anxiety can be treated with medication; hence, a referral to a psychiatrist would be appropriate if the anxiety lasts more than a week and interferes with the patient's performance in rehabilitation. Those who continue to experience anxiety from phobias despite desensitization therapy and medication should be referred to a psychologist for a more in-depth exploration of their fears. A referral to a psychologist is indicated if the anxiety seems to be a deeply rooted characteristic of the patient's personality.

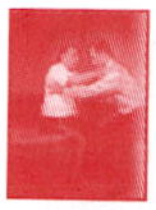

Evidence Summary Box 2.3

Research Examining the Effects of Cognitive Therapy versus Antidepressants for Depression

Reference	Subjects	Design/ Intervention	Duration	Results	Comments
Beck,[73] 2004	Depressed (nonbipolar and nonpsychotic) or dysthymic outpatients 72.7% female; Mean age = 27.1	Randomized treatment-outcome study comparing two groups: cognitive therapy (N = 18) and cognitive therapy plus antidepressant treatment (amitriptyline) (N = 15)	12 weeks of therapy and/or medication in a clinic	Cognitive group became depressed again during a one year period following intervention vs 18% of the cognitive plus antidepressant group, a non-significant difference ($p > .05$)	Small sample size and both treatment groups contained cognitive therapy. Five more patients relapsed in the cognitive group than the cognitive plus antidepressant group
Blackburn and Moorhead,[74] 2000	Depressed (nonbipolar and nonpsychotic) or dysthymic outpatients 64% female; Mean age = 43.7	Randomized treatment-outcome study comparing two groups: cognitive therapy (N = 22) and antidepressant treatment (amitriptyline or clomipramine) (N = 20)	12.9 weeks of therapy or medication in a hospital	21% of the cognitive group became depressed again during a 2-year period following intervention vs 78% of the antidepressant group, a significant ($p < .05$) difference	Cognitive therapy for patients with mild to moderate depression should be considered before referral to a psychiatrist for antidepressants
Miller et al,[75] 1985	Depressed (nonbipolar and nonpsychotic) or dysthymic outpatients 73.9% female; Mean age = 36.8	Randomized treatment-outcome study comparing two groups: cognitive therapy (N = 14) and antidepressant treatment (N = 17)	15 weeks of therapy or medication in a hospital	46% of the cognitive group became depressed again after a one-year period following intervention vs 82% of the antidepressant group, a significant ($p < .05$) difference	Cognitive therapy for patients with mild to moderate depression should be considered before referral to a psychiatrist for antidepressants
Bowers,[76] 1990	Depressed (nonbipolar and nonpsychotic) or dysthymic outpatients 80% female; Mean age = 36.2	Randomized treatment-outcome study comparing two groups: cognitive therapy (N = 10) and antidepressant treatment (N = 10)	4.2 weeks of therapy or medication in a hospital	20% of the cognitive group became depressed again after a 1-year period following intervention vs 80% of the antidepressant group, a significant ($p < .05$) difference	Cognitive therapy for patients with mild to moderate depression should be considered before referral to a psychiatrist for antidepressants
Gloaguen et al,[77] 1998	Patients with (N = 2765) nonbipolar and nonpsychotic major depression or dysthymia	78 controlled clinical trials. Pre- and posttests of the Beck Depression Inventory. Meta-analysis using Hedges and Olkin d +	Ranged from 4 to 79.3 weeks of therapy	Cognitive therapy was more effective than antidepressants ($p < 0.0001$), no intervention, and a group of miscellaneous therapies ($p < 0.01$), but equal to behavioral therapy	Limitation: Between-trial homogeneity was not met for two groups, the miscellaneous therapies and the placebo, so the comparison of cognitive therapy and these groups should be made cautiously

Box 2.4 Commonly Prescribed Antianxiety Medications

Alprazolam (Xanax)
Baclofen (Lioresal)
Buspirone hydrochloride (BuSpar)
Carisoprodol (Soma)
Clorazepate dipotassium (Tranxene, Gen-Xene)
Chlordiazepoxide (Librium, Mitran, Reposans-10)
Chlorzoxazone (Paraflex, Remular-S)
Cyclobenzaprine hydrochloride (Flexeril)
Dantrolene sodium (Dantrium)
Diazepam (Diastat, Valium)
Estazolam (Prosom)
Flurazepam hydrochloride (Dalmane)
Hydroxyzine hydrochloride (Vistaril)
Hydroxzine pamoate
Lithium carbonate (Eskalith, Lithobid)
Lithium citrate
Lorazepam (Ativan)
Meprobamate (Equanil, Mittown)
Methocarbamol (Robaxin)
Midazolam hydrochloride (Versed)
Oxazepam (Serax)
Temazepam (Restoril)
Tizanidine hydrochloride (Zanaflex)
Triazolam (Halcion)
Zaleplon (Sonata)
Zolpidem tartrate (Ambien)

Note: Brand names are shown in parentheses.

A social work referral can be helpful if the patient's anxiety results from a lack of necessary resources or involves family members.

Acute Stress Disorder (ASD) and Posttraumatic Stress Disorder (PTSD)

People who were disabled as a result of a traumatic event (e.g., a violent crime, abuse, an accident, a natural disaster, or war) or individuals who have witnessed such are at risk for *posttraumatic stress disorder* (PTSD) or *acute stress disorder* (ASD). Both are specific forms or subsets of anxiety disorders. The *Diagnostic and Statistical Manual of Mental Disorders* differentiates between both disorders in terms of the duration of the disorder and its symptoms. **Acute stress disorder** (ASD) involves symptoms that must range in duration between 2 days to a maximum of 4 weeks. PTSD is differentiated as *acute* PTSD if symptoms last more than but less than 3 months and as *chronic* PTSD if symptoms last beyond 3 months or longer. Both ASD and PTSD, however, must result from exposure to a traumatic event, and PTSD can be qualified with the term "with delayed onset" if symptoms first occur at least half a year after the traumatic event. Research notes that PTSD is an expected outcome for a certain percentage of patients experiencing even mild traumas.[78,79]

Among the symptoms exhibited are one or more of the following: reexperiencing the traumatic event; numbing of responsiveness to, or reduced involvement with the external world; and/or a variety of autonomic, dysphoric, or cognitive symptoms. The reexperiencing of the event is described as recurrent, painful, and consisting of intrusive recollections, dreams and nightmares, and, on rare occasions, dissociative states during which the individual may act as if reliving the actual traumatic event. This may last only several minutes or occur for hours or even days. The numbing of responsiveness, also called psychic numbing or emotional anesthesia, is expressed by complaints of feeling detached or estranged from others, a loss of ability or interest in previously enjoyable activities, or the lack of any emotions or feelings. Cognitive symptoms may include impairment of memory, concentration, and task completion ability. Patients may experience excessive autonomic arousal resulting in hyper-alertness, anticipatory anxiety, an exaggerated startle response, constant scanning of the environment, the perception of people and objects that are not real (i.e., hallucinations), or difficulty falling and remaining asleep.[80] Following this state of hypervigilance, the patient may experience a denial reaction marked by a diminution of responsiveness to the environment. Survival guilt may be present in those cases in which others were harmed or killed during a catastrophic event.

Additional associated features that should alert the physical therapist to the presence of PTSD are increased irritability, hostile behavior, constant tension, chronic free-floating anxiety, muscle tension, sexual and social difficulties, and somatic stress symptoms. Box 2.5 summarizes some of the prominent behavioral features of PTSD.

Not everyone who experiences trauma develops PTSD. The triple vulnerability model postulates that three vulnerabilities need to be present to develop an anxiety disorder: (1) a biological vulnerability; (2) a generalized psychological vulnerability (existing from past experiences of lost control over unpredictable events); and (3) a specific psychological vulnerability that links anxiety to specific situations.[81] Keane and Barlow have proposed an explanation for how PTSD develops based on the triple vulnerability model.[82] They suggest that during a traumatic event, a person experiences alarm and other intense emotions. If the event and resultant emotions are perceived to be unpredictable and beyond the person's control, the person is more likely to develop PTSD. If the event is perceived to be predictable and within the person's control, it is less likely that PTSD will occur.

Chronic pain frequently occurs concurrently with PTSD, and the occurrence of both disorders tends to negatively affect the treatment outcome for each.[83] Similar processes such as avoidance, fear, anxiety, oversensitivity, and

Box 2.5 Behavioral Features (Warning Signs) of Possible Posttraumatic Stress Disorder (PTSD)

Any one of the following behaviors:

- Recurrent, intrusive recollection of traumatic event
- Intrusive and distressing dreams of event
- Dissociative states (behaving as if reliving event; can last for several seconds or minutes)
- Amnesia of events

More than one of the following behaviors:

- Psychic numbing (lack of interest in social or physical environment or activities; significantly lowered participation in social or physical environment)
- Unable to feel emotions (e.g., intimacy, love, sexuality, anger)
- Disturbed sleep patterns
- Hypervigilance
- Exaggerated startle response
- Ongoing level of irritability
- Heightened difficulty with concentration

catastrophizing (i.e., interpreting an experience as overly threatening), may act to maintain both conditions. Given the high comorbidity of PTSD and chronic pain, physical therapists should examine patients with PTSD for the existence of chronic pain. The *Yale Multidimensional Pain Inventory* or the *McGill Pain Questionnaire* can be administered.[84,85] PTSD may be examined using the *Clinician Administered PTSD Scale Revised* or the *Posttraumatic Stress Disorder Checklist*.[86,87] Examination should also include the patient's beliefs, self-efficacy, level of anxiety sensitivity, coping style, expectations, and degree of behavioral and cognitive avoidance in order to understand the mechanisms that may maintain these conditions. See Chapter 28 for a more detailed discussion of instruments designed to measure pain.

The main desired outcome of treatment for PTSD should be engagement in healthy, satisfying, necessary, activities. The physical therapist can help patients to build positive self-efficacy through cognitive restructuring, development of healthy coping skills, and learning to use the relaxation response—all in a predictable, safe environment. Techniques used to help decrease catastrophizing and avoidance include situational exposure exercises (mentioned earlier) and interoceptive exposure exercises (such as running in place or spinning in a chair).[88] Interoceptive exposure exercises help patients cope with uncomfortable physiological sensations that may prevent participation in activities. Finally, the therapist should provide the patient education regarding how PTSD and pain can facilitate each other and result in avoidance. As participation in healthy activities increases, co-occurring disorders—such as depression, anxiety, panic, and substance abuse—may decrease, and a higher quality of life may ensue for the patient with PTSD.

Depression

Depression refers to feelings of despair and hopelessness, negative shifts in perception, and decreased interest in activities that once provided pleasure. A person may have a depressed personality (referred to as dysthymia) and therefore experience sadness throughout his or her entire life. As in most cases of depression, a person may have one or more episodes of depression, before and after which a normal mood exists. A certain degree of depression is normal in response to life's events, but when depression lasts 2 or more weeks and affects occupational and social functioning, it is considered to be *major depression*. Depression may occur as a biochemical imbalance in the brain, which may be triggered by stress, or in response to internal conflicts or life events. For example, the rate of depression in people with spinal cord injury is five times higher than that of the general population.[89]

Women with disabilities are more prone to depression (30 percent) than women without disabilities (8 percent), men with disabilities (26 percent), and the general population (7 percent) according to *Healthy People 2010*.[13] Other researchers support the finding that women with disabilities tend to experience depression more commonly than their male counterparts. In their analysis of 443 women with disabilities, Hughes et al found depression to be a frequently occurring secondary condition (51 percent of the sample scored in the mildly depressed range or higher on the Beck Depression Inventory-II [BDI-II]).[90] Fifty-nine percent of women with spinal cord injury were found to be clinically depressed, compared to a rate of 4.5 to 9.3 percent of women in the United States at any given time.[91] This high rate of depression among disabled women may be due to the combination of being a woman and having a disability, since both are risk factors for depression. Women are more than twice as likely to have a depressive episode than men due to economic, social, psychological, and biological factors.[92] Female socialization experiences and gender-based roles may also increase their vulnerability to depression. Depression in women has been linked to experiences of abuse and poverty, lack of social support, reduced mobility, chronic pain, lower educational levels, and lower levels of perceived control.[93]

If untreated, depression can spiral into greater severity and may result in suicide; 15 percent of people who are depressed commit suicide each year.[18] Depression may begin with loss, such as the onset of a physical disability, divorce, death, or the departure of a close friend. As a result of such losses, patients may become appropriately

Table 2.4 Signs and Symptoms Associated with Mild, Moderate, and Severe Depression

Mild Depression	Moderate Depression	Severe Depression
Anger	Decreased self-esteem	Anguish
Anxiety	Despair	Change in appetite and weight
Decreased concentration	Despondence	Decreased sex drive
Depressed mood	Excessive guilt	Desperation
Indecisiveness	Fearfulness	Feeling overwhelmed
Intrusive thoughts	Inadequacy	Helplessness
Irritability	Sensitivity	Hopelessness
Lethargy		Insomnia or excessive sleep
Loneliness		Recurrent thoughts of suicide
Neediness		Worthlessness
Sadness		

sad and mournful. If patients reach out to friends and express their feelings, they can alleviate feelings of loneliness and isolation that commonly occur in response to loss. However, if patients do not take steps to express their feelings, the downward spiral of depression may continue. Over time, patients may lose interest in activities and remain at home. They may lack the energy or motivation to attend to their responsibilities, and feelings of guilt may ensue. A decrease in role participation usually leads to decreased self-esteem and feelings of worthlessness. Eventually, people stop caring about their hygiene. They may avoid social contact and become increasingly lonely. At this point, staying in bed becomes a welcome alternative to dealing with the outside world and the painful feelings it may incur.

Depression and Rehabilitation

Given the signs and symptoms of depression (Table 2.4) and its associated behaviors (Table 2.5), depression may negatively affect the outcome of treatment. Depressed patients may have difficulty getting out of bed and may not be motivated to attend therapy. If they do attend treatment, they may display *psychomotor retardation* and lack energy and interest; they may also verbalize self-deprecating remarks, feel criticized, and believe that they are progressing inadequately. It may be difficult for physical therapists to leave depressed patients unattended while working with others because the depressed patient may not engage in the prescribed exercises. Patients may feel guilty that they are in the hospital instead of taking care of their children, working to earn money for their family, or engaging in other life roles.

Depression usually affects performance negatively. Depressed patients may not want to make gains in rehabilitation because of decreased motivation and lack of pleasure in life. They may believe that they are unable to progress in rehabilitation as a result of low self-esteem or feelings of hopelessness. Such patients may also have difficulty asserting themselves because of feelings of worthlessness and an inability to express anger. When people feel worthless or have low self-esteem, they may feel unworthy of having or voicing an opinion. Depression may result from anger turned inwards. Instead of expressing anger in the moment, depressed patients may turn their anger against themselves or repress it. People who experience this type of depression may not have been allowed to express hostility in the past.

Depressed patients often become immobilized because they have difficulty making decisions. They may weigh the pros and cons of each choice and become overwhelmed. They may be unable to concentrate on one thought long enough to make decisions. Sometimes depressed patients experience the opposite; when they attempt to execute a decision they may have no thoughts at all (referred to as *thought blocking*). Consequently, they may need one to 2 minutes to think about and answer questions.

Treating Patients with Depression

Depressed patients require assistance with motivation. Physical therapists can facilitate motivation by providing encouragement, emphasizing strengths, offering positive feedback, addressing values, and mobilizing guilt into goal acquisition. Empowering patients by providing activities that offer opportunities for self-control and success have been shown to decrease depression.[94,95]

Depressed patients experience a narrowing of perception. They have difficulty seeing alternate solutions to

Table 2.5 Behaviors Associated with Mild, Moderate, and Severe Depression

Mild Depression	Moderate Depression	Severe Depression
Being easily frustrated	Crying	Decreased interest in all activities
Difficulty planning ahead	Feeling pessimistic about the future	Lack of personal hygiene
Obsessing about tasks	Having difficulty making decisions	Staying in bed all day
Sitting alone	Making frequent self-deprecating remarks	Suicide (or suicide attempt)
	Over dependence	
	Reacting strongly to criticism	
	Reporting psychosomatic symptoms	
	Ruminating about problems	
	Ruminating about the past	
	Social withdrawal	

problems or simple tasks and often feel there is no solution to obstacles. They may perceive their condition as terminal when there is no justification for such a belief. Because of these distortions, it is important to offer reality checks—such as pointing out their strengths when they feel worthless. Cognitive therapy can be used to correct ongoing pessimism by challenging negative thought patterns.

If given choices about their treatment, depressed patients may become ambivalent and unable to decide upon a course of action. As a result, they may do nothing. Physical therapists should choose treatment that provides the patient with opportunities for progressive success experiences, avoiding feelings of failure. When reluctant patients perceive that they can succeed in therapy instead of giving up, their chances of continuing treatment increase. Progress made in physical rehabilitation can alleviate depression, as patients report feeling better after having succeeded in an activity they believed they could not accomplish.

Perhaps the most valuable information that a physical therapist can offer depressed patients is that depression will not last forever. Patients will eventually become better through the combination of therapy and possible medication management. Depression can cause an activity or life role that once seemed effortless—such as being a partner in a relationship—to become arduous. It is important for the patient to understand that this does not mean that the relationship caused the depression; more likely, the role of partner has become more difficult to carry out because of depression.

Families often experience a depressed family member as lazy, obstinate, or uncaring, and may not recognize that he or she is suffering from an illness. Depression can be just as disabling as a physical illness. Families need to be educated that depression, like physical disability, causes decreased functioning and requires treatment. Recovery from depression does not have a specific timeline. Each patient's situation is unique, as is the recovery period. Most patients cannot "snap out of it" as many family members desire.

When to Make a Referral for Depression

If depression is suspected, the physical therapist should determine if the patient is currently being treated for depression or has received treatment in the past. If the patient has never been treated for depression and is experiencing suicidal ideation (see section on Suicide below) or symptoms of depression that markedly impair life roles, the therapist should refer the patient to a psychiatrist for possible medication management. Medication can enable patients to attend therapy, more readily discuss problems, and express repressed feelings. Being familiar with the names of medications used to treat depression may help therapists identify patients with depression, especially if a psychiatric diagnosis is not indicated in their chart. Frequently prescribed antidepressant medications are listed in Box 2.6.

Patients with less severe symptoms who are not suicidal can be referred to a psychologist for verbal therapy. If a patient's depression seems to be caused by family turmoil, a referral to a social worker for family intervention can be made. Patients who have difficulty verbalizing their feelings can be referred to a creative arts therapist to facilitate expression through nonverbal means—such as music, dance, art, or drama. A referral to an occupational therapist can be made to help patients regain function in daily life roles that have been disrupted by depression.

Suicide

Each year there are more than 35,000 cases of suicide reported in the United States and 65,000 additional cases

Box 2.6 Commonly Prescribed Antidepressant Medications

Amitriptyline hydrochloride (Elavil)
Amoxapine (Asendin)
Bupropion (Wellbutrin)
Celexa (Lexapro)
Desipramine hydrochloride (Norpramin)
Doxepin hydrochloride (Sinequan, Zonalon)
Fluoxetine (Prozac, Sarafem)
Fluvoxamine (Luvox)
Imipramine hydrochloride (Tofranil)
Imipramine pamoate
Isocurboxazid (Marplan)
Maprotiline (Ludiomil)
Nefazodone (Serzone)
Nortriptyline hydrochloride (Aventyl, Pamelor)
Paroxetine (Paxil)
Sertraline (Zoloft)
Phenelzine (Nardil)
Protriptyline (Vivactil)
Tranylcypromine (Parnate)
Trazodone (Desyrel)
Trimipramine maleate (Surmontil)
Venlafaxine (Effexor)

Note: Brand names are shown in parentheses.

that may go unreported due to complications regarding the cause of death.[26] More people lose their lives to suicide than to any other cause, with the exception of cancer and cardiovascular disease. Suicide is often a result of poor social support, low self-esteem, ineffective coping skills, and the inability to see a solution to difficult situations. Risk factors include serious illness, previous suicide attempts, family history of suicide, alcohol and substance abuse/dependence, loss of a loved one through rejection or death, prolonged depression, and financial difficulties.

Recognizing the warning signs of possible suicide risk is important for its prevention. The most frequent signs of suicide risk include:

- Direct comments about suicide, such as, "I just want to die"
- Indirect comments about suicide, such as, "My mother will not have to worry about me anymore"
- A plan to commit suicide
- Writing a suicide note
- Preoccupation with death
- A sudden flight into happiness or relief after a long depression
- Excessive risk taking (e.g., driving while inebriated) and a careless attitude
- Final preparations (e.g., composing a will, giving away personal possessions, repairing broken relationships, or writing revealing letters)
- Self-hatred
- Changes in personal appearance, eating habits, sexual drive, sleep patterns, menstrual cycle, behavior (e.g., inability to concentrate or disinterest in activities), or personality (e.g., withdrawal, anxiousness, sadness, irritability, apathy, indecisiveness, or fatigue)
- A recent loss accompanied by an inability to stop grieving

The most important thing for a physical therapist to do when suspecting that a patient is suicidal is to prevent him or her from carrying out the act. This usually involves obtaining help from a mental health professional, preferably a physician with the knowledge and ability to admit the person to a hospital if needed. It is important not to leave the patient alone while waiting for help. During this period, the following should take place:

- Ask patients if they are thinking of hurting or killing themselves.
- Listen to patients without expressing shock, without discrediting what they say, and without devaluing their feelings; take all suicide threats seriously even if you do not believe them at the time.
- Respond to patients with empathy and understanding; tell them how much you care about them and that you will be available to help them.
- Help patients think of alternatives; offer choices based on your knowledge about the patient's life, rather than generic answers that are easy to offer when under pressure.
- Alert family members, friends, and significant others to the patient's suicide risk; all of these individuals may help prevent the patient from trying to commit suicide; suicidal ideation does not go away in a day; additional help is required from all possible sources over time.

Substance Abuse

Substance abuse occurs when an individual demonstrates a dysfunctional pattern of drug and/or alcohol use characterized by recurrent and significant adverse consequences. Substances may include, but are not limited to, alcohol, amphetamines, caffeine, marijuana, cocaine, hallucinogens, inhalants, opioids, or sedatives.[9]

Substance Abuse and Rehabilitation

If clients come to the clinic under the influence of drugs or alcohol, they may be inappropriate, argumentative, irritable, disinhibited, stubborn, illogical, or angry and will have difficulty following treatment plans (see Table 2.6 and Box 2.7). They may also disturb other clients, some of whom may be in their own substance abuse recovery. For these reasons, intoxicated clients should be escorted out of the treatment area and referred back to their substance abuse programs, with a call to their substance abuse provider describing the

Box 2.7 Behaviors Associated with Substance Abuse

- Associating only with other substance abusers
- Cheating
- Compulsive use of drugs
- Decreased ability to manage stress
- Decreased ability to manage time
- Difficulty holding a job
- Discontinuation of usual activities
- Drug seeking and using behaviors
- Falling
- Inability to control drug use
- Inability to fulfill major life roles
- Isolation
- Lying
- Not paying one's bills
- Poor hygiene
- Spending all money on drugs
- Staying up all night
- Stealing

incident that occurred. If they are not currently engaged in a substance abuse program, a referral should be made.

If patients are not under the influence during treatment, but are using drugs or alcohol at home, they may miss treatment sessions or may come to rehabilitation tired, hungry, or late. They may have poor concentration and irritable moods resulting from hangovers. They may experience recurring injuries from falls. Often, patients will not comply with treatment and fail to complete their home exercises or forget to take their prescribed medications. When prescribed medications are ingested along with illegal substances, adverse drug reactions can occur. Patients may lack insight about the extent of their abuse and the trouble that it produces in their lives. They may mask feelings such as anger, guilt, anxiety, or depression through the numbing effect of the substance, but try to present themselves as though they are fine.

Patients in denial commonly do not perceive their need for physical rehabilitation, often neglect to follow precautions, and frequently attempt to obtain discharge before completing rehabilitation goals. Their low frustration tolerance causes them to quit treatment easily. Whether they are actively using substances or not, patients who have abused substances may have cognitive deficits that inhibit their ability to follow or remember instructions. They may experience family discord and lose family support, thus finding themselves homeless. Patients with a history of chronic alcohol abuse tend to have poor balance resulting from changes in the cerebellum and peripheral nerves.[96] To maintain balance, they develop a stereotypic, wide-based gait. Such factors should be considered during gait examination and training. Despite their gruff demeanor, patients that abuse substances can be overly sensitive, easily hurt, suffer from low self-esteem, and easily stressed once they are no longer abusing substances. These patients tend to have poor boundaries. They can be intrusive, flirtatious, or deal-seeking in order to obtain what they want, such as alcohol, cigarettes, or extra medication.

Treating Patients Who Abuse Substances

Physical therapists can help patients in recovery by providing opportunities that allow them to gain control over their lives again. Such assistance may include opportunities to practice setting boundaries, regulating emotions, and tolerating frustration. Physical therapists can emphasize healthy activities that provide pleasure and decrease cravings. Stress management, time management, activities of daily living (ADLs), and social skills are usually necessary skills to promote recovery.

Education on Substance Abuse

Physical therapists, patients, and patients' family members should be aware that substance abuse is an illness. Like physical or mental illness, it causes a decrease in function, requires skilled intervention for recovery, results in decreased role performance, and can affect anyone. Patients with a diagnosis of substance abuse usually cannot stop using drugs and alcohol on their own. They need help, and recovery is a life-long process that includes developing skills to manage cravings, dealing with stress in healthy ways, expressing feelings, participating in 12-step programs, and engaging in drug-free activities.

When to Make a Referral for Substance Abuse

If the patient is going through withdrawal, the physical therapist should immediately refer the patient to a physician. Signs of withdrawal can include sweating, impaired sleep, seizures, impaired motor coordination, faulty judgment, anxiety, shaking, slurred speech, fluctuating levels of consciousness, and visual and tactile hallucinations. After stabilizing the patient, the physician may transfer him or her to a detoxification unit. If the patient is not experiencing withdrawal and is not already in a substance abuse treatment program, physical therapists can make a referral to an appropriate treatment center. Such treatment centers include 28-day inpatient rehabilitation centers, long-term (1 to 1.5 years) inpatient therapeutic communities, 12-step programs for community-dwelling outpatients, and dual diagnosis programs for patients who have also been diagnosed with mental illness.

Patients who have been abusing substances for long periods of time should be referred to a nutritionist for proper dietary regulation. Physical therapy patients who have been abusing substances can be referred to occupational therapists to address regulating emotions, setting

Table 2.6 **Signs and Symptoms Associated with Substance Abuse/Dependence**

Physiological		Psychological		Behavioral
Abnormal blood pressure	Peripheral neuropathy	Cognitive deficits	Isolation	Alcohol on breath
Abnormal pupillary response	Perspiration	Denial	Loneliness	Belligerence
Bulging ocular veins	Poor concentration	Depression	Low frustration tolerance	Decreased role performance
Chills	Psychomotor disturbances	Disinhibition	Low self-esteem	Drug paraphernalia
Cravings	Red nose	Disturbances in interpersonal behavior	Paranoia	Impaired judgment
Enlarged heart	Sensory losses	Disturbances of perception	Poor boundaries	Impulsivity
Gastrointestinal bleeding	Shiny ears	Emotional lability	Thought disturbances	Irritability
Hallucinations	Sleep disturbances	Grandiosity	Triggers	Poor hygiene
Hyperactivity	Tolerance	Intense emotions		Violence
Hypertension	Ulcers			
Liver damage	Visible track marks			
Loss of consciousness	Withdrawal			
Malnutrition	Yellow, brittle nails, hair and teeth			
Nervousness				

and maintaining appropriate boundaries, tolerating frustration, managing time, obtaining social skills, and regaining necessary activities of daily living. Occupational therapists also can help patients learn that healthy activities can be pleasurable, through task groups in which patients choose, engage in, and discuss healthy activities. A social work referral can be made if the patient requires community integration, family intervention, or social supports.

Agitation and Violence

Physical therapists may believe that patients will not demonstrate sexual, aggressive, or violent behaviors, yet most have witnessed such behaviors at least once. Therapists should learn how to predict violence, identify signs of escalation, manage aggressive patients, and verbally respond to threats. Violence is not always predictable, but the more therapists understand its signs, the better equipped they will be to handle a dangerous situation.

An initial step involves recognizing the early signs of agitation. Agitation usually does not diminish on its own. Instead, it may build to a verbal altercation or physical act. Some signs of agitation may include clenching fists, pacing back and forth, making angry facial expressions, grunting, groaning, swearing, tapping a foot, spitting, refusing to engage in therapy, throwing objects, and banging weights or other therapeutic equipment.

After observing signs of agitation, physical therapists should identify the source of the agitation in order to better control it. While many situations can cause agitation, it is important to remember that events that agitate one person may have no effect on another; levels of frustration vary from person to person. People with Alzheimer's disease may become agitated because they cannot recall the names of familiar objects or remember familiar motor plans. They may believe that family members are lying to them, deceiving them, or attempting to place them in a nursing home. People can become agitated as a result of physical pain, memory failure, hunger, fatigue, and dependency on others. Temporal lobe injury, psychosis, and the side effects of certain mediations can cause agitation. People with personality disorders who have difficulty managing anger and who have experienced an upsetting event can easily become agitated.

Addressing the underlying circumstance causing the agitation may help to defuse it. If the source of agitation is unknown, the physical therapist should acknowledge to the patient, in a non-accusatory manner, that he or she seems upset. Many people are unaware of their agitation and calm down once it is brought to their attention. The therapist can then encourage the patient to verbally express why he or she feels upset. Therapists can also attempt to redirect patient anger into more productive channels and help alter their perspective regarding the disturbing issue.

Violence also can happen without warning. Many therapists working on inpatient units have been bitten, kicked, punched, or scratched. Patients may feel that they are being forced to participate in therapy they do not need, or that they are being treated like children. They may believe that staff members have assumed control over their lives. To avoid humiliating the patient, therapists can use a client-centered therapy approach in which patients are offered respect and included in goal setting and treatment planning.

If efforts to defuse the patient's agitation do not work and he or she becomes violent, the physical therapist should remove all other patients from the area, then leave and call for help. After an act of violence, members of the rehabilitation team should examine what occurred to learn from the incident, prevent a future recurrence, and provide support and education to those involved. In reviewing the incident, the physical therapist should address the following questions:

- What was the patient's potential for aggression?
- What were the signs of escalating anger?
- Did the patient have a history of violence? If so, under what circumstances?
- How did therapists and patients respond to the aggressor before, during, and after the act?
- What could have been done differently during the incident?

In addition to managing an agitated or violent patient, physical therapists need to recognize when a patient is undergoing abuse. It is estimated that 10 percent of women with disabilities experience sexual, physical, or disability-related violence.[97] Abuse has been related to decreased social support, increased social isolation, and elevated levels of depression and stress.[96] Women with disabilities may be even more susceptible to abuse, due to their dual minority status as people with disabilities and as women. As compared to women without disabilities, women having disabilities experienced longer periods of abuse and abuse from a greater number of perpetrators.[98] Nosek et al have identified several factors that predict with 80 percent accuracy whether or not a woman has experienced abuse within the past year. These include decreased mobility, social isolation, depression, and a lack of education. Examination for abuse should be considered for women with disabilities.[99] Nosek et al developed a four-item screening tool, the *Abuse Assessment Screen—Disability* (AAS-D), that examines sexual, physical, and disability-related abuse in the past year.

Hypersexuality

Hypersexuality is a state of heightened sexual arousal that may be accompanied by verbal or physical aggression. These behaviors can be caused by mania, childhood sexual abuse, or brain damage. Patients may desire attention, to provoke, to exert power over others, to impress others, or to show off. Verbal signs of hypersexuality can include whistling; verbalizing sexual desires or asking for physical closeness, phone numbers, or dates. Physical behaviors include staring, pinching, brushing up against another's body, touching, kissing, exposing genitalia, masturbating, and blocking another's exit from a room.

There are several ways to proceed when a patient exhibits hypersexual behavior. If the therapist feels threatened, he or she should leave the area and obtain assistance. If the patient's hypersexual behavior is a newly observed behavior, the therapist can describe the behavior to the patient and firmly state that it is inappropriate and will not be tolerated. If the therapist believes that the patient is exhibiting symptoms of mania or hypomania, referral should be immediately made to a psychiatrist. Holding a multidisciplinary team conference may help the patient understand that hypersexual behaviors are not tolerated in the clinic.

Psychosocial Wellness

According to Donatelle and Davis, wellness is a dynamic process in which people attempt to fully develop their emotional, social, environmental, physical, spiritual, and intellectual health.[100] Donatelle and Davis describe a well individual as someone who can forgive themselves and others, learn from mistakes, appreciate all things both grand and small, develop a realistic sense of self and the environment, achieve a balance in life roles and daily activities, respect others and maintain healthy relationships, feel a sense of life satisfaction, understand one's needs and express emotions appropriately, and function in his or her community. Achieving this definition of wellness may require substantial effort for someone with a disability who may experience multiple barriers to wellness.

Barriers to Wellness for People with Disabilities

Healthy People 2010 has identified gaps and disparities in the health and wellness of Americans with disabilities.[13] They found that 56 percent of Americans with disabilities did not engage in physical leisure activity, only 10 percent participated in one organized health activity, 68 percent maintained a weight considered to be unhealthy, and 33 percent smoked cigarettes. Barriers to wellness for people with disabilities include stress, low self-esteem, multiple secondary conditions, and decreased social support.

Women with disabilities experience higher levels of *stress* than do males with disabilities, possibly owing to higher incidences of poverty, violence, abuse, chronic health problems, and social isolation.[92] Economic disadvantage may be due to stress-inducing factors such as earning a lower income, having less access to disability benefits from public programs, having less education than their male counterparts with disabilities, and having a higher likelihood of being unemployed or unmarried.[101] People with spinal cord injury (SCI) report a higher level of perceived stress than the general population, and women with SCI tend to have a higher level of perceived stress than men with SCI.[102]

Social Support

Social support is critical in maintaining or achieving psychosocial wellness. Social support is defined as the availability of other persons in the environment who can offer emotional support, financial or material help, a listening ear, guidance, or encouragement. Social support has been associated with increased self-esteem, coping, and adjustment for individuals with disabilities. Evidence suggests that social support plays a strong preventative and palliative role in a wide range of physical and medical conditions. Rintala et al found that the amount of social support was directly related to a sense of life satisfaction and well-being in patients with spinal cord injury.[103] Hardy et al and Kaplan found that high social support was predictive of a return to vocational functioning after rehabilitation.[104,105]

Researchers have suggested that failure to recover from depression stemming from disability may correlate to a lack of adequate social support. Social isolation is a frequently encountered condition associated with disability. Physical restrictions such as pain and mobility limitations may discourage connections with others. The combination of diminished social opportunities, negative societal perceptions, and multiple environmental barriers may result in isolation and a lack of emotional intimacy.

Social support can be used to enhance treatment and promote patient compliance. The physical therapist can use adaptive equipment and environmental devices to improve a patient's access to social networks and socialization. Appendix C contains several internet resources regarding assistive technology, disability periodicals and research, and information needed to assure access to housing, employment, recreational facilities, health and social services, transportation, and support groups.

Wellness in Rehabilitation

Psychosocial wellness requires that patients experience success in both short-term rehabilitation activities and long-term relationships and roles. Short-term rehabilitation activities should engage the patient in functional skills (e.g., functional mobility) and meaningful events that foster socialization (e.g., playing wheelchair basketball with other patients). Long-term relationships and roles include being a spouse, parent, worker, and friend. Readjustment to these long-term roles can be facilitated by psychologists, social workers, and occupational therapists. Both short-term rehabilitation activities and long-term relationships and roles should provide a sense of contentment, happiness, and well-being. Physical therapists can provide opportunities for patients to choose and engage in meaningful activities that promote psychosocial wellness.

Patients who spend a great deal of time dwelling on the past and worrying about the future are unable to be fully cognizant of the present moment. The ability to become absorbed in the present moment can decrease anxiety concerning the past or future—the patient's emotional energy is focused on his or her immediate activities. Each instance in which a patient can focus on the present offers him or her the power to change, to break through old habits, to view circumstances differently, and to recognize available choices. Physical therapists can help patients remain focused on the present moment by selecting activities that are both meaningful to and congruent with the patient's goals for rehabilitation.

Having a daily balance of work, leisure, and social activities is important to sustain psychosocial wellness. Any psychological or physical impairment can disrupt this balance. In a study of the relationship between depression and leisure participation in people with SCI, Loy et al found that patients without depression had wider repertoires and higher levels of leisure activity than patients with depression.[106] Therapists can help patients engage in leisure activities through the use of activity interest surveys and schedules. Activity interest surveys are used to gather information about the types of leisure pursuits patients previously engaged in, which leisure pursuits they currently hold interest in, and which leisure activities they would like to pursue in the future.

A negative outlook inhibits psychosocial wellness. Physical therapists can help patients with negative perspectives to positively alter their expectations through goal setting, identifying optimistic options, using cognitive–behavioral techniques that challenge the validity of negative perceptions, or referring the patient to a psychologist for longer term intervention.

Integrating Psychosocial Factors into Rehabilitation: Case Example

Bill, a 19-year-old who was training to be an Olympic gymnast, sustained a SCI in a motorcycle accident. Bill had developed a strong social support system and participated in a variety of extracurricular activities. He was engaged to be married, participated on his college's gymnastic team, and worked as an athletic counselor in the summer camp he had attended since age seven. The SCI he sustained caused a loss of function from his chest down.

All of Bill's energy is now focused on getting through each day. He does not view himself as able to work or attend school. The accident has changed his expectations for the future, his outlook on life, his environmental challenges, and his social support system. His depression was compounded by his broken marriage engagement, and Bill no longer meets his friends for social events; in fact, he rarely leaves his home other than to attend rehabilitation. Just when he was becoming independent of his parents, Bill has now become dependent upon them again. He observes his younger sisters and brothers progressing in their lives and feels stagnant, angry, depressed, and ashamed. His self-esteem, which was once high, is now severely diminished and he has lost his familiar identity.

As part of his rehabilitation, the therapist should provide a safe way for Bill to express his anger; referral to a psychologist is also warranted. The therapist can help him to better understand his physical limitations and capabilities. Based on Bill's strengths and limitations, the therapist should help him to redefine interests that could emerge into new roles and a new identity. For instance, it might be helpful if Bill could identify a meaningful activity that could take the place of his athletic training (such as coaching a children's gymnastic team). Information about college and distance-learning could also be beneficial. The therapist also can assist Bill and his family in the understanding of SCI and reasonable expectations for the future.

Suggestions for Rehabilitative Intervention

Table 2.7 offers a list of behaviors that suggest inappropriate and pathologic response patterns to disability. This list is not meant to be fully inclusive, but rather indicates areas requiring further consideration. It is important to understand that even mild expressions of pathological response patterns can become chronic and worsen in severity over time. Table 2.8 identifies patient behaviors that warrant a mental health consult.

Human reactions, response patterns, and the adaptation process are variable and individualistic. Each patient must be approached uniquely and treatment goals should incorporate the patient's individual personality characteristics, responses, and needs. An important component of rehabilitation is the patient–practitioner relationship. Physical therapists can establish a therapeutic atmosphere of communication, understanding, and cooperation with patients—which can serve as the foundation necessary to produce positive rehabilitation outcomes. Therapists can sometimes forget the powerful influence they have in setting the tone of this interaction. The very structure and

Table 2.7 Behaviors Suggesting Pathological Response Patterns

Grieving	Depression	Damaged Self-Esteem	Heightened Possibility for Suicide	Heightened Possibility for Violence
Grieving for actual or perceived impairment of functioning or actual loss is normal and expected, but the following might serve as clues to a more severe reaction: Denial of problem or its severity Exaggeration or idealizing the loss Obsession with the past or the preloss state Obsession with guilt related to loss Regression Difficulty with concentration Loss of interest in activities and events Lability of mood Inability to discuss loss Fear of being left alone Acting out behaviors (tantrums, suicidal gestures, promiscuity) Angry stance	Flat affect (showing little emotion) Very low energy levels Manic energy and behavior Psychomotor retardation (slowing down of movement and action) Ruminating about negative thoughts Change in eating and sleeping patterns (insomnia or hypersomnia) Regression Social withdrawal Self-destructive behaviors Loss of interest in environment, people, and events Self-blame and self-criticism	Isolation from social sphere Self-destructive behavior Inability to sustain eye contact Inability to accept praise Judgmental attitude Self-deprecating and self-critical Unwarranted pessimism Unconcern for appearance Unconcern for personal safety	Depression Giving away possessions Hoarding/hiding medications or potential weapons Writing suicide note Updating will Verbalizing loneliness or hopelessness Statements regarding benefit of release of pain, absence, and so forth Intrusiveness of such thoughts	Low threshold for anger Depression High anxiety state Motoric agitation Self-mutilation Oversensitive Argumentative Inability to express feelings Fears of abandonment Highly dependent Disassociative states

atmosphere of service delivery and the personality and type of communication given by the practitioner exert a strong influence on patient participation and response to rehabilitation efforts.

Optimizing Patient Involvement

Patients should be involved as fully as possible in their own treatment. This includes involvement in goal setting and treatment planning, as well as in the ongoing evaluation of progress. Patient cooperation is also dependent on the therapist's clear explanation of the patient's situation, possible interventions, and expected outcomes. Relating to the patient as a partner in therapy can engender cooperation and trust in the therapeutic relationship. When patients feel a heightened sense of control and ability (i.e., locus of control), feelings of despair and helplessness can be mitigated.

Therapists should also maintain a receptive ear to patient concerns and encourage communication. Listening carefully to patients in a nonjudgmental manner will allow them to reveal concerns and issues they may otherwise feel uncomfortable discussing. Clear and articulate communication, however, can be disrupted by emotion, uncertainty, or power discrepancies that exist when patients become passive recipients of service. While it may sometimes appear easier to do for patients than to witness their struggle—particularly when patients assume a passive role in rehabilitation—promoting self-reliance and independence fosters patients' engagement and responsibility in their recovery. Allowing patients to maintain a passive role fosters helplessness, dependency, and slows progress in the long term.

Table 2.8 Patient Behaviors Warranting a Mental Health Consult

Regression	Regression involves reverting to earlier, more immature patterns of functioning. This may be more commonly observed in children but might be observed in adults as well. For example, children may revert back to sucking their thumb, or may appear to have lost their toilet training skills. Regression in adults may generally be seen in lost skills and abilities and/or even in the extreme behavior of reverting to taking a fetal position.
Disorientation	Disorientation is confusion as to time, place, activity, self-identity, or identity of others. Occasional, transient disorientation is not wholly uncommon in the average person, yet persistence in frequency or duration of occurrence is cause for examination and intervention. Any more extreme confused behaviors and thought processes need to be carefully examined.
Delusional thinking	Delusional thinking refers to faulty and mistaken beliefs and, although related to inaccurate interpretation of environment, is distinguished by the persistence of this belief system. This can run the gamut from delusions of grandeur or of persecution, to delusions about the nature and scope of a disability. These delusions hold up and persist in the face of contrary information.
Inaccurate interpretation of environment	This is the broadest category in this list, but fortunately is also the most readily understood category. Clearly when a patient significantly misinterprets and misunderstands the objective situation and reality about them, it is probably most readily noted by non-mental health practitioners in its many expressions. This should draw attention and intervention, not only in its extreme form of a psychotic break, but also in its minor form of small, repeated episodes of misinterpretations.
Inappropriate affect	Affect refers to the mood state displayed by the patient, where feelings such as joy, sadness, fear, and so forth are reflected in body language, facial expression, and verbalizations. Inappropriate affect can be seen in an affective expression alien to the situation; for example, demonstrating and expressing joy upon hearing bad news. It also refers to a spilt between displayed affect and verbalization; for example, the verbal expression of mourning and condolence offered while smiling brightly and jumping for joy.
Hypo- or hypervigilance	Hypovigilance can be noted in a patient being oblivious to his or her surroundings and the events around them, socially, as well as physically. Hypervigilance refers to an intense focus and alertness to social and physical surrounds. Each of these have different ramifications and meaning to the mental health team. Suffice it to say that a consult is suggested as either extreme is approached.
Mood swings	We all experience changes in mood, yet hopefully, most of the time these changes are relatively appropriate reactions to external determinants, such as the receipt of news and information or to changing occurrences and circumstances in our environment. Although changeable, moods are generally persistent and stable. When mood shifts either to extremes and/or with some frequency, it suggests either instability or that mood is being driven predominantly by internal rather than external factors.
Self-destructive behaviors	Any self-destructive behavior, particularly ones that persist, are cause for serious concern. Self-destructive behaviors can run the gamut from subtle, difficult to detect signs to very clear and frightening overt signs. Subtle signs can include noncompliance with treatment regimen, poor self-maintenance activities such as not eating, overeating, diminishment of personal care, and hygiene, or carelessness in negotiating the environment. Clearer signs can include self-inflicted wounds and suicidal ideation and expressions.
Normal behaviors taken to extremes	Normal human behavior enjoys a wide latitude of response repertoire before drawing attention as being out of expected bounds. This latitude must usually be extended further when dealing with someone undergoing a more extreme, traumatic, or stressful experience. Someone confronted with a disability would be expected to naturally focus their attention, concerns, and anxiety around this issue. The level of focus on a left leg given by someone preparing to have that leg amputated would be considered obsessive in a healthy ambulatory person, yet normal here. Care in judgment is required by the clinician when determining behavior expressions. That said, issues such as obsessiveness, extreme distractibility, immobilization in the face of routine decisions, and unexpected egocentricity or self-denigration may require a consult. An overly compliant patient, an extremely calm patient, as well as an overly contentious, argumentative, or extremely anxious or hysterical patient also promotes concern. Any response (verbal or behavioral) that appears unwarranted to the stimuli should draw attention. Overreactions in opposite directions or any behavior which appears to be at an extreme, using reasonable judgment, deserves attention.

Use of Jargon and Labels

Patient–therapist communication should be characterized by simple and easy to understand language that matches the cognitive level of the patient. The use of scientific jargon and labels should be avoided when speaking with patients, as it impedes patient understanding and emotionally distances patients from therapists. Similarly, when patients hear therapists referring to fellow patients by their diagnosis, they receive the message that patients are nothing more than disabilities. Such practice should be avoided and, instead, therapists should use language that reflects respect for the patient's dignity and unique life circumstances.

Rehabilitation Team Members' Self-Awareness

Finally, and perhaps most importantly, therapists need to be aware of their own feelings, motivations, and responses. Such self-awareness is critical for therapists to understand their own reactions to patients. It is normal for people to respond to others based on conscious or unconscious memories. Sometimes patients can remind therapists of significant others, such as siblings, parents, spouses, or employers. However, when therapists react to patients based on unconscious associations to others, they can misperceive patient needs and respond inappropriately. For example, unconscious reactions to patients can cause therapists to become overprotective or, at the other extreme, become frustrated with patients without recognizing that their own reactions have more to do with other relationships than with the patient at hand. Generally, when therapists feel a heightened sense of emotion in response to a particular patient it may often serve as a cue that such emotions stem from unconscious associations to others. When this occurs, it is important for therapists to step back and evaluate their own feelings in order to discern the connection between their reaction to the patient and how the patient may be triggering unconscious emotions.

The converse is also true; patients will respond to therapists based on their own unconscious associations with significant others who have similar personality characteristics to those of the therapist. Therapists must be aware of this normal phenomenon and refrain from responding emotionally to the patient's unconscious associations. Rather, the therapist should continue to build a respectful relationship with the patient that, in time, will demonstrate to the patient that his or her first impressions were misperceptions.

Summary

It is important for physical therapists to identify and understand the individual psychosocial factors that enhance or inhibit the rehabilitation of their patients, and intervene accordingly. Successful intervention depends on:

- Achieving a complete psychosocial understanding of each patient including personality styles and coping skills.
- Understanding how to recognize the common defense mechanisms that patients use in rehabilitation.
- Understanding the stages of psychosocial adaptation to disability and helping patients progress in their own adjustment.
- Understanding how to identify anxiety, depression, and substance abuse. Understanding how to address these problems with patients and make appropriate referrals to other treatment team members.
- Using a client-centered approach to rehabilitation whereby therapists demonstrate respect, empathy, and compassion.
- Empowering patients and families through psychosocial education, and wellness and prevention techniques.
- Helping patients develop treatment goals that match their current needs, values, and level of functioning.
- Collaborating with patients and other treatment team members in the identification and implementation of appropriate interventions.
- Utilizing a team approach and making referrals as necessary.

Acknowledgments

The editors wish to acknowledge and graciously thank Dr. Sharon A. Gutman and Dr. Anne Hiller Scott for the vision, expertise, and wise insights they provided as guest editors of this chapter.

Questions for Review

1. Identify five psychosocial factors and state how each factor may influence rehabilitation.
2. Give examples of interventions for each psychosocial factor that may impair rehabilitation.
3. Identify the different mental health professionals who can treat patients with psychosocial issues and state their roles.
4. Describe the steps used to calm an agitated patient.
5. Describe a method for managing a violent patient and how to analyze an act of violence after it has occurred.
6. List signs of and methods to address hypersexuality.
7. List and describe the phases of psychosocial adaptation to disability.
8. Discuss three coping strategies that have been found effective in the psychosocial adaptation to chronic disability and illness.
9. Describe five common defense mechanisms that patients use in response to disability.
10. State the signs and symptoms of posttraumatic stress disorder.

11. Describe how to recognize when normal reactions of grieving and depression have become pathological.
12. Describe several ways to optimize patient involvement in the rehabilitation process and promote self-reliance.
13. State the importance of client-centered therapy and techniques to achieve this type of interaction.
14. Describe the general adaptation syndrome.

Case Study

The patient is a 68-year-old Caucasian female, admitted to an inpatient unit 2 days after sustaining a hip fracture from falling down her basement stairs. Prior to her fall, she was in fair health but was experiencing declining eyesight, poor short-term memory, and osteoporosis. Her hip fracture has placed her at high risk for further deconditioning and loss of function. The patient's husband had suffered a prolonged illness; the patient cared for him during the last 5 years until he passed away. She has a son whom she rarely sees, as he is married with children and living in another part of the country. Her best friend now lives in Florida and the rest of her friends have died. The patient is embarrassed to be seen in public in a wheelchair.

Given the deaths of her husband and friends, and given her recent accident, the patient is now very anxious about her own mortality for the first time in her life. She is preoccupied with her husband's death since he was so much a part of her life. She feels that she has no future and nothing to look forward to. She no longer knows who she is and longs to "be reunited with" her husband.

GUIDING QUESTIONS

1. Identify the psychosocial factors apparent in this case study.
2. What relevant questions about the patient remain unanswered?
3. How might the patient's emotional condition affect rehabilitation?
4. List the patient's assets and limitations.
5. Establish reasonable goals that are measurable and time-specific.
6. Formulate an approach to plan of care.
7. Identify appropriate referrals to other team members.

References

1. Webster's New World Dictionary of American English, ed 2. Prentice-Hall, Upper Saddle River, NJ, 1988.
2. Vaillant, GE: Adaptation to Life. Little, Brown, Boston, 1977.
3. Wickramasekera, I, et al: Applied psychophysiology: A bridge between the biomedical model and the biopsychosocial model in family medicine. Prof Psychol Res Pr 27:221, 1996.
4. Lieberman, A, Lieberman, MB, and Reichberg Lieberman, B: Psychosocial concomitants to disability and rehabilitation. In: O'Sullivan, SB, Schmitz, TJ: Physical Rehabilitation: Assessment and Treatment, ed 4. FA Davis, Philadelphia, 2001, p 19.
5. Siegel, B: Love, Medicine and Miracles. Harper Collins, New York, 1988.
6. Doskoch, P: Happy ever laughter. Psychol Today 29:32, 1996.
7. Watts, R: Trauma counseling and rehabilitation. J Appl Rehab Counseling 28:8, 1997.
8. Gleckman, AD, and Brill, S: The impact of brain injury on family functioning: Implications for subacute rehabilitation programs. Brain Inj 9:385, 1995.
9. American Psychiatric Association: Diagnostic and Statistical Manual of Mental Disorders, 4th ed. Text Revision. American Psychiatric Association, Washington, DC, 1994.
10. Moore, D, and Li, L: Substance abuse among applicants for vocational rehabilitation services. J Rehabil 60:48, 1994.
11. Friedland, J, and McColl, M: Disability and depression: Some etiological considerations. Soc Sci Med 34:395, 1992.
12. Turner, RJ, and Beiser, M: Major depression and depressive symptomatology among the physically disabled: Assessing the role of chronic stress. J Nerv Ment Dis 178:343, 1990.
13. U.S. Department of Health and Human Services. Healthy People 2010: Understanding and Improving Health, ed 2. Washington, DC: US Government Printing Office, November 2000.
14. Paolucci, S, et al: Post stroke depression and its role in rehabilitation of inpatients. Arch Phys Med Rehabil 80:985, 1999.
15. Kreuter, M, et al: Partner relationships, functioning, mood, and global quality of life in persons with spinal cord injury and traumatic brain injury. Spinal Cord 36:252, 1999.
16. Meara, J, et al: Use of the GDS-geriatric depression scale as a screening instrument for depressive symptomatology in patients with Parkinson's disease and their careers in the community. Age Ageing 28:35, 1999.
17. Denollet, J: Personality and coronary heart disease: The type-D scale-16. Ann Behav Med 20(3):209, 1998.
18. Nemeroff, CB: The neurobiology of depression. Sci Am June:42, 1998.
19. Heinemann, A, et al: Substance abuse by persons with recent spinal cord injuries. Rehabil Psychol 35:217, 1990.
20. Zegans, J: The embodied self: Integration in health and illness. Adv J Inst Advance Health 7(3):29, 1991.
21. Benson, H: The Relaxation Response, HarperCollins, New York, 1974.
22. Livneh, H, and Antonak, RF: Psychosocial Adaptation to Chronic Illness and Disability. Aspen, Gaithersburg, MD, 1997.
23. Keany, KC, and Glueckauf, RL: Disability and value changes: An overview and analysis of acceptance of loss theory. Rehabil Psychol 38:199, 1993.
24. Jacobson, AM, et al: Adherence among children and adolescents with insulin-dependent diabetes mellitus over a four-year longitudinal follow-up: I. The influence of patient coping and adjustment. J Pediatr Psychol 15:511, 1990.
25. Grzesiak, RC, and Hicok, DA: A brief history of psychotherapy and physical disability. Am J Psychother 48:240, 1994.
26. Donatelle, RJ, and Davis, LG: Access to Health, ed 6. Allyn and Bacon, Needham Heights, MA, 2000.

27. Strobe, W, and Strobe, MS: Bereavement and Health: The Psychological and Physical Consequences of Partner Loss (The Psychology of Social Issues). Cambridge University Press, New York, 1987.
28. Burke, ML, et al: Current knowledge and research on chronic sorrow: A foundation for inquiry. Death Stud 16:231, 1992.
29. Lindgren, CL, et al: Chronic sorrow: A lifespan concept. Sch Inq Nurs Pract 6:27, 1992.
30. Selye, H: The general adaptation syndrome and the disease of adaptation. J Clin Endocrinol Metab 6:117, 1946.
31. Heinrichs, SC, et al: Anti-stress action of a corticotropin-releasing factor antagonist on behavioral reactivity to stressors of varying type and intensity. Neuropsychopharmacology 11:179, 1994.
32. Theorell, T, et al: "Person Under Train" incidents: Medical consequences for subway drivers. Psychosom Med 54:480, 1992.
33. Breznitz, S: The seven kinds of denial. In Breznitz (ed): The Denial of Stress. International Universities Press, New York, 1983, p 257.
34. Taylor, SE, and Aspinwell, LG: Psychosocial aspects of chronic illness. In Costa, PT, and VandenBox, GR (eds): Psychological Aspects of Serious Illness: Chronic Conditions, Fatal Diseases, and Clinical Care. American Psychological Association, Washington, DC, 1990, p 7.
35. Rodin, G, et al: Depression in the Medically Ill: An Integrated Approach. Brunner/Mazel, New York, 1991.
36. Levin, HS, and Grossman, RG: Behavioral sequelae of closed head injury. Arch Neurol-Chicago 35:720, 1978.
37. Brooks, N: Behavioral abnormalities in head injured patients. Scand J Rehabil Med Supplement 17:41, 1988.
38. Mairs, N: Waist High in the World. Beacon Press, Boston, 1996.
39. Hermann, M, and Wallesch, CW: Depressive changes in stroke patients. Disabil Rehabil 15:55, 1993.
40. Davidhizer, R: Disability does not have to be the grief that never ends: Helping patients adjust. Rehabil Nurs 22(1):32, 1997.
41. Kabat-Zinn, J: The power of breathing: Your unsuspected ally in the healing process. In: Full Catastrophe Living: The Wisdom of Your body and Mind to Face Stress, Pain, and Illness. Delacorte, New York, 1991, p 47.
42. Trieshman, RB: Spinal Cord Injuries: Psychological, Social and Vocational Rehabilitation, ed 2. Demos, New York, 1988.
43. Bramble, K: Body image. In Lubkin, IM (ed): Chronic Illness: Impact and Interventions, ed 3. Jones and Bartlett, Boston, 1995, p 285.
44. Neff, W (ed): Rehabilitation Psychology. American Psychological Association, Washington, DC, 1971.
45. Freidman, HS, and Booth-Kewley, S: The 'disease-prone personality': A meta-analytic view of the construct. Am Psychol 42:539, 1987.
46. Lerman, C, and Glanz, K: Stress, coping, and health behavior. In: Glanz, K, Lewis, FM, Rimer, BK (ed): Health Behavior Education. Jossey-Bass, San Francisco, 1997, p 113.
47. Selye, H: Stress. In: Health and Disease. Butterworth: Reading, MA, 1976.
48. Stone, AA, and Porter, MA: Psychological coping: Its importance for treating medical problems. Mind/Body Medicine 1(1):46, 1995.
49. Tate, D, et al: Coping with the late effects—differences between depressed and nondepressed polio survivors. Am J Phys Med Rehabil 73:27, 1994.
50. Krause, JS, and Rohe, DE: Personality and life adjustment after spinal cord injury: An exploratory study. Rehabil Psychol 43:118, 1998.
51. Radomski, M: Assessing context: Personal, social, and cultural. In Trombly, CA, Radomski, M (eds.): Occupational Therapy for Physical Dysfunction, ed 5. Lippincott Williams & Wilkins, Baltimore, 2002, p 213.
52. Adahan, M: Calm Down: Taking Control of Your Life. Targum Press, Southfield, Michigan, 1995.
53. Gale, B: Veterinary update: Pets keep people healthy. Vet Econ Summer, 1999, p 3.
54. Webster, G, et al: Relationship and family breakdown following acquired brain injury: The role of the rehabilitation team. Brain Inj 13:593, 1999.
55. Steinhauer, PD: Developing resiliency in children from disadvantaged populations. In National Forum on Health Secretariat (eds.): Canada Health Action—Building the Legacy. Vol. 1. Determinants of Health: Children and Youth. Editions MultiMondes, Sainte-Foy, Canada, 1997, p 51.
56. King, G: Turning points and protective processes in the lives of people with chronic disabilities. Qual Health Res 13(2):184, 2003.
57. Gorman, LM, et al: Psychosocial Nursing Handbook for the Nonpsychiatric Nurse. Williams & Wilkins, Baltimore, 1989, p 51.
58. Holmes, T, and Rahe, R: The Social Readjustment Scale. J Psychosom Res 11:213, 1967.
59. Kanner, AD, et al: Comparison of two modes of stress management: Daily hassles and uplifts versus major life events. J Behav Med 4:1, 1981.
60. Tusek, D: Guided imagery: A powerful tool to decrease length of stay, pain, anxiety, and narcotic consumption. J Invas Cardiol 11:265, 1999.
61. Tiernan, P: Independent nursing interventions: Relaxation and guided imagery in critical care. Crit Care Nurse 14(5):47, 1994.
62. Early, MB: Mental Health Concepts and Techniques for the Occupational Therapy Assistant, ed 3. Lippincott Williams & Wilkins, Baltimore, 2000.
63. Precin, P: Living Skills Recovery Workbook. Butterworth-Heinemann, Woburn, MA, 1999.
64. Walker, LG, and Eremin, O: Psychoneuroimmunology: New fad or the fifth cancer treatment modality? Am J Surg 170:2, 1995.
65. Tusek, D, et al: Effect of guided imagery and length of stay, pain and anxiety in cardiac surgery patients. J Cardiovasc Manage 10:22, 1999.
66. Scheufele, PM: Effects of progressive relaxation and classical music on measurements of attention, relaxation, and stress responses. J Behav Med 23(2):207, 2000.
67. Benson, H, et al: Decreased blood pressure in pharmacologically treated hypertensive patients who regularly elicited the relaxation response. Lancet 1(7852):289, 1974.
68. Rossman, ML: Guided Imagery for Self-Healing: An Essential Resource for Anyone Seeking Wellness. New World Library, Novato, CA, 2000.
69. Dossey, BM: Holistic modalities & healing moments. Am J Nurs 98(6):44, 1998.
70. Eisenman, A, and Cohen, B: Music therapy for patients undergoing regional anesthesia. AORN J 62:947, 1991.
71. White, J: Music therapy: An intervention to reduce anxiety in the myocardial infarction patient. Clin Nurs Specialist 6:58, 1992.
72. Burns, D: The Feeling Good Handbook. Plume, New York, 1990.
73. Beck, AT: Cognition and Psychotherapy ed 2. Springer, New York, 2004.
74. Blackburn, IM, and Moorhead, S: Update in cognitive therapy for depression. J Cogn Psychother 14(3):305, 2000.
75. Miller, IW, et al: Cognitive/behavioural therapy and pharmacotherapy with chronic, drug-refractory depressed inpatients: A note of optimism. Behav Psychother 13(4):320, 1985.
76. Bowers, WA: Treatment of depressed in-patients: Cognitive therapy plus medication, relaxation plus medication, and medication alone. Br J Psych 156:73, 1990.
77. Gloaguen, V, et al: A meta-analysis of the effects of cognitive therapy in depressed patients. J Affect Disord 49:59, 1998.
78. Mayou, RA, and Smith, KA: Posttraumatic symptoms following medical illness and treatment. J Psychosom Res 43:121, 1997.
79. Bryant, RA, and Harvey, AG: Avoidant coping style and PTS following motor vehicle accidents. Behav Res Ther 33:631, 1995.
80. Herman, JL: Trauma and Recovery. Basic Books, New York, 1992.
81. Barlow, DH: Unraveling the mysteries of anxiety and its disorders from the perspective of emotion theory. Am Psychol 55:1247, 2000.
82. Keane, TM, and Barlow, DH: Posttraumatic stress disorder. In Barlow, DH, (ed): Anxiety and Its Disorders. Guilford Press, New York, 2002, p 418.
83. Geisser, ME, et al: The relationship between symptoms of posttraumatic stress disorder and pain, affective disturbance and disability among patients with accident and non-accident related pain. Pain 66:207, 1996.
84. Kerns, RD, et al: West Haven-Yale multidimensional pain inventory (WHYMPI). Pain 23:345, 1985.
85. Melzack, R: McGill Pain Questionnaire: Major properties and scoring methods. Pain 1:277, 1975.

86. Blake, DD, et al: A clinician rating scale for assessing current and lifetime PTSD: the CAPS-1. Behav Ther 13:187, 1990.
87. Weathers, FW, et al: The PTSD Checklist (PCL): Reliability, validity, and diagnostic utility. Annual Meeting of the International Society for Traumatic Stress Studies, San Antonio, Texas, 1993.
88. Otis, JD, et al: An examination of the relationship between chronic pain and post-traumatic stress disorder. J Rehabil Res Dev 40(5):397, 2003.
89. Boekamp, JR, et al: Depression following a spinal cord injury. Int J Psychiatr Med 26(3):329, 1996.
90. Hughes, RB, et al: Characteristics of depressed and nondepressed women with physical disabilities. Arch Phys Med Rehabil 86(3):473, 2005.
91. Hughes, RB, et al: Depression and women with spinal cord injury. Top Spinal Cord Inj Rehabil 7(1):16, 2001.
92. McGrath, E, et al: Women and Depression: Risk Factors and Treatment Issues: Final Report of the American Psychological Association's National Task Force on Women and Depression. American Psychological Association, Washington, DC, 1990.
93. Warren, LW, and McEachren, L: Psychosocial correlates of depressive symptomatology gin adult women. J Abnormal Psychol 92:151, 1983.
94. Neville, A: The model of human occupation and depressions. Am Occup Ther Assoc Mental Health Special Interest Section Newslett 8(1):1, 1985.
95. Seligman, ME: Helplessness: On Depression, Development and Death. Freeman, San Francisco, 1975.
96. Heinemann, AW: Substance Abuse and Physical Disability. Haworth, New York, 1993.
97. McFarlane, et al: Abuse Assessment Screen-Disability (AAS-D): Measuring frequency, type, and perpetrator of abuse toward women with physical disabilities. J Women's Health Gend Based Med 10:861, 2001.
98. Nosek, MA, et al: National study of women with physical disabilities: Final report. Sex Disabil 19(1):5, 2001.
99. Nosek, MA, et al: Vulnerabilities for abuse among women with disabilities. Sex Disabil 19:177, 2001.
100. Jacobs, K, and Jacobs, L: Quick reference dictionary for occupational therapy. Slack, Thorofare, NJ, 2001.
101. Nosek, MA, and Hughes, RB: Psychosocial issues of women with physical disabilities: The continuing gender debate. RCB 46(4):224, 2003.
102. Rintala, DH, et al: Perceived stress in individuals with spinal cord injury. In Krotoski, DM, Mosek, MA, and Turk, MA (eds): Women with Physical Disabilities: Achieving and Maintaining Health and Well-being. Brookes, Baltimore, 1996, p 223.
103. Rintala, DH, et al: Social support and the well-being of persons with spinal cord injury living in the community. Rehabil Psychol 37:155, 1992.
104. Hardy, C, et al: The role of social support in the life stress/injury relationship. Sport Psychologist 5:128, 1991.
105. Kaplan, SP: Psychosocial adjustment three years after traumatic brain injury. Clin Neuropsychol 5:360, 1991.
106. Loy, DP, et al: Dimensions of leisure and depression symptoms after spinal cord injury. Annu Ther Recreat 11:43, 106, 2002.

Supplemental Readings

Armstrong, MJ, and Fitzgerald, MH: Culture and disability studies: An anthropological perspective. Rehabil Educ 10:247, 1996.
Benson, H: Timeless Healing: The Power and Biology of Belief. Fireside, New York, 1997.
Benson, H, and Friedman, R: Harnessing the power of the placebo effect and renaming it 'remembered wellness.' Annu Rev Med 47:193, 1996.
Boersma, K, and Linton, SJ: Screening to identify patients at risk: Profiles of psychological risk factors for early intervention. Clin J Pain 21(1):38, 2005.
Brenes, GA, et al: The influence of anxiety on the progression of disability. J Am Geriatr Soc 53(1):34, 2005.
Carlson, J: Evaluating patient motivation in physical disabilities practice settings. Am J Occup Ther 51:347, 1996.
Drench, ED, et al: Psychosocial Aspects of Health Care. Prentice Hall (Pearson Education, Inc.), Upper Saddle River, NJ, 2003.
Elfstrom, M, et al: Relations between coping strategies and health-related quality of life in patients with spinal cord lesion. J Rehabil Med. 37(1):9, 2005.
Falvo, D: Medical and Psychosocial Aspects of Chronic Illness and Disability, 3rd ed. Jones and Bartlett Publishers, Sudbury, MA, 2005.
Fordyce, WE, and Brockway, JA: Psychological Assessment and Management. In Kottke, FJ, and Lehmann, JF: Krusen's Handbook of Physical Medicine and Rehabilitation, 4th ed., Philadelphia: WB Saunders, 1990, p 153.
Greenberger, D, and Padesky, C: Mind Over Mood. Guilford Press, New York, 1995.
Hedaya, RJ: Understanding Biological Psychiatry. Norton, New York, 1995.
Helfrich, C, et al: Volition as narrative: Understanding motivation in chronic illness. Am J Occup Ther 48:311, 1994.
Hughes, RB, et al: Stress and women with physical disabilities: Identifying correlates. Women Health Issue 15(1):14, 2005.
Kemp, JK: Psychological care of the older rehabilitation patient. Geriatr Rehabil 9:841, 1993.
Kolt, GS, and Anderson, MB (eds): Psychology in the Physical and Manual Therapies. Churchill Livingstone, NY, 2004.
Miller, JF: Coping with Chronic Illness: Overcoming Powerlessness, 3rd ed. FA Davis, Philadelphia, 2000.
Moldover, JE, et al: Depression after traumatic brain injury: a review of evidence for clinical heterogeneity. Neuropsychol Rev 14(3):143, 2004.
Rytsala, HJ, et al: Functional and work disability in major depressive disorder. J Nerv Ment Dis Mar 193(3):189, 2005.
Solet, JM: Optimizing personal and social adaptation. In: Trombly, CA, Vining Radomski, M (eds): Occupational Therapy for Physical Dysfunction, 5th ed. Lippincott Williams & Wilkins, Baltimore, 2002, p 761.
Spector, E: Cultural Diversity in Health and Illness, 4th ed. Appleton & Lange, Stanford, CT, 1996.
Yerxa, EJ: The social and psychological experience of having a disability: Implications for Occupational Therapists. In Pedretti, LW, and Early, MB (eds): Occupational Therapy: Practice Skills for Physical Dysfunction, 5th ed. Mosby, St. Louis, 2001, p 470.

Appendix A: Holmes-Rahe Social Readjustment Scale

Rank	Life Event	Mean Value
1	Death of spouse	100
2	Divorce	73
3	Marital separation	65
4	Jail term	63
5	Death of close family member	63
6	Personal injury or illness	53
7	Marriage	50
8	Fired at work	47
9	Marital reconciliation	45
10	Retirement	45
11	Change in health of family member	44
12	Pregnancy	40
13	Sex difficulties	39
14	Gain of new family member	39
15	Business readjustment	39
16	Change in financial state	38
17	Death of close friend	37
18	Change to different line of work	36
19	Change in number of arguments with spouse	35
20	Mortgage over $10,000	31
21	Foreclosure of mortgage or loan	30
22	Change in responsibilities at work	29
23	Son or daughter leaving home	29
24	Trouble with in-laws	29
25	Outstanding personal achievement	28
26	Wife begin or stop work	26
27	Begin or end school	26
28	Change in living conditions	25
29	Revision of personal habits	24
30	Trouble with boss	23
31	Change in work hours or conditions	20
32	Change in residence	20
33	Change in schools	20
34	Change in recreation	19
35	Change in church activities	19
36	Change in social activities	18
37	Mortgage or loan less than $10,000	17
38	Change in sleeping habits	16
39	Change in number of family get-togethers	15
40	Change in eating habits	15
41	Vacation	13
42	Christmas	12
43	Minor violations of the law	11

From Holmes, T, and Rahe, R,[58] with permission.

Appendix B: The Hassles Scale

Directions: Hassles are irritants that can range from minor annoyances to fairly major pressures, problems, or difficulties. They can occur few or many times.

Listed in the center of the following pages are a number of ways in which a person can feel hassled. First, circle the hassles that have happened to you *in the past month.* Then look at the numbers on the right of the items you circled. Indicate by circling a 1, 2, or 3 how *severe* each of the *circled* hassles has been for you in the past month. If a hassle did not occur in the last month, do *not* circle it.

Hassles	Severity		
	1. Somewhat Severe	2. Moderately Severe	3. Extremely Severe
(1) Misplacing or losing things	1	2	3
(2) Troublesome neighbors	1	2	3
(3) Social obligations	1	2	3
(4) Inconsiderate smokers	1	2	3
(5) Troubling thoughts about your future	1	2	3
(6) Thoughts about death	1	2	3
(7) Health of a family member	1	2	3
(8) Not enough money for clothing	1	2	3
(9) Not enough money for housing	1	2	3
(10) Concerns about owing money	1	2	3
(11) Concerns about getting credit	1	2	3
(12) Concerns about money for emergencies	1	2	3
(13) Someone owes you money	1	2	3
(14) Financial responsibility for someone who does not live with you	1	2	3
(15) Cutting down on electricity, water, etc.	1	2	3
(16) Smoking too much	1	2	3
(17) Use of alcohol	1	2	3
(18) Personal use of drugs	1	2	3
(19) Too many responsibilities	1	2	3
(20) Decisions about having children	1	2	3
(21) Non-family members living in your house	1	2	3
(22) Care for pet	1	2	3
(23) Planning meals	1	2	3
(24) Concerned about the meaning of life	1	2	3
(25) Trouble relaxing	1	2	3
(26) Trouble making decisions	1	2	3
(27) Problems getting along with fellow workers	1	2	3
(28) Customers or clients give you a hard time	1	2	3
(29) Home maintenance (inside)	1	2	3
(30) Concerns about job security	1	2	3
(31) Concerns about retirement	1	2	3
(32) Laid-off or out of work	1	2	3
(33) Do not like current work duties	1	2	3
(34) Do not like fellow workers	1	2	3

(continued)

	Severity		
	1. Somewhat Severe	2. Moderately Severe	3. Extremely Severe
(35) Not enough money for basic necessities	1	2	3
(36) Not enough money for food	1	2	3
(37) Too many interruptions	1	2	3
(38) Unexpected company	1	2	3
(39) Too much time on hands	1	2	3
(40) Having to wait	1	2	3
(41) Concerns about accidents	1	2	3
(42) Being lonely	1	2	3
(43) Not enough money for health care	1	2	3
(44) Fear of confrontation	1	2	3
(45) Financial security	1	2	3
(46) Silly practical mistakes	1	2	3
(47) Inability to express yourself	1	2	3
(48) Physical illness	1	2	3
(49) Side effects of medication	1	2	3
(50) Concerns about medical treatment	1	2	3
(51) Physical appearance	1	2	3
(52) Fear of rejection	1	2	3
(53) Difficulties with getting pregnant	1	2	3
(54) Sexual problems that result from physical problems	1	2	3
(55) Sexual problems other than those resulting from physical problems	1	2	3
(56) Concerns about health in general	1	2	3
(57) Not seeing enough people	1	2	3
(58) Friends or relatives too far away	1	2	3
(59) Preparing meals	1	2	3
(60) Wasting time	1	2	3
(61) Auto maintenance	1	2	3
(62) Filling out forms	1	2	3
(63) Neighborhood deterioration	1	2	3
(64) Financing children's education	1	2	3
(65) Problems with employees	1	2	3
(66) Problems on job due to being a woman or man	1	2	3
(67) Declining physical abilities	1	2	3
(68) Being exploited	1	2	3
(69) Concerns about bodily functions	1	2	3
(70) Rising prices of common goods	1	2	3
(71) Not getting enough rest	1	2	3
(72) Not getting enough sleep	1	2	3
(73) Problems with aging parents	1	2	3
(74) Problems with your children	1	2	3
(75) Problems with persons younger than yourself	1	2	3
(76) Problems with your lover	1	2	3
(77) Difficulties seeing or hearing	1	2	3
(78) Overloaded with family responsibilities	1	2	3
(79) Too many things to do	1	2	3
(80) Unchallenging work	1	2	3
(81) Concerns about meeting high standards	1	2	3
(82) Financial dealings with friends or acquaintances	1	2	3
(83) Job dissatisfactions	1	2	3

	Severity		
	1. Somewhat Severe	2. Moderately Severe	3. Extremely Severe
(84) Worries about decisions to change jobs	1	2	3
(85) Trouble with reading, writing, or spelling abilities	1	2	3
(86) Too many meetings	1	2	3
(87) Problems with divorce or separation	1	2	3
(88) Trouble with arithmetic skills	1	2	3
(89) Gossip	1	2	3
(90) Legal problems	1	2	3
(91) Concerns about weight	1	2	3
(92) Not enough time to do the things you need to do	1	2	3
(93) Television	1	2	3
(94) Not enough personal energy	1	2	3
(95) Concerns about inner conflicts	1	2	3
(96) Feel conflicted over what to do	1	2	3
(97) Regrets over past decisions	1	2	3
(98) Menstrual (period) problems	1	2	3
(99) The weather	1	2	3
(100) Nightmares	1	2	3
(101) Concerns about getting ahead	1	2	3
(102) Hassles from boss or supervisor	1	2	3
(103) Difficulties with friends	1	2	3
(104) Not enough time for family	1	2	3
(105) Transportation problems	1	2	3
(106) Not enough money for transportation	1	2	3
(107) Not enough money for entertainment and recreation	1	2	3
(108) Shopping	1	2	3
(109) Prejudice and discrimination from others	1	2	3
(110) Property, investments, or taxes	1	2	3
(111) Not enough time for entertainment and recreation	1	2	3
(112) Yardwork or outside home maintenance	1	2	3
(113) Concerns about news events	1	2	3
(114) Noise	1	2	3
(115) Crime	1	2	3
(116) Traffic	1	2	3
(117) Pollution			
HAVE WE MISSED ANY OF YOUR HASSLES? IF SO, WRITE THEM IN BELOW.			
(118) ______________________			
ONE MORE THING: HAS THERE BEEN A CHANGE IN YOUR LIFE THAT AFFECTED HOW YOU ANSWERED THIS SCALE? IF SO, TELL US WHAT IT WAS.			

From Kanner, AD, et al.,[59] with permission.

Appendix C: Internet Resources for Improving Community Accessibility

Independent Living Centers—http://www.senioroutlook.com
United Advertising Publications. Searches over 40,000 apartment communities for people with disabilities. Includes virtual tours, searches by distance, photos and floor plans. Contains information on insurance, storage, home mortgages, moving, types of housing facilities and a glossary of housing terms. Updated weekly.

Links to Centers for Independent Living—http://www.abledata.com
Includes information on and links to periodicals and research on disability, assistive technology and lists of health care professionals.

The Design Linc—http://www.designlinc.com/centers3.htm
Provides product information and design tips for families, consumers, and therapists designing for people with disabilities.

CHAPTER

3

LEARNING OBJECTIVES

1. Identify what a value is and how it directs human behavior.
2. Recognize how humans acquire values.
3. Identify how values influence the choices of patients, clients, and health professionals.
4. Distinguish between value-directed behavior that enhances healing and value-directed behavior that is likely to interfere with healing.
5. Describe examples of ethical distress that accompany health care provided by managed care organizations.
6. Learn a clinical reasoning process to aid in resolving ethical dilemmas.

Influence of Values on Patient Care: Foundation for Decision Making

Carol M. Davis, PT, EdD, MS, FAPTA

OUTLINE

Initially, one might question the logic of including a chapter on values in a text related to management of adult rehabilitation patients. The fact is that the entire book is devoted to educating the reader about the proper decisions to make in the rehabilitation process, and values play a critical role in most decision making. It is therefore important to consider this aspect of decision making.

Providing an operating definition of a *value* is something of a challenge. Many interpretations have been offered, and different authors have provided a variety of definitions.[1–5] For the purposes of this chapter, a **value** is defined as an inner force that provides the standards by which choices are made. For example, if people value the safety of their lives, among other acts, they will probably choose to wear a seat belt while driving or riding in an automobile. That choice is guided by the importance they place on their safety, or by their value of safety.

Because values are internal and difficult to measure, they have not been studied as vigorously as other aspects of human behavior. One cannot see a value; one can only feel it working. Values play a particularly important role in influencing our choices. The importance of this influence is emphasized when one considers that *knowing* the right thing to do and *doing* it are two separate phenomena. The first has to do with knowledge or cognition, the second with values or attitudes. This text is aimed at teaching the "knowing" aspect; this chapter, however, is devoted to elucidating the value aspect in choosing.

Most choices are value based; some decisions seem more difficult to make than others. Difficulty may arise when the therapist must resolve a values dilemma, when two seemingly equal goals or choices compete with one another. Difficulty also may arise when the therapist's values conflict with the values of the patient, the patient's family, colleagues, the larger health care system, and/or society. This chapter further defines values, describes how we acquire our values, and illustrates the influence values have on decisions. In addition, the influence that patient's values have on therapists' decisions is explored; examples of common difficult decisions in rehabilitation are provided. The **ethical distress** that can occur when providing care while working with a for-profit-business or managed care organization is explored. Value issues inherent in the process of delegating care to supportive staff as the role of the physical therapist becomes further refined as a diagnostician are also explored. Finally, the role communication plays in the process of making difficult choices is discussed.

Process of Decision Making

How choices are made is different from *what* choices are made. The latter can be viewed as the answer or the solution; the former describes a process. Decision making or choosing in rehabilitation is sometimes composed of nothing more than a reactive, instinctive stimulus–response effort, or haphazard trial-and-error guessing. But more often, making the right decision, choosing the best alternative, results from professionally educated problem solving. One type of problem solving in health care is termed **clinical reasoning**. Even before the therapist first sees a patient, the process of clinical reasoning begins. On reviewing patient information, hypotheses are generated and various questions are asked in sequence to examine the patient's problem fully and, inevitably, to decide on the diagnosis that will guide physical therapy treatment. Further reasoning results in a decision about the most appropriate treatment for this particular person at this point in time, whenever possible verified by evidence in the literature.

The greater part of professional education in health care is devoted to developing good clinical reasoners. The best instructors bravely refuse to give the "right" answer and encourage students to learn the process of discovery. In this way, students rise above the technical level of training. They are encouraged to become professionals capable of responding to complex patient situations by carefully reading the literature, questioning, touching, testing, and listening with the "third ear" to what is said as well as to what is left unsaid.

Problem solving is fundamental to our daily lives as humans. We often do not realize we are problem solving because the process is so habitual, so subconscious. Just deciding what to have for breakfast can involve an intricate multistep process:

What shall I have for breakfast?
What's in the kitchen?
Cereal, eggs, bacon, pancakes, juice, toast.
How hungry am I?
Starved!
How much time do I have?
Thirty minutes.
What did the scale say?
Five pounds over.
That does it; juice and dry toast!

The answer to this problem solving process was based on identifying the importance of one value over others. The fact that the scale revealed 5 excess pounds became a determining factor for making the final choice. Another person might have made the same choice but for a different reason:

How much time do I have?
5 minutes.
No time to eat! I'll have toast and juice and eat it on the way!

Most choices result from prioritizing values. The more we know about our values, the more we learn and understand our science, and the more we know about the facts of the situation, the easier it is to make a decision that seems best.[1]

Deciding what to eat for breakfast is a decision making process of a different sort than deciding whether a patient is a good candidate to receive a transfemoral (above-knee) prosthesis. The differences are important. The first, what to eat, is a personal choice; the second, whether to recommend a prosthesis, is a professional decision. The first is a choice that bears little consequence for the chooser if the less-than-best decision is made. However, the decision about the prosthesis has profound consequence for another person if the less-than-best decision is made. What to eat for breakfast is more accurately viewed as a value preference or a **nonmoral value** choice; the prosthesis decision is made up largely of several moral- and value-laden decisions. **Moral values**, such as justice, honesty, compassion, and integrity, all reflect a way of relating to human beings; thus moral values carry more importance than value preferences, because humans are more important than food, music, or what we wear.[2,6]

When we study to become professionals, part of the professional socialization process involves the adoption of values that usually overlap with our personal values. At times, however, they might conflict with them. Professional responsibility, we learn, requires that we put the patient's needs before our own and act in ways that show we deserve the patient's trust.[7,8] Let us take a closer look at what a value is and how we obtain our personal and professional values.

Values and Valuing

A value cannot be seen directly, and it cannot be measured. Values are constructs (moral schemes) that are made up of beliefs, emotions, and attitudes about what is best and what is not good.[3] We can view values only indirectly by asking people what they value, or even more important, by watching another person's behavior. Values are reflected in our actions, especially the pattern of our actions over time. Thus one might say, "I value honesty," but we might wonder how much that's true when the person knowingly cheats on income tax returns. Another value obviously has priority over honesty for this person.

At times values cooperate, and at other times conflict with each other. A dilemma exists when we have difficulty choosing which value should have priority. For example, respect for life is the central value for advocates of a woman's right to choose abortion as well as for those opposed to abortion. The difference in opinion and belief of these two groups is not over the value of life, but the importance of the mother's life over the fetus' life above all considerations. Reproductive freedom advocates emphasize the primacy of the mother's choice for the quality of her life and resist outside interference to her right to choose. The right to life activists value the life of the unborn fetus who requires an advocate.[6] Resolving dilemmas involves a special form of clinical reasoning that will be explained later.

People are not born with values, but they are born with instincts and needs. Values are acquired from those who socialize us, primarily parents and family, and, for many, religion. The initial learning of values takes the form of "following the rules" that parents believe will minimize personal pain and conflict, maximize pleasure and meaning, and promote harmony and peace in the home. In recent years, it can be said that television, video games, film, and music have played an increasingly large part in forming the values of adolescents and young adults.

Adolescents, as a part of natural maturation, test the values of the home by breaking rules and trying forbidden behaviors. This process marks the beginning of a transformation in which value-based rules followed to avoid punishment become internalized and, on reflection, are adopted as one's own. Most people end up with a set of values very similar to that of their parents. However, for some, the difference in the way they prioritize their values causes a distancing between themselves and certain family members. One example of children prioritizing their values differently from their parents is the son or daughter who is the first in four generations not to study law, or the child who decides not to go to college at all.

The values of health professionals take on a different priority from the values of people in other careers whose primary satisfaction in work comes not from helping people directly but largely from working with ideas or inanimate objects. Likewise, although physical therapists as a group seem to display a consistent set of values, it might be conjectured that one of the key differences that distinguishes profoundly different specialists—for example, physical therapists whose practice focuses on sports-related injuries (i.e., patients who are well but injured), from those devoted to caring for seriously ill brain-injured patients—is the way that the specialist prioritizes values. The physical therapist working with sports injuries expresses different interests and focuses professional goals on a population with needs very different from those of brain-injured patients. The different choices made in preferred patient populations may stem from different values as well as different needs and interests.[6]

We make our most meaningful choices based on what attracts us and leads us to growth and self-fulfillment, a life of happiness and meaning.[3] Being aware of our values helps us to make informed and consistent choices that lead to personal and professional satisfaction. This is part of the process physical therapists undergo as they search out a specialty area of interest following their first few years in clinical practice.

Code of Ethics

The set of moral norms adopted by a professional group to direct value-laden choices in a way consistent with professional responsibility is termed a **code of ethics** (Box 3.1). Most codes of ethics of the professions are composed of statements that have at their core one of four value principles—**autonomy, beneficence,** nonmaleficence, and **justice**—and three rules that follow from these four principles: (1) veracity, (2) **confidentiality** and privacy, and (3) **fidelity**[9] (Box 3.2). One might follow their code without internalizing it, just as small children follow the "rules of the house." For the code of ethics to function as a set of professional values, one must reflect on it and decide that it, indeed, forms a values complex around which one is willing to organize professional choices. Thus, as was previously stated, reflection is necessary to the internalization of values to make them truly one's own.[3–5] The choices that then follow this internalization are likely to be consistent with one's basic beliefs, show coherence, be authentic or genuine, and be adequate to the task of decision making. Those who make the smoothest transitions into professional practice are likely to be those whose personal values and priorities significantly overlap with the values inherent in their chosen professional practice. Given that one's basic human survival needs are met, the more one reflects on one's choices and on which choices result in a good and meaningful life, the more one is apt to experience consistent reward from opportunities.[3]

The Values of Patients as a Factor in Care

Patients come to physical therapy as whole persons in need of professional help and guidance. All people can be viewed as possessing five areas of need that comprise the whole: the physical, the intellectual, the emotional, the social, and the spiritual.[6] It could be said that a more meaningful and peaceful life results when choices are made that respond equally to the demands of all four quadrants of need. Central to the work of Carl Jung is the belief that a healthy personality results from achieving a *balance* between thinking and feeling and between intuition and sensation.[10]

Patients come to physical therapy at various stages in their lives and with a unique history of having made thousands of choices. Over time the therapist comes to realize that some patients display a life pattern of meaningful, consistent, well thought out choices; others reveal a life of capricious, noncentered, unorganized value-based behavior. Often patients' risky choices have directly or indirectly brought them to therapy; for example, the young patient with quadriplegia who drove into a tree while drunk. Many patient problems in movement and function that are

Box 3.1 Code of Ethics of the American Physical Therapy Association

Preamble
This Code of Ethics sets forth principles for the ethical practice of physical therapy. All physical therapists are responsible for maintaining and promoting ethical practice. To this end, the physical therapist shall act in the best interest of the patient/client. This Code of Ethics shall be binding on all physical therapists.

Principle 1
A physical therapist shall respect the rights and dignity of all individuals and shall provide compassionate care.

Principle 2
A physical therapist shall act in a trustworthy manner towards patients/clients, and in all other aspects of physical therapy practice.

Principle 3
A physical therapist shall comply with laws and regulations governing physical therapy and shall strive to effect changes that benefit patients/clients.

Principle 4
A physical therapist shall exercise sound professional judgment.

Principle 5
A physical therapist shall achieve and maintain professional competence.

Principle 6
A physical therapist shall maintain and promote high standards for physical therapist practice, education, and research.

Principle 7
A physical therapist shall seek only such remuneration as is deserved and reasonable for physical therapy services.

Principle 8
A physical therapist shall provide and make available accurate and relevant information to patients/clients about their care and to the public about physical therapy services.

Principle 9
A physical therapist shall protect the public and the profession from unethical, incompetent, and illegal acts.

Principle 10
A physical therapist shall endeavor to address the health needs of society.

Principle 11
A physical therapist shall respect the rights, knowledge, and skills of colleagues and other health professionals.

Adopted by the House of Delegates, June 2000. (From the American Physical Therapy Association, with permission.)

Box 3.2 Moral Principles and Rules that Form the Foundations of Health Care Ethics[9]

Principles

1. **Autonomy:** The patient's right to choose for one's life, and to voice that choice for as long as possible.
2. **Beneficence:** Doing what is best for one's patient. Contrasts with paternalism or patronizing. Beneficence is a moral obligation of all health care practitioners. We must act with beneficence when we are aware of the facts and the patient is at significant risk of harm or loss and our action is needed to prevent that harm or loss. We must act with beneficence if the benefit to the patient outweighs the potential harm to the health care practitioner.
3. **Nonmaleficence:** Do no harm. Do not injure, disable, or kill a person, or undermine a person's reputation, property, or privacy.
4. **Justice**
   Fairness
   Distributive—equal distribution to all members of a group
   Compensatory—making up for past injustice (affirmative action)
   Procedural—first come, first served, alphabetical order, and so forth

Ethical Rules that Follow These Principles

1. **Veracity**—Tell the truth, do not lie.
   From the principles of autonomy and beneficence.
   Key ethical issue is how much of the truth to tell in view of beneficence.
2. **Confidentiality and Privacy**
   From the principle of beneficence.
   Health care practitioners are morally obliged to keep confident all information concerning patients even if not requested specifically, except when to do so would bring harm to innocent people or to the patient.
   Patients have the right to keep private any information not relevant to their care.
3. **Fidelity**
   From the principle of beneficence.
   Health care practitioners' actions and treatments will remain faithful to their patient and to their colleagues, even when they disagree with their colleagues.

encountered in rehabilitation are not the result of "fate," but result from a lifetime of choices that placed other values and needs at a higher priority than physical health, or than the prevention of illness and injury. The more physical therapists become aware of how much control people actually have over their state of wellness and health, the more difficult it becomes for some therapists to remain nonjudgmental about their patients. It is exceedingly difficult for some clinicians, for example, to remain nonjudgmental while treating a chronic smoker for emphysema or a tremendously obese patient for hip and knee joint problems.[11]

It is important, however, to remember that we are morally and ethically bound to give to all patients the highest quality of care as free from judgment and bias as possible. This is where balance in all of our areas of need helps us. If our needs are being met in all five areas (physical, intellectual, emotional, social, and spiritual), we feel less frustrated and irritated by personal stress and can remain centered and better able to remain nonjudgmental and can set more adequate boundaries with compassion. Patients, with all their frailties, can be seen as separate from us, doing the best for themselves that they can.[6]

When a reflex wave of judgment and criticism starts to make its way into the conversation with a patient, it helps to breathe deeply, center yourself, and adopt the value-neutral attitude of *curiosity*. Remember none of us can literally put ourselves into the shoes of our patients, so as soon as we think we know better, and are ready to admonish our patients, it is better to stop, breathe, and say, "I'm *curious*. What made you decide to do that?" And then be quiet and listen to try to understand without judging.

To be "centered" is to experience one's energy concentrated in the middle and balanced so that no one area's needs predominate. When we feel centered, we feel balanced, just as the balanced karate expert stands with his or her weight so distributed that blows coming in any direction can be absorbed and pushed away without loss of balance. If, for example, our emotional needs are not being met, we often feel unbalanced or uncentered. We either spend energy repressing or expressing the stress of loneliness, need for attention, or irritability. On the other hand, when our five areas of need are equally attended to, we feel centered and thus can feel whole in every part. Centered energy and consciousness then allow us to free our attention away from our needs and toward the patient's needs, and we can be therapeutically present.

When we need nothing more than to assist our patients in healing, whatever they choose to do can be viewed with greater objectivity. When we, ourselves, "need" our patients to get better, to thank us, to praise us, to acknowledge our skill and intellect because those common human emotional needs are not being met outside the clinic, we are more likely to judge our patients when they fail to meet our needs.[6]

The Influence of Values on the Primary Goal of Patient Care

When health practitioners experience feelings of criticism and negative judgment toward a patient, they must be aware of it and consciously work not to let it affect their behavior. The primary goal of health practitioners is to help *all* people recover or maintain their health so that day to day they may function at the most autonomous level possible. If the primary goal is to achieve optimal health and healing, certain values seem to promote that goal more than others. One way to ascertain values that promote health and healing is to describe behavior between a therapist and patient that does the very opposite, or that interferes with health and healing. Putting yourself in the place of the patient, what therapist behaviors would *interfere* with your progress toward getting well or healing? Table 3.1 presents a sample list of very obvious behaviors that would detract from a patient's ability to function optimally in a therapeutic setting. Also included is a list of possible negative values that might underlie each of these behaviors.[11]

Behaviors and underlying values that *facilitate* healing might be described as the exact opposite of those that detract from healing[11] (Table 3.2). These therapist behaviors help restore a patient's hope, promote progress toward recovery, and assist with achieving the highest possible level of independent function.

Many of us who would read the list of negative behaviors (see Table 3.1) that detract from healing would respond, "I'd never behave in such a way with my patients!" But, in fact, a huge gap exists between knowing the right thing to do, wanting to do it, and actually doing it.

Essential to a "therapeutic use of self" is the capacity to feel **compassion** for those who suffer. Compassion is quite different from **pity**, where a person feels sorry for those who are less fortunate. The compassion of the mature health professional is fueled by imagination, or the ability to envision what is possible from the other person's perspective.[6,12] Imaginative understanding involves **self-transposal** (a cognitive attempt to put oneself in the place of another) at the least and **empathy** (a complex type of **identification** with another's experience) at the most.[6] As healers, therapists must not block but, rather, must allow empathy to occur, a momentary "crossing over" into the patient's frame of reference. Thus, compassion is a very personal, intimate experience that is built on "trust, honesty, and the time and willingness to listen (p 189)."[12]

Let us examine some patient care situations that require professional choice that may result in a less-than-optimal prioritizing of our professional and personal values.

Table 3.1 Therapist Behaviors and Possible Underlying Values that Detract from the Healing Process

Therapist Behaviors that Interfere or Detract from the Healing Process	Negative Values that Might Underlie Each Behavior
1. Acting cool or aloof, obviously paying more attention to other patients.	1. a. Prejudice: to prejudge or to classify a person as belonging to a larger group and thus to believe things about that person that one believed about the larger group. b. Indifference: lack of interest or concern: aloofness, detachment.
2. Overly criticizing you (the patient) so that you feel as if nothing you do is right.	2. a. Prejudice. b. Perfectionism: the doctrine that the perfection of moral character is a person's highest good and that freedom from imperfection is attainable. c. Lack of flexibility.
3. Treating you as an object rather than as a person with feelings of pain, worry, and insecurity.	3. Depersonalization: to detract from an individual's uniqueness; to fail to honor a person's individuality.
4. Treating you as if you were a child, incapable of really understanding anything that is said.	4. Patronizing: to adopt an air of condescension.
5. Being unable or unwilling to help you in your exercises; leaving you alone most of the time.	5. a. Indifference. b. Prejudice.
6. Making fun of you in your presence and behind your back.	6. Depersonalization.
7. Telling others things you have shared in confidence.	7. Breaking confidentiality; not keeping another person's trust private and secret.
8. Not letting you work on your own.	8. Fostering dependence.
9. More often than not guessing about what is best for you. Admitting he or she "is not sure" what to do, but "let us not let that stop us."	9. Failure to recognize and to act on one's limits of knowledge.
10. Always fitting you in as if everything else in the therapist's life is more important than you are.	10. Placing self-interest over patient's needs.

Value-Laden Situations in Rehabilitation

What would you do, and *why*, if this situation happened to you? Joyce, a 22-year-old college student, was referred to physical therapy following surgical removal of her left leg owing to osteogenic sarcoma. Other than generalized weakness from chemotherapy, surgery, and bed rest and incisional pain and soreness, she was in "good health" on her arrival to the rehabilitation center.

You have been treating her for several weeks, having begun therapy from her admission to the rehabilitation center where you work. Preoperative training was given in the acute setting. You have assisted her with pre-prosthetic training, strengthening, prosthetic training and acceptance, and gait training. She has been progressing well.

Joyce is intelligent and inquisitive, yet somewhat stubborn. Two weeks before discharge you notice an increasing tendency on her part to be careless and to take unnecessary risks, like hopping on one foot rather than donning her prosthesis. In addition, she admits to thinking that her daily strengthening exercises are stupid and that, after discharge, she may just throw the prosthesis away and depend on a wheelchair. Even crutches are too much bother.

You feel confused and frustrated. You have invested a great deal of energy into the successful rehabilitation of this person and her behavior at this point seems ignorant

Table 3.2 Therapist Behaviors and Possible Underlying Values that Facilitate the Healing Process

Therapist Behaviors that Facilitate or Promote the Healing Process	Positive Values that Might Underlie Each Behavior
1. Offering you (the patient) the same amount of attention offered other patients, so it balances out from day-to-day.	1. Justice: the quality of impartiality or fairness.
2. Accepting your weaknesses along with your strengths and verbally reinforcing the desired behaviors.	2. Unconditional positive regard; acceptance.
3. Always treating you as a person with feelings and being sensitive to those feelings each day.	3. a. Respect: the act of giving particular attention to a person; worthy of high regard. b. Compassion: sympathetic consciousness of another's situation and the desire to be of effective help in relieving a painful situation.
4. Explaining things at your level, not oversimplifying or making things too complex.	4. a. Respect. b. Accurate and sensitive communication.
5. Always reachable yet never fostering dependence; encouraging independent activity.	5. a. Autonomy: a quality or state of self-governance; independence. b. Dignity: the quality of being worthy, honored, esteemed; to have distinction as a person.
6. Never using humor inappropriately, never laughing *at* you, but encouraging you to be able to laugh, sometimes even at yourself.	6. Appropriate humor, nondefensive humor.
7. Always keeping your confidence.	7. Confidentiality: keeping another person's trust private and secret.
8. Fostering your own independent activity without letting you feel stranded.	8. Autonomy.
9. Realizing when the advice of someone else is needed and asking for help in a timely fashion.	9. Recognizing the limits to one's knowledge, knowing when to get help or to refer; honesty.
10. Making you feel special, cherished, and unique; showing individual concern for you and your progress.	10. a. Compassion. b. Sensitivity to your uniqueness.

and manipulative. Her refusal to cooperate with your suggestions angers you; you feel that her basic laziness in requesting a wheelchair existence represents settling for a quality of life that is less than optimal and selfish. You feel as if you have failed to help her realize her full potential, as well as overstressed with the demands of your work.

Once the patient care day has begun, therapists seldom find or take the time to reflect on the larger issues, those that hover on the fringe of the work consciousness. Instead, therapists tend to focus on the immediate situation in front of them, quickly gathering data and problem solving as they go. Joyce's growing problem of reluctance could be viewed as a peripheral issue at first, one the therapist hoped would pass without needing to be confronted. But as her discharge date comes closer, the therapist is forced to respond to what appears to be regressive behavior.

The therapist's responses may reveal one or more of several thoughts and feelings. Especially when under stress, one may become impatient and angry and lecture Joyce to "grow up." The therapist may feel personal failure and frustration and, in a condescending way, let her know far more reward was expected for the efforts placed in her successful rehabilitation. These are often reactive, automatic, emotion-based responses based on a value of, or need for, spontaneous honesty and the right to express feelings regardless of the impact that the expression may have on others. The therapist is unhappy and wants the situation to change but does not know how to change it, so the therapist displays poor impulse control and aggressively "lets off steam."

As "human" as this choice may seem, more mature behavior is required of health professionals. No longer may we claim the luxury of a spontaneous outburst, for the impact of the therapist's outburst rarely solves value-based problems and often creates larger ones. Obviously, this is not conducive to healing.

On reflection, one realizes that Joyce's regressive behavior may likely reveal inner conflict, fear, and/or depression. From Joyce's point of view, it is not difficult to come to some understanding that a person under these circumstances might be afraid and might see a safer existence in a wheelchair. Stopping to breathe, and then acting on the value of compassion, sustained by empathy and self-transposal, elevates the problem-solving process from *reaction* to a *professional choice* to sit down and to discuss this issue comprehensively with Joyce, referring her to the social worker for psychological support and counseling, if necessary.

Nonjudgmental concern and understanding are foundations of healing. In addition, health professionals caring for adults must accept that occasionally they will encounter a patient who is unwilling to cooperate with their suggestions and who resists their attempts to offer therapeutic care and advice. With the value of patient autonomy in mind, the professional's role is not to assume a paternalistic stance indicating "I know what's better for you than you do," but instead to outline as clearly, creatively, and accurately as possible the predictable results of the choices the patient is making. Patients must have control over their own lives to the greatest extent possible.[6,7] But in the end, we cannot and should not force patients to undergo treatment when they have simply refused. It is their autonomous right to refuse care and we must honor that.

These guidelines exist in their purest sense when therapists are treating adult patients who are not suffering from confusion, mental or intellectual disorders, or significant depression. With children or adults who are experiencing the conditions mentioned, therapists must aim for the greatest extent of autonomous choice possible and focus appropriate attention on parents and family caregivers.

Beneficence versus Benevolence: The Ethic of Care

Mary Romanello, a physical therapist, and her colleague wrote an interesting piece entitled, "The 'Ethic of Care' in Physical Therapy Practice and Education: Challenges and Opportunities,"[13] in which she reinforces the point made earlier, that an ethic of caring goes beyond simple beneficence, doing what is good because that is our duty, or benevolence, being kind because that is also our duty. Caring for our patients involves something greater than this.

> *But benevolence falls short of an ethic of care that allows health care practitioners 'to truly and consistently connect with, be with, and attend to and do for their patients.' A relational ethic of care is a critical component of physical therapy that compels practitioners to construct this relationship with patients as subjects, rather than objects of the healing encounter. Benevolence is an important virtue, but it is not a sufficient ethic to guide practitioners in today's work climates. The ethic of care goes beyond benevolence to build a relationship based on the needs and goals that arise out of the physical therapist-patient relationship.*[p 21]

The authors stress the distinction between one's ethical duty to not harm a patient and one's deeper role in the relational ethic of care. Although the authors do not use the terms, basically they make a recommendation for elevating moral sensitivity (the ability to understand how one's actions may affect another) and moral judgment (the ability to analyze a situation and make a good moral decision) to moral action based on an ethic of care. The importance of developing the skill of listening and paying attention and the relevance of individual patient-centered care is stressed. The caring relationship must always be at the heart of all that we do in rehabilitation. This demands time and energy that the current health care climate is not willing to give easily. But the patient–practitioner relationship is primary and we must "expect to deal with risks that produce conflict and guilt."[13, p 23] Experience alone will not foster an ethic of care. Clinicians and clinical educators must teach directly about this moral philosophy, and point it out in case studies and in clinical practice. "How to consider a patient's wants, needs, concerns, and values can be interwoven with the teaching of evaluation and therapeutic exercise skills so students learn to combine an ethic of care with their scientific knowledge in order to put the patient's interests before their own."[13, p 25]

Resolving Ethical or Moral Dilemmas in Practice

Ethical *situations* differ from ethical *problems*, and both differ from an ethical *dilemma*. Ethical *situations* are with us every day. An example would be the situation where a physical therapist is cautioned to be careful about documenting accurate charges for patients to avoid overcharging. It is unethical for physical therapists to charge more for treatments than is listed (see Box 3.1, Principle 7).

An ethical *problem* occurs when a physical therapist is confronted with an ethical temptation, but clearly understands the right thing to do. An example would be a patient's offer of a gift of a vacation for two to the Caribbean to a physical therapist in gratitude for the excellent treatment given. The Code of Ethics clearly outlines how this would be a breach of ethical behavior (Box 3.1, Principle 4) by affecting sound professional judgment. It would be very difficult not to treat that patient with special regard in the future. Likewise an ethical problem occurs when "management" requires that a clinician treat more patients in a day than is possible and still maintain quality care. Clinicians feel very guilty for running from one patient to the next, with no opportunity to establish the kind of relationship required to facilitate meeting personal goals, or spending the time required to individualize care. Patients are not well-served when the quantity of patients seen or the profit of the practice takes precedence over the quality of patient care and the professional service of the practice. We know the importance of therapeutic relationships, and when we sacrifice them for profit, we are responding to an ethical problem in an unethical way. But this does not constitute a true dilemma, for loyalty to our patients must take precedence over our employers.[14] This is discussed in more detail later in this chapter.

A special kind of clinical reasoning is required when one confronts a true moral or **ethical dilemma**. In the presence of an ethical dilemma, when the best action eludes us, it helps to reflect in a systematic way, and then consult with a fellow professional or someone skilled in dilemma resolution (Box 3.3).[6] In resolving moral or ethical dilemmas in health care, the best decision usually results only when the facts or context of the situation are delineated as clearly and as precisely as possible. Whether you decide to resolve the dilemma *teleologically* (deciding what the best outcome would be [for the greatest number, for example]) or *deontologically* (weighing the two or more values that seem to be fighting with each other, and deciding which is the "higher" or "more moral" action in this particular case with these particular facts), the best decision can be made only with careful thought. Box 3.3 outlines a process of reasoning that can guide you in resolving ethical dilemmas in your practice. You should be able to justify your final decision by explaining both your ethical reasoning process and your conscious weighing of one value over another in this situation. A well-reasoned moral decision is always a combination of one's personal values system (discernment) guided by one's professional values or the values of health care.

Let's take a rather simple but familiar example in physical therapy. A 90-year-old man had recently had a revision of his transtibial (below knee) amputation to a transfemoral (above knee) amputation. The surgeon requested the physical therapist teach the patient exercises for home, but not to prepare him for a new transfemoral prosthesis because the literature indicated that his age did not permit a successful outcome with a prosthesis. The physical therapist knew the patient well, and disagreed with the physician's decision. The patient had exercised all his life and had excellent cardiopulmonary fitness. Can you identify the values at war with each other in this dilemma? The dilemma was between beneficence (doing what is good for the patient) and autonomy (the patient clearly hoped to get a new limb), versus fidelity to the physician colleague. After discussing this with a supervisor, and with the supervisor's support, the therapist fabricated a pylon. This allowed the patient to successfully begin ambulation. The therapist invited the surgeon to watch the patient in the parallel bars, and based on this new information, the surgeon facilitated the process of securing a new limb. Hence by using creative clinical reasoning, what seemed to be an either/or situation (an ethical dilemma) was turned into a "third way" resolution for the good of the patient.

Sometimes this is not possible, however. Sometimes a dilemma just has to be resolved with weighing all of the facts and values, and choosing the highest or most right alternative, given the context of the situation. An example is reluctantly agreeing to honor an older patient's autonomous request to remain at home in spite of the fact that health care professionals and family members have clear evidence that the patient's balance is compromised and it is just a matter of time until a fall and injury occur.

Box 3.3 Solving the Ethical Dilemma[6]

Ethical dilemmas occur when two or more ethical principles conflict with each other in a given situation and it is unclear what the best or highest moral action would be. This problem solving process can be applied in the search for the best alternative.

1. **Gather all of the facts** that can be known about the situation.
2. **Decide which ethical principles or rules are involved,** such as beneficence, autonomy, non-maleficence, justice, confidentiality, veracity, or fidelity. Is self-interest a factor on the part of the health professional?
3. **Clarify your professional duties** in this situation; for example, do no harm, obey the law, tell the truth, stand up for one's colleagues even when you disagree. Do the Code of Ethics and Guide to Professional Conduct speak to this particular issue?
4. **Describe the general nature of the outcome that would be most desired, or the consequences of a poor action.** What seems to be most important of all in this situation?
5. **Describe the practical features** of this situation. What are the disputed facts? Does the law instruct here? What are the wishes of the people involved? What about resources available? What is the main risk here? How certain can we be of the truth and the completeness of the facts that are known? What are the predominant values of the people involved?

When all of the pertinent aspects that go into this particular decision are laid out before you, then **you must use your discernment to decide which action is the highest moral alternative.** Most often simply asking, "What is best for my patient?" is the simplest route. But there are times when beneficence is not the best alternative, when it can be shown that others would suffer by acting on what is best for your patient. Self-interest, acting on what benefits you before considering the needs of your patient, is almost never a justifiable moral choice. Exceptions might be argued for a professional who must act on behalf of his or her child, parent, or spouse in an emergency situation, for example.

The dilemma is between the patient's autonomy and nonmaleficence, above all do (or allow) no harm.

Reactive versus Proactive Decision Making

Reactive care, characterized by on-the-spot problem solving and decision making, is an unavoidable part of rehabilitation. However, the greater the number of our decisions that are based on reaction rather than on proaction or well thought out alternatives, the more idiosyncratic, inconsistent, and erratic our behavior will seem. It was suggested that to stop, breathe, and center is a useful way to avoid reactive judgment. Stopping to breathe will help bring about more proactive decisions, rather than reactive ones. Part of professional responsibility is to anticipate possible problems and to think through alternatives in advance. Likewise, the more that therapists base their decisions on scientific evidence and the more that they reflect on the values behind alternative choices, the more apt they are to experience consistent, scientific-based decisions reflective of the highest professional care. These decisions are inevitably more conducive to healing.

Value Decisions and Managed Care

Corporate health care, managed competition, capitation, and prepaid health organizations (PPOs) in many cases have been limiting patient access to physical and occupational therapists, and limiting the therapists' choice of and duration of reimbursed treatments. Under managed care, physical therapists have both professional obligations to treat patients and may also have contractual obligations to managed care organizations (MCOs). It is important that health care professionals be able to carefully analyze their patients' needs and use sound moral reasoning and ethical dilemma resolution skills to decide on appropriate care when there is a shortage of professional care available, or when there is inadequate reimbursement for needed care.[14]

Remember that until recently, managed care corporations had no moral obligations to their clients, the patients. Managed care is a business only. In the eyes of the law, MCOs do not practice health care. The primary duty of the health care professional is always to the patient, and secondarily to the business contract. This can result in *ethical distress* when you know the best thing to do, but are prohibited from doing it by the organization within which you practice.[15] For example, if the six visits provided by an MCO under a capitation agreement do not suffice to reach the anticipated goals set with the patient at the initial examination, the health care professional risks being held liable for abandonment if he or she discharges the patient prematurely with the comment, "Your MCO told me I had to stop care." *The business cannot dictate to a health professional when to discontinue treatment.*[15] MCOs do not tell professionals when to stop care, but simply when they will no longer pay for care. Professionals are obligated to provide needed care. Likewise, professionals have the right to maintain an adequate financial base of practice, and thus should seek private reimbursement or other reimbursement from the patient, and work diligently to reverse inadequate payment decisions by lobbying insurance groups and by conducting and publishing the research needed to show reasonable time frames for efficacious care.

Case law now indicates that the court's expectations are for the professional to continue to serve the patient pro bono, or without compensation.[15] Thus each practice needs to develop a policy or guide outlining how it will determine the incidents and limits of pro bono care, and beyond that, the care of the patient who cannot pay but requires treatment should be transferred to colleagues who have *pro bono* capacity at that time.[15]

When health care as a service is managed as if it were a business, where profit is the primary reason for its existence, a conflict is bound to emerge. The foundational ethic of business is *buyer beware*. Business exists to make a profit, and will go to great lengths to convince consumers that they need what business is selling. On the other hand, the professions were created to provide a service to those in need, and thus the foundational ethic of the professions is, *primum non nocere*—above all, do no harm.[8] It is easy to see how these foundational ethical principles are fundamentally in conflict with each other.

We have seen the concept of facilitating the *healing of the whole patient or client* all but disappear from health care in the United States. When business executives have their eyes on the bottom line and dictate to health care professionals *who they can treat, for how long, and what is reasonable to charge,* they strip health professionals of their ethical foundations. The very definition of a profession's autonomy requires that professionals are the only ones who can make those judgments, and they are morally obligated to make them free from interference, not with profit or self-interest in mind, but with the intent to provide service for those in need.[8]

It is important that health professionals stay current with local, state, and federal guidelines on health care practice and reimbursement, and learn how to identify and resolve the ethical dilemmas that result in these unstable times. Some predict that the negative impact of business on health care will become even more restrictive to providing quality care before improvements begin. But benefits have occurred as a result of this shift toward managed care. The current trend has resulted in greater cost containment, which is absolutely necessary, as well as a greater shift of the burden of care to patients and their families. This has resulted in more responsibility on the part of patients for their own health, and for preventative habits and maintenance of their own care.[6]

Above and beyond all trends and reimbursement mechanisms, when the interests of the patient and the professional collide, always remember that ethically beneficence and autonomy must outweigh self-interest[8] (see Box 3.2). If professionals were engaged only in business, there would be no dilemma. But health care professionals are bound by codes of ethics of service, not profit, that mandate advocacy for patients who come to them because they have both the education and the commitment to help them. To use patients for our own benefit beyond service literally destroys the profession.[8]

Values Inherent in Delegating to Supportive Personnel

A majority of states now provide direct access to the services of physical therapists. As the profession of physical therapy advances to assume more autonomous responsibility for the prevention, diagnosis, and management of problems within the human movement system, the role of the professional becomes more centered on diagnosis and planning for appropriate treatment, and health and community education. In day-to-day patient care it is becoming more important to delegate treatment to others who are qualified to carry out care at less expense to the patient. What values and principles can guide us so that we know when we can delegate safely and wisely? Watts[16] suggests that there is a way to make these decisions based on task analysis and recognition of the qualifications of various supportive personnel involved in patient care. In patient care circumstances where the consequences of action are predictable with certainty, the stability of the situation indicates that change is unlikely to occur rapidly, the basic indicators of treatment are readily observable and nonambiguous, and the criticality of methods used is not severe, it is likely that care can be safely delegated to an assistant or family member. The values behind appropriate and cost-effective delegation of care are beneficence, nonmaleficence, and justice. Beneficence, or doing good for the patient, can be justified only when others are not harmed by your action. Many times physical therapists continue with treatment of a patient that could be carried out by a physical therapist assistant or in a home program, while other patients wait to be examined and evaluated to begin care. The physical therapist is the only professional who can examine and diagnose, and then plan treatment based on that diagnosis, yet the waiting patients are given lower priority. This situation is an example of violating the moral principle of distributive justice.[17]

Value Decisions in Triage Situations

Triage situations always involve value priorities. A decision as simple as who to see first of three new inpatient referrals requires a value-based choice. What factors seem important in making the decision among these three new patients?

1. An 80-year-old, frail elderly woman with osteoporosis admitted following surgery to repair a fractured hip. Room 300.
2. A 30-year-old man with severe low back pain secondary to possible herniated disk. Room 201.
3. A 53-year-old woman who had a mild heart attack three weeks ago, admitted for cardiac rehabilitation. Room 302.

How would you decide, at 8 AM, which of these three patients to see first? What facts seem to make a difference? The patient's age? His or her location in the hospital (closest vs farthest away from where you are now)? Your existing patient load and schedule? Your subconscious or conscious aversion to certain patients, such as those with low back pain, worker's compensation patients, or elderly patients? If our primary goal in rehabilitation is to help patients recover their health so that they might function at the highest, most independent level possible, how can we use this goal to help direct our choices?

Putting the patient's needs first by way of autonomy and beneficence seems to be critical to this decision. The therapist's choice should not be based solely on personal convenience or self-interest. What additional facts are needed?[1,6] Putting oneself in the place of the patient, one comes to realize that the existence of certain factors requires our immediate attention. One factor that readily comes to mind that demands immediate consideration is responding to patients in pain. Pain can totally consume one's attention and will take immediate priority in our choices. Responding first to patients in severe discomfort seems very important in sequencing the order of treatments. The therapist needs to find out which of these three individuals may have had a difficult night and is most in need of attention for relief of pain.

Summary

Professional rehabilitative care requires clinical decision making that is proactive, evidence-based, and demonstrates a consistent, conscious value of choosing behavior that is conducive to healing. Clinicians must become "informed reasoners"[2] who have systematically gathered the facts, have recognized potential choices and values dilemmas, and have taken the time to weigh which choice is most conducive to the healing process.

Central to this process is the courage to confront seemingly peripheral factors that therapists are tempted to hope will go away, as well as the willingness to put oneself in the place of the patient. Pellegrino[18] cautions us not to be so egocentric as to treat others simply as we would like to be treated. Instead, he suggests that the Golden Rule of health care should be *the right of each patient to voice his or her needs or preferences*. The health care professional, after all, would expect similar sensitivity if he or she were to assume the role of the patient.

Finally, sensitive and accurate communication is required. In health, people feel alive by their connectedness to the world, and in illness they feel cut off, fragmented, and uninterested in the world. The therapist's role as a healer then becomes one of entering the patient's context of meaning. By using human-to-human skills of listening accurately to words and feelings; by communicating trust, truth, respect, interest, and caring; by explaining in ways that are relevant and intelligible to the patient; and by being sensitive to the patient's values, the perception of the therapist as the patient's advocate in the world is facilitated. In other words, the therapist helps the patient do what is necessary to feel once more alive in the world, connected, and hopeful of recovery to a meaningful life. Even in the face of chronic debilitating disease, terminal illness, or irreversible paralysis, there is a sense that the therapist can help patients feel reconnected to the possibility of a life with meaning.

The behaviors that enhance the therapeutic moment flow out of placing the person and the meaning of what is wrong central to any and all attempts to offer help. Behaviors that emerge from valuing a patient's humanity—sensitive and accurate listening, respect, trust, compassion, and problem solving, to name a few—work to reinforce autonomy and dignity and to restore a patient's hope and personal control of his or her life as therapists simultaneously apply their scientific knowledge and skill.[11] This is what is required of health care professionals in day-to-day patient care. To do less is to render less than compassionate, professional help. Reflecting, coming to know with greater confidence the best or right thing to do, and consistently doing it, results in a professional life of growth and meaning. These actions, one by one, weave a cloak of integrity that supports the professional mantle of responsibility that health professionals accept at their graduation. Thus not only do we grow as individuals, our profession grows and we are better able to contribute to the meaningful growth of our patients and of our society.

Questions for Review

1. A person's values are difficult to identify. How can one know what a person values?
2. How are values related to behavior?
3. A belief is not a value, but beliefs direct our values. If a person believes fairness is good, what values can you predict the individual will hold?
4. What is the difference between a moral and a nonmoral value?
5. What four personal values make up most codes of ethics in the professions?
6. Give an example of a nonmoral value choice and a moral value choice.
7. What is the difference between behavior that agrees with a code of ethics and behavior that is value-based?
8. What is our obligation as health professionals when a patient of sound mind refuses to take our suggestions and recommendations for healing? What are the two primary values involved in this dilemma?
9. What role does communication play in making value-based decisions in rehabilitation?
10. What is our obligation to the patient when his or her insurance no longer covers our care and the agreed upon goals have not been met?
11. Describe the essential difference between moral beneficence and moral caring.

Case Study

You are a physical therapist specializing in hand therapy and have been working for 5 years. You have decided that the time is right to establish a practice of your own, and have spent considerable time cultivating referrals from local orthopedists. Unfortunately, your practice is still in the red, and you have not been able to pay yourself a salary, yet. Managed care has shifted your referral base to more primary care physicians who hesitate to refer for specialty care.

One patient, for whom you created a wrist and hand splint, begins to regain function sooner than expected. You call the referring physician, an orthopedist who refers most of your patients to you, to inform him that you need to remove the splint, because it is actually hindering the healing process. The physician is on vacation, and you are unable to reach his colleague covering for him. So after a thorough examination, you remove the splint, give the patient precise instructions for a home exercise program, and ask the patient to return for physical therapy three times a week for 3 weeks. You send a copy of your notes to the vacationing physician. When the physician returns to the office, he reads your correspondence and immediately calls you and says, "Who gave you the authority to remove the splint from this patient's hand? I want you to call the patient and tell him that you made a mistake, to put the splint back on, and send him to me immediately. I will remove it if I feel it should come off." He then bangs the phone down in your ear.

GUIDING QUESTIONS

Note: Box 3.1 can serve as a guide to your problem solving.

1. List the facts affecting this situation.
2. Identify the elements of the dilemma and values at war with each other (ethical principles involved).
   - On the one hand:
   - On the other hand:
3. List your professional duties.
4. List the practical features that impact this situation.
5. Come to a final decision that you can justify because you are acting on the higher value in this situation.

This case also appears in Davis, CM: When the interests of PT and patient collide: Habits of thought. PT Magazine January: 71, 1995.

References

1. Purtilo, RB, and Cassel, CK: Ethical Dimensions in the Health Professions. Saunders, Philadelphia, 1981.
2. Wehlage, G, and Lockwood, AL: Moral relativism and values education. In: Purpel, D, and Ryan, K (eds): Moral Education: It Comes with the Territory. McCutchen, Berkeley, CA, 1976, p 330.
3. Morrill, RL: Teaching Values in College. Jossey-Bass, San Francisco, 1980.
4. Beck, C: A philosophical view of values and value education. In Hennessy, T (ed): Values and Moral Development. Paulist Press, New York, 1976, p 13.
5. Raths, LE: Values and Teaching. Charles E. Merrill, Columbus, OH, 1966.
6. Davis, CM: Patient Practitioner Interaction: An Experiential Manual for Developing the Art of Health Care, ed 3. Slack, Thorofare, NJ, 1998.
7. Pellegrino, ED: What is a profession? J Allied Health 12:161, 1983.
8. Pellegrino, ER: Altruism, self interest and medical ethics. In Mapes, TA, and Zembang, JS (eds): Biomedical Ethics, ed 3. McGraw-Hill, New York, 1991, p 113.
9. Beauchamp, TL, and Childress, JF: Principles of Biomedical Ethics, ed 3. Oxford University Press, New York, 1989.
10. Jung, CG: The Structure and Dynamics of the Psyche. Pantheon, New York, 1960.
11. Davis, CM: The influence of values on patient care. In Payton, OD (ed): Psychosocial Aspects of Clinical Practice. Churchill Livingstone, New York, 1986, p 119.
12. Pence, GE: Can compassion be taught? J Med Ethics 9:189, 1983.
13. Romanello M, and Knight-Abowitz K: The "ethic of care" in physical therapy practice and education: challenges and opportunities. J Phys Ther Educ 14(3):20, 2000.
14. Pellegrino, ED: The commodification of medical and health care: The moral consequences of a paradigm shift from a professional to a market ethic. J Med Philos 24(3):243, 1999.
15. Scott, R: Challenges in professional ethics. Symposium of Annual Scientific Meeting, American Physical Therapy Association, San Diego, CA, June, 1997.
16. Watts N: Task analysis and division of responsibility in physical therapy. Phys Ther 51:23, 1971.
17. Pellegrino, ED: Personal communication, March, 1995.
18. Pellegrino, ED, and Tomasma, DC: A Philosophical Basis of Medical Practice. Oxford University Press, New York, 1981.

Supplemental Readings

Blackmer, J: Ethical issues in rehabilitation medicine. Scand J Rehabil Med 32(2):51, 2000.

Caplan, A: Moral Matters/Ethical Issues in Medicine and the Life Sciences. John Wiley, New York, 1995.

Clancy, CM, and Brody, H: Managed care. Jekyll or Hyde? JAMA 273:338, 1995.

Curtin, LL: Why good people do bad things. Nursing Management 27:63, 1996.

Galambos, C: Resolving ethical conflicts in a managed care environment. Health Soc Work 24(3):191, 1999.

Hall, RT: An Introduction to Health Care Organizational Ethics. Oxford University Press, New York, 2000.

Hall, K: Medical decision-making: An argument for narrative and metaphor. Theor Med Bioeth 23(1):55, 2002.

Healy, TC: Ethical decision making: Pressure and uncertainty as complicating factors. Health Soc Work 28 (4):293, 2003.

Kirschner, KL, Stocking, C, Wagner, LB, Foye, SL, and Siegler, M: Ethical issues identified by rehabilitation clinicians. Arch Phys Med Rehabil 82:S2-8, 2001.

Oddo, AR: Healthcare ethics: A patient-centered decision model. J Bus Ethics 29:125, 2001.

Palermo, BJ: Capitation on trial. California Medicine 7:25, 1996.

Robinson, JC: The politics of managed competition: Public abuse of the private interest. J Health Polit Policy Law 28:341, 2003.

Rodwin, MA: Medicine, Money and Morals. Oxford University Press, New York, 1993.

Scott, R: Professional Ethics: A Guide for Rehabilitation Professionals. Mosby, St. Louis, 1998.

Seedhouse, D: Commitment to health: A shared bond between professions. J Interprof Care 16(3):249, 2002.

Sharp, HM: Ethical decision-making in interdisciplinary team care. Cleft Palate Craniofac J 32:495, 1995.

Ucke, KT: Ethical implications of caring in rehabilitation. Nurs Clin North Am 33(2):253, 1998.

Ulrich, CM, Soeken, KL, and Miller, N: Ethical conflict associated with managed care: Views of nurse practitioners. Nurs Res 52(3):168, 2003.

Welie, JV: The relationship between medicine's internal morality and religion. Christian Bioethics 8(2):175, 2002.

Zwerner, AR: Capitation empowers doctors. California Medicine 7:29, 1996.

SECTION TWO

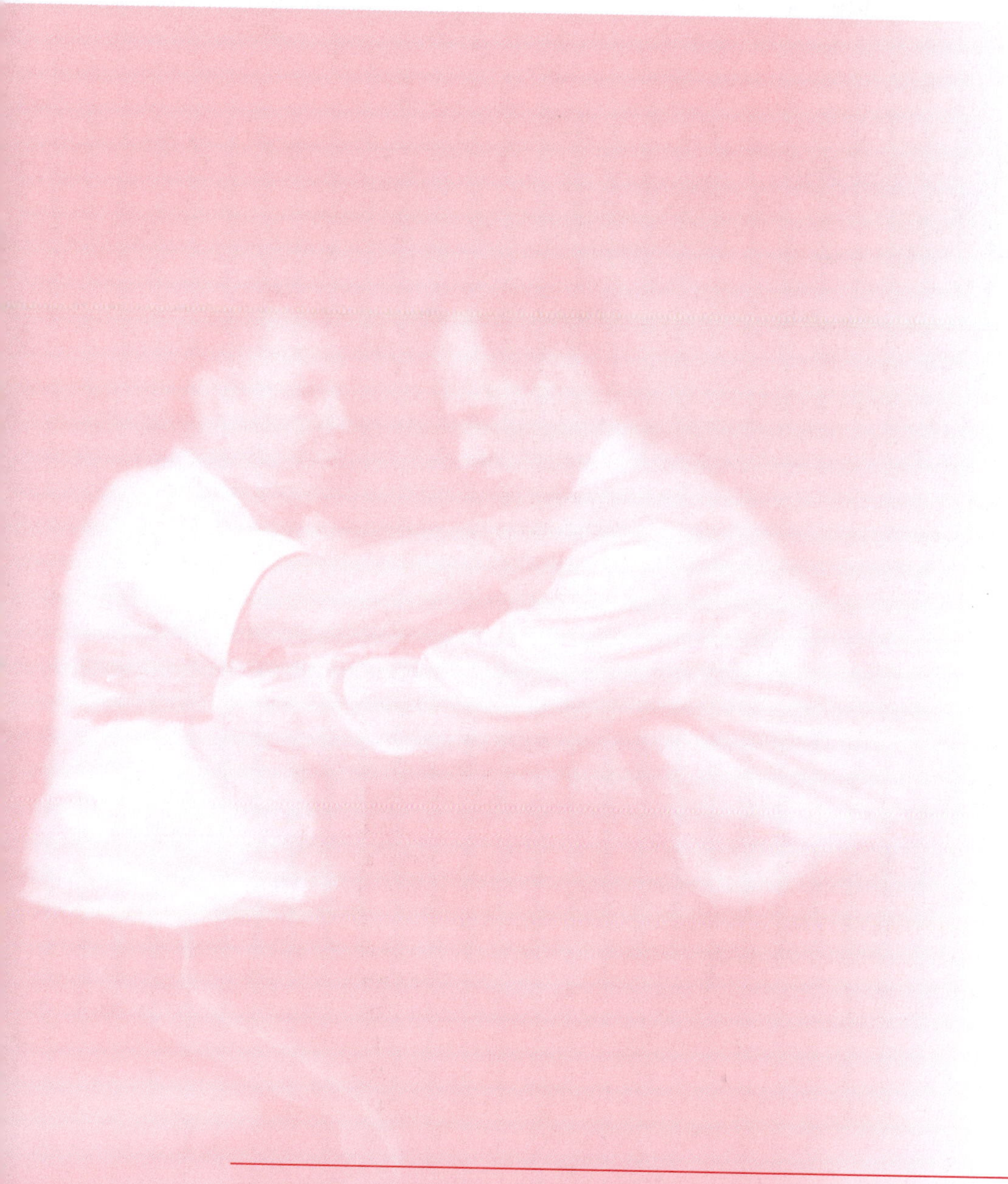

Examination

CHAPTER

4

LEARNING OBJECTIVES

1. Describe the rationale for including vital sign measures in the patient examination.
2. Explain the relevance of vital signs data in clinical judgments related to assigning a diagnostic label, determining the prognosis, and establishing a plan of care.
3. Recognize the importance of vital signs data in determining physiological response to treatment and evaluating patient progress.
4. Describe the procedure for monitoring temperature, pulse, respiration, and blood pressure.
5. Differentiate between normal and abnormal values or ranges for each vital sign.
6. Identify the normative variations in vital signs and the factors that influence these changes.
7. Identify the clinical application of pulse oximetry in screening for hypoxemia.
8. Describe the recommended elements for documentation of vital signs data.

Vital Signs

Thomas J. Schmitz, PT, PhD

OUTLINE

Examination of body temperature, pulse rate, respiratory rate, and blood pressure provide the physical therapist with important information about the status of the cardiovascular/pulmonary system. Owing to their importance as indicators of the body's physiological status and response to physical activity, environmental conditions, and emotional stressors, they are collectively referred to as **vital signs**. In addition, although not considered a primary vital sign, **pulse oximetry** is an important related measure that provides information on arterial blood oxygen saturation levels. Pulse oximetry data allow the therapist to screen and monitor for *hypoxemia* often associated with pulmonary disorders that impair ventilation of the lungs (e.g., pneumonia, chronic obstructive pulmonary disease [COPD], anemia, respiratory muscle weakness, and circulatory impairments).

The Guide to Physical Therapist Practice includes examination of vital signs (e.g., blood pressure, heart rate, respiratory rate) in the cardiovascular/pulmonary systems review for each of the four major categories of practice patterns. Vital signs are also identified among the tests and measures used to characterize or quantify circulatory status. Pulse oximetry is included in the ventilation and respiration/gas exchange category of tests and measures for each of the cardiovascular/pulmonary practice patterns.[1]

Also referred to as *cardinal signs*, vital signs provide quantitative measures of the status of the cardiovascular/pulmonary system and reflect the function of internal organs. Variations in vital signs are a clear indicator that some change in the patient's physiological status has occurred. Taken at rest and during and after exercise, these measures also provide important data on aerobic capacity and endurance. Together with other examination data, vital sign measures assist the physical therapist in making clinical judgments to[1]:

1. Assign a diagnostic label and classify patient findings within a specific practice pattern.
2. Determine the prognosis and plan of care (POC), including identification of anticipated goals and expected outcomes, and selection of specific interventions.
3. Evaluate patient progress through reexamination at periodic intervals during an episode of care.
4. Evaluate the effectiveness of selected interventions in achieving anticipated goals and expected outcomes (changes in impairment, functional limitations, and disabilities and changes in health, wellness, and fitness).
5. Determine if a referral to another practitioner is warranted.

The physical therapist's clinical judgment will determine which vital signs should be measured and the frequency of measurement for an individual patient within a specific context (e.g., self-paced ambulation on level surfaces vs stair climbing). Although taking vital sign measures may be delegated to a physical therapist assistant (PTA) or other support personnel, the physical therapist will evaluate and determine the significance of the data.

Normative data for vital signs measures are presented in Table 4.1. These data represent average values for the age-specific population from which they were derived. Normative values provide the physical therapist with a general reference for comparison during evaluation of clinical findings. However, normative values should be used cautiously as a global reference, as considerable discrepancy exists in the literature about the exact boundaries of the range of normal values. It is also important to note that *normal* values are specific to an individual. Some individuals typically display values different from those represented by normative figures. This illustrates the importance of monitoring vital signs as a serial process. Vital sign measurements yield the most useful information when performed and recorded at *periodic intervals over time* as opposed to a single measurement taken at a given point in time. Serial recording allows changes in patient status or response to treatment to be monitored over time and can indicate an acute change in physiological status at a specific point in time (e.g., response to an exercise test).

Situations may arise when an abnormally high or low value for a vital sign is obtained. It is important to maintain a calm professional demeanor and not adversely react to the information. If repeated measures are required, calmly explain to the patient that you obtained a high or low value and that you want to confirm accuracy.[2]

Alterations in Vital Signs Data

Overview of Influential Variables

Several lifestyle patterns (modifiable) and patient characteristics (nonmodifiable) influence vital sign measures. Lifestyle patterns include, but are not limited to, caffeine intake, tobacco use, diet, alcohol consumption, response to stress, obesity, physical activity level, medications, and use of illegal drugs.[3] Patient characteristics include hormonal status, age, gender, and family history. Other variables that affect vital sign measures include time of day, time of the month (menstrual cycle), general health status, and pain. Information about lifestyle patterns and patient characteristics is gathered from the patient history, the systems review, and tests and measures. Factors identified as modifiable should become the focus of patient-related instruction (e.g., current condition, risk factor reduction, health promotion). Specific factors influencing each vital sign are addressed in greater detail later in the chapter.

Table 4.1 **Normative Vital Signs Values by Age**

Age	Temperature (F°)	Temperature (C°)	Pulse (beats/minute)	Respiratory Rate (breaths/minute)	Blood Pressure (mm Hg)
Newborn	98.6–99.8	37–37.6	70–190	25–50	S: 50–52 D: 25–30
3 years	98.5–99.5	36.9–37.5	80–125	20–30	S: 78–114 D: 46–78
10 years	97.5–98.6	36.4–37	70–110	16–22	S: 90–120 D: 56–84
16 years	97.6–98.8	36.4–37.1	55–100	15–20	S: 104–120 D: 60–84
Adult	96.8–99.5	36–37.5	60–90	12–20	S: 95–119 D: 60–79
Older Adult	96.5–97.5	35.9–36.3	60–90	15–22	S: 90–140 D: 60–90

D = Diastolic; S = Systolic.
Adapted from Fitzgerald, MA,[7, p 39] with permission.

Culture and Ethnicity

As with any physical therapy test or measure, the influence of culture and ethnicity on vital sign measures can vary from a subtle to a marked impact. For example, a patient who appears anxious or hostile during examination of vital signs may be displaying a response to stress typically shared by others who have a deep-seated distrust of American health care practices. This situation would clearly affect the accuracy of the vital sign measures. *Culture* refers to an integration of learned behaviors (not biologically inherited) characteristic of a society. It is a set of shared behavioral standards that includes fundamental values, beliefs, and customs, including those related to health care and illness.[4] *Ethnicity* is defined as an affiliation with a group of people who share a common cultural origin or background, or common racial, national, religious, linguistic, or cultural characteristics.[5] Recent demographic changes in the United States have created greater societal diversity and have heightened the need for health care providers to address these issues during examination procedures and treatment interventions. Culture and ethnicity directly impact the attitudes held by an individual toward health care.[6] Metzgar[5] and Fitzgerald[7] offer the following general suggestions for interaction with a culturally diverse patient population:

1. Stereotypes should be avoided. Although a patient may share characteristics with others of the same culture, each patient will also have unique, individual differences.
2. Respect cultural inferences and individual differences in beliefs and attitudes toward health care.
3. Focus on developing the patient's trust and rapport.
4. Remain aware that one's own personal values and beliefs may distort the examination of a patient from a different background.
5. Be cautious not to interpret ethnic or cultural preferences in dress, manner, and physical appearance as abnormal behavior or psychological disorder.

For additional information on the impact of cultural diversity in health care, the reader is referred to the work of Spector,[6] Purnell and Paulanka,[8] Lynch and Hanson,[9] Galanati,[10] Luckman and Nobels,[11] and Huff and Kline.[12]

Patient Observation

Prior to a formal examination of vital signs, careful systematic observation of the patient can reveal important preliminary data. Observation alone will not provide definitive diagnostic information; however, when combined with data from vital sign measures, it will provide important clues for directing further screening and/or examination procedures. Lewis[3] offers the following general strategies to guide the therapist's observations:

- Signs of immediate patient distress or discomfort are typically evident by observation of facial expressions, use of accessory muscles for breathing, an irregular breathing pattern, and frequent positional changes.
- Clues about nutritional status may be indicated by obesity or the presence of **cachexia**, a state of ill health, appearance of malnutrition, and wasting associated with many chronic diseases.
- Skin color changes will indicate if **cyanosis** is present. Color changes in the mucous membranes are associated with **central cyanosis**. These membranes are normally pink and shiny irrespective of skin color. Central cyanosis is indicative of marked arterial desaturation. **Peripheral cyanosis** is observed as skin color changes in the earlobes, nose, lips, and toes. It is usually transient, occurs secondary to vasoconstriction, and is typically relieved by warming the area.
- The skin should be observed for changes in texture and hair growth. Patients with diabetes mellitus or atherosclerosis typically lack hair growth on the legs and display thickening of the nails of the fingers and toes. Skin texture also varies with age and poor nutritional status.
- *Diaphoresis* (profuse perspiration) often indicates that the body is working to compensate for a reduced cardiac output. It is associated with a variety of diagnostic categories including myocardial infarction, **hypotension**, and shock.
- Abnormal sitting postures may be suggestive of pain or structural abnormalities of the pectoral or vertebral regions that may interfere with respiratory patterns.
- Use of accessory muscles of breathing may be indicative of cardiac or pulmonary impairments.
- Peripheral extremities should be observed for the presence of edema or **clubbing**. Clubbing is a bulbous swelling at the distal fingers and toes accompanied by a loss of the normal angle between the nailbed and the skin. It develops gradually over time and is associated with diagnoses imposing long-standing **hypoxia** and cyanosis such as congenital heart defects and pulmonary disorders. Peripheral edema is typically associated with right heart failure or venous insufficiency.

During this initial observation, use of well-structured, impairment-specific questions will assist development of an initial database of patient information. Depending on individual patient needs, data may be gathered from the patient, family member, or caregiver. Box 4.1 presents a sample of clinical indicators that typically warrant monitoring of vital signs. Below each clinical indicator are sample guiding statements or questions designed to facilitate history taking during initial observation of the patient. Associated tests and vital sign measures of most immediate interest are also included.

Measuring Body Temperature

Body temperature represents a balance between the heat produced or acquired by the body and the amount lost. Because humans are warm-blooded, or *homoiothermic*, body

Box 4.1 Sample of Clinical Indicators that Typically Warrant Determination of Vital Sign Measures

Below each clinical indicator are sample guiding statements or questions designed to facilitate history taking during initial observation of the patient prior to, or during, gathering of vital sign data. If warranted by the clinical indicator, specific areas of needed observation and vital sign measures *beyond the standard* are noted.

Clinical Indicator
Dyspnea (shortness of breath, breathlessness, uncomfortable awareness of one's sensation of breathlessness).

Sample Statements or Questions
- Obtain a description of the dyspnea.
- What provokes it?
- What alleviates it?
- Does the dyspnea have a sudden or gradual onset?
- Does position affect it?
- Does time of day affect it?
- Review medications patient is taking.

Clinical Indicator
Fatigue (weakness) and syncope.

Sample Statements or Questions
- Obtain a description of the fatigue (weakness) and syncope.
- What provokes the onset?
- What alleviates the fatigue and syncope?
- Review medications patient is taking.

Clinical Indicator
Chest pain (discomfort).

Sample Statements or Questions
- Obtain a description of the chest discomfort.
- Where is the discomfort located?
- Identify the severity of the discomfort on a scale of 1 to 10.
- What provokes the discomfort?
- What alleviates it?
- Has the discomfort occurred before?
- Does rest stop the discomfort?
- Does the discomfort radiate (move) in any direction?
- Is the discomfort sudden or gradual in onset?
- Review medications patient is taking.

Clinical Indicator
Irregular heartbeat (palpitations).

Sample Statements or Questions and Specific Vital Sign Measure
- Obtain a description of the palpitations.
- Identify heart rhythm.
- Does the patient sense skipped beats or experience a sensation that the heart is racing?
- What provokes and alleviates the irregular heartbeat?
- Review medications the patient is taking.

Clinical Indicator
Cyanosis.

Areas of Needed Observation
- Central cyanosis: observed by inspecting the mucous membranes; indicates a shunting of deoxygenated blood to the arterial circulation.
- Peripheral cyanosis: observed by examining the extremities; associated with a vasoconstriction in response to cold and is usually not a serious clinical manifestation.

Clinical Indicator
Intermittent claudication (leg pain that occurs with activity or rest).

Sample Statements or Questions and Specific Vital Sign Measures
- Obtain a description of the leg pain.
- Locate site of pain.
- Examine femoral, popliteal, and pedal pulses.
- Examine skin color and temperature of legs.
- What provokes the pain?
- What alleviates the pain?
- Examine severity of the pain on a scale of 1 to 10.
- Examine quality of the pain.
- Review medications the patient is taking.

Clinical Indicator
Pedal edema (swelling of the feet and lower legs).

Areas of Needed Observation and Specific Vital Sign Measures
- Examine femoral, popliteal, and pedal pulses.
- Examine skin condition and color.
- Observe edema. Note the extent of edema in the tissue (i.e., from toes to ankle). To determine pitting edema, gently touch edematous tissue. In 15-second intervals, observe how long it takes the skin to return to a normal state. A time interval of 0 to 15 seconds is 1+ edema, 16 to 30 seconds is 2+ edema, 31 to 45 seconds is 3+ edema, and greater than 46 seconds is 4+ edema. Pitting edema can also be examined by depth using a small ruler such that 1+ edema = 2 mm depth, 2+ edema = 4 mm depth, 3+ edema = 6 mm depth, and 4+ edema = 8 mm or greater depth.

Adapted from Lewis, PS,[3] with permission.

temperature remains relatively constant, despite changes in the external environment. This is in contrast to cold-blooded, or *poikilothermic*, animals (such as reptiles) in which body temperature varies with that of their environment.

The Thermoregulatory System

The purpose of the thermoregulatory system is to maintain a relatively constant internal body temperature. This system

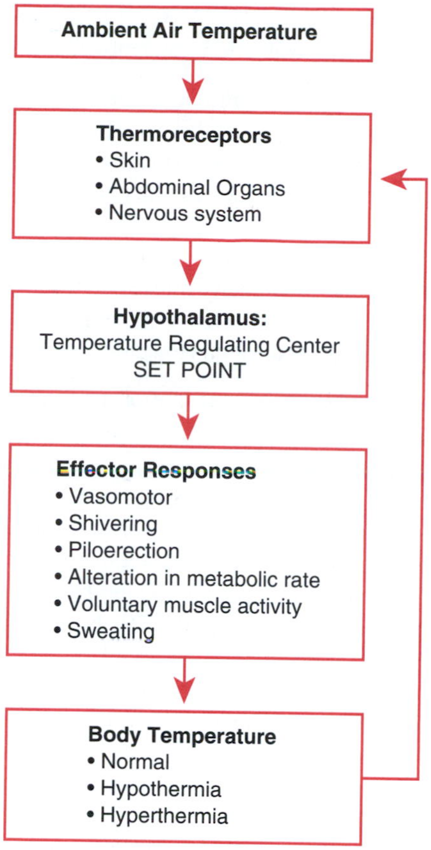

Figure 4.1 Thermoregulatory responses. The thermoreceptors provide input regarding changes in body temperature that signal the preoptic nucleus of the hypothalamus. This physiological thermostat compares incoming signals of actual body temperature with the set point value. If body temperature is lower than the set point value, heat gain mechanisms are implemented. If body temperature is higher than the set point value, heat loss mechanisms are implemented.[13–16]

monitors and acts to maintain temperatures that are optimal for normal cellular and vital organ function. The thermoregulatory system consists of three primary components: the thermoreceptors, the regulating center, and the effector organs (Fig. 4.1).[13–16]

Thermoreceptors

The thermoreceptors provide input to the temperature-regulating center located in the hypothalamus. The regulating center is dependent on information from thermoreceptors to achieve constant temperatures. Once this information reaches the regulatory center, it is compared with a "set point" standard or optimal temperature value. Depending on the contrast between the "set" value and incoming information, mechanisms may be activated either to conserve or dissipate heat.[14]

Peripheral and central thermoreceptors provide afferent temperature input to the regulating center. The peripheral receptors, composed primarily of free nerve endings, have a high distribution in the skin (cutaneous thermoreceptors). They are also located in the abdominal organs and nervous system.[13,14] The cutaneous thermoreceptors demonstrate a larger distribution of cold to warmth receptors and are sensitive to rapid changes in temperature.[15] Signals from these receptors enter the spinal cord through afferent nerves and travel to the hypothalamus via the lateral spinothalamic tract.

The central thermoreceptors are located in the hypothalamus and are sensitive to temperature changes in blood perfusing the hypothalamus. These cells also can initiate responses to either conserve or dissipate heat. They are particularly sensitive to core temperature changes and monitoring body warmth.[15]

Regulating Center

The temperature-regulating center of the body is located in the hypothalamus. The hypothalamus functions to coordinate the heat production and loss processes, much like a thermostat, ensuring an essentially constant and stable body temperature. By influencing the effector organs, the hypothalamus achieves a relatively precise balance between heat production and heat loss. In a healthy individual, the hypothalamic thermostat is set and carefully maintained at 98.6° ± 1.8°F (37° ± 1°C).[15] In situations in which input from thermoreceptors indicates a drop in temperature below the "set" value, mechanisms are activated to conserve heat. Conversely, a rise in temperature will activate mechanisms to dissipate heat. Mechanisms to dissipate heat are particularly important during strenuous exercise. Figure 4.2 summarizes the primary physiological adjustments to exercise or increases in environmental temperature that occur during heat acclimation (the physiological adaptations that improve tolerance to heat). These responses are activated through hypothalamic control over the effector organs. Input to the effector organs is transmitted through nervous pathways of both the somatic and autonomic nervous systems.[13–19]

Effector Organs

The effector organs respond to both increases and decreases in temperature. The primary effector systems include vascular, metabolic, skeletal muscle responses (shivering), and sweating. These effector systems function either to increase or to dissipate body heat.

Conservation and Production of Body Heat

When body temperature is lowered, mechanisms are activated to conserve heat and increase heat production. The following are descriptions of heat conservation and production mechanisms.

Vasoconstriction of Blood Vessels. The hypothalamus activates sympathetic nerves, an action that results in vasoconstriction of cutaneous vessels throughout the body. This significantly reduces the lumen of the vessels and decreases blood flow near the surface of the skin where the blood would normally be cooled. Thus the amount of heat lost to the environment is decreased.

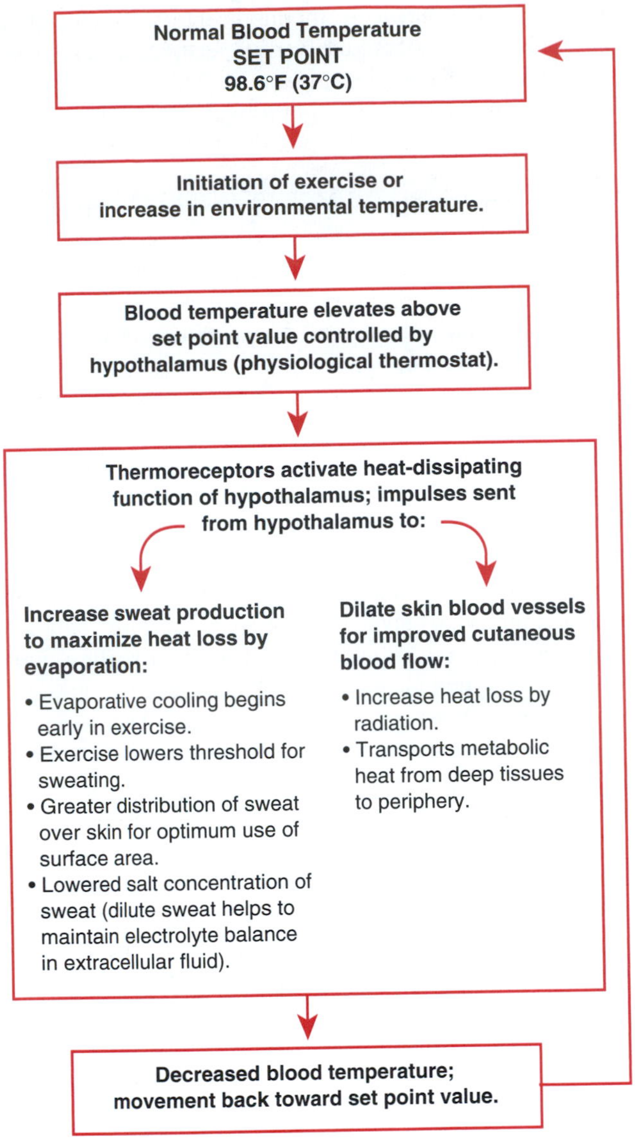

Figure 4.2 Physiological adjustments during heat acclimation. Increased body temperature activities heat dissipation to maintain normal body temperature.

Decrease (or Abolition) of Sweat Gland Activity. To reduce or to prevent heat loss by evaporation, sweat gland activity is diminished. Sweating is totally abolished with cooling of the hypothalamic thermostat below approximately 98.6°F (37°C).[14,15]

Cutis Anserina or Piloerection. Also a response to cooling of the hypothalamus, this heat conservation mechanism is commonly described as "gooseflesh." The term *piloerection* means "hairs standing on end." Although of less significance in humans, this mechanism functions to trap a layer of insulating air near the skin and decrease heat loss in lower mammals with greater hair covering.

The body also responds to decreased temperature with several mechanisms designed to produce heat. These mechanisms are activated when the body thermostat falls below approximately 98.6°F (37°C).[14] The following are descriptions of heat production mechanisms.

Shivering. The primary motor center for shivering is located in the posterior hypothalamus. This area is activated by cold signals from the skin and spinal cord. In response to cold, impulses from the hypothalamus activate the efferent somatic nervous system causing increased tone of skeletal muscles. As the tone gradually increases to a certain threshold level, shivering (involuntary muscle contraction) is initiated and heat is produced. This shivering reflex can be at least partially inhibited through conscious cortical control.[14]

Hormonal Regulation. The function of hormonal influence in thermal regulation is to increase cellular metabolism, which subsequently increases body heat. Increased metabolism occurs through circulation of two hormones from the adrenal medulla: *norepinephrine* and *epinephrine*. Circulating levels of these hormones, however, are of greater significance in maintaining body temperature in infants than in adults. Heat production by these hormones can be increased in an infant by as much as 100 percent, as opposed to 10 to 15 percent in an adult.[14]

A second form of hormonal regulation involves increased output of thyroxine by the thyroid gland. Thyroxine increases the rate of cellular metabolism throughout the body. This response, however, occurs only as a result of prolonged cooling, and heat production is not immediate.[15] The thyroid gland requires several weeks to hypertrophy before increased demands for thyroxine can be achieved.

Loss of Body Heat

Excess heat is dissipated from the body through four primary methods: radiation, conduction, convection, and evaporation.

Radiation. The transfer of heat by electromagnetic waves from one object to another is accomplished by radiation. This heat transfer occurs through the air between objects that are not in direct contact. Heat is lost to surrounding objects that are colder than the body (e.g., loss of heat to a wall or surrounding room objects). As depicted in Figure 4.3, a person without clothing in a room maintained at normal temperature loses approximately 60 percent of total heat loss to radiation.[14]

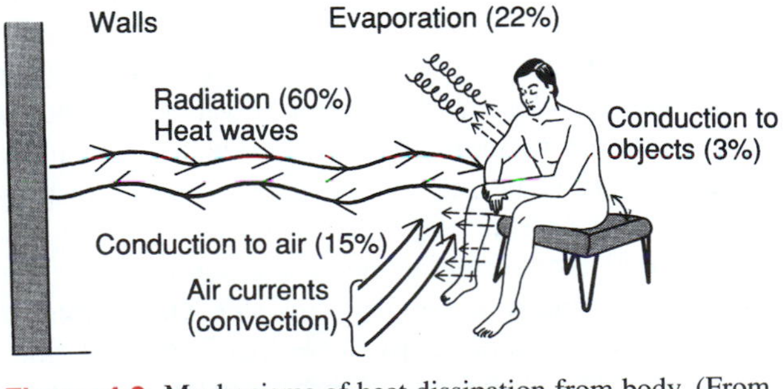

Figure 4.3 Mechanisms of heat dissipation from body. (From Guyton, AC, et al,[14, p 576] with permission.)

Conduction. The transfer of heat from one object to another through a liquid, solid, or gas takes place by conduction. This type of heat transfer requires direct molecular contact between two objects, as when a person is sitting on a cold surface, or when heat is lost in a cool swimming pool. Heat is also lost by conduction to air.

Convection. The transfer of heat by movement of air or liquid (water) is achieved by convection. This form of heat loss is accomplished secondary to conduction. Once the heat is conducted to the air, the air is then moved away from the body by convection currents. Use of a fan or a cool breeze provides convection currents. Heat loss by convection is most effective when the air or liquid surrounding the body is continually moved away and replaced.

Evaporation. Dissipation of body heat by the conversion of a liquid to a vapor occurs by evaporation. This form of heat loss occurs on a continual basis through the respiratory tract and through perspiration from the skin. Evaporation provides the major mechanism of heat loss during heavy exercise. Profuse sweating provides a significant cooling effect on the skin as it evaporates. In addition, this cooling of the skin functions to further cool the blood as it is shunted from internal structures to cutaneous areas.

Abnormalities in Body Temperature

Increased Body Temperature

An elevation in body temperature is generally believed to assist the body in fighting disease or infection. Pyrexia is the elevation of normal body temperature, more commonly referred to as fever. Hyperpyrexia and hyperthermia are terms that describe an extremely high fever, generally above 106°F (41.1°C).[20] The primary clinical manifestations of hyperthermia are presented by body system in Table 4.2.

Pyrexia occurs when the "set" value of the hypothalamic thermostat rises. This elevation is caused by the influence of **pyrogens** (fever-producing substances). Pyrogens are secreted primarily from toxic bacteria or are released from degenerating body tissue.[16] The effects of these pyrogens result in fever during illness. As a result of the new, higher thermostat value, the body responds by activating its heat conservation and production mechanisms. These mechanisms raise body temperature to the new, higher value over a period of several hours. Thus a fever, or **febrile** state, is produced.

The clinical signs and symptoms of a fever vary with the level of disturbance of the thermoregulatory center, and with the specific stage of the fever (onset, course, or termination). These signs and symptoms may include general malaise, headache, increased pulse and respiratory rate, chills, piloerection, shivering, loss of appetite **(anorexia)**, pale skin that later becomes flushed and hot to the touch, nausea, irritability, restlessness, constipation, sweating, thirst, coated tongue, decreased urinary output, weakness, and insomnia.[13,21] With higher elevations in temperature (hyperpyrexia), disorientation, confusion, convulsions, or coma may occur. These latter symptoms are more common in children younger than 5 years of age and are believed to be related to the immaturity of the nervous system.

Table 4.2 Primary Clinical Manifestations of Hyperthermia Presented by Body System

System	Effects
Cardiovascular	Heart rate may increase by 8.5 beats/min for each 33.8°F (1°C) rise in temperature during fever, and up to 25 beats/min in other forms of hyperthermia. Decreased perfusion and high metabolic rate promote metabolic acidosis.
Nervous	Febrile seizures occur in 2–4% of young children with high temperatures. Hypoxia and decreased perfusion result in sleepiness and confusion in lower-grade fevers and in delirium, stupor, or coma in extreme hyperthermia.
Respiratory	Increased metabolic rate and activation of heat loss mechanisms induces hypoxia and respiratory alkalosis.
Renal	Increased metabolic rate and dehydration promote electrolyte imbalances and accumulation of metabolic wastes in the blood (azotemia). Thermal injury to muscle may cause rhabdomyolysis (release of myoglobin), which obstructs renal tubules.
Hematologic	Dehydration results in hemoconcentration. Disseminated intravascular coagulation can occur secondary to tissue injury.

From Hansen, MJ,[9 p 223] with permission.

Specific stages have been identified describing the course of a fever:

- The *prodromal phase* is the period just prior to temperature elevation; nonspecific symptoms may be experienced such as a slight headache, muscles aches, general malaise, or loss of appetite.
- *Invasion* or *onset* is the period from either gradual or sudden rise until the maximum temperature is reached; symptoms include chills, shivering, and pale appearance of skin.
- *Stationary phase* (*fastigium* or *stadium* [course]) is the point of highest elevation of the fever. Once maximum

Box 4.2 Types of Fever

Intermittent: Body temperature alternates at regular intervals between periods of fever and periods of normal temperatures.
Remittent: Elevated body temperature that fluctuates more that 3.6°F (2°C) within a 24-hour period but remain above normal.
Relapsing: Periods of fever are interspersed with normal temperatures that last at least one day; also called *recurrent* fever.
Constant: Body temperature is constantly elevated with fluctuations less than 3.6°F (2°C)

temperature is reached, it remains relatively stable. Fever is sustained; skin may be warm and appear flushed.

- *Defervescence* (termination, resolution) identifies the period during which the fever subsides and temperatures move toward normal. This drop in temperature can occur suddenly (crisis) or gradually (lysis); sweating is typically initiated during this phase.

Common types of fever, presented in Box 4.2, include *intermittent*, *remittent*, *relapsing*, and *constant*.[22,23]

Lowered Body Temperature

Exposure to extreme cold produces a lowered body temperature called **hypothermia**. With prolonged exposure to cold there is a decrease in metabolic rate, and body temperature gradually falls. As cooling of the brain occurs, there is a depression of the thermoregulatory center. The function of the thermoregulatory center becomes seriously impaired when body temperature falls below approximately 94°F (34.4°C) and is completely lost with temperatures below 85°F (29.4°C).[14] Therefore, the body's heat regulatory and protection mechanism is lost. Symptoms of hypothermia include decreased pulse and respiratory rates, cold and pale skin, cyanosis, decreased cutaneous sensation, depression of mental and muscular responses, and drowsiness, which may eventually lead to coma. If hypothermia is left untreated, the progression of these symptoms may lead to death. The primary clinical manifestations of hypothermia are presented by body system in Table 4.3.

Table 4.3 Primary Clinical Manifestations of Hypothermia Presented by Body System

System	Effects
Cardiovascular	Decreased perfusion results from increased blood viscosity and denaturation (loss of function) of serum proteins. Vasoconstriction further decreases peripheral perfusion, promoting injury of peripheral tissues with freezing (frostbite). Lactic acidosis develops. First **tachycardia** then **bradycardia** is the typical cardiac rhythm. Decreased cardiac perfusion produces electrocardiographic changes, including Osborne (J) waves following the QRS complex, and lengthening of the PR, QRS, and QT intervals. Blood pressure drops. Atrial and ventricular dysrhythmias are induced by myocardial hypoxia. Asystole occurs at temperatures below 82.4°F (28°C).
Nervous	Hypothalamic heat gain mechanisms are activated early, including vasoconstriction, shivering, and increased metabolic rate. Shivering stops with moderate hypothermia as muscles stiffen. Stupor and coma occur with reduced cerebral perfusion. Pupils become nonreactive, and reflexes disappear. Response to pain decreases. Electroencephalogram may be flat with severe hypothermia.
Respiratory	Respiratory rate is initially increased but soon decreases as oxygen consumption declines. Arterial blood gas values obtained from hypothermic patients are unreliable. A 50% decrease in CO_2 production occurs with a decrease of 46.4°F (8°C) in temperature. Bronchorrhea and cough suppression are apparent at first, followed by pulmonary edema. Hypothermia shifts the oxyhemoglobin dissociation curve to the left, decreasing oxygen delivery to tissues.
Renal	Cold-induced diuresis occurs. Renal acid excretion is impaired. Glycosuria and electrolyte imbalances develop.
Hematologic	Hematocrit increases 2% for each 33.8°F (1°C) decline in temperature, contributing to hypercoagulability. Cold directly inhibits the clotting cascade. Production of thromboxane B_2 by platelets declines, and thrombocytopenia results from bone marrow suppression and hepatic sequestration.

From Hansen, MJ,[9 p 227], with permission.

Factors Influencing Body Temperature

A statistical average or normal temperature of 98.6°F (37°C) taken orally has been established for body temperature in an adult population. However, body temperature is most accurately presented as a range. A range of values is more representative of normal body temperature because certain everyday circumstances (e.g., time of day) or activities (e.g., exercise) influence the body's temperature. In addition, some individuals typically run a *slightly higher* or *lower* body temperature than the statistical average. Therefore, deviations from the average will be apparent from individual to individual, as well as between measures taken from a single subject under varying circumstances.

Time of Day

The term **circadian rhythm** describes a 24-hour cycle of normal variations in body temperature. Certain predictable and regular changes in temperature occur on a daily basis. Body temperature tends to be lowest between 4 and 6 AM, and highest between 4 and 8 PM. These regular changes in body temperature are influenced significantly by both digestive processes and the level of skeletal muscle activity. For individuals who work at night, this pattern is usually inverted.[14,15]

Age

Compared with adults, infants demonstrate a higher normal temperature owing to the immaturity of the thermoregulatory system (see Table 4.1). Infants are particularly susceptible to environmental temperature changes, and their body temperature will fluctuate accordingly. Young children also average higher normal temperatures because of the heat production associated with increased metabolic rate and high physical activity levels. Elderly populations tend to demonstrate lower than average body temperatures, owing to a variety of factors, including lower metabolic rates, decreased subcutaneous tissue mass (which normally insulates the body against heat loss), decreased physical activity levels, and inadequate diet.

Emotions/Stress

Stimulation of the sympathetic nervous system causes increased production of epinephrine and norepinephrine with a subsequent increase in metabolic rate.

Exercise

The effects of exercise on body temperature are an important consideration for physical therapists. Strenuous exercise significantly increases body temperature because of increased metabolic rate. Active muscle contractions are an important and potent source of heat production. During exercise, body temperature increases are proportional to the relative intensity of the workload. Vigorous exercise can increase the metabolic rate by as much as 20 to 25 times that of the basal level.[15]

Menstrual Cycle

Increased levels of progesterone during ovulation cause body temperature to rise 0.5° to 0.9°F (0.3° to 0.5°C). This slight elevation is maintained until just prior to the initiation of menstruation, at which time it returns to normal levels.

Pregnancy

Because of increased metabolic activity, body temperature remains elevated by approximately 0.9°F (0.5°C). Temperature returns to normal after parturition.

External Environment

Generally, warm weather tends to increase body temperature, and cold weather decreases body temperature. Environmental conditions influence the body's ability to maintain constant temperatures. For example, in hot, humid environments the effectiveness of evaporative cooling is severely diminished because the air is already heavily moisture laden. Other forms of heat dissipation are also dependent on environmental factors such as movement of air currents (convection). Clothing also can be an important external consideration because it can function both to conserve and to facilitate release of body heat. The amount and type of clothing is important. To dissipate heat, absorbent, loose-fitting, light-colored clothing is most effective. To conserve heat, several layers of lightweight clothing to trap air and to insulate the body are recommended.

Measurement Site

Body temperatures vary among body parts. Rectal and tympanic (ear) membrane temperatures are from 0.5° to 0.9°F (0.3° to 0.5°C) higher than oral temperatures; axillary temperatures are approximately 1.1°F (0.6°C) lower than oral temperatures. The normative value for oral temperature in a healthy adult population is generally considered 98.6°F (37.0°C) and for rectal and tympanic membrane temperatures the value is 99.5°F (37.5°C). Being an external measure, the axillary normative value is somewhat lower at 97.6°F (36.5°C).

Ingestion of Warm or Cold Foods

Oral temperatures will be affected by oral intake, including smoking. Patients should refrain from smoking or eating for at least 15 minutes (preferably 30 minutes) prior to an oral temperature reading.

Types of Thermometers

Glass Mercury Thermometers

Traditionally, temperatures have been taken via a glass thermometer, which consists of a glass tube with a bulbous tip filled with mercury. Once the bulb is in contact with body heat, the mercury expands and rises in the glass column to register body temperature. Reflux of mercury down the tube is prevented by a narrowing of the base. The device must be shaken vigorously to return the mercury to the bulb before the next use. Today, the use of glass mercury thermometers in patient care settings has been largely replaced by electronic thermometers. However, they remain in use in the home care setting.

Glass thermometers are calibrated in centigrade (Celsius [C]) scale, Fahrenheit (F) scale, or both. The range is from approximately 93° to 108°F (34° to 42.2°C), with slight variations among different manufacturers. The calibrations are in degrees and tenths of a degree. As such, each long line represents a full degree and each short line indicates 0.1° on the centigrade thermometer and 0.2° on the Fahrenheit thermometer. When recording temperatures, it is common practice to round the fractions of degrees to the nearest whole number (one tenth of a degree on the Fahrenheit scale). If a situation occurs that requires changing a temperature reading from one scale to the other, a conversion formula can be used. To convert centigrade into Fahrenheit, multiply the centigrade value by 9/5 and add 32 ($F = [9/5 \times C°] + 32°$). To change from Fahrenheit into centigrade, subtract 32 from the Fahrenheit value and multiply by 5/9 ($C = [F - 32°] \times 5/9$). Table 4.4 presents a comparison of Fahrenheit and centigrade temperature values.

The distal tip (bulb) of the glass mercury thermometer is used for insertion and is long and slender or has a more blunt, round shape (Fig. 4.4). The long slender shape is used for oral temperatures and is designed with a larger surface area to maximize tissue contact with the oral

Table 4.4 Comparison of Fahrenheit and Centigrade Temperature Values

Fahrenheit	Centigrade
93.2	34.0
95.0	35.0
96.8	36.0
97.7	36.5
98.6	37.0
99.5	37.5
100.4	38.0
101.3	38.5
102.2	39.0
104.0	40.0
105.8	41.0
107.6	42.0
109.4	43.0
111.2	44.0

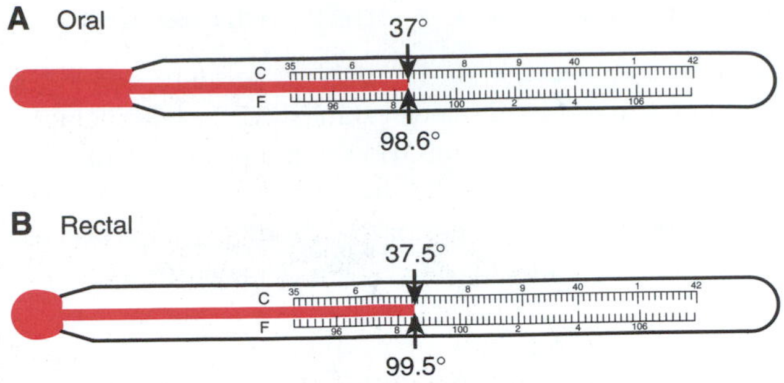

Figure 4.4 Shape of tips (bulbs) on mercury glass thermometers. The long slender shape (*A*) is for oral use and the blunt round shape (*B*) is for rectal measures.

mucosa. The more blunted, round-shaped bulb is for rectal temperatures and is designed to minimize trauma to the rectal mucosa. The oral thermometer can also be used for axillary temperatures. The tips of mercury glass thermometers may also be color-coded (*blue* for oral and *red* for rectal).

Electronic Thermometers

Electronic thermometers are widely used in patient care settings. They provide a rapid (several second), highly accurate measure of body temperature. Standard oral electronic thermometers consist of a portable battery-operated unit, an attached probe, and plastic disposable probe covers (Fig. 4.5). The units provide a digital display of body temperature. An important advantage of these thermometers is the low chance of cross-infection, as long as the probe covers are used only once.

Hand-held electronic oral thermometers are also commercially available. These units are typically about 5

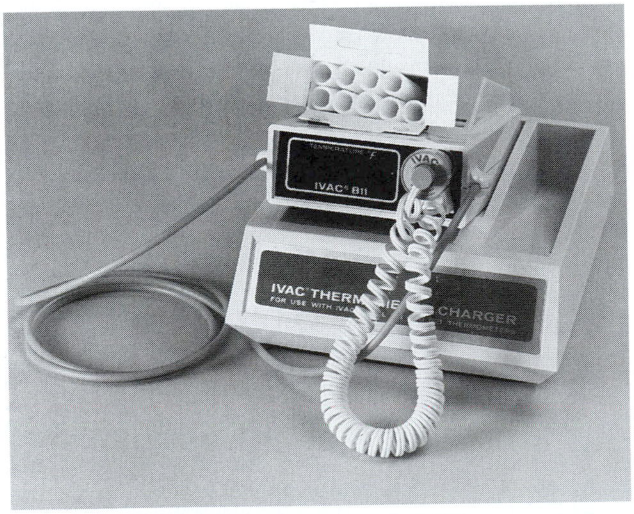

Figure 4.5 Standard electronic oral thermometer. Components include a battery-powered unit with a digital display, a probe, and disposable probe covers. (Courtesy of IVAC Corporation, San Diego, CA 92121.)

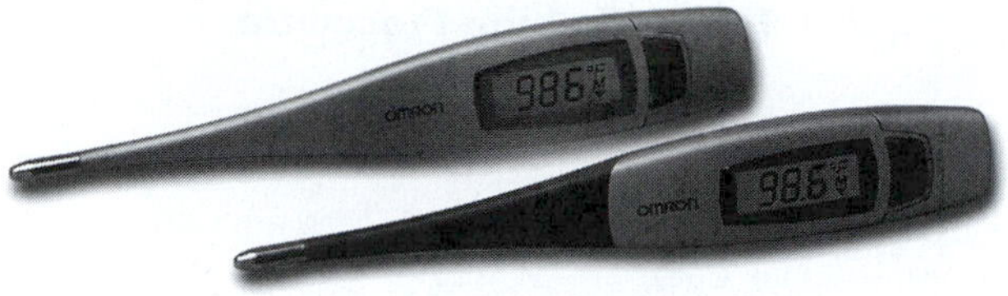

Figure 4.6 Hand-held electronic oral thermometer. (Courtesy of Omron, Inc, Vernon Hills, IL 60061.)

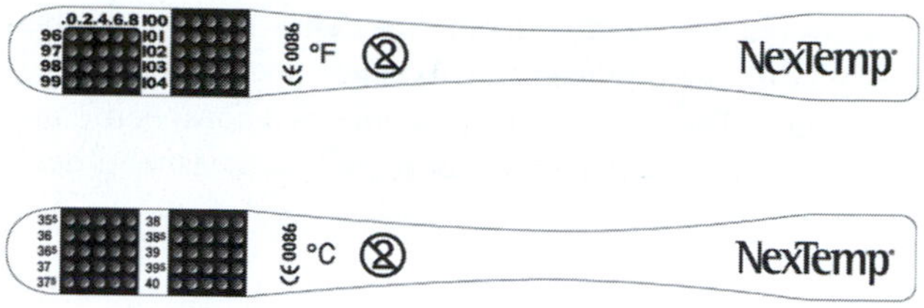

Figure 4.8 Disposable single-use thermometer in Fahrenheit (*top*) and Centigrade (*bottom*) scales. (Courtesy of Medical Indicators, Inc, Pennington, NJ 08534.)

inches in length with a tapered design (Fig. 4.6). One end of the device is narrow and serves as the probe. The opposite end is broad and houses the battery. These thermometers also provide a flashed, digital display of body temperature. Many models allow use with disposable covers and some have memory capabilities.

Another type of electronic thermometer is the tympanic (infrared) thermometer. These thermometers measure body temperature through a sensor probe placed in the ear that detects infrared radiation from the tympanic membrane.[23–26] This location provides an important reflection of core temperature because the tympanic membrane receives its blood supply from a tributary of the internal carotid artery that supplies the hypothalamus (temperature-regulating center). These hand-held portable thermometers include an ear probe (with disposable covers) and provide a digital display of body temperature within several seconds (Fig. 4.7). They are particularly useful with infants older than 2 months and children who may have difficulty remaining still while using other types of monitoring and in emergency situations where rapid temperature values are required.[24] A tympanic thermometer should never be used in the presence of a draining or infected ear.[25]

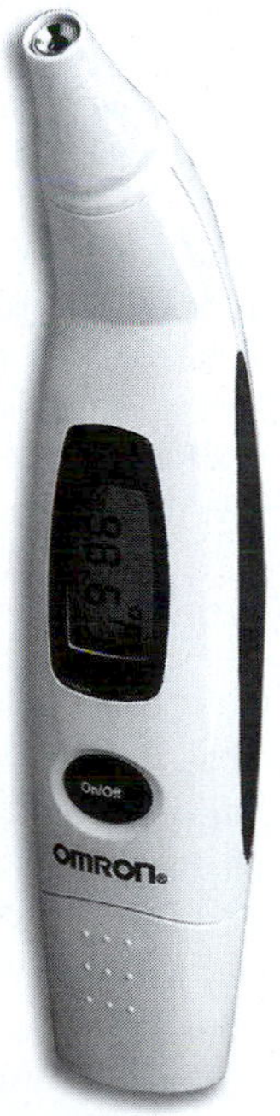

Figure 4.7 A tympanic thermometer incorporates a sensor that detects infrared radiation from the tympanic membrane (eardrum) and converts the warmth into a digital temperature reading. (Courtesy of Omron, Inc, Vernon Hills, IL 60061.)

Other variations of electronic thermometers include earlobe clips and finger sleeve or clip sensors. Digital nipple-shaped pacifier designs are also available for monitoring oral temperatures of infants.

Disposable Single-Use Thermometers

These devices are used in a similar fashion to the glass mercury thermometer because they are placed under the tongue. They consist of a thin plastic strip with a series of raised calibrated dots impregnated with a temperature-sensitive chemical (Fig. 4.8). The dots change color to indicate the temperature. After the thermometer is removed from the mouth, the dots are examined for color changes to determine the temperature reading (Fig 4.9). They are available in both Fahrenheit and Celsius scales and are disposed of after use. Although most commonly used for oral temperatures, disposable thermometers can also be used to obtain axillary temperatures, and some are available with covers (sheaths) containing semirigid stays that allow use for rectal measures.

Temperature-Sensitive Strips

Heat-sensitive strips (tape, patches, or disks) provide a general measure of body surface temperature. They also respond to body temperature by changing color and are

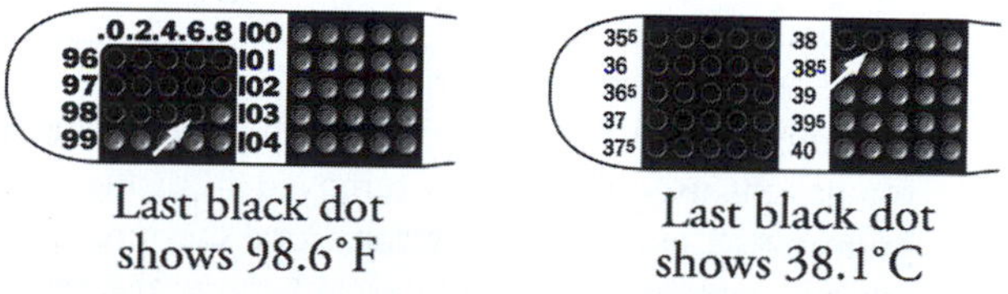

Figure 4.9 The chemical dots on the disposable single-use thermometers change color from green to black to reflect the temperature (Fahrenheit, *left* and centigrade, *right*). The green dots turn black from left to right. The last dot to turn black indicates the temperature. Note there are two grids of dots on each scale (*left* and *right*). Values that fall in the right grid indicate fever is present. In the example on the right, 38.1°C (100.5°F) represents fever. (Courtesy of Medical Indicators, Inc, Pennington, NJ 08534.)

more frequently used with children. They must be applied to dry skin. The forehead and abdomen are common placement sites. The temperature readings are nonspecific and are usually confirmed with a more precise measure if deviations are noted.

Procedure for Measuring Body Temperature

For purposes of establishing baseline data and determining response to treatment, physical therapists generally use oral monitoring. Oral temperatures are contraindicated for patients with *dyspnea* or who are mouth breathers, have had oral surgery, or have a history of epilepsy or are prone to seizures. They also should not be used with infants or small children or patients who are irrational, unconscious, or uncooperative. In situations in which oral temperatures may be contraindicated and an electronic unit with an alternative sensor (e.g., earlobe clip, finger sleeve) is unavailable, an axillary measure may be substituted.

Several preliminary activities apply universally to any examination of body temperature. These include:

- Wash hands. Hand washing is "one of the most important measures for preventing transmission of pathogens in health-care facilities."[27, p 2] The Centers for Disease Control and Prevention (CDC) recommends vigorous hand washing for at least 15 seconds covering all surfaces of the hand and fingers.[27] See Box 4.3 for hand washing procedure.[23–25,28]
- Don plastic gloves. Gloves should be worn if indicated or appropriate (e.g., medical asepsis, infection control).
- Inform the patient. A thorough explanation of the procedure and rationale should always be provided in terms appropriate to the patient's understanding.
- Ensure the patient's understanding, safety, and comfort.

Measuring Oral Temperature: Electronic Thermometer

A. Assemble equipment.

1. An electronic thermometer with disposable probe covers or sheaths.
   Note: Some electronic thermometers are stored in a charging base to ensure readiness and optimal charge for patient use. The unit is removed from the base prior to use. Hand-held electronic oral thermometers are self-contained with an internal battery; the proximal end houses the digital display and battery and the distal end serves as the temperature probe.

B. Procedure

1. Turn on the power unit.
2. Grasp the temperature probe with the thumb and forefinger and attach the disposable cover over the probe until it snaps or locks in place (some probes have a proximal button that releases the probe cover after temperature reading is complete). If one is using a small hand-held electronic unit, the distal end is covered with a plastic sheath.
3. Ask patient to open his or her mouth, and place the covered probe at the posterior base of the tongue to the right or left of the frenulum in the sublingual pocket. This placement positions the tip of the thermometer over superficial blood vessels that reflect core body temperature. Instruct the patient to close the lips (not teeth) around the thermometer. Continue

Box 4.3 Hand Washing Procedure

Equipment

1. Warm running water
2. Soap (most facilities provide liquid soap from a dispenser at the sink)
3. Paper towels

Procedure

1. Remove jewelry as microorganisms can accumulate in the irregular surfaces. A wristwatch may be pushed up to midforearm level. *Note*: If paper towels are dispensed via a lever or circular wheel device, advance ample toweling prior to washing hands. This will eliminate contact with the dispensing mechanism once the hands are washed.
2. Turn on water using faucet, foot or knee pedal control and adjust the temperature to warm (some faucets have infrared sensors that turn on in response to motion detection). Running water assists with removal of microorganisms and a warm temperature removes less protective oils from the hands than hot water. The force of the water should not cause splashing that can promote the transfer of microorganisms. Do not lean against the sink to avoid contact with a potentially contaminated area.
3. Wet hands and distal forearms under running water keeping the hands lower than the elbows so water flows toward fingertips. This technique allows the water to flow from the least contaminated area (distal forearms) to the potentially most contaminated area (hands).
4. Apply soap to hands. Using firm circular motions and sufficient lather, vigorously rub the palms and dorsum of hands, fingers, and areas between fingers. Interlace the fingers and thumbs of hands during washing. Wash each hand for 15 to 30 seconds using firm friction and a generous amount of soap. Carefully clean under and around fingernails as these sites frequently harbor microorganisms. Avoid contact with the sides of the sink during washing.
5. Rinse forearms and hands thoroughly keeping the hands lower than the elbows.
6. Dry hands thoroughly with a paper towel with finger tips pointing down. The hands should be dried wiping from the finger tips toward the forearm. This technique minimizes the chance of recontamination of the cleaned area.
7. Turn off the water. If a foot or knee pedal control is not available, a clean paper towel should be used to turn off the faucet.

to hold the probe in place as the weight of the probe may displace it from the sublingual pocket.[24]

4. Hold the probe in the sublingual pocket until an audible beep is heard (several seconds).The beep indicates maximum temperature has been reached. Remove the probe from the patient's mouth and note the temperature reading on the digital display for recording.
5. Remove the probe cover over a waste receptacle for disposal. If available on the unit, use the probe release mechanism; if a plastic sheath cover is used, use a clean paper towel for removal (cover sheath with paper towel, place thumb and forefinger proximally on probe over paper towel, and slide fingers distally).
6. Return thermometer to battery pack or appropriate storage area.
7. Wash hands.

Measuring Oral Temperature: Glass Mercury Thermometer

A. Assemble equipment.

1. Clean oral glass mercury thermometer
2. Clean tissue to wipe thermometer
3. Watch (or wall clock)

B. Procedure

1. Remove the thermometer from storage in disinfectant solution, rinse under cold water, and dry with tissue using a firm rotary motion wiping from the bulb toward the fingers.
2. Hold the thermometer between the thumb and forefinger at the end of the stem (opposite the bulb). Holding the thermometer horizontally at eye level (required to obtain an accurate reading), rotate until the column of mercury is clearly visible. Note the level of the column. The reading should be below 95°F (35°C) before placing the thermometer in the patient's mouth. If the value is higher, "shake down" the thermometer until the mercury is below 95°F (35°C). While holding the thermometer securely, use quick, downward snapping motions of the wrist, which will effectively lower the column.
3. Ask the patient to open his or her mouth, and place the bulb of the thermometer at the posterior base of the tongue to the right or left of the frenulum in the sublingual pocket. Instruct the patient to close the lips (not teeth) around the thermometer to hold it in place.
4. Leave the glass mercury thermometer in place for 3 to 5 minutes.
5. Remove the thermometer.
6. Using a clean tissue, wipe the thermometer away from the fingers (toward the bulb) using a firm rotary motion.
7. Hold the thermometer at eye level, rotate until the mercury is clearly visible, and read the highest point on the scale to which the mercury has risen for recording.
8. Wash the thermometer in tepid soapy water and return to the storage container.
9. Wash hands.

Measuring Axillary Temperature: Glass Mercury Thermometer

A. Assemble equipment.

1. Clean the oral glass mercury thermometer
   Note: Axillary temperatures can also be measured with electronic thermometers as well as disposable single-use thermometers.
2. Clean tissue to wipe thermometer
3. A towel to dry axillary region (moisture will conduct heat).
4. Watch (or wall clock)

B. Procedure

1. Expose the axilla and ensure area is dry. If any moisture is present, the area should be gently towel dried with a patting motion (vigorous rubbing will increase temperature of the area).
2. Remove thermometer from storage in disinfectant solution, rinse under cold water, and dry with tissue using a firm rotary motion, wiping from the bulb toward the fingers.
3. Hold the thermometer horizontally at eye level and rotate until the column of mercury is clearly visible; note the level of mercury. If necessary, shake the thermometer until the mercury is below 95°F (35°C).
4. Place the bulb of the thermometer in the center of the axillary region between the trunk and upper arm (Fig. 4.10). The patient's upper extremity should be placed tightly across the chest to keep the thermometer in place (asking the patient to move the hand toward the opposite shoulder is often a useful direction). If the patient is disoriented or very young, the thermometer must be held in place.
5. Leave thermometer in place for 10 minutes (more time is required for the mercury to expand when measuring axillary temperature).
6. Remove the thermometer.
7. Using a clean tissue, wipe the thermometer away from the fingers (toward the bulb) using a firm rotary motion.
8. Hold the thermometer at eye level, rotate until the mercury is clearly visible, and read the highest point on the scale to which the mercury has risen for recording.
   Note: Generally, a temperature reading is assumed an oral measure unless otherwise noted. Axillary values are designated by a circled A after the temperature or the designation "AT" for *axillary temperature* (e.g., 95°F AT). Similarly, the designation RT (*rectal temperature*) or a circled R after the value indicates a rectal measure (e.g., 99°F ®).

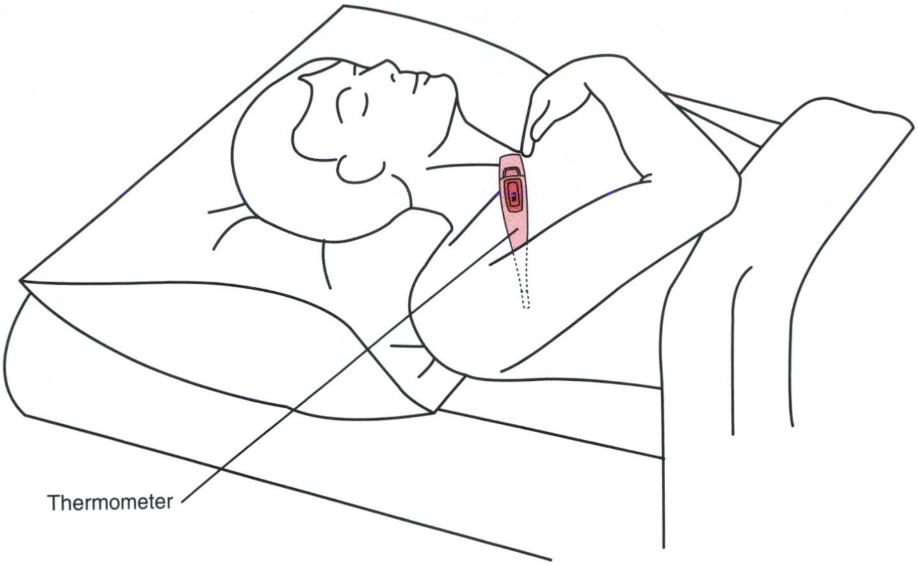

Figure 4.10 Positioning for monitoring axillary temperature. Placing the patient's arm across chest holds the thermometer in place near the vascular supply to the axilla.

9. Wash the thermometer in tepid soapy water and return to the storage container.
10. Wash hands.

Measuring Tympanic Membrane Temperature: Tympanic (Infrared) Thermometer

A. Assemble equipment

1. Tympanic thermometer (many units include a storage base and protective cap that fits over the probe tip)
2. Disposable probe covers

B. Procedure

1. Attach the disposable cover to the probe, holding it with the thumb and forefinger (ensure the firm circular collar of the cover engages with the base by gently pushing it down; do not touch the plastic film of the probe cover).
2. Turn the patient's head to one side. Pulling on the pinna (auricle) may help straighten the ear canal and provide better access. For an adult, the pinna is pulled up and back; for a child it is pulled down and back.[25,29]
3. Insert the probe snugly into the ear canal. A firm gentle pressure should be used; avoid forcing the probe too deeply. The probe should seal the opening of the ear canal. To ensure accurate reading, the probe should be angled anteriorly toward the jawline, as if approaching the patient from behind.[24]
4. Press the button that activates the thermometer. The temperature is usually displayed within 2 seconds. Some units provide an audible beep or flashing light when the maximum temperature is reached.
5. Gently remove the probe from the ear. Eject or remove the probe cover over a waste receptacle for disposal. Manual removal of probe cover should be done using a clean paper towel or tissue.
6. Return tympanic thermometer to storage base.
7. Wash hands.

Monitoring Pulse

The *pulse* is the wave of blood in the artery created by contraction of the left ventricle during a cardiac cycle (one complete cycle of cardiac muscle contraction and relaxation). With each contraction, blood is pumped into an already full aorta. The inherent elasticity of the aortic walls allows expansion and acceptance of the new supply. The blood is then forced out and surges through the systemic arteries. It is this wave or surge of blood that is felt as the pulse. The strength or amplitude of the pulse reflects the amount of blood ejected with each myocardial contraction (stroke volume).

Peripheral pulses are those located in the periphery of the body that can be felt by palpating an artery over a bony prominence or other firm surface. Examples of peripheral pulses include the radial, carotid, and popliteal pulses. The *apical pulse* is a central pulse located at the apex of the heart that is typically monitored using a stethoscope.

Pressure changes in the large arteries during the cardiac cycle are reflected in the normal arterial waveform (Fig. 4.11 [top]). The lowest point of pressure occurs during ventricular **diastole**, while the highest point occurs during ventricular **systole** (peak ejection). The notch on the descending slope of the pulse wave represents closure of the aortic valve and is not palpable.[30] A healthy adult heart beats an average of 70 times per minute, a rate that provides continuous circulation of approximately 5 to 6 liters

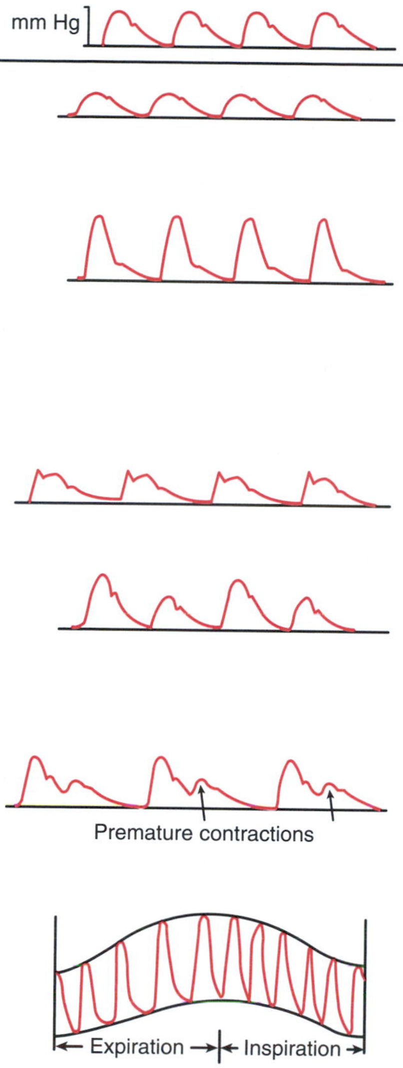

NORMAL — The pulse pressure is about 30–40 mm Hg. The pulse contour is smooth and rounded. (The notch on the descending slope of the pulse wave is not palpable.)

SMALL, WEAK PULSES — The pulse pressure is diminished, and the pulse feels weak and small. The upstroke may feel slowed, the peak prolonged. Causes include (1) decreased stroke volume, as in heart failure, hypovolemia, and severe aortic stenosis; and (2) increased peripheral resistance, as in exposure to cold and severe congestive heart failure.

LARGE, BOUNDING PULSES — The pulse pressure is increased and the pulse feels strong and bounding. The rise and fall may feel rapid, the peak brief. Causes include (1) an increased stroke volume, a decreased peripheral resistance, or both, as in fever, anemia, hyperthyroidism, aortic regurgitation, arteriovenous fistulas, and patent ductus arteriosus; (2) an increased stroke volume due to slow heart rates, as in bradycardia and complete heart block; and (3) decreased compliance (increased stiffness) of the aortic walls, as in aging or atherosclerosis.

BISFERIENS PULSE — A bisferiens pulse is an increased arterial pulse with a double systolic peak. Causes include pure aortic regurgitation, combined aortic stenosis and regurgitation, and, though less commonly palpable, hypertrophic cardiomyopathy.

PULSUS ALTERNANS — The pulse alternates in amplitude from beat to beat even though the rhythm is basically regular (and must be for you to make this judgment). When the difference between stronger and weaker beats is slight, it can be detected only by sphygmomanometry. Pulsus alternans indicates left ventricular failure and is usually accompanied by a left-sided S^3.

BIGEMINAL PULSE — This is a disorder of rhythm that may masquerade as pulsus alternans. A bigeminal pulse is caused by a normal beat alternating with a premature contraction. The stroke volume of the premature beat is diminished in relation to that of the normal beats, and the pulse varies in amplitude accordingly.

PARADOXICAL PULSE — A paradoxical pulse may be detected by a palpable decrease in the pulse's amplitude on quiet inspiration. If the sign is less pronounced, a blood-pressure cuff is needed. Systolic pressure decreases by more than 10 mm Hg during inspiration. A paradoxical pulse is found in pericardial tamponade, constrictive pericarditis (though less commonly), and obstructive lung disease.

Figure 4.11 Normal (*top*) and abnormal pulses, as reflected in the arterial waveforms. (From Bates, B,[30, p 308] with permission.)

of blood through the body. The pulse can be palpated wherever a superficial artery can be stabilized over a bony surface. In monitoring the pulse, specific attention is directed toward determining three parameters: *rate*, *rhythm*, and *volume*.

Rate

The pulse *rate* (or *frequency*) is the number of pulsations (peripheral pulse waves) per minute. **Bradycardia** is an abnormally slow pulse rate, less than 60 beats per minute. **Tachycardia** is an excessively high pulse rate, greater than 100 beats per minute. *Palpitation* refers to the sensation of a rapid or irregular pulse rate perceived by the patient without actually palpating a peripheral pulse. Multiple factors will influence the pulse rate including age, gender, emotional status, stress, and physical activity level. Body size and stature also influence pulse rate. Tall, thin individuals generally have a slower pulse rate than those who are obese or have stout frames.

Rhythm

The pulse *rhythm* is the pattern of pulsations and the intervals between them. In a healthy individual, the rhythm is regular and indicates the time intervals between pulse beats are essentially equal. *Arrhythmia* or *dysrhythmia* refers to an irregular rhythm in which pulses are not evenly spaced. An irregular rhythm may present as premature, late, or missed pulse beats, or random, irregular beats in either a predictable or unpredictable pattern.[22,29] Irregular rhythms are often associated with conduction abnormalities or an impulse originating from a site other than the SA node.[24]

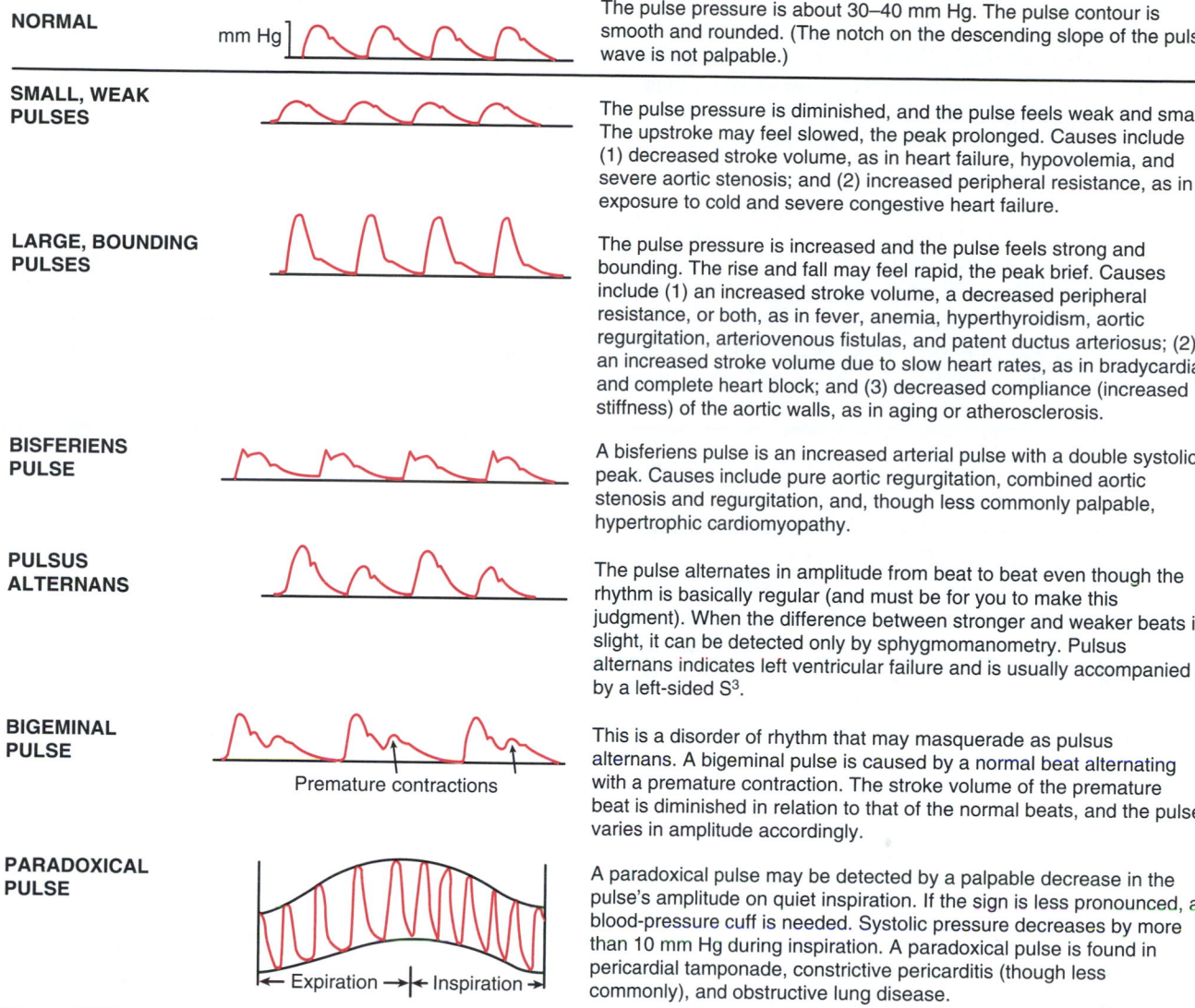

Quality

The *quality* (also called *amplitude* or *volume*) of the pulse refers to the amount of force created by the ejected blood against the arterial wall during each ventricular contraction. In examining the quality of the pulse, the therapist is determining the feel of the blood as it passes through a vessel. The quantity (volume) of blood within the vessel produces the force of the pulse. Normally, the pulse volume of each beat is the same. The force of the pulse is greater with a higher blood volume, and weaker with a lower blood volume. The volume is examined by how easily the pulse can be obliterated. A normal pulse is described as full or strong can be palpated using moderate pressure of the fingers over a bony landmark. With lower volumes, the pulse is *small,* is easily obliterated, and termed **weak** or **thready**. With an increased volume the pulse is *large,* difficult to obliterate, and is termed a **bounding** (or *full*) pulse; a feeling of high tension is noted. A numerical scale is often used to document the quality (strength) of the pulse (Table 4.5).

In addition to rate, rhythm, and quality, the feel of the arterial wall under the examiner's fingertips should be determined. Normally, a vessel will feel smooth, elastic, soft, flexible, and relatively straight. With advancing age, vessels may demonstrate sclerotic changes. These changes frequently cause the vessels to feel twisted, hard, or cord-like, with decreased elasticity and smoothness.

Several other important terms are used to describe variations in pulse. The term **bigeminal** is used to describe an abnormality in pulse rhythm where two beats occur in rapid succession (double systolic peak). **Pulsus alterans (alternating pulse)** is marked by a fluctuation in amplitude between beats (weak and a strong), with minimal change in overall rhythm. A normal pulse beat is followed by a premature beat of diminished amplitude. A **paradoxical pulse (pulsus paradoxus)** is a decreased amplitude of the pressure wave detected during quiet inspiration with a return to full amplitude on expiration; it is often associated with obstructive lung disease. Figure 4.11 provides a schematic illustration of normal (top) and common alterations in arterial pulse waveforms.

Table 4.5 Numerical Scale for Grading Pulse Quality (Strength)

Grade	Pulse	Description
0	Absent	No perceptible pulse even with maximum pressure
1+	Thready	Barely perceptible; easily obliterated with slight pressure; fades in and out
2+	Weak	Difficult to palpate; slightly stronger than thready; can be obliterated with light pressure
3+	Normal	Easy to palpate; requires moderate pressure to obliterate
4+	Bounding	Very strong; hyperactive; is not obliterated with moderate pressure

Factors Influencing Pulse

Essentially, any factor that alters the metabolic rate will also influence HR. Several factors are of particular importance when considering pulse rate.

Age

Fetal pulse rates average 120 to 160 beats per minute. The pulse rates for a newborn range between 70 and 190, with an average of 120 beats per minute. Pulse rate gradually decreases with age until it stabilizes in adulthood (see Table 4.1). The adult pulse rate range is generally considered to be between 60 and 90 beats per minute; however, in highly trained athletes the resting value may be considerably lower. This lowered resting value occurs because the effectiveness of each cardiac contraction is 40 to 50 percent greater in the trained versus untrained individual.[16]

Gender

Men and boys typically have slightly lower pulse rates than women and girls.

Emotions/Stress

Responses to a variety of emotions (e.g., grief, fear, anger, excitement, anxiety, or pain) activate the sympathetic nervous system, with a resultant increase in pulse rate. The stress inducing effects of moderate to severe pain will also elevate pulse rate.

Exercise

Oxygen demands of skeletal muscles are significantly increased during physical activity. At rest, only 20 to 25 percent of the available muscle capillaries are open.[14,15] During vigorous exercise, extensive vasodilation causes all capillaries to open. The HR increases to provide additional blood flow to muscles and to meet the increased oxygen requirement. For physical therapists, monitoring a patient's pulse rate is an important method of evaluating response to exercise. Typically, the pulse rate will increase as a function of the intensity of the activity. A linear relationship exists between pulse rate and intensity of workload. To use the pulse rate effectively, both the patient's resting and predicted maximal HRs must be determined. Maximum HR values can be determined by a maximal graded exercise test, whenever possible, or by using a formula. Age-adjusted HR (maximum HR [HR_{max}] equals 220 minus age) or the Karvonen Formula are examples. Generally, pulse rates during a 15- to 30-minute therapeutic exercise program for a healthy individual should not exceed 60 to 90 percent of predicted HR_{max}. Lower exercise intensities are indicated for individuals with low fitness levels.[15] (See Chapter 16.)

In examining pulse rate response to exercise, level of aerobic fitness also must be considered. Both resting and submaximal exercise HRs are typically lower in trained individuals. In response to an identical exercise intensity, a sedentary person's HR will demonstrate greater acceleration when compared with a trained individual. Although the metabolic requirements of an activity are the same, the lower HR response in a trained individual occurs as a result of a more efficient (increased) stroke volume owing to greater cardiac strength and efficiency. The linear relationship between pulse rate and workload exists for both trained and untrained individuals. However, the rate of rise will differ. When compared with a sedentary person, the trained individual will achieve a higher work output and greater oxygen consumption before reaching a specified submaximal HR.

Medications

The impact of medications on pulse rate is particularly important for patients with cardiac disease and **hypertension**. Beta-blockers are a category of drug that block the sympathetic beta receptors and decrease both resting HR and HR response to exercise.[15] They are commonly used in the treatment of angina pectoris, arrhythmias, hypertension, and the acute phase of myocardial infarction. Some commonly prescribed beta blockers include digitalis, nadolol, and atenolol. Patients taking beta-blockers typically experience early fatigue with exercise, and an alternative measure to pulse monitoring, such as Ratings of Perceived Exertion (RPE scale), should be considered to monitor exercise intensity.[31]

Systemic or Local Heat

During periods of fever, HR will increase. The body will attempt to dissipate heat by vasodilation of peripheral vessels. HR will increase to shunt blood flow to cutaneous areas for cooling. Local applications of thermal modalities (such as a hot pack) may also elevate HR in order to provide increased circulation to cutaneous areas secondary to arteriolar and capillary dilation.

Pulse Sites

A peripheral pulse can be monitored at a variety of sites on the body. A superficial artery located over a bone or other firm surface is easiest to palpate. Table 4.6 identifies

Table 4.6 Pulse Sites, Locations, and Indications for Use

Pulse Site	Location	Indication for Use
Temporal	Over temporal bone; superior and lateral to the eye.	When radial pulse inaccessible; often used with infants; used by anesthesiologists for monitoring during surgical interventions.
Carotid	On either side of the lower neck, below the jaw, fingers over thyroid cartilage between the trachea and medial border of sternocleidomastoid; pressure should not be applied bilaterally or high on the neck to avoid stimulation of the carotid sinus and a subsequent reflex drop in pulse rate.	During shock or cardiac arrest, often used with infants; used to monitor cranial circulation; easily accessible if other peripheral pulses difficult or too weak to locate.
Brachial	Distal medial aspect of the humerus, the biceps can be gently pushed laterally during palpation, or medially in the antecubital fossa; elbow should be slightly flexed and supported to avoid contraction of biceps.	During cardiac arrest; used routinely to monitor blood pressure.
Radial	Distal radius at base of the thumb, lateral to tendon of the flexor carpi radialis.	Most common site for peripheral pulse monitoring; easy to locate and easily accessible.
Femoral	Inferior to the inguinal ligament, midway between the anterior superior iliac spine and the symphysis pubis; typically monitored in supine.	During cardiac arrest; used to monitor lower extremity circulation.
Popliteal	Inferior aspect of popliteal fossa; popliteal artery is deep and at times may be difficult to palpate; typically monitored in prone with knee flexed to relax hamstrings and popliteal fascia; can also be accomplished in supine.	Used to monitor lower extremity circulation; weak or absent popliteal pulse may indicate impaired flow or blockage in femoral artery.
Pedal (dorsalis pedis)	Dorsal, medial aspect of foot, lateral to the tendon of the extensor hallicus longus; ankle should be slightly dorsiflexed; some individuals have congenitally nonpalpable pedal pulses.	Used to monitor circulation to feet; weak or absent pulse may be indicative of arterial disease or occlusion.

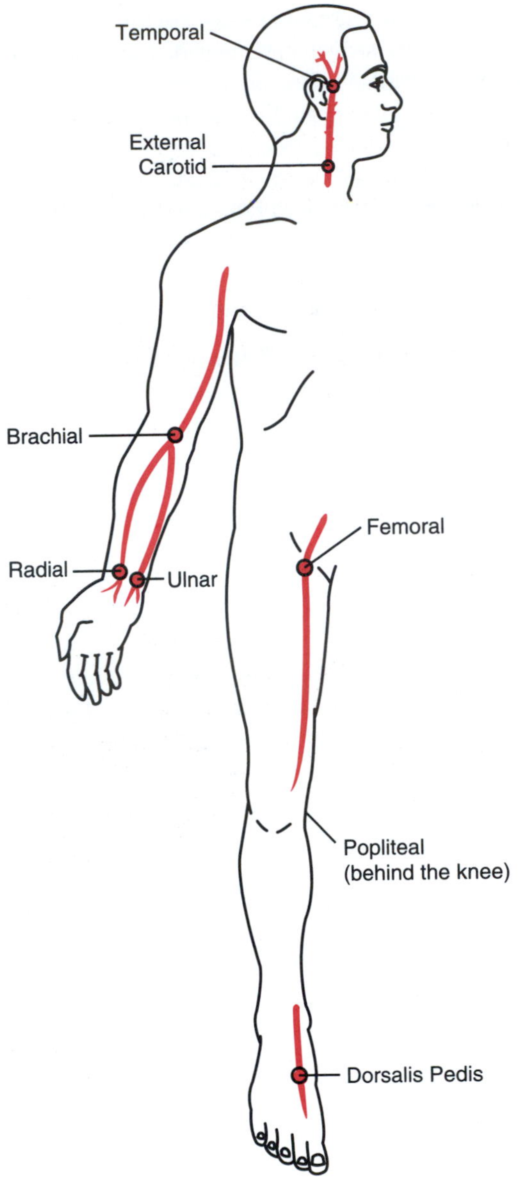

Figure 4.12 Common sites for monitoring peripheral pulses. Site selection will be influenced by patient condition and reasons for monitoring pulse.

common peripheral pulse sites, their locations, and some general indications for their use.[22,24,29,32] Pulse sites are illustrated in Figure 4.12.

The apical (central) pulse is monitored by auscultation (listening), using a stethoscope directly over the apex of the heart or by placing the hand over the chest to feel the pulsations. In infants, the apical pulse can be felt with the fingertips. Apical pulses are used when other sites are inaccessible (e.g., medical or surgical contraindications) or difficult to locate and palpate and are generally done by auscultation. The apical pulse is typically used to monitor the effects of cardiac medications designed to alter HR and rhythm.[23]

Procedure for Monitoring Pulse

Peripheral pulses are monitored by palpation using the first three fingers or the index and third finger of one hand.[24] The thumb should not be used because it has its own pulse that will interfere with monitoring. Generally, a light pressure is used initially to locate the pulse and then more firm pressure is used when determining the rate, rhythm, and quality. The fingertips should be moved gently over the selected site until the strongest pulsation is found. To monitor resting values, the patient should be resting quietly for at least 5 minutes prior to the pulse measurement.

As it is the most common site, the procedure for measuring the radial pulse follows. With few modifications, the same procedure can be followed for monitoring at other pulse site locations.

Measuring Radial Pulse

A. Assemble equipment.

1. Watch (or wall clock) with a second hand

B. Wash hands (see Box 4.3).

C. Procedure

1. Explain procedure and rationale in terms appropriate to the patient's understanding.
2. Ensure patient understanding, safety, and comfort.
3. The patient's wrist should be in a neutral position relative to flexion and extension and the forearm supported in pronation. If measuring from supine, the forearm can be supported across the patient's chest or at his or her side with partial flexion of the elbow. From a sitting position, the forearm can rest across the patient's thigh, supported by a pillow or the therapist's arm. This relaxed positioning of the upper extremity generally facilitates artery palpation.
4. Place the first three fingers squarely and firmly over the radial pulse; use only enough pressure to feel the pulse accurately. If the pressure is too great, it will occlude the artery.
5. Once the strongest pulsation is located, note the position of the second hand on the watch or clock. The first pulsation should be counted as zero to avoid overestimating.[24] Determine the *rate* (number of pulsations per minute) by counting the pulse for 30 seconds and multiplying by 2; if any irregularities are noted, a full 60-second count should be taken to improve accuracy. Note the *rhythm* (time intervals between pulse beats) and the *quality* (force) of the pulse.
6. Wash hands.

Measuring Apical Pulse

A. Assemble equipment.

1. Watch (or wall clock) with a second hand
2. Stethoscope

3. Antiseptic wipes for cleaning earpieces and diaphragm of stethoscope before and after use

B. Wash hands (see Box 4.3).

C. Procedure

1. Explain the procedure and rationale in terms appropriate to the patient's understanding. Indicate there will be a request to remain quiet during monitoring to avoid interference with auscultation.
2. Assure patient understanding, safety, and comfort. Apical pulses are typically monitored with the patient either supine or sitting.
3. Use antiseptic wipe to clean the earpieces and diaphragm of the stethoscope.
4. Expose the sternum and chest.
5. Locate the site where pulse will be monitored; the apical pulse is located approximately 3.5 inches (8.9 cm) to the left of the midsternum, in the fifth intercostal space, within an inch of the midclavicular line drawn parallel to the sternum. These landmarks are guides to locating the apical pulse. In some individuals, a stronger pulse may be noted by altering placement of the stethoscope (e.g., placement in the fourth or sixth intercostal space).
6. Place the earpieces of the stethoscope (tilting slightly forward) into ears. The tubes of the stethoscope should not be crossed and should hang freely.
7. Place the flat disk diaphragm of the stethoscope over the apex of heart and locate the point where the apical pulse is heard most clearly. This is called the *point of maximal impulse (PMI)*. If the rhythm is regular, count the pulse for 30 seconds and multiply by 2. If any irregularities are noted, a full 60-second count should be taken. The pulse will be heard as a "lubb-dubb." The "lubb" represents closure of the atrioventricular (tricuspid and mitral) valves. The "dubb" represents closure of the semilunar (aortic and pulmonic) valves.
8. Wash hands and clean the stethoscope. If the same examiner is using the stethoscope again, it is not necessary to clean the earpieces; the diaphragm should always be cleaned.

Measuring Apical–Radial Pulse

Monitoring the apical–radial pulse involves two examiners simultaneously measuring the pulse at two separate locations: (1) the apical pulse at the apex of the heart; and (2) the radial pulse at the wrist. The values from the two different sites are then compared. Typically, the apical and radial pulse values are the same. However, in some situations (e.g., variations in stroke volume or vascular occlusion) blood pumped from the heart may not be reaching the distal site causing a weak or imperceptible radial pulse. For example, if the heart contracts prematurely, the ventricles have insufficient time to fill, resulting in a diminished stroke volume and creating an imperceptible pulse in the radial artery.[16] On the other hand, stroke volume may be normal with a weak or imperceptible radial pulse, suggesting a more peripheral problem such as impaired flow or blockage within a vessel. In either situation, there is a deficit in the number of radial pulses when compared with the number of apical pulses.[16] This is called a **pulse deficit**, defined as the difference between the rate of radial and apical pulses. The value of this measure is that it provides important information about the cardiovascular system's ability to perfuse the body.

Electronic Heart Rate Monitoring

In recent years, considerable advances have been made in the design, features, accuracy, computer interface capabilities, and information storage capacity of heart rate monitors (HRMs). In addition to monitoring HR, some HRMs provide data on HR variability (calculation of the time between pulses), real time display of percentage of maximum HR, and estimates of maximal oxygen uptake (VO_{2max}).[33] HRMs with computer interface capabilities allow data to be downloaded to a computer for analysis and storage using HR software programs. This provides a permanent record and sequential data on exercise performance. Most models allow programming of a prescribed exercise HR range with an audible and visible warning when the HR is outside of the predetermined range. Some models include a talking feature that "speaks" HR information through headphones. Memory capabilities allow storage of exercise information over a variable number of exercise sessions.

HRMs, also referred to as *pulse monitors* and *pulse meters,* consist of two basic elements: (1) a sensor that transmits data; and (2) a monitor that incorporates a receiver, microprocessor, and display.[34] One style of HRM integrates sensors into a chest strap that provides wireless transmission of signals to a monitor worn as a wristwatch (Fig. 4.13A). Another style of HRM replaces the chest strap with a fingertip sensor directly on a wrist (Fig. 4.13B) or a worn around-the-neck monitor (Fig 4.13C). HR data are recorded when a fingertip is placed in contact with the sensor. Still other HRMs incorporate a lead wire with a distal sensor housed in an earlobe clip, fingertip cover, or finger sleeve (Fig, 4.13 D, E, and F). Some HRMs are equipped with more than one type of sensor. This feature allows selection of a sensor appropriate to the activity. For example, an earlobe clip or chest strap would be preferable to a finger sleeve for monitoring an activity that involved upper extremity movement.

HRMs have gained expanded use in prescribed exercise and training programs because they provide a practical, accurate method of continual pulse monitoring as well as being lightweight, comfortable, and easy to use.[34] In recent years, many types of exercise training devices (e.g., treadmills, stairclimbers, bicycles) incorporate HRMs directly into the unit design using a metal hand-grip sensor device.

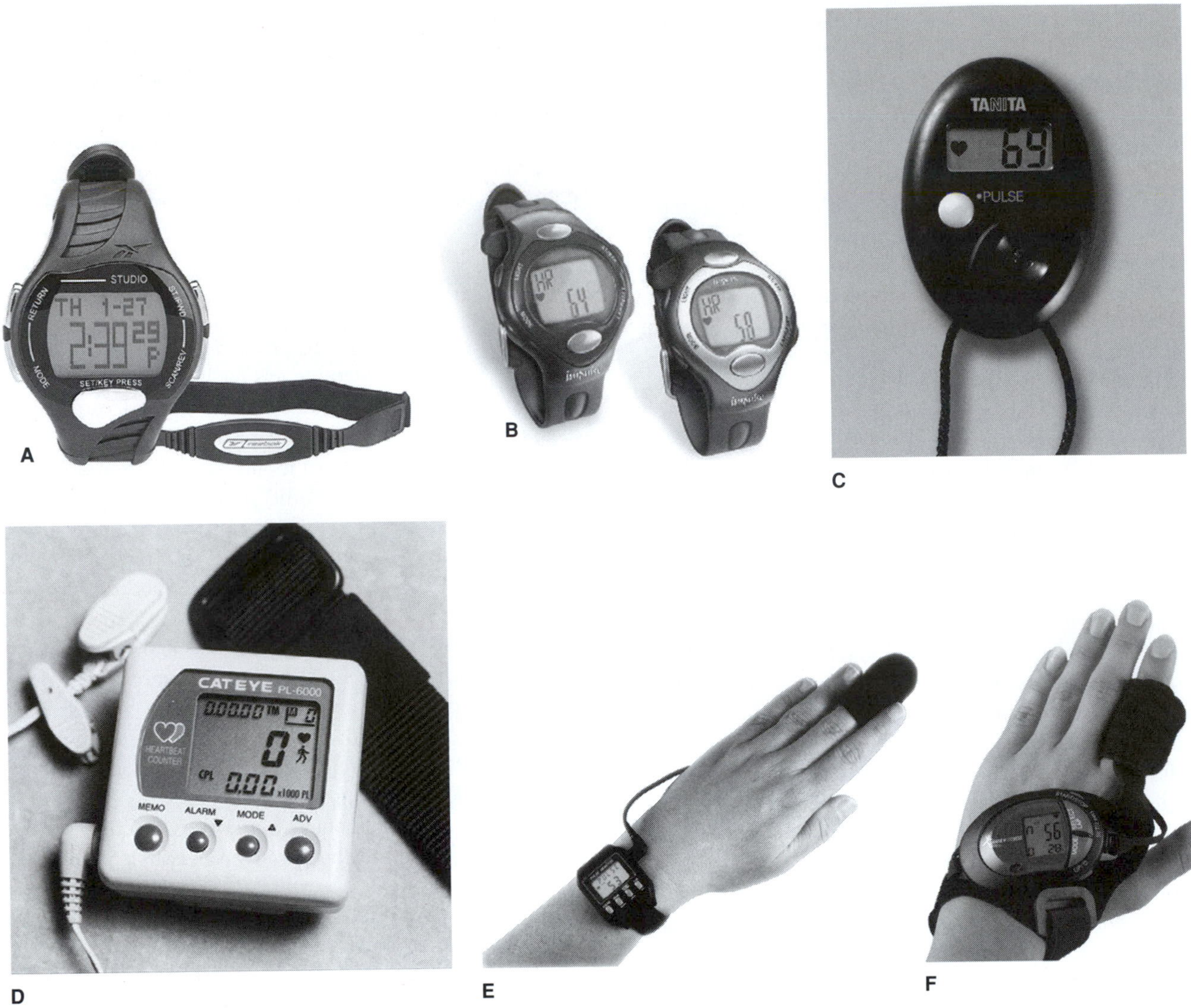

Figure 4.13 Heart rate monitors. (*A*) Wrist monitor with chest strap transmitter worn directly on the skin and positioned at heart level. (Courtesy of Sports Beat, Inc, Deer Park, NY 11729.) (*B*) Example of wrist monitors with two fingertip sensors above and below LCD; the index and middle finger are placed on contact points to obtain HR. (Courtesy of Sports Beat, Inc, Deer Park, NY 11729.) (*C*) Monitor with neck strap and fingertip sensor. (Courtesy of Tanita Corporation of America, Arlington Heights, IL 60005.) (*D*) This HRM incorporates a belt-clip design, includes a universal mounting strap allowing attachment to exercise equipment, a lead wire and earlobe clip sensor. (Courtesy of Source Distributors, Inc, Dallas, TX 75229.) (*E*) Wrist monitor with lead wire and fingertip sensor. (Courtesy of Mark of Fitness, Inc, Shrewsbury, NJ 07702.) (F) Heart rate monitor worn on dorsum of hand with finger sleeve sensor. (Courtesy of Mark of Fitness, Inc, Shrewsbury, NJ 07702.)

Other HRM features are available and differ with the model and manufacturer. Among the more common features are multifunction wrist monitors (time, stopwatch, alarm clock, lap timer, and calendar), illuminated and large-number LCD displays (some with a zoom feature that doubles the size of information on the screen), bar graph memory displays of previous training sessions, and estimates of calories burned and energy expended during exercise. HRMs can interface with a personal computer (PC) either wirelessly using infrared signals (Fig 4.14A) to transfer data, or by placing the wrist monitor in an interface unit connected to the PC to launch the transfer of data (Fig. 4.14B).

Telemetry is the science of remote measurement that includes both gathering data from a distant source and transmitting the data electronically. Telemetric HRMs are not new and have been available since 1983.[35] Since that time, continued research has led to greater and more advanced applications of telemetry in health care. For example, in 1998 NASA designed a sophisticated telemetry system to ground monitor astronauts' vital signs data from space. This technology led to the development of the *Patient Monitoring System* that involves having the patient continually wear a small transmitter that delivers vital signs data to a central location where multiple patients can be monitored simultaneously.[15]

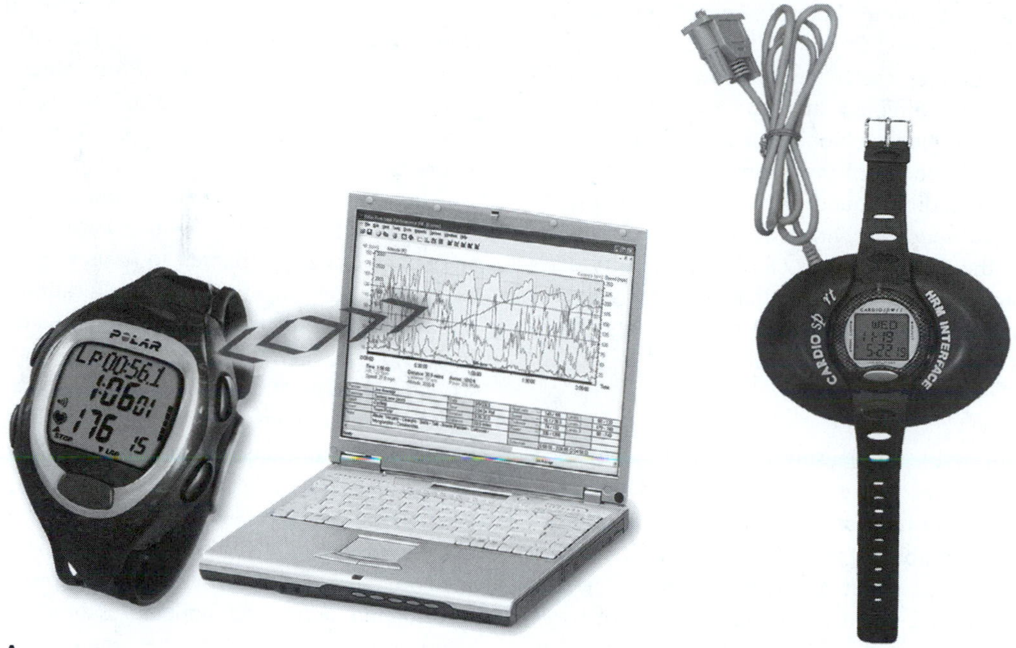

A B

Figure 4.14 (*A*) Schematic depiction of wireless transmission of data from wrist monitor to computer via infrared signals. (Courtesy of Polar Electro, Inc, Lake Success, NY 11042.) (*B*) Heart rate monitor in computer interface unit. (Courtesy of Sports Beat, Inc, Deer Park, NY 11729.)

Gandsas et al applied telemetric technology to examine the efficacy of using a low-cost approach to transmitting vital signs data from an aircraft to a ground medical facility. Enacting an in-flight simulated medical emergency, vital sign data were collected with a monitoring device and transmitted using a lap top computer, an airline seat-back telephone, and the Internet. All data were received without corruption with a maximum delay of 1 second. The authors suggest that during an actual in-flight emergency, patient data could potentially be delivered to an assigned medical facility, as well as to the physician's desktop computer anywhere in the world irrespective of the geographical location of the aircraft.[36] Another area of research involves developing uniform standards of communication for transmission of data from vital signs monitoring equipment directly to clinical information systems currently in use in many healthcare settings.[37]

For additional information on HR monitoring devices, the reader is referred to review articles by Achten and Jeukendrup[33] and Thivierge and Leger.[38] A number of studies have also addressed the accuracy of specific HRMs manufactured by individual companies.[39–45] Many investigators have used electrocardiogram (ECG) data as the "gold standard" for comparison with HR data obtained from the device under study. In reviewing the literature on HRMs, it is important to note that innovations in HRMs evolve very rapidly. Data presented for a given monitoring device at a specific point in time cannot be generalized to more recent models produced by the same manufacturer.

Related Measures

Doppler Ultrasound

Doppler ultrasound (DUS) is a noninvasive instrument used to examine pulses that are extremely weak or faint, obliterated by even slight pressure, or when arterial flow is severely compromised. DUS is based on the principle that high-frequency ultrasound waves directed at a moving interface (i.e., blood flowing through a vessel) will cause a change in the wave frequency reflective of the velocity of the moving interface (called the *Doppler effect*). In essence, the DUS measures how sound waves are reflected off moving blood cells. The resultant frequency change caused by the movement alters the pitch of the sound waves as they are reflected back to the examiner. The change in pitch heard by the examiner provides important information about the blood flow through a vessel.

Several models of DUS units are available. The essential elements include the ultrasound unit, a handheld probe (piezoelectric crystal) that transmits and receives sound waves, and earpieces that look similar to those on a stethoscope or a small speaker to amplify the sound. Passed gently over the skin surface above an artery using ample coupling gel, the probe transmits high-frequency sound waves to an artery. The waves are disturbed by movement of the red blood cells, reflected back to the probe and transformed into an amplified audible sound.[46] Mohr and Young[47] offer the analogy that this is, "rather like the [way a] police microwave transmitter bounces energy off passing cars to estimate their speed."[p 26]

The audible sound represents the difference in frequency between the waves directed at the vessel and those reflected back by motion of blood cells; the frequency is proportional to the velocity of the moving red blood cells. The absence of an audible sound indicates no detection of movement and, subsequently, no perfusion. Using a computer interface, the flow measures can be graphically displayed and stored. It should be noted that while the specific characteristics of the reflected sounds are not diagnostic, they can assist in identifying abnormal flow.[48,49]

Pulse Oximetry

Pulse oximetry provides a measure of arterial blood oxygenation that is updated with each pulse wave.[50] Oxygen is carried in the blood in two forms: (1) dissolved in arterial plasma; and (2) combined with hemoglobin.[15] Arterial plasma transports only about 3 percent of the oxygen in blood and is measured as PaO_2 (partial pressure of oxygen).The greater amount of oxygen (~ 97%) is carried by hemoglobin and measured as S_aO_2 (arterial hemoglobin oxygen saturation). Pulse oximetry measures arterial blood oxygen saturation as a noninvasive intervention. Oxygen saturation via pulse oximetry is reported as SpO_2[51–53] and can be measured at any adequately perfused peripheral pulse.

Normal oxygen saturation levels are between 96 percent and 100 percent. In general, saturation levels below 90 percent are considered significant and warrant additional testing beyond the data provided by pulse oximetry (e.g., arterial blood gas analysis), as well as mark the potential need for administration of supplemental oxygen.[52,54] *Hypoxemia* is a term used to describe deficient oxygenation of the blood. *Hypoxia* is a diminished supply of oxygen available to body tissues, and *anoxia* is the complete lack of oxygen, a condition that can be sustained for only a very brief period.[51]

Alterations in heart function (e.g., arrhythmias, decreased HR) typically reduce cardiac output and the amount of oxygen delivered to tissues. Examples of other conditions that impact oxygen saturation levels include impaired ability of the lungs to oxygenate blood, anemia (reduction in hemoglobin molecules available to carry oxygen), hypoventilation (e.g., bronchitis, emphysema), and diffusion impairments that impact blood-gas exchange (e.g., alveolar fibrosis, interstitial fluid).[51]

The pulse oximeter provides data on the percent of oxygen that is combined with hemoglobin (SpO_2). The electronic units are relatively small (Fig. 4.15A and B), easy to use and transport, and provide the therapist with immediate information about the patient's saturation levels.[54] The monitor provides a digital percentage of the amount of hemoglobin saturated with oxygen, displays a pulsatile waveform and pulse rate with an audible signal indicating each pulsation. The patient interface is provided by a lead wire and sensor that attaches to the unit. The sensor is placed over a pulsating arteriolar vascular bed.[53] Several types of sensors are available, including adhesive fingertip and forehead (Fig. 4.16A and B) as well as nasal, earlobe, and foot styles. The sensors contain two light sources (red and infrared) and a photodetector (Fig. 4.17). The dual light source is used because oxygenated and deoxygenated hemoglobin have different patterns of light absorption.[55]

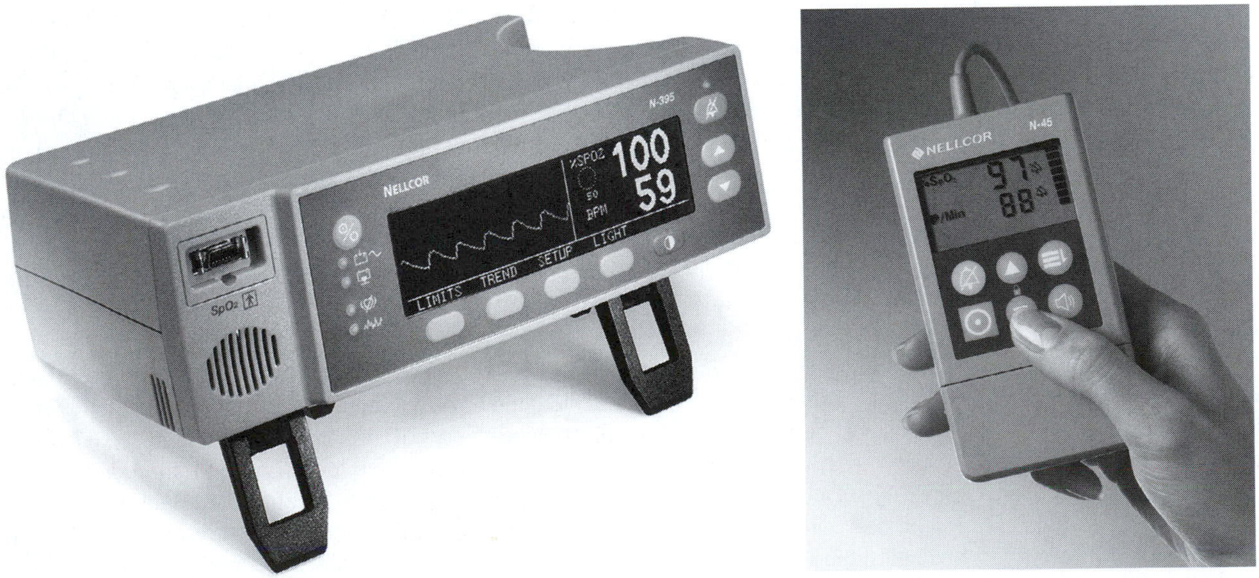

A B

Figure 4.15 Pulse oximeters provide data on arterial blood oxygen saturation as well as pulse rate. (*A*) Standard pulse oximetry unit. (*B*) Portable handheld pulse oximeter. (Courtesy of Nellcor Puritan Bennett, Inc, Pleasanton, CA 94588.)

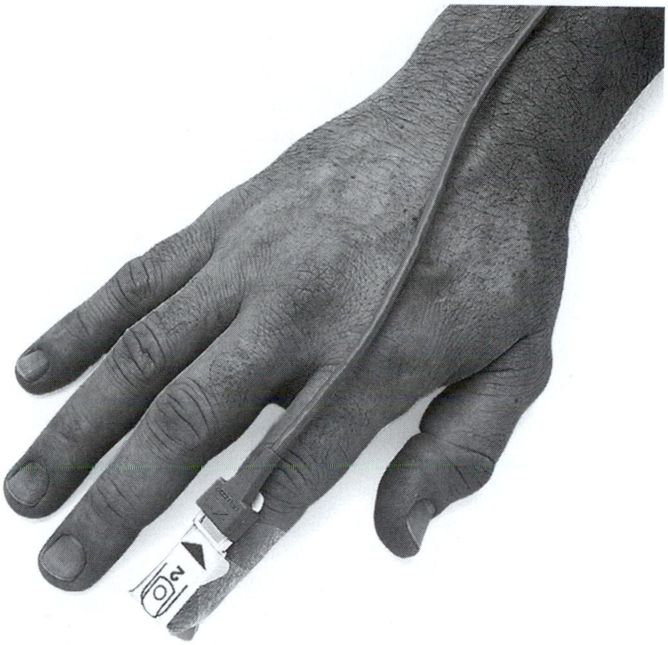

A

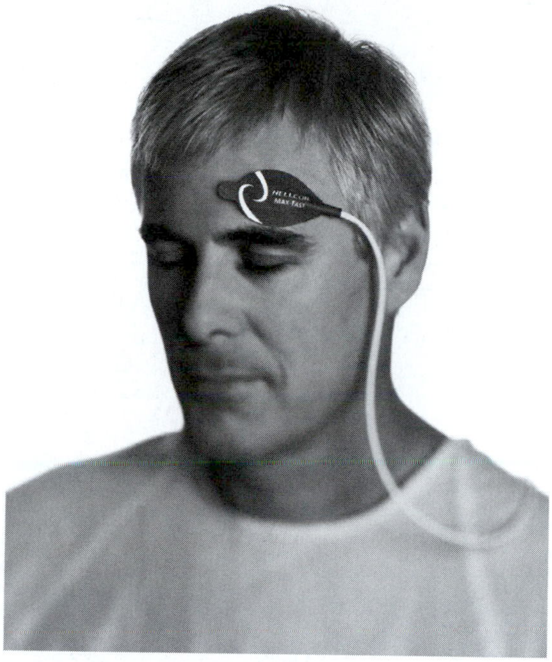

B

Figure 4.16 Oximetry sensors. (*A*) The fingertip (transmission) sensor and (*B*) forehead (reflectance) sensor. (Courtesy of Nellcor Puritan Bennett, Inc., Pleasanton, CA 94588.)

The ratio of the amount of each light absorbed during systole and diastole allows quantification of an oxygen saturation measurement (SpO_2).[53,55]

Perhaps the most important use of pulse oximetry in patient management is that it assists with (1) early identification of hypoxemia; (2) monitoring patient tolerance to activity; and (3) evaluating patient response to treatment.

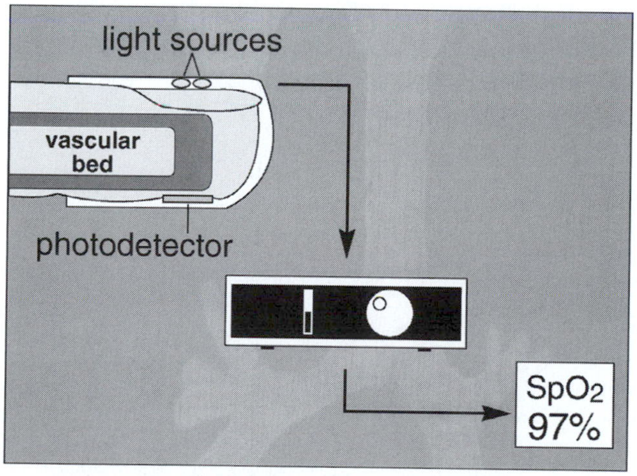

Figure 4.17 Cross-sectional drawing of a fingertip oximetry sensor illustrating the dual light sources, photodetector, schematic connection to oximeter and hypothetical oxygen saturation measurement output. *Note*: In the fingertip (transmission) sensors, the light sources are positioned opposite the photodetector. In the forehead (reflectance) sensors, the light sources and photodetector are positioned on one side of the sensor. (Courtesy of Nellcor Puritan Bennett, Inc., Pleasanton, CA 94588.)

Pulse oximetry measures may be done continuously, intermittently to generate a series of values over time, or as a single measure at a given point in time (e.g., as an initial screening tool or for low-risk patients). The measurement pattern will be determined within the context of the patient history and examination findings. Telemetry oximetry monitoring allows continuous communication of SpO_2 data from remote locations.[53]

Monitoring Respiration

The primary function of respiration (movement of air into and out of the lungs) is to supply the body with oxygen for metabolic activity and to remove carbon dioxide. The respiratory system consists of a series of branching tubes and brings atmospheric oxygen into contact with the gas exchange membrane of the lungs in the alveoli. Oxygen is then transported throughout the body via the cardiovascular system. *External respiration* is the exchange of oxygen and carbon dioxide between the alveoli of the lungs and the blood. *Internal respiration* is the exchange of oxygen and carbon dioxide between the circulating blood and body tissues.

The Respiratory System

The entire pathway that transports air from the environment extends from the mouth and nose down to the alveolar sacs. Figure 4.18 illustrates an overview of the respiratory

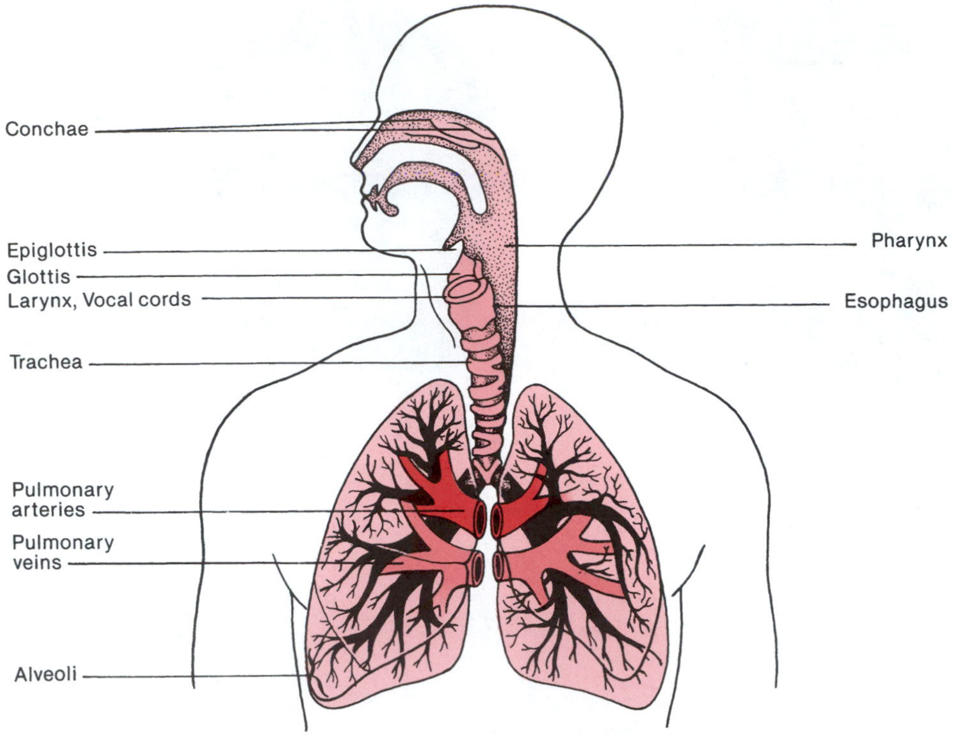

Figure 4.18 The respiratory pathways. (From Guyton, AC and Hall, JE,[14, p 316] with permission.)

system. The upper respiratory airways include the nose, mouth, pharynx, and larynx. Air enters the body by way of the nose and mouth and is then moved to the pharynx, where it is warmed, filtered, and humidified. The pharynx serves as a common pathway for both air and food. Inspired air is then moved to the larynx, which contains the epiglottis, vocal cords, and cartilaginous structures. The anatomical arrangement of the larynx and pharyngeal muscles provides the critical function of protecting the lungs from entry of foreign particles, as well as assists with phonation (production of vocal sounds) and coughing, which is the primary physiological mechanism for clearing the airways. The *laryngopharynx* is the area where solid and liquid food intake is separated from inspired air. It is also the site of bifurcation into the larynx and esophagus. The pharyngeal muscles close the glottis during swallowing to protect the lungs from aspiration. If a foreign body passes the glottis and enters the tracheobronchial tree, the cough reflex is initiated to clear the air passage. Immediately below the thyroid cartilage of the larynx ("Adam's apple") is the site for emergency opening to the tracheal air pathway.[14,51,56,57]

The trachea is approximately 4 to 5 inches (11 to 13 cm) long and continues from the cartilaginous structures of the neck into the thorax. At the level of the carina (Fig. 4.19), the trachea divides into two mainstem bronchi. The carina contains the majority of cough receptors and is located approximately between the sternum and manubrium at the second intercostal space. The right and left mainstem bronchi are asymmetrical in size and shape and continue into the lower respiratory tract further subdividing into the respiratory bronchioles where gas exchange begins. However, gas exchange primarily occurs in the alveolar ducts and the large surface area provided by the alveoli. The bronchioles, alveolar ducts, and alveoli (alveolar sacs) comprise the functional zones of the respiratory

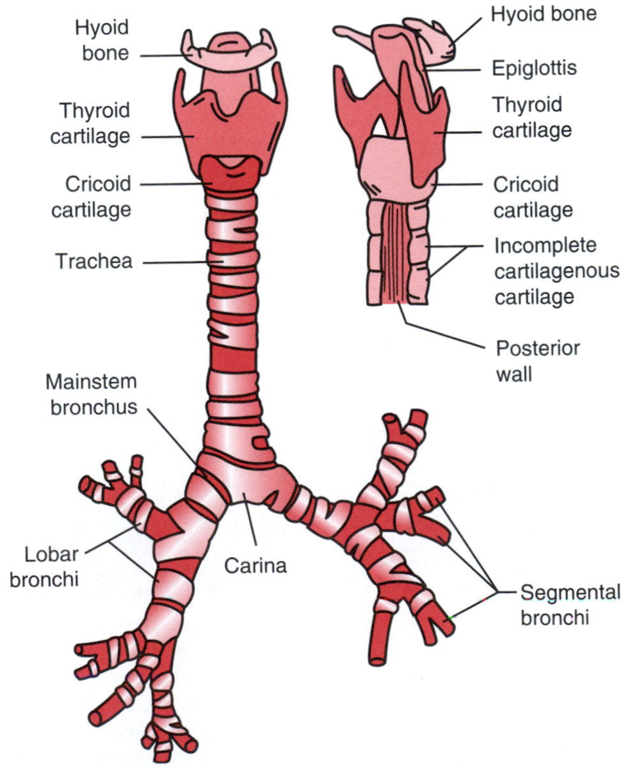

Figure 4.19 Structure of cartilaginous airways, including the trachea and major bronchi. (From Henderson, BS,[57, p 388] with permission.)

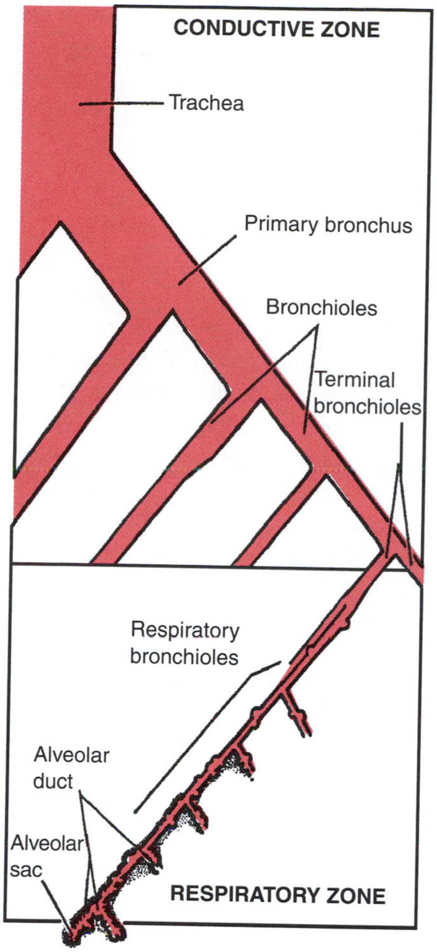

Figure 4.20 Schematic illustration of the functional zones of the respiratory tract. The top area from the trachea to the terminal bronchioles is called the "conductive zone" because these airways transport (conduct) inhaled air to and from the respiratory zone. The bottom area of the illustration represents the areas where air exchange takes place. The air exchange occurs in progressively increasing increments in the respiratory bronchioles, alveolar ducts, and alveolar sacs. Collectively these areas constitute the "respiratory zone." (From Henderson, BS,[57, p 389] with permission.)

tract for air exchange (Fig. 4.20). The airways do not contribute to air exchange and comprise **the anatomical dead space.**[14,51,55,56]

Inspiration

Inspiration is initiated by contraction of the diaphragm and intercostal muscles. During contraction of these muscles, the diaphragm moves downward and the intercostals lift the ribs and sternum up and outward. The thoracic cavity is thus increased in size and allows for lung expansion. Normal inspiration lasts 1 to 1.5 seconds.[22]

Expiration

During relaxed breathing, expiration is essentially a passive process. Once the respiratory muscles relax, the thorax returns to its resting position, and the lungs recoil. This ability to recoil occurs because of the inherent elastic properties of the lungs. Normal expiration lasts 2 to 3 seconds.[22]

Regulatory Mechanisms

Regulation of respiratory function involves multiple components of both neural and chemical control and is closely integrated with the cardiovascular system. Breathing is controlled by the **respiratory center**, which lies bilaterally in the pons and medulla. The respiratory muscles are controlled by motor nerves whose cell bodies are located in this area. The respiratory center provides control of both the **rate** and the **depth** of breathing in response to the metabolic needs of the body.[58]

Both *central* and *peripheral* chemoreceptors influence respiration. *Central* chemoreceptors located in the respiratory center are sensitive to changes in either carbon dioxide or hydrogen ion levels of arterial blood. An increase in either carbon dioxide levels or hydrogen ions will stimulate breathing.[16] *Peripheral* chemoreceptors are located at the bifurcation of the carotid arteries (carotid bodies) and in the arch of the aorta (aortic bodies). These receptors are sensitive to the partial pressure of oxygen (PaO_2) in the arterial blood. When PaO_2 levels in arterial blood drop, afferent impulses carry this information to the respiratory center. Motor neurons to the respiratory muscles are stimulated to increase **tidal volume** (amount of air exchanged with each breath) or, with very low oxygen levels, to increase the respiratory rate as well. These peripheral chemoreceptors cause an increase in respiration only when PaO_2 levels fall to approximately 60 mm Hg (from a normal level of about 90 to 100 mm Hg). This is because the receptors are sensitive only to PaO_2 levels in plasma and not to the total oxygen in blood.[16,58]

Respiration also is influenced by a protective stretch mechanism called the *Hering-Breuer reflex*. Pulmonary stretch receptors throughout the walls of the lungs detect the amount of stretch imposed by entering air.[59] When overstretched, these receptors send impulses to the respiratory center to inhibit further inspiration and increase the duration of expiration. Impulses stop at the end of expiration so that another inspiration can be initiated.[16,51] In adults, this reflex is rarely demonstrated and would likely not be activated until tidal volume reached higher than 1.5 liters.[16] However, evidence suggests the Hering-Breuer reflex has a significant impact on the breathing pattern of neonates.[60] Respiration is also stimulated by vigorous movements of joints and muscle (exercise) and is strongly influenced by voluntary cortical control.

Factors Influencing Respiration

Multiple factors can alter normal, relaxed, effortless respiration. As with temperature and pulse, any influence that increases the metabolic rate also will increase the respiratory rate (RR). Increased metabolism and subsequent demand for oxygen will stimulate increased respiration. Conversely, as metabolic demands diminish, respirations also will decrease. Several influencing factors are of particular importance when examining respiration. These include age, body size, stature, exercise, and body position.

Age

The RR of a newborn is between 25 and 50 breaths per minute. The rate gradually slows until adulthood, when it ranges between 12 and 20 breaths per minute. In elderly individuals, the RR increases owing to decreased elasticity of the lungs and decreased efficiency of gas exchange. Other factors associated with normal ageing that impact respiratory function include weakening of respiratory muscles, deterioration of alveolar walls, decreased thoracic mobility, and decreased lung volumes.[61]

Body Size and Stature

Men generally have a larger vital capacity than women, adults larger than adolescents and children. Tall, thin individuals generally have a larger vital capacity than stout or obese individuals. With larger lung capacity there is also a lower RR.

Exercise

RR and depth will increase with exercise as a result of increased oxygen demand and carbon dioxide production.

Body Position

The recumbent position can significantly affect respiration and predispose the patient to stasis of fluids. Among the influential factors that limit normal lung expansion when lying down are compression of the chest against the supporting surface and pressure from abdominal organs against the diaphragm. Both of these factors cause increased resistance to breathing. Difficult recumbent breathing is common during the late stages of pregnancy as the fetus shifts the diaphragm upward,[24] as well as in patients with congestive heart failure (CHF).

Environment

Exposure to pollutants such as gas and particle emissions, asbestos, chemical waste products, or coal dust can diminish the ability to transport oxygen. Other common offending pollutants include high ozone concentrations, sulfur dioxide, and carbon monoxide.[19] These respiratory irritants typically increase mucus production. High altitudes also impact the respiratory system owing to reduced air mass (i.e., the partial pressure of oxygen in inspired air is low). This means there is less oxygen molecules per liter of air, causing a reduction in arterial blood oxygen levels. This typically results in shortness of breath and reduced tolerance to activity. Hyperventilation, tachycardia, and pulmonary edema (accumulation of fluid in alveolar walls) can also occur at high altitudes.[19,24,62,63]

Emotions/Stress

Stress as well as emotions can result in an increased rate and depth of respirations owing to stimulation of the sympathetic nervous system.

Pharmacological Agents

Essentially any drug that depresses central nervous system (CNS) function will result in respiratory depression. Narcotic agents (e.g., morphine, meperidine hydrochloride [Demerol]) will decrease the rate and depth of respirations. Other categories of CNS depressant agents include barbiturates (e.g., phenobarbitol [Nembutal], secobarbital [Seconal]), benzodiazepines (e.g., Ativan, Diazepam), neuroleptics (e.g., Thorazine, haloperidol, clozapine) opiates, muscle relaxants, tricyclic antidepressants, and anticonvulsants. Conversely, bronchodilators decrease airway resistance and residual volume with a resultant increase in vital capacity and airflow. Common bronchodilator medications include Albuterol (Ventolin, Proventil), metaproterenol (Alupent), terbutaline (Brethine, Brethaire) and bitolterol (Tornalate).[64]

Parameters of Respiration

In examining respiration, four parameters are considered: *rate, depth, rhythm,* and *sound*. The *rate* is the number of breaths per minute. Either inspirations or expirations are counted, but not both. The normal adult RR is 12 to 20 per minute. The rate should be counted for 30 seconds and multiplied by 2. If any irregularities are noted, a full 60-second count is indicated.

The *depth* of respiration refers to the amount (volume) of air exchanged with each breath. Normally, the depth of respirations is consistent, producing a relatively even, uniform movement of the chest. The normal adult tidal volume is approximately 500 mL of air. The depth of respiration is determined by observation of chest movements and is usually described as *deep* or *shallow,* depending on whether the amount of air exchanged is greater or less than normal. With deep breaths, a large volume of air is exchanged; with shallow respirations, a small amount of air is exchanged, typically with minimal lung expansion or chest wall movement.

The *rhythm* refers to the regularity of inspirations and expirations. Normally, there is an even time interval between respirations. The respiratory rhythm is described as *regular* or *irregular*.

The *sound* of respirations refers to deviations from normal, quiet, effortless breathing. Although some respiratory sounds are audible, accurate identification requires auscultation (listening with a stethoscope placed directly against the chest wall). Normal (vesicular) breath sounds are heard primarily during inspiration and sound relatively smooth and soft.[55] Common abnormal (adventitious) sounds of breathing include:

- *Wheezing,* which is a continuous whistling sound produced by air passing through a narrowed airway such as a bronchi or bronchiole, is often compared to the whistling produced when stretching the neck of a balloon and allowing air to escape slowly through the narrowed passageway. It may be heard on both inspiration and expiration, but is more prominent on expiration. Wheezing is a common symptom of asthma, is also seen in CHF, and can result from an airway obstruction.

- **Stridor** is a harsh, high-pitched crowing sound that occurs with upper airway obstructions resulting in narrowing of the glottis or trachea. It is apparent in patients with tracheal stenosis or presence of a foreign object.
- **Crackles** (also called *rales*) are rattling or bubbling sounds that occur owing to secretions in the air passages of the respiratory tract. The sound is often compared to that of rustling a cellophane bag. Crackles may be heard with the ear but are most accurately determined using a stethoscope; apparent in patients with CHF.
- **Sigh** is a deep inspiration followed by a prolonged, audible expiration. Occasional sighs are normal and function to expand alveoli; frequent sighs are abnormal and may be indicative of emotional stress.
- **Stertor** is a snoring sound owing to partial obstruction (e.g., secretions) in the upper airway (e.g., trachea, large bronchi).

Patterns of Respiration

Examination of the rate, rhythm, and depth allows the therapist to determine the *pattern* of respiration. Not all patients will present with a distinct pattern of respiration. However, several patterns occur with sufficient frequency that uniform terminology has developed methods for their identification. Common respiratory patterns are presented in Figure 4.21.

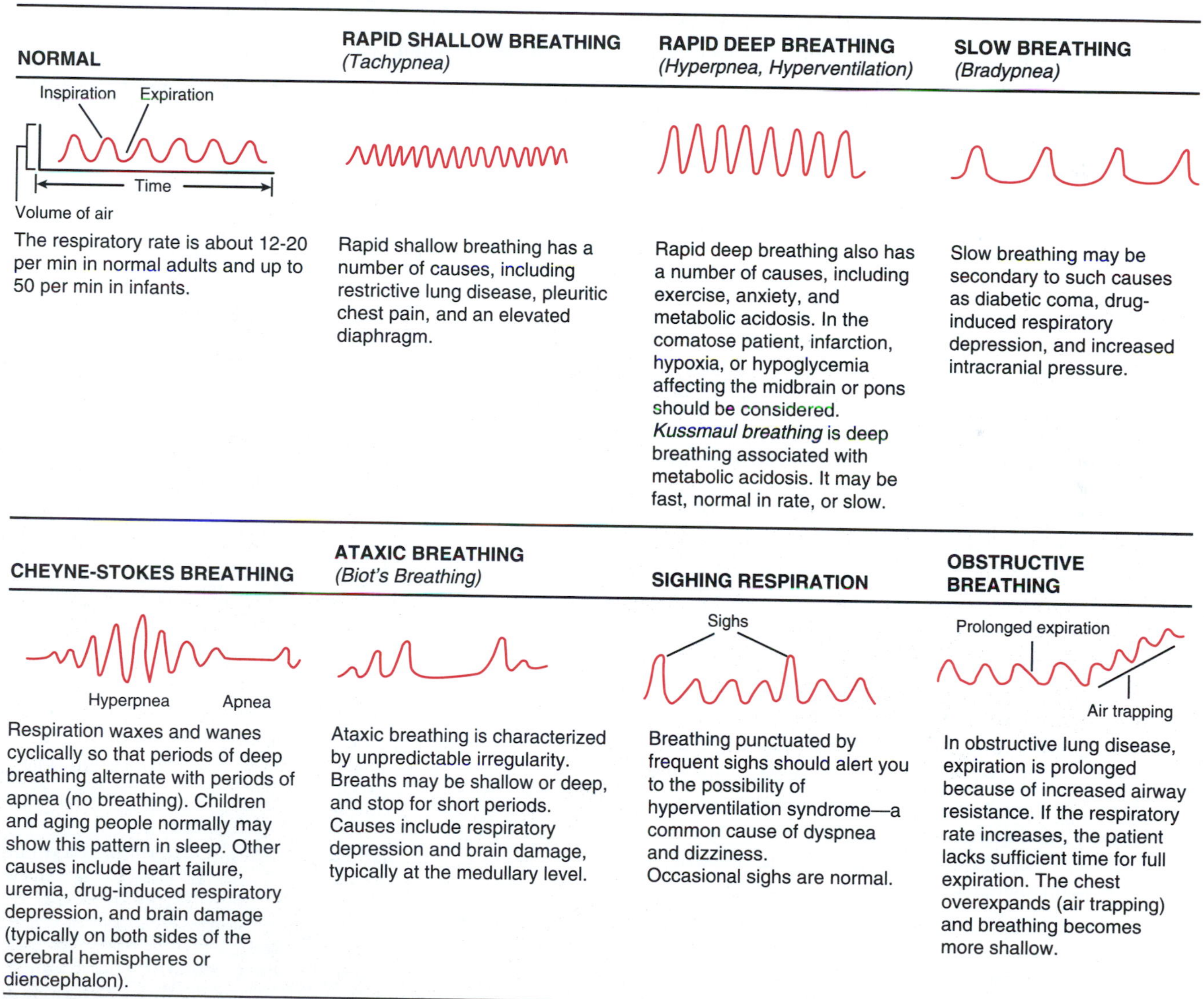
NORMAL
Inspiration
Expiration
Time
Volume of air
The respiratory rate is about 12-20 per min in normal adults and up to 50 per min in infants.
RAPID SHALLOW BREATHING
(Tachypnea)
Rapid shallow breathing has a number of causes, including restrictive lung disease, pleuritic chest pain, and an elevated diaphragm.
RAPID DEEP BREATHING
(Hyperpnea, Hyperventilation)
Rapid deep breathing also has a number of causes, including exercise, anxiety, and metabolic acidosis. In the comatose patient, infarction, hypoxia, or hypoglycemia affecting the midbrain or pons should be considered. Kussmaul breathing is deep breathing associated with metabolic acidosis. It may be fast, normal in rate, or slow.
SLOW BREATHING
(Bradypnea)
Slow breathing may be secondary to such causes as diabetic coma, drug-induced respiratory depression, and increased intracranial pressure.
CHEYNE-STOKES BREATHING
Hyperpnea
Apnea
Respiration waxes and wanes cyclically so that periods of deep breathing alternate with periods of apnea (no breathing). Children and aging people normally may show this pattern in sleep. Other causes include heart failure, uremia, drug-induced respiratory depression, and brain damage (typically on both sides of the cerebral hemispheres or diencephalon).
ATAXIC BREATHING
(Biot's Breathing)
Ataxic breathing is characterized by unpredictable irregularity. Breaths may be shallow or deep, and stop for short periods. Causes include respiratory depression and brain damage, typically at the medullary level.
SIGHING RESPIRATION
Sighs
Breathing punctuated by frequent sighs should alert you to the possibility of hyperventilation syndrome—a common cause of dyspnea and dizziness. Occasional sighs are normal.
OBSTRUCTIVE BREATHING
Prolonged expiration
Air trapping
In obstructive lung disease, expiration is prolonged because of increased airway resistance. If the respiratory rate increases, the patient lacks sufficient time for full expiration. The chest overexpands (air trapping) and breathing becomes more shallow.

Figure 4.21 Normal (*top left*) and abnormal respiratory patterns. When examining respiratory patterns, consider rate, rhythm, and depth of the patient's breathing. Describe what is seen in these terms. Note that below each descriptor of abnormal breathing pattern are more traditional terms, such as tachypnea, hyperpnea, and hyperventilation. It is important to understand what these traditional terms mean. However, for purposes of documentation, simpler descriptions (such as "rapid, shallow breathing") are recommended. (Adapted from Bates, B,[30, p 256] with permission.)

Eupnea is the term used to describe a normal breathing pattern of 12 to 20 times per minute in an adult (see Table 4.1 for age appropriate variations). **Hyperventilation** is an abnormally fast rate and depth of respiration often associated with anxiety, emotional stress, and panic disorders. A common response to an acute episode is to have the patient rebreathe into a paper bag, which replaces some of the lost carbon dioxide (*hypocapnia*). Prolonged hyperventilation may be caused by CNS or pulmonary disorders. **Hypoventilation** is a reduction in the rate and depth of respirations. This decrease in the amount of air entering the lungs causes an increase in arterial carbon dioxide levels.

Difficult or labored breathing is called *dyspnea*. Patients with dyspnea require increased, noticeable effort to breathe, and often appear as if struggling to get air into the lungs. In an effort to increase effectiveness of respiration, accessory muscles such as the intercostals and abdominals are often active. The intercostals assist in raising the ribs to expand the thoracic cavity; the abdominals assist function of the diaphragm. Additional muscles that may provide accessory functions in respiration are the sternocleidomastoid, pectoralis major and minor, scalenes, and the subclavius. Use of accessory muscles to breathe is referred to as **costal** or **thoracic breathing.** Dyspnea is sometimes accompanied by pain and nasal flaring (to bring in more oxygen). Acute episodes may be brought on by blockage of an air passage, infection of the respiratory tract, or trauma to the thorax. Long-standing dyspnea is a hallmark of the chronic obstructive pulmonary diseases (COPD) such as asthma or bronchitis. Therapists often instruct patients with COPD in a breathing technique called *pursed-lip breathing* to help prevent small airway collapse. Air is inhaled slowly through the nose and slowly exhaled through pursed lips.

Orthopnea is difficult or labored breathing (dyspnea) when the patient is lying down that is relieved by moving to a sitting or standing position. The change in positioning causes gravity to lower abdominal organs, allowing increased room for chest expansion. Orthopnea is a characteristic symptom of heart failure and also may be seen with asthma, advanced emphysema, and pulmonary edema. **Tachypnea** is an abnormally fast RR, usually greater that 24 breaths per minute. This pattern is seen with respiratory insufficiency and fever as the body attempts to rid itself of excess heat. During fever, RR may increase as much as 4 per minute with each 1°F (0.6° C) increase in temperature.[23] **Bradypnea** is an abnormally slow RR, usually 10 breaths or fewer per minute. Bradypnea is associated with impairment of the respiratory control center as may occur with increased intracranial pressure (tumor), drug intake (narcotics) or metabolic disorder. **Apnea** is the absence of respirations and is usually transient. If sustained for longer than several minutes, brain damage and death may occur.

Because respiration is under both voluntary (cortical) and involuntary control, it is important that the patient is unaware that respiration is being examined. Once aware of the examination, characteristics of the breathing pattern will likely be altered. This is a normal reaction to being observed. It is often recommended that respirations be observed immediately after taking the pulse. After monitoring the pulse, the fingers can remain in place at the pulse site, and respirations can be monitored without drawing the patient's conscious attention to his or her breathing pattern. Ideally, respiration should be examined with the chest exposed. If this is not possible, or if respirations cannot be easily observed through clothing, maintain fingers on the radial pulse site and place the patient's arm across the chest. This will allow limited palpation without drawing conscious input from the patient. Chapter 15 provides a more thorough discussion of the respiratory examination.

Procedure for Monitoring Respiration

A. Assemble equipment

1. Watch (or wall clock) with a second hand

B. Wash hands (see Box 4.3)

C. Procedure

1. Ensure patient safety and comfort. Respirations are typically monitored with the patient either supine or sitting.
   Note: The patient should be in a quiet resting position for at least 5 minutes prior to monitoring respirations.
2. Expose chest area; if area cannot be exposed and respirations are not readily observable, place patient's arm across chest and keep fingers positioned as if continuing to monitor the radial pulse.
3. As the patient breathes, observe the rise and fall of the chest; note the amount of effort required or audible sounds produced during breathing (normally, respiration is effortless and silent).
4. Using the second hand of a watch or clock, determine the rate by counting respirations (either inspirations or expirations, but not both) for 30 seconds and multiply by 2.
5. Identify the rhythm (regularity of inspirations and expirations); note deviations from normal uninterrupted, even spacing. If any irregularities are noted, count for a full 60 seconds to accommodate the fluctuations and ensure an accurate count.
6. Observe the depth of respiration; determine if a small, large, or approximately normal volume of air is inspired. Observe involvement of accessory muscles which suggests weakness in the primary muscles of breathing (diaphragm and external intercostal muscles); if difficult to observe, palpation of chest wall excursion can be used to identify depth of respiration. Record as shallow, deep, or normal.
   Note: Chest wall excursion can also be determined by circumferential chest measures using a tape measure

at specific bony landmarks. Three common landmarks for circumferential chest measures are: (1) the sternal angle of Luis; (2) the xiphoid process; and (3) midway between the xiphoid process and the umbilicus.

7. If indicated, determine the sound of breathing using a stethoscope.
8. Return clothing if chest has been exposed.
9. Wash hands.

Monitoring Arterial Blood Pressure

Blood pressure (BP) refers to the force the blood exerts against a vessel wall. It is measured in millimeters of mercury (mm Hg) and recorded in the form of a fraction (e.g., 119/79). The top number indicates systolic pressure, the bottom indicates diastolic pressure. Because liquid flows only from a higher to a lower pressure, the pressure is highest in the arteries, lower in the capillaries, and lowest in veins.[14,15]

Inasmuch as the heart is an intermittent pulsatile pump, pressure is measured at both the highest and lowest points of the pulse. These points are represented by the systolic (ventricular contraction) and diastolic (ventricular relaxation) pressures. The **systolic pressure** is the highest pressure exerted by the blood against the arterial walls. The **diastolic pressure** (which is constantly present) is the lowest pressure. The elastic properties of the arterial walls allow for expansion and recoil in response to the changing volume of circulating blood during the cardiac cycle. The mathematical difference between the systolic and diastolic pressures is called the **pulse pressure.** For example, a systolic pressure of 119 mm Hg and a diastolic pressure of 79 mm Hg result in a pulse pressure of 40 mm Hg.

BP is a function of two primary elements: (1) cardiac output (amount of blood flow); and (2) peripheral resistance (impediment to blood flow within a vessel) that the heart must overcome. The relationship between blood pressure (BP) and cardiac output (CO) and peripheral resistance (R) is expressed in the equation: $BP = CO \times R$. Additional factors that contribute to this relationship include the diameter and elasticity of vessel walls, blood volume, and blood viscosity.[26]

Blood Pressure Regulation

The *vasomotor center* is located bilaterally in the lower pons and upper medulla. It transmits impulses through sympathetic nerves to all vessels of the body. The vasomotor center is tonically active, producing a slow, continual firing in all vasoconstrictor nerve fibers. It is this slow, continual firing that maintains a partial state of contraction of the blood vessels and provides normal *vasomotor tone.*[18] The vasomotor center assists in providing the stable arterial pressure required to maintain blood flow to body tissue and organs. This occurs because of its close connection to the cardiac controlling center in the medulla (because changes in cardiac output will influence BP). In addition, the vasomotor and cardiac controlling centers require input from afferent receptors.

Afferent input regarding BP is provided primarily by *baroreceptors* and *chemoreceptors*. The *baroreceptors* (pressoreceptors) are stimulated by stretch of the vessel wall from alterations in pressure. These receptors have a high concentration in the walls of the internal carotid arteries above the carotid bifurcation and in the walls of the arch of the aorta. Baroreceptors located in the *carotid sinuses* of the carotid arteries monitor BP to the brain. Baroreceptors in the *aortic sinuses* of the aortic arch are responsible for monitoring BP throughout the body.

In response to an increase in BP, the baroreceptor input to the vasomotor center results in an inhibition of the vasoconstrictor center of the medulla and excitation of the vagal center.[14] This results in a decreased HR, decreased force of cardiac contraction, and vasodilation, with a subsequent drop in BP. The baroreceptor input during a lowering of BP would produce the opposite effects.

The *chemoreceptors* are stimulated by reduced arterial oxygen concentrations, increases in carbon dioxide tension, and increased hydrogen ion concentrations. These receptors lie close to the baroreceptors. Those located in the carotid artery are called *carotid bodies,* and on the aortic arch they are termed *aortic bodies*. Impulses from these receptors travel to the brain (cardioregulatory and vasomotor centers) via afferent pathways in the vagus and glossopharyngeal nerves. Efferent impulses from these centers, in response to alterations in BP, will alter HR, strength of cardiac contractions, and size of blood vessels.[16,65]

Factors Influencing Blood Pressure

Many factors influence pressure. As with all vital signs, BP is represented by a range of normal values and will yield the most useful data when monitored over a period of time. Several important factors that should be considered when examining BP include blood volume, diameter and elasticity of arteries, cardiac output, age, exercise, and arm position.

Blood Volume

The amount of circulating blood in the body directly affects pressure. Blood loss (e.g., hemorrhage) will cause pressure to drop, and can result in **hypovolemic shock** from inadequate tissue perfusion. Conversely, an increase in the amount of circulating blood (e.g., blood transfusion) will cause the pressure to rise. Reduced fluid volume, as may occur with diarrhea or inadequate oral intake (dehydration), will also lower BP; excess fluid, as occurs with congestive heart failure, will increase pressure.[24] Essentially, any situation causing a shift (increase or decrease) in body fluids (intravascular, interstitial, or intracellular) will alter BP.[24] Bladder distension may also contribute to BP elevation.

Diameter or Elasticity of Arteries

The size (diameter) of the vessel lumen will provide either increased peripheral resistance (vasoconstriction) or decreased resistance (vasodilation) to cardiac output. The elasticity of the vessel wall also influences resistance. Normally, the expansion and recoil properties of the arterial walls provide a continuous, smooth flow of blood into the capillaries and veins between heartbeats. With age, these properties are diminished. Thus, there is a higher resistance to blood flow with resultant *increase* in systolic pressure. Because the flexibility and recoil properties are diminished, there is a *lower* diastolic pressure. A characteristic feature of arteriosclerosis is reduced vessel wall compliance in response to fluctuations in pressure.

Cardiac Output

When increased amounts of blood are pumped into the arteries, the walls of the vessels distend, resulting in a higher BP. With lower cardiac output, less blood is pushed into the vessel, and there is a subsequent drop in pressure.

Age

BP varies with age (see Table 4.1). It normally rises gradually after birth and reaches a peak during puberty. By late adolescence (18 to 19 years), adult BP is reached. For many years, the normal adult BP was considered 120/80 mm Hg. In 2003, new BP guidelines were presented in the Seventh Report of the Joint National Committee on Prevention, Detection, Evaluation, and Treatment of High Blood Pressure: The JNC 7 Report (Table 4.7).[66] The new recommendations recognize the high prevalence of hypertension that affects about 50 million individuals in the United States and 1 billion people worldwide. Hypertension is a primary risk factor for myocardial infarct, heart failure, stroke, and kidney disease. The earlier normal adult BP value of 120/80 mm Hg now falls into the new category of prehypertension (systolic pressure: 120 to 139; diastolic pressure: 80 to 89). A BP value of 119/79 mm Hg or below is the new adult standard. The JNC 7 Report recommends implementation of expansive and effective measures to prevent further increases in the prevalence of hypertension.[66]

Table 4.7 Classification of Blood Pressure for Adults Ages 18 Years and Older

BP Classification	Systolic BP (mm Hg)	Diastolic BP (mm Hg)
Normal	<120	<80
Prehypertension	120–139	80–89
Hypertension		
Stage 1	140–159	90–99
Stage 2	≥160	≥100

From Chobanian, AV, et al[66] with permission.

For older adults, the rise in blood pressure values is primarily because of the degenerative effects of arteriosclerosis. Small arteries and arterioles lose their elasticity, the walls of the vessels become thick and hard rendering them unable to yield to the pressure exerted by blood flow, and the lumen gradually narrows and may eventually become blocked. This results primarily in an increase in systolic pressure. Because the vessel walls gradually lose the ability to recoil with decreased pressure, diastolic pressure also increases.

Exercise

Physical activity will increase cardiac output, with a consequent linear increase in BP. Greater increases are noted in systolic pressure owing to proportional changes in pressure gradient of peripheral vessels. This means that although cardiac output during exercise is high, vasodilation reduces peripheral resistance to maintain a relatively low diastolic pressure. BP increases are proportional to the intensity of the workload.

Valsalva Maneuver

The **Valsalva maneuver** is an attempt to exhale forcibly with the glottis, nose, and mouth closed. It causes an increase in intrathoracic pressure with an accompanying collapse of the veins of the chest wall. There is a subsequent decrease in blood flow to the heart, a decreased venous return, and a drop in arterial BP. This maneuver serves to internally stabilize the abdominal and chest wall during periods of rapid and maximum exertion such as lifting a heavy object. When the breath is released, the intrathoracic pressure decreases, and venous return is suddenly reestablished as an "overshoot" mechanism to compensate for the drop in BP. In turn, there is a marked increase in HR and arterial BP. This rapid rise in arterial pressure causes vagal slowing of the HR (bradycardia). Although the Valsalva maneuver can temporarily enhance muscle function via the internal stabilization, it has an indirect undesirable effect by increasing BP and should be avoided by individuals with cardiac impairment.[15,18]

CLINICAL NOTE: A common misconception concerning the Valsalva maneuver is that it directly increases HR and BP. As described above, it is the body's recovery mechanism of suddenly increasing venous return that causes this increase. The subsequent drop in BP due to the Valsalva maneuver may result in seeing "black dots" and the feeling of dizziness that often accompanies straining while lifting a heavy object.

Postural (Orthostatic) Hypotension

Associated with prolonged immobility and periods of bed rest, *postural (orthostatic) hypotension* is a sudden drop in BP that occurs when movement to upright postures (sitting or standing) is initiated. The positional change causes a gravitational blood pooling in the lower extremity veins. Venous return and cardiac output are reduced with a resultant cerebral hypoperfusion. This triggers an episode of lightheadedness or even loss of consciousness. In response to positional changes under normal circumstances, BP is maintained by reflex vasoconstriction (baroreceptors), which increases HR. After a period of inactivity, postural hypotension should be anticipated and requires a gradual acclimation to the upright position until normal reflex control returns. Other predisposing factors for postural hypotension include exercise, drugs such as antihypertensives and vasodilators, reduction in baroreceptor response with aging, the Valsalva maneuver, and **hypovolemia** (abnormally low volume of circulating blood).[67,68] As a useful precaution, any patient restricted to a recumbent position for even short periods should be considered at risk for postural hypotension. These events can be minimized by use of external pressure supports such as abdominal binders or full-length elastic stockings (elastic bandages can also be used effectively) and a very gradual acclimation to upright postures. Should postural hypotension occur during treatment, the patient should be reclined from upright and the legs elevated.

Arm Position

BP may vary as much as 20 mm Hg by altering arm position. For consistency of measures, the patient should be sitting with the arm in a horizontal, supported position at heart level. If patient condition or the type of activity precludes these positions, alterations should be carefully documented. As with other vital signs, factors such as fear, anxiety, or emotional stress also will cause an increase in BP.

Other Risk Factors

High BP is also associated with high sodium intake, obesity and being overweight, a sedentary lifestyle, heavy alcohol consumption, pregnancy, gender, and age (until age 55 men have a greater risk for high BP than women, between 55 and 75 years of age the relative risks are comparable, after age 75 women are at greater risk), race (African Americans are at greater risk as compared Caucasians), and heredity (parental history of high BP places the individual at greater risk). In addition, some medications can either increase BP or interfere with antihypertensive drugs. These drugs include steroids, nonsteroidal anti-inflammatory agents, diet pills, cyclosporine, erythropoietin, tricyclic antidepressants, monoamine oxidase inhibitors, and some oral contraceptives.[69]

Equipment Requirements

A noninvasive or *indirect* measure of BP is used by physical therapists. In critical care settings, invasive or *direct* measures of BP are obtained by placing a thin catheter directly into an artery. The equipment required for taking

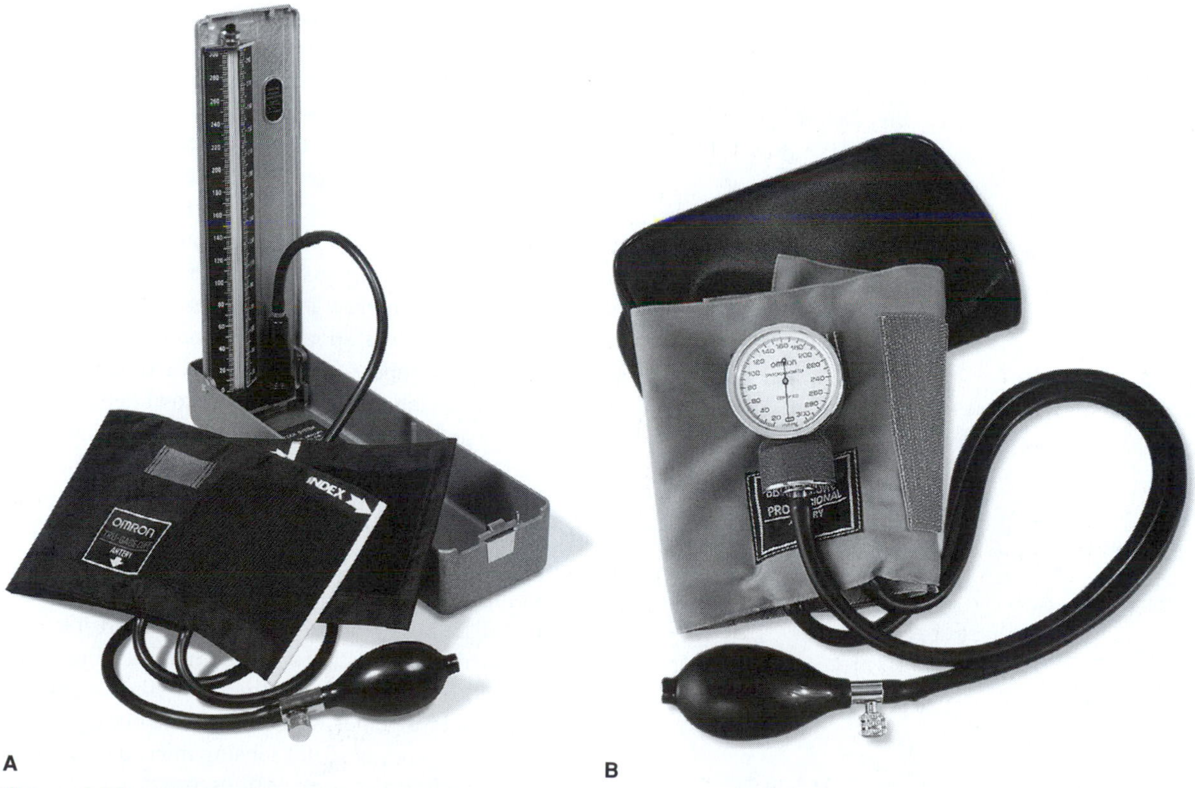

A B

Figure 4.22 Sphygmomanometers. (*A*) Mercury gauge manometers have a vertical glass tube containing liquid mercury with a 300 mm Hg scale marked in 2-mm increments. (*B*) Aneroid manometers consist of a circular glass-covered 300 mm Hg gauge in 2-mm increments with needle marker. (Courtesy of Omron, Inc, Vernon Hills, IL 60061.)

blood pressure using the more common noninvasive auscultatory (listening) method includes a *sphygmomanometer* and a *stethoscope*. The sphygmomanometer (frequently referred to as a *blood pressure cuff*) consists of a flat, airtight, inflatable, latex bladder. The bladder is covered with a cotton or nylon sleeve that extends beyond the length of the bladder. There are two tubes that extend from the cuff. One is attached to a rubber bulb that has a valve used to maintain or to release air from the cuff. The second tube is attached to a pressure manometer (portion of sphygmomanometer that registers the pressure reading).

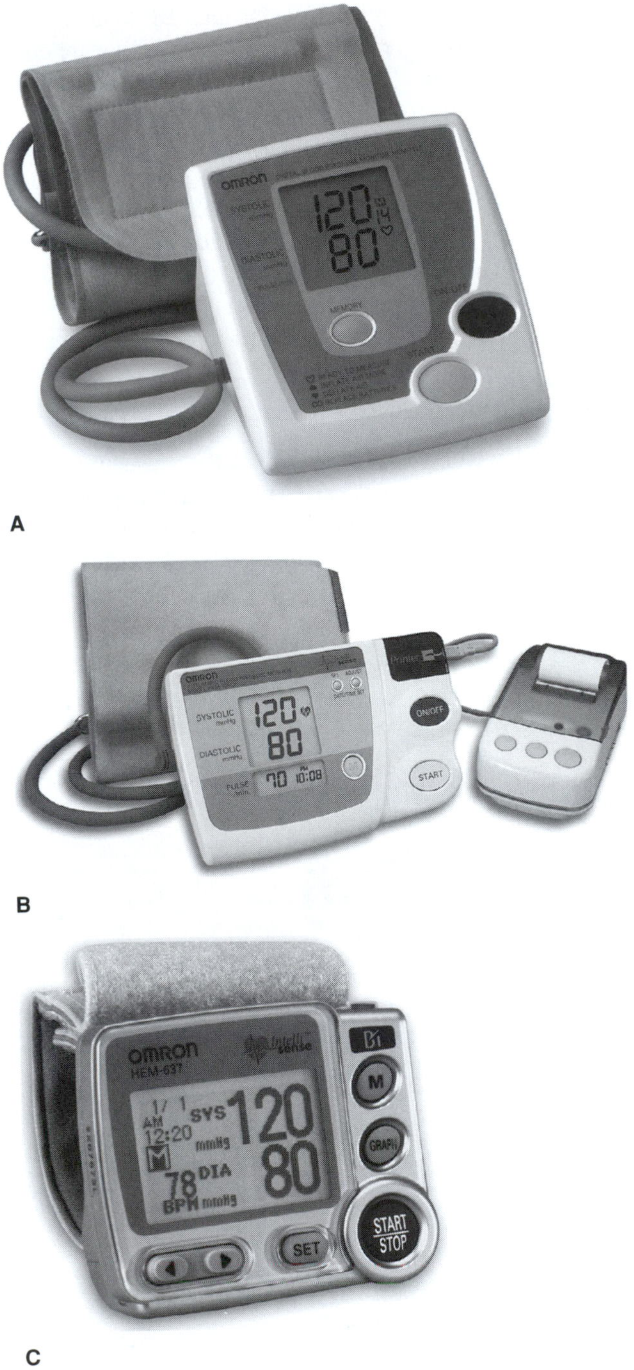

Figure 4.23 Electronic sphygmomanometers. (*A*) Arm cuff monitor. (*B*) Arm cuff monitor with printer that provides a hard copy record of blood pressure and pulse readings in either numerical or bar graph format. (*C*) Wrist monitor. (Courtesy of Omron, Inc, Vernon Hills, IL 60061.)

BP cuffs are typically secured on the patient's extremity by a Velcro™ closure. They come in a variety of sizes. The bladder within the cuff should be long enough to encircle 80 percent of the arm. Obtaining a cuff of appropriate size is important. Cuffs that are too narrow will show inaccurately high readings; cuffs that are too wide will show inaccurately low readings.[66,70]

The manometer registers the BP reading. Manometers are termed either *mercury* or *aneroid* (Fig. 4.22A and B). The mercury manometer registers BP on a mercury-filled calibrated cylinder. At the uppermost portion of the mercury column is a convex curve called the *meniscus*. A reading is obtained by viewing the meniscus at *eye level*. If not observed directly at eye level, an inaccurate reading will be obtained. The aneroid manometer registers BP by way of a circular calibrated dial and needle.

Electronic sphygmomanometers are also available. These are self-inflating battery-powered units; some models are equipped with an AC adapter as well as storage capacity. They provide a rapid digital display of blood pressure and many also monitor pulse. They are particularly useful and practical for patients requiring frequent self-monitoring. A stethoscope is not required because during automated inflation and deflation the diastolic and systolic pressures are recorded. Electronic sphygmomanometers are easy to use; once the cuff is in place all that is required is to activate the start button (Fig. 4.23).

To monitor BP with a mercury or aneroid sphygmomanometer, an acoustic stethoscope is used to listen to the sounds over the artery as pressure is released from the cuff. By a combination of listening through the stethoscope and watching the manometer, the BP reading is obtained. A stethoscope amplifies and carries body sounds to the examiner's ears. Proximally, it consists of two rubber or plastic earpieces attached to narrow metal tubing that projects laterally from the earpieces about 1 inch and then downward about 6 inches. The tubes are connected by a flexible, semicircular metal spring mechanism; the total length of a stethoscope is approximately 30 inches. These metal tubes are referred to as *binaurals* (designed for use in both ears). The semicircular spring provides tension to maintain position of the earpieces in the examiner's ears during use. The metal tubes then either (1) insert into fork-shaped rubber or plastic tubing that joins to form a single lumen and attach to the head distally (Fig. 4.24, left); or (2) insert into two separate rubber or plastic tubes that do not join (Fig. 4.24, right) and lead individually directly to the diaphragm (the two tubes are held together with small metal clasps).

There are two types of distal sensing microphones (also called *head* or *chestpiece*) on stethoscopes: a *bell-shape* (Fig. 4.25, left) and a *flat disk diaphragm* (Fig. 4.25, right). Stethoscopes may have only one type of head; others have a combination design with one side bell-shaped and the

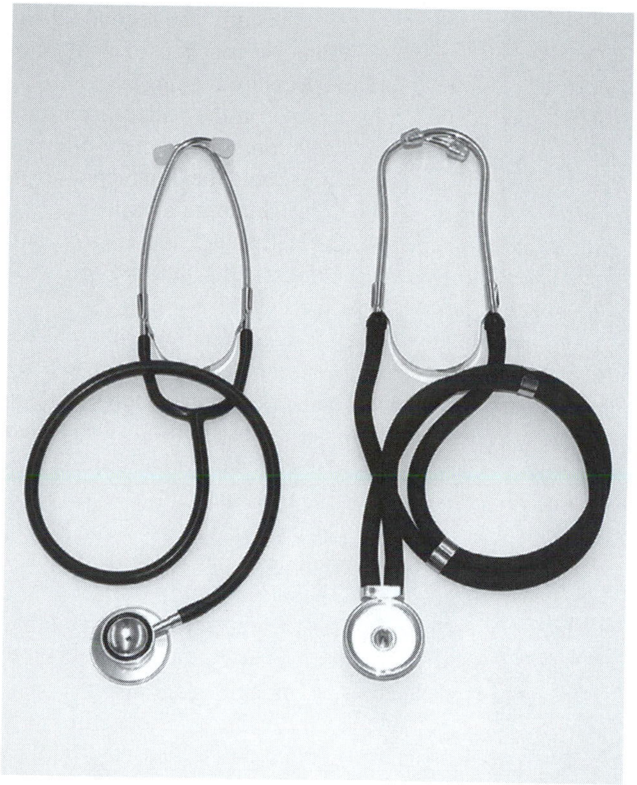

Figure 4.24 Stethoscopes. Standard acoustic stethoscope with a single tube leading to diaphragm (*left*) and Sprague Rappaport type stethoscope with two separate tubes leading to diaphragm (*right*).

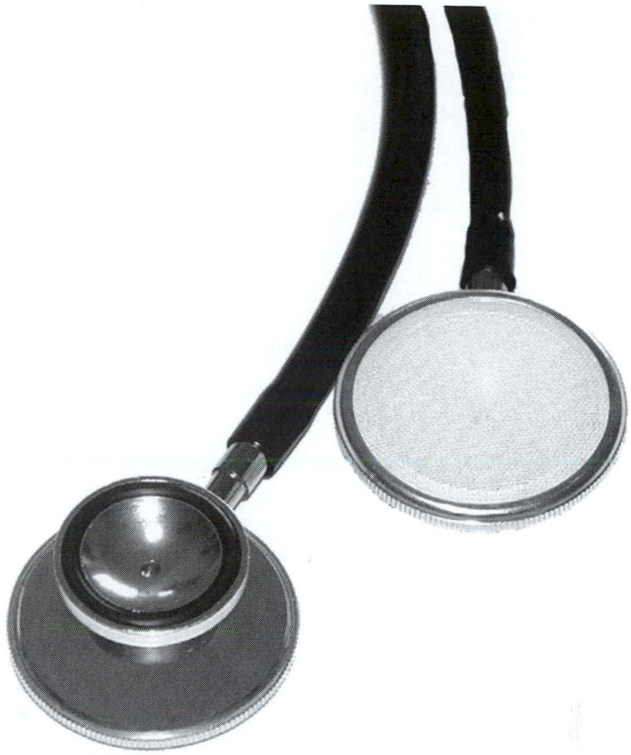

Figure 4.25 Combination design stethoscope head with one side bell-shaped (*left*) to auscultate low-frequency sounds and the opposite side a flat disk diaphragm (*right*) for high-frequency sounds.

other a flat disk. The bell-shape amplifies low-frequency sounds such as those produced in blood vessels and are generally recommended for determining BP. The flat disk diaphragm is more useful for high-frequency sounds such as heart and lung sounds. Another type of sensor incorporates both high- and low-frequency capabilities of the two shapes into a single-sided unit that eliminates the need to turn the head over. To hear low-frequency sound (bell-shape), light pressure of the examiner's fingers is used; firm pressure allows high-frequency sounds to be heard.

Electronic (battery-powered) stethoscopes (Fig. 4.26A) provide higher levels of amplification with volume control, and dual-frequency sound filtering; some are available with interchangeable removable heads. A design variation for prehospital Emergency Medical Service (EMS) personnel provides higher amplification levels by replacing the earpieces with a headset (Fig. 4.26B). The headset is designed to block out noise in a moving ambulance allowing the paramedic to hear low breath and heart sounds and to monitor BP.

Disposable stethoscopes are also available for use in high-risk settings where minimizing the risk of cross-infection is essential.

Korotkoff's Sounds

When measuring BP, a series of sounds is heard through the stethoscope called **Korotkoff's sounds**. The bell side of the stethoscope is used for auscultation because Korotkoff's sounds are low-frequency. Initially when pressure is applied through the cuff around the patient's arm, the blood flow is occluded and no sound is heard through the stethoscope. As the pressure is gradually released, a series of five phases of sounds can be identified.

The therapist should be alert for the presence of an **auscultatory gap** especially in patients with BP above normal values (hypertension). An auscultatory gap is the temporary disappearance of sound normally heard over the brachial artery between phase 1 and 2 and may cover a range of as much as 40 mm Hg. Not identifying this gap may can lead to an underestimation of systolic pressure and overestimation of diastolic pressure.

- **Phase I:** The first clear, faint, rhythmic tapping sound that gradually increases in intensity is heard. The period when blood initially flows through the artery is recorded as *systolic pressure*. This represents the highest pressure in the arterial system during ventricular contraction. *Be alert for an auscultatory gap.*
- **Phase II:** A murmur or swishing sound is heard as artery widens and more blood flows through artery.
- **Phase III:** Sounds become crisp, more intense, and louder; blood is now flowing relatively unobstructed.
- **Phase IV:** Sound is distinct, abrupt muffling; soft blowing quality. "In children less than 13 years old, pregnant

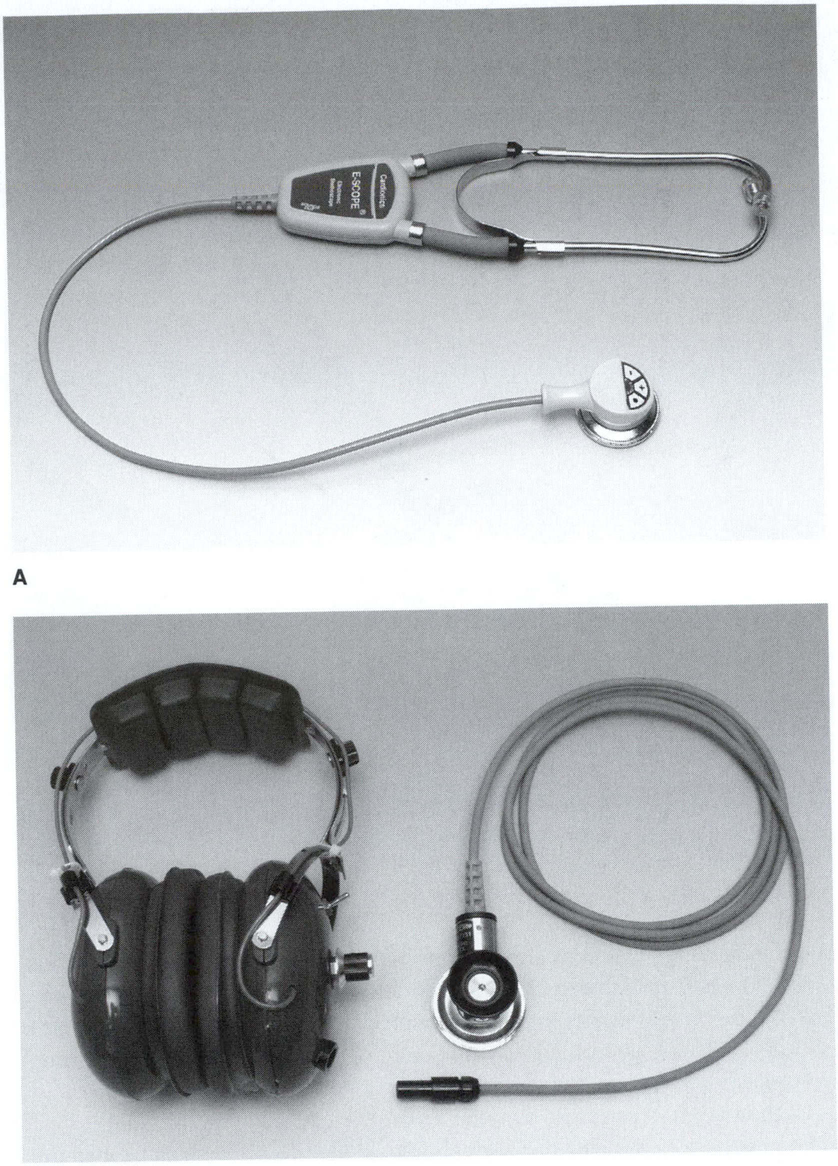

Figure 4.26 Electronic stethoscopes. (*A*) Standard electronic stethoscope and (*B*) electronic stethoscope with headset to block out environmental noise designed for use by Emergency Medical Service (EMS) personnel. (Courtesy of Cardionics, Inc, Webster, TX 77598.)

women, and patients with high cardiac output or peripheral vasodilatation, sounds are often heard at levels far below those at which muffling occurs, sometimes to levels approaching 0 mm Hg. In these situations, for practical purposes, muffling should be used to indicate diastolic pressure, but both muffling (phase IV) and disappearance (phase V) should be recorded."[70, p 6]

- **Phase V:** Last sound is heard; is recorded as *diastolic pressure* in adults.

The American Heart Association recommends use of the fifth phase as the most accurate index of diastolic pressure in adult populations.[70] A BP reading with a systolic pressure of 117 and a second diastolic reading of 76 would be recorded as 117/76. In specific instances (as noted above) where both phase IV and V are recorded as diastolic pressures, three numbers are documented. For example, a systolic pressure of 117, a phase IV reading of 78 and a phase V value of 76 would be recorded as 117/78/76.

A primary consideration in determining BP is that it should be done in a minimal amount of time. The BP cuff acts as a tourniquet. As such, venous pooling and considerable discomfort to the patient will occur if the cuff is left in place too long. The brachial artery is the most common site for BP monitoring and will be described in detail. A description for monitoring lower extremity BP is also presented.

Procedure for Measuring Brachial Blood Pressure

A. Assemble equipment

1. A stethoscope. A bell-shaped head is preferred; however, a diaphragm can also be used effectively.

2. A sphygmomanometer with a blood pressure cuff (size of cuff should be appropriate for size of extremity). In adults, the width of the bladder should be 40 percent of the arm circumference (measurement can be made using a tape measure midway between the acromion and olecranon processes) and should be long enough to encircle at least 80 percent of the arm. In children, the bladder should be long enough to completely encircle the entire arm.[66,70]
3. Antiseptic wipes for cleaning earpieces and head of stethoscope before and after use.

B. Wash hands (see Box 4.3)

C. Procedure

1. Explain procedure and rationale in terms appropriate to the patient's understanding. Indicate there will be a request to remain quiet during monitoring to avoid interference with auscultation.
   Note: As with other vital sign measures, BP is monitored after the patient has been in a relaxed quiet setting for a period of time as activity or physical exertion will cause an elevation in measurements.
2. Assist the patient to the desired position (the sitting position is recommended). If a supine position is used, the arm should be at the patient's side and slightly elevated to the middle of the trunk. If measuring BP in standing (e.g., monitoring postural hypotension) ensure the arm is supported at heart level.
3. Ensure patient understanding, safety, and comfort.
4. Use antiseptic wipe to clean the earpieces and head of stethoscope.
5. Expose the patient's arm; the midpoint of the arm should be at heart level with the elbow slightly flexed. With the patient in a seated position, the upper extremity should be supported on a treatment table or other appropriate surface.
6. Wrap the deflated cuff snuggly and evenly around the patient's bare arm approximately 1 inch (2.5 cm) above the antecubital fossa; the center of cuff should be in line with the brachial artery (Fig. 4.27). Avoid rolling up a garment sleeve as this will create a tourniquet effect.
7. Ensure the aneroid gauge is easily visible; a mercury manometer must be on a level surface at eye level. Check that the sphygmomanometer registers zero.
   Note: The first time BP is measured on a patient, an estimation of the systolic pressure should be made. This will ensure that during the actual measure, an adequate level of cuff inflation is used. The procedure is as follows: (a) locate and palpate the radial artery on the distal forearm of the cuffed upper extremity; (b) close the valve of the BP cuff (turn clockwise); (c) while continuing to monitor the pulse, rapidly inflate the BP cuff to 30 mm Hg above the level at which the radial pulse is no longer felt; (d) note the pressure value on the gauge; this is the estimate of maximum pressure required to measure systolic pressure for the individual patient; and (e) allow air to release quickly.

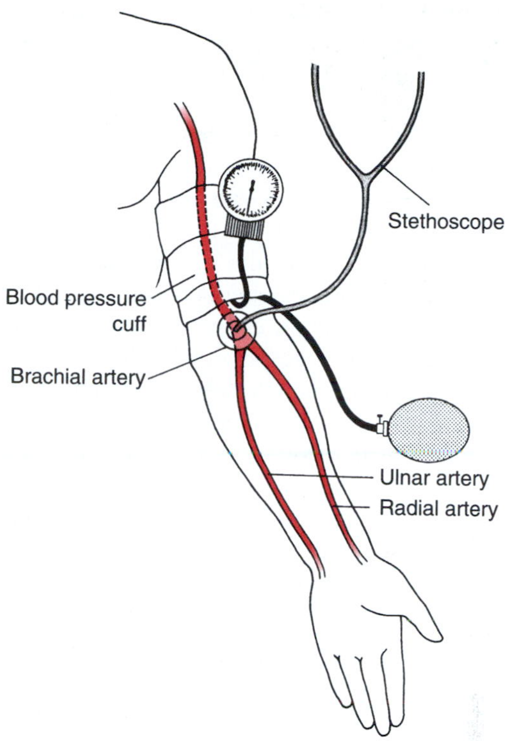

Figure 4.27 Placement of blood pressure cuff and stethoscope for monitoring brachial artery blood pressure.

8. Place the earpieces of the stethoscope (tilting slightly forward) into ears; the tubes of the stethoscope should not be crossed and should hang freely; use the low-frequency bell side of stethoscope head.
9. Locate and palpate the brachial artery slightly above and medial to the antecubital fossa. Place the head of the stethoscope firmly over the artery at the lower border of the BP cuff (see Fig. 4.27). Sufficient pressure should be used to avoid gapping between circumference of stethoscope head and skin.
   Note: In situations where the pulse is extremely weak and undetectable, Doppler ultrasound may be substituted for use of the stethoscope.
10. Close the valve of the BP cuff (turn clockwise), and inflate the cuff to the estimated level previously determined or until the manometer registers approximately 20 to 30 mm Hg above the anticipated systolic pressure.
11. Release the valve carefully, allowing air out slowly; air should be released at a rate of 2 to 3 mm Hg per heartbeat. Listen for the appearance of Korotkoff sounds.
12. Watch the manometer closely and note the point at which the first sound is heard (a mercury manometer must be viewed at eye level); this is the point

where blood first begins to flow through the artery and represents the systolic pressure (phase I). Deflections in the dial or column of mercury will now be noted.
Note: If Korotkoff sounds are difficult to hear, have the patient raise the cuffed arm overhead and make a fist several times. With the arm still overhead, inflate the cuff to 50 mm Hg above anticipated systolic pressure; return the arm to heart-level rapidly and continue measurement in usual manner.[70]

13. Continue to release air carefully. Note when the sound first becomes muffled (phase IV) and the value on the manometer when the sound disappears (phase V); this is recorded as the diastolic pressure.
14. Allow remainder of air to release quickly.
Note: After a minimum 30-second interval, The American Heart Association recommends repeating the BP measurement and averaging the two values.[70]
15. Clean the head and earpieces of stethoscope with antiseptic wipes. If the same examiner is using the stethoscope again, it is not necessary to clean the earpieces. However, the head of the stethoscope should always be cleaned between patients.

Procedure for Measuring Popliteal (Thigh) Blood Pressure

Measurement of popliteal BP is indicated in situations where comparisons between the upper and lower extremity is warranted, such as peripheral vascular disease. They also are used when upper extremity pressures are contraindicated, such as following trauma or surgery. Essentially, the procedure is the same as that for determining pressure at the brachial artery, with the following variations:

1. The patient is placed in a prone position; alternately, the supine position may be used. The knee is placed in slight flexion to facilitate placement of stethoscope in popliteal space. In comparison to the brachial artery, the popliteal artery usually yields higher systolic pressure owing to use of the larger bladder; diastolic values are approximately the same or slightly lower.
2. Expose the thigh area using appropriate draping procedures.
3. Locate the popliteal artery by palpation (posterior knee).
4. Wrap the deflated cuff snuggly and evenly around the patient's midthigh (a wide cuff is used; use guidelines for cuff size described for brachial BP). The center of the bladder should be directly over the popliteal artery.
Note: As described for brachial BP, a palpatory estimate of maximum pressure required to measure systolic pressure can be made using the popliteal or dorsalis pedis artery.
5. Proceed with auscultating the pressure as for the brachial artery.

Recording Results

For purposes of physical therapy documentation, many therapists include vital signs data directly within the narrative format of their note. Using the SOAP (Subjective, Objective, Assessment, Plan) format, vital sign data is included in the *objective section*. In the Patient/Client Management Model described in the Guide to Physical Therapist Practice[1] these data are included in *Tests and Measures*. The most important element in recording this information is that it allows easy comparison from one entry to the next. The date, time of day, patient position, examiner's name, and equipment used should all be clearly indicated. For example, assume a vital signs examination provided the following data: Temperature: 98.9°F, taken orally; a pulse of 84 beats per minute (bpm), with fluctuations between weak and strong beats; a respiratory rate of 16 per minute, with a regular rhythm and unlabored quality; and a BP reading of 122/84 mm Hg in sitting and 120/86 mm Hg standing. A sample format for including these data as a component of narrative documentation is presented in Box 4.4.

The nursing section of the medical record is an important source of vital signs data. Here, data is typically provided in graph form with time represented on the horizontal axis and the measured values on the vertical axis. The visual record allows easy identification of data trends reflective of normal variations or a response to disease or therapeutic intervention.[24] For the therapist practicing in facilities where such forms are used, familiarity with the specific recording system is important. Several methods are used to differentiate vital sign entry; they generally include some variation of open and closed circles, connecting lines, color codes, or other symbols to differentiate among temperature, HR, RR, and BP data. Modifications of this type of form also may be useful for documenting response to physical therapy treatment.

Box 4.4 Elements of Documentation for Vital Signs Data

Patient Name: __________	**Therapist:** __________
Date:	(date of examination)
Time:	(time of day examination performed)
Position:	(sitting)
Equipment:	(electronic thermometer; mercury manometer)*
Temp:	98.9°F (oral)
HR:	84/min; alternating quality (weak/strong)
RR:	16/min; regular, deep, unlabored
BP:	122/84 mm Hg (sitting) 120/80 mm Hg (standing)

* If equipment includes identification numbers, they should be included in documentation.

BP = blood pressure; HR = heart rate; RR = respiratory rate; Temp = temperature.

Summary

Values obtained from monitoring vital signs provide the physical therapist with important information about the patient's physiological status. Results from these measures assist in establishing and maintaining a database of values for an individual patient. They also assist in formulating clinical judgments for determining the diagnosis and prognosis, designing the plan of care, and establishing and evaluating effectiveness of selected treatment interventions.

The procedure for measuring each vital sign has been presented. Because multiple factors influence vital signs, the most useful data are obtained when measures are taken at periodic intervals rather than as single measure in time. Sequential measures allow changes in patient status or response to treatment to be monitored over time, as well as indicate an acute change in status at a specific point in time.

For purposes of physical therapy documentation, vital signs data are typically included within the narrative format of the note. Use of a graph to record this information may prove a useful adjunct to the physical therapy record. Regardless of the system of documentation selected, of critical importance is that it allows easy comparison of serial entries over time.

Questions for Review

1. Together with other examination data, vital sign measures help guide clinical judgments about what elements of the patient/client management model?
2. Prior to a vital signs examination, what preliminary data can be obtained by a careful systematic observation of the patient?
3. Explain why vital sign values are more useful when monitored as a serial process as compared to measurement at a single point in time?
4. Describe the primary mechanisms by which the body conserves and produces heat; differentiate the four primary heat loss mechanisms: radiation, conduction, convection, and evaporation.
5. Describe the procedure for determining both oral and axillary temperatures.
6. Define pulse rate, rhythm, and volume.
7. What factors influence the pulse?
8. Describe the procedure for monitoring the radial pulse.
9. What is a pulse deficit? What information does it provide?
10. What parameters are addressed when monitoring respiration? Define each.
11. What factors influence respiration?
12. Describe the Valsalva maneuver. Identify its influence on HR and BP during and after the maneuver.
13. Describe the procedure for monitoring respiration.
14. What factors influence BP?
15. What are the five phases of Korotkoff's sounds?
16. When monitoring brachial BP, what guidelines are used to determine the appropriate cuff size? How does a cuff that is too narrow or too wide effect BP measures?
17. Describe the procedure for determining blood pressure using a stethoscope and sphygmomanometer.

Case Study

EMERGENCY ROOM ADMISSION

A 24-year-old man was separated from his skiing group due to an unexpected and violent snowstorm. The situation was complicated by his being in an unfamiliar area without electronic communication. A 2-day helicopter search located him after approximately 48 hours of exposure to temperatures that ranged between 10° and 20°F. The emergency team initiated intravenous fluid replacement (to help restore fluid and electrolyte balance) en-route to the hospital.

HISTORY

As reported by his parents, medical history is unremarkable except for the usual childhood diseases. He had recently relocated to the area because of a desire to be a competitive skier (an activity he has enjoyed all his life). He works as an accountant for a local investment firm.

ADMITTING DIAGNOSIS

Hypothermia and frostbite of the toes, thumb, and index and middle fingers, bilaterally.

Blood pressure: Systolic pressure is 45 mm Hg; diastolic not perceptible.
Pulse: Decreased rate, small, weak carotid pulse (12 bpm); peripheral pulses not perceptible.
Respiratory rate: 6 breaths per minute; respirations barely perceptible.
Temperature: 82°F (rectal).
Cognition: Depressed, unresponsive.
Deep tendon reflexes: Absent.

Cutaneous sensation: Unresponsive to all sensory modalities, including pain.
Integument: Marked skin color changes; bluish gray appearance of earlobes, lips, fingers, and toes.

PHYSICAL THERAPY

The patient is now in the Intensive Care Unit (ICU) and a referral has been made to physical therapy requesting "examination and treatment."

GUIDING QUESTIONS

1. Describe the body system responses to hypothermia as presented by the clinical features of the case.
2. Considering this patient is unresponsive and cyanotic, what would be the most appropriate pulse to monitor? Provide a brief rationale for your answer.
3. The function of the thermoregulatory center becomes seriously impaired when body temperature falls below approximately _______ and is completely lost with temperatures below _______.
4. Extremes in environmental temperature have a large impact on the body's ability to maintain constant temperatures. What type of clothing can best assist in protecting the body from low environmental temperatures?

References

1. American Physical Therapy Association: Guide to physical therapist practice. Phys Ther 81:1, 2001.
2. Grabbe, LL: Physical assessment skills. In Morton, PG (ed): Health Assessment, ed 2. FA Davis, Philadelphia, 1995, p 16.
3. Lewis, PS: Cardiovascular assessment. In Ruppert, SD, et al (eds): Dolan's Critical Care Nursing: Clinical Nursing Through the Nursing Process, ed 2. FA Davis, Philadelphia, 1991, p 151.
4. Tripp-Reimer, T, Johnson, R, and Sorofman, B: Cultural dimensions in gerontological nursing. In Stanley, M, and Beare, PG: Gerontological Nursing, ed 2. FA Davis, Philadelphia, 1999, p 21.
5. Metzgar, ED: The health history. In Morton, PG (ed): Health Assessment, ed 2. FA Davis, Philadelphia, 1995, p 3.
6. Spector, RE: Cultural Diversity in Health and Illness, ed 6. Pearson Education, Upper Saddle River, NJ, 2004.
7. Fitzgerald, MA: Nursing Health Assessment: Concepts and Activities. FA Davis, Philadelphia, 1995.
8. Purnell, LD, and Paulanka, BJ (eds): Transcultural Health Care: A Culturally Competent Approach, ed 2. FA Davis, Philadelphia, 2003.
9. Lynch, EW, and Hanson, MJ (eds): Developing Cross-Cultural Competence: A Guide for Working with Young Children and Their Families, ed 2. Brookes, Baltimore, 1998.
10. Galanti, G: Caring for Patients from Different Cultures, ed 3. University of Pennsylvania Press, Philadelphia, 2003.
11. Luckman, J, and Nobles, ST: Transcultural Communication in Health Care. Delmar Thomson Learning, Albany, NY, 2000.
12. Huff, RM, and Kline, MV: Promoting Health in Multicultural Populations: A Handbook for Practitioners. SAGE Publications, Thousand Oaks, CA, 1999.
13. Hansen, M: Pathophysiology: Foundations of Disease and Clinical Intervention. WB Saunders, Philadelphia, 1998.
14. Guyton, AC, and Hall, JE: Human Physiology and Mechanisms of Disease, ed 6. WB Saunders, Philadelphia, 1997.
15. McArdle, WD, Katch, FI, and Katch, VL: Exercise Physiology: Energy, Nutrition, and Human Performance, ed 5. Lippincott Williams & Wilkins, Philadelphia, 2001.
16. Guyton, AC, and Hall, JE: Textbook of Medical Physiology, ed 10. WB Saunders, Philadelphia, 2000.
17. Lemons, DE, Riedel, G, and Downey, JA: Thermoregulation and the effects of thermomodalities. In Gonzalez, EG, Myers, SJ, Edelstein, JE, Lieberman, JS, and Downey, JA: Downey & Darling's Physiological Basis of Rehabilitation Medicine, ed 3. Butterworth Heinemann, Boston, 2001, p 507.
18. McArdle, WD, Katch, FI, and Katch, VL: Essentials of Exercise Physiology, ed 2. Lippincott Williams & Wilkins, Philadelphia, 2000.
19. Powers, SK, and Howley, ET: Exercise Physiology, ed 4. McGraw-Hill, New York, 2001.
20. Thomas, CL (ed): Taber's Cyclopedic Medical Dictionary, ed 19. FA Davis, Philadelphia, 2001.
21. Goodman, CC, and Kelly Snyder, TE: Infectious disease. In Goodman, CC, Boissonnault, WG, and Fuller, KS (eds): Pathology: Implications for the Physical Therapist, ed 2. WB Saunders, Philadelphia, 2003, p 194.
22. Kozier, B, et al: Fundamentals of Nursing: Concepts, Process, and Practice, ed 6. Prentice Hall Health, Upper Saddle River, NJ, 2000.
23. Taylor, C, Lillis, C, and LeMone, P: Fundamentals of Nursing: The Art and Science of Nursing Care, ed 4. Lippincott Williams & Wilkins, 2001.
24. Craven, RF, and Hirnle, CJ (eds): Fundamentals of Nursing: Human Health and Function, ed 3. Lippincott Williams & Wilkins, NewYork, 2000.
25. Smith, SF, Duell, DJ, and Martin, BC: Clinical Nursing Skills: Basic to Advanced Skills, ed 5. Prentice Hall Health, Upper Saddle River, NJ, 2000.
26. Perry, AG, and Potter, PA: Clinical Nursing Skills and Techniques, ed 5. Mosby, Philadelphia, 2002.
27. Centers for Disease Control and Prevention (CDC): Guidelines for Hand Hygiene in Health-Care Settings: Recommendations of the Healthcare Infection Control Practices Advisory Committee and the HICPAC/SHEA/APIC/IDSA Hand Hygiene Task Force. MMWR 2002; 51 (No. RR-16), CDC, Department of Health and Human Services, Atlanta, GA, 2002.
28. Wilkins, F: Infection Control. In Daniels, R (ed): Nursing Fundamentals: Caring and Clinical Decision Making. Delmar Learning, Clifton Park, NY, 2004, p 507.
29. Rayman, SM: Health assessment. In Daniels, R (ed): Nursing Fundamentals: Caring and Clinical Decision Making. Delmar Learning, Clifton Park, NY, 2004, p 545.
30. Bates, B: A Guide to Physical Examination and History Taking, ed. 5. Lippincott, Philadelphia, 1991.
31. Stevens, J, and MacAuley, D: Older exercise participants. In Kolt, GS, and Snyder-Mackler, L (eds): Physical Therapies in Sport and Exercise. Churchill Livingstone, Philadelphia, 2003. p 483.
32. Moore, KL, and Dalley, AF: Clinically Oriented Anatomy (ed. 4). Lippincott Williams & Wilkins, Philadelphia, 1999.
33. Achten, J, and Jeukendrup, AE: Heart rate monitoring: Applications and limitations. Sports Med 33(7):517, 2003.
34. Boudet, G, and Chaumoux, A: Ability of new heart rate monitors to measure normal and abnormal heat rate. J Sports Med Phys Fitness 41: 546, 2001.
35. Laukkanen, RMT, and Virtanen, PK: Heart rate monitors: State of the art. J Sports Sci 16:S3, 1998.
36. Gandsas, A, et al: In-flight continuous vital signs telemetry via the Internet. Aviat Space Envir Md 71(1):68, 2000.
37. Sims, AJ, Pay, DA, and Watson, BG: An architecture for the automatic acquisition of vital signs by clinical information systems. IEEE T Inf Technol B 4(1):74, 2000.
38. Thivierge, M, and Leger, L: Critical review of heart rate monitors. Can Assoc Health Phys Educ Rec J 55(3):26, 1989.
39. Crouter, SE, Albright, C, and Bassett, DR, Jr: Accuracy of polar S410 heart rate monitor to estimate energy cost of exercise. Med Sci Sports Exerc 36(8):1433, 2004.

40. Leger, L, and Thivierge, M: Heart rate monitors: Validity, stability, and functionality. Physician Sports Med 16:143, 1988.
41. Godsen, R, Carroll, T, and Stone, S: How well does Polar Vantage XL Heart Rate Monitor estimate actual heart rate? Med Sci Sports Exerc, Suppl, 23(4):S14, 1991.
42. Terbizan, DJ, Dolezal, BA, and Albano, C: Validity of seven commercially available heart rate monitors. Meas Phys Educ Exerc Sci 6(4):243, 2002.
43. Macfarlane, DJ, Fogarty, BA, and Hopkins, WC: The accuracy and variability of commercially available heart rate monitors. N Zeal J Sports Med 17(4):51, 1989.
44. Seaward, BL, et al: The precision and accuracy of a portable heart rate monitor. Biomed Instrum Technol 24(1):37, 1990.
45. Treiber, FA, et al: Validation of a heart rate monitor with children in laboratory and field settings. Med Sci Sports Exerc 21(3):338, 1989.
46. Patterson, GK: Vascular evaluation. In Sussman, C, and Bates-Jensen, BM (eds): Wound Care: A Collaborative Practice Manual for Physical Therapists and Nurses. Aspen Publishers, Gaithersburg, MD, 2001, p 177.
47. Mohr, JP, and Young, WL: Anatomy and physiology of the vascular supply to the brain. In Gonzalez, EG, Myers, SJ, Edelstein, JE, Lieberman, JS, and Downey, JA: Downey & Darling's Physiological Basis of Rehabilitation Medicine, ed 3. Butterworth Heinemann, Boston, 2001, p 17.
48. Roberts, JM: Vascular assessment. In Merriman, LM, and Turner, W (eds): Assessment of the Lower Limb, ed 2. Churchill Livingstone, Philadelphia, 2002, p 79.
49. Myers, BA: Wound Management: Principles and Practice. Prentice Hall, Upper Saddle River, NJ, 2004.
50. Howell, M: Pulse oximetry: An audit of nursing and medical staff understanding. Br J Nurs 11(3):191, 2002.
51. Cottrell, GP: Cardiopulmonary Anatomy and Physiology for Respiratory Care Practitioners. FA Davis, Philadelphia, 2001.
52. Berry, BE, and Pinard, AE: Assessing Tissue Oxygenation. Critical Care Nurse 22(3):22, 2002.
53. Clinical Monograph: Monitoring Oxygen Saturation with Pulse Oximetry. Nellcor Pruitan Bennett, Inc, Pleasanton, CA, 2001. Retrieved September 25, 2004, from http://www.nellcor.com.
54. Massery, M, and Cahalin, LP: Physical therapy associated with ventilatory pump dysfunction and failure. In DeTurk, WE, and Cahalin, LP: Cardiovascular and Pulmonary Physical Therapy: An Evidence-Based Approach. McGraw-Hill, New York, 2004, p 593.
55. Weinberger, SE: Principles of Pulmonary Medicine, ed 4. WB Saunders, Philadelphia, 2004.
56. Collins, SM, and Cocanour, B: Anatomy of the cardiopulmonary system. In DeTurk, WE, and Cahalin, LP: Cardiovascular and Pulmonary Physical Therapy: An Evidence-Based Approach. McGraw-Hill, New York, 2004, p 73.
57. Henderson, BS: Anatomy and physiology of the respiratory system. In Ruppert, SD, et al (eds): Dolan's Critical Care Nursing: Clinical Management Through the Nursing Process, ed 2. FA Davis, Philadelphia, 1996, p 387.
58. Goodman, CC: The respiratory system. In Goodman, CC, Boissonnault, WG, and Fuller, KS (eds): Pathology: Implications for the Physical Therapist, ed 2. WB Saunders, Philadelphia, 2003, p 553.
59. Schelegle, ES, and Green, JF: An overview of the anatomy and physiology of slowly adapting pulmonary stretch receptors. Respir Physiol 125:17, 2001.
60. Hassan, A, et al: Volume activation of the Hering Breuer inflation reflex in the newborn infant. J Appl Physiol 90:763, 2001.
61. Certo, C: Cardiopulmonary Rehabilitation of the Geriatric Patient and Client. In Lewis, CB: Aging: The Health-Care Challenge, ed 4. FA Davis, Philadelphia, 2002, p 143.
62. Robergs, RA, and Keteyian, SJ: Fundamentals of Exercise Physiology for Fitness, Performance, and Health. McGraw-Hill, New York, 2003.
63. Arnheim, DD, and Prentice, WE: Principles of Athletic Training, ed 9. McGraw-Hill, New York, 1997.
64. Woo, TM: Drugs Affecting the Respiratory System. In Wynne, AL, Woo, TM, and Millard, M: Pharmacotherapeutics for Nurse Practitioner Prescribers. FA Davis, Philadelphia, 2002, p 311.
65. Gilman, S, and Newman, SW: Manter and Gatz's Essentials of Clinical Neuroanatomy and Neurophysiology, ed. 10. FA Davis, Philadelphia, 2003.
66. Chobanian, AV, et al. Seventh report of the Joint National Committee on Prevention, Detection, Evaluation, and Treatment of High Blood Pressure: The JNC 7 report. JAMA 289(19):2560, 2003.
67. Goodman, CC: The cardiovascular system. In Goodman, CC, Boissonnault, WG, and Fuller, KS (eds): Pathology: Implications for the Physical Therapist, ed 2. WB Saunders, Philadelphia, 2003, p 367.
68. Gould, BE: Pathophysiology for the Health Related Professions. WB Saunders, Philadelphia, 1997.
69. American Heart Association. Heart and Stroke Facts. American Heart Association, Dallas, TX, 1992-2003. Retrieved September 25, 2004, from http://www.americanheart.org.
70. Perloff, D, et al: Human Blood Pressure Determination by Sphygmomanometry. American Heart Association, Dallas, TX, 2001. Retrieved September 16, 2004, from http://www.americanheart.org.

Supplemental Readings

American Heart Association: BLS [Basic Life Support] for Healthcare Providers. American Heart Association, Dallas, TX, 2001.

Attin, M, et al: An educational project to improve knowledge related to pulse oximetry. Am J Crit Care 11(6):529, 2002.

Brack, T, Jubran, A, and Tobin, MJ: Dyspnea and decreased variability of breathing in patients with restrictive lung disease. Am J Respir Care Med 165:1260, 2002.

Carroll, M: An evaluation of temperature measurement. Nursing Standard 14(44):39, 2000.

Chauhan, A, et al: Role of respiratory function in exercise limitation in chronic heart failure. Chest 118(1):53, 2000.

Cottin, F, Papelier, Y, and Escourrou, P: Effects of exercise load and breathing frequency on heart rate and blood pressure variability during dynamic exercise. Int J Sports Med 20:232, 1999.

Crouter, SE, Albright, C, and Bassett, DR: Accuracy of polar S410 heart rate monitor to estimate energy cost of exercise. Med Sci Sports Exerc 36(8):1433, 2004.

Eastwood, PR, Hillman, DR, and Finucane, KE: Inspiratory muscle performance in endurance athletes and sedentary subjects. Respirology 6:95, 2001.

Edmonds, ZV, et al: The reliability of vital sign measurements. Ann Emerg Med 39:233, 2002.

Evans, D, Hodgkinson, B, and Berry, J: Vital signs in hospital patients: A systematic review. Int J Nurs Stud 38:643, 2001.

Giuliano, KK, et al: Temperature measurement in critically ill adults: A comparison of tympanic and oral methods. Am J Crit Care 9(4):254, 2000.

Halberg, F, et al: Engineering and governmental challenge: 7-day/24 hour chronobiologic blood pressure and heart rate screening; Part I. Biomed Instrum Technol 36(2):89, 2002.

Jensen BN, et al: Accuracy of digital tympanic, oral, axillary, and rectal thermometers compared with standard rectal mercury thermometers. Eur J Surg 166(11):848, 2000.

Kocoglu, H, et al: Infrared tympanic thermometer can accurately measure the body temperature in children in an emergency room setting. Int J Pediatr Otorhinolaryngol 65(1):39, 2002

Lavietes, MH, et al: Inspiratory muscle weakness in diastolic dysfunction. Chest 126(3):838, 2004.

Lucia, A, et al: Breathing pattern in highly competitive cyclists during incremental exercise. Eur J Appl Physiol 79:512, 1999.

Mattu, GS, Heran, BS, and Wright, JM: Comparison of the automated non-invasive oscillometric blood pressure monitor (BpTRU) with the auscultatory mercury sphygmomanometer in a paediatric population. Blood Press Monit 9(1):39, 2004.

Mattu, GS, Perry, TL, and Wright, JM: Comparison of the oscillometric blood pressure monitor (BPM-100_{Beta}) with the auscultatory mercury sphygmomanometer. Blood Press Monit 6(3):153, 2001.

Miura, K: Strategies for prevention and management of hypertension throughout life. J Epidemiol 14(4):112, 2004.

O'Brien, E, et al: Blood pressure measuring devices: Recommendations of the European Society of Hypertension. BMJ 322:531, 2001

Piergiuseppe, A, et al: Exercise hyperpnea in chronic heart failure: Relationships to lung stiffness and expiratory flow limitation. J Appl Physiol 92:1409, 2002.

Reppert, SM, and Weaver, DR: Coordination of circadian timing in mammals. Nature 418:935, 2002.

Smith, LS: Reexamining age, race, site, and thermometer type as variables affecting temperature measurement in adults: A comparison study. BMC Nurs 2(1):1, 2003.

Smith, LS: Using low-tech thermometers to measure body temperatures in older adults: A pilot study. J Gerontol Nurs 29(11):26, 2003.

Terathongkum, S, and Pickler, RH: Relationships among heart rate variability, hypertension, and relaxation techniques. J Vasc Nurs 22(3):78, 2004.

Terbizan, DJ, Dolezal, BA, and Albano, C: Validity of seven commercially available heart rate monitors. Measure Phys Educ Exer Sci 6(4):243, 2002.

Vercueil, L, et al: Breathing pattern in patients with Parkinson's disease. Resp Physiol 118:163, 1999.

Wilhelm, FH, Roth WT, and Sackner, MA: The LifeShirt: An advanced system for ambulatory measurement of respiratory and cardiac function. Behav Modif 27(5):671, 2003.

Zeller A, et al: Blood pressure and heart rate of students undergoing a medical licensing examination. Blood Press 13(1):20, 2004.

CHAPTER

5

Examination of Sensory Function

Thomas J. Schmitz, PT, PhD

LEARNING OBJECTIVES

1. Understand the purpose(s) of performing a sensory examination.
2. Understand the relationship between preliminary mental status screening tests and tests for sensory integrity.
3. Describe the classification and function of the receptor mechanisms involved in the perception of sensation.
4. Identify the spinal pathways that mediate sensation.
5. Understand the guidelines for administering an examination of sensory function.
6. Describe the testing protocol for each sensory modality.
7. Using the case study example, apply clinical decision-making skills to application of sensory examination data.

OUTLINE

Sensory Integration

If all of the sensory stimuli which enter the central nervous system were allowed to bombard the higher centers of the brain, the individual would be rendered utterly ineffective. It is the brain's task to filter, organize, and integrate a mass of sensory information so that it can be used for the development and execution of the brain's functions.[1, p 25]

—*A. Jean Ayers, PhD*

The human system is continually inundated with sensory information from a variety of environmental inputs as well as from movement, touch, awareness of the body in space, sight, sound, and smell. "In all higher order motor behaviors, the brain must correlate sensory inputs with motor outputs to accurately assess and control the body's interaction with the environment."[2, p 32] **Sensory integration** is the ability of the brain to organize, interpret, and use sensory information. This integration provides an internal representation of the environment that informs and guides motor responses.[2] These sensory representations provide the foundation on which motor programs for purposeful movements are planned, coordinated, and implemented.[3] Ayers defined *sensory integration* as "the neurological process that organizes sensation from one's own body and from the environment and makes it possible to use the body effectively within the environment."[4, p 11] In an intact system, sensory integration occurs automatically without conscious effort.

Sensory integration is a theory developed by A. Jean Ayers, an occupational therapist whose work focused on examining the manner in which sensory integration develops, identifying patterns of dysfunction in children with learning disorders, and developing intervention strategies to improve processing of sensory information. The theory purports that disordered sensory integration directly impacts both motor and cognitive learning and that interventions designed to enhance sensory integration will improve learning.[1] Bundy and Murray[5] suggest the value of the theory lies in its usefulness in: (1) explaining behaviors of individuals with impaired sensory integration functions, (2) establishing a plan of care (POC) to address specific impairments, and (3) predicting expected outcomes of the selected interventions.

Sensation and Movement

Motor learning and motor performance are inextricably linked to *sensation*. As a motor task is practiced, the individual learns to anticipate and correct or modify movements based on sensory input organized and integrated by the central nervous system (CNS). The CNS uses this information to influence movement by both feedback and feedforward control. Feedback control uses sensory information received *during the movement* to monitor and adjust output. Feedforward control is a proactive strategy that uses sensory information obtained from experience. Signals are sent in *advance of movement* allowing for anticipatory adjustments in postural control or movement.[3,6] The primary role of sensation in movement is to: (1) guide selection of motor responses for effective interaction with the environment and (2) adapt movements and shape motor programs through feedback for corrective action. Sensation also provides the important function of protecting the organism from injury. See Chapter 8 for a more detailed discussion of CNS control of motor function.

Sensory Integrity

The term *somatosensation* (somatosensory) refers to sensation received from the skin and musculoskeletal system (as opposed to that from specialized senses such as sight or hearing). Examination of sensory function involves testing sensory integrity by determining the patient's ability to interpret and discriminate among incoming sensory information. The sensory examination is based on the premise that within the intact human system, sensory information is taken in from the body and the environment; the CNS then processes and integrates the information for use in planning and organizing behavior. This premise is more aptly termed a *theoretical construct* (a concept that represents an *unobservable* event). We cannot *directly* observe CNS processing, integration of sensory information, or the motor planning process. However, our current knowledge of CNS function and motor behavior provides evidence that these unobservable events do occur. We *can* observe impairments in motor behavior, but can only *hypothesize* that they truly result from faulty sensory integration mechanisms.[5]

The *Guide to Physical Therapist Practice* defines sensory integrity as "the intactness of cortical sensory processing, including proprioception, pallesthesia, stereognosis, and topognosis."[7, p 690] Sensory integrity is included among the list of 24 categories of tests and measures that may be used by physical therapists during patient examination and is included in all practice patterns (i.e., musculoskeletal, neuromuscular, cardiovascular/pulmonary, and integumentary).

Box 5.1 presents examples of pathologies, impairments, functional limitations, disabilities, risk factors, and health, wellness, and fitness needs associated with changes in sensory integrity.

This chapter focuses primarily on examination of somatosensory integrity of the trunk and extremities as well as screening for cranial nerve integrity; testing approaches for examining *cranial nerve integrity* and *reflex testing* are addressed in Chapter 8. As the CNS analyzes and uses all sensory input to identify movement errors and initiate corrective responses, examination of sensory function typically precedes examination of motor function. This sequence assists the physical therapist in differentiating the impact of sensory impairments on motor function.

Clinical Indications

Indications for examination of sensory function are based on the history and systems review (including a *sensory screening* described later in this chapter). This includes "information provided by the patient/client, family, significant other, or caregiver; symptoms described by the patient/client; signs observed and documented during the systems review; and information derived from other sources and records."[7, p 98] These data may indicate the existence of pathology (or risk of pathology) resulting in sensory changes that may impose impairments, functional limitations, or disability (see Box 5.1).

Sensory dysfunction may be associated with any pathology or injury affecting either the peripheral nervous system (PNS) or CNS, or with a combined involvement of both systems. Deficits may occur at any point within the system including the sensory receptors, peripheral nerves, spinal nerves, spinal cord nuclei and tracts, brainstem,

Box 5.1 Examples of Pathologies, Impairments, Functional Limitations, Disabilities, Risk Factors and Health, Wellness, and Fitness Needs Associated with Changes in Sensory Integrity

I. Pathology/pathophysiology (disease, disorder, or condition) in the following systems:
- Cardiovascular (e.g., cerebral vascular accident, peripheral vascular disease)
- Endocrine/metabolic (e.g., diabetes, rheumatological disease)
- Integumentary (e.g., burn, frostbite, lymphedema)
- Multiple Systems (e.g., AIDS, Guillain-Barré syndrome, trauma)
- Musculoskeletal (e.g., derangement of joint; disorders of bursa, synovia, and tendon)
- Neuromuscular (e.g., cerebral palsy, developmental delay, spinal cord injury)
- Pulmonary (e.g., respiratory failure, ventilatory pump failure)

II. Impairments in the following categories:
- Circulation (e.g., numb feet)
- Integumentary integrity (e.g., redness under orthotic)
- Muscle performance (e.g., decreased grip strength)
- Orthotic, protective, and supportive devices (e.g., wears ankle foot orthosis)
- Posture (e.g., forward head)

III. Functional limitations in the ability to perform actions, tasks, or activities in the following categories:
- Self-care (e.g., inability to put on trousers while standing because of loss of feeling in foot)
- Home management (e.g., difficulty with sorting change because of numbness)
- Work (job/school/play) (e.g., inability as a day care provider to change child's diaper because of loss of finger sensation, inability to operate cash register because of clumsiness)
- Community/leisure (e.g., inability to drive car because of loss of spatial awareness, inability to play guitar because of hyperesthesia)

IV. Disability, that is, the inability or restricted ability to perform actions, tasks, or activities of required roles within the individual's sociocultural context, in the following categories:
- Self-care
- Home management
- Work (job/school/play)
- Community/leisure

V. Risk factors for impaired sensory integrity:
- Lack of safety awareness in all environments
- Risk-prone behaviors (e.g., working without protective gloves)
- Smoking history
- Substance abuse

VI. Health, wellness, and fitness needs:
- Fitness, including physical performance (e.g., inadequate balance to compete in dancing competition, limited perception of arms and legs in space during ballroom dancing)
- Health and wellness (e.g., inadequate understanding of role of proprioception in balance)

From American Physical Therapy Association,[7, p 98] with permission.

thalamus, and sensory cortex.[8] Examples of conditions that generally demonstrate some level of sensory impairment include pathology, disease, or injury to the peripheral nerves such as trauma (e.g., fracture) that can sever, crush, or damage a nerve; metabolic disturbances (diabetes, hypothyroidism, alcoholism); infections (Lyme disease, leprosy, human immunodeficiency virus [HIV]); impingement or compression (arthritis, carpal tunnel syndrome); burns; toxins (lead, mercury, chemotherapy); and nutritional deficits (vitamin B_{12}). Sensory impairments are also associated with injury to nerve roots or spinal cord, cerebral vascular accident (CVA), transient ischemic attack (TIA), tumors, multiple sclerosis, and brain injury or disease. These examples, which are not all-inclusive, indicate the wide spectrum of injuries, disease, and pathologies that may present with some element of sensory deficit.

Pattern (Distribution) of Sensory Impairment

Examination of sensory function contributes critical information to establishing a physical therapy diagnosis and prognosis, identifying anticipated goals and expected outcomes, and developing a POC. A seminal feature of the examination involves determining the *pattern* (specific boundaries) of sensory involvement. Pattern identification is accomplished using knowledge of skin segment innervation by the dorsal roots and peripheral nerves (Figs. 5.1 and 5.2). The term **dermatome** (or *skin segment*) refers to the skin area supplied by one dorsal root.[9]

CLINICAL NOTE: Considerable variation exists in the clinical presentation of sensory impairments. This variability is typically associated with the nervous system involved (CNS vs PNS), the type of injury, pathology, or disease as well as the severity, extent, and duration of involvement.

During the review of systems, asking the patient to carefully describe the pattern or distribution of symptoms (e.g., tingling, numbness, diminished, or absent sensation) provides the therapist with preliminary information to help guide the examination and to assist in identifying the

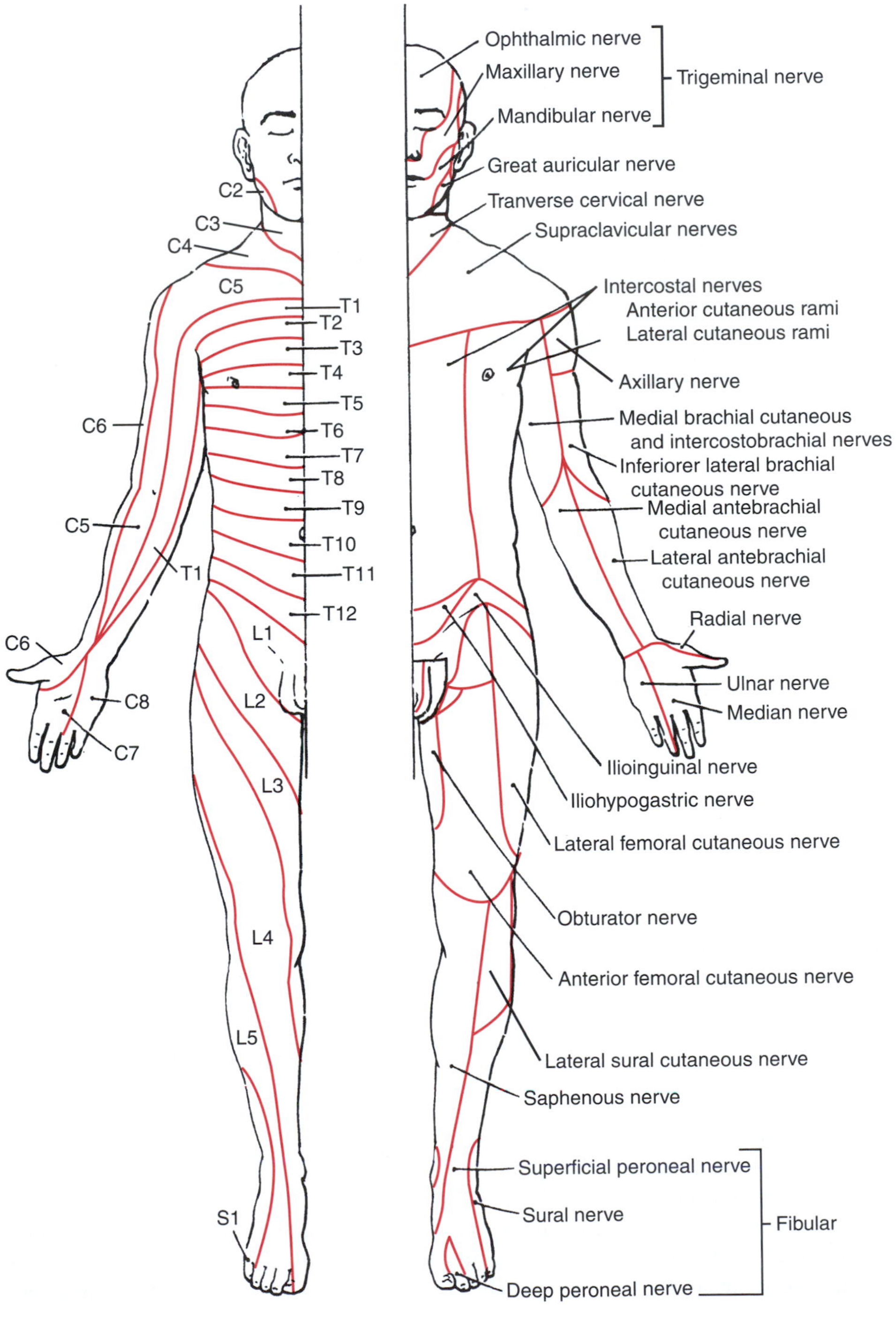

Figure 5.1 Anterior view of skin segment innervation by dorsal roots (*left*) and peripheral nerves (*right*). (From Gilman, S, and Newman, SW,[9, p 43] with permission.)

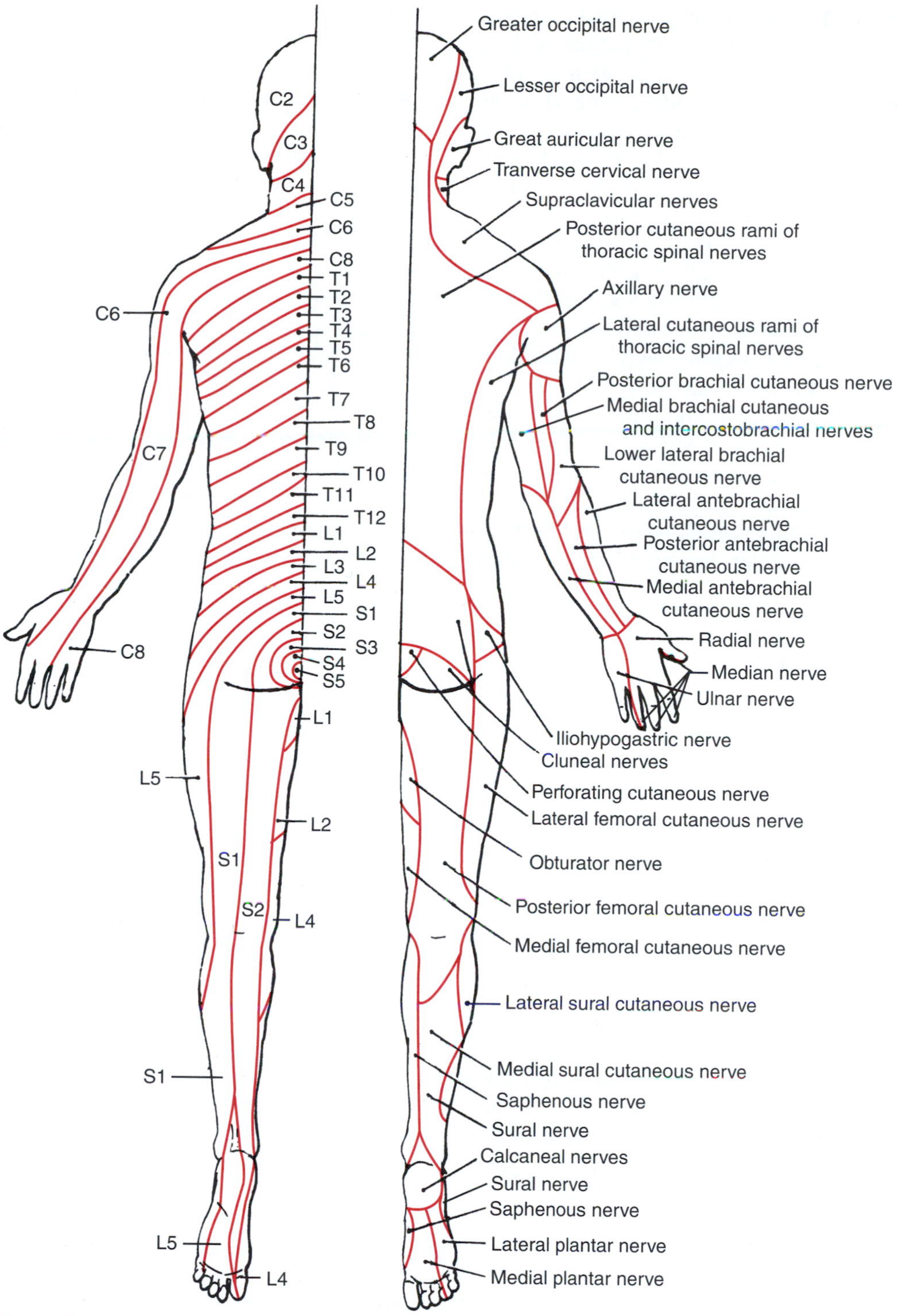

Figure 5.2 Posterior view of skin segment innervation by dorsal roots (*left*) and peripheral nerves (*right*). (From Gilman, S, and Newman, SW,[9, p 44] with permission.)

dermatome(s) and nerve(s) involved. Peripheral nerve injuries generally present sensory impairments that parallel the distribution of the involved nerve and correspond to its pattern of innervation. For example, if a patient presents with complaints of numbness on the ulnar half of the ring finger, the little finger, and the ulnar side of the hand, the therapist would be alerted to carefully address ulnar nerve (C8 and T1) integrity during the sensory examination. Complaints of sensory disturbances on the palmar surface of the thumb and the palmar and distal dorsal aspects of the index, middle, and the radial half of the ring finger would be indicative of median nerve (C6–8 and T1) involvement.

Other patterns of sensory loss may be associated with specific pathology. For example, with peripheral neuropathy (e.g., diabetes), sensory loss is often an early symptom and presents in a "glove and stocking" distribution (referring to the typical involvement of the hands and feet). In contrast, multiple sclerosis frequently presents with an unpredictable or scattered pattern of sensory involvement.

Spinal cord injury (SCI) often presents with a more diffuse pattern of sensory involvement below the lesion level that is typically bilateral, although not necessarily symmetrical. Examination of sensory function following SCI provides critical data that reflect the degree of neurological impairment. Together with other tests and measures, sensory data contribute to determining the relative completeness of the injury, the existence of *zones of partial preservation* (areas distal to a complete lesion that retain partial innervation), symmetry or asymmetry of the lesion, and the presence of sacral sensation below the neurological level of lesion (a defining feature of an incomplete lesion).

Spinal Cord Tracts

Examination of sensory function also provides data that reflect the integrity of the spinal cord tracts that carry somatosensory and special sense (e.g., sight, hearing) information. For example, contralateral loss or impairment of pain and temperature perception is suggestive of lesions in the anterolateral tracts. Deficits in discriminative sensations such as vibration and two-point discrimination suggest lesions of the dorsal column.

Evidence of both sensory and motor loss is usually indicative of nerve root involvement (recall that the dorsal and ventral roots converge to form the spinal nerves). CNS lesions (e.g., CVA, brain injury) may produce significant sensory impairments characterized by a diffuse pattern of involvement (e.g., head, trunk, and limbs) and can result in significant motor dysfunction (sensory ataxia) and impairment of fine motor control and motor learning, as well as present a significant threat of injury to anesthetic limbs (e.g., an inability to determine the temperature of bath water).

Age-Related Sensory Changes

Alterations in sensory function occur with normal aging and should be clearly differentiated from those associated with specific illness, disease, or pathology. In recent years there has been a gradual expansion of interest in and information about the causes and consequences of age-related sensory changes. This has been evident through the expanding body of literature devoted to the neuroscience of aging and its impact on function and quality of life of older adults.[10–34] *Generations*, the Journal of the American Society of Aging, has devoted an entire issue to "Aging and the Senses" (Vol. XXVII; No. 1, Spring, 2003). The topics addressed are specific age-related changes in vision, hearing, and the somatosensory system; treatment, prevalence, and risk factor information; as well as the role of public policy and public health in addressing age-related sensory loss. *Healthy People 2010*,[35] published by the United States Department of Health and Human Services, presents a comprehensive health promotion and wellness agenda for the first decade of the 21st century. The goals of *Healthy People 2010* are to: (1) increase quality and years of healthy life and (2) eliminate health disparities. The first goal draws national attention to an expanding population of older adults and the impact of age (including changes in sensation such as vision and hearing) on health improvement and health promotion strategies. Decreased acuity of many sensations occurs and is considered a characteristic finding with aging.[36–40] The exact morphology of diminished sensation with age has not been completely established. However, several neurological changes have been identified and suggest potential explanations.

Over the lifespan neurons are replaced at a declining rate and this may account for the decline of average weight of the brain with aging. Although a feature of Alzheimer's disease, normal aging does not produce a significant loss in the number of cortical neurons.[40] Other changes in the brain include degeneration of neurons with presence of replacement gliosis, lipid accumulation in the neurons, loss of myelin, and development of neurofibrils (masses of small, tangled fibrils) and plaques on the cells.[40–42] There is also a decrease in the number of enzymes responsible for synthesis of dopamine, norepinephrine, and to a lesser degree acetylcholine,[43] as well as depletion of the neuronal dendrites in the aging brain.[43,44]

Electrophysiological studies have identified a gradual reduction in conduction velocity of sensory nerves with advancing age,[45–47] and this may reflect degenerative changes in myelin sheaths or loss or reduction in size of sensory axons.[45,48] Evoked potentials provide a quantitative measure of sensory function and have been found to decrease in amplitude with age.[27] A reduction in the number of Meissner's corpuscles[49] has also been identified. These corpuscles, responsible for touch detection, are limited to hairless areas and become sparse, take on an irregular distribution, and vary in size and shape with age.[49,50] Age-related changes in morphology and decreased concentrations of Pacinian corpuscles, responsive to rapid tissue movement (e.g., vibration), have also been reported.[51]

Degenerative changes in myelin have been documented in both the central and peripheral nervous systems.[28,40,45] In a review of the literature on the effects of normal aging on myelin and nerve fibers, Peters[40] suggests that

(1) age-associated cognitive decline is more likely due to widespread damage to myelin sheaths of cortical neuron axons than to actual loss of these neurons and (2) the resulting changes in conduction velocity alter the normal timing of neuronal circuits.

In the PNS, a decrease in the distance between the nodes of Ranvier has been associated with advancing age.[52] This finding may be related to a slowing of saltatory conduction identified by some authors.[41,53] Destruction of myelin sheaths has been linked to a reduced expression of primary myelin proteins, axonal atrophy, and to reduced expression and axonal transport of cytoskeletal proteins.[28] As compared to younger subjects, lower sensory nerve conduction velocities have been documented for both the median[45,46] and sural[46] nerves in older subjects.

Documented changes in sensory integrity with aging include changes in response to tactile[24,54,55] and vibratory stimuli,[10,19,22,56] decreased two-point discrimination,[57] and decreased acuity of joint position sense (proprioception).[30,58] Impaired postural control has been demonstrated by reduced performance in timed balance tests[16,17,26,59] as well as increased postural sway.[11,20,60] Age-related reduced efficiency in motor planning has also been documented.[61]

These changes frequently appear in the presence of age-related visual or hearing losses that impair compensatory capabilities. In addition, some medications may further influence the distortion of sensory input. This combination of sensory changes may pose a variety of functional limitations for the elderly individual such as postural instability, exaggerated body sway, balance problems, wide-based gait, diminished fine motor coordination, tendency to drop items held in the hand, and difficulty in recognizing body positions in space. Evidence Summary Box 5.2 provides an overview of research data exploring age-related sensory changes.

CLINICAL NOTE: In addition to age-related sensory changes, functional limitations may be exacerbated by muscle weakness associated with a reduction in the number and size of skeletal muscle fibers and overall cross-sectional area of muscle.

Preliminary Considerations

Accuracy of data from examination of sensory function relies on the patient's ability to respond to application of multiple somatosensory stimuli. Use of several easily administered preliminary tests will provide sufficient data to determine the patient's ability to concentrate on, and respond to, the battery of sensory test items. The two general categories of preliminary tests include the patient's (1) arousal level, attention span, orientation, and cognition[62] and (2) memory, hearing, and visual acuity. These preliminary tests are typically considered with sensory involvement associated with CNS lesions.

Arousal, Attention, Orientation, and Cognition

A necessary first step is to determine the patient's arousal level for participation in the test protocol. **Arousal** is the physiological readiness of the human system for activity.[7] It is described by using traditionally accepted key terms and definitions to identify the patient's level of consciousness. These terms include *alert*, *lethargic*, *obtunded*, *stupor*, and *coma* and represent a continuum of physiological readiness for activity; they are defined as follows[62]:

- *Alert.* The patient is awake and attentive to normal levels of stimulation. Interactions with the therapist are normal and appropriate.
- *Lethargic.* The patient appears drowsy and may fall asleep if not stimulated in some way. Interactions with the therapist may get diverted. Patient may have difficulty in focusing or maintaining attention on a question or task.
- *Obtunded.* The patient is difficult to arouse from a somnolent state and is frequently confused when awake. Repeated stimulation is required to maintain consciousness. Interactions with the therapist may be largely unproductive.
- *Stupor* (semicoma). The patient responds only to strong, generally noxious stimuli and returns to the unconscious state when stimulation is stopped. When aroused, the patient is unable to interact with the therapist.
- *Coma* (deep coma). The patient cannot be aroused by any type of stimulation. Reflex motor responses may or may not be seen.

Reliable information about the integrity of the somatosensory system can be obtained from patients who are alert. Reliability is proportionally reduced in patients with lethargy and nonexistent in patients who are obtunded, stuporous, or comatose.

Attention is selective awareness of the environment or responsiveness to a stimulus or task without being distracted by other stimuli.[6,9,62] Attention can be examined by asking the patient to repeat items on a progressively more challenging list. These repetition tasks can begin with two or three items and gradually progress to longer lists. For example, the patient might be asked to repeat a series of numbers, letters, or words. Another approach to examining attention is to ask the patient to spell words backwards (e.g., book, fork, bottle, garden). The task can be made more challenging by using progressively longer words. Individuals with a high attention span will be able to perform the task. Attention deficits will be apparent when the order of letters is confused.[62]

Orientation refers to the patient's awareness of time, person, and place. In medical record documentation the

Evidence Summary Box 5.2
Research Exploring Age-Related Changes in Sensory Function

Reference	Purpose	Subjects/Design	Results	Conclusions/Comments
Stuart, et al,[10] 2003	To determine if vibrotactile sensibility of several skin surfaces deteriorated equally with advanced age.	Two groups of healthy adults, mean age 20.2 years and 68.6 years, respectively. Four skin sites (palmar surface or the tip of the middle finger, volar surface of the forearm, lateral aspect of the shoulder, cheek caudal to the zygomatica) tested bilaterally for vibration detection thresholds at two frequencies (30 Hz and 200 Hz).	Significant differences were found between the young ($N = 22$) and old ($N = 22$) group. Thresholds were elevated in the old group for both frequency and site, except at the fingertip. Similar effects were found within the old group (those aged 75.90 compared to those aged 65.74).	Confirms that vibration sensitivity decreases in the elderly. The lack of significant deterioration in the fingertips reflects the importance of this area in manipulating and exploring the environment and the resultant plasticity in this area; relatively small sample size.
Tran, et al,[12] 1997	To examine the effect of aging on motion detection and perception.	46 visually normal (visual acuity 20/40) subjects aged 19–92 years. Motion detection was tested objectively via infrared oculography and motion perception was tested via subjects' use of a computer joystick.	Motion detection and perception both showed age-related deterioration.	No relationship was found between detection and perception, suggesting that these two pathways are distinct. Age-related deterioration of motion detection and perception may be related to function of these pathways; relatively small sample size.
Benjuya, et al,[13] 2004	To identify the shift to reliance on visual and somatosensory modalities that takes place during aging as a means for maintaining postural stability.	Two groups of healthy subjects, one group containing 20 subjects, mean age 26.6 (young [Y]), the other containing 32 with a mean age of 77.8 (old [O]). Subjects were tested using a force plate (center of pressure [COP], sway) and surface EMG (dominant leg musculature). Balance was tested for 20 seconds under 4 conditions: (1) eyes open, wide base (EO, WB); (2) eyes closed (EC, WB); (3) EO, narrow base (NB); and (4) EC, NB.	Significant increases found in COP path, sway, and muscle contraction from Y to O under condition 1. Consistently higher values for these data in the O group for condition 2. The O group significantly increased muscle contraction from EO to EC, but most did not have a significant increase in sway, as did group Y. Significant changes found in condition 3 from Y to O in sway and contraction. Similar changes found in condition 4.	Reduction of visual input had a greater impact on postural sway in Y group. EMG showed the O group used a soleus and tibialis anterior co-contraction pattern to control body sway. Older subjects exhibited a tendency to utilize muscular contraction strategies rather than rely on sensory input to control postural sway; relatively small sample size.
Stones, et al,[17] 1986	*Experiment 1:* To determine if (1) age dependency in balance is greater with EO than with EC; (2) correlations of respiratory function are greater with EO; and (3) balance with EO shows greater sensitivity to physical fitness training. *Experiment 2:* To determine if (1) minimally sighted	*Experiment 1:* One-year longitudinal study with two waves; 225 subjects, men and women aged 50 to 82 (mean 62.8) years. More than 50% of the sample participated in a formal exercise program (wave one, wave two, both) consisting of flexibility and endurance training. Balance on one leg was tested for a maximum of 60 seconds. Two measures of respiratory function were taken as well (forced vital capacity, 1-second forced expiratory volume).	*Experiment 1:* EO balance tests showed more age-dependent results than EC tests. EO test showed high relationships with respiratory function and improved with exercise. EO tests found to be more reliable. *Experiment 2:* No significant relationship was found with respect to age. No significant difference was found between those born blind and those with acquired blindness.	EO balance tests give more valid indication of normal postural control skills than EC tests. Postural control may improve with fitness training. Balance skills are lower in subjects with blindness compared to those with some sight, but both are significantly lower than skills seen in sighted subjects; large sample size used for data collection.

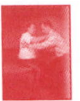

Evidence Summary Box 5.2

Evidence Summary: Research Exploring Age-Related Changes in Sensory Function (continued)

Reference	Purpose	Subjects/Design	Results	Conclusions/Comments
	subjects would have an advantage over blind subjects due to some visual input; and (2) test if balance is better in subjects who acquired blindness as opposed to those born blind.	*Experiment 2*: 22 subjects, either fully blind (15 subjects), or minimally sighted (7 subjects, maximum vision 20%). Ages ranged from 19 to 84 (mean 52.7). Balance was tested with the unipedal balance task.	Minimally sighted subjects had longer balance times than blind subjects.	
Valentijn, et al,[18] 2005	To examine the longitudinal relationship between sensory function and cognitive function after 6-year follow-up in the Maastricht Aging Study.	All participants recruited from the Maastricht Aging Study. 418 individuals (214 men, 204 women) aged 55 and older (mean 65.9). 27 received an intervention to improve sight or hearing. Cognitive measures included the Visual Verbal Learning Test, the Stroop Color Word Test, the Concept Shifting Task, the Verbal Fluency Test, and the Letter-Digit Substitution Test. Sensory measures included: Visual acuity—Landolt-C optotype chart; Auditory acuity—pure tone auditory thresholds.	A change in visual acuity was associated with change in most cognitive measures. Change in hearing acuity was associated with change in memory performance.	These results suggest strong connections between auditory and visual domains and cognitive performance. This supports the need to screen older individuals for sensory deficits so that such deficits will not be confused with cognitive problems; large sample size used for data collection.
Wells, et al,[19] 2003	To determine how much age affects plantar vibration sensation, and to find if these changes depend on frequency and location of the vibration.	12 participants, 6 in a young age group (mean age 26 years), 6 in an older age group (mean age 88 years 8 months). Vibrotactile thresholds were determined for 4 different frequencies at 55 locations at the footsole. Subjects were tested in an unloaded position (laying face down). Testing locations were divided into three groups according to threshold values (toes, arch/ball, lateral border/heel) for purposes of comparison.	Acuity loss was found in elderly persons at frequencies of 50 Hz and higher. The greatest acuity loss was found in the lateral border/heel, followed by the arch/ball, then the toes.	More callused areas showed decreased sensitivity to vibrotactile sense, corroborating earlier investigations that suggest thickening of the skin leads to decreased reception. Decreased vibration sensation may have a detrimental effect on gait; relatively small sample size.
Hughes, et al,[20] 1996	To examine the relationship of postural sway to sensorimotor impairment, functional performance, and self-reported disability.	Cross-sectional cohort study of 100 community-dwelling elderly (mean age 77.2) unable to climb stairs step-over-step. Postural sway (path length, area) was measured using a force platform, 2 trials EO, 2 trials EC. LE strength was measured at the plantarflexors, dorsiflexors, knee flexors and extensors, and hip abductors, along	All measures of postural sway were significantly positively correlated with tibialis latency except EC path length. Area measures were significantly positively correlated with strength indices. Ankle ROM did not have an effect on results. Subjects with impaired sensation had greater sway	These findings suggest that postural sway more likely provides a picture of sensorimotor problems rather than functional abilities. However, this study cannot be generalized to all elderly patients, as all subjects were moderately functionally impaired; relatively large sample size used for data collection.

(continued)

Evidence Summary Box 5.2

Evidence Summary: Research Exploring Age-Related Changes in Sensory Function (continued)

Reference	Purpose	Subjects/Design	Results	Conclusions/Comments
		with tibialis anterior latency after unexpected perturbation of support surface. Ankle dorsiflexion ROM was measured. Ankle proprioception and vibration detection (tuning fork at head of first metatarsal) were measured. Functional performance was measured using functional reach, timed 10-m walk, chair rise, Duke Functional Mobility Skills, and 6-minute walk. Disability was measured using the Falls Efficacy Scale and the MOS-SF36.	with eyes closed. There was no correlation between measures of sway and any measures of functional performance, and very weak correlations were present with measures of disability.	
Wiles, et al,[22] 1991	To collect data from a large cohort of the normal healthy population and produce age related charts of normative data.	1365 healthy volunteers, range 8–91 years. Vibration perception threshold was measured bilaterally at the thumbs, great toes, and over medial malleoli using a hand-held biothesiometer.	Age proved to be the major determinant of vibration thresholds.	These results agree with previous studies that upper and lower extremities exhibit a decrease in vibration sensation after the age of 50; large sample size used for data collection.
Prioli, et al,[25] 2005	To verify the coupling between visual information and body sway in active and sedentary elders.	48 participants were divided into three groups of 16: active elderly (AE), sedentary elderly (SE), and young adults (YA). Subjects were asked to maintain stance in a moving room consisting of three walls and a ceiling. The walls were covered with vertical stripes. The room moved forward and backward either continuously (1.1 cm displacement, 0.69 cm/sec peak velocity) or discretely (2 sec. of displacement, 2.6 cm, 1.3 cm/sec).	While the visual manipulation affected sway in all three groups, the results indicated that the coupling between visual information and body sway was stronger for AE and SE. SE swayed more than AE and YA under discrete conditions.	Changes in elderly postural control might not be due to visual cues from the environment, but how these cues are integrated in order to produce appropriate motor activity. SE were more susceptible to visual manipulation; possibly because they have problems solving a conflicting sensory situation; relatively small sample size.
Gustafson, et al,[26] 2000	To evaluate the change in balance performance in active healthy elderly people in a follow up study 7 years after 30 subjects participated in a study to evaluate the effect of physical training on balance.	17 out of 30 original subjects, mean age of 80.5 years. The original subjects participated in an exercise program consisting of endurance and balance training. The current study had the following components: questionnaire (addressing health habits, vision and hearing, medical history, and activity level); static balance tests (Romberg tests, one legged stance); walking tests (30-m normal and heel-to-toe); and dynamic posturography (sensory organization test [SOT] and movement coordination test [MCT]).	All subjects reported their activity levels to be equal or less than that during the original study. 11 subjects reported balance and vertigo problems. The group had significantly impaired static balance results in 4 of 6 tests compared with the original study (Sharpened Romberg). Time required to walk 30-m had increased significantly. Most dynamic posturography scores had not changed significantly (some MCT changes).	More difficult static balance tests (Sharpened Romberg, one-legged stance) are needed for examining balance in healthy elderly people. There is a need for research concerning how and when different aspects of balance change during aging. While few changes are seen in body sway and SOT from the ages of 73–80, there are changes in difficult static balance tests and MCT.

Evidence Summary Box 5.2

Evidence Summary: Research Exploring Age-Related Changes in Sensory Function (continued)

Reference	Purpose	Subjects/Design	Results	Conclusions/Comments
Bouche, et al,[46] 1993	To study the effects of age on the peripheral nervous system and determine risk factors (RF) that may adversely affect nerve fibers.	59 physically active subjects over 60 years of age and 23 healthy young subjects. All subjects underwent a neurological examination consisting of a sensory examination and a tendon reflex examination, EMG readings using a concentric needle electrode of the tibialis anterior (TA), first dorsal interosseous (FDI), and extensor carpi radialis (ECR). Median and common peroneal nerves were investigated using surface electrodes in order to determine nerve conduction velocities. A laboratory investigation of the elderly subjects consisted of screening for potential causes of peripheral neuropathy of various origins.	The subjects were divided into 5 groups (1, young subjects; 2, younger than 80, without RF; 3, older than 80, without RF; 4, younger than 80, with RF; and 4 older than 80, with RF). 29 elderly subjects were considered to have risk factors. Proprioception impairment, absence of ankle reflexes, and reported sensory system changes clearly increased with age. EMG amplitude decrease was shown in patients over 80. Decrease in nerve conduction velocity was found with increased age, especially after the age of 80. Group number too small to allow statistical analysis of RF.	Age-dependent sensory changes are a result of alterations of the peripheral sensory receptors, muscle and tendon structural changes, and changes in the peripheral nerves. Age-related changes in muscles are known to be caused by myopathic and neurogenic processes; relatively small sample size.
Bohnannon, et al,[59] 1984	To establish a relationship between timed balance performance and age both with EO and EC (increased reliance on proprioceptive input)	184 subjects aged 20 to 79, with 30 or more members in each age decade. Subjects had no vestibular deficits or dysfunction of the trunk and lower extremities. Subjects performed the following balance activities: 1) balancing on two legs, feet 8 inches apart, then together, with EO and then EC and 2) balancing on each leg, eyes open and then eyes closed. Trials were allowed a maximum time of 30 seconds.	All subjects, though some elderly required more than one trial, balanced for 30 seconds in all two-legged stance trials (both EO and EC). For one-legged stance, the mean balance time diminished with age. All subjects under 45 balanced on one leg for 30 seconds with EO. No subject older than 70 could balance more than 13 seconds.	The duration that individuals can stand on one leg is highly related to age. Inability to maintain balance for 30 seconds (EO or EC) while feet are together can be considered abnormal in patients aged 20 to 79. The limited number of subjects prevents use of these results as true normative values for balance. Expectations for balance test results should be age specific.
Kenshalo, Sr., 1986*	To examine several modes of somatosensory acuity and determine location where losses can be demonstrated and whether these losses are site specific.	27 young (ages 19 to 31) and 21 elderly (ages 55 to 84) subjects. Absolute thresholds were measured for six modes of cutaneous sensation (tactile, through single ramp-and-hold skin indentation, vibration at 40 and 250 Hz, temperature increase and decrease, and noxious heat). Tests were performed at the thenar eminence and plantar surface of foot.	Elderly persons were significantly less sensitive than young individuals to mechanical stimuli at both sites. No significant differences were found for thermal stimuli, except that elderly feet were less sensitive to warmth than young feet.	There was no increase in deficits found with increasing age; relatively small sample size.

* Kenshalo, Sr., DR: Somesthetic sensitivity in young and elderly humans. J Gerontol 41(6):732, 1986.

Evidence Summary Box 5.2 prepared by Stephen A. Caronia.

Box 5.3 Sample Questions for Examining Orientation

A series of simple questions is posed to the patient. The questions are designed to determine the patient's understanding of recognition of who he or she is, location including the present facility (the name of hospital or clinic), the present time, and the passage of time.

Person

- What is your name?
- Do you have a middle name?
- How old are you?
- When were you born?

Place

- Do you know where you are right now?
- What kind of a place is this?
- Do you know what city and state we are in?
- What city or town do you live in?
- What is your address at home?

Time

- What is today's date?
- What day of the week is it?
- What time is it?
- Is it morning or afternoon?
- What season is it?
- What year is it?
- How long have you been here?

From Nolan, MF,[62, p 26] with permission.

results of this mental status screening are often abbreviated "oriented × 3," referring to the three parameters of time, person, and place. If a patient is not fully oriented to one or more domains, the notation would read "oriented × 2 (time)" or "oriented × 1 (time, place)." With partial orientation entries, it is customary to include the *domains of disorientation* within parentheses. Box 5.3 presents sample questions for examining orientation.[9,62,63]

Cognition is defined as the process of knowing and includes both awareness and judgment.[6]

Nolan[62] suggests three areas for testing cognition-dependent functions: (1) fund of knowledge, (2) calculation ability, and (3) proverb interpretation. **Fund of knowledge** is defined as the sum total of an individual's learning and experience in life, which will be highly variable and different for each patient. Detailed information about premorbid knowledge base is often not available. However, a number of general categories of information can be used to test this cognitive function. Sample questions might include[62]:

- Who became president after Kennedy was shot?
- Who is the current vice president of the United States?
- Which is more—a gallon or a liter?
- In what country is the Great Pyramid?
- What would you add to your food to make it sweeter?
- In what state would you find the city of Boston?
- From where do the space shuttles take off?
- What are the elements that make up water and salt?
- Can you name a car made by General Motors?
- Who is Charles Dickens?

Calculation ability examines foundational mathematical abilities.[62,63] Two associated terms are **acalculia** (inability to calculate) and **dyscalculia** (difficulty in accomplishing calculations).[62] This cognitive screening can be administered either verbally or in written format. The patient is asked to mentally perform a series of calculations when provided with mathematical problems. The test should be initiated with simple problems and progress to the more difficult. Adding and subtracting are generally easier than multiplication and division. An alternative approach is to provide written mathematical problems and ask the patient to fill in the answer (e.g., 4 + 4 = ____; 10 + 22 = ____; 46 × 8 = ____; 13 × 7 = ____; 4 × 3 = ____; 6 × 6 = ____; and so forth).

Proverb interpretation examines the patient's ability to interpret use of words outside of their usual context or meaning. This is a sophisticated cognitive function. During the screening, the patient should be asked to describe the meaning of the proverb. Several sample proverbs are[62,63]:

- People who live in glass houses shouldn't throw stones.
- A rolling stone gathers no moss.
- A stitch in time saves nine.
- The early bird catches the worm.
- The dog that trots about finds the bone.
- The empty wagon makes the most noise.
- Every cloud has a silver lining.
- Grass doesn't grow on a busy street.

Memory, Hearing, and Visual Acuity

Also related to the ability to respond during sensory testing is the status of the patient's memory and hearing function as well as visual acuity.

Memory

Both long- and short-term memory should be examined. Impairments of short-term memory will be the most disruptive to collecting sensory information owing to patient difficulties in remembering and following directions. Long-term (remote) memory can be examined by requesting information on date and place of birth, number of siblings, date of marriage, schools attended, historical facts, and so forth. Short-term memory can be addressed by verbally providing the patient with a series of words or numbers. For example, a series of words might include "car, book, cup"; use of numbers could include a seven-digit list; a short sentence could also be used to test short-term memory. The sequence should be repeated immediately by the patient to ensure understanding of the task. Individuals with normal memory function should be able to recall the list 5 minutes[9] later and at least two of the items from the list after 30 minutes.[62]

Hearing

A gross examination of hearing can be made by observing the patient's response to conversation. Note should be made of how alterations in voice volume and tone influence patient response.

Visual Acuity

A gross visual examination can be made by use of a standard Snellen chart mounted on the wall or visual acuity cards for use at bedside. If the patient uses corrective lenses, they should be worn during testing. Visual acuity is typically recorded at 20 feet (6 m) from the Snellen chart (standard eye chart). This distance (20 feet [6 m]) is then placed over the size of the type the individual is able to read comfortably. For example, on a continuum of visual acuity 20/20 is considered excellent and 20/200 is considered poor acuity.[9]

Peripheral field vision can be examined by sitting directly in front of the patient with outstretched arms. The index fingers should be extended and gradually brought toward the midline of the patient's face. The patient is asked to identify when the therapist's approaching finger is first seen. Differences between right and left visual field should be noted carefully. Depth perception may be grossly checked by holding two pencils or fingers (one behind the other) directly in front of the patient. The patient is asked to identify the foreground object.

Because tests of sensory integrity require a verbal response to the stimulus, patients with arousal, attention, orientation, cognitive, or short-term memory impairments generally cannot be accurately tested. However, impairments in vision, hearing, or speech will not adversely affect test results if appropriate adaptations are made in providing instructions and indicating responses (e.g., signaling with either one or two fingers during tests for two-point discrimination, pointing to an area of stimulus contact, mimicking joint position sense or awareness of movement with the contralateral extremity, or object identification by selecting from a group of items during tests for stereognosis).

Classification of the Sensory System

Several different schemes have been proposed for categorizing the sensory system. Among the more common is classification by the type (or location) of *receptors* and the *spinal pathway* mediating information to higher centers.

Sensory Receptors

Sensory receptors (sensory nerve endings) are located at the distal end of an afferent nerve fiber. Once stimulated, they give rise to perception of a specific sensation. Sensory receptors are highly sensitive to the type of stimulus for which they were designed (termed *receptor specificity*). This specificity of nerve fiber sensitivity to a single modality of sensation is called the *labeled line principle*.[64] This means that individual tactile sensations are perceived when specific types of receptors are stimulated. For example, in response to touch, selective activation of Merkel discs and Ruffini endings generate the sensation of steady pressure in the cutaneous area above the active receptors.[65]

It should be noted that the term *modality* has a specific meaning within the context of sensation. Modality "defines a general class of stimulus, determined by the type of energy transmitted by the stimulus and the receptors specialized to sense that energy."[65, p 413] Each type of sensation perceived (e.g., vision, hearing, taste, touch, smell, pain, temperature, proprioception) is referred to as a modality of sensation.

The three divisions of sensory receptors include those that mediate the (1) superficial, (2) deep, and (3) combined (cortical) sensations.[9]

Superficial Sensation

Exteroceptors are responsible for the superficial sensations.[66] They receive stimuli from the external environment via the skin and subcutaneous tissue. Exteroceptors are responsible for the perception of pain, temperature, light touch, and pressure.[9,66]

Deep Sensation

Proprioceptors are responsible for the deep sensations. These receptors receive stimuli from muscles, tendons, ligaments, joints, and fascia,[63] and are responsible for position sense[67] and awareness of joints at rest, movement awareness (kinesthesia), and vibration.

Combined Cortical Sensations

The combination of both the superficial and deep sensory mechanisms makes up the third category of combined sensations. These sensations require information from both the exteroceptive and proprioceptive receptors, as well as intact function of cortical sensory association areas. The cortical combined sensations include stereognosis, two-point discrimination, barognosis, graphesthesia, tactile localization, recognition of texture, and double simultaneous stimulation.

Spinal Pathways

Sensations also have been classified according to the system by which they are mediated to higher centers. Sensations are mediated by either the *anterolateral spinothalamic system* or the *dorsal column-medial lemniscal system*.[66–70]

Anterolateral Spinothalamic

This system initiates self-protective reactions and responds to stimuli that are potentially harmful in nature. It contains slow-conducting fibers of small diameter, some of which are unmyelinated. The system is concerned with transmission of thermal and nociceptive information, and mediates pain, temperature, crudely localized touch, tickle, itch, and sexual sensations.

Dorsal Column–Medial Lemniscal System

The dorsal column is the system involved with responses to more discriminative sensations. It contains fast-conducting fibers of large diameter with greater myelination. This system mediates the sensations of discriminative touch and pressure sensations, vibration, movement, position sense, and awareness of joints at rest. The two systems are interdependent and integrated so as to function together.

Types of Sensory Receptors

The sensory receptors frequently are divided according to their structural design and the type of stimulus to which they preferentially respond. These divisions include (1) *mechanoreceptors*, which respond to mechanical deformation of the receptor or surrounding area; (2) *thermoreceptors*, which respond to changes in temperature; (3) *nociceptors*, which respond to noxious stimuli and result in the perception of pain; (4) *chemoreceptors*, which respond to chemical substances and are responsible for taste, smell, oxygen levels in arterial blood, carbon dioxide concentration, and osmolality (concentration gradient) of body fluids; and (5) *photic (electromagnetic) receptors*, which respond to light within the visible spectrum.[8,9,66,69,71]

The perception of pain is not limited to stimuli received from nociceptors, because other types of receptors and nerve fibers contribute to this sensation. High intensities of stimuli to any type of receptor may be perceived as pain (e.g., extreme heat or cold and high-intensity mechanical deformation).

The general classification of sensory receptors is presented in Box 5.4.[63,64,72,73] Note that this list also includes the receptors responsible for electromagnetic (visual) and chemical stimuli.

Cutaneous Receptors

Cutaneous sensory receptors are located at the terminal portion of the afferent fiber. These include free nerve endings, hair follicle endings, Merkel's discs, Ruffini endings, Krause's end-bulbs, Meissner's corpuscles, and Pacinian corpuscles. The density of these sensory receptors varies for different areas of the body. For example, there are many more tactile receptors in the fingertips than in the back. These areas of higher receptor density correspondingly display a higher cortical representation in somatic sensory area I. Receptor density is a particularly important consideration in interpreting the results of a sensory examination for

Box 5.4 Classification of Sensory Receptors

I. Mechanoreceptors
- A. Cutaneous sensory receptors
  1. Free nerve endings
  2. Hair follicle endings
  3. Merkel's discs
  4. Ruffini endings
  5. Krause's end-bulbs
  6. Meissner's corpuscles
  7. Pacinian corpuscles

II. Deep Sensory Receptors
- A. Muscle receptors
  1. Muscle spindles
  2. Golgi tendon organs
  3. Free nerve endings
  4. Pacinian corpuscles
- B. Joint receptors
  1. Golgi-type endings
  2. Free nerve endings
  3. Ruffini endings
  4. Paciniform endings

III. Thermoreceptors
- A. Cold
  1. Cold receptors
- B. Warmth
  1. Warmth receptors

IV. Nociceptors
- A. Pain
  1. Free nerve endings
  2. Extremes of stimuli*

V. Electromagnetic Receptors
- A. Vision
  1. Rods
  2. Cones

VI. Chemoreceptors
- A. Taste
  1. Receptors of taste buds
- B. Smell
  1. Receptors of olfactory nerves in olfactory epithelium
- C. Arterial oxygen
  1. Receptors of aortic and carotid bodies
- D. Osmolality
  1. Probably neurons of supraoptic nuclei
- E. Blood CO_2
  1. Receptors in or on surface of medulla and in aortic and carotid bodies
- F. Blood glucose, amino acids, fatty acids
  1. Receptors in hypothalamus

*Extremes of stimuli to other sensory receptors will be perceived as pain.

Adapted from Waxman, SG,[63] Guyton, AC, and Hall, JE,[64] Fitzgerald, MJT,[72] and Fredericks, CM.[73]

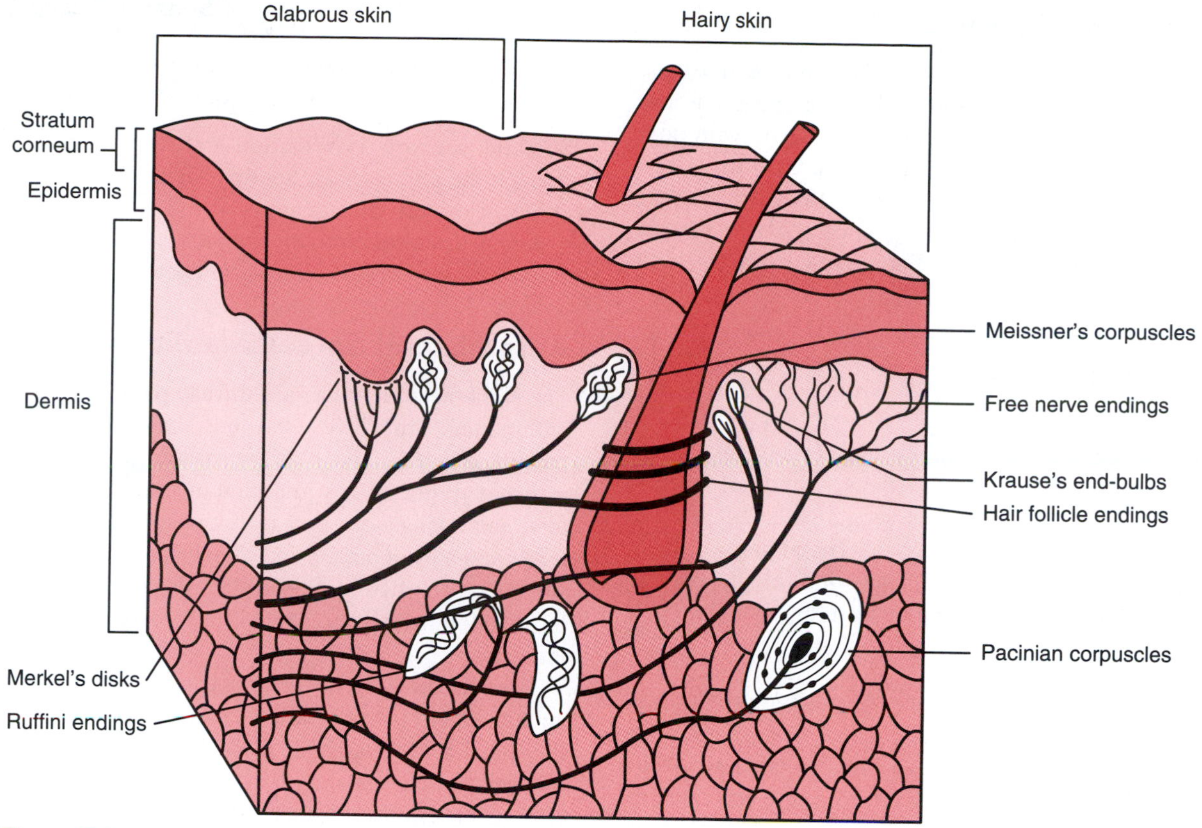

Figure 5.3 The cutaneous sensory receptors and their respective locations within the various layers of skin (epidermis, dermis, and the subcutaneous layer).

a given body surface. Figure 5.3 illustrates the cutaneous sensory receptors and their respective locations within the various layers of skin.

Free Nerve Endings

These receptors are found throughout the body. Stimulation of free nerve endings result in the perception of pain, temperature, touch, pressure, tickle, and itch sensations.[9,63]

Hair Follicle Endings (Hair End-Organs)

At the base of each hair follicle a free nerve ending is entwined. The combination of the hair follicle and its nerve provides a sensitive receptor. These receptors are sensitive to mechanical movement and touch.[67,74]

Merkel's Discs

These touch receptors are located below the epidermis in hairless smooth (glabrous) skin with a high density in the finger tips. They are sensitive to low-intensity touch, as well as to the velocity of touch, and respond to constant indentation of the skin. They provide for the ability to perceive continuous contact of objects against the skin and are believed to play an important role in both two-point discrimination and localization of touch.[66,67,74]

Ruffini Endings

Located in the deeper layers of the dermis, these encapsulated endings are involved with the perception of touch and pressure. They are slowly adapting and particularly important in signaling continuous skin deformation such as tension or stretch; they are also found in joint capsules and assist with joint position sense.[64]

Krause's End-Bulb

These low-threshold mechanical receptors are located in the dermis. They are believed to have a contributing role in the perception of touch and pressure.[74]

Meissner's Corpuscles

Located in the dermis, these encapsulated nerve endings contain many branching nerve filaments within the capsule. They are rapidly adapting and in high concentration in the fingertips, lips, and toes, areas that require high levels of discrimination. These receptors play an important role in discriminative touch (e.g., recognition of texture) and movement of objects over skin.[64,67]

Pacinian Corpuscles

These receptors are located in the subcutaneous tissue layer of the skin and in deep tissues of the body (including tendons and soft tissues around joints). They are stimulated by rapid movement of tissue and are quickly adapting. They play a significant role in the perception of deep touch and vibration.[75]

Deep Sensory Receptors

The deep sensory receptors are located in muscles, tendons, and joints[63,64,68] and include both muscle and joint receptors. They are concerned primarily with posture, position sense, proprioception, muscle tone, and speed and direction of movement. The deep sensory receptors include the muscle spindle, Golgi tendon organs, free nerve endings, Pacinian corpuscles, and joint receptors.

Muscle Receptors

Muscle Spindles

The muscle spindle fibers (intrafusal fibers) lie in a parallel arrangement to the muscle fibers (extrafusal fibers). They monitor changes in muscle length (Ia and II spindle afferent endings) as well as velocity (Ia ending) of these changes. The muscle spindle plays a vital role in position and movement sense and in motor learning.

Golgi Tendon Organs

These receptors are located in series at both the proximal and distal tendinous insertions of the muscle. The Golgi tendon organs function to monitor tension within the muscle. They also provide a protective mechanism by preventing structural damage to the muscle in situations of extreme tension. This is accomplished by inhibition of the contracting muscle and facilitation of the antagonist.

Free Nerve Endings

These receptors are within the fascia of the muscle. They are believed to respond to pain and pressure.

Pacinian Corpuscles

Located within the fascia of the muscle, these receptors respond to vibratory stimuli and deep pressure.

Joint Receptors

Golgi-Type Endings

These receptors are located in the ligaments, and function to detect the rate of joint movement.

Free Nerve Endings

Found in the joint capsule and ligaments, these receptors are believed to respond to pain and crude awareness of joint motion.

Ruffini Endings

Located in the joint capsule and ligaments, Ruffini endings are responsible for the direction and velocity of joint movement.

Paciniform Endings

These receptors are found in the joint capsule and primarily monitor rapid joint movements.

Pathways for Transmission of Somatic Sensory Signals

Somatic sensory information enters the spinal cord through the dorsal roots. Sensory signals are then carried to higher centers via ascending pathways from one of two systems: the *anterolateral spinothalamic system* or the *dorsal column–medial lemniscal system.*

Anterolateral Spinothalamic Pathway

The spinothalamic tracts are diffuse pathways concerned with nondiscriminative sensations such as pain, temperature, tickle, itch, and sexual sensations. This system is activated primarily by mechanoreceptors, thermoreceptors, and nociceptors, and is composed of afferent fibers that are small diameter and slowly conducting. Sensory signals transmitted by this system do not require discrete localization of signal source or precise gradations in intensity.

After originating in the dorsal roots, the fibers of the spinothalamic pathway immediately cross and ascend up the spinal cord through the medulla, pons, and midbrain to the ventroposterolateral (VPL) nucleus of the thalamus (Fig. 5.4). Axons of the VPL neurons project to the somatosensory cortex via the internal capsule.[69,75]

Compared with the dorsal column–medial lemniscal system, the anterolateral spinothalamic pathways make up a cruder, more primitive system. The spinothalamic tracts are capable of transmitting a wide variety of sensory modalities. However, their diffuse pattern of termination results in only crude abilities to localize the source of a stimulus on the body surface, and poor intensity discrimination.[63]

The three major tracts of the spinothalamic system include the (1) *anterior (ventral) spinothalamic tract,* which carries the sensations of crudely localized touch and pressure; (2) the *lateral spinothalamic tract,* which carries pain and temperature; and (3) the *spinoreticular tract,* which is involved with diffuse pain sensations.[63]

Dorsal Column–Medial Lemniscal Pathway

This system is responsible for the transmission of discriminative sensations received from specialized mechanoreceptors. Sensory modalities that require fine gradations of intensity and precise localization on the body surface are mediated by this system. Sensations transmitted by the dorsal column–medial lemniscal pathway include discriminative touch, **stereognosis**, tactile pressure, **barognosis**, *graphesthesia,* recognition of texture, kinesthesia, **two-point discrimination**, proprioception, and vibration.

This system is composed of large, myelinated, rapidly conducting fibers. After entering the dorsal column the

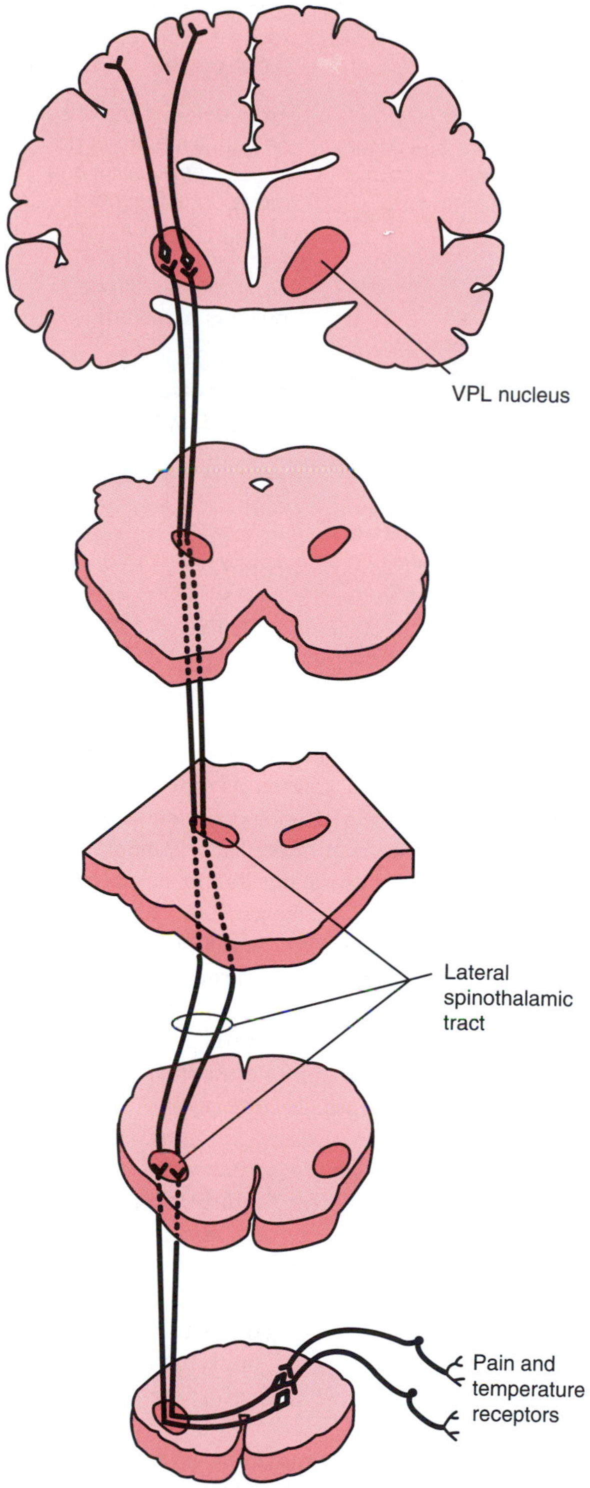

Figure 5.4 Anterolateral spinothalamic tract carrying pain and temperature.

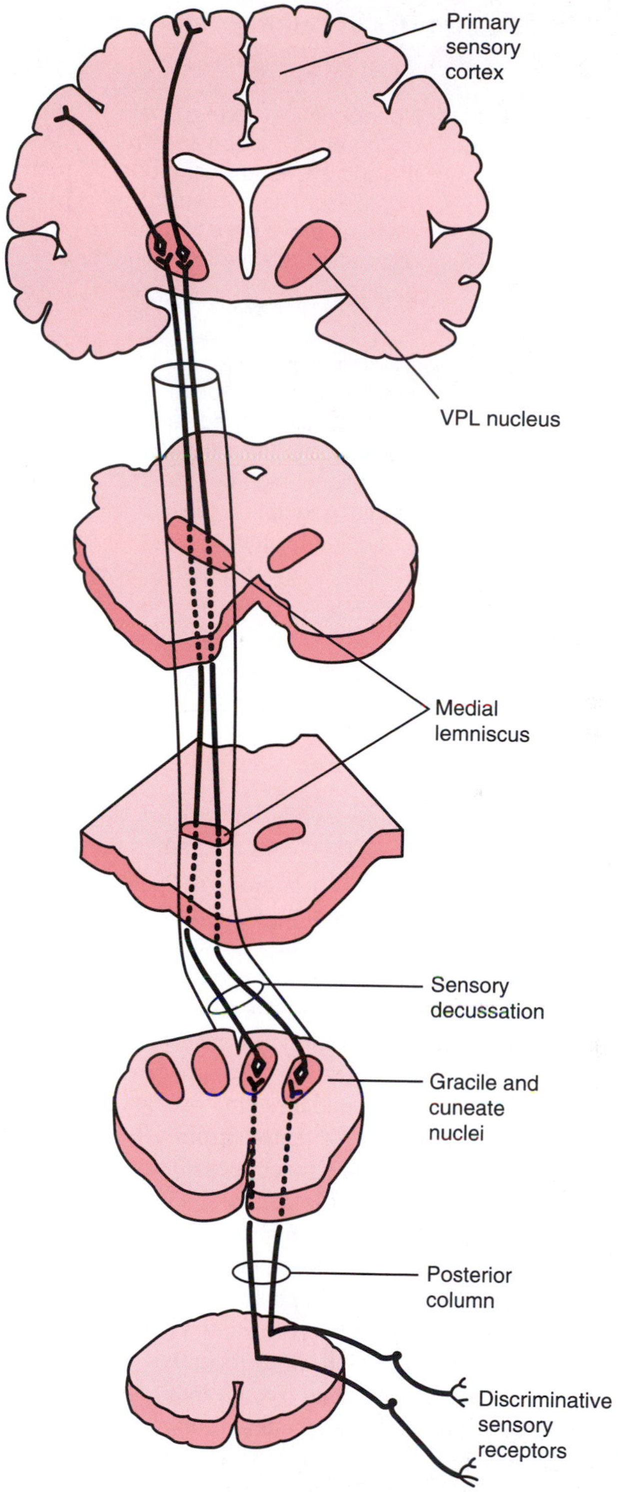

Figure 5.5 Dorsal column–medial lemniscal tract carrying discriminative sensations such as kinesthesia and touch.

fibers ascend to the medulla and synapse with the dorsal column nuclei (nuclei gracilis and cuneatus). From here they cross to the opposite side and pass up to the thalamus through bilateral pathways called the *medial lemnisci*. Each medial lemniscus terminates in the ventral posterolateral thalamus. From the thalamus, third-order neurons project to the somatic sensory cortex. Projection to sensory association areas in the cortex allows for the perception and interpretation of the combined cortical sensations (Fig. 5.5).[63,64,66,75] Table 5.1 presents a comparison of the most salient features of each ascending pathway.

Table 5.1 Features of Pathways for Transmission of Somatic Sensory Signals

Pathway	Type of Sensation	Afferent Fibers	Origin	Projection
Anterolateral spinothalamic	Nondiscriminative (e.g., pain, temperature); broad spectrum of sensory modalities; crude localization; poor intensity discrimination; poor spatial orientation relative to origin of stimulus	Small-diameter, slowly conducting	Skin: mechanoreceptors, thermoreceptors, nociceptors	From dorsal roots of spinal nerves, synapse at dorsal horns, fibers cross and move up spinal cord, through medulla, pons, and midbrain to the ventroposterolateral nucleus of thalamus
Dorsal column –medial lemniscal	Discriminative (e.g., stereognosis, two-point discrimination); precise localization; fine intensity gradations; high degree of spatial orientation relative to origin of stimulus	Large, rapidly conducting	Skin, joints, tendons: specialized mechanoreceptors	From dorsal roots of spinal nerves, ascend to medulla, synapse with dorsal column nuclei, cross to contralateral side and ascend to thalamus; then project to sensory cortex.

Somatosensory Cortex

The most complex processing of sensory information occurs in the somatosensory cortex which is divided into three main divisions: S-I, S-II, and the posterior parietal cortex (Fig. 5.6A). The primary somatosensory (S-I) area occupies a lateral strip called the postcentral gyrus (posterior to the central sulcus) and includes four distinct areas: Brodmann's areas 3a, 3b, 1, and 2. SI neurons identify the location of stimuli as well as discern the size, shape, and texture of objects. At the superior aspect of the lateral sulcus is the secondary somatosensory cortex (S-II), which is innervated by neurons from S-I. S-II projects to the insular cortex that innervates the temporal lobe, believed important in tactile memory. The posterior parietal lobe is behind S-I and consists of areas 5 and 7. Area 5 integrates tactile input from mechanoreceptors of the skin with proprioceptive input from muscles and joints. Area 7 integrates stereognostic and visual information from visual, tactile, and proprioceptive input.[67,68,75,76] These processing areas analyze and integrate somatosensory information and contribute to motor performance by (1) determining the initial position required before a movement occurs, (2) error detection as movement occurs, and (3) identification of movement outcomes which helps to shape learning.

Animal models have provided considerable insight into the function of the cortical association areas. Complete removal of area S-I of the somatosensory system produces deficits in position sense and the ability to determine the size, texture, and shape of objects. Temperature and pain perception are diminished but not abolished. Owing to reliance on input from S-I, removal of S-II results in severe impairment of the perception of both shape and texture of objects. Animal models have also shown reduced ability to learn new discriminative tasks, which are based on the shape of an object. Insult to the posterior parietal cortex presents profound impairments in attending to sensory input from the contralateral side of the body.[76]

The sensory homunculus (somatotopic map) represents a cross-sectional view through the postcentral gyrus and identifies the relative size of the cortex devoted to specific body parts (Fig. 5.6B). Note that certain areas of the body are exaggerated such as the hand, face, and mouth owing to greater innervation density of the skin. The relative size of body parts represents both the *density* of sensory input from the body region as well as the *importance* of sensory information from the area as it relates to function.[75,76] For example, the relative size of the foot is reflective of its importance in locomotion; the relative size of the index finger reflects its role in fine motor skills. In contrast, cortical areas for the trunk and back are small, implying a lower receptor density and reduced role in sensory perception related to function.

Using two-point discrimination as an example, Bear et al provide an extraordinary illustration of how our ability to perceive a stimulus varies remarkably across the body:

> *Two-point discrimination varies at least twentyfold across the body. Fingertips have the highest resolution. The dots of Braille are 1 mm high and 2.5 mm apart; up to six dots make a letter. An experienced Braille reader can scan an index finger across a page of raised dots and read about 600 letters per minute, which is roughly as fast as someone reading aloud.*

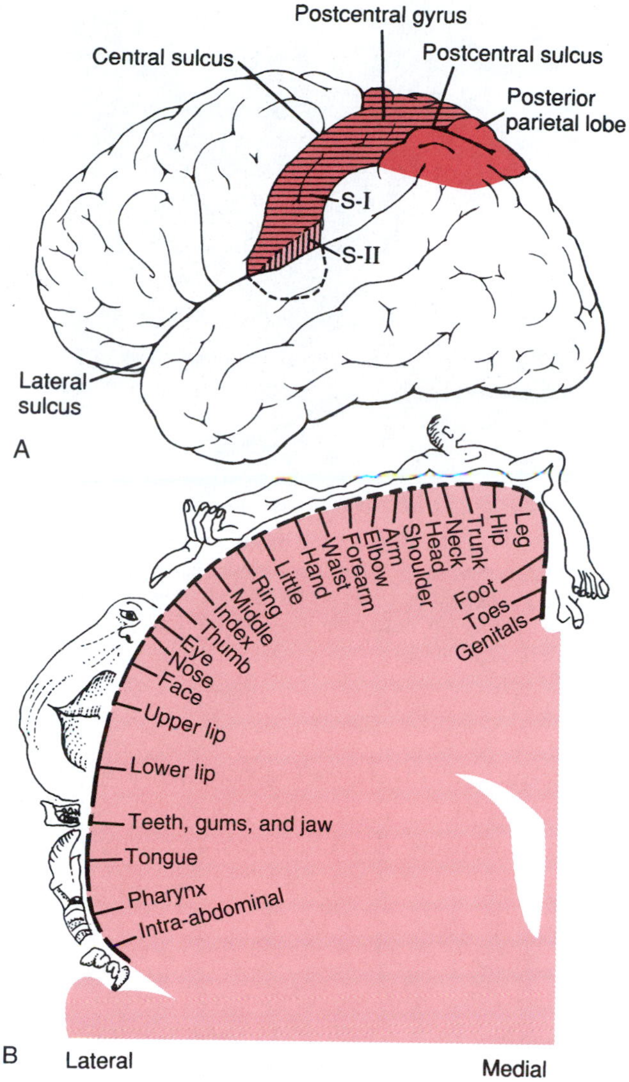

Figure 5.6 (*A*) The somatosensory cortex has three main divisions: The primary (S-I) and secondary (S-II) areas, and the posterior parietal lobe. (*B*) The sensory homunculus. Areas of the body used for tactile discrimination are represented by large areas of cortical tissue, such as the lips, tongue, and fingers. Areas with reduced cortical representation, such as the trunk, are reflective of body parts with lesser roles in sensory perception. (From Kandel, ER, and Jessell, TM: Touch. In Kandel, ER, Schwartz, JH and Jessel, TM: Principles of Neural Science, ed 3. Appleton and Lange, Norwalk, CT, 1991 with permission, pp 368 [*A*] and 372[*B*]).

There are several reasons the fingertip is so much better than, for example, the elbow for Braille reading: (1) There is a much higher density of mechanoreceptors in the skin of the fingertip than on other parts of the body; (2) the fingertips are enriched in receptor types that have small receptive fields; (3) there is more brain tissue (and thus more raw computing power) devoted to the sensory information of each square millimeter of fingertip than elsewhere; and (4) there may be special neural mechanisms devoted to high-resolution discriminations.[75, p 402]

Screening

An important component of physical therapy intervention is to accurately and efficiently meet individual patient needs. Together with information from the history and review of systems, screenings assist the therapist in proficiently identifying the needed tests and measures and setting priorities within the examination process. Screenings consist of a series of brief tests that provide the therapist an "overview" of the system of interest (e.g., sensation, muscle strength). Within this context, screenings are conducted to[7,77]:

- Determine the need for further or more detailed examination
- Determine in a timely manner if referral to another health care practitioner is warranted
- Focus the search for the origin of symptoms to a specific location or body part
- Identify system-related impairments that contribute to functional limitations or disability

CLINICAL NOTE: The term screening is also used in another context. It additionally refers to identification of individuals or groups who are not currently receiving physical therapy services but may be at risk for a health problem.[7] *Examples might include identification of risk factors for low back injury, diabetes, obesity, or falls in the elderly. Physical therapy interventions associated with this type of screening typically involve prevention strategies, fitness promotion, and health promotion and wellness programs*[78] *designed to meet the needs of an individual client or target population.*

To perform a sensory screening, several easily tested (i.e., requiring little or no specialized equipment) modalities of sensation are selected. It is important to select modalities from each of the general categories of sensations. For example, the therapist might select pain and light touch (superficial), kinesthesia and vibration (deep), and two-point discrimination or stereognosis (combined).

The sensory screening is performed by using the selected modalities to test randomly over somewhat large surface areas. For example, several applications of each stimulus might be distributed over the upper and lower extremities and trunk. The information gathered assists the therapist in clinical decision making. If sensory impairments are identified it may (1) indicate the need for more detailed testing, (2) help narrow the origin of symptoms, or (3) provide insight into the cause of functional limitations.

As mentioned earlier, screening tests for mental status (arousal, attention, orientation, cognition, and memory), vision, and hearing acuity should be performed prior to the sensory examination.

Preparation for Administering the Sensory Examination

Prior to initiating the examination of sensory function, the testing environment should be identified and prepared, needed equipment gathered, and consideration given to patient preparation (i.e., what information and instruction will be provided).

Testing Environment

The sensory examination should be administered in a quiet, well-lighted treatment area. Depending on the number of body areas to be tested, either a sitting or recumbent position may be used. If full body testing is indicated, both prone and supine positions will be required and use of a treatment table is recommended to allow examination of each side of the body.

Equipment

To perform a sensory examination the following equipment and materials are used:

1. *Pain*. A large-headed or safety pin or a large paper clip that has one segment bent open (providing one *sharp* and one *dull* end). The sharp end of the instrument should not be sharp enough to risk puncturing the skin. If a large-headed or safety pin is used, the sharp end may be further blunted by a light sanding. Commercially available single-use protected neurological pins may also be used (Fig. 5.7).

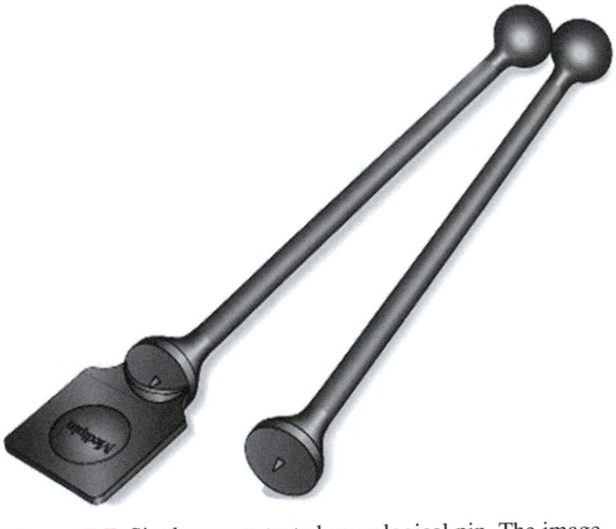

Figure 5.7 Single use protected neurological pin. The image on the *left* shows the pin prior to use with the protective cap intact (although schematically presented to allow visualization of pin location). On the *right*, the protective cap is removed and the pin exposed. On the opposite end of the pin is a smooth rounded surface used to randomly intersperse application of a dull stimulus. After use, the point is destroyed by compressing it against a hard surface and disposed of in a biohazard receptacle. (Courtesy of US Neurologicals, Kirkland, WA 98033.)

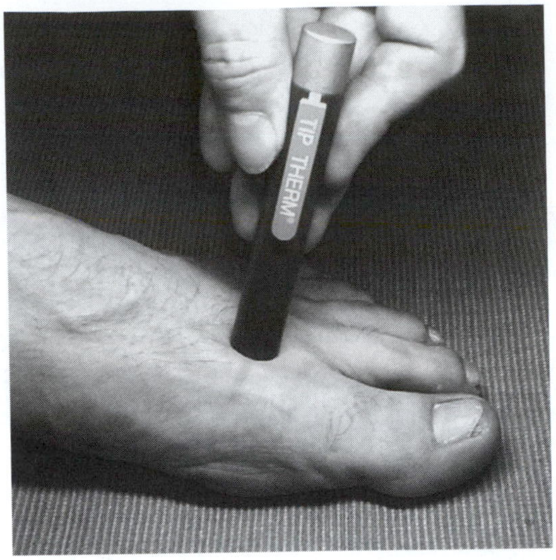

Figure 5.8 The Tip Therm® is a thermal instrument designed for patient monitoring of gross temperature perception of the feet. The instrument is 4 inches (100 mm) long with a .59 inch (15 mm) diameter. (Courtesy of Tip-Therm® GmbH, Düsseldorf, Germany.)

2. *Temperature*. Two standard laboratory test tubes with stoppers.

CLINICAL NOTE: The Tip Therm® is an early detection tool for identification of changes in thermal perception designed for monitoring polyneuropathy associated with diabetes (Fig. 5.8). It provides a method for patients to test temperature sensitivity of their feet independently. It provides only a gross estimate of temperature perception; however, its convenience, low cost, and patients' ability to use it are important characteristics. The tool can be used many times, requires no energy, and makes use of the special characteristics of synthetic material and metal. One end is metal and the opposite side is synthetic material. Both materials are essentially at room temperature; however, the metal end takes more heat from the body (metal has a higher conductivity than the synthetic end). As a result, the metal end is perceived as warm and the synthetic end as cooler.

3. *Light touch*. A camel hair brush, a piece of cotton, or a tissue.
4. *Vibration*. Tuning fork and earphones (if available, to reduce auditory clues). Tuning forks are made of steel or magnesium alloy and grossly resemble a two-pronged fork. When the tines are stuck against a surface (usually the palm of the examiner's hand) the fork resonates at a specific pitch (e.g., 128, 256, or 512 Hz) determined by the length of the two U-shaped prongs (tines).
5. *Stereognosis* (*object recognition*). A variety of small commonly used articles such as a comb, fork, paper clip, key, coin, pencil, and so forth.

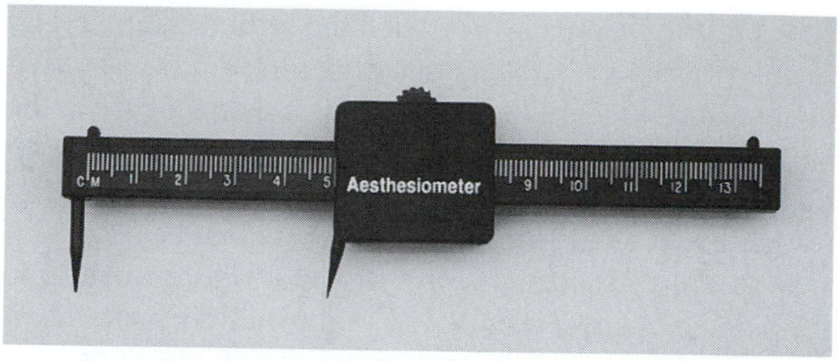

Figure 5.9 A hand-held aesthesiometer provides a quantitative measure of two point-point discrimination. The two-point threshold is determined by gradually bringing the moveable tips closer together as it is sequentially applied to the patient's skin. The scale is calibrated to the nearest 0.1 cm and measures up to 14 cm.

6. *Two-point discrimination*. Several instruments are available to measure two-point discrimination. A two-point discrimination aesthesiometer (Fig. 5.9) is a small hand-held instrument designed to measure the shortest distance that two points of contact on the skin can be distinguished. It consists of a small ruler with two moveable (sliding) tips coated with vinyl. The vinyl coverings help to minimize the impact of temperature on perception of contact. Some instruments also have a third tip allowing ease of alternating from two points to a single point of contact during testing. If used on an uneven body surface, care should be taken not to allow the "ruler" portion of the instrument to make contact with the skin. *Note*: The term *aesthesiometer* is not specific to this instrument; it is used to describe any number of instruments designed to examine touch perception.

   For finer gradations in measurement (e.g., fingertips), small circular disks can be used to measure two-point discrimination (Fig. 5.10). These instruments typically allow quantification of two-point discrimination from 1 to 25 mm.

   Electrocardiogram (ECG) calipers[79] with the tips sanded to blunt the ends[80] and a small ruler have also been used to measure two-point discrimination.

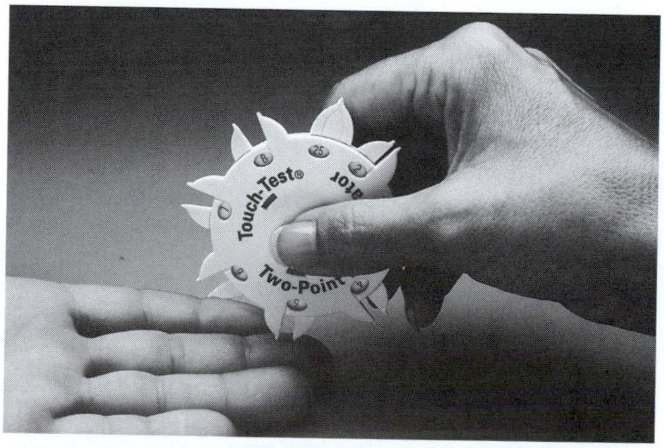

Figure 5.10 This circular two-point discrimination instrument consists of two joined plastic rotating disks with rounded tips placed at standard testing intervals. (Courtesy of North Coast Medical, Inc, Morgan Hill, CA 95037.)

7. *Recognition of texture*. Samples of fabrics of various textures such as cotton, wool, or silk (approximately 4 × 4 inches [10 × 10 cm]).

Patient Preparation

A full explanation of the purpose of the testing should be provided. The patient also should be informed that cooperation is necessary to obtain accurate test results. It is of considerable importance that the patient be requested *not to guess* if uncertain of the correct response.

During the examination, the patient should be in a comfortable, relaxed position. Preferably, the tests should be performed when the patient is well rested. Considering the high level of concentration required, it is not surprising that fatigue has been noted to affect results of some sensory tests adversely.[79]

Note: A "trial run" or demonstration of each test should be performed just prior to actual administration. This will orient the patient to the sensation being tested, what to anticipate, and what type of response is required. The importance of this initial trial should not be underestimated. If a practice trial is inadequately or not performed, what appears to be a sensory impairment may in reality only be a reflection of the patient's lack of understanding of the testing protocol or how to respond to a stimulus.

Some method of occluding the patient's vision during the testing should be used (vision should not be occluded during the explanation and demonstration). Visual input is prevented because it may allow for compensation of a sensory deficit and thus decrease the accuracy of test results. The traditional methods of occluding vision are by use of a fabric blindfold (such as those worn by travelers to sleep on an airplane), a small folded towel, or by asking the patient to keep the eyes closed. These methods are practical in most instances. However, in situations of CNS dysfunction, a patient may become anxious or disoriented if vision is occluded for a long period of time. In these situations, a small screen or folder may be preferable as a visual barrier. Whatever method is used, it should be removed between the tests while directions and demonstrations are provided.

CLINICAL NOTE: Impaired sensation is a contraindication or precaution for use of some physical agents because the end range of intensity or duration is frequently associated with the patient's subjective report of how the intervention feels (i.e., patient tolerance).

The Sensory Examination

The superficial (exteroceptive) sensations are usually examined first, inasmuch as they consist of more primitive responses, followed by the deep (proprioceptive), and then the combined cortical sensations. If a test indicates impairment of the superficial responses, some impairment of the more discriminative (deep and combined) sensations also will be noted and may be a contraindication to further testing (e.g., lack of touch sensation would be a contraindication for testing stereognosis). That is, the primary modality of sensation (touch) must be sufficiently intact to permit meaningful testing of cortical sensory function (ability to identify objects placed in the hand).

For each sensory test, the following data will be generated:

- The modality tested
- The quantity of involvement or body surface areas affected (pattern identification)
- The degree or severity of involvement (e.g., absent, impaired, or delayed responses)
- Localization of the exact boundaries of the sensory impairment
- The patient's subjective feelings about changes in sensation
- The potential impact of sensory loss on function (i.e., functional limitation, disability)

Knowledge of skin segment (dermatome) innervation by the dorsal roots and peripheral nerve innervation (see Figs. 5.1 and 5.2) is required for making sound, accurate diagnostic and prognostic judgments. They serve as critical references during testing as well as provide a framework for documenting results.

Sensory tests are typically performed in a distal to proximal direction. This progression will conserve time, particularly when dealing with localized lesions involving a single extremity, where deficits tend to be more severe distally. It is generally not necessary to test every segment of each dermatome; testing general body areas is sufficient. However, once a deficit area is noted, testing must become more discrete and the exact boundaries of the impairment should be identified. A skin pencil may be useful to mark the boundaries of sensory change directly. This information should be transferred later to a sensory examination form, graphically presented on a dermatome chart, and peripheral nerve involvement identified. This form will then be entered in the medical record. Figure 5.11 presents a sample Sensory Examination Form. Most clinicians find it challenging to create a single documentation form applicable to the variety of patients seen in a given practice settings (with the exception of specialized centers or clinics). However, the following are common elements of sensory examination forms: (1) dermatome chart to graphically display findings; (2) some variation of a grading scale (e.g., 1—intact; 2—decreased; and so forth) to score patient perception of individual modalities; and (3) a section for narrative comments.

Most often the dermatome charts are completed using a color code (i.e., each color represents a different sensory modality). The colors used to plot each sensation are then coded by the examiner directly on the form (see Fig. 5.11). In many instances hatch marks of varying density are used to represent gradations in sensory impairment (i.e., the closer together, the greater the sensory impairment). With this method, a completely colored-in area indicates no response to a given sensation. With varied or "spotty" sensory loss it is not uncommon that more than one dermatome chart is required to completely depict all test findings. With use of several dermatome charts, the sensation(s) represented should appear in bold print at the top of each page.

Figure 5.11 provides the foundational elements of documentation typically included for sensory examinations. It should be modified or expanded to meet the needs of a given population or facility. It is also not uncommon for therapists to included sensory testing data within the body of a narrative or progress report.

During testing, the application of stimuli should be applied in a random, unpredictable manner with variation in timing. This will improve accuracy of the test results by avoiding a consistent pattern of application, which might provide the patient with "clues" to the correct response. During application of stimuli, consideration must be given also to skin condition. Scar tissue or callused areas are generally less sensitive and will demonstrate a diminished response to sensory stimuli. Recall that a trial test is performed to instruct the patient in what to expect and how to respond to application of the specific stimuli; and that patient vision is occluded during testing.

The following sections present the individual sensory tests. The tests are subdivided for superficial, deep, and combined cortical sensations. Table 5.2 presents terminology used to describe common sensory impairments.

CLINICAL NOTE: Hands should always be washed prior to and after patient contact. Hand washing is "one of the most important measures for preventing transmission of pathogens in health-care facilities."[81, p 2] *The Centers for Disease Control and Prevention (CDC) recommends vigorous hand washing for at least 15 seconds, covering all surfaces of the hand and fingers.*[81] *See Chapter 4 (Box 4.3) for hand washing procedure.*

Superficial Sensations

Pain Perception

This test is also referred to as *sharp/dull discrimination* and indicates function of protective sensation. To test pain awareness, the sharp and dull end of a large-headed or safety pin, a reshaped paper clip (the segment pulled away from the body of the paper clip provides a sharp end), or a single-use protected neurological pin (see Fig. 5.6) is used. The instrument should be carefully cleaned before administering the test and disposed of immediately afterward (owing to the protective cap on the neurological pin,

This form provides a record of the type, severity, and location of sensory impairments. It should be used in conjunction with additional dermatome sheets, if needed, to graphically outline the exact boundaries of the impairment. The designations P and D may be added to the grading key to indicate either a proximal (P) or a distal (D) location of the impairment on a limb or body part. The dermatome chart should be color coded and filled in using varying density hatch marks (higher density for more severe areas of impairment). Indicate the color used for documentation in the box titled Color Code (a different color should be used for each sensation). Separate notation should be made for examination of the face and identification of peripheral nerve involvement. Abnormal responses should be briefly described in the comments section.

Patient Name: ______________________________ Date: ____________

Examiner: ______________________________

ANTERIOR

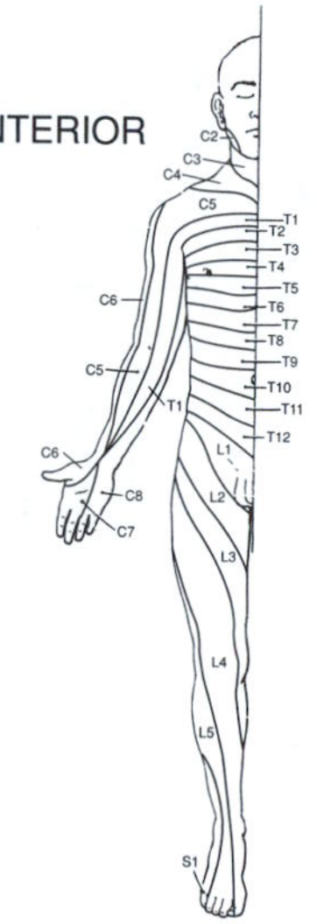

Sensations	Upper Extremity		Lower Extremity		Trunk		Comments
	Right	Left	Right	Left	Right	Left	
Pain							
Temperature							
Touch							
Vibration							
Two-Point Disc							
Kinesthesia							
Proprioception							
Stereognosis							

Note: Areas shaded indicate sensation not typically tested for corresponding body part.

Key to Grading
1. Intact: normal accurate response
2. Decreased: delayed response
3. Exaggerated: increased sensitivity or awareness of stimulus after removed
4. Inaccurate: inappropriate perception of stimulus
5. Absent: no response
6. Inconsistent or ambiguous: response inadequate to determine function accurately

P = Proximal; D = Distal

Color Code

Color	Sensation

POSTERIOR

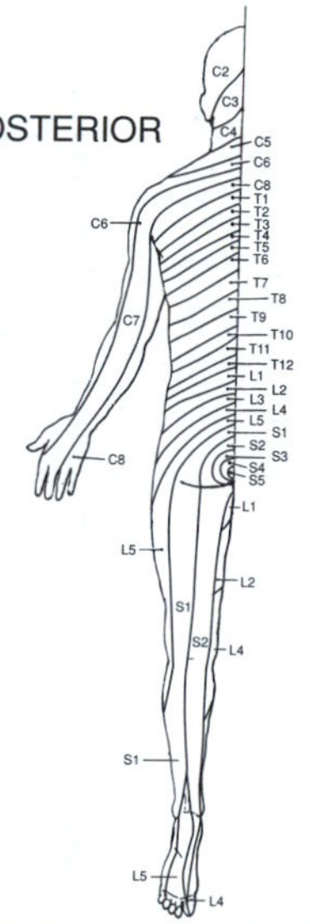

Indicate Peripheral Nerve Involvement:

Figure 5.11 Sample Sensory Examination Form.

Table 5.2 Terminology Describing Common Sensory Impairments

Abarognosis	Inability to recognize weight
Allesthesia	Sensation experienced at a site remote from point of stimulation
Allodynia	Pain produced by a non-noxious stimulus (e.g., touch)
Analgesia	Complete loss of pain sensitivity
Astereognosis	Inability to recognize the form and shape of objects by touch (synonym: tactile agnosia)
Atopognosia	Inability to localize a sensation
Causalgia	Painful, burning sensations, usually along the distribution of a nerve
Dysesthesia	Touch sensation experienced as pain
Hypalgesia	Decreased sensitivity to pain
Hyperalgesia	Increased sensitivity to pain
Hyperesthesia	Increased sensitivity to sensory stimuli
Hypesthesia	Decreased sensitivity to sensory stimuli
Pallanesthesia	Loss or absence of sensibility to vibration
Paresthesia	Abnormal sensation such as numbness, prickling, or tingling, without apparent cause
Thalamic syndrome	Vascular lesion of the thalamus resulting in sensory disturbances and partial or complete paralysis of one side of the body, associated with severe, boring-type pain; sensory stimuli may produce an exaggerated, prolonged, or painful response
Thermanalgesia	Inability to perceive heat
Thermanesthesia	Inability to perceive sensations of heat and cold
Thermhyperesthesia	Increased sensitivity to temperature
Thermhypesthesia	Decreased temperature sensibility
Thigmanesthesia	Loss of light touch sensibility

cleaning is not required). The sharp and dull end of the instrument is randomly applied perpendicularly to the skin. To avoid summation of impulses, the stimuli should not be applied too close to each other or in too rapid a succession. To maintain a uniform pressure with each successive application of stimuli, the pin or reshaped paper clip should be held firmly and the fingers allowed to "slide" down the pin or paper clip once in contact with the skin. This will avoid the chance of gradually increasing pressure during application. The instrument used to test pain perception should be sharp enough to deflect the skin, but not puncture it.

Response

The patient is asked to verbally indicate *sharp* or *dull* when a stimulus is felt. All areas of the body may be tested.

Temperature Awareness

This test determines the ability to distinguish between warm and cool stimuli. Two test tubes with stoppers are required for this examination; one should be filled with warm water and the other with crushed ice. Ideal temperatures for cold are between 41°F (5°C) and 50°F (10°C) and for warmth, between 104°F (40°C) and 113°F (45°C). Caution should be exercised to remain within these ranges, because exceeding these temperatures may elicit a pain response and consequently inaccurate test results. The side of the test tube should be placed in contact with the skin (as opposed to only the distal end). This technique provides sufficient surface area contact to determination the temperature. The test tubes are randomly placed in contact with the skin area to be tested. All skin surfaces should be tested.

Response

The patient is asked to reply *hot* or *cold* after each stimulus application.

CLINICAL NOTE: The clinical usefulness of thermal testing may be problematic. Nolan[79] points out that the tests are extremely difficult to duplicate on a day-to-day basis owing to rapid changes in temperature once the test tubes are exposed to room air. Although it is a simple test to perform, determining changes over time is not practical unless a method of monitoring the temperature of the test tubes is used.[79]

Touch Awareness

This test determines perception of tactile touch input. A camel-hair brush, piece of cotton (ball or swab), or tissue is used. The area to be tested is lightly touched or stroked. Examination of finer gradations of light touch can be quantified using monofilaments (see later section titled Quantitative Sensory Testing and Specialized Testing Instruments).

Response

The patient is asked to indicate when he or she recognizes that a stimulus has been applied by responding "yes" or "now."

Note: A quantitative score for pain perception, temperature, and light touch awareness can be obtained by dividing the number of *correct responses* by the *number of stimuli* applied (normal response would be 100 percent).[82] Also, inability to verbally communicate does not necessary preclude obtaining accurate data. For example, having the patient hold up one or two fingers might be used for dichotomous responses (yes/no; hot/cold). Other options might include nodding the head, pointing to index cards containing printed responses; or using hand gestures to indicate recognition of a stimulus.

Pressure Perception

The therapist's fingertip or a double-tipped cotton swab is used to apply a firm pressure on the skin surface. This pressure should be firm enough to indent the skin and to stimulate the deep receptors. This test can also be administered using the thumb and fingers to squeeze the Achilles tendon.[79]

Response

The patient is asked to indicate when an applied stimulus is recognized by responding "yes" or "now."

Deep Sensations

The deep sensations include **kinesthesia, proprioception,** and **vibration**. Kinesthesia is the awareness of movement. Proprioception includes position sense and the awareness of joints at rest. Vibration refers to the ability to perceive a rapidly oscillating or vibratory stimuli. Although these sensations are closely related, they are examined individually.

Kinesthesia Awareness

This test examines *awareness of movement*. The extremity or joint(s) is moved passively through a relatively small range of motion (ROM). Small increments in ROM are used as joint receptors fire at specific points throughout the range. The therapist should identify the ROM being examined (e.g., initial, mid-, or terminal range). As discussed, a trial run or demonstration of the procedure should be performed prior to actual testing. This will ensure that the patient and the therapist agree on terms to describe the direction of movements.

Response

The patient is asked to describe verbally the direction and range of movement in terms previously discussed with the therapist (up, down, in, out, and so forth) while the extremity is in *motion*. The patient may also respond by simultaneously duplicating the movement with the opposite extremity. This second approach, however, is usually impractical with proximal lower extremity joints, owing to potential stress on the low back. During testing, movement of larger joints is usually discerned more quickly than that of smaller joints. The therapist's grip should remain constant and minimal (fingertip grip over bony prominences), to reduce tactile stimulation.

Proprioceptive Awareness

This test examines *joint position sense* and *the awareness of joints at rest*. The extremity or joint(s) is moved through a ROM and held in a static position. Again, small increments of range are used. The words selected to identify the ROM examined should be identified to the patient during the practice trial (e.g., initial, mid-, or terminal range). As with kinesthesia, caution should be used with hand placements to avoid excessive tactile stimulation.

Response

While the extremity or joint(s) is held in a static position by the therapist, the patient is asked to describe the position verbally or to duplicate the position of the extremity or joint(s) with the contralateral extremity.

Vibration Perception

This test requires a tuning fork that vibrates at 128 Hz.[79] The ability to perceive a vibratory stimulus is tested by placing the base of a vibrating tuning fork on a bony prominence (such as the sternum, elbow, or ankle). The tuning fork base (the "handle" of the fork) is held between the examiner's thumb and index finger. The tines are then briskly hit against the open palm of the examiner's opposite hand to initiate the vibration. Care must be taken not to touch the tines, as this will stop the vibration. The base of the fork in then placed over a bony prominence. If vibration sensation is intact, the patient will perceive the vibration. If there is impairment, the patient will be unable to distinguish between a vibrating and nonvibrating tuning fork. Therefore, there should be a random application of vibrating and nonvibrating stimuli.

Auditory clues can pose a challenge in obtaining accurate test results. Typically it is easy to hear the sound of the tines making vigorous contact with the examiner's hand to initiate the vibration. If the sound is not heard, it provides an easy indicator to the patient that the next application will be nonvibrating. To minimize this effect, the vibration can be initiated for *every* stimulus application; however, when a nonvibrating stimulus is desired, brief contact of the therapist's fingers on the tines will stop the vibration prior to placement on the skin. This, though, does not solve the problem of the auditory cues generated during application of a vibrating stimulus. The best solution is use of sound occlusive earphones (the type often worn by airport ground workers). Unfortunately, such earphones are seldom available in a clinic setting.

Response

The patient is asked to respond by verbally identifying or otherwise indicating if the stimulus is vibrating or nonvibrating each time the fork makes contact.

Combined Cortical Sensations

Stereognosis Perception

This test determines tactile object recognition. A variety of small, easily obtainable, and culturally familiar objects of

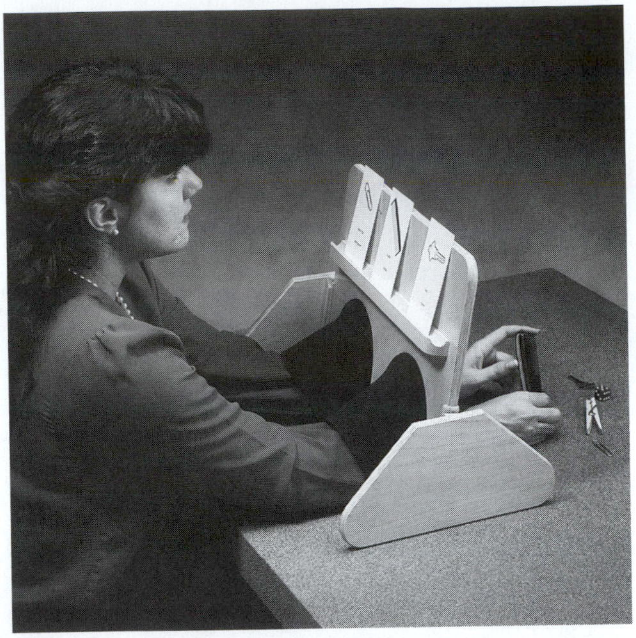

Figure 5.12 A sensory testing shield can be used for examining stereognosis in the presence of speech or language impairments. In this simulation, the subject manipulates the object without the use of visual input. Following manipulation, the subject points to the matching object pictured on the ledge of the testing shield. (Courtesy of North Coast Medical, Inc, Morgan Hill, CA 95037.)

differing size and shape are required (e.g., keys, coins, combs, safety pins, pencils, and so forth). A single object is placed in the hand, the patient manipulates the object, and then identifies the item verbally. The patient should be allowed to handle several sample test items during the explanation and demonstration of the procedure.

Response

The patient is asked to name the object verbally. For patients with speech impairments, sensory testing shields can be used (Fig. 5.12). Alternately, the item manipulated can be identified from a group of images presented after each test.

Tactile Localization

This test addresses the ability to localize touch sensation on the skin. It examines the ability to identify the specific point of application of a touch stimulus (e.g., tip of ring finger, lateral malleus, and so forth) and not simply the perception of touch. Tactile localization is typically not tested in isolation and frequently examined in combination with similar tests such as pressure perception or touch awareness. Using a cotton swap or fingertip, the therapist touches different skin surfaces. After each application of a stimulus the patient is given time to respond.

Response

The patient is asked to identify the location of the stimuli by pointing to the area or by verbal description. The patient's eyes may be open during the response component of this test. The distance between the application of the stimulus and the site indicated by the patient can be measured and recorded. Accuracy of localization over various parts of the body may be compared to determine the relative sensitivity of different areas.

Two-Point Discrimination

This test determines the ability to perceive two points applied to the skin simultaneously. It is a measure of the smallest distance between two stimuli (applied simultaneously and with equal pressure) that can still be perceived as two distinct stimuli. Two-point discrimination values vary for different individuals and body parts. As this sensory function is most refined in the distal upper extremities, this is the typical site for testing. It is believed to contribute to precision grip movements and instrumental activities of daily living (IADL).[83]

Two-point discrimination is among the most practical and easily duplicated tests for cutaneous sensation. Some years ago, a series of classic two-point discrimination studies were conducted by Nolan.[84–86] The purpose of his research was to establish normative data on two-point discrimination for young adults. His sample consisted of 43 college students ranging in age from 20 to 24 years. Values from Nolan's studies for the upper and lower extremities as well as the face and trunk are presented in Appendix A. The results from these studies should be used cautiously, inasmuch as they relate to a specific population. They should not be generalized for interpreting data from older or younger patients. Normative data for two-point discrimination values have also been documented by Desrosiers et al,[87] Shimokata and Kuzuya,[88] Hermann et al,[89] and Richards et al.[90]

As mentioned earlier, the aesthesiometer (see Fig. 5.9) and the circular two-point discriminator (see Fig. 5.10) are among the most common devices used for measurement. Two reshaped paper clips can also be used; however, this requires the assistance of a second examiner to measure the distance between the two points using a small ruler. During the test procedure the two tips of the instrument are applied to the skin simultaneously with tips spread apart. To increase the validity of the test, it is appropriate to alternate the application of two stimuli with the random application of only a single stimulus. With each successive application, the two tips are gradually brought closer together until the stimuli are perceived as one. The smallest distance between the stimuli that is still perceived as two distinct points is measured.

Response

The patient is asked to identify the perception of "one" or "two" stimuli.

Double Simultaneous Stimulation

Double simultaneous stimulation (DSS) examines the ability to perceive a simultaneous touch stimulus on opposite sides of the body; proximally and distally on a single extremity; or proximally and distally on one side of the body. The therapist simultaneously (and with equal pressure) touches: (1) identical locations on opposite sides of the body, (2) proximally and distally on opposite sides of the body, and (3) proximal and distal locations on the same side of the body. The term *extinction phenomena* describes a situation in which only the proximal stimulus is perceived, with "extinction" of the distal.

Response
The patient verbally states when he or she perceives a touch stimulus and the number of stimuli felt.

Several additional tests for the combined (cortical) sensations include graphesthesia (traced finger identification), recognition of texture, and barognosis (recognition of weight). However, these tests are usually not performed if stereognosis and two-point discrimination are found to be intact.

Graphesthesia (Traced Figure Identification)

The ability to recognize letters, numbers, or designs traced on the skin is examined using a fingertip or the eraser end of a pencil. A series of letters, numbers, or designs is traced on the palm of the patient's hand. During the practice trial, agreement should be reached about the orientation of the tracings. (For example, the bottom of the traced figures will always be oriented toward the base of the patient's hand [wrist].) Between each separate drawing the palm should be gently wiped with a soft cloth to clearly indicate a change in figures to the patient. This test is also a useful substitute for stereognosis when paralysis prevents grasping an object.

Response
The patient is asked to identify verbally the figures drawn on the skin. For patients with speech or language impairments, the figures can be selected (pointed to) from a series of line drawings.

Recognition of Texture

This test examines the ability to differentiate among various textures. Suitable textures may include cotton, wool, or silk. The items are placed individually in the patient's hand. The patient is allowed to manipulate the sample texture.

Response
The patient is asked to identify the individual textures as they are placed in the hand. They may be identified by name (e.g., silk, cotton) or by texture (e.g., rough, smooth).

Barognosis (Recognition of Weight)

For recognition of weight, a set of discrimination weights consisting of small objects of the same size and shape but of graduated weight is used (Fig. 5.13). The therapist may choose to place a series of different weights in the same hand one at a time, place a different weight in each hand simultaneously, or ask the patient to use a fingertip grip to pick up each weight.

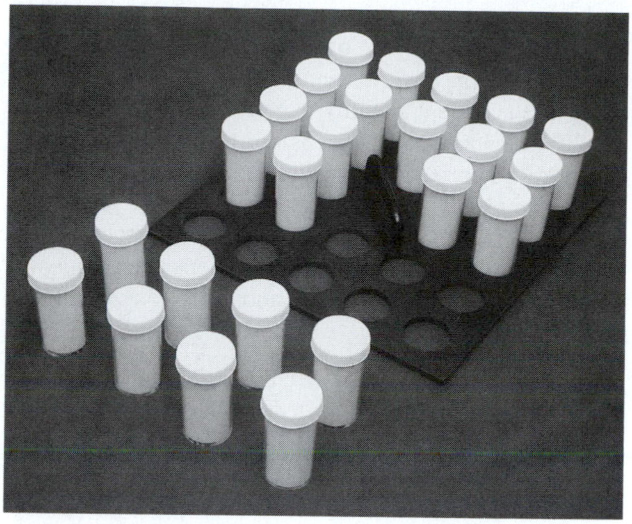

Figure 5.13 Discrimination weights are identical in size, shape, and texture. The only distinguishing feature is their variation in weight. (Courtesy of Lafayette Instruments, Lafayette, IN 47903.)

Response
The patient is asked to identify the comparative weight of objects in a series (i.e., to compare the relative weight of the object with the previous one); or when the objects are placed (or picked up) in both hands simultaneously the patient is asked to compare the weight of the two objects. The patient responds by indicating that the object is "heavier" or "lighter."

Reliability

Reliability is an important parameter of any test or measure. However, few systematic reports addressing the reliability of traditional sensory tests appear in the literature. This is likely due to the inability to accurately quantify test results. In an important early reliability study by Kent[91] the upper limbs of 50 adult patients with hemiplegia were tested for sensory and motor deficits. Three sensory tests were administered and then repeated by the same examiner within 1 to 7 days. Results revealed a high reliability for both stereognosis ($r = 0.97$) and position sense ($r = 0.90$). A lower reliability was reported for two-point discrimination, with correlation coefficients ranging from 0.59 to 0.82, depending on the body area tested.

Although limited published data are available related to reliability measures, several approaches can be used to improve this aspect of the tests, including (1) use of consistent guidelines for completing the tests; (2) administration of the tests by trained, skillful examiners; and (3) subsequent retests performed by the same individual. It also should be noted that the reliability of sensory tests will be further influenced by the patient's understanding of the test procedure and the patient's ability to communicate results.

With developing advances in technology allowing quantitative approaches to collecting sensory testing data, greater emphasis on reliability will follow. Additional research related to standardization of testing protocols and identification of normative data for various age groups will improve the overall reliability and interpretation of test results for patient care.

Quantitative Sensory Testing and Specialized Testing Instruments

With the expanding availability of specialized testing systems and instruments, quantitative sensory testing (QST) has gained considerable clinical and research interest. This is clearly evident from the expanding body of literature on this topic.[92–106] QST allows quantification of the level of stimuli required for perception of a sensory modality. Although sufficient data are not available to predict the ultimate integration of QST instrumentation into clinical practice, preliminary information suggests its potential usefulness. This section provides a brief overview of selected QST devices and is certainly not all-inclusive. The Internet provides a rich source of information on this developing technology and instrumentation

TSA-II Thermal Sensory Analyzer + VSA 3000 (Medoc, Ltd, Durham, NC)

This computer-controlled system (Fig. 5.14) is capable of generating and recording a response to repeatable vibratory and thermal stimuli (i.e., warmth, cold, heat- or cold-induced pain). For testing thermal sensation, a "thermode" capable of heating or cooling is placed on the patient's skin (Fig. 5.15). The patient is asked to respond to the stimulus by pushing a response button. A sensory threshold is recorded and a computer comparison to age-matched normative data is generated. The system includes hand and foot (Fig. 5.16) support vibratory stimulators as well as a hand-held vibrating units (see Fig 5.14). A variety of report formats can be generated; a sample is presented in Figure 5.17. Several examples of clinical applications include neuropathies (e.g., diabetic, metabolic, cancer), compression injuries, and pharmacological trials.

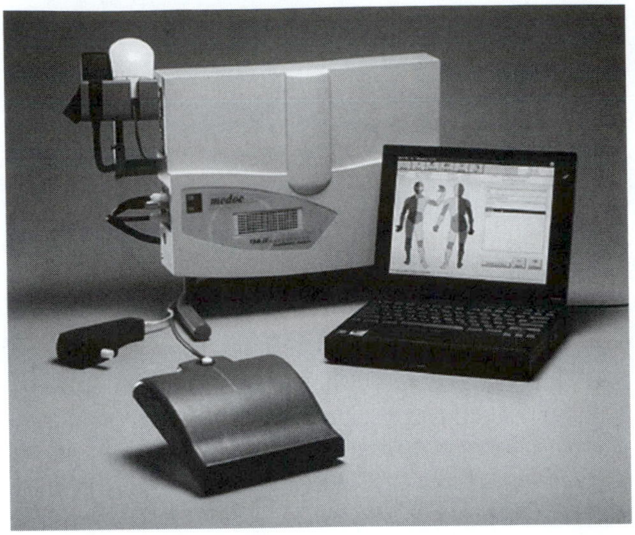

Figure 5.14 TSA-II Thermal Sensory Analyzer + VSA 3000. This system provides quantitative measures of both thermal and vibratory stimuli using a variety of patient interfaces. Note the small hand-held vibratory unit on the far left. (Courtesy of Medoc, Ltd, Durham, NC 27707.)

von Frey Aesthesiometer (Somedic Sales AB, Hörby, Sweden)

Monofilaments are not new to examination of sensory function and are actually considered a classic tool for measuring touch-evoked potentials (Fig. 5.18). They are designed to detect very small changes in touch threshold. The filaments are available as sets, in various sizes (i.e., thicknesses), with each mounted on a handle. The force required to bend the monofilament increases from 0.026 g for the first handle to 100 g for the last (pressure range of between 5 g/mm^2 and 178 g/mm^2). The filaments are applied individually to the patient's skin until it bends; each filament providing a specific amount of force (thicker filaments are used if the thinner are not perceived). With vision occluded, the patient responds "yes" when a stimulus is felt. The filaments are held perpendicular to the skin

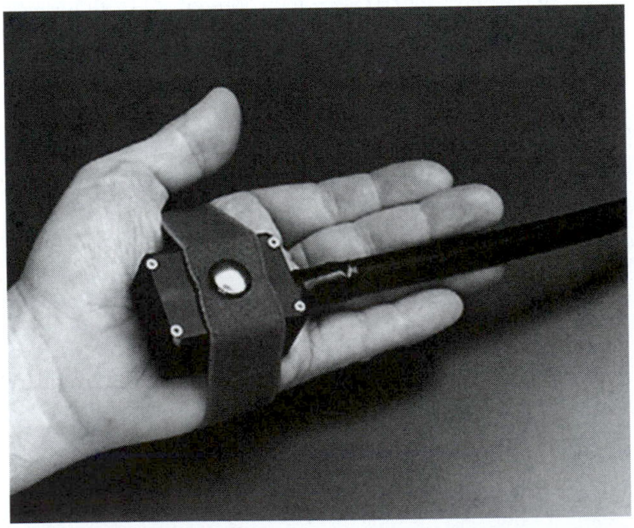

Figure 5.15 Thermode placed in hand for measuring perception of thermal stimuli. (Courtesy of Medoc, Ltd, Durham, NC 27707.)

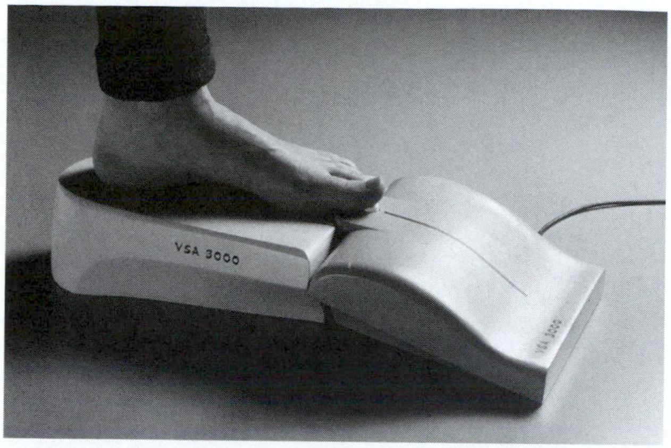

Figure 5.16 Foot support vibratory stimulator. (Courtesy of Medoc, Ltd, Durham, NC 27707.)

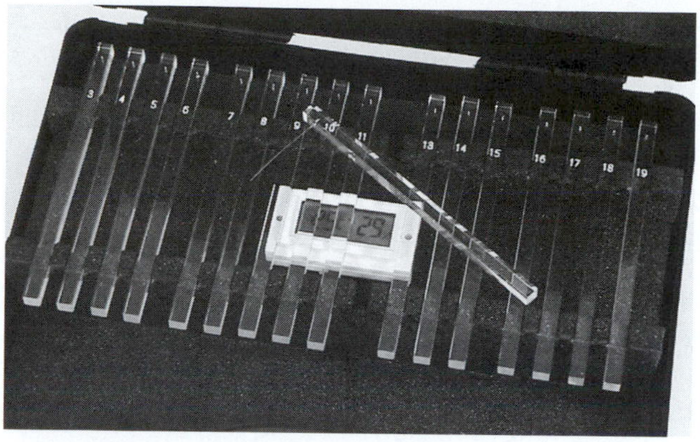

Figure 5.18 von Frey Aesthesiometer. This set contains 17 monofilaments mounted on plexiglass handles. (Courtesy of Somedic Sales AB, Hörby, Sweden.)

and application is usually repeated three times at each testing site.[82] Monofilaments are frequently used in hand rehabilitation clinics; other examples of clinical applications include neuropathies (e.g., diabetic) and peripheral nerve injuries.

Touch-Test Sensory Evaluator (North Coast Medical, Inc, Morgan Hill, CA)

Individual monofilaments are also available in increments ranging from 0.008 to 300 grams (Fig. 5.19). These instruments are convenient and can be carried in a pocket. The handle opens to a 90° angle for testing; when folded it protects the monofilament when not in use.

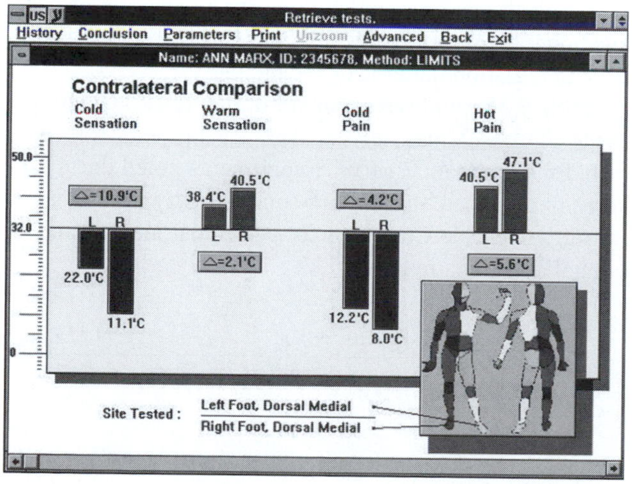

Figure 5.17 Computer-generated data from thermal testing that presents a comparison between the two sides of the body. Note the data for the right foot presents consistently higher threshold values than that of the left. Values are generated for each foot as well as the total difference between the feet. All values are in Celsuis. Conversions for the temperature scale on the left border are: 32°C = 89.6°F and 50°C = 122°F. (Courtesy of Medoc, Ltd., Durham, NC 27707.)

Rydel-Seiffer 64/128 Hz Graduated Tuning Fork (US Neurologicals, Kirkland, WA)

This qualitative tuning fork contains small scaled weights on the distal ends of the two prongs converting it from 128 to 64 Hz (Fig. 5.20). The two triangles move closer together and their intersection moves upward as the intensity of vibration decreases. The intensity where the patient no longer perceives the vibration is recorded as the number adjacent to the intersection of the triangles. This instrument allows more sensitive and specific testing for detecting sensory changes as compared to qualitative tuning forks and has demonstrated high inter- and intratester reliability.[107]

Rolltemp (Somedic Sales AB, Hörby, Sweden)

This instrument is used as a screening tool for determining changes in perception of thermal sensation (Fig. 5.21). The rollers are housed in a storage unit to maintain temperature. The individual rollers are placed in contact with the skin to provide a gross estimate of temperature perception.

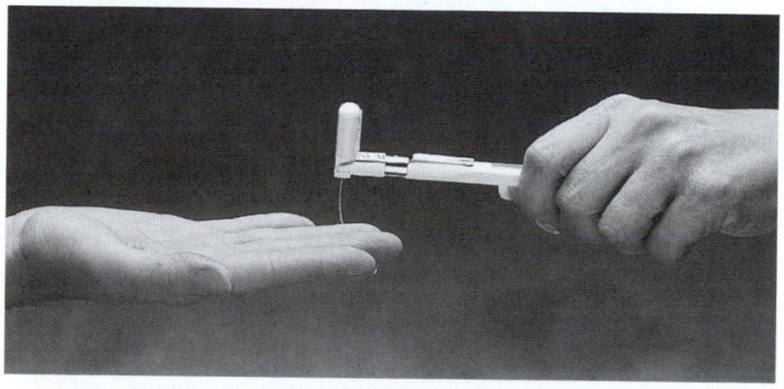

Figure 5.19 Individual monofilament. (Courtesy of North Coast Medical, Inc, Morgan Hill, CA 95037.)

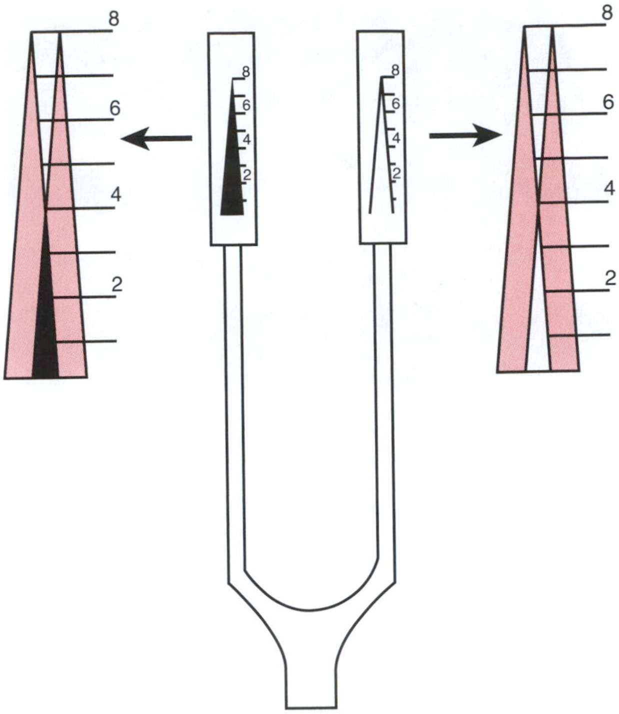

Figure 5.20 Schematic illustration of the Rydel-Seiffer tuning fork. (Courtesy of US Neurologicals, Kirkland, WA, 98033.)

Bio-Thesiometer (Bio-Medical Instrument Co, Newbury, OH)

This instrument is designed to measure threshold perception of a vibratory stimulus (Fig. 5.22). The stimulus is applied using a hand-held device applied to the skin. Intensity of stimulation can be preset or gradually increased until the threshold is reached (or gradually lowered until not longer felt).

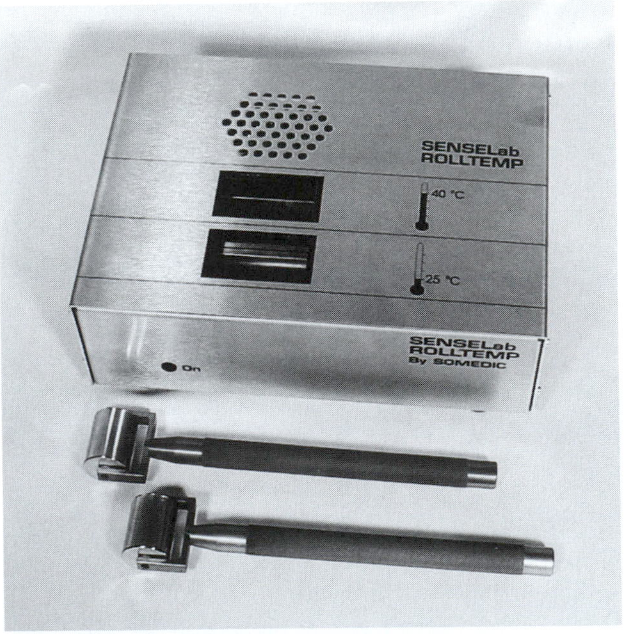

Figure 5.21 The Rolltemp provides a quick screening tool for thermal sensation. The rollers are mounted on handles and stored upright in the two square insertion points on the storage unit. One roller is maintained at 40°C (104°F); the other at 25°C (77°F). (Courtesy of Somedic Sales AB, Hörby, Sweden.)

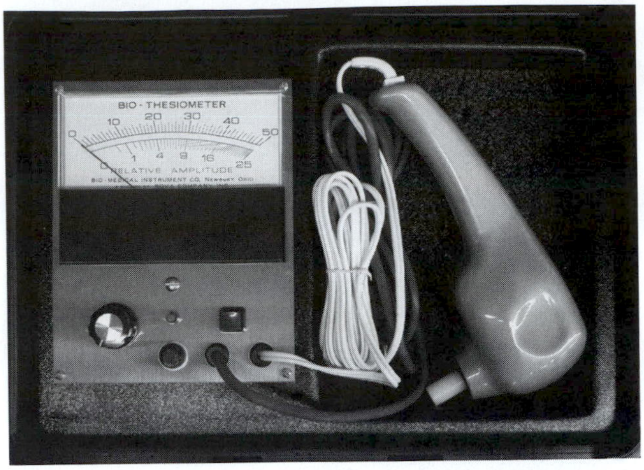

Figure 5.22 Bio-Thesiometer for measuring perception of vibratory stimulus. (Courtesy of Bio-Medical Instrument Co, Newbury, OH, 44065.)

Cranial Nerve Screening

Screening tests for the cranial nerves provide information about location of dysfunction within the brainstem as well as identification of cranial nerves that require more detailed examination. Data generated may include function of muscles innervated by the cranial nerves; visual, auditory, sensory, and gag reflex integrity; perception of taste; swallowing characteristics; eye movements; and constriction and dilation patterns of the pupils.

Table 5.3 provides a summary of the functional components of the cranial nerves. Box 5.5 presents screening tests for each cranial nerve. Impairments noted during the screening indicate that a more comprehensive examination is warranted. See Chapter 8 for additional information on cranial nerve examination.

Sensory Integrity Within the Context of Treatment

Learning a motor behavior is dependent on the patient's ability to take in sensory information from the body and the environment (sensory intake), process it (sensory integration), and use it to plan and organize behavior (output). When patients experience impairment in processing sensory intake, deficits typically occur in planning and organizing behavior. This produces behaviors that may interfere with successful motor learning and motor function.

Table 5.3 Functional Components of the Cranial Nerves

Number	Name	Components	Function
I	Olfactory	Afferent	Olfaction (smell)
II	Optic	Afferent	Vision
III	Oculomotor	Efferent	
		Somatic	Elevates eyelid Turns eye up, down, in
		Visceral	Constricts pupil Accommodates lens
IV	Trochlear	Efferent (somatic)	Turns the adducted eye down and causes intorsion (inward rotation) of eye
V	Trigeminal	Mixed	
		Afferent	Sensation from face Sensation from cornea Sensation from anterior tongue
		Efferent	Muscles of mastication Dampens sound (lensor tympani)
VI	Abducens	Efferent (somatic)	Turns eye out.
VII	Facial	Mixed	
		Afferent	Taste from anterior tongue
		Efferent (somatic)	Muscles of facial expression Dampens sound (stapedius)
		Efferent (visceral)	Tearing (lacrimal gland) Salivation (submandibular and sublingual glands)
VIII	Vestibulocochlear	Afferent	Balance (semicircular canals, utricle, saccule) Hearing (organ of Corti)
IX	Glossopharyngeal	Mixed	
		Afferent	Taste from posterior tongue Sensation from posterior tongue Sensation from oropharynx
		Efferent	Salivation (parotid gland)
X	Vagus	Mixed	
		Afferent	Thoracic and abdominal viscera
		Efferent	Muscles of larynx and pharynx Decreases heart rate Increases GI motility
XI	Spinal accessory	Efferent	Head movements (sternocleidomastoid and trapezius)
XII	Hypoglossal	Efferent	Tongue movements and shape

From Nolan, MF,[62, p 44] with permission.
GI, gastrointestinal.

The POC designed for a patient with impaired sensation is typically guided by one of two approaches, the *Sensory Integration Approach* and the *Compensatory Approach*. The selection of a treatment model is based on a complete data set of information from all examinations together with the established prognosis and diagnosis. The treatment approach depicted in Figure 5.23 is based largely on the Sensory Integration Model developed by Ayers.[1,108–112] The basic premise of this approach is that specific treatment techniques can enhance sensory integration (CNS processing) with a resultant change in motor performance.

Using the Sensory Integration Approach, data obtained from the examination of sensory function informs development of a POC to enhance opportunities for *controlled* sensory intake within a framework of meaningful functional skills (see Chapter 13). During treatment, the patient is provided guided practice in planning and organizing motor behaviors using both *intrinsic* feedback (from the movement itself) and *augmented* feedback (cues planned by the therapist). This approach is designed to improve the ability of the CNS to process and integrate information and promote motor learning. The reader is referred to the work of Ayers[1,108–112] and Bundy and Murray[5] for a detailed presentation of both the theory and practice of the Sensory Integration Model.

Box 5.5 Screening Tests for Cranial Nerves[9,62]

Cranial nerve I: Examine olfactory acuity using non-noxious odors such as lemon oil, coffee, cloves or tobacco.

Cranial nerve II: Examine visual acuity using a Snellen chart; both central and peripheral vision are tested.

Cranial nerves III, IV, and VI: Determine equality and size of pupils; reaction to light; presence of strabismus (loss of ocular alignment); ability of eyes to follow a moving target without head movement; presence of ptosis of eyelid.

Cranial nerve V: Sensory tests of face (sharp/dull discrimination, light touch); open and close jaw against resistance; jaw jerk reflex.

Cranial nerve VII: Examine any asymmetry of face at rest and during voluntary contraction.

Cranial nerve VIII: Test auditory acuity using a vibrating tuning fork (Weber test) placed on vertex of skull or forehead, patient indicates on which side the tone is louder; rub fingers together at a distance and gradually bring toward patient, note distance when first heard; alter volume of conversation; Rinne test (air bone conduction) vibrating tuning fork placed on mastoid process, then near external ear canal, note hearing acuity.

Cranial nerve IX: Examine taste on posterior one-third of tongue; examine gas reflex.

Cranial nerve X: Examine swallowing; observe uvula and soft palate for any asymmetry (tongue depressor).

Cranial nerve XI: Examine strength of the sternocleidomastoid and trapezius muscles.

Cranial nerve XII: With tongue protruded, examine ability to move tongue rapidly from side to side.

The Compensatory Approach is a more traditional intervention that focuses on patient education to accommodate to the limitations imposed by the sensory deficit. The therapist's role is to assist the patient in achieving optimum functional capacity, minimizing functional limitations, protecting anesthetic limbs, and creating appropriate environmental adaptations to enhance safety and function. Guided by this approach, the therapist instructs the patient in practical strategies such as testing bath water with a thermometer or body part with intact sensation before entering; not going barefoot; regularly checking insensitive skin areas for cuts or bruises (particularly important for patients with diabetes); adaptations ("compensations" for the sensory loss) that can include substituting vision for absent tactile cues when carrying objects; wearing heat-resistant gloves when working in the kitchen; using a rolling cart in kitchen or other work space to transport items from one area to another; and arranging kitchen supplies to eliminate need for access to storage areas directly over the stove.

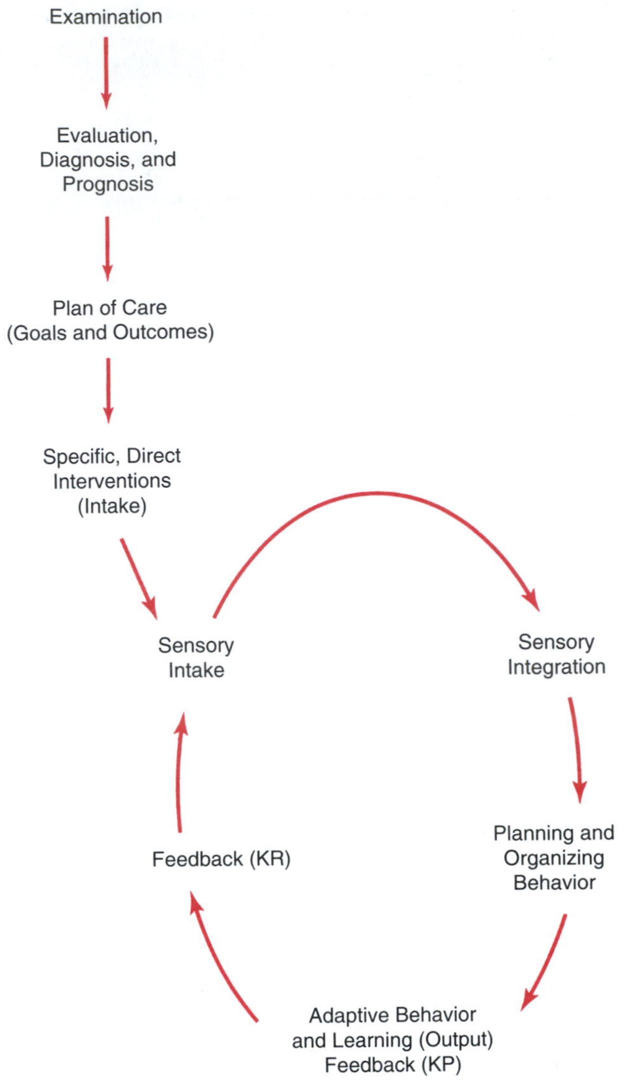

Figure 5.23 Elements of patient management for sensory impairment. KP refers to knowledge of performance (feedback about the quality of movement produced) and KR refers to knowledge of result (feedback about the end result or outcome of the movement). (Adapted from Bundy, AC, and Murray, EA,[5, p 5])

Summary

Examination of sensory function provides important information about the integrity of the somatosensory system. Findings from the examination assist in making clinical judgments about diagnosis, prognosis, identifying goals and outcomes, and establishing the POC. Periodic reexamination provides critical data on changes in patient status and in determining progress toward anticipated goals and expected outcomes. Individual tests for each sensory modality have been presented. Reliability of these test procedures can be improved by careful adherence to consistent guidelines, administration of tests by trained individuals, and subsequent retests performed by the same examiner. Documentation of test results should address the type(s) of sensation affected, the quantity and degree of involvement, and localization of the exact boundaries of the sensory deficits. Finally, it should be emphasized that additional research related to sensory testing is warranted. Further development of QST techniques, standardized protocols, reliability measures, and additional normative data will significantly improve the clinical applications of data obtained from the examination of sensory function.

Questions for Review

1. Define sensory integrity.
2. Identify six impairments or functional limitations that would warrant (or indicate the need for) an examination of sensory function.
3. Describe the preliminary screening tests used to determine mental status for each of the following areas: arousal, attention, orientation, and cognition.
4. Identify the seven types of *cutaneous* receptors, their location, and types of stimuli to which they respond.
5. Identify the four types of *muscle* receptors, their location, and types of stimuli to which they respond.
6. Identify the four types of *joint* receptors, their location, and types of stimuli to which they respond.
7. Identify the sensations mediated by the (A) anterolateral spinothalamic system and the (B) dorsal column–medial lemniscal system.
8. Describe the type of data generated from examination of sensory function and how it is used by the physical therapist.
9. Describe the equipment required to administer a sensory examination.
10. What is meant by a screening? Explain how and why you might perform a screening for sensory integrity.
11. Explain why impaired sensation is a contraindication or precaution for use of some physical agents.
12. Identify the information you would provide the patient prior to administration of sensory tests.
13. For each of the three groups of sensations (superficial, deep, and combined cortical) describe each sensory test, providing both the test protocol and directions for patient response.
14. Describe the method(s) you would use to record the results of sensory testing.

Case Study

A 61-year-old woman presents for outpatient physical therapy. She arrives in a rented wheelchair accompanied by her son. On initial meeting, the patient greets you with a verbal "hello" and a handshake. The son speaks for his mother and recounts that she has been complaining of a burning feeling in her feet and difficulty ambulating.

The son indicates that his mother took an early retirement four years ago from her position as an elementary school teacher. This was a position she had held and enjoyed for 25 years. Her children encouraged the retirement. Their mother had frequently complained about difficulty keeping up with the teaching responsibilities and that the work had become "just too much" for her.

She has four other grown children who all live in the same suburban community. The patient lives alone in a two-bedroom apartment in a building with an elevator and level entrance to the lobby. She was widowed 6 years ago. The children recently decided that a wheelchair should be used for shopping and other outdoor travel as she had stumbled and fallen twice while walking on a level sidewalk.

You thank the son for the information and move the patient into a treatment room to begin your examination.

GUIDING QUESTIONS

1. After explaining the reasons for conducting a thorough examination, you start with a brief mental status examination. Describe how you would examine: *attention, fund of knowledge*, and *memory*.
2. Your preliminary screening tests indicate that cognitive function is grossly intact and that there are no abnormal cranial nerve findings. You plan to continue your examination with the following: manual muscle test, gait analysis and determination of coordination, sensation, and functional status. Identify which tests or measures you would complete first and provide a rationale to substantiate your choice.
3. The first portion of your sensory examination includes perception of pain and temperature. Describe the test protocol for each and identify the ascending pathway that mediates pain and temperature.
4. Your findings for pain and temperature indicate both are intact. You now progress to test proprioception and vibration. Describe the test protocol for each.
5. The test findings indicate severe loss of proprioception and vibration in the lower extremities (distal more than proximal). What receptors are responsible for these sensory modalities? Where are the receptors located? Identify the ascending pathway that mediates proprioception and vibration. What are the functional implications of the findings?

References

1. Ayers, JA: Sensory Integration and Learning Disabilities. Western Psychological Services, Los Angeles, 1972.
2. Byl, NN: Multisensory control of upper extremity function. Neurology Report (now JNPT) 26(1):32, 2002.
3. Ghez, C, and Krakauer, J: The organization of movement. In Kandel, ER, Schwartz, JH, and Jessell, TM: Principles of Neural Science, ed. 4. McGraw-Hill, New York, 2000, p 653.
4. Ayers, AJ: Sensory Integration and Praxis Tests (SIPT Manual). Western Psychological Services, Los Angeles, 1989.
5. Bundy, AC, and Murray, EA: Sensory integration: A. Jean Ayres' theory revisited. In Bundy, AC, Lane, SJ, and Murray, EA: Sensory Integration: Theory and Practice, ed 2. FA Davis, Philadelphia, 2002, p 3.
6. Iyer, MB, and Pedretti, LW: Evaluation of sensation and treatment of sensory dysfunction. In Pedretti, LW, and Early, MB (eds): Occupational Therapy: Practice Skills for Physical Dysfunction, ed 5. CV Mosby, St. Louis, 2001, p 422.
7. American Physical Therapy Association: Guide to physical therapist practice. Phys Ther 81:1, 2001.
8. Aminoff, MJ, et al: Clinical Neurology, ed 3. Appleton & Lange, Stamford, CT, 1996.
9. Gilman, S, and Newman, SW: Manter and Gatz's Essentials of Clinical Neuroanatomy and Neurophysiology, ed 10. FA Davis, Philadelphia, 2003.
10. Stuart, M. et al: Effects of aging on vibration detection thresholds at various body regions. BMC Geriatr 3(1):1, 2003.
11. Woollacott, MH, Shumway-Cook, A, and Nashner, LM: Aging and posture control: Changes in sensory organization and muscular coordination. Int J Aging Hum Dev 23(2):97, 1986.
12. Tran, DB, et al: Age-related deterioration of motion perception and detection. Graefes Arch Clin Exp Ophthalmol 236(4):269, 1998.
13. Benjuya, N, Melzer, I, and Kaplanski, J: Aging-induced shifts from a reliance on sensory input to muscle cocontraction during balanced standing. J Gerontol 59A(2):166, 2004.
14. Fukunaga, A, Uematsu, H, and Sugimoto, K: Influences of aging on taste perception and oral somatic sensation. J Gerontol A Biol Sci Med Sci 60A(1):109, 2005.
15. McClenaghan, BA, et al: Special characteristics of aging postural control. Gait Posture 4:112, 1996.
16. Iverson, BD, et al: Balance performance, force production, and activity levels in noninstitutionalized men 60 to 90 years of age. Phys Ther 70(6):348, 1990.
17. Stones, MJ, and Kozma, A: Balance and age in the sighted and blind. Arch Phys Med Rehabil 68(2):85, 1987.
18. Valentijn, SA, et al: Change in sensory functioning predicts change in cognitive functioning: Results from a 6-year follow-up in the Maastricht aging study. J Am Geriatr Soc 53(3):374, 2005.
19. Wells, C, et al: Regional variation and changes with ageing in vibrotactile sensitivity in the human footsole. J Gerontol A Biol Sci Med Sci 58(8):680, 2003.
20. Hughes, MA, et al: The relationship of postural sway to sensorimotor function, functional performance, and disability in the elderly. Arch Phys Med Rehabil 77(6):567, 1996.
21. Merchut, MP, and Toleikis, SC: Aging and quantitative sensory thresholds. Electromyogr Clin Neurophysiol 30:293, 1990.
22. Wiles, PG, et al: Vibration perception threshold: Influence of age, height, sex, and smoking, and calculation of accurate centile values. Diabet Med 8:157, 1990.
23. de Neeling, JN, et al: Sensory thresholds in older adults: Reproducibility and reference values. Muscle Nerve 17:454, 1994.
24. Gescheider, GA, et al: The effects of aging on information-processing channels in the sense of touch: 1. Absolute sensitivity. Somatosens Mot Res 11:345, 1994.
25. Prioli, AC, Freitas Junior, PB, and Barela, JA: Physical activity and postural control in the elderly: Coupling between visual information and body sway. Gerontology 51(3):145, 2005.
26. Gustafson AS, et al: Changes in balance performance in physically active elderly people aged 73–80. Scand J Rehabil Med 32(4):168, 2000.
27. Onofri, M, et al: Age-related changes of evoked potentials. Neurophysiol Clin 31(2):83, 2001.
28. Verdu, E, et al: Influence of aging on peripheral nerve function and regeneration. J Peripher Nerv Syst 5(4):191, 2000.
29. Helme, RD, Meliala, A, and Gibson, SJ: Methodologic factors which contribute to variations in experimental pain threshold reported for older people. Neurosci Lett 361:1-3:144, 2004.
30. Hurley, MV, Rees, J, and Newham, DJ: Quadriceps function, proprioceptive acuity and functional performance in healthy young, middle-aged and elderly subjects. Age Ageing 27(1):55, 1998.
31. Ulfhak, B, Bergman, E, and Fundin BT: Impairment of peripheral sensory innervation in senescence. Auton Neurosci 96(1):43, 2002.
32. Hofer, SM, Berg, S, and Era, P: Evaluating the interdependence of aging-related changes in visual and auditory acuity, balance, and cognitive functioning. Psychol Aging (2):285, 2003.
33. Takekuma, K, et al: Age and gender differences in skin sensory threshold assessed by current perception in community-dwelling Japanese. J Epidemiol 10(1 Suppl):S33, 2000.
34. Woollacott, M, and Shumway-Cook, A: Attention and the control of posture and gait: A review of an emerging area of research. Gait Posture 16(1):1, 2000.
35. U.S. Department of Health and Human Services. Healthy People 2010: Understanding and Improving Health. 2nd ed. Washington, DC: US Government Printing Office, November 2000.
36. Jackson-Wyatt, O: Brain function, aging, and dementia. In Umphred, DA (ed): Neurological Rehabilitation, ed 4. CV Mosby, St. Louis, 2001, p 790.
37. Hopper, CR: Sensory and sensory integrative development. In Bonder, BR, and Wagner, MB (eds): Functional Performance in Older Adults, ed 2. FA Davis, Philadelphia, 2001, p 121.
38. Hills, GA: The changing realm of the senses. In Lewis, CB (ed): Aging: The Health Care Challenge, ed 4. FA Davis, Philadelphia, 2002, p 83.
39. Gallman, RL, and Elfervig, LS: The aging sensory system. In Stanley, M, and Gauntlett Beare, P (eds): Gerontological Nursing, ed 2. FA Davis, Philadelphia, 1999, p 93.
40. Peters, A: The effects of normal aging on myelin and nerve fibers: A review. J Neurocytol 31:581, 2002.
41. Adams, RD, and Victor, M: Principles of Neurology, ed 6. McGraw-Hill, New York, 1996.
42. Gould, B: Pathophysiology for the Health Related Professions, ed 2. WB Saunders, Philadelphia, 2002.
43. Price, DL: Aging of the brain and dementia of the Alzheimer type. In Kandel, ER, Schwartz, JH, and Jessell, TM: Principles of Neural Science, ed. 4, McGraw-Hill, New York, 2000, p 1149.
44. Craik, RL: Sensorimotor changes and adaptation in the older adult. In Guccione, AA (ed): Geriatric Physical Therapy. CV Mosby, Philadelphia, 1993, p 71.
45. Dorfman, LJ, and Bosley, TM: Age-related changes in peripheral and central nerve conduction in man. Neurology 29(1):38, 1979.
46. Bouche, P. et al: Clinical and electrophysiological study of the peripheral nervous system in the elderly. J Neurol 240(5):263, 1993.
47. Taylor, PK: Nonlineal effects of age on nerve conduction in adults. J Neurol Sci 66:223, 1984.
48. Downie, AW, and Newell, DJ: Sensory nerve conduction in patients with diabetes mellitus and controls. Neurology 11:876, 1961.
49. Bolton, CF, et al: A quantitative study of Meissner's corpuscles in man. Neurology 16:1, 1966.
50. Matsuoka, S, et al: Quantitative and qualitative studies of Meissner's corpuscles in human skin, with special reference to alterations caused by aging. J Dermatol 10(3):205, 1983.
51. Verrillo, RT: Age related changes in the sensitivity to vibration. J Gerontol 35:185, 1980.
52. Lascelles, RG, and Thomas, PK: Changes due to age in internodal length in the sural nerve of man. J Neurol Neurosurg Psychiatry 29:40, 1966.
53. Lewis, CB, and Bottomley, JM: Geriatric Physical Therapy: A Clinical Approach. Appleton & Lange, Norwalk, CT, 1994.
54. Woodward, KL: The relationship between skin compliance, age, gender, and tactile discriminative thresholds in humans. Somatosens Mot Res 10(1):63, 1993.

55. Thornbury, JM, and Mistretta, CM: Tactile sensitivity as a function of age. J Gerontol 36:34, 1981.
56. Muijser, H: The influence of spatial contrast on the frequency-dependent nature of vibration sensitivity. Percept Psychophys 48(5):431, 1990.
57. Gellis, M, and Pool, R: Two-point discrimination distances in the normal hand and forearm. Plast Reconstr Surg 59:57, 1977.
58. Skinner HB, Barrack, RL, and Cook, SD: Age-related decline in proprioception. Clinic Orthopaedics Related Res 184:208, 1984.
59. Bohannon, RW, et al: Decrease in timed balance test scores with aging. Phys Ther 64(7):1067, 1984.
60. Baloh, RW, et al: Comparison of static and dynamic posturography in young and older normal people. J Am Geriatr Soc 42(4):405, 1994.
61. Labyt, E, et al: Influence of aging on cortical activity associated with a visuo-motor task. Neurobiol Aging 25(6):817, 2004.
62. Nolan, MF: Introduction to the Neurologic Examination. FA Davis, Philadelphia, 1996.
63. Waxman, SG: Correlative Neuroanatomy, ed 24. New York, Lange Medical Books/McGraw-Hill, 2000.
64. Guyton, AC, and Hall, JE: Textbook of Medical Physiology, ed 10. WB Saunders, Philadelphia, 2000.
65. Gardner, EP, and Martin, JH: Coding of sensory information. In Kandel, ER, Schwartz, JH, and Jessell, TM: Principles of Neural Science, ed. 4, McGraw-Hill, New York, 2000, p 411.
66. Kiernan, JA: Barr's The Human Nervous System: An Anatomical Viewpoint, ed 8. Lippincott Williams & Wilkins, Philadelphia, 2005.
67. Kingsley, RE: Concise Text of Neuroscience, ed 2. Lippincott Williams & Wilkins, Philadelphia, 2000.
68. Lundy-Ekman, L: Neuroscience: Fundamentals for Rehabilitation, ed 2. WB Saunders, Philadelphia, 2002.
69. Afifi, AK, and Bergman, RA: Functional Neuroanatomy: Text and Atlas, ed 2. Lange Medical Books/McGraw-Hill, New York, 2005.
70. Jacobs, SE, and Lowe, DL: Somatic senses I: The anterolateral system. In Cohen, H (ed): Neuroscience for Rehabilitation, ed 2. Lippincott Williams & Wilkins, Philadephia, 1999, p 77.
71. Gardner, EP, Martin, JH, and Jessel, TM: The bodily senses. In Kandel, ER, Schwartz, JH, and Jessell, TM: Principles of Neural Science, ed. 4, McGraw-Hill, New York, 2000, p 430.
72. Fitzgerald, MJT: Neuroanatomy: Basic and Clinical, ed 3. WB Saunders, Philadelphia, 1996.
73. Fredericks, CM: Basic sensory mechanism and the somatosensory system. In Fredericks, CM, and Saladin, LK (eds): Pathophysiology of the Motor Systems: Principles and Clinical Presentations. FA Davis, Philadelphia, 1996, p 78.
74. Petty, NJ: Principles of Neuromusculoskeletal Treatment and Management: A Guide for Therapists. Churchill Livingstone, New York, 2004.
75. Bear, MF, Connors, BW, and Paradiso, MA: Neuroscience: Exploring the Brain, ed 2. Lippincott Williams & Wilkins, Philadelphia, 2001.
76. Gardner, EP, and Kandel, ER: Touch. In Kandel, ER, et al (eds): Principles of Neural Science, ed 4. McGraw-Hill, New York, 2000, p 451.
77. Janos, SC, and Boissonnault, WG: Upper quarter screening examination. In Boissonnault, WG (ed): Primary Care for the Physical Therapist: Examination and Triage. WB Saunders, Philadelphia, 2005, p 138.
78. Green, LW, and Kreuter, MW: Health Program Planning: An Educational and Ecological Approach, ed 4. McGraw-Hill, New York, 2005.
79. Nolan, MF: Clinical assessment of cutaneous sensory function. Clin Manage Phys Ther 4:26, 1984.
80. Werner, JL, and Omer, GE: Evaluating cutaneous pressure sensation of the hand. Am J Occup Ther 24:347, 1970.
81. Centers for Disease Control and Prevention (CDC): Guidelines for Hand Hygiene in Health-Care Settings: Recommendations of the Healthcare Infection Control Practices Advisory Committee and the HICPAC/SHEA/APIC/IDSA Hand Hygiene Task Force. MMWR 2002; 51 (No. RR-16), CDC, Department of Health and Human Services, Atlanta, GA, 2002.
82. Bentzel, K: Assessing abilities and capacities: Sensation. In Trombly, CA, and Radomski, MV (eds): Occupational Therapy for Physical Dysfunction, ed 5. Lippincott Williams & Wilkins, Philadelphia, 2002, p 159.
83. Gutman, SA, and Schonfeld, AB: Screening Adult Neurologic Populations: A Step-By-Step Instruction Manual. AOTA Press, Bethesda, MD, 2003.
84. Nolan, MF: Limits of two-point discrimination ability in the lower limb in young adult men and women. Phys Ther 63:1424, 1983.
85. Nolan, MF: Quantitative measure of cutaneous sensation: Two-point discrimination values for the face and trunk. Phys Ther 65:181, 1985.
86. Nolan, MF: Two-point discrimination assessment in the upper limb in young adult men and women. Phys Ther 62:965, 1982.
87. Desrosiers, J, et al: Hand sensibility of healthy older people. J Am Geriatr Soc 44(8):974, 1996.
88. Shimokata, H, and Kuzuya, F: Two-point discrimination test of the skin as an index of sensory aging. Gerontology 41(5):267, 1995.
89. Hermann, RP, Novak, CB, and Mackinnon, SE: Establishing normal values of moving two-point discrimination in children and adolescents. Dev Med Child Neurol 38(3):255, 1996.
90. Richards, PM, Persinger, MA, and Michel, RN: Ontogeny of two-point discrimination for fingers and toes in children (ages 7 through 15 years). Percept Mot Skills 86(3 Pt 2):1259, 1998.
91. Kent, BE: Sensory-motor testing: The upper limb of adult patients with hemiplegia. J Am Phys Ther Assoc 45:550, 1965.
92. Boivie, J: Central pain and the role of quantitative sensory testing (QST) in research and diagnosis. Eur J Pain 7(4):339, 2003.
93. Cheng, WY, et al: Quantitative sensory testing and risk factors of diabetic sensory neuropathy. J Neurol 246(5):394, 1999.
94. Chong, PS, and Cros, DP: Technology literature review: Quantitative sensory testing. Muscle Nerve 29(5):734, 2004.
95. Gibbons, C, and Freeman, R: The evaluation of small fiber function-autonomic and quantitative sensory testing. Neurol Clin 22(3):683, 2004.
96. Granot, M, Sprecher, E, and Yarnitsky, D: Psychophysics of phasic and tonic heat pain stimuli by quantitative sensory testing in healthy subjects. Eur J Pain 7(2):139, 2003.
97. Greenspan, JD, et al: Allodynia in patients with post-stroke central pain (CPSP) studied by statistical quantitative sensory testing within individuals. Pain 109(3):357, 2004.
98. Hagander, LG, et al: Quantitative sensory testing: Effect of site and pressure on vibration thresholds. Clin Neurophysiol 111(6):1066, 2000.
99. Hayes, KC, et al: Clinical and electrophysiologic correlates of quantitative sensory testing in patients with incomplete spinal cord injury. Arch Phys Med Rehabil 83(11):1612, 2002.
100. Lundstrom, R: Neurological diagnosis—aspects of quantitative sensory testing methodology in relation to hand-arm vibration syndrome. Int Arch Occup Environ Health 75(1-2):68, 2002.
101. Polianskis, R, Graven-Nielsen, T, and Arendt-Nielsen, L: Computer-controlled pneumatic pressure algometry—a new technique for quantitative sensory testing. Eur J Pain 5(3):267, 2001.
102. Rommel, O, et al: Quantitative sensory testing, neurophysiological and psychological examination in patients with complex regional pain syndrome and hemisensory deficits. Pain 93(3):279, 2001.
103. Rosenberg, D, Conolley, J, and Dellon, AL: Thenar eminence quantitative sensory testing in the diagnosis of proximal median nerve compression. J Hand Ther 14(4):258, 2001.
104. Samuelsson, L, and Lundin, A: Thermal quantitative sensory testing in lumbar disc herniation. Eur Spine J 11(1):71, 2002.
105. Shy, ME, et al: Therapeutics and Technology Assessment Subcommittee of the American Academy of Neurology: Quantitative sensory testing: Report of the Therapeutics and Technology Assessment Subcommittee of the American Academy of Neurology. Neurology 60(6):898, 2003.
106. Ziegler, D, et al: Validation of a novel screening device (NeuroQuick) for quantitative assessment of small nerve fiber dysfunction as an early feature of diabetic polyneuropathy. Diabetes Care 28(5):1169, 2005.
107. Pestronk, A, et al: Sensory exam with a quantitative tuning fork: Rapid, sensitive and predictive of SNAP amplitude. Neurology 62(3):461, 2004.
108. Ayers, JA: Tactile functions: Their relation to hyperactive and perceptual motor behavior. Am J Occup Ther 18:83, 1964.

109. Ayers, JA: Interrelations among perceptual-motor abilities in a group of normal children. Am J Occup Ther 20:288, 1966.
110. Ayers, JA: Improving academic scores through sensory integration. J Learn Disabil 5:338, 1972.
111. Ayers, JA: Cluster analysis of measures of sensory integration. Am J Occup Ther 31:362, 1977.
112. Ayers, JA: Sensory Integration and the Child. Western Psychological Services, Los Angeles, 1979.

Supplemental Readings

Allen, GL, et al: Aging and path integration skill: Kinesthetic and vestibular contributions to wayfinding. Percept Psychophys 66 (1):170, 2004.

Bril, V, and Perkins, BA: Comparison of vibration perception thresholds obtained with the Neurothesiometer and the CASE IV and relationship to nerve conduction studies. Diabet Med 19(8):661, 2002.

Gilman, S: Joint position sense and vibration sense: Anatomical organisation and assessment. J Neurol Neurosurg Psychiatry 73:473, 2002.

Ingram, HA, et al: The role of proprioception and attention in a visuomotor adaptation task. Exp Brain Res 132(1):114, 2000.

Kamei, N, et al: Effectiveness of Semmes-Weinstein monofilament examination for diabetic peripheral neuropathy screening. J Diabet Compl 19(1):47, 2005.

Kastenbauer, T, et al: The value of the Rydel-Seiffer tuning fork as a predictor of diabetic polyneuropathy compared with a neurothesiometer. Diabet Med 21(6):563, 2004.

Liu, W, et al: Noise-enhanced vibrotactile sensitivity in older adults and patients with stroke and patients with diabetic neuropathy. Arch Phys Med Rehabil 83: 71, 2002.

Nardone, A, et al: Loss of large-diameter spindle afferent fibres is not detrimental to the control of body sway during upright stance: Evidence from neuropathy. Exp Brain Res 135(2):155, 2000.

Paisley, AN, et al: A comparison of the Neuropen Against standard quantitative sensory-threshold measures for assessing peripheral nerve function. Diabet Med 19(5):400, 2002.

Speers, RA, Kuo, AD, and Horak, FB: Contributions of altered sensation and feedback responses to changes in coordination of postural control due to aging. Gait Posture 16(1):20, 2002.

Viswanathan, V, et al: Early recognition of diabetic neuropathy: Evaluation of a simple outpatient procedure using thermal perception. Postgrad Med J 78:541, 2002.

Appendix A: Two-point Discrimination Values for Healthy Subjects 20–24 Years of Age

Two-Point Discrimination Values for the Upper Extremities of Healthy Subjects 20 to 24 Years of Age ($N = 43$)

Skin Region	$\bar{X}$ (mm)	s
Upper—lateral arm	42.4	14.0
Lower—lateral arm	37.8	13.1
Mid—medial arm	45.4	15.5
Mid—posterior arm	39.8	12.3
Mid—lateral forearm	35.9	11.6
Mid—medial forearm	31.5	8.9
Mid—posterior forearm	30.7	8.2
Over first dorsal interosseous muscle	21.0	5.6
Palmar surface—distal phalanx, thumb	2.6	0.6
Palmar surface—distal phalanx, long finger	2.6	0.7
Palmar surface—distal phalanx, little finger	2.5	0.7

Two-Point Discrimination Values for the Lower Extremities of Healthy Subjects 20 to 24 Years of Age ($N = 43$)

Skin Region	$\bar{X}$ (mm)	s
Proximal—anterior thigh	40.1	14.7
Distal—anterior thigh	23.2	9.3
Mid—lateral thigh	42.5	15.9
Mid—medial thigh	38.5	12.4
Mid—posterior thigh	42.2	15.9
Proximal—lateral leg	37.7	13.0
Distal—lateral leg[a]	41.6	13.0
Medial leg	43.6	13.5
Tip of great toe	6.6	1.8
Over 1–2 metatarsal interspace	23.9	6.3
Over 5th metatarsal	22.2	8.6

[a] $n = 41$

Two-Point Discrimination Values For the Face and Trunk of Healthy Subjects 20 to 24 Years of Age ($N = 43$)

Skin Region	$\bar{X}$ (mm)	s
Over eyebrow	14.9	4.2
Cheek	11.9	3.2
Over lateral mandible	10.4	2.2
Lateral neck	35.2	9.8
Medial to acromion process	51.1	14.0
Lateral to nipple	45.7	12.7[a]
Lateral to umbilicus	36.4	7.3[b]
Over iliac crest	44.9	10.1[c]
Lateral to C7 spine	55.4	20.0[b]
Over inferior angle of scapula	52.2	12.6[b]
Lateral to L3 spine	49.9	12.7[b]

[a] $n = 26$
[b] $n = 42$
[c] $n = 33$

From Nolan, MF,[84–86] with permission of the American Physical Therapy Association.

CHAPTER

6

Musculoskeletal Examination

D. Joyce White, PT, DSc

LEARNING OBJECTIVES

1. Identify the purposes of performing a musculoskeletal examination.
2. Describe the components of a musculoskeletal examination.
3. Identify questions that should be included in a patient interview.
4. Describe the procedures used to selectively test specific tissue types in a musculoskeletal examination.
5. Identify additional procedures that often complement a musculoskeletal examination.
6. Using the case study examples, apply clinical decision making skills in evaluating musculoskeletal examination data.

OUTLINE

The musculoskeletal system includes bones; muscles with their related tendons and synovial sheaths; bursa; and joint structures such as cartilage, menisci, capsules, and ligaments. Acute injuries or chronic conditions that disrupt the anatomy or physiology of musculoskeletal tissues can greatly affect a patient's function by causing impairments such as pain, inflammation, swelling, structural deformity, restricted joint movement, joint instability, and muscle weakness. Examples of diagnoses that result in direct impairment of the musculoskeletal system include fracture, rheumatoid arthritis, osteoarthritis, joint dislocation, tendinitis, bursitis, muscle strain/rupture, and ligament sprain/rupture.

Many pathological conditions that initially affect other body systems such as the neurological, cardiovascular, or pulmonary systems can result in secondary or indirect impairment of the musculoskeletal system. This often occurs when patients' activities are restricted by the condition—perhaps as a result of confinement for a period of time to a bed or wheelchair—or the patient moves the upper or lower extremities in an inefficient or stress-causing pattern. Diagnoses that can cause indirect impairments of the musculoskeletal system included traumatic brain injury, cerebral vascular accident, cerebral palsy, spinal and peripheral nerve injury, burns, and myocardial infarction, just to name a few.

Both direct and indirect musculoskeletal impairments can contribute to functional limitation and disability that affect a patient's ability to perform certain tasks and roles in society. By considering the few examples of diagnoses that cause direct and indirect musculoskeletal impairments provided in the preceding text, one can appreciate how often physical therapists and other health professionals encounter clinical problems of the musculoskeletal system. Administering musculoskeletal tests and measures is almost always a major component of an initial patient examination.

This chapter discusses the purposes of, and provides a general framework for, conducting a musculoskeletal examination. The principles and components of a musculoskeletal examination, together with how to organize and integrate the data with those of other body systems, are emphasized. Other resources are available that provide detailed musculoskeletal testing procedures of specific body regions.[1–5]

Purpose of the Musculoskeletal Examination

Evaluation of data from the musculoskeletal examination contributes to establishing a diagnosis and prognosis, setting goals and outcomes, and developing and implementing a plan of care. A musculoskeletal examination is also an important component of evaluating treatment outcomes both periodically during the treatment process and at the conclusion of therapy. The purposes of performing a musculoskeletal examination include the following:

1. To determine the presence or absence of impairments, functional limitations, and disability involving muscles, bones, and related joint structures.
2. To identify the specific tissues that are causing/contributing to the impairment, functional limitation, or disability.
3. To determine baseline status.
4. To help formulate appropriate anticipated therapeutic goals, expected outcomes, and plan of care.
5. To evaluate the effectiveness of rehabilitation, medical, or surgical management.
6. To identify risk factors to prevent the development or worsening of impairments, functional limitations, or disabilities.
7. To determine orthotic and adaptive equipment necessary for functional performance of occupational and recreational activities.
8. To motivate the patient.

Examination Procedures

Patient History and Interview

Prior to beginning the physical examination it is important to gain as much information as possible about the patient's current condition and past medical history. This information will help to direct and focus the examination to an area and system of the body. Information on symptoms and functional ability will help to establish a baseline against which treatment effectiveness can be judged. It will also enable the examination and treatment of the patient to be conducted safely.

Typically, most of this information is obtained by interviewing the patient. However, utilizing other information sources can be very efficient and provide objectivity and details to supplement an interview. If the patient is hospitalized in an acute care or rehabilitation setting, the medical records including admission reports, progress notes, medication sheets, surgical summaries, body imaging reports, and laboratory test results, should be available and sought out. Referral summaries from previous medical care settings that review prior treatment approaches and discuss functional status may also be included. Other members of the health care team can be consulted for their input.

Outpatients often arrive with only a general diagnosis from a referring physician, or may be self-referred. In such cases it will be helpful to ask the patient to complete a medical history form prior to the examination process. A medical history form should include space for the patient to note the chief problem and date of onset; diagnostic tests performed for the problem; name and date of all surgeries; all medications currently being taken; a checklist of common medical conditions the patient may have experienced; brief family medical history; and patient's age, occupation, and lifestyle questions pertaining to smoking, alcohol use, and exercise. Figure 6.1 provides an example of a medical history form.

A thorough understanding of the patient's medical background is critical for selection and safe application of examination and treatment procedures. For example, a history of a myocardial infarction would cause the therapist to limit and more closely monitor the patient during muscle performance testing. A history of diabetes mellitus would cause the therapist to suspect and test for potentially compromised peripheral vascular and peripheral nervous systems, and to possibly avoid the use of heat modalities during treatment. Even if a patient completes a medical history form, it is important for the therapist to review and clarify the information with the patient. Sometimes important medical background data is inadvertently forgotten as the patient focuses on current problems. Verbally reviewing the information with the patient may jog the patient's memory.

After reviewing the information gained from medical records, other health care providers, and the patient-completed medical history form, the therapist is ready to begin the patient interview. Ideally, the patient interview should be conducted in a quiet, well-lit room that offers a measure of privacy. To encourage good communication, the therapist and patient should be at a similar eye level, facing each other, with a comfortable space between them—about 3 feet apart is customary in the United States. The patient should have the therapist's undivided attention; telephone calls and other interruptions should be avoided. The therapist may wish to have paper and pen available to record particular dates and information that is easily forgotten, but the interview should flow as an active conversation, not a dictation session. Repeated practice greatly improves the therapist's ability to listen, direct the interview, and establish a positive working relationship with the patient.

Over the course of the interview the therapist gains information about the patient's current complaints including onset, location, type and behavior of symptoms, current medications, previous treatments, secondary medical problems, and medical history. The patient's age and gender should be noted; some conditions are more common in particular age groups and genders. Often, detailed information about a patient's occupation, recreational activities, and social/living situation are required to understand the cause of the impairments, functional limitations, and to develop a relevant plan of care that focuses on the patient's goals. Open-ended, objective questions that do not promote biased answers should be used. For example, instead of asking "Is your right knee painful?" the therapist should ask, "Where are your symptoms located?" The therapist should carefully guide the interview to keep it focused on pertinent information and conclude in a timely manner. All

The purpose of this questionnaire is to assist us in providing you with quality care by obtaining a better understanding of your total health status. This questionnaire is part of your confidential medical record.

NAME: ____________________ DATE: __________

CHIEF PROBLEM OR COMPLAINT: ____________________

REFERRING MD: ____________________ DATE OF NEXT MD VISIT: __________

MEDICATIONS: Please list *all* medications currently being taken, along with the dosage, if known, and frequency.

1. ____________________ 4. ____________________

2. ____________________ 5. ____________________

3. ____________________ 6. ____________________

SURGERY: Please list *all* surgeries and approximate date.

1. ____________________ DATE: __________

2. ____________________ DATE: __________

3. ____________________ DATE: __________

4. ____________________ DATE: __________

DIAGNOSTIC TESTS: Please check tests for current problem only.

X-rays: __________ CT Scan: __________ MRI: __________ Bone Scan: __________

EMG: __________ Blood Test: __________ Myelogram: __________ Others: __________

OCCUPATION: ____________________

LIFE STYLE: Non Smoker: ____ Smoke ____/day

No Alcohol: ____ Alcohol ____/day or ____/week

No Exercise: ____ Exercise ____/day or ____/week

FAMILY HISTORY: Mother, Father, siblings: Alive and healthy: __________

If deceased, cause of death: ____________________

Figure 6.1 An example of a medical history recording form. (Courtesy of North Andover Physical Therapy Associates, North Andover, MA.)

(*continued*)

DO YOU HAVE, OR HAVE YOU HAD, ANY OF THE FOLLOWING: Please check *All* that apply.

___ High blood pressure
___ Heart problems
___ Heart palpitations, murmur
___ Chest pain

___ Shortness of breath
___ Coughing

___ Difficulty sleeping lying flat
___ Lung problems
___ Asthma
___ Allergies

___ Ulcers
___ Recent weight gain or loss
___ Nausea, vomiting
___ Bowel or bladder changes
___ Loss of appetite

___ Sexual dysfunction
___ Abnormal or painful menstruation
___ Pelvic inflammatory disease
___ Currently pregnant
___ Date of last mammogram:_____

___ Blood in urine
___ Incontinence

___ Seizures
___ Head trauma
___ Paralysis
___ Loss of consciousness
___ Headaches

___ Numbness or tingling
___ Dizziness
___ Balance problems

___ Arthritis

___ Hot or cold intolerance
___ Diabetes
___ Low blood sugar
___ Thyroid problems

___ Tumors ___ Cancer
___ Bleeding or bruising
___ Dialysis
___ Blood transfusion

___ Rashes
___ Scars
___ Changes in hair or nails

___ Wear eye glasses, contacts
___ Changes in vision
___ Blurred or double vision

___ Difficulty swallowing
___ Ear pain
___ Vocal changes
___ Ringing in ears

___ Dentures
___ Major dental work
___ Difficulty eating

___ Varicose veins
___ Muscle cramps
___ Joint or muscle pain

___ Psychiatric or psychological care

___ Fractures (broken bones)
Where?____________________
___ Problem requiring orthopedic shoes
___ Hip or ankle problem
___ Unusual illness as child

Please check if you have ever been in a motor vehicle accident _____

Figure 6.1 continued

questions should use conversational language rather than medical terminology so the questions are easily understood by the patient. The therapist should ask one question at a time and be sure to obtain a response before proceeding to other questions. Follow-up inquiries may be needed to clarify initial answers. It is important for the therapist to keep an open mind during the interview and not rush to conclusions about the patient's symptoms and diagnosis.

The following sequence is suggested as a way of organizing the interview. Similar information on general patient interviewing, that includes slight variations in format, can be found in texts by Talley and O'Connor,[6] Hertling and Kessler,[1] and Paris.[7]

Opening Question

The interview should begin with a general question such as "What brings you to physical therapy today?" or "What seems to be the problem?" If the patient is hospitalized the question may need to be rephrased to avoid having the patient retell the medical history to every health care provider. "I see from your medical chart that you fractured your hip and underwent a surgical repair yesterday. Is that what happened?" The patient should be given the opportunity to present the story. After the patient has concluded his or her statement, it is appropriate to say, "That's good. Now I have an idea of the problem. I have some other questions I need to ask to help me understand your problem better." Depending on the information provided by the patient, some of the following questions may be asked.

Onset of Symptoms

"How did this pain (swelling, limitation, problem, and so forth) begin?" The therapist must know if the onset was sudden (e.g., caused by trauma such as a fall, blow, or skiing or automobile accident). Specific information about the patient's body position at the time of trauma and the mechanism of injury will help to identify the structures involved. If the onset was more gradual or insidious, a systemic condition or chronic biomechanical problem may be more likely. A congenital onset is also a possibility.

Location of the Symptoms

"Where is your pain? Can you point to the location?" A body chart (Fig. 6.2) can be used to help identify and document the specific location of symptoms. The patient (or therapist with the patient's direction) can darken the involved area on the body chart using a pen or pencil.

Often the location of the symptoms coincides with the location of the lesion. This is more likely if the lesion is in superficial and distal tissues. For example, a lesion in a superficial tendon near the ankle will usually cause pain over the tendon site. Lesions in deeper, more proximal

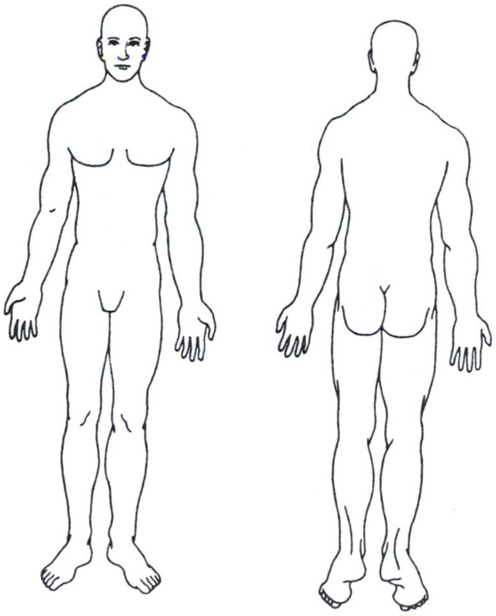

Figure 6.2 This body chart can supplement the patient's verbal description of the location of the pain. (From Dyrek, DA,[190, p 74] with permission.)

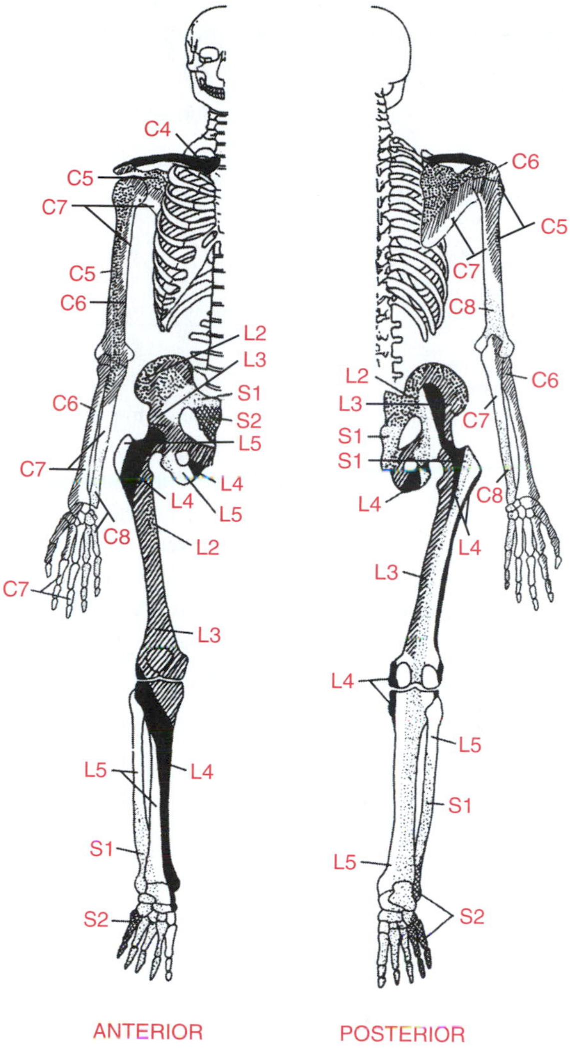

Figure 6.3 Sclerotomes. (From Hertling, D and Kessler, RM,[1, p 52] with permission.)

tissues often refer pain distally following *sclerotome* (Fig. 6.3) or dermatome patterns (see Chapter 5).

Referred pain may be perceived as originating from any or all tissues innervated by the same segmental spinal level in which the lesion is located. For example, pain due to osteoarthritis of the hip is often felt in the anterior groin and thigh along the sclerotomes or dermatomes for L2 and L3. Considerable individual variation has been noted in dermatome and sclerotome patterns.[8]

"Has the pain changed in location? Spread to other areas? Become more focused?" Pain that is spreading usually indicates a worsening condition, while more focused symptoms indicate improvement. Changes in symptoms in relationship to varying body positions, activities, and treatments should be noted.

Quality of the Symptoms

"How severe is the pain? Is the pain sharp? Dull? Throbbing?" A simple yet effective way to document pain

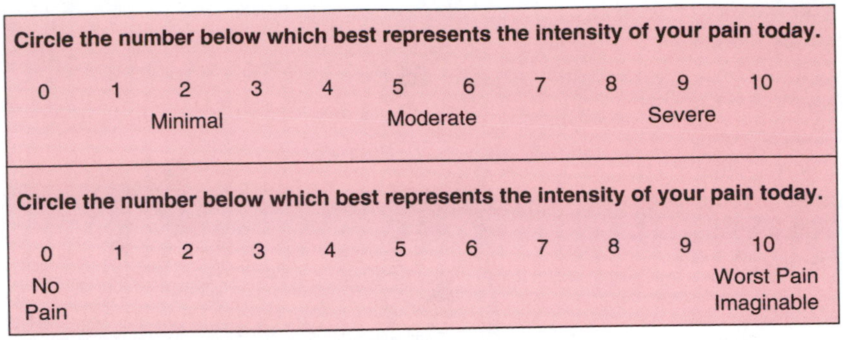
Circle the number below which best represents the intensity of your pain today.
0 1 2 3 4 5 6 7 8 9 10
Minimal
Moderate
Severe
Circle the number below which best represents the intensity of your pain today.
0 1 2 3 4 5 6 7 8 9 10
No Pain
Worst Pain Imaginable

Figure 6.4 Two types of numerical pain rating scales.

severity is to ask the patient to rate his or her pain from 0 (no pain) to 10 (most severe pain imaginable) as illustrated in the numerical pain rating scale presented in Figure 6.4. A visual analog scale (Fig. 6.5) or thermometer pain scale (Fig. 6.6) can also be used if preferred. A checklist of adjectives like that found in the McGill-Melzack Pain Questionnaire [9] can clarify symptoms further (Fig. 6.7).

The adjectives used to describe pain may have diagnostic implications. Dull, aching pain may indicate muscle or joint lesions. Numbness, tingling, shooting pain, or burning sensations may indicate nervous system involvement. Deep, throbbing pain, or coolness in a body region may indicate vascular problems. Weakness, clumsiness, or incoordination may suggest muscle and possibly peripheral or central nervous system dysfunction.

Behavior of the Symptoms

"What makes your symptoms increase? Decrease?" Symptoms from musculoskeletal conditions typically vary in response to rest, activity, and body positions that either increase or decrease mechanical stress placed on the involved tissue. The behavior of the symptoms helps to establish a diagnosis and determine which treatment techniques are more likely to be effective. For example, pain from overuse syndromes such as tendonitis will decrease with rest, whereas joint stiffness caused by osteoarthritis often increases following rest. If a patient reports that the sitting position reduces back pain, then the therapist will probably have more success in relieving the pain using back flexion rather than extension exercises.

Symptoms that do not vary with a change in activity or body position are rarely due to musculoskeletal lesions, and in fact are a "red flag" for more serious conditions such as space-occupying tumors and pathologies involving internal organs. Often patients will report that "nothing helps the pain." This statement should be fully explored with follow-up questions such as "Is your pain better or worse in the morning when you wake up from sleeping? Does your pain vary if you sleep on your back versus on your stomach?"

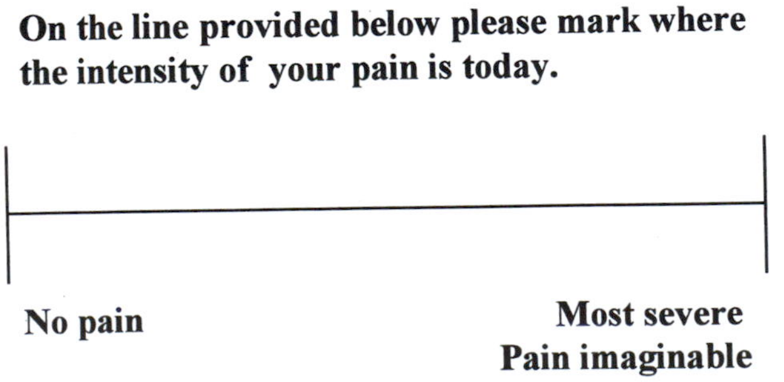
On the line provided below please mark where the intensity of your pain is today.
No pain
Most severe Pain imaginable

Figure 6.5 Visual analog pain rating scale. The line is usually 3.9 in (10 cm) in length. The patient's mark is measured from the left (no pain) end of the scale and is recorded in centimeters.

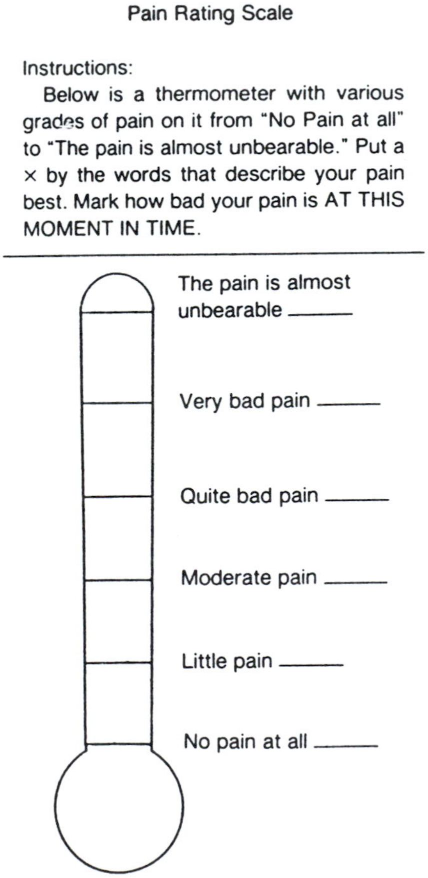

Below is a thermometer with various grades of pain on it from "No Pain at all" to "The pain is almost unbearable." Put a × by the words that describe your pain best. Mark how bad your pain is AT THIS MOMENT IN TIME.
The pain is almost unbearable

Figure 6.6 Thermometer pain rating scale. (From Brodie, DJ, et al: Evaluation of low back pain by patient questionnaires and therapist assessment. J Orthop Sport Phys Ther 11:528, 1990, with permission.)

Look carefully at the twenty groups of words. If any word in any group applies to *your pain*, please circle that word – but do not circle more than *one word in any one group* – so you must choose the *most suitable word* in that group.

In groups that do not apply to your pain, there is no need to circle *any* word – just leave them as they are.

Group 1 Flickering Quivering Pulsing Throbbing Beating Pounding	*Group 2* Jumping Flashing Shooting	*Group 3* Pricking Boring Drilling Stabbing Lancinating	*Group 4* Sharp Gritting Lacerating	*Group 5* Pinching Pressing Gnawing Cramping Crushing
Group 6 Tugging Pulling Wrenching	*Group 7* Hot Burning Scalding Searing	*Group 8* Tingling Itching Smarting Stinging	*Group 9* Dull Sore Hurting Aching Heavy	*Group 10* Tender Taut Rasping Splitting
Group 11 Tiring Exhausting	*Group 12* Sickening Suffocating	*Group 13* Fearful Frightful Terrifying	*Group 14* Punishing Gruelling Cruel Vicious Killing	*Group 15* Wretched Blinding
Group 16 Annoying Troublesome Miserable Intense Unbearable	*Group 17* Spreading Radiating Penetrating Piercing	*Group 18* Tight Numb Drawing Squeezing Tearing	*Group 19* Cool Cold Freezing	*Group 20* Nagging Nauseating Agonizing Dreadful Torturing

Figure 6.7 The McGill Melnack Pain Questionnaire. Patients are asked to circle only those words that best describe their pain; to leave out any category that is not suitable; and to use only a single word in each appropriate category (i.e., the one that best applies). The first 10 groups of words are somatic (describing what the pain feels like), 11–15 are affective, 16 is evaluative, and 17–20 miscellaneous. (From Wells, PE, et al: Pain Management in Physical Therapy. Appleton & Lange, Norwalk, CT, p 14 with permission.)

Behavior of Symptoms During the Last 48 Hours

It is important to understand the behavior of the symptoms during the past few days, not just at the current moment. Sometimes symptoms suddenly worsen or disappear at the time of the physical examination. A more accurate picture of the situation is told if the time frame spans 48 hours. "Are the symptoms getting better, worse, or staying the same?" The answer to this question will help the therapist judge the effectiveness of future treatment. If the patient's pain has been steadily worsening over the last 48 hours and treatment stabilizes the pain, then the treatment may be deemed helpful. However, if the patient reports that the pain has been steadily improving over the last 48 hours and treatment stabilizes the pain, then the treatment may be deemed as detrimental.

Previous Care

"What previous care has been sought for the problem? Who else (e.g., physician, therapist, chiropractor) has treated the problem? What tests and treatments did they perform? What have you done to relieve the problem?" From these and similar questions, all previous exercises, physical modalities, manual treatments, medications, injections, orthotics, and surgical procedures should be delineated. The answers to these questions help the therapist decide if further medical referrals are needed, and focus on the most effective treatment for the condition. For example, a patient who fell 3 days ago is experiencing severe ankle pain and swelling. The patient borrowed a friend's crutches and has been self-treating the ankle with ice and elevation. The therapist would recommend that the patient be examined by a physician and have radiographs taken to rule out a fracture prior to physical therapy intervention. As another scenario, if a patient has been treated previously by two physical therapists with ultrasound and had no improvement, then other treatments should be considered.

Specific Medical History

"Has this problem occurred before? How was it treated? How was it resolved?" Many musculoskeletal problems tend to recur with continued occupational, recreational, and daily activities if underlying biomechanical abnormalities, weaknesses, joint laxity, or tightness persist. Information about previous successful and unsuccessful treatments for similar past problems can help in treatment planning for the current problem.

General Medical History

A brief history should be obtained concerning medical problems and prior surgeries involving other body regions and systems. Conditions involving the cardiac, respiratory, neurological, vascular, metabolic, endocrine, gastrointestinal, genital urinary, visual, and dermatological systems should be noted. Having a patient complete a medical history form prior to the examination is an efficient means of obtaining this information, but the information should also be verified during the interview. Therapists also need to be aware of other conditions that mimic signs and symptoms often attributable to the musculoskeletal system. For example, inflammation of the gallbladder (cholecystitis) may result in right shoulder pain. However, shoulder pain related to cholecystitis typically will not increase with shoulder movements or resisted isometric testing of shoulder musculature, as would occur in the presence of musculoskeletal conditions. Patients with cholecystitis would likely have additional symptoms such as upper abdominal discomfort, bloating, belching, nausea, and intolerance of fried foods. Knowledge of systemic human pathology allows the therapist to recognize conditions requiring additional physician evaluation and intervention. Boissonnault[10] and Goodman and Snyder[11] have provided useful references to assist physical therapists in screening for medical conditions.

Medications

The type, frequency, dose, and effect of medications the patient is taking should be noted. The use of analgesic or anti-inflammatory medications may reduce the intensity of symptoms at the time of the examination. Changes in the use of these medications may make it difficult to determine the effects of physical therapy treatment. The secondary effects of some medications may necessitate the modification of examination and treatment techniques. For example, prolonged use of corticosteroids is associated with osteopenia (reduced bone mass) and reduced tensile strength of ligaments. The therapist may need to limit manual force applied through the lever of long bones to prevent fracture or ligament tear. The use of anticoagulants may make the patient susceptible to contusions and hemarthrosis. Such patients should be closely monitored for bruising and joint swelling. The amount of force used in exercise and manual therapies may need to be reduced.

Social History and Occupational, Recreational, and Functional Status

Questions in this area might include: "What type of work do you do in and outside of the home? How has this problem affected your ability to perform your job? Care for your children? Play golf? Dress? Bathe?" and so forth. Certain occupational and recreational activities may contribute to the problem or interfere with recovery. Figure 6.8 presents questions that can be used to quantify the effects of the problem on function. Strategies (e.g. joint preservation techniques) and use of assistive devices may need to be considered to allow performance of necessary tasks. Medical insurance companies often make treatment reimbursement decisions based on a patient's functional status as related to the medical problem.

"Do you have to climb stairs to get into your house? To reach the bedroom? Bathroom?" Characteristics of the home environment may determine whether a patient dependent on an ambulatory assistive device needs instruction in stair activities prior to returning home. The condition of floors, size of halls and doorways, placement of furniture, and bathroom facilities will need to be considered for a patient using a wheelchair. A more detailed discussion of examination of the environment including the home, workplace, and community can be found in Chapter 12.

"Do you live alone?" It is helpful to understand the patient's living situation to determine if others are available to assist with exercise programs, ambulation, and transfer activities. Some patients have responsibility for the care of children, elderly parents, or a disabled spouse or sibling. These responsibilities may need to be restructured to allow time for rest and recovery.

"Do you use tobacco products? Alcohol? Recreational drugs?" Cigarette smoking has been associated with decreased bone density,[12,13] greater spinal disk degeneration,[14] increased low back pain,[15–17] and increased upper and lower extremity musculoskeletal disorders.[18,19] Use of alcohol and recreational drugs can lead to risk-taking behaviors resulting in increased incidence of injuries, or difficulty in safely performing functional activities and home exercise programs. Therapists may wish to advise a patient to reduce the use of these substances and refer the patient to appropriate social services or self-help organizations for counseling.

Anticipated Goals, Expected Outcomes, and Time Frame of Recovery

"What do you hope will be the outcome of this therapy? When do you anticipate returning home? To work? To playing football?" and so forth as appropriate. These questions enable the therapist and patient to discuss and determine mutually agreed upon anticipated goals and expected outcomes. The therapist should not presume what issues are important to the patient. Answers to these questions help the therapist to determine whether the patient has realistic expectations or will need further patient education concerning his or her condition and typical recovery. For example, an elderly patient who suffered a fractured hip yesterday and is currently hospitalized may expect to remain in the acute care hospital for 2 weeks until he or she can independently ambulate and be independent in self-care. More realistic goals given current health insurance practices may need to be discussed, such as discharge from the hospital in 3 or 4 days to a rehabilitation or extended care facility for further nursing care, physical and occupational therapy, or discharge home with home health aides, visiting nurses, and home care physical and occupational therapists.

What percentage of your normal work activities are you able to perform?

0% 10% 20% 30% 40% 50% 60% 70% 80% 90% 100%

What percentage of your normal home activities are you able to perform?

0% 10% 20% 30% 40% 50% 60% 70% 80% 90% 100%

What percentage of your normal recreational activities are you able to perform?

0% 10% 20% 30% 40% 50% 60% 70% 80% 90% 100%

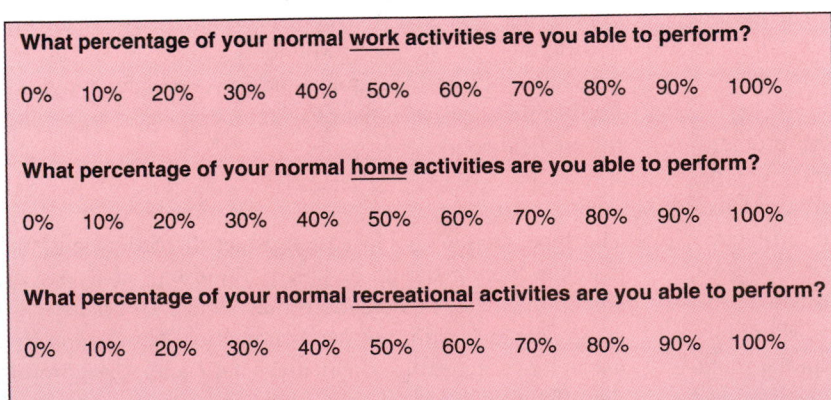

Figure 6.8 Questions used to rate a patient's function. The patient circles the percent of activity that he or she is able to perform.

Concluding Question

When the therapist has finished obtaining the above information, one final type of open-ended question needs to be asked. "Is there anything else you wish to tell me?" or "Is there anything else you think I should know concerning your condition that I have not asked about?" Most likely the patient will respond by saying that he or she has no further information to offer and believes you understand the problem clearly. Sometimes, though, a patient may take this opportunity to clarify a previous point or share a concern that is adding stress to his or her life. Without this type of question at the conclusion of the interview, important information that may impact treatment and recovery may be lost.

The information elicited with the questions listed above may be supplemented with additional questions based on the specific region of the body being examined and suspected etiologies. The physical therapist's knowledge of anatomy, kinesiology, pathokinesiology, physiology, and pathophysiology, as well as the physical presentation and progression of musculoskeletal conditions, provide the appropriate background on which to base and develop patient interview questions.

Mental Status

During the interview, the patient's orientation to person, place, and time as well as general arousal state and cognitive and communication abilities should be noted. If deficits in these areas are present, the examination may need to be modified to gain accurate information. The use of simple words, concise instructions, and task demonstrations may be helpful. Distractions in the environment should be kept to a minimum. Communication difficulties may be overcome through the use of foreign language interpreters, gestures, drawings, and language boards. Changes in medications, upright positioning, and access to natural light via windows and skylights may improve patient arousal and orientation to time. Depending on the type of deficit, the patient may benefit from an evaluation by a neurologist, neuropsychologist, speech-language pathologist, and/or occupational therapist.

Vital Signs

If a patient's medical record or interview suggests a compromised cardiovascular system, heart rate, blood pressure, and respiratory rate should be determined prior to beginning other physical examination procedures (see Chapter 4). Patients getting out of bed for the first time following recent surgery or prolonged bed rest should routinely have vital signs taken to establish baseline values prior to movement.

Observation/Inspection

Observation begins with the therapist's first contact with the patient, whether at bedside in the case of hospitalized patients, or in the waiting room for outpatients. The patient's general posture and ability to perform functional tasks—change bed position, transfer from sitting to standing, ambulate to the examining room—provides information about the severity of symptoms, willingness to move, range of joint motion, and muscle strength. This information, although preliminary, helps to focus and individualize the physical examination. For example, a patient with a shoulder disorder who uses the upper extremity to push off from a chair during transfers, stands with level bilateral shoulder height, and has an alternating arm swing during gait, would be expected to have milder symptoms, tolerate a more extensive examination, and have a greater range of motion (ROM) and muscle function than a patient who stands with an elevated scapula and protectively cradles the upper extremity during transfers and gait. If functional difficulties and gait abnormalities are noted, detailed functional status (see Chapter 11) and gait (see Chapter 10) examinations would be performed later.

To perform the physical examination and inspect specific areas of the body, the patient must be suitably dressed. Observation of the shoulders, elbows, or spine will require males to remove their shirt and females to wear only a bra or loose hospital gown that can be draped to expose the upper extremity and back. To observe the lower extremities, patients should undress from the waist down, wearing only undergarments or shorts.

Once the patient is in the privacy of an examining room and appropriately disrobed, the therapist begins a careful inspection of the body region implicated in the interview as well as biomechanically related areas. The lower extremities and lumbar region, being intricately involved in weightbearing activities, should be inspected as a functional unit. Likewise, conditions involving the shoulder require the examination of the cervical and thoracic regions, and vice versa. Visual inspection should focus on bone, soft tissue structures, skin, and nails. The therapist should view the body region anteriorly, posteriorly, and laterally. Often palpation, which is discussed in the next section, is combined with observation.

Bone shafts and joints are judged against normative models for symmetry, comparing one side of the body to the other. Contour and alignment should be considered. Common causes of changes in bone contour include acute fractures, callus formation or bone angulation owing to healed fractures, congenital variations, or bone hyperplasia at tendon insertions, and arthritis. Alignment differences can be due to the above conditions as well as muscle and soft tissue tightness, muscle weakness, muscle and ligament laxity, and joint dislocation.

Often a gross screening examination is performed to assist in determining postural alignment. From an *anterior* view both eyes, shoulders (acromion processes), iliac crests, anterior superior iliac spines, greater trochanters of the femur, patellae, and ankle malleoli should be horizontally level. Waist angles should be symmetrical. Patellae

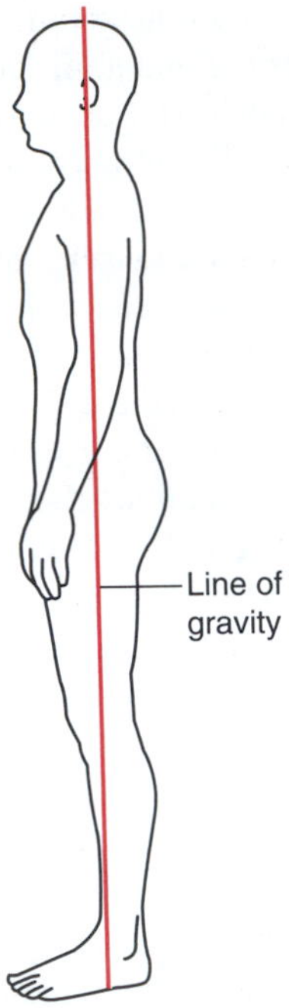

Figure 6.9 The location of the line of gravity from the lateral view. (From Levangie, PK, and Norkin, CC,[20, p 410] with permission.)

and feet should face anteriorly. *Laterally* the line of gravity should bisect the external auditory meatus, acromion process, greater trochanter, lie just posterior to the patella and approximately 2 inches anterior to the lateral malleolus (Fig. 6.9).[20]

The cervical and lumbar spine should exhibit moderate lordotic curves, and the thoracic spine a moderate kyphotic curve. From a *posterior* view the ear lobes, shoulders, inferior angles of the scapula, iliac crests, posterior superior iliac spines, greater trochanters, buttock and knee creases, and malleoli should be level. The spine should be straight, with the medial borders of the scapula equidistant from the spine bilaterally. Varus and valgus deformities of the knee and calcaneus should be noted.

The size and contour of soft tissue structures should be inspected and compared bilaterally. An increase in size may indicate soft tissue edema, joint effusion, or muscle hypertrophy. A decrease in size often indicates muscle atrophy. A loss of soft tissue continuity can suggest a muscle rupture. Cysts, rheumatoid nodules, ganglia, and gouty tophi can all change soft tissue contour. *Clubbing,* a rounded increase in soft tissue in distal fingers and toes, is believed to be caused by chronic hypoxemia and is typically associated with cardiovascular diseases, respiratory diseases, or neurovascular abnormalities.[6] Skin color and texture provide important clues to pathological conditions. *Cyanosis,* a blue discoloration of the skin and nail bed, indicates a lack of oxygen and excessive carbon dioxide in superficial blood vessels.[6] Inspection of the tongue for cyanosis helps determine if the poor perfusion is due to central or peripheral causes. *Pallor* is noted with a decrease in blood flow or blood hemoglobin—for example, in situations such as peripheral vasoconstriction, shock, internal bleeding, and anemia. *Erythema,* a localized redness, usually indicates increased blood flow and inflammation. Generalized redness can suggest fever, sunburn, or carbon monoxide poisoning. Yellow skin tone may be due to increased carotene intake, or liver disease. Brown, highly pigmented, hairy areas sometimes overlay bony defects such as spina bifida. Open wounds should be measured and diagrammed in patient records. New scars will be red, and older scars will be white in color. Skin tissue thickenings such as *calluses* can indicate chronic overloading and stress. Thin, glossy skin with decreased elasticity and hair loss is often found with peripheral nerve lesions or neurovascular disorders.

Palpation

It is suggested that palpation immediately follow or be integrated with observation, and occur prior to other testing procedures. Often other procedures will aggravate the patient's condition, making it more difficult to localize tenderness if palpation is performed later. The information gained from palpation will also help direct the therapist to choose additional appropriate testing procedures.

Palpation requires detailed knowledge of anatomy and a systematic approach. All structures on one body surface should be palpated before proceeding to another surface. For example, all structures on the anterior surface of the patient should be palpated before beginning to palpate structures on the posterior surface. The uninvolved side is palpated first to acquaint the patient with the procedure and, in some cases, to serve as a normative model for comparison. The therapist should develop a system of moving from superior to inferior structures, medial to lateral, or superior and then inferior from a joint line. Which direction the therapist moves is not important, but the palpation process should be consistent and thorough.

Bone, soft tissue structures, and the skin are palpated by varying the therapist's tactile pressure and using various parts of the hands. Light tactile pressure allows palpation of superficial tissues like the skin, whereas more pressure is needed to palpate deeper structures like bone. Usually the fingertips are used for palpation, but large, deeper structures such as the greater trochanter of the femur or borders of the scapula are easier to locate using the entire surface of the hand. Rolling the skin and soft tissue between the fingertips and thumb helps the therapist judge myofascial mobility. Changes in skin temperature may be easier to detect using the posterior surface of the therapist's hand. When moving from one area to another, the therapist's hand should stay in firm contact with the skin whenever possible to prevent a tickling sensation. The fingers should not "crawl" or "walk" across the skin.

During palpation the therapist seeks feedback from the patient to help localize painful structures. Some lesions in deep or proximal structures will refer symptoms to other body areas, but localized tenderness often helps to implicate particular structures. Localized skin temperature should be noted: cool temperatures suggest reduced circulation, whereas warmth indicates increased circulation and often inflammation. Skin and soft tissue density and extensibility should be considered. Often muscle spasms and adhesions in skin and connective tissue can be found with palpation. The quality (amplitude) of peripheral pulses will provide gross information on arterial blood supply. Bilateral edema in the ankles and legs that forms pits with tactile pressure (termed *pitting edema*) can indicate cardiac failure, liver, or renal conditions. Unilateral pitting edema is typically associated with obstruction of returning circulation.

Anthropometric Characteristics

Abnormalities noted during observation and palpation may be further documented with anthropometric measurements. Using a cloth or flexible plastic tape measure, limb lengths are measured from one bony landmark to another and compared bilaterally. For example, true leg length is commonly measured from the anterior superior iliac spine to the medial malleolus.

Circumferential measurements help substantiate joint effusion, edema, and muscle hypertrophy and atrophy. Typically, these measurements are taken at specified distances (inches or centimeters) above or below a bony landmark so they can be reliably reproduced during subsequent measurements. For example, circumference measurements of the upper arm should be taken at noted distances distal to the acromion process of the scapula or proximal to the olecranon process of the ulna. If measurements are needed of the hands or feet, volumetric measurements can be taken by submerging the distal extremity in a container of water and noting the volume of water that is displaced.

Range of Motion

Joints and their related structures are examined by performing active and passive joint motions. Joint motion is a necessary component of most functional tasks. Numerous studies have identified the ROM needed to walk on level surfaces,[21–24] descend stairs,[25–27] rise from a chair,[28–30] eat with a spoon,[31,32] and perform many upper extremity activities.[33–35] Careful examination of joint motion for range, end-feel, effect on symptoms, and pattern of restriction help identify and quantify impairments causing functional limitations, and determine which structures need treatment.

Active Range of Motion

The examination of joint motion begins by testing **active range of motion (AROM)**. Active motion is the unassisted voluntary movement of a joint. The patient is asked to move a body part through the osteokinematic motions at the involved and other biomechanically related joints. **Osteokinematics** refers to the gross angular motions of the shafts of bones. These motions are described as occurring in the three cardinal planes of the body: flexion and extension in the sagittal plane, abduction and adduction in the frontal plane, and medial and lateral rotation in the transverse plane. For example, in an examination of the hip the patient would be asked to move the hip into flexion, extension, abduction, adduction, and medial and lateral rotation. Often flexion and extension of the knee, as well as flexion, extension, rotation, and lateral flexion of the lumbar spine are tested, as knee and spine motions can impact hip function. Some therapists prefer to have the patient move in functional, combined motions rather than straight plane motions. For example, a patient would be asked to reach a hand behind the head to test shoulder abduction and medial rotation simultaneously rather than perform isolated, individual motions.

Active motion is a good screening procedure to further focus the physical examination. The amount, quality, and pattern of motion, as well as the occurrence of pain and crepitus should be noted. Often active ROM is visually estimated, but if more objective and accurate measurements are needed, a goniometer should be used. Normal ROM varies among individuals and is influenced by factors such as age,[36–41] gender,[42–46] and measurement methods.[47–51] Ideally, to determine if ROM is impaired, the ROM values should be compared with those obtained with the same measurement methods from people of the same age and gender. Studies that provide normative values by age and gender have been summarized by Norkin and White.[52] However, when particular values are not available, the therapist may need to compare ROM values to those of the patient's contralateral extremity or to average adult values from sources such as the American Academy of Orthopedic Surgeons[53,54] and the American Medical Association.[55] If the patient can complete active ROM easily, without presenting pain or other symptoms, then further passive testing of that motion is usually unnecessary.

If, however, the amount of active motion is less than normal the therapist will not be able to isolate the cause without further testing. Capsule, ligament, muscle and soft tissue tightness, joint surface abnormalities, and muscle weakness are all capable of causing limitations in active ROM. Pain during active ROM may be due to the contracting, stretching, or pinching of contractile tissues such as muscles, tendons, and their attachments to bone, or due to the stretching or pinching of noncontractile tissues such as ligaments, joint capsules, and bursa.[56] Variations in the quality and pattern of active motion can result from central and peripheral nervous system disorders and metabolic conditions, in addition to disorders involving musculoskeletal structures. So, although active motion is an effective screening procedure, positive findings require a variety of additional tests to identify the underlying etiology and thus enable effective treatment.

Passive Range of Motion

Passive motions are movements performed by the therapist without the assistance of the patient. The term **passive range of motion (PROM)** typically refers to the amount of osteokinematic motion available when the patient's joint is moved without the patient's assistance. Normally, passive ROM is slightly greater than active ROM because joints have a small amount of motion at the end of the range that is not under voluntary control. This additional range helps to protect joint structures by allowing the joint to absorb extrinsic forces. Passive ROM is examined not only for amount of motion, but also for the motion's effect on symptoms, the type of tissue resistance felt by the therapist at the end of the motion (end-feel), and pattern of limitation.

Passive range of osteokinematic motions depends on the integrity of joint surfaces and the extensibility of the joint capsule, ligaments, muscles, tendons, and soft tissue. Limitations in passive ROM may be due to bone or joint abnormalities or tightness of soft tissue structures. Because the therapist provides the muscle force needed to perform passive ROM, rather than the patient, passive ROM (unlike active ROM) does not depend on the patient's muscle strength and coordination.

Pain during passive ROM is often due to moving, stretching, or pinching of noncontractile structures. Pain occurring at the end of passive ROM may be due to stretching contractile structures, as well as noncontractile structures. Pain during passive ROM is not due to the active shortening (contracting) of muscle and the resulting pull on tendon and bone attachments. By comparing which motions (active vs passive) cause pain, and noting the location of the pain, the therapist can begin to determine which injured tissues are involved.

For example, on examination a patient is found to have limited and painful active knee flexion. This pain and limitation may be due to a lesion in the hamstring muscles (including tendons and bone attachments), the quadriceps muscles (including patella tendon and bone attachments), tibiofemoral and patellofemoral joint surfaces, meniscus, joint capsule, collateral and cruciate ligaments, or various anterior and posterior bursa. If the patient had similar pain and limitation during passive ROM, the quadriceps muscles, tibiofemoral and patellofemoral joint surfaces, meniscus, joint capsule, collateral and cruciate ligaments, or various anterior bursa may be involved. The hamstring muscles would not be implicated as these structures are put on slack and relieved of tension during passive knee flexion. Careful consideration of patient history, observation and palpation findings, and the results of additional tests such as end-feel determination, capsular versus noncapsular joint limitation patterns, accessory joint motion tests, and ligament stress tests will help to isolate the involved structures. These additional tests are discussed later in this chapter. If, however, passive knee flexion ROM were now normal and pain free as compared to painful during active flexion, a lesion in the hamstring muscles would be likely. The performance of resisted isometric muscle contractions would be used to confirm the presence of a lesion in the hamstring muscles.

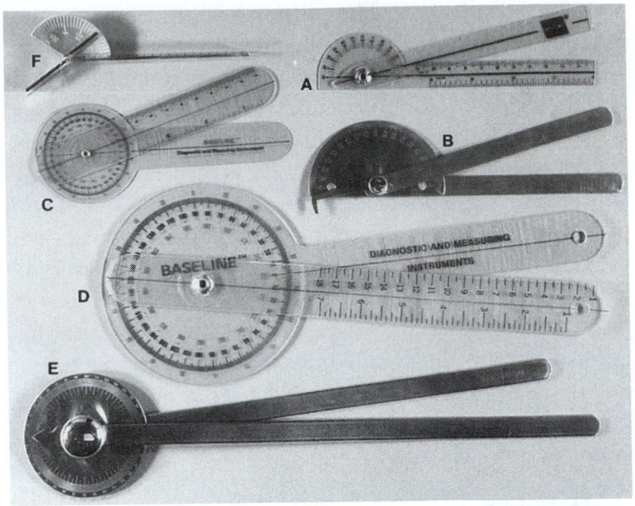

Figure 6.10 A variety of metal and plastic universal goniometers in different sizes and shapes. All universal goniometers have a central "body" with a protractor and fulcrum to center over the patient's joint, as well as two "arms" to align with the patient's body parts. (From Norkin, CC, and White, DJ,[52, p 22] with permission.)

In the clinical setting, passive ROM is usually measured with **universal goniometers** (Fig. 6.10) or less frequently with **inclinometers** (Fig. 6.11), tape measures, and flexible rulers. Visual estimates should not be used because they are less accurate than measurements taken with universal goniometers.[57,58] Both the beginning and the end of the motion are measured and recorded so as to clearly indicate the ROM (Fig. 6.12A and B)

Using the most common notation system, the 0 to 180° system, all motions except rotation begin in anatomical

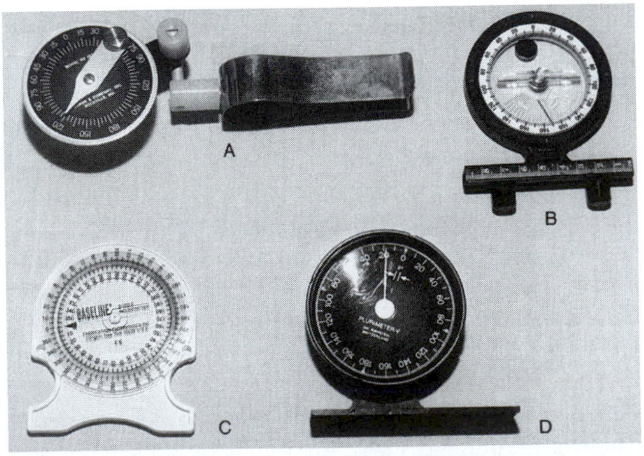

Figure 6.11 Several inclinometers or gravity-dependent goniometers. Each uses a weighted pointer or bubble to indicate the position of the goniometer relative to gravity. (From Norkin, CC, and White, DJ,[52, p 25] with permission.)

A

B

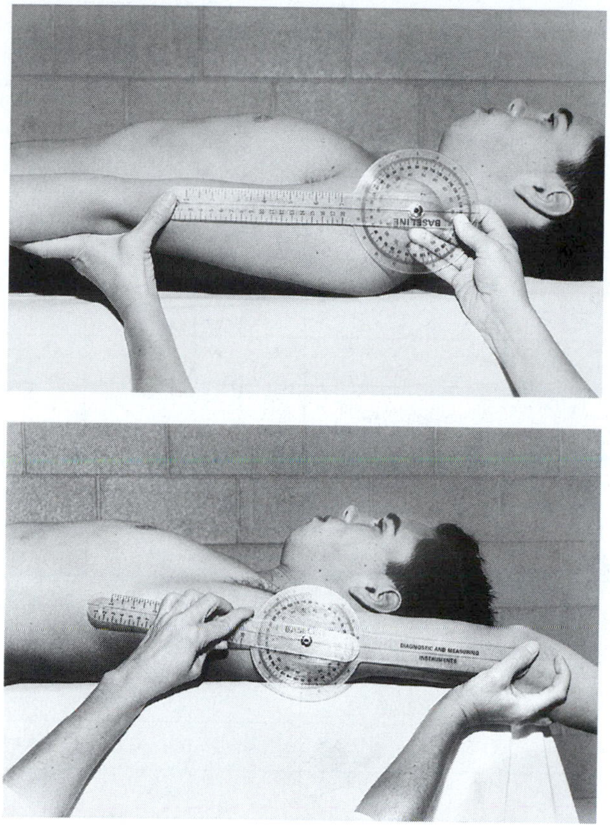

Figure 6.12 Measurement of the beginning (A) and end (B) of shoulder flexion ROM. The universal goniometer is moving from 0° toward 180° during the motion. (From Norkin, CC, and White, DJ,[52] with permission.)

position at 0° and progress toward 180°. For example, a motion that begins at 0° and ends at 135° would be recorded as 0 to 135°. A ROM that does not start with 0° or ends prematurely indicates joint **hypomobility**. Joint **hypermobility** at the beginning of the range is noted by the inclusion of a zero (the normal starting position) between the starting and ending measurements. For example, if the elbow joint has 5° of hypermobility in extension and 140° of flexion, it would be recorded as 5—0—140°. Hypermobility at the end of the ROM is denoted with an excessive ending measurement as compared to normal values. Measurement results are incorporated into narrative reports or recorded on specialized forms (Fig. 6.13). Texts by Norkin and White,[52] Clarkson,[59] and Reese and Bandy[60] provide detailed descriptions of goniometric measurement procedures.

ROM measurements taken with a universal goniometer of the extremity joints generally have good to excellent reliability. Reliability does vary depending on the joint and motion being measured. Reliability studies that include ROM measurements of elbow motions with a universal goniometer are presented in Evidence Summary Box 6.1. ROM measurements of upper extremity joints have been found to be more reliable than measurements of the lower extremity[47,62,68] and spine.[69–71] In an often quoted study, Boone et al[62] found the average standard deviation between measurements made on the same subjects by different testers to be 4.2° for upper extremity motions and 5.2° for lower extremity motions. These differences in reliability have been attributed to difficulties in measuring complex as compared to simple hinged joints, in palpating bony landmarks, and in moving heavy body parts.[62,72] The use of standardized positions, stabilization of the body part proximal to the joint being tested, use of bony landmarks to align the goniometer, and repeated testing conducted by the same therapist (rather than multiple therapists) all help to improve the validity and reliability of goniometric measurements.[47,58,73]

End-Feel

The end of each motion at each joint is limited from further movement by particular anatomical structures. The type of structure that limits a joint motion has a characteristic feel, that may be detected by the therapist performing the passive ROM. This feeling, which is experienced by the therapist as resistance, or a barrier to further motion, is called the **end-feel**. Cyriax and Cyriax,[56] Kaltenborn,[74] and Paris[75] have described a variety of normal (physiological) and abnormal (pathological) end-feels. A summary of the types of end-feels has been adapted from the work of these authors. Normal end-feels are generally described as *soft, firm,* or *hard* (Table 6.1). A soft end-feel has a gradual increase in resistance as muscle, skin, and subcutaneous tissues are compressed between body parts.[76] A firm end-feel has a more abrupt increase in resistance as compared to a soft end-feel. Firm end-feels include varying amounts of creep, or give, depending on whether the barrier to the end of the motion is the stretching of muscle, capsule, or ligament tissue. The firm end-feel with the most creep would be the rubbery resistance offered by the stretch of muscle tissue, and the least amount of creep would be provided by the stretch of ligament tissue. The firm end-feel created by the stretch of a joint capsule usually has a moderate amount of creep. A hard end-feel is abrupt; there is an immediate stop to movement as when bone contacts bone.

End-feels are considered to be abnormal when they occur sooner or later in the ROM than is typical, or if they are not the type of end-feel that is normally found for that joint motion. Abnormal end-feels have been associated with more pain than normal end-feels.[77] Many abnormal, pathological end-feels have been described, but most can be categorized as variations of soft, firm, and hard end-feels (Table 6.2). An abnormal end-feel that cannot be categorized as soft, firm, or hard, is an *empty end-feel*. This term describes the inability of the therapist to detect any anatomical barrier to the end of the ROM. Rather, the patient through verbal nor nonverbal cues indicates that no further motion should occur, usually because of pain.

The ability to determine the type of end-feel is important in helping the therapist identify the limiting structures and choose a focused and effective treatment. Developing

Range of Motion—Lower Extremity

Patient's Name ______________________________ Date of Birth ______________

Left				Right		
			Date			
			Examiner's Initials			
			Hip			
			Flexion			
			Extension			
			Abduction			
			Medial Rotation			
			Lateral Rotation			
			Knee			
			Flexion			
			Ankle			
			Dorsiflexion			
			Plantarflexion			
			Inversion—Tarsal			
			Eversion—Tarsal			
			Inversion—Subtalar			
			Eversion—Subtalar			
			Inversion—Midtarsal			
			Eversion—Midtarsal			
			Great Toe			
			MTP Flexion			
			MTP Extension			
			MTP Abduction			
			IP Flexion			
			Toe			
			MTP Flexion			
			MTP Extension			
			MTP Abduction			
			PIP Flexion			
			DIP Flexion			
			DIP Extension			
			Comments:			

Figure 6.13 Range of motion recording form for the lower extremity. (From Norkin, CC, and White, DJ,[52, p 390] with permission.)

Evidence Summary Box 6.1

Outcome Studies on Reliability of Using Universal Goniometer to Measure Elbow Range of Motion

Reference	Subjects	Design/Intervention/Duration	Results	Comments
Hellebrandt et al,[61] 1949	77 patients	Repeated measures design AROM 1 highly experienced PT tester 8 average experienced PT testers 2 trials by same tester, time between trials not defined	Highly experienced tester had mean difference between trials of 1.0° for flexion and 0.1° for extension. Sig difference between trials for flexion	High intratester reliability. Sig difference not clinically important. No data on elbow motions for average-experienced testers
Boone et al,[62] 1978	12 healthy males 26–54 years	Repeated measures design AROM Standardized method 4 PT testers with 5–20 years of experience 3 trials by each tester in one session 1 weekly session for 4 weeks (4 sessions total)	No sig difference between 3 trials by each tester in one session so session means used in intra- and intertester calculations. Sig difference between testers Intratester $r = 0.94$ SD = 0.2° Intertester $r = 0.88$ SD = 2.6°	High intra- and intertester reliability. Intratester reliability higher than intertester reliabilty
Rothstein et al,[47] 1983	12 patients had elbow measured	Repeated measures design, blinded PROM; method not standardized. 12 PT testers with 1–4 years experience 3 types of universal goniometer: large metal, large plastic, small plastic 2 trials per goniometer per tester 2 testers evaluated each patient.	Single trial: Intratester reliability $r =$ .95 – .99 ICC = .86. – .99 Intertester reliability $r =$ .89 – .97 ICC = .85 – .95 Mean of 2 trials: Intertester reliability $r =$ .94 – .97 ICC = .89 – .96	High intra- and intertester reliability. Intratester reliability slightly higher than intertester reliability. Minimal improvement in intertester reliability by using mean of 2 trials versus score from single trial (differences in ICC no. 0.12)
Grohmann,[63] 1983	1 healthy adult	Repeated measures design, blinded Elbow held in 2 fixed positions: 1 obtuse and 1 acute angle. 40 PT student testers used over-the-joint and lateral methods to measure each position 1 trial daily for 4 days	No sig difference between methods	No difference in using over-the-joint method or lateral method of measuring elbow position
Walker et al,[44] 1984	4 healthy adults, 60 years	Repeated measures design, blinded. AROM 4 testers Each tester performed 5 trials on each subject in one day.	Intratester reliability $r = 81$	High intratester reliability
Fish and Wingate,[64] 1985	1 healthy adult	Repeated measures design, blinded 46 PT student testers measured with 2 instruments: plastic and steel goniometers 3 conditions: ALIGN = elbow in fixed position with landmarks noted, ASSIGN = elbow in fixed position with no landmarks, PROM = full range of passive flexion	ALIGN plastic SD = 1.8° – 2.1° ALIGN steel SD = 2.0° – 2.6° ASSIGN plastic SD = 2.5° – 3.0° ASSIGN steel SD = 2.5° – 3.4° PROM plastic SD = 3.4° – 3.8° PROM steel SD = 3.9° – 4.2°	Variability of scores increased as standardization of measurements decreased

(continued)

Evidence Summary Box 6.1

Outcome Studies on Reliability of Using Universal Goniometer to Measure Elbow Range of Motion (continued)

Reference	Subjects	Design/Intervention/Duration	Results	Comments
Greene and Wolf,[66] 1989	20 healthy adults (10 males, 10 females) 18–55 years	Repeated measures design. AROM 1 PT tester 2 instruments: universal goniometer and pendulum goniometer 3 trials per instrument in a session 3 sessions within 2 weeks	Universal goniometer within-sessions: Flexion: ICC = .94; SD = 1.2°; 95%CI = 3.0°; Extension: ICC = .95; SD = 1.0°; 95%CI = 1.9°; Both instruments had sig difference between sessions. Low correlation (r =.11 – .21) and sig difference between instruments within-sessions	High intratester reliability with universal goniometer in one session. 95% of time reliability within 2–3° if taken by same tester in one session. Different instruments should not be used interchangeably.
Goodwin et al,[65] 1992	23 healthy females, 18–31 years	Repeated measures design. AROM 3 experienced testers. 3 instruments: universal goniometer, fluid goniometer, electrogoniometer. Landmarks noted on skin. 3 trials per instrument by each tester in a session. 2 sessions 4 weeks apart.	Universal goniometer intratester reliability between sessions: r = .61 – .92 ICC = .56 – .91. Difference in means between sessions = 0.9°; Average difference in means between testers = 5.1°; Sig differences and interactions between goniometers, testers, and sessions	Moderate to high intratester reliability between 2 sessions 4 weeks apart, depending on tester. Differences between sessions smaller than differences between testers. Different instruments should not be used interchangeably.
Armstrong et al,[67] 1998	38 patients with history of surgery for upper extremity injury. 19 males, 19 females 14–72 years	Repeated measures design. AROM 5 testers of varying experience. 2 instruments: universal goniometer and electrogoniometer. 2 trials per instrument by each tester on same day	Universal goniometer: Intratester reliability for flexion: ICC = .55 – .98, mean difference between trials = 3.2°; 95%CI = 5.9° Extension: ICC = .45 – .98, mean difference = 3.5°; 95%CI = 6.6° Intertester reliability for flexion: ICC = .58 – .62, mean difference = 6.4°; 95%CI = 9.2°; Extension: ICC = .58 – .87, mean difference = 7.0°; 95%CI = 8.9°	Moderate to high intratester reliability. Moderate intertester reliability. 95% of time reliability within 6.7° if taken by same tester, and 9° if taken by different testers.

AROM = active range of motion; CI = confidence interval; ICC = intraclass correlation coefficient; PROM = passive range of motion; PT = physical therapist; r = Pearson's correlation coefficient; sig = significant.

this ability takes practice and sensitivity. Passive ROM, particularly toward the end of the motion, must be performed slowly and carefully. Secure stabilization of the bone proximal to the joint being tested is critical in preventing multiple joints and structures from moving and interfering with determination of the end-feel.[78,79]

Capsular Patterns of Restricted Motion

Cyriax and Cyriax[56] initially described characteristic patterns of restricted joint ROM due to diffuse, intra-articular inflammation involving the entire joint capsule. These patterns of restricted motion, which usually involve multiple motions at a joint, are called **capsular patterns.** The restrictions do not involve the loss of a fixed number of degrees, but rather the loss of a proportion of one motion relative to another. Capsular patterns vary from joint to joint. Table 6.3 presents common capsular patterns as described by Cyriax and Cyriax[56] and Kaltenborn.[74] Although therapists have been using capsular patterns in clinical decision making for many years, studies are needed to test the hypotheses regarding the cause of capsular patterns and to determine the capsular pattern for each joint.[80,81]

Hertling and Kessler,[1] expanding on Cyriax's work, have suggested that capsular patterns are due to one of two

Table 6.1 Normal End-Feels

End-Feel	Structure	Example
Soft	Soft tissue approximation	Knee flexion (contact between soft tissue of posterior leg and posterior thigh)
Firm	Muscular stretch	Hip flexion with the knee straight (passive elastic tension of hamstring muscles
	Capsular stretch	Extension of metacarpophalangeal joints of fingers (tension in the anterior capsule)
	Ligamentous stretch	Forearm supination (tension in the palmar radioulnar ligament of the inferior radioulnar joint, interosseous membrane, oblique cord)
Hard	Bone contacting bone	Elbow extension (contact between the olecranon process of the ulna and the olecranon fossa of the humerus)

From Norkin, CC, and White, DJ,[52, p 8] with permission.

Table 6.2 Abnormal End-Feels

End-Feel		Examples
Soft	Occurs sooner or later in the ROM than is usual, or in a joint that normally has a firm or hard end-feel; Feels boggy.	Soft tissue edema Synovitis
Firm	Occurs sooner or later in the ROM than is usual, or in a joint that normally has a soft or hard end-feel	Increased muscular tonus Capsular, muscular, ligamentous shortening
Hard	Occurs sooner or later in the ROM than is usual, or in a joint that normally has a soft or firm end-feel. A bony grating or bony block is felt.	Chondromalacia Osteoarthritis Loose bodies in joint Myositis ossificans Fracture
Empty	No real end-feel because pain prevents reaching end of ROM. No resistance is felt except for patient's protective muscle splinting or muscle spasm.	Acute joint inflammation Bursitis Abscess Fracture Psychogenic disorder

From Norkin, CC, and White, DJ,[52, p 9] with permission.

general situations: (1) joint effusion or synovial inflammation or (2) relative capsular fibrosis. Joint effusion or synovial inflammation results in a capsular pattern of limitation by distending the entire joint capsule, causing the joint to maintain a position that allows the greatest intra-articular volume. Pain triggered by stretching the capsule, and muscle spasms that protect the capsule from further stretch, inhibit movement and cause a capsular pattern of restricted motion. The other general situation that causes capsular patterns is relative capsular fibrosis, seen in the resolution of acute capsular inflammation, chronic low-grade capsular inflammation, and immobilization of a joint. These conditions cause a decrease in the extensibility of the entire capsule from an increase in collagen content of the capsule relative to the mucopolysaccharide content, or from internal changes in the collagen tissue.

To plan an effective treatment, the therapist must determine whether the capsular pattern is caused by joint effusion/synovial inflammation or capsular fibrosis. If joint effusion or synovial inflammation is present, treatment methods typically focus on resolving the acute inflammation with rest, cold modalities, compression, elevation, joint mobilization using grade 1 sustained and grade 1 and 2 oscillations, gentle ROM exercise, and anti-inflammatory medications. Capsular fibrosis, a more chronic condition, can be treated with heat modalities, joint mobilization using grade 3 sustained stretch and grade 3 and 4 oscillations, passive stretching procedures, and more vigorous ROM exercises. Patient history, observation, palpation, and careful determination of end-feels will help establish the cause of the capsular pattern.

Noncapsular Patterns of Restricted Motion

Restricted passive ROM that is not proportioned similarly to a capsular pattern is called a **noncapsular pattern** of restricted motion.[1,56] Noncapsular patterns usually involve only one or two motions of a joint, in contrast to capsular patterns, which involve all or most motions of a joint. Noncapsular patterns are caused by conditions involving structures other than the entire joint capsule. Internal joint derangement, adhesion of a part of a joint capsule, and extracapsular lesions such as ligament shortness, muscle strain, and muscle shortness are examples of conditions that can result in noncapsular patterns. For instance, shortness of the iliopsoas muscle will result in the noncapsular pattern of limited passive hip extension; the passive range

Table 6.3 Capsular Patterns of Extremity Joints

Shoulder (glenohumeral joint)	Maximum loss of external rotation Moderate loss of abduction Minimum loss of internal rotation
Elbow complex	Flexion loss is greater than extension loss
Forearm	Full and painless Equally restricted in pronation and supination in presence of elbow restrictions
Wrist	Equal restrictions in flexion and extension
Hand	
Carpometacarpal joint I	Abduction and extension restriction
Carpometacarpal joints II-V	Equally restricted in all directions
Upper extremity digits	Flexion loss is greater than extension loss
Hip	Maximum loss of internal rotation, flexion, abduction Minimal loss of extension
Knee (tibiofemoral joint)	Flexion loss is greater than extension loss
Ankle (talocrural joint)	Plantarflexion loss is greater than extension loss
Subtalar joint	Restricted varus motion
Midtarsal joint	Restricted dorsiflexion, plantarflexion, abduction, and medial rotation
Lower extremity digits	
Metatarsalphalangeal joint I	Extension loss is greater than flexion
Metatarsalphalangeal joints II-V	Variable, tend toward flexion restriction
Interphalangeal joints	Tend toward extension restriction

From Dyrek, DA,[190, p 72] with permission. Capsular patterns are from Cyriax[56] and Kaltenborn.[74]

of other hip motions will not be affected. This is in contrast to the capsular pattern of the hip caused by diffuse joint effusion or capsular fibrosis, in which there is loss of passive internal rotation, flexion, and abduction.

The sole recognition of a noncapsular pattern is not enough to direct appropriate treatment. Information gained from the patient history, observation, palpation, active and passive ROM, end-feels, resisted isometric muscle tests, joint mobility tests, and special tests must be integrated to determine the most likely cause of the noncapsular pattern. For example, both chronic shortness and acute strain of the iliopsoas muscle may result in a noncapsular pattern of limited passive hip extension. However, those conditions will present differently in terms of patient history, pain during active and passive ROM, end-feel, and resisted isometric muscle tests, and will require different treatment approaches.

Accessory Joint Motions

If passive ROM is found to be limited or painful, an examination of arthrokinematic motions in indicated. **Arthrokinematics** refers to the motion of joint surfaces. These motions, often called **accessory** or **joint play motions**, are used to determine joint mobility and integrity. MacConaill and Basmajian[82] describe accessory joint motions as slides (or glides), spins, and rolls. A **glide (slide)** is a translatory motion of one surface sliding over another. A **roll** is a rotary motion similar to the bottom of a rocking chair rolling over the floor. A **spin** is a rotary motion around a fixed point or axis.

Accessory motions usually occur in combination with each other and result in angular movement of the bone shaft, or osteokinematic motion. Kaltenborn[74] refers to the combination of translatory glide and the rotary motion of rolling as **roll-gliding**. The combination of a roll and glide allows for increased ROM by postponing the joint compression and separation that would occur at either side of the joint during a pure rolling motion. The direction of the rolling and gliding components of roll-gliding depends on whether a concave or convex joint surface is moving. If a concave joint surface is moving, the gliding component occurs in the same direction as the rolling or angular movement of the shaft of the bone (Fig. 6.14). For example, during flexion of the knee with the femur fixed, the shaft of the tibia rolls posteriorly while the joint surface of the tibia also glides posteriorly. If a convex joint surface is moving, the gliding component occurs in the direction opposite to the rolling or angular movement of the shaft of the bone. As an example, during abduction of the glenohumeral joint, the shaft and humeral head roll cranially, while the contacting articular surface of the humeral head glides caudally. In the human body, roll-gliding is by far the most frequently occurring arthrokinematic motion, although there are several instances of pure spin motions. An example of a spin joint motion would be supination and pronation of the radius at the humeroradial joint.

Normal arthrokinematic (accessory) motions are necessary for full and symptom-free osteokinematic motions. The careful examination of accessory motions helps to

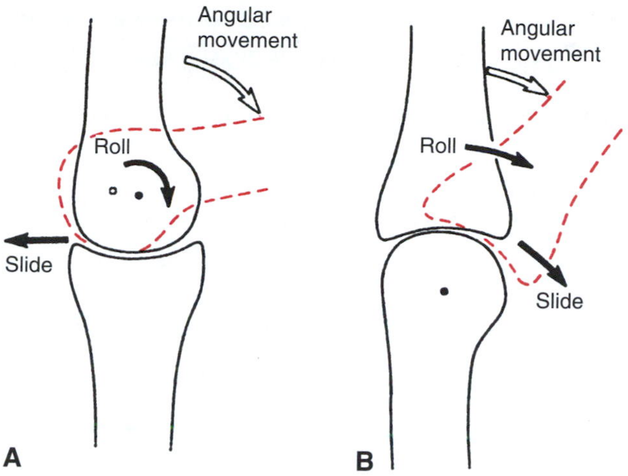

Figure 6.14 Diagrammatic representation of the concave-convex rule. (A) If the joint surface of the moving bone is convex, sliding is in the opposite direction of the angular movement of the bone. (B) If the joint surface of the moving bone is concave, sliding is in the same direction as the angular movement of the bone. (From Kisner, C, and Colby, LA,[83, p 219], with permission.)

more specifically locate and treat the source of impaired osteokinematic motions. Accessory motions cannot be performed actively by the patient because these motions are not under voluntary control. Rather, they are tested passively by the therapist. The accessory motions most commonly tested are translatory motions: glides that are parallel to the joint surfaces, and *distractions* and *compressions* that are perpendicular to the joint surfaces. Kaltenborn,[74] Kisner and Colby,[83] and Hertling and Kessler[1] describe specific testing and treatment techniques that focus on accessory motions—usually under the topic of **joint mobilization**. Careful attention must be given to general patient positioning, specific joint positioning, relaxation of surrounding muscles, stabilization of one joint surface, and mobilization of the other joint surface.

Accessory joint motions are examined for amount of motion, effect on symptoms, and end-feel. The ranges of accessory motions are very small and cannot be measured with goniometers or standard rulers. Rather, they are typically compared to the same motion on the contralateral side of the patient's body, or compared to the therapist's past experience in testing people of similar age and gender as the patient. Accessory motions are assigned a joint play mobility grade of 0 to 6 (Table 6.4).[74] These mobility grades have implications for treatment as follows[1,84]:

- Grades 0 and 6: Joint mobilization is not indicated. Surgery should be considered.
- Grades 1 and 2: Joint mobilization to increase the extensibility of joint structures is indicated. Heat modalities prior to mobilization and ROM exercises after mobilization should be considered.
- Grade 3: Joint mobilization is not needed, as findings are normal.

Table 6.4 Accessory Joint Motion Grades

Grade	Joint Status
0	Ankylosed
1	Considerable hypomobility
2	Slight hypomobility
3	Normal
4	Slight hypermobility
5	Considerable hypermobility
6	Unstable

Adapted from Wadsworth, CT: Manual Examination and Treatment of the Spine and Extremities. Williams & Wilkins, Baltimore, 1988, p 13, with permission.

- Grades 4 and 5: Joint mobilization to increase joint extensibility is not indicated. Taping, bracing, strengthening exercises, and education regarding posture and positions to be avoided should be considered.

The testing of accessory motions puts stress on specific anatomical structures. A change in symptoms during the performance of an accessory motion helps to implicate particular structures. Distraction stresses the entire joint capsule and numerous ligaments surrounding and supporting the joint. Glides stress a specific part of the joint capsule and particular ligaments, depending on the direction of the glide and joint. Compression applies force to intracapsular structures such as meniscus, bone, cartilage, and projections of the synovial lining of the joint capsule into the joint space. Accessory motions are of such a small magnitude that they do not stress surrounding muscles. Angular changes in joint position that typically occur during osteokinematic ROM movements more effectively change the length of muscle tissue. Normal and abnormal end-feels noted during passive accessory motions are characterized as soft, firm, and hard. Similar to end-feels noted during passive osteokinematic motions, they help determine the limiting structures and appropriate treatment.

Muscle Performance

Muscle performance is the ability of a muscle to do work.[85] **Linear work** is defined as force multiplied by distance, while **rotational work** is defined as torque (force multiplied by perpendicular distance from the axis of rotation) multiplied by arc of movement. Usually during a musculoskeletal examination, a component of muscle performance—muscle strength—is tested. *Muscle strength,* as described in the *Guide to Physical Therapist Practice,*[85] is the force exerted by a muscle or group of muscles to overcome a resistance in one maximal effort. Clinical methods of determining muscle strength include manual muscle testing, hand-held dynamometry, and isokinetic dynamometry. Depending on the patient, other characteristics related to muscle performance may also be tested. *Muscle power* is work produced per unit of time, or the product of strength and speed. **Muscle endurance** is the ability of the muscle to contract repeatedly over time. In addition to these quantitative measures, the patient's qualitative response in terms of changes in pain during resisted isometric testing is important in identifying musculotendinous lesions.

Resisted Isometric Testing

During the performance of active and passive ROM testing, a patient may complain of pain. The patient history, location of pain, and the pattern of painful motions may suggest a lesion in contractile tissues such as muscle or tendons and their insertions into bone, or involvement of inert tissues such as the joint surfaces, joint capsule, or ligaments. Resisted isometric testing can be used to further clarify which type of tissue, contractile or inert, is involved. *Increased pain* during a resisted isometric contraction, caused by shortening of the muscle and pulling on the tendon, helps to confirm the involvement of contractile tissues. Sometimes more pain is felt when the contraction is released and lengthening occurs; this would still be considered a positive finding for a lesion in contractile tissues. The *lack of pain* during resisted isometric testing, pain noted with limited accessory joint motions, a capsular pattern of joint restriction, or particular end-feels during passive ROM and accessory joint motions help to confirm the involvement of inert tissues. For example, bicipital tendinitis would be painful during resisted isometric testing of elbow flexion and shoulder flexion. An adhesive capsulitis of the glenohumeral joint would be painless during these same maneuvers.

Resisted isometric testing must be performed carefully to stress particular contractile tissue while avoiding stress to surrounding inert tissue. The therapist should place the patient's joint in a position midway through the ROM, so that minimal tension is put on inert structures. The body part proximal to the joint being tested must be well stabilized by the therapist to allow the patient to relax and avoid extraneous muscle substitutions. Then the patient is asked to hold this position while the therapist gradually applies resistance. Joint movement is strictly avoided. Although some compression of articular surfaces will occur during the isometric contraction, this does not usually present a problem in interpreting the results. However, a bursa located deep to the musculotendinous tissue will also be compressed. Although bursae are not considered to be connective tissue, pain will be felt during the isometric contraction if a bursa is inflamed. Fortunately, treatment for bursitis is similar to treatment for musculotendinous strains and inflammation.

In addition to determining the absence or presence of pain during the resisted isometric testing, the therapist should also note the strength of the muscle contraction. If weakness is found, more extensive testing of muscle strength should be performed using manual muscle testing or dynamometers. Muscle weakness may be due to many causes, including pathologies involving upper motor neurons, peripheral nerves, neuromuscular junctions, muscles, and tendons. Pain, fatigue, and disuse atrophy can also cause weakness. The pattern of muscle weakness will help to identify the site of the pathology and direct treatment. The patient history and the results of sensory, coordination, motor control, cardiopulmonary, and electromyography testing will help clarify findings as well.

Table 6.5 Results of Resisted Isometric Testing

Findings	Possible Pathologies
Strong and painless	There is no lesion or neurological deficit involving the tested muscle and tendon.
Strong and painful	There is a minor lesion of the tested muscle or tendon.
Weak and painless	There is a disorder of the nervous system, neuromuscular junction, or a complete rupture of the tested muscle or tendon, or disuse atrophy.
Weak and painful	There is a serious, painful pathology such as a fracture or neoplasm. Other possibilities include an acute inflammatory process that inhibits muscle contraction, or a partial rupture of the tested muscle or tendon.

Cyriax and Cyriax[56] and others[1,2] have suggested using the results of resisted isometric testing to determine the type of pathology. The strength of the muscle contraction as well as its effect on pain are used to categorize the findings (Table 6.5). A study by Franklin et al[86] indicates that the conditions related to the finding of "weak and painful" need to be expanded to include not only serious pathologies, but relatively minor muscle damage and inflammation such as that induced by eccentric isokinetic exercise. Intratester and intertester reliability of resisted isometric testing have been examined to determine diagnostic categories for the shoulder and knee.[87,88]

Manual Muscle Testing

Manual muscle testing (MMT) was developed by Wright[89] and Lovett[90] beginning in 1912 as a means of testing and grading muscle strength based on gravity and manually applied resistance. Over the years others have described various MMT methods, but the two methods most frequently used in the United States are those proposed by Daniels and Worthingham,[91,92] and Kendall and

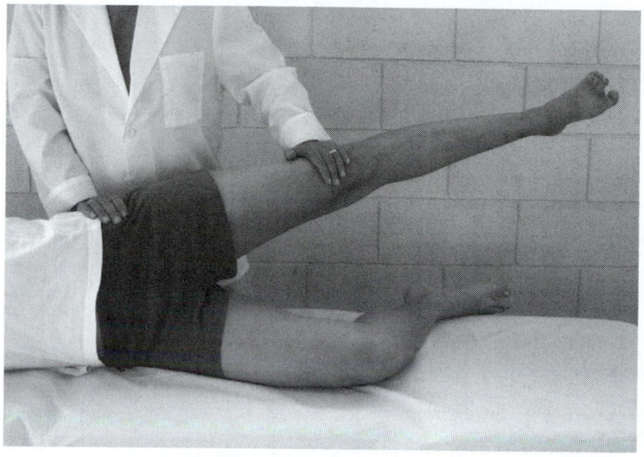

Figure 6.15 Manual muscle testing of the left hip abductors (gluteus medius and minimus) for grades greater than *Fair.* The limb has moved against gravity into hip abduction, and is now holding the position against the therapist's resistance.

Kendall in their classic 1949 work entitled *Muscles: Testing and Function*. Recent textbooks describing these methods have been authored by Hislop and Montgomery[92] and Kendall et al.[93] Both methods, based on the work by Wright and Lovett, use arc of motion, gravity, and manually applied resistance by the therapist to test and determine muscle grades. Generally, the patient is positioned so that the muscle or muscle group being tested has to hold or move against the resistance of gravity. If this is well tolerated, the therapist applies manual resistance gradually to the distal end of the body part in which the muscle inserts, and in a direction opposite to the torque produced by the muscle(s) being tested (Fig. 6.15).

In recent editions, both methods recommend applying manual resistance in the form of a **break test** in which the patient holds a joint position until the therapist gradually overpowers the patient and an eccentric contraction begins to occur. Both methods suggest that the break test occurs at the end of the ROM when testing one-joint muscles, and at mid-range when testing two-joint muscles. In the case of weaker muscles that cannot hold or move well against gravity, the patient is repositioned and attempts to move the body part through a gravity-minimized (horizontal) plane of motion. During all testing, stabilization of the body part on which the muscle originates and careful avoidance of substitution by other muscle groups are emphasized. Results can be noted in a narrative report or on standardized recording forms (Fig. 6.16).

Although there are many similarities, there are some differences between these two popular MMT methods. Kendall and associates[93] propose to examine individual muscles insofar as practical, whereas the Daniels and Worthingham[91,92] method examines muscle groups that perform particular joint motions. Some testing positions are similar but others vary between the two methods, with Daniels and Worthingham providing more instruction and emphasis on gravity-minimized positioning for weaker muscle groups. Daniels and Worthingham recommend that the patient move through the arc of motion when testing both against gravity or with gravity minimized. Kendall and associates have the patient move through an arc of motion only when testing with gravity minimized; otherwise the patient is positioned against gravity at the middle or end of the ROM and asked to hold the position.

Both methods use a grading system based on the work of Lovett with categories of Normal, Good, Fair, Poor, Trace, and Zero. However, Kendall and associates suggest a 0 to 100 percent or a 0 to 10 scale; Daniels and Worthingham suggest a 0 to 5 scale (Table 6.6). If numerical scoring is used, it is important to clarify which scale is being used by noting the score followed by a slash indicating the maximal value of the scale. For example, a grade of *Fair* strength should be noted as 3/5 if using a 0 to 5 scale, or 5/10 if using a 0 to 10 scale. It is important to note that these numerical scales indicate ordinal data, as the intervals between the numbers do not represent equal units of measure. The MMT grades of *Good* and *Normal* typically encompass a large range of a muscle's strength, while the grades of *Fair, Poor,* and *Trace* include a much narrower range. Sharrard,[94] counting alpha motor neurons in spinal cords of individuals with poliomyelitis at the time of autopsy, found that muscles previously receiving a grade of *Good* had 50 percent of their innervated motor neurons, while muscles graded as *Fair* had only 15 percent of their motor neurons. Beasley[95] noted that patients with poliomyelitis were graded as having *Good, Fair,* and *Poor* knee extension when they had on average only 43, 9, and 3 percent of the knee extension force of normal subjects, respectively. Andres and associates,[96] in a study of four muscle groups in patients with amyotrophic lateral sclerosis, found that the muscles were often graded as *Normal* until up to 50 percent of strength was lost.

The concurrent validity of MMT with muscle strength measured by hand-held dynamometers (described in the following section) and strain gauges has been supported by many research studies. Schwartz and co-workers[97] studied 24 muscle groups in 122 patients with spinal cord injury and noted correlation coefficients ranging from .59 to .94 between strength measured with MMT grades and hand-held dynamometry. Other investigators have reported similar findings.[96,98,99] However, several researchers have noted a wide range of strength values within a MMT grade and an overlap in strength values between adjacent MMT grades, especially in the grades of *Good* and *Normal*.[97,99,100] MMT has been shown to be less sensitive in detecting strength deficits in stronger muscles than in weaker muscles. Although more costly and time consuming than MMT, hand-held dynamometry can be used to improve objectivity and sensitivity as needed. When muscles are strong enough to move against gravity and the dynamometer's lever arm, isokinetic dynamometry may also be used.

DOCUMENTATION OF MUSCLE EXAMINATION

LEFT				RIGHT		
3	2	1	Date of Examination / Examiner's Name	1	2	3
			NECK			
			Capital extension			
			Cervical extension			
			Combined extension (capital plus cervical)			
			Capital flexion			
			Cervical flexion			
			Combined flexion (capital plus cervical)			
			Combined flexion and rotation (Sternocleidomastoid)			
			Cervical rotation			
			TRUNK			
			Extension—Lumbar			
			Extension—Thoracic			
			Pelvic elevation			
			Flexion			
			Rotation			
			Diaphragm strength			
			Maximal inspiration less full expiration (indirect intercostal test) (inches)			
			Cough (indirect forced expiration) (F, WF, NF, O)			
			UPPER EXTREMITY			
			Scapular abduction and upward rotation			
			Scapular elevation			
			Scapular adduction			
			Scapular adduction and downward rotation			
			Shoulder flexion			
			Shoulder extension			
			Shoulder scaption			
			Shoulder abduction			
			Shoulder horizontal abduction			
			Shoulder horizontal adduction			
			Shoulder external rotation			
			Shoulder internal rotation			
			Elbow flexion			
			Elbow extension			
			Forearm supination			
			Forearm pronation			
			Wrist flexion			
			Wrist extension			
			Finger metacarpophalangeal flexion			
			Finger proximal interphalangeal flexion			
			Finger distal interphalangeal flexion			
			Finger metacarpophalangeal extension			
			Finger abduction			
			Finger adduction			
			Thumb metacarpophalangeal flexion			
			Thumb interphalangeal flexion			

*After Hislop and Montgomery

Figure 6.16 An example of a manual muscle testing recording form. (From Hislop, HJ, and Montgomery, J,[92, p 7] with permission.)

Table 6.6 Manual Muscle Testing Grades

Grades	Grade Abbreviations	0–5 Scale	0–10 Scale	Criteria
Normal	N	5	10	Full available ROM, against gravity, strong manual resistance
Good Plus	G+	4+	9	Full available ROM, against gravity, nearly strong manual resistance
Good	G	4	8	Full available ROM, against gravity, moderate manual resistance
Good Minus	G−	4−	7	Full available ROM, against gravity, nearly moderate manual resistance
Fair Plus	F+	3+	6	Full available ROM, against gravity, slight manual resistance
Fair	F	3	5	Full available ROM, against gravity, no resistance
Fair Minus	F−	3−	4	At least 50% of ROM, against gravity, no resistance
Poor Plus	P+	2+	3	Full available ROM, gravity minimized, slight manual resistance
Poor	P	2	2	Full available ROM, gravity minimized, no resistance
Poor Minus	P–	2−	1	At least 50% of ROM, gravity minimized, no resistance
Trace Plus	T+	1+		Minimal observable motion (less than 50% ROM), gravity minimized, no resistance
Trace	T	1	T	No observable motion, palpable muscle contraction, no resistance
Zero	0	0	0	No observable or palpable muscle contraction

Generally, intratester reliability of MMT has been found to be good among trained therapists using established methods, with correlation coefficients ranging from .63 to .98.[101–103] The results of studies on intertester reliability of MMT vary more widely, but findings can be summarized. Several investigators[103–107] report complete agreement between testers who examined the same patient to be the lowest, ranging from 28 to 75 percent. Using a 0–5 scale, agreement between testers within a half grade (plus or minus) was better, ranging from 50 to 97 percent. Using a 0–10 scale, agreement between testers within plus or minus one full grade was high, ranging from 89 to 100 percent. Correlation coefficients for intertester reliability ranged from .11 to .94.[97,103,104,108] Training to standardize testing positions, stabilization, and grading criteria resulted in higher agreement and correlation coefficients between testers. Global strength scores that average MMT results from multiple muscle groups also resulted in higher reliability.[103,108]

To improve reliability, grade definitions modified from Kendall et al,[93] Hislop and Montgomery,[92] and Hines[109] are presented with specific criteria in Table 6.6. Although grades *Zero* through *Fair* are based on objective criteria, grade *Fair+* through *Normal* depend on the therapist's subjective opinion of what is minimal, moderate, and maximal resistance. A *Normal* grade is typically equated with the normal strength for that muscle given the patient's age, gender, and body size. It should be noted that there is considerable variability in the amount of resistance that normal muscles can hold against; for example, large muscles in the lower extremity will normally hold against considerably more force than small muscles of the hand. The application of resistance throughout the arc of motion (**make test** or active resistance test) in addition to resistance at only one point in the arc of motion (**break test**) may help in judging a muscle's strength.

Hand-held Dynamometry

Hand-held dynamometers (HHD) are portable devices, placed between the therapist's hand and the patient's body, that measure mechanical force at the point of application (Fig. 6.17).

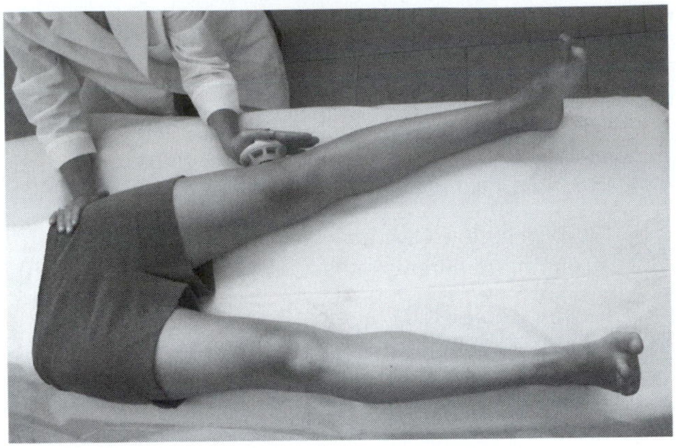

Figure 6.17 Measurement of the strength of the left hip abductors with a hand-held dynamometer. The hand-held dynamometer measures force at the point of application, which should be converted to torque.

Patients are typically asked to push against the therapist in a maximal isometric contraction (make test), or hold a position until the therapist overpowers the muscle producing an eccentric contraction (break test). The force measured by the dynamometer will vary depending on the method of applying the resistance (make or break test), the patient's body position in relationship to gravity, joint angle, dynamometer placement on the patient (lever arm), stabilization to prevent muscle substitution, and the therapist's strength.[110–112] Although force values determined with make and break tests are highly correlated, break tests usually result in greater force values than make tests,[113,114] so they should not be used interchangeably. To avoid the effect of the weight of the moving body segment on force measurements, it is recommended that muscle groups be tested in gravity-minimized positions. For example, to test the strength of the hip abductors the patient would be positioned supine so that the muscle action would pull in a horizontal plane relative to the ground (Fig. 6.17). Soderberg[112] provides detailed information on recommended positions and procedures for HHD. The joint should also be positioned at an easily reproducible angle so that muscle length remains constant. The dynamometer is applied perpendicular to the body segment at an established location on the patient's body. When muscles contract they produce **torque** which creates angular joint motion. The therapist must be strong enough to resist the patient's torque to ensure an isometric (make test), or if desired an eccentric contraction (break test). If the therapist is unable to provide adequate resistance, the dynamometer can be attached to a fixed surface[115,116] or an isokinetic dynamometer can be used with the speed set to 0°/sec.

Normative force values for particular muscle groups by patient age and gender have been reported,[117–121] but therapists must be careful to replicate the normative study's methods to ensure appropriate comparisons. Some authors have also included regression equations to take into account body weight and height.[117,118] Most normative studies have reported results in units of force such as pounds, newtons, or kilogram-force. However, these force values will vary depending on the length between the dynamometer's location on the patient's body to the axis of motion, or lever arm. A better method of comparison across people would be to use torque.[112,122] To determine torque, the measured force is multiplied by the distance between the dynamomter's location and the joint axis. Examples of units of torque are foot-pounds, Newton-meters, or kgf-meters.

For patients with unilateral conditions, it may be helpful to compare results to that of the uninvolved extremity. Andrews et al[118] found no statistically significant difference in force between the dominant and nondominant lower extremities using a hand-held dynamometer, but did find a difference between the dominant and nondominant upper extremities. In general, differences were between 0 and 4.5 pounds or between 0 and 11.2 percent of the average forces generated. Phillips and associates[117] found statistically significant differences in force between sides in a variety of upper and lower extremity muscle groups ranging from 0.2 to 8.0 percent. Sapega[123] has recommended that a difference in muscle force between sides of greater than 20 percent probably indicates abnormality, while a difference of 10 to 20 percent possibly indicates abnormality.

Muscle forces measured with HHD have been compared to forces measured with isokinetic dynamometers to evaluate concurrent validity. Most studies have found good to excellent validity with correlation coefficients ranging from .78 to .98.[124–126] Several investigators have reported that HHD underestimates strength in large muscle groups such as the knee extensors,[127,128] or when forces are greater than 196 to 250 Newtons.[124,129]

Depending on the study, hand-held dynamometers have demonstrated good to excellent intratester reliability, and poor to excellent intertester reliability.[18,25,113,128,130–136] Several reviews of such reliability studies are available.[112,137,138] Reliability seems to be better when testing the upper extremities than when testing the lower extremities and trunk,[131,133] in particular, the measurements of ankle dorsiflexion and hip abduction.[117,118,128,131] Agre et al.[130] found the standard deviation of the repeated measurements expressed as a percentage of the mean force measurements (coefficient of variation of replication) to be 5.1 to 8.3 percent for the upper extremity muscle groups, and 11.3 to 17.8 percent for the lower extremity muscle groups. Wang and associates[134] reported coefficient of variation of replication ranging from 4.2 to 7.4 percent for three lower extremity muscle groups. Researchers believe some of the error in using hand-held dynamometers is due to off-center loading of the dynamometer, difficulties in positioning and stabilization, and limitations in the strength and experience of the therapists.

Isokinetic Dynamometry

An *isokinetic dynamometer* is a stationary, electromechanical device that control the velocity of a moving body segment by resisting and measuring the patient's effort so that the body segment cannot accelerate beyond the preset angular velocity (Fig. 6.18). For example, the velocity of a Biodex System 3 Pro isokinetic dynamometer in concentric mode can be set from 0 to 500°/sec, and the resistance, measured in torque, can be monitored from 0 to 500 ft-lbs or 0-680 Newton-meters.[139] Speeds of 60, 120, and 180°/sec are commonly tested in relatively sedentary patients, and faster speeds may be warranted in athletes. Isokinetic dynamometers can be used to measure the torque produced during isometric contractions (if the velocity is set to 0°/sec), concentric contractions, and in some models eccentric contractions. Isokinetic dynamometers, although expensive and cumbersome, are especially helpful in examining the performance of large, strong muscle groups. In such situations, manual muscle testing and hand-held dynamometers are often insensitive to muscle performance abnormalities.[95,111] Muscle groups acting at the knee, shoulder, back and to a lesser extent the elbow and ankle are the ones most frequently tested with isokinetic devices.

Isokinetic dynamometers measure torque and ROM as a function of time. Muscle performance characteristics most often noted are peak (maximal) torque, and less frequently peak torque/body weight (Nm/kg), and average torque. Work measurements can be derived from the angular displacement and torque values. Power, which is work per unit time, also can be determined. Endurance (muscle fatigue) can also be measured. One common method of measuring endurance is to note the time required for peak torque to decrease by 50 percent.[123,140] Peak torque ratios of reciprocal (agonist-antagonist) muscle groups such as the hamstrings/ quadriceps and external/internal rotators of the shoulder have been noted. However, careful corrections for the weight of the limb (gravity effects) are necessary to arrive at an accurate relationship.[141–144] If gravity corrections are not utilized, the muscles assisted by gravity will exhibit erroneously high torque values, whereas the muscles that resist gravity will exhibit erroneously low torque values.

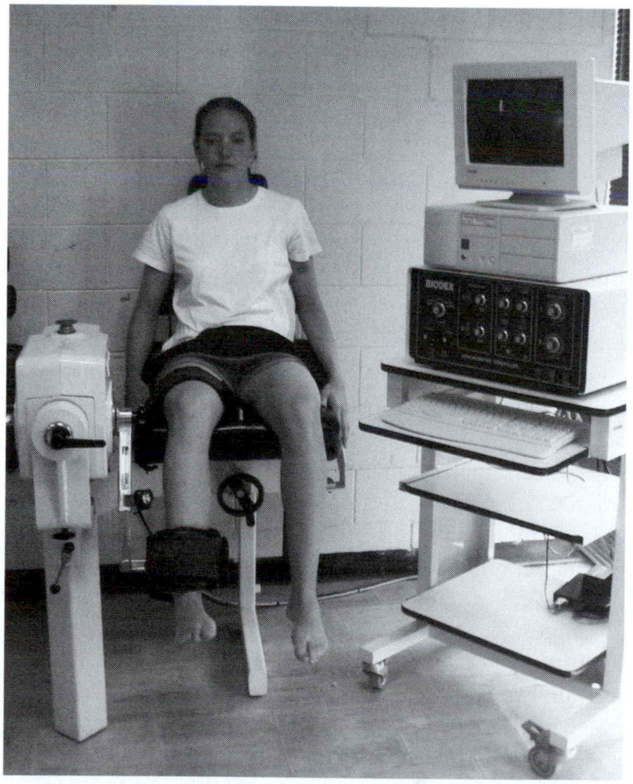

Figure 6.18 An isokinetic dynamometer is being used to measure muscle performance characteristics of the right knee extensors (quadriceps). Peak torque is the most frequently noted characteristic.

It has been suggested that submaximal patient effort can be detected by the increased variability of repeated measures of peak torque, average torque, and slope to peak torque in isometric and concentric contractions.[145–147] However, research in this area has produced conflicting findings and demonstrated large errors in classifying effort into maximal and submaximal categories.[143,148–150] Many factors such as patient pain, fear, or fatigue, and damp settings, preload forces, mechanical artifact, and acceleration and deceleration rampings can affect the variability of torque measurements. The use of isokinetic dynamometer records to form clinical opinions of patient effort is not advised until further research is conducted.

To ensure the validity of isokinetic dynamometry measurements, calibration of the equipment is necessary and should be performed each day of testing, at the same speed and damp setting to be used during testing.[143] Proper alignment of joint axis and machine axis, stabilization of proximal body parts, and gravity correction are needed. Several practice trials of the motion to acquaint the patient with the equipment and testing protocol is helpful, and at least one to three maximal test repetitions should be performed prior to recording measurements.[151,152] It is important to note that torque values will vary with type of muscle contractions (isometric, concentric, eccentric) and changes in velocity settings, joint angle, patient position, test trials, rest intervals, patient feedback, and preload, damp, and ramping machine settings. For example, concentric contractions will result in lower torque values than isometric contractions in the same muscle group, while eccentric contractions will result in higher torque values than isometric contractions. Faster velocity settings during concentric contractions will result in lower torque values than slower velocity settings. All of these factors must be kept constant in order to effectively use repeat testing data to judge patient progress. Keating and Matyas,[153] Rothstein,[143] Davies et al,[154] and Gaines and Talbot[155] have presented information to improve the validity and reliability of isokinetic testing. Peak torque and work measurements in a variety of healthy and patient populations have shown good to excellent reliability for concentric contractions, and poor to good reliability for eccentric contractions.[151,156–166] Reciprocal (agonist–antagonist) ratios have shown less reliability than peak torque measurements.[166]

Normative data on adults[166–173] and children[174–179] can provide a reference for evaluating and interpreting patient data. However, comparisons with published data are appropriate only when identical procedures are used and tested populations are similar. Patient age, gender, weight, height, and athletic participation can affect recorded values. Out of necessity, the involved extremity is often compared to the contralateral extremity. Generally, studies have found no statistically significant difference between dominant and nondominant sides in torque measurements for muscles surrounding the knee joint,[170,174,180–182] elbow,[175,179] and shoulder.[175] Alternatively, some studies have found differences due to side dominance for certain motions at the elbow and shoulder especially in highly skilled male athletes.[179,183,184] A difference of at least 10 percent in torque values between opposing sides of the body has been suggested as an indicator of impairment.[185,186] Others have noted imbalances of more than 10 percent between sides of the body in healthy populations.[187,188] Further research is needed to establish the magnitude of difference between opposite limbs that would indicate impairment.[153] At the present time it seems appropriate to use the guidelines provided by Sapega,[123] suggesting that a difference in muscle force between sides of greater than 20 percent probably indicates abnormality, while a difference of 10 to 20 percent possibly indicates abnormality.

Special Tests

After completing the patient interview, observation, palpation, and examination of ROM, accessory motions, and muscle performance, the therapist may suspect the nature of the pathology. Special tests, designed to focus on specific conditions in a particular region of the body, may be helpful in confirming the diagnosis. A therapist would ordinarily choose to perform only those tests indicated by previous findings that are relevant to the area of the body being examined. False-positive and false-negative results are possible. However, a positive test finding in conjunction with other aspects of the examination would be highly suggestive of pathology. There are many special tests presented in the work of Cailliet,[188] Hoppenfeld,[4] Magee,[2] Richardson and Inglarsh,[3] and Tomberlin and Saunders.[5]

One category of special tests is used to determine the integrity of ligaments in supporting a joint. These **ligamentous instability tests**, also called ligament stress tests, are performed by the therapist on a relaxed, passive patient. These maneuvers are often similar to tests of accessory or joint play motions. If possible, results should be compared with those from the uninvolved, contralateral joint. The amount of laxity is usually graded from I to IV (Table 6.7).[189]

Table 6.7 Grading of Ligamentous Instability Tests

Grades	Amount of Movement
I	0–5 mm
II	6–10 mm
III	11–15 mm
IV	>15 mm

Although these tests focus on ligament integrity, capsular integrity as well as dynamic muscle support may influence the results. Examples of ligamentous instability tests include the Lachman test, which examines injury to the anterior cruciate ligament; the drawer test, which examines anterior and posterior knee instability; and varus and valgus stress tests at the knee. In addition to ligament instability tests, there are more general tests that examine joint subluxation and dislocation. These tests are often called **apprehension tests** because the patient is placed in a vulnerable joint position while being monitored for apprehension. For example, to test for a history of an anterior subluxation or dislocation of the glenohumeral joint, the shoulder is positioned in 90° of abduction and moved toward external rotation.

The length of muscles that cross and act at one joint can usually be examined in the process of testing passive ROM. However, some muscles cross and act at two or more joints. Some special tests examine the length of these muscles. The Thomas test,[52,93] which examines the length of one and two joint hip flexors; the Ober test,[52,93] which focuses on the length of the tensor fascia lata; and the Bunnel-Littler test,[3,4] which determines the role of the lumbricles, interossei, extensor digitorum, and joint capsule in limited flexion of the proximal interphalangeal joints of the hand, are examples of special muscle length tests.

Numerous special tests address common conditions affecting the integrity of muscle and tendon structures. These tests typically stretch or contract the inflamed or injured structure, resulting in pain if the tests are positive. For example, the Finkelstein test[4] is used to examine inflammation of the tendons of the abductor pollicis longus and extensor pollicis brevis by stretching these structures. The tennis elbow test[4] has the patient isometrically contract the extensor carpi radialis muscles against manual resistance. Often the therapist will have previously noted pain, limitation, and possibly weakness during ROM and muscle performance; special tests are used to clarify these earlier findings.

Another category of special tests reproduces the symptoms caused by compression of peripheral nerves or diminished blood flow. For example, the test for carpal tunnel syndrome places the wrist in full flexion for 60 to 90 seconds to reproduce the numbness and tingling caused by compression of the median nerve by the transverse carpal ligament.[188] Homan's sign utilizes ankle dorsiflexion, knee extension, and deep palpation to elicit calf pain. It is suggestive of deep vein thrombophlebitis; however diagnostic reliability is limited.[4]

Additional Tests and Measures

Depending on examination findings, other procedures may be indicated. Many of these additional examination procedures are discussed in detail in other chapters of this book. For example, patient complaints of paresthesia or difficulty in muscle performance often indicate neurological involvement that calls for testing of superficial and proprioceptive sensations (see Chapter 5), reflexes and motor tone (see Chapter 8), coordination (see Chapter 7), or nerve conduction velocity (see Chapter 9). These tests, in conjunction with muscle performance results, help to identify conditions affecting peripheral nerves, spinal nerve roots, and the central nervous system. Therapists must distinguish peripheral nerve versus nerve root patterns of sensory and motor innervation. References on manual muscles testing, such as those by Kendall et al,[93] and Hislop and Montgomery[92] provide extensive information on innervation patterns. Figure 6.19 presents muscle testing recording forms that are helpful in recognizing impaired innervation patterns. Myotomes and deep tendon reflexes that are often included as part of a musculoskeletal examination are shown in Tables 6.8 and 6.9. Upper motor neuron lesions usually result in hyperreflexia, whereas lower motor neuron lesions involving the spinal nerve root or peripheral nerves usually cause hyporeflexia of deep tendon reflexes.

Impairments in ROM, accessory joint motions, and motor performance may impact activities of daily living, and occupational and recreational activities. In such cases the examination of gait (see Chapter 10), functional abilities (see Chapter 11), and environmental surroundings (see Chapter 12) is often appropriate. Sometimes findings indicate the need for additional testing by other health professionals such as physician specialists, psychologists, speech-language pathologists, and occupational therapists.

Evaluation of Examination Findings

At the conclusion of the musculoskeletal examination, all pertinent historical, subjective, and physical findings are evaluated to establish a diagnosis upon which treatment is based. A diagnosis has been defined as a label encompassing a cluster of signs and symptoms, syndromes, or categories.[85] The specific tissues causing the impairments should be identified so that treatment can be focused and effective. The therapist must have a thorough understanding of the pathologies commonly affecting the body segment under consideration.[190] The symptoms and clinical manifestations of these pathologies are compared to the current examination findings to establish a diagnosis.

Table 6.8 Myotomes

	Upper Quarter Myotomes	
Level	**Action to Be Tested**	**Muscle**
C5	Shoulder abduction	Deltoid
C5, C6	Elbow flexion	Biceps
C7	Elbow extension	Triceps
C8	Ulnar deviation	Flexor carpi ulnaris Extensor carpi ulnaris
T1	Digit abduction/adduction	Interossei
	Lower Quarter Myotomes	
Level	**Action to Be Tested**	**Muscle**
L2, L3	Hip flexion	Iliopsoas
L3, L4	Knee extension	Quadriceps
L5	Ankle dorsiflexion	Anterior tibialis
	Extension of great toe	Extensor hallicus longus
S1	Plantarflexion	Gastrocnemius

From Dyrek, DA,[190, p 76] with permission.

Table 6.9 Deep Tendon Reflexes

	Root Level	Muscle	Peripheral Nerve
Upper quarter:	C5–6	Biceps	Musculocutaneous
	C5–6	Brachioradialis	Radial
	C7	Triceps	Radial
Lower quarter:	L3–4	Quadriceps	Femoral
	S1	Gastrocnemius	Sciatic (tibial)

The degree of reflex activity is graded on a 0 to 4 scale. Grades are awarded based on a predicted response and comparison of responses between body halves.

0 = no reflex response
1 = minimal response } normal range
2 = moderate response } normal range
3 = brisk, strong response } normal range
4 = clonus

From Dyrek, DA,[190, p 76] with permission.

SPINAL NERVE AND MUSCLE CHART

NECK, DIAPHRAGM AND UPPER EXTREMITY

Name Date

PERIPHERAL NERVES

KEY ⟶ D. = Dorsal Prim. Ramus
V. = Vent. Prim. Ramus
P.R. = Plexus Root
S.T. = Superior Trunk
P. = Posterior Cord
L. = Lateral Cord
M. = Medial Cord

SPINAL SEGMENT

Group	Muscle	Muscle Strength Grade	Cervical (D.) 1-8	Cervical (V.) 1-8	Cervical (V.) 1-4	Phrenic (V.) 3, 4, 5	Long Thor. (P.R.) 5, 6, 7, (8)	Dor. Scap (P.R.) 4, 5	N. to Subcl. (S.T.) 5, 6	Suprascap (S.T.) 4, 5, 6	U. Subscap. (P.) (4), 5, 6, (7)	Thoracodor (P.) (5), 6, 7, 8	L. Subscap. (P.) 5, 6, (7)	Lat. Pect. (L.) 5, 6, 7	Med. Pect. (M.) (6), 7, 8, T1	Axillary (P.) 5, 6	Musculocu. (L.) (4), 5, 6, 7	Radial (P.) 5, 6, 7, 8, T1	Median (L.M.) 5, 6, 7, 8, T1	Ulnar (M.) 7, 8, T1	C1	C2	C3	C4	C5	C6	C7	C8	T1
	HEAD & NECK EXTENSORS		•																		1	2	3	4	5	6	7	8	1
Cervical nerves	INFRAHYOID MUSCLES				•																1	2	3						
Cervical nerves	RECTUS CAP ANT. & LAT.				•																1	2							
Cervical nerves	LONGUS CAPITIS				•																1	2	3	(4)					
Cervical nerves	LONGUS COLLI			•																		2	3	4	5	6	(7)		
Cervical nerves	LEVATOR SCAPULAE				•			•															3	4	5				
Cervical nerves	SCALENI (A. M. P.)			•																			3	4	5	6	7	8	
Cervical nerves	STERNOCLEIDOMASTOID				•																(1)	2	3						
Cervical nerves	TRAPEZIUS (U. M. L.)				•																	2	3	4					
Cervical nerves	DIAPHRAGM					•																	3	4	5				
Brachial Plexus – Root	SERRATUS ANTERIOR						•																		5	6	7	8	
Brachial Plexus – Root	RHOMBOIDS MAJ & MIN							•																4	5				
Brachial Plexus – Trunk	SUBCLAVIUS								•																5	6			
Brachial Plexus – Trunk	SUPRASPINATUS									•														4	5	6			
Brachial Plexus – Trunk	INFRASPINATUS									•														(4)	5	6			
Brachial Plexus – P Cord	SUBSCAPULARIS										•		•												5	6	7		
Brachial Plexus – P Cord	LATISSIMUS DORSI											•														6	7	8	
Brachial Plexus – P Cord	TERES MAJOR												•												5	6	7		
Brachial Plexus – L	PECTORALIS MAJ (UPPER)													•											5	6	7		
Brachial Plexus – M&L	PECTORALIS MAJ (LOWER)													•	•											6	7	8	1
Brachial Plexus – M&L	PECTORALIS MINOR														•											(6)	7	8	1
Axil.	TERES MINOR															•									5	6			
Axil.	DELTOID															•									5	6			
Musculo-cutan	CORACOBRACHIALIS																•									6	7		
Musculo-cutan	BICEPS																•								5	6			
Musculo-cutan	BRACHIALIS																•								5	6			
Radial	TRICEPS																	•								6	7	8	1
Radial	ANCONEUS																	•									7	8	
Radial – Lat.M	BRACHIALIS (SMALL PART)																	•							5	6			
Radial – Lat.M	BRACHIORADIALIS																	•							5	6			
Radial – Lat.M	EXT CARPI RAD L																	•							5	6	7	8	
Radial – Lat.M	EXT CARPI RAD B																	•								6	7	(8)	
Radial – Post Inter	SUPINATOR																	•							5	6	(7)		
Radial – Post Inter	EXT DIGITORUM																	•								6	7	8	
Radial – Post Inter	EXT DIGITI MINIMI																	•								6	7	8	
Radial – Post Inter	EXT CARPI ULNARIS																	•								6	7	8	
Radial – Post Inter	ABD POLLICIS LONGUS																	•								6	7	8	
Radial – Post Inter	EXT POLLICIS BREVIS																	•								6	7	8	
Radial – Post Inter	EXT POLLICIS LONGUS																	•								6	7	8	
Radial – Post Inter	EXT INDICIS																	•								6	7	8	
Median	PRONATOR TERES																		•							6	7		
Median	FLEX CARPI RADIALIS																		•							6	7	8	
Median	PALMARIS LONGUS																		•							(6)	7	8	1
Median	FLEX DIGIT SUPERFICIALIS																		•								7	8	1
Median – A Inter	FLEX DIGIT PROF I & II																		•								7	8	1
Median – A Inter	FLEX POLLICIS LONGUS																		•							(6)	7	8	1
Median – A Inter	PRONATOR QUADRATUS																		•								7	8	1
Median	ABD POLLICIS BREVIS																		•							6	7	8	1
Median	OPPONENS POLLICIS																		•							6	7	8	1
Median	FLEX POLL BREV (SUP. H)																		•							6	7	8	1
Median	LUMBRICALES I & II																		•							(6)	7	8	1
Ulnar	FLEX CARPI ULNARIS																			•							7	8	1
Ulnar	FLEX DIGIT. PROF. III & IV																			•							7	8	1
Ulnar	PALMARIS BREVIS																			•							(7)	8	1
Ulnar	ABD DIGITI MINIMI																			•							(7)	8	1
Ulnar	OPPONENS DIGITI MINIMI																			•							(7)	8	1
Ulnar	FLEX DIGITI MINIMI																			•							(7)	8	1
Ulnar	PALMAR INTEROSSEI																			•								8	1
Ulnar	DORSAL INTEROSSEI																			•								8	1
Ulnar	LUMBRICALES III & IV																			•							(7)	8	1
Ulnar	ADDUCTOR POLLICIS																			•								8	1
Ulnar	FLEX POLL BREV. (DEEP H.)																			•								8	1

SENSORY

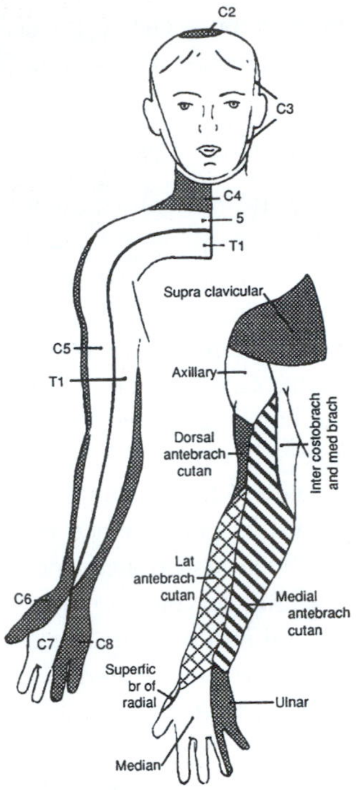

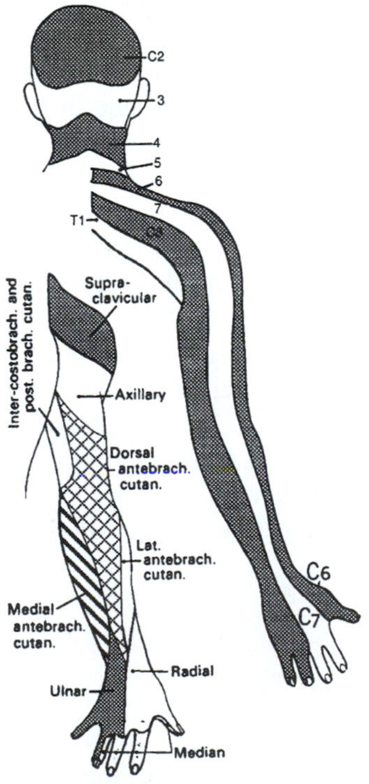

Dermatomes redrawn from Keegan and Garrett Anat Rec 102. 409. 437. 1948
Cutaneous Distribution of peripheral nerves redrawn from *Gray's Anatomy of the Human Body.* 28th ed

Figure 6.19 A manual muscle testing recording form that aids in determining the site or level of a nerve lesion. (From Kendall, FP, McCreary, EK, and Provance, PG,[93, p 393] with permission.)

Musculoskeletal Practice Patterns listed in the *Guide to Physical Therapist Practice*[85] can assist in categorizing diagnoses into common clusters, and provide information on prognosis, anticipated goals and expected outcomes, and interventions (see Appendix A in Chapter 1).

Sometimes the evaluation process does not yield an identifiable diagnosis; not all patients present with textbook-perfect symptoms. In such cases, a provisional diagnosis and the alleviation of symptoms and impairments become the basis for treatment. In other instances, the evaluation may indicate the presence of two or more conditions. The therapist should then prioritize and focus initially on the condition causing the most serious impairments, functional limitations, and disability.

The evaluation should clearly determine the baseline for the patient's symptoms, impairments, functional limitations, and disabilities. This information becomes the basis of the clinical problem list and guides development of anticipated goals and expected outcomes. The results of future examinations can be compared to this baseline to evaluate the effectiveness of treatment.

In addition to establishing a diagnosis and baseline data, the evaluation of findings should ascertain etiological factors. Unless the underlying causes of the condition are recognized and treated, chronic problems can be expected.[1] The therapist must not only direct attention to the specifically involved tissues, but must also think more broadly of physiological units of function and biomechanics. For example, a patient with a sprain of the medial collateral ligament of the knee may initially respond well to treatment consisting of compression elastic wrapping, ice, elevation, reduced activity, and a protective non-weightbearing crutch gait. However, if the condition is partially due to abnormal foot pronation, the resumption of normal weightbearing activities may cause reinjury unless the alignment of the foot and leg is improved with orthotics. Similarly, a patient with tendinitis of the supraspinatus muscle may react well to rest, modalities applied to the tendon, and gentle glenohumeral ROM exercises, but often also requires eventual strengthening of the rotator cuff, trapezius, and serratus anterior muscles, as well as lengthening of the posterior and inferior glenohumeral capsule to restore normal scapulohumeral rhythm and prevent recurrent subacromial impingement of the supraspinatus tendon.

Other information that impacts the prognosis and course of treatment should be determined during the evaluation process. The mode and mechanism of onset must be established. Was the onset sudden, gradually acquired, or congenital? Generally, the prognosis is better for a condition caused by a well-defined event than for a congenital condition or one with an insidious, gradual onset. The mode and mechanism of onset also provide clues to help develop strategies for prevention of reoccurring episodes of the injury or condition.

Finally, an analysis of the examination findings should establish the stage of the patient's condition. The stage, whether acute, subacute, or chronic, can indicate how well the patient will tolerate mechanical loads such as those imposed by daily activities or by a therapist during treatment.[190] The *acute stage* is usually defined as occurring up to the first 48 to 72 hours after onset. The *subacute stage* may continue up to 2 weeks to several months after onset. Typically, conditions are considered in the *chronic stage* after 3 to 6 months. Another way of defining the stages, which is probably more relevant to treatment planning, focuses on tissue inflammation and the repair process.[1] Conditions in an acute inflammation stage will show signs and symptoms of inflammation associated with hyperemia, increased capillary permeability with protein and plasma leakage, and an influx of granulocytes and other defensive cells. These signs and symptoms include swelling, elevated skin temperature at the lesion site, and pain at rest that worsens with ROM and resisted isometric contractions that even minimally stress the involved tissues. The chronic inflammation stage produces signs and symptoms associated with attempts at tissue repair, including an increase in the number of fibrocytes and the presence of granulation tissue; the patient will now have minimal or no swelling and elevated temperature at the lesion site. Pain tends to occur only at the extremes of ROM when the end-feel is reached, or with a moderate to maximal amount of isometric resistance. Tissues in an acute stage will often not tolerate mechanical loading from daily, recreational, occupational, or therapeutic activities. The force, frequency, and duration of treatment procedures must be monitored closely so as not to increase inflammation and worsen the condition. In contrast, tissues in the chronic stage will usually tolerate and require treatment procedures involving more mechanical loading, frequency, and duration to effect positive changes in the tissues. The stage of the condition also adds prognostic information. Typically, an acute condition will show more spontaneous improvement over a shorter period of time than a chronic condition. A chronic condition usually requires a longer period of treatment to promote a smaller improvement in status.

Summary

The musculoskeletal examination provides important information concerning the status of bones, articular cartilage, joint capsules, ligaments, and muscles. The examination process begins with a review of the patient's medical records and a detailed interview. Careful observation, palpation, and ROM, accessory joint motion, and muscle performance tests are typically performed. Depending on the findings, special tests particular to the body region under examination may need to be included. Examination of the peripheral and central nervous system, gait, functional ability, and the environment is often required. At the conclusion of this process, all findings must be evaluated to determine the diagnosis, baseline status, etiological factors, mode of onset, and stage (acute, subacute, or chronic) of the condition. At this point the prognosis, anticipated goals, expected outcomes, and plan of care can be developed.

Questions for Review

1. Identify the components of a musculoskeletal examination. Describe the appropriate sequence of performing these procedures. Provide a rationale for your response.
2. What information should be obtained during a patient interview? Why is this information important?
3. What are the three types of normal end-feels? What types of tissue contribute to these end-feels?
4. Provide an example of a capsular and a noncapsular pattern of restriction at a joint of your choice. What would cause these two different patterns?
5. Compare and contrast osteokinematic and arthrokinematic motions. Give three examples of each type of motion. How do arthrokinematic motions combine to produce osteokinematic motion in a typical synovial joint in which the moving joint surface is concave? convex?
6. Distinguish between muscle performance, strength, endurance, work, and power.
7. Discuss the implications of a finding of pain versus no pain, and strength versus weakness during the performance of resisted isometric testing.
8. Describe the criteria for the manual muscle testing grades of *Zero, Poor, Fair, Good,* and *Normal.* Compare and contrast the criteria for the grades of *Poor minus, Poor,* and *Poor plus.*
9. What are the advantages and disadvantages of using manual muscle testing, hand-held dynamometers, and isokinetic dynamometers to determine muscle strength?
10. What summary information should be determined from evaluation of the musculoskeletal examination findings to develop a clinical problem list, goals, outcomes, prognosis, and plan of care?

Case Studies

CASE STUDY 1

A 45-year-old man enters the outpatient physical therapy department with a complaint of right shoulder pain of 1 week's duration. The pain began Monday morning following a weekend of scraping and painting his house. The patient describes his pain as aching and troublesome; his pain is a 6 on a pain scale of 0 to 10. He reports that he is married, and having difficulty in home maintenance activities such as lawn mowing. He is able to perform only 30 percent of his normal home and recreational activities. The therapist decides to conduct a musculoskeletal examination.

While palpating the shoulder region, increased tenderness and skin temperature in the region of the bicipital groove of the right anterior shoulder is noted. Active ROM of the right shoulder reveals increased pain and some limitations during shoulder flexion, abduction, and extension; all other active motions are pain free and within normal ROM limits. Passive shoulder motions are pain free with normal ROM, except for shoulder extension, which is limited and causes an increase in pain toward the end of motion.

GUIDING QUESTIONS

1. What are the purposes of a musculoskeletal examination?
2. What additional information should be gathered during the interview?
3. What is a capsular pattern of limitation? Does this patient have a capsular pattern of limitation for the glenohumeral joint?
4. The therapist suspects the presence of bicipital tendinitis. Do the findings during testing of active and passive ROM support this diagnosis? Explain.
5. What additional tests should be performed to selectively examine contractile tissue and help to support or repudiate the diagnosis of bicipital tendinitis? Provide a rationale for your selection.

CASE STUDY 2

A 14-year-old girl is referred for outpatient physical therapy 12 weeks after sustaining midshaft fractures of her left tibia and fibula from a bicycle accident. Her long leg cast was removed yesterday. The fracture is reported to be well healed. The patient reports her left knee and ankle are stiff and painful when she tries to bend them. She also describes her left leg as weak. At this time she is ambulating with two crutches, weightbearing as tolerated, with hopes of progressing off the crutches as soon as possible.

GUIDING QUESTIONS

1. On observation, the patient's left thigh and calf appear to be thinner than the right. How can this observation

be objectively measured and documented? Why might the patient's left leg be thinner than the right?

2. Passive ROM for left knee flexion is 10 to 70°. The end-feel for left knee flexion is firm. What is an end-feel? What are the three general types of normal end-feels? What tissues could be causing a firm end-feel for knee flexion in this patient?
3. What accessory joint motion should be examined considering the limitation in passive knee flexion ROM? Apply the concave–convex rules for determining the direction of the glide given the shape of the joint surfaces. The accessory joint motion was found to be very hypomobile. What grade should the accessory joint motion be given?
4. The therapist conducts a manual muscle test of the left lower extremity. What three factors are important in determining manual muscle testing grades? What would be the criteria for a manual muscle testing grade of *Fair*?
5. In addition to observing, palpating, and testing active ROM, passive ROM, accessory joint motions, and muscle performance, what other testing procedures would be important to include in the examination of this patient?

References

1. Hertling, D, and Kessler, RM: Management of Common Musculoskeletal Disorders: Physical Therapy Principles and Methods, ed 3. Lippincott, Philadelphia, 1996.
2. Magee, DJ: Orthopedic Physical Assessment, ed 4. WB Saunders, Philadelphia, 2002.
3. Richardson, JK, and Iglarsh, ZA: Clinical Orthopaedic Physical Therapy. WB Saunders, Philadelphia, 1994.
4. Hoppenfeld, S: Physical Examination of the Spine and Extremities. Prentice-Hall, Englewood Cliffs, NJ, 1976.
5. Tomberlin, JP, and Saunders, HD: Evaluation, Treatment, and Prevention of Musculoskeletal Disorders, Vol 2, ed 3. Saunders Group, Minnesota, 1994.
6. Talley, N, and O'Connor, S: Clinical Examination: A Guide to Physical Diagnosis. Williams & Wilkins, Baltimore, 1988.
7. Paris, SV: The Spine. Course notes, Boston, MA, 1976.
8. Keegan, JJ, and Garrett, FD: The segmental distribution of the cutaneous nerves in the limbs of man. Anat Rec 102:430, 1948.
9. Melzack, R: The McGill pain questionnaire: Major properties and scoring methods. Pain 1:277, 1975.
10. Boissonnault, WG: Examination in Physical Therapy Practice: Screening for Medical Disease. Churchill Livingstone, New York, 1991.
11. Goodman, CC, and Snyder, TK: Differential Diagnosis in Physical Therapy, ed 2. WB Saunders, Philadelphia, 1995.
12. Slemenda, CW, et al: Long-term bone loss in men: Effects of genetic and environmental factors. Ann Intern Med 117:286, 1992.
13. Hopper, JL, and Seeman, E: The bone density of female twins discordant for tobacco use. N Engl J Med 330:387, 1994.
14. Battie, MC, et al: Smoking and lumbar intervertebral disc degeneration: An MRI study of identical twins. Spine 16:1016, 1991.
15. Deyo, RA, and Bass, JE: Lifestyle and low-back pain: The influence of smoking and obesity. Spine 14:501, 1989.
16. Heliovaara, M, et al: Determinants of sciatica and low-back pain. Spine 16:608, 1991.
17. Boshuizen, JC, et al: Do smokers get more back pain? Spine 18:35, 1993.
18. Ekberg, K, et al: Case-control study of risk factors for disease in the neck and shoulder area. Occup Environ Med 51:262, 1994.
19. Brage, S, and Bjerkedal, T: Musculoskeletal pain and smoking in Norway. J Epidemiol Community Health 50:166, 1996.
20. Levangie, PK , and Norkin, CC: Joint Structure and Function: A Comprehensive Analysis, ed 4. FA Davis, Philadelphia, 2005.
21. Murray, MP: Gait as a total pattern of movement. Am J Phys Med 46:290, 1967.
22. Ostrosky, KM, et al: A comparison of gait characteristics in young and old subjects. Phys Ther 74:637, 1994.
23. Kuster, M, Sakurai, S, and Wook, GA: Kinematic and kinetic comparison of downhill and level walking. Clin Biomech 10:79, 1995.
24. Kerrigan, DC: Gender differences in joint biomechanics during walking: Normative study in young adults. Am J Phys Med Rehabil 77:2, 1998.
25. Livingston, LA, et al: Stairclimbing kinematics on stairs of differing dimensions. Arch Phys Med Rehabil 72:398, 1991.
26. Johnson, RC, and Smidt, GL: Hip motion measurements for selected activities of daily living. Clin Orthop 72:205, 1970.
27. Laubenthal, KN, Smidt, GL, and Kettelkamp, DB: A quantitative analysis of knee motion during activities of daily living. Phys Ther 52:34, 1972.
28. Rodosky, MW, Andriacchi, TP, and Andersson, GB: The influence of chair height on lower limb mechanics during rising. J Orthop Res 7:266, 1989.
29. Ikeda, ER, et al: Influence of age on dynamics of rising from a chair. Phys Ther 71:473, 1991.
30. Janssen, GM, Bussmann, HBJ, and Stam, HJ: Determinants of the sit-to-stand movement: A review. Phys Ther 82:866, 2002.
31. Safee-Rad, R, et al: Normal functional range of motion of upper limb joints during performance of three feeding activities. Arch Phys Med Rehabil 71:505, 1990.
32. Packer, TL, et al: Examining the elbow during functional activities. Occup Ther J Res 10:323, 1990.
33. Morrey, BF, et al: A biomechanical study of normal functional elbow motion. J Bone Joint Surg Am 63:872, 1981.
34. Ryu, J, et al: Functional ranges of motion of the wrist joint. J Hand Surg 16A:409, 1991.
35. Matsen, FA: et al: Practical Evaluation and Management of the Shoulder. WB Saunders, Philadelphia, 1994.
36. Boone, DC, and Azen, SP: Normal range of motion of joints in male subjects. J Bone Joint Surg Am 61:756, 1979.
37. Bell, RD, and Hoshizaki, TB: Relationship of age and sex with range of motion: Seventeen joint actions in humans. Can J Appl Sci 6:202, 1981.
38. Roach, KE, and Miles, TP: Normal hip and knee active range of motion: The relationship to age. Phys Ther 71:656, 1991.
39. Schwarze, DJ, and Denton, JR: Normal values of neonatal limbs: An evaluation of 1000 neonates. J Res Pediatr Orthop 13:758, 1993.
40. Moll, JMH, and Wright,V: Normal range of spinal mobility. Ann Rheum Dis 30:381, 1971.
41. Youdas, JW, et al: Normal range of motion of the cervical spine: An initial goniometric study. Phys Ther 72:770, 1992.
42. Allander, E, et al: Normal range of joint movement in shoulder, hip, wrist and thumb with special reference to side: A comparison between two populations. Int J Epidemiol 3:253, 1974.
43. Beighton, P, et al: Articular mobility in an African population. Ann Rheum Dis 32:23, 1973.
44. Walker, JM, et al: Active mobility of the extremities in older subjects. Phys Ther 64:919, 1984.
45. Escalante, A, et al: Determinants of hip and knee flexion range: Results from the San Antonio Longitudinal Study of Age. Arthritis Care Res 12:8, 1999.
46. Boon, AJ, and Smith, J: Manual scapular stabilization: Its effect on shoulder rotation range of motion. Arch Phys Med Rehabil 81:978, 2000.

47. Rothstein, JM, et al: Goniometric reliability in a clinical setting: Elbow and knee measurements. Phys Ther 63:1611, 1983.
48. Ekstrand, J, et al: Lower extremity goniometric measurements: A study to determine their reliability. Arch Phys Med Rehabil 63:171, 1982.
49. Sabari, JS, et al: Goniometric assessment of shoulder range of motion: Comparison of testing in supine and sitting positions. Arch Phys Med Rehabil 79:64, 1998.
50. Kebaetse, M, McClure, P, and Pratt, NA: Thoracic position effect on shoulder range of motion, strength, and three-dimensional scapular kinematics. Arch Phys Med Rehabil 80:945, 1999.
51. Simoneau, GG, et al: Influence of hip position and gender on active hip internal and external rotation. J Orthop Sports Phys Ther 28:158, 1998.
52. Norkin, CC, and White, DJ: Measurement of Joint Motion: A Guide to Goniometry, ed 3. FA Davis, Philadelphia, 2003.
53. American Academy of Orthopaedic Surgeons: Joint Motion: A Method of Measuring and Recording. AAOS, Chicago, 1965.
54. Greene, WB, and Heckman, JD (ed): American Academy of Orthopaedic Surgeons: The Clinical Measurement of Joint Motion: AAOS, Chicago, 1994.
55. American Medical Association: Guide to the Evaluation of Permanent Impairment, ed 3. AMA, Milwaukee, 1990.
56. Cyriax, JH, and Cyriax, PJ: Illustrated Manual of Orthopaedic Medicine. Butterworth, London, 1983.
57. Low, JL: The reliability of joint measurement. Physiotherapy 62:227, 1976.
58. Watkins, MA, et al: Reliability of goniometric measurements and visual estimates of knee range of motion obtained in a clinical setting. Phys Ther 71:90, 1991.
59. Clarkson, HM: Musculoskeletal Assessment: Joint Range of Motion and Manual Muscle Strength, ed 2. Lippincott Williams & Wilkins, Philadelphia, 2000.
60. Reese, NB, and Bandy, WD: Joint Range of Motion and Muscle Length Testing. WB Saunders, Philadelphia, 2002.
61. Hellebrandt, FA, Duvall, EN, and Moore, ML: The measurement of joint motion: Part III - Reliability of goniometry. Phys Ther Rev 29:302, 1949.
62. Boone, DC, et al: Reliability of goniometric measurements. Phys Ther 58:1355, 1978.
63. Grohmann, JL: Comparison of two methods of goniometry. Phys Ther 63:922, 1983.
64. Fish, DR, and Wingate, L: Sources of goniometric error at the elbow. Phys Ther 65:1666.1985.
65. Goodwin, J, et al: Clinical methods of goniometry: A comparison study. Disabil Rehabil 14:10, 1992.
66. Greene, BL, and Wolf, SL: Upper extremity joint movement: Comparison of two measurement devices. Arch Phys Med Rehabil 70:288, 1989.
67. Armstrong, AD, et al: Reliability of range-of-motion measurement in the elbow and forearm. J Shoulder Elbow Surg 7:573, 1998.
68. Pandya, S, et al: Reliability of goniometric measurements in patients with Duchenne muscular dystrophy. Phys Ther 65:1339, 1985.
69. Tucci, SM, et al: Cervical motion assessment: A new, simple and accurate method. Arch Phys Med Rehabil 67:225, 1986.
70. Burdett, RG, Brown, KE, and Fall, MP: Reliability and validity of four instruments for measuring lumbar spine and pelvic positions. Phys Ther 66:677, 1986.
71. Nitschke, JE, et al: Reliability of the American Medical Association Guides' model for measuring spinal range of motion. Spine 24:262, 1999.
72. Gajdosik, RL, and Bohannon, RW: Clinical measurement of range of motion: Review of goniometry emphasizing reliability and validity. Phys Ther 67:1987.
73. Ekstrand, J, et al: Lower extremity goniometric measurements: A study to determine their reliability. Arch Phys Med Rehabil 63:171, 1982.
74. Kaltenborn, FM: Manual Mobilization of the Joints: The Extremities, ed 5. Olaf Norlis Bokhandel, Oslo, 1999.
75. Paris, S: Extremity Dysfunction and Mobilization. Institute Press, Atlanta, 1980.
76. Riddle, DL: Measurement of accessory motion: Critical issues and related concepts. Phys Ther 72:865, 1992.
77. Petersen, CM, and Hayes, KW: Construct validity of Cyriax's selective tension examination: Association of end-feels with pain at the knee and shoulder. J Orthop Sports Phys Ther 30:512, 2000.
78. Chesworth, BM, et al: Movement diagram and end-feel reliability when measuring passive lateral rotation of the shoulder in patients with shoulder pathology. Phys Ther 78:593, 1998.
79. Hayes, KH, and Petersen, CM: Reliability of assessing end-feel and pain and resistance sequence in subjects with painful shoulders and knees. J Orthop Sports Phys Ther 31:432, 2001.
80. Hayes, KW, Petersen, C, and Falconer, J: An examination of Cyriax's passive motion tests with patients having osteoarthritis of the knee. Phys Ther 74:697, 1994.
81. Fritz, JM, et al: An examination of the selective tissue tension scheme, with evidence for the concept of a capsular pattern of the knee. Phys Ther 78:1046, 1998.
82. MacConaill, MA, and Basmajian, JV: Muscles and Movement: A Basis for Human Kinesiology, ed 2. Robert E Krieger, New York, 1977.
83. Kisner, C, and Colby, LA: Therapeutic Exercise: Foundations and Techniques, ed 4. FA Davis, Philadelphia, 2003.
84. Edmond SL: Manipulations and Mobilization: Extremity and Spinal Techniques. CV Mosby, St. Louis, 1993.
85. American Physical Therapy Association: Guide to Physical Therapist Practice; ed. 2. Phys Ther 81:1, 2001.
86. Franklin, ME, et al: Assessment of exercise-induced minor muscle lesions: The accuracy of Cyriax's diagnosis by selective tension paradigm. J Orthop Sports Phys Ther 24:122, 1996.
87. Pellecchia, CL, Paolino, J, and Connell, J: Intertester reliability of the Cyriax evaluation in assessing patients with shoulder pain. J Orthop Sports Phys Ther 23:34, 1996.
88. Hayes, KW, and Peterson, CM: Reliability of classifications derived from Cyriax's resisted testing in subjects with painful shoulders and knees. J Orthop Sports Phys Ther 33:235, 2003.
89. Wright W: Muscle training in the treatment of infantile paralysis. Boston Med Surg J 167:567, 1912.
90. Lovett, R: Treatment of Infantile Paralysis. Blakiston's Son & Co., Philadelphia, 1917.
91. Daniels, L, and Worthingham, C: Muscle Testing: Techniques of Manual Examination, ed. 5. WB Saunders, Philadelphia, 1986.
92. Hislop, HJ, and Montgomery, J: Daniels and Worthingham's Muscle Testing: Techniques of Manual Examination, ed 7. WB Saunders, Philadelphia, 2002.
93. Kendall, FP, McCreary, EK, and Provance, PG: Muscles Testing and Function, ed 4. Williams & Wilkins, Baltimore, MD, 1993.
94. Sharrard, WJW: Muscle recovery in poliomyelitis. J Bone Joint Surg Br 37:63, 1955.
95. Beasley, WC: Quantitative muscle testing: Principles and application to research and clinical services. Arch Phys Med Rehabil 42:398, 1961.
96. Andres, PL, et al: A comparison of three measures of disease progression in ALS. J Neurol Sci 139-S:64, 1996.
97. Schwartz, S: Relationship between two measures of upper extremity strength: Manual muscle test compared to hand-held myometry. Arch Phys Med Rehabil 73:1063, 1992.
98. Aitkens, S, et al: Relationship of manual muscle testing to objective strength measurements. Muscle Nerve 12:173, 1989.
99. Bohannon, RW: Measuring knee extensor muscle strength. Am J Phys Med Rehabil 80:13, 2001.
100. Noreau, L, and Vachon, J: Comparison of three methods to assess muscular strength in individuals with spinal cord injury. Spinal Cord 36:716, 1998.
101. Wadsworth, CT, et al: Intrarater reliability of manual muscle testing and hand-held dynametric muscle testing. Phys Ther 67:1342, 1987.
102. Florence, JM, et al: Intrarater reliability of manual muscle test (Medical Research Council scale) grades in Duchenne's muscular dystrophy. Phys Ther 72:115, 1992.
103. Barr, AE, et al: Reliability of testing measures in Duchenne or Becker muscular dystrophy. Arch Phys Med Rehabil 72:315, 1991.
104. Frese, E, et al: Clinical reliability of manual muscle testing: Middle trapezius and gluteus medius muscles. Phys Ther 67:1072, 1987.
105. Silver, M, et al: Further standardization of manual muscle test for clinical study: Applied in chronic renal disease. Phys Ther 50:1456, 1970.

106. Iddings, DM, et al: Muscle testing: Part 2. Reliability in clinical use. Phys Ther Rev 41:249, 1961.
107. Lilienfeld, AM, et al: A study of the reproducibility of muscle testing and certain other aspects of muscle scoring. Phys Ther Rev 34:279, 1954.
108. Escolar, DM, et al: Clinical evaluator reliability for quantitative and manual muscle testing measures of strength in children. Muscle Nerve 24:787, 2001.
109. Hines, TF: Manual Muscle Examination. In Licht, S, and Johnson, EW (eds): Therapeutic Exercise, ed 2. Waverly Press, Baltimore, MD, 1965.
110. Smidt, GL, and Rodger, MW: Factors contributing to the regulation and clinical assessment of muscular strength. Phys Ther 62:1283, 1982.
111. Mulroy, SJ, et al: The ability of male and female clinicians to effectively test knee extension strength using manual muscle testing. J Orthop Sport Phys Ther 26:192, 1997.
112. Soderberg, GL: Handheld Dynamometry for Muscle Testing. In Reese, NB: Muscle and Sensory Testing. WB Saunders, Philadelphia, 1999, p 378.
113. Bohannon, RW: Make tests and break tests of elbow flexor muscle strength. Phys Ther 68:193, 1988.
114. Stratford, PW, and Balsor, BE: A comparison of make and break tests using a hand-held dynamometer and the Kin-Com. J Orthop Sports Phys Ther 19:28, 1994.
115. Ford-Smith, CD, et al: Reliability of stationary dynamometer muscle strength testing in community-dwelling older adults. Arch Phys Med Rehabil 82:1128, 2001.
116. Nadler, SF, et al: Portable dynamometer anchoring station for measuring strength of the hip extensors and abductors. Arch Phys Med Rehabil 81:1072, 2000.
117. Phillips, BA, et al: Muscle force measured using “break” testing with a hand-held myometer in normal subjects aged 20 to 69 years. Arch Phys Med Rehabil 81:653, 2000.
118. Andrews, AW, et al: Normative values for isometric muscle force measurements obtained with hand-held dynamometers. Phys Ther 76:248, 1996.
119. Bohannon, RW: Upper extremity strength and strength relationships among young women. J Orthop Sport Phys Ther 8:128, 1986.
120. Backman, E, et al: Isometric muscle force and anthropometric values in normal children aged between 3.5 and 15 years. Scand J Rehabil Med 21:105, 1989.
121. Van der Ploeg, RJO, et al: Hand-held myometry: Reference values. J Neurol Neurosurg Psychiatry 54:244, 1991.
122. Magnusson, PS: Clinical strength testing. Rehab Management Dec-Jan:38, 1993.
123. Sapega, AA: Muscle performance evaluation in orthopaedic practice. J Bone Joint Surg 72A(10):1562, 1990.
124. Visser, J, et al: Comparison of maximal voluntary isometric contraction and hand-held dynamometry in measuring muscle strength of patients with progressive lower motor neuron syndrome. Neuromuscul Disord` 13:744, 2003.
125. Brinkmann, JR: Comparison of a hand-held and fixed dynamometer in measuring strength of patients with neuromuscular disease. J Orthop Sports Phys Ther 19:100, 1994.
126. Bohannon, RW: Hand-held compared with isokinetic dynamometry for measurement of static knee extension torque (parallel reliability of dynamometers). Clin Phys Physiol Meas 11:217, 1990.
127. Reinking, MF, et al: Assessment of quadriceps muscle performance by hand-held, isometric, and isokinetic dynamometry in patients with knee dysfunction. J Orthop Sport Phys Ther 24:154, 1996.
128. Kilmer, DD, et al: Hand-held dynamometry reliability in persons with neuropathic weakness. Arch Phys Med Rehabil 78:1364, 1997.
129. Beck, M, et al: Comparison of maximal voluntary isometric contractions and Drachman’s hand-held dynamometry in evaluating patients with amyotrophic lateral sclerosis. Muscle Nerve 22:1265, 1999.
130. Agre, JC, et al: Strength testing with a portable dynamometer: Reliability for upper and lower extremities. Arch Phys Med Rehabil 68:454, 1987.
131. Bohannon, RW, and Andrews, AW: Interrater reliability of hand-held dynamometry. Phys Ther 67:931, 1987.
132. Riddle, DL, et al: Intrasession and intersession reliability of hand-held dynamometer measurements taken on brain-damaged patients. Phys Ther 69:182, 1989.
133. Moreland, J, et al: Interrater reliability of six tests of trunk muscle function and endurance. J Orthop Sport Phys Ther 26:200, 1997.
134. Wang, CY, Olson, SL, and Protas, EJ: Test-retest strength reliability: Hand-held dynamometry in community-dwelling elderly fallers. Arch Phys Med Rehabil 83:811, 2002.
135. Ottenbacher, KJ, et al: The reliability of upper- and lower-extremity strength testing in a community survey of older adults. Arch Phys Med Rehabil 83:1423, 2002.
136. Hayes, K, et al: Reliability of 3 methods for assessing shoulder strength. Shoulder Elbow Surg 11:33, 2002.
137. Bohannon, RW: Intertester reliability of hand-held dynamometry:A concise summary of published research. Percept Mot Skills 88(3 Pt 1):899, 1999.
138. Sloan, C: Review of the reliability and validity of myometry with children. Phys Occup Ther Pediatr 22:79, 2002.
139. System 3: Biodex Medical Systems, Inc, Shirley, NY, 11967. Retrieved June 22, 2004 from http://www.biodex.com.
140. Cybex 6000 Testing and Rehabilitation System Users Guide (Revision-D), Cybex, Inc, Ronkonkoma, NY, 1991.
141. Keating, JL, and Matyas, TA: Method-related variations in estimates of gravity correction values using electromechanical dynamometry: A knee extension study. J Orthop Sports Phys Ther 24:142, 1996.
142. Kellis, E, and Baltzopoulos, V: Gravitational moment correction in isokinetic dynamometry using anthropometric data. Med Sci Sports Exerc 28:900, 1996.
143. Rothstein, JM, et al: Clinical uses of isokinetic measurements: Critical issues. Phys Ther 67:1840, 1987.
144. Winter, DA, et al: Errors in the use of isokinetic dynamometers. Eur J Appl Physiol 46:397, 1981.
145. Lin, PC, et al: Detection of submaximal effort in isometric and isokinetic knee extension tests. J Orthop Sports Phys Ther 24:19, 1996.
146. Bohannon, RW: Differentiation of maximal from submaximal static elbow flexor efforts by measurement variability. Am J Phys Med Rehabil 66:213, 1987.
147. Kishino, ND, et al: Quantification of lumbar function. Spine 10:921, 1985.
148. Robinson, ME, et al: Variability of isometric and isotonic leg exercise: Utility for detection of submaximal efforts. J Occup Rehabil 4:163, 1994.
149. Murray, MP, et al: Maximum isometric knee flexor and extensor contractions: Normal patterns of torque versus time. Phys Ther 57:637, 1977.
150. Hazard, RG, et al: Lifting capacity: Indices of subject effort. Spine 17:1065, 1992.
151. Johnson, J, and Siegel, D: Reliability of an isokinetic movement of the knee extensors. Res Q 49:88, 1978.
152. Mawdsley, RH, and Knapik, JJ: Comparison of isokinetic measurements with test repetitions. Phys Ther 62:169, 1982.
153. Keating, JL, and Matyas, TA: The influence of subject and test design on dynamometric measurements of extremity muscles. Phys Ther 76:866, 1996.
154. Davies, GJ, et al: Assessment of strength. In Malone, TR, et al (eds): Orthopedic and Sports Physical Therapy, ed 3. CV Mosby, St. Louis, 1997, pp 225.
155. Gaines, JM, and Talbot, LA: Isokinetic strength testing in research and practice. Biol Res Nurs 1:57, 1999.
156. Molnar, GE, et al: Reliability of quantitative strength measurements in children. Arch Phys Med Rehabil 60:218, 1979.
157. Tredinnick, TJ, and Duncan, PW: Reliability of measurements of concentric and eccentric isokinetic loading. Phys Ther 68:656, 1988.
158. Morris-Chatta, R, et al: Isokinetic testing of ankle strength in older adults: Assessment of inter-rater reliability and stability of strength over six months. Arch Phy Med Rehabil 75:1213, 1994.
159. Emery, CA, Maitland, ME, and Meeuwisse,WH: Test-retest reliability of isokinetic hip adductor and flexor muscle strength. Clin J Sports Med 9:79, 1999.
160. Ayalon, M et al: Reliability of isokinetic strength measurements of the knee in children with cerebral palsy. Dev Med Child Neurol 42:398, 2000.

161. Pohl, PS, et al: Reliability of lower extremity isokinetic strength testing in adults with stroke. Clin Rehabil 14:601, 2000.
162. Hsu, AL, Tang, PF, and Jan, MH: Test-retest reliability of isokinetic muscle strength of the lower extremities in patients with stroke. Arch Phys Med Rehabil 83:1130, 2002.
163. Quittan, M, et al: Isokinetic strength testing in patients with chronic heart failure—a reliability study. Int J Sports Med 22:40, 2001.
164. van Meeteren, J, Roebroek, ME, and Stam, HJ: Test-retest reliability in isokinetic muscle strength measurements of the shoulder. J Rehabil Med 34:91, 2002.
165. Plotnikoff, NA, and MacIntyre, DL: Test-retest reliability of glenohumeral internal and external rotator strength. Clin J Sports Med 12:367, 2002.
166. Kramer, JF, and Ng, LR: Static and dynamic strength of the shoulder rotators in healthy, 45 to 75 year-old men and women. J Orthop Sports Phys Ther 24:11, 1996.
167. Cahalan, TD, et al: Quantitative measurements of hip strength in different age groups. Clin Orthop 246:136, 1989.
168. Murray, MP, et al: Strength of isometric and isokinetic contractions: Knee muscles of men aged 20 to 86. Phys Ther 60:412, 1980.
169. Smith, SS, et al: Quantification of lumbar function, Part I: Isometric and multispeed isokinetic trunk strength measures in sagittal and axial planes in normal subjects. Spine 10:757, 1985.
170. Neder, JA, et al: Reference values for concentric knee isokinetic strength and power in nonathletic men and women from 20 to 80 years old. J Orthop Sports Phys Ther 29:116, 1999.
171. Gajdosik, R, Vander Linden, DW, and Williams, AK: Concentric isokinetic torque characteristics of the calf muscles of active women aged 20 to 84 years. J Orthop Sports Phys Ther 29:181, 1999.
172. Hulens, M, et al: Assessment of isokinetic muscle strength in women who are obese. J Orthop Sports Phys Ther 32:347, 2002
173. Aniansson, A, et al: Muscle function in 75-year-old men and women. A longitudinal study. Scand J Rehabil Med Suppl 9:92, 1983.
174. Holmes, JR, and Alkerink, GJ: Isokinetic strength characteristics of the quadriceps femoris and hamstring muscles in high school students. Phys Ther 64:914, 1984.
175. Weltman, A, et al: Measurement of isokinetic strength in prepubertal males. J Orthop Sports Phys Ther 9:345, 1988.
176. Henderson, RC, et al: Knee flexor-extensor strength in children. J Orthop Sports Phys Ther 18:559, 1993.
177. Ramos, E, et al: Muscle strength and hormonal levels in adolescents: Gender related differences. Int J Sports Med 19:526, 1998.
178. Kellis, S, et al: Prediction of knee extensor and flexor isokinetic strength in young male soccer players. J Orthop Sports Phys Ther 30:693, 2000.
179. Ellenbecker, TS, and Roetert, EP: Isokinetic profile of elbow flexion and extension strength in elite junior tennis players. J Orthop Sports Phys Ther 33:79, 2003.
180. Grace, TG, et al: Isokinetic muscle imbalance and knee-joint injuries. J Bone Joint Surg Am 66:734, 1984.
181. Hageman, PR, et al: Effects of speed and limb dominance on eccentric and concentric isokinetic testing of the knee. J Orthop Sports Phys Ther 10:59, 1988.
182. Lucca, JA, and Kline, KK: Effects of upper and lower limb preference on torque production in the knee flexors and extensors. J Orthop Sports Phys Ther 11:202, 1989.
183. Aquino Mde, A, et al: Isokinetic assessment of knee flexor/extensor muscular strength in elderly women. Rev Hosp Clin Fac Med Sao Paulo 57:131, 2002.
184. Hinton, RY: Isokinetic evaluation of shoulder rotational strength in high-school baseball pitchers. Am J Sports Med 16:274, 1988.
185. Perrin, DH, et al: Bilateral isokinetic peak torque, torque acceleration energy, power, and work relationships in athletes and nonathletes. J Orthop Sports Phy Ther 9:184, 1987.
186. Mira, AJ, et al: A critical analysis of quadriceps function after femoral shaft fracture in adults. J Bone Joint Surg Am 62:61, 1980.
187. LoPresti, C, et al: Quadriceps insufficiency following repair of the anterior crucitate ligament. J Orthop Sports Phys Ther 9:245, 1988.
188. Cailliet, R: Soft Tissue Pain and Disability, ed 3. FA Davis, Philadelphia, 1996.
189. Paulos, LE: Knee and leg: Soft-tissue trauma. In American Academy of Orthopedic Surgeons: Orthopedic Knowledge Update 2, 1987.
190. Dyrek, DA: Assessment and Treatment Planning Strategies for Musculoskeletal Deficits. In O'Sullivan, SB, and Schmitz, TJ (eds): Physical Rehabilitation: Assessment and Treatment, ed 3. FA Davis, Philadelphia, 1994, p 61.

CHAPTER

7

Examination of Coordination

Thomas J. Schmitz, PT, PhD

LEARNING OBJECTIVES

1. Understand the purposes of performing a coordination examination.
2. List the types of data generated from the examination.
3. Describe the common coordination impairments associated with lesions of the cerebellum, basal ganglia, and dorsal column–medial lemniscal pathway.
4. Explain the primary age-associated changes that impact coordination.
5. Discuss the purpose of screenings within the context of the coordination examination of motor function.
6. Provide a rationale for the preliminary patient observation prior to performing a coordination examination.
7. Identify the motor task requirements and movement capabilities addressed during a coordination examination.
8. Differentiate between tests used to examine nonequilibrium and those used to address equilibrium coordination.
9. Explain the testing protocol for performing a coordination examination.
10. Using the case study example, apply clinical decision making skills to application of coordination examination data.

OUTLINE

Motor control is "the ability of the central nervous system to control or direct the neuromotor system in purposeful movement and postural adjustment by selective allocation of muscle tension across appropriate joint segments."[1, p 688] Components of motor control include normal muscle tone and postural response mechanisms, selective movement, and coordination.[2]

Coordination is the ability to execute smooth, accurate, controlled motor responses. The ability to produce these responses is dependent on somatosensory, visual, and vestibular input as well as a fully intact neuromuscular system from the motor cortex to the spinal cord.[3] Coordinated movements are characterized by appropriate speed, distance, direction, timing, and muscular tension. In addition, they involve appropriate synergistic influences (muscle recruitment), easy reversal between opposing muscle groups (appropriate sequencing of contraction and relaxation), and proximal fixation to allow distal motion or maintenance of a posture.[4] Schmidt and Lee define coordination as the "behavior of two or more degrees of freedom in relation to each other to produce skilled activity."[5, p 463] *Coordination impairments* are characterized by awkward, extraneous, uneven, or inaccurate movements.

Two terms often associated with coordination are dexterity and agility.[1] *Dexterity* refers to skillful use of the fingers during fine motor tasks.[6] *Agility* refers to the ability to rapidly and smoothly initiate, stop, or modify movement while maintaining postural control.

There are several general types of coordination. *Intralimb* coordination refers to movements occurring within a single limb[7–10] (e.g., alternately flexing or extending the elbow; use of one upper extremity [UE] to brush the hair;

or motor performance of a single lower extremity [LE] during a gait cycle). *Interlimb* coordination refers to the integrated performance of two or more limbs working together[7,11–15] (e.g., alternately flexing one elbow while extending the other; bilateral UE tasks as required during sliding transfers or dressing activities; or between limb movements of the LEs and/or UEs during walking). *Visual motor* coordination[16–18] refers to the ability to integrate both visual and motor abilities with the environmental context to accomplish a goal (e.g., tracing over a zigzag line, writing a letter, riding a bicycle, or driving an automobile). A subcategory of visual motor coordination with important implications for ADL is *eye–hand* coordination[19–21] such as required for using eating utensils, personal hygiene, or reaching for a visual target (e.g., a book from a shelf). Eye–hand coordination is perhaps more aptly termed *eye–hand–head* coordination because movement of the head is typically required for the eyes to fixate on a target or object.

Physical therapists are frequently involved in management of patients with coordination impairments. Data from the examination of coordination inform the therapist about existing impairments. These impairments are often associated with functional limitations that are related to, and indicative of, the type, extent, and location of central nervous system (CNS) pathology.[22] Some CNS lesions present very classic and stereotypical impairments, but others are much less predictable. Several examples of diagnoses that typically demonstrate coordination impairments include traumatic brain injury, Parkinson's disease, multiple sclerosis, Huntington's disease, cerebral palsy, Sydenham's chorea, cerebellar tumors, vestibular pathology, and some learning disabilities.

The *Guide to Physical Therapist Practice*[1] includes coordination (together with dexterity and agility) as a subcategory of Motor Function (Motor Control and Motor Learning) among the list of 24 categories of tests and measures that may be used by physical therapists during patient examination. In addition, the *Guide to Physical Therapist Practice*[1] includes coordination among the tests and measurements identified for: all Musculoskeletal Practice Patterns, Neuromuscular Practice Patterns A–H, and Cardiovascular/Pulmonary Practice Pattern D.

The purposes of performing a coordination examination of motor function are to determine the:

1. Muscle activity characteristics during voluntary movement
2. Ability of muscles or groups of muscles to work together to perform a task or functional activity
3. Level of skill and efficiency of movement
4. Ability to initiate, control, and terminate movement
5. Timing, sequencing, and accuracy of movement patterns
6. Effects of therapeutic and pharmacological intervention on motor function over time

In addition, data from the coordination examination assist the therapist with establishing the diagnosis of underlying impairments, functional limitations, and disability; assist with establishing anticipated goals to remediate impairments and formulating expected outcomes to remediate functional limitations and disability; and support decision making in establishing a prognosis and determining specific, direct interventions.

Overview of the Motor System

The motor system can be grossly divided into *peripheral* and *central* elements. The peripheral somatic motor system includes muscles, joints, and their sensory and motor innervation.[23] The central elements can be divided into three hierarchical levels to assist understanding their organization as well as delineating the contribution of each neuroanatomical structure. However, this does not imply a strictly top-down control of coordinated movement as each level of the nervous system can influence other levels (above and below) depending on task demands (i.e., flexible hierarchical theory). Bear et al provide a practical description of the three hierarchical levels relative to their functional contributions to motor control as follows: "The highest level, represented by the association areas of the neocortex and basal ganglia of the forebrain, is concerned with *strategy*: the goal of the movement and the movement strategy that best achieve the goal. The middle level, represented by the motor cortex and cerebellum, is concerned with *tactics*: the sequences of muscle contractions, arranged in space and time, required to smoothly and accurately achieve the strategic goal. The lowest level, represented by the brain stem and spinal cord, is concerned with *execution*: activation of the motor neuron and interneuron pools that generate the goal-directed movement and make any necessary adjustments of posture."[23, p 466]

The motor system can also be viewed as having a parallel arrangement. For example, information is conveyed not only from the motor cortex to the spinal cord but also directly from premotor areas as well. Although the cerebellum and basal ganglion are involved in movement, they have no direct output to the spinal cord. Instead, their effect on movement is provided via connections to the motor cortex.[24]

The critical role of sensory input on the motor system cannot be overemphasized. The integration of sensory input provides an internal representation of the environment that informs and guides motor responses.[4] These sensory representations provide the foundation on which motor programs for purposeful movements are planned, coordinated, and implemented.[3] Sensory input to the motor system guides selection and adaptation of motor responses as well as shapes motor programs for corrective action. For example, the somatosensory system provides the needed information to adjust walking when moving from a smooth surface to an uneven terrain; to maintain standing balance on a moving bus; or to make the required adjustments

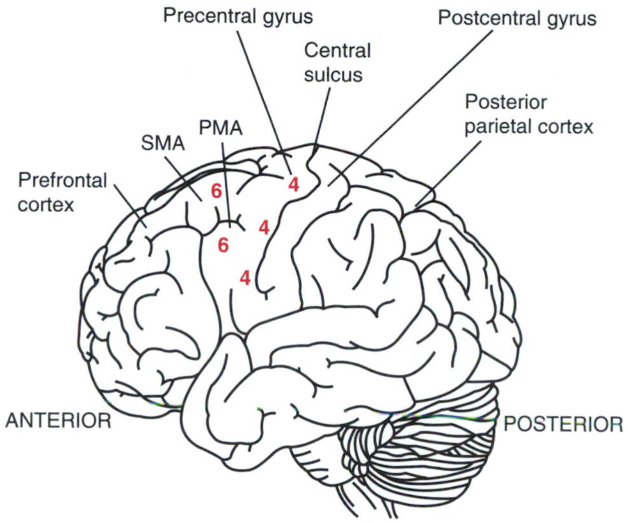

Figure 7.1 Primary areas of motor cortex involved in coordinated movement.

when throwing a ball from a stable sitting surface (chair) versus an unstable one (therapy ball). To rule out sensory impairments as a contributing factor to coordination impairments, sensory testing (see Chapter 5) should always *precede* the coordination examination.

The Motor Cortex

The principal brain area involved in motor function is the motor cortex, which comprises cortical (Brodmann's) areas 4 and 6 located in a demarcated area of the frontal lobe called the precentral gyrus (Fig. 7.1). However, planning coordinated movement to accomplish a task involves many areas of the neocortex as it requires knowledge of the body's position in space, the location of the intended target, selection of an optimum movement strategy (i.e., which joints, muscles, or body segments will be used), memory storage until time of execution, and specific instructions to implement the movement strategy selected (where to move or what to do).[23,25]

Brodmann's area 4 is designated the *primary motor cortex (PMC)* as it is the most specific cortical motor area containing the largest concentration of corticospinal neurons.[26] It lies anterior to the central sulcus on the precentral gyrus and controls contralateral voluntary movements. Brodmann's area 6 lies just anterior to area 4 and is subdivided into the superiorly placed *supplementary motor area (SMA)* and the inferiorly positioned *premotor area (PMA)*.[27] The SMA gives rise to axons that directly innervate motor units involved in initiation of movement, simultaneous bilateral grasping movements, sequential tasks, and orientation of the eyes and head. The PMA provides input to the reticulospinal neurons innervating motor units that control trunk and proximal limb movements and contributes to anticipatory postural changes.[23,28,29] Stimulation of area 4 typically results in uncomplicated movements of a single joint while stimulation to the premotor areas (area 6) evokes more intricate coordinated movements involving multiple joints.[25]

The somatotopic organization of the motor cortex is very similar to the sensory cortex. The motor homunculus schematically illustrates the amount of cortical area devoted to motor control of a given body part or region (Fig. 7.2). Beginning on the lateral aspect of the homunculus, the mouth and face areas are represented; moving upward are areas devoted to the hands, trunk, LEs, and feet. Note that areas requiring finer gradations of control such as the fingers, hand, and face (including muscles of speech) occupy a disproportionately larger representation (approximately half) in the motor cortex. The SMA and PMA are similarly somatotopically organized.

The motor cortex receives information from three primary sources: the *somatosensory cortex* (peripheral receptive fields), the *cerebellum,* and the *basal ganglia.* Somatosensory input is relayed directly to the primary motor cortex from the thalamus (e.g., cutaneous tactile sensations, joint and muscle receptors). The thalamus also relays information to the motor areas from the cerebellum and the basal ganglia. These connections allow for integration of motor control functions of the motor cortex, cerebellum, and basal ganglia (i.e., to carry out the appropriate course of motor action).[30]

Descending Motor Pathways

The most important descending pathway of the motor system is the corticospinal (pyramidal) tract which transmits signals from the motor cortex directly to the spinal cord. It is among the longest and largest CNS tracts. It originates primarily in areas 4 and 6 and passes through the internal capsule and the brainstem. The majority of fibers then cross to the opposite side in the medulla and descend through the lateral corticospinal tracts of the spinal cord. The fibers that do not cross at the medulla form the ventral corticospinal tracts, but the majority of these eventually cross to the opposite side in the cervical or upper thoracic regions. All fibers of the corticospinal tract terminate on the interneurons of the cord gray matter. The corticospinal tract is concerned with skilled, fine motor control, especially of the distal limbs.[30,31] The other major descending motor pathways used to control neurons innervating muscle include:

- Corticobulbar tract: Some fibers project directly to motor cranial nerve (CN) nuclei (e.g., trigeminal, facial, hypoglossal), and others to the reticular formation before reaching cranial nerve nuclei.
- Tectospinal tract: This relatively small tract projects to motor neurons in the cervical cord; fibers influence neurons innervating neck muscles as well as the spinal accessory nucleus (CN XI); important in guiding head movements during visual motor tasks.
- Reticulospinal tract (medial and lateral): Projects to the anterior horn of the spinal cord; important influence on muscle tone and reflex activity via influence on muscle

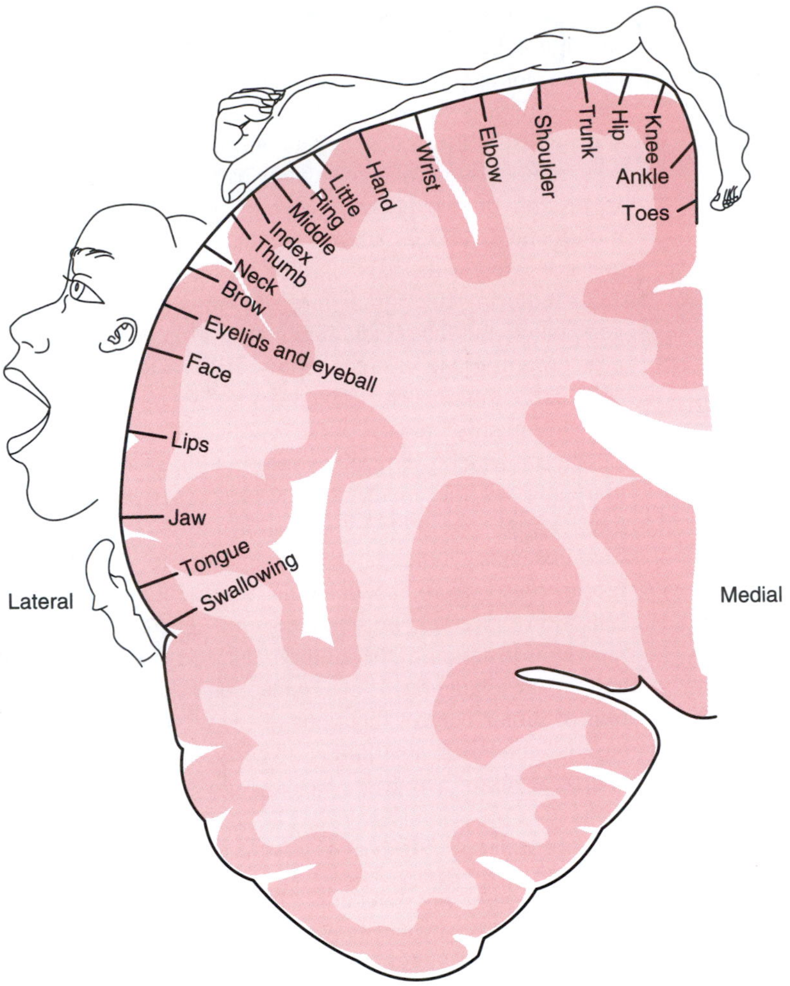

Figure 7.2 The motor homunculus indicates the somatotrophic organization of the motor cortex. The relative size of body parts reflects the proportion of the motor cortex devoted to controlling that area.

spindle activity (increasing or decreasing sensitivity); the pontine (medial) reticulospinal tract facilitates extension of the LEs (excitation of extensor motoneurons) augmenting antigravity reflexes of the spinal cord; important influence on posture and gait. The medullary (lateral) reticulospinal tract has the reverse effect (excitation of flexor motoneurons).

- Vestibulospinal tracts (medial and lateral): The lateral vestibulospinal tract descends to all levels of the spinal cord; important contributions to postural control and movements of the head (facilitates axial extensors; inhibits axial flexors). The medial vestibulospinal tract projects primarily to the ipsilateral cervical spinal cord; also involved in coordinated head and eye movements.
- Rubrospinal tract: This tract merges with the corticospinal tract in the cervical region. Its role in human motor control is considered insignificant. It is believed that during primate evolution the role of this tract was completely taken over by the corticospinal tract.

Cerebellum

The primary function of the cerebellum is regulation of movement, postural control, and muscle tone. Although all of the mechanisms of cerebellar function are not clearly understood, lesions have been noted to produce typical patterns of impaired motor function and balance, and decreased muscle tone (see section titled *Cerebellar Pathology*).

Several theories of function of the cerebellum in motor activity have been established. Among the more widely held is that the cerebellum functions as a *comparator* and *error-correcting mechanism*.[25,32] The cerebellum compares the commands for the *intended* movement transmitted from the motor cortex with the *actual* motor performance of the body segment. This occurs by a comparison of information received from the cortex with that obtained from peripheral feedback mechanisms (termed *feedforward control*). The motor cortex and brainstem motor structures provide the commands for the intended motor response (internal feedback).[32] Peripheral feedback during the motor response is provided by muscle spindles, Golgi tendon organs, joint and cutaneous receptors, the vestibular apparatus, and the eyes and ears (external feedback). This feedback provides continual input regarding posture and balance, as well as position, rate, rhythm, and force of slow movements of peripheral body segments. If the input from the feedback systems does not compare appropriately (i.e., movements deviate from the intended command), the cerebellum supplies a corrective influence. This effect is achieved by corrective signals sent to the cortex, which, via motor pathways, modifies or corrects the ongoing movement (e.g., increasing or decreasing the level of activity of specific muscles). The cerebellum also functions to modify cortical commands for subsequent movements.[32,33]

This CNS analysis of movement information, determination of level of accuracy, and provision for error correction is referred to as a **closed-loop system**. Schmidt and Lee define this model as, "a control system employing feedback, a reference for correctness, a computation of error, and subsequent correction in order to maintain a desired state."[5, p 462] It should be noted that not all movements are controlled by this system. Stereotypical movements (e.g., gait activities) and rapid, short-duration movements, which do not allow sufficient time for feedback to occur, are believed to be controlled by an **open-loop system** defined as "a control system with preprogrammed instructions to an effector that does not use feedback information and error-detection processes."[5, p 466] In this system, control originates centrally from a **motor program**, which is a memory or preprogrammed pattern of information for coordinated movement. The motor system then follows the established pattern largely independent of feedback or error-detection mechanisms. Motor programs can be called up in their entirety, modified, or reassembled in a new order. They provide the important function of freeing higher executive levels from attending to all aspects of a motor response.

Basal Ganglia

The basal ganglia are a group of nuclei located at the base of the cerebral cortex. The three main nuclei of the basal ganglia include the *caudate nucleus*, the *putamen*, and the *globus pallidus*. These nuclei have close anatomical and functional connections with two other subcortical nuclei that are also frequently considered as part of the basal ganglia: the *subthalamic nucleus* and the *substantia nigra*.[22,24]

Although the influences of the basal ganglia on movement are not understood as clearly as those of the cerebellum, there is evidence that the basal ganglia play an important role in several complex aspects of movement and postural control. These include the initiation and regulation of gross intentional movements, planning and execution of complex motor responses, facilitation of desired motor responses while selectively inhibiting others, and the ability to accomplish automatic movements and postural adjustments.[30,34–36] In addition, the basal ganglia play an important role in maintaining normal background muscle tone. This is accomplished by the inhibitory effect of the basal ganglia on both the motor cortex and lower brainstem. The basal ganglia also are believed to influence some aspects of both perceptual and cognitive functions.[34]

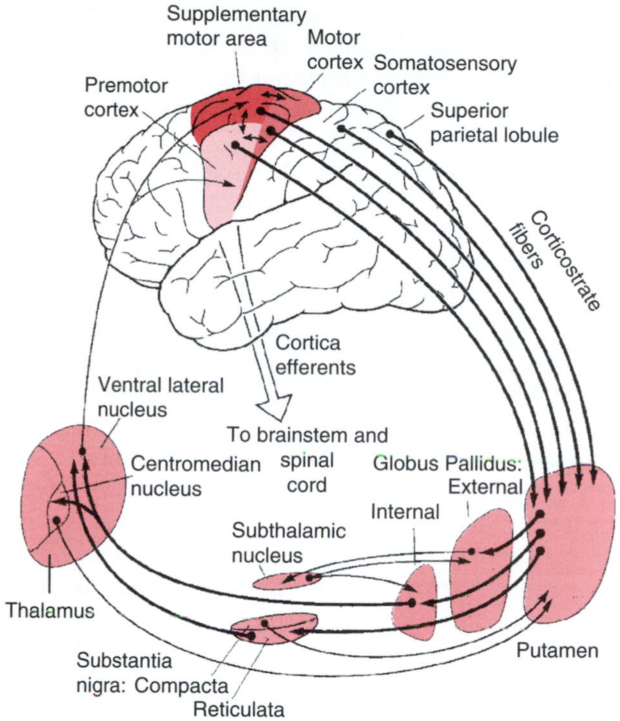

Figure 7.3 The motor circuit of the basal ganglia provides a subcortical feedback loop from the motor and somatosensory areas of the cortex, through portions of the basal ganglia and thalamus, and back to the cortical motor areas (premotor cortex, supplementary motor area, and motor cortex). (From Ghez, C, and Gordon, J,[37, p 548] with permission.)

The motor portion of the basal ganglia assumes a somatotopic organization. The anatomical positioning of the basal ganglia provides insight into its contribution to motor performance. The areas of the brain associated with movement (primary motor cortex, supplementary motor area, premotor area, and the somatosensory cortex) form dense projections to the motor portion of the putamen. Output of this pathway forms the *motor circuit* of the basal ganglia, which is directed back to the supplementary motor area and the premotor area. These two areas and the primary motor cortex are all interconnected, and each has descending projections to the brainstem motor centers and spinal cord. This anatomical arrangement indicates that the influence of the basal ganglia on motor function is indirect and mediated by descending projections from the cortical motor areas.[34,35,37] Figure 7.3 schematically illustrates the motor circuit of the basal ganglion.

Dorsal Column–Medial Lemniscal Pathway

Regulation of movement is dependent on sensory afferent information. Peripheral somatosensory receptors and pathways provide information about the status of the environment, the status of the body, as well as the status of the body in relation to the environment.[5] This information is encoded and conveyed to various parts of the CNS. The data are processed based on peripheral feedback and memory, which leads to selection (or modification) of a movement strategy appropriate to the task demands and environmental conditions.

The dorsal column–medial lemniscal pathway is particularly important to coordinated movement as it is responsible for the afferent transmission of discriminative sensations. Sensory modalities that require fine gradations of intensity and precise localization on the body surface are mediated by this system. Sensations transmitted by the dorsal column–medial lemniscal pathway include discriminative touch, stereognosis, tactile pressure, barognosis, graphesthesia, recognition of texture, kinesthesia, two-point discrimination, proprioception, and vibration.

This system is composed of large, myelinated, rapidly conducting fibers. After entering the dorsal column the fibers ascend to the medulla and synapse with the dorsal column nuclei (nuclei gracilis and cuneatus). From here they cross to the opposite side and pass up to the thalamus through bilateral pathways called the *medial lemnisci*. Each medial lemniscus terminates in the ventral posterolateral thalamus. From the thalamus, third-order neurons project to the somatic sensory cortex.

Features of Coordination Impairments

As the cerebellum, basal ganglia, and dorsal column–medial lemniscal pathway provide input to, and act together with, the cortex in the production of coordinated movement, lesions in any of these areas impact higher level processing and execution of coordinated motor responses. Although it is incorrect to assign all problems of incoordination to one of these sites, lesions in these areas are responsible for many characteristic motor deficits seen in adult populations. The following sections present an overview of common clinical features associated with lesions in each of these areas.

Cerebellar Pathology

A number of specific motor impairments that impact coordinated movement are associated with cerebellar pathology.[38–44] Many of these impairments either directly or indirectly influence the patient's ability to execute accurate, smooth, controlled movements. The motor deficits identified emphasize the crucial influence of the cerebellum on equilibrium, posture, muscle tone, and initiation and force of movement. **Ataxia** is perhaps the most common term used to describe motor impairments of cerebellar origin. Cerebellar ataxia is a general, comprehensive term used to describe loss of muscle coordination as a result of cerebellar pathology. Ataxia may affect gait, posture, and patterns of movement and is linked to difficulty initiating movement as well as errors in the rate, rhythm, and timing of responses.

Perlman[41] provides an adept summary of the motor impairments associated with each of the major anatomic regions of the cerebellum as follows: "The cerebellum has three anatomic divisions that account for the three types of dysfunction commonly seen: (1) the midline (vermis, paleocerebellum), which underlies titubation, truncal ataxia, orthostatic tremor, and gait imbalance; (2) the hemispheres (neocerebellum – right controlling the right side of the body and left controlling the left side), which contribute to limb ataxia (e.g., dysdiadochokinesia, dysmetria, and kinetic tremor), dysarthria, and hypotonia; and (3) the posterior (flocculonodular lobe, archicerebellum), which also influences posture and gait as well as causing eye movement disorders (e.g., nystagmus, vestibulo-ocular reflex disruption)."[41, p 216]

The following motor impairments are manifestations of cerebellar pathology.

Asthenia is generalized muscle weakness associated with cerebellar lesions.

Dysarthria is a disorder of the motor component of speech articulation. The characteristics of cerebellar dysarthria are referred to as **scanning speech** (often described as having a *one-word-at-a-time* quality). This speech pattern is typically slow, and may be slurred, hesitant, with prolonged syllables and inappropriate pauses. Word use, selection, and grammar remain intact, but the melodic quality of speech is altered.[32,33]

Dysdiadochokinesia is an impaired ability to perform rapid alternating movements. This deficit is observed in movements such as rapid alternation between pronation and supination of the forearm. Movements are irregular, with a rapid loss of range and rhythm especially as speed is increased.[33]

Dysmetria is an inability to judge the distance or range of a movement. It may be manifested by an overestimation **(hypermetria)** or an underestimation **(hypometria)** of the required range needed to reach an object or goal. **Dyssynergia (movement decomposition)** describes a movement performed in a sequence of component parts rather than as a single, smooth activity. For example, when asked to touch the index finger to the nose, the patient might first flex the elbow, then adjust the position of the wrist and fingers, further flex the elbow, and finally flex the shoulder. **Asynergia** is the loss of ability to associate muscles together for complex movements.

Gait ataxia involves ambulatory patterns that typically demonstrate a broad base of support. Upright stance stability is often poor and the arms may be held away from the body to improve balance (high guard position). Stepping patterns are irregular in direction and distance.[40] Initiation of forward progression of a lower extremity may start slowly, and then the extremity may unexpectedly be flung rapidly and forcefully forward and audibly hit the floor.[45] Gait patterns tend to be generally unsteady (postural instability), irregular, and staggering, with deviations from an intended forward line of progression (veering to one side; swaying or pitching in different directions).

Hypotonia is a decrease in muscle tone. It is believed to be related to the disruption of afferent input from stretch receptors and/or lack of the cerebellum's facilitatory efferent influence on the fusimotor system. A diminished resistance to passive movement will be noted, and muscles may feel abnormally soft and flaccid. Diminished deep tendon reflexes also may be noted.[32]

CLINICAL NOTE: After testing the patellar tendon jerk with a reflex hammer in a normal subject, the knee typically returns immediately to the resting state. With cerebellar pathology, the knee may oscillate six to eight times before returning to rest.[32]

Nystagmus is a rhythmic, quick, oscillatory, back-and-forth movement of the eyes. It is typically apparent as the eyes move away from midline to fix on an object in either the medial or lateral field (i.e., extremes of temporal or nasal vision).[46] The patient has difficulty holding the gaze on the object in the peripheral field. An involuntary drift back to midline with immediate return to the object may be observed.[47] Nystagmus causes difficulty with accurate fixation and vision and is believed linked to the cerebellum's influence on synergy and tone of the extraocular muscles.

Rebound phenomenon, originally described by Holmes, is the loss of the check reflex,[45] or check factor, which functions to halt forceful active movements when resistance is eliminated. Normally, when application of resistance to an isometric contraction is suddenly removed, the limb will remain in approximately the same position by action of the opposing muscle(s). For example, in applying resistance to an isometric contraction in the middle range of elbow flexion and then releasing it without warning, the intact subject will "check" or stop the motion quickly through activation of the opposing triceps as well as feedback regarding joint position and force required to prevent further motion. With cerebellar involvement, the patient is unable to stop the motion, and the limb will move suddenly when resistance is released. The patient may strike himself or herself or other objects when the resistance is removed.

Tremor is an involuntary oscillatory movement resulting from alternate contractions of opposing muscle groups. Different types of tremors are associated with cerebellar lesions. An **intention**, or **kinetic**, **tremor** occurs during voluntary motion of a limb and tends to increase as the limb nears its intended goal or speed is increased.[32] Intention tremors are diminished or absent at rest. **Postural (static) tremor** may be evident by back-and-forth oscillatory movements of the body while the patient maintains a standing posture. Postural tremors also may be observed as up-and-down oscillatory movements of a limb when it is held against gravity. *Titubation* typically refers to rhythmic oscillations of the head (side-to-side, forward-and-backward, or they may have a rotary component); however, the term is also less frequently used to refer to axial involvement of the trunk.

In addition to these characteristic clinical features of cerebellar involvement, a greater length of time may also be required to initiate voluntary movements (delayed reaction time). Difficulty may also be observed in stopping or changing the force, speed, or direction of movement.[24] Motor learning will also be affected. Recall that the cerebellum compares the intended movement (internal feedback) with the actual movement (external feedback). For subsequent movements, the cerebellum generates corrective signals to reduce the errors (feed-forward control). Lack of this feed-forward control is responsible for deficits in motor learning and coordination.

Basal Ganglia Pathology

Patients with lesions of the basal ganglia typically demonstrate several characteristic motor deficits. These include (1) poverty and slowness of movement; (2) involuntary, extraneous movement; and (3) alterations in posture and muscle tone.[28,35] Thus, patients with basal ganglia involvement present on a continuum of motor behavior from severely diminished as seen in advanced Parkinson's disease to excessive extraneous movements apparent with Huntington's disease.[35] The following motor impairments are manifestations of basal ganglia pathology.[48–56]

Akinesia is an inability to initiate movement and is seen in the late stages of Parkinson's disease. This deficit is associated with assumption and maintenance of fixed postures (freezing episodes). A tremendous amount of mental concentration and effort is required to perform even the simplest motor activity.

Athetosis is characterized by slow, involuntary, writhing, twisting, "wormlike" movements. Frequently, greater involvement in the distal UEs is noted[57]; this may include fluctuations between hyperextension of the wrist and fingers and a return to a flexed position, combined with rotary movements of the extremities. Many other areas of the body may be involved, including the neck, face, tongue, and trunk. The phenomena are also referred to as athetoid movements. Pure athetosis is relatively uncommon and most often presents in combination with spasticity, tonic spasms, or chorea. Athetosis can be a clinical feature of some forms of cerebral palsy.

Bradykinesia is a decreased amplitude and velocity of voluntary movement. It may be demonstrated in a variety of ways, such as a decreased arm swing; slow, shuffling gait; difficulty initiating or changing direction of movement; lack of facial expression; or difficulty stopping a movement once begun; characteristic of Parkinson's disease.

Chorea is characterized by involuntary, rapid, irregular, and jerky movements involving multiple joints. Choreiform movements demonstrate irregular timing, are most apparent in the UEs, and cannot be voluntarily inhibited; associated with Huntington's disease.[58]

Choreoathetosis is a term used to describe a movement disorder with features of both chorea and athetosis.

Dystonia (dystonic movements) involves sustained involuntary contractions of agonist and antagonist muscles[27,35] causing abnormal posturing (*dystonic* posture) or twisting movements. Most common in trunk and extremity musculature but also may affect the neck, face, and vocal cords. Torsion spasms also are considered a form of dystonia, with spasmodic torticollis being the most common.[45]

Hemiballismus is characterized by large-amplitude sudden, violent, flailing motions of the arm and leg of one side of the body. Primary involvement is in the axial and proximal musculature of the limb. Hemiballismus results from a lesion of the contralateral subthalamic nucleus.[22,24] Associated terms include **hyperkinesis**, which is abnormally increased muscle activity or movement; and **hypokinesis**, which is a decreased motor response especially to a specific stimulus.

Rigidity is an increase in muscle tone causing greater resistance to passive movement. It tends to be more pronounced in the flexor muscles of the trunk and extremities causing functional limitations in such activities as dressing, transfers, speech, eating, and postural control.[59]

Two types of rigidity may be seen: *leadpipe* and *cogwheel*. **Leadpipe rigidity** is a uniform, constant resistance felt by the examiner as the extremity is moved through a range of motion (ROM). **Cogwheel rigidity** is considered a combination of the leadpipe type with tremor. It is characterized by a series of brief relaxations or "catches" as the extremity is passively moved.

Tremor is an involuntary, rhythmic, oscillatory movement observed at rest **(resting tremor)**. Resting tremors typically disappear or decrease with purposeful movement, but may increase with emotional stress. Tremors associated with basal ganglia lesions (e.g., Parkinson's disease) are frequently noted in the distal upper extremities in the form of a "pill-rolling" movement, where it looks as if a pill is being rolled between the first two fingers and the thumb. Motion of the wrist, and pronation and supination of the forearm, may be evident. Tremors also may be apparent at other body parts as well, such as the jaw; characteristic of Parkinson's disease. Table 7.1 provides a summary of common coordination impairments associated with pathology of the cerebellum and basal ganglia.

Dorsal Column–Medial Lemniscal Pathology

Coordination impairments associated with dorsal column–medial lemniscal (DCML) lesions are somewhat less characteristic than those produced by either cerebellar or basal ganglia pathology. Lesion of the DCML typically result in coordination and equilibrium impairments related to the patient's lack of joint position sense and awareness of movement, and impaired localized touch sensation. Recall that this ascending pathway carries the peripheral (external) feedback required for feedforward control. It mediates sensations critical to coordinated movement such as proprioception, kinesthesia, and discriminative touch.

Disturbances of gait are a common finding with DCML pathology. The gait pattern is usually wide-based and swaying, with uneven step lengths and excessive lateral displacement. The advancing leg may be lifted too high and then dropped abruptly with an audible impact. Watching the feet during ambulation is typical and is indicative of a proprioceptive loss. Another common deficit seen with DCML pathology is dysmetria. As mentioned, this is an impaired ability to judge the required distance or range of movement and may be noted in both the upper and lower extremities. It is manifested by the inability to place an extremity accurately or to reach a target object. For example, in attempting to lock a wheelchair brake, the patient may inaccurately judge (overestimate or underestimate) the required movement needed to reach the brake handle. Fine motor skills may also be impaired owing to alterations in discriminative tactile and object recognition abilities.

Because vision can assist in guiding movements, maintaining balance, as well as improve accuracy of discriminative tasks, visual feedback can be an effective mechanism to compensate partially for DCML pathology. Thus, coordination and/or balance problems will be exaggerated when vision is occluded or when the patient's eyes are closed. The inability to maintain standing balance with the feet together when the eyes are closed is termed a positive **Romberg sign** and is usually indicative of proprioceptive loss. Visual guidance will also reduce the manifestations of dysmetria and diminished tactile perception. However, some noticeable slowing of movements may be observed as visually guided motions are generally more accurate when speed of movement is reduced.

Age-Related Changes Impacting Coordinated Movement

Alteration in the ability to execute smooth, accurate, controlled motor responses occurs with normal aging. The importance of understanding the basis of these changes is reflected in the expanding body of literature devoted to examining various aspects of motor performance in older adults.[60–77] This section presents an overview of the most salient age-associated changes impacting coordinated movement. Evidence Summary Box 7.1 presents specific findings from studies exploring the impact of advancing age on coordinated movement. For a more comprehensive perspective on the physiological, neurological, and musculoskeletal changes associated with aging, the reader is referred to the work of Bottomley and Lewis,[78] Spirduso et al,[79] and Lewis.[80]

Table 7.1 Common Coordination Impairments Associated with Pathology of the Cerebellum and Basal Ganglia

Cerebellar Pathology	
Asthenia	Generalized muscle weakness
Asynergia	Loss of ability to associate muscles together for complex movements
Delayed reaction time	Increased time required to initiate voluntary movement
Dysarthria	Disorder of the motor component of speech articulation
Dysdiadochokinesia	Impaired ability to perform rapid alternating movements
Dysmetria	Inability to judge the distance or range of a movement
Dyssynergia	Movement performed in a sequence of component parts rather than as a single, smooth activity; decomposition
Gait disorders	Ataxic pattern; broad base of support; postural instability; high-guard position of UEs
Hypotonia	Decrease in muscle tone
Hypermetria	Overestimation of distance or range needed to accomplish a movement
Hypometria	Underestimation of distance or range needed to accomplish a movement
Nystagmus	Rhythmic, quick, oscillatory, back-and-forth movement of the eyes
Rebound phenomenon	Inability to halt forceful movements after resistive stimulus removed; patient unable to stop sudden limb motion
Tremor	Involuntary oscillatory movement resulting from alternate contractions of opposing muscle groups
• Intention (kinetic)	Oscillatory movement during voluntary motion; increases as the limb nears target; diminished or absent at rest
• Postural (static)	Exaggerated oscillatory movement of the body in standing posture or of a limb held against gravity
Titubation	Rhythmic oscillations of the head; axial involvement of the trunk
Basal Ganglia Pathology	
Akinesia	Inability to initiate movement; associated with fixed postures
Athetosis	Slow, involuntary, writhing, twisting, "wormlike" movements; frequently greater involvement in distal UEs
Bradykinesia	Decreased amplitude and velocity of voluntary movement
Chorea	Involuntary, rapid, irregular, jerky movements involving multiple joints; most apparent in UEs
Choreoathetosis	Movement disorder with features of both chorea and athetosis
Dystonia (dystonic movements)	Sustained involuntary contractions of agonist and antagonist muscles
Hemiballismus	Large-amplitude sudden, violent, flailing motions of the arm and leg of one side of the body
Hyperkinesis	Abnormally increased muscle activity or movement
Hypokinesis	Decreased motor response especially to a specific stimulus
Rigidity	Increase in muscle tone causing greater resistance to passive movement; greater in flexor muscles
• Leadpipe	Uniform, constant resistance as limb is moved
• Cogwheel	Series of brief relaxations or "catches" as limb is passively moved
Tremor (resting)	Involuntary, rhythmic, oscillatory movement observed at rest

Evidence Summary Box 7.1

Research Exploring Age-Related Changes in Motor Coordination

Reference	Purpose	Subjects/Design	Results	Conclusions/Comments
Capranica, L,[62] 2004	To examine variations in homolateral interlimb coordination across the life-span; To determine whether in-phase (pairing wrist extension with ankle dorsiflexion; and wrist flexion with foot plantarflexion) and antiphase (pairing wrist flexion with ankle dorsiflexion; and wrist extension with ankle plantarflexion) coordination and frequency influence performance differently in young/old populations.	77 subjects divided into 4 age groups: children (25, mean 10 years); adults (16, mean 22.9 years); young/old (21, mean 67.6 years); old (15, mean 78.9 years). Subjects were seated on a table with the elbow and knee flexed to 90°. Subjects performed flexion and extension movements around the wrist and ankle at a 1:1 ratio for 60 seconds (homolateral). Movement was tested in-phase (iso-directional) and antiphase (noniso-directional). Each test was performed at 3 metronome paced frequencies: 80, 120, 180 bpm. Total time of correct movement was recorded by one observer.	Age showed a significant effect on time of correct execution, except for insignificant changes from young/old to old. Most older adults shifted to in-phase mode within 10 seconds when performing antiphase mode regardless of frequency. Older subjects displayed increased trial-to-trial variability.	Age, mode of coordination, and movement frequency should be considered during examination of coordination; authors suggest additional research is warranted to determine if interlimb coordination can be more successfully maintained in older adults; moderate sample size.
Desrosiers, J, et al,[63] 1995	To develop normative data for the TEMPA (a UE performance test for the elderly); To assist clinicians using this test to differentiate between normal and pathological UE performance. To correlate UE performance with personal variables, including age.	360 subjects, 60 years and older, stratified for age by decade. The TEMPA administered together with a battery of tests measuring gross and manual dexterity. The TEMPA consists of 13 items designed to test multiple aspects of UE performance. Each task is measured based on length of execution, functional rating, and task analysis. Functional rating is based on a 4-level scale according to independence; task analysis quantifies difficulties according to five dimensions related to UE skill. An interview was used to determine variables potentially related to UE performance.	All subjects obtained perfect scores in the functional rating and task analysis sections of the TEMPA. The length of most tasks increased significantly with age exponentially. Variability within length of execution increased with age as well. Age, self-perceived health, and current activity level were the best predictors of UE performance. Women performed tasks related to dexterity faster than men, while men performed tasks related to grip strength faster than women. There were some correlations between the sensibility tests and performance on the TEMPA.	In subjects who are active, it is difficult to tell whether their UE performance is better because they are active, or they are active because of better UE performance. Endurance is not related to the TEMPA because the tasks are generally short and not repeated. This study may not be representative of all healthy elderly people, and is certainly not representative of the elderly who have pathology affecting the UE; large sample size.
Hartley, AA,[64] 2001	To explore the possibility of an age-related reduction in the ability to generate and execute 2 similar motor programs.	22 younger adults (mean 19 years) and 22 older adults (mean 76.2 years). Self-report of health status administered together with a test for spatial acuity. Several training trials conducted. *Color-judgment*	Task 2 reaction times increased for all subjects as stimulus onset time decreased, more so for older adults than for younger adults, when both tasks required a manual	The authors note that findings can be interpreted several ways. Increases in task 2 reaction times with short stimulus onset times may occur owing to factors stemming from Task 1 that affect processing prior to response

Evidence Summary Box 7.1

Research Exploring Age-Related Changes in Motor Coordination (continued)

Reference	Purpose	Subjects/Design	Results	Conclusions/Comments
		task—letter X presented on a computer screen in white, after 500 msec color changed to yellow or blue. Subjects identified the change by pressing a key, stimulus remained until key was pressed or after 1500 msec. *Tone-judgment task*—procedure identical except that stimulus was a 200-msec tone. *Letter-alone task*—similar to color judgment task, except that X changes to the letter B or D. Identification was either signified by a manual response (key press) or oral response (saying the name of the letter). *Dual task testing*—task 1: tone/color discrimination; task 2: manual/oral response to letter-identification task; stimulus onset time varied (50, 150, 500, or 1000 msec) after color changed or tone sounded.	response. Reaction times increased more when task 1 was color discrimination (both tasks required visual input).	selection in Task 2 can begin. There may be a limited capacity for generating similar motor responses, a capacity that is reduced in older adults. While reaction times increased when both stimuli were visual, this was not due to aging. Relatively small sample used for data collection.
McGibbon, CA, and Krebs, DE,[69] 2000	To explore if aging in healthy adults affects the kinematic coordination of the lower trunk during gait, and examine if these changes are modulated by age-related changes in kinematic gait parameters (walking speed, range of movement). To examine if alterations in sagittal plane lower trunk coordination with aging is a result of flexor/extensor muscle coordination.	93 healthy subjects divided into two groups, 49 age <50, 44 age ≥ 50. Subjects performed several level-surface walking trials at self-selected speed, for 10 m, barefoot. Force plates detected GRF; 11 body segments tracked using LEDs. Segment 3-D movements were recorded, and segment mass, COM, and mass movement-of-inertia were computed. Angular velocity and phase shift angles were observed in the sagittal plane.	Young subjects walked faster per unit height than did older subjects. Low back flexion ROM was high in young subjects. Gait speed increased moderately with age overall. Phase shift significantly increased with age (elderly subjects lead pelvic motion with their trunks). Gait speed and low back ROM do not significantly account for changes in phase shift. Older subjects transferred more eccentric muscle energy between body segments.	Data suggest a reversal in phase relationship of the trunk occurs with aging, which indicates a reversal in muscle lengthening and shortening sequence in the low back musculature. The trunk leading strategy employed by the elderly resulted in an increase in mechanical energy demands of the low back musculature; moderate sample size.
Seilder-Dobrin, RD, et al,[72] 1998	To determine whether elderly persons exhibit reciprocal phasing of muscle activity and scale EMG burst amplitude in the same manner as young people.	7 subjects (mean age 72.3 years) 7 subjects (mean age 24.3 years). Subjects grasped a lever with the elbow over a pivot point, rotations produced by elbow flexion and extension displayed on a computer. Home position was 50° from full elbow extension, target position 30° of elbow flexion. Visual input	Elderly missed required time window more frequently at each load level. Too fast: too slow time ratio was similar for both groups, elderly were slightly more prone to being too slow. No difference in the average time of counted trials. Significant age difference	Elderly group proved to be less accurate overall in attaining movement goal. Elderly group showed decreased ability to produce controlled, stable movements, as illustrated by the increased time spent in acceleration. Elderly subjects employed co-contraction as a means of stabilization; small sample size.

(*continued*)

Evidence Summary Box 7.1

Research Exploring Age-Related Changes in Motor Coordination (continued)

Reference	Purpose	Subjects/Design	Results	Conclusions/Comments
		removed by placing a cover over arm and lever. Movement paced by a metronome (800 msec target time for each phase). 3 blocks of 50 trials; each trial block had a different load applied to arm (no load, .75 kg, 1.5 kg). EMG electrodes placed at the biceps brachii and medial head of the triceps. 650 msec–980 msec was the required time window for the trial to be counted.	for acceleration/ deceleration phase ratio (elderly achieved peak velocity later in motion than did the younger group). Agonist contraction was prolonged in the elderly, elderly were more likely to co-contract.	
Serrien, DJ, et al,[73] 2000	To investigate age-related modifications in in-phase and antiphase coordinative movements and determine their relative stability. To determine if differences in performance between homologous/nonhomologous limbs exist in older adults.	8 younger (mean age 24 years) and 8 older (mean age 75 years) participants in good health, involved in daily activities and hobbies. Subjects seated in a chair; limbs attached to levers that allow sagittal plane movement. Subjects asked to perform cyclical flexion and extension movements for two limbs at the elbow and knee at a pace provided by a metronome. Six performance conditions included: homologous (upper/lower extremities), homolateral (right/left side), and heterolateral (right UE/left LE, left UE/right LE). In-phase and antiphase movements were included. Interlimb coordination determined by joint angle between the two moving limbs. Deviation from the intended angle and the peak of flexion/extension was measured (accuracy), and within trial variability was measured (stability). Cycle duration and amplitude were measured.	Accuracy and stability did not differ between young and older adults for homologous conditions; they deteriorated for the older adults during homolateral and heterolateral condition, more strongly for antiphase movement. Quality of performance was similar for young adults on nondominant side, decreased for older adults. Older adults produced slower cycles than young adults. Young adults increased amplitude during antiphase, while it remained the same for older adults. Temporal and spatial variability were increased for older adults. 25% of trials by older adults displayed a transition to in-phase movement when antiphase was initially required.	Older adults displayed decreases in performance depending on limb combination and coordination mode. These modifications can be a result of (1) deficits in afferent information processing for steering coordinated behavior and (2) declines in cognitive regulation, emerging from a deterioration of inhibitory mechanisms and reduced attentional monitoring of sensory feedback. Movement slowing may be an adaptive strategy to cope more successfully with more demanding task requirements, or related to the fact that older adults rely more on visual cues, adding temporal constraints to adjustment processes; small sample size.
Shkuratova, N, et al,[74] 2004	To determine if older people adapt stepping behavior differently than young people in response to various balance perturbations during locomotion. To examine whether changes in gait parameters are	20 healthy older adults (mean 71.5 years) and 20 young adults (mean 25.3 years). Performance compared between groups in the following tasks: (1) straight line walking at preferred speed; (2) straight line walking at fast speed; (3) figure-of-eight walking at preferred speed; and (4) figure-of-eight walking while performing a secondary motor	Young adults increased their walking speed and stride length to a greater extent than did older adults when changing from preferred speed to fast speed. All subjects significantly decreased their walking speed, stride length, and cadence when changing from straight line walking to walking and turn-	Reduced speed and stride length and increased double support time in older adults are usually interpreted as age related adaptations to produce gait that is safer and less destabilizing. Older adults are usually more cautious and opt for greater stability; small sample size.

Evidence Summary Box 7.1

Research Exploring Age-Related Changes in Motor Coordination (continued)

Reference	Purpose	Subjects/Design	Results	Conclusions/Comments
	task specific and vary according to types of perturbations encountered.	task (transferring coins from one pocket to another). Stride length, cadence, speed, and double support time were measured using the Clinical Stride Analyzer. Walkways were marked with strips of blue tape 150 mm apart. Subjects were instructed to stay within the lines in order to appropriately challenge balance.	ing. Both groups significantly decreased stride length and increased cadence when changing to dual-task walking. Older adults showed higher cadence rates and reduced stride length compared to young adults. Both groups transferred a similar number of coins. Older adults, in general, had a higher double support time in all conditions than young adults.	
Sparrow, WA, et al,[75] 2005	To determine whether older individuals have more absolute error and greater metabolic and cognitive cost when performing the same task as younger adults. To determine whether aging would affect the capacity to learn interlimb coordination tasks with extended practice.	8 healthy older men (mean 73.1 years) and 8 healthy young men (mean 23.3 years) participated. Two arm-and-hand ergonometers were positioned side-by-side allowing the inside handle to be moved independently. Two metronome-paced conditions were measured: antiphase movement (180° difference, in opposite directions) and relative 90° phase (one hand follows the other by a quarter cycle). A reaction time task was given by asking subjects to press a button after hearing a sound, done alone and during the cycling task. Oxygen consumption and carbon dioxide production were measured continuously. A retention test was done 1 week after the trials.	In the relative phase condition, the older adults were consistently farther from the target coordination and as practice progressed they shifted even further from the desired phase. Young adults were consistently accurate in the antiphase movements, while older adults were inaccurate but improved with practice. Older adults had greater difficulty producing the relative phase pattern, and had greater errors in performance than young adults. Variability was greater for older adults and did not improve with practice. There was no age effect on oxygen consumption, but older adults had significantly higher heart rates. The younger group displayed a greater decrease in oxygen consumption and heart rate from acquisition trials to retention trials. Older adults displayed a significantly greater reaction time while cycling for both conditions.	Cognitive declines and the dynamic stability of antiphase movement (demanding less cognitive and metabolic energy) caused the older group to be attracted to antiphase coordination. The older adults displayed less capacity to modify relative timing from cycle-to-cycle. Older adults performed the tasks economically in terms of oxygen consumption, however may avoid novel motor tasks due to negative feelings associated with elevated heart rate. Motor performance was more attention demanding for the older adults, inhibiting their ability to divide attention across multiple tasks. To minimize the metabolic and cognitive cost of learning new motor skills, older adults may fall into preferred stable, low energy movement patterns; small sample size.
Shinohara, M, et al[a], 2004	To examine if changes in indices of finger interaction during maximal force production	12 young (mean 28.9 years) and 12 elderly (mean 82.1 years) subjects participated; all subjects were healthy and right-handed. An apparatus with	Peak maximal force production was higher at the PP than at the DP for all subjects. Elderly subjects produced less force than	Age is associated with both a larger loss of muscle force by the intrinsic hand muscles and a diminished ability to stabilize important performance variables

(continued)

Evidence Summary Box 7.1

Research Exploring Age-Related Changes in Motor Coordination (continued)

Reference	Purpose	Subjects/Design	Results	Conclusions/Comments
	(MVC) associated with aging are accompanied by changed coordination of fingers in multi-finger accurate, submaximal, force production tasks.	loops attached to sensors was used to detect finger force production at the distal and proximal phalanges. First, the subjects produced a brief, maximal force 1 finger at a time and with all 4 fingers together. Then, subjects were required to press with one finger such that the force signal shown on a computer screen followed a ramp line from 0 to the peak force shown in the first test. Finally, subjects used all 4 fingers to trace an on-screen ramp line. Each test was conducted with force applied at the distal phalanx and proximal phalanx.	young subjects. Reduction in maximal force was more prominent at the PP compared to the DP. Normalized error indices for ramped output measures were twice as large for older subjects than for younger subjects. Variance for individual fingers and 4-finger measures was higher in elderly adults as compared to younger subjects at both sites.	during accurate force production; small sample size.

Evidence Summary Box 7.1 prepared by Stephen A. Caronia.

[a]Shinohara, M, et al: Finger interaction during accurate multi-finger force production tasks in young and elderly persons. Exp Brain Res 156:282, 2004.

COM = Center of mass; DP = distal phalanx; GRF = ground reaction force; LED = light-emitting diode; MVC = maximum voluntary contraction; PP = proximal phalanx; UE = upper extremity.

Decreased strength. Diminished strength is a well-documented finding in older adults.[81–85] Several factors are believed to contribute to loss of strength, reduced muscle mass (decreased cross-sectional area), and decreased function. These include a loss of alpha motor neurons (decreased number of functional motor units), loss or atrophy of fast twitch fibers (most notably type IIb), reduced number and diameter of muscle fibers,[86] diminished oxidative capacity of exercising muscle, and a subsequent reduction in ability to produce torque.[87] In general, there appears to be a greater loss of strength in antigravity muscles of the back and LEs (e.g., latissimus dorsi, hip extensors, quadriceps) as compared to the UE and greater loss in proximal than distal muscles.[78,88]

Slowed reaction time. Older adults typically move more slowly. This is particularly evident for tasks that require both speed and accuracy; speed will decrease to ensure greater accuracy (speed–accuracy trade-off).[5] In general, the time interval between application of a stimulus and initiation of movement is increased.[89] This finding is also linked to degenerative changes in the motor unit. In addition, *premotor time* (time interval between onset of a stimulus and initiation of a response) and *movement time* (time interval between the initiation of movement and the completion of movement) are lengthened with normal aging.[90] Some evidence suggests that reaction times are slower in sedentary vs active elderly persons,[91] and that delayed reaction times are more often seen in fine motor vs gross motor activities.[92]

Decreased ROM. The majority of investigators examining subjects from various age groups have found a reduced ROM in older adults.[93–95] Decreases in ROM with advancing age have been found for wrist flexion and extension, hip and shoulder rotation,[93] small decreases (5° or less) were found in mean active hip and knee motions,[94] and James and Parker[95] found consistent declines in both active and passive ROM for 10 LE joints in a population of 80 healthy adults older than 70 years of age. Increased joint tightness tends to be most evident toward the end ROM and may impact the overall skill in coordinated movement. Decrease ROM has been linked to biologic aging of joint surfaces,[95] degenerative changes in collagen fibers, dietary deficiencies, and sedentary lifestyle.[78]

Postural changes. The lateral view of normal postural alignment is represented by a straight line projecting through the ear, acromion, greater trochanter, posterior patella, and lateral malleolus. Common postural changes seen with aging include forward head, rounded shoulders (kyphosis), altered lordotic curve (either flattened or exaggerated), and a slight increase in hip and knee flexion.[80] The base of support may also be widened. Diminished strength and ROM as well as inactivity and prolonged sitting may contribute to poor postural alignment. Of particular importance is the potential loss of ability to fully accomplish preparatory postural adjustments prior to execution of a movement.

Impaired balance (postural control). Decreased balance and increased postural sway (oscillating movements of body over feet during relaxed standing) both occur with advancing age.[96–99] A reduction in postural limits of stability (LOS) and functional reach magnitude has also been documented.[100–102] However, Robinovitch and Cronin[103] found that elderly subjects with impaired LOS lacked awareness of their limitations and as a result tended to plan movements that resulted in a loss of balance.

A variety of task-dependent coordinated movement changes have also been linked to advancing age, including slowing of eye–hand coordination,[104] elbow flexion,[61,72] and aiming movements[66]; performance regression in coordinated interlimb,[73,75] dual-task,[64,68] and homolateral hand and foot movements[62]; changes in multisegmental,[71,76] head–trunk,[105] and lower trunk coordination[69]; and increased time requirements for activities of daily living (ADLs).[63]

Changes in skilled motor performance are a predictable aspect of normal aging. However, this information should not negate or undermine the importance of treatment strategies to improve functional performance and quality of life. An important consideration in treatment planning is that the aging neuromuscular system maintains its physiologic adaptive response to training stimuli.[106] Physical therapy intervention is highly effective in promoting and sustaining a more successful approach to aging.[107–114] This is a particularly important concern as the population ages. Estimates from the U.S. Census Bureau indicate that by 2010 approximately 13 percent of the population will be 65 or older and by 2020 the number will increase to 16.3 percent.[115]

CLINICAL NOTE: The identified changes impacting coordinated movement in the older adult may be accentuated further by alterations in sensation (see Chapter 5), perceptual impairments (see Chapter 29), and diminished vision and hearing acuity. Knowledge of these anticipated age-related changes will improve the therapist's ability to establish effective communication to optimize patient performance as well as assist with interpretation of test results. The potential presence of these changes has important implications for how the therapist communicates with, and provides directions to, the patient during the coordination examination. Sensitive and accurate communication is central to the role of the physical therapist. Because elderly patients typically experience some changes in sensory function, communication skills that enhance the therapeutic interaction should be adopted. This involves conveying information in a language or context that is meaningful and intelligible to the patient and communicates trust, respect, and compassion. DeMont and Peatman[116] suggest several important strategies to improve communication with elderly patients (Box 7.2).

Screening

Screenings are a series of brief tests that provide the therapist an "overview" of the area of interest (e.g., sensation, ROM, strength). Recall that screenings are used to: (1) determine the need for further or more detailed examination; (2) rule out or differentiate specific system involvement; (3) determine if referral to another health care practitioner is warranted; (4) focus the search for the origin of symptoms to a specific location or body part; and (5) identify system-related impairments that contribute to functional limitations or disability.[1,117] In combination with the information from the history and review of systems, screenings assist the therapist in proficiently identifying the needed tests and measures and assist in setting priorities within the examination process.

An important starting point for identification of areas to be screened is consideration of all potential (possible) contributing factors to an observed functional limitation. For example, observation of a coordination impairment imposing functional limitations on dressing abilities would certainly direct the therapist's attention to consider its' origin. However, prior to a detailed systematic examination of all systems, screenings can quickly and efficiently direct the therapist's attention to:

- Areas grossly intact that can subsequently be "ruled out" as contributing to the functional limitation; additional examination of these areas is likely not warranted.
- Areas suspected of contributing to the clinical problem (screening findings are abnormal); further examination is indicated.
- Identification of the need for referral to another practitioner (e.g., occupational therapist for management of a perceptual deficit).

For example, ROM, strength, and level of function of the sensory system have direct implications for successful execution of coordinated movements. It may be likely that formal examination of these areas has already been accomplished prior to a coordination examination. If not, however, screening of these areas is indicated.

CLINICAL NOTE: An initial screening of ROM, strength, and sensation prior to the coordination examination will improve validity because impairments in any of these areas may influence the ability to produce smooth, accurate, controlled motor responses. However, it is also important to note that coordination impairments may occur in the presence of normal ROM, strength, and intact sensation.

Box 7.2 Strategies to Improve Communication with Elders

1. Do not stereotype. Do not assume a level of decreased mental function or confusion. Posture, gesture, and facial expressions can be deceiving.
2. Be aware of, and adapt to, any age-related physical limitations that an elder may possess. Consider the sensory deficits in sight, hearing, speech, and reaction time, which may be barriers to communication.
3. Secure the elder's attention by eye contact or a gentle touch.
4. Identify yourself when greeting an elder.
5. Request information from each elder on how best to communicate, e.g., "Should I speak louder?" or "Would you like your glasses?"
6. Ask each individual what form of address is preferred. Do not use generic or pet names such as "Grampa" or "Mama." Each individual has a unique identity.
7. Request permission to adjust the volume of the television or radio or to change the amount or angle of light.
8. Maintain eye contact.
9. Do not pretend to understand an elder's response. Request confirmation or clarification of a message you do not understand.
10. Avoid speaking to elders as if they were children. Do not use a singsong voice, baby talk, or give orders.
11. Do not ignore individuals or talk about them in the presence of others as if they were not there.
12. Respect an elder's routines and control of his or her life. Schedule and keep appointments at mutually agreed-on times.

From DeMont, ME and Peatman, NL,[116, p 24] with permission.

Examples of Screenings

By virtue of their purpose (i.e., providing quickly and efficiently obtained information), screenings are generally performed with the patient seated on a firm surface. Although to fully screen some areas (e.g., the hip) or if several different screenings are planned in sequence, the supine position may be preferable. If abnormal findings are identified during screening, it is a clear indication for more detailed testing.

Range of Motion

Generally, ROM screenings involve active movements. The patient is asked to selectively move different joints and body segments actively through their available range. For example, the patient might be asked to flex, abduct, and then extend the shoulder; flex and extend the elbow; flex, extend, or circumduct (flexion–abduction–extension–adduction) the wrist; flex and extend the knee; plantarflex, dorsiflex, and circumduct the ankle, and so forth. To minimize time required in providing verbal directions, the therapist may opt to sit directly in front and perform the movements while directing the patient to "mirror" the movements. Alternately, functional movements can be used that combine motions of several joints. For example, the patient might be asked to individually place each hand on the back or top of the head, to reach as high as possible toward the ceiling with each (or both) UE, to place each hand on the small of the back, reach down to touch the ankle, and so forth.

Using careful observation and knowledge of normative ROM values, the therapist makes a gross determination of whether the ROM is *within normal limits* (WNL); if functional movements are used, the designation is *within functional limits* (WFL). If complete, active, painless ROM is available, additional testing is likely not necessary. If active ROM is incomplete or painful, a more detailed examination is needed to determine the cause and extent of the screening findings.[118]

Strength

Typically the ROM screening will precede the strength screening so some information about strength will already be gathered. If the patient performed active ROM movements against the resistance of gravity, a logical assumption is that gross strength is at least a fair grade (ability to move through the ROM against the resistance of gravity). The screening will then be directed toward further refining this estimate using application of manual resistance. Although standard manual muscle testing positions[119,120] are not used for screening, adherence to foundational principles is indicated. Segments proximal to those being screened should be stabilized; resistance is applied at the distal end of the moving segment and at a 90° angle (perpendicular) to the primary axis of movement.

From the sitting position, the patient might be asked to raise the knee toward the ceiling to test hip flexion with application of resistance on the distal femur; to extend the knee to test knee extension strength with resistance on the distal leg; to bring the hand toward the shoulder to test elbow flexion strength with resistance applied on the distal forearm; and so forth.

Sensation

To perform a sensory screening, several easily tested (i.e., requiring little or no specialized equipment) modalities of sensation are selected. Modalities from each of the general categories of sensations should be selected. For example, the therapist might select pain and light touch (superficial), kinesthesia and vibration (deep), and two-point discrimination or stereognosis (combined). For modalities such as pain and light touch, the sensory screening is performed by using the selected modalities to screen randomly over somewhat large surface areas. For example, several applications of each stimulus might be distributed over the upper and lower extremities and trunk. For sensations such as kinesthesia or proprioception, screening should include selected joints and movements of both the upper and lower extremities.

Features of Coordination Tests

Gross and Fine Motor Movements

Coordination tests generally can be divided into two main categories: *gross motor* and *fine motor movements*. Gross motor tests include body posture, balance, and extremity movements involving large muscle groups. Examples of gross motor activities include crawling, kneeling, standing, walking, and running. Fine motor tests address movements concerned with utilization of small muscle groups that involve skillful, controlled manipulation of objects. Examples of fine motor activities include finger dexterity tasks such as buttoning a shirt, typing, or handwriting.

Nonequilibrium and Equilibrium (Balance) Tests

Coordination tests can be further subdivided into nonequilibrium and equilibrium tests. *Nonequilibrium* tests address both static and mobile components of movements when the patient is in a sitting position. These tests involve both gross and fine motor activities. *Equilibrium* tests consider both static and dynamic components of posture and balance when the patient is in an upright standing position. They involve primarily gross motor activities and require observation of the body in both static (stationary) and dynamic (body in motion) postures.

Equilibrium or balance (postural stability) coordination tests identify impairments associated with the two primary goals of the postural control system, *stability* and *function*. Balance involves the complex interaction of (1) the sensory afferent system (including various joint and muscle receptors as well as tactile sensations such as those of the feet and toes) involved in identification of body position and control; (2) the motor effector system involved in execution of the motor response; and (3) integrated CNS control processes. Other components of balance include: *reactive postural control* (response to external forces such as perturbations acting on the body), *proactive (anticipatory) postural control* (anticipatory response to destabilizing forces imposed on the body's own movements such as when lifting a heavy object), and *adaptive postural control* (modification of sensory and motor systems relative to task or environmental demands)[59] as well as vision, weight distribution, and postural orientation and alignment (see Chapter 8 for a more detailed discussion of postural control and balance). As multiple systems are involved in balance, analysis of equilibrium coordination responses will guide selection of additional tests and measures to allow determination of the origin of symptoms.

Motor Task Requirements

Coordination tests address patient capabilities in four basic motor task requirements, including mobility, stability (static postural control), controlled mobility (dynamic postural control), and skill. *Mobility* refers to initial movement occurring within a functional pattern. Examples of mobility impairments include insufficient motor unit activity to initiate a contraction, problems sustaining a movement, and difficulty moving against gravity. *Stability* (static postural control) is the ability to maintain a steady position in a weightbearing, antigravity posture. Impairments present as instability or increased postural sway in sitting or standing (inability to maintain a posture), episodes of loss of balance, and risk of falls. *Controlled mobility* (dynamic postural control) is the ability to alter a position or change positions while maintaining stability. Impairments in controlled mobility include difficulty maintaining balance during weight shifting or rocking within a posture (e.g., sitting), and the inability to assume a posture independently (e.g., inability to move to sitting from a supine position). This latter activity requires movement against gravity through a large ROM. *Static dynamic control* is a variation of controlled mobility and refers to the ability to shift weight onto one limb and free the contralateral limb for nonweightbearing dynamic activities. The inability to lift one upper or lower limb off the supporting surface from a quadruped position is an example of impaired static dynamic control. *Skill* refers to highly coordinated movement that allows interaction with the environment. Examples of skill-level impairments include an inability to stabilize proximal limb segments while distal segments move; and movements that are inconsistent, require increased effort, and lack appropriate direction and timing. In addition, skill impairments impose limitations on precise control of movement, maintenance of movement for extended periods, and the ability to combine several movement sequences.

Movement Capabilities

The coordination examination focuses on movement capabilities in five main areas:

(1) *Alternate* or *reciprocal motion*, which is the ability to reverse movement between opposing muscle groups;

(2) *Movement composition,* or synergy, which involves movement control achieved by muscle groups acting together;
(3) *Movement accuracy* is the ability to gauge or judge distance and speed of voluntary movement;
(4) *Fixation or limb holding,* addresses the ability to hold the position of an individual limb or limb segment; and
(5) *Equilibrium (postural stability),* which is the ability to maintain balance in response to alterations in center of gravity and/or base of support.

The progression of difficulty of coordination tests (gradual increases in challenge to the patient) typically utilizes the following sequence: (1) unilateral tasks; (2) bilateral symmetrical tasks; (3) bilateral asymmetrical tasks; and (4) multilimb tasks (these constitute the highest level of difficulty). Table 7.2 presents a summary of motor task requirements and movement capabilities addressed during the examination of coordination.

Preparation for Administering the Coordination Examination

Prior to initiating the coordination examination, the testing environment should be identified and prepared, needed equipment gathered, and consideration given to patient preparation (i.e., what information and instruction will be provided).

Testing Environment

The coordination examination should be administered in a quiet, well-lighted treatment area sufficiently large to accommodate walking activities included in the equilibrium portion of the tests. Ideally, the room should be equipped with two standard chairs and a mat or treatment table. A watch or clock with a second hand should be available for timed components of the examination as well as a method of occluding vision (an inexpensive blindfold used for sleeping works well).

Patient Preparation

The coordination examination should be administered when the patient is well rested. A full explanation of the purpose of the testing should be provided. Each coordination test should be described and demonstrated individually by the therapist before actual testing. Such demonstrations should be attended to carefully, as lack of clarity will negatively impact motor responses. Because testing procedures require mental concentration and some physical activity, fatigue, apprehension, or fear may adversely influence test results.

Preliminary Observation

Observation is an essential skill in clinical decision making. Accurate and careful patient observation provides a rich source of preliminary information prior to performing a coordination examination. Inasmuch as treatment intervention will be directed, at least in part, toward improving functional performance and activity levels, initial observations should logically focus here. Depending on the practice setting environment, the patient might be observed performing any number of functional activities such as bed mobility, self-care routines (e.g., dressing, combing hair, brushing teeth), transfers, eating, writing, changing position from lying or sitting to standing, maintaining a standing position, walking, and so forth. Use of appropriate patient guarding techniques is indicated during the initial observation. While observing the patient, general information can be obtained that will assist in localizing specific areas of impairment. This information will include:

Table 7.2 Motor Task Requirements and Movement Capabilities Addressed During the Examination of Coordination

Motor Task Requirements	Movement Capabilities
• *Mobility:* initial movement within a functional pattern	• Alternate or reciprocal motion: reversing movement between opposing muscle groups
• *Stability:* static postural control; ability to maintain a steady position in a weightbearing, antigravity posture	• Movement composition (synergy): movement control achieved by muscle groups acting together
• *Controlled mobility:* dynamic postural control; ability to alter a position or change positions while maintaining stability; *static dynamic control* (variation of controlled mobility): weight shifting onto one limb to free opposite limb for non-weightbearing dynamic activities	• Movement accuracy: gauging or judging distance and speed of voluntary movement • Fixation (limb holding): holding position of individual limb or limb segment
• *Skill:* highly coordinated movement that allows interaction with the environment (e.g., gait)	• Equilibrium (postural stability): maintaining balance in response to alterations in center of gravity and/or base of support

- General level of skill in each activity (amount of assistance or assistive devices required)
- The occurrence of extraneous movements, oscillations, swaying, or unsteadiness
- Number of extremities involved (unilateral and/or bilateral)
- Distribution of motor impairment: proximal and/or distal musculature
- Situations or occurrences that alter (increase or decrease) impairments
- Amount of time required to perform an activity
- Level of safety

From this initial observation, the therapist will be guided in selecting the appropriate tests for the general areas of impairment noted. Table 7.3 and Box 7.3 present sample tests appropriate for examining nonequilibrium and equilibrium coordination, respectively. It should be noted that a single test is often appropriate to examine several different movement capabilities simultaneously to conserve time. The tests presented (Table 7.3 and Box 7.3) are intended as samples and are not all-inclusive. Other activities may be developed that are equally effective in examining a particular impairment and may be more appropriate for an individual patient. As noted above, performance in any variety of functional skills (e.g., self-care routines, wheelchair propulsion, transfers, dressing, and so forth) is also an effective means of examining many aspects of movement capabilities (e.g., alternate or reciprocal motion, movement composition, movement accuracy, and so forth).

The two subdivisions of coordination tests presented here (nonequilibrium and equilibrium) have traditionally been used for providing structure and organization to administration of the tests. However, it should be noted that the "nonequilibrium" division is somewhat of a misnomer in that elements of posture and balance (equilibrium-based) are required during these tests (i.e., maintaining an upright sitting posture). In addition, equilibrium demands can be heightened using unsupported sitting postures. Although each subdivision places particular emphasis on certain movement capabilities, there will clearly be overlap between findings from the two subdivisions. Table 7.4 includes selected impairments and suggested tests appropriate for the clinical problem.

In addition to the specific tests presented in Table 7.3 and Box 7.3, gait analysis measures also add important data to the coordination examination. A systematic gait analysis will assist with the diagnosis of movement impairments by identifying:

- Characteristics of initiation and control of movement
- Abnormalities in muscle tone
- Influence of abnormal synergistic patterns and nonintegrated reflexes
- Control of sequential timing of muscular activity
- Control of body movements as a whole and of body segments in relation to each other
- Deviations from normal posture and motion (e.g., leaning, lurching, or excessive or diminished motion at a specific joint)
- Quality of movement termination
- Impact of environmental constraints
- Characteristics of dual task performance (e.g., walking while bouncing a ball)

Standardized gait instruments and functional balance measures are particularly useful (1) in identifying coordinated movement impairments associated with a skill-level motor task (i.e., highly coordinated movement allowing interaction with environment); (2) making decisions about the differences between the patient's performance and the parameters of normal gait; and (3) providing data to inform decisions about the underlying mechanisms responsible for producing the movement impairments. Although not all-inclusive, the following list of gait instruments are among those more commonly used in clinical settings: the Get Up and Go Test (GUG),[121] the Timed Up and Go Test (TUG),[122] the Functional Independence Measure (FIM),[123–125] The Sickness Impact Profile,[126,127] the Physical Performance and Mobility Examination (PPME),[128] the Performance-Oriented Mobility Assessment (POMA),[129,130] the Gait Assessment Rating Scale (GARS),[131] the Dynamic Gait Index,[59] the Walky-Talkie Test,[132] the Berg Balance Scale (BBS),[133–135] and a timed walking test.[136]

These gait instruments are described elsewhere in the text. More detailed information can be found in Chapters 8, 10, and 11.

The Coordination Examination

Guided by information from the preliminary observation of functional activities, tests should be selected (see Table 7.3 and Box 7.3) to address the required movement capabilities of interest for the individual patient. Generally, nonequilibrium tests are completed first, followed by the equilibrium tests. Attention should be directed to carefully guarding the patient during testing; use of a safety belt may be warranted. During testing, the following questions can be used to help direct the therapist's observations. The findings should be included in the comment section of the coordination examination form.

- Are movements direct, precise, and easily reversed?
- Do movements occur within a reasonable or normal amount of time?
- Does increased speed of performance affect quality of motor activity?
- Can continuous and appropriate motor adjustments be made if speed and direction are changed?
- Can a position or posture of the body or specific extremity be maintained without swaying, oscillations, or extraneous movements?

Table 7.3 Nonequilibrium Coordination Tests[a]

1. Finger-to-nose	The shoulder is abducted to 90° with the elbow extended. The patient is asked to bring the tip of the index finger to the tip of his or her nose. Alterations may be made in the initial starting position to observe performance from different planes of motion.
2. Finger-to-therapist's finger	The patient and therapist sit opposite each other. The therapist's index finger is held in front of the patient. The patient is asked to touch the tip of his or her index finger to the therapist's index finger. The position of the therapist's finger may be altered during testing to observe ability to change distance, direction, and force of movement.
3. Finger-to-finger	Both shoulders are abducted to 90° with the elbows extended. The patient is asked to bring both hands toward the midline and approximate the index fingers from opposing hands.
4. Alternate nose-to-finger	The patient alternately touches the tip of his or her nose and the tip of the therapist's finger with the index finger. The position of the therapist's finger may be altered during testing to observe ability to change distance, direction, and force of movement.
5. Finger opposition	The patient touches the tip of the thumb to the tip of each finger in sequence. Speed may be gradually increased.
6. Mass grasp	An alternation is made between opening and closing fist (from finger flexion to full extension). Speed may be gradually increased.
7. Pronation/supination	With elbows flexed to 90° and held close to body, the patient alternately turns the palms up and down. This test also may be performed with shoulders flexed to 90° and elbows extended. Speed may be gradually increased. The ability to reverse movements between opposing muscle groups can be examined at many joints. Examples include active alternation between flexion and extension of the knee, ankle, elbow, fingers, and so forth.
8. Rebound test	The patient is positioned with the elbow flexed. The therapist applies sufficient manual resistance to produce an isometric contraction of biceps. Resistance is suddenly released. Normally, the opposing muscle group (triceps) will contract and "check" movement of the limb. Many other muscle groups can be tested for this phenomenon, such as the shoulder abductors or flexors, elbow extensors, and so forth.
9. Tapping (hand)	With the elbow flexed and the forearm pronated, the patient is asked to "tap" the hand on the knee.
10. Tapping (foot)	The patient is asked to "tap" the ball of one foot on the floor without raising the knee; heel maintains contact with floor.
11. Pointing and past pointing	The patient and therapist are opposite each other, either sitting or standing. Both patient and therapist bring shoulders to a horizontal position of 90° of flexion with elbows extended. Index fingers are touching or the patient's finger may rest lightly on the therapist's. The patient is asked to fully flex the shoulder (fingers will be pointing toward ceiling) and then return to the horizontal position such that index fingers will again approximate. Both arms should be tested, either separately or simultaneously. A normal response consists of an accurate return to the starting position. In an abnormal response, there is typically a "past pointing," or movement beyond the target. Several variations to this test include movements in other directions such as toward 90° of shoulder abduction or toward 0° of shoulder flexion (finger will point toward floor). Following each movement, the patient is asked to return to the initial horizontal starting position.
12. Alternate heel-to-knee; heel-to-toe	From a supine position, the patient is asked to touch the knee and big toe alternately with the heel of the opposite extremity.
13. Toe to examiner's finger	From a supine position, the patient is instructed to touch the great toe to the examiner's finger. The position of finger may be altered during testing to observe ability to change distance, direction, and force of movement.
14. Heel on shin	From a supine position, the heel of one foot is slid up and down the shin of the opposite LE.
15. Drawing a circle	The patient draws an imaginary circle in the air with either UE or LE (a table or the floor also may be used). This also may be done using a figure-eight pattern. This test may be performed in the supine position for the LE.
16. Fixation or position holding	UE: The patient holds arms horizontally in front (sitting or standing). LE: The patient is asked to hold the knee in an extended position (sitting).

[a]Tests should be performed first with eyes open and then with eyes closed. Abnormal responses include a gradual deviation from the "holding" position and/or a diminished quality of response with vision occluded. Unless otherwise indicated, tests are performed with the patient in a sitting position.
LE = Lower extremity; UE = upper extremity.

Box 7.3 Equilibrium Coordination Tests

1. Standing, comfortable posture with normal base of support (BOS).
2. Standing, feet together (narrow BOS).
3. Standing in tandem position, with one foot directly in front of the other (toe of one foot touching heel of opposite foot).
4. Standing on one foot.
5. Arm position may be altered in each of the above postures (i.e., arms at side, over head, hands on waist, and so forth).
6. Perturbations: displace balance unexpectedly (while carefully guarding patient).
7. Standing, functional reach: forward trunk flexion with UE reach.
8. Standing, laterally flex trunk to each side.
9. Standing: eyes open (EO) to eyes closed (EC); inability to maintain an upright posture without visual input is referred to as a positive Romberg sign.
10. Standing in tandem position eyes open (EO) to eyes closed (EC) (Sharpened Romberg).
11. Tandem walking, placing the heel of one foot directly in front of the toe of the opposite foot.
12. Walking along a straight line drawn or taped to the floor, or place feet on floor markers while walking.
13. Walk sideways, backward, or cross-stepping.
14. March in place.
15. Alter speed of ambulatory activities; observe patient walking at normal speed, as fast as possible, and as slow as possible.
16. Stop and start abruptly on command while walking.
17. Walk and pivot on command (turn 90, 180, or 360°).
18. Walk in a circle, alternate directions.
19. Walk on heels or toes.
20. Walk with horizontal and vertical head turns on command.
21. Step over or around obstacles.
22. Stairclimbing with and without using handrail; one step at-a-time, step-over-step.
23. Jumping jacks
24. Sitting on a therapy ball: alternate flexing and extending the knees (coordinated movement with upright balance).

- Are placing movements of both upper and lower extremities exact?
- Does occluding vision alter the quality of motor activity?
- Is there greater involvement proximally or distally?
- Is there greater involvement on one side of body versus the other?
- Does the patient fatigue rapidly?
- Is there a consistency of motor response over time?

Recording Test Results

A generally accepted format for recording results from coordination tests has not been established and approaches to documentation vary considerably among institutions and individual therapists. Owing to the nature of the tests and the wide variation in types and severity of deficits, observational coordination forms are not highly standardized. However, an exception to this are the UE standardized tests addressing specific components of manual dexterity through the use of functional or work-related tasks. Some of these tests originally were developed to assist with determining if an individual had the needed manual skills required for specific employment tasks. Several examples of these tests are presented in the section titled *Standardized Instruments: Upper Extremity Coordination*.

Several options are available for recording results from a comprehensive examination of coordination. A coordination examination form is frequently useful to provide a composite picture of the areas of impairment noted. These forms are often developed within clinical settings. They may be general (a sample is presented in Table 7.5), or they may be specific to a given group of patients, such as those with brain injuries.[137] In general, these forms lack reliability testing. However, they do provide a systematic method of data collection and documentation. In addition, use of the same form for periodic reexamination facilitates ease of comparison of changes over time. These forms frequently include some type of rating scale in which level of performance is weighted using an arbitrary scale. An example of such a scale follows:

4 Normal performance is demonstrated.
3 Movement is accomplished with only slight difficulty.
2 Moderate difficulty is demonstrated in accomplishing activity; movements are arrhythmic, and performance deteriorates with increased speed.
1 Severe difficulty is noted: movements are very arrhythmic; significant unsteadiness, oscillations, and/or extraneous movements are noted.
0 Patient unable to accomplish activity.

A score from the rating scale would then be assigned to each component of the coordination examination. An advantage of using rating scales is that they provide a mechanism for quantifying patient performance based on subjective ratings. Several inherent limitations exist in using such scales. Often the descriptions are not reflective of exact patient performance. Alternatively, the rating scale may not be defined adequately or detailed appropriately, thus decreasing reliability of repeated or interexaminer testing. Frequently, coordination forms include a comments section. This component of the form allows for additional narrative descriptions of patient performance. Using a combination of a rating scale and narrative comments or summary will ensure that all coordination impairments are adequately documented.

Measuring the length of time required to complete a motor or functional task provides an important quantitative measure of movement capability. Because accomplishing

Table 7.4 Sample Tests for Selected Coordination Impairments

Impairment	Sample Test
Dysdiadochokinesia	Finger-to-nose Alternate nose-to-finger Pronation/supination Knee flexion/extension Walking, alter speed or direction
Dysmetria	Pointing and past pointing Drawing a circle or figure eight Heel on shin Placing feet on floor markers; sitting, standing
Dyssynergia	Finger-to-nose Finger-to-therapist's finger Alternate heel-to-knee Toe-to-examiner's finger
Hypotonia	Passive movement Deep tendon reflexes
Tremor (intention)	Observation during functional activities (tremor will typically increase as target is approached or movement speed increased) Alternate nose-to-finger Finger-to-finger Finger-to-therapist's finger Toe-to-examiner's finger
Tremor (resting)	Observation of patient at rest; limb or jaw movements Observation during functional activities (tremor will diminish significantly or disappear with movement)
Tremor (postural)	Observation of steadiness of normal posture; sitting, standing
Asthenia	Fixation or position holding (upper and lower extremity) Application of manual resistance to determine ability to hold
Rigidity	Passive movement Observation during functional activities Observation of resting posture(s)
Bradykinesia	Walking, observation of arm swing and trunk motions Walking, alter speed and direction Request that a movement or gait activity be stopped abruptly Observation of functional activities: timed tests
Disturbances of posture	Fixation or position holding (upper and lower extremity) Displace balance unexpectedly in sitting or standing (perturbation) Standing, alter base of support (e.g., one foot directly in front of the other; standing on one foot)
Disturbances of gait	Walk along a straight line Walk sideways, backward March in place Alter speed and direction of ambulatory activities Walk in a circle

Table 7.5 **Coordination Examination Form**

Patient Name: ______________________ Examiner: ______________________ Date: __________

PART I: NONEQUILIBRIUM COORDINATION TESTS

Key to Grading

5 Normal Performance

4 Minimal Impairment: Able to accomplish; slightly less than normal speed; requires supervision/minimal contact guarding

3 Moderate Impairment: Able to accomplish activity; movements are slow, awkward, and unsteady; requires moderate contact guarding

2 Severe Impairment: Able only to initiate activity without completion; requires maximal contact guarding

1 Activity Impossible

Notations should be made under comments section if:

- Lack of visual input renders activity impossible or alters quality of performance
- Verbal cuing is required to accomplish activity
- Alterations in speed affect quality of performance
- Excessive amount of time required to complete activity
- Changes in arm position alters sitting balance
- Extraneous movements, unsteadiness, or oscillations noted in head, neck, or trunk
- Fatigue alters consistency of response
- Performance impacts patient safety

Grade: Left	Coordination Test	Grade: Right	Comments
	Finger-to-nose		
	Finger-to-therapist's finger		
	Finger-to-finger		
	Alternate nose-to-finger		
	Finger opposition		
	Mass grasp		
	Pronation/supination		
	Rebound phenomenon		
	Tapping (hand)		
	Tapping (foot)		
	Pointing and past-pointing		
	Alternate heel-to-knee; heel-to-toe		
	Toe-to-examiner's finger		
	Heel-on-shin		
	Drawing a circle (hand)		
	Drawing a circle (foot)		
	Fixation/position holding (UE)		
	Fixation/position holding (LE)		

(*continued*)

Table 7.5 **Coordination Examination Form** (continued)

Patient Name: ____________________ Examiner: ____________________ Date: __________

PART II: EQUILIBRIUM COORDINATION TESTS

Key to Grading

5 Normal Performance
4 Minimal Impairment: Able to accomplish activity; slightly less than normal speed; requires supervision/minimal contact guarding
3 Moderate Impairment: Able to accomplish activity; movements are slow, awkward, and unsteady; requires moderate contact guarding
2 Severe Impairment: Able only to initiate activity with difficulty; unable to complete; safety concerns; requires maximal contact guarding
1 Activity Impossible

Notations should be made under comments section if:

- Lack of visual input renders activity impossible or alters quality of performance
- Verbal cuing is required to accomplish activity
- Alterations in speed affect quality of performance
- Excessive amount of time required to complete activity
- Changes in arm position alters standing balance/postural stability
- Extraneous movements, unsteadiness, or oscillations noted in head, neck, or trunk
- Fatigue alters consistency of response
- Performance impacts patient safety

Grade	Coordination Test	Comments
	Standing in a normal comfortable posture	
	Standing, feet together (narrow base of support)	
	Standing on one foot	
	Standing, with one foot directly in front of the other in tandem position (toe of one foot touching heel of opposite foot)	
	Standing, forward trunk flexion and return to neutral	
	Standing, laterally flex trunk to each side	
	Standing: eyes open (EO) to eyes closed (EC) (*Romberg Test*)	
	Standing in tandem position: EO to EC (*Sharpened Romberg Test*)	
	Walk at normal speed	
	Walk as fast as possible	
	Walk as slow as possible	
	Walk: stop and start abruptly	
	Walk and pivot (turn 90, 180, or 360°)	
	Walking, placing the heel of one foot directly in front of the toe of the opposite foot (tandem walking)	

	Walking along a straight line drawn or taped to the floor	
	Walking, placing feet on floor markers	
	Walk: sideways	
	Walk: backwards	
	Walk: cross-stepping	
	Walk: in a circle, alternate directions	
	Walk: on heels	
	Walk: on toes	
	March in place	
	Walk with horizontal and vertical head turns	
	Step over or around obstacles	
	Stairclimbing with handrail	
	Stairclimbing without handrail	
	Stairclimbing: one step at-a-time	
	Stairclimbing: step-over-step	

an activity in a reasonable amount of time is a component of performance, the length of time required to accomplish certain activities is recorded by use of a stopwatch. Using time as a measure of performance has important implications for both function and safety. For example, assume a patient with multiple sclerosis who uses a wheelchair plans to return to school but requires 2.5 hours to complete dressing activities. The time element here would not be considered functional, especially if attempting to make an early morning class. Consider also an ambulatory patient with an ataxic gait unable to cross a street in the allotted time provided by the traffic signal. This time requirement presents a considerable patient safety issue and, as such, would also not be considered functional.

Some standardized measurement tools have been developed based on timed activities (e.g., Timed Up and Go test[122]). However, timed performance measures may be incorporated into any variety of motor or functional tasks.

Periodic videotaping of patient performance has been used effectively to document coordination impairments as well as monitor progress over time. For some patients they can provide the basis for suggestions about altering movement strategies to improve function and direct attention to safety precautions. Viewed in sequence over time, videotapes can also impact patient motivation to attain further gains. Videotapes have also been used to determine the impact of medications on coordinated movement via pre- and post-intervention recordings (e.g., patients with Parkinson's disease).

CLINICAL NOTE: It is also not uncommon for therapists to document data from the coordinaation examination directly within the body of a narrative note or within the objective section of a SOAP note.

Quantitative Coordination Testing and Specialized Testing Instruments

CATSYS System

The *CATSYS System* (Danish Product Development, Ltd, Denmark) is a Windows®-based testing system that allows quantification of several types of coordination impairments.[138–141] The system interfaces with a computer via a small data logger box (serial cable). The data logger records information from four sensors including a:

- Tremor Pen™ for documenting tremor intensity and frequency
- Reaction time hand-held switch activated by the thumb
- Touch recording plate for measuring pronation/supination and finger-tapping
- Force platform for measuring postural sway

Normative data are available and the system allows comparison of inter- and intrapatient data over time. This system has been used to document movement dysfunction associated with neurodegenerative pathology as well those associated with neurotoxic exposure (e.g., mercury poisoning).[142]

Postural Sway Analyzer

The *Postural Sway Analyzer* (Neuro-Test Inc, Pasadena, CA 91117) measures postural sway (a component of equilibrium coordination) using a computerized head-tracking monitor. A sound-generating stylus is embedded in a lightweight headset placed on the patient's head. Two microphones mounted 14.2 inches (36 cm) apart on the extended arm of a tripod are placed 13.7 inches (35 cm) from the patient's head. The microphones record the horizontal path and movement speed of the sonic (sound) source. The mean speed of sway is recorded as cm/s.[143–145] A large sway path would be indicative of postural instability.

Choice Reaction Time Analyzer

The *Choice Reaction Time Analyzer* (Neuro-Test Inc, Pasadena, CA 91117) is a computerized instrument that allows monitoring of both simple reaction time (SRT) and choice reaction time (CRT). Reaction times are measured from the time a stimulus appears on the screen to the time a response in recorded by pressing one of two small key pads labeled "A" and "S" (pressing a keypad stops the timed measure). For example, in measuring SRT, the patient may be asked to press keypad "A" as quickly as possible each time the color blue appears (note that the color blue here is an arbitrary example, as any number of letters, colors, objects, and so forth can serve as the target stimulus; items can also be presented at various angle orientations [i.e., sideways, up-side-down, and so forth]). For CRT, the subject responds differentially by pressing either the "A" or the "S" key in response to two separate target stimuli. For example, the patient may be instructed to press keypad "A" as quickly as possible each time an inverted number "2" appears and keypad "B" each time the number "2" appears in its normal orientation.[146–148]

Dynamic Posturography

Multiple dynamic posturography systems are commercially available. This sophisticated instrumentation includes a dynamic platform (both linear and angular movement), a moving visual surround screen, and a computer interface. The dynamic platform imposes postural perturbations and the surround screen (sway referenced) presents visual conflict. Both the platform and surround screen are patient referenced via hydraulic mechanisms. Posturography provides quantitative data on balance control and postural stability (direction and amplitude of postural sway).

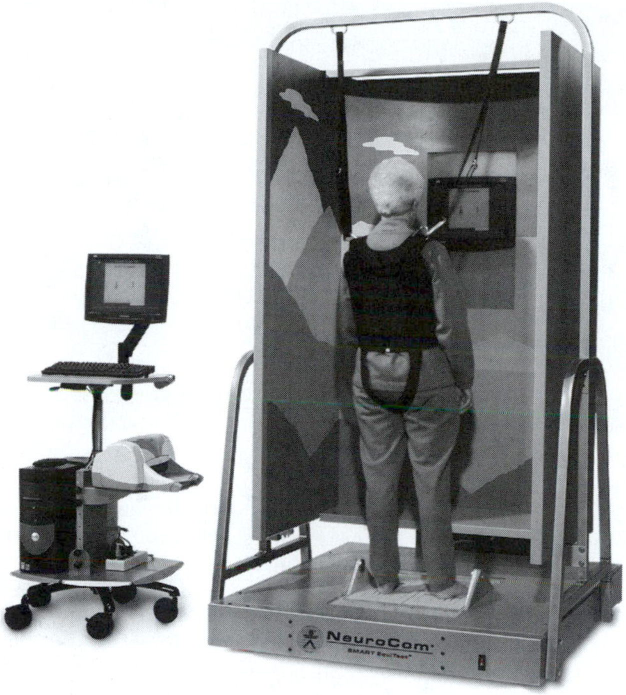

Figure 7.4 SMART EquiTest® (Courtesy of NeuroCom® International, Inc, Clackamas, OR 97015.)

An example of a posturography instrument is the *SMART EquiTest®* (NeuroCom® International, Inc, Clackamas, OR 97015). The system (Fig. 7.4) includes a dynamic force plate (18 × 18 inches [46 × 46 cm]) with both rotational and translation capabilities allowing measurement of vertical forces exerted by the patient's feet. The patient stands on the force plate and is surrounded by a visual environment. A safety harness is worn by the patient that attaches to a stationary bar. The system is designed for both patient examination as well as for balance training using visual biofeedback. The parameters can be altered such that both the support surface and the visual environment can be either stable or dynamic. The dynamic support surface is intended to simulate the challenges imposed by daily activities (normal conditions that change proprioceptive input). See Chapter 8 for additional information on posturography.

Standardized Instruments: Upper Extremity Coordination

Several standardized tests are available to examine arm–hand and eye–hand coordination as well as fine motor dexterity of the fingers through use of function-based skills or activities. Many of these tests were originally designed to predict employment success for jobs requiring manipulation of small parts such as might be required for assembly-line work. The vast majority of tests are scored based both on time required for completion and quality (accuracy) of results.

Most of these standardized tests include an examiner's manual containing normative data to assist with interpretation of test results. Adherence to the prescribed method of administration is particularly important when using standardized tests. Any deviations from the established protocol will affect the validity and reliability of the measures and consequently make comparisons with published norms invalid. The skill of the examiner is another important consideration. The tests should be administered by an individual knowledgeable about testing guidelines and interpretation of results. Subsequent retests should be performed by the same individual. These standardized tests are useful in providing objective measures of patient progress over time. The following is a description of several of these tests.

The *Jebsen-Taylor Hand Function Test* (Sammons Preston Rolyan, Bolingbrook, IL 60440) examines hand and finger coordination using seven subtests of functional skills: writing; card turning; picking up small objects; simulated feeding; stacking; picking up large, lightweight objects; and picking up large, heavy objects (Fig. 7.5). The test is easy to construct, administer, and score (commercially available test kits contain all materials together with instructions in a tote bag). Normative data are included relating to age, gender, maximum time, and hand dominance. The test allows examination of hand function in seven common activities of daily living.[149–153]

The *Minnesota Manual Dexterity Test* (Lafayette Instrument Co, Lafayette, IN 47903) was designed to select personnel for semiskilled operations requiring coordinated arm/hand/finger movements as well as eye–hand coordination such as required for handling small tools or assembly materials that do not require differentiating size or shape (Fig. 7.6). The test includes placing and turning tasks and requires use of a board with wells and round disks. Normative data are available. An expanded variation of this test is the Minnesota Rate of Manipulation Test, which includes five operations: placing, turning, displac-

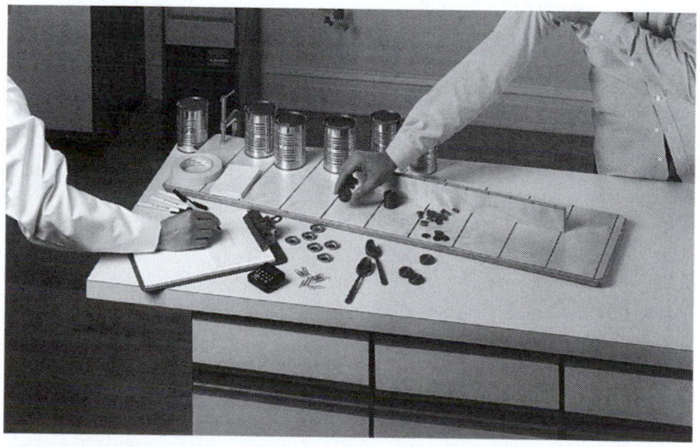

Figure 7.5 The Jebsen-Taylor Hand Function Test includes a subset of seven functional tasks allowing examination of a broad range of skills requiring coordinated movement of the hand and fingers. Common items are used such as spoons, paper clips, cans, pencils, and so forth. (Courtesy of Sammons Preston Rolyan, Bolingbrook, IL 60440-3593.)

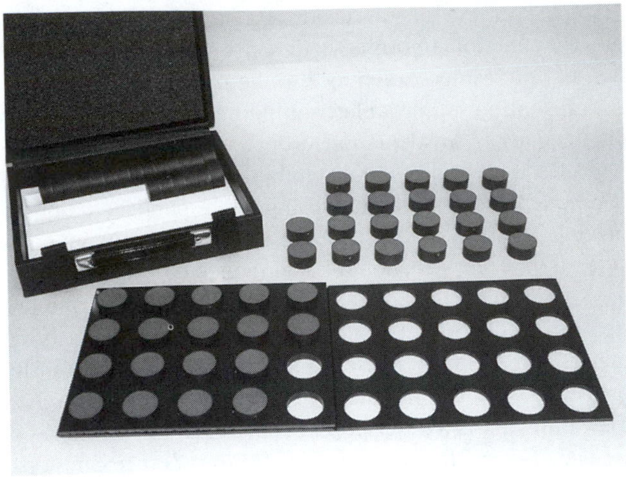

Figure 7.6 Minnesota Manual Dexterity Test consists of two operations: *placing* and *turning*. Following a practice trial, scores are based on the time required to complete each of four trials for each operation.

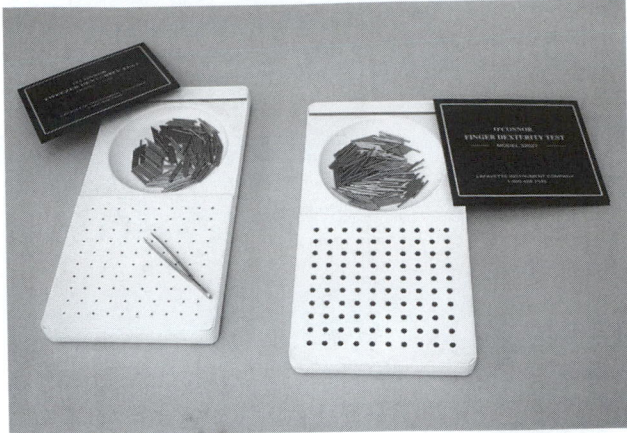

Figure 7.8 The O'Connor Tweezer (*left*) and Finger Dexterity (*right*) Tests examine fine motor coordination. Each board is 11 × 5.5 inches (28 cm × 14 cm) with 100 holes and shallow wells to hold the pins. The black covers slide through grooved channels to keep pins in place during storage.

ing, one-hand turning and placing, and two-hand turning and placing.[153–155]

The *Purdue Pegboard* (Lafayette Instrument Co, Lafayette, IN 47903) test addresses both gross coordination of the arm/hand/fingers as well as fine coordination (dexterity) of the fingers by placement of pins, collars, and or washes on a pegboard (Fig. 7.7).[153,156] There are several subtests, including right-hand prehension, left-hand prehension, prehension test with both hands, and assembly. The test has been used to select personnel for industrial jobs that require manipulative skills. Normative values are available, and both unilateral and bilateral coordinated movement can be examined. This test requires use of a testing board, pins, collars, and washers. The Purdue Pegboard was found to high test–retest reliability in persons with multiple sclerosis.[157]

The *Crawford Small Parts Dexterity Test* (Harcourt Assessment, San Antonio, TX 78270) uses the manipulation of small tools to examine motor performance. The test uses pins, collars, and screws as well as a board into which these small objects fit. Use of tweezers is required both to place the pins in holes and to place a collar over the pin. The screws must be placed with the fingers and screwed in with a screwdriver. This test has been used in prevocational testing. Normative data are available. This test is scored by time.[153]

The *O'Connor Tweezer Test* (Fig. 7.8, *left*) and *Finger Dexterity Test* (Fig. 7.8, *right*) examine the ability to rapidly manipulate small objects (Lafayette Instrument Co,

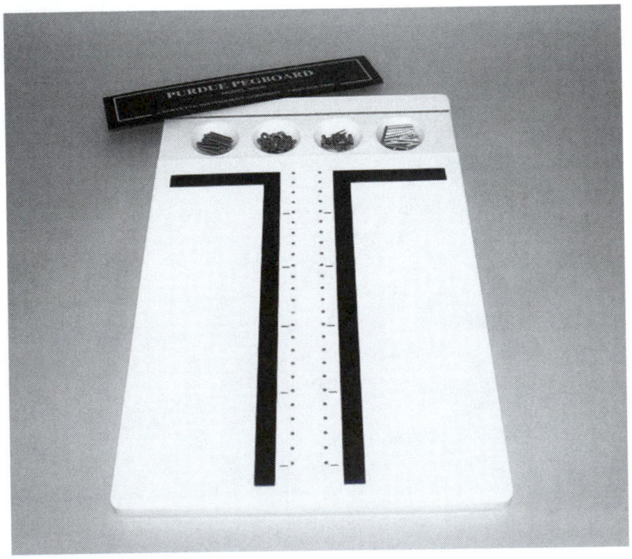

Figure 7.7 The Purdue Pegboard Test includes a pegboard equipped with pins, collars, and washers. Scores are based on the number of assemblies completed within either a 30- or 60-second period.

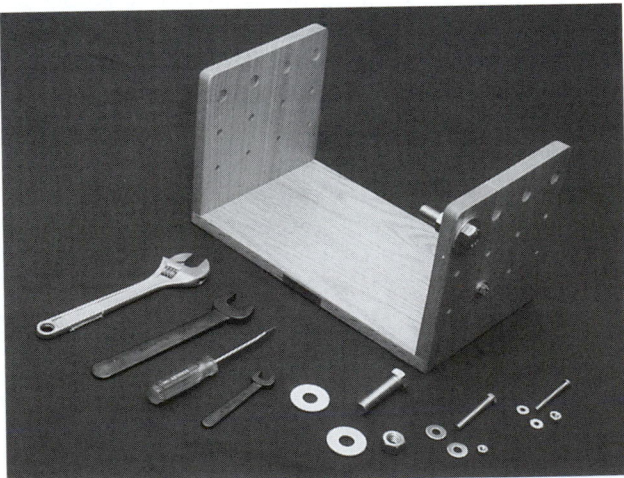

Figure 7.9 The Hand Dexterity Tool Test utilizes ordinary tools for removing and remounting the nuts and bolts. The test is timed from initiation of task (picking up first tool) until the last bolt is secured. (Courtesy of Lafayette Instrument Co, Lafayette, IN 47903.)

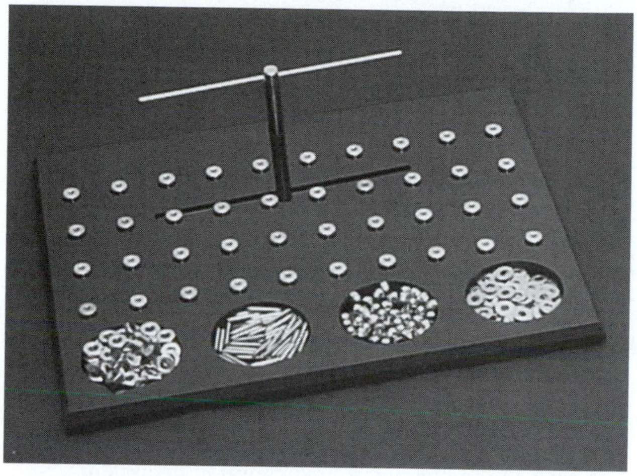

Figure 7.10 The Roeder Manipulative Aptitude Test is scored by counting the number of nuts and washers assembled within the allotted time. (Courtesy of Lafayette Instrument Co, Lafayette, IN 47903.)

Lafayette, IN 47903). The Tweezer Test emphasizes eye–hand and fine motor dexterity by requiring the subject to use a tweezers to place a single pin in each 1/16-inch diameter hole. The Finger Dexterity Test also addresses fine motor dexterity through manual placement of three pins per hole. Both of these tests were originally developed to predict successful employment for assembly-line work requiring rapid manipulation of small parts (e.g., assembling miniature components of watches).

The *Hand Tool Dexterity Test* (Fig. 7.9) utilizes ordinary tools to examine coordinated movement of arm/hand/fingers during a functional task. The test frame consists of a flat board to which two side uprights are attached. The test requires disassembly of the nuts and bolts on one upright using the appropriate tools and reassembling them on the opposite upright. The test is timed and normative data are available.

The *Roeder Manipulative Aptitude Test* (Fig. 7.10) measures arm–hand–finger coordination (including thrusting and twisting) as well as eye–hand coordination. The test materials consist of a high-density plastic board with four wells for washers, rods, caps, and nuts; a T-bar for placement of washer–nut assemblies; and rows of sockets for installing nuts. The test protocol includes four timed operations: dominant hand rod–cap assembly and T-bar washer–nut assembly using both hands, right hand, and left hand. Normative data are available.

Other standardized and commercially distributed tests are available. Selection of standardized instruments should be based on: (1) the intended movement capabilities to be examined such as reciprocal motion, movement composition, reaction time, or accuracy; and (2) the required tasks needed to fully explore coordinated movement for an individual patient (i.e., unilateral tasks, bilateral symmetrical tasks, or bilateral asymmetrical tasks). In addition, careful consideration should be made of criteria used for standardization of the testing instrument and the availability of normative data to assist interpretation of findings.

Summary

An examination of coordination provides the physical therapist with important information related to motor performance. Findings provide information about the underlying origin of impairments (although some clinical findings may not be attributable to a single area of CNS involvement). Data from the coordination examination also assist with establishing anticipated goals and expected outcomes, determining a plan of care, and identifying the effectiveness of treatment interventions. Because observational coordination tests are not highly standardized, there is a potential for error and misinterpretation of results. Sources of potential error can be reduced by the use of well-defined rating scales, administration of tests by skilled examiners, and subsequent retesting performed by the same therapist.

A variety of traditional observational coordination tests have been identified. Although the tests have been presented individually for clarity, most can be used to examine more than one type of movement capability. Documentation should include the type, severity, and location of the impairments as well as factors that alter the quality of performance. Emphasis has been placed on the variety of influences that affect movement capabilities. As such, test results must be considered with respect to findings from other examinations such as sensation, ROM, muscle strength, and muscle tone.

Questions for Review

1. What type(s) of data are generated from the coordination examination?
2. What roles do the cerebellum, basal ganglia, and the dorsal column–medial lemniscal pathway play in coordinated movement?
3. Identify and describe the common coordination impairments associated with pathology of the cerebellum, basal ganglia, and the dorsal column–medial lemniscal pathway.
4. What predictable aspects of normal aging impact coordinated movement?
5. Assume you are about to initiate a coordination examination. What screenings would be appropriate and why; and in what order would you perform the screenings?
6. Identify, differentiate, and describe the *motor task requirements* and *movement capabilities* addressed within a coordination examination.

7. Explain the purpose of a preliminary observation of the patient prior to the coordination examination. What types of activities should be observed? What information should be gathered?
8. Differentiate between the types of activities included in equilibrium versus nonequilibrium coordination tests. Why is the term "nonequilibrium" considered something of a misnomer as a subdivision of coordination tests?
9. What data can a systematic gait analysis add to the examination of coordination?
10. What questions related to patient performance should be considered during a coordination examination to help direct the therapist's observations?

Case Study

The patient is a 62-year-old man with a 5-year history of Parkinson's disease. Since the time of the diagnosis, he reports a progressive decline in functional activity level. With encouragement from his wife and children, he took an early retirement 3 years ago from his career as a commercial airline pilot. He lives with his wife of 38 years in a one-level suburban home. His four adult children all live in neighboring communities.

Initial examination reveals the following:

- Movements are decreased and slowed.
- A uniform, constant resistance is felt as the extremities are moved passively; patient reports an overall feeling of "stiffness."
- Involuntary, rhythmic, oscillatory movements of the distal upper extremities are noted at rest.
- Regular incidence of falls (two to three times per week) is reported; standing balance is easily displaced with tendency to fall stiffly; patient has difficulty changing direction of movement or stopping a movement.
- Patient has difficulty alternating distal UE movements required for buttoning shirts, using eating utensils, and writing.
- Patient has difficulty making movement transitions, such as standing up from a chair or rolling from prone to supine.

The patient's medication is about to be changed from L-dopa alone to a combination of L-dopa with carbidopa (Sinemet). The physical therapy referral is for examination prior to the change in medication to document baseline function. Following the medication change, the examination will be repeated and treatment initiated.

GUIDING QUESTIONS

1. Identify the terms used to describe the following features of basal ganglia disorders: (a) decreased and slowed movement; (b) a uniform constant resistance to passive movement; and (c) involuntary, rhythmic, oscillatory movements of the distal upper extremities at rest.
2. What general movement impairments would be evident in the presence of bradykinesia?
3. Identify the nonequilibrium coordination tests appropriate for examining the patient's movement capabilities in performing alternating distal UE movements.
4. Identify the equilibrium coordination tests appropriate for examining the patient's altered postural reactions and balance.
5. Describe a plan for documenting findings from the examination.

References

1. American Physical Therapy Association: Guide to physical therapist practice. Phys Ther 81:1, 2001.
2. Preston, LA: Motor control. In Pedretti, LW, and Early, MB (eds): Occupational Therapy: Practice Skills for Physical Dysfunction, ed 5. CV Mosby, St. Louis, 2001, p 360.
3. Ghez, C, and Krakauer, J: The organization of movement. In Kandel, ER, Schwartz, JH, and Jessell, TM (eds): Principles of Neural Science, ed. 4, McGraw-Hill, New York, 2000, p 653.
4. Byl, NN: Multisensory control of upper extremity function. Neurology Report (now JNPT) 26(1):32, 2002.
5. Schmidt, RA, and Lee, TD: Motor Control and Learning: A Behavioral Emphasis, ed 4. Human Kinetics, Champaign, IL, 2005.
6. Wiesendanger, M, and Serrien, DJ: Toward a physiological understanding of human dexterity. News Physiol Sci 16:228, 2001.
7. Weiss, P, and Jeannerod, M: Getting a grasp on coordination. News Physiol Sci 13:70, 1998.
8. Carson, RG, Riek, S, and Byblow, WD: The timing of intralimb coordination. J Mot Behav 31(2):113, 1999.
9. Field-Fote, EC, and Tepavac, D: Improved intralimb coordination in people with incomplete spinal cord injury following training with body weight support and electrical stimulation. Phys Ther 82(7), 2002.
10. Ridderikkoff, A, et al: Mirrored EMG activity during unimanual rhythmic movements. Neurosci Lett 381(3):228, 2005.
11. Cauraugh, JH, and Summers, JJ: Neural plasticity and bilateral movements: A rehabilitation approach for chronic stroke. Prog Neurobiol 75(5):309, 2005.
12. Donker, SF, Daffertshofer, A, and Beek, PJ: Effects of velocity and limb loading on the coordination between limb movements during walking. J Mot Behav 37(3):217, 2005.
13. Rose, DK, and Winstein, CJ: The co-ordination of bimanual rapid aiming movements following stroke. Clin Rehabil 19(4):452, 2005.
14. Pellecchia, GL, and Turvey, MT: Cognitive activity shifts the attractors of bimanual rhythmic coordination. J Mot Behav 33(1):9, 2001.
15. Debaere, F, et al: Brain areas involved in interlimb coordination: A distributed network. Neuroimage 14(5):947, 2001.

16. de Jong, BM, et al: The distribution of cerebral activity related to visuomotor coordination indicating perceptual and executional specialization. Brain Res Cogn Brain Res 8(1):45, 1999.
17. Campos, TF, et al: Diurnal variation in a visual-motor coordination test in healthy humans. Biol Rhythm Res 32(2):255, 2003.
18. Chen, Y, Ding, M, and Kelso, JAS: Task-related power and coherence changes in neuromagnetic activity during visuomotor coordination. Exp Brain Res 148(1):105, 2003.
19. Gribble, PL, et al: Hand-eye coordination for rapid pointing movements. Arm movement direction and distance are specified prior to saccade onset. Exp Brain Res 145(3):372, 2002.
20. Snyder, LH, et al: Eye-hand coordination: Saccades are faster when accompanied by a coordinated arm movement. J Neurophysiol 87(5):2279, 2002.
21. Tseng, Y, Scholz, JP, and Schoner, G: Goal-equivalent joint coordination in pointing: Affect of vision and arm dominance. Motor Control 6(2):183, 2002.
22. Gilman, S, and Newman, SW: Manter and Gatz's Essentials of Clinical Neuroanatomy and Neurophysiology, ed 10. FA Davis, Philadelphia, 2003.
23. Bear, MF, Connors, BW, and Paradiso, MA: Neuroscience: Exploring the Brain, ed 2. Lippincott Williams & Wilkins, Philadelphia, 2001.
24. Nolte, J: The Human Brain: An Introduction to Its Functional Anatomy, ed 5. CV Mosby, St. Louis, 2002.
25. Krakauer, J, and Ghez, C: Voluntary movement. In Kandel, ER, Schwartz, JH, and Jessell, TM: Principles of Neural Science, ed. 4, McGraw-Hill, New York, 2000, p 756.
26. Mihailoff, GA, and Haines, DE: Motor system II: Corticofugal systems and the control of movement. In Haines, DE (ed): Fundamental Neuroscience, ed 2. Churchill Livingstone, New York, 2002, p 387.
27. Kingsley, RE: Concise Text of Neuroscience, ed 2. Lippincott Williams & Wilkins, Philadelphia, 2000.
28. Lundy-Ekman, L: Neuroscience: Fundamentals for Rehabilitation, ed 2. WB Saunders, Philadelphia, 2002.
29. Martin, JH: Neuroanatomy: Text and Atlas, ed 3. McGraw Hill, New York, 2003.
30. Guyton, AC, and Hall, JE: Textbook of Medical Physiology, ed 10. WB Saunders, Philadelphia, 2000.
31. Afifi, AK, and Bergman, RA: Functional Neuroanatomy: Text and Atlas, ed 2. Lange Medical Books/McGraw-Hill, New York, 2005.
32. Ghez, C, and Thach, WT: The cerebellum. In Kandel, ER, Schwartz, JH, and Jessell, TM (eds): Principles of Neural Science, ed. 4, McGraw-Hill, New York, 2000, p 832.
33. Melnick, ME, and Oremland, B: Movement dysfunction associated with cerebellar problems. In Umphred, DA (ed): Neurological Rehabilitation, ed. 4. CV Mosby, St. Louis, 2001, p 717.
34. Melnick, ME: Basal ganglia disorders: Metabolic, hereditary, and genetic disorders in adults. In Umphred, DA (ed): Neurological Rehabilitation, ed. 4. CV Mosby, St. Louis, 2001, p 661.
35. DeLong, MR: The basal ganglia. In Kandel, ER, Schwartz, JH, and Jessell, TM (eds): Principles of Neural Science, ed. 4. McGraw-Hill, New York, 2000, p 853.
36. Porter, LL: Motor 2: Higher centers. In Cohen, H (ed): Neuroscience for Rehabilitation, ed 2. Lippincott Williams & Wilkins, Philadelphia, 1999, p 243.
37. Ghez, C, and Gordon, J: Voluntary Movement. In Kandel, ER, Schwartz, JH, and Jessell, TM et al (eds): Essentials of Neural Science and Behavior. Appleton & Lange, E. Norwalk, CT, 1995, p 529.
38. Hudson, CC, and Krebs, DE: Frontal plane dynamic stability and coordination in subjects with cerebellar degeneration. Exp Brain Res 132(1):103, 2000.
39. Joyal, CC, et al: Effects of midline and lateral cerebellar lesions on motor coordination and spatial orientation. Brain Res 739(1-2):1, 1996.
40. Palliyath, S, et al: Gait in patients with cerebellar ataxia. Mov Disord 13(6):958, 1998.
41. Perlman, SL: Cerebellar ataxia. Curr Treat Options Neurol 2(3):215, 2000.
42. Salman, MS: The cerebellum: It's about time! But timing is not everything—New insights into the role of the cerebellum in timing motor and cognitive tasks. J Child Neurol 17:1, 2002.
43. Serrien, DJ, and Wiesendanger, M: Grip-load force coordination in cerebellar patients. Exp Brain Res 128(1–2):76, 1999.
44. Verleger, R, et al: Consequences of altered cerebellar input for the cortical regulation of motor coordination, as reflected in EEG potentials. Exp Brain Res 127(4):409, 1999.
45. Waxman, SG: Correlative Neuroanatomy, ed 24. New York, Lange Medical Books/McGraw-Hill, 2000.
46. Gutman, SA: Quick Reference Neuroscience for Rehabilitation Professionals: The Essential Neurologic Principles Underlying Rehabilitation Practice. Slack, Thorofare, NJ, 2001.
47. Fuller, KS: Introduction to central nervous system disorders. In Goodman, CC, Boissonnault, WG, and Fuller, KS (eds): Pathology: Implications for the Physical Therapist, ed 2. WB Saunders, Philadelphia, 2003, p 977.
48. Alberts, JL, et al: Disruptions in the reach-to-grasp actions of Parkinson's patients. Exp Brain Res 134(3):353, 2000.
49. Almeida, QJ, Wishart, LR, and Lee, TD (eds): Bimanual coordination deficits with Parkinson's disease: The influence of movement speed and external cueing. Mov Disord 17(1):30, 2002.
50. Byblow, WD, et al: Bimanual coordination in Parkinson's disease: Deficits in movement frequency, amplitude, and pattern switching. Mov Disord 17(1):20, 2002.
51. Nowak, DA, and Hermsdorfer, J: Coordination of grip and load forces during vertical point-to-point movements with a grasped object in Parkinson's disease. Behav Neurosci 116(5):837, 2002.
52. Poizner, H, et al: The timing of arm-trunk coordination is deficient and vision-dependent in Parkinson's patients during reaching movements. Exp Brain Res 133(3):279, 2000.
53. van den Berg, C, et al: Coordination disorders in patients with Parkinson's disease: A study of paced rhythmic forearm movements. Exp Brain Res 134(2):174, 2000.
54. Gordon, AM, et al: Coordination of prehensile forces during precision grip in Huntington's disease. Exp Neurol 163(1):136, 2000.
55. Quinn, L, et al:Altered movement trajectories and force control during object transport in Huntington's disease. Mov Disord 16(3):469, 2001.
56. Serrien, DJ, Burgunder, KM, and Wiesendanger, M: Control of manipulative forces during unimanual and bimanual tasks in patients with Huntington's disease. Exp Brain Res 143(3):328, 2002.
57. Ma, TP: The basal nuclei. In Haines, DE (ed): Fundamental Neuroscience, ed 2. Churchill Livingstone, New York, 2002, p 405.
58. Kiernan, JA: Barr's The Human Nervous System: An Anatomical Viewpoint, ed 8. Lippincott Williams & Wilkins, Philadelphia, 2005.
59. Shumway-Cook, A, and Woollacott, MH: Motor Control: Theory and Practical Applications, ed 2. Lippincott Williams & Wilkins, Philadelphia, 2001.
60. Briggs, RV, et al: Balance performance among noninstitutionalized elderly women. Phys Ther 69(9):748, 1989.
61. Buchman, AS, et al: Effect of age and gender in the control of elbow flexion movements. J Mot Behav 32(4):391, 2000.
62. Capranica, L, et al: Field evaluation of cycled coupled movements of hand and foot in older individuals. Gerontology 50(6):399, 2004.
63. Desrosiers, J, et al: Upper extremity performance test for the elderly (TEMPA): Normative data and correlates with sensorimotor parameters. Arch Phys Med Rehabil 76(12):1125, 1995.
64. Hartley, AA: Age differences in dual-task interference are localized to response-generation processes. Psychol Aging 16(1):47, 2000.
65. Ketcham, CJ, Dounskaia, NV, and Stelmach, GE: Age-related differences in the control of multijoint movements. Motor Control 8(4):422, 2004.
66. Ketcham, CJ, et al: Age-related kinematic differences as influenced by task difficulty, target size, and movement amplitude. J Gerontol B Psychol Sci Soc Sci 57(1):P54, 2002.
67. Larsson, L, and Ramamurthy, B: Aging-related changes in skeletal muscle: Mechanisms and interventions. Drugs Aging 17(4):303, 2000.
68. Lindenberger, U, Marsiske, M, and Baltes, PB: Memorizing while walking: Increase in dual-task costs from young adulthood to old age. Psychol Aging 15(3):417, 2000.
69. McGibbon, CA, and Krebs DE: Age-related changes in lower trunk coordination and energy transfer during gait. J Neurophysiol 85(5):1923, 2001.

70. Prioli, AC, Freitas Junio, PB, and Barela JA: Physical activity and postural control in the elderly: Coupling between visual information and body sway. Gerontology 51(3):145, 2005.
71. Sediler, RD, Alberts, JL, and Stelmach, GE: Changes in multi-joint performance with age. Motor Control 6(1):19, 2002.
72. Seidler-Dobrin, RD, He, J, and Stelmach, GE: Coactivation to reduce variability in the elderly. Motor Control 2(4):314, 1998.
73. Serrien, DJ, Swinnen, SP, and Stelmach, GE: Age-related deterioration of coordinated interlimb behavior. J Gerontol B Psychol Sci Soc Sci 55(5):P295, 2000.
74. Shkuratova, N, Morris, ME, and Huxham, F: Effects of age on balance control during walking. Arch Phys Med Rehabil 85(4):582, 2004.
75. Sparrow, WA, et al: Aging effects on the metabolic and cognitive energy cost of interlimb coordination. J Gerontol A Biol Sci Med Sci 60(3):312, 2005.
76. Williams, K, Haywood, K, and VanSant, A: Changes in throwing by older adults: A longitudinal investigation. Res Q Exerc Sport 69(1):1, 1998.
77. Wu, T, and Hallett, M: The influence of normal human ageing on automatic movements. J Physiol 562(Pt 2):605, 2005.
78. Bottomley, JM, and Lewis, CB: Geriatric Rehabilitation: A Clinical Approach, ed 2. Prentice-Hall, Upper Saddle River, NJ, 2003.
79. Spirduso, WW, Francis, KL, and MacRae, PG: Physical Dimensions of Aging, ed 2. Human Kinetics, Champaign, IL, 2005.
80. Lewis, CB: Aging: The Health-Care Challenge, ed 4. FA Davis, Philadelphia, 2002.
81. Hurley, BF: Age, gender, and muscular strength. J Gerontol A Biol Sci Med Sci 50A:41, 1995.
82. Frontera, WR, et al: A cross-sectional study of muscle strength and mass in 45 to 78-year-old men and women. J Appl Physiol 71:644, 1991.
83. Harries, UJ, and Bassey, EJ: Torque-velocity relationships for the knee extensors in women in their 3rd and 7th decades. Eur J Appl Physiol 60:187, 1990.
84. Kallman, DA, Plato, CC, and Tobin, JD: The role of muscle loss in the age-related decline of grip strength: Cross-sectional and longitudinal perspectives. J Gerontol A Biol Sci Med 45: M82, 1990.
85. Lindle, RS, et al: Age and gender comparisons of muscle strength in 654 women and men aged 20-93 yr. J Appl Physiol 83(5):1581, 1997.
86. Bortz, WM: Disuse and aging. JAMA 248:1203, 1982.
87. Craik, RL: Sensorimotor changes and adaptation in the older adult. In Guccione, AA (ed): Geriatric Physical Therapy. Mosby-Year Book, St. Louis, 1993, p 71.
88. Grimby, G, et al: Morphology and enzymatic capacity in arm and leg muscles in 78–81 year old men and women. Acta Physiol Scand 115(1):125, 1982.
89. Stelmach, GE, and Worthingham, CJ: Sensory motor deficits related to postural stability. Clin Geriatr Med 1:679, 1985.
90. Welford, AT: Between bodily changes and performance: Some possible reasons for slowing with age. Exp Aging Res 10:73, 1984.
91. Spirduso, WW: Physical fitness, aging, and psychomotor speed: A review. J Gerontol 35:850, 1980.
92. Weiss, AT: Between bodily changes and performance: Some possible reasons for slowing with age. Exp Aging Res 10:73, 1984.
93. Allander, E, et al: Normal range of joint movements in shoulder, hip, wrist and thumb with special reference to side: A comparison between two populations. Int J Epidemiol 3(3):253, 1974.
94. Roach, KE, and Miles, TP: Normal hip and knee active range of motion: The relationship to age. Phys Ther 71(9):656, 1991.
95. James, B, and Parker, AW: Active and passive mobility of lower limb joints in elderly men and women. Am J Phys Med Rehabil 68(4):162, 1989.
96. DiFabio, RP, and Emasithi, A: Aging and the mechanisms underlying head and postural control during voluntary motion. Phys Ther 77:458, 1997.
97. Woollacott, MH, and Tang, PF: Balance control during walking in the older adult: Research and its implications. Phys Ther 77:646, 1997.
98. Woollacott, MH: Changes in posture and voluntary control in the elderly: Research findings and rehabilitation. Top Geriatr Rehabil 5:1, 1990.
99. Pyykko, I, et al: Postural control in elderly subjects. Age Ageing 19:215, 1990.
100. King, MB, Judge, JO, and Wolfson, L: King, MB, et al: Functional base of support decreases with age. J Gerontol 49(6):M258, 1994.
101. Duncan, PW, et al: Functional reach: Predictive validity in a sample of elderly male veterans. J Gerontol 47(3):M93, 1992.
102. Weiner, DK, et al: Functional reach: A marker of physical frailty. J Am Geriatr Soc 40(3):203, 1992.
103. Robinovitch, SN, and Cronin, T: Perception of postural limits in elderly nursing home and day care participants. J Gerontol A Biol Sci Med Sci 54(3):B124, 1999.
104. Ruff, RM, and Parker, SB: Gender- and age-specific changes in motor speed and eye-hand coordination in adults: Normative values for the finger tapping and grooved pegboard tests. Percept Mot Skills 76:1219, 1993.
105. Keshner, EA: Head-trunk coordination in elderly subjects during linear anterior-posterior translations. Exp Brain Res 158:213, 2004.
106. Vandervoort, AA: Aging of the human neuromuscular system. Muscle Nerve 25(1):17, 2002.
107. Barry, BK, and Carson, RG: The consequences of resistance training for movement control in older adults. J Gerontol A Biol Sci Med Sci 59(7):730, 2004.
108. Jette, AM, et al: Exercise—it's never too late: The strong-for-life program. Am J Public Health 89(1):66, 1999.
109. King, MB, et al: The Performance Enhancement Project: Improving physical performance in older persons. Arch Phys Med Rehabil 83(8):1060, 2002.
110. King, MB, et al: Reliability and responsiveness of two physical performance measures examined in the context of a functional training intervention. Phys Ther 80(1):8, 2000.
111. Islam, MM, et al: Effects of combined sensory and muscular training on balance in Japanese older adults. Prev Med 39(6):1148, 2004.
112. Ramsbottom, R, et al: The effect of 6 months training on leg power, balance, and functional mobility of independently living adults over 70 years old. J Aging Phys Act 12(4):497, 2004.
113. Rubenstein, LZ, et al: Effects of a group exercise program on strength, mobility, and falls among fall-prone elderly men. J Gerontol A Biol Sci Med Sci 55(6):M317, 2000.
114. Toraman, NF, Erman, A, and Agyar, E: Effects of multicomponent training on functional fitness in older adults. J Aging Phys Act 12(4):538, 2004.
115. United States (US) Census Bureau: US Interim Projections by Age, Sex, Race, and Hispanic Origin (Table 2a), 2004. Retrieved July 14, 2005 from http://www.census.gov/ipc/www/usinterimproj/.
116. DeMont, ME, and Peatman, NL: Communication, values, and the quality of life. In Guccione, AA (ed): Geriatric Physical Therapy. Mosby-Year Book, St. Louis, 1993, p 21.
117. Janos, SC, and Boissonnault, WG: Upper quarter screening examination. In Boissonnault, WG (ed): Primary Care for the Physical Therspist: Examination and Triage. WB Saunders, Philadelphia, 2005, p 138.
118. Norkin, CC, and White, DJ: Measurement of Joint Motion: A Guide to Goniometry, ed 3. FA Davis, Philadelphia, 2003.
119. Hislop, HJ, and Montgomery, J: Daniels and Worthingham's Muscle Testing, ed 7. WB Saunders, Philadelphia, 2002.
120. Kendall, FP, et al: Muscles Testing and Function with Posture and Pain, ed 5. Lippincott Williams & Wilkins, Philadelphia, 2005.
121. Mathias, S, et al: Balance in elderly patients: The "get-up and go" test. Arch Med Rehabil 67:387, 1986.
122. Podsiadlo, D, and Richardson, S: The timed "up and go": A test of basic functional mobility for frail elderly persons. J Am Geriatr Soc 39:142, 1991.
123. Granger, CV, et al: Functional assessment scales: A study of persons with multiple sclerosis. Arch Phys Med Rehabil 71:870, 1990.
124. Granger, CV, et al: Advance in functional assessment for medical rehabilitation. Top Geriatr Rehabil 1:59, 1986.
125. Keith, RA, et al: The functional independence measure. Adv Clin Rehabil 1:6, 1987.
126. Bergner, M, et al: The sickness impact profile: Development and final revision of a health status measure. Med Care 19:787, 1981.
127. Follick, MJ, et al: The sickness impact profile: A global measure of disability in chronic low back pain. Pain 21:67, 1985.

128. Winograd, CH, et al: Development of a physical performance and mobility examination. J Am Geriatr Soc 42:743, 1994.
129. Tinetti, M, et al: A fall risk index for elderly patients based on number of chronic disabilities. Am J Med 80:429, 1986.
130. Tinetti, M, and Ginter, S: Identifying mobility dysfunctions in elderly patients: Standard neuromuscular examination or direct assessment? JAMA 259:1190, 1988.
131. Wolfson, L, et al: Gait assessment in the elderly: A gait abnormality rating scale and its relation to falls. J Gerontol 45:M12, 1990.
132. Rose, D: Fall Proof: A Comprehensive Balance and Mobility Training Program. Human Kinetics, Champaign IL, 2003.
133. Berg, K, et al: Measuring balance in the elderly: Preliminary development of an instrument. Physiother Can 41:304, 1989.
134. Berg, K, et al: A comparison of clinical and laboratory measures of postural balance in an elderly population. Arch Phys Med Rehabil 73:1073, 1992.
135. Berg, K, et al: Measuring balance in the elderly: Validation of an instrument. Can J Public Health 83(Suppl 2):S7, 1992.
136. Harada, N, et al: Physical therapy to improve functioning of older people in residential care facilities. Phys Ther 75:830, 1995.
137. Cruz, VW: Evaluation of coordination: A clinical model. Clin Manage Phys Ther 6:6, 1986.
138. Despres, C, Lamoureux, D, and Beuter, A: Standardization of a neuromotor test battery: The CATSYS system. Neurotoxicology 21(5):725, 2000.
139. Edwards, R, and Beuter, A: Sensitivity and specificity of a portable system measuring postural tremor. Neurotoxicol Teratol 19(2):95, 1997.
140. Edwards, R, and Beuter, A: Indexes for identification of abnormal tremor using computer tremor evaluation systems. IEEE Trans Biomed Eng 46(7):895, 1999.
141. Orsnes, GB, and Sorensen, PS: Evaluation of electronic equipment for quantitative registration of tremor. Acta Neurol Scand 97(1):36, 1998.
142. Netterstrom, B, Guldager, B, and Heeboll, J: Acute mercury intoxication examined with coordination ability and tremor. Neurotoxicol Teratol 18(4):505, 1996.
143. Kilburn, KH, Warshaw, RH, and Hanscom, B: Are hearing loss and balance dysfunction linked in construction iron workers? Br J Ind Med 49(2):138, 1992.
144. Kilburn, KH, Warshaw, RH, and Hanscom, B: Balance measured by head (and trunk) tracking and a force platform in chemically (PCB and TCE) exposed and referent subjects. Occup Environ Med 51(6):381, 1994.
145. Gerr, F, Letz, R, and Green, RC: Relationships between quantitative measures and neurologist's clinical rating of tremor and standing steadiness in two epidemiological studies. Neurotoxicology 21(5):753, 2000.
146. Anstey, KJ, et al: Biomarkers, health, lifestyle, and demographic variables as correlates of reaction time performance in early, middle, and late adulthood. Q J Exp Psychol A 58(1):5, 2005.
147. Kilburn, KH, et al: An examination of factors that could affect choice reaction time in histology technicians. Am J Ind Med 15(6):679, 1989.
148. Miller, JA, et al: Choice (CRT) and simple reaction times (SRT) compared in laboratory technicians: Factors influencing reaction times and a predictive model. Am J Ind Med 15(6):687, 1989.
149. Jebson, RH, et al: An objective and standardized test of hand function. Arch Phys Med Rehabil 50:311, 1969.
150. Hackel, ME, et al: Changes in hand function in the aging adult as determined by the Jebsen test of hand function. Phys Ther 72:373, 1992.
151. Mathiowetz, V: Role of physical performance component evaluations in occupational therapy functional assessment. Am J Occup Ther 47:228, 1993.
152. Taylor, N, et al: Evaluation of hand function in children. Arch Phys Med Rehabil 54:129, 1973.
153. Asher, IE: Occupational Therapy Assessment Tools: An Annotated Index, ed 2. The American Occupational Therapy Association, Bethesda, MD, 1996.
154. Gloss, DS, and Wardle, MG: Use of the Minnesota Rate of Manipulation Test for disability evaluation. Percept Mot Skills 55(2):527, 1982.
155. Surrey, LR, et al: A comparison of performance outcomes between the Minnesota Rate of Manipulation Test and the Minnesota Manual Dexterity Test. Work 20(2):97, 2003.
156. Mathiowetz, V, et al: The Purdue pegboard: Norms for 14- to 19-year-olds. Am J Occup Ther 40:174, 1986.
157. Gallus, J, and Mathiowetz, V: Test-retest reliability of the Purdue Pegboard for persons with multiple sclerosis Am J Occup Ther 57(1):108, 2003.

Supplemental Readings

Adamovish, SV, et al: Hand trajectory invariance in reaching movements involving the trunk. Exp Brain Res 138(3):288, 2001.
Allum, JH, et al: Differences between trunk sway characteristics on a foam support surface and on the Equitest ankle-sway-referenced support surface. Gait Posture 16(3):264, 2002.
Camicioli, R, Panzer, VP, and Kaye, J: Balance in the healthy elderly: Posturography and clinical assessment. Arch Neurol 54(8):976, 1997.
Carson, RG, et al: Role of peripheral afference during acquisition of a complex coordination task. Exp Brain Res 144(4):496, 2002.
Debaere, F, et al: Brain areas involved in interlimb coordination: A distributed network. Neuroimage 14(5):947, 2001.
Debaere, F, et al: Changes in brain activation during the acquisition of a new bimanual coordination task. Neuropsychologia 42(7):855, 2004.
Dounskaia, N, Van Gemmert, AW, and Stelmach, GE:Dounskaia, N, et al: Interjoint coordination during handwriting-like movements. Exp Brain Res 135(1):127, 2000.
Exner, C, Koschack, J, and Irle, E: The differential role of premotor frontal cortex and basal ganglia in motor sequence learning: Evidence from focal basal ganglia lesions. Learn Mem 9(6):376, 2002.
Gianna-Poulin, C, et al: Dynamic posturography in humans imagining a fixed spatial reference. Acta Otolaryngol 124(8):937, 2004.
Hay, L, and Redon, C: Development of postural adaptation to arm raising. Exp Brain Res 139(2):224, 2001.
Henriques, DY, and Crawford, JD: Role of eye, head, and shoulder geometry in the planning of accurate arm movements. J Neurophysiol 87(4):1677, 2002.
Krebs, DE, McGibbon, CA, and Goldvasser, D: Analysis of postural perturbation responses. IEEE Trans Neural Syst Rehabil Eng 9(1):76, 2001.
Krisnamoorthy, V, et al: Muscle modes during shifts of the center of pressure by standing persons: Effect of instability and additional support. Exp Brain Res 157:18, 2004.
Leiguarda, R, et al: Disruption of spatial organization and interjoint coordination in Parkinson's disease, progressive supranuclear palsy, and multiple system atrophy. Mov Disord 15(4):627, 2000.
Nardone, A, et al: Postural coordination in elderly subjects standing on a periodically moving platform. Arch Phys Med Rehabil 81(9):1217, 2000.
Pelz, J, Hayhoe, M, and Loeber, R: The coordination of eye, head, and hand movements in a natural task. Exp Brain Res 139(3):266, 2001.
Scholz, JP, et al: Understanding finger coordination through analysis of the structure of force variability. Biol Cybern 86: 29, 2002.
Shields, RK, et al: Proprioceptive coordination of movement sequences in humans. Clin Neurophysiol 116(1):87, 2005.
Speers, RA, Kuo, AD, and Horak, FB: Contributions of altered sensation and feedback responses to changes in coordination of postural control due to aging. Gait Posture 16(1):20, 2002.
Spirduso, WW, et al: Quantification of manual force control and tremor. J Mot Behav 37(3):197, 2005.
Tseng, Y, Scholz, JP, and Schoner, G: Goal-equivalent joint coordination in pointing: Affect of vision and arm dominance. Motor Control 6:183, 2002.
Wiesendanger, M, and Serrien, DJ: Neurological problems affecting hand dexterity. Brain Res Brain Res Rev 36(2–3):161, 2001.

CHAPTER

8

LEARNING OBJECTIVES

1. Identify the purposes and components of the examination of motor function: motor control and motor learning.
2. Describe the examination process and specific measures of motor function.
3. Describe common deficits associated with disorders of motor function.
4. Discuss factors that influence the complexity of the motor examination and evaluation process.
5. Discuss factors that influence determination of the physical therapy diagnosis.
6. Using the case study example, apply clinical decision making skills in evaluating motor function data.

Examination of Motor Function: Motor Control and Motor Learning

Susan B. O'Sullivan, PT, EdD

OUTLINE

Overview of Motor Function

Motor control evolves from a complex set of neural, physical, and behavioral processes that govern posture and movement. Some movements have a genetic basis and emerge through processes of normal growth and development. Examples of these include the reflex patterns that predominate during much of early life. Other movements, termed **motor skills**, are learned through interaction and exploration of the environment. Practice and feedback are important variables in defining motor learning and motor skill development. Sensory information about movement is used to guide and shape the development of the motor program. A **motor program** is defined as "an abstract representation that, when initiated, results in the production of a coordinated movement sequence."[1, p 466] A **motor plan** (*complex motor program*) is an idea or plan for purposeful movement that is made up of several component motor programs. **Motor memory** (*procedural memory*) involves the recall of motor programs or subroutines and includes information on (1) initial movement conditions; (2) how the movement felt, looked, and sounded (sensory consequences); (3) specific movement parameters; and (4) outcome of the movement (knowledge of results). The term **neuroplasticity** refers to the capacity of the brain to adapt to injury through mechanisms of repair and change. Neuroplasticity includes "a continuum from short-term changes in the efficiency or strength of synaptic connections to long-term structural changes in the organization and numbers of connections among neurons."[2, p 92] As learning progresses there is a shift from short-term to long-term memory processes. Memory allows for continued access of this information for repeat performance or modification of existing patterns of movement.

Motor skills are acquired and modified by actions of the central nervous system (CNS) through processes of **motor learning**. Motor learning is defined as "a set of internal processes associated with practice or experience leading to relatively permanent changes in the capability for skilled behavior."[1, p 466] The CNS organizes and integrates vast amounts of sensory information. **Feedback** is response-produced information received during or after the movement and is used to monitor output for corrective actions. **Feedforward**, the sending of signals in advance of movement to ready the sensorimotor systems, allows for anticipatory adjustments in postural activity. Processing of information by the CNS is both serial and parallel, leading to the production of coordinated movement. **Coordination** is the ability to execute smooth, accurate, and controlled motor responses. **Coordinative structures** (synergistic units) are the "functionally specific units of muscles and joints that are constrained by the nervous system to act cooperatively to produce an action."[3, p 416]

Different motor control theories have been proposed to explain the cooperative actions of the CNS that allow accommodation of movement to the specific demands of the task and the environment. Two of the major ones are dynamical systems theory and hierarchical theory. *Dynamical systems control theory* is based on a distributed model of motor control. A basic concept of this theory is that units of the CNS are organized around specific task demands (termed *task systems*). The entire CNS may be necessary for complex tasks, whereas only small portions may be needed for simple tasks. Command levels vary depending on the specific task executed. Thus, the highest level of command may not be required in the execution of some simple movements.[4] *Hierarchical control theory* is based on organization of the CNS into higher, middle, and lower levels with top-down control. The highest level components include the association cortex and portions of the basal ganglia which function to organize sensorimotor information and are responsible for decision making. Middle level components include the sensorimotor cortex, cerebellum, basal ganglia, and brainstem. These areas shape and define the specific motor programs and initiate commands. The lowest level component is the spinal cord, which executes the commands, translating them into the final muscle actions. In hierarchical theory, initial decision making for acquisition of a skill requires activation of the highest level. As skill learning progresses, control is systematically shifted to lower level processing responsible for motor programming.[1]

Damage to the CNS interferes with motor function processes. Lesions affecting areas of the CNS can produce specific, recognizable deficits that are consistent among patients (e.g., patients with upper motor neuron syndrome). Individual differences in CNS plasticity, recovery, and functional outcomes can be expected. In conditions with widespread damage to the CNS (e.g., traumatic brain injury) the resultant problems in motor function are numerous, complex, and difficult to delineate. An accurate picture of the scope of deficits may not be readily apparent on initial examination. A process of reexamination over time will generally yield an understanding of the patient's performance capabilities and deficits. The comprehensive examination focuses on delineation of impairments, functional limitations, and disabilities. Those impairments that directly impact on function should be clearly identified. Anticipated goals, expected outcomes, and plan of care (POC) can then be effectively developed.

Examination of Motor Function

An examination of motor function involves three components: (1) patient history, (2) a review of relevant systems, and (3) specific tests and measures that allow formulation of the diagnosis, prognosis, and plan of care.[5]

Patient History

During the patient/client history, information is gathered on: (1) general demographics; (2) social history; (3) employment/work (job/school/play); (4) living environment; (5) general health status; (6) social/health habits; (7) family history; (8) medical/surgical history; (9) current condition(s)/chief complaint(s); (10) functional status and activity level; (11) medications; and (12) other clinical tests. Information is obtained from the patient and other interested persons (family members, significant others, and caregivers). If the patient is unable to communicate accurate and meaningful information, as is frequently the case with injury to the brain, data must be gathered from other sources (e.g., family members, caregivers). A review of the medical record can be used to verify and triangulate data obtained from personal communications. Often, the medical record of a patient with pronounced deficits in motor function (e.g., the patient with traumatic brain injury) is filled with volumes of data that can be unwieldy and difficult to sort through. The therapist can benefit from the application of a framework to identify and classify problems. The disablement model, focusing on impairments, functional limitations, and disabilities, provides such a useful framework and is an important element of the American Physical Therapy Association's *Guide to Physical Therapist Practice*.[5] (See Chapter 1.)

Systems Review

A systems review serves the purpose of a screening examination; that is, a brief or limited examination of body systems. The physical therapist can then use this information to identify potential problems that will require more extensive testing. For example, screening examinations for posture and tone may reveal significant impairments and functional limitations. More detailed tests and measures are then required to delineate the exact nature of the problems uncovered. Sometimes screening examinations reveal problems in communication and/or cognition that preclude further testing. For example, a patient with stroke and severe communication and cognitive impairments will be unable to follow directions and cooperate with many individual tests of physical function. The therapist will document this in the medical record as *unable to test at the present time due to severe communication/cognitive deficits*.

Tests and Measures

Specific parameters of dyscontrol should be closely examined using appropriate tests and measures. If the test accurately measures the parameter of performance being examined, it is said to have *validity*. Validity can be established through construct, content, and criterion-based validity (concurrent, predictive, and prescriptive). The *reliability* of an instrument is reflected in the consistency of results obtained by a single examiner over repeat trials (intrarater reliability) or among multiple examiners (interrater reliability). *Sensitivity* refers to the proportion of times that a method of analysis correctly identifies an abnormality as being present (true positive). *Specificity* refers to the proportion of times that a method of analysis correctly identifies an abnormality as being absent (true negative). Therapists should select standardized methods and instruments with established validity and reliability, consistent with the American Physical Therapy Association's goal of evidence-based practice (EBP).

An examination of motor function is a multifaceted process that requires a number of different specific tests and measures. Instruments can be qualitative, utilizing observations of complex aspects of performance. Insights and understanding of patterns of movement or postures are developed from inductive reasoning (formulating generalizations from specific observations). The experienced therapist or expert clinician is far more efficient in reaching decisions about qualitative performance than the novice therapist.[6,7] Quantitative instruments use objective measurement as a way of examining performance. Documentation constraints imposed by the health care system and third-party payers increasingly emphasize objective instruments as proof of the need for services and the effectiveness of services. However, many aspects of motor function are not easily measured. For example, motor learning is not directly measurable but rather is inferred from measures of performance, retention, generalizability, and adaptability. Thus these constructs are used to infer changes in the CNS that occur with learning. The therapist must be sensitive to the nature of the variables being examined and identify appropriate measures that provide a meaningful analysis of patient function. It is not likely that any one measure will provide all of the data needed for the examination of motor function.

Reexaminations are performed to determine if goals and outcomes are being met, and if the patient is benefiting from the plan of care. Interventions can then be modified or redirected as appropriate. Successful achievement of anticipated goals and expected outcomes is an indication for discharge and referral for follow-up or additional services. Reexamination is also an important quality assurance measure.

Elements of the Motor Function Examination

Mental Status

An examination of mental status includes (1) level of consciousness; (2) orientation; (3) attention; (4) memory; and (5) executive or higher cognitive functions (e.g., calculating abilities, abstract thinking, constructional ability). Mental state reflects the mood and thoughts of an individual. Abnormalities can occur with neurological disease (e.g., frontal lobe disease, traumatic brain injury) or psychiatric illness (e.g., panic attacks, depression following stroke). Cognitive deficits can range from orientation and memory deficits to poor judgment; distractibility; and difficulties in information processing, abstract reasoning, and learning, to name just a few. Patients with deficits across many or all areas of cognitive function demonstrate diffuse or multifocal pathology (e.g., Alzheimer's disease, chronic brain syndrome). Patients with deficits in only one or a few areas of testing typically demonstrate focal deficits (e.g., stroke). The physical therapist may be one of the first professionals to interact with the patient and should be able to screen for cognitive deficits and initiate appropriate referrals. A detailed examination by a neuropsychologist, occupational therapist, and/or speech-language pathologist is usually necessary to obtain a complete and accurate picture of these deficits. See Chapter 29 for a more complete discussion. Lack of attention to the patient's mental status by the physical therapist can render the results of other motor function tests in a patient with brain damage invalid and unreliable.

Consciousness

Examination of consciousness and arousal is important in determining the degree to which an individual is able to respond. The *ascending reticular activating system* (ARAS) includes core neurons in the brainstem terminating in the locus coeruleus and raphe nuclei cells. It functions to arouse and awaken the brain and control sleep–wake cycles. Lesions in the brainstem are associated with sleep and coma, whereas high levels of activity are associated with extreme excitement (high arousal). The *descending reticular activating system (DRAS)* is composed of the pontine reticulospinal tract, which assists in spinal cord antigravity reflexes (extensor tone) and the medullary reticulospinal pathways, which have the opposite effect of decreasing extensor tone.[8]

Five different levels of consciousness have been identified. Full **consciousness** is a state of alertness or awareness and implies orientation to person, place, and time. An alert patient is clearly awake and responds fully and appropriately when spoken to or to varying stimuli. There is awareness of self and the environment. **Lethargy** refers to a general slowing of motor processes, including speech and movement. The lethargic patient appears drowsy but when questioned can open the eyes and respond briefly. The patient easily falls asleep if not continually stimulated and does not fully appreciate the environment. Attempts to communicate with the patient are difficult owing to deficits in maintaining focus. The therapist should speak in a loud voice while calling the patient's name. Questions should be simple and directed toward the individual (e.g., How are you feeling?). **Obtundation** refers to dulled or blunted sensitivity. The obtunded patient is difficult to arouse from sleeping and once aroused, appears confused. Attempts to interact with the patient are generally nonproductive. The patient responds slowly and demonstrates little interest or awareness of the environment. The therapist should shake the patient gently as if awakening someone from sleep and again use simple questions. **Stupor** refers to a state of semiconsciousness. The patient lacks responsiveness, and can be aroused only by intense stimuli (e.g., painful stimuli such as sharp pressure, pinch, or rolling a pencil across the nail bed). The patient demonstrates little in the way of voluntary verbal or motor responses. Mass movement responses may be observed in response to painful stimuli or loud noises. The unconscious patient is said to be in a **coma** and cannot be aroused. The eyes remain closed and there are no sleep/wake cycles. The patient does not respond to repeated painful stimuli and is ventilator dependent. Reflex reactions may or may not be seen, depending on the location of the lesion(s) within the CNS.[9]

Clinically the patient can progress from one level of consciousness to another. For example, with an intracranial bleed, the swelling and mass effect compress the brain, resulting in decreasing levels of consciousness. The patient progresses from consciousness, to lethargy, to stupor, and finally to coma. If medical interventions are successful, recovery is evidenced by a reverse progression. True coma is generally time limited. Patients emerge into a *vegetative state,* characterized by return of irregular sleep/wake cycles and normalization of the so-called vegetative functions—respiration, digestion, and blood pressure control. Current efforts are focused on using the term *minimally conscious state* to refer to this state. The patient may be aroused, but remains unaware of his or her environment. There is no purposeful attention or cognitive responsiveness. The term *persistent vegetative state* is used to describe individuals who remain in a vegetative state 1 year or longer after traumatic brain injury and 3 months or more for anoxic brain injury. This is caused by severe brain injury.

The *Glasgow Coma Scale (GCS)* is the gold standard used to document level of consciousness. Three areas of function are examined: eye opening, best motor response, and verbal response (Chapter 22, Table 22.4). Total GCS scores range from a low of 3 to a high of 15. A total score of 8 or less is indicative of severe brain injury and coma; a score between 9 and 12 is indicative of moderate brain injury, whereas a score from 13 to 15 is indicative of mild brain injury.[10]

Examination of the pupillary size and reaction can also reveal important information about the unconscious patient. Pupils that are bilaterally small may be indicative of damage to the sympathetic pathways in the hypothalamus or metabolic encephalopathy. Pinpoint pupils are suggestive of a hemorrhagic pontine lesion or narcotic overdose (e.g., morphine, heroin). Pupils that are fixed in midposition and slightly dilated are suggestive of midbrain damage while large bilaterally fixed and dilated pupils suggest severe anoxia or drug toxicity (e.g., tricyclic antidepressants). If only one pupil is fixed and dilated, temporal lobe herniation with compression of the oculomotor nerve and midbrain is likely.[9]

Orientation

Orientation is examined with respect to (1) *time* (What day/month/season/year is it?, What is the time of day?); (2) *place* (Where are you? What city/state are we in? What is the name of this place?) and (3) *person* (What is your name? How old are you? Where were you born? What is the name of your wife/husband?). The therapist records the accuracy of the patient's responses. Findings are documented in the medical record as: Patient is alert and oriented times 3 (time, person, place) or times 2 (person, place) depending on the domains correctly identified. An additional domain that can be examined is *circumstance* (What happened to you? What kind of a place is this? Why do people come here?). To answer these last questions correctly, the individual must be able to take in, store, and recall new information. This may be severely disrupted in the patient with traumatic brain injury. Disorientation is also common with in the patient with delirium or advanced dementia.

Attention

Attention is the capacity of the brain to process information from the environment or from long-term memory. An individual with intact *selective attention* is able to screen and process relevant sensory information about both the task and the environment while screening out irrelevant information. The complexity and familiarity of the task determines the degree of attention required. If new or complex information is presented, concentration and effort are increased. Patients who are inattentive will have difficulty concentrating. Attention deficits are typically seen in individuals with delirium, brain injury, dementia, mental retardation, or performance anxiety.

Selective attention can be examined by asking the patient to attend to a particular task. For example, the therapist asks the patient to repeat a short list of numbers forwards or backwards (*digit span test*). The therapist documents the number of digits the patients is able to recall. Normally individuals can recall seven forward and five backward numbers. For patients with communication impairments, the therapist can read a list of items while the patient is asked to identify or signal each time a particular item is mentioned. *Sustained attention* (or vigilance) is examined by determining how long the patient is able to maintain attention on a particular task (time on task). *Alternating attention* (attention flexibility) is examined by requesting the patient to alternate back and forth between two different tasks (e.g., add the first two pairs of numbers, then subtract the next two pairs of numbers). Requesting the patient to perform two tasks simultaneously is used to determine *divided attention*. For example, the patient talks while walking (*Walkie–Talkie Test*), or walks while locating an object placed to the side (simulated grocery shopping). Documentation should include the specific component of attention examined, any slowness or hesitation in the response, the duration and frequency of episodes of inattention, the environmental conditions that contribute to or hinder attention abilities, and the amount of required redirection (verbal cueing) to the task.[11,12]

Memory

Memory is the process of registration, retention, and recall of past experience, knowledge, and ideas. **Declarative memory** events (explicit memory) involves the conscious recollection of facts and events. **Motor memory** information (procedural or implicit memory) involves recall of movements or motor information and storage of motor programs, subroutines, or schema. The length of time required from initial acquisition into memory also distinguishes types of memory. **Immediate memory** (immediate recall) refers to the immediate registration and recall of information after an interval of a few seconds (e.g., repeat after me). **Short-term memory, STM** (recent memory) refers to the capability to remember current, day-to-day events (e.g., what was eaten for breakfast, date), learn new material, and retrieve material after an interval of minutes, hours, or days. **Long-term memory, LTM** (remote memory) refers to the recall of facts or events that occurred years before (e.g., birthdays, anniversary, historic facts). It includes items an individual would be expected to know.

A simple test for memory involves presenting the patient with a short list of words of unrelated objects (e.g., pony, coin, pencil) and asking the patient to repeat those words immediately after presentation (immediate recall) and again 5 minutes after presentation (STM). LTM can be determined by having the patient recall events or persons from his or her past (Where were you born? Where did you go to school? Where do/did you work?). The patient's fund of general knowledge can also be examined (Who is the president? Who was president during World War II?). The questions selected should represent sensitivity to the cultural and educational background of the patient. It is important to consider that memory may be influenced by attention, motivation, rehearsal, fatigue, and other factors.[12] The *Mini-Mental Status Examination (MMSE)* provides a valid and reliable quick screen of cognitive function.[13]

Patients with **amnesia** typically demonstrate pronounced memory deficits. **Anterograde amnesia** (*post-traumatic amnesia, PTA*) refers to the inability to learn new material acquired after a brain insult. **Retrograde amnesia** refers to the inability to remember previous learning acquired prior to a brain insult. Patients with **delirium** (*acute confusional state*) typically demonstrate impairments in immediate and STM along with confusion, agitation, disorientation, and usually illusions or hallucinations. Patients with **dementia** demonstrate broad-based memory impairments and learning. Significant memory deficits are also seen in patients with diffuse encephalopathies, bilateral temporal lesions, and Korsakoff's psychosis (thiamine deficiency). Certain drugs can improve memory (e.g., CNS stimulates, cholinergic agents) while other drugs can degrade memory (e.g., benzodiazepines, anticholinergic drugs).[9] Patients who demonstrate difficulty retrieving information will often relate that the information is on the "tip of their tongue" (the *tip of the tongue phenomenon*). Various different strategies can be used to facilitate recall of information (e.g., prompting, rehearsal, and repetition). If attention and memory are impaired, instructions during the examination should be kept simple and brief (one-level commands vs two- or three-level commands). The therapist should structure or choose an environment in which distractions are reduced (i.e., a closed environment) to ensure maximum performance during the examination. Demonstration and positive feedback can assist the patient to understand what is expected, and can be used to motivate and improve performance. Use of any memory-enhancing strategy during an examination should be carefully documented in the patient's chart.[11]

Higher Cognitive Functions

An examination of higher cognitive functions typically includes (1) information and vocabulary; (2) calculating ability; (3) abstract thinking; and (4) constructional ability.[12]

The patient's grasp of information and ability to communicate should be ascertained. The therapist should listen carefully to spontaneous speech during the initial examination sessions. The patient's understanding of spoken language can be determined using simple tests. Word comprehension can be determined by varying the difficulty of commands, from one-stage to two or three (Point to your nose; Point to your right hand and lift your left hand). Repetition and naming can be tested (Repeat after me: Name the parts of a watch). Reading comprehension and writing ability can also be examined.

Patients can demonstrate problems with articulation (**dysarthria**), evidenced by speech errors, difficulties with timing, vocal quality, pitch, volume, and breath control. Problems of fluency, word flow without pauses or breaks, should be noted. Speech that flows smoothly but contains errors, neologisms (nonsense words), paraphasias (misuse of words), and circumlocutions (word substitution) is indicative of **fluent aphasia** (i.e., Wernicke's aphasia). The patient typically demonstrates deficits in auditory comprehension with well-articulated speech marked by word substitutions. Speech that is slow and hesitant with limited vocabulary and impaired syntax is indicative of **nonfluent aphasia** (i.e., Broca's aphasia). Articulation is labored and word finding difficulties are apparent. In some settings, especially the acute hospital setting, the physical therapist may be the first to become aware of communication deficits. Referral to a speech-language pathologist is indicated for comprehensive examination and evaluation. See Chapter 30 for a thorough discussion of this topic.

To ensure the validity of the physical therapy examination, it is necessary to identify an appropriate means of communicating with the patient. Consultation with the speech-language pathologist is essential. This may include simplifying instructions, using written instructions, or using alternate forms of communication such as gestures, pantomime, or communication boards. A common error is to assume that the patient understands the task at hand when he or she really has no idea what is expected. To ensure accuracy of testing, frequent checks for comprehension should be performed throughout the examination. For example, the use of message discrepancies (saying one thing and gesturing another) can be used to test the patient's level of understanding.

Calculating ability can be tested by asking the patient to perform arithmetical calculations, ranging from simple addition (what is 2 + 4?) to more difficult calculations (e.g., multiplication—what is 4 times 4?). The *Serial 7 Test* is also commonly used. The patient is instructed to start with 100 and subtract 7 and keep on subtracting 7. More functional tests involving the use of money can also be used (How much change should you get for an item that costs 59 cents if you give the clerk a dollar bill?). Impaired calculation can be indicative of diffuse encephalopathy or psychiatric disease.[9]

Abstract thinking can be examined by having the patient provide interpretations to common proverbs (e.g., Explain what is meant by "People in glass houses shouldn't throw stones" or "A stitch in time saves nine"). The therapist documents if the patient is able to provide a correct interpretation. Patients with difficulty in abstract thinking will typically answer by providing concrete or physical interpretations (e.g., "It means stones are heavier than glass"). An alternate test is to have the patient describe similarities or differences between objects (e.g., an orange and an apple, a horse and a donkey, skirt and trousers). Impaired performance can be indicative of frontal lobe or diffuse encephalopathy or psychiatric illness.

Constructional ability is the ability to copy figures. Testing is typically done by the occupational therapist who may use a series of paper-and-pencil tasks of increasing difficulty. The patient is asked to copy figures of varying shapes and sizes or to draw the face of a clock. Impairments in constructional ability are seen in patients with parietal lobe damage and dementia.

Arousal

Balanced interaction of the autonomic and somatic systems allows for reactive yet stable responses of an individual. Sympathetic nervous system (SNS, *the alarm system*) activity allows actions to be initiated to protect the individual under varying circumstances. Stimulation of the SNS results in (1) hyperalertness; (2) increased heart rate (HR); (3) increased blood pressure (BP); (4) increased respiratory rate (RR); (5) increased blood flow to muscles; (6) depressed digestive functions; and (7) mobilized glucose reserves. Motor systems become engaged in carrying out defensive commands, producing **fight or flight responses** (e.g., the aroused patient with traumatic brain injury may hit or bite). Dilated pupils and increased sweating may also be evident, depending upon the degree of arousal. Stimulation of the parasympathetic nervous system produces the opposite responses: slowing of HR, BP, RR, and so forth.[8]

Whereas a certain level of arousal is necessary for optimal motor performance, very low or high levels cause deterioration in motor performance. This is referred to as the **inverted-U theory (Yerkes-Dodson law)**.[14] Excess levels of arousal can also yield unexpected responses. Patients at either end of an arousal continuum (either very high or very low) may not respond at all or may respond in an unpredictable manner. This phenomenon may explain the reactions of patients who are labile and lack homeostatic controls for normal function. Examination of baseline homeostatic levels should, therefore, precede other elements in the patient suspected of autonomic instability (e.g., the patient with brain injury).[15,16]

Critical components for baseline examination include (1) a representative sampling of ANS responses, including HR, BP, RR, pupil dilation, and sweating; (2) a determination of patient reactivity, including the degree and rate of response to sensory stimulation; and (3) a determination of compensatory mechanisms in response to physiological stressors. Careful monitoring during a motor performance examination assists in defining homeostatic stability. Specific guidelines for the examination of vital functions can be found in Chapter 4.

Sensory Integrity and Integration

Sensory information is a critical component of motor function. It provides the necessary feedback for determination of initial position before a movement, error detection during the movement, and movement outcomes necessary to shape further learning.[1] A *closed-loop system* of motor control is defined as "a control system employing feedback, a reference of correctness, computation of error, and subsequent correction in order to maintain a desired state."[1, p 462] A variety of feedback sources are used to monitor movement including visual, vestibular, proprioceptive, and tactile inputs. The term **somatosensation** (or somatosensory inputs) is sometimes used to refer to sensory information received from the skin and musculoskeletal systems. The CNS analyzes all available movement information, determines error, and institutes appropriate corrective actions as necessary. Thus, a thorough sensory examination of each of these systems is an important first step in the examination of motor function. See Chapter 5 for a complete discussion of this topic. The primary role of closed-loop systems in motor control appears to be the monitoring of constant states such as posture and balance, and the control of slow movements, or those requiring a high degree of precision or accuracy. Feedback information is also essential during learning of new motor skills. Patients who have deficits in any movement-monitoring sensory system may be able to compensate with other sensory systems. For example, the patient with major proprioceptive losses can use vision as an error-correcting system to maintain a stable posture. When vision is also impaired, however, postural instability becomes readily apparent. Significant sensory losses and inadequate compensatory shifts to other sensory systems may result in severely disordered movement responses. The patient with proprioceptive losses and severe visual disturbances such as diplopia (commonly seen in the patient with multiple sclerosis) may be unable to maintain a stable posture at all. An accurate examination, therefore, requires that the therapist not only look at each individual sensory system but also at the overall sensory interaction and integration and the adequacy of compensatory adjustments. Postural tasks, balance, slow (ramp) movements, tracking tasks, or new motor tasks provide the ideal challenge in which to test feedback control mechanisms and closed-loop processes.

An *open-loop system* of motor control is a "control system with preprogrammed instructions to an effector that does not use feedback information and error-detection processes."[1, p 466] Movements emerge from learned motor programs or schema that contain "a rule, concept, or relationship formed on the basis of experience."[1, p 467] Rapid and skilled movement sequences or well-learned movements can thus be completed without the benefit of sensory feedback. Absence of sensation degrades movement quality, as evidenced from sensory deafferentation studies. A more likely theory for everyday motor function is a hybrid motor control system in which the CNS utilizes both closed- and open-loop control processes to produce skilled movement.

Joint Integrity, Postural Alignment, and Mobility

Joint range of motion (ROM) and soft tissue flexibility are important elements of motor function. Limitations restrict the normal coordinated action of muscles as well as alter the biomechanical alignment of body segments and posture. Long-standing immobilization results in contracture, a fixed resistance resulting from fibrosis of tissues surrounding a joint, and restricted movement. The resultant compensatory movement patterns are frequently dysfunctional, producing additional stresses and strains on the musculoskeletal system. They are also more energy costly and can significantly limit functional mobility. For example, shortening of the gastrocnemius muscles results in a toe walking gait pattern; tightness of the hip adductors results in a scissoring gait pattern. Changes in alignment secondary to muscle tightness alter postural control. For example, in standing anterior pelvic tilting and flexion of the hips and knees are typically the result of hip flexor tightness. Posterior pelvic tilting is associated with kyphosis and forward head in sitting and is typically the result of hamstring tightness. Abnormalities in alignment that alter the center of mass within the base of support place increased demands on the postural control system. For example, the patient with stroke will stand with the weight displaced over the sound leg and away from the affected limb. This patient will be limited in the use of normal postural control strategies. Thus, an examination of the musculoskeletal system is important to complete before examination of other elements of the neurological examination.

Tone

Tone is defined as the resistance of muscle to passive elongation or stretch when an individual attempts to maintain muscle relaxation. It represents the degree of residual contraction in normally innervated, resting muscle, or steady-state contraction. Tone is due to a number of factors, including (1) physical inertia, (2) intrinsic mechanical-elastic stiffness of muscle and connective tissues, and (3) reflex muscle contraction (tonic stretch reflexes).[17] It excludes resistance to passive stretch from fixed contracture. Because muscles rarely work in isolation, the term *postural tone* is preferred by some clinicians to describe a pattern of muscular tension that exists throughout the body and affects groups of muscles. Tonal abnormalities are categorized as **hypertonia** (increased above normal resting levels), **hypotonia** (decreased below normal resting levels), or **dystonia** (impaired or disordered tonicity).

Abnormal Tone

Spasticity

Spasticity is a hypertonic motor disorder characterized by velocity-dependent resistance to passive stretch. Thus the larger and quicker the stretch, the stronger the resistance of the spastic muscle. During rapid movement, initial high resistance (spastic catch) may be followed by a sudden inhibition or letting go of the limb (relaxation) in response to a stretch stimulus, termed **clasp-knife response**. Chronic spasticity is associated with contracture, abnormal posturing and deformity, functional limitations, and disability.

Spasticity arises from injury to corticospinal pathways (pyramidal tracts) and occurs as part of **upper motoneuron (UMN) syndrome**. Loss of inhibitory control on lower motor neurons results in disordered spinal segmental reflexes, including increased alpha motoneuron excitability, increased spindle (Ia) and flexor reflex afferent excitability, altered synaptic activity, decreased presynaptic Ia inhibition, and so forth.[18] The signs and symptoms of UMN syndrome include hyperactive stretch reflexes, involuntary flexor and extensor spasms, clonus, Babinski's sign, exaggerated cutaneous reflexes, and loss of precise autonomic control. Dyssynergic movement patterns also occur, including coactivation of agonist and antagonist muscle groups, abnormal timing, paresis, loss of dexterity, and fatigability.[19] **Clonus** is characterized by cyclical, spasmodic alternation of muscular contraction and relaxation in response to sustained stretch of a spastic muscle. Clonus is common in the plantar flexors, but may also occur in other areas of the body such as the jaw or wrist. The **Babinski sign** is dorsiflexion of the great toe with fanning of the other toes on stimulation of the lateral sole of the foot.[20]

Rigidity

Rigidity is a hypertonic state characterized by increased uniform resistance that persists throughout the whole ROM and is independent of the velocity of movement **(leadpipe rigidity)**. It is associated with lesions of the basal ganglia system (*extrapyramidal syndromes*) and is seen in Parkinson's disease. Rigidity is the result of excessive supraspinal drive (upper motor neuron facilitation) acting on alpha motor neurons; spinal reflex mechanisms are normal.[21] Patients demonstrate stiffness, inflexibility, and significant functional limitation. **Cogwheel rigidity** refers to a hypertonic state with superimposed rachetlike jerkiness and is commonly seen in upper extremity movements (e.g., wrist or elbow flexion and extension) in patients with Parkinson's disease. It may represent the presence of tremor superimposed on rigidity. Tremor, bradykinesia, and loss of postural stability are also associated motor deficits in patients with Parkinson's disease.

Hypotonia

Hypotonia and **flaccidity** are the terms used to define decreased or absent muscular tone. Resistance to passive movement is diminished, stretch reflexes are dampened or absent, and limbs are easily moved (floppy). Hyperextensibility of joints is common. **Lower motor neuron (LMN) syndrome** results from lesions that affect the anterior horn cell and peripheral nerve (e.g., peripheral neuropathy, cauda equina lesion, radiculopathy). It produces symptoms of decreased or absent tone, decreased or absent reflexes, paresis, muscle fasciculations and fibrillations with denervation, and neurogenic atrophy. Mild decreases in tone along with asthenia can also be seen in cerebellar lesions. Temporary states of flaccidity or hypotonia, termed *spinal shock* or *cerebral shock* depending on the location of the lesion, can be seen with UMN lesions (e.g., hemiplegia, tetraplegia, paraplegia). The duration of the CNS depression that occurs with shock is highly variable, lasting days or weeks. It is typically followed by the development of spasticity and classic UNM signs.

Dystonia

Dystonia is a hyperkinetic movement disorder characterized by disordered tone and involuntary movements involving large portions of the body. The movements are similar to athetoid movements, with typical twisting or writhing motions. *Dystonic posturing* refers to sustained abnormal postures caused by co-contraction of muscles that may last for several minutes, hours, or permanently. Dystonia results from a CNS lesion (commonly in the basal ganglia) and can be inherited (primary idiopathic dystonia), associated with neurodegenerative disorders (Wilson's disease, Parkinson's disease on excessive L-dopa therapy), or metabolic disorders (amino acid or lipid disorders). Dystonia can affect only one part of the body (*focal dystonia*) as seen spasmodic torticollis (wry neck) or isolated writer's cramp. *Segmental dystonia* affects two or more adjacent areas (e.g., torticollis and dystonic posturing of the arm).[20,22]

Decorticate and Decerebrate Rigidity

Significant brain lesions can result in coma with decorticate or decerebrate rigidity. **Decorticate rigidity** (abnormal flexor response) refers to sustained contraction and posturing of the upper limbs in flexion and the lower limbs in extension. The elbows, wrists, and fingers are held in flexion with shoulders adducted tightly to the sides while the legs are held in extension, internal rotation, and plantarflexion. **Decerebrate rigidity** (abnormal extensor response) refers to sustained contraction and posturing of the trunk and limbs in a position of full extension. The elbows are extended with shoulders adducted, forearms pronated, and wrist and fingers flexed. The legs are held in stiff extension with plantarflexion. Decorticate rigidity is indicative of a corticospinal tract lesion at the level of diencephalon (above the superior colliculus), while decerebrate rigidity indicates a corticospinal brainstem lesion between the superior colliculus and vestibular nucleus. **Opisthotonus** is strong and sustained contraction of the extensor muscles of the neck and trunk. The patient assumes a rigid hyperextended posture. All of these postures are associated with exaggerated and severe forms of spasticity.

Examination of Tone

An examination of tone consists of (1) initial observation of resting posture and palpation, (2) passive motion testing, and (3) active motion testing. Variability of tone is common. For example, patients with spasticity can vary in their presentation from morning to afternoon, day to day, or even hour to hour depending on a number of factors including (1) volitional effort and movement, (2) stress and anxiety, (3) position and interaction of tonic reflexes, (4) medications, (5) general health, (6) environmental temperature, and (7) state of CNS arousal or alertness. In addition, urinary bladder status (full or empty), fever and

Table 8.1 Typical Patterns of Spasticity in Upper Motor Neuron Syndrome

Upper Limbs	Actions	Muscles Affected
Scapula	Retraction, downward rotation	Rhomboids
Shoulder	Adduction and internal rotation, Depression	Pectoralis major, Latissimus dorsi, Teres major, Subscapularis
Elbow	Flexion	Biceps, Brachialis, Brachioradialis
Forearm	Pronation	Pronator teres, Pronator quadratus
Wrist	Flexion, adduction	F. carpi radialis
Hand	Finger flexion, clenched fist thumb, adducted in palm	F. dig. profundus/sublimis, Add. pollicis brevis, F. pollicis brevis
Lower Limbs	**Actions**	**Muscles Affected**
Pelvis	Retraction (hip hiking)	Quadratus lumborum
Hip	Adduction (scissoring) Internal rotation Extension	Add. Longus/brevis Add. Magnus, Gracilis Gluteus maximus
Knee	Extension	Quadriceps
Foot and ankle	Plantarflexion Inversion Equinovarus Toes claw (MP ext., PIP flex, DIP ext) Toes curl (PIP, DIP flex)	Gastroc-soleus Tibialis posterior Long toe flexors Ext. Hallucis longus Peroneus longus
Hip and knee (prolonged sitting posture)	Flexion Sacral sitting	Iliopsoas Rectus femoris, Pectineus Hamstrings
Trunk	Lateral flexion with concavity Rotation	Rotators Internal/external obliques
COG forward (prolonged sitting posture)	Excessive forward flexion Forward head	Rectus abdominis, External obliques Psoas minor

The form and intensity of spasticity may vary greatly, depending upon the CNS lesion site and extent of damage. The degree of spasticity can fluctuate within each individual (i.e., due to body position, level of excitation, sensory stimulation, and voluntary effort). Spasticity predominates in antigravity muscles (i.e., the flexors of the upper extremity and the extensors of the lower extremity). If left untreated, spasticity can result in movement deficiencies, subsequent contractures, degenerative joint changes, and deformity.

Adapted from Mayer NH, Esquenazi A, Childers MK: Common patterns of clinical motor dysfunction. Muscle and Nerve 6:S21, 1997.

infection, and metabolic and/or electrolyte imbalance can also influence tone. The therapist should therefore consider the impact of each of these factors in arriving at a determination of tone. Repeat testing and a consistent approach to examination is necessary to improve the accuracy and reliability of test results.

Initial observation of the patient can reveal abnormal posturing of the limbs or body. Careful inspection should be made regarding the position of the limbs, trunk, and head. With spasticity, posturing in fixed, antigravity positions is common; for example, the upper extremity is held fixed against the body in flexion, adduction, and supination with elbow and wrist/finger flexion. In the supine position, the lower extremities are held in extension, adduction with plantarflexion, and inversion (Table 8.1). Limbs that appear floppy and lifeless (e.g., a lower extremity rolled out to the side in external rotation) may indicate hypotonicity. *Palpation* of the muscle belly may yield additional information about the resting state of muscle. Consistency, firmness, and turgor should all be examined. Hypotonic muscles will feel soft and flabby, whereas hypertonic muscles will feel taut and harder than normal.

Passive motion testing reveals information about the responsiveness of muscles to stretch. Because these responses should be examined in the absence of voluntary control, the patient is instructed to relax, letting the therapist support and move the limb. During a passive motion test, the therapist should maintain firm and constant manual contact, moving the limb in all motions. When tone is normal, the limb moves easily and the therapist is able to alter direction and speed without feeling abnormal resistance. The limb is responsive and feels light. Hypertonic limbs generally feel stiff and resistant to movement, while flaccid limbs feel heavy and unresponsive. Older adults may find it difficult to relax; their stiffness should not be mistaken for hypertonicity. Varying the speed of movement is an important determinant of spasticity. Faster movements will intensify the resistance to passive motion. Clonus, a phasic stretch response, is examined using a quick stretch stimulus that is then maintained. For example, ankle clonus is tested by sudden dorsiflexion of the foot and maintaining the foot in dorsiflexion. The presence of a clasp-knife response should also be noted. All limbs and body segments are examined, with particular attention given to those identified as problematic in the initial observation. Comparisons should be made between upper and lower limbs and right and left extremities. Documentation should include a determination of whether the tonal abnormalities are symmetrical or asymmetrical. Asymmetrical tonal abnormalities are always indicative of neurological dysfunction.[9] Comparison to the unaffected side in patients with stroke should be performed. It is also important to remember that measurement of tone in one position does not ensure that measurement will be the same in other positions or during functional activities. A change in position such as sitting up or standing up substantially alters the requirements for postural support (postural tone).

A qualitative determination of the degree of tone should be made. Therapists need to be familiar with the wide range of normal and abnormal tonal responses to develop an appropriate frame of reference to grade tone. Tone is graded on a 0 to 4+ scale:

0 No response (flaccidity)
1+ Decreased response (hypotonia)
2+ Normal response
3+ Exaggerated response (mild to moderate hypertonia)
4+ Sustained response (severe hypertonia)

Spastic hypertonia can be graded using the Modified Ashworth Scale, a subjective, 5-point ordinal scale.[23,24] This scale remains the "gold standard" by which other tests are validated, and has been shown to have good intrarater reliability (0.84) and good interrater reliability (0.83) (see Table 8.2). Problems with use of the scale can include (1) inability to detect small changes and (2) limited application; can be used for extremity testing only.

Table 8.2 Modified Ashworth Scale for Grading Spasticity

Grade	Description
0	No increase in muscle tone.
1	Slight increase in muscle tone, manifested by a catch and release or by minimal resistance at the end of the ROM when the affected part(s) is moved in flexion or extension.
1+	Slight increase in muscle tone, manifested by a catch, followed by minimal resistance throughout the remainder (less than half) of the ROM.
2	More marked increase in muscle tone through most of the ROM, but affected part(s) easily moved.
3	Considerable increase in muscle tone, passive movement difficult.
4	Affected part(s) rigid in flexion or extension.

From Bohannon, R and Smith, M,[24 p 207] with permission.

Special tests that can also be used to examine spasticity include the *pendulum test*.[25] With the patient seated or lying with knees flexed over the end of a table, the patient's knee is fully extended and allowed to drop and swing like a pendulum. A normal and hypotonic limb will swing freely for several oscillations. Hypertonic limbs are resistant to the swinging motion and will quickly return to the initial dependent starting position. The pendulum test has been quantified using an isokinetic dynamometer for lower extremity testing with high test–retest reliability. Relative angle of reversal can be determined.[26] EMG response to stretch can also be documented for various velocities of stretch. The detailed and lengthy setup limits this method to largely the research environment. A *myotonometer* is a handheld computerized electronic device developed by Leonard and co-workers[27,28] that can be used to measure muscle tone. It provides quantitative measurements of force and displacement of muscle tissue and is able to detect small changes in both extremity and postural tone.

The therapist's documentation of tone abnormalities should include a determination of: (1) the body segments demonstrating abnormal tone, (2) the type of abnormality present (e.g., velocity dependent uniform, clasp-knife), (3) the presence of asymmetries, and (4) factors that modify tone. Of great importance is a description of the effects of tone on active movement, posture, and function.

Reflex Integrity

Deep Tendon Reflexes

A **reflex** is an involuntary, predictable, and specific response to a stimulus dependent on an intact reflex arc (sensory receptor, afferent neuron(s), efferent neuron(s), and responding muscle(s) or gland). The deep tendon reflex (DTR) results from stimulation of the stretch-sensitive IA afferents of the neuromuscular spindle producing muscle contraction via a monosynaptic pathway. It is tested by tapping sharply over the muscle tendon with a standard reflex hammer or with the tips of the therapist's fingers. To ensure adequate response, the muscle is positioned in midrange and the patient is instructed to relax. Stimulation can result in observable movement of the joint (brisk or strong responses). Weak responses may be evident only with palpation (slight or sluggish responses with little or no joint movement). The quality and magnitude of responses should be carefully documented. Reflexes are graded on a 0 to 4+ scale:

0 No response
1+ Present but depressed, low normal
2+ Average, normal
3+ Increased, brisker than average; possibly but not necessarily abnormal
4+ Very brisk, hyperactive, with clonus; abnormal

Table 8.3 presents an overview of the examination of DTR reflexes.

Table 8.3 Examination of Deep Tendon Reflexes

Myotatic Reflexes (Stretch)	Stimulus	Response
Jaw (CN V)	Patient is sitting, with jaw relaxed and slightly open. Place finger on top of chin; tap downward on top of finger in a direction which causes the jaw to open.	Jaw rebounds and closes
Biceps Musculocutaneous nerve (C5, C6)	Patient is sitting with arm flexed and supported. Place thumb over the biceps tendon in the cubital fossa, stretching it slightly. Tap thumb or directly on tendon.	Slight contraction of elbow flexors.
Brachioradialis (supinator) Radial nerve (C5, C6)	Patient is sitting with arm flexed onto the abdomen. Place finger on the radial tuberosity and tap finger with hammer.	Slight contraction of elbow flexors, slight wrist extension or radial deviation
Triceps Radial nerve (C6, C7)	Patient is sitting with arm supported in abduction, elbow flexed. Palpate triceps tendon just above olecranon. Tap directly on tendon.	Slight contraction of elbow extensors
Finger flexors Median nerve (C6–T1)	Hold hand in neutral position. Place finger across palmar surface of distal phalanges of four fingers and tap.	Slight contraction of finger flexors
Hamstrings Tibial branch, sciatic nerve (L5, S1, S2)	Patient is prone with knee semiflexed and supported. Palpate tendon at the knee. Tap on finger or directly on tendon.	Slight contraction of knee flexors
Quadriceps (patellar, knee jerk) Femoral nerve (L2, L3, L4)	Patient is sitting with knee flexed, foot unsupported. Tap tendon of quadriceps muscle between the patella and tibial tuberosity.	Slight contraction of knee extensors
Achilles (ankle jerk) Tibial (S1–S2)	Patient is prone with foot over the end of the plinth or sitting with knee flexed and foot held in slight dorsiflexion. Tap tendon just above its insertion on the calcaneus. Maintaining slight tension on the gastrocnemius-soleus group improves the response.	Slight contraction of plantarflexors

If DTRs are difficult to elicit, responses can be enhanced by specific reinforcement maneuvers. In the *Jendrassik maneuver,* the patient hooks together the fingers of the hands and strongly pulls them apart. While this pressure is maintained, lower extremity reflexes are tested. Maneuvers that can be used to reinforce responses in the upper extremities include squeezing the knees together, clenching the teeth, or making a fist with the contralateral extremity.[20] The use of any reinforcing maneuvers to elicit responses in patients with hyporeflexia should be carefully documented.

DTRs are increased in UMN syndrome (e.g., stroke) and decreased in LMN syndrome (e.g., peripheral neuropathy, nerve root compression), cerebellar syndrome, and muscle disease. Reflex spread (the extension of the response beyond the muscle normally expected to contract) is indicative of UMN syndrome. Because each DTR arises from specific spinal segments, an absent reflex can be used to identify the level of a spinal lesion (e.g., radiculopathy).[20]

Superficial Cutaneous Reflexes

Superficial cutaneous reflexes are elicited with a light stroke applied to the skin. The expected response is brief contraction of muscles innervated by the same spinal segments receiving the afferent inputs from the cutaneous receptors. A stimulus that is strong may produce irradiation of cutaneous signals with activation of protective withdrawal reflexes. Cutaneous reflexes include the plantar reflex, confirming toe signs (Chaddock), and abdominal reflexes. The *plantar reflex* is tested by applying a stroking stimulus on the sole of the foot along the lateral border and up across the ball of the foot. A normal response consists of flexion of the big toe; sometimes the other toes will demonstrate a downgoing response, or no response at all. An abnormal response (positive Babinski sign) consists of dorsiflexion (upgoing) of the big toe, with fanning of the lateral four toes. It is indicative of a corticospinal (UMN) lesion. The *Chaddock sign* is elicited by stroking around the lateral ankle and up the lateral dorsal aspect of the foot. It also produces dorsiflexion of the big toe and is considered a confirmatory toe sign. The *abdominal reflex* is elicited with brisk, light strokes over the skin of the abdominal muscles. A localized contraction under the stimulus is produced, with a resultant deviation of the umbilicus toward the area stimulated. Each quadrant should be tested in a diagonal direction. Umbilical deviation in a superior/lateral direction indicates integrity of spinal segments T8 to T9. Umbilical deviation in an inferior/lateral direction indicates integrity of spinal segments T10 to T12. Loss of response is abnormal and indicative of pathology (e.g., thoracic spinal cord injury). Asymmetry from side to side is highly significant with respect to neurological disease. Abdominal reflexes may be absent with in patients with obesity, or abdominal surgeries.[9] Table 8.4 presents an overview of the examination of superficial cutaneous reflexes.

Table 8.4 Examination of Superficial Cutaneous Reflexes

Superficial Reflexes (Cutaneous)	Stimulus	Response
Plantar (S1, S2)	With blunt object (key or wooden end of applicator stick), stroke the lateral aspect of the sole, moving from the heel to the ball of the foot, curving medially across the ball of the foot.	Normal response is flexion (plantarflexion) of the great toe, and sometimes the other toes (negative Babinski sign). Abnormal response, termed a **positive Babinski sign**, is extension (dorsiflexion) of the great toe with fanning of the four other toes (indicates UMN lesions).
	Alternate stimuli for plantar (for sensitive feet): • Chaddock: stroke lateral ankle and lateral aspect of foot. • Oppenheim: stroke down tibial crest	Same as for plantar.
Abdominal reflexes above umbilicus = T8–T10 below umbilicus = T10–T12	Position patient in supine, relaxed. Make brisk, light stroke over each quadrant of the abdominals from the periphery to the umbilicus.	Localized contraction under the stimulus, causing the umbilicus to move toward the stimulus. Masked by obesity. Can be absent in both UMN and LMN disorders.

Primitive and Tonic Reflexes

Primitive and *tonic reflexes* are normally present during infancy and become integrated by the CNS at an early age. Once integrated, these reflexes are not generally recognizable in adults in their pure form. They may continue, however, as adaptive fragments of behavior, underlying normal motor control.[29–31] Adult patients with brain injury (e.g., stroke, traumatic brain injury) may exhibit primitive and tonic reflexes affecting voluntary movement control and posture.[32,33] Patients who exhibit these reflexes typically present with extensive brain damage and other UMN signs. Obligatory and sustained responses that dominate motor behavior are always considered pathological in the adult.

Reflexes important to examine in the patient suspected of abnormal reflex activity include flexor withdrawal, traction, grasp, tonic neck, tonic labyrinthine, positive support, and associated reactions. *Flexor withdrawal reflex* is generally the simplest to observe and is judged by appearance of an overt movement response. *Tonic neck reflexes,* on the other hand, bias the musculature and may not be visible through overt movement responses. In fact, movement is rarely produced but rather posture is typically influenced through tonal adjustments. Thus the term "tuning reflexes" is an appropriate description of their function. Abnormal postures should be examined for their reflex dependence (e.g., the patient with brain injury exhibits excessive extensor tone in supine but not in side lying). To obtain an accurate examination, the therapist must be concerned with several factors. The patient must be positioned appropriately to allow for the expected response. An adequate test stimulus is essential, including both an adequate magnitude and duration of stimulation. Keen observation skills are needed to detect what may be subtle movement changes and abnormal responses. Palpation skills can assist in identifying tonal changes not readily apparent to the eye. Objective scoring of responses is essential. A reflex scoring key from Capute et al[34,35] is:

0+ Absent
1+ Tone change: slight, transient with no movement of the extremities
2+ Visible movement of extremities
3+ Exaggerated, full movement of extremities
4+ Obligatory and sustained movement, lasting for more than 30 seconds

Table 8.5 presents an overview of the examination of primitive and tonic reflexes.

Cranial Nerve Integrity

There are 12 pairs of cranial nerves (CN), all distributed to the head and neck with the exception of CN X (vagus), which is distributed to the thorax and abdomen. CNs I, II, and VIII are purely sensory and carry the special senses of smell, vision, hearing, and equilibrium. Cranial nerves III, IV, and VI are purely motor and control pupillary constriction and eye movements. Cranial nerves XI and XII are also purely motor, innervating the sternocleidomastoid, trapezius, and tongue muscles. Cranial nerves V, VII, IX, and X are mixed, containing both motor and sensory fibers. Motor functions include chewing (V), facial expression (VII), swallowing (IX, X), and vocal sounds (X). Sensations are carried from the face and head (V, VII, IX), alimentary tract, heart, vessels, and lungs (IX, X), and tongue, mouth, and palate (VII, IX, X). Parasympathetic secretomotor fibers (ANS) are carried in CN III for control of smooth muscles in the eyeball, VII for control of salivary and lacrimal glands, IX to the parotid salivary gland, and X to the heart, lungs, and most of the digestive system.

An examination of cranial nerve function should be performed with suspected lesions of the brain, brainstem, and cervical spine. Deficits in olfactory function (CN I) should be suspected with lesions of the nasal cavity, and anterior/inferior cerebrum. Lesions of the optic pathways (optic nerve [CN II], optic chiasma, optic tract, lateral geniculate body, superior colliculus) and visual cortex may produce visual deficits. Midbrain (mesencephalic) lesions may result in deficits of CNs III and IV (oculomotor, trochlear). Pontine lesions may involve several CNs, including V (ophthalmic, maxillary, and mandibular branches) and VI (abducens). Nuclei of CNs VII (facial) and VIII (vestibular and cochlear branches) are located at the junction of the pons and medulla. Lesions affecting the medulla may involve IX (glossopharyngeal), X (vagus), XI (spinal accessory), and XII (hypoglossal). The spinal root of XI is found in the upper five cervical segments.[8] The CNs, their function, clinical tests, and possible abnormal findings are presented in Table 8.6.

Muscle Performance

Strength and Power

Muscle performance is "the capacity of a muscle or a group of muscles to generate forces."[5, p 688] **Muscle strength** is "the measurable force exerted by a muscle or group of muscles to overcome a resistance in one maximal effort."[5, p 688] Isotonic contractions involve active shortening of muscles, and eccentric contractions involve active lengthening of muscles. Isometric contractions produce high levels of tension for holding contractions without overt movement. **Muscle power** is "work produced per unit of time or the product of strength and speed."[5, p 688] Muscle performance depends on a number of interrelated factors including length–tension characteristics, viscoelasticity, velocity, and metabolic adequacy (fuel storage and delivery). Of equal importance are the integrated actions of the CNS (neuromuscular control factors) including (1) the number and type of motor units recruited, (2) firing rate, (3) timing/sequencing, and (4) postural stabilization.

Patients with neurological dysfunction and impairments in motor control pose unique challenges for the examination of muscle performance. Weakness (*paresis*) or

Table 8.5 Examination of Primitive and Tonic Reflexes

Primitive/Spinal Reflexes	Stimulus	Response
Flexor withdrawal	Noxious stimulus (pinprick) to sole of foot. Tested in supine or sitting position.	Toes extend, foot dorsiflexes, entire LE flexes uncontrollably. Onset: 28 weeks gestation. Integrated: 1–2 months.
Crossed extension	Noxious stimulus to ball of foot of LE fixed in extension; tested in supine position.	Opposite LE flexes, then adducts and extends. Onset: 28 weeks gestation. Integrated:1–2 months.
Traction	Grasp forearm and pull up from supine into sitting position.	Grasp and total flexion of the UE. Onset: 28 weeks gestation. Integrated: 2–5 months.
Moro	Sudden change in position of head in relation to trunk; drop patient backward from sitting position.	Extension, abduction of UEs, hand opening, and crying followed by flexion, adduction of arms across chest. Onset: 28 weeks gestation. Integrated: 5–6 months.
Startle	Sudden loud or harsh noise.	Sudden extension or abduction of UEs, crying. Onset: birth. Integrated: persists.
Grasp	Maintained pressure to palm of hand (palmar grasp) or to ball of foot under toes (plantar grasp).	Maintained flexion of fingers or toes. Onset: palmar, birth; plantar, 28 weeks gestation. Integrated: palmer, 4–6 months; plantar, 9 months.
Tonic/Brainstem Reflexes	**Stimulus**	**Response**
Asymmetrical tonic neck (ATNR)	Rotation of the head to one side.	Flexion of skull limbs, extension of the jaw limbs, "bow and arrow" or "fencing" posture. Onset: birth. Integrated: 4–6 months.
Symmetrical tonic neck (STNR)	Flexion or extension of the head.	With head flexion: flexion of UEs, extension of LEs; with head extension: extension of UEs, flexion of LEs. Onset: 4–6 months. Integrated: 8–12 months.
Symmetrical tonic labyrinthine (TLR or STLR)	Prone or supine position.	With prone position: increased flexor tone/flexion of all limbs; with supine: increased extensor tone/extension of all limbs. Onset: birth. Integrated: 6 months.
Positive supporting	Contact to the ball of the foot in upright standing position.	Rigid extension (co-contraction) of the LEs. Onset: birth. Integrated: 6 months.
Associated reactions	Resisted voluntary movement in any part of the body.	Involuntary movement in a resting extremity. Onset: birth–3 months. Integrated: 8–9 years.

LE = lower extremity; UE = upper extremity.

Table 8.6 Examination of Cranial Nerve Integrity

Cranial Nerve	Function	Test	Possible Abnormal Findings
I Olfactory	Smell	Test sense of smell on each side (close off other nostril): use common, nonirritating odors.	Anosmia (inability to detect smells), seen with frontal lobe lesions
II Optic	Vision	Test visual acuity. Central: Snellen eye chart; test each eye separately (covering other eye); test at distance of 20 ft.	Blindness, myopia (impaired far vision), presbyopia (impaired near vision)
		Test peripheral vision (visual fields) by confrontation.	Field defects: homonymous hemianopsia
II, III Optic and oculomotor	Pupillary reflexes	Test pupillary reactions (constriction) by shining light in eye light; if abnormal, test near reaction.	Absence of pupillary constriction
		Examine pupillary size/shape.	Anisocoria (unequal pupils) Horner's syndrome, CN III paralysis
III, IV, VI Oculomotor, trochlear, and abducens	Extraocular movements	Test saccadic (patient is asked to look in each direction) and pursuit eye movements (patient follows moving finger).	Strabismus (eye deviates from normal conjugate position) Impaired eye movements Double vision
III	Medial, superior and inferior rectus: inferior oblique; turns eye up, down, in.	Observe position of eye. Test eye movements.	Strabismus: eye pulled outward by CN VI Eye cannot look upward, downward, inward movements.
	Elevates eyelid.		May see ptosis, pupillary dilation.
IV	Superior oblique: turns eye down when adducted.	Test eye movements.	Eye cannot look down when eye is adducted.
VI	Lateral rectus: turns eye out.	Observe position of eye. Test eye movements.	Esotropia (eye pulled inward) Eye cannot look out.
V Trigeminal Ophthalmic, maxillary, mandibular divisions	Sensory: face Sensory: cornea	Test pain, light touch sensations: forehead, cheeks, jaw (eyes closed). Test corneal reflex: touch lightly with wisp of cotton.	Loss of facial sensations, numbness with CN V lesion Trigger area with trigeminal neuralgia Loss of corneal reflex ipsilaterally (blinking in response to corneal touch)
	Motor: muscles of mastication	Palpate temporal and masseter muscles. Observe spontaneous movements. Have patient clench teeth, hold against resistance.	Weakness, wasting of muscles When opened, deviation of jaw to ipsilateral side
VII Facial	Facial expression	Test motor function facial muscles. Raise eyebrows, frown. Show teeth, smile. Close eyes tightly. Puff out both cheeks.	Paralysis: Inability to close eye, Drooping corner of mouth, Difficulty with speech articulation Unilateral LMN: Bell's palsy (PNI) Bilateral LMN: Guillain-Barré Unilateral UMN: stroke

(continued)

Table 8.6 Examination of Cranial Nerve Integrity (continued)

Cranial Nerve	Function	Test	Possible Abnormal Findings
	Taste to anterior two thirds of tongue	Apply saline solution and sugar solution using a cotton swab.	Incorrectly identifies solution.
VIII Vestibulocochlear (acoustic)	Vestibular function	Test balance: vestibulospinal function (VSR). Test eye–head coordination: vestibular ocular reflex (VOR).	Vertigo, dysequilibrium Gaze instability with head rotations, nystagmus (constant, involuntary cyclical movement of the eyeball)
	Cochlear function	Test auditory acuity.	Deafness, impaired hearing, tinnitus
		Test for lateralization (Weber test): place vibrating tuning fork on top of head, mid-position; check if sound heard in one ear, or equally in both.	Unilateral conductive loss: sound lateralized to impaired ear Sensorineural loss: sound heard in good ear
		Compare air and bone conduction (Rinne test): place vibrating tuning fork on mastoid bone, then close to ear canal; sound heard longer through air than bone.	Conductive loss: sound heard through bone is equal to or longer than air Sensorineural loss: sound heard longer through air
IX Glossopharyngeal	Sensory to posterior one third of tongue, pharynx, middle ear	Apply saline solution and sugar solution. Not typically tested	Incorrectly identifies solution.
IX, X Glossopharyngeal and vagus	Phonation Swallowing	Listen to voice quality. Examine for difficulty in swallowing glass of water.	Dysphonia: hoarseness denotes vocal cord weakness; nasal quality denotes palatal weakness. Dysphagia
	Palatal, pharynx control	Have patient say "ah"; observe motion of soft palate (elevates) and position of uvula (remains midline).	Paralysis: palate fails to elevate (lesion of CN X); asymmetrical elevation with unilateral paralysis
	Gag reflex	Stimulate back of throat lightly on each side.	Absent reflex: lesion of CN IX; possibly CN X
XI Spinal accessory	Motor function: Trapezius muscle Sternocleidomastoid	Examine bulk, strength. Shrug both shoulders upward against resistance. Turn head to each side against resistance.	LMN: atrophy, fasciculations, ipsilateral weakness Inability to shrug ipsilateral shoulder; shoulder droops Inability to turn head to opposite side UMN: weakness of ipsilateral sternocleidomastoid and contralateral trapezius
XII Hypoglossal	Tongue movements	Listen to patient's articulation. Examine resting position of tongue. Examine tongue movements: ask patient to protrude tongue, move side-to-side.	Dysarthria (seen with lesions of CN X or CN XII, also V, VII) Atrophy or fasciculations of tongue (LMN, ALS) Impaired movements, deviation to weak side UMN lesion: tongue deviates away from side of cortical lesion

From O'Sullivan S, and Siegelman R,[133, p 88] with permission.

absence of muscle strength (*plegia*) is seen in patients with UMN syndrome along with spasticity, hyperactive reflexes, and so forth. Patients may present with *hemiplegia* (one-sided paralysis), paraplegia (lower extremity paralysis) or *tetraplegia* ([quadriplegia] paralysis of all four limbs). Weakness of muscles in patients UMN lesions is a primary or direct impairment with force production impaired in the agonist muscle. Altered recruitment and decreased motor unit firing rates have been identified.[36–40] Patients with stroke show up to a 50 percent decrease in motor units of affected extremities within 2 months after insult.[41] Muscle performance is also influenced by the presence of other impairments including spasticity, disordered synergistic activity/mass patterns of movements (positive signs), and/or profound sensory deficit. Researchers investigating strength changes in patients with stroke have also found impairments in strength on the supposedly normal extremities, suggesting bilateral effects of ipsilateral lesions of the cerebral cortex.[42] These findings cast doubt as to the validity of using the uninvolved side as a reference for normal control in patients with hemiplegia. Strength can also be negatively influenced by disuse (an indirect impairment).

Atrophy is the loss of muscle bulk (wasting). It can occur as a result of the loss of functional mobility (*disuse atrophy*), LMN disease (*neurogenic atrophy*), or protein-calorie malnutrition. The therapist should visually inspect the muscles, comparing and contrasting their size and contour. Muscles that look flat or concave are indicative of atrophy. Comparisons should be made between and within limbs. Is the atrophy unilateral or bilateral? Multiple limbs? Proximal or distal? *Fasciculations* are random, spontaneous twitching of muscle fibers that are visible through the skin. If present with atrophy, LMN disease is indicated. Girth measurements or volumetric displacement measures (e.g., hands or feet) can be used to confirm visual inspection findings.[9]

The clinical examination of muscle strength and power utilizes standardized methods and protocols (e.g., manual muscle testing [MMT], hand-held dynamometers, instrumented isokinetic systems). See Chapter 6 for a thorough discussion of this topic. Analysis of muscle timing including amplitude, duration, waveform, and frequency can be obtained using EMG (see Chapter 9). Analysis of functional performance also yields important data about muscle performance.

Strength testing measures (MMTs) were originally developed to examine motor function in patients with polio (a LMN disease). Their usefulness in the clinical examination of patients with UMN lesions has been questioned.[43,44] Strength testing using standardized protocols may be appropriate for some patients with UMN syndrome, but not for others. Appropriate criteria are therefore critical in determining whether the standards of validity and reliability are met. First and foremost, the therapist must consider the patient's movement capabilities. Individual joint movements, mandated by standardized MMT procedures and isokinetic protocols, may not be possible in the presence of UMN lesion with stereotypic abnormal movement patterns, abnormal coactivation, spasticity, and abnormal posturing. These barriers to normal movement have been termed *active restraint*. The prescribed test positions may also be precluded by the presence of abnormal reflex activity (e.g., supine testing influenced by presence of the tonic labyrinthine reflex). Muscle and soft tissue changes in viscoelasticity (e.g., contracture) offer a form of *passive restraint* and may also preclude the use of standardized testing. In these instances, the decision should be made not to use standardized MMTs. An estimation of strength can be made from observations of active movements during performance of functional tasks. For example, shallow knee bends or sit-to-stand transfers can be used to examine the strength of hip extensors and knee extensors. Standing heel-rises or toe-rises can be used to examine the strength of foot-ankle muscles (dorsiflexors, plantarflexors). Documentation should clearly indicate that UMN involvement precluded use of standardized MMT procedures and that estimates of strength are based on observations during performance of functional tasks.

Movements can be graded using the following ordinal scale:

0 Zero (0)	No evidence of contraction by vision or palpation
1 Trace (T)	Slight contraction, no motion
2 Poor (P)	Movement through complete ROM in gravity-minimized position
3 Fair (F)	Movement through complete ROM against gravity
4 Good (G)	Movement through complete ROM against gravity; able to hold against moderate resistance; can be broken (break test) at end range
5 Normal (N)	Movement through complete ROM against gravity; able to hold against maximum resistance; cannot be broken at end range

If MMT is to be used, therapists should utilize standardized positions. If a modified position is required (e.g., the patient lacks full ROM or adequate stabilization), it should be carefully documented. *Substitutions* (muscle actions that compensate for specific muscle weakness) should be identified, eliminated whenever possible, and carefully documented. For example, the patient with spinal cord injury typically presents with common muscle substitutions (e.g., wrist extensors are used to close the fingers using tenodesis grasp). Knowledge of common substitutions is very helpful when working with this patient group. Reliability of MMT in the clinical setting has been low. In one study, the investigators found the percentage of therapists, obtaining the same muscle grade, only ranged from 50 to 60 percent. Factors that influence the reproducibility of the results include difficulty with determining the magnitude of resistive force (subjectivity of good and normal grades), differences in testing method, differences in force application (point, line of force, speed), duration of the contraction, patient factors (cooperation, fatigue), therapist factors (experience, instructions, volume of commands, interactions with patient), and environment (distracting influences).[45] It is important to note that generalizability of strength measurements taken in one position to performance of functional tasks is problematic.

Hand-held dynamometers are small portable devices that measure mechanical force; they have been incorporated clinically into manual muscle testing procedures. The therapist reads the exact amount of force applied to the muscle during tests for good and normal grades instead of estimating the amount of resistance. High intra- and intertester reliability scores have been reported.[46–50] Limitations in their use include difficulty in stabilizing both the limb and device, controlling the rate of muscle tension development, and applying sufficient force for a break test. These may be influential factors in reports that indicate the portable dynamometer is less reliable for testing lower extremity muscle groups.[50]

The use of an *isokinetic dynamometer* allows the therapist to monitor many important parameters of motor control, including velocity of muscle shortening or lengthening, peak torque at varying speeds, and ROM or arc of excursion as a function of time. Rate of tension development (time to peak torque) and shape of the torque curve can also be determined. Concentric and eccentric contractions and reciprocal agonist/antagonist relationships can be analyzed. This is especially important for an understanding of functional performance.[51] See Chapter 6 for a more complete discussion.

Patients with stroke typically demonstrate a variety of deficits on testing with an isokinetic dynamometer, including (1) decreased torque development; (2) decreased limb excursion; (3) extended times to peak torque development and the time peak torque is held; (4) increased time intervals between reciprocal contractions; and (5) problems in torque development at higher speeds.[52,53] For example, many patients with stroke are unable to develop tension above 70 to 80° per second. When this value is compared to the speed needed for normal walking (100° per second), reasons for gait difficulties become readily apparent. Normative data, when available, can provide an appropriate reference for evaluating and interpreting patient data.

Endurance

Muscle endurance is "the ability to sustain forces repeatedly or to generate forces over a period of time."[5, p 688] An examination of muscle endurance is important in determining functional capacity. **Fatigue** has been defined as "the failure to generate the required or expected force during sustained or repeated contractions."[54, p 463] Although fatigue is protective and serves a useful function in guarding against overwork and injury, it is a serious problem for some individuals. For example, patients with postpolio syndrome or chronic fatigue syndrome may experience significant restrictions in their functional activities and work as a result of debilitating fatigue. Other groups of individuals who may also experience limitations as a result of fatigue include those with multiple sclerosis, amyotrophic lateral sclerosis, Duchenne muscular dystrophy, and Guillain-Barré syndrome.[55–59]

An examination of fatigue begins with routine questioning during the initial interview and is followed up with more specific functional tests as indicated. Self-assessments using a questionnaire are the preferred format rather than performance-based tests, which are likely to fatigue the patient. The patient should be asked questions pertaining to the frequency and severity of fatigue episodes, and the circumstances surrounding the onset and cessation of fatigue. Precipitating activities should be identified within the context of habitual daily activity. It is important to document the *fatigue threshold,* defined as "that level of exercise that cannot be sustained indefinitely."[60, p 691] In most cases, the onset of fatigue is gradual, not abrupt, and dependent on the intensity and duration of the activity attempted. Additional factors that can influence fatigue include health status, environmental context (e.g., stressful environment), and temperature (e.g., heat stress in the patient with multiple sclerosis). The therapist should carefully document the patient's level of performance, including independence, modified independence, or level of assistance required (minimal, moderate, or maximal). Perceived level of fatigue can be documented using a visual analog scale or the Borg Scale for *Ratings of Perceived Exertion.*[61] The *Modified Fatigue Impact Scale (MFIS)* is a useful instrument initially developed to assess quality-of-life problems related to fatigue in patients with multiple sclerosis. It includes questions on the cognitive and social domains, as well as physical performance (see Chapter 19, Appendix B).[62]

Exhaustion is defined as the limit of endurance, beyond which no further performance is possible. Most patients can report with great accuracy the point at which exhaustion is reached. Of concern with some patients is **overwork weakness (injury)**, defined as "a prolonged decrease in absolute strength and endurance due to excessive activity of partially denervated muscle."[63, p 22] For example, patients with postpolio syndrome may experience weakness following strenuous activity that is not recovered with ordinary rest. They report having to spend the entire next day or two in bed following an exhaustive exercise session. It is therefore important to document the type, length, and effectiveness of rest attempts. *Delayed onset muscle soreness (DOMS)* is common in patients with overwork weakness, peaking between 1 and 5 days post-activity.

Examination of muscle fatigue can include both volitional and electrically elicited fatigue tests using an isokinetic dynamometer. This equipment permits quantification of torque outputs. Patients are asked to perform repetitive, submaximal isokinetic contractions. A drop-off of peak torque by 50 percent can be used as an index of fatigue. Electrically induced fatigue tests can also be used to examine muscle performance and may provide a more reliable measure in individuals with low motivation or who have a disorder of central drive (e.g., stroke). The muscle is stimulated with groups of electrical pulses (pulse trains) and percentage of decline in force production is measured.[64–66] Timed performance on functional tasks (e.g., timed self-care tasks; time to walk a particular distance, 6-minute walk test) also provide objective and reproducible measures of endurance.

Voluntary Movement Patterns

Voluntary movement patterns utilize functionally linked muscles or **synergies** that are constrained by the CNS to act cooperatively to produce an action. The CNS is able to reduce the **degrees of freedom**, defined as the number of separate independent dimensions of movement that must be controlled by engaging these cooperative units of muscle action.[1] Synergistic movements are defined by precise spatial and temporal organization. Coordination involves control of speed, distance, direction, rhythm, and levels of muscle tension. In individuals with normal motor control, the patterns of coordination are numerous and variable, including patterns of single limb and multiple limb coordination, bilateral (bimanual) coordination, symmetrical, asymmetrical, or reciprocal limb patterns coordinated with appropriate proximal stabilization and postural support. Movements are also appropriately timed with events in the environment (*coincident timing*). (See Chapter 7.)

Abnormal Synergistic Patterns

Synergistic organization of movement may be disturbed in cases of UMN syndrome. **Abnormal mass synergies** are defined as obligatory, highly stereotyped mass patterns of movement. Selective movement control (isolated joint movements) becomes severely disordered or disappears completely. For example, patients with stroke may demonstrate obligatory flexion synergies and extension synergies (see Chapter 18, Table 18.6). Abnormal synergies are highly predictable and characteristic of middle stages of stroke recovery.[32,33]

The examination of abnormal synergies is both qualitative and quantitative. The therapist observes whether voluntary movement can be initiated, completed, and how the movement is carried out. If movement is stereotypical, what muscle groups are linked together? How strong are the linkages between muscle groups? Are there linkages between upper and lower limbs? Are the movements influenced by other components of UMN syndrome—primitive reflexes? spasticity? paresis? position? For example, does elbow, wrist, and finger flexion always occur when shoulder flexion is initiated? Is head turning used to initiate or reinforce upper extremity flexion? Therapists also need to identify when these patterns occur, under what circumstances, and what variations are possible. As CNS recovery progresses, the synergy patterns become more variable and may reemerge only under conditions of stress or fatigue. Lessening of synergy dominance and emergence of selective movement control are evidence of sequential recovery in patients with stroke. The *Fugl-Meyer Post-Stroke Assessment of Physical Performance* provides an objective and quantifiable measure of synergistic dominance and recovery after stroke[67] (see Chapter 18, Appendix A).

Table 8.7 presents a summary of the differential diagnosis comparing upper motor neuron and lower motor neuron syndromes. Table 8.8 presents a summary of the differential diagnosis comparing the major types of motor control disorders.

Functional Task Analysis

Examination at the functional level focuses on observation and classification of functional abilities and the identification of functional limitations. Performance-based measures yield important information about motor function. Numerous instruments are available with quantitative scoring systems (e.g., the Functional Independence Measure [FIM]). See Chapter 11 for a thorough discussion.

Qualitative analysis of functional tasks provides important information about the complex nature of these skills and the patient's level of motor control. Performance is observed through careful task analysis. The therapist interprets the observed behaviors by comparing them to a reference of normative behaviors. Interpretations are made about the nature of the motor performance and the possible links between documented impairments and performance difficulties. For example, the patient with acute stroke typically sits up from supine using primarily the sound side. The affected extremities lag behind, not well integrated into the movement pattern. The final sitting position is often asymmetrical with most of the weight borne on the sound side and the affected upper extremity held in an abnormally flexed and adducted position. It is important to document these qualitative findings as they provide important data necessary for developing an effective plan of care (POC) to improve motor function. The worksheet presented Box 8.1 provides a series of questions that can be used to facilitate functional task analysis.

Functional mobility skills (FMS) important to analyze include (1) bed mobility (e.g., rolling from side to side, bridging and scooting, moving from supine to sit and sit to supine); (2) sitting skills (e.g., moving in the posture, reaching); (3) transfer skills (e.g., moving from sit-to-stand and stand-to-sit), transfers from one surface to another (e.g., bed to wheelchair, wheelchair to car and so forth); (4) standing skills (e.g., maintenance of posture, moving in the posture, reaching, stepping); (5) walking; and (6) stair climbing. Control can also be examined in other postures including prone-on-elbows, quadruped (hands and knees), kneeling, half-kneeling, and standing up from the floor. It is important to note that there is considerable variability in motor performance of FMS across the lifespan.[68–72] Changes are influenced by such factors as changing body dimensions, age, health, level of physical activity, and so forth. Thus, the

Table 8.7 **Differential Diagnosis: Comparison of Upper Motor Neuron (UMN) and Lower Motor Neuron (LMN) Syndromes**

	UMN Lesion	LMN Lesion
Location of lesion, Structures involved	Central nervous system cortex, brainstem, corticospinal tracts, spinal cord	Cranial nerve nuclei/nerves Spinal cord: anterior horn cell, spinal roots Peripheral nerve
Diagnosis/Pathology	Stroke, traumatic brain injury, spinal cord injury	Polio, Guillain-Barré, Peripheral nerve injury, Peripheral neuropathy, Radiculopathy
Tone	Increased: hypertonia Velocity dependent	Decreased or absent: hypotonia, flaccidity Not velocity dependent
Reflexes	Increased: hyperreflexia, clonus Exaggerated cutaneous and autonomic reflexes, +Babinski	Decreased or absent: hyporeflexia Cutaneous reflexes decreased or absent
Involuntary movements	Muscle spasms: flexor or extensor	With denervation: fasciculations
Strength	Weakness or paralysis: ipsilateral (stroke) or bilateral (SCI) Corticospinal: contralateral if above decussation in medulla; ipsilateral if below Distribution: never focal	Ipsilateral weakness or paralysis Limited distribution: segmental or focal pattern, root-innervated pattern
Muscle bulk	Disuse atrophy: variable, widespread distribution, especially of antigravity muscles	Neurogenic atrophy: rapid, focal distribution, severe wasting
Voluntary movements	Impaired or absent: dyssynergic patterns, obligatory mass synergies	Weak or absent if nerve interrupted

From O'Sullivan S, and Siegelman R,[133, p 94] with permission.

activities of rolling over and sitting up may vary considerably between two adults of different size, age, or health.

Control observed during functional skills can be documented according to the nature of the task: (1) mobility, (2) static postural control, (3) dynamic postural control, and (4) skill (see Table 13.2, Categories of Motor Skills). **Mobility** is the ability to move from one position to another independently and safely.[2] Common characteristics of normal mobility include the ability to move the body while maintaining postural control. Deficits in *initial mobility* range from failure to initiate or sustain movements to poorly controlled movement. At the very lowest level, the impaired patient is only able to roll partially over to side lying and exhibits poorly sustained and controlled movements. At the highest end, the patient is asked to stand up and walk across the room. The impaired patient exhibits difficulty standing up (may require several attempts) but once up is able to walk with only a few abnormal gait characteristics. Key elements the therapist should observe and document include (1) the initiation and control of movements; (2) the sensory, motor, and cognitive strategies required and overall coordination; (3) movement termination; and (4) environmental constraints that must be considered.

Static postural control (*static equilibrium, static balance, or stability*) is the ability to maintain postural stability and orientation with the center of mass (COM) over the base of support (BOS) and the body at rest. For example, the patient demonstrates stability in sitting or standing if he or she is able to maintain the posture with minimum sway, no loss of balance, and no handhold. Key elements the therapist should observe and document include (1) the base-of-support (BOS); (2) the position and stability of the center-of-mass (COM) within the BOS; (3) the degree of postural sway; (4) the degree of stabilization from upper or lower extremities (e.g., handhold, hooked legs); (5) number of episodes of loss of balance (LOB) and direction; (6) the degree of external assistance required; and (7) fall safety risk.

Dynamic postural control (*dynamic equilibrium, dynamic balance, or controlled mobility*) is the ability to maintain postural stability and orientation with the COM over the BOS while parts of the body are in motion. Thus an individual is able to weight shift or rock back and forth

Table 8.8 Differential Diagnosis: Comparison of Major Types of Central Nervous System Disorders

Location of Lesion	Cerebral cortex Corticospinal tracts	Basal ganglia	Cerebellum	Spinal cord
Diagnosis/ Pathology	Stroke	Parkinson's disease	Tumor, stroke	Trauma, tumor, vascular insult: complete, incomplete SCI
Sensation	Impaired or absent: depends on lesion location; contralateral sensory loss	Not affected	Not affected	Impaired or absent below the level of lesion
Tone	Hypertonia/spasticity velocity-dependent; clasp-knife Initial flaccidity: cerebral shock	Leadpipe rigidity: increased, uniform resistance Cogwheel rigidity: increased, rachet-like resistance	Normal or may be decreased	Hypertonia/ spasticity below the level of the lesion Initial flaccidity: spinal shock
Reflexes	Hyperreflexia	Normal or may be decreased	Normal or may be decreased	Hyperreflexia
Strength	Contralateral weakness or paralysis: hemiplegia or hemiparesis Disuse weakness in chronic stage	Disuse weakness in chronic stage	Normal or weak: asthenia	Impaired or absent below the level of the lesion: paraplegia or paraparesis; tetraplegia or tetraparesis
Muscle Bulk	Normal during acute stage; disuse atrophy in chronic stage	Normal or disuse atrophy	Normal	Disuse atrophy
Involuntary Movements	Spasms	Resting tremor	None	Spasms
Voluntary Movements	Dyssynergic: abnormal timing, co-activation, fatigability	Bradykinesia: slowness of movement Akinesia: absence of movement	Ataxia: intention tremor dysdiadochokinesia dysmetria dyssynergia nystagmus	Above level of lesion: intact (normal) Below level of lesion: impaired or absent
Postural Control	Impaired or absent, depends on lesion location Impaired balance	Impaired: stooped (flexed) Impaired balance	Impaired: truncal ataxia Impaired balance	Impaired below level of lesion Impaired balance
Gait	Impaired: gait deficits due to abnormal weakness, synergies, spasticity, timing deficits	Impaired: shuffling, festinating gait	Impaired: ataxic gait deficits, wide-based, unsteady	Impaired or absent: depends on level of lesion

From O'Sullivan S, and Siegelman R,[133, p 94] with permission.
SCI = spinal cord injury.

Box 8.1 Functional Task Analysis Worksheet

Task analysis begins with an appreciation of normal movements. An examination and evaluation of the patient's task performance is completed and a comparison of the differences is made. Critical skills include accurate observation, recognition and interpretation of movement deficiencies, determination of how underlying impairments relate to the movement deficiencies observed, and determination of what needs be altered and how. The following questions can be used as a guide for qualitative functional task analysis.

A. What are the normal requirements of the functional task being observed?
   1. What is the overall movement sequence (motor plan)?
   2. What are the initial conditions required? Starting position and initial alignment?
   3. How and where is the movement initiated?
   4. How is the movement executed?
   5. What are the musculoskeletal components required for successful completion of the task?
   6. What are the motor control strategies required for successful completion of the task? Is this a mobility activity? Stability activity? Skill activity?
   7. What are the requirements for timing, force, and direction of movements?
   8. What are the requirements for balance?
   9. How is the movement terminated?
   10. What are the environmental constraints that must be considered?

B. How successful is the patient's overall movement in terms of outcome?
   1. Was the overall movement sequence completed?
   2. What components of the patient's movements are normal? Almost normal?
   3. What components of the patient's movements are abnormal?
   4. What components of the patient's movements are missing? Delayed?
   5. If abnormal, are the movements compensatory and functional? Noncompensatory and nonfunctional?
   6. What are the underlying impairments that constrain or impair the movements?
   7. Do the movement errors increase over time? Is fatigue a constraining factor?
   8. Is this a mobility level activity? Are the requirements met?
   9. Is this a stability level activity? Are the requirements met for static and dynamic control?
   10. Is this a skill level activity? Are the requirements met?
   11. Are balance requirements met? Is patient safety evident throughout the task?
   12. What environmental factors constrain or impair the movements?
   13. Can the patient adapt to changing task and environmental demands?
   14. What difficulties do you expect this patient will have with other functional tasks?
   15. What difficulties do you expect this patient will have in other environments?

Adapted from Task Force of the Neurology Section of APTA: A Compendium for Teaching Professional Level Neurologic Content, Neurology Section, American Physical Therapy Association, (APTA), Alexandria, VA, 2000.

or side to side in a posture (e.g., in sitting or standing) without losing control. The ability to shift weight onto one side and free a limb for non-weightbearing dynamic activity is also evidence of dynamic postural control (sometimes called *static-dynamic control*). The initial weight shift and redistributed weightbearing places increased demands for stability on the support segments while the dynamic limb challenges control. For example, a patient with traumatic brain injury is positioned in quadruped and demonstrates difficulty when asked to lift either an upper or lower limb, or lift the opposite upper and lower limbs together. In sitting, the patient with stroke is unable to reach forward and to the affected side with the sound limb without losing balance and falling over. Key elements the therapist should observe and document include (1) the degree of postural stability maintained by the weightbearing segments; (2) the range and degree of control of the dynamic movements; and (3) level and type of assistance required (e.g., verbal cues, manual cues, guided movement).

Skill is the ability to consistently perform coordinated movement sequences for the purposes of investigation and interaction with the physical and social environment. Proximal segments stabilize while distal segments are free for skilled function (e.g., manipulation or transport). Skills are learned, and are the direct result of practice and experience. Key elements the therapist should observe and document include (1) response orientation and direction of movements (correct movement response); (2) precision, control, and consistency of movements (continuous and appropriate motor adjustments, steadiness); (3) control of movement speed and timing including reaction time, movement time; and (4) economy of effort. Motor skills can be discrete, continuous, or serial. Kicking a ball is an example of a discrete skill, with a recognizable beginning and end. Walking is a continuous skill (no recognizable beginning and end), and playing a piano represents a serial skill (a series of discrete actions put together). A skilled individual is able to adapt movements easily to the specific environments in which they occur. Thus, control of walking is evident in the clinic as well as in the home environment. A movement skill performed in a stable, nonchanging environment is called a **closed motor skill**, while a movement skill performed in a variable, changing environment is called an **open motor skill**. A skilled individual is also able to perform simultaneous movement tasks *(dual task control)*. For example, the individual is able to stand or walk while holding or manipulating an object (e.g., bouncing or throwing a ball).[73]

The qualitative analysis of functional skills can be enhanced by the use of video equipment or still photographs. Patient responses are recorded, providing a permanent record of motor performance and allowing the therapist the opportunity to compare responses over time. Recordings made at 3 or 6 weeks of recovery can be compared easily without reliance on the therapist's memory or written notes. Accuracy of observations can be improved. A therapist who is closely involved in assisting or guarding during performance may not be attentive enough to observe all movement parameters (e.g., when assisting the patient with traumatic brain injury with severe ataxia). Depending on equipment capabilities, videotapes can be viewed repeatedly at different speeds to determine control during different tasks and at different body segments. For example, a patient's performance in a task such as sitting up from supine can be observed first at regular speeds, then at slow motion speeds. Stop-action or freezing a frame can be used to isolate a problematic point in the movement sequence. This may be helpful, particularly for the inexperienced therapist, in improving both the quality and reliability of observations. Repeat trials on a functional performance test may needlessly tire the patient while yielding a decrease in performance. Sequential recordings over the course of rehabilitation provide visual documentation of patient progress and can be an important motivational and educational tool in therapy for use with the patient and family.[74] Reliability of recordings for intersession comparisons can be improved by the following measures. Placement of equipment should be planned in advance to achieve the best location and should be consistently placed over subsequent sessions. Use of a tripod can improve the stability of the recording. Verbal descriptions of the performance during each trial can be edited directly onto a videotape or documented in a written summary.[75]

Postural Control and Balance

Postural orientation involves control of the relative positions of body parts by skeletal muscles with respect to each other and gravity. **Balance** is the condition in which all the forces acting on the body are balanced such that the center of mass (COM) is within the stability limits, the boundaries of the base of support (BOS). The overall goals of the postural control system, stability and function, are achieved through integrated CNS systems of control. *Reactive postural control* occurs in response to external forces acting on the body (e.g., perturbations) displacing the COM or moving the BOS (e.g., moveable platform, therapy ball). Feedback systems provide the sensory inputs required to initiate corrective responses. *Proactive (anticipatory) postural control* occurs in anticipation of internally generated, destabilizing forces imposed on the body's own movements (e.g., catching a weighted ball).[2] An individual's prior experiences allow the various elements of the postural control system to be pretuned or readied for upcoming movements using feedforward mechanisms. Postural requirements vary depending on the characteristics of the task and the environment. *Adaptive postural control* allows the individual to appropriately "modify sensory and motor systems in response to changing task and environmental demands."[2, p 1] Balance emerges from a complex interaction of (1) sensory (afferent) systems responsible for the detection of body position and motion, (2) motor (effector) systems responsible for the execution of motor responses, and (3) CNS integration processes. An examination of balance must therefore focus on each of these three areas.

Postural Alignment and Weight Distribution

Normal postural alignment in standing can be examined by observing skeletal alignment using a plumb or weighted line. More sophisticated analysis can be achieved using motion analysis systems with light emitting signals, photography, and electromyography. In standing, the COM occurs at a point about two thirds of the body height above the BOS. Static posture in standing is examined by positioning the patient with the feet apart, normal stance width. When viewed from the side (sagittal plane alignment) the plumb line is positioned just in front of the lateral malleolus. The vertical *line of gravity (LOG)* is expected to fall close to most joint axes: slightly anterior to the ankle and knee joints, at or slightly posterior to the hip joint, through midline of the trunk, just anterior to the shoulder joint, and through the external auditory meatus.[76] Natural spinal curves are present but flattened in upright stance depending on the level of postural tone, lumbar and cervical lordosis, and thoracic or dorsal kyphosis. The pelvis is held in neutral position, with no anterior or posterior tilt. When viewed from the front or back (frontal plane analysis), the feet are positioned equidistant from the plumb line. The examiner looks for equal weight distribution between feet and symmetry and of the trunk and extremities. Normal alignment minimizes the need for active muscle contraction during standing. Muscles that are tonically active at low levels during quiet stance include tibialis anterior and gastrocnemius-soleus; tensor fascia latae, gluteus medius, and iliopsoas; and abdominals and erector spinae.[77] In sitting when viewed from the side, head and trunk are vertical. Natural spinal curves are present and the pelvis is maintained in a neutral position. When viewed from the front or back, the trunk and head are held in a midline orientation with symmetrical weightbearing on both lower extremities (buttocks, thighs, and feet).

Limits of stability (LOS) are defined as the maximum distance an individual is able or willing to lean in any direction without loss of balance or changing the BOS. Thus in standing an individual can shift forward and backward or side to side without losing balance or taking a step. In normal individuals, the anteroposterior (AP) LOS in standing is approximately 12 degrees while the medial–lateral (ML) LOS is approximately 16° from side to side (normal stance width, 4 inches). LOS is influenced by individual characteristics such as height and foot length for AP LOS and distance between the feet and height for ML LOS.[78] The midpoint of LOS is termed the *COM alignment*. *Steadiness* refers to the ability to maintain a given posture with minimum movement (sway).[79] During standing, an individual normally exhibits small range postural shifts (*postural sway*), cycling intermittently from side-to-side and from heel-to-toe. *Sway envelope* refers to the path of the body's movement during standing. During walking, there are minimal COM movements up and down and side-to-side, resulting in a smooth sinusoidal curve. In sitting, the BOS is larger and COM lower (just above the support base), resulting in greater LOS.

Postural sway can be examined using visual inspection with the patient standing against a postural grid.[80] More sophisticated instrumentation, posturography, utilizes forceplate to measure ground reaction forces, either center of force (COF) measures or center of pressure (COP) measures. COF is calculated using only vertical forces, and COP is calculated using both vertical and horizontal shear forces. The weight of each foot is determined, forces calculated, and converted into a visual image (Fig. 8.1). Audio signals are available on some devices. Software allows analysis of data and typically includes protocols that can be used for training. Measures of the initial stance position (center of alignment), mean sway path, total excursion (LOS), and the zone of stability can be obtained and are valid and reliable measures of postural control.[81,82] Using this information, the therapist can objectively determine the patient's postural symmetry, which is a reflection of the amount of weight placed on each foot. Patients with asymmetry may present with the COP positioned away from midline. For example, the patient with stroke typically stands with most of the weight on the sound limb. Steadiness can be determined by using postural sway measures. A large sway path is evidence of postural unsteadiness. For example, the patient with ataxia typically demonstrates hypermetric responses, with excessive sway, uncoordinated movements, and limited postural steadiness. The patient with Parkinson's disease presents with the opposite problem, hypometric responses with diminished sway and excessive stabilization.[83] Dynamic stability can be determined by using LOS information. Patients with deficits in motor control (e.g., the patient with stroke) typically have reduced LOS. LOS and COM alignment are also typically altered in other pathological states (e.g., muscle weakness, skeletal deformity, and tonal abnormalities). Reexamination following training using force platform biofeedback has been used to demonstrate the effectiveness of training using such devices.[79,84,85]

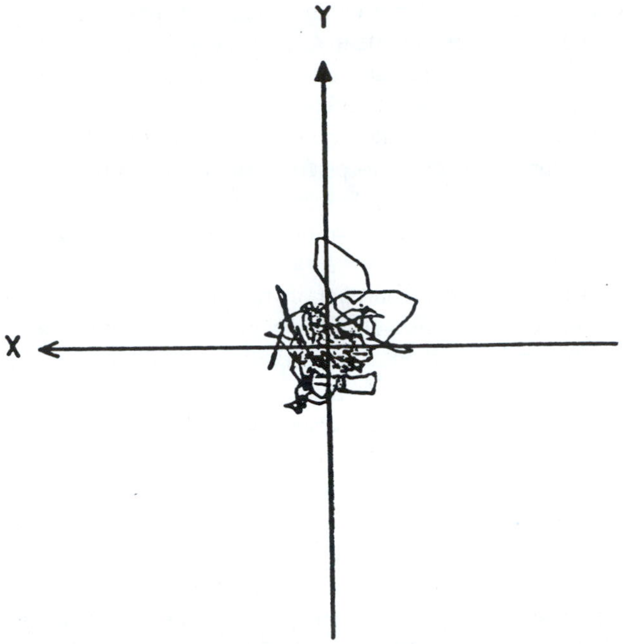

Figure 8.1 Postural sway. Recording of the movement of the center of pressure for 60 seconds in a subject standing on a balance platform. Values: mean amplitude of sway path in inches = .13 × .15 Y; length of path = 32.2; velocity = .45 in/sec. (From Smith, L, et al: Brunnstrom's Clinical Kinesiology, ed 5. FA Davis, Philadelphia, 1996, p 406, with permission.)

Sensory Organization

The sensory systems (vision, somatosensory, and vestibular) provide the CNS with important information about postural control and balance, including information about the results of our own actions and the surrounding environment. The CNS integrates these inputs and initiates both goal-directed conscious actions as well as automatic, unconscious adjustments in our posture and movements. Each individual sensory system provides unique and important information and no one system provides all the information needed.

The visual system serves an important source of information for our ability to perceive our movements and detect the relative orientation of the body parts and orientation of the body in space. This ability has been termed **visual proprioception**.[86] Two separate functional visual systems have been identified. Various different names have been used: (1) *focal vision* (cognitive or explicit vision) and (2) *ambient vision* (sensorimotor or implicit vision). Focal vision plays a major role in localizing features in the environment and in our conscious reaction to visual events. In contrast, ambient vision utilizes the entire visual field to provide information on the localizing features about the environment and to guide movements using largely nonconscious awareness.[1] Thus each visual system has unique functional significance. For example, the patient with brain injury who has a condition called optic ataxia can recognize an object (focal vision) but cannot use visual information to accurately guide his or her hand to the object (impaired ambient vision). The opposite occurs in a patient with visual agnosia. The patient cannot recognize common objects, but can use the ambient visual system to reach and grab an object. Vision also contributes to righting reactions of the head, trunk, and limbs (optical righting reactions).

Visual acuity (focal vision) can be examined using a Snellen eye chart. A distance acuity poorer than 20/50 will have a significant effect on postural stability.[87] Whereas focal vision is detected by the central retina only, ambient vision is detected by the entire visual field (central and peripheral vision). Patients with loss of peripheral vision (e.g., a patient with stroke and hemianopsia or a patient with glaucoma) may demonstrate deficits in visual proprioception and functional performance. Peripheral vision can be examined using the *confrontation method*. The patient sits in front of the therapist and is instructed to focus gaze on the therapist's nose. The therapist then slowly brings a target (moving finger or pencil) slowly into the patient's field of view from the right or left side. The patient is instructed to indicate (point or declare) when and where the target is detected. Ambient vision can be examined by instructing the patient to navigate across the busy physical therapy gym. The ability to navigate safely, localize features in the environment, and anticipate changes necessary to avoid obstacles and successfully reach the target area are determined. Patients with stroke who exhibit topographical disorientation will have difficulty navigating their environment and understanding the relationship of one place to another.

Somatosensory inputs include the cutaneous and pressure sensations from the body segments in contact with the support surface (e.g., the feet in standing or buttocks, thighs, and feet in sitting) and muscle and joint proprioception throughout the body. They provide information about the relative orientation and movement of the body in relation to the support surface. Cutaneous sensation (touch and pressure) of the feet/ankles and proprioception of the feet/ankles and hips are particularly important in maintaining upright standing balance. Sensory examination of the extremities and trunk is therefore essential (examination techniques are discussed fully in Chapter 5).

The semicircular canals (SCCs) of the vestibular system detect angular acceleration and deceleration forces acting on the head whereas the otolith organs detect linear acceleration and orientation of the head with reference to gravity. The SCCs are sensitive to fast (phasic) movements of the head, and the otoliths respond to slow head movements and position. The vestibular system functions to stabilize gaze during head movements (via the vestibulo-ocular reflex [VOR]), and to assist in the regulation of postural tone and postural muscle activation. Tests for vestibular function include positional and movement testing. The patient is observed for symptoms of vestibular dysfunction (e.g., dizziness, vertigo, nystagmus).[88] See Chapter 24 for a complete discussion of this topic.

CNS Integration

Sensory integration by the CNS is flexible; although all inputs are important, the CNS weights the various inputs. During quiet stance, defined as a stable support surface and surroundings, all inputs contribute to the maintenance of posture. For intact adults under these conditions, the CNS places greater weight on somatosensory inputs. Somatosensory inputs assume a major role when platform perturbations are introduced. If somatosensory inputs are impaired (e.g., the patient with peripheral neuropathy) or if somatosensory conflicting information is introduced (e.g., standing on dense foam), vision assumes a greater role. If both somatosensory and visual inputs are impaired or distorted, vestibular inputs, which are referenced to gravity, are critical to resolve sensory conflict.[78] Balance responses are therefore task and context dependent and are triggered by availability and accuracy of specific sensory inputs. Because these inputs are redundant, stable balance can be maintained with visual impairment, on unstable surfaces, or in sensory conflict situations. However, if more than one sensory system is deficient, substantial deficiencies in balance control will be evident.[89] In addition, the cognitive system plays an important role in interpreting the information and planning an effective responses. Patients with impairments in cognition or attention demonstrate increased fall risk.

The Clinical Test for Sensory Interaction in Balance (CTSIB) is based on the work of Nashner[90,91] and can be used to determine the effectiveness of an individual to utilize different sensory inputs. It examines body sway during quiet standing under six different sensory test conditions (Fig. 8.2). Dynamic posturography equipment provides a moving platform that introduces mechanical perturbations (sliding or tilting movements). A moving visual surround screen is sway referenced and introduces visual conflict. Both the surround and force plate are referenced to the patient by means of hydraulic mechanisms. Test condition 1 provides accurate somatosensory, visual, and vestibular information and is the baseline reference. Each of the other five conditions systematically varies sensory inputs, increasing the level of sensory conflict and postural difficulty.

- Condition 1: Eyes Open, Stable Surface (EOSS)
- Condition 2: Eyes Closed, Stable Surface (ECSS)
- Condition 3: Visual Conflict with Moving Surround, Stable Surface (VCSS)
- Condition 4: Eyes Open, Moving Surface (EOMS)
- Condition 5: Eyes Closed, Moving Surface (ECMS)
- Condition 6: Visual Conflict with Moving Surround, Moving Platform (VCMS)

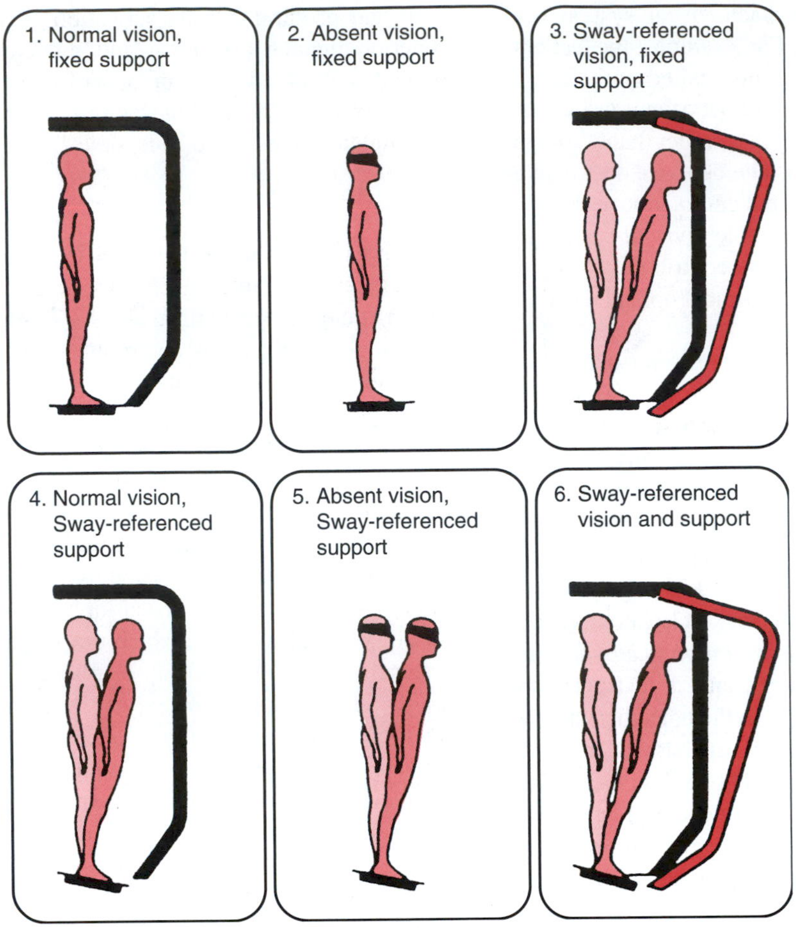

Figure 8.2 The sensory organization test.

Conditions 1 to 3 are all performed with the patient standing on a stable support surface, providing accurate somatosensory inputs. Visual inputs are varied: condition 1 uses EO, condition 2 uses EC, and condition 3 uses a moving visual surround (screen) referenced to body sway, thus providing inaccurate visual information. Conditions 4 through 6 repeat the visual conditions but with an altered support surface (moving platform) that provides inaccurate somatosensory information. In conditions 5 and 6 maintenance of posture depends on availability and accuracy of vestibular inputs. Thus, patients with vestibular dysfunction will demonstrate maximum instability in conditions 5 and 6. Patients who are visually dependent for postural control will demonstrate instability in conditions 2, 3, 5, and 6. Patients who are surface dependent will demonstrate instability in conditions 4, 5, and 6.[2] Each condition is maintained for 30 seconds. If the patient is able to stand for the required 30 seconds, the test is progressed to the next sensory condition. If the patient is unsuccessful on the first attempt, a second trial can be given. The CTSIB is scored by observing changes in the amount and direction of postural sway. A numerical scoring system can be used[92,93]:

1 Minimal sway
2 Mild sway
3 Moderate sway
4 Fall

Posturography equipment provides a printed bar graph indicating how well the patient performed during each of the six conditions in terms of postural sway. Ratios comparing one condition to another can provide information regarding reliance on one sensory system over another. Additional analyses of motor coordination using EMG can provide information about the relative level of individual muscle activity as well as overall muscle recruitment patterns.

In the absence of sophisticated posturography equipment, an alternate version of the CTSIB (Sensory Organization Test) can be used in clinical or home settings to identify if the use of sensory information is normal or abnormal. The test requires an individual stand quietly in each of the six different sensory test conditions. Dense foam is used instead of the moving platform to provide the inaccurate somatosensory information. A dome head piece is used instead of a moving surround screen to provide inaccurate visual information required in conditions 3 and 6.[92] A simplified version, the *M-CTSIB*, using only four conditions (1, 2, 4, and 5) has been recommended for older, community dwelling adults, omitting the dome head piece. The same posture should be adopted in each of the conditions, i.e., feet shoulder-width apart and arms folded across chest. Time in balance (30 seconds each trial, 120 seconds total time) and increased sway or loss of balance are recorded. Subjective complaints of the patient (e.g., nausea, dizziness) and postural strategies used are also documented. The test is stopped if the patient alters the posture (widens or moves feet, opens eyes, unfolds arms) or loses balance, requiring manual assistance. Three trials are given and the average time in balance is documented.[94]

Motor Strategies

In observational studies of infants and young children and lesioned animals (decerebration experiments), righting and equilibrium reactions comprise the postural reflex mechanism. Automatic righting reactions (RR) orient the head in space (optical RR, labyrinthine RR, body-on-head RR) and the body in relation to the head and support surface (neck-on-body RR, body-on-body RR). Equilibrium reactions include tilting reactions, and parachute or protective reactions. In normal adults, however, postural adjustments are far more complex and demonstrate a high degree of adaptability in response to both task and environmental context demands.

Postural adjustments vary from the simple stretch responses to the activation of specific motor strategies (synergistic patterns of movement). Muscles closest to the BOS are particularly important to the maintenance of balance. As the LOS is reached with a COM disturbance, the magnitude of the postural response is increased. In standing, the *ankle strategy* involves shifting the COM forward and back by moving the body as a relatively fixed pendulum about the ankle joints. Muscles are activated in a distal-to-proximal sequence. With forward sway, gastrocnemius is activated first, followed by hamstrings, then paraspinal muscles. With backward sway, the anterior tibialis is activated first, followed by quadriceps, then abdominals. The ankle strategy is a commonly used strategy when disturbances are small and well within the LOS. The *hip strategy* involves shifts in the COM by flexing or extending at the hips. It has a proximal pattern of muscle activation. With forward sway abdominals are activated first, followed by quadriceps. With backward sway, paraspinal muscles are activated first, followed by hamstrings. With lateral destabilization, hip abductors provide primary control. The hip strategy is typically recruited with larger and faster disturbances of the COM or when standing on a BOS that is narrower than the length of the feet. These strategies have been termed *fixed-support strategies,* in that the COM is controlled over a fixed BOS.[90,91,95,96]

Change-in-support strategies are defined as movements of the lower or upper limbs to make a new contact with the support surface.[97] The *stepping strategy* realigns the BOS under the COM by using rapid steps or hops in the direction of the displacing force, for example, forward or backward steps. In instances of lateral destabilization, the individual takes a side step or a cross step to bring the BOS back under the COM. The stepping strategies are typically recruited in response to fast, large postural perturbations (Fig. 8.3). Change-in-support movements of the upper limb can also assist in stabilizing the COM over the BOS, and serve a protective function in absorbing impact and protecting the head in a fall event. Grasping movements assist in extending the BOS and stabilizing posture. These reactions were found to be prevalent in destabilization situations, occurring in 85 percent of trials. Stepping strategies were also frequent, leading researchers to suggest that change-in-support strategies should not be viewed as strategies of last resort. They are often initiated well before the COM nears or exceeds the LOS, contrary to the traditional view.[96]

While these strategies have been investigated individually as distinct movement patterns, research has also shown that during normal balance combinations of strategies are used.[95]

In sitting, the BOS is comprised of the thighs and buttocks and the feet if in contact with the support surface. Postural strategies to maintain balance include movement of the trunk about the hips. Backward sway elicits primary responses in hip flexors along with activity of the abdominals and neck flexors. In forward sway, extensor muscles of the hips are activated along with the extensors of the

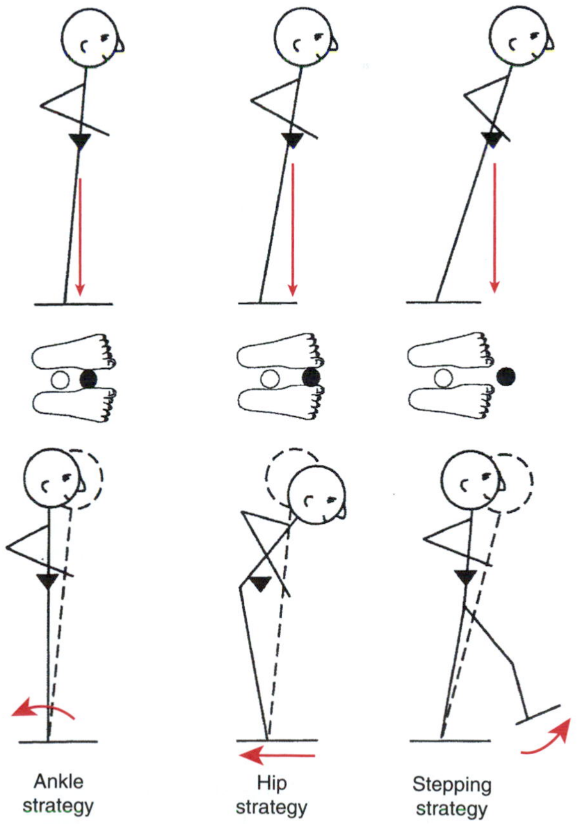

Figure 8.3 Strategies for correcting balance perturbations.

neck and trunk. If the feet are in contact, tibialis anterior is recruited during forward reaching movements of the arm and the gastrocnemius is recruited to brake forward movements and return the body to erect sitting.[98] Somatosensory inputs from backward rotation of the pelvis may have an important role in triggering the postural strategies in sitting.[99] In frontal plane movements, activity of the hip abductors and adductors along with the quadratus lumborum is important.

An examination of motor strategies should first begin with the musculoskeletal elements (ROM, postural tone, and strength). Weakness and limited ROM in the ankles will affect successful use of an ankle strategy, whereas weakness and limited ROM about the hips will influence the hip strategy. Limitations of neck ROM can be expected in patients with primary vestibular disorders. Available motor strategies in response to destabilizations (anteroposterior, medial–lateral) should be determined.

Dynamic posturography provides the ideal way to study motor strategies. The *Movement Coordination Test (MCT)* developed by Nashner and co-workers[96] provides information about postural responses to control the COM when the platform moves, including symmetry of weight-bearing and forces generated, latency of postural responses, amplitude of response in relation to the stimulus size, and strategy utilized (ankle or hip). EMG monitoring can reveal specific muscle activation patterns and latencies. The main disadvantage is that the equipment is expensive and not portable. Correlation with performance during functional tasks (walking) is also lacking.

The therapist needs to determine and document if the motor strategies are (1) present and normal, (2) present but limited or delayed, (3) present but inappropriate for the particular context or situation, (4) abnormal, or (5) absent.[91] Differences in responses can be seen by systematically varying sensory inputs and the size and type of perturbations. Both reactive and anticipatory postural strategies should be examined. For example, the patient can be asked to raise the arms overhead or lift a weighted ball. The destabilizing effects of voluntary movement and strategies used to maintain position should be documented. Finally, the ability to adapt postural strategies should be examined. For example, the patient can be asked to stand first with normal stance width, then with a narrowed BOS. The ability to improve performance with repeat practice trials should be documented.

Functional Balance Tests

Functional tests of balance focus on the maintenance of posture (static balance), balance during weight shifting or voluntary movement (dynamic balance), balance responses to manual perturbations, and functional mobility (gait) (Table 8.9). Examples of static balance tasks in standing include double limb stance, single limb stance (SLS), tandem stance (heel-toe position), and the Romberg test. Dynamic balance tasks include sit-to-stand (STS) and sit down (SIT); reaching movements; turning, and step-ups. Walking tasks include timed walking, walking with commands to turn direction (180° or 360° turns), turn the head (side to side or up and down), or stop and start. Scoring can vary from a simple subjective scale (impaired or intact) to a scale with specific criterion descriptions for successful performance. Table 8.10 presents an example of scale of functional balance grades with descriptors that can be used to define control in both sitting and standing. The objectivity of measurements can be increased by using timed performance. For example, a stopwatch can be used to document time in balance during a 30-second trial of a single limb stance.[100,101]

Standardized tests of balance are available that examine functional performance. It is important to consider instruments with established reliability, validity, and sensitivity. A summary of functional balance instruments discussed in this chapter is presented in Evidence Summary Box 8.2.

The Romberg Test

The Romberg Test is used to determine proprioceptive contributions to upright balance. The patient is instructed to stand with feet together, eyes open (EO) unaided for 20 to 30 seconds. If the patient falls with EO, the test is over. The patient is then asked to stand with eyes closed (EC). In

Table 8.9 Functional Balance Grades

Normal	Patient able to maintain steady balance without handhold support (static). Patient accepts maximal challenge and can shift weight easily within full range in all directions (dynamic).
Good	Patient able to maintain balance without handhold support, limited postural sway (static). Patient accepts moderate challenge; able to maintain balance while picking object off floor (dynamic).
Fair	Patient able to maintain balance with handhold support; may require occasional minimal assistance (static). Patient accepts minimal challenge; able to maintain balance while turning head/trunk (dynamic).
Poor	Patient requires handhold support and moderate to maximal assistance to maintain position (static). Patient unable to accept challenge or move without loss of balance (dynamic).

Evidence Summary Box 8.2
Functional Balance Test

Instrument	Content	Validity	Reliability	Comments
The Balance Scale (Berg Balance Scale) Berg[108] 1989 Equipment needed: chairs with and without arms, stopwatch, ruler, 6-inch step	Multitask test of 14 balance tasks common in everyday living: 6 static balance items; 8 dynamic balance items Focuses on: • Maintenance of position • Postural adjustment to voluntary movement Items 1–5 = tests of basic balance ability Scoring: 5-point ordinal scale (graded 0–4) with specific task criteria for levels ranging from I > D; some items timed Max score = 56	Content validity: expert consensus (health professionals and geriatric patients). Concurrent validity: correlation with Tinetti Balance Sub test = .91 Barthel Mobility = .67 TUG = .76 Predictive: of falls in the elderly (hospitals, long-term care, community)	Reliability (ICC) Interrater = .98 Intrarater = .99 Individual items ranged from .71 to .99 Internal consistency (Cronbach's alpha) = .96	High degree of agreement of raters Strong internal consistency Simple, easy to administer (15–20 min.); comprehensive Requirements: able to stand independently Does not include items on gait or reaction to external stimulus/uneven surface Provides baseline, and outcome data; scores of 45 or below are predictive of falls in the elderly
Tinetti Performance Oriented Mobility Assessment (POMA) Tinetti[115,116] 1986 Equipment needed: chair, walkway; patient can use usual walking aid	Multitask test: Balance sub-test: 9 items (4 static; 5 dynamic) Gait subtest: 8 items Focuses on: • Maintenance of position • Postural response to voluntary movement • Postural response to perturbation • Gait mobility Scoring: some items graded can/cannot perform; some 3-point scale with specific task criteria Max score = 28	Content validity: expert consensus Concurrent validity: correlation with Berg = .91 Barthel index = .76 Predictive of falls in the elderly (long-term care)	Reliability (ICC) Interrater = .85 Lacks intrarater reliability testing	High degree of agreement of raters Simple, easy to administer (15 min) Requirements: able to stand and walk independently Some scoring criteria vague; difficult to detect small changes Provides baseline data; predictive of falls in elderly: > 24 low risk 19–24 mod risk 18 > high risk
Timed Up and Go (TUG) Podsiadlo and Richardson[121] 1991 Get Up and Go Test: Mathias, Nayak, Issacs[120] 1986 Equipment needed: stopwatch, armchair, measured walkway patient can use AD	Single task test: stand-up, walk 3 m (10 ft), turn around, and return to chair Focuses on: functional mobility Scoring: timed test Uses 1 practice/3 trials for average score	Content validity: expert consensus Concurrent validity: Berg = .81 Barthel = .78	Reliability (ICC) Interrater = .99 Intrarater = .98	High degree of agreement of raters Simple, easy to administer, quick screen (< 3 min) Requirements: able to stand and walk independently Provides baseline and outcome data; Predictive of falls in elderly: < 10 sec. = independent 20 – 29 sec. = normal for frail elderly or disabled patients > 30 sec. = dependent in mobility skills and most ADL

(continued)

Evidence Summary Box 8.2

Functional Balance Test (continued)

Instrument	Content	Validity	Reliability	Comments
Functional Reach (FR) Duncan et al[102] 1990 Equipment needed: level yardstick mounted on wall at shoulder height	Single task test: Examines forward UE reach with shoulder at 90° flexion, feet still Focuses on: • Postural responses related to voluntary UE movement • Examines Limits of Stability (LOS) Scoring: distance in inches Uses 1 practice/3 trials for average score	Content validity: expert consensus Concurrent validity: Duke mobility = .65 Gait speed = .71	Reliability (ICC) Interrater = .98 Intrarater = .92	High degree of agreement of raters Simple, easy to administer, quick screen (5 min) Requirements: • able to stand independently • requires adequate shoulder ROM FR affected by age and height Provides baseline and outcome data; Predictive of falls in the elderly
Mulitdirectional Reach Test (MDRT) Newton[106] 2001 Equipment needed: yardstick, wall	Single task test: Examines UE reach with shoulder at 90° flexion, feet still—forwards, sidewards, and backwards Focuses on: • Postural responses related to voluntary UE movements • Examines Limits of Stability (LOS) Scoring: distance in inches Uses 1 practice/3 trials for average score			Same as for FR
Timed Walking Test Murray et al[123] 1966 Equipment needed: measured walkway (e.g., 50-ft/15.2 m), stopwatch, tape Tape markers at 10, 60, and 70 foot marks (3, 18, and 21 m); measured zones for acceleration, target speed, and deceleration AD can be used as needed	Single, continuous test item Compares self-paced, preferred gait speed and fast speed Focuses on • overall gait speed (distance over time) • ability to adapt gait speed • can calculate stride length Uses 1 practice/3 trials for average score			Simple, easy to administer, quick screen (3 min) Requirements: independent ambulation, for mod. to high functioning adults Provides screening, baseline and outcome data; results reported as time taken (seconds) or speed (distance/sec.) Use of AD is associated with slower gait speeds Age-related norms: • healthy young adults = 1.2–1.5 m/s • older adults = 0.9–1.3 m/s

AD = Assistive devices; D = dependent; I = independent.

Table 8.10 Functional Reach (FR) Reference Values (NORMS) By Age

Age	Men (inches)	Women (inches)
20–40 Age	16.7 (± 1.9)	14.6 (± 2.2)
41–69	14.9 (± 2.2)	13.8 (± 2.2)
70–87	13.2 (± 1.6)	10.5 (± 3.5)

From Duncan, P, et al.[102]

a negative test there is only minimal sway. If the test is positive, the patient is able to stand with EO but demonstrates increased instability or falls with EC. It is important to tell the patient you are prepared to catch him or her in event of a fall. A positive Romberg test is indicative of a loss of proprioception that can occur with posterior column lesions in the spinal cord (e.g., cervical spondylosis, tumor, degenerative spinal cord disease, tabes dorsalis) and peripheral neuropathy. If unsteadiness occurs in standing with EO (e.g., the patient with cerebellar ataxia or vestibular dysfunction) the Romberg test is not appropriate.[20] In the sharpened Romberg test, the feet are placed in tandem (heel–toe position) and the EO to EC conditions imposed.

Functional Reach and Multidirectional Reach Test

The Functional Reach Test (FR) was developed by Duncan and co-workers to provide a quick screen of balance problems in older adults.[102–104] It is the maximal distance one can reach forward beyond arm's length while maintaining a fixed BOS in the standing position. The test uses a level yardstick mounted on the wall and positioned at the height of the patient's acromion. The patient stands sidewards next to the wall (without touching), feet normal stance width and weight equally distributed on both feet. The shoulder is flexed to 90° and elbow extended with the hand fisted. An initial measurement is made of the position of the 3rd metacarpal along the yardstick. For forward reach, the patient is instructed to lean as far forward as possible without losing balance or taking a step. A second measurement is taken also using the 3rd metacarpal for reference. This measurement is then subtracted from the initial measurement. See Table 8.10 for normative values of FR. The *Multidirectional Reach Test (MDFR)* developed by Newton evolved from the earlier FR and measures how far an individual can reach in the forward, backward, and lateral directions.[105–107] For backward reach, the test position is the same as FR with the yardstick position reversed to detect posterior movements. For lateral reach, the patient faces away from the wall and reaches sideways to the right (and then to the left) as far as possible. One practice trial is allowed before the start of three test trials. The therapist records functional reach in inches for all three trials and then averages the three trials. The amount of reach is influenced by several factors, including the size and height of the individual, gender, age, and health. The movement strategy used during a reach test should be documented (i.e., ankle or hip strategy, trunk rotation, scapular protraction). See Table 8.11 for normative values of MDRT.

The Berg Balance Scale

The Berg Balance Scale (BBS) developed by Berg and coworkers[108–110] is an objective measure of static and dynamic balance abilities. The scale consists of 14 functional tasks commonly performed in everyday life. The items range from sitting or standing unsupported, to movement transitions (sit-to-stand, stand-to-sit), variations in standing position (EO/EC), feet together, forward reach, retrieving an object from the floor, turning, standing on one foot) to placing the foot on a stool. Scoring uses a five-point ordinal scale, with scores ranging from 0 to 4. Descriptive criteria are provided for scoring each level: a score of 4 is used to indicate that the patient *performs independently and meets time and distance criteria,* and a score of 0 is used for *unable to perform* (see Appendix A). A maximum score of 56 points is possible. The BBS was originally developed for use with elderly patients with stroke in the acute rehabilitation setting and has been shown to be a sensitive measure of recovery. Balance scale scores have also been shown to be useful in predicting falls in the elderly[111,112] and evaluating changes in patients undergoing physical therapy.[113] A scores of 45 or below is associated with a high fall risk and each one-point drop in scores ranging from 54 to 36 is associated with a 6 to 8 percent increase in fall risk.[112] The BBS is a sensitive measure for low-functioning older adults.[111–113] The first five items are considered basic balance items while the last nine items

Table 8.11 Multidirectional Reach Test (MDRT) Reference Values

REACH-MDRT	Mean (inches) Standard Deviation Mean Age, 74	Above Average (inches)	Below Average (inches)
Forward	8.9 ± 3.4	>12.2	<5.6
Backward	4.6 ± 3.1	>7.6	<1.6
Right lateral	6.2 ± 3.0	>9.4	<3.8
Left lateral	6.6 ± 2.8	>9.4	<3.8

From Newton, R.[106]

are considered more advanced balance tasks. The *modified Berg Balance Scale (M-BBS)* excludes the basic balance items and utilizes only the advanced balance items (items 6 to 14). The maximum score of the M-BBS is 36. It can be useful to test the balance of higher-functioning, community-dwelling individuals.[114]

Performance-Oriented Mobility Assessment (POMA)

The *Performance-Oriented Mobility Assessment (POMA)* developed by Tinetti[115,116] provides a brief, and reliable measure of both static and dynamic balance. Items are organized into two subtests of balance and gait. Balance test items include sitting balance, sit-to-stand, standing balance (nudged or perturbed, EC, turning 360°), and stand-to-sit. Gait test items include initiation of gait, path, missed step (trip or loss of balance), turning, and timed walk. Some items are scored on a two-point scale (can/cannot perform), some on a three-point (0 to 2) scale, and some items are timed (see Appendix B). The original POMA I scale has a total possible score of 28. It was developed for use with the frail elderly, especially nursing home residents with a propensity to fall.[117] Patients who score less than 19 are considered at high risk for falls while those who score between 19 and 24 are at moderate risk for falls. A revised form, the POMA Ia, includes five additional items and was designed for use as a predictor of falls among community dwelling elderly (with a total possible score of 40). The POMA II was developed as an outcome measure in a frailty and injury prevention trial (the Yale FICSIT trial) with a total possible score of 54.[118,119]

Timed Get Up and Go Test

The *Get Up and Go (GUG) Test* developed by Mathias et al[120] is a quick measure of dynamic balance and mobility. The patient is seated comfortably in a firm chair with arms and back resting against the chair. The patient is then instructed to rise, stand momentarily, and then walk 3 m (10 ft) toward a wall at normal walking speed, turn without touching the wall, return to the chair, turn, and sit down. Tape is used to mark the walking distance and turning point. Performance on the original GUG test is scored using a five-point ordinal scale ranging from 1, Normal (no risk of falls) to 2, Very Slightly Abnormal; 3, Mildly Abnormal (increased risk of falls); 4, Moderately Abnormal; and 5, Severely Abnormal (high risk of falls). If an assistive device is required, the type is recorded. Efforts by Podsiadlo and Richardson[121] to improve the objectivity and reliability resulted in the *Timed Up and Go Test (TUG)*. Timing with a stopwatch begins when the patient is instructed with "go" and ends when the patient returns to the start position in the chair. Research indicates that most adults can complete the test in less than 10 seconds. Scores of 11 to 20 seconds are considered within normal limits for frail elderly or individuals with a disability; scores over 30 seconds are indicative of impaired functional mobility. The Timed Up and Go Test provides a reliable quick screening measure; abnormal scores warrant additional comprehensive examination.

Timed Walking Test

A *timed walking test* is an important part of the examination of postural control and functional mobility.[122] The patient is asked to walk at his or her *preferred speed* over a set distance clearly marked on the floor (e.g., 10-m walk test [33 ft] or 50-ft walk test [15 m]). The patient is then asked to walk again at *maximum speed,* as fast as possible. Time is measured using a stopwatch. The results are reported in speed (meters/second or feet/second) or less commonly in total time taken (seconds). Comparisons are made between the two trials. Gait speed has been shown to be a sensitive measure of functional performance. There is a wide range of normal gait speeds reported, ranging from 1.2 to 1.5 m/sec (4 to 5 ft/sec) in healthy young adults. Gait speeds decrease in older adults (0.9 to 1.3 m/sec or 3 to 4.25 ft/sec), in individuals with a disability, and those requiring assistive devices.[123] Distance tests (e.g., the *3-, 6-,* or *12-Minute Walk Test*) can also be used to document functional mobility.[124–126] The patient is instructed to walk at a comfortable pace. During the test the patient can stop to rest or use an assistive device as needed. The total distance achieved during the preselected timed segment of walking is recorded along with average gait velocity, number of rests, number of deviations from a 15-inch wide gait path, and number of episodes of loss of balance (LOB). Other parameters can also be documented, including BOS, step width, stride length, cadence, trunk and extremity movements, and exertional intolerance (heart rate, chest pain, shortness of breath, Rating of Preceived Exertion [RPE]). See Chapter 10 for a complete description of gait analysis. Gait abnormalities should be carefully documented. Inconsistency and irregularity of stepping and movements, weaving, staggering, widely spaced steps, and arms held out to the side in guard position are all indicative of decreased balance control.[127]

The *Gait Assessment Rating Scale (GARS)* developed by Wolfson et al[128] has been used to document gait abnormalities in the elderly and to identify those at risk for falls. The *Dynamic Gait Index* developed by Shumway-Cook[2] includes variations in speed (slow, fast), head turning (looking right, left, up, and down), turning (pivot turn, 360° turn), stepping over an obstacle, stepping around obstacles, stair climbing, picking an object up from the floor, and alternate step-ups on a stool. The Dynamic Gait Index appears sensitive in predicting likelihood for falls with older adults and in individuals with vestibular dysfunction. Whitney found a moderate correlation between the Dynamic Gait Index and the Berg Balance Scale when testing individuals with vestibular and balance dysfunction.[129] The *Walkie-Talkie Test* can be used to determine attentional demands.[94] The therapist walks alongside the patient while walking and begins a conversation. Questions posed should require more than "yes" or "no" answers. The test is positive if the patient has increased difficulty walking while talking (slows down, staggers or loses balance) or has to stop walking in order to talk. The introduction of secondary task interference through dual tasking (i.e., reaching for objects, carrying an object) also reveals important information about cognitive function and attentional demands of postural control.[130]

The Balance Efficacy Scale

The *Balance Efficacy Scale (BES)* is a self-report measure that examines how confident an individual feels while performing items of daily functional mobility and ADL tasks both with or without assistance (handhold). The 18 items on the test include getting out of a chair, walking up or down a flight of 10 stairs, getting out of bed, getting in and out of a shower or bathtub, walking on uneven ground, standing on one leg, and reaching for an object. Individuals are asked to consider how confident they feel, today, that they could complete each of the tasks without losing balance. Scoring of each item is based on a range of responses from 0 percent (not confident at all) to 100 percent (absolutely confident), with scoring points at 10 percent increases. As this is a measure of perceived confidence, it should not be administered after a performance test that might jeopardize perceptions if difficulties become apparent. Items scored below 50 percent indicate low confidence and may serve as a focus for intervention.[94]

Motor Learning

Learning is a complex process that requires spatial, temporal, and hierarchical organization within the CNS. Changes in the CNS are not directly observable, but rather are inferred from improvement in performance as a result of practice or experience. Individual differences in learning are expected and influence both the rate and degree of learning possible. Motor learning abilities among individuals vary across three main foundational categories of abilities: cognitive abilities, perceptual speed ability, and psychomotor ability.[131] Differences occur as a result of both genetics and experience. The therapist should be sensitive to such factors as alertness, anxiety, memory, speed of processing information, speed and accuracy of movements, uniqueness of the setting, and so forth. In addition, patients may vary in their learning potential according to the pathology present, the number and type of impairments, and general health status and co-morbidities. Although most skills can be learned through practice or experience, the therapist should be sensitive to the patient's underlying capabilities (abilities) that support certain skills. For example, some patients with spinal cord injury are not able to learn to manage curbs using "wheelies" because of the difficulty of the task, their residual abilities, and general health status.

Performance Changes

One measure of motor learning is improvements in performance that result from practice or experience. Performance criteria are established and used for comparison to determine the success of learning outcomes. The therapist must select appropriate response outcome and response production measures of motor skill performance (Table 8.12). For example, an individual recovering from stroke is able to demonstrate functional independence in transfers after a series of training sessions. Improvement in functional scores (e.g., FIM scores) documents changes in the level of assistance needed. Qualitative changes in performance when compared to the criterion skill can also be used to document motor learning. Thus the movement is performed with improved coordination, indicative of changes in spatial and temporal organization. Error scores can be used to document accuracy of movement. Thus, therapists can report the number and type of errors (constant, variable) that occur within a given practice session and across practice sessions. A decrease in the frequency of errors is consistent with improvements in learning. One common measurement problem in skill learning is the *speed–accuracy trade-off.* Typically initial practice sessions are characterized by slowed performance in order to improve movement accuracy. As learning progresses, performance speed can be increased once accuracy demands are satisfied. Thus number of errors should be considered along with speed of performance. For tasks that require speed, the number of errors and time to complete the task can be added and then divided by two to achieve a *speed-accuracy score.*[3] Reduced effort and concentration are indicative of learning and should be documented. Whereas a high degree of cognitive monitoring is necessary in early learning (cognitive stage), performance in the associative and autonomous stages of motor learning is characterized by reduced cognitive monitoring and increasing automaticity.[132] As learning progresses, performance is increasingly characterized by persistence and consistency. Thus the acquired skills are observed for more than one performance trial and trial-to-trial variability decreases.

Practice Observations

The number of practice trials or practice time required to achieve skill mastery can be documented. Practice observations can be misleading in that performance is not always an accurate reflection of learning. It is possible to practice enough to temporarily improve performance but not retain the learning. Conversely, factors such as fatigue, anxiety, poor motivation, boredom, or drugs can cause performance to deteriorate while learning may still occur. Thus the patient who is fatigued or stressed performs very poorly during scheduled treatment but returns after the weekend rested and calm, and is able to perform the task with ease. *Performance plateaus,* defined as a leveling off of performance after a period of steady improvement, characterize normal practice and can be expected to occur. During plateaus, learning may still be going on. Typically these are temporary steady states and performance will begin to show improvement again. Plateaus can also be the result of *ceiling effects,* a high level of performance in which further improvement cannot be detected by limitations in the performance measure. *Floor effects* are a low level

Table 8.12 **Response Outcome and Response Production Measures of Motor Skill Performance**

Category	Examples of Measures	Performance Examples
1. Response outcome measures	Time to complete a movement (MT) in seconds, minutes, or hours	Amount of time to walk a set distance (e.g., the 6-Meter or 10-Meter Walk Test) Total time to complete a functional task (e.g., dressing or bathing)
	Time to initiate a response (RT) in seconds or minutes	Amount of time required to initiate sit-to-stand transfers
	Distance	Distance completed (e.g., 6-Minute Walk Test or 3-Minute Walk Test)
	Change in score of performance instrument	FIM score changes (e.g., from 3/Mod Assist to 5/No Helper after 4 weeks of gait training)
	Type of error in performing criterion task	Error in overall program selection (e.g., patient with stroke incorrectly transfers to the sound side when asked to transfer to the affected side) Error in program execution (e.g., patient with TBI gets distracted and lost in the middle of a transfer)
	Amount of error in performing criterion movement	Constant error (CE): the average error of a set of scores from a target value (e.g., patient exhibits a Functional Reach of 6 inches; mean for age [72 years, women] ≥13.8 inches) Variable error (VE): the standard deviation of a set of scores from an average score; measures consistency of responses (e.g., group of patients exhibit a Functional Reach SD of 5 inches; average SD is 3.4 inches)
	Number of successful attempts	Number of successful attempts (e.g., Sit-to-Stand transfers 4 out of 10 total attempts) Percentage of successful attempts (e.g., 40%)
	Time on/off target	Number of second/minutes patient is able to maintain stability in sitting or standing (e.g., 2 min)
	Time on/off balance	Number of seconds BOS is within COM (e.g., dynamic posturography)
	Trials to completion	Number of trials required until correct response obtained (e.g., 10 practice trials required for independent w/c to mat transfers)
2. Response production measures	Limb displacement, trajectory	Distance limb(s) traveled to produce response (e.g., observational/kinematic gait analysis)
	Velocity	Speed limb(s) moved while performing response, (e.g., observational or instrumental motion analysis, isokinetic dynamometry)
	Acceleration	Acceleration/deceleration pattern while moving (e.g., observational or instrumental motion analysis, isokinetic dynamometry)
	Joint angle	Angle of each joint during movement (e.g., observational analysis, electrogoniometry)
	Electromyography (EMG)	Patterns, timing of muscle activity (e.g., time at which the gastrocnemius initially fires)

(continued)

Table 8.12 Response Outcome and Response Production Measures of Motor Skill Performance (continued)

Category	Examples of Measures	Performance Examples

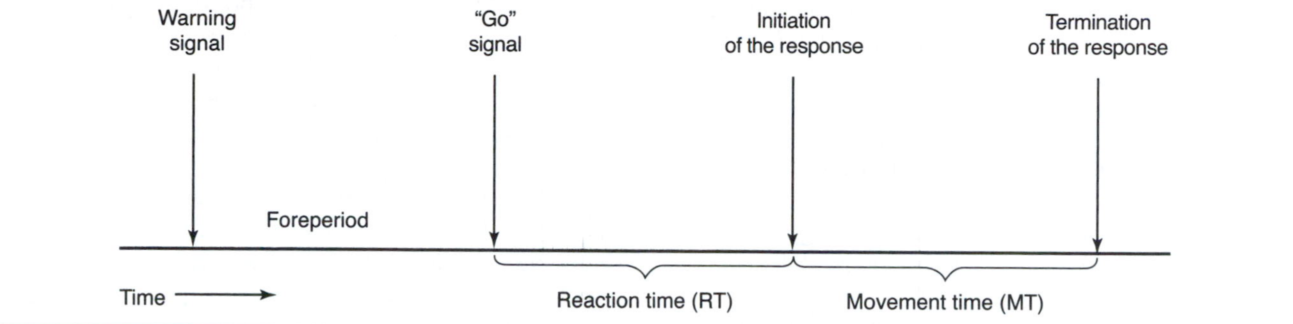

BOS = base of support; COM = center of mass; FIM = Functional Independence Measure; SD = standard deviation; TBI = traumatic brain injury.

Reaction time (RT) = the interval between the initial presentation of a stimulus/command to move and the initiation of a movement response.

Movement time (MT) = the interval between the initiation of movement and the completion of movement.

Adapted from Magill, R: Motor Learning Concepts and Applications, ed 4. WCP Brown & Benchmark, Madison, WI, 1993, p 17, with permission.

of performance in which further decreases cannot be detected by limitations in the performance measure. They can affect a determination of negative learning.[1]

The patient who is able to engage in active introspection and self-evaluation of performance and reach decisions independently about how to improve performance demonstrates an important element of learning. Some physical therapists over-emphasize guided movements and errorless practice. Although this may be important for safety reasons, lack of exposure to performance errors may preclude the patient from developing capabilities for self-evaluation. In an era of fiscal responsibility and limitations on the amount of physical therapy sessions allowed, many patients are able to learn only the very basic skills while in active rehabilitation. Much of the necessary learning of functional skills occurs after discharge and during outpatient episodes of care. The therapist cannot possibly structure practice sessions to meet all of the functional challenges the patient may face. The acquisition of independent problem solving/decision making skills ensures that the final goal of rehabilitation—independent function—can be achieved. The therapist needs to evaluate this very important function.

Retention Tests

More reliable inferences about learning can be made through the use of retention tests and transfer tests. **Retention** refers to persistence of a motor skill, an acquired capability for performance (habit), and is a function of motor memory. A *retention test,* defined as "a performance test administered after a retention interval for the purposes of assessing learning,"[1, p 467] provides an important measure of learning. The learner is asked to demonstrate the skill after a period of no practice (*retention interval*). Retention intervals can be of varying lengths. For example, a patient who is seen only once a week in an outpatient clinic is asked to demonstrate a skill practiced the previous week. Performance after the retention interval is compared to performance on the initial practice session. A *difference score* can be determined, that is, the difference in performance scores from the end of the original acquisition phase and the beginning of the retention phase. Performance typically shows a slight initial decrease but should return to original performance levels within relatively few practice trials if learning has occurred (termed *warm-up decrement*). It is important not to provide any verbal cueing or knowledge of results during the retention trial. This same patient may have been given a home exercise program (HEP) that includes daily practice of the desired skill. If upon return to the clinic some weeks later, performance of the desired skill has not been maintained or has deteriorated, the therapist might reasonably conclude that the patient has not been diligent with the HEP and learning has not been retained.

Transfer Tests

Transfer is defined as "the gain (or loss) in the capability for performance in one task as a result of practice or experience on some other task."[1, p 436] Learning obtained from the criterion task enhances (*positive transfer*) or detracts from (*negative transfer*) learning on other tasks. For example, the patient with stroke practices feeding skills using the non-affected upper extremity. Performance on the feeding task using the affected upper extremity is then evaluated. The therapist makes a determination as to the effectiveness of the prior practice (e.g., number and frequency of practice trials, time, effort) on performance using the affected extremity. Transfer of learning is greatest when tasks are similar, that is, have similar stimuli and similar responses.

Generalizability is defined as the "extent to which practice on one task contributes to the performance of other, related skills."[1, p 316] Thus the individual is able to apply a learned skill to the learning of other similar tasks. Individuals who learn to transfer from wheelchair to platform mat can apply that learning to other variations of transfers (e.g., wheelchair to car, wheelchair to tub). The number of practice trials, time, and effort required to perform these new types of transfers should be evaluated and are typically reduced from that required to learn the initial skill.

Resistance to contextual change is also an important measure of learning. This is the adaptability required to perform a motor task in altered environmental situations. Thus an individual who has learned a skill (e.g., walking with a cane) should be able to apply that learning to new and variable environments (e.g., walking at home, walking outdoors, walking downtown on a busy street). The therapist documents how successful the individual is in performing the skill in the new and varying environments. The patient who is able to perform the skill in only one type of environment, for example, the patient with traumatic brain injury who is only able to function within a tightly controlled, clinic environment (*closed environment*), demonstrates limited and largely nonfunctional skills in other environments. This patient is not likely to return home independent in the community environment (*open environment*), and will likely require placement in an assisted living (structured) setting.

Learning Styles

Individuals vary in their *learning style,* defined as their characteristic mode of gaining, processing, and storing information. Learning styles differ according to a number of factors, including personality characteristics, reasoning styles (inductive vs deductive), initiative (active vs passive), and so forth. Some individuals utilize an analytical/objective learning style. They process information in a step-by-step order and learn best with factual information and structure. Other individuals are more intuitive/global learners. They tend to process information all at once, and learn best when information is personalized and presented in the context of practical, real-life examples. They may have difficulty in ordering steps and comprehending details. Some individuals rely heavily on visual processing and demonstration to learn a task. Others depend more on auditory processing, talking themselves through a task. Individual characteristics and preferences are best determined by talking with the patient and family, using careful listening and observation skills. The medical record may also provide information concerning relevant premorbid history (e.g., educational level, occupation, interests). A thorough understanding of each of these factors allows the therapist to appropriately structure the learning environment and therapist–patient interactions.

Evaluation

Evaluation refers to the clinical judgments therapists make based on the data gathered from the examination.[5] Numerous factors influence the judgments therapists make when working with patients with impairments of motor function, including complexity and understanding of the nervous system, clinical findings, psychosocial considerations, and overall physical function and health. Therapists evaluate data in terms of severity of problems (impairments, functional limitations, disability), and level of chronicity. Therapists must also consider the consequences of failure to intervene appropriately when the patient is at risk for additional problems. Potential discharge placement and resources also influence evaluation of the data and development of the plan of care. There is a clear need for the therapist to focus on those problems that directly impact on function and can be successfully remediated.

Diagnosis

The physical therapy diagnosis is determined from evaluation of examination findings and is based on a cluster of signs, symptoms, or categories. The *Guide to Physical Therapist Practice,*[5] a consensus document developed by expert physical therapy clinicians, identifies diagnostic categories and preferred practice patterns that delineate appropriate interventions (see Chapter 1, Appendix A). For example, Impaired Motor Function and Sensory Integrity Associated with Acquired Nonprogressive Disorders of the Central Nervous System includes patients with traumatic brain injury, cerebrovascular accident, tumor, and so forth.[5, p 365] The reader is referred to this document for comparison and refinement of his or her own practice. Novice therapists can gain understanding and insights into the complex practice issues facing therapists who work with patients with impairments in motor function.

Summary

Examination of motor function is a challenging, multifaceted process, critically related to the therapist's ability to accurately determine and categorize findings. An understanding of normal motor control and motor learning mechanisms is essential to this process. Determining the causative factors responsible for abnormal movement patterns and behaviors must be based on comparison of expected or normal responses (norm-referenced behaviors) with the patient's abnormal ones. This can best be achieved by a systematic and thorough approach to examination. Emphasis should be on the use of valid, reliable, and responsive measurement tools.

Examination of systems yields valuable information about the integrity of individual components (e.g., neuromuscular, musculoskeletal, cognitive, and so forth). However, it is important to remember that normal motor control and motor learning is achieved through the integrated action of the CNS. The therapist must therefore also focus on integrated function evidenced through an examination at the functional level. Success in rehabilitation is also dependent on our ability to understand the learning abilities of the patient and potential training strategies important for cognitive engagement and practice. Our theoretical understanding of the CNS, motor control, and motor learning processes is both incomplete and imperfect. Therapists must, therefore, be constantly aware of the changing knowledge base in neuroscience and in neurological rehabilitation to incorporate new ideas into their examination and intervention plan.

Questions for Review

1. What are the components of the examination of motor function? How can the components be structured (ordered) to improve validity and reliability of results?
2. Describe the examination of consciousness and arousal, and cognition. How can deficits in each of these areas influence the motor function examination?
3. What tests can be used for a screening examination of motor function of the cranial nerves?
4. The presence of abnormal tone, reflexes, or synergy may impair normal movement. How can each be examined?
5. Describe the reasons, both pro and con, for using strength testing (MMT) in patients with neurological dysfunction.
6. Lesions of the dorsal columns/lemniscal system can result in decreased discriminative touch and proprioception. In the lower extremities how can these losses contribute to deficits in balance, coordination, and gait? What are the expected deficits, and how can each be examined?
7. Describe two functional balance measures. What aspects of balance do they examine?
8. Following neurological injury, functional mobility skills are typically impaired. What are the components of functional task analysis?
9. Differentiate between the use of performance observations and retention tests in providing evidence of motor learning.
10. Discuss factors that can influence the examination and evaluation of the patient with motor function deficits.

Case Study

The patient is a 17-year-old female who is 6 months post-motor vehicle accident (MVA). At the time of admission to the hospital, she was comatose and decerebrate. CT scan revealed intracranial bleeding into the right occipital horn. She received a tracheostomy and a gastrostomy. Two months post-MVA, she was transferred to a *long-term care facility* specializing in traumatic brain injury.

On initial admission she was able to open her eyes to verbal and tactile stimuli but was unable to visually track. She withdrew her upper and lower extremities in response to stimulation but was not able to move them on command. She was alert but confused, and was unable to carry on a conversation. ROM was within normal limits (WNL) except for right elbow flexion (20 to 100°) and right knee flexion (10 to 110°). She demonstrated increased tone (Modified Ashworth Scale 3) in her left upper extremity (LUE), 4 in her right upper extremity (RUE), and 4 in both lower extremities (BLEs). She exhibited 4+ bilateral ankle clonus. She was unable to sit unsupported. During supported sitting in the wheelchair, her head and trunk control was poor, with persistent posturing to the left side.

She is now 6 months post-MVA and is currently being examined for transfer to active rehabilitation status.

PHYSICAL THERAPY EXAMINATION FINDINGS

Consciousness/Arousal

Fully awake; responds appropriately to varying stimuli.
Oriented to person; some confusion with orientation to place and time.
Can become agitated with minimal stimulation, especially when tired.

Cognition/Behavior

Demonstrates difficulty with concentration and attention.
Able to follow simple instructions (one- or two-level commands) but occasionally forgets what is asked of her.
Reaction time is slowed as the number of choices is increased.
Easily forgets what she is doing.

Sensory Integrity

Aware of sensory input (pinprick, vibration, light touch) to all extremities.
Unable to discern common objects placed in either hand for stereognosis discrimination.

Joint Integrity and Mobility

RLE: plantarflexion contracture (40 to 50°)
flexion contractures at the hip (10 to 120°) and knee (10 to 120°)
RUE: flexor contracture at the elbow (10 to 110°)
Full PROM in the LUE and LLE.

Tone

Increased bilaterally (R > L).
On Modified Ashworth Scale: RUE and RLE 3; LUE and LLE 2.

Reflex Integrity

Hyperactive, 3+ DTRs RUE, RLE.
3+ bilateral ankle clonus.

Cranial Nerve Integrity

Dysphagia and dysphonia are present.

Muscle Performance

Strength is decreased in the RUE, RLE, and trunk (unable to test with MMT).
She is unable to sustain R knee extension during standing.

Voluntary Movement Patterns

RUE moves in partial range, obligatory mass flexor synergy pattern only.
RLE moves in flexor and extensor synergy patterns with no variation.
LUE and LLE demonstrate full voluntary control with isolated joint movements. Coordination is decreased. Unable to reach directly to an object that is held out to her and demonstrates foot placement problems with the LLE in sitting or in standing.
Demonstrates problems with coordinating limb and trunk movements.

Postural Control and Balance

Demonstrates good head control in all positions.
Sitting: can sit independently for up to 5 minutes. Demonstrates difficulty in maintaining weight equally on both buttocks. Tends to list to the right side while placing weight primarily on her left buttock. Able to reach to the left and forward; demonstrates loss of balance (LOB) with minimal reaching to right.
Standing: able to stand in parallel bars with minimal assistance 1 for up to 2 minutes. Has to be reminded to place weight on RLE. Tends to lose her balance easily if she moves quickly; associated with brief episodes of dizziness and vertigo.

Functional Mobility Skills

Rolling: requires supervision and occasional minimal assistance with rolling to the right; she requires maximal assist when rolling to the left.
Supine-to-sit: able to come to sitting by rolling to the L side and pushing up with her LUE; requires minimal assistance.
Transfers: able to perform stand pivot transfers with minimal assistance of 1.
Gait: does not initiate ambulation on her own. Can ambulate the length of the parallel bars (2 m or 6 ft) with maximal assistance of 2 persons. Requires posterior splint to stabilize R knee.
Propels wheelchair by using the LUE and both feet for pushing; requires supervision for safety.

Motor Learning

Demonstrates profound deficits in short-term memory; unable to remember new information presented during therapy. Her memory for events and learning prior to the MVA is good.

GUIDING QUESTIONS

Based on your evaluation of the data presented in the case history and the physical therapy examination, answer the following questions:

1. Categorize the patient's level of consciousness upon admission to the long-term care facility using the Glasgow Coma Scale (Table 22.4).
2. Categorize the patient's problems in terms of:
   (a) direct impairments
   (b) indirect impairments
   (c) functional limitations
3. Prioritize the problems; establish anticipated goals and expected outcomes.
4. Determine the physical therapy diagnosis using the preferred practice patterns identified by the *Guide to Physical Therapist Practice*[5] (Chapter 1, Appendix A).

References

1. Schmidt, R, and Lee, T: Motor Control and Learning, ed 4. Human Kinetics, Champaign, IL, 2005.
2. Shumway-Cook, A, and Woollacott, M: Motor Control: Theory and Practical Applications, ed 2. Lippincott Williams & Williams, Philadelphia, 2001.
3. Magill, R: Motor Learning—Concepts and Applications, ed 4. WCB Brown & Benchmark, Madison, WI, 1993.
4. Bernstein, N: The Coordination and Regulation of Movements. Pergamon Press, New York, 1967.
5. American Physical Therapy Association. Guide to Physical Therapist Practice, ed 2. American Physical Therapy Association, Alexandria, VA, 2001.
6. Riolo, L: Skill differences in novice and expert clinicians in neurologic physical therapy. Neurology Report 20:60, 1996.

7. Jensen, G, et al: Expertise in Physical Therapy Practice. Butterworth Heinemann, Boston, 1999.
8. Bear, M, Connors, B, and Paradiso, M: Neuroscience—Exploring the Brain, ed 2. Lippincott Williams & Wilkins, Philadelphia, 2001.
9. Bickley, L, and Szilagyi, P: Bates' Guide to Physical Examination and History Taking, ed 8. Lippincott Williams & Wilkins, Philadelphia, 2003.
10. Jennett, B, and Bond, M: Assessment of outcome after severe head injury: A practical scale. Lancet 1:480, 1975.
11. Zoltan, B: Vision, Perception, and Cognition: A Manual for the Evaluation and Treatment of the Neurologically Impaired Adult, ed 3. Slack, Thorofare, NJ, 1986.
12. Strub, R, and Black, F. The Mental Status Examination in Neurology, ed 4. FA Davis, Philadelphia, 2000.
13. Folstein, M: Mini-mental state: A practical method for grading the cognitive state of patients for the clinician. J Psychiatr Res 12:189, 1975.
14. Yerkes, R, and Dodson J: The relation of strength of stimulus to rapidity of habit-formation. J Comp Neurol Psychol 18:459, 1908.
15. Wilder, J: Basimetric approach (law of initial value) to biological rhythms. Ann NY Acad Sci 98:1211, 1961.
16. Stockmeyer, S: Clinical decision making based on homeostatic concepts. In Wolf, S (ed): Clinical Decision Making in Physical Therapy. FA Davis, Philadelphia, 1985, p 79.
17. Katz, R, and Rymer, Z: Spastic hypertonia: Mechanisms and measurement. Arch Phys Med Rehabil 70:144, 1989.
18. Burke, D: Spasticity as an adaptation to pyramidal tract injury. In Waxman, S (ed): Advances in Neurology, Vol. 47: Functional Recovery in Neurological Disease. Raven Press, New York, 1988.
19. Dobkin, B: Neurologic Rehabilitation. FA Davis, Philadelphia, 1996.
20. Fuller, G: Neurological Examination Made Easy, ed 3. Churchill Livingstone, New York, 2004.
21. Jankovic, J: Pathophysiology and clinical assessment of motor symptoms in Parkinson's disease. In Koller, W (ed): Handbook of Parkinson's Disease. Marcel Dekker, New York, 1987, p 99.
22. Jankovic, J, and Fahn, S: Dystonic syndromes. In Jankovic, J, and Tolosa, E (eds): Parkinson's Disease and Movement Disorders. Urban & Schwarzenburg, Baltimore, 1988, p 283.
23. Ashworth, B: Preliminary trial of carisoprodol in multiple sclerosis. Practitioner 192:540, 1964.
24. Bohannon, R, and Smith, M: Interrater reliability of a modified Ashworth scale of muscle spasticity. Phys Ther 67:206, 1987.
25. Bajd, T, and Vodovnik, L: Pendulum testing of spasticity. J Biomech Eng 6:9, 1984.
26. Bohannon, R: Variability and reliability of the pendulum test for spasticity using a Cybex II Isokinetic Dynamometer. Phys Ther 67:659, 1987.
27. Leonard, C, Stephens, J, and Stroppel, S: Assessing the spastic condition of individuals with upper motoneuron involvement: Validity of the Myotonometer. Arch Phys Med Rehabil 82:1416, 2001.
28. Leonard, C, et al: Myotonometer intra- and inter-rater reliabilities. Arch Phys Med Rehab 2003.
29. Easton, T: On the normal use of reflexes. Am Sci 60:591, 1972.
30. Hellebrandt, F, et al: Methods of evoking the tonic neck reflexes in normal human subjects. Am J Phys Med 35:144, 1956.
31. Hellebrandt, F, and Waterland, J: Expansion of motor patterning under exercise stress. Am J Phys Med 41:56, 1962.
32. Brunnstrom, S: Movement Therapy in Hemiplegia. Harper & Row, New York, 1970.
33. Bobath, B: Abnormal Postural Reflex Activity Caused by Brain Lesions. Heinemann, London, 1965.
34. Capute, A, et al: Primitive Reflex Profile. University Park Press, Baltimore, 1978.
35. Capute, A, et al: Primitive reflex profile: A pilot study. Phys Ther 58:1061, 1978.
36. Gowland, C, et al: Agonist and antagonist activity during voluntary upper-limb movement in patients with stroke. Phys Ther 72:624, 1992.
37. Bourbonnais, D, et al: Abnormal spatial patterns of elbow muscle activation in hemiparetic human subjects. Brain 112:85, 1989.
38. Rosenfalck, A, and Andreassen, S: Impaired regulation of force and firing pattern of single motor units in patients with spasticity. J Neurol Neurosurg Psychiatry 43:907, 1980.
39. Knuttsson, E, and Martensson, A: Dynamic motor capacity in spastic paresis and its relation to prime mover dysfunction, spastic reflexes and antagonist co-activation. Scand J Rehabil Med 12:93, 1980.
40. Sahrmann, S, and Norton, B: The relationship of voluntary movement to spasticity in the upper motor neuron syndrome. Ann Neurol 2:460, 1977.
41. Bourbonnais, D, and Vanden Noven, S: Weakness in patients with hemiparesis. Am J Occup Ther 43:313, 1989.
42. Watkins, M, et al: Isokinetic testing in patients with hemiparesis. Phys Ther 64:184, 1984.
43. Rothstein, J, et al: Commentary. Is the measurement of muscle strength appropriate in patients with brain lesions? Phys Ther 69:230, 1989.
44. Bohannon, R: Is the measurement of muscle strength appropriate in patients with brain lesions? Phys Ther 69:225, 1989.
45. Frese, E, et al: Clinical reliability of manual muscle testing: Middle trapezius and gluteus medius muscles. Phys Ther 67:1072, 1987.
46. Riddle, D, et al: Intrasession and intersession reliability of hand-held dynamometer measurements taken on brain-damaged patients. Phys Ther 69:182, 1989.
47. Bohannon, R: Test–retest reliability of hand-held dynamometry during a single session of strength assessment. Phys Ther 66:206, 1986.
48. Bohannon, R, and Andrews, A: Interrater reliability of handheld dynamometry. Phys Ther 67:931, 1987.
49. Agre, J, et al: Strength testing with a portable dynamometer: Reliability for upper and lower extremities. Arch Phys Med Rehabil 68:454, 1987.
50. Kloos, A: Measurement of muscle tone and strength. Neurology Report 16:9, 1992.
51. Rothstein, J, et al: Clinical uses of isokinetic measurements. Phys Ther 67:1840, 1987.
52. Griffin, J, et al: Sequential isokinetic and manual muscle testing in patients with neuromuscular disease: A pilot study. Phys Ther 66:32, 1986.
53. Kozlowski, B: Reliability of isokinetic torque generation in chronic hemiplegic subjects. Phys Ther 64:714, 1984.
54. Edwards, R: Physiological analysis of skeletal muscle weakness and fatigue. Clin Sci Mol Med 54:463, 1978.
55. Curtis, C, and Weir, J: Overview of exercise responses in healthy and impaired states. Neurology Report 20:13, 1996.
56. Wade, C, and Forstch, J: Exercise and Duchenne muscular dystrophy. Neurology Report 20:20, 1996.
57. Costello, E, et al: Exercise prescription for individuals with multiple sclerosis. Neurology Report 24:13, 1996.
58. Bassile, D: Guillain-Barré syndrome and exercise guidelines. Neurology Report 24:31, 1996.
59. McDonald, M: Exercise and postpolio syndrome. Neurology Report 24:37, 1996.
60. Bigland-Richie, B, and Woods, J: Changes in muscle contractile properties and neural control during human muscular fatigue. Muscle Nerve 7:691, 1984.
61. Borg, G: Psychophysical bases of perceived exertion. Med Sci Sports Exerc 14:377, 1982.
62. Fisk, J, et al: The impact of fatigue on patients with multiple sclerosis. J Can Sci Neurol 21:9, 1994.
63. Bennett, R, and Knowlton, G: Overwork weakness in partially denervated skeletal muscle. Clin Orthop 12:22, 1958.
64. Barnes, S: Isokinetic fatigue curves at different contractile velocities. Arch Phys Med Rehabil 62:66, 1981.
65. Binder-Macleod, S, and Synder-Mackler, L: Muscle fatigue: Clinical implications for fatigue assessment and neuromuscular electrical stimulation. Phys Ther 73:902, 1993.
66. McDonnell, M, et al: Electrically elicited fatigue test of the quadriceps femoris muscle. Phys Ther 67:941, 1987.
67. Fugl-Meyer, A: The post-stroke hemiplegic patient, I: A method for evaluation of physical performance. Scand J Rehabil Med 7:13, 1975.
68. VanSant, A: Life span development in functional tasks. Phys Ther 70:788, 1990.

69. Shenkman, M, et al: Whole-body movements during rising to standing from sitting. Phys Ther 70:638, 1990.
70. VanSant, A: Rising from a supine position to erect stance: Description of adult movement and a developmental hypothesis. Phys Ther 68:185, 1988.
71. Green, L, and Williams, K: Differences in developmental movement patterns used by active vs sedentary middle-aged adults coming from a supine position to erect stance. Phys Ther 72:560, 1992.
72. Richter, R, et al: Description of adult rolling movements and hypothesis of developmental sequences. Phys Ther 69:63, 1989.
73. Gentile, A: Skill acquisition: Action, movement and neuromotor processes. In Carr, J, et al (eds): Movement Science: Foundations for Physical Therapy in Rehabilitation. Aspen, Rockville, MD, 1987, p 93.
74. Pink, M: High speed video applications in physical therapy. Clin Manage 5:14, 1985.
75. Lewis, A: Documentation of movement patterns used in the performance of functional tasks. Neurology Report 16:13, 1992.
76. Norkin, C, and Levangie, P: Joint Structure and Function: A Comprehensive Analysis, ed 2. FA Davis, Philadelphia, 2002.
77. Smith, L, et al: Brunnstrom's Clinical Kinesiology, ed 5. FA Davis, Philadelphia, 1996.
78. Nashner, L: Sensory, neuromuscular, and biomechanical contributions to human balance. In Duncan, P (ed): Balance. American Physical Therapy Association, Alexandria, VA, 1990, p 5.
79. Nichols, D: Balance retraining after stroke using force platform biofeedback. Phys Ther 77:553, 1997.
80. Horak, F: Clinical measurement of postural control in adults. Phys Ther 67:1881, 1987.
81. Goldie, P, et al: Force platform measures for evaluating postural control: Reliability and validity. Arch Phys Med Rehabil 70:510, 1989.
82. Liston, R, and Brouwer, B: Reliability and validity of measures obtained from stroke patients using the Balance Master. Arch Phys Med Rehabil 77:425, 1996.
83. Horak, F, et al: Postural perturbations: New insights for treatment of balance disorders. Phys Ther 77:517, 1997.
84. Dettman, M, et al: Relationships among walking performance, postural stability, and functional assessments of the hemiplegic patient. Am J Phys Med 66:77, 1987.
85. Dickstein, R, et al: Foot-ground pressure pattern of standing hemiplegic patients: Major characteristics and patterns of movement. Phys Ther 64:19, 1984.
86. Lee, DN, and Lishman, JR: Visual proprioceptive control of stance. J Hum Mov Stud 1:87, 1975.
87. Brandt, T, et al: Visual acuity, visual field and visual scene characteristics affect postural balance. In Igarash, M, and Black, F (eds): Vestibular and Visual Control on Posture and Locomotor Equilibrium. Karger, Basel, 1985.
88. Herdman, S: Vestibular Rehabilitation, ed 2. FA Davis, Philadelphia, 2000.
89. Horak, F, et al: Postural strategies associated with somatosensory and vestibular loss. Exp Brain Res 82:167, 1990.
90. Nashner, L: Adaptive reflexes controlling human posture. Exp Brain Res 26:59, 1976.
91. Nashner, L, and McCollum, G: The organization of human postural movements: A formal basis and experimental synthesis. Behav Brain Sci 9:135, 1985.
92. Shumway-Cook, A, and Horak, F: Assessing the influence of sensory interaction on balance: Suggestion from the field. Phys Ther 66:1548, 1986.
93. Cohen, H, et al: A study of CTSIB. Phys Ther 73:346, 1993.
94. Rose, D: Fall Proof—A Comprehensive Balance and Mobility Training Program. Human Kinetics, Champaign IL, 2003.
95. Horak, F, and Nashner, L: Central programming of postural movements: Adaptation to altered support-surface configuration. J Neurophysiol 55:1369, 1986.
96. Nashner, L: Fixed patterns of rapid postural responses among leg muscles during stance. Exp Brain Res 30:13, 1977.
97. Maki, B, and McIlron, W: The role of limb movements in maintaining upright stance: The "change-in-support" strategy. Phys Ther 77:488, 1977.
98. Dean, C, and Shepherd, R: Task-related training improves performance of seated reaching tasks following stroke: A randomized controlled trial. Stroke 28:722, 1997.
99. Forssberg, H, and Hirschfeld, H: Postural adjustments in sitting humans following external perturbations: Muscle activity and kinematics. Exp Brain Res 97:515, 1994.
100. Lee, W, et al: Quantitative and clinical measures of static standing balance in hemiparetic and normal subjects. Phys Ther 68:970, 1988.
101. Bohannon, R, et al: Decrease in timed balance test scores with aging. Phys Ther 64:1967, 1984.
102. Duncan, P, et al: Functional reach: A new clinical measure of balance. J Gerontol 45:M192, 1990.
103. Duncan, P, et al: Functional reach: Predictive validity in a sample of elderly male veterans. J Gerontol 47:M93, 1992.
104. Weiner, D, et al: Functional reach: A marker of physical frailty. J Am Geriatr Soc 40:203, 1992.
105. Newton, R: Balance screening of an inner city older adult population. Arch Phys Med Rehabil 78:587, 1997.
106. Newton, R: Validity of the multi-directional reach test: A practical measure for limits of stability in older adults. J Gerontol Med Sci 56A: M248, 2001.
107. Newton, R: Balance screening of an inner city older adult population. Arch Phys Med Rehabil 78:587, 1997.
108. Berg, K, et al: Measuring balance in the elderly: Preliminary development of an instrument. Physiother Can 41:304, 1989.
109. Berg, K, et al: A comparison of clinical and laboratory measures of postural balance in an elderly population. Arch Phys Med Rehabil 73:1073, 1992.
110. Berg, K, et al: Measuring balance in the elderly: Validation of an instrument. Can J Public Health 83 (Suppl 2):S7, 1992.
111. Berg, K, et al: The Balance Scale: Reliability assessment for elderly residents and patients with an acute stroke. Scand J Rehabil Med 27:27, 1995.
112. Thorbahn, L, and Newton, R: Use of the Berg Balance Test to predict falls in elderly persons. Phys Ther 76:576, 1996.
113. Harada, N, et al: Physical therapy to improve functioning of older people in residential care facilities. Phys Ther 75:830, 1995.
114. Harada N, et al: Screening for balance and mobility impairment in elderly individuals living in residential care facilities. Phys Ther 75:462, 1995.
115. Tinetti, M, et al: A fall risk index for elderly patients based on number of chronic disabilities. Am J Med 80:429, 1986.
116. Tinetti, M, and Ginter, S: Identifying mobility dysfunctions in elderly patients: Standard neuromuscular examination or direct assessment? JAMA 259:1190, 1988.
117. Tinetti, M: Factors associated with serious injury during falls by ambulatory nursing home residents. J Am Geriatr Soc 35:644, 1987.
118. Tinetti, M, et al: Risk factors for falls among elderly persons living in the community. N Engl J Med 319:1701, 1988.
119. Tinetti, M, et al: Yale FISCIT: Risk factor abatement strategy for fall prevention. J Am Geriatr Soc 41:315, 1993.
120. Mathias, S, et al: Balance in elderly patients: The "Get-up and go" test. Arch Phys Med Rehabil 67:387, 1986.
121. Podsiadlo, D, and Richardson, S: The timed "Up and Go": A test of basic mobility for frail elderly persons. J Am Geriatr Soc 39:142, 1991.
122. Cunha, I, et al: Performance-based gait tests for acute stroke patients. Am J Phys Med Rehabil 81:838, 2002.
123. Murray, M, et al: Comparison of free and fast speed walking patterns of normal men. Am J Phys Med 45:8, 1966.
124. Sadaria, K, and Bohannon, R: The 6-Minute Walk Test: A brief review of literature. Clin Exerc Physiol. 3:127, 2001.
125. Harada N, Chiu, V, and Stewart, A: Mobility-related function in older adults: Assessment with a 6-minute walk test. Arch Phys Med Rehbil 80:837, 1999.
126. Miller, P, et al: Measurement properties of a standardized version of the Two-Minute Walk Test for individuals with neurological dysfunction. Physiother Can, 54: 241, 2003.
127. Guralnick, J, et al: Lower-extremity function over the age of 70 years as a predictor of subsequent disability. N Engl J Med 332:556, 1995.
128. Wolfson, L, et al: Gait assessment in the elderly: A gait abnormality rating scale and its relation to falls. J Gerontol 45:M12, 1990.
129. Whitney S, Wrisley, D, and Furman, J: Concurrent validity of the Berg Balance Scale and the Dynamic Gait Index in people with vestibular dysfunction. Physiother Res Int 8:178, 2003.

130. Abernethy, B: Dual-task methodology and motor skills research: Some applications and methodological constraints. J Hum Mov Studies 14:101, 1988.
131. Ackerman, P: Individual differences in skill learning: An integration of psychometric and information processing perspectives. Psychol Bull 102:3, 1988.
132. Fitts, P, and Posner, M: Human Performance. Brooks/Cole, Belmont, CA, 1969.
133. O'Sullivan, S, and Siegelman, R: National Physical Therapy Examination Review & Study Guide, International Educational Resources, Ltd, Evanston, IL, 2005.

Supplemental Readings

Bickley, L, and Szilagyi, P: Bates' Guide to Physical Examination and History Taking, ed 8. Lippincott Williams & Wilkins, Philadelphia, 2003.

Fuller, G: Neurological Examination Made Easy, ed 3. Churchill Livingstone, New York, 2004.

Gilman, S (ed): Clinical Examination of the Nervous System. McGraw-Hill, New York, 2000.

Strub, R, and Black, F: The Mental Status Examination in Neurology, ed 4. FA Davis, Philidelphia, 2000.

Appendix A: Berg Balance Scale

1. Sitting to standing

Instructions: *Please stand up, try not to use your hands for support.*

( ) 4 able to stand without using hands and stabilizes independently
( ) 3 able to stand independently using hands
( ) 2 able to stand using hands after several tries
( ) 1 needs minimal aid to stand or stabilize
( ) 0 needs moderate or maximal assist to stand

2. Standing unsupported

Instructions: *Please stand for 2 minutes without holding.*

( ) 4 able to stand safely 2 minutes
( ) 3 able to stand 2 minutes with supervision
( ) 2 able to stand 30 seconds unsupported
( ) 1 needs several tries to stand unsupported 30 seconds
( ) 0 unable to stand 30 seconds without support

3. Sitting with back unsupported but feet supported on floor or on a stool

Instructions: *Please sit with arms folded for 2 minutes.*

( ) 4 able to sit safely and securely 2 minutes
( ) 3 able to sit 2 minutes with supervision
( ) 2 able to sit 30 seconds
( ) 1 able to sit 10 seconds
( ) 0 unable to sit without support 10 seconds

4. Standing to sit

Instructions: *Please sit down.*

( ) 4 sits safely with minimal use of hands
( ) 3 controls descent by using hands
( ) 2 uses back of legs against chair to control descent
( ) 1 sits independently, but has uncontrolled descent
( ) 0 needs assistance to sit

5. Transfers

Instructions: *Arrange chairs for a pivot transfer. Ask the patient to transfer one way toward a seat without armrests and one way toward a seat with arms. You may use two chairs or a bed/mat and a chair.*

( ) 4 able to transfer safely with minor use of hands
( ) 3 able to transfer safely with definite need of hands
( ) 2 able to transfer with verbal cuing and/or supervision
( ) 1 needs one person to assist
( ) 0 needs two people to assist or supervise to be safe

6. Standing unsupported with eyes closed

Instructions: *Please close your eyes and stand still for 10 seconds.*

( ) 4 able to stand 10 seconds safely
( ) 3 able to stand 10 seconds with supervision
( ) 2 able to stand 3 seconds
( ) 1 unable to keep eyes closed for 3 seconds but stands safely
( ) 0 needs help to keep from falling

7. Standing unsupported with feet together

Instructions: *Place your feet together and stand without holding.*

( ) 4 able to place feet together independently and stand safely 1 minute
( ) 3 able to place feet together independently and stand with supervision for 1 minute
( ) 2 able to place feet together independently but unable to hold for 30 seconds
( ) 1 needs help to assume the position but can stand for 15 seconds, feet together
( ) 0 needs help to assume the position and unable to stand for 15 seconds

8. Reaching forward with outstretched arm while standing

Instructions: *Lift arm to 90°. Stretch out your fingers and reach forward as far as you can. (Clinician places a ruler at the tips of the outstretched fingers—subject should not touch the ruler when reaching.) Distance recorded is from the fingertips with the subject in the most forward position. The subject should use both hands when possible to avoid trunk rotation.*

( ) 4 can reach forward confidently 20–30 cm (10 inches)
( ) 3 can reach forward safely 12 cm (5 inches)
( ) 2 can reach forward safely 5 cm (2 inches)
( ) 1 reaches forward but needs supervision
( ) 0 loses balance when trying, requires external support

9. Pick up object from the floor from a standing position

Instructions: *Pick up the shoe slipper which is placed in front of your feet.*

( ) 4 able to pick up the slipper safely and easily
( ) 3 able to pick up the slipper but needs supervision
( ) 2 unable to pick up the slipper, but reaches 2–5 cm (1–2 inches) from the slipper and keeps balance independently

( ) 1 unable to pick up and needs supervision while trying
( ) 0 unable to try/needs assistance to keep from losing balance/falling

10. Turning to look behind over your left and right shoulders while standing
Instructions: *Turn and look directly behind you over toward the left shoulder. Repeat to the right. Examiner may pick an object to look at directly behind the subject to encourage a better twist.*
( ) 4 looks behind from both sides and weight shifts well
( ) 3 looks behind one side only, other side shows less weight shift
( ) 2 turns sideways only but maintains balance
( ) 1 needs close supervision or verbal cuing
( ) 0 needs assistance while turning

11. Turn 360°
Instructions: *Turn completely around in a full circle, pause, then turn a full circle in the other direction.*
( ) 4 able to turn 360° safely in 4 seconds or less
( ) 3 able to turn 360° safely, one side only, 4 seconds or less
( ) 2 able to turn 360° safely, but slowly
( ) 1 needs close supervision or verbal cuing
( ) 0 needs assistance while turning

12. Place alternate foot on step or stool while standing unsupported
Instructions: *Place each foot alternately on the step stool. Continue until each foot has touched the step stool 4 times.*
( ) 4 able to stand independently and safely and complete 8 steps in 20 seconds
( ) 3 able to stand independently and complete 8 steps >20 seconds
( ) 2 able to complete 4 steps without aid with supervision
( ) 1 able to complete >2 steps needs minimal assistance
( ) 0 needs assistance to keep from falling/unable to try

13. Standing unsupported one foot in front
Instructions: *Demonstrate to subject. Place one foot directly in front of the other. If you feel that you cannot place your foot directly in front, try and step far enough ahead that the heel of your forward foot is ahead of the toes of your other foot. To score three points, the length of the step should exceed the length of the other foot and the width of the stance should approximate the subject's normal stance width.*
( ) 4 able to place foot tandem independently and hold 30 seconds
( ) 3 able to place foot ahead of the other independently and hold 30 seconds
( ) 2 able to take a small step independently and hold 30 seconds
( ) 1 needs help to step but can hold 15 seconds
( ) 0 loses balance while stepping or standing

14. Standing on one leg
Instructions: *Stand on one leg as long as you can without holding*
( ) 4 able to lift leg independently and hold >10 seconds
( ) 3 able to lift leg independently and hold 5–10 seconds
( ) 2 able to lift leg independently and hold >2 seconds
( ) 1 tries to lift leg unable to hold 3 seconds but remains standing independently
( ) 0 unable to try or needs assistance to prevent fall

________ **TOTAL SCORE (Maximum 56)**

Appendix B: Performance-Oriented Assessment of Mobility I–POMA I (Tinetti)

BALANCE

Instructions: Subject is seated in hard armless chair. The following maneuvers are tested.

1. Sitting balance
- 0 = leans or slides in chair
- 1 = leans in chair slightly or slight increased distance from buttocks to back of chair
- 2 = steady, safe, upright

2. Arising
- 0 = unable without help or loses balance
- 1 = *able* but uses arm to help *or* requires more than two attempts or excessive forward flexion
- 2 = *able* without use of arms in one attempt

3. Immediate standing balance (first 5 seconds)
- 0 = unsteady marked staggering, moves feet, marked trunk sway or grabs object for support
- 1 = steady but uses walker or cane *or* mild staggering but catches self without grabbing object
- 2 = steady without walker or cane or other support

4. Side-by-side standing balance
- 0 = unsteady
- 1 = unsteady, but wide stance (medial heels more than 4 inches apart) or uses cane, walker or other support
- 2 = narrow stance without support

5. Pull test (subject at maximum position as above, examiner stands behind and exerts mild pull back at wrist)
- 0 = begins to fall
- 1 = staggers, grabs, but catches self
- 2 = steady

6. Turn 360°
- 0 = unsteady (grabs, staggers)
- 1 = steady but steps discontinuous
- 2 = steady and steps continuous

7. Able to stand on one leg for 5 seconds (pick one leg)
- 0 = unable or holds onto any object
- 1 = some staggering, swaying or moves foot slightly
- 2 = able

8. Tandem stand
- 0 = unable to stand with one foot in front of other or begins to fall
- 1 = some staggering, swaying, moves arms, or moves foot slightly
- 2 = able to tandem stand 5 seconds

9. Reaching up—Examiner holds 5-pound weight at height of subject's fully extended reach
- 0 = unable or holds onto any object
- 1 = some staggering, swaying or moves foot slightly
- 2 = able

10. Bending over (place 5-pound weight on floor and ask subject to pick it up)
- 0 = unable or is unsteady
- 1 = able and is steady

10a. Time required_______seconds

11. Sit down
- 0 = unsafe (misjudged distance; falls into chair)
- 1 = uses arms or not a smooth motion
- 2 = safe, smooth motion

11a. Timed rising

Time required to rise from chair three times _____ seconds

Total Balance Subtest: 21 points

Timed items: 10, 11

GAIT

Instructions: *Subject stands with examiner. Walks down 15 foot walkway (measured). Ask subject to walk down walkway, turn and walk back. Subject should use customary walking aid.*

1. Initiation of gait (immediately after told to "go")
- 0 = any hesitancy or multiple attempts to start
- 1 = no hesitancy

2. Path (estimated in relation to line on floor or rug). Observe excursion of one foot over middle 10 feet of course.
- 0 = marked deviation
- 1 = mild/moderate deviation or uses walking aid
- 2 = straight without walking aid

3. Missed step (trip or loss of balance)
- 0 = yes and inappropriate attempt to recover balance
- 1 = yes, but appropriate attempt to recover
- 2 = no

4. Turning (while walking)
0 = staggers, unsteady
1 = discontinuous, but no staggering, or uses walker or cane
2 = steady, continuous without walking aid

5. Timed walk performed after 1–7 complete (measure out 15 foot walkway)
a) Ask subject to walk at normal pace _____ seconds
b) Ask subject to walk as "fast as feels safe" ______seconds

6. Step over obstacle (to be assessed in a separate walk with a block placed on course)
0 = begins to fall or unable
1 = able but uses walking aid or some staggering but catches self
2 = able and steady
Total Gait Subtest: 9 points
Timed items: 5

_________ **TOTAL SCORE (Maximum = 30 points)**

CHAPTER

9

Electromyography and Nerve Conduction Velocity Tests

Leslie G. Portney, DPT, PhD, FAPTA
Serge H. Roy, PT, ScD
John L. Echternach, PT, EdD, ECS, FAPTA

LEARNING OBJECTIVES

1. Describe the instrumentation system used to record the electromyographic (EMG) signal for clinical and kinesiological uses.
2. Describe the general methodology used to perform an EMG and nerve conduction velocity (NCV) examination.
3. Describe the characteristics of normal and abnormal EMG potentials.
4. Describe the EMG signal and NCV findings typically seen with neuromuscular disorders.
5. Discuss the implications of clinical EMG findings for goal setting and treatment planning.
6. Discuss the relationship between the EMG signal and force with different types of muscle contractions.
7. Discuss procedural, technical, and physiological considerations for interpreting clinical and kinesiological EMG data.
8. Describe the uses of kinesiological EMG data for evaluation of movement.
9. Using the case study examples, apply clinical decision making skills in evaluating EMG data.

OUTLINE

Luigi Galvani presented the first report on electrical properties of muscles and nerves in 1791.[1] He demonstrated that muscle activity was a direct result of neuronal stimulation and recorded potentials from muscle fibers in states of voluntary contraction in frogs. In the mid-1800s Du Bois-Reymond was the first to describe the muscle membrane potential and subsequently the first to detect the electrical manifestations of voluntary muscle contraction in man.[2] Duchenne made considerable advancements in the technique soon thereafter; however, most of the developments were disregarded until the early part of the twentieth century, when instrumentation was developed to make recording such activity reliable and valid.[3] Today, clinical **electromyography (EMG)** is used to evaluate the scope of neuromuscular disease or trauma, and kinesiological electromyography is used to study muscle function.

As an examination procedure, clinical EMG involves the detection and recording of electrical potentials from skeletal muscle fibers. **Nerve conduction velocity (NCV)** tests determine the speed with which a peripheral motor or sensory nerve conducts an impulse. Together with other clinical examinations, these two electrodiagnostic procedures can provide information about the extent of nerve injury and/or muscle disease. These two forms of testing, sometimes referred to as **electroneuromyography (ENMG)**, can contribute valuable information leading to a diagnosis and prognosis as well as assist with establishing anticipated goals and expected outcomes for patients with musculoskeletal and neuromuscular disorders.

Kinesiological EMG is used to study muscle activity and establish the role of various muscles in specific activities. Although the concepts are the same, the focus of kinesiological EMG is quite different from that of clinical EMG in terms of instrumentation requirements and data analysis techniques. Basmajian and DeLuca[4] have provided a thorough review of literature in this area. More recently, standards for the recording, processing, and reporting of surface EMG signal information for kinesiological applications were reported following recommendations from the International Society of Electrophysiology and Kinesiology (ISEK) and a European partnership.[5,6] Selective topics in the use of surface EMG signals in the occupational setting are also available in the literature.[7,8]

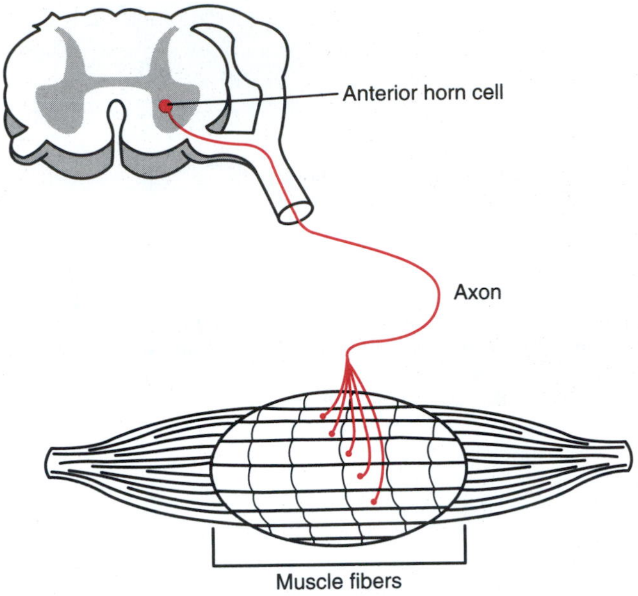

Figure 9.1 The motor unit is composed of one anterior horn cell, one axon, its neuromuscular junction and all the muscle fibers innervated by that axon.

Concepts of Electromyography (EMG)

EMG is the recording of the electrical activity of muscle and in essence, the study of motor unit activity. Motor units are composed of one anterior horn cell, one axon, its neuromuscular junctions, and all the muscle fibers innervated by that axon (Fig. 9.1). The single axon conducts an impulse to all its muscle fibers, causing them to depolarize at relatively the same time. This depolarization produces electrical activity that is manifested as a *motor unit action potential (MUAP)* and recorded and displayed graphically as the EMG signal. Instrumentation for recording EMG potentials requires a three-phase system: an input phase that includes electrodes to pick up electrical potentials from contracting muscle; a processor phase, during which the small electrical signal is amplified; and an output phase, in which the electrical signal is converted to visual and/or audible signals so that the data can be displayed and analyzed (Fig. 9.2).

Instrumentation and Signal Characteristics

Detecting the EMG Signal: Electrodes

An **electrode** is a transducer; a device for converting one form of energy into another. Several types of electrodes can be used to record the EMG signal. *Surface electrodes* are used frequently when performing a NCV test and in

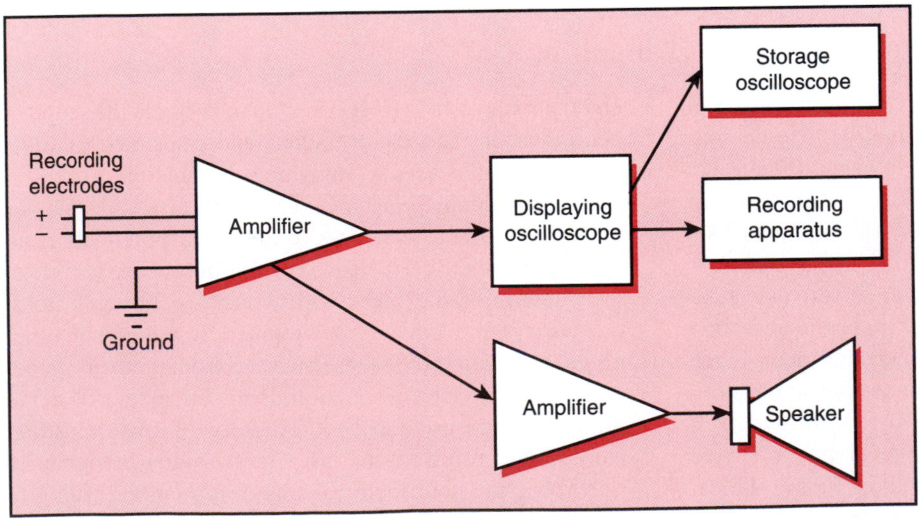

Figure 9.2 The EMG recording system. (Adapted from Echternach, J,[56, p 4] with permission.)

some kinesiological investigations. They are generally considered adequate for monitoring large superficial muscles or muscle groups. Surface electrodes cannot be used for clinical EMG examinations. They are not considered selective enough to record activity accurately from an individual **motor unit** or from specific small or deep muscles, unless special recording procedures using multielectrode arrays and spatial filtering techniques are utilized.[9,10] *Fine-wire indwelling electrodes* can be used for kinesiological study of small and deep muscles. Needle electrodes are necessary to record single motor unit potentials for clinical EMG.

In addition to a *recording electrode* (either surface or needle), a *ground electrode* must be applied to provide a mechanism for canceling out the interference effect of external electrical noise such as that caused by fluorescent lights, broadcasting facilities, elevators, and other electrical apparatus. The ground electrode is a surface electrode that is attached to the skin near the recording electrodes, but usually not over muscle.

The simplest surface EMG electrode is configured as a small metal disc, commonly made of silver/silver chloride, which is typically 3 to 5 millimeters (mm) in diameter contained within a casing that can be affixed to the surface of the skin with adhesive collars or tape. Electrode gel is applied beneath these electrodes to facilitate the conduction of electrical potentials. Other surface electrodes are self-adhesive and pre-gelled (Fig. 9.3). Two of these electrodes are applied to the skin overlying the appropriate muscle, to achieve bipolar recording, where they are typically arranged in a longitudinal direction parallel to the muscle fibers (Fig. 9.4). Often, some skin preparation is necessary to reduce skin resistance, which can interfere with the quality of recording.[11] This may include washing, rubbing with alcohol, and abrading the superficial skin layer to remove dead, dry skin cells.

Improvements in surface electrode technology have resulted in the *active electrode* which achieves bipolar recording from a single sensor containing preamplifiers

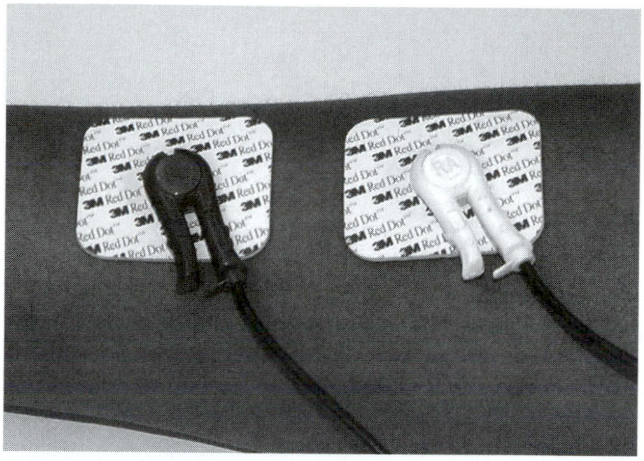

Figure 9.4 Two surface electrodes applied to the skin overlying a muscle to achieve a bipolar reading.

and signal conditioners at the detection site. Active electrodes are typically configured with a fixed interelectrode separation of 1 or 2 cm (Fig. 9.5) and attached to the skin using a double-sided adhesive interface (Fig. 9.6). Active electrodes have the advantage of not requiring skin preparation, and they minimize signal artifacts that can result from movement of the leads. Their fixed interelectrode distance also minimizes modifications in signal amplitude and spectral content which can occur when this distance is allowed to vary, as for instance when silver/silver chloride disc electrodes move with respect to each other during limb movement and stretching of the skin.[6,12]

Fine-wire indwelling electrodes were introduced in the early 1960s for kinesiological study of small and deep

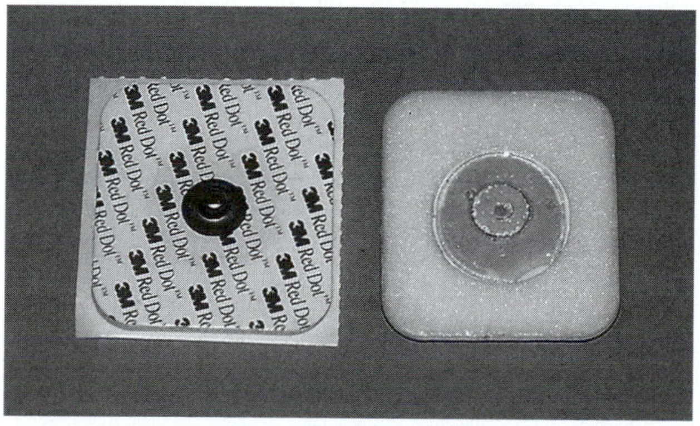

Figure 9.3 Surface electrodes are available with a self-adhering surface. The thin protective backing (*left,* backing in place) is removed prior to use (*right,* backing removed). Note the small circular well (*right*) containing the electrode gel.

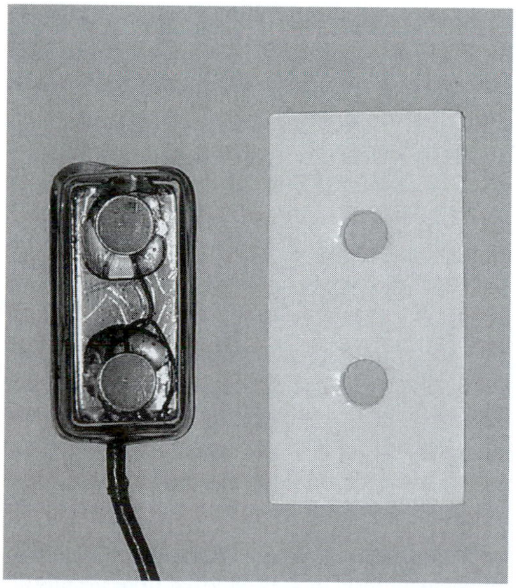

Figure 9.5 Active electrodes (*left*) are configured with a fixed interelectrode separation of 1 or 2 cm. A small double-sided adhesive strip with electrode openings (*right*) is used for attachment to skin surface.

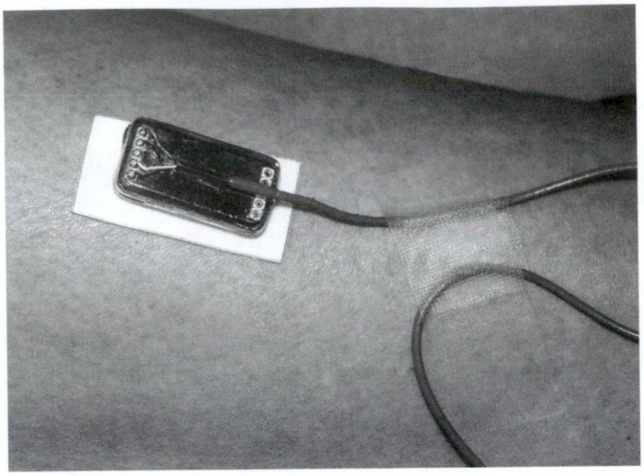

Figure 9.6 Active electrode attached to skin using a double-sided adhesive strip.

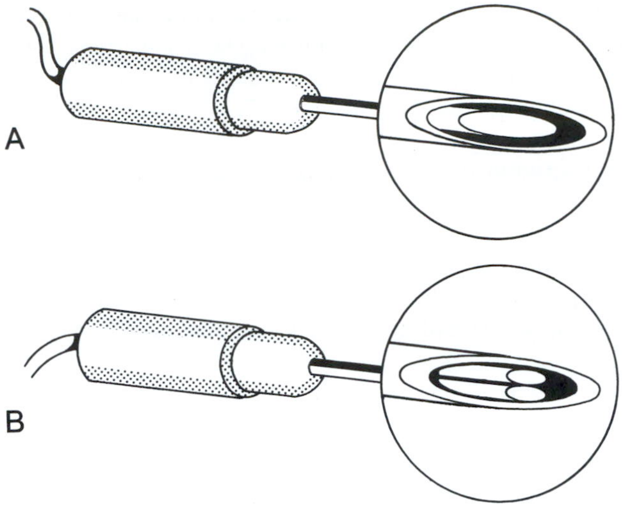

Figure 9.8 Concentric needle electrodes, showing single (*A*) and bipolar (*B*) wire configurations.

muscles.[13] The electrodes are made with two strands of small-diameter wire (approximately 100 μm). These are coated with a polyurethane or nylon insulation and threaded through a hypodermic needle. The tips of the wires are bared for 1 to 2 mm and bent back against the needle shaft (Fig. 9.7). The needle is inserted into the muscle belly and immediately withdrawn, leaving the wires embedded in the muscle. Because of the small diameter of these wires, which are as thin as a hair, subjects cannot feel the presence of the wires in the muscle. The wires form a bipolar electrode configuration that can record from a localized area and are capable of picking up single motor unit potentials. Fine-wire electrodes are necessary for monitoring activity from deep muscles, such as the soleus, or small or narrow muscles, such as the finger flexors. They may not be as useful for larger muscles because they sample motor unit activity from such a small area of the muscle.

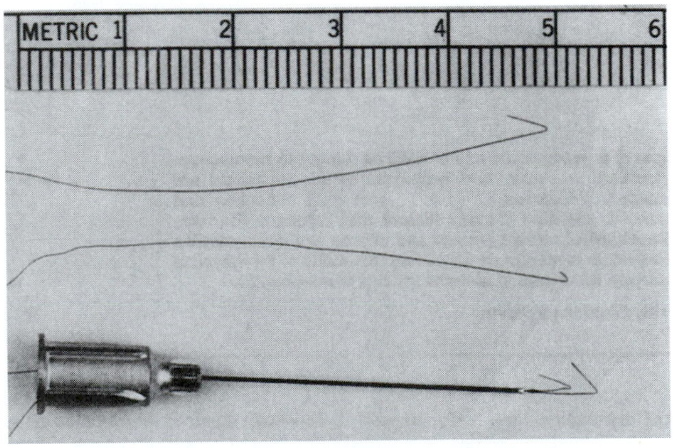

Figure 9.7 Fine-wire indwelling electrode: 27-gauge hypodermic needle through which two strands of polyurethane-coated wire are threaded. Insulation is removed from the tips of the wires, and hooks are created to keep the wires imbedded while the needle is removed from the muscle. (From Soderberg, GL, and Cook, TM: Electromyography in biomechanics. Phys Ther 64:1814, 1984, with permission.)

A needle electrode is required for clinical EMG, so that single motor unit potentials can be recorded from different parts of a muscle. The first studies of motor unit activity were done in 1929 by Adrian and Bronk,[14] who used a *concentric (coaxial) needle electrode.* This type of electrode consists of a stainless steel cannula, similar to a hypodermic needle, through which a single or double wire of platinum or silver is threaded (Fig. 9.8). The cannula shaft and wire are insulated from each other, and only their tips are exposed. The wire and the needle cannula act as electrodes, and the difference in potential between them is recorded. The bare tip of the platinum wire is considered to be the active electrode and the cannula acts as the reference electrode.

Another commonly used approach for clinical EMG involves the use of a *monopolar needle electrode,* which is composed of a single fine needle, insulated except at the tip (Fig. 9.9). A second surface electrode placed on the skin near the site of insertion serves as the *reference electrode.* These electrodes are less painful than concentric electrodes because they are smaller in diameter. Because monopolar configurations record much larger potentials than bipolar, the type of electrode should be specified to avoid misinterpretation of data relative to the size of potentials and the

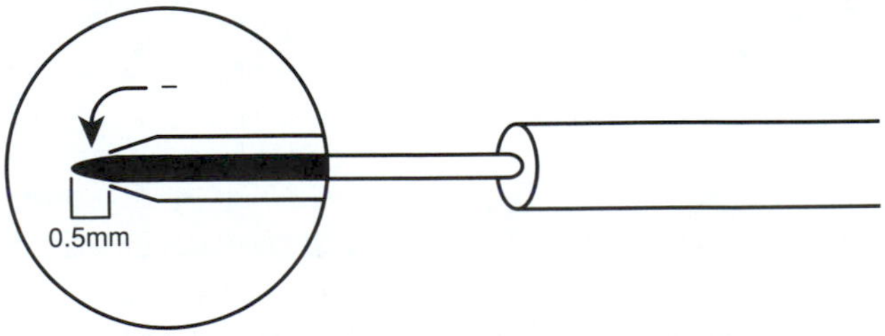

Figure 9.9 The monopolar needle electrode is a single finely sharpened needle, insulated except for the 0.5-mm tip.

area of recording. Clinical EMG can also be used to record from single muscle fibers.[15] *Single-fiber needle electrodes* are concentric, but have wires 25 micrometers (μm) in diameter (as compared to 0.1 mm for standard concentric electrode wires).

Needle electrodes are not useful for kinesiological studies because of the discomfort caused by the needle remaining in the muscle during contraction. Fine-wire electrodes are inappropriate for use in clinical EMG because the examiner has neither good control over placement of the electrode, nor the ability to move the electrode within the muscle once it is placed. Ultrasound imaging has recently been used with great success in helping to guide the placement of fine-wire electrodes in deeply situated muscles, such as the iliopsoas.[16] Guidelines for insertion of electrodes have been published[17,18] and anatomical references should always be consulted to ensure accurate and safe placement when using needles. Because they pierce the skin, all needle and fine-wire electrodes must be sterilized. Clinical studies are done almost exclusively with commercially available sterile disposable needle electrodes.

The Myoelectric Signal

This section contains foundational information about EMG that pertains to both kinesiological and clinical use but is not specific to either use. Later sections on each of these applications address more specific considerations.

EMG electrodes convert the bioelectric signal resulting from muscle or nerve depolarization into an electrical potential capable of being processed by an *amplifier*. It is the difference in electrical potential between the two recording electrodes that is processed.

The unit of measurement for difference of potential is the *volt* (V). The amplitude, or height, of potentials is usually measured in microvolts (1 $\mu V = 10^{-6}$ V) or in millivolts (1mV $= 10^{-3}$ V). The greater the difference in potential recorded by the electrodes, the greater the amplitude, or voltage, of the electrical potential. The amplitude of a MUAP is usually measured from peak to peak (i.e., from the highest to the lowest point). The *duration* of the potential is a measure of time from onset to cessation of the electrical potential. Typical peak-to-peak ranges for MUAP amplitude are 5 μV to 5 mV; duration varies from 2 to 14 msec.[4]

The Motor Unit Action Potential (MUAP)

It is important to understand the process by which a MUAP is transmitted to an amplifier in order to understand how such potentials can be interpreted. Because of the dispersion of the fibers in a single motor unit, the muscle fibers from several motor units may be interspersed with one another (Fig. 9.10). Therefore, when one motor unit contracts, the depolarizing fibers are not necessarily close together. Consequently, a needle, wire, or surface electrode cannot be situated precisely within or over any one motor unit.

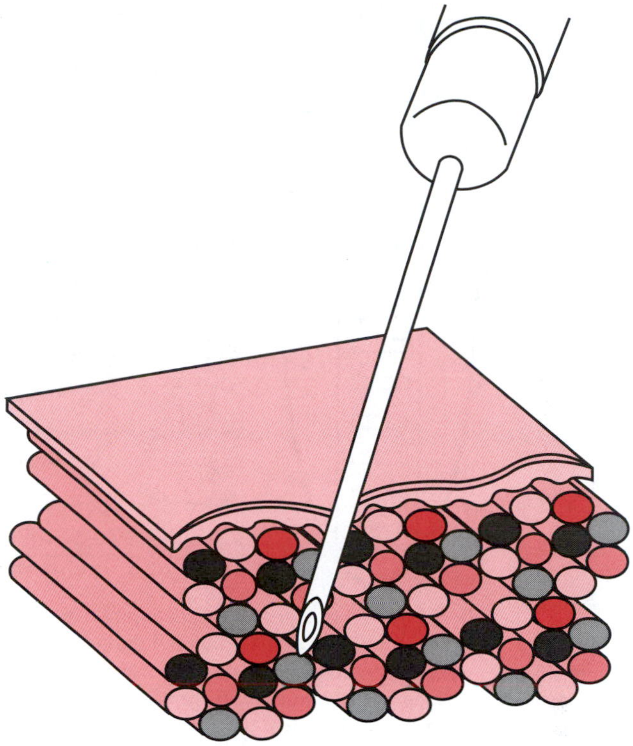

Figure 9.10 Cross-sectional view of muscle belly with needle electrode inserted. Differently shaded fibers represent different motor units.

All the fibers of a single motor unit contract almost synchronously, and the electrical potentials arising from them travel through body fluids as a result of the excellent conducting properties of the electrolytes surrounding the fibers. This process is called *volume conduction*. The electrical activity will flow through the conducting medium, the *volume conductor*, in all directions, not just in the direction of the inserted needle, wire, or the surface electrodes on the skin. Fibrous tissue, fat, and blood vessels act as insulation against the flow. Therefore, the actual pattern of the flow of electrical activity within the volume conductor is not predictable. The signals that do reach the electrode are transmitted to the amplifier. All others are simply not recorded, although they are present. The activities produced by all the individual fibers contracting at any one time are summated, because they reach the electrode almost simultaneously. Electrodes only record potentials they pick up, without differentiating their origin. Therefore, if two motor units contract at the same time, from the same or adjacent muscles, the activity from fibers of both units will be summated and recorded as one large potential when using surface electrodes.

Myoelectric signals recorded from a multielectrode array as a function of time (Fig. 9.11) is a way to demonstrate that the EMG signal is generated from the point of innervation of the muscle and propagates in opposing directions until it dies at the tendinous zones of the muscle fibers. Figure 9.11 demonstrates how this technique can be

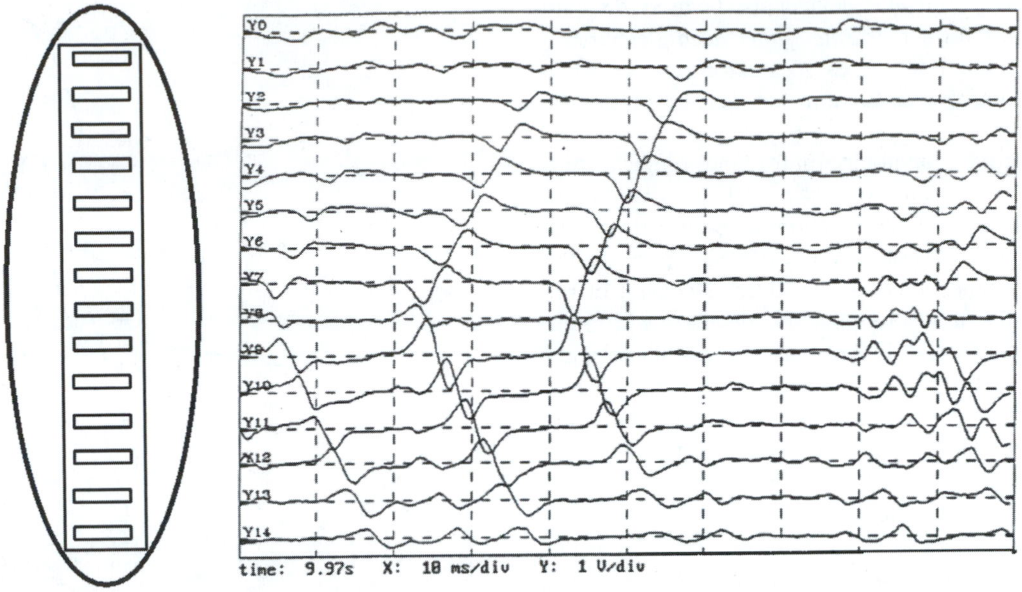

Figure 9.11 Illustration of recording from a multielectrode array demonstrating the propagation of the motor unit action potential during a voluntary isometric contraction of the biceps brachii sustained at constant force. The drawing on the left illustrates how the array was positioned on the surface over the muscle. Each EMG channel (numbered Y0 to Y14) is a differential recording from two consecutive parallel detection "bars" or electrodes. The EMG data indicate the presence of an innervation zone at channel Y8 and tendinous zones at approximately Y1 (proximal) and Y13 (distal). The time delay between successive EMG waveforms represents the conduction velocity of the EMG signal.

used as a means of estimating muscle fiber conduction velocity, locating the innervation and tendinous zones, and noninvasively identifying individual MUAPs.[9,10,19,20] A recent literature review summarizes the basic principles of operation of linear electrode arrays as well as current kinesiological and clinical applications.[21]

Variables that Affect the MUAP

What variables, then, influence how much electrical activity is recorded by the electrodes, and consequently, the amplitude and shape of the recorded potential? First, the proximity of the electrodes to the fibers that are firing will affect the amplitude and duration of the recorded potential. Fibers that are further away will contribute less to the recorded potential. The tissue between the electrode and active muscle fibers also acts as a low-pass filter, attenuating the higher frequency components of the signal.[2] Second, the number and size of the fibers in the motor unit will influence the potential's size. A larger motor unit will produce more activity. Third, the distance between the fibers will affect the output, because if the fibers are very spread out, less of their total activity is likely to reach the electrodes. The size of the electrodes may also be a consideration. If the recording surface is larger, the electrodes will pick up from a larger area, making the size of the recorded signal greater. Therefore, to record from smaller muscles, a smaller electrode should be used.

The distance between the electrodes is another major factor affecting the size of the recorded potential. Greater electrode spacing will increase the surface, width, and depth of the recording area. Because voltage is dependent on the difference in potential between the electrodes, the greater the distance, the greater the voltage, or amplitude. There is, of course, a critical limit to this distance above which the electrodes will not be able to record a valid signal. Lynn et al[22] have theoretically shown that any active fiber at a depth of approximately half of the interelectrode spacing will dominate the surface EMG signal. Furthermore, the recording from fibers at a depth of more than 1.5 times the interelectrode spacing will be obliterated by inadequate signal-to-noise ratio. Some surface electrode assemblies, such as active EMG electrodes, have been developed in which the two electrodes are fixed within a casing, so that interelectrode distance is standardized. Concentric needle electrodes have a fixed distance between the wires and the needle shaft; this distance never changes, even when the electrode is moved. Fine-wire indwelling electrodes are the least reliable in this aspect, because there is little control over the interwire distance within the muscle. The wires are often prone to change position within the muscle after repeated contractions, a situation that may compromise the validity of the signals.

The shape, size, and duration of the recorded motor unit potential is actually a graphic representation of the electrical

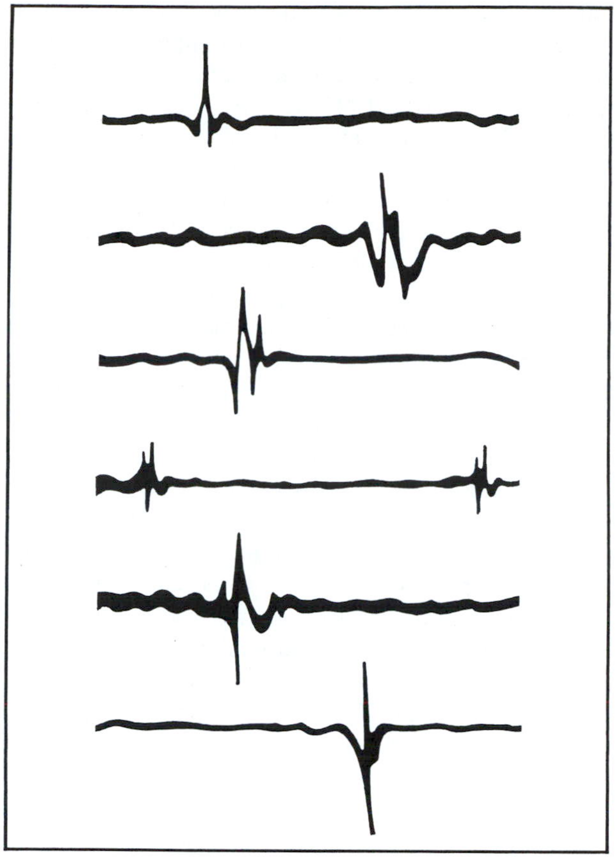

Figure 9.12 Single motor unit potentials as seen on an oscilloscope.

activity being picked up by the electrodes, relative to the structure of the motor unit and the electrode placement (Fig. 9.12). Therefore, with a given electrode placement, each motor unit potential will look distinctly different. The implications of this process for repeated EMG testing should be evident. It is impossible to recognize a motor unit potential as the same one if electrodes have been reinserted or moved, because the spatial and temporal relationships between the electrodes and the muscle fibers cannot be validly duplicated. This holds true for surface electrodes as well, although reapplication of surface electrodes has been shown to be more reliable than reinsertion of wire electrodes.[23]

Cross-Talk

Another important consideration is the ability of electrodes to record activity selectively from a single muscle. Because of volume conduction, electrical activity from nearby contracting muscles, other than the muscle of interest, may reach the electrodes and be processed simultaneously. There is no way to distinguish this activity by looking at the output signal. Careful electrode placement and spacing and choice of size and type of electrode will help control such *cross-talk* or electrical overflow.[4] Empirical evidence from the research literature has identified cross-talk between lower leg muscles as high as nearly 20 percent.[24]

Recent innovations using a three-bar electrode can eliminate the presence of cross-talk through a process referred to as *double-differentiation* (DD).[25] As shown in Figure 9.13A, the EMG is recorded in two ways: first, using the bipolar signal from bars 1 and 3 (single differentiation [SD]), and second, by subtracting the SD signal from electrode bars 1 and 2 from the SD signal from electrode bars 2 and 3. Figure 9.13B shows that there is a difference between the SD and DD signals when recording from wrist flexors during wrist extension. The fact that the DD signal is near baseline indicates that the SD recording is cross-talk from wrist extensors. During wrist flexion, shown in Figure 9.13C, no cross-talk is present, as the SD and DD signals are similar in magnitude.

Telemetry

When EMG recordings are considered for environments in which it is not practical to have the subject tethered, **telemetry** of the EMG signal via radio frequency transmitter and receiver is an option.[2] Typically, a small battery-powered transmitter combines the EMG signal with an FM radio signal. This combined signal is then broadcast at the

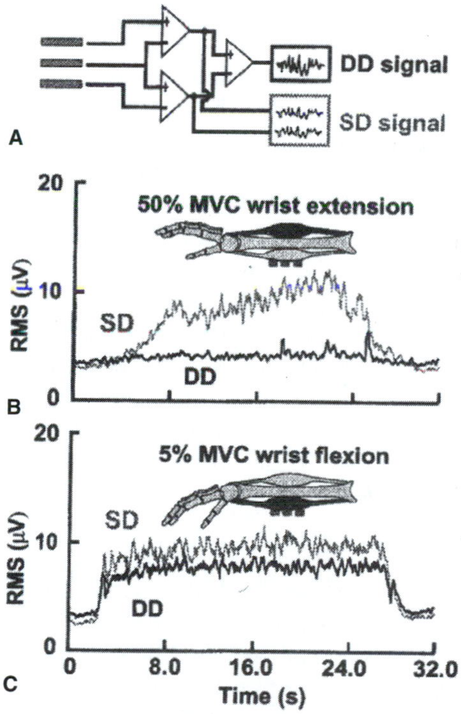

Figure 9.13 Illustration of the double differential technique to eliminate the presence of cross-talk. (*A*) Surface EMG is recorded from flexor carpi ulnaris muscle using both single-differentiated (between electrode bars 1 and 3) and double-differentiated signals (the difference between 1–2 and 2–3). The activity is recorded during wrist extension (*B*), showing cross-talk with single-differentiated signal, and during wrist flexion (*C*), showing no cross-talk, as single- and double-differentiated signals are of nearly equal magnitude. (Adapted from DeLuca, CJ,[12, p 135] with permission.)

FM carrier frequency to the receiver. The receiver, in turn, demodulates the FM signal to recover the EMG information. The power output of the transmitter and the *sensitivity* of the receiver determine the range of the telemetry link. Although transmitter range is more than adequate for most indoor applications (30 m or more), a far more serious limiting factor is the directionality of the transmitting antenna. Multiple antennas or omnidirectional antennas are used to alleviate this problem.

The decision to invest in telemetered EMG systems must be made by considering the significant added expense versus the advantage of greater freedom of movement of the subject. A recent alternative, still under development, is *portable data loggers*. These are small battery-operated devices worn on the person that provide on-board storage of multichannel EMG data (via magnetic or digital tape or a digital signal processing card). The stored data can then be downloaded after acquisition to a mainframe system for analysis.

Artifacts

The EMG signal should be a true representation of motor unit activity occurring in the muscle of interest. Unfortunately, many excess signals, or **artifacts** can be recorded and processed simultaneously with the EMG signal. An artifact is any unwanted electrical activity that arises outside of the tissues being examined. These artifacts can be of sufficient voltage to distort the output signal markedly. Electromyographers will usually observe the output signal on an oscilloscope or computer screen to monitor artifacts. Some newer commercial devices have built-in artifact suppression circuitry, or produce an audible signal and/or LED display to indicate the presence of an artifact such as 60-cycle interference in near real-time. A recent review summarizes methods for reducing noise, artifact, and interference in recorded EMG signals.[26] Recommendations in the review emphasize the need to first reduce artifact and interference at the source, through appropriate skin preparation and instrumentation. Various signal processing techniques are described for noise reduction that can be applied afterward, including band pass filtering, adaptive noise-cancellation filters, and wavelet transform filters.

Movement Artifact

All electrodes are composed of a metallic detecting surface that is in contact with an electrolyte. This electrolyte may be the oils and moisture on the skin, the conductive electrode gel placed between a surface electrode and the skin, or it may be the tissue fluids surrounding an inserted needle or fine-wire electrode. An ion exchange occurs at the interface between the electrode and electrolyte, and this is recorded as a bioelectric event when a difference of potential exists between the two electrodes. If no muscle activity is present, therefore, and the ionization that exists at each electrode–electrolyte interface is stable, then no difference of potential exists, resulting in electrical silence.

If, however, some disturbance occurs at one or both electrode–electrolyte interfaces, so as to produce a difference of potential, a low-frequency signal will be recorded that does not represent EMG activity. This signal is called *movement artifact*. It may result from movement of the skin beneath a surface electrode, pressure on or movement of the electrodes, or movement of a needle or fine-wire electrode within a contracting muscle. For example, if hamstring muscle activity is being monitored during an activity in the sitting position, pressure on the electrodes on the posterior aspect of the thigh may cause movement artifact. Some form of padding under the thigh, placed proximal and distal to the electrodes, can help alleviate this pressure. The use of a conductive electrolytic gel or emulsifying agent applied between the metal contact and the skin, or the use of silver/silver chloride electrodes, may also decrease such artifacts.[27] Most movement artifact occurs at signal frequencies below 10 to 20 hertz (Hz), causing minimal interference with the amplitude of the signal, but creating a wavy baseline. These artifacts can usually be eliminated with firm fixation of the electrodes and proper high-pass filtering of the signal to attenuate frequencies below a specified frequency, such as 20 Hz (see discussion of frequency response in the next section).

Movement of electrode cables can also cause a high-voltage, high-frequency artifact as a result of disturbance in the electromagnetic field that surrounds the conducting lead wires. These artifacts produce wide, large-amplitude spikes, and are not easily filtered. Active electrodes eliminate this problem by placing the preamplification stage as close as possible to the detection surface. This signal is then fed to the EMG amplifier on a low impedance section of the circuit. For nonactive electrodes used during activities requiring broad movements, cables should be taped down as much as possible, either to a table or chair, or along the limb itself, to avoid artifacts caused by cable movement.

Power Line Interference

The human body acts as an antenna, attracting electromagnetic energy from the surrounding environment. This energy is most commonly drawn from power lines and electrical equipment operating under an alternating current at 60 cycles per second (60 Hz) in the United States, and possibly at other frequencies internationally. An artifact caused by this interference current resembles a sine wave and can cause a constant hum in the recorded signal if it is not eliminated through appropriate amplification techniques. A 60-Hz signal can occur if electrode attachments become loose, or if electrodes are broken or frayed. Electrode wires often break beneath the protective tubing that connects the electrode itself to the lead wire. If raw data are not monitored, this condition may not be noticed. Other equipment in the area also may be the source of electrical interference. Diathermy equipment, electrical stimulators, cell phones, fluorescent lights, radios, and vibrators are examples of devices that generate electrical noise. Sometimes, using isolated power lines will help with this situation. A *notch filter* can be used to remove 60-Hz signals, although this will also eliminate some of the EMG signal within that frequency range.

Electrocardiogram

A third type of artifact, from the electrocardiogram, or ECG can occur when electrodes are placed on the trunk, upper arm, or upper thigh. If the EMG is being analyzed for frequency characteristics, this signal will provide significant interference. Correct application of the ground electrode and use of an amplifier with appropriate characteristics should help reduce these potentials, but may not be able to eliminate them. Their amplitude will vary depending on placement of electrodes. Electrocardiogram artifacts are generally regular, however, and their effect may be successfully attenuated. One such effective high pass filtering technique was described recently for removal of ECG artifact from EMG signals recorded from trunk muscles.[28]

Other Sources

In addition to the main sources of artifact and noise described earlier, other sources are present that result predominantly from the inherent limitations of the electronic hardware used to acquire and process the EMG signal. Electronic amplifiers used to amplify and condition the EMG signal are a source of broad band, low-level noise (i.e., less than 1.5 μV RMS in a well-designed amplifier when bipolar electrodes are shorted to ground). This noise level is not typically problematic during moderate or high-level contractions where it would typically comprise only 1 to 2 percent of the EMG amplitude, and therefore maintain a relatively high signal-to-noise ratio. For very low force level contractions, noise due to the instrumentation and electrode-skin interface may be a concern, and filtering techniques described above may be warranted.[26]

Amplifying the EMG Signal

Differential Amplifier

Before the motor unit potential can be visualized, it is necessary to amplify the inherently small EMG signal. An amplifier converts the electrical potential recorded by electrodes to a voltage signal large enough to be displayed. This electrical potential is composed of the EMG signal from muscle contraction and unwanted *noise* from static electricity in the air and power lines. To control for the unwanted part of the signals, the recording electrodes each transmit electrical potentials to two sides of a *differential amplifier,* each electrode supplying input to one side. The difference in potential between each input and ground is processed in opposite directions. The difference between these signals is amplified and recorded, hence the name of the amplifier. If the two electrodes receive equal signals, no activity is recorded. Noise is transmitted to both ends of the amplifier as a *common mode signal*. The noise, being equal at both ends of the amplifier, is cancelled out when the difference of potential between the two sides is recorded. The signals that are common to both inputs are generally the unwanted signals from interference.

Common Mode Rejection Ratio

In reality, however, the noise is not eliminated completely in a differential amplifier. Some of the recorded voltage will include noise. The *common mode rejection ratio (CMRR)* is a measure of how much the desired signal voltage is amplified relative to the unwanted signal. A CMRR of 1000:1 indicates that the wanted signal is amplified 1000 times more than the noise. The CMRR may also be expressed in decibels (dB) (1000:1 = 60 dB). The higher this value, the better. A good differential amplifier should have a CMRR exceeding 100,000:1.

Signal-to-Noise Ratio

Noise also can be internally generated by the electronic components of an amplifier, including resistors, transistors, and integrated circuits. This noise is often manifested as a hissing sound on a speaker and shows on a screen (oscilloscope) as a "fattened" baseline. The factor that reflects the ability of the amplifier to limit this noise relative to the amplified signal is the *signal-to-noise ratio,* or the ratio of the wanted signal to the unwanted signal.

Gain

This characteristic refers to the amplifier's ability to amplify signals. The gain refers to the ratio of the output signal level to the input level. A higher gain will make a smaller signal appear larger on the display. The gain is often larger for clinical EMG where individual motor units must be distinctly visible and their amplitude measured.

Input Impedance

Impedance is a resistive property, opposing current flow, such as that occurring in alternating current circuits (such as an amplifier). It is analogous to resistance, which is exhibited by direct circuits. Electrodes provide one source of impedance and are affected by such variables as electrode material, electrode size, length of the leads, and the electrolyte. If the electrode impedance is too great, the signal will be attenuated. Electrode impedance can be reduced by using larger electrodes of good conductivity with shorter leads. Fine-wire and needle electrodes generally have much greater impedance than surface electrodes because of their much smaller surface area.

Body tissues, including adipose tissue, blood, and skin, also provide a source of resistance to the electrical field. Resistance and impedance are measured in units called ohms (Ω). Skin impedance can be measured with an ohmmeter and its value reduced by proper preparation. Most researchers have reported acceptable skin impedance under 20,000 Ω, although with proper preparation and good electrodes, resistance can usually be reduced to between 1000 and 5000 Ω. Some skin areas, such as those with darker pigments or those that are more exposed, generally have higher impedance. Skin impedance obviously is a concern only with surface electrodes.

Impedance is also present at the input of an amplifier. The muscle action potential is effectively divided into voltage changes at the electrode and amplifier input terminals. Because of the direct relationship between voltage and impedance (based on Ohm's law), if the impedance at the amplifier is greater than the impedance at the electrode, the voltage drop will be greater at the amplifier and the recorded potential will more accurately represent the true signal voltage. If the electrode impedance is too great, the voltage will drop at the source of the signal and less of the electrical energy will be transmitted to the amplifier. Therefore, the amplifier input impedance should be substantially greater (at least 1000 times) than the impedance recorded at the electrodes. An input impedance of 1 megaohm ($1\ M\Omega = 10^6\Omega$) is acceptable for surface electrodes, but should be greater with fine-wire and needle electrodes. Active electrodes use amplifiers with high input impedance (>100 MΩ) to compensate for the unwanted noise and signal attenuation that is produced by the high resistance of the skin. Because skin resistance contributes to the impedance measured at the electrodes, greater input impedance decreases the need for skin preparation with surface electrodes.

Frequency Bandwidth

The EMG waveforms processed by an amplifier are actually the summation of signals of varying frequencies, measured in *hertz* (1 Hz = 1 cycle per second). A MUAP can be likened to a piano chord, which is composed of many notes, each at a different frequency (sound). If we vary the notes, the chord will sound different. Similarly, the shape and amplitude of an action potential are, in part, a function of the frequencies that compose the waveform. Amplifiers usually have variable filters that can be adjusted to limit the range of frequencies they will process. The main reason for using filters is to reduce noise.

The *frequency bandwidth* delineates the highest and lowest frequency components that will be processed, or the upper and lower cutoff frequencies. If the full ranges of frequencies that make up the major portion of a waveform are not processed, the potential will be distorted. Amplifiers should be able to respond to signals between 10 and 10,000 Hz to accurately record nerve and muscle potentials for clinical EMG.[29]

For kinesiological purposes, however, where specific waveform characteristics are not of major interest, lower bandwidths are used. The frequency content of an EMG signal is inversely proportional to the interelectrode separation distance. Consequently, the frequency spectrum extends from 10 to 500 Hz for most surface electrodes, and from 10 to 1000 Hz for fine-wire electrodes. Limiting signals to these frequency ranges by a filter is helpful for reducing the effects of low- and high-frequency artifacts.

Displaying the EMG Signal

The amplified signal must be displayed in a useful fashion. The form of output used is dependent on the type of information desired and instrumentation available.

Computers sample and store EMG data for display and analysis. Data may be stored in *analog* (i.e., as a continuous varying signal) or in *digital* form (i.e., the continuous signal is converted into a series of numbers, each of which represents the amplitude of the signal at a particular instant in time). The conversion process is referred to as analog-to-digital (A-to-D) conversion, and the device that performs this task is called an A-to-D converter. The process involves sampling the signal at a frequency of at least 1 KHz, and converting it into numerical form with a 10- or 12-bit A-to-D converter, or higher. A 10-bit converter divides the signal into 2^{10} (or 1028) discrete levels, and a 12-bit converter divides the signal into 2^{12} (or 4096) discrete levels. When working with A-to-D converters, it is necessary to specify the sampling rate for EMG data acquisition. An important rule, referred to as the *Nyquist sampling rate*, is to select a sampling rate that is at least twice the highest frequency component of the signal. Because surface EMG signals may have frequency components as high as 300 to 500 Hz, a sampling rate of at least 1000 Hz should be selected. If the sampling rate is specified lower than the Nyquist rate, the signal will be distorted and information will be lost.

The electrical signal can be displayed visually on a cathode ray oscilloscope or computer monitor for analysis. The motor unit potential can also be converted into sound in the same way that a radio signal is processed. For the same reason that every motor unit potential will look different, it will also sound different. Normal and abnormal potentials have distinctive sounds that are helpful in distinguishing them. These will be described in the next section.

Several types of recorders have been used in kinesiological study. Graphic recorders, such as pen or chart recorders, provide a permanent written record of the output. These recorders rarely have a full-scale bandwidth greater than 60 Hz, but are more useful for integrated or averaged waveforms. An oscilloscope is often used in conjunction with a pen recorder to allow visual inspection of raw signals for artifacts. With the advent of computer workstations and digital processors, pen and chart recorders are not commonly used today.

Unlike graphic recorders, machine-interpretable recorders, such as FM magnetic tape recorders or digital recorders, store information in a form that cannot be read or analyzed without a machine interface. The advantage of the FM tape recorder is that it can store the EMG signal in its original analog form. When using FM recorders, it is important to be aware that the bandwidth of the tape recorder is directly proportional to the tape speed. Therefore, a recording speed must be selected that provides a bandwidth adequate for the signal being recorded. Second, FM recorders have an input dynamic range (typically ± 1 V) that cannot be exceeded; otherwise that portion of the waveform that exceeds the input dynamic range will be clipped. This means that the investigator must adjust the gain of the amplifier appropriately. Too large a gain will result in distortion of the signal due to clipping. Inadequate gain will result in poor signal-to-noise ratio.[11]

Digital recorders can store data on digital magnetic tape or disc following A-to-D conversion of the signal. Their primary advantages are that they avert the noise and distortion problems of FM recorders and they provide data in a digital format that can be directly input to a computer for analysis and display. The fidelity of the digitally recorded data is dependent primarily on the performance of the A-to-D converter.

Clinical EMG

The EMG Examination

EMG examines the integrity of the neuromuscular system, including upper and lower motor neurons, the neuromuscular junction, and muscle fibers. Testing usually involves observation of muscle action potentials from several muscles in different stages of muscle contraction. The EMG signal is only part of a complete examination, however, which will include a thorough understanding of the patient's history and clinical findings. For example, the therapist might also examine muscle strength, pain, reflexes, sensory function, and the presence of atrophy as well as functional abilities in extremity and trunk musculature. This clinical examination will suggest which muscles and/or nerves should be tested.

Insertional Activity

Initially, the patient is asked to relax the muscle to be examined during insertion of the needle electrode. Insertion into a contracting muscle is uncomfortable, but bearable. At this time, the electromyographer will observe a spontaneous burst of potentials, which is possibly caused by the needle breaking through muscle fiber membranes. This is called *insertional activity* and normally lasts less than 300 msec.[30] This activity is also seen during examination as the needle is repositioned in the muscle. It usually stops when the needle stops moving. Insertional activity can be described as normal, reduced, absent, increased, or prolonged. Absent insertional activity can be an indication to the examiner that the electrode is either not in muscle tissue or that it is in fibrotic muscle tissue. Increased or prolonged activity may be an indication of unstable or excitable membranes and occurs when muscle is actively denervating or muscle tissue is inflamed. It is considered a measure of muscle excitability and may therefore be markedly reduced in fibrotic muscles or exaggerated when denervation or inflammation is present (Fig. 9.14).

The Muscle at Rest

Following cessation of insertional activity, a normal relaxed muscle will exhibit electrical silence, which is the absence of electrical potentials. Observation of silence in the relaxed state is an important part of the EMG examination. Potentials arising spontaneously during this period are significant abnormal findings. It is often difficult for a patient to relax sufficiently to observe complete electrical silence. However, the potentials seen will be distinct motor unit potentials, whereas *spontaneous potentials* can be differentiated by their distinct characteristics related to amplitude, shape, frequency, waveform, and sound.

One exception to finding no activity in normal resting muscle occurs when the needle is in the motor end-plate region. Such activity may be reflected as a constant low-amplitude noise (10 to 20 mV) or higher amplitude intermittent spikes which are biphasic, short duration 100- to 300-mV potentials. This activity disappears by repositioning the needle slightly. Also the patient frequently reports that there is less discomfort from the needle electrode

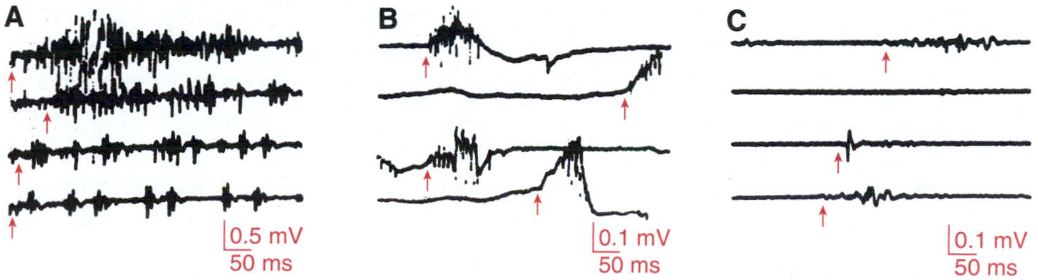

Figure 9.14 Increased (*A*), normal (*B*), and decreased (*C*) insertion activity induced by movements of the needle electrode (*arrows*). The tracings were obtained from the first dorsal interosseus in a patient with tardy ulnar palsy (*A*), tibialis anterior in a control subject (*B*), and fibrotic deltoid of a patient with severe dermatomyositis (*C*). (From Kimura, J,[30, p 231] with permission.)

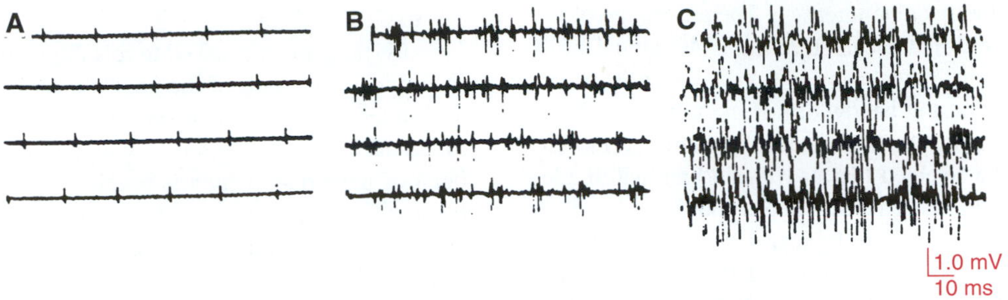

Figure 9.15 Normal recruitment of the triceps brachii in a 44-year-old healthy man. Activity was recorded during minimal contraction (*A*) where single motor unit activity is evident, during moderate contraction (*B*) when motor units are recruited, and during maximal contraction (*C*) when an interference pattern is visible. (From Kimura, J,[30, p 241] with permission.)

when repositioned. Some authors have reported that end-plate potentials may be excessive in denervated muscle.[30]

Normal Motor Unit Action Potentials

After observing the muscle at rest, the patient is asked to contract the muscle minimally (Fig. 9.15). This weak voluntary effort should cause individual motor units to fire. These motor unit potentials are examined with respect to amplitude, duration, shape, sound, and frequency (Fig. 9.16). These five parameters are the essential characteristics that distinguish each normal and abnormal potential. Finally, the patient is asked to increase levels of contraction progressively to a strong effort, allowing determination of recruitment patterns.

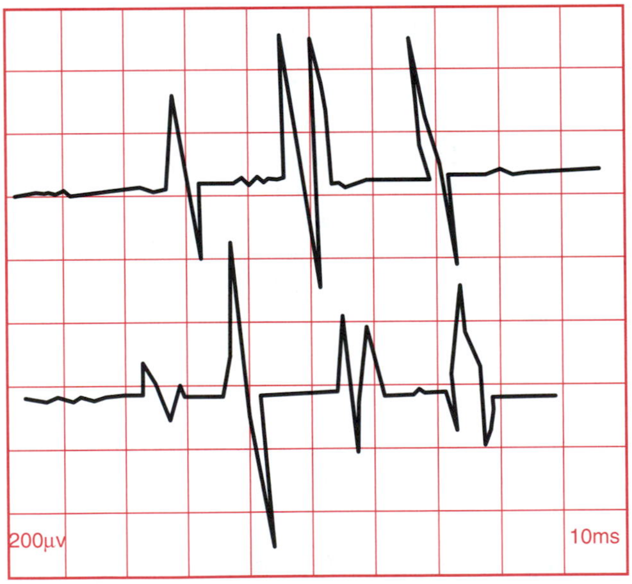

Figure 9.16 Illustration of a waveform (normal motor units). Characteristics of normal motor units include:

- *Voltage (amplitude)*: 100 µV to 4000 to 5000 µV (4 to 5 µV)
- *Duration*: 2 to 17 msec; most are 8 to 12 msec
- *Waveform*: Mono- to four-phase, most are bi- or triphasic; more than four is polyphasic
- *Frequency*: 1 to 60/sec, highly variable depending on individual muscles
- *Sound*: Clear, sharp, thump, or plunk. Duration and proximity to needle electrode determine sharpness of sound

(From Echternach, J,[56, p 62] with permission.)

A motor unit potential is actually the summation of electrical potentials from all the fibers of that unit close enough to the electrodes to be recorded. The amplitude (voltage) is affected by the number of fibers involved or by the motor unit territory. The duration and shape are functions of the distance of the fibers from the recording electrodes, the more distant fibers contributing to terminal phases of the potential.

In normal muscle, the peak-to-peak amplitude of a single MUAP, recorded with a concentric needle, may range from 100 µV to 5 mV. The amplitude is determined primarily by a limited number of fibers located close to the electrode tip. Therefore, motor units must be sampled from different sites in a muscle to determine the amplitude of motor units in that muscle accurately.

The total duration, measured from initial baseline deflection to return to baseline, will normally range from 2 to 17 msec, with the largest number being 8 to 12 msec. Duration is a function of the synchrony with which individual muscle fibers fire within a motor unit. This characteristic is affected by the conduction velocity of the axon terminals and by the length of muscle fibers. Duration can be affected significantly by electrical activity originating in fibers distant to the electrode. The *rise time* of the potential, measured from the initial positive peak to the following negative peak, provides an indication of the distance between the electrode and the contracting motor unit. A normal unit close to the electrode should have a rise time between 100 and 200 microseconds (µs). Distant discharges will have a longer rise time, and will not be useful for determining motor unit properties. The sharper the MAUP in appearance and the clearer the sound on the speaker (a sharp thump or plunk) the closer that MAUP is to the recording electrode.

The number of phases in a normal motor unit can be from one to four phases. The typical shape of an MUAP is diphasic or triphasic, with a *phase* representing a section of a potential above or below the baseline. It is not abnormal to observe small numbers of *polyphasic potentials,* having five or more phases, in normal muscle. However, when polyphasic potentials represent more than 10 percent of a muscle's output, it may be an abnormal finding.

The normal motor unit will fire up to 15 times per second with strong contraction. The identifying sound is a clear, distinct thump. Gradually increasing the force of contraction will allow the electromyographer to observe the pattern of recruitment in the muscle. With greater effort, increasing numbers of motor units fire at higher frequencies, until the individual potentials are summated and can no longer be recognized, and an *interference pattern* is seen (see Fig. 9.15). This is the normal finding with a strong contraction. Highest amplitudes for interference patterns typically vary between 2 and 5 mV.

One of the disadvantages of conventional testing methods is that examination of single motor unit potentials can be made only during weak voluntary effort, essentially restricting the analysis to low-threshold type I motor units. An interesting alternative involves the use of *automatic quantitative assessment*, which further analyzes the interference pattern by determining the number of directional changes of the waveform that do not necessarily cross the baseline.[31,32] These data are processed by a computer to display the number of reversals and the intervals between reversals within a given time period. Such ratios can vary between normal and pathological conditions, allowing for greater diagnostic precision in the differentiation of primary muscle disease and neurogenic lesions.[33,34] This approach allows the electromyographer to observe the behavior of motor units even during maximal effort, when individual potentials cannot be delineated.

An electromyographer, therefore, examines insertion activity, as well as activity with the muscle at rest and in states of minimal, moderate, and maximal contraction. The needle electrode is moved to different areas and depths of each muscle to sample different muscle fibers and motor units. This is necessary because of the small area from which a needle electrode will pick up electrical activity, and because the effects of pathology may vary within a single muscle. Up to 25 different points within a muscle may be examined by moving and reinserting the needle electrode.

Abnormal Potentials

Spontaneous Activity

Because a normal muscle at rest exhibits electrical silence, any activity seen during the relaxed state can be considered abnormal. Such activity is termed spontaneous because it is not produced by voluntary muscle contraction. Four types of spontaneous potentials have been identified: *fibrillation potentials, positive sharp waves, fasciculation potentials*, and *repetitive discharges.*

Fibrillation Potentials. Fibrillation potentials are believed to arise from spontaneous depolarization of a single muscle fiber. This theory is supported by the small amplitude and duration of the potentials. They are not visible through the skin. Fibrillation potentials are classically indicative of lower motor neuron disorders, such as peripheral nerve lesions, anterior horn cell disease, radiculopathies, and polyneuropathies with axonal degeneration. They are also found to a lesser extent in myopathic diseases such as muscular dystrophy, dermatomyositis, polymyositis, and myasthenia gravis.

Fibrillation potentials are biphasic spikes with the initial phase being in the positive direction and their spikes may vary in amplitude from 10 to 300 μV (can be larger, up to 600 μV) with an average duration of 2 msec (Fig. 9.17). Their sound is a high-pitched click, which has been likened to rain falling on a roof or wrinkling tissue paper. Fibrillation potentials have been recorded at frequencies of up to 30 per second.

Positive Sharp Waves. Positive sharp waves have been observed in denervated muscle at rest, usually accompanied by fibrillation potentials. However, they are also reported in primary muscle disease, especially muscular dystrophy and polymyositis. The waves are typically biphasic, with a sharp initial positive deflection (below baseline) followed by a slow negative phase (see Fig. 9.17). The negative phase is of much lower amplitude than the positive phase, and of much longer duration, sometimes up to 100 msec. The peak-to-peak amplitude may be variable, with voltages from 50 μV up to 2mV. The discharge frequency may range from 2 to 100 per second with 10 per second being common. The sound has been described as a dull thud. Positive

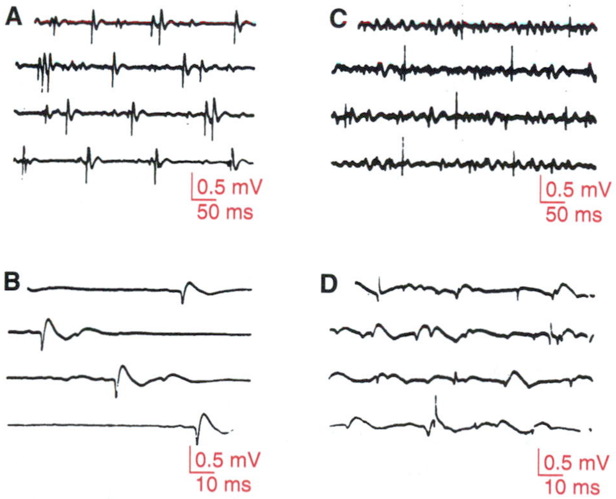

Figure 9.17 Spontaneous activity of the anterior tibialis in a 68-year-old woman with amyotrophic lateral sclerosis. Positive sharp waves (*A, B*) have a consistent configuration with a sharp positive deflection followed by a long-duration, low-amplitude negative deflection (*B*). Fibrillation potentials (*C, D*) are low-amplitude biphasic spikes. (From Kimura, J,[30, p 256] with permission.)

sharp waves are recorded when the tip of the recording electrode is in contact with the depolarized muscle membrane.[35]

Evidence indicates that fibrillation potentials and positive sharp waves may also be present with upper motor neuron lesions, creating a need for alternative explanations for their occurrence.[36] Researchers have observed both types of potentials in patients with spinal cord lesions and attributed their occurrence to the lack of some trophic factor from higher centers to the anterior horn cell. The occurrence of the denervation activity with central involvement supports the assumption of a transsynaptic degeneration of alpha-motoneurons. Berman suggests that spinal cord trauma can cause loss of motor axons in regions several segments caudal to the site of injury.[37] This interpretation may have implications for the design of rehabilitation strategies. Speilholz[38] postulated that these findings may also explain the observation of fibrillations and positive sharp waves with myopathies, and that the presence of these potentials indicates that muscle disease also affects the neuron. A similar hypothesis was formulated to explain the finding of spontaneous potentials in patients who had sustained a cerebral vascular accident.[39,40]

Investigators have also demonstrated spontaneous potentials in normal muscles of healthy subjects, primarily in muscles of the feet.[41] They have suggested that pathological changes involving axonal loss, segmental demyelination, and collateral sprouting may be associated with aging or mechanical trauma to the feet. Dimitru has recently question the rate of occurrence and the types of abnormal potentials seen in normal individuals; however, he also stresses the importance of care in the interpretation the electromyographic findings.[42] These findings have important clinical implications because interpretation of EMG signal patterns is necessary for accurate patient evaluation.

Fasciculations. Fasciculations are spontaneous potentials seen with irritation or degeneration of the anterior horn cell, chronic peripheral nerve lesions, nerve root compression, and muscle spasms or cramps. They are believed to represent the involuntary asynchronous contraction of a bundle of muscle fibers or a whole motor unit. Although their origin is not clearly known, there is evidence that the spontaneous discharge originates in the spinal cord or anywhere along the path of the peripheral nerve, causing contraction of the muscle fibers.[43]

Fasciculations are often visible through the skin, seen as a small twitch. They are not by themselves a definitive abnormal finding, however, because they are also seen in normal individuals,[44] particularly in calf muscle, eyes, hands, and feet.[45] When seen with other abnormal factors, such as fibrillations and positive sharp waves, fasciculations do contribute information indicating pathology. These potentials have been found in amyotrophic lateral sclerosis and progressive spinal muscular atrophy. Findings of fasciculation potentials in these conditions should be widespread and found in several

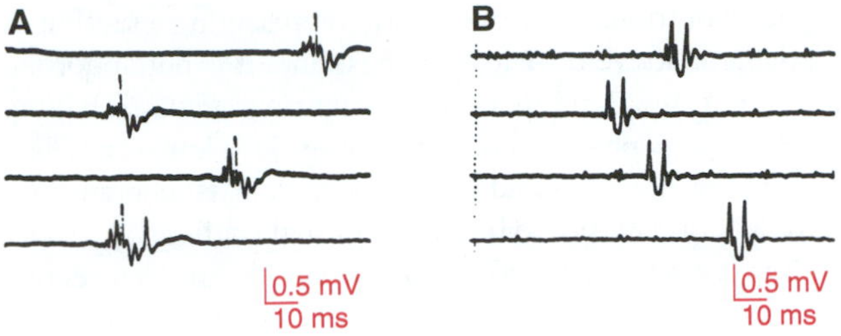

Figure 9.18 Fasciculation potentials in two patients with polyneuropathy. Recordings were obtained from the tibialis anterior in both patients, showing a very polyphasic potential of long duration (*A*) and a double-peaked, complex discharge (*B*). Fasciculation potentials are not always abnormal in waveform, as shown here, and are usually indistinguishable in shape from voluntarily activated motor unit potentials. (From Kimura, J,[30, p 260] with permission.)

locations and more than one extremity. Rosenfeld has pointed out that in amyotrophic lateral sclerosis that fibrillation potentials should also be found before a diagnosis can be made.[46] The amplitude and duration of these potentials may be similar to a motor unit potential (Fig. 9.18). They may also be polyphasic. Their firing rate is usually irregular, up to 50 per second. Their sound has been described as a low-pitched thump.

Myotonic and Complex Repetitive Discharges. Complex repetitive discharges, previously called bizarre high-frequency discharges, may be seen with lesions of the anterior horn cell and peripheral nerves, and with myopathies. The discharge is characterized by an extended train of potentials of with the same or nearly the same waveform (Fig. 9.19A). The feature that distinguishes these discharges from other spontaneous potentials is their regular and repetitive waveform. The frequency usually ranges from 5 to 100 impulses per second. The amplitude can vary from 50 μV to

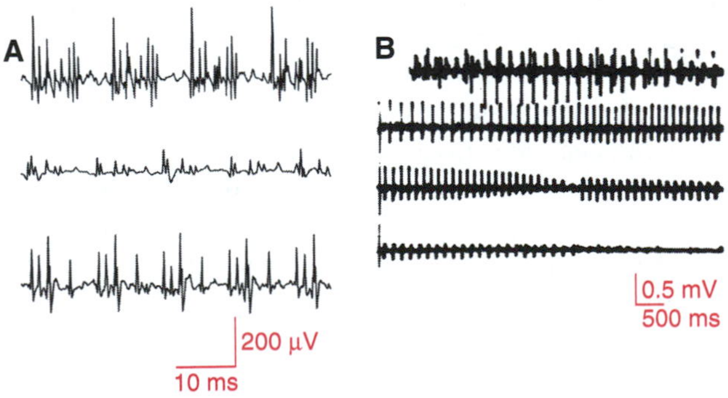

Figure 9.19 (*A*) Three examples (A–C) of complex repetitive discharges. Note how the same potentials appear in the same repetitive groups (symmetrical pattern). The minor differences between discharges is due to baseline irregularities. (From Dumitru, D, Amato, AA, and Zwarts, M,[69, p 277] with permission.). (*B*) Repetitive discharge from the right anterior tibialis in a 39-year-old man with myotonic dystrophy. The waxing and waning quality of these discharges is evident (asymmetrical pattern). (From Kimura, J,[30, p 254] with permission.)

1 mV, and duration may be up to 100 msec. Myotonic repetitive discharges that increase and decrease in amplitude in a waxing and waning fashion are found in myotonic disorders such as myotonic dystrophy as well as other myopathies (Fig. 9.19B). The sound is highly characteristic and sounds like a "dive-bomber." High-frequency discharges are probably triggered by movement of the needle electrode within unstable muscle fibers, or by volitional activity.

Abnormal Voluntary Potentials

Polyphasic potentials are generally considered abnormal, and are elicited on voluntary contraction, not at rest. By definition, polyphasic potentials are motor unit potentials with five or more phases. They are typical of myopathies, peripheral nerve involvement and nerve root compression. In primary muscle disease (myopathies), these potentials are generally of smaller amplitude than normal motor units, and of shorter duration and have been described by some as myopathic potentials. These multiphasic changes occur because of the decrease in the number of active muscle fibers within the individual motor units due to pathology. Although the entire unit will fire during voluntary contraction, fewer fibers are available in each unit to contribute to the total voltage and the duration of the potential.

The polyphasic configuration may be a result of slight asynchrony of firing of muscle fibers within a motor unit. This phenomenon is probably due to the difference in the length of the terminal branches of the axon extending to each individual fiber. The effects of this are normally not seen because the time differences are so slight. When some fibers are no longer contracting, or a delay in conduction is found in the terminal branches, these differences become more apparent, resulting in a fragmentation of the motor unit potential (Fig. 9.20).

Polyphasic potentials may also be seen during degeneration and after regeneration of a peripheral nerve. As some muscle fibers become reinnervated, they will generate action potentials with voluntary contraction. However, there are significantly fewer fibers acting than were present in the original unit, and these fibers will clearly reflect asynchronous depolarization. These polyphasic potentials are also much smaller in amplitude and duration than normal units, and they have been termed *nascent motor units*. Although polyphasic potentials are generally considered an abnormal finding, they are a positive finding in patients with regenerating peripheral nerve lesions because they indicate reinnervation.

Some forms of neuropathic involvement, such as chronic peripheral nerve lesions, peripheral neuropathies, and anterior horn cell disease, will result in a change in motor unit territory of an intact motor unit by collateral sprouting of axons to fibers of denervated motor units, forming *"giant" motor units*. Many electromyographers no longer use this terminology, preferring to call these potentials simply larger than normal motor unit potentials. In the early stages of this process these sprouts are of small diameter and have

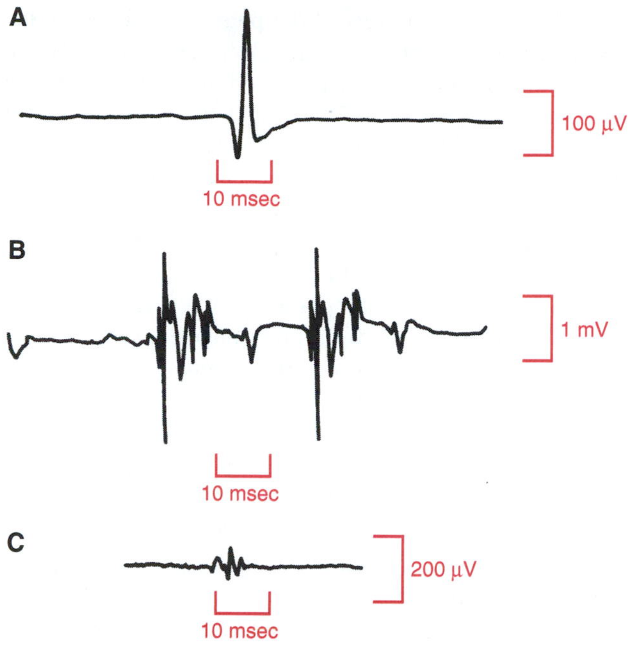

Figure 9.20 Motor unit action potentials. (*A*) Normal potential. (*B*) Long-duration polyphasic potential (shown twice). (*C*) Short-duration, low-amplitude, polyphasic potential. (From Aminoff, MJ: Electromyography in Clinical Practice, ed 3. Churchill Livingstone [Elsevier], New York, 1997, p 74, with permission.)

slow conduction velocities, resulting in a dispersion in the recorded potential, which increases the amplitude and duration and results in a polyphasic shape. These potentials may be seen in post-polio syndrome.[47–49] If this situation is sufficiently prevalent, the interference pattern may be incomplete. The amplitude of these potentials is greater than 5 mV in small muscles such as the intrinsic muscles of the hands and feet. In other muscles, amplitudes of 3 or more millivolts could be considered as larger than normal. Duration of these motor units is 4 to 5 msec up to 25 to 30 msec. Other characteristics are similar to normal motor units.

Single-Fiber EMG

Some properties of muscle can be examined using extracellular recordings from individual muscle fibers within the same motor unit using a technique called *single fiber electromyography (SFEMG)*. This procedure was developed to study neuromuscular transmission in the end-plate region in patients with myasthenia gravis, and has proven to be a useful adjunct to the EMG examination in patients with myopathies, myasthenic syndromes, and motor neuron disease.[50]

SFEMG requires the use of a small electrode (25 μm in diameter), which is inserted via a steel canula. During a slight voluntary contraction, recordings are taken from a single site. Because consecutive discharges from a single fiber have reproducible properties, timed measurements are able to accurately record the potentials. To determine neuromuscular transmission, the electrode is positioned to record from two fibers in the motor unit. A trigger is used to control the tracings of these potentials, allowing the measurement of latency between the two discharges. This latency, called *jitter*, represents the variable conduction time across the neuromuscular junction. For normal muscle contraction, mean values for jitter fall between 5 and 60 μsec. In a patient with myasthenia gravis, normal and increased values for jitter have been recorded. Impulse blocking can occur as well, with intermittent failure of some axons.[50] This basically experimental technique has been used in studies of myasthenia gravis, for example, to evaluate the effectiveness of drug therapy looking for changes in the jitter measurement. If a drug is effective, the mean jitter value changes toward normal or lower values.[51]

SFEMG has also been used to determine changes in muscle morphology as a function of *fiber density*, by counting the number of spikes in a single muscle fiber potential. With conditions causing changes in the organization of motor units, such as myopathies or reinnervation, fiber density will appear higher than normal.

Macro EMG

Another specialized technique, called *macro EMG*, is used to determine the overall status of the motor unit. Using a modification of the SFEMG electrode, recordings are made from as many fibers from one motor unit as possible. Two channels of EMG signals are recorded, one from the needle cannula, and the other as a difference of potential between the needle tip and the cannula. Using timed recordings and averaging techniques, the peak-to-peak amplitude and area of the macro EMG signal will reflect the number and size of the muscle fibers within the entire motor unit.

With normal muscle, the macro EMG motor unit potentials will differ in shape from one motor unit to another.[52] With myopathy, the macro EMG potential is decreased. Studies of patients with post-polio syndrome have identified dramatic increases in motor unit size, often more than 20 times normal.[48,53]

Nerve Conduction Tests

Hodes et al[54] first developed the technique for calculating the conduction velocity of the ulnar nerve in 1948. Dawson and Scott[55] further refined the procedure a year later, recording nerve potentials from the ulnar and median nerves through the skin at the wrist. This EMG technique has since become a valuable tool for identifying abnormalities and lesions of peripheral nerves, as well as localizing the site of involvement.

NCV tests involve direct stimulation to initiate an impulse in motor or sensory nerves. The *conduction time* is measured by recording the *evoked potential* either from the muscle innervated by the motor nerve or from the sensory nerve itself. NCV can be tested on any peripheral nerve that is superficial enough to be stimulated through the skin at two different points. The most commonly tested motor nerves are the ulnar, median, fibular (peroneal), tibial, radial, femoral, and sciatic nerves. Commonly tested sensory nerves include the median, ulnar, radial, sural, and superficial fibular nerves. Complete guidelines for performing NCV tests are available in comprehensive references.[56,57]

Instrumentation

Whereas EMG techniques record the spontaneous or volitional potentials of motor units, nerve conduction measurements involve evoked potentials, produced by direct electrical stimulation of peripheral nerves. The instrumentation, therefore, includes a stimulator in addition to all the components of the EMG system already described (Fig. 9.21).

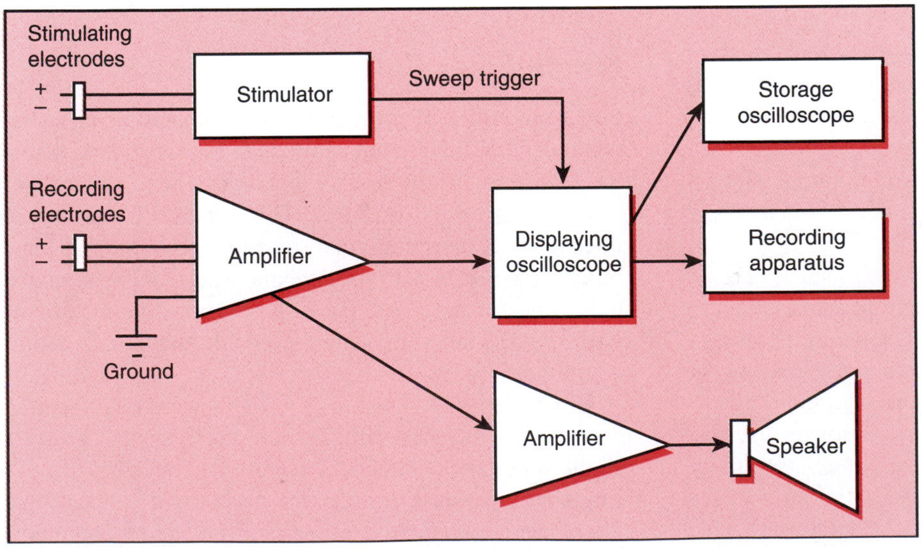

Figure 9.21 Instrumentation required for nerve conduction studies includes a stimulator in addition to all the components of the EMG system already described. (From Echternach, J,[56, p 4] with permission.)

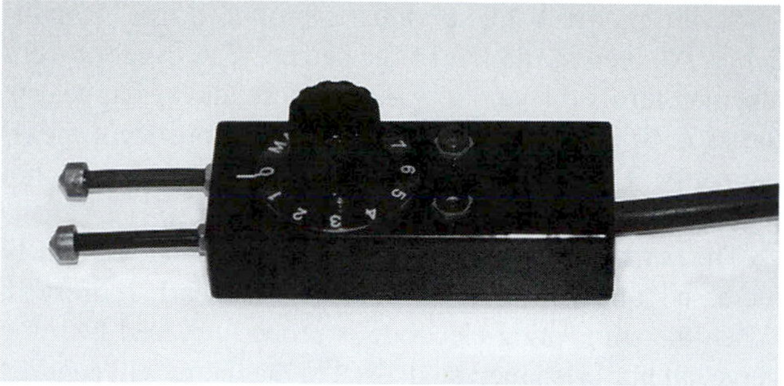

Figure 9.22 Nerve conduction velocity bipolar stimulating electrode.

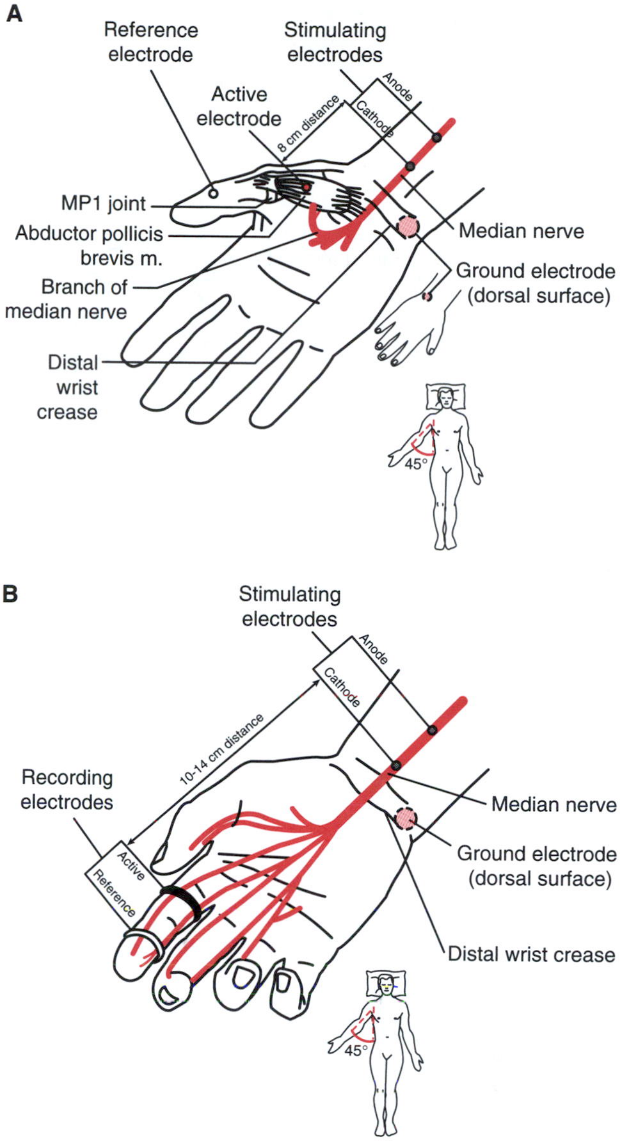

Figure 9.23 (*A*) Body position of subject receiving median nerve conduction study showing location of recording and distal stimulating electrodes and ground. (From Nelson, RM, et al: Clinical Electrotherapy, ed 3. Appleton & Lange, Stamford, CT, 1999, p 529, with permission.) (*B*) Body position and location of recording, stimulating, and ground electrodes for antidromic median sensory nerve conduction study. (From Nelson, RM, et al: Clinical Electrotherapy, ed 3. Appleton & Lange, Stamford, CT, 1999, p 534, with permission.)

The *stimulating electrode* is typically a two-pronged bipolar electrode with the cathode (−) and the anode (+) extending from a plastic casing (Fig. 9.22). A needle electrode can also be used to stimulate the nerve. The stimulus is provided by a square-wave generator with pulses typically delivered at a duration of 0.1 msec and a frequency of 1 pulse per second (Fig. 9.23A and B). The intensity of the stimulus needed to effectively stimulate the nerve will vary with the nerve and the individual patient. Most stimulators will deliver a stimulus up to 300 V, or 5 and 40 mA.[30] These intensities are considered safe for most patients. With a cardiac pacemaker, however, grounding should be checked and stimulation should be a sufficient distance from the pacemaker.[58] With indwelling cardiac catheters or central venous pressure lines, nerve conduction studies are contraindicated, because the electrical current may directly reach the cardiac tissue.

A trigger mechanism is incorporated into the recording system, so that the sweep seen on the screen is triggered by the stimulator. The sweep begins when the stimulus is delivered, producing a stimulus artifact on the screen with each successive stimulus. This allows the measurement of time from stimulus onset to subsequent motor or sensory response. The sweep makes one complete excursion across the screen for each pulse put out by the stimulator.

Motor Nerve Conduction Velocity Testing

Stimulation and Recording

Recording potentials directly from a peripheral nerve makes monitoring of purely sensory or motor fibers impossible. Therefore, to isolate the potentials conducted by motor axons of a mixed nerve, the evoked potential is recorded from a distal muscle innervated by the nerve under study. Although the stimulation of the nerve will evoke sensory and motor impulses, only the motor fibers contribute to the contraction of the muscle. For example to test the ulnar nerve, the test muscle is typically the abductor digiti minimi. Other examples are the following: for the median nerve, the abductor pollicis brevis; for the fibular nerve, the extensor digitorum brevis; and for the tibial nerve, the abductor hallicus or abductor digiti minimi.

Small surface electrodes are usually used to record the evoked potential from the test muscle, although needle electrodes may be used when responses are very weak. The *recording electrode* is placed over the belly of the test muscle. Accurate location of this electrode is important to the accuracy of the test, and the belly of the muscle should be carefully palpated, preferably against slight resistance. A second electrode, the *reference electrode,* is taped over the tendon of the muscle, distal to the active electrode. The

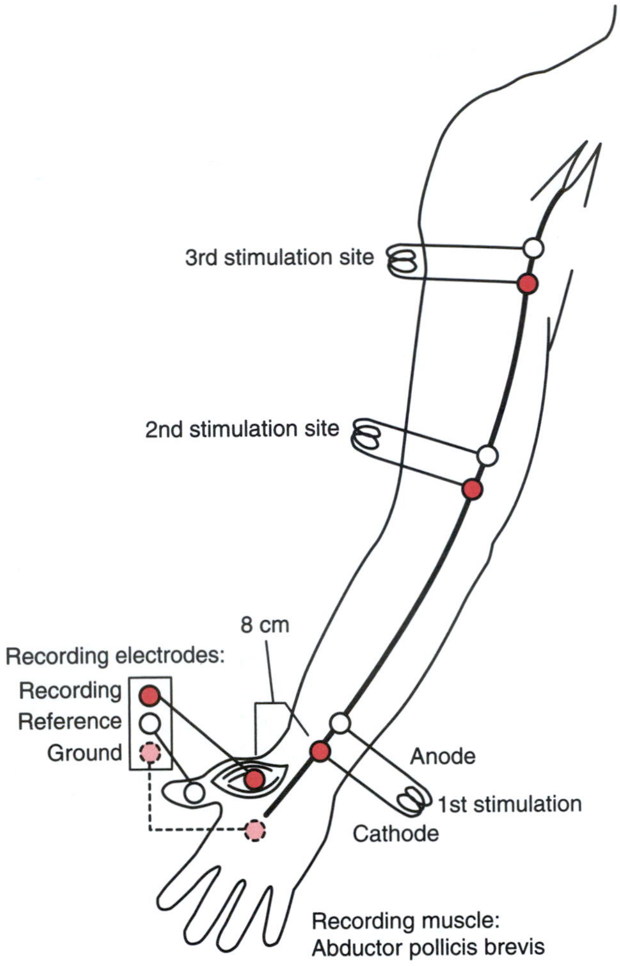

Figure 9.24 Sites of stimulation for motor nerve conduction study of the median nerve. (From Echternach, J,[56, p 34] with permission.)

skin may be cleaned with alcohol to reduce skin resistance before applying electrodes. A ground electrode is placed over a neutral area between the electrodes and the stimulation sites, usually over the dorsum of the hand or foot, or over the wrist or ankle.

For the purposes of illustration, the test procedure for the motor NCV of the median nerve will be described (Fig 9.24). The technique is basically the same for all nerves, except for the sites of stimulation and placement of the electrodes. The recording electrode is taped over the belly of the test muscle, the abductor pollicis brevis, and the reference electrode is taped over the tendon at the proximal phalanx just distal to the metacarpophalangeal joint. The stimulating electrode is placed over the median nerve at the wrist (at a measured distance usually at 8cm. from the recording electrode), just proximal to the distal crease on the volar surface, with the cathode directed toward the recording electrodes. The *cathode* is the stimulating electrode (usually black) and the *anode* is the inactive electrode (usually red). It is important that the cathode be directed toward the recording electrodes to stimulate depolarization toward the muscle (orthodromic conduction).

At the moment the stimulus is produced, the *stimulus artifact* is seen at the left of the screen. The trigger mechanism controls this and it will, therefore, always appear in the same spot on the screen, facilitating consistent measurements. This spike is purely mechanical and does not represent any muscle activity.

The stimulus intensity starts out low and is slowly increased until the evoked potential is clearly observed. When the stimulating electrode is properly placed over the nerve, all muscles innervated distal to that point will contract and the patient will see and feel his hand "jump." The intensity is then increased until the evoked response no longer increases in size. At that time, the intensity is increased further to be sure that the stimulus is *supramaximal*. Because the intensity must be sufficient to reach the threshold of all motor fibers in the nerve, a supramaximal stimulus is required. It is also essential that the cathode be properly placed over the nerve trunk so that the stimulus reaches all the motor axons.

As in the EMG signal, the potentials seen on the screen represent the electrical activity detected by the recording electrode. The signal will represent the difference in electrical potential between the recording and reference electrodes. When the supramaximal stimulus is applied to the median nerve at the wrist, all the axons in the nerve will depolarize and begin conducting an impulse, transmitting the signal across the motor end plate, initiating depolarization of the muscle fibers. During these events, the two recording electrodes do not record a difference in potential because no activity is taking place beneath the electrodes. When the muscle fibers begin to depolarize, the electrical potentials are transmitted to the electrodes through the volume conductor, and a deflection is seen on the oscilloscope. This is the evoked potential, which is called the *M wave*. The M wave is also referred to as the MAP (motor action potential) or CMAP (compound motor action potential). The M wave represents the summated activity of all motor units in the muscle that responded to stimulation of the nerve trunk. The amplitude of this potential is, therefore, a function of the total voltage produced by the contracting motor units. The initial deflection of the M wave is the negative portion of the wave, above the baseline. To complete the example of the median nerve, two other sites would be stimulated, where the median nerve crosses the elbow (Fig. 9.24) and in the axilla (not shown). Although motor NCV tests can be performed on these more proximal segments of the nerve trunk, these areas are tested less frequently than the distal-most site.

Calculation of Motor Nerve Conduction Velocity

The point at which the M wave leaves the baseline indicates the time elapsed from the initial propagation of the nerve impulse to the depolarization of the muscle fibers beneath the electrodes. This is called the response *latency*. The latency is measured in milliseconds from the stimulus artifact to the onset of the M wave. This time alone is not a valid measurement of nerve conduction because it incorporates other events besides pure nerve conduction—namely, transmission across the myoneural junction and generation of the muscle action potential. There is also evidence that the distal segments and terminal branches of axons to individual muscle fibers conduct at slower rates than the main axon.[59] Therefore, these extraneous factors must be eliminated from the calculation of the motor NCV, so that the measurement reflects only the speed of conduction within the nerve trunk.

To account for these distal variables, the nerve is stimulated at a second, more proximal point. This will produce a response similar to that seen with distal stimulation. The stimulus artifact will appear in the same spot on the screen, but the M wave will originate in a different place because the time for the impulses to reach the muscle would, obviously, be longer. Subtraction of the *distal latency* from the *proximal latency* will determine the conduction time for the nerve trunk segment between the two points of stimulation. **Conduction velocity (CV)** is determined by dividing the distance between the two points of cathodal stimulation (measured along the surface) by the difference between the two latencies (velocity = distance/time).

$$\text{CV} = \text{Conduction distance}/(\text{Proximal latency} - \text{Distal latency})$$

Conduction velocity is always expressed in meters per second (m/sec), although distance is usually measured in centimeters and latencies in milliseconds. These units must be converted during calculation.

To compute the motor NCV for the test illustrated in Figure 9.24, the proximal and distal latencies are determined by measuring the time from the stimulus artifact to the initial M wave deflection, according to the calibration scale, or sweep speed. The conduction time is calculated by taking the difference between these latencies. *Conduction distance* is then determined by measuring the length of the nerve between the two points of stimulation. For example:

Proximal latency: 7 msec
Distal latency: 2 msec
Conduction distance: 300 mm or 30 cm
CV = 30 cm / (7 msec − 2 msec) = 30 cm/5 msec = 60 m/sec

Interpretation of the motor NCV is made in relation to normal values, which are usually expressed as mean values, standard deviations, and ranges. Normal values have been determined by many investigators in different laboratories. Even so, average values seem to be fairly consistent. The motor NCV for the upper extremity has a fairly wide range, with values reported from 50 to 70 m/sec. The average normal value is about 60 m/sec. For the lower extremity, the average value is about 50 m/sec. Distal latencies and average normal amplitudes of M waves are also found in such tables, but these must be viewed with caution, because technique, electrode setup, instrumentation, and patient size can affect these values.

The nerves that are most commonly studied in the upper extremity are the ulnar, median, and radial nerves. Other nerves that have been studied are the axillary, musculocutaneous, long thoracic, and suprascapular nerves. The nerves that have been studied in the lower extremity include the tibial, fibular (peroneal), and femoral nerves. The sciatic nerve can be examined also using special techniques. The reader is referred to more comprehensive discussions for complete details about the techniques for studying these nerves and for tables of normal values.[56,57]

It is important to note that the value calculated as the conduction velocity is actually a reflection of the speed of the fastest axons in the nerve. Although all axons are stimulated at the same point in time, and supposedly fire at the same time, their conduction rates vary with their size. Not all motor units will contract at the same time; some receive their nerve impulse later than others. Therefore, the initial M wave deflection represents the contraction of the motor unit, or units, with the fastest conduction velocity. The curved shape of the M wave is reflective of the progressively slower axons reaching their motor units at a later time.

The M wave can also provide useful information about the integrity of the nerve or muscle. Three parameters should be examined: amplitude, shape, and duration. Any change occurring in these characteristics is called *temporal dispersion*. These parameters reflect the summated voltage over time produced by all the contracting motor units within the test muscle. Therefore, if the muscle is partially denervated, fewer motor units will contract after nerve stimulation. This will cause the M wave amplitude to decrease. Duration may change depending on the conduction velocity of the intact units. Similar changes may also be evident in myopathic conditions, in which all motor units are intact, but fewer fibers are available in each motor unit.

The shape of the M wave can also be variable. Deviation from a smooth curve need not be abnormal, and it is often useful to compare the proximal and distal M waves with each other as well as with the contralateral side if indicated. They should be similar. In abnormal conditions, changes in shape may be the result of a significant slowing of conduction in some axons, repetitive firing, or asynchronous firing of axons after a single stimulus.

Sensory Nerve Conduction Velocity Testing

Sensory neurons demonstrate the same physiological properties as motor neurons, and NCV can be measured in a similar way. However, some differences in technique are necessary to differentiate between sensory and motor axons. Although sensory fibers can be tested using *orthodromic conduction* (physiological direction) or *antidromic*

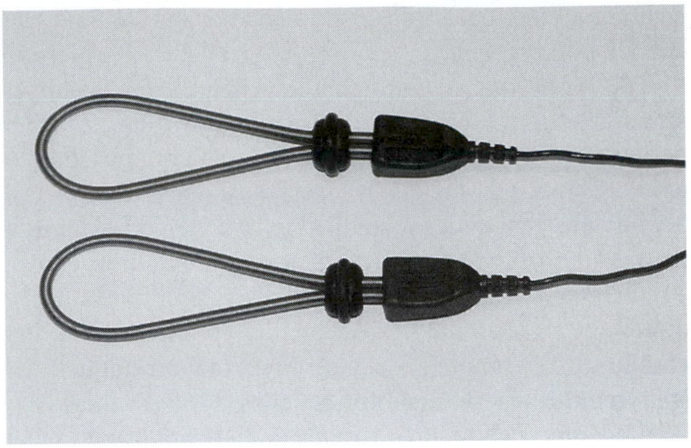

Figure 9.25 Ring electrodes.

conduction (opposite to normal conduction), antidromic measurements appear to be more common. For the same reason that motor axons are examined by recording over muscle, sensory axons are either stimulated or recorded from digital sensory nerves. This eliminates the activity of the motor axons from the recorded potentials.

Stimulation and Recording

The stimulating electrode used for motor NCV tests can be used for sensory NCV tests, or the stimulus may be provided by ring electrodes (Fig. 9.25) placed around the base of the middle of the digit innervated by the nerve. The recording electrodes can be surface or needle electrodes. Surface electrodes are placed over the nerve trunk, where it is superficial to the skin. The active electrode is placed distally, and a ground electrode is usually set between the stimulating and recording electrodes (orthodromic technique).

The electrode positions can be reversed, measuring antidromic conduction. If electrode sites are consistent, the latencies should be essentially equivalent in both directions. Orthodromic stimulation of fingertips appears to be more uncomfortable than stimulation of the nerve trunk. Also the amplitude of the response is much larger when antidromic recording is done.

Sensory potentials for the median and ulnar nerves can be recorded antidromically by stimulating at the wrist, elbow, and upper arm. Typically the sensory study of these nerves is limited to stimulation at the wrist. Other sensory nerves can be studied in the upper extremity, which include the superficial radial nerve, the medial and lateral antibrachial cutaneous nerves and the dorsal branch of the ulnar nerve. In lower extremities, the sensory nerves most commonly studied are the sural nerve and the superficial fibular (peroneal) nerves. Other nerves that have been studied include the lateral femoral cutaneous nerve and the saphenous nerve.

Calculation of Sensory Nerve Conduction Velocity

Latencies historically are usually measured from the stimulus artifact to the peak of the evoked potential, rather than to the initial deflection, because of the uneven baseline seen with sensory tests (Fig. 9.26). The baseline is more uneven because sensory tests require much greater amplifier sensitivity than do motor tests, and this allows more "noise" to interfere with recording. Advances in the technology of recording have resulted in the ability to measure the latency of sensory potentials to where to leave the baseline however, many examiners continue to measure to the peak of the evoked potential therefore it is important to know when looking at a report of a test which method the examiner used. Although sensory NCV can be determined in the same way as motor NCV (dividing distance by difference between latencies), often latencies are sufficient measurements, because terminal branching does not seem to be a significant limitation. Therefore, the latency essentially represents sensory nerve conduction activity only.

Normal sensory NCV ranges between 40 and 75 m/sec. Amplitude, measured with surface electrodes, may be 10 to 120 μV, and duration should be short, less than 2 msec. Sensory evoked potentials are usually sharp, not rounded like the M wave. Sensory NCVs have been found to be slightly faster than motor NCVs because of the larger diameter of sensory nerves.[60]

H Reflex

The **H reflex** (named for Hoffmann[61]) is a useful diagnostic measure for radiculopathy and peripheral neuropathy. Its most common application is in testing the integrity of the sensory and motor monosynaptic pathways of S1 nerve roots, and to a lesser extent at C6 and C7.[62] A submaximal stimulus is applied to the tibial nerve at the popliteal fossa, and a motor response is recorded from the medial portion of the soleus muscle. The action potentials travel along the IA afferent neurons toward the spinal cord, synapsing onto alpha-motoneurons within the anterior horn. The consequent activation of the motor neuron leads to an impulse traveling peripherally to the response muscle, resulting in a muscle contraction. Because the stimulus causes impulses to travel both distally and proximally within a mixed motor and sensory neuron, the latency of this response is a measure of the integrity of both sensory and motor fibers.

Because the initial phase of the H reflex is the afferent arc along IA fibers, its response is linked to the presence of muscle spindles. Muscles with slow-twitch fibers contain an abundance of muscle spindles and are able to demonstrate the H reflex most consistently. Therefore, the soleus muscle, composed predominantly of slow-twitch fibers, is most often used. Sabbahi and Khalil[63] have also demonstrated the H reflex in the flexor carpi radialis muscle to test the median nerve.

The H-reflex response latency is a function of age and leg length, according to the equation:

$$\text{H-reflex latency} = 0.46\ (\text{leg length [cm]}) + 9.14 + 0.1\ (\text{Age [yr]})$$

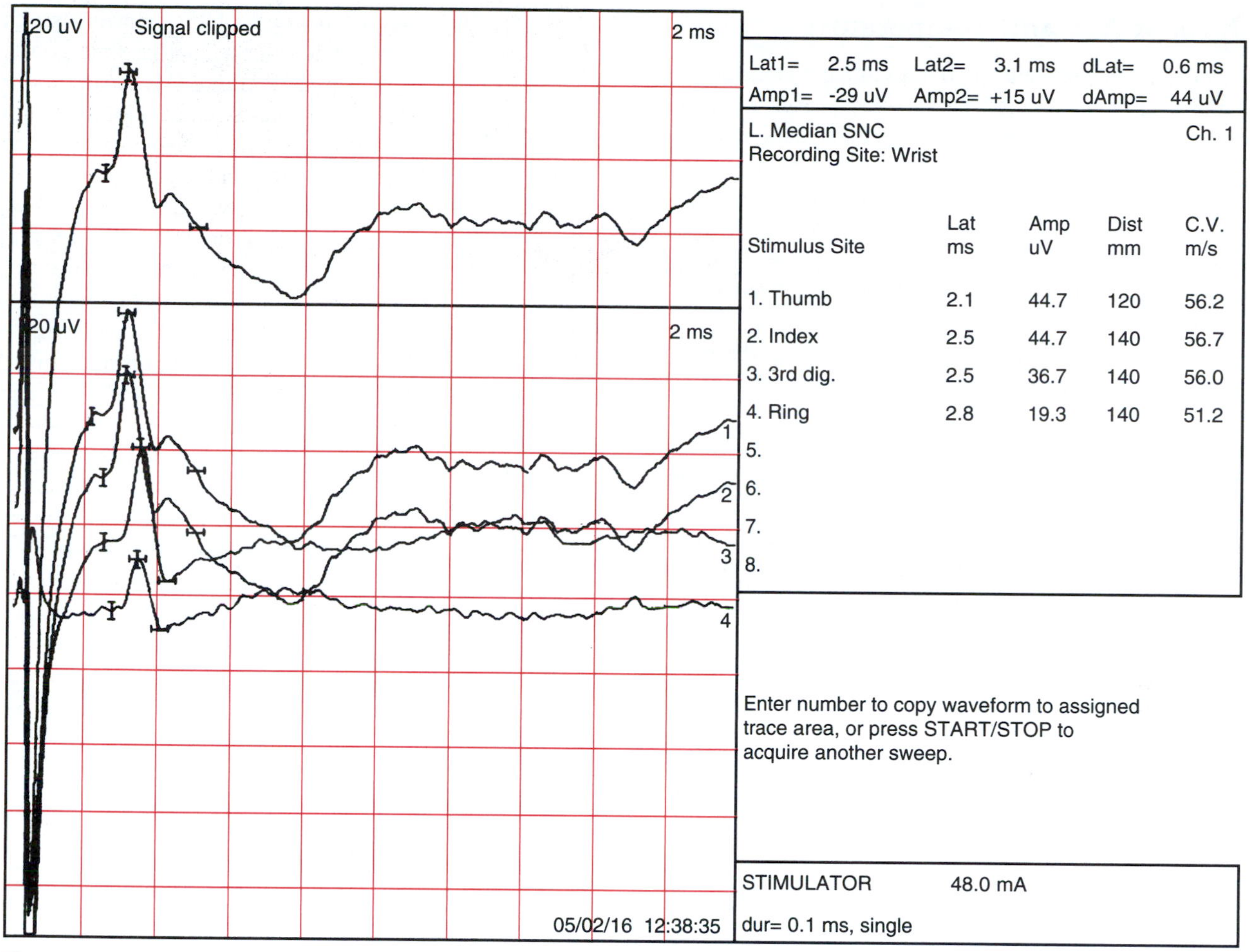

Figure 9.26 Sensory test of median nerve done antidromically on a normal elderly subject.

A normal response falls within ± 5.5 msec of this calculated latency. An average response is 29.8 msec (± 2.74 msec).[64] A slowed latency is indicative of abnormal dorsal root function, often from a herniated disc or impingement syndrome. Because of this central involvement, the peripheral motor and sensory NCV would not be affected. This latency may also identify nerve root compression prior to obvious EMG changes. The H-reflex latency is elicited using fixed stimulus parameters, resulting in a stable response from trial to trial. Latency can be affected by facilitatory and inhibitory techniques, reflecting the excitability of the motor neuron pool; however, the response will be more variable.[65]

The F Wave

The **F wave** was first described by Magladery and McDougal in 1950.[66] It is elicited by the supramaximal stimulus of a peripheral nerve at a distal site, leading to both orthodromic and antidromic impulses. While the orthodromic impulse travels to the distal muscle, the antidromic response travels to the anterior horn cell. This impulse is thought to reverberate; that is, the axon hillock is depolarized, leading to depolarization of dendrites, which in turn depolarizes the axon hillock once again, generating an orthodromic volley back to the muscle. No synapse is involved, so the F wave is not considered a reflex, but only a measure of motor neuron conduction.

The F wave is a useful supplement to nerve conduction and EMG measures, and is most helpful in the diagnosis of conditions where the most proximal portion of the axon is involved, such as Guillain-Barré syndrome, thoracic outlet syndrome, brachial plexus injuries, and radiculopathies with more than one nerve root involved.[56] The F response has also been used in pharmacological studies of spasticity, as a measure of alpha motor neuron excitability.[67,68]

The latency of the F wave is normally approximately 30 seconds in the upper limb and less than 60 seconds in the lower limb. This total time includes the M wave elicited as part of the motor NCV. Only a small percent of motor neurons actually participate in the F response.[69] Because it is an inconsistent response, it must be calculated on the basis of at least 10 successive trials.

Effects of Age and Temperature

Age and temperature are the two most influential factors that can cause variations in conduction velocity. Nerve conduction is slowed considerably in infants and young children, and less so in elderly individuals. At birth, the motor NCV is approximately one half of normal adult values, gradually increasing until reaching adult rates around 5 years of age.[70] Motor and sensory conduction velocities have been shown to decrease slightly after age 35, with larger, significant differences noted after age 70.[71,72]

Lower temperature can also decrease motor and sensory conduction velocities significantly.[73] Decrements of 1.8°F (1°C) in intramuscular temperature have been correlated with changes of 2 to 2.4 m/sec in conduction velocity. It is advisable to warm a cool limb before examination to stabilize the limb's temperature. The examination room should be a warm environment and if the patient's limbs feel cool then skin temperatures should be measured. If the temperature is less than 35°C in the upper extremity or 32°C in the lower extremity then the extremity should be warmed or an appropriate correction formula for cool limbs should be used.

Reporting the Results of the Clinical EMG Examination

The performance of reliable and valid EMG examinations requires extensive experience and expertise with biomedical instrumentation, as well as a thorough understanding of neuromuscular anatomy and pathology. The material presented here, however brief, is intended to provide sufficient background for the reader to intelligently utilize information from an EMG report and to apply these data to other aspects of patient care specifically related to prognosis, goal setting, and treatment planning. With this in mind, it seems appropriate to review how such reports are presented.

The EMG report is typically found in a patient's chart or medical record. The essential data include (1) the specific muscle or muscles tested, including side of the body and the innervation of these muscles; (2) the response seen during electrode insertion; (3) the response at rest (spontaneous activity, specifying type of potentials or electrical silence); and (4) responses with voluntary contraction (motor unit potentials and recruitment) (Fig. 9.27). The data provided should relate to the five parameters of electrical potentials previously described: amplitude, duration, shape, sound, and frequency.

Reports of nerve conduction measurements should include (1) location of recording and stimulating electrodes; (2) the calculated velocity in meters per second; (3) the distal latency and distance between recording and stimulating electrodes; and (4) the amplitude and duration of the M wave or evoked sensory potential (Fig. 9.28). Comments should follow the data, stating the impression or implications of findings.

It is extremely important to stress here that diagnoses are not made solely on the basis of EMG data. EMG findings are considered together with data from other appropriate examination procedures to provide a complete picture of the patient's disorder. These include a history, laboratory tests, as well as physical therapy examinations (e.g., manual muscle testing, examination of sensory function, range of motion, pain, and so forth). Electrodiagnostic (e.g., EMG/NCV) findings will often provide objective evidence to support clinical observations.

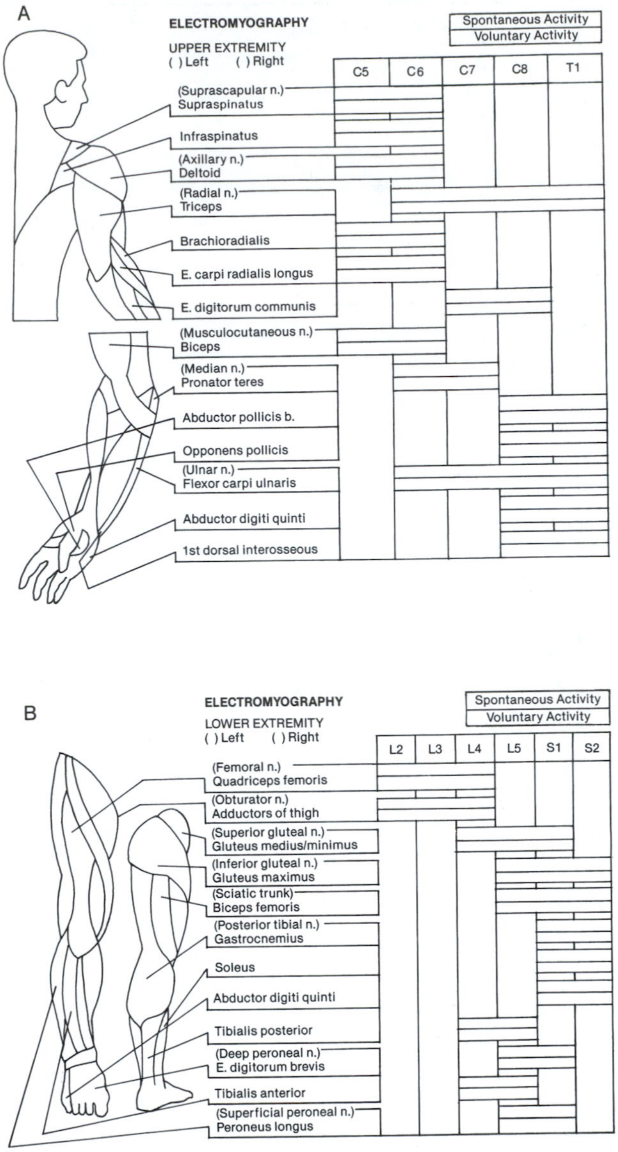

Figure 9.27 Sample report form for EMG. This pictorial form demonstrates the relative position and peripheral nerve and root innervation of the commonly tested upper extremity and lower extremity muscles. Information about spontaneous and voluntary activity can be recorded for each muscle. (From Brumback, RA, et al: Pictorial report form for needle electromyography. Phys Ther 63:224, 1983, with permission.)

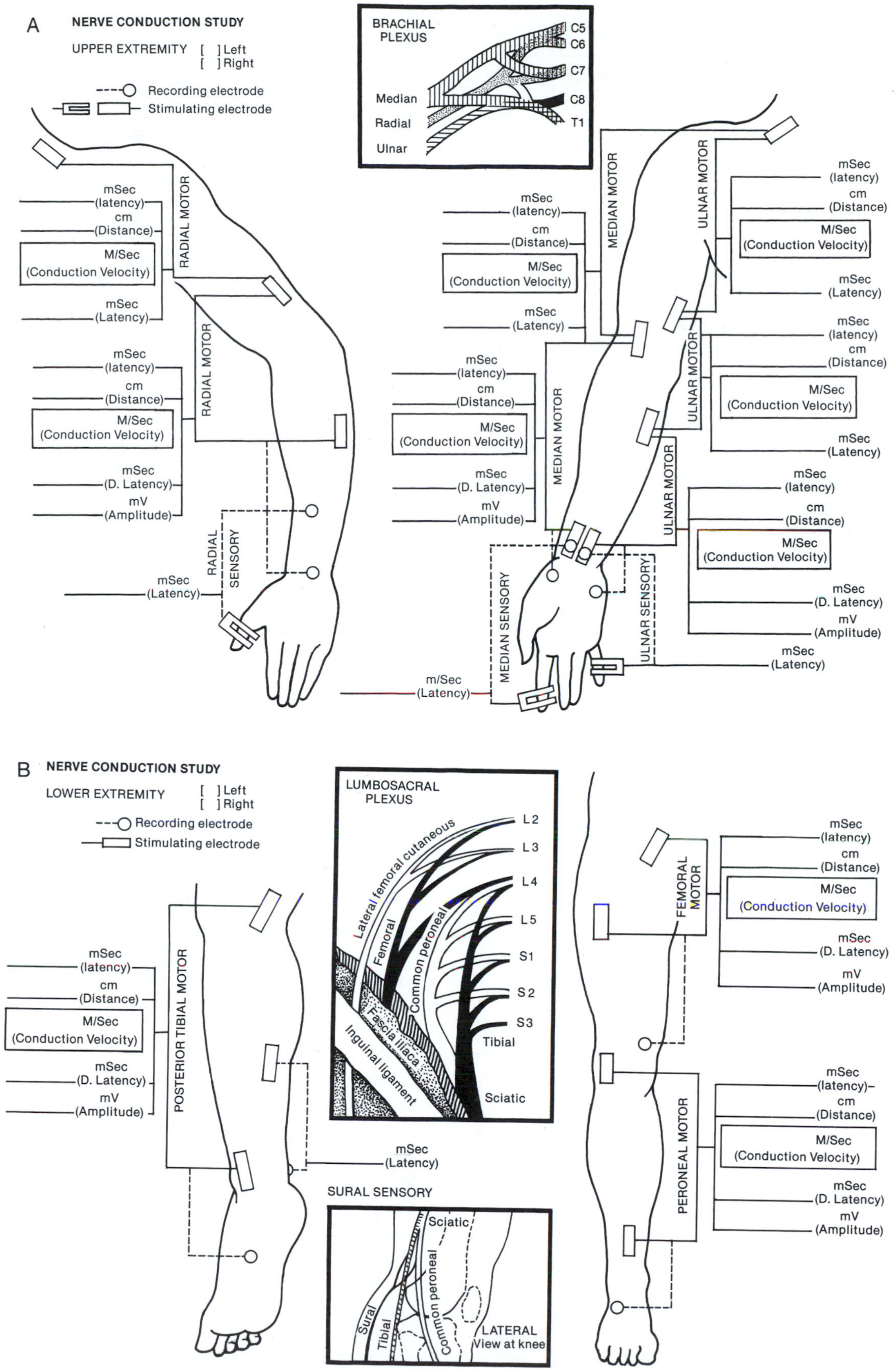

Figure 9.28 Sample report form for nerve conduction studies, containing listings of latencies, electrode distances, potential amplitudes, and calculated conduction velocities, followed by interpretation. Forms for upper and lower extremity show relationship of anatomy to nerve conduction velocity data. (From Brumback, RA, et al: Pictorial report form for nerve conduction studies. Phys Ther 61:1457, 1981, with permission.)

Clinical Implications of EMG Tests

Typical findings with neurogenic or myogenic disorders can be described. The following discussion focuses on selected disorders that typify EMG and NCV results, and their implications for evaluation and treatment planning.

Disorders of the Peripheral Nerve

Electrophysiological findings usually correlate with clinical signs in patients with neuropathic involvement. Some differences exist between types of neuropathies in terms of relative onset of sensory and motor symptoms and nerve conduction changes. EMG findings are usually significant only if axonal damage is a factor. Often, electrophysiological changes in sensory conduction are seen before clinical manifestations such as definable sensory changes or motor weakness. In many neuropathic conditions sensory nerves are affected before motor nerves and EMG findings are unremarkable. The sensory NCV test may then provide the most helpful information. Clinicians may find such information useful in following progression or remission of an existing condition.

Peripheral Nerve Lesions

Lesions of the peripheral nerve fall into three categories: neurapraxia, axonotmesis, and neurotmesis or class 1, class 2, or class 3 nerve injury. These lesions may be due to traumatic injury or entrapment. Such disorders typically cause weakness and atrophy of all muscles innervated distal to the lesion. Sensory findings may occur first, but may not be as definitive as motor deficits in localizing the site of the lesion. EMG data can assist in the identification, diagnosis, and prognosis of such cases.

Neurapraxia

A *neurapraxia* (class 1) involves some form of local compression or blockage, which stops or slows conduction across that point in the nerve. Conduction above and below the blockage is usually normal. Compression disorders (e.g., Bell's palsy [facial nerve], Saturday night palsy [radial nerve compression in spiral groove], pressure over the peroneal nerve at the fibula head, carpal tunnel syndrome [median nerve entrapment]) are the most common causes of neurapraxic lesions. NCV tests can detect evidence of demyelinization prior to axonal degeneration, which may occur with long-standing compression. Nerve conduction measurements will usually reveal increased latencies across the compressed area, but normal conduction velocity above and below. In acute conditions with no denervation, the EMG signal will reveal no spontaneous activity. This should be considered a positive prognostic sign. The interference pattern may be decreased or absent if there is severe blockage.

Axonotmesis

With *axonotmesis* (class 2) the neural tube is intact, but axonal damage has occurred, with Wallerian degeneration distal to the lesion. This may be a progressive condition as a result of long-standing neurapraxia, or it may occur from a traumatic lesion. The deficit in NCV will depend partly on the number of axons affected. If the larger diameter fibers remain intact, the conduction velocity may be normal. However, M-wave amplitude will be decreased because fewer motor units are contracting. Fibrillation potentials and positive sharp waves are typically seen on EMG 2 to 3 weeks after denervation, depending on the distance of the axon from the cell body.

Neurotmesis

Neurotmesis (class 3) involves total loss of axonal function, with disruption of the neural tube. Conduction ceases below the lesion. A conduction velocity test cannot be performed because no evoked response can be elicited. Recovery is dependent on proper orientation of axons as they regenerate. Spontaneous potentials will appear with the muscle at rest, and no activity is produced with attempted voluntary contraction.

Regeneration of peripheral nerves will be signaled by the presence of small polyphasic potentials (nascent units) with voluntary contraction. These may be seen before clinical recovery is evident through the results of other examination procedures, such as the manual muscle test. After clinical recovery is established, polyphasic potentials may persist, often as larger than normal (giant) potentials, as a result of collateral sprouting. Rehabilitation goals for patients with peripheral nerve injuries can be influenced by results of serial EMG findings. Evidence of regeneration will suggest that motor function is improving and treatment plans should address minimal exercise for the weak and easily fatigued muscles. Positive signs of regeneration will also help in setting realistic outcomes for functional recovery.

Polyneuropathies

Polyneuropathies typically result in sensory changes, distal weakness, and hyporeflexia. Neuropathies can be related to general medical conditions, such as diabetes, alcoholism, renal disease, or malignancies; they may result from infections, such as leprosy or Guillain-Barré syndrome; and they may be associated with metabolic abnormalities, such as malnutrition or the toxic effects of drugs or chemicals.

Neuropathic conditions may be manifested as primarily axonal damage or primarily demyelination of axons and are generally a mixture of both with one or the other being predominant. With axonal lesions, recruitment will be severely affected. A partial interference pattern may be observed with maximal effort, or single motor unit potentials may still be identifiable (Fig. 9.29). The motor unit duration and amplitude may be decreased. Fibrillation

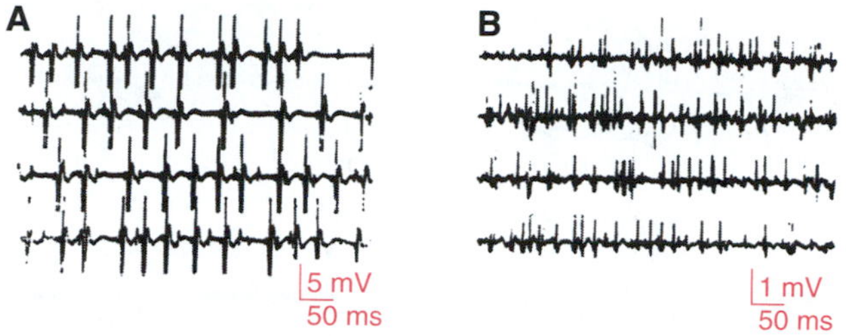

Figure 9.29 Large amplitude, long duration motor unit potentials from the first dorsal interosseus (*A*) compared with relatively normal motor unit potentials from orbicularis oculi (*B*) in a patient with polyneuropathy. Note discrete single unit interference pattern during maximal voluntary contraction. (From Kimura,[30, p 267] with permission.)

potentials, positive sharp waves, and fasciculations are typically seen (see Fig. 9.17).

With demyelinization, nerve conduction measurements will often provide the most useful data. Sensory fibers may be affected before motor fibers, and significant slowing of sensory conduction velocity may be seen. The evoked potential will typically be reduced in amplitude.

Motor Neuron Disorders

Motor neuron disorders most commonly involve degenerative diseases of the anterior horn cells. These include poliomyelitis, and diseases that are characterized by degeneration of both upper and lower motor neurons, such as amyotrophic lateral sclerosis, progressive muscular atrophy, and progressive bulbar palsy. Spinal muscular atrophies are another classification of motor neuron disease. The reader is referred to comprehensive texts to review clinical features of these diseases.

Diseases of the anterior horn cell are classically indicated by fibrillation potentials and positive sharp waves (see Fig. 9.17), and by reduced recruitment with voluntary contraction, due to loss of motor neurons. When single MUAPs can be seen with maximal effort by the patient the resulting activity is called a single motor unit pattern. Motor NCV may be slowed, depending on the distribution of degeneration among motor fibers, but sensory evoked potentials are unaffected. Newer techniques for estimation of the number of motor units in a muscle have allowed electromyographers to examine the progressive nature of many motor neuron diseases.[74–76]

Al-Shekhlee and Katirji[77] have reported on a small series of cases of West Nile virus infection who presented with acute paralytic poliomyelitis. Their report focused on the usefulness of EMG and NCV testing in these patients revealing both focal and widespread changes associated with their West Nile Virus infection. Depending on the timing of the EMG examination some patients showed wide spread fibrillation potentials.

Polyphasic motor unit potentials of increased amplitude and duration are often seen later in the course of motor neuron disease, due primarily to collateral sprouting and reinnervation. This is a typical finding in post-polio syndrome and amyotrophic lateral sclerosis, where enlarged motor units are found in partially denervated muscle.[78,79] Macro EMG has shown signs of reinnervation in these groups,[48,53] although denervation often continues and has been found in affected and supposedly unaffected limbs.[80] Individuals with post-polio syndrome often exhibit functional decline many years after their acute episode. These individuals experience new muscle weakness and atrophy in extremities, bulbar and respiratory muscles, and excessive fatigue. This syndrome appears to manifest when the reinnervation process crosses a critical threshold, whereby remaining neurons cannot support all their muscle fibers.[80]

Myopathies

In primary muscle diseases, such as muscular dystrophy and limb girdle myopathies, the motor unit remains intact, but degeneration of muscle fibers is evident. Therefore, the number of fibers innervated by one axon is diminished. Motor nerve conduction is typically normal, although the amplitude of the M wave will be decreased because fewer muscle fibers per motor unit are responding to stimulation. Sensory nerve potentials and neuromuscular transmission are normal. In the early stages, the EMG examination shows prolonged insertion activity, perhaps due to the instability of the muscle membrane of degenerating muscle fibers. Fibrillations and positive sharp waves are also seen, sometimes with repetitive discharges. Voluntary contraction typically elicits short-duration, low-amplitude potentials, some of which maybe polyphasic reflecting random loss of muscle fibers. Less than maximal effort will require early recruitment, and an interference pattern is evoked because more motor units are needed to create the necessary tension within the muscle (Fig. 9.30). The total amplitude of the interference pattern, however, will be diminished. Use of single-fiber EMG, macro EMG, and motor unit estimation have been used to identify the course of myopathic disease.[32]

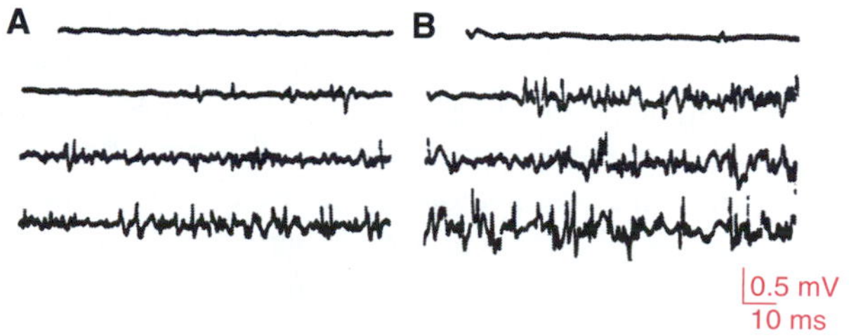

Figure 9.30 Low-amplitude, short-duration motor unit potentials recorded during minimal voluntary contraction from the biceps brachii (*A*) and tibialis anterior (*B*) in a 7-year-old boy with Duchenne's dystrophy. A high number of discharging motor units during minimal contraction reflects early recruitment. (From Kimura, J,[30, p 268] with permission.)

In advanced stages of muscular dystrophy, when contractile tissue is replaced by fibrous and other tissues, no electrical potentials may be seen at all. On insertion, the needle will meet some resistance as it enters the fibrotic tissue. Motor nerve conduction measurements will also be impossible under such conditions because no evoked potential can be elicited.

Because most myopathies are progressive, clinicians will find EMG and motor NCV findings helpful in documenting the extent of deterioration over time. EMG will help delineate the distribution of the involvement, assisting the therapist in focusing treatment and planning adaptations for functional activities.

Myotonia

Myotonia is a disorder characterized by delayed relaxation of previously contracted muscle. It results in pathological muscle stiffness. Myotonia dystrophica exhibits EMG changes typical of myopathy as well. Myotonic disorders do not have a known etiology, although research suggests that a defect in the sarcolemmal membrane causes after-depolarization following activation of the muscle membrane.[81]

As a part of the generalized membrane abnormality, myotonia may result in mildly slowed motor NCV, and a marked reduction in motor unit activity and strength.[82,83] The typical EMG response in myotonia, however, is the persistence of high-frequency repetitive discharges with alternately increasing and decreasing amplitude (see Fig. 9.19B). This "waxing and waning" is a distinctive feature, producing the classic "dive-bomber" sound. These trains of potentials can discharge at frequencies up to 150 pulses per second. The myotonic discharge follows voluntary contraction or may be provoked by needle insertion or movement. Myotonic symptoms can be abolished or lessened pharmacologically. The finding of myotonic potentials is not specifically diagnostic since these potentials can be found in subjects who do not have myotonia.

Myasthenia Gravis

Myasthenia gravis and myasthenic syndrome are disorders of neuromuscular transmission characterized by weakness following repetitive contractions, and recovery following rest or administration of an anticholinesterase. Myasthenia gravis is thought to be an autoimmune disorder, often associated with other immunological diseases.[30] It is characterized by weakness and excessive fatigability, and frequently manifested by weakness and fatigability of the ocular muscles or palatal and pharyngeal muscles.

Myasthenic syndrome often is associated with small "oat" cell carcinoma of the bronchus, and is more prevalent in males. Weakness and fatigability primarily affect the lower extremities, particularly the pelvic girdle and thigh muscles.[30]

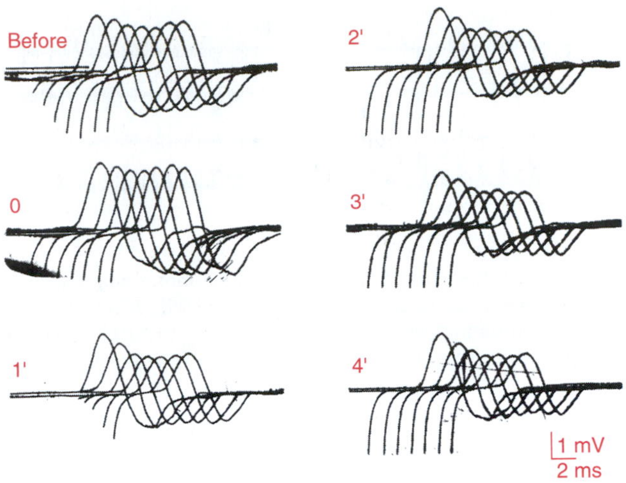

Figure 9.31 Decremental evoked motor responses before and after voluntary exercise in a patient with generalized myasthenia gravis. The median nerve was stimulated at the rate of three shocks per second for seven shocks in each train. The M wave was recorded from the thenar muscles. Comparing the amplitude of the last response with the amplitude of the first, the decrement was 25 percent at rest. (From Kimura, J,[30, p 191] with permission.)

Myasthenic disorders demonstrate normal EMG characteristics at rest, although fibrillation potentials and positive sharp waves may be present in severely affected muscles, indicating loss of innervation. Motor unit potentials will appear normal at first and then progressively decrease in amplitude with continued effort. Repetitive stimulation during a motor nerve conduction test will cause progressive decreases in the amplitude of the M wave (Fig. 9.31). Pharmacological intervention often will normalize the response. Specific protocols are available when using repetitive stimulation to evaluate these problems.

Radiculopathy

Nerve root involvement, or radiculopathy, is not an uncommon condition at all spinal levels. EMG can often assist in identifying this condition, determining the etiology for radiating pain, persistent weakness, hyporeflexia, and fasciculations. Sensory symptoms accompany motor signs, and may range from mild paresthesias to complete loss of sensation.

The fundamental feature in the determination of motor nerve root involvement is the delineation of the distribution of abnormal findings within muscles receiving their peripheral innervation from the same myotome. For example, abnormal potentials seen in the extensor muscles of the hand may suggest involvement of the radial nerve. However, if the biceps brachii is examined (musculocutaneous nerve), as well as the opponens pollicis (median nerve), and these muscles also exhibit some abnormal EMG potentials, the common feature could be considered the C6 nerve root. These findings would have significant implications for treatment planning in terms of addressing the cause of muscle weakness or fatigue.

EMG abnormalities are those typical of neuropathic involvement. Compression of a nerve root can result in irritation or degeneration of nerve fibers. If the lesion is of sufficient severity and duration, the EMG signal will show increased insertion activity, fibrillation potentials, and positive sharp waves at rest, as well as low-amplitude polyphasic potentials. In later stages, high-amplitude polyphasic potentials may appear, reflecting reinnervation. Polyphasic potentials have been documented within 1 to 3 weeks of the onset of radicular symptoms,[84] perhaps resulting from inflammation, causing activation of two to three motor units that appear as a single potential. Electrodiagnostic examination has shown that patients with cervical or lumbosacral radiculopathy will often have abnormalities in paraspinal muscles as well.[85]

EMG is especially valuable in differentiating between disorders of the peripheral nerve trunk and more proximal involvement. It may be more useful than NCV studies, which may not show any remarkable changes at distal segments of these peripheral nerves unless diffuse degeneration has occurred. The F wave and the H reflex have been shown to be clinically useful in the examination of radiculopathy, independent of clinical EMG testing.[86] For example, even with normal distal EMG signals, if the H reflex is diminished and the F wave is normal, that would be evidence of dorsal root involvement.

Kinesiological EMG

In addition to being a standard method for neuromuscular examination, surface EMG can also be used as a kinesiological tool to examine muscle function during specific, purposeful tasks or therapeutic regimens. For this purpose, the therapist looks at patterns of muscle response, onset, and cessation of activity, muscle fatigue, and the level of muscle response in relation to effort, type of muscle contraction, and position. With the growing need for evidence-based practice, kinesiologic EMG presents an objective means for documenting the effect of treatment on muscle impairments. The therapist should have a basic understanding of kinesiologic EMG to critically consider methods and data analysis procedures in published studies. Many professional journals and societies exist for clinicians and researchers with a common interest centered on the use of EMG signals for kinesiological studies.

While the principles of recording and instrumentation are the same for clinical and kinesiological EMG, several additional factors must be considered when interpreting kinesiological EMG data.

Surface and Fine-Wire Recording

As described, surface and fine-wire indwelling electrodes are used in kinesiological study, although surface electrodes are used more. Once a muscle is selected for study, its size and location must be considered in choosing and applying or inserting electrodes. Based on previous discussions of volume conduction and the factors affecting the motor unit potential, the following determinations must be made: (1) electrode size, (2) interelectrode distance, (3) location of electrode sites (including the ground), and (4) skin preparation (for some surface electrodes). There is currently no agreement on the preferred configuration and dimensions of a surface EMG electrode, although researchers have attempted to promote standardization.[25,87,88]

Smaller muscles obviously require the use of smaller electrodes, with a small interelectrode distance. If electrodes are too far apart, even on larger muscles, activity from nearby muscles may be recorded. This cross-talk would confound interpretation of the output by making activity look greater than it actually was. The ground electrode should be located reasonably close to the recording electrodes, preferably on the same side of the body. Skin should be prepared to reduce impedance, although newer amplifiers may have sufficient input impedance to make this unnecessary.

Locating Electrode Sites

Criteria for location of electrode sites are not universally accepted. Fine-wire electrodes should be inserted into the muscle belly using guidelines similar to those used for clinical EMG. For surface electrodes, Basmajian and DeLuca[4] and DeLuca[25] recommend placing the electrodes in the region halfway between the center of the innervation zone and the furthest tendon. Many investigators and clinicians have found it efficient to use palpation for locating surface electrode sites over the muscle belly, if the subject can voluntarily contract the muscle to facilitate this process. However, if repeated measurements are attempted, requiring reapplication of surface electrodes, this method may be unreliable. When electrodes are not oriented to the muscle in the same way with repeated testing, the output will look different, even with identical levels of contraction.

Some investigators have used electrical stimulation of motor points to locate optimal electrode sites. Some have marked the skin with indelible solutions to be able to relocate electrodes. Still others have used body landmarks and measured specific distances to standardize application sites (Fig. 9.32). Basmajian and Blumenstein[89] provide guidelines for placement of surface electrodes for use with biofeedback that can be useful for kinesiological study as well, but do not adjust locations for variation in body parameters and muscle bulk. Verification of surface electrode placement is usually attempted using manual muscle testing procedures to see if the EMG signal responds when appropriate resistance is applied. The technique is only partially effective, however, because muscles cannot effectively be isolated.

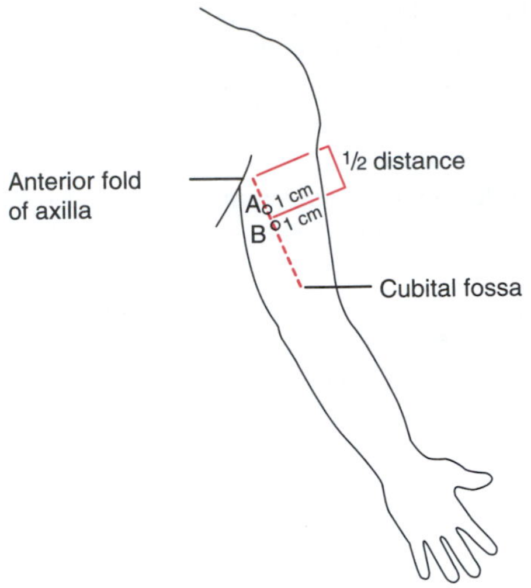

Figure 9.32 Example of standardized electrode placement for the biceps brachii. A line is drawn from the anterior axillary fold to the center of the cubital fossa, and a point marked at the center of this line. Electrodes are then placed 1 cm above and below this point along this line.

The distance between electrodes must also be standardized so that repeated EMG analysis is valid. The best way to achieve this is to use electrodes that have their bipolar detection surfaces fixed as a single unit. If interelectrode separation is altered from session to session, the same level of contraction may produce higher or lower amplitude readings, or different frequency content. DeLuca[25] recommended that the surface EMG electrode be standardized such that the detection surfaces are arranged as two parallel "bars" 1 cm apart, 1 cm long, and 1 to 2 mm wide.[25] Others, particularly among the European community, recommend similar arrangements where separation between the detection surfaces is 20 mm.[6]

When using surface electrodes, the therapist must also consider problems related to the displacement of skin overlying muscle during movement. The spatial relationship between the electrodes and the muscle can change greatly as a muscle contracts through its range. This will, of course, affect the EMG signal. The electrode sites should be determined with this in mind. Such problems are often seen when monitoring the biceps brachii, sternocleidomastoid, or scapula muscles, for instance. Electrodes should be applied to the skin with the limb or body part positioned as it will be during the procedure.

When placement criteria are specified, researchers have shown fairly good test–retest reliability for surface electrodes,[23,90] although submaximal contractions have demonstrated better reproducibility than maximal contractions.[91] Reapplication of indwelling electrodes is less reliable than that of surface electrodes because of the difficulty in consistently placing a needle within muscle tissue on reinsertion.[23,92] Reapplication of surface EMG electrodes on different days or test sessions is also less reliable than when reliability is determined without removing the electrodes.[93]

Signal Processing

Technology has advanced sufficiently today that microcomputers are now readily applied to the processing of conditioned signals, including integration and display. Personal computers can be easily adapted to interface with EMGs of all types. The EMG signal can be stored, averaged, and sampled in a variety of ways to permit detailed and complete analysis. Digital techniques are becoming more common than analog techniques but they require A-to-D conversion. All analog processing schemes can be replaced by a digital equivalent.

Quantification

For clinical EMG, the raw signal is displayed to allow visual examination of the size and shape of individual muscle and nerve potentials. For kinesiological EMG, however, the therapist is generally interested in looking at overall muscle activity during specific activities, and quantification of the signal is often desired to describe and compare changes in the magnitude and pattern of muscle response.

Rectification and Linear Envelope

The EMG signal can be manipulated electronically in several ways to facilitate quantification, and to eliminate problems of processing raw data (Fig. 9.33). Through a process called *rectification,* both the negative and positive portions of the raw signal appear above the baseline; the signal is then full-wave rectified. The rectified signal can be "smoothed" through low-pass filtering to produce a *linear envelope*, which describes a curve outlining the peaks of the full-wave rectified signal.[29] With the correct type of filter and cut-off frequency, the linear envelope profile closely follows muscle tension.[94] Many authors and electronic equipment companies call this an "integrated" signal, but that is a misnomer, because the linear envelope is a moving average of the EMG output over time.

Integration

Another type of signal conditioning is produced through mathematical *integration* of the EMG signal over the time of the contraction. Its units (mV*s) represent the area under the full-wave-rectified signal.[29] The integrated EMG (IEMG) signal is produced either through digital signal processing or through the accumulation of electrical energy on a capacitor, or condenser. IEMG can be processed in several ways (see Fig. 9.33). The simplest method is integration throughout the period of muscular activity. The total accumulated activity can be determined for a series of contractions or a single contraction. The slope of the curve, or ramp, is a direct function of the amount of electrical energy being processed.

Alternatively, the condenser can be set to discharge at predetermined intervals based on time or voltage amplitude. Time intervals can be set so that the capacitor resets

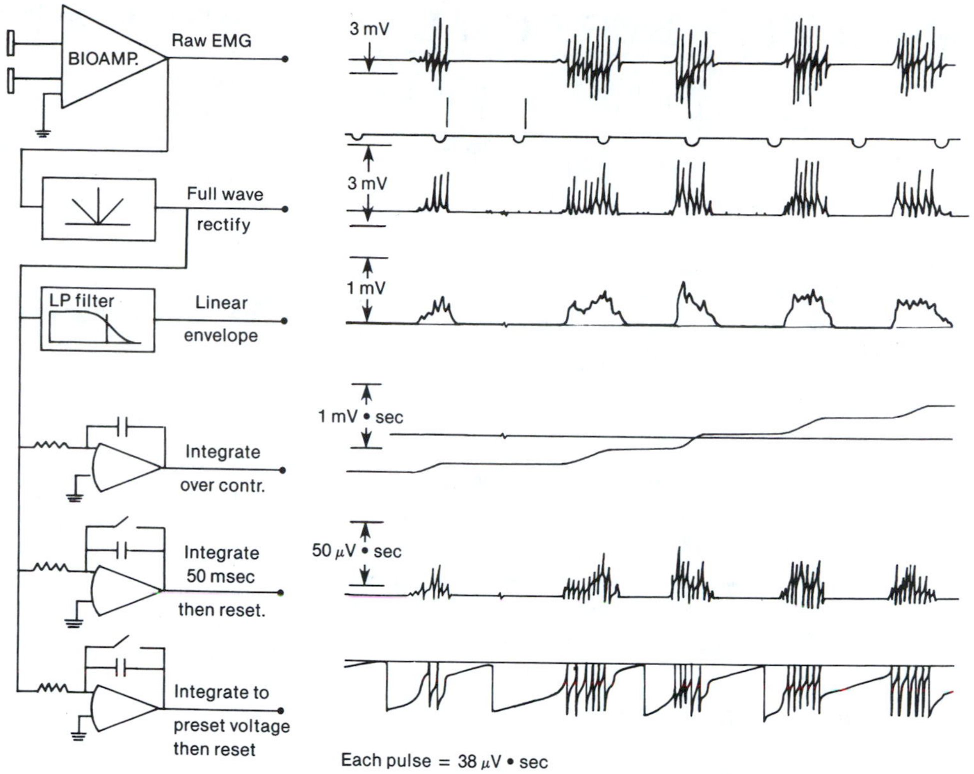

Figure 9.33 Illustration of the raw EMG and several methods of signal processing. The raw EMG was full-wave rectified and expressed as a linear envelope and integrated data. (From Winter, DA: Biomechanics of Human Movement. John Wiley & Sons, New York, 1979, p 140, with permission.)

to zero on a regular basis, within periods as small as 200 msec or as long as 10 seconds. The height of each peak, or ramp, then represents the accumulated activity over that time interval. Integration can also be based on a preset voltage level. When the condenser reaches this voltage, it resets to zero, without regard to time. If the EMG signal is very weak, the condenser may continue to collect electrical energy for indefinite periods until its discharge threshold is finally reached. The frequency with which the condenser resets is an indication of the level of EMG activity. Each ramp can also be depicted as a pulse, and the frequency of pulses can be counted to determine the level of activity (see Fig. 9.33).

Average EMG

Closely related to the IEMG is the average EMG, which is the time integral of the full-wave-rectified signal divided by the integration period. This parameter provides a single number with which to report the general level of activity of any given muscle over a predetermined time, such as a period of movement. For example, Kellis[95] studied the effect of fatigue on agonist and antagonist EMG patterns at the knee during 90° of dynamic knee extension. He averaged the EMG within arcs of 10 to 35°, 36 to 55°, and 56 to 80° to characterize differences in EMG at shortened, middle, and lengthened ranges.

Cycle-to-cycle averages of EMG profiles, such as during walking, running, or cycling, can be obtained through ensemble averaging. The full-wave-rectified and linear envelope EMG signals are averaged for each cycle, where each cycle is normalized to 100 percent. To illustrate this, MacIntyre and Robinson[96] studied patterns of the quadriceps muscles in female runners diagnosed with patellofemoral pain syndrome. Linear envelope EMG signals from vastus medialis, vastus lateralis, and rectus femoris were recorded as each subject ran on a treadmill at 80 percent of their normal running pace. Each stride period was normalized to 100 percent, then the linear envelopes for 10 trials were ensemble averaged to achieve a mean ensemble for each muscle from each subject.

Root-Mean-Square

The root-mean-square (RMS), an electronic average, represents the square root of the average of the squares of the current or voltage over the whole cycle. The RMS provides a nearly instantaneous output of the power of the EMG signal.[29] This EMG parameter is considered by some researchers to be the preferred estimate of muscle tension.[2]

Frequency Parameters

A method of signal processing commonly used to interpret changes in the EMG signal resulting from fatigue or abnormalities in the neuromuscular system is to analyze the *frequency spectrum* of the signal by Fourier analysis. Because any continuous signal can be represented as a summation of sine and cosine waveforms of different frequencies, an interference pattern can be decomposed into its different frequency components. With localized fatigue (i.e., fatigue from within the muscle, rather than central), there is a reduction in the high-frequency components of the spectrum, and

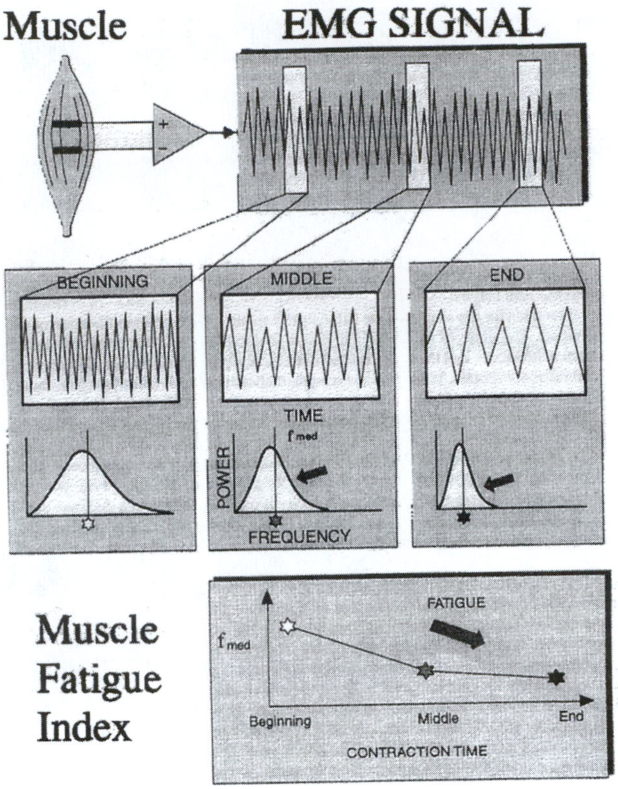

Figure 9.34 Diagrammatic explanation of the change to the EMG signal and its frequency spectrum that occurs as a result of localized fatigue. The upper panel represents the EMG signal sampled at the beginning, middle, and end of a sustained contraction. Each sample "window" of data is analyzed to calculate the frequency spectrum, as illustrated by the POWER versus FREQUENCY plot in the center panel. The median frequency, or midpoint of the spectrum, is indicated as a vertical line and star in each of the three figures. These three median frequency data points are plotted as a function of contraction time in the lower panel. The Muscle Fatigue Index is represented by the decay in EMG median frequency. (From DeLuca, CJ,[12, p 135] with permission.)

an increase in the low-frequency components (Fig. 9.34). This frequency shift may be monitored by tracking a statistical parameter, such as the median frequency. The median frequency is defined as the frequency that divides the frequency spectrum into two parts of equal area, as illustrated in Figure 9.34. The *muscle fatigue index* is represented by the decay in the median or mean frequency during a sustained contraction. Caution must be observed in calculating this index for activities that are nonisometric or nonisotonic. This is because classical techniques for computing median and mean frequency, such as Fourier analysis, require that the signal is mathematically *stationary.* Changes in muscle length, muscle force, and electrode position during nonisometric or nonisotonic contractions can produce a nonstationary signal. Therefore, dynamic contractions are not typically amenable to localized examination of fatigue on the basis of median or mean frequency parameters. Recently developed techniques using time–frequency analysis and wavelet analysis have been successful in measuring spectral compression of the signal associated with localized fatigue.[97] However, the activities being monitored are typically limited to cyclic or repetitive movement where changes in the biomechanics of the activity are more or less predictable.[97] This work is still under development in various research laboratories and too premature for routine clinical use.

Timing of Muscle Activity

A number of different computer-based analysis procedures have been described for quantifying latencies and amplitude of EMG signals during purposeful activities. The timing of a muscle's response is often of interest to determine the latency of responses between different muscles, or relative to some other parameter (e.g., the command to move) or specific task components. Measurement of EMG onset to determine muscle activation time requires knowledge of the amount of noise present. An epoch of noise must be recorded before the EMG signal is activated to estimate the noise level. Figure 9.35 provides an example of EMG signal activation for a slowly increasing isometric contraction.[25] The top trace represents the raw EMG signal and the bottom trace the RMS value. The amplitude of the noise is represented by the shaded area in the lower RMS time plot. This area was calculated as ± 2 standard deviations of the mean value, thus capturing approximately 95 percent of the amplitude of the noise signal. The raw signal is not sufficient to mark a clear differentiation between noise and EMG. Using the RMS value, however, the specific time at which the EMG signal exceeds this noise level for a minimally defined amount of time (e.g., at least 20 msec) can be determined. This can be considered the "on" time of the muscle, indicated as t_0 in Figure 9.35.[25] This differentiation is essential to an accurate appraisal of EMG activity.

Normalization

For many studies, the quantified EMG signal is used to compare activity between sessions, muscles, or subjects. Because of the variability inherent in the EMG signal, and interindividual differences in anatomy and movement, however, it is not reasonable to compare the EMG activity of one muscle to another, or from one person to another. Therefore, some form of normalization is necessary to validate these comparisons. This is usually done by first recording the EMG of a muscle during a maximal voluntary isometric contraction (MVIC), or some known submaximal level of contraction, and then expressing all other EMG values as a percentage of this contraction. This *control value* serves as a standard against which all comparisons can be made, even if test values exceed the control. In this way subjects and muscles can be compared, and activity on different days can be correlated by repeating the control contraction at each test session. This helps

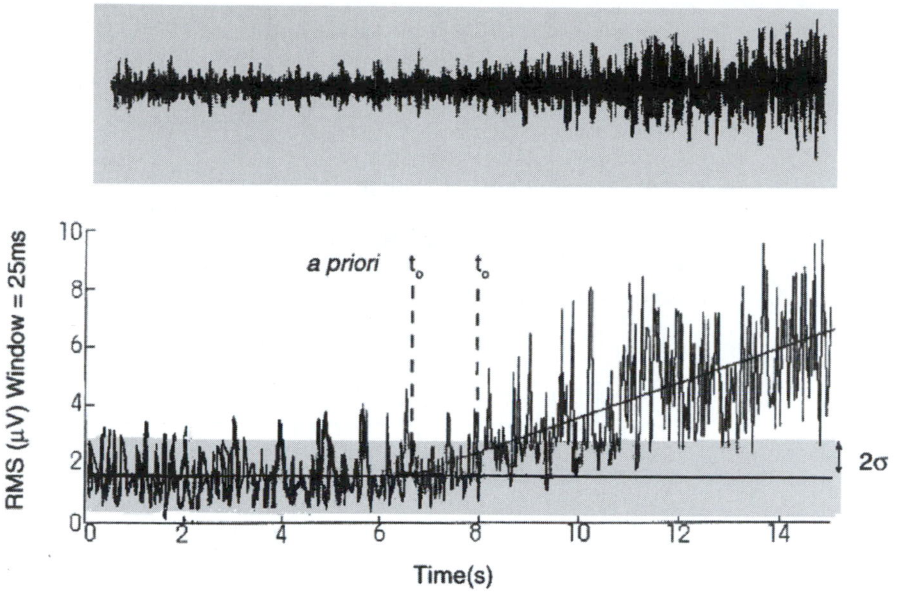

Figure 9.35 Example of background noise before initiation of EMG signal activation (t_0) from the erector spinae muscles during slowly increasing isometric extension of the trunk. The raw EMG signal is presented in the upper trace. The shaded area in the lower trace represents 2 standard deviations from the average RMS before initiation at t_0. Muscle initiation is identified as the time when the RMS signal exceeds a threshold of 2 standard deviations of the background signal. (Adapted from DeLuca, CJ,[12, p 135] with permission.)

eliminate some of the problems related to reapplication of electrodes as well.

Other methods of normalization have included using a series of submaximal contractions,[98] contractions during defined reference tasks,[99] or one of the tasks being tested.[100] Although no standard method has been developed for this normalization, most investigators use MMT positions, resisting isometric contractions either manually or against some fixed resistance. In a comparison of various normalization methods, Knutson et al[101] found that an MVIC provided the greatest reproducibility.

When using dynamic movements, this issue becomes cloudier. Because the changing muscle length through a movement alters the length–tension relationships and consequently the EMG activity, a static contraction may not be a reasonable "control" condition when examining movement. Researchers have shown that measurements of dynamic EMG will vary with different normalization procedures, suggesting that it is more appropriate to normalize EMG activity over specific arcs of movement.[102] For example, investigators have looked at maximal activity through a range of motion, and quantified the EMG within arcs of 10 or 30°. This maximal EMG within each arc is then used as the control value, and EMG measured during the test activity is normalized as a percentage of this value at the same angle.

The Relationship Between the EMG Signal and Force

The relationship between the EMG signal and muscle tension has been studied since 1952.[103,104] It is generally accepted that a direct relationship exists between the EMG signal and muscular effort, but this relationship must be discussed in terms of muscle length and type of contraction.

Isometric Contractions

Several early studies have demonstrated that when muscles contract while maintaining a constant length, EMG signal amplitude varies directly with muscle tension. Many investigators have documented a linear relationship between muscle tension and IEMG.[104–106] Others have reported curvilinear relationships.[106–108] The linear slope or the degree of nonlinearity seems to vary with the muscle tested, the joint position or muscle length, the electrode placements, and the method of measurement of force.[106,107,109] DeLuca[25] adds that when the detection volume of the electrode is much smaller than the cross-sectional area of the active muscle (e.g., in large muscles), newly recruited motor units located close to the muscle will contribute proportionally greater increases to the EMG signal than to the muscle force. This effect will therefore result in a curvilinear relationship between EMG amplitude and force. Conversely, when the detection area of the electrode is closer to the active cross-sectional area of the muscle, an approximate one-to-one relationship between the EMG amplitude and force will result, thereby producing a linear relationship.

Although methods vary among studies, they all support the general conclusion that an increase in EMG output is observed with increasing muscle tension, as long as the muscle length does not change (i.e., during an isometric contraction). When muscle length is varied, however, this relationship between EMG amplitude and tension does not hold. Generally, less EMG amplitude is seen with greater tension as a muscle is lengthened and, conversely, greater EMG amplitude is seen with decreased tension as a muscle is shortened (Fig. 9.36).[88] Theoretically, therefore, we can assume that fewer motor units are needed to produce the same level of tension in the lengthened position.

If it is impossible for the investigator to constrain the test contractions to isometric conditions, EMG signal processing

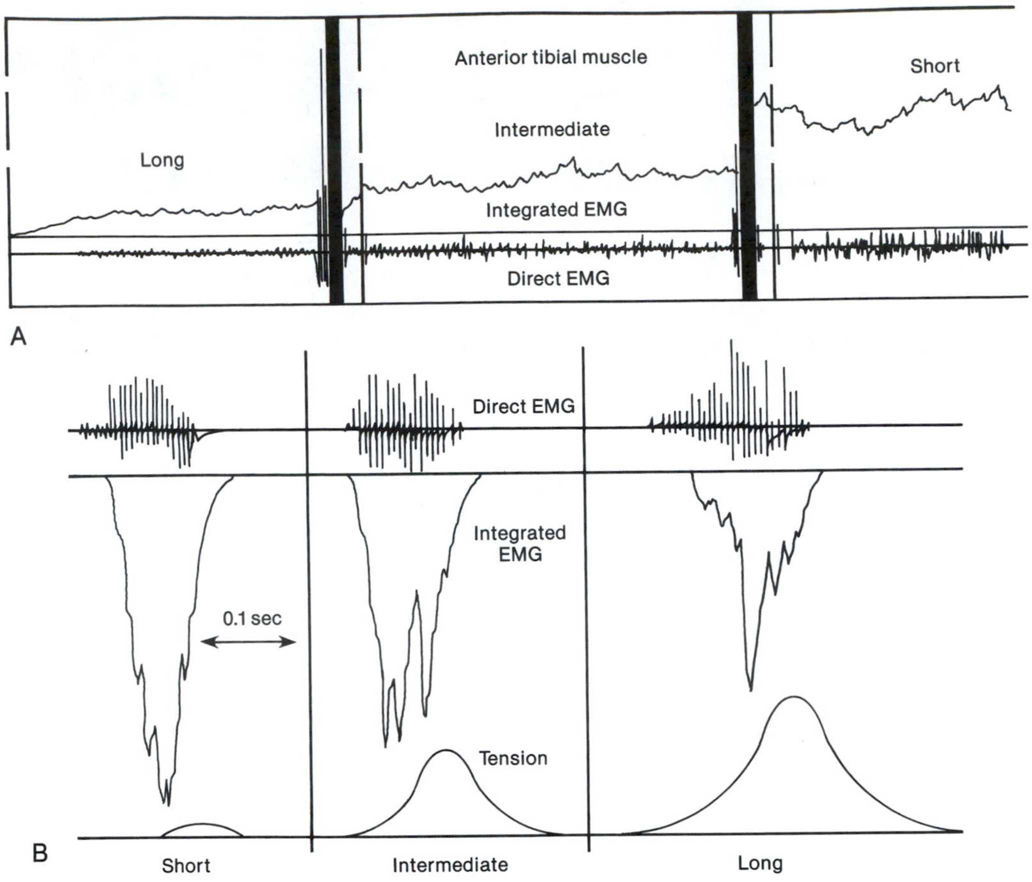

Figure 9.36 (*A*) Maximal voluntary isometric contraction of the anterior tibialis of a normal subject with the muscle at different lengths. Note the rise in EMG activity as the muscle is progressively shortened. The integrated EMG is really a linear envelope. (*B*) EMG activity of the triceps brachii of a cineplastic amputation, illustrating the same effect. (From Inman, VT, et al,[104, p 193] with permission.)

for estimation of muscle force should be limited to portions of the activity that are near isometric. Furthermore, if the anisometric activity is cyclical, such as during gait or cycling, then a fixed epoch in the period of the contraction should be chosen for analysis, and all comparisons should be made for this epoch.[25]

Isotonic Contractions

The relationship between EMG signals and force is further confounded during isotonic contractions, which are defined as contractions producing average constant force or torque.[29] When muscle length continually changes during movement, several factors must be considered. The force–length relationship of the muscle varies throughout the contraction, thereby constantly altering the motor unit activity in proportion to tension. The axis of rotation of the joint changes as the limb moves through its range, so as to change the moment arm and resulting force components. The movement of the skin over the muscle and the variation in shape of the muscle as it contracts will also affect the spatial relationship between the electrodes and muscle fibers, and change the amount of electrical activity actually recorded at different muscle lengths. It is difficult, therefore, to validly quantify muscle activity when movement is occurring.

The EMG–force relationship has also been examined in terms of eccentric and concentric contractions. Eccentric, or lengthening, contractions utilize elastic elements and metabolic processes more efficiently than concentric contractions. Therefore, for the same amount of muscle tension, an eccentric contraction will require fewer motor units (i.e., less overall EMG activity) than a concentric contraction.

The rate of muscle shortening is another consideration. During eccentric contractions, the level of EMG activity remains constant for a given load, independent of the velocity of the contraction.[110] Concentric EMG activity, on the other hand, is greater for a given force as velocity is increased, and probably reflects a need for greater recruitment to accommodate for a faster contraction time. However, only when velocity is kept constant is the EMG proportional to tension.[110] Therefore, with isotonic movement at uncontrolled velocity, the EMG signal will not be a direct reflection of muscle tension. This is an important point when we consider clinical applications of EMG signals.

Muscle Fatigue

When a muscle exhibits localized fatigue after a sustained contraction, one might expect to see a decrease in overall EMG output. The opposite is generally observed initially, however. Typically, an increase in EMG amplitude is seen initially as a muscle fatigues. In an attempt to maintain the level of active tension in the muscle, additional motor units are recruited, and active motor units fire at increasing rates to compensate for the decreased force of contraction of the fatigued fibers. After maximal contraction, when the entire motor unit pool is supposedly recruited, force declines and EMG amplitude stays constant and eventually declines. The presence of constant EMG amplitude suggests that the maximal number of motor units is still contracting. Eventually, however, as the contraction continues, the contractile elements within the muscle will fail and EMG activity will simultaneously start to decrease. EMG indications of fatigue can occur very quickly, within the first several seconds of both submaximal and maximal contractions.

Researchers have observed both linear[105,107] and nonlinear[106,111] EMG–force relationships during fatiguing contractions. The slope of this relationship varies with the degree of fatigue. Studies have also demonstrated a relationship between predominance of fiber type within a muscle and its EMG fatigue characteristics.[106] Muscles composed of primarily type I (slow-twitch) fibers fatigue at a slower rate and demonstrate only small increases in EMG signal amplitude.

Frequency Analysis

EMG evidence of localized muscle fatigue may also be quantified by frequency analysis of the EMG signal during constant-force isometric contractions. It has been proposed that spectral indices of fatigue are a more direct representation of localized fatigue than amplitude parameters.[2,112] The spectral modification to the signal appears as compression toward lower frequencies is accompanied by a skewing of the power density spectrum. Essentially, the high-frequency components of the signal are diminished and there is a gradual increase in the low-frequency components of the spectrum.[112]

Using shifts in EMG median frequency to determine whether a muscle is exhibiting local fatigue has at least two advantages over mechanical indices of fatigue: (1) it provides a noninvasive, muscle-specific measure of fatigue and (2) spectral EMG indices of fatigue change continuously from the initiation of a sustained contraction and do not require the subject to expend considerable effort for long periods of time.

Researchers have been able to document muscle fatigue during specific tasks using this technique.[113–117] By measuring frequency shifts in the electrical potentials of an impaired muscle during treatment, a therapist can determine whether the muscle is being sufficiently exercised.[4,112,118] If the frequency spectrum does not change over time, then synergists may be responsible for the force being generated, rather than the involved muscle. If a decrease in the frequency is seen at first, and the frequency then abruptly levels off without a decrease in output force, the involved muscle may have stopped participating, and other muscles may have taken over to generate the force. Such a technique could be helpful in discriminating which muscles are truly contributing the force output that is measured over a joint. Of course, appropriate instrumentation for recording and analysis must be available. These types of data will not be analyzed with conventional EMG units or biofeedback devices. More and more commercially available EMG systems, however, include spectral analysis as a component of their analysis software.

The EMG Signal and Muscle Strength

The above factors are of great significance for interpreting EMG amplitude during activities that require muscles to operate at different lengths or speeds, or that utilize different types of contractions. Those who use EMG signals to study muscle function during activities are often tempted to make statements regarding the muscle's "strength." Although this term is used clinically, it must be used with caution. Strength is a construct that must be defined as torque or force produced under a specific set of conditions. Clinicians must be very careful, therefore, about concluding that a muscle is "working harder" or that a muscle is "stronger" just because the EMG activity is greater. Within a single session, when electrode positions remain constant, the position of the limb, the type of contraction, and the speed of movement will affect the level of EMG activity recorded.

The significance of these factors becomes apparent when comparisons are made between isometric exercises performed at different joint angles. The recorded EMG activity from a single muscle positioned at different points in the range may have varied amplitudes, but may in fact represent contractions of similar tension levels. Therefore, the EMG signal, which is a recording of motor unit activity, must be distinguished from muscle tension, which is a function of contractile processes. Therapists often use the term "optimal" to describe a biomechanical advantageous position for a muscle; however, EMG signals could be lower at this optimal position because fewer motor units are required to create a given level of force. Greater EMG activity may actually indicate that a muscle's efficiency is decreased.

Therapists should also be cognizant of the fact that EMG signals can represent the activity of individual muscles, whereas the force or torque measured across a joint may represent the resultant interaction of agonists, antagonists, and synergists. Adjacent muscles make differential contributions to the strength, stability, and coordination of a contraction. The EMG signals from the agonists may not necessarily be a valid representation of activity around a joint. Therefore, EMG data cannot be expected to provide direct information about an individual muscle's "strength."

Muscle Tone

Therapists must also resist the temptation to make inferences about muscle tone based on EMG activity. Normal muscle "tonus" refers to resting tension within a muscle due to the elastic and viscoelastic properties of muscle fibers. Tone also reflects the level of gamma input to the muscle spindle, or readiness of a muscle to contract. Essential to a definition of tone is the fact that even though a relaxed muscle shows no electrical activity on EMG, it still maintains a passive state of tone. Therefore, tone is not a function of motor unit activity, and cannot be measured by the EMG signal. This means that when the term spasticity is used to indicate a state of hypertonia, it actually refers to the potential for an overactive muscle response to a stimulus, and not motor unit activity per se. Just as in a normal muscle at rest, a "relaxed" spastic muscle will exhibit electrical silence. This is true of the rigid muscles of patients with parkinsonism as well.[119]

Movement Patterns

Kinesiological EMG helps us interpret the role of muscles in various movements, specifically related to amplitude, timing, and changes in the power spectrum. When used in combination with biomechanical measures (e.g., force or torque instrumentation, three-dimensional motion analysis systems, foot switches, electrogoniometers, video), these studies provide a rich understanding of muscle function. With an appreciation for the concepts of recording and of the limitations of interpretation previously discussed, the therapist will find EMG a valuable clinical tool to help validate intervention.

It is impossible to provide a comprehensive review of these applications; however, it is useful to consider some examples to illustrate the utility and limitations of EMG methodology.

EMG and Exercise

Motor Learning

EMG has been used to document changes in motor unit recruitment patterns with skill acquisition and coordination. Studies in motor learning have looked at EMG activity over time to determine how muscle activity changes as skill improves. Researchers have shown changes in premovement electrical activity, in sequential firing of various muscles, and other myotemporal variations with motor learning.[120,121] Bernardi et al[122] examined the median frequency power spectrum recorded from biceps and triceps as subjects learned to control levels of force during elbow flexion. They found that repeated functional use of the muscle resulted in slower, prolonged recruitment of motor units in the agonist muscle, allowing a more precise and accurate control of force increments. The authors suggested that these findings have significant implications for rehabilitation, reinforcing the concepts of plasticity of motor unit control according to the functional demands imposed on the muscle.[123]

Principles of Exercise

Many exercise principles are based on anatomical and biomechanical considerations, providing the foundation for assumptions that guide our choices of interventions. EMG data allow us to determine whether these assumptions should be supported. For example, the concepts of co-contraction and joint stability are often applied to specific exercises. Santello and McDonagh[124] documented co-contraction of ankle musculature during jumps from different heights, suggesting that this pattern was responsible for increasing ankle joint stiffness as fall height was increased. Hefzy et al[125] saw co-contraction with hamstrings and quadriceps muscles during a maximal lunge activity.

Therapeutic concepts such as co-contraction must be operationally defined, however. For example, Isear et al[126] looked at quadriceps and hamstring muscles during an unloaded squat in healthy individuals, measuring EMG signals during 30° arcs through the range. They found minimal hamstring activity (4 to 12 percent MVIC) as compared to quadriceps activity (22 to 68 percent MVIC). They suggested that the low hamstring activity reflected low demand placed on the hamstrings to counteract anterior shear forces acting on the proximal tibia. So is this co-contraction? How much activity must be present in a group of muscles around a joint for "co-contraction" to be present? Must all the muscles be equally active? Other important considerations for this question include the difficulty in interpreting EMG when the force of the antagonist is not measurable, velocity of movement is variable, position changes, and cross-talk may be evident.[127]

Consideration of concepts of muscle function must include a discussion about the roles of agonist and antagonist. Is a muscle an antagonist by virtue of being attached on the opposite side of a joint, or is it defined by its action? Can a muscle normally considered an antagonist be a synergist? These questions cause us to consider aspects of motor control that are not clearly understood. For instance, in a study of triceps brachii activation during elbow flexion and extension, Garland et al[128] showed that the same motor units were activated whether the muscle was functioning as an agonist or antagonist, controlling both acceleration and deceleration of the movement.

The closed-chain exercise is another concept that has been used to reinforce the application of increased weight bearing and facilitation of co-contraction around a joint. In 1993, Lutz et al[129] demonstrated that a closed kinetic chain exercise produced significantly greater compression forces at the knee with muscle co-contraction, compared to open-chain activities at similar angles, which produced maximal shear forces and minimal co-contraction. These benefits have been supported in other investigations as well. For example, in a comparison of the squat, leg press, and open knee extension, Escamilla et al[130] found that the squat generated approximately twice as much hamstring activity as the leg press and knee extensions. Quadriceps muscle activity was greatest in the closed-chain activity when the knee was near full flexion, and in the open-chain activity when the knee was near full extension. The open-chain movement produced more rectus femoris activity, whereas the closed chain produced more vasti muscle activity. The authors suggest that an understanding of these results can help in choosing appropriate exercises for rehabilitation and training.

In a study of patients with patellofemoral dysfunction, improvements in peak torque were observed in patients who had performed either open- or closed-chain exercises, but only the closed-chain group showed significant improvement in functional status.[131] An important contrast to these findings was demonstrated in a study of upper extremity tasks, where no difference in EMG signals was found between open- and closed-chain activities, suggesting that load was more of an issue in determining muscle activity than the boundary of the task.[132] This type of conflict illustrates the need to consider specific measurement methods and activities before generalizations are drawn.

Proximal stability is also an issue that lends itself readily to EMG investigation. For instance, researchers have examined synergistic shoulder activity elicited during maximal hand grip. Sporrong et al[133] examined four shoulder muscles—the supraspinatus, infraspinatus, the middle portion of the deltoid, and the descending part of the trapezius—with EMG in adducted and flexed arm positions in healthy subjects. They demonstrated that shoulder activity was greatest with the arm elevated during grip, suggesting that the stabilizing function of the shoulder was an important consideration during manual tasks. In another example, Krebs et al[134] examined EMG activity during gait with and without a cane in an 85-year-old man with a left-instrumented femoral head prosthesis. They found highest acetabular contact pressures at the posterosuperior acetabulum, just prior to peak EMG amplitude, during late stance phase. Their data identified a small area of high acetabular and femoral head stress during gait, and suggested that muscle activity, rather than solely body weight, drives hip loading. Therefore, therapeutic goals to limit hip loads should include reduction in both hip muscle contraction and weightbearing in late stance.

Neuromuscular Dysfunction

EMG has also been a useful adjunct for investigating elements of motor control in patients who have experienced neuromuscular dysfunction. For example, many researchers have compared motor activity in patients with hemiplegia and control subjects, with varying results. Levin and Hui-Chan[135] studied the co-contraction ratio between plantar and dorsiflexors, and found an inverse correlation with force in paretic dorsiflexors. They also established that the EMG output was reproducible over time, suggesting that this type of testing could be useful for tracking change with treatment.

Gowland et al[136] looked at upper extremity tasks in patients with hemiplegia, and found that the inability to perform these tasks was due to inadequate recruitment of the agonist muscle, not increased activity of the antagonist. A similar outcome was obtained in a study of knee EMG signals during isometric and isokinetic exercises, where co-contraction was low or absent, and was similar for patients and control subjects.[137] These findings support aiming treatment at improving recruitment of the agonist, rather than concentrating on inhibition of the antagonist. A contradictory finding was obtained in a study of isometric wrist extension and flexion, where researchers found increased antagonist activity with decreased agonist activity in the paretic arm, concluding that intervention should address decreasing antagonist activity. Once again, we must be cautious in drawing any generalizations. Perhaps the most important message these findings provide is the need to attend to potential methodological and physiological differences that might account for conflicting results. As with any other research method, the consumer must consider the samples studied, the instrumentation used, the muscles selected, and the operational definitions of the activities, to determine whether direct comparisons are warranted.

Pain-Related Muscle Impairments

Clinical research has demonstrated the usefulness of incorporating EMG parameters, such as activation time, amplitude, and median frequency, into a classification scheme for musculoskeletal pain disorders. By understanding the interaction between pain and motor performance, clinicians can directly address motor impairments that will impact function. For example, Madeleine et al[138] examined mechanisms leading to chronic neck and shoulder pain during upper extremity activities. They found shifts in patterns of muscle synergy and higher EMG frequency components, suggesting altered motor unit recruitment with painful conditions. Wadsworth and Bullock-Saxton[139] studied competitive swimmers, comparing those with unilateral shoulder injuries and noninjured athletes, to determine differences in shoulder EMG patterns with pathology. They demonstrated significant variation or delays in muscle activation with injury, indicating that temporal recruitment patterns are related to injury of the scapular rotators, interfering with consistency of movement. They were also able to identify muscle function deficits on the unaffected side. These outcomes suggest intervention strategies that focus on functional tasks, and the need to examine the effect of injury on other joints as part of these tasks.

Patellofemoral pain has also been a major topic of interest for EMG researchers. Questions regarding the most effective exercises, or the role of various knee muscles during functional activities, lend themselves to EMG study. Many clinical approaches to this problem have focused on the ratio of activity between the vastus medialis oblique and vastus lateralis. Interestingly, in studies of isometric exercises (even with hip adduction),[140] sitting and standing,[141] weight-bearing and non-weightbearing activities,[142] and running,[96] several researchers have found no difference between symptomatic and nonsymptomatic subjects. Clinicians have also tried to document the effect of specific interventions for improving knee strength. For instance, Werner et al[143] studied the effects of taping on patients with patellar hypermobility, and found significant increases in knee extensor torque after taping. In terms of general exercise positions, studies have shown us that the vastus medialis is more active during a quadriceps setting exercise than during a straight leg raise in subjects with healthy and painful knees.[144,145] These data provide a useful guide for making intervention choices.

EMG research has been used extensively to study paraspinal muscle impairment in patients with low back pain.[115,118] Declines in mean and median frequency have been identified in those with chronic low back pain, indicative of increased fatigability.[146–148] These same parameters have been used to establish the success of exercise programs as well.[149] Functional activities, such as gait, have also demonstrated differences in those with low back pain, including greater lumbar muscle activity during swing, as compared to normals, in whom these muscles are relatively silent.[150]

Summary

EMG provides a powerful tool for documenting the role of muscle in physical activity, and for determining the integrity of the neuromuscular system. Despite its common use in movement research, however, therapists must use EMG measurements wisely, recognizing its limitations as a measurement tool. Interpretation of the EMG signal must account for the effect of velocity and acceleration, type of muscle contraction, instrumentation, and a host of anatomical, physiological, and neurogenic factors that can influence the output signal.[11] EMG can show that a muscle is working, but not why it is working, and it can only be interpreted as a measure of motor unit activity. EMG cannot determine that a treatment is "effective" in the sense of achieving expected outcomes. EMG by itself cannot provide information as to whether a muscle has gotten stronger or weaker, or if it is hypertonic or hypotonic. Under most circumstances, with repeated testing over short time periods, small changes will be difficult to identify. These must be determined through clinical examination. But the EMG signal can provide information that may increase efficacy during treatment. It is a form of feedback for the therapist that can be invaluable in situations where overt movement or muscle contraction is not observable.

Kinesiological literature abounds with studies concerning the use of EMG signals to examine muscle function under different conditions.[4] Therapists should be familiar with this body of literature in order to interpret and utilize EMG data. One must be critical of EMG studies, however, because many of them demonstrate methodological faults that can invalidate findings. In addition, the results of EMG studies may not always be generalized to a specific patient, and should not be considered the "correct" responses in all cases. Obviously, the therapist's clinical judgment must prevail when observing responses of individual patients.

The clinician is encouraged to explore the uses of EMG signals in any situation where response of superficial muscles is of interest. As long as the limitations of interpretation of EMG signals are kept in mind, this tool can be a major adjunct to patient examination and therapeutic intervention.

Questions for Review

1. What are the basic components of a recording system for EMG and NCV tests?
2. What are the stages in a clinical EMG examination?
3. Describe how motor and sensory nerve conduction velocities are calculated.
4. What are the typical EMG and NCV findings with peripheral nerve lesions, myopathy, and motor neuron disease?
5. What are the possible causes of movement artifact? How can these effects be reduced or eliminated?
6. Describe four types of signal processing for EMG.
7. What is the effect of changing muscle length on the relationship between EMG and force?
8. What types of changes are seen in the EMG signal when a muscle fatigues?
9. Assume you are including EMG to monitor muscle response as a component of a treatment program. What considerations are important for setting up your procedure in terms of:
   - Choice and placement of electrodes?
   - Type of contractions?
   - Patient position?
   - Timing of activities?
   - How the EMG will be interpreted?

Case Study 1

It is widely recognized that muscle dysfunction can result from direct neuromuscular injury, pain, or disuse. Some muscles may compensate for this deficit, resulting in a relative alteration in their EMG activity during sustained tasks that cause localized fatigue. A case report is described to provide an example of how surface EMG signal measurements were used to determine paraspinal muscle impairment in a patient with low back pain (LBP).

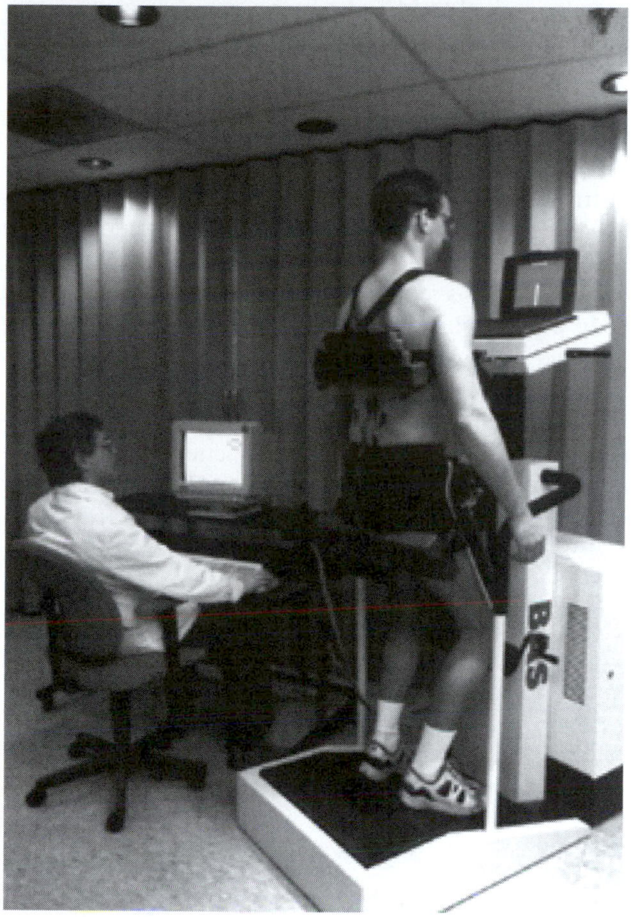

Figure 9.37 The Back Analysis System used for acquiring EMG signals and force during sustained isometric extension of the trunk. A subject is shown positioned in the postural restraint apparatus with six surface EMG electrodes positioned bilaterally on the lower back. The subject's task is to produce a trunk extension torque against the scapular pad according to a target force set on the visual feedback display facing him. The EMG signals are automatically sampled and analyzed from a computer workstation shown in front of the operator. The test results are compared to a database for classification of back muscle impairment. (Courtesy of Neuromuscular Research Center, Boston University, Boston, MA.)

PATIENT DESCRIPTION

The patient, a 36-year-old man with subacute, nonspecific lower back pain (LBP), was initially examined by his general practitioner and was treated with rest for several days, a home program of stretching exercise, cold packs as needed, and a prescription for a nonsteroidal anti-inflammatory drug (NSAID). The patient was in otherwise good health with no history of neurological disorders or serious musculoskeletal injuries. The onset of his back pain symptoms occurred 6 weeks before the EMG testing. The patient did not associate this episode of LBP with a specific triggering event, but indicated that he has had LBP off and on for more than 8 years. Previous examinations using radiographic imaging procedures have been unremarkable. At the time of his EMG, which was conducted as part of a clinical research study, the patient reported pain symptoms bilaterally in the lower lumbar region and upper buttock area which was most severe on arising in the morning or while standing. At the time of the EMG, the patient completed a self-report of pain intensity (6/10 using the Visual Analog Scale) and pain-related function (38 percent using the Oswestry Disability Scale[151]).

MEASUREMENT PROCEDURE

A surface EMG-based dynamometer, referred to as the Back Analysis System (BAS), was used to acquire and process the surface EMG signals. The technique is described in detail in previous reports,[152] and is based on monitoring the change in fatigue indices from EMG signals acquired simultaneously from a lumbar electrode array during a sustained isometric extension of the trunk. The efficacy of the technique has been described in recent review articles[115,118] and in specific research publications. The BAS was used to monitor treatment progression in patients with subacute and chronic LBP undergoing work-hardening rehabilitation,[116] in patients with chronic LBP while in remission,[148] and in competitive rowers with subacute and chronic LBP.[153]

The BAS device, depicted in Figure 9.37, includes the following key components: (1) an adjustable test frame to maintain static posture and isolate the paraspinal muscles; (2) a torque feedback system to maintain constant muscle force; and (3) an EMG acquisition and processing system designed for near-real-time display of EMG median frequency and RMS. With the patient positioned in the device as illustrated in the figure, six active surface EMG electrodes were placed at anatomical locations corresponding to contralateral longissimus thoracis (L1 spinal level), iliocostalis lumborum (L2 spinal level), and multifidus (L5 spinal level) muscles. A padded strap, connected at each end to a noncompliant force transducer, was placed across the scapular region for the subject to push against during the test contractions. A monitor was positioned in front of the subject to provide force feedback and a target force level, which was set according to the test protocol.

The test protocol began with a set of warm-up and training exercises in the BAS device. The patient practiced the task of exerting isometric trunk extension at targeted force levels using the feedback display to guide them. After these preliminary trials were successfully completed, the patient was instructed to exert several attempts at producing a maximal voluntary contraction in trunk extension. After a brief rest period, the subject was instructed to follow a "staircase" protocol in which he had to exert a series of sustained isometric trunk extensions in the device at force levels set at 20, 50, 70, and 90 percent of his ideal body weight, respectively. Ideal body was calculated from a weight table established for men and women according to frame size.[154] The use of ideal body weight to standardize the protocol task was adopted to eliminate the confounding effects of subject motivation when previous test contractions were based on the maximal voluntary contraction. Each contraction was sustained for 30 seconds. A rest period of 15 seconds was provided between each contraction.

RESULTS

Using the "staircase" protocol described, results showed altered neuromuscular control of paraspinal muscles for the patient (Fig. 9.38A) as compared to a control subject (Fig. 9.38B) matched for age, sex, ideal body weight, and strength. The results are displayed for the force (lower plot), the EMG median frequency (MF), and the EMG and root mean square (RMS). EMG data from the six electrode sites are plotted separately.

The example demonstrates that despite the ability of the two subjects to produce similar forces, there are obvious differences in neuromuscular control and/or muscle fatigability. A consistent pattern of increasing RMS with increasing force was seen in the control subject, whereas in the patient with LBP, the changes in RMS with force were highly variable and asymmetric. Similar results were apparent for the median frequency curves. For the control subject, the MF decreased more rapidly as the force increased, and the pattern was highly symmetric and well

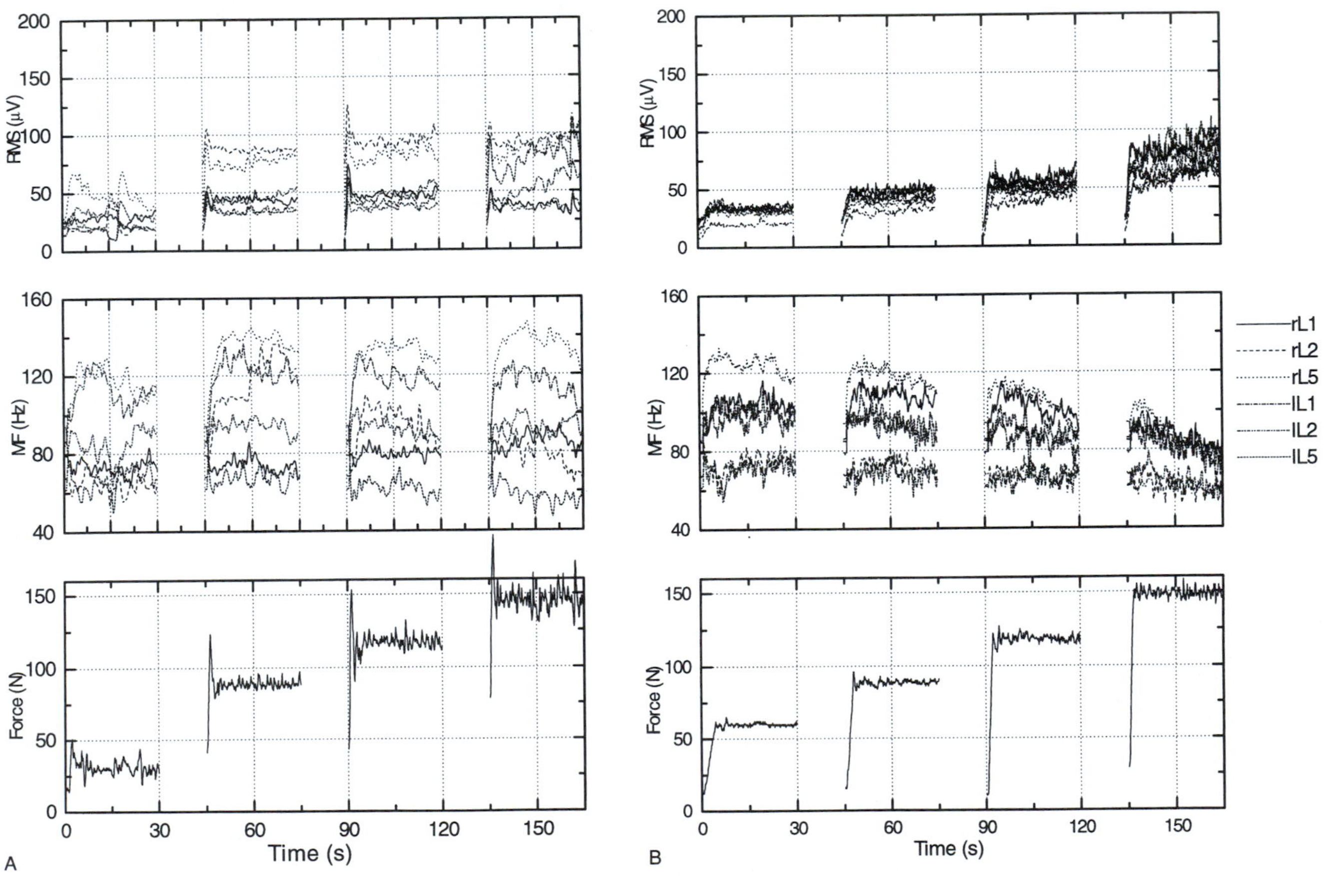

Figure 9.38 Examples of RMS, median frequency (MF) and force data recorded during a "staircase" protocol in the Back Analysis System in (*A*) a patient with subacute LBP and (*B*) a control subject without LBP. The staircase protocol requires the subject to sustain a constant-force isometric contraction for progressively higher target force levels. In this instance, the subjects were tested at 20, 50, 70, and 90 percent of their ideal body weight. Each contraction was held for 30 seconds. (From Roy, SH, and Oddsson, LI: Classification of paraspinal muscle impairments by surface electromyography. Phys Ther 78:838, 1998, with permission.)

ordered in contralateral muscle groups. In contrast, in the patient with LBP, the MF appeared to stay more or less constant for most muscles, decreasing slightly near the end of the contraction at the higher force levels.

SIGNIFICANCE

In this instance, the lack of a gradual, orderly fatigue response in the patient with LBP may represent a characteristic loss of the ability of paraspinal muscles to produce greater forces as needed when external loads or torque is increased. Based on large-scale clinical trials, it has been proposed that these differences in EMG measurements reflect a characteristic signature of pain-related impairments that is likely the result of muscle inhibition and avoidance behavior. The hypothesis for this model of impairment is that in the presence of pain, muscles respond by reducing their level of activity and thereby accommodate a lesser share of the mechanical loads displaced across the joints they support.[155] As a result, normal patterns of muscle activity among synergistic muscles become recognizably altered, the so-called favoring of muscle use.

The examination and treatment of LBP-related impairments have always assumed a common role among physical therapists. Treatment approaches to LBP disorders are based for the most part on reversing and preventing recurrence of the musculoskeletal components to LBP, with the expectation that such change will lead to improved function and reduced disability. Back pain specialists have traditionally relied on a variety of qualitative and quantitative methods to characterize the musculoskeletal integrity of the spinal complex and identify related impairments. Paraspinal muscle impairments have been quantitatively determined by the use of dynamometers in an attempt to supplement standard clinical examination procedures and provide greater objectivity. The measurements are based entirely on mechanical output, such as torque, velocity, or displacement of the trunk. Consequently, they share a common flaw: The kinematic and force variables can be cognitively perceived by the subject and purposefully altered in a manner that compromise validity. Therefore maximal physical performance capability cannot be completely isolated from factors related to motivation and secondary gain.

The developers of the BAS propose that muscle performance objectivity is enhanced by specifying that the test be limited to the performance of submaximal, constant-force, isometric contractions in which the duration of the contraction is predetermined.[148] Furthermore, the useful information from the EMG signals is not derived from a single muscle group or a single parameter, but rather is the result of the concurrent behavior or mapping of many coactive muscle groups. It is assumed that the subject is likely to be unaware of, and cannot volitionally control, parameters derived from such a measurement scheme.

GUIDING QUESTIONS

1. What do you consider to be the minimal requirements for an examination procedure to be meaningful?
2. How well does the EMG procedure described in the case satisfy these requirements?
3. Specifically, how would the information derived from the results of the EMG be used to guide therapeutic intervention?
4. How else might this EMG testing technique be used to describe other kinds of muscle impairments associated with LBP?

Case Study 2

PATIENT DESCRIPTION

The patient is a 64-year-old woman who fell and fractured her elbow ten months ago. The fractures that occurred as a result of this fall were described as a combination of a "y" shaped transcondylar fracture and an olecranon type II fracture. Initial medical/surgical treatment was joint reconstruction by pinning and plates. It was noted that the patient had a diagnosis of osteoporosis prior to falling.

After a period of immobilization, the patient noted a marked loss of motion particularly supination of the forearm and flexion of the elbow and complained of significant elbow discomfort. Physical therapy was initiated with the general goals of improving function and gaining range of motion (ROM). The patient continued to complain of significant elbow joint discomfort and pain. She also expressed dissatisfaction with her progress in physical therapy and requested further treatment from the surgeon for pain relief and increased ROM. The patient had 0° of supination and 90° of pronation. Elbow ROM was 30 to 65° which limited function of simple tasks such as bringing an eating utensil to her mouth. Following a consult with the surgeon, a decision was made to insert a total elbow joint replacement arthroplasty. X-ray films taken prior to surgery revealed significant heterotopic bone formation which was felt to be interfering with the patient's ROM and was perhaps the source of pain.

Following the total joint replacement, the patient made slow but steady progress. The surgeon's note states that the patient was reporting good progress. Elbow flexion ROM was now 20 to 110°. The patient continued to have 0° of supination with 90° of pronation. The patient at this time also reported no complaints of pain but was now reporting paresthesias in the ulnar nerve distribution. Muscle function was reported as being intact.

Table 9.1 NCV Results: Median Nerve

Site	Latency	Amplitude	Velocity
Wrist	4.0 msec	4.2 mV	
Elbow	7.2 msec	4.2 mV	63 m/sec
Sensory II	2.4 msec	47 μV	
Sensory III	2.4 msec	47 μV	

A follow-up visit had the patient reporting weakness in her hand and atrophy was noted in the ulnar intrinsic muscle. The patient had persistent numbness and a referral was made for electrophysiologic testing. A brief clinical examination done prior to the electrophysiologic testing revealed numbness in the ulnar nerve distribution. The patient had weakness in the ulnar nerve distribution and manual muscle testing of the first dorsal interosseous was 0/5, abductor digiti minimi 0/5, flexor digitorum profundus to the fifth digit was 2−/5, and the flexor carpi ulnaris was graded as 2−/5. Atrophy of the intrinsic muscles of the hand was obvious. The patient had a positive Tinel sign over the ulnar nerve at the elbow proximal to the cubital tunnel. ROM for elbow flexion was limited to 20 to 110°. Supination was 0, pronation was 0 to 90 degrees. The patient also had marked reduction in shoulder motion and abduction and flexion were 0 to 60°. Wrist extension was 0°.

TEST RESULTS

Tables 9.1 and 9.2 show the results of the nerve conduction velocity testing of the median and ulnar nerves. The right median nerve showed a borderline normal distal motor latency, normal distal sensory latencies, normal amplitudes of motor and sensory responses and normal conduction velocity. Examination of the right ulnar nerve presented difficulties because no response was obtained in the recording from the first dorsal interosseous or the abductor digiti minimi when stimulating the ulnar nerve at the wrist and elbow. Also no sensory response could be obtained in the hand in the ulnar nerve distribution. The ulnar nerve study was done by recording from the flexor digitorum profundus (ulnar nerve portion) by stimulating the ulnar nerve above and below the elbow. This revealed a very small amplitude response with a normal condition velocity across the elbow of 60 m/sec. Increasing the length of the segment examined across the elbow by stimulating in the upper arm and below the elbow revealed a conduction velocity of 50 m/sec. The motor response recorded was markedly reduced in amplitude and the waveform was dispersed. Recordings were made using needle electrodes.

An EMG examination was also performed. Table 9.3 summarizes the results of this examination. EMG findings in the abductor pollicis brevis were normal. No activity could be recorded in the first dorsal interosseous. In the abductor digiti minimi the patient showed a few highly polyphasic potentials that were of low amplitude. In the flexor digitorum profundus (ulnar portion), the patient was able to generate polyphasic potentials that were both large and small. The interference pattern was never better than one third of normal. The recruitment of motor units was a problem. The flexor carpi ulnaris also revealed polyphasic potentials that were large and small. Recruitment was incomplete and the interference pattern was never better than 1/3 of normal. There was no significant amount of spontaneous activity found in any of the ulnar innervated muscles on this examination.

GUIDING QUESTIONS

1. Based on a review of the electrophysiological examination results, characterize the function of the median and ulnar nerves.
2. What is the possible cause?

Table 9.2 NCV Results: Ulnar Nerve

Site	Latency	Amplitude	Velocity
Wrist	0		
B/Elbow	3.9 msec	200 μV	
A/Elbow	6.0 msec	155 μV	6 m/sec
U/Arm	7.1 msec	150 μV	[50 m/sec]

Comments: Needle recording from FDP(V) Waveform dispersed.

Table 9.3 EMG Results

Muscle	Spontaneous Activity	Voluntary Activity	Pattern
APB	0	NMU	Normal
1st DI	0	0	0
ADM	0	Small polys	Marked decrease
FDP (ulnar)	0	Polys—large and small	1/3 N
FCU	0	As above	1/3 N

ADM = abductor digiti minimi; APB = abductor pollicis brevis; FCU = flexor carpi ulnaris; FDP = flexor digitorum profundus; 1st DI = first dorsal interosseous.

References

1. Green, RM: Commentary on the Effect of Electricity on Muscular Motion. Elizabeth Licht, Cambridge, 1953.
2. Medved, V: Measurement of Human Locomotion, CRC Press, Boca Raton, FL, 2001.
3. Geddes, LA, and Baker, LE: Principals of Applied Biomedical Instrumentation. John Wiley & Sons, New York, 1968.
4. Basmajian, JV, and DeLuca, CJ: Muscles Alive, ed 2. Williams & Wilkins, Baltimore, 1985.
5. Merletti, R, and Hermens, HJ: Detection and conditioning of the surface EMG signal. In Merletti, R, and Parker, P (eds): Electromyography: Physiology, Engineering, and Noninvasive Applications. Institute of Electrical and Electronics Engineers (IEEE, Inc), John Wiley & Sons, Hoboken, NJ, 2004, p 107.
6. Hermens, H, and Freriks, B (eds): SENIAM 5: The State of the Art on Sensors and Sensor Placement Procedures for Surface Electromyography: A Proposal for Sensor Placement Procedures. Roessingh Research and Development, Enschede, Netherlands, 1997.
7. Soderberg, GL: Selected Topics in Surface Electromyography for Use in the Occupational Setting. US Department of Health and Human Services, Public Health Service, Centers for Disease Control, Washington, DC, NIOSH, Publication No. 91–100, 1992.
8. Kumar, S, and Mital, A: Electromyography in Ergonomics. Taylor & Francis Ltd, Bristol, PA, 1996.
9. Reucher, H, et al: Spatial filtering of noninvasive multielectrode EMG: Part I—Introduction to measuring technique and applications. IEEE Trans Biomed Eng 34:98, 1987.
10. Reucher, H, et al: Spatial filtering of noninvasive multielectrode EMG: Part II—Filter performance in theory and modeling. IEEE Trans Biomed Eng 34:106, 1987.
11. Gerleman, DG, and Cook, TM: Instrumentation. In Soderberg, GL (ed): Selected Topics in Surface Electromyography for Use in the Occupational Setting: Expert Perspectives. U.S. Department of Health and Human Services, Public Health Service, Centers for Disease Control, Washington, DC, NIOSH, Publication No. 91–100, 1992, p 44.
12. DeLuca, CJ: The use of surface electromyography in biomechanics. J Appl Biomech 13:135, 1997.
13. Basmajian, JV, and Stecko, G: A new bipolar electrode for electromyography. J Appl Physiol 17:849, 1962.
14. Adrian, ED, and Bronk, DW: The discharge of impulses in motor nerve fibers. J Physiol (Lond) 67:119, 1929.
15. Nelson, RM, et al: Comparison of motor unit action potentials using monopolar vs. concentric needle electrodes in the middle deltoid and abductor digiti minimi muscles. Electromyogr Clin Neuophysiol 43(8):459, 2003.
16. Andersson, E, et al: EMG activities of the quadratus lumborum and erector spinae muscles during flexion-relaxation and other motor tasks. Clin Biomech 11:392, 1996.
17. Perotto, A, and Delagi, E: Anatomical Guide for the Electromyographer: The Limbs and the Trunk, ed 3. Charles C Thomas, Springfield, IL, 1996.
18. Geiringer, SR: Anatomic Localization for Needle Electromyography. Mosby-Year Book, St. Louis, 1999.
19. Merletti, RM, and Roy, SH: Myoelectric and mechanical manifestations of muscle fatigue in voluntary contractions. J Orthop Sports Phys Ther 24:342, 1996.
20. Merletti, R, et al: Modeling of surface myoelectric signals. Part II: Model based interpretation of EMG signals. IEEE Trans Biomed Eng 46(7):821, 1999.
21. Merletti, R, et al: The linear electrode array: A useful tool with many applications. J Electromyogr Kinesiol 13:37, 2003.
22. Lynn, PA, et al: Influences of electrode geometry on bipolar recordings of the surface electromyogram. Med Biol Eng Comput 16:651, 1978.
23. Komi, PV, and Buskirk, ER: Reproducibility of electromyographic measurements with inserted wire electrodes and surface electrodes. Electromyography 10:357, 1970.
24. DeLuca, CJ, and Merletti, R: Surface myoelectric signal cross-talk among muscles of the leg. Electroencephalogr Clin Neurophysiol 69:568, 1988.
25. Broman, H, et al: A note on non-invasive estimation of muscle fiber conduction velocity. IEEE Trans Biomed Eng, 32:341, 1985.
26. Clancy, EA, et al: Sampling, noise reduction, and amplitude estimation issues in surface electromyography. J Electromyogr Kinesiol 12:1, 2002.
27. Kingma, YJ, et al: Improved Ag/AgCl pressure electrodes. Med Biol Eng Comput 21:351, 1983.
28. Redfern, MS: Elimination of EKG contamination of torso electromyographic signals. In Asfour, SS (ed): Trends in Ergonomics/human Factors IV. Elsevier Science, North-Holland, Amsterdam, 1987.
29. Ad Hoc Committee of the International Society of Electrophysiological Kinesiology: Units, Terms and Standards in the Reporting of EMG Research. Department of Medical Research, Rehabilitation Institute of Montreal, Montreal, 1980.
30. Kimura, J: Electrodiagnosis of Diseases of Nerve and Muscle: Principles and Practice, ed 2. FA Davis, Philadelphia, 1989.
31. McGill, KC, and Dorfman, LJ: Automatic decomposition electromyography (ADEMG): Validation and normative data in brachial biceps. Electroencephalogr Clin Neurophysiol 61:453, 1985.
32. Liguori, R, et al: Electromyography in myopathy. Neurophysiol Clin 27:200, 1997.
33. Fuglsang-Frederiksen, A, et al: Electrical muscle activity during a gradual increase in force in patients with neuromuscular diseases. Electroencephalogr Clin Neurophysiol 57:320, 1984.
34. Hausmanowa-Petrusewicz, I, and Kopec, J: EMG parameters changes in the effort pattern at various load in dystrophic muscle. Electromyogr Clin Neurophysiol 24:121, 1984.
35. Terebuh, BM, and Johnson, EW: Electrodiagnosis (EDX) consultation including EMG examination. In Johnson, EW, and Pease, WS (eds): Practical Electromyography. Williams & Wilkins, Baltimore, 1997, p 1.
36. Cruz Martinez, A: Electrophysiological study in hemiparetic patients. Electromyography, motor conduction velocity, and response to repetitive nerve stimulation. Electromyogr Clin Neurophysiol 23:139, 1983.

37. Berman, SA, et al: Injury zone denervation in traumatic quadriplegia in humans. Muscle Nerve 19:701, 1996.
38. Spielholz, NI, et al: Electrophysiological studies in patients with spinal cord lesions. Arch Phys Med Rehabil 53:558, 1972.
39. Brown, WF, and Snow, R: Denervation in hemiplegic muscles. Stroke 21:1700, 1990.
40. Johnson, EW, et al: Sequence of electromyographic abnormalities in stroke syndrome. Arch Phys Med Rehabil 56:468, 1975.
41. Falck, B, and Alaranta, H: Fibrillation potentials, positive sharp waves and fasciculation in the intrinsic muscles of the foot in healthy subjects. J Neurol Neurosurg Psychiatry 46:681, 1983.
42. Dumitri, D, et al: Prevalence of denervation in paraspinal and foot intrinsic musculature. Am J Phys Med Rehabil 80(7):482, 2001.
43. Wettstein, A: The origin of fasciculations in motoneuron disease. Ann Neurol 5:295, 1979.
44. Wenzel, S, et al: Surface EMG and myosonography in the detection of fasciculations: A comparative study. J Neuroimaging 8:148, 1998.
45. Van der Heijden, A, et al: Fasciculation potentials in foot and leg muscles of healthy young adults. Electroencephalogr Clin Neurophysiol 93:163, 1994.
46. Rosenfeld, J: Fasciculations without fibrillations: The dilemma of early diagnosis. Amyotroph Lateral Scler Other Motor Neuron Disord Suppl 1:S53-6, 2000.
47. Rodriquez, AA, et al: Electromyographic and neuromuscular variables in post-polio subjects. Arch Phys Med Rehabil 76:989, 1995.
48. Stalberg, E, and Grimby, G: Dynamic electromyography and muscle biopsy changes in a 4-year follow-up: Study of patients with a history of polio. Muscle Nerve 18:699, 1995.
49. Roeleveld, K, et al: Motor unit size estimation of enlarged motor units with surface electromyography. Muscle Nerve 21:878, 1998.
50. Stalberg, E: Needle electromyography. In Johnson, EW, and Pease, WS (eds): Practical Electromyography. Williams & Wilkins, Baltimore, 1997, p 89.
51. Meriggioli, MN, and Rowin, J: Single fiber EMG as an outcome measure in myasthenia gravis: Results from a double blind, placebo-controlled trial. J Clin Neurophsiol 20(5):382. 2003.
52. Stalberg, E, and Fawcett, PRW: Macro EMG changes in healthy subjects of different ages. J Neurol Neurosurg Psychiatry 45:870, 1982.
53. Luciano, CA, et al: Electrophysiologic and histologic studies in clinically unaffected muscles of patients with prior paralytic poliomyelitis. Muscle Nerve 19:1413, 1996.
54. Hodes, R, et al: The human electromyogram in response to nerve stimulation and the conduction velocity of motor axons. Arch Neurol Psychiatry 60:340, 1948.
55. Dawson, GD, and Scott, JW: The recording of nerve action potentials through the skin in man. J Neurosurg Psychiatry 12:259, 1949.
56. Echternach, JL: Introduction to Electromyography and Nerve Conduction Testing, ed 2. Slack, Thorofare, NJ, 2003.
57. Johnson, EW, and Pease, WS: Practical Electromyography, ed 3. Williams & Wilkins, Baltimore, 1997.
58. Association of Electromyography and Electrodiagnosis Medicine (AEEM): Professional Practice Committee Guidelines in Electrodiagnostic Medicine. Muscle & Nerve 22: Suppl 8, 1999.
59. Trojaborg, W: Motor nerve conduction velocities in normal subjects with particular reference to the conduction in proximal and distal segments of median and ulnar nerves. Electroencephalogr Clin Neurophysiol 17:314, 1964.
60. Dawson, GD: The relative excitability and conduction velocity of sensory and motor nerve fibers in man. J Physiol (Lond) 131:436, 1956.
61. Hoffman, P: Uber die beziehungen der sehnen reflexe zur wilkurlichen bewegung und zum tonus. Z Biol 68:351, 1918.
62. Gersh, MR: Electrotherapy in Rehabilitation. FA Davis, Philadelphia, 1992.
63. Sabbahi, MA, and Khalil, M: Segmental H-reflex studies in upper and lower limbs of healthy subjects. Arch Phys Med Rehabil 71:216, 1990.
64. Braddom, RL, and Johnson, EW: Standardization of H-reflex and diagnostic use in S1 radiculopathy. Arch Phys Med Rehabil 55:161, 1974.
65. Abbruzese, M, et al: Changes in central delay of soleus H-reflex after facilitory or inhibitory conditioning in humans. J Neurophysiol 65:1598, 1991.
66. Magladery, JW, and McDougal, JB: Electrophysiological studies of nerve and reflex activity in normal man. I. Identification of certain reflexes in the electromyogram and the conduction velocity of peripheral nerve fibers. Bull Johns Hopkins Hosp 86:265, 1950.
67. Milanov, I, and Georgiev, D: Mechanisms of trizanidine action on spasticity. Acta Neurol Scand 89:274, 1994.
68. Nance, PW: A comparison of clonidine, cyproheptadine and baclofen in spastic spinal cord injured patients. J Am Paraplegic Soc 17:150, 1994.
69. Dumitru, D, Amato, AA, and Zwarts,M: Electrodiagnostic Medicine, ed 2. Hanley & Belfus, Philadelphia, 2001.
70. Gamstorp, I: Normal conduction velocity of ulnar, median and peroneal nerves in infancy, childhood and adolescence. Acta Paediatrica 146(Suppl):68, 1963.
71. Buchthal, F, and Rosenfalck, A: Evoked action potentials and conduction velocity in human sensory nerves. Brain Res 3:1, 1966.
72. Norris, AH, et al: Age changes in the maximum conduction velocity of motor fibers of human ulnar nerves. J Appl Physiol 5:589, 1953.
73. Halar, EM, et al: Nerve conduction studies in upper extremities: Skin temperature corrections. Arch Phys Med Rehabil 64:412, 1983.
74. McComas, AJ: Motor-unit estimation: The beginning. J Clin Neurophysiol 12:560, 1995.
75. Daube, JR: Estimating the number of motor units in a muscle. J Clin Neurophysiol 12:585, 1995.
76. Doherty, T, et al: Methods for estimating the numbers of motor units in human muscles. J Clin Neurophysiol 12:565, 1995.
77. Al-Shekhlee, A, and Katirji, B: Electrodiagnotic features of acute paralytis poliomyelitis associated with West Nile virus infection. Muscle Nerve 29(3):376, 2004.
78. McComas, AJ, et al: Early and late losses of motor units after poliomyelitis. Brain 120:1415, 1997.
79. Bromberg, MB, et al: Motor unit number estimation, isometric strength, and electromyographic measures in amyotrophic lateral sclerosis. Muscle Nerve 16:1213, 1993.
80. Dulakas, MC: Pathogenetic mechanisms of post-polio syndrome: Morphological, electrophysiological, virological and immunological correlations. Ann NY Acad Sci 753:167, 1995.
81. Rowland, LP: Pathogenesis of muscular dystrophies. Arch Neurol 33:315, 1976.
82. Chisari, C, et al: Sarcolemmal excitability in myotonic dystrophy: Assessment through surface EMG. Muscle Nerve 21:543, 1998.
83. Orizio, C, et al: Muscle surface mechanical and electrical activities in myotonic dystrophy. Electromyogr Clin Neurophysiol 37:231, 1997.
84. Colachis, SC, et al: Polyphasic motor unit action potentials in early radiculopathy: Their presence and ephaptic transmission as an hypothesis. Electromyogr Clin Neurophysiol 32:27, 1992.
85. Czyrny, JJ, and Lawrence, J: The importance of paraspinal muscle EMG in cervical and lumbosacral radiculopathy: Review of 100 cases. Electromyogr Clin Neurophysiol 36:503, 1996.
86. Toyokura, M, et al: Follow-up study on F-wave in patients with lumbosacral radiculopathy: Comparison between before and after surgery. Electromyogr Clin Neurophysiol 36:207, 1996.
87. Hermens, HJ, et al: European Applications of Surface Electromyography. Second General SENIAM Workshop, Stockholm, 1997.
88. Hermens, HJ, et al: European Activities on Surface Electromyography. First General SENIAM Workshop, Torino, Italy, 1996.
89. Basmajian, JV, and Blumenstein, R: Electrode Placement for EMG Biofeedback. Williams & Wilkins, Baltimore, 1980.
90. Graham, GP: Reliability of electromyographic measurements after surface electrode removal and replacement. Percept Mot Skills 49:215, 1979.
91. Yang, JF, and Winter, DA: Electromyography reliability in maximal and submaximal isometric contractions. Arch Phys Med Rehabil 64:417, 1983.
92. Kadaba, MP, et al: Repeatability of phasic muscle activity: Performance of surface and intramuscular wire electrodes in gait analysis. J Orthop Res 3:350, 1985.
93. Viitasalo, JH, and Komi, PV: Signal characteristics of EMG with special reference to reproducibility of measurements. Acta Physiol Scand 93:531, 1975.

94. Winter, DA: The Biomechanics and Motor Control of Walking, ed 2. University of Waterloo Press, Waterloo, Canada, 1991.
95. Kellis, E: The effects of fatigue on the resultant joint moment, agonist and antagonist electromyographic activity at different angles during dynamic knee extension efforts. J Electromyogr Kinesiol 9:191, 1999.
96. MacIntyre, DL, and Robertson, DG: Quadriceps muscle activity in women runners with and without patellofemoral pain syndrome. Arch Phys Med Rehabil 73:10, 1992.
97. Perry, J, and Bekey, GA: EMG-force relationships in skeletal muscle. Crit Rev Biomed Eng 7:22, 1981.
98. Bonato, P: Time-frequency parameters of the surface myoelectric signal for assessing muscle fatigue during cyclic dynamic contractions. IEEE Trans Biomed Eng 48(7):745, 2001.
99. Winkel, J, and Bendix, T: Muscular performance during seated work evaluated by two different EMG methods. Eur J Appl Physiol 55:167, 1986.
100. Janda, DH, et al: Objective evaluation of grip strength. J Occup Med 29:569, 1987.
101. Knutson, LM, et al: A study of various normalization procedures for within day electromyographic data. J Electromyography Kinesiol 4:47, 1994.
102. Kellis, E, and Baltzopoulos, V: The effects of normalization method on antagonistic activity patterns during eccentric and concentric isokinetic knee extension and flexion. J Electromyogr Kinesiol 6:235, 1996.
103. Lippold, OCJ: The relation between integrated action potentials in a human muscle and its isometric tension. J Physiol (Lond) 117:492, 1952.
104. Inman, VT, et al: Relation of human electromyogram to muscular tension. Electroencephalogr Clin Neurophysiol 4:187, 1952.
105. Edwards, RG, and Lippold, OCJ: The relation between force and integrated electrical activity in fatigued muscle. J Physiol (Lond) 132:677, 1956.
106. Woods, JJ, and Bigland-Ritchie, B: Linear and non-linear surface EMG/force relationships in human muscles. Am J Phys Med Rehabil 62:287, 1983.
107. Vredenbregt, J, and Rau, G: Surface electromyography in relation to force, muscle length and endurance. In Desmedt, JE (ed): New Developments in Electromyography and Clinical Neurophysiology, Vol 1. Karger, Basel, 1973, p 606.
108. Zuniga, EN, and Simons, DG: Nonlinear relationship between averaged electromyogram potential and muscle tension in normal subjects. Arch Phys Med Rehabil 50:613, 1983.
109. Lawrence, JH, and DeLuca, CJ: Myoelectric signal vs. force relationship in different human muscles. J Appl Physiol 54:1653, 1983.
110. Bigland, B, and Lippold, OCJ: The relation between force, velocity and integrated electrical activity in human muscles. J Physiol (Lond) 123:214, 1954.
111. Petrofsky, JS, et al: Evaluation of the amplitude and frequency components of the surface EMG as an index of muscle fatigue. Ergonomics 25:213, 1982.
112. DeLuca, CJ: Myoelectrical manifestations of localized muscular fatigue in humans. Crit Rev Biomed Eng 11:251, 1985.
113. Kuorinka, I: Restitution of EMG spectrum after muscular fatigue. Eur J Appl Physiol 57:311, 1988.
114. Huijing, PA, et al: Triceps source EMG spectrum changes during sustained submaximal isometric contractions at different muscle lengths. Electromyogr Clin Neurophysiol 26:181, 1986.
115. Roy, SH, et al: Classification of back muscle impairment based on the surface electromyographical signal. J Rehabil Res Dev 34:405, 1997.
116. Roy, SH, et al: Spectral electromyographic assessment of back muscles in patients with low back pain undergoing rehabilitation. Spine 20:38, 1995.
117. Oddsson, LI, et al: Development of new protocols and analysis procedures for the assessment of LBP by surface EMG techniques. J Rehabil Res Dev 34:415, 1997.
118. Roy, SH, and Oddsson, LI: Classification of paraspinal muscle impairments by surface electromyography. Phys Ther 78:838, 1998.
119. Shimazu, H, et al: Rigidity and spasticity in man: Electromyographic analysis with reference to the role of the globus pallidus. Arch Neurol 6:10, 1962.
120. Vorro, J, and Hobart, D: Kinematic and myoelectric analysis of skill acquisition: I. 90cm subject group. Arch Phys Med Rehabil 62:575, 1981.
121. Hobart, DJ, et al: Modifications occurring during acquisition of a novel throwing task. Am J Phys Med 54:1, 1975.
122. Bernardi, M, et al: Force generation performance and motor unit recruitment strategy in muscles of contralateral limbs. J Electromyogr Kinesiol 9:121, 1999.
123. Bernardi, M, et al: Motor unit recruitment strategy changes with skill acquisition. Eur J Appl Physiol 74:52, 1996.
124. Santello, M, and McDonagh, MJ: The control of timing and amplitude of EMG activity in landing movements in humans. Exp Physiol 83:857, 1998.
125. Hefzy, MS, et al: Co-activation of the hamstrings and quadriceps during the lunge exercise. Biomed Sci Instrum 33:360, 1997.
126. Isear Jr, JA, et al: EMG analysis of lower extremity muscle recruitment patterns during an unloaded squat. Med Sci Sports Exerc 29:532, 1997.
127. Kellis, E: Quantification of quadriceps and hamstring antagonist activity. Sports Med 25:37, 1998.
128. Garland, SJ, et al: Motor unit activity during human single joint movements. J Neurophysiol 76:1982, 1996.
129. Lutz, GE, et al: Comparison of tibiofemoral joint forces during open-kinetic-chain and closed-kinetic-chain exercises. J Bone Joint Surg Am 75:732, 1993.
130. Escamilla, RF, et al: Biomechanics of the knee during closed kinetic chain and open kinetic chain exercises. Med Sci Sports Exerc 30:556, 1998.
131. Stiene, HA, et al: A comparison of closed kinetic chain and isokinetic joint isolation exercise in patients with patellofemoral dysfunction. J Orthop Sports Phys Ther 24:136, 1996.
132. Blackard, DO, et al: Use of EMG analysis in challenging kinetic chain terminology. Med Sci Sports Exerc 31:443, 1999.
133. Sporrong, H, et al: Hand grip increases shoulder muscle activity: An EMG analysis with static hand contractions in 9 subjects. Acta Orthop Scand 67:485, 1996.
134. Krebs, DE, et al: Hip biomechanics during gait. J Orthop Sports Phys Ther 28:51, 1998.
135. Levin, MF, and Hui-Chan, C: Ankle spasticity is inversely correlated with antagonist voluntary contraction in hemiparetic subjects. Electromyogr Clin Neurophysiol 34:415, 1994.
136. Gowland, C, et al: Agonist and antagonist activity during voluntary upper-limb movement in patients with stroke. Phys Ther 72:624, 1992.
137. Davies, JM, et al: Electrical and mechanical output of the knee muscles during isometric and isokinetic activity in stroke and healthy adults. Disabil Rehabil 18:83, 1996.
138. Madeleine, P, et al: Shoulder muscle co-ordination during chronic and acute experimental neck-shoulder pain: An occupational pain study. Eur J Appl Physiol 79:127, 1999.
139. Wadsworth, DJ, and Bullock-Saxton, JE: Recruitment patterns of the scapular rotator muscles in freestyle swimmers with subacromial impingement. Int J Sports Med 18:618, 1997.
140. Laprade, J, et al: Comparison of five isometric exercises in the recruitment of the vastus medialis oblique in persons with and without patellofemoral pain syndrome. J Orthop Sports Phys Ther 27:197, 1998.
141. Thomee, R, et al: Quadriceps muscle performance in sitting and standing in young women with patellofemoral pain syndrome and young healthy women. Scand J Med Sci Sports 6:233, 1996.
142. Karst, GM, and Willett, GM: Onset timing of electromyographic activity in the vastus medialis oblique and vastus lateralis muscles in subjects with and without patellofemoral pain syndrome. Phys Ther 75:813, 1995.
143. Werner, S, et al: Effect of taping the patella on concentric and eccentric torque and EMG of knee extensor and flexor muscles in patients with patellofemoral pain syndrome. Knee Surg Sports Traumatol Arthrosc 1:169, 1993.
144. Soderberg, GL, and Cook, TM: An electromyographic analysis of quadriceps femoris muscle setting and straight leg raising. Phys Ther 63:1434, 1983.
145. Soderberg, GL, et al: Electromyographic analysis of knee exercises in healthy subjects and in patients with knee pathologies. Phys Ther 67:1691, 1987.

146. Kankaanpaa, M, et al: Back and hip extensor fatigability in chronic low back pain patients and controls. Arch Phys Med Rehabil 79:412, 1998.
147. Mannion, AF, et al: The use of surface EMG power spectral analysis in the evaluation of back muscle function. J Rehabil Res Dev 34:427, 1997.
148. Roy, SH, et al: Lumbar muscle fatigue and chronic lower back pain. Spine 14:992, 1989.
149. Mooney, V, et al: Relationships between myoelectric activity, strength, and MRI of lumbar extensor muscles in back pain patients and normal subjects. J Spinal Disord 10:348, 1997.
150. Arendt-Nielsen, L, et al: The influence of low back pain on muscle activity and coordination during gait: A clinical and experimental study. Pain 64:231, 1996.
151. Fairbank, JC, et al: The Oswestry low back pain disability questionnaire. Physiotherapy 66:271, 1980.
152. DeLuca, CJ: Use of the surface EMG signal for performance evaluation of back muscles. Muscle Nerve 16:210, 1993.
153. Roy, SH, et al: Fatigue, recovery, and low back pain in varsity rowers. Med Sci Sports Exerc 22:463, 1990.
154. Society of Actuaries and Association of Life Insurance Medical Directors of America: Build Study, 1979. Metropolitan Life Insurance Company, New York, 1983.
155. Rainville, J, et al: Altering beliefs about pain and impairment in a functionally oriented treatment program for chronic low back pain. Clin J Pain 9:196, 1993.

Supplemental Readings

Aminoff, MJ: Electromyography in Clinical Practice, ed 3. Churchill Livingstone, New York, 1997.

Barboi, AC, and Barkhaus, PE: Electrodiagnostic testing in neuromuscular disorders. Neurol Clin 22(3):619.41, 2004.

Beck RB, et al: A technique to track individual motor unit action potentials in surface EMG by monitoring their conduction velocities and amplitudes. IEEE Trans Biomed Eng 52(4):622, 2005.

Chemali, KR, and Tsao, B: Electrodiagnostic testing of nerves and muscles: When, why, and how to order. Cleve Clin J Med 72(1):37, 2005.

Cho, SC, Siao Tick Chong, P, and So, YT: Clinical utility of electrodiagnostic consultation in suspected polyneuropathy. Muscle Nerve 30(5):659, 2004.

Daube JR: Electrodiagnostic studies in amyotrophic lateral sclerosis and other motor neuron disorders. Muscle Nerve 23(10):1488, 2000.

Haghighi, SS, Baradarian, S, and Bagheri, R: Sensory and motor evoked potentials findings in patients with thoracic outlet syndrome. Electromyogr Clin Neurophysiol 45(3):149, 2005

Havton, LA, Hotson, JR, and Kellerth, JO: Partial peripheral motor nerve lesions induce changes in the conduction properties of remaining intact motoneurons. Muscle Nerve 24(5): 662, 2001.

Kimura, J: Electrodiagnosis in Diseases of Nerve and Muscle: Principles and Practice. Oxford University Press, New York, 2001.

Lee, DH, Claussen, GC, and Oh, S: Clinical nerve conduction and needle electromyography studies. J Am Acad Orthop Surg 12(4):276, 2004.

Leis, AA, and Trapani, VC: Atalas of Electromyography. Oxford University Press, New York, 2000.

Lo, YL, et al: Pectoral nerve conduction studies: Technique in healthy subjects and evaluation of brachial plexopathy. Arch Phys Med Rehabil 86(8):1702, 2005.

Nandedkar, SD, et al: Some observations on fibrillations and positive sharp waves. Muscle Nerve 23(6):888, 2000.

Nelson, RM, Hayes, KW, and Currier, DP: Clinical Electrotherapy, ed 3. Appleton & Lange, Stamford, CT, 1999

Nobuta, S, et al: Clinical results in severe carpal tunnel syndrome and motor nerve conduction studies. J Orthop Sci 10(1):22, 2005

Perry, JD. Electrodiagnosis in musculo-skeletal disease. Best Pract Res Clin Rheumatol 9(3):453, 2005.

Puri, V, et al: Brachial plexopathy: A clinical and electrophysiological study. Electromyogr Clin Neurophysiol 44(4):229, 2004.

Rayegani, SM, et al: Palmar cutaneous branch of the median nerve conduction study. Electromyogr Clin Neurophysiol 45(1):29, 2005.

Shipe, C, and Zivkovic, SA: Electrodiagnostic evaluation of motor neuron disorders. Am J Electroneurodiagnostic Technol 44(1):30, 2004.

Wee, AS: Ulnar nerve stimulation at the palm in diagnosing distal ulnar nerve entrapment. Electromyogr Clin Neurophysiol 45(1):47, 2005.

CHAPTER

10

LEARNING OBJECTIVES

1. Define the terms used to describe normal gait.
2. Define reliability, validity, sensitivity, and specificity in relation to gait analysis.
3. Describe the variables that are examined in each of the following types of gait analyses: kinematic qualitative analysis, kinematic quantitative analysis, and kinetic analysis.
4. Describe and provide examples of some of the most commonly used types of gait profiles.
5. Compare and contrast the advantages and disadvantages of kinematic qualitative and kinematic quantitative gait analyses.
6. Using the case study example, apply clinical decision making skills in evaluating gait analysis data.

Examination of Gait

Cynthia C. Norkin, PT, EdD
With contributions by Sandra J. Olney, BSc (P&OT) MEd, PhD

OUTLINE

One of the major purposes of the rehabilitative process is to help patients achieve as high a level of functional independence as possible within the limits of their particular impairments. Human ambulation, or gait, is one of the basic components of independent function commonly affected by either disease processes or injury. Consequently, the desired outcome of most physical therapy interventions is to either restore or improve a patient's ambulatory status. Although there are many specific reasons for performing a gait analysis, all of them require some information about the gait performance of either an individual or a group of people with a particular disability. This information is needed to serve one or more of the following purposes that are applicable to either individual persons, or to a disability group: (1) to gain an understanding of the gait characteristics of a particular disorder; (2) to assist movement diagnosis; (3) to inform treatment selection; and (4) to evaluate the effectiveness of treatment. Because there are multiple approaches to gait analysis, ranging from very simple to extremely complex, the therapist must carefully consider how information obtained from a gait analysis is to be used. General as well as specific clinical indications for conducting a gait analysis may be found in the *Guide to Physical Therapist Practice,* some of which are included below.[1]

Purposes of Gait Analysis

1. To assist with understanding the gait characteristics of a particular disorder. This includes:
   - Obtaining accurate descriptions of gait patterns and gait variables typical of different conditions
   - Identifying and describing gait deviations present, or typically present in specific disorders
   - Determining balance, endurance, energy expenditure, and safety
   - Determining the functional ambulation capabilities of the patient in relation to functional ambulation demands of the home, community, and work environments
   - Classifying the severity of disability
   - Predicting a patient's future status
2. To assist with movement diagnosis by:
   - Identifying and describing gait deviations and describing the differences between a patient's performance and the parameters of normal gait
   - Analyzing gait deviations and identifying the mechanisms responsible for producing them
   - Examining balance, endurance, energy expenditure, and safety and determining their impact on gait
3. To inform selection of intervention(s) by guiding the therapist in:

- Proposing appropriate treatment of impairments that may improve gait performance
- Determining the need for adaptive, assistive, orthotic, prosthetic, protective, or supportive devices or equipment

4. To evaluate the effectiveness of treatment and guide the therapist in:
   - Determining how interventions such as therapeutic exercise, endurance activities, developmental activities, strengthening or stretching, electrical stimulation, balance training, surgical procedures, and medication will affect gait
   - Determining the effectiveness and fit of devices or equipment selected in providing joint protection and support, correcting deviations and dysfunctions, reducing energy expenditure, and promoting safe locomotive function.

Many examples illustrating these purposes are found in the literature: descriptions of the differences between a patient's performance and the parameters of normal gait,[2–11] identification of the mechanisms causing dysfunction,[12] determination of either the need for or the effectiveness of a prosthetic device,[12] comparison of the effects of different types of assistive devices,[13] determination of either the need for or the effectiveness of an orthotic device,[14–19] determination of the effects of treatment interventions,[20,21] determination of energy expenditure,[13] and prediction of future status.[22,23]

Selection of Approach to Gait Analysis

The type of gait analysis that is selected depends not only on the purpose of the analysis, but also on the type of equipment available and the experience, knowledge, and skills of the therapist. The type of equipment necessary for performing a specific type of gait analysis, in turn, depends on the purpose of the analysis, equipment availability, and the amount of time the therapist can expend. Equipment used in a gait analysis may be either as simple as a pencil, paper, and stopwatch,[24] or as complex as an electronic imaging system with force plates embedded in the floor.[25,26] To select the appropriate method, the therapist must be aware of the types of analyses available and be able to determine which methods are reliable and valid. Much of the information about gait characteristics of particular disorders, as well as the mechanisms responsible for producing them, has been achieved in clinical research settings using complex instrumentation often not available for general patient use. However, if a therapist understands the gait characteristics typical of a particular disorder, the mechanisms that are usually responsible, and the effectiveness of appropriate interventions, simpler gait analysis methods can be identified that may be even more useful in addressing specific purposes.

Regardless of the method, a gait analysis of individual patients should provide accurate, reliable, and valid data that can be used as a basis for describing present status (performance limitations and strengths), planning and implementing interventions, evaluating effectiveness and progress over time, evaluating outcomes, and in some instances, for predicting future status.

Reliability

Reliability, as applied to gait analysis, refers to the level of consistency of either a measuring instrument (e.g., footswitches, force plates, motion analysis systems, electrogoniometers) or a method of analysis (e.g., observational gait analysis checklists, ambulation profiles, and formulas for measuring stride length). To determine if a measuring instrument is reliable, the measurements obtained from successive and repeated use of the instrument must be consistent. For example, if an electrogoniometric measurement of a known angle of 60° consistently measures 60° on every Monday morning for 2 months, the instrument is said to be reliable. However, if the measurement obtained were 60° on the first Monday morning, 30° on the second and 40° on the third, the instrument would have very low reliability. Two types of reliability may be referred to: relative (association) or absolute (concordance). Relative reliability uses statistical techniques that are correlational[27]; they detect the existence of a relationship between sets of data. The statistical techniques used by absolute reliability can detect the magnitude of differences between measures.

Unlike more tightly controlled scientific conditions, the measures used in gait for determining reliability reflect all of the variability present in the measurement process. This includes trial-to-trial or day-to-day performance variation of the subject, as well as differences in the way the tester carries out the test. To make the best possible determination of the reliability of an instrument, one must rule out factors other than the instrument that could influence the measurement (e.g., that a subject has not injured a knee between successive measurements or that the placement of the instrument had not changed).

To determine whether an analysis method has both relative and absolute reliability, two different forms of reliability need to be determined: *intratester* and *intertester reliability.* The intratester reliability of an analysis method can be determined by examining the consistency of the results obtained when one individual uses a particular method repeatedly. For example, a therapist uses a particular method to examine a student physical therapist's gait. The therapist repeats the examination at 2-week intervals for 8 weeks and obtains the same results each time. In this instance, the method would be considered as having high intratester reliability because the results obtained by the same person are consistent over time. However, this example is strictly hypothetical, as factors other than the therapist's skill, such as fatigue, time of day, and other variables, may affect performance and must be controlled in any analysis.

Intertester reliability is determined by examining the consistency of the data obtained from repeated analyses performed by a number of different persons. If the results obtained by numerous examiners are in agreement both relatively and absolutely, and no significant differences in the results exist among testers, the method has high intertester reliability.

Sensitivity and Specificity

Sensitivity and specificity are important considerations when selecting a method of analysis. **Sensitivity**, as it relates to gait analysis, refers to the proportion of times that a method of analysis correctly identifies a gait abnormality or condition when that abnormality or condition is actually present. **Specificity** refers to the proportion of times that a method of analysis correctly identifies the abnormality as being absent when it truly is absent.[28] Additional information about these parameters will be available as more sophisticated statistical treatment of gait findings becomes common practice.

Validity

Validity refers to the degree that a measurement reflects what it is supposed to measure. There are several types of validity. They include:

- *Construct validity*—determined through logical argumentation based on theoretical research evidence (the ability of an instrument to measure an abstract concept or construct).
- *Content validity*—determined by providing evidence that the measuring instrument contains all relevant elements of a construct and no extraneous elements. In this instance, the test developer might justify the test by demonstrating that all items in the test were correlated with each other.
- *Criterion-based validity*—established by comparisons of either one instrument with another or with data obtained from other forms of testing.
- *Concurrent validity*—the inference is justified by comparisons between the results of a specific test (gait analysis) and another test (functional test) taken at approximately the same time.
- *Predictive validity*—validity is determined by the capability of the instrument to predict future events, such as falls.

It is difficult to imagine a method of measuring or analyzing gait that is not inherently valid for gait itself. However, gait is not a single construct, but a complex process that mirrors the complexity of human performance. Using a fairly simple approach, one can ask if a particular measure is valid for the specific purpose identified. Examining the tools described below, one may reflect on the purposes of gait analysis identified earlier, and ask if the tool being considered would be valid for that purpose.

By examining the literature, the therapist may determine if the reliability and validity of an instrument or method of analysis has been established. If the instrument or method has not been tested, therapists may wish to incorporate methods such as repeated testing within the context of a research study to confirm reliability.

Gait Terminology

The Gait Cycle

The largest unit used to describe gait is called a *gait cycle,* which has both spatial (distance) and temporal (time) parameters. In normal walking, a gait cycle begins when the heel of the reference extremity contacts the supporting surface and ends when the heel of the same extremity contacts the ground again. In some abnormal gaits, the heel may not be the first part of the foot to contact the ground, so the gait cycle may be considered to begin when some other portion of the reference extremity contacts the ground. The cycle ends when that same portion of the extremity contacts the ground again. The gait cycle is divided into two phases, *stance* and *swing,* and two periods of *double support.* In normal gait the *stance phase,* which constitutes 60 percent of the gait cycle, is defined as the interval in which the foot of the reference extremity is in contact with the ground. For example, if the right lower extremity (LE) is the reference extremity, the left LE will be in the swing phase when the right LE is in its stance phase. A single gait cycle contains right and left stance phases. The *swing phase,* which constitutes 40 percent of the gait cycle, is that portion in which the reference extremity does not contact the ground. Therefore, a single gait cycle includes both right and left swing phases. The term *double support time* refers to the two intervals in a gait cycle in which body weight is transferred from one foot to the other and both right and left feet are in contact with the ground at the same time (Fig. 10.1). Each of these variables may be measured in time, for example, *stance time* (right and left) *swing time* (right and left), *double support time,* and *cycle time.*

Two steps, a right step and a left step, comprise a *stride,* and a stride is equal to a gait cycle. *Step* and stride may be defined in two dimensions: distance and time. *Step length* is the distance from the point of heel strike of one extremity to the point of heel strike of the opposite extremity, whereas *stride length* is the distance from the point of heel strike of one extremity to the point of heel strike of the same extremity. *Stride time* and *step time* refer to the length of time required to complete a step and a stride, respectively (Fig. 10.2).

Phases of Gait

Traditionally, each phase of gait (stance and swing) has been divided into the following units: stance (heel strike, footflat, midstance, heel-off, and toe-off) and swing (acceleration, midswing, and deceleration). The Los Amigos Research and Education Institute, Inc. (LAREI) of Rancho Los Amigos National Rehabilitation Center has developed different terminology in which the subdivisions have been redefined and named as follows: stance (initial contact, loading response, midstance, terminal stance, and preswing) and swing (initial swing, midswing, and terminal swing).[29,30]

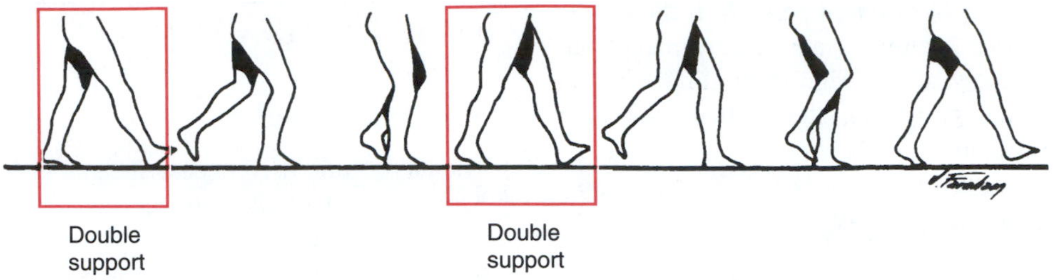

Figure 10.1 Double support is defined as the period in which some portion of the feet of both extremities are in contact with the supporting surface at the same time. Two periods of double support occur within the single gait cycle. One period occurs early in the stance phrase of the reference extremity and the other occurs late in the stance phase of the reference extremity. (From Levangie, P, and Norkin, C,[38, p 439] with permission.)

The similarities and differences between the two terminologies are presented in Table 10.1.

Angular rotations at the joints in each portion of both swing and stance phases, as well as muscle activity and function, are presented in Tables 10.2 to 10.7. Familiarity with ranges and patterns of motion associated with normal gait provides the therapist a basis of comparison to identify deviations from these normative standards. Familiarity with the muscle activity and function associated with normal gait allows the therapist to analyze causes of the deviations.

Types of Gait Analyses

The types of analyses in use today can be classified under two broad categories: **kinematic** and **kinetic**. Kinematic gait analysis is used to describe movement patterns without regard for the forces involved in producing the movement. A kinematic gait analysis consists of a description of movement of the body as a whole and/or body segments in relation to each other during gait. Kinematic gait analysis can be either *qualitative* or *quantitative*. Kinetic gait analysis is used to determine the forces involved in gait. In some instances, both kinematic and kinetic gait variables may be examined in one analysis. In addition to examining kinematic and kinetic variables, physiological variables such as heart rate, oxygen consumption, and energy cost may be considered.

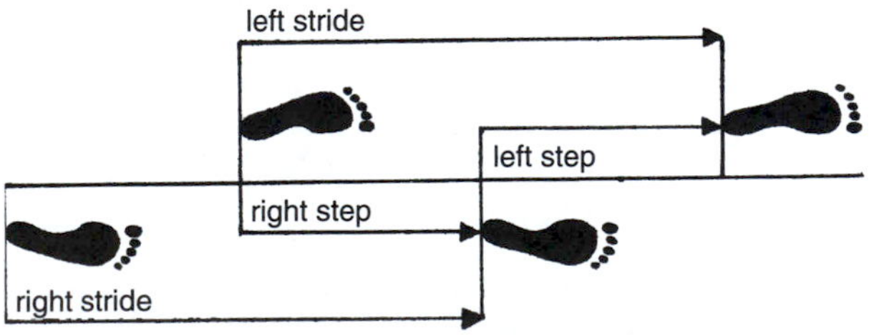

Figure 10.2 A right stride and a left stride. Right stride length is the distance between the point of contact of the right heel (at the lower left corner of the diagram) and the next contact of the right heel. Left stride length is the distance between the point of contact of the left heel (at the top left of the diagram) to the point of contact at the next left heel. Each stride contains two steps, but only both steps in the left stride are labeled. The left stride contains a right step and a left step. The right step length (shown in the middle of the diagram) is the distance between the left heel contact to the point of the right heel contact. Left step length is the distance between the right heel contact and the next left heel contact. Step and stride times refer to the amount of time required to complete a step and to complete stride, respectively.

Kinematic Qualitative Gait Analysis

The most common method used in clinical settings is a *qualitative gait analysis*. This method usually requires only a small amount of equipment and a minimal amount of time. The primary variable examined in a qualitative kinematic analysis is *displacement,* which includes a description of patterns of movement, deviations from normal body postures, and joint angles at specific points in the gait cycle.

Observational Gait Analysis (OGA)

The Rancho Los Amigos Observational Gait Analysis (OGA) system is probably the most common OGA system used by physical therapists.[29,30] Podiatrists have developed their own unique OGA system.[31] The Rancho Los Amigos OGA method involves a systematic examination of the movement patterns of the following body segments at each point in the gait cycle: ankle, foot, knee, hip, pelvis, and trunk. The system uses a recording form comprising 48 descriptors of common gait deviations such as toe drag, excessive plantarflexion and dorsiflexion, excessive varus or valgus at the knee or foot, hip hiking, and trunk flexion. The observing therapist must determine whether or not a deviation is present and note the occurrence and timing of the deviation on the special form.[30]

Considerable training and practice are necessary to develop the observational skills needed for performing any OGA. Therapists who wish to learn the Rancho method can learn independently by studying the Rancho Los Amigos Observational Gait Analysis Handbook.[30] Separate forms for recording gait analyses that focus on specific body areas such as the knee or hip are available as well as a form for a full body analysis, which is shown in Figure 10.3. Practice gait film strips useful for developing and improving one's observational skills as well as for learning how to use the recording forms may be obtained by writing to LAREI,

Table 10.1 Gait Terminology

Traditional	Rancho Los Amigos	Traditional	Rancho Los Amigos
Stance Phase		*Swing Phase*	
Heel strike: The beginning of the stance phase when the heel contacts the ground. The same as initial contact.	Initial contact: The beginning of the stance phase when the heel or another part of the foot contacts the ground.	Acceleration: The portion of beginning swing from the moment the toe of the reference extremity leaves the ground to the point when the reference extremity is directly under the body.	Initial swing: The portion of swing from the point when the reference extremity leaves the ground to maximum knee flexion of the same extremity.
Foot flat: Occurs immediately following heel strike, when the sole of the foot contacts the floor. This event occurs during loading response.	Loading response: The portion of the first double support period of the stance phase from initial contact until the contralateral extremity leaves the ground.	Midswing: Portion of the swing phase when the reference extremity passes directly below the body. Midswing extends from the end of acceleration to the beginning of deceleration.	Midswing: Portion of the swing phase from maximum knee flexion of the reference extremity to a vertical tibial position.
Midstance: The point at which the body passes directly over the reference extremity.	Midstance: The portion of the single limb support stance phase that begins when the contralateral extremity leaves the ground and ends when the body is directly over the supporting limb.	Deceleration: The swing portion of the swing phase when the reference extremity is decelerating in preparation for heel strike.	Terminal swing: The portion of the swing phase from a vertical position of the tibia of the reference extremity to just prior to initial contact.
Heel off: The point following midstance at which time the heel of the reference extremity leaves the ground. Heel off occurs prior to terminal stance.	Terminal stance: The last portion of the single limb support stance phase that begins with heel rise and continues until contralateral extremity contacts the ground.		
Toe off: The point following heel off when only the toe of the reference extremity is in contact with the ground.	Preswing: The portion of stance that begins the second double support period from the initial contact of the contralateral extremity to lift off of the reference extremity.		

Rancho Los Amigos National Rehabilitation Center, 7601 East Imperial Highway, Downey, CA 90242.

A biomechanical gait analysis form for podiatrists, described by Southerland,[31] is presented in Figure 10.4. This form is used in conjunction with a static quantitative analysis which includes measurements of range of motion (ROM) of all joints from the hip to the toes, as well as measurements of limb length. Detailed information is also collected on both the dorsal and plantar surfaces of the feet such as callus formation and corns. The examiner is expected to document abnormalities such as hallux valgus and hammer toes. The dynamic qualitative component of the analysis uses a shorthand system for recording the details of the OGA. The acronym GHORT (gait, homunculus, observed, relational, and tabular) is used to assist in recording information gathered from the observational analysis (Fig. 10.5). An example of the recording method is shown in Figure 10.6. Following completion of the dynamic portion, the rater's qualitative impressions of the patient's gait are compared with the results of the static analysis to verify the accuracy of the findings and determination of the causes of abnormal function. The author states that after the first five analyses, a new rater's results are the same or similar to other raters; however, the author did not reference any reliability and/or validity studies.[31] In general, these protocols provide the therapist with a systematic approach to OGA by directing the observer's attention to a specific joint or body segment during a given point in the gait cycle.

The advantages of OGAs are that they require little or no instrumentation, are inexpensive to use, and can yield general descriptions of gait variables. The disadvantages

Table 10.2 Ankle and Foot: Stance Phase, Sagittal Plane Analysis

Portion of Phase	Normal Motion[30]	Normal Moment	Normal Muscle Activity	Result of Weakness	Possible Compensation
Heel strike to foot flat	0–15 degrees plantarflexion	Plantarflexion	Pretibial group acts eccentrically to oppose plantarflexion moment and thereby to prevent foot slap by controlling plantarflexion.	Lack of ability to oppose the plantarflexion moment causes the foot to slap the floor.	To avoid foot slap and to eliminate the plantarflexion moment, the foot may be placed flat on the floor or placed with the toes first at initial contact.
Foot flat through midstance	15 degrees plantarflexion to 10 degrees dorsiflexion	Plantarflexion to dorsiflexion	Gastrocnemius and soleus act eccentrically to oppose the dorsiflexion moment and to control tibial advance.	Excessive dorsiflexion and uncontrolled tibial advance.	To avoid excessive dorsiflexion, the ankle may be maintained in plantarflexion.
Midstance to heel off	10–15 degrees dorsiflexion	Dorsiflexion	Gastrocnemius and soleus contract eccentrically to oppose the dorsiflexion moment and control tibial advance.	Excessive dorsiflexion and uncontrolled forward motion of tibia.	The ankle may be maintained in plantarflexion. If the foot is flat on the floor, the dorsiflexion moment is eliminated and a step-to gait is produced.
Heel off to toe off	15 degrees dorsiflexion to 20 degrees plantarflexion	Dorsiflexion	Gastrocnemius, soleus, peroneus brevis, peroneus longus, flexor hallicus longus contract to plantarflex the foot.	No roll off. Decreased contralateral step.	Whole foot is lifted off the ground.

Table 10.3 Ankle and Foot: Swing Phase, Sagittal Plane Analysis

Portion of Phase	Normal Motion	Normal Moment	Normal Muscle Action	Result of Weakness	Possible Compensation
Acceleration to midswing	Dorsiflexion to neutral	None	Dorsiflexors contract to bring the ankle into neutral and to prevent the toes from dragging on the floor.	Foot drop and/or toe dragging.	Hip and knee flexion may be increased to prevent toe drag, or the hip may be hiked or circumducted. Sometimes vaulting on the contralateral limb may occur.
Midswing to deceleration	Neutral	None	Dorsiflexion	Foot drop and/or toe dragging.	Hip and knee flexion may be increased to prevent toe drag. The swing leg may be circumducted, or vaulting may occur on the contralateral side.

Table 10.4 Knee: Stance Phase, Sagittal Plane Analysis

Portion of Phase	Normal Motion	Normal Moment	Normal Muscle Action	Result of Weakness	Possible Compensation
Heel strike to foot flat	Flexion 0–15°	Flexion	Quadriceps contracts initially to hold the knee in extension and then eccentrically to oppose the flexion moment and control the amount of flexion.	Excessive knee flexion because the quadriceps cannot oppose the flexion moment.	Plantarflexion at ankle so that foot flat instead of heel strike occurs. Plantarflexion eliminates the flexion moment. Trunk lean forward eliminates the flexion moment at knee and therefore may be used to compensate for quadriceps weakness.
Foot flat through midstance	Extension 15–5°	Flexion to extension	Quadriceps contracts in early part, and then no activity is required.	Excessive knee flexion initially.	Same as above in early part of midstance. No compensation required in later part of phase.
Midstance to heel off	5° of flexion to 0° (neutral)	Flexion to extension	No activity required.		None required.
Heel off to toe off	0–40° flexion	Extension to flexion	Quadriceps required to control amount of knee flexion.		

are that the observational method, being dependent on both the therapist's training and observational skills, is subjective, has only low to moderate reliability, and validity has not been demonstrated.[32] Difficulties involved in observing and making accurate judgments about motions occurring simultaneously at numerous body segments, and inadequate training in OGA methods are thought to contribute to the low reliability. Also, therapists differ in their observational skills. A drawback to using the Rancho Los Amigos OGA technique is that reliability and validity of the method have not been published.

If therapists decide to use an OGA method, they should seriously consider using a camcorder that has the capability of slowing or stopping motion. A visual record is especially important when using the Rancho Los Amigos format because of the time involved in examining a large number of variables at six different body parts. Most patients cannot walk continuously for the length of time required to complete a detailed, full-body observational analysis. Furthermore, the observers cannot rate or score a large number of variables while a subject is walking. Videotape records of a patient's initial performance

Table 10.5 Knee: Swing Phase, Sagittal Plane Analysis

Portion of Phase	Normal Motion	Normal Moment	Normal Muscle Action	Result of Weakness	Possible Compensation
Accleration to midswing	40–60° flexion	None	Little or no activity in quadriceps. Biceps femoris (short head), gracilis, and sartorius contract concentrically.	Inadequate knee flexion.	Increased hip flexion, circumduction, or hiking.
Midswing	60–30° extension	None			
Deceleration	30–0° extension	None	Quadriceps contracts concentrically to stabilize knee in extension, in preparation for heel strike.	Inadequate knee extension.	

Table 10.6 Hip: Stance Phase, Sagittal Plane Analysis

Portion of Phase	Normal Motion	Normal Moment	Normal Muscle Action	Result of Weakness	Possible Compensation
Heel strike to foot flat	30° flexion	Flexion	Erector spinae, gluteus maximus, hamstrings.	Excessive hip flexion and anterior pelvis tilt owing to inability to counteract flexion moment.	Trunk leans backward to prevent excessive hip flexion and to eliminate the hip flexion moment.
Foot flat through midstance	30° flexion to 5° (neutral)	Flexion to extension	Gluteus maximus at beginning of period to oppose flexion moment, then activity ceases as moment changes from flexion to extension.	At the beginning of the period, excessive hip flexion and anterior pelvic tilt owing to inability to counteract flexion moment.	At beginning of the period, subject may lean trunk backward to prevent excessive hip flexion; however, once the flexion moment changes to an extension moment, the subject no longer needs to incline the trunk backward.
Midstance to heel-off		Extension	No activity.	None.	None required.
Heel-off to toe-off	10° of hyperextension to neutral	Extension	Illiopsoas, adductor, magnus, and adductor longus.	Undetermined.	Undetermined.

that can be replayed in slow motion allow therapists the time needed to make judgments about gait events.

Although the use of videotape may provide an opportunity for the observers to determine the reliability of their scoring, reliability will probably remain in the low to moderate range unless therapists are knowledgeable about normal gait parameters and variables, and are adequately trained to use the measuring instrument. Russell et al[33] found that when observers were trained in the scoring of a Gross Motor Function Measure (GMFM), a significant improvement occurred following training compared with the observers' pretraining scoring of the videotape. On the other hand, Eastlack et al[34] found only low to moderate interrater reliability among 54 practicing physical therapists who rated 10 gait variables while observing the videotaped gait of three patients. These therapists had reported they were comfortable performing observational gait analyses. The lack of agreement among raters found in this study, as well as the rater's lack of knowledge of normal gait parameters and terminology, has serious implications for patient treatments based on the results of observational gait analyses.[34] Krebs[35] argues that OGA is impossible to perform in a clinical setting. However, in a recent study using OGA, physical therapists were able to make accurate and reliable judgments of scored push-off power in the videotaped gait of subjects following stroke. This study suggests that focused analysis on specific gait parameters may be more reliable than general analyses.[36]

If OGA is used, it should be used in conjunction with quantitative measures. Videotape or film can provide a permanent record of the patient's gait. Videography may also

Table 10.7 Hip: Swing Phase, Sagittal Plane Analysis

Portion of Phase	Normal Motion	Normal Moment	Normal Muscle Activity	Result of Weakness	Possible Compensation
Acceleration to midswing	20–30° flexion	None	Hip flexor activity to initiate swing illiopsoas, rectus, femoris, gracilis, sartorius, tensor fascia lata.	Diminished hip flexion causing an inability to initiate the normal forward movement of the extremity and to raise the foot off the floor.	Circumduction and/or hip hiking may be used to bring the leg forward and to raise the foot high enough to clear the floor.
Midswing to deceleration	30° flexion to neutral	None	Hamstrings.	A lack of control of the swinging leg. Inability to place limb in position for heel strike.	

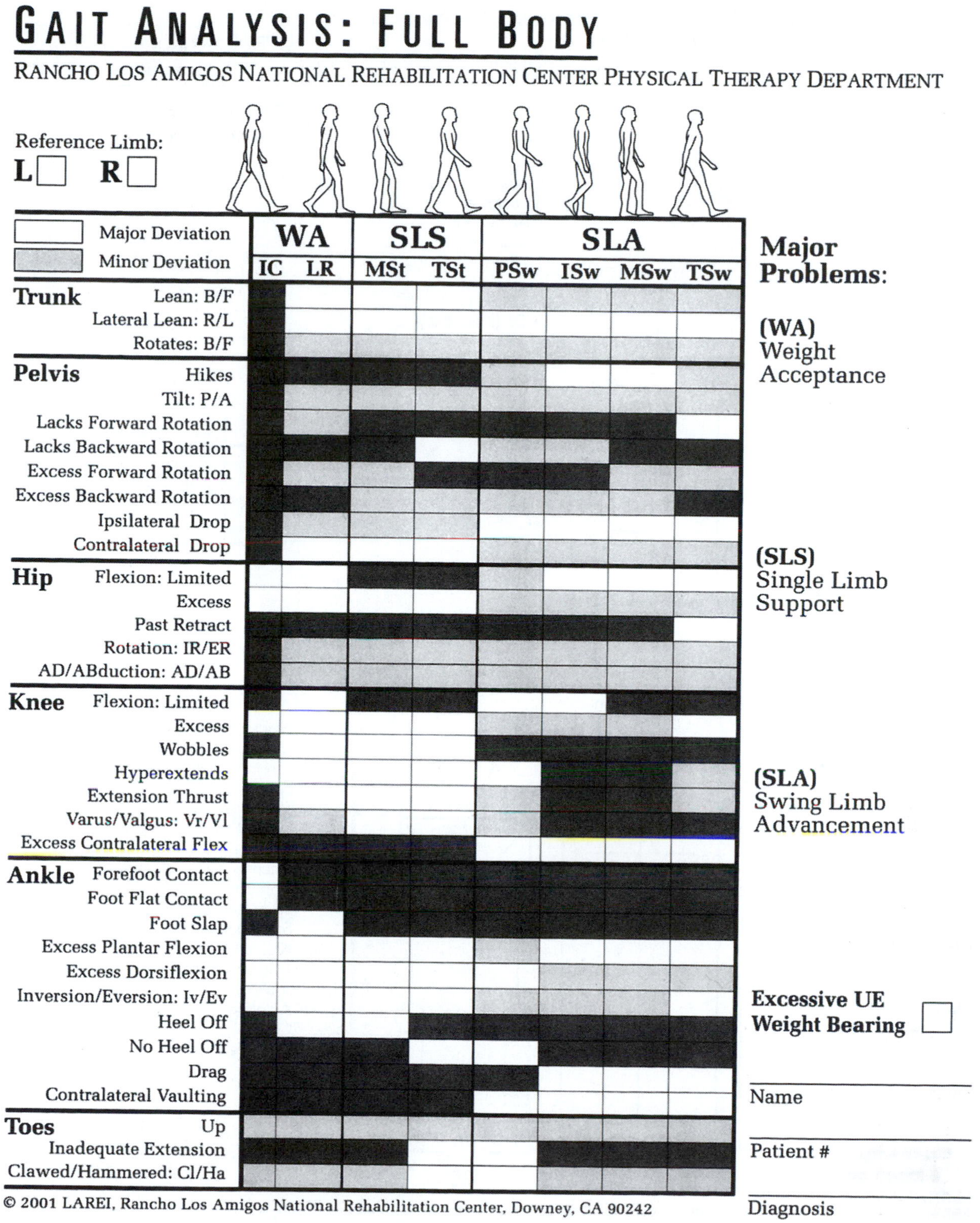
GAIT ANALYSIS: FULL BODY
RANCHO LOS AMIGOS NATIONAL REHABILITATION CENTER PHYSICAL THERAPY DEPARTMENT
Reference Limb:
L R
Major Deviation
Minor Deviation
WA
SLS
SLA
IC LR
MSt TSt
PSw ISw MSw TSw
Trunk
Lean: B/F
Lateral Lean: R/L
Rotates: B/F
Pelvis
Hikes
Tilt: P/A
Lacks Forward Rotation
Lacks Backward Rotation
Excess Forward Rotation
Excess Backward Rotation
Ipsilateral Drop
Contralateral Drop
Hip
Flexion: Limited
Excess
Past Retract
Rotation: IR/ER
AD/ABduction: AD/AB
Knee
Flexion: Limited
Excess
Wobbles
Hyperextends
Extension Thrust
Varus/Valgus: Vr/Vl
Excess Contralateral Flex
Ankle
Forefoot Contact
Foot Flat Contact
Foot Slap
Excess Plantar Flexion
Excess Dorsiflexion
Inversion/Eversion: Iv/Ev
Heel Off
No Heel Off
Drag
Contralateral Vaulting
Toes
Up
Inadequate Extension
Clawed/Hammered: Cl/Ha
Major Problems:
(WA) Weight Acceptance
(SLS) Single Limb Support
(SLA) Swing Limb Advancement
Excessive UE Weight Bearing
Name
Patient #
Diagnosis
© 2001 LAREI, Rancho Los Amigos National Rehabilitation Center, Downey, CA 90242

Figure 10.3 Full Body Gait Analysis Form. (From Observational Gait Analysis Handbook,[30] with permission.)

be used to examine joint ROM at the hip, knee, and ankle, by taking goniometric measurements directly from the screen. Stuberg et al[37] found no significant differences between goniometric measurements taken from videotaped gait and measurements taken from film for 10 children with cerebral palsy and 9 normal children. Examples of the process involved in an OGA will be presented in the following section.

Examination of Variables

The purpose of this section is to introduce the process involved in an OGA. The first step in the process involves

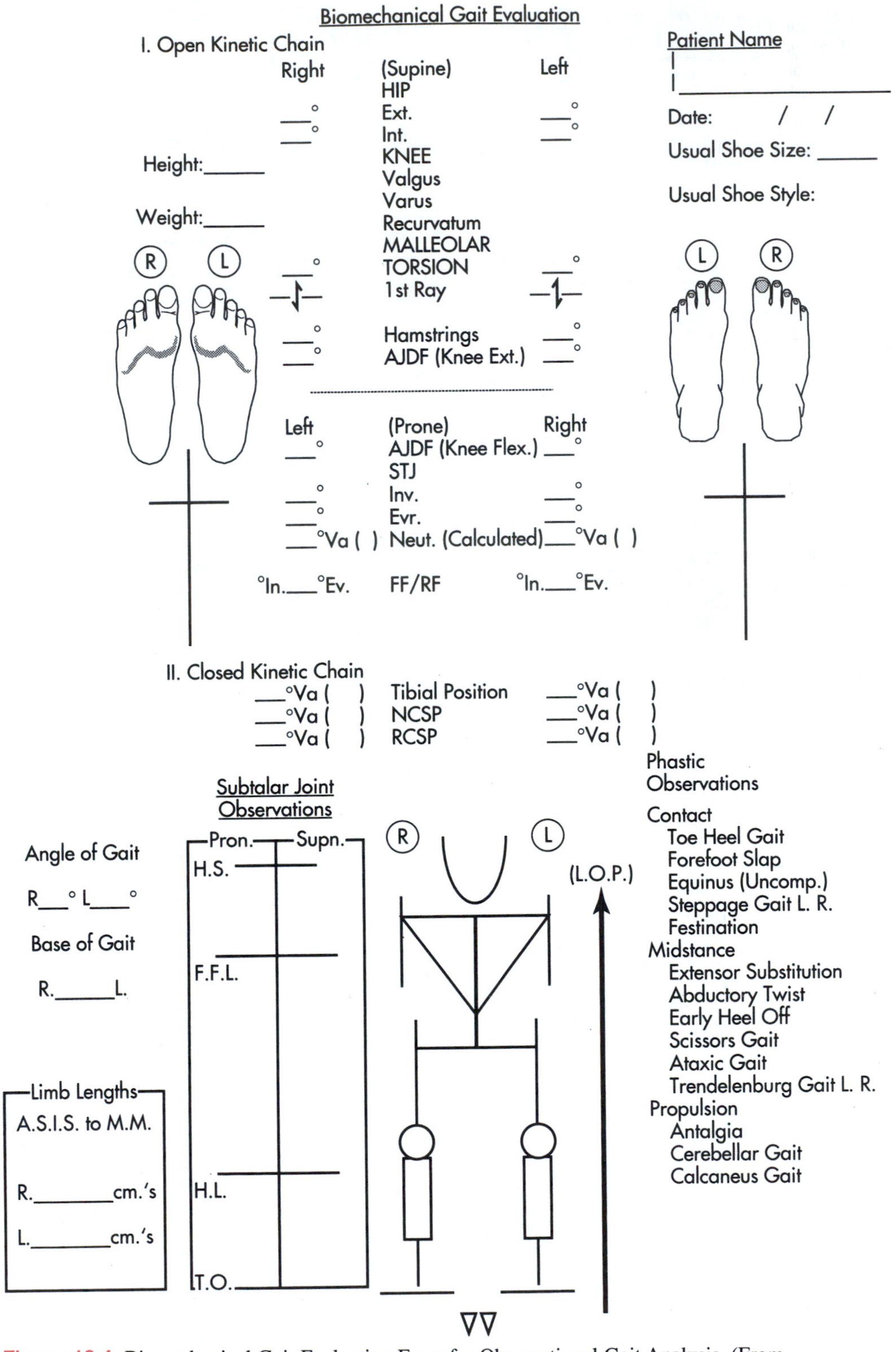

Figure 10.4 Biomechanical Gait Evaluation Form for Observational Gait Analysis. (From Sutherland, CC,[31, p 155] with permission.)

the identification and accurate description of the patient's gait pattern and any existing deviations. The second step involves a determination of the causes of the deviations. To properly identify and describe a patient's gait, the therapist must have good knowledge of gait terminology and an accurate mental picture of normal gait postures and normal displacements of the body segments in each portion of the two phases of gait, and in each plane of analysis (sagittal, coronal, and transverse). To determine the causes of a patient's gait pattern and specific deviations, the therapist must

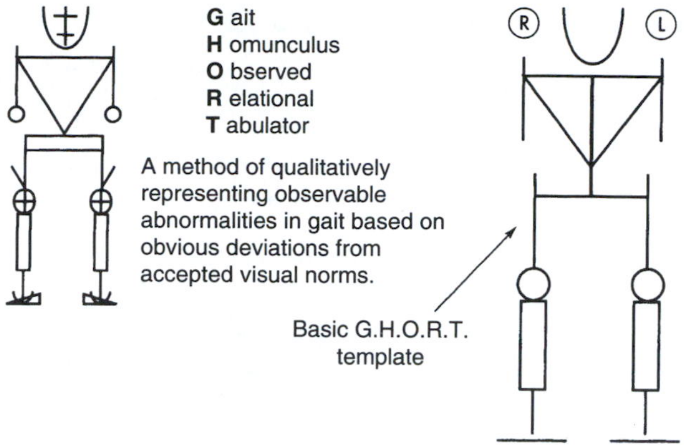

G ait
H omunculus
O bserved
R elational
T abulator
A method of qualitatively representing observable abnormalities in gait based on obvious deviations from accepted visual norms.
Basic G.H.O.R.T. template
R
L

Figure 10.5 GHORT. (From Sutherland, CC,[31, p 159] with permission.)

understand the normal roles and functions of muscles during gait and the normal forces involved.[26,29,38] Deviations from normal occur because of an inability to perform the tasks of walking in a normal fashion. For example, a patient with paralysis of the dorsiflexors (which causes a foot drop) cannot attain the normal neutral position of the ankle necessary to complete the task of clearing the floor during the swing phase. Therefore, the patient must find some other method of clearing the floor. The patient could compensate for the inability to dorsiflex the ankle by some method such as increasing the amount of hip and knee flexion above the normal amount, by circumduction of the entire limb, or by hiking the hip. The type of compensation that a particular individual selects depends on the specific disability. Increased hip and knee flexion may be used if the patient has an isolated problem in the ankle and adequate muscle strength and ROM in the extremity. Circumduction or hip hiking may be used if the patient has either a stiff knee or extensor thrust,

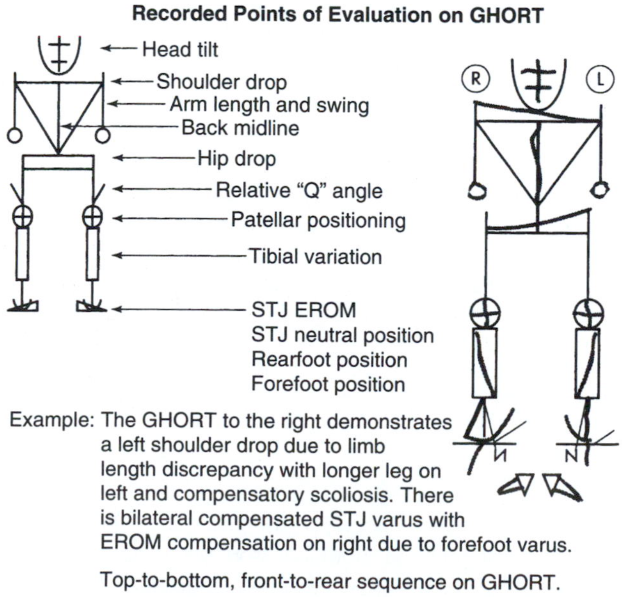

Shoulder drop
Arm length and swing
Back midline

Relative "Q" angle
Patellar positioning
Tibial variation

Rearfoot position
Forefoot position
Example: The GHORT to the right demonstrates a left shoulder drop due to limb length discrepancy with longer leg on left and compensatory scoliosis. There is bilateral compensated STJ varus with EROM compensation on right due to forefoot varus.
Top-to-bottom, front-to-rear sequence on GHORT.

Figure 10.6 Recording points of Evaluation on GHORT. (From Sutherland, CC,[31, p 164] with permission.)

which prevents use of increased knee flexion to raise the plantarflexed foot above the floor.[6] The therapist must be aware that patients may use a variety of methods to compensate for joint or muscle deficits.

Review of Kinematic and Kinetic Parameters of Normal Gait

Tables 10.2 to 10.7 provide a review of the normal sagittal plane joint displacements, moments of force, and muscle activity and function, as well as the results of isolated muscle weaknesses and possible compensations. Tables 10.8 to 10.14 present some of the common deviations observed in a sagittal plane analysis and probable causes for the deviations. Tables 10.15 and 10.16 provide sample gait analysis recording forms. If the reader decides to use the gait analysis recording forms presented in this text, reliability tests should be conducted because these forms are presented only as guides and have not been evaluated.

In Tables 10.2 to 10.7, the phase of gait, the normal joint displacements, moments of force, and muscle activity are presented in the first four columns, and the effects of muscle weakness and possible compensations are presented in the last two columns (the reader should be aware that only the effects of isolated muscle weaknesses and associated compensations are presented). The purpose of the tables is to identify components of normal gait that must be considered when observing gait and to provide an example of how to proceed with an analysis of the causes of an atypical gait pattern or particular deviation.

Tables 10.8 to 10.14 present some of the common gait deviations, as well as possible causes and analyses. Notice that the sample recording form presented in Table 10.16 is formatted in the same manner as Tables 10.8 to 10.14. Therefore, the clinician can use the sample analyses presented in the tables as guides.

Directions for Performing an OGA

Directions for performing an OGA for the sagittal and coronal planes are presented below.

1. Select the area in which the patient will walk and measure the distance that you want the patient to cover.
2. Position yourself to allow an unobstructed view of the subject. If filming, the cameras should be positioned to view the patient's LEs and feet as well as the head and trunk from both the sagittal and coronal perspectives.
3. Select the joint or segment to be observed first (e.g., ankle and foot), and mentally review the normal displacement patterns and muscle functions.
4. Select either a sagittal plane observation (view from the side) or a coronal plane observation (view from the front and/or back).
5. Observe the selected segment during the initial part of the stance phase and make a decision about the position of the segment. Note any deviations from the normal pattern.
6. Observe either the same segment during the next part of the stance phase or another segment at the initial part of

Table 10.8 Common Deviations, Ankle and Foot: Stance Phase, Sagittal Plane Analysis

Portion of Phase	Deviation	Description	Possible Causes	Analysis
Initial contact	Foot slap	At heel strike, forefoot slaps the ground.	Flaccid or weak dorsiflexors or reciprocal inhibition of dorsiflexors; atrophy of dorsiflexors.	Look for low muscle tone at ankle. Look for steppage gait (excessive hip and knee flexion) in swing phase.
	Toes first	Toes contact ground instead of heel. The tip-toe posture may be maintained throughout the phase, or the heel may contact the ground.	Leg length discrepancy; contracted heel cord; plantarflexion contraction; spasticity of plantarflexors; flaccidity of dorsiflexors; painful heel.	Compare leg lengths and look for hip and/or knee flexion contractures. Analyze muscle tone and timing of activity in plantarflexors. Check for pain in heel.
	Foot flat	Entire foot contacts the ground at heel strike.	Excessive fixed dorsiflexion; flaccid or weak dorsiflexors; neonatal/proprioceptive walking.	Check range of motion at ankle. Check for hyperextension at the knee and persistence of immature gait pattern.
Midstance	Excessive positional plantarflexion	Tibia does not advance to neutral from 10 degrees plantarflexion.	No eccentric contraction of plantarflexors; could be due to flaccidity/weakness in plantarflexors; surgical overrelease, rupture, or contracture of Achilles tendon.	Check for spastic or weak quadriceps; hyperextension at the knee; hip hyperextension; backward- or forward-leaning trunk. Check for weakness in plantarflexors or rupture of Achilles tendon.
	Heel lift in midstance	Heel does not contact ground in midstance.	Spasticity of plantarflexors.	Check for spasticity in plantarflexors, quadriceps, hip flexors, and adductors.
	Excessive positional dorsiflexion	Tibia advances too rapidly over the foot, creating a greater than normal amount of dorsiflexion.	Inability of plantarflexors to control tibial advance. Knee flexion or hip flexion contractures.	Look at ankle muscles, knee and hip flexors, range of motion, and position of trunk.
	Toe clawing	Toes flex and "grab" floor.	Could be due to a plantar grasp reflex that is only partially integrated; could be due to positive supporting reflex; spastic toe flexors.	Check plantar grasp reflex, positive supporting reflexes, and range of motion of toes.
Push-off (heel-off to toe-off)	No roll-off	Insufficient transfer of weight from lateral heel to medial forefoot.	Mechanical fixation of ankle and foot. Flaccidity or inhibition of plantarflexors, inverters, and toe flexors. Rigidity/cocontraction of plantarflexors and dorsiflexors. Pain in forefoot.	Check range of motion at ankle and foot. Check muscle function and tone at ankle. Look at dissociation between posterior foot and forefoot.

the stance phase. Progress through the same process as in number 5.

7. Repeat the process described in number 6 until you have completed an observation of all segments in the sagittal and coronal planes. Remember to concentrate on one segment at a time in one part of the gait cycle. Do not jump from one segment to another or from one phase to another.
8. Always perform observations on both sides (right and left). Although only one side may be involved pathologically, the other side of the body may be affected.

Table 10.9 Common Deviations, Ankle and Foot: Swing Phase, Sagittal Plane Analysis

Portion of Phase	Deviation	Description	Possible Causes	Analysis
Swing	Toe drag	Insufficient dorsiflexion (and toe extension) so that forefoot and toes do not clear floor.	Flaccidity or weakness of dorsiflexors and toe extensors. Spasticity of plantarflexors. Inadequate knee or hip flexion.	Check for ankle, hip, and knee range of motion. Check for strength and muscle tone at hip, knee, and ankle.
	Varus	The foot is excessively inverted.	Spasticity of the invertors. Flaccidity or weakness of dorsiflexors and evertors. Extensor pattern.	Check for muscle tone invertors and plantarflexors. Check strength of dorsiflexors and evertors. Check for extensor pattern of the lower extremity.

Table 10.10 Common Deviations, Knee: Stance Phase, Sagittal Plane Analysis

Portion of Phase	Deviation	Description	Possible Causes	Analysis
Initial contact (heel strike)	Excessive knee flexion	Knee flexes or "buckles" rather than extends as foot contacts ground.	Painful knee; spasticity of knee flexors or weak or flaccid quadriceps. Short leg on contralateral side.	Check for pain at knee; tone of knee flexors; strength of knee extensors; leg lengths; anterior pelvic tilt.
Foot flat	Knee hyperextension (genu recurvatum)	A greater than normal extension at the knee.	Flaccid/weak quadriceps and soleus compensated for by pull of gluteus maximus. Spasticity of quadriceps. Accommodation to a fixed ankle plantarflexion deformity.	Check for strength and muscle tone of knee and ankle flexors, and range of motion at ankle.
Midstance	Knee hyperextension (genu recurvatum)	During single limb support, tibia remains in back of ankle mortice as body weight moves over foot. Ankle is plantarflexed.	Same as above.	Same as above.
Push-off (heel-off to toe-off)	Excessive knee flexion	Knee flexes to more than 40° during push-off.	Center of gravity is unusually far forward of pelvis. Could be due to rigid trunk, knee/hip flexion contractures; flexion-withdrawal reflex; dominance of flexion synergy in middle recovery from CVA.	Look at trunk posture, knee and hip range of motion, and flexor synergy.
	Limited knee flexion	The normal amount of knee flexion (40°) does not occur.	Spastic/overactive quadriceps and/or plantarflexors.	Look at tone in hip, knee, and ankle muscles.

CVA = cerebrovascular accident.

Table 10.11 Common Deviations, Knee: Swing Phase, Sagittal Plane Analysis

Portion of Phase	Deviation	Description	Possible Causes	Analysis
Acceleration to midswing	Excessive knee flexion	Knee flexes more than 65°	Diminished preswing knee flexion, flexor-withdrawal reflex, dysmetria.	Look at muscle tone in hip, knee, and ankle. Test for reflexes and dysmetria.
	Limited knee flexion	Knee does not flex to 65°	Pain in knee, diminished range of knee motion, extensor spasticity. Circumduction at the hip.	Assess for pain in knee and knee range of motion. Test muscle tone at knee and hip.

An additional (blank) sample recording form for OGA is presented in Appendix A. Another (completed) sample recording form for OGA is presented in Appendix B with therapist entries as they might appear following completion of the gait analysis.

OGA in Neuromuscular Disorders

The gait patterns of individuals with neuromuscular deficits are influenced primarily by abnormalities in muscle tone and synergistic organization, influences of nonintegrated early reflexes, and a decrease in influence of righting and

Table 10.12 Common Deviations, Hip: Stance Phase, Sagittal Plane Analysis

Portion of Phase	Deviation	Description	Possible Causes	Analysis
Heel strike to foot flat	Excessive flexion	Flexion exceeding 30°	Hip and/or knee flexion contractures. Knee flexion caused by weak soleus and quadriceps. Hypertonicity of hip flexors.	Check hip and knee range of motion and strength of soleus and quadriceps. Check tone of hip flexors.
Heel strike to foot flat	Limited hip flexion	Hip flexion does not attain 30°	Weakness of hip flexors. Limited range of hip flexion. Gluteus maximus weakness.	Check strength of hip flexors and extensors. Analyze range of hip motion.
Foot flat to midstance	Limited hip extension	The hip does not attain a neutral position.	Hip flexion contracture, spasticity in hip flexors.	Check hip range of motion and tone of hip muscles.
	Internal rotation	An internally rotated position of the extremity.	Spasticity of internal rotators. Weakness of external rotators. Excessive forward rotation of opposite pelvis.	Check tone of internal rotators and strength of external rotators. Measure range of motion at both hip joints.
	External rotation	An externally rotated position of the extremity.	Excessive backward rotation of opposite pelvis.	Assess range of motion at both hip joints.
	Abduction	An abducted position of the extremity.	Contracture of the gluteus medius. Trunk lateral lean over the ipsilateral hip.	Check for abduction pattern.
	Adduction	An adducted position of the lower extremity.	Spasticity of hip flexors and adductors such as seen in spastic diplegia. Pelvic drop to contralateral side.	Assess tone of hip flexors and adductors. Test muscle strength of hip abductors.

Table 10.13 Common Deviations, Hip: Swing Phase, Sagittal Plane Analysis

Portion of Phase	Deviation	Description	Possible Causes	Analysis
Swing	Circumduction	A lateral circular movement of the entire lower extremity consisting of abduction, external rotation, adduction, and internal rotation.	A compensation for weak hip flexors or a compensation for the inability to shorten the leg so that it can clear the floor.	Check strength of hip flexors, knee flexors, and ankle dorsiflexors. Check range of motion in hip flexion, knee flexion, and ankle dorsiflexion. Check for extensor pattern.
	Hip hiking	Shortening of the swing leg by action of the quadratus lumborum.	A compensation for lack of knee flexion and/or ankle dorsiflexion. Also may be a compensation for extensor spasticity of swing leg.	Check strength and range of motion at knee, hip, and ankle. Also check muscle tone at knee and ankle.
	Excessive hip flexion	Flexion greater than 20–30 degrees.	Attempt to shorten extremity in presence of foot drop. Flexor pattern.	Check strength and range of motion at ankle and foot. Check for flexor pattern.

balance reactions, dissociation among body parts, and incoordination. If proximal stability (co-contraction of the postural muscles of the trunk) is threatened by atypically low, high, or fluctuating muscle tone, controlled mobility is lost. In gait, a loss of control over the sequential timing of muscular activity may result in asymmetrical step and stride lengths. In addition, deviations from normal posture and motion may occur such as forward or backward trunk leaning, excessive flexion or extension at the hip and knee in the stance phase, and diminished dorsiflexion or excessive plantarflexion.

In the presence of multiple muscle involvement or neurological deficits that affect balance, coordination, and muscle tone, the deviations observed and the analysis of

Table 10.14 Common Deviations, Trunk: Stance, Sagittal Plane Analysis

Portion of Phase	Deviation	Description	Possible Causes	Analysis
Stance	Lateral trunk lean	A lean of the trunk over the stance extremity (gluteus medius gait/Trendelenburg gait).	A weak or paralyzed gluteus medius on the stance side cannot prevent a drop of pelvis on the swing side, so a trunk lean over the stance leg helps compensate for the weak muscle. A lateral trunk lean over the affected hip also may be used to reduce force on hip if a patient has a painful hip.	Check strength of gluteus medius and assess for pain in the hip.
	Backward trunk lean	A backward leaning of the trunk, resulting in hyperextension at the hip (gluteus maximus gait).	Weakness or paralysis of the gluteus maximus on the stance leg. Anteriorly rotated pelvis.	Check for strength of hip extensors. Check pelvic position.
	Forward trunk lean	A forward leaning of the trunk, resulting in hip flexion.	Compensation for quadriceps weakness. The forward lean eliminates the flexion moment at the knee. Hip and knee flexion contractures.	Check for strength of quadriceps.
		A forward flexion of the upper trunk.	Posteriorly rotated pelvis.	Check pelvic position.

Table 10.15 Gait Analysis Recording Form

Fixed Postures Observed During Gait					
Patient's Name		**Age**		**Sex**	
Head	Tilt	To the right	________	To the left	________
		Forward	________	Backward	________
Trunk	Lean	To the right	________	To the left	________
		Forward	________	Backward	________
Pelvis	Tilt	To the right	________	To the left	________
		Anterior	________	Posterior	________
Hip	Flexion	On the right	________	On the left	________
		Bilateral	________		
	Extension	On the right	________		
		Bilateral	________		
	Abduction	On the right	________	On the left	________
		Bilateral	________		
	Adduction	On the right	________	On the left	________
		Bilateral	________		
	External rotation	On the right	________		
		Bilateral	________		
	Internal rotation	On the right	________	On the left	________
		Bilateral	________		
Knee	Flexion	On the right	________	On the left	________
		Bilateral	________		
	Extension	On the right	________	On the left	________
		Bilateral	________		
	Hyperextension	On the right	________	On the left	________
		Bilateral	________		
	Valgum	On the right	________	On the left	________
		Bilateral	________		
	Varum	On the right	________	On the left	________
		Bilateral	________		
Ankle/foot	Dorsiflexion	On the right	________	On the left	________
		Bilateral	________		
	Plantarflexion	On the right	________	On the left	________
		Bilateral	________		
	Varus	On the right	________	On the left	________
		Bilateral	________		
	Valgus	On the right	________	On the left	________
		Bilateral	________		
	Pes planus	On the right	________	On the left	________
		Bilateral	________		
	Pes cavus	On the right	________	On the left	________
		Bilateral	________		

these deviations will be more complex than indicated in the tables. Examples of gait patterns observed in association with spasticity and with hypotonus follow.

An individual with spasticity (e.g., an individual with diplegic cerebral palsy) may have a posteriorly tilted pelvis, forward flexion of the upper trunk, protracted scapulae, and somewhat excessive neck extension. Excessive hip flexion, with adduction and internal rotation (scissoring) may be observed during stance and may be accompanied by either excessive knee flexion or hyperextension. If excessive knee flexion occurs during stance, dorsiflexion at the ankle may be exaggerated during late stance/preswing to advance the tibia over the ankle and clear the toes and forefoot from the ground after push-off (heel-off to toe-off).

In other individuals with hypertonia, hyperextension at the knee occurs in stance and may be accompanied by plantarflexion and inversion at the ankle and foot. Electromyographic (EMG) recordings may show prolonged activity in the quadriceps and in the gastrocnemius-soleus muscle groups. The hamstrings, gluteal, and dorsiflexor muscle groups may be reciprocally inhibited.

In individuals with low muscle tone (hypotonia) in the trunk, proximal stability (tonic extension and co-contraction of axial muscles) is diminished. The pelvis may be anteriorly tilted so that the upper trunk is slightly extended. The

Table 10.16 Recording Form for Observational Gait Analysis

Patient's name__________________________ Age________ Sex ________ Height ________ Weight ______
Diagnosis ____
Footwear ______________ Assistive devices ____
Date ________________ Therapist ____

DIRECTIONS: Place a check in the space opposite the deviation if the deviation is observed.

		Stance										Swing						Possible	
Body Segment	**Deviation**	**HS**		**FF**		**MST**		**HO**		**TO**		**ACC**		**MSW**		**DEC**		**Cause**	**Analysis**
Ankle and foot	None	R	L	R	L	R	L	R	L	R	L	R	L	R	L	R	L		
Observations	Foot flat																		
In the sagittal plane	Foot slap																		
	Heel off																		
	No heel off																		
	Excessive plantarflexion																		
	Excessive dorsiflexion																		
	Toe drag																		
	Toe clawing																		
	Contralateral vaulting																		
Observations in the frontal plane	Varus																		
	Valgus																		
Knee	None																		
Observations in the sagittal plane	Excessive flexion																		
	Limited flexion																		
	No flexion																		
	Hyperexten-sion																		
	Genu recurvatum																		
	Diminished extension																		
Observations in the frontal plane	Varum																		
	Valgum																		
Hip	None																		
Observations in the sagittal plane	Excessive flexion																		

(*continued*)

Table 10.16 Recording Form for Observational Gait Analysis (Continued)

			Stance				Swing			Possible	
Body Segment	**Deviation**	**HS**	**FF**	**MST**	**HO**	**TO**	**ACC**	**MSW**	**DEC**	**Cause**	**Analysis**
	Limited flexion										
	No flexion										
	Diminished extension										
Observations in the frontal plane	Abduction Adduction										
	External rotation										
	Internal rotation										
	Circumduction										
	Hiking										
Pelvis	None										
Observations in sagittal plane	Anterior tilt										
	Posterior tilt										
	Increased backward rotation										
	Increased forward rotation										
	Limited backward rotation										
	Limited forward rotation										
	Drops on contralateral side										
Trunk	None										
Observations in frontal plane	Backward rotation										
	Lateral lean										
	Forward rotation										
	Backward lean										
	Forward lean										

ACC = acceleration; DEC = deceleration; FF = foot flat; HO = heel off; HS = heel strike; MST = midstance; MSW = midswing; TO = toe off.

scapulae may be retracted and the head may be forward. During stance, the hip may be flexed and the knee may be hyperextended, accompanied by plantarflexion at the ankle. The foot may be pronated with the majority of body weight borne on the medial border. Frequently, these individuals show diminished longitudinal trunk rotation and sluggish trunk balance reactions. They tend to rely on protective extension reactions of the limbs to maintain balance. The staggering or stepping reactions of the lower extremities may be pronounced, stride length and step length may be uneven, and gait may be wide based and unsteady.

Although the gait patterns in neurological gait may be complex and an analysis of the causes may be difficult, a detailed OGA can provide valuable data. Generally, to analyze gait patterns in persons who have sustained neurological damage, the following preliminary questions must be asked:

1. What is the influence of abnormal tone (hypertonicity and hypotonicity) on position and movement?
2. How does the position of the head influence muscle tone, position, and movement?
3. How does weightbearing influence muscle tone, position, and movement?
4. What is the influence of abnormal (obligatory) synergistic activity on position and movement?
5. What is the influence of weakness (paresis) on position and movement?
6. What is the influence of coordination deficits on position and movement?
7. What is the influence of impaired balance reactions on position and movement?

Ambulation Profiles and/or Scales

Profiles and rating scales constitute types of gait analyses that often include both qualitative (observational) and quantitative (spatial and temporal) measures. Profiles and scales are used for a variety of reasons, for example, examination of ambulation skills,[39] determination of the patient's need for assistance, identification of a change in a patient's status, screening for identification of the patient's need for physical therapy,[40] and identification of elderly individuals who are at risk for falling.[22] Gait analyses of one type or another may be either the sole focus of a profile, or the gait analysis may constitute only a small portion of a broad examination profile that includes balance skills as well as other functional activities. One particular advantage of some of these profiles is that subordinate gait skills such as standing balance may be examined in individuals who may not be able to walk unassisted. Since many of these profiles were developed for use with specific populations, comparative data may be available to the therapist.

The following profiles have been selected for review in this chapter because they are in current use and have been examined for reliability and/or validity: the Functional Ambulation Profile (FAP),[39] the Emory Functional Ambulation Profile (EFAP) and the Modified Emory Functional Ambulation Profile (mEFAP),[41] the Iowa Level of Assistance Score,[42] the Functional Independence Measure (FIM),[43] the Functional Independence Measure (FIM) plus the Functional Assessment Measure (FAM) or the (FIM + FAM),[44] the Functional Independence Measure for Children (WeeFIM),[45] the Gait Abnormality Rating Scale (GARS)[46] and the Modified GARS (GARS-M),[22] the Dynamic Gait Index, Berg Balance Scale,[23] and the Fast Evaluation of Mobility, Balance, and Fear (FEMBAF).[47]

Functional Ambulation Profile and Modifications

The *Functional Ambulation Profile (FAP),* developed by Arthur J. Nelson PT, PhD, FAPTA, is designed to examine gait skills on a continuum from standing balance in the parallel bars to independent ambulation.[39] A stopwatch is used to measure the amount of time required either to maintain a position or perform a task. The test consists of three phases. In the first phase, the patient is asked to perform the following three tasks in the parallel bars: bilateral stance, uninvolved leg stance, and involved leg stance. In the second phase, the patient is asked to transfer weight from one extremity to another as rapidly as possible. In the third phase, the patient is asked to walk 20 ft (6 m) in the parallel bars, with an assistive device, and, if possible, independently.

A more recent version of the FAP developed at Emory University is called the *Emory Functional Ambulation Profile (EFAP).* This profile differs from the original FAP in that five environmental challenges have been added which the individual may negotiate with or without the use of orthotics or assistive device. The modified Emory Functional Ambulation Profile (mEFAP) incorporates manual assistance into the EFAP. Subtasks include 16.4-ft (5 m) walks on a hard floor and on a carpeted floor, rising from a chair and completing a 9.8-ft (3 m) walk and sitting back down (timed get up and go test), negotiating through a standardized obstacle course and ascending and descending five stairs.

Iowa Level of Assistance Scale

The *Iowa Level of Assistance Scale* examines four functional tasks (one of which involves gait): getting out of bed, standing from bed, ambulating 15 ft (4.57 m), and walking up and down three steps. The patient's performance on the tasks is rated according to the following seven levels: (1) not tested for safety reasons; (2) activity attempted but not completed; (3) maximum assistance (therapist applies three or more points of contact); (4) moderate assistance (therapist applies two points of contact); (5) minimal assistance (therapist provides one point of contact); (6) standby assistance (no therapist contact but therapist not comfortable leaving patient); and (7) independence (therapist comfortable leaving room).

Functional Independence Measure

The *Functional Independence Measure (FIM)* is the result of a project funded by The National Institute of Handicapped Research, which was conducted in order to develop a

Table 10.17 The Functional Independence Measure (FIM™) Instrument Seven-Point Scoring System for Locomotion–Version 5.1

LOCOMOTION: WALK/WHEELCHAIR: Includes walking, once in a standing position, or if using a wheelchair, once in a seated position, on a level surface. Performs safely. Indicate the most frequent mode of locomotion (Walk or Wheelchair). If both are used about equally, code: "Both."

NO HELPER

7 Complete Independence—Subject *walks* a minimum of *150* ft (50 m) without assistive devices. Does not use a wheelchair. Performs safely.

6 Modified Independence—Subject *walks* a minimum of *150* ft (50 m) but uses a brace (orthosis) or prosthesis on leg, special adaptive shoes, cane, crutches, or walkerette; takes more than reasonable time or there are safety considerations.

If not walking, subject operates manual or motorized wheelchair independently for a minimum of *150* ft (50 m); turns around; maneuvers the chair to a table, bed, toilet; negotiates at least a 3% grade; maneuvers on rugs and over door sills.

5 Exception (Household Ambulation)—Subject walks only short distances (a minimum of *50* ft or 17 m) *independently* with or without a device. Takes more than reasonable time, or there are safety considerations, or operates a manual or motorized wheelchair independently only short distances (a minimum of *50* ft or 17 m).

HELPER

5 Supervision

If walking, subject requires standby supervision, cueing, or coaxing to go a minimum of *150* ft (50 m).

If not walking, requires standby supervision, cueing, or coaxing to go a minimum of *150* ft (50 m) in wheelchair.

4 Minimal Contact Assistance—Subject performs 75% or more of locomotion effort to go a minimum of *150* ft (50 m).

3 Moderate Assistance—Subject performs 50% to 74% of locomotion effort to go a minimum of *150* ft (50 m).

2 Maximal Assistance—Subject performs 25% to 49% of locomotion effort to go a minimum of *50* ft (17 m). Requires assistance of one person only.

1 Total Assistance—Subject performs less than 25% of effort, or requires assistance of two people, or does not walk or wheel a minimum of *50* ft (17 m).

Comment: If the subject requires an assistive device for locomotion: wheelchair, prosthesis, walker, cane, AFO, adapted shoe, etc., the Walk/Wheelchair score can never be higher than level 6. The mode of locomotion (Walk or Wheelchair) must be the same on admission and discharge. If the subject changes mode of locomotion from admission to discharge (usually wheelchair to walking), record the admission mode and scores based on the *more frequent mode of locomotion at discharge*.

From The Uniform Data System for Medical Rehabilitation, a division of UB Foundation Activities, Inc (UDS_{MR} SM). Guide for the Uniform Data Set for Medical Rehabilitation (Including the FIM™ Instrument), Version 5.1, Buffalo: UDSMR, 1997, with permission.

Guide for a Uniform Data Set for Medical Rehabilitation.[48] The FIM is designed to examine a patient's progress during inpatient rehabilitation. The FIM is now proprietary, and the FIM™ is the trademark of the Uniform Data System for Medical Rehabilitation, a division of the University of Buffalo Foundation Activities, Inc. The FIM Locomotion: Walk/Wheelchair Guide is the portion of the Guide for the Uniform Data Set (Including the FIM™ instrument) related to gait (Table 10.17). A study designed to evaluate the accuracy of clinical judgments of patient functioning found that bias and poor judgment of a patient's functional level played a significant role in 50 rehabilitation professionals' ratings of patient functioning. The authors of the study suggested that blind ratings of the FIM and training in eliminating bias would improve accuracy.[49]

Functional Assessment Measure

The 12-item *Functional Assessment Measure (FAM)* was developed by a multidisciplinary group of clinicians at Santa Clara Valley Medical Center, San Jose, CA,[44] to provide a measure of disability that reflected the communication, psychosocial adjustment, and cognitive functions of the populations of individuals who sustained traumatic brain injury (TBI) and stroke, respectively. The FAM uses a seven-point rating scale modeled after the FIM to examine the individual's level or degree of independence, amount of assistance required, use of adaptive or assistive

Table 10.18 The Functional Assessment Measure (FAM) Items

1. Swallowing	7. Emotional Status
2. Car Transfer	8. Adjustment to Limitations
3. Community Access	9. Employability
4. Reading	10. Orientation
5. Writing	11. Attention
6. Speech Intelligibility	12. Safety Judgment

The 12 items of the FAM are not designed to stand alone but to be added to the 18 items of the FIM to produce the FIM + FAM.

Courtesy of Santa Clara Valley Medical Center (1998). The Functional Assessment Measure. The Center for Outcome Measurement in Brain Injury. Retrieved August 23, 2004 from http://tbims.org/combi/FAM.

devices, and percentage of tasks completed successfully (Table 10.18).

The 12 items of the FAM have been added to the 18-item FIM to produce the FIM + FAM with the intent of providing more detailed data for TBI and stroke population groups. The FIM and FIM + FAM total scales are psychometrically similar measures of global disability whereas the BI, FIM, and FIM + FAM motor scales are similar measures of physical disability.[50] However, in a study of 376 stroke patients in Canadian inpatient rehabilitation units who were concurrently given the FIM and the FAM, the results of a Rasch analysis showed that in the motor domain only the FAM community access item was more difficult than the FIM items. In the cognitive domain, the only FAM item that extended the range of the FIM was the one assessing employability. In light of the results, the authors from the University of Buffalo concluded that adding the FAM items to the FIM reduced test efficiency and provided only minimal protection against ceiling effects of the FIM.[51]

Functional Independence Measure for Children

The original version of the *Functional Independence Measure for Children (WeeFIM)* consisted of 18 items involving the following 6 subscales: (1) self-care, (2) sphincter control, (3) transfers, (4) locomotion, (5) communication, and (6) social cognition. The WeeFIM^{R} is designed to measure the need for assistance and the severity of disability in children between the ages of 6 months and 7 years. The WeeFIM II^{SM} system is an online pediatric outcomes management system, which documents functional performance in children and adolescents with either acquired or congenital disabilities in all types of settings (inpatient, outpatient, and community). Data from users of the FIM and WeeFIM have been reported for a number of years to the CIHI National Rehabilitation Reporting System at the University of Buffalo, Foundation Activities Inc.[43]

Gait Abnormality Rating Scale and Modifications

The *Gait Abnormality Rating Scale (GARS)* was designed to identify patients living in nursing homes who were at risk for falling. Time, space, and resources are often very limited in nursing homes, and the only expenses involved in administering the GARS included purchase of a camcorder and videotapes and the therapist's time to film, review, and rate the videotapes. The test developers selected 16 features of the gait cycle and a scoring system, in which the features are scored on a 0 to 3 rating scale (0 = normal, 1 = mildly impaired, 2 = moderately impaired, and 3 = severely impaired). Because the GARS scores correlated well with walking speed, stride length, and with risk of falling, the instrument appears to be a valid predictor of the history of falling when used with nursing home residents. Arm-swing amplitude, upper and LE synchrony, and guardedness best distinguished fallers from other subjects. However, the GARS does not provide information regarding the type of falls (trips, slips, losing balance) sustained by this population.[52] Therefore, it is not helpful in determining the cause of the falls.

The *Modified GARS (GARS-M),* which is a modified seven-item version of the GARS, contains the following variables: (1) variability, (2) guardedness, (3) staggering, (4) foot contact, (5) hip ROM, (6) shoulder extension, and (7) arm–heel strike synchrony. These variables were selected for inclusion because they were found to be the most reliable in the original GARS. Scoring is the sum of the seven items; the total score represents a rank ordering for risk of falling based on the number of gait abnormalities recognized and the severity of any abnormality identified. A higher score is associated with a more abnormal gait. The GARS-M has been deemed a good predictor for persons at risk for falls.[22]

Shumway-Cook et al[23] examined the following four instruments in an attempt to develop a model for predicting the likelihood of falls among community-dwelling elderly (65 years of age and older): (1) *Balance Self Perceptions Test,* (2) *Berg Balance Scale,* (3) mobility (timed walking at self-paced preferred speed and at fast speed for 50 feet [15.2 m]), and (4) the *Dynamic Gait Index*. The Balance Self Perceptions Test is a self-rating of the degree to which balance and perceived risk for falls interfere with daily activities. The Berg Balance Scale is a performance-based measure of balance and mobility, in which subjects are rated on a 0 to 4 scale (0 = cannot perform to 4 = normal performance) on 14 different tasks (see Chapter 8, Appendix A). The *50-foot walk test* for mobility is timed, and mean speed is calculated for both self-paced and fastest speed. The Dynamic Gait Index is designed to examine the ability to adapt gait to changes in task demands. Performance is rated on a 0 to 3 scale (0 = poor to 3 = excellent). Individuals are rated on eight different tasks including gait on even surfaces, gait while changing speeds, gait and head turns in a vertical or horizontal direction, stepping over obstacles, and gait with pivot turns and steps. Although the Dynamic Gait Index was included as one of the factors that predicted a risk of falling, the final model included only the Berg Balance Scale and history of falling, with the Berg Balance Scale being the best single predictor of fall status. Patients who have high scores on the Berg Balance Scale have a relatively low fall risk, while patients with a score of 40 or less (total possible score is 56) have a high risk for falls and would appear to be candidates for physical therapy.[23]

Fast Evaluation of Mobility Balance and Fear

The *Fast Evaluation of Mobility Balance and Fear (FEMBAF)* is another instrument designed to identify risk factors, functional performance, and factors that hinder mobility. It consists of a 22-item risk factor questionnaire and an 18-item performance component, which includes, among other measures, stair climbing and descending, stepping over an obstacle, and one-legged standing.

Kinematic Quantitative Gait Analysis

Kinematic quantitative gait analysis is used to obtain information on spatial and temporal gait variables, as well as motion patterns. The data obtained through these analyses are quantifiable and therefore provide the therapist with baseline data that can be used to plan treatment programs and evaluate progress toward goals or goal attainment. The fact that the data are quantifiable is important because third-party payers are demanding that therapists use measurable parameters when examining patient function, establishing treatment strategies, and documenting the outcomes of a plan of care. However, data derived from qualitative observations may be necessary to determine degrees of motor impairment, and to check the validity of the quantitative variables measured. For example, examination of spatial and temporal variables is necessary for the interpretation of kinetic and EMG data. Therefore, both qualitative and quantitative kinematic gait analyses should be performed to provide a more comprehensive picture of an individual's gait.

Spatial and temporal measures may be critical factors in determining a patient's independence in ambulation. For example, a patient may need to attain a certain gait speed to cross a local street within the time allotted by a crossing light, or a patient may need to walk a certain distance to shop in the local supermarket. Therapists need to survey the community to determine the distances and time requirements for accessing stores and public buildings prior to making a judgment about a patient's functional ambulation status. Robinett and Von Dran[53] found that target goals on a sample of gait analysis forms were low compared to distance and velocity requirements for crossing the street found in a community survey. Walsh et al[54] found that individuals at 1 year post total knee arthroplasty achieved more than 80 percent of the normal walking speeds of their age and gender-matched counterparts. However, for 62 percent of the females and 25 percent of the males, the normal walking speed attained would not be sufficient to cross a street intersection safely.

Spatial and Temporal Variables

The variables measured in a quantitative gait analysis are listed and described in Table 10.19. Because spatial and temporal variables are affected by a number of factors such as age,[55–59] gender,[60,61] height and weight,[62,63] level of physical activity,[64,65] and level of maturation,[66] attempts have been made to take some of these factors into account. Ratios, such as stride-length divided by functional LE length, may be used to normalize for differences in patients' leg lengths. Step length divided by the subject's height may be used in an attempt to normalize differences among patients' heights. In an attempt to control for both height and weight, body weight is divided by standing height to yield the **body mass index (BMI)**. Other ratios are used to assess symmetry, for example, right swing time divided by left swing time and swing time divided by stance time. Sutherland et al[66] list the ratio of pelvic span to ankle spread as one of the determinants of mature gait in children.

Measurement of Variables

The techniques and equipment required for measurement of spatial and temporal variables range from simple to complex. The time requirements also vary, and the therapist must be familiar with different methods of examining these variables in order to select the method most appropriate to each situation. Prior to selecting a method of measurement, the therapist must understand the variable in question and how that variable is related to the patient's gait.

Simple Methods of Measuring Spatial and Temporal Variables

Determining of the distance completed within a set time frame is one of the simplest methods used to measure spatial variables. An example of this simple method is the *6-Minute Walk Test*. In this test, the distance covered by subjects walking at a comfortable pace for 6 minutes is determined. Schenkman et al used the 6-minute walk test to examine the physical performance of patients with Parkinson's disease.[67] This simple test, used in combination with other physical performance and impairment measures (i.e., ROM and muscle force), could be used to either monitor decline or evaluate improvement associated with treatment interventions. Mossberg found the 6-minute walk test a reliable measurement of functional ambulation (distance walked) of patients with acquired brain injury.[68] For individuals with limited endurance, a 3-Minute Walk Test may be used in place of the 6-minute test.[69]

Measurement of spatial variables such as degree of foot angle, width of base of support, step length, and stride length also can be determined simply and inexpensively by recording the patient's footprints during gait. Simple methods of recording footprints include either the application of paints, ink, or chalk to the bottom of the patient's foot or shoe or the attachment of inked pads or other markers. For example, a felt-tipped marker may be taped to the back of a patient's shoe. Using these methods, measurements of

Table 10.19 Gait Variables: Quantitative Gait Analysis

Variable	Description
Speed **Free speed** **Slow speed** **Fast speed**	A scalar quantity that has magnitude but not direction. A person's normal walking speed. A speed slower than a person's normal speed. A rate faster than normal.
Cadence	The number of steps taken by a patient per unit of time. Cadence may be measured in centimeters as the number of steps per second $$\text{Cadence} = \frac{\text{number of steps}}{\text{time}}$$ A simple method of measuring cadence is by counting the number of steps taken by the patient in a given amount of time. The only equipment necessary is a stopwatch, paper, and pencil.
Velocity **Linear velocity** **Angular velocity** **Walking velocity**	A measure of a body's motion in a given direction. The rate at which a body moves in a straight line. The rate of motion in rotation of a body segment around an axis. The rate of linear forward motion of the body. This is measured in either centimeters per second or meters per minute. To obtain a person's **walking velocity**, divide the distance traversed by the time required to complete the distance. $$\text{Walking velocity} = \frac{\text{distance}}{\text{time}}$$ Walking velocity may be affected by age, level of maturation, height, sex, type of footwear, and weight. Also, velocity may affect cadence, step, stride length, and foot angle as well as other gait variables.
Acceleration **Angular acceleration**	The rate of change of velocity with respect to time. Body acceleration has been defined by Smidt and Mommens[2] as the rate of change of velocity of a point posterior to the sacrum. Acceleration is usually measured in meters per second per second (m/s^2). The rate of change of the angular velocity of a body with respect to time. Angular acceleration is usually measured in radians per second per second ($radians/s^2$).
Stride time	The amount of time that elapses during one stride: that is, from one foot contact (heel strike if possible) until the next contact of the same foot (heel strike). Both stride times should be measured. Measurement is usually in seconds.
Step time	The amount of time that elapses between consecutive right and left foot contacts (heel strikes). Both right and left step times should be measured. Measurement is in seconds.
Stride length	The linear distance between two successive points of contact of the same foot. It is measured in centimeters or meters. The average stride length for normal adult males is 1.46 meters. The average stride length for adult females is 1.28 meters.
Swing time	The amount of time during the gait cycle that one foot is off the ground. Swing time should be measured separately for right and left extremities. Measurement is in seconds.
Double support time	The amount of time spent in the gait cycle when both lower extremities are in contact with the supporting surface. Measured in seconds.
Cycle time (stride time)	The amount of time required to complete a gait cycle. Measured in seconds.
Step length	The linear distance between two successive points of contact of the right and left lower extremities. Usually a measurement is taken from the point of heel contact at heel strike of one extremity to the point of heel contact of the opposite extremity. If a patient does not have a heel strike on one or both sides, the measurement can be taken from the heads of the first metatarsals. Measured in centimeters or meters.
Width of walking base (step width)	The width of the walking base (base of support) is the linear distance between one foot and the opposite foot. Measured in centimeters or meters.[7]
Foot angle (degree of toe out or toe in)	The angle of foot placement with respect to the line of progression. Measured in degrees.[7]

(continued)

Table 10.19 Gait Variables: Quantitative Gait Analysis (continued)

Variable	Description
Bilateral stance time (for the FAP)	The length of time up to 30 seconds that a person can stand upright in the parallel bars bearing weight on both lower extremities.
Uninvolved stance time (for the FAP)	The length of time up to 30 seconds that an individual can stand in the parallel bars while bearing weight on the uninvolved lower extremity (involved extremity is raised off the supporting surface).
Involved stance time (for the FAP)	The length of time up to 30 seconds that an individual can stand in the parallel bars on the involved lower extremity (uninvolved lower extremity is raised off the supporting surface).
Dynamic weight transfer rate (for the FAP)	The rate at which an individual standing in the parallel bars can transfer weight from one extremity to another. Measured in seconds from the first lift-off to the last lift-off.
Parallel bar ambulation (for the FAP)	Length of time required for an individual to walk the length of the parallel bars as rapidly as possible. Two trials are averaged to obtain this measurement. Measurement is in seconds.

FAP = Functional Ambulation Profile.

step length, stride length, step width, and foot angle may be obtained.

Another way of obtaining step length and stride length data is by placing a grid pattern on the floor.[70] A strip of masking tape about 1 ft (30 cm) wide and 32 ft (10 m) long is laid down in a straight line. The tape is marked off in 1-in. (3 cm) increments for its entire length, and the segments are numbered consecutively so that the patient's heel strikes can be identified. The therapist then calls out the heel strike locations from the numbers on the grid pattern into a tape recorder.

For most methods of determining stride and step lengths, temporal variables such as cadence, velocity, and stride times may be calculated if the elapsed time for the subject to walk a measured distance (d) is obtained using a stopwatch. **Cadence** (c) can be determined by dividing the number of steps (n) taken during the walking trial by the elapsed time (tn) between the first and last heel strikes using the following formula $c = n/tn$. **Velocity** (v) can be calculated by taking the total distance (d) between the first and last heel strikes and dividing it by the elapsed time (td) for the distance ($v = d/td$). To obtain a normal walking speed, the patient should be allowed to take a few steps prior to the beginning of any measurements.

Todd and co-workers tested 84 normal children (41 girls and 43 boys) ages 13 months to 12 years, and analyzed data from more than 200 other children ages 11 months to 16 years. A two-dimensional gait graph was developed using the data that provides a visual record of a child's walking performance. While the gait graph is similar in appearance to graphs used for height and weight, it shows norms for gait dimensions of cadence and stride length adjusted by height (Fig. 10.7).

Instruments for Examining Variables

Accelerometers. The Step Watch Activity Monitor 3™ (SAM) is a commercially available instrument that records the number of strides taken in 1-minute intervals during daily activities for up to 15 consecutive days (CYMA Corp, Seattle, WA 98115). The SAM includes a sensor (custom accelerometer) that measures 7.5 × 50 × 20 mm and weighs approximately 1.3 ounces (Fig. 10.8). The battery provides up to 4 to 5 years of continual use.[71] The case is

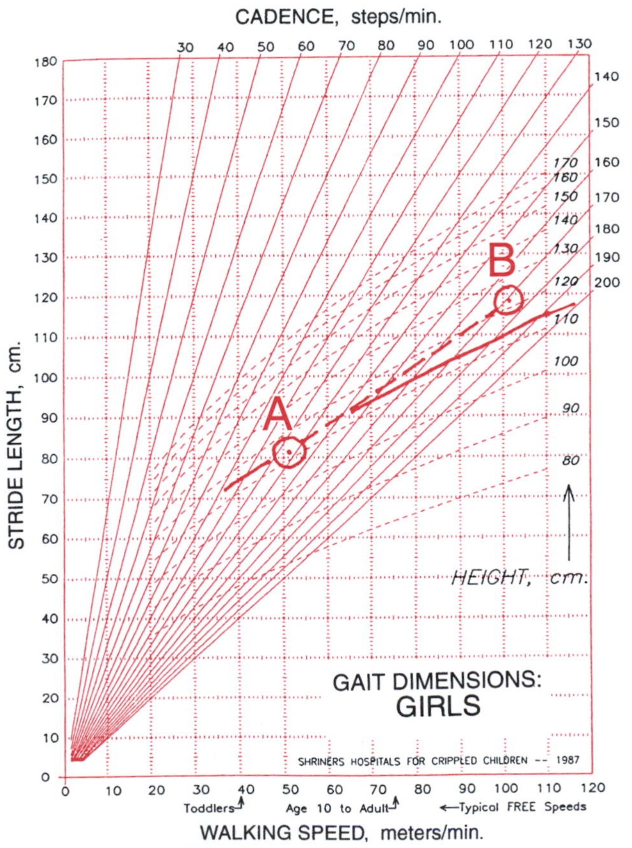

Figure 10.7 The solid line on the gait graph represents normal parameters for height. The dashed line represents data plotted for a normal 6-year-old girl whose height was 114 cm. A similar chart is available for boys. (From Todd, FN, et al,[59, p 201] with permission.)

Evidence Summary Box 10.1

Studies using the Step Watch Activity Monitor 3™ (SAM) as a Component of Data Collection

References	Subjects	Design	Results	Comments
Maluf, KS and Mueller, MJ[133] 2003	30 subjects: 10 subjects without diabetes; 10 subjects with diabetes and peripheral neuropathy (DMPN); and 10 subjects with DMPN plus plantar ulcers (DMPN + U)	Cross-sectional with matched groups	Validity: mean absolute error of 1.07 (SD 3.07%) for healthy obese subjects and 1.75 for diabetic subjects; reliability for daily strides measured during 2 consecutive 7-day periods (ICC = 0.97); subjects with diabetes were less active than control subjects; cumulative stress was lower in subjects with a history of recurrent ulcers compared to subjects with or without DMPN who had never developed a plantar ulcer.	Need for a larger number of subjects to further explore the relationship between stress and plantar ulcer formation.
Hartsell, H, et al[132] 2002	10 healthy adults (24–68 years) wearing an athletic shoe for a distance of 530 m over flat ground and up and down stairs; same subjects walked and climbed stairs wearing a fiberglass total contact cast (TCC) with a rubberized rockerbottom sole	Repeated measures used to determine accuracy of SAM under varying conditions	The mean percent error for the SAM for flat surface walking was 0.136% for the athletic shoe and 0.206% for the TCC; the SAM undercounted the number of steps taken by the subject during stair climbing while wearing either type of foot wear but percent error considered small and not clinically important.	Although using only healthy subjects was a limitation of the study, the subjects' gait with a cast was similar to the gait of patients when casted.
Resnick, B, et al.[130] 2001	30 subjects with a mean age of 86 (SD = 6.1); 4 subjects wore the SAM for extended periods and kept diaries of activities which supported the SAM data	Repeated measures 60 one-minute walks while 2 observers counted steps	Overall step counting accuracy of 96% for SAM.	Subjects reported that SAM was comfortable to wear and researchers reported that it was easy to use, valid, and was a reliable measure of activity in older adults.

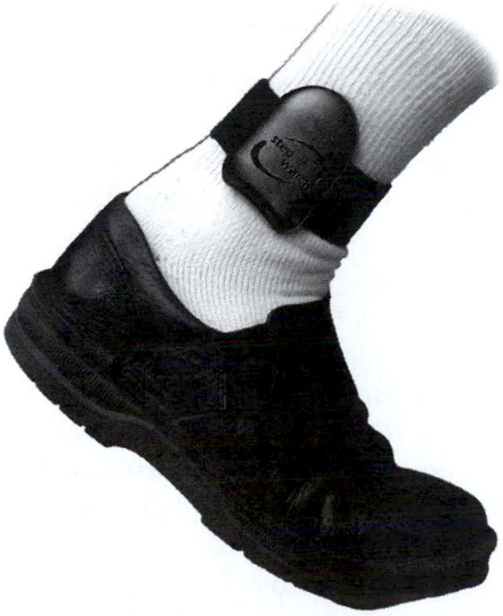

Figure 10.8 The Step Watch Activity Monitor 3® (SAM) is a pager-sized instrument worn at the ankle for long term monitoring of gait function. (Courtesy of CYMA Corp, Mountlake Terrace, WA 98043.)

contoured to fit just above the lateral malleolus and is attached by an elastic strap. A personal computer is used to set up the SAM for monitoring, and also for downloading data to a computer file. Box 10.1 presents a summary of studies using the Step Watch 3 Step Activity Monitor (SAM) as a component of data collection.

Triaxial accelerometers have been attached to the trunk in order to measure mean acceleration, cadences, step, and stride lengths.[72,73] Acclerometers have also been attached to the head and pelvis to determine acceleration patterns of the head and pelvis while subjects walked on different surfaces.[74]

Gyroscopes. *Gyroscopes* are another type of instrument that may be used for the estimation of spatial and temporal gait parameters. The gyroscope measures the Coriolis acceleration of a vibrating triangular prism. The signal from the prism is proportional to the angular velocity. The instruments are light, portable, and relatively inexpensive. A single uniaxial gyroscope attached on the skin surface of the lower leg can provide data for calculating cadence, number of steps, and estimating stride length and walking speed. Tong and Granat suggested that usage of gyroscopes could be a viable alternative to foot sensors for determining temporal and spatial gait parameters because gyroscopes can capture information during swing as well as stance.[75]

Instrumented Systems for Determining Spatial and Temporal Gait Parameters

Examples of instrumented systems for measuring spatial and temporal variables include two types of walkways: The GAITMAT II™ and The GAITRite,® and two types of footswitch systems: the Krusen Limb Monitor and the Stride Analyzer. (Manufacturer contact information for motion analysis equipment is presented in Appendix C.)

Walkways. *GAITMAT II*™(EQ, Inc, Chalfont, PA 18914) is a commercially available walkway with embedded pressure-sensitive switches that open and close in response to contact with the patient's feet. The time of openings and closures of the switches are recorded by a computer that provides information on individual footprints, step and stride length, base of support, and step, swing, stance, single support and double support times for each extremity. The main advantage of this system is that the patient is unencumbered by equipment attached to either the feet or body.

Bowen and colleagues found that the GAITMAT II™ was able to detect decreases in velocity and increases in the percentage of double support in dual-task compared to single-task conditions in 11 patients with stroke.[76] In another study, variations in scoring increased among raters as subjects' walking patterns became more abnormal.[77]

The *GAITRite®* (CIR Systems, Inc., Clifton, NJ 07012) is another commercially available walkway system. The 14-foot portable walkway in this system contains 16,128 switches embedded between two sheets of vinyl. Spatial and temporal parameters can be measured, as well as dynamic pressure mapping of footprints during walking. The pressure parameters measured include peak pressure, pressure time, and sectional integrated pressure overtime. The walkway system can be used with or without shoes, orthoses, or walking aids, and the GAITRite software is capable of calculating spatial and temporal parameters and displaying them in graphs and tables.

Footswitches and Footswitch Systems. Foot switches are pressure-sensitive switches placed either on the patient's feet or the inside or outside of the shoes. The switches do not require a walkway, but the patient usually has to carry a data collection device. Foot switches consist of transducers and a semiconductor and are used to signal such events as heel strike. One type of foot switch device used to examine both temporal and loading variables is the *Krusen Limb Load Monitor.*[78] This device consists of a pressure-sensitive force plate that can be worn in a patient's shoe. It can be connected to a strip chart recorder to yield a permanent record of temporal and distance gait variables.[78]

The *Stride Analyzer* (B & L Engineering, Tustin, CA 92780) is a footswitch system with special insoles containing four-pressure sensitive switches placed under the heel, at the heads of the first and fifth metatarsals, and at the great toe. The parameters measured by this system include stride length, velocity, cadence, cycle time, single and double limb support time, swing time, and stance time. These measurements are recorded automatically and the information is transmitted to a computer that analyzes the data. The computer can also provide graphic displays of foot–floor contact patterns. Times are presented in seconds, and as a percentage of the gait cycle. The computer analysis also includes a percentage of normal using a built-in database (Appendix D).

The advantages of the Stride Analyzer system are that measurements from both feet are available, the system is easy to move from place to place, and, because it has been used by a large number of physical therapists with different populations, data comparisons are possible.[13,19,40,79–84,89] Several of the recent studies in which the Stride Analyzer was used are included in Table 10.20.[90–92] The sample studies appear to indicate that the Stride Analyzer is suitable for use with various age groups as well as for patients with neurological or orthopedic problems.

Electrogoniometers. Joint displacement can be measured relatively simply by using an electrogoniometer. The electrogoniometer is composed of two rigid links connected by a potentiometer that converts movement into an electrical signal that is proportional to the degree of movement. The rigid links or arms of the electrogoniometer are attached to the proximal and distal limb segments. According to Perry,[29] electrogoniometers, which cost approximately $3000, are the most convenient and least costly means of measuring knee and ankle motion during walking.

Methods of Gait Analysis for Kinematic and Kinetic Variables

Motion Analysis Systems

Imaging-based systems are the most sophisticated and expensive methods of determining joint displacement and patterns of motion. In computerized motion analysis systems, markers placed on body segments such as the knee, ankle, and hip are tracked by automated systems. Generally, two major types of motion analysis systems are available: systems that use active markers and systems that use passive markers. Active markers are generally *light-emitting diodes (LEDs)* that flash at given frequencies. Passive markers require an external source of illumination that may be provided by external light sources (e.g., Peak System) or a ring of infrared emitting diodes located around the lens of the camera (e.g., Vicon). In the latter case, the diodes on the camera pick up the infrared light reflected by the markers that they can "see," which means that a large number of cameras are necessary for obtaining unrestricted views of markers.

Table 10.20 Studies Using the Stride Analyzer

Authors	Purpose	Method	Variables	Subjects	Results
Evans, MD, Goldie, PA, and Hill, KD[84] 1997	To obtain intersession estimates of error for time and distance parameters of gait.	Stride Analyzer	Velocity, cadence, stride length, gait cycle duration, single support time, and double limb support time	Thirty-one patients with stroke who were four months post-stroke and involved in inpatient rehabilitation	Patients would have to increase gait velocity by more than 6.8 m/min. or decrease velocity more than 6.8 m/min. before it could be assumed with 95% confidence that genuine change beyond limits of error had occurred. Alternative strategies such as serial measurements may be required for measuring changes in velocity.
Harada, N, et al[40] 1995	To identify persons for referral for physical therapy evaluation.	Stride Analyzer, Berg Balance Scale, Tinetti Performance Oriented Mobility Assessment and the Tinetti Fall Efficiency Scale	Velocity	Fifty-three patients with stroke living in two residential facilities	A combination of the Berg Balance Scale results and gait velocity yielded the highest sensitivity level of 91% and therefore might be the best combination for screening. The sensitivity of gait velocity was 80% and the specificity was 89%.
Powers, CM, et al[79] 1996	To establish the relationship between isometric muscle force and temporal/spatial gait characteristics for individuals with below knee amputations.	Stride Analyzer	Velocity, cadence, and stride length	Fifteen males and seven females with below knee amputations	Mean walking speed was limited to 59% of normal. Hip extensor torque of the residual limb was the only predictor for both free speed and fast gait. Cadence was equal to 83% of normal. Hip abductor torque of the sound limb was the only predictor of cadence for free and fast speed. Stride length was 69% of normal.
Powers, CM, et al[81] 1997	To compare stride characteristics and joint motion in subjects with patellofemoral pain with and without patellar taping.	Stride Analyzer Vicon Motion Analyzer System	Velocity, stride length and cadence Sagittal plane joint motion of the pelvis, hip, knee and ankle	Fifteen female subjects with the diagnosis of patellofemoral pain	No significant differences were found in gait velocity or cadence between the taped and untaped trials. Patellar taping resulted in a small but significant increase in knee flexion loading response. The increase in knee flexion could help with shock absorption at heel strike.
Powers, CM, et al[82] 1997	To determine the influence of pain and muscle weakness on gait variables in subjects with patellofemoral pain.	Stride Analyzer Vicon Motion Analysis System Lido Dynamometer Visual Analog Pain Scale	Velocity, stride length and cadence Sagittal plane joint motion of the hip, knee and ankle Isometric knee extensor torque Knee pain	Nineteen female subjects with a diagnosis of patellofemoral pain and 19 female subjects without patellofemoral pain	The primary compensation in the patellofemoral pain group was a decrease in walking speed which was a function of decreased stride length and cadence. Knee extensor torque was the only predictor of gait function with increased torque correlating with improved stride characteristics.

(continued)

Table 10.20 Studies Using the Stride Analyzer (continued)

Authors	Purpose	Method	Variables	Subjects	Results
		Functional Assessment Questionnaire	Patellofemoral joint symptoms		
Von Schroeder, HP, et al[3] 1995	To compare gait parameters and patterns in patients with stroke and controls.	3-D Motion Analysis	Joint motion at ankle, knee, hip and pelvis		
		Surface EMG Stride Analyzer	Muscle timing Velocity, cadence, stride length, gait cycle time, double support time, single limb support and swing phase time	Forty-nine ambulatory patients with stroke and 24 age-matched controls	Patients walked significantly slower than control subjects. The patients had decreased cadence, increased cycle time, and increased double support time. The unaffected limb had significantly more time spent in stance and single limb support.

When the systems were first developed, visualization of passive markers was problematic, but now markers are automatically tracked and thousands of computations are performed by computer. However, passive marker systems require many cameras, are expensive, and require training to operate the hardware and software.[25]

The two most important problems that still exist with both active and passive marker systems concern skin movement over the skeleton and the need to improve accuracy of derivation of joint centers. In the future, magnetic resonance imaging (MRI) should prove valuable in locating the exact joint centers. At the present time, LEDs for the active systems are expensive, and Sutherland suggests that in the future it may be possible to use radiofrequency active emitters to replace LEDs.[25]

The following two commercially available systems use active markers: Optotrak® (Northern Digital, Inc, Waterloo, Ontario, Canada N2VIC5) and the Selspot System (Selcom, Inc, Southfield, MI 48075). Systems that use passive markers include Peak Motus® (Peak Performance Technologies, Inc, Centennial, CO 80112), Ariel Performance Analysis System® (Ariel Dynamics, Inc, San Diego, CA 92111), OrthoTrak,® (Motion Analysis Corp, Santa Rosa, CA 95403), Vicon Motion Analysis System® (Vicon Motion Systems, Oxford, UK OX20JB), and ELITE® (Bioengineering Technology Systems, Garbagnate Milanese, Italy 20024).

Peak Motus®

The Peak Motus®, when used with the 3-D Gait Analysis Module, provides information on displacement for right and left hip, knee, and ankle joint centers of rotation as well as joint angles for hip, knee, ankle, and pelvic motions. This system is able to measure kinetic variables as well as spatial and temporal variables. Figure 10.9 provides an example of passive marker placement on a subject, as well as a graph of linear velocities of the shoulder, hip, and knee, and angular velocities of the shoulder, elbow, and knee. In Figure 10.10, the degrees of motion for the ankle and knee are plotted against time. In Figure 10.11, stick figures are shown with accompanying knee angles. Peak Motus® systems are able to synchronize analog data, such as signals from force platforms and EMG electrodes with kinematic motion data.

Ariel Performance System®

The Ariel Performance Analysis System® (APAS), when used with the APAS/Gait module, is able to perform kinematic analysis, as well as use input from force plates for inverse dynamic analyses. Obstruction of markers by body segments, skin/soft tissue motion, marker vibration, and improper placement of markers in relation to the joint center of motion can introduce potential errors. Owing to the use of passive markers, these video-based systems are especially susceptible to errors caused by marker obstruction when markers are in close proximity to one another.

Vicon Motion Analysis System®

The Vicon Motion Analysis System® is also able to incorporate kinetic data. The Vicon Data Station synchronizes signals from the Vicon cameras, and provides for direct integration of data from devices such as force plates and EMG systems.

OrthoTrak

OrthoTrak® is a fully automated 3-D clinical gait measurement, evaluation, and database management system, which is able to integrate kinematic analysis with EMG and force plate data. The system is also able to capture head, trunk, arms, and shoulder measurements.

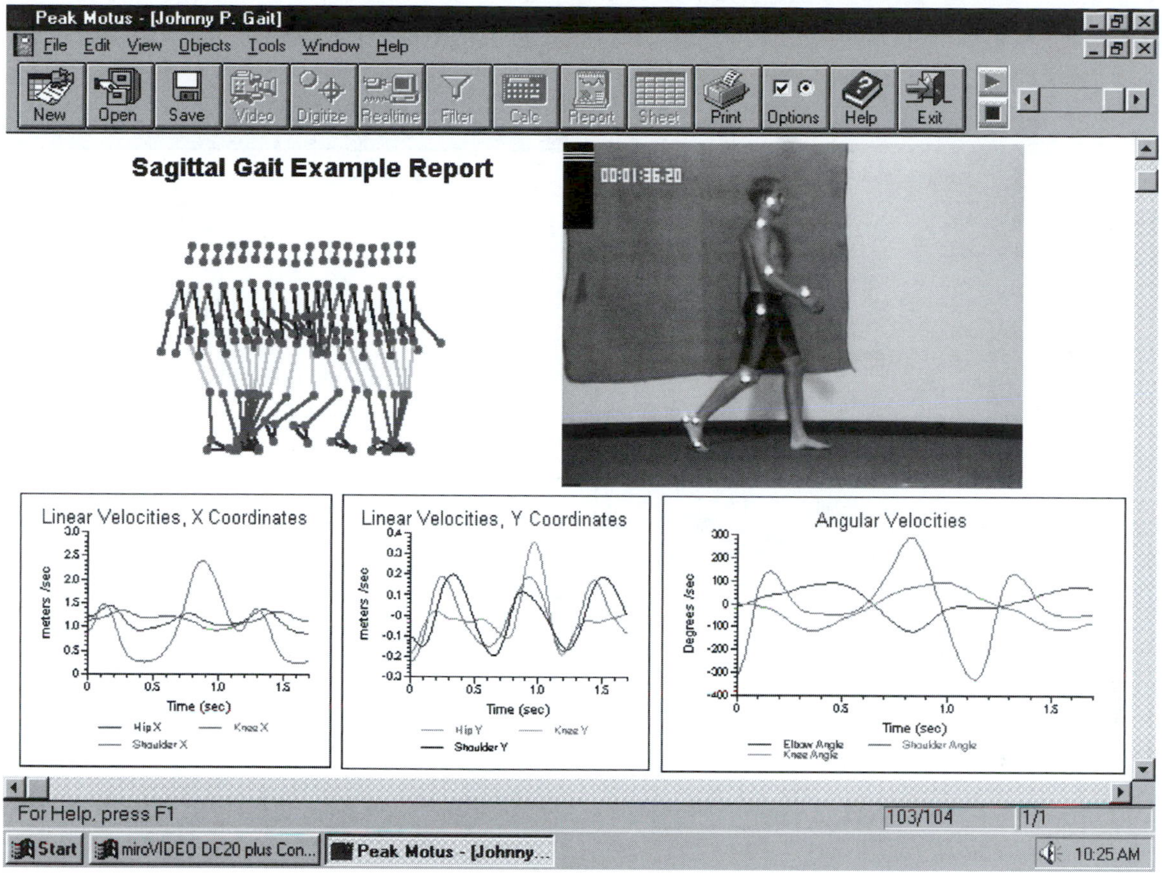

Figure 10.9 A typical computer screen from an automated video-based motion-analysis system. Marker placement on the individual whose gait is being analyzed can be seen in the video image at the right upper side of the screen. Computer-generated stick figure representations of the person's gait are shown in the left upper side of the screen. The bottom half of the screen provides linear and angular velocities. (Courtesy of Peak Performance Technologies, Inc, Centennial, CO 80112.)

ELITEplus®

The ELITEplus® motion analyzer system uses passive markers, up to eight high-sensitivity video cameras, and either a visible or infrared light source. A video image processor digitizes the analog signal, recognizes individual markers, and computer software calibrates, captures, and displays the data. Force platform and EMG data may be gathered simultaneously. Sampling rates are 50 to 120 frames/sec and system accuracy 1/2800 of the field view. Used with GAITEL acquisition and processing software, clinically relevant kinematic and kinetic variables can be calculated and reports produced automatically.

Motion analysis systems are continually evolving with the incorporation of new features and options, including simultaneous acquisition and processing of force plate and EMG data. EMG is used to identify the particular portion of the gait cycle in which the muscle activity occurs. An example of how EMG is used in combination with a motion analysis system (Vicon) is presented in Figure 10.12. The figure shows the EMG output and ROM on the graph while the computer generated figures provide a visual image. The differences in muscle activity among the three types of walking patterns are easily seen in the graphs. The deviations from normal ROM at the knee are also easy to identify. A careful observation of the figures in the extension thrust pattern shows an extension thrust of the knee immediately after initial contact and excessive plantarflexion at the ankle both at heel strike and throughout the gait cycle. Refer to Chapter 9 for a more detailed discussion of EMG.

New Developments in Motion Analysis

Two examples of current developments in motion analysis systems include an ultrasonic gait analysis system and a magnetic system. Huitema and colleagues[85] describe an ultrasonic motion analysis system capable of measuring spatial and temporal gait parameters. The system consists of a small ultrasonic receiver attached to both shoes of a walking subject, and a stationary transmitter placed on the floor. Comparison data obtained from foot contact switches on four healthy subjects walking on the floor showed that by applying two relative thresholds to the speed graph of the foot, heel strike and toe-off could be reliably generated by the ultrasonic system.[85]

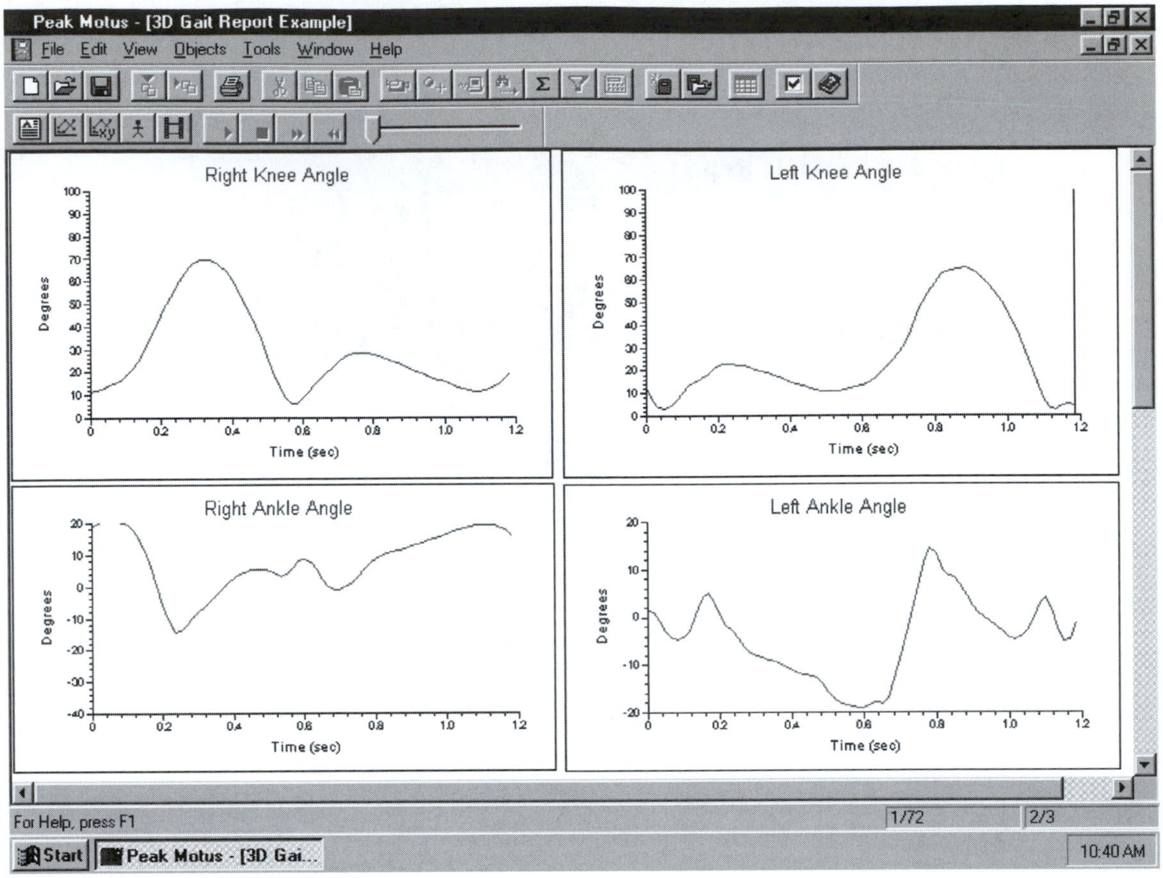

Figure 10.10 A typical computer-generated graph from a motion-analysis system. The graph shows knee and ankle range-of-motion patterns, which are plotted against time for both lower extremities. (Courtesy of Peak Performance Technologies, Inc, Centennial, CO 80112.)

The Flock of Birds® is an electromagnetic motion analysis system produced by Ascension Technology Corporation in Burlington, Vermont. The Flock of Birds system uses pulsed direct current tracking to simultaneously track one to four sensors without delay or lag. Tracking is unrestricted without any line of the sight restrictions that sometimes are used to analyze the timing and peak found in passive marker systems.

Based on the history of gait analysis, one may expect that many of the older motion analysis systems will continue to evolve and more innovative methods of quantifying human gait will be created. However, the most important issues for rehabilitation professionals is how reliable and valid the information is, and how information can be used to fulfill the four purposes for gait analysis as described in the *Guide for Physical Therapist Practice.*[1] Tables 10.21 and 10.22 present studies illustrating how current motion analysis systems are being used by researchers. The tables include the purpose of the study, motion analysis system used, variables measured, and relevant results.

The primary advantages of time and distance measures are that they can be determined simply and inexpensively, and that they yield objective and reliable baseline data that can be used to formulate anticipated goals and expected outcomes, and to evaluate the patient's progress. For example, gait patterns displayed by patients with arthritis often are characterized by a reduced rate and range of knee motion compared with those of normal subjects, and they have a slower than normal gait velocity. Brinkmann and Perry[93] found that following joint replacement the rate and range of knee motion and gait velocity increased above preoperative levels, but did not reach normal levels. Usually, increases in measures such as cadence and velocity indicate improvement in a patient's gait. However, comparisons with normal standards are appropriate only if the goal of treatment is to restore a normal gait pattern (e.g., for a patient recovering from a meniscectomy). Comparison with normative standards may not be appropriate for a patient who has had a cerebral vascular accident. The appropriate norms for examining the gait of a patient with hemiplegia may be either a population of patients with hemiplegia who are of similar age, gender, and involvement, or the patient's pretreatment gait. Few disadvantages exist regarding kinematic quantitative gait analysis, except for the possible expense involved in instrumentation, and the fact that a certain amount of uncertainty exists about how to normalize for leg length,

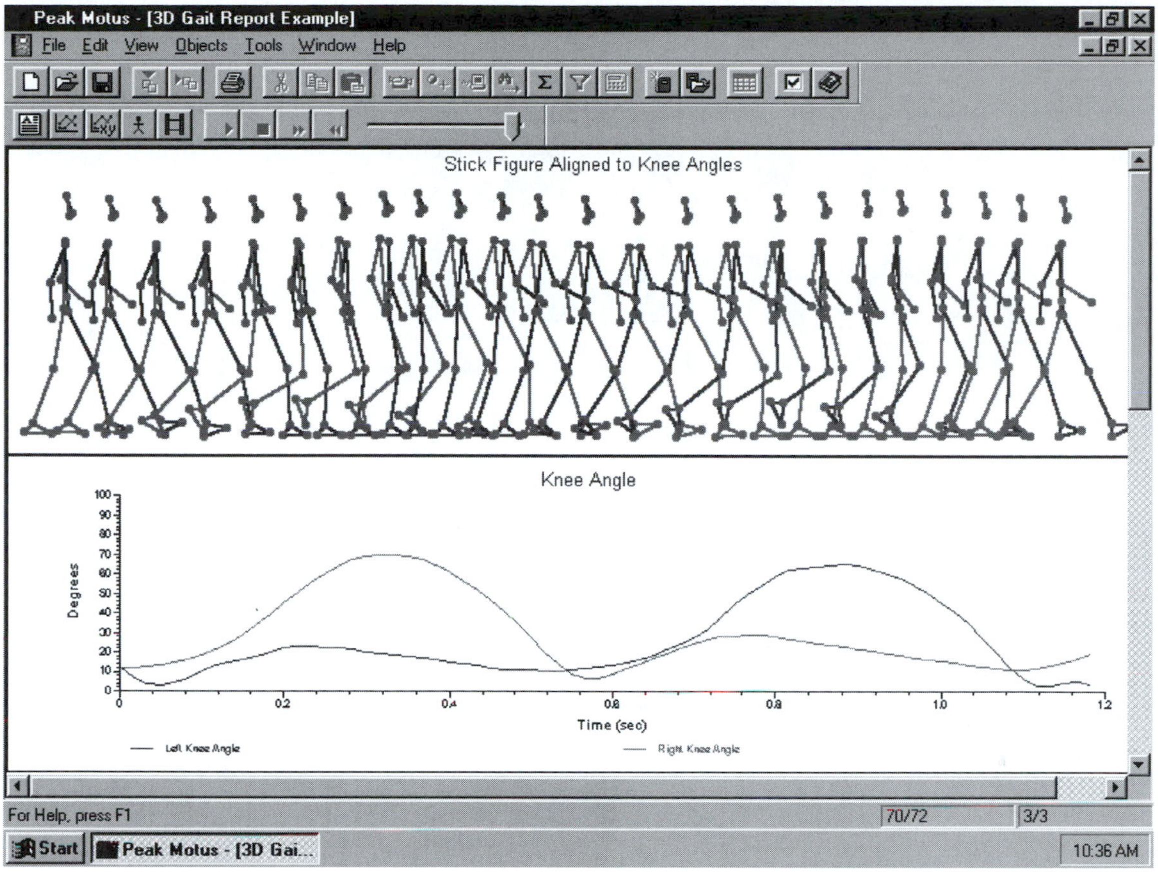

Figure 10.11 Another format for presentation of the data from a motion-analysis system is computer-generated stick figure representations of one complete gait cycle. In this particular case, the pattern of knee motion is graphically presented below the stick figures. (Courtesy of Peak Performance Technologies, Inc, Centennial, CO 80112.)

height, age, gender, weight, level of maturation, and disability. Temporal and distance determinants should be used as an integral part of, or in conjunction with, both observational and kinetic analyses to provide a complete picture of gait. A sample recording form for time and distance variables is presented in Table 10.23.

Therapists must be extremely cautious when selecting a norm or standard by which to measure patient progress. Significant age, gender, weight, and activity level related differences have been found in both temporal and distance measures.[55,94,95] Hinman et al found that the oldest group (63 to 102 years) of 289 subjects had a significantly slower self-selected walking speed and smaller step length in comparison to the younger group. Age was a significant determinant of walking speed after age 62, but height was a significant determinant prior to age 62.[94] Step length has been found to be significantly shorter and the double support stance period significantly increased in an elderly sample compared to a database of young adults.[55] Chou and colleagues found a number of gender differences in kinematic and kinetic gait variables. For example, females had shorter stride lengths and narrower step widths, a more anteriorly tilted pelvis, greater hip flexion and internal rotation, greater knee valgus, and smaller ankle joint moment compared to males. Some of these changes were attributed to the females' wider pelvises.[96]

McGibbon and Krebs[64] found a healthy group of elderly subjects had a slower gait speed and step length, decreased late-stance ankle plantarflexion angle, increased late-stance peak eccentric knee power absorption, and early-stance peak concentric hip extensor power generation compared to young adults. Bohannon et al[57] found that gender, body weight, and nondominant hip flexor strength were the best predictors of both comfortable and maximum gait speed for a group healthy men women ages 50 to 79 years. However, these variables accounted for only a small percentage of the variance in gait speed. Furthermore, muscle strength correlated more highly with maximal gait speed than with comfortable speed.

The interpretation of motion patterns obtained through motion analysis systems usually involves comparisons of an individual's data with a mean curve for normal subjects using one standard deviation (SD) for boundaries. Sutherland and co-workers[97] suggest that motion patterns cannot be fully analyzed without consideration of all points along the curve. They propose the use of prediction

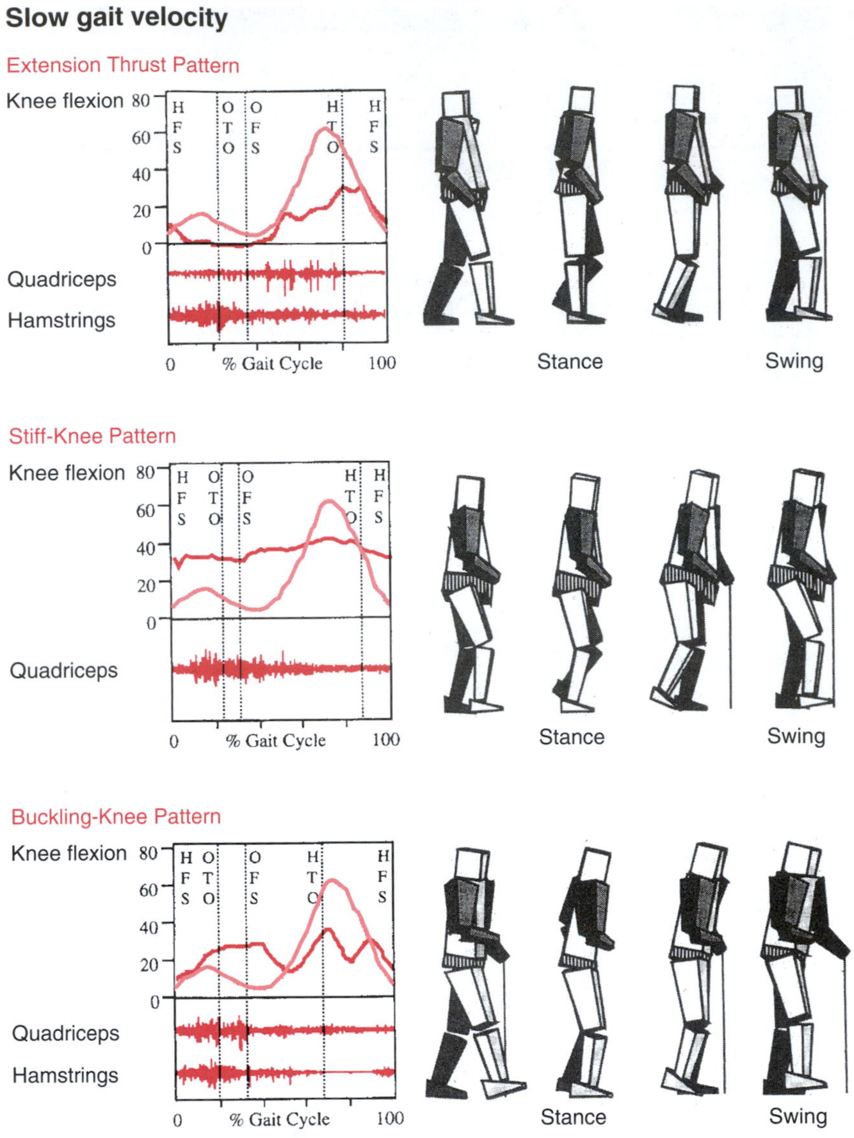

Figure 10.12 Graphs and EMG data for motion of the knee in the sagittal plane for one gait cycle of the three motion patterns. Each patient represents only one of the three motion patterns (extension thrust, stiff knee and buckling knee) associated with a slow gait velocity. The solid dark red line indicates the motion pattern and the lighter red line represents the normal. HFS, foot strike (initial contact) on the hemiplegic side; OTO, toe-off on the contralateral (unaffected) side; OFS, foot strike (initial contact) on the contralateral (unaffected) side; HTO, toe-off on the hemiplegic side. (From De Quervain, IAK, et al,[6] with permission.)

regions (multiples of the SD above and below the mean curve of data for each point in the gait cycle) (Fig. 10.13). Within a prediction region, if any point along the curve of joint motion falls outside of the defined region, the patient's gait is considered to be abnormal.

Gait Pattern Classification

Identification of gait parameters that deviate widely from a norm is a fairly simple outcome of gait analysis. However, identification of groups or clusters of gait deviations that characterize a known disorder is more complicated and represents one of the very urgent needs in gait analysis. In an attempt to classify gait disorders, a number of statistical techniques are being used for both kinematic and kinetic gait variables. The *bootstrap technique*[98] is used to establish the boundaries (prediction regions) about the mean curve for healthy control subjects in order to establish the limits of normal variability. *Discriminant analysis* is being used to recognize gait patterns of healthy people and persons with gait deviations. *Principal components analysis* is useful to reduce the large quantities of data acquired in a gait analysis to a set of features that accurately describes gait patterns. *Cluster analysis* is used to place subjects in homogeneous groups, or clusters, based on specified input parameters.

Normalcy Index

Principal components analysis was used to develop a *Normalcy Index (NI),* which was able to quantify the amount of deviation in a subject's gait compared to the gait of an average unimpaired person. The *NI* has been found to be sensitive enough to distinguish unimpaired subjects from idiopathic toe walkers and to distinguish between plegic and uninvolved limbs of hemiplegic subjects. However, the gait pathology of nonindependent walkers

Table 10.21 **Studies Addressing Specific Disorders and Movement Diagnosis Using Motion Analysis Systems**

Authors	Purpose	Motion Analysis Method	Variables	Subjects	Relevant Results
Kim, CM, and Eng, JJ[86] 2004	To understand whether the magnitude or pattern of 3D kinematic and kinetic profiles relate to gait performance	OptoTrak[1] force platform	Joint angles, moments and powers	20 individuals with chronic stroke	Many highly related variables: sagittal plane paretic side hip power generation, nonparetic side ankle power generation; frontal plane paretic side hip power generation, nonparetic side ankle power generation.
Neptune, RR, Zajac, FE, Kautz SA[87] 2004	To understand the contribution of individual muscles to support and forward progression of the body	Optoelectronic system[2] force platform; SIMM[3]	Simulated muscle forces, joint angles, moments and powers	5 healthy males	Uniarticular knee and hip extensor muscles are critical to body support in early stance; redistribution of segmental power by muscles is critical to forward progression of trunk and legs.
Schwartz, MH, Novacheck, TF, Trost, J[88] 2000	To objectively diagnose clinical change in hip function	Vicon 370 motion analysis system[4]	Joint angles, moments, powers	6 children with cerebral palsy; 23 normal control subjects	A hip function diagnostic index was developed using principal component analysis. Variables included maximum pelvic tilt, a hip moment timing variable, max hip extension, H3 (pull-off) power.
Maurer, BT, et al[89] 1993	To diagnose ankle equinus deformity	Custom-built Podiatric Telefactor Motion Analysis Systeme[5]; force platform	Ankle angle, moment, distance of ankle to center of pressure in transverse plane, ankle angle	22 persons with varied equinus disorders aged 5–34 years; 9 able-bodied, aged 23–28 years	Preliminary data showed protocol to be useful in diagnosing nature of equinus and evaluating treatment effectiveness.

Table 10.22 Studies Addressing Selection of Intervention or Effectiveness of Treatment Using Motion Analysis Systems

Authors	Purpose	Motion Analysis Method	Variables	Subjects	Relevant Results
Park, ES, Park, CI, Kim JY[13] 2001	To inform selection of anterior vs posterior walkers for children with spastic diplegic cerebral palsy	Vicon 370 motion analysis system[4]	Spatiotemporal, joint angles	10 spastic diplegic cerebral palsied children average age 9 years	Flexion angles of trunk, hip and knee were lower with posterior walker; posterior walker has more upright positioning.
Thomas, SS, et al[90] 2002	To inform choice of three possible ankle-foot orthosis configurations for stair locomotion in children with spastic hemiplegia	Vicon 370 motion analysis system with Vicon Clinical Manager[4]	Joint angles hip knee and ankle of both limbs in stair ascent and descent	19 children with spastic hemiplegia age 9 ± 3 years	Hinged AFO provided greatest dorsiflexion during stance; all reduced plantarflexion in comparison to barefoot; the use of any AFO did not impair stair ambulation.
Teixeira-Salmela, LF, et al[91] 2001	To evaluate effectiveness of strengthening and conditioning on gait of subjects with stroke	Peak Motus 2D motion analysis system[6]	Joint angles, moments and powers, work of major muscle groups	13 subjects chronic stroke (6 females, 7 males, age 67 ± 9.2 years)	Subjects were able to generate higher levels of powers and positive work by the ankle plantar flexor and hip flexor/extensor muscles.
Schwartz, MH, et al[92] 2004	To evaluate effectiveness of gait analysis and surgery on gait of children with CP	Vicon 370/512 motion analysis system[4]	16 clinically relevant kinematic parameters	135 children with CP who had gait analysis and surgery between 1994 and 2002.	79% of subjects improved on a predominance of outcome measures; only 7% of subjects worsened.

[1]Northern Digital, Inc, Ontario N2V 1C5 Canada
[2]Computerized Functional Testing Components, Chicago, IL
[3]MusculoGraphics, Inc, Santa Rosa, CA
[4]Oxford Metrics, Ltd, Botley, Oxford, UK
[5]Podiatric Telefactor Motion Analysis System
[6]Peak Performance Technologies, Inc, Centennial, CO

Table 10.23 Gait Analysis Recording Form: Temporal and Spatial Measures

Patient's name ______________________ Age ________ Sex ________
Height ________ Weight ________

Diagnosis ______________________

Ambulatory aids: Yes ________ No ________

Type: Crutch(es) ________ Cane(s): R ________ Walker: ________
L ________

Other: ________

Date											
Therapist's initials											
Distance walked (distance from first to last heel strike)											
Elapsed time (time from first to last heel strike)											
Walking velocity (distance walked divided by elapsed time)											
Left stride length (distance between two consecutive left heel strikes)											
Right stride length (distance between two consecutive right heel strikes)											
Left step length (distance between a right heel strike and the next consecutive left heel strike)											
Right step length (distance between a left heel strike and the next consecutive right heel strike)											
Step length difference (difference between right and left step lengths)											
Cadence (total number of steps taken divided by the elapsed time)											
Width of walking base (perpendicular distance between right and left heel strike)											
Left foot angle (angle formed between a line bisecting the left foot and the line of progression)											
Right foot angle (angle formed between a line bisecting the right foot and the line of progression)											
Right stride length to right lower extremity length (right stride length divided by right lower extremity length)											
Left stride length to left lower extremity length (left stride length divided by left lower extremity length)											

The therapist may obtain averages for stride and step lengths, width of walking base, and foot angles.

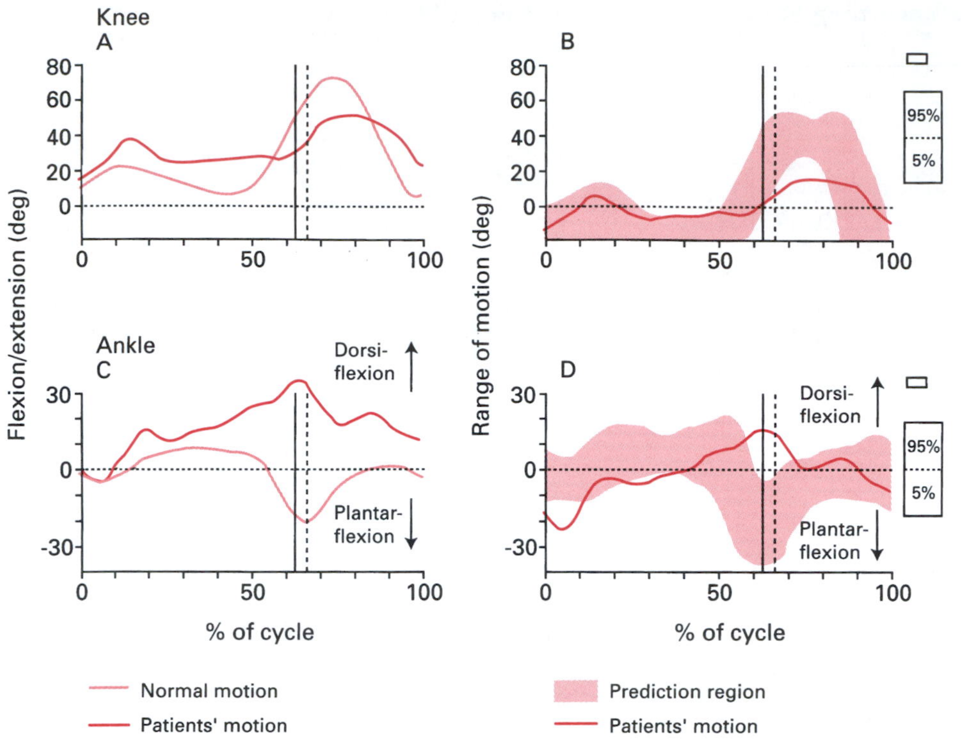

Figure 10.13 Prediction regions (Sutherland, DH, et al,[97] with permission.)

was not well categorized. The authors suggested that perhaps the inclusion of kinetic variables along with kinematic variables might be helpful.

The principal components method derived the NI by assigning weighted factors inversely proportional to the amount of variation exhibited by each gait measure in the unimpaired population. However, since the data come from a motion analysis system they are subject to the same sources of error such as soft tissue artifacts and marker misplacement.[99]

Cluster Analysis

Cluster analysis is a commonly used statistical technique in the social sciences, but only relatively recently has been used to create an objective classification system of gait patterns. Cluster analysis has been used to classify gait patterns of patients with stroke based on spatial and temporal parameters for each phase of the gait cycle and identified the following four clusters of gait patterns: fast, moderate, flexed, and extended. The authors suggested that clinicians could use critical parameters to categorize patients with CVA, so that intervention programs could be more specifically targeted to underlying impairments.[100]

Kinetic Gait Analysis

Variables

Kinetic gait analyses are directed toward examination and analysis of the forces involved in gait, including ground reaction forces, joint torques, center of pressure (CoP), center of mass (CoM), mechanical energy, moments of force, power, support moments, work, joint reaction forces, and intrinsic foot pressure (Table 10.24). Although in the past kinetic gait analyses have been used primarily for research purposes, at the present time they are being used clinically as well.

The instrumentation required to examine kinetic variables is complex and expensive because derivation of kinetics requires knowledge of all of the forces on the part of the body analyzed (e.g., the foot or the thigh). The analysis usually starts with the forces being applied to the foot, which is determined by a force plate embedded in the floor. These plates contain load transducers that measure the **center of pressure (CoP)**, **center of mass (CoM)** and ground reaction forces during gait. Typically, the force plates are based on either strain gage or piezoelectric technology.

Calculation of kinetic variables at the ankle requires knowledge of the forces acting on the foot, mass, and location of the CoM (derived from standard anthropometric tables), and knowledge about the acceleration of the CoM. Once this knowledge is obtained, equations can be set up to solve for the net forces and net moments occurring at the ankle, at that particular instant in time, in order for the foot to have moved with those particular accelerations. When solutions are found for forces and moments at the ankle, similar equations can be applied to the adjacent proximal segment (the lower leg). One then knows, for each instant in time, whether the dominant internal moment is being caused by the dorsiflexors or the plantarflexors. If the internal moment for each instant in time is multiplied by the net angular velocity between the ankle and the lower

Table 10.24 Gait Variables: Kinetic Gait Analysis

Ground reaction forces	Vertical, anterior-posterior, and medial-lateral forces created as a result of foot contact with the supporting surface. These forces are equal in magnitude and opposite in direction to the force applied by the foot to the ground. Ground reaction forces are measured with force platforms in newtons (N) or pound force.
Pressure	Pressure = force per unit area. In gait analysis the pressure parameter that is usually measured is the pressure distribution under the foot.
Center of Pressure (COP)	The point of application of the resultant force. Movement of the COP as a function of time is used as a measure of stability of a subject who is either standing or walking on a force plate.
Torque (moment of force)	The turning or rotational effect produced by the application of a force. The greater the perpendicular distance from the point of application of a force from the axis of rotation, the greater the turning effect, or torque, produced. Torque is calculated by multiplying the force by the perpendicular distance from the point of application of the force and the axis of rotation. Torque = force × perpendicular distance or moment arm

leg, the result is knowledge of the net power being produced by the muscles across the ankle. Concentric contractions add power to the limb (power generation), and eccentric contractions reduce the power (power absorption). The most important periods of power generation of the work of walking occur through concentric contraction of the ankle plantarflexors at push-off, the hip flexors during push-off and the short period immediately following, and the hip extensors in the early stance phase. Variations in these expected patterns are particularly useful in examining deficiencies and in determining treatment goals.

The **ground (floor) reaction force (GRF)** is defined as the net vertical and shear or horizontal forces acting between the foot and the supporting surface. The force is three-dimensional and can be resolved into three components: vertical, anterior–posterior, and medial–lateral. Each component varies throughout the gait cycle and is affected by velocity, cadence, and body mass. The averaged wave forms of the vertical and anterior–posterior force components, presented as a percentage of body

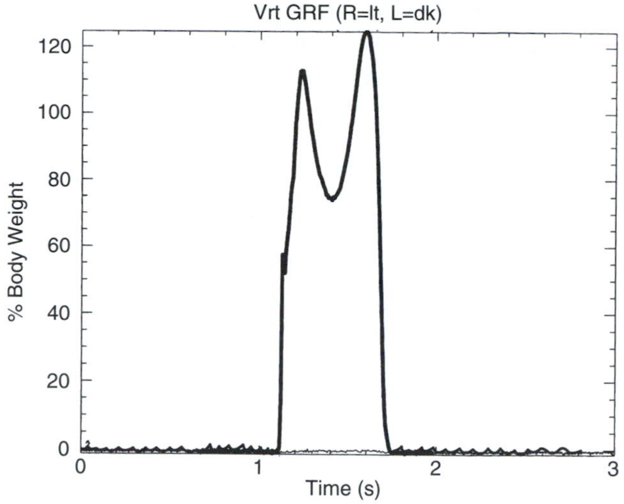

Figure 10.14 The computer-generated graph of the vertical component of the ground-reaction force was obtained using a force plate. (Courtesy of Dr. David Krebs, Motion Analysis Laboratory, MGH Institute of Health Professions, Boston, MA 02129.)

weight, show consistent patterns across normal subjects for loading rate, peak force, average force, and unloading rate. The anterior–posterior force has a characteristic negative phase followed by a positive phase. The negative phase represents deceleration, and the positive phase represents deceleration of the body mass. The vertical force waveform shows a characteristic double hump (Fig. 10.14). The medial–lateral force waveforms are variable even in normal individuals.

Instruments for Measuring Kinetic Variables

Force Plate Technology

Force plate technology, such as that produced by both Kistler Instrument Corporation and Advanced Mechanical Technology, Inc (AMTI), is capable of measuring the ground reaction force (GRF) as well as calculating the CoM, *acceleration, velocity, displacement, power,* and *work.* A graphic display is possible showing the waveforms of the GRF. Kistler Instrument Corp also markets a treadmill called the Gaitway. The treadmill is capable of measuring the GRF and CoP during both walking and running. In addition to graphical presentation and statistical functions, the treadmill system can calculate temporal and spatial parameters.

Cook et al[11] used a force plate to investigate the effect of a knee flexion restriction (using a brace) and walking speed on the GRF. The authors concluded that the application of a brace to restrict knee flexion for the purpose of protection after injury, or while surgically repaired structures were healing, may actually increase the stress on both the braced and unbraced limbs.

Hesse et al[5] compared the trajectories of the CoP and the CoM in 10 healthy and 14 subjects with hemiparesis.

They found that the healthy subjects showed no differences in the behavior of the CoP, CoM, temporal parameters, and step length when initiating gait with either the right or left extremity. In comparison, patients with hemiparesis showed pronounced asymmetric behavior depending on which limb was the starting limb (affected vs nonaffected). While patients who initiated gait with the affected limb were similar to healthy subjects, patients who started gait with the nonaffected limb showed inconsistent movement of the CoP and were incapable of producing directional movement of the body's CoM. Therefore, therapists should be cautioned about promoting that type of gait initiation because the affected leg may be too weak to support starting gait with the unaffected leg. Rossi et al[7] investigated the CoM, CoP, and GRF in a study of gait initiation in patients with transtibial amputations. These authors found that the patients consistently loaded the intact limb more than the prosthetic limb regardless of which limb initiated gait.[7]

Force plates may be used either as part of, or in combination with, motion analysis systems, and may be used with temporal-distance analysis systems, as well as in conjunction with EMG and electrogoniometry, for a comprehensive analysis of kinematic and kinetic gait variables.

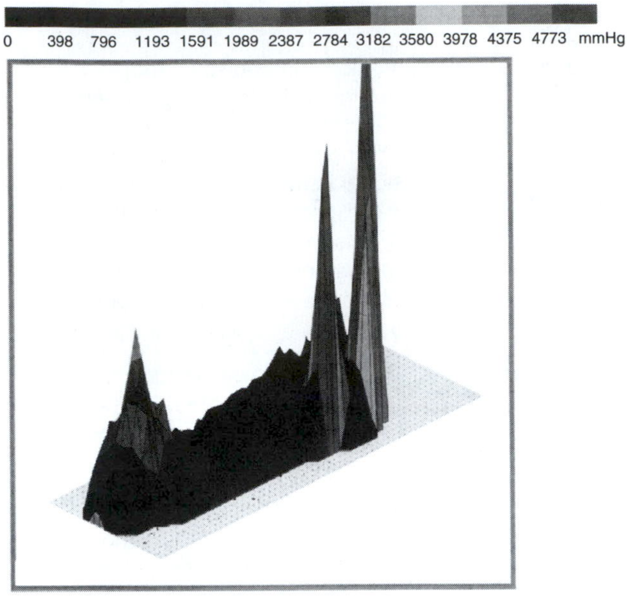

Figure 10.15 Magnitude and location of peak pressure during one complete left foot strike. The highest pressures are shown on the heel, first metatarsal head and great toe. (Courtesy of Tekscan, Inc, South Boston, MA 02129.)

Plantar Pressure Measurement Systems

Pressure measurement systems may also be used with force plates. Pressure is equal to force divided by area, and is measured by pressure sensors. Therefore, pressure is equal to the force on the sensor divided by the area of the sensor. Plantar pressure measurements are most commonly in gait analysis to determine the pressure distribution under the foot: foot-to-ground contact, foot-to-shoe contact, and shoe-to-ground contact. Pressure measurements may be used to determine orthotic efficacy, ulceration risk in diabetes, and for regulating weight bearing following surgery. Many different types of measurement techniques have been developed for measuring contact pressures. Tekscan Inc (Boston, MA 02127) has a system called the *F-Scan® Bipedal In-Shoe Plantar Pressure/Force Measurement System* that measures bipedal plantar pressures using paper-thin disposable pressure sensors placed in a patient's shoes. The sensor is ultrathin, flexible, and trimmable with 960 sensing locations distributed across the entire plantar surface. An example of the type of information obtained from the F-scan system is presented in Figure 10.15. Reliability of the F-scan system was determined by Randolph and colleagues to be sufficient for the purpose of designing corrective measures to relieve excessive pressures on the foot.[101] Birke and co-workers used the F-scan system to compare the effectiveness of a wedge shoe with a short leg walker and other type shoes in relieving plantar pressure.[102] Another system produced by Tekscan, Inc (Boston, MA 02127) is called *Mat-Scan System,®* which is a pressure-sensing floor mat that allows the clinician to identify barefoot pressures. Mueller et al[103] used the *F-Scan Bipedal In-Shoe Plantar Pressure/Force Measurement System* in the management of patients with neuropathic ulcers or metatarsalgia. Armstrong et al[104] found that patients found to have high plantar pressures and wounds greater than 3.12 in. (8 cm) took significantly longer to heal than other patients. Wertsch et al[105] described a portable insole plantar pressure measurement system that also could be used to study cane cadence and residual limb pressures of below-knee prosthesis.

EMED Pedar® (Novel Electronics, Inc, St Paul, MN 55105) in-shoe planter pressure measurement system is another type of pressure measurement system. Insoles placed between the shoe and sock are comprised of a matrix of 99 capacitance sensors. Warren and co-workers used this type of sensor system, combined with EMG, to describe the temporal patterns of plantar pressures and lower leg muscle activities over a wide range of treadmill walking speeds in normal subjects.[106]

Simple hand-held dynamometers and isokinetic systems can be used to obtain static and dynamic peak torques prior to obtaining temporal and distance measures. Connelly and Vandervoort[65] found that decreases in isometric and dynamic quadriceps strength led to significant decreases in fast-paced and self-selected speed.

Methods for Measuring Energy Costs During Gait

Walking at constant speed is a cyclical activity that requires the body to add energy by means of concentric contractions, and remove energy by means of eccentric contractions. These energy transfers and exchanges are cleverly designed to make walking efficient. Generally, conditions that affect either the motor control of gait and posture or conditions that affect joint and muscle structure and function will increase the energy cost of gait.[107–111] The type of footwear,[112] use of assistive devices, and speed of gait affect energy expenditure as well.[23] Energy expenditure is an important consideration in gait analyses, particularly in neurological conditions in which muscular resources are low. There are three general approaches in determining energy costs: *physiological measurement, mechanical energy analysis,* and *heart rate data.* The selection of a particular approach should be based on the purpose of taking the measure and the relative importance of test characteristics outlined at the beginning of this chapter.

Physiological Energy Cost Measures

Physiological cost measures estimate the heat (energy) produced by a subject at rest and during exercise by indirect calorimetry, based on the assumption that all energy-using reactions of the body depend on oxygen uptake. The most common method of measuring oxygen uptake during walking is open-loop spirometry in which exhaled air is sampled and analyzed for its oxygen content, classically using the Douglas bag method.[107] More recently, stationary or moving metabolic carts or lightweight portable devices perform breath-by-breath oxygen and carbon dioxide analysis. Two parameters of prime interest are *oxygen cost* and *oxygen rate.* One may be interested in the oxygen cost or energy expenditure per unit of distance walked (in mL/kg/m), which relates to the physiological work involved in the task and reflects gait efficiency. Alternatively the oxygen rate, or energy expenditure per unit of time (in mL/kg/min), reflects the power of walking and is interpreted using knowledge of walking speed.[108,113]

Physiological cost analysis methods are most useful in comparing the energy cost of walking with normal values or an individual's maximum capacity, and for determining the effects on energy costs of interventions such as the use of orthoses. Physiological cost analyses reflect overall costs of walking with respect to distance or time, but they cannot discern the possible causes. If insight into the particular movements is needed, mechanical energy analysis can be helpful.

Mechanical Energy Cost Determination

There are two methods of obtaining mechanical energy costs. In the first method, kinematic data alone are required, using estimates of masses of body parts and of locations of the centers of mass of these parts. By employing a spatial motion analysis system with basic equations of motion and anthropometric constants for masses of body parts, the potential energy and translational and rotational kinetic energy levels of each body part can be calculated. The differences between values obtained at each time increment indicate energy cost. Various equations are used to combine the costs across body parts to yield the total body cost. The large head-arms-and-trunk segment shows excellent energy exchanges between kinetic and potential types, providing the body with energy efficiency. When the body is at its highest position (mid-stance), it is also moving most slowly, but as the head-arms-and-trunk "roll down the hill" into initial contact of the foot, this potential energy is changed into kinetic energy, and the head-arms-and-trunk picks up speed. In this way, a great deal of energy is saved and the movement is efficient. However, if the person walks very slowly or very quickly, or has a stiff knee and has to lift one side of the body excessively to clear the floor, the energies are no longer complementary in size and/or shape; less energy exchange can take place.[114] These modes of walking are less efficient than normal walking.

The second method of obtaining mechanical energy costs uses a kinetic approach. Briefly stated, the energy changes in a body part between subsequent instants in time are calculated (1) from the products of the forces on each end of the joint and the velocity of the point of application and (2) from the muscle powers, which are the products of each muscle moment and the angular velocity of the body part. In some cases, the muscle is adding energy to the part (generation), and, in other cases, it is absorbing energy. There are a number of different methods of handling the calculations of mechanical energy, exchanges, and transfers but a sound approach is described by McGibbon and colleagues.[115]

Heart Rate Data

A third general approach to determining the relative energy cost of gait is by measuring the heart rate (HR) during ambulation. Relative energy consumption has been found to be highly correlated with HR and absolute level of energy consumption has been found to be highly correlated with HR and maximum walking speed. The most accurate way to determine HR is to use a telemetry system that produces beat-by-beat information as well as electrocardiographic activity. Many inexpensive heart rate monitors are also available and some are designed to download stored information to a computer (see Chapter 4). HR responses to ambulation can also be determined by palpation of the radial or carotid arteries, though somewhat more error may be present.

HR measures have been shown to be adequately sensitive for some applications. For example, simple measures of HR and maximum ambulatory velocity allowed accurate prediction ($r = 0.89$) of energy consumption in 35 children with myelomeningocele.[113] However, Herbert and colleagues[109] found no difference in HR between children with transtibial amputations and those with intact lower extremities even though energy consumption was 15 percent higher in the children with amputations. Perhaps because the conditions were more disparate, Waters and co-workers found that in patients with hip arthrodesis

Table 10.25 Salient Features of Studies Examining Various Methods of Gait Analysis

Author(s)	Method of Gait Analysis Studied	Subjects/Parameters	Findings/Conclusions
Nelson, AJ[39] 1974	FAP	31 patients with neurological deficits	High interrater and intrarater reliability.
Titianova, EB, et al[126] 2003	FAP	Comparison between individuals who were approximately 6 months post-stroke and healthy individuals	FAP scores relate well to the patient's gait variations and variations in functional outcome, but only at an unhurried gait speed.
Wolf, SL, Catlin, PA, Gage, K[41] 1999	EFAP	28 patients who had sustained a stroke	High interrater reliability, construct, and concurrent validity.
Baer, HR, and Wolf, SL[127] 2001	MEFAP	26 patients who were between 16 and 66 days post-stroke	High interrater reliability and test–retest reliability for the timed portion of the profile. The mEFAP provided clear and specific functional information and was sensitive to changes in the amount of time taken to complete ambulation tasks.
Shields, RK, et al[42] 1995	Iowa Level of Assistance Scale	Patients following total hip or knee replacements	Highly reliable, valid, and responsive.
Hawley, CA, et al[128] 1999	FIM + FAM	Psychometric analysis of 2268 FIM + FAM examinations of 965 patients from 11 brain injury centers	Use of untransformed ratings should be adequate for most clinical and research purposes in comparable samples of patients with head injury.
Donaghy, S, and Wass, PJ[129] 1998	FIM + FAM	53 severely involved survivors of traumatic brain injury (40 men, 13 women)	Motor items in the FIM + FAM have better reliability than the cognitive items. ICCs in the good to excellent range for 29 of the 30 items and for all subscales except psychosocial adjustment.
Ottenbacher, KJ, et al[45] 1997	Functional Independence Measure for Children (WeeFIM)	205 children (11 to 87 months of age) diagnosed with cerebral palsy, developmental disabilities, mental retardation, Down syndrome, and other cognitive impairments	Agreement and stability of the WeeFIM was found to be excellent across trained raters and time.
Van Swearingen, JM, et al[22] 1996	GARS-M	52 community-dwelling elderly residents	Reliable and valid and could be used to predict persons at risk for falls.
Shumway-Cook, A, et al[23] 1997	Berg Balance Scale	Community dwelling elderly persons	Sensitivity of 91% (20 of the 22 fallers correctly classified) and a specificity of 82% (18 of the 22 nonfallers correctly classified).
Di Fabio, RP, and Seay, R[47] 1997	FEMBAF	35 community-dwelling elders (4 men, 31 women), mean age: 79.9 years	Valid and reliable measurement of risk factors, functional performance, and factors that hinder mobility.
Brandes, M, and Rosenbaum, D[131] 2004	SAM	Comparisons between the percentage of locomotion monitored by the DynaPort activity of daily living monitor and the number of steps determined by the SAM	High concurrent validity ($r = 0.95$).

(continued)

Table 10.25 Salient Features of Studies Examining Various Methods of Gait Analysis (continued)

Author(s)	Method of Gait Analysis Studied	Subjects/Parameters	Findings/Conclusions
Coleman, KL, et al[71] 1999	SAM	45 subjects with diabetic neuropathy	Average deviation of the SAM count from 2 observers using the hand-held tally counters was 0.54% for the first trial and 0.65% for the second trial.
Moe-Nilssen, R[72] 1998	Triaxial accelerometer	19 healthy students	High absolute test–retest repeatability for 2-feet standing; relative reliability low owing to restricted range of values (ICC >.56); for one-foot standing, reliability highest in mediolateral direction (ICC = .84); reliability of walking tests ICC values ranged from .79 to .94.
Henriksen, M, et al[73] 2004	Triaxial accelerometer	6 men, 14 women (mean age = 35.2; range 18–57)	Measurement error values were very low (0.007–0.01 for mean acceleration to 1.644 step/min for cadences). Reliability was high with ICC values ranging from .77 to .96.
Tong, K, and Granat, MH[75] 1999	Gyroscopes	Data from a uniaxial gyroscope (ENC-05EA, Murata, Japan) was compared with simultaneous data produced from the Vicon Motion Analysis System. 2 pairs of force sensing resistors placed under the feet of 9 young (mean age = 21 years) and 11 elderly subjects (mean age = 79 years)	Good correlations were found between the signals from the motion analysis system and the gyroscope.
Aminian, K et al[134] 2004	Gyroscopes	New algorithm based upon wavelet transformation to detect toe-off and heelstrike from angular velocity	Good agreement (r >0.99) was found between actual gait events detected by foot sensors and events detected by gyroscopes. No significant differences were noted between sensors and gyroscope for gait cycle and stance times, stride length, and velocity.
Pomeroy, VM, et al[77] 2004	GAITMAT II	5 raters determined the spatiotemporal parameters of 19 stroke patients	8 of the 17 parameters tested showed significant differences between raters.
Bliney, B, Morris, M, Webster, K[135] 2003	GAITRite and Stride Analyzer	25 healthy adults walking at fast and slow speeds	Strong concurrent validity and test–retest reliability, but best at preferred and fast speeds.
McDonough, AL, et al[136] 2001	GAITRite	GAITRite system compared to paper and pencil recordings and video	High correlation between measures of cadence, walking speed, right and left step and stride lengths, and step times.
Titianova, AEB, and Tarka, IM[137] 1995	GAITRite	Relationship between the FAP, type of stroke, patient's functional disability, and spatial and temporal variables. Compared footprint parameters to the FAP in 62 healthy subjects	Found GAITRite easy to use, suitable for repetitive measurements and quick to report information on temporal, spatial, and footprint parameters.

(continued)

Table 10.25 Salient Features of Studies Examining Various Methods of Gait Analysis (continued)

Author(s)	Method of Gait Analysis Studied	Subjects/Parameters	Findings/Conclusions
Nelson, AJ, et al[138] 2002	GAITRite	People with early stage Parkinson's disease and healthy controls at preferred speed, but not at fast speed	Discriminated between groups (patient group attained a significantly lower FAP score). ICCs for all variables were 0.92 and higher, except base of support (ICC = 0.80). At fast walking speed all variables had ICCs of 0.91 or higher, except swing and single support time (ICC = 0.89) and base of support (ICC = 0.79).
Van Uden, CJT, and Besser, MP[139] 2004	GAITRite	21 healthy subjects (19–59 years)	At preferred walking speed, ICCs for all variables were 0.92 and higher except base of support (ICC = 0.80). At fast walking speed, all variables had ICCs above 0.89 except base of support (ICC = 0.79).
Menz, HB, et al[140] 2004	GAITRite	30 healthy young people (22–40 years) and 31 older people (76–87 years)	Test–retest reliability for both groups for walking speed, cadence, and step length were excellent (ICC between 0.82 and 0.92 and coefficients of variation (CVs) between 1.4% and 3.5%). Base of support and toe in/out angles had high ICCs, but were associated with higher CVs (8.3%–17.7%) in young people and 14.3%–33% in older subjects.
Besser, M, et al[141] 1996	Ariel Performance System	Skeleton with 9 passive markers placed on the pelvis and left LE. Joint angles were measured with an electronic inclinometer.	For most trials, the APAS and GaitLab™ hip and knee flexion and extension angle measurements agreed with the inclinometer, but occasionally large nonsystematic disagreements of up to 18.6° occurred. The only consistent error was with hip abduction and adduction using the APAS software (32–97°). Not unexpected, because the system calculates angles using marker-to-marker vectors and no marker can be placed on the actual center of the hip joint.
Wilson, DJ, et al[142] 1997	Ariel Performance System	Reconstructed angular estimates of the Ariel Performance System	Mean errors were consistently within the range of + or −1°.

EFAP = Emory Functional Ambulation Profile; FAM = Functional Assessment Measure; FAP = Functional Ambulation Profile; FEMBAF = Fast Evaluation of Mobility, Balance, and Fear; FIM = Functional Independence Measure; FIM + FAM = Functional Independence Measure (FIM) plus the Functional Assessment Measure (FAM); GARS-M = Modified Gait Abnormality Rating Scale; ICC = Intraclass Correlation Coefficient; MEFAP = Modified Emory Functional Ambulation Profile; SAM = Step Activity Monitor.

oxygen consumption was 32 percent greater than normal and that HR was significantly greater than normal.[107]

An energy index based on HR called the *Physiological Cost Index (PCI)* was developed specifically to determine the relative costs of walking per unit of distance walked.[116] Calculated as the difference between the walking HR and the resting HR divided by the average speed, it is expressed in beats per meter.

Some researchers have found oxygen uptake measures to be more repeatable and less variable than PCI.[117–119] In one study, oxygen cost was found to be considerably more reliable than PCI, indicating somewhat low PCI sensitivity.[118]

Ijzerman and Nene[120] concluded that subtracting baseline heart rate when calculating the PCI is probably not useful because it increased within-subject variability. It is possible that the PCI has better repeatability with unimpaired subjects.[121] Despite somewhat questionable variability and sensitivity in persons with disabilities, it has been used successfully to distinguish between the cost of walking versus wheelchair leg-wheeling and arm-wheeling[122] in persons with motor limitations, to demonstrate the positive effects of a slider shoe in a single case study of a person with stroke,[123] and to show that increasing the lateral rigidity of a mechanical orthosis for achieving reciprocal walking in patients with high level paraplegic produces a very positive effect on the energetics, namely a 30 percent reduction in PCI.[124] Recently a *Total Heart Beat Index* has been developed which shows promise of greater reproducibility than the PCI, and readers should watch for reports examining its reliability and sensitivity.[125] Table 10.25 presents an overview of the salient features of studies examining various methods of gait analysis.

Summary

An overview of some methods for kinematic and kinetic gait analyses has been presented in this chapter. Many of the common variables examined in gait analyses have been defined and described, and examples of studies using gait analyses have been presented. Observational gait analysis and time and distance variables have been emphasized, because they appear to be the most common types of analyses used in the clinical setting. A brief overview of some of the motion analysis systems has been provided. Readers are encouraged to investigate the capabilities of individual motion analysis systems, and to consult the gait literature for reliability and validity studies regarding these systems. The ability to perform a gait analysis that accurately describes a patient's gait will provide important quantifiable information necessary for optimal treatment planning.

Questions for Review

1. Describe each of the three different types of gait analyses (kinematic qualitative, kinematic quantitative, and kinetic).
   - List the variables examined in each of the three types of gait analyses.
   - Select one variable from each type of analysis and describe a method of analysis for each variable selected.
2. Explain intratester and intertester reliability and how they relate to gait analysis.
3. Compare the advantages and disadvantages of a kinematic qualitative gait analysis with the advantages and disadvantages of a kinematic quantitative analysis.
4. Using the model presented in Tables 10.1 to 10.11, perform an OGA that includes both identification of observed deviations and an analysis to determine the causes of the deviations.
5. Which type of gait analysis would be appropriate for examining velocity and cadence? Stride length? Peak plantar pressures? Ground reaction forces? Describe the analysis system you selected and justify your reason for selecting that particular system or method of analysis.
6. How quickly must one walk to cross a street before the typical traffic light changes?
7. Explain validity and how it relates to gait analysis. Give an example of each of the different types of validity.
8. How could a gait analysis of temporal parameters be used to demonstrate a patient's progress or lack of progress?

Case Study

HISTORY

This 65-year-old woman is 5 days post right total hip arthroplasty. The surgery was performed following a femoral neck fracture incurred during a fall on the ice in front of her home. She has had daily bedside physical therapy for the past 3 days and now is independent in transfers. However, she needs to be independent in walking before she goes home.

She has a past history of diabetes mellitus (onset age 50), which is controlled with daily insulin injections. She denies any history of "heart problems." She does not participate in any regular exercise program and spends a great deal of time sitting during her work as a seamstress. She is alert and oriented to time and place and has a pleasant demeanor. She is 5 feet 3 inches tall, and weighs 160 pounds.

Passive Rom Examination

Goniometric Assessment (ROM): Lower Extremities			
	Range of Motion (Degrees)	Left	Right
Hip	Flexion	WFL	0–40
	Extension	WFL	0–10
	Abduction	WFL	0–20
	Adduction	WFL	0–10
	Medial Rotation	WFL	Not tested
	Lateral Rotation	WFL	0–20
Knee	Flexion	WFL	0–120
Ankle	Dorsiflexion	WFL	0–15
	Plantarflexion	WFL	0–45
	Inversion	WFL	0–5
	Eversion	WFL	0–20

WFL = within functional limits; upper extremities: all ROM measurements are WFL.

Manual Muscle Test (MMT)

		Lower Extremities	
		Left	Right
Hip	Flexion	G	F
	Extension	G−	P
	Abduction	G−	P
	Adduction	G	F+
	Lateral Rotation	G	G−
	Medical Rotation	G	G−
Knee	Flexion	G	G−
	Extension	G−	G−
Ankle	Dorsiflexion	G	P
	Plantarflexion	G−	G−
	Inversion	G−	F
	Eversion	G	F+
Toes	Flexion	G−	G−
	Extension	G	P

MMT Upper Extremities: all muscle grades are within the G to G− range.

SENSATION

Right Lower Extremity

Deficits noted primarily along the medial aspect of right foot and two medial toes. Numeric values refer to the Sensation Scale below.

Sensory Examination

	Medial Aspect R Foot	Two Medial Toes
Sharp/dull	5	5
Light touch	5	5
Temperature	5	5
Propioceptive sensation	4	4

Sensation Scale

1. Intact: normal, accurate
2. Decreased: delayed response
3. Exaggerated: increased sensitivity
4. Inaccurate: inappropriate perception of stimuli
5. Absent: no response
6. *Inconsistent or ambiguous*

INSPECTION

Patient has an ulcer on the medial aspect of the right plantar surface which is 0.7 × 6.0 cm in diameter and 1.5 mm deep.

FUNCTIONAL ASSESSMENT

Transfers
  FIM level = 7
Activities of daily living
  Eating: FIM = 7
  Bathing: FIM = 7
  Dressing: FIM = 7

GUIDING QUESTIONS

1. Develop a physical therapy problem list.
2. Complete the sample OGA form based on the information presented (see Appendix A).
3. Present your recommendations for physical therapy intervention.

References

1. American Physical Therapy Association: Guide to physical therapist practice. Phys Ther 81:1, 2001.
2. Mueller, MJ, et al: Differences in gait characteristics of patients with diabetes and peripheral neuropathy compared with age-matched controls. Phys Ther 74:299, 1994.
3. Von Schroeder, HP, et al: Gait parameters following stroke: A practical assessment. J Rehabil Res Dev 32:25, 1995.
4. Walker, SC, et al: Gait pattern alteration by junctional sensory substitution in healthy and in diabetic subjects with peripheral neuropathy. Arch Phys Med Rehabil 78:853, 1997.
5. Hesse, S, et al: Asymmetry of gait initiation in hemiparetic stroke subjects. Arch Phys Med Rehabil 78:719, 1997.
6. De Quervain, IAK, et al: Gait pattern in the early recovery period after stroke. J Bone Joint Surg 78A:10:1506, 1996.
7. Rossi, SA, et al: Gait initiation of persons with below-knee amputations: The characterization and comparison of force profiles. J Rehabil Res 32:120, 1995.
8. Roth, EJ, et al: Hemiplegic gait: Relationships between walking speed and other temporal parameters. Am J Phys Med Rehabil 76:128, 1997.
9. Al Zahrani, KS, and Bakheit, AM: A study of the gait characteristics of patients with chronic osteoarthritis of the knee. Disabil Rehabil 24:275, 2002.
10. Kim, CM, and Eng, JJ: The relationship of lower-extremity muscle torque to locomotor performance in people with stroke. Phys Ther 83:49, 2003.
11. Cook, TM, et al: Effects on restricted knee flexion and walking speed on the vertical ground reaction force during gait. Phys Ther 25:236, 1997.
12. Postema, K, et al: Energy storage and release of prosthetic feet. Part 1: Biomechanical analysis related to user benefits. Prosth Orthot Int 21:17, 1997.
13. Park, ES, Park, CI, and Kim, JY: Comparison of anterior and posterior walkers with respect to gait parameters and energy expenditure of children with spastic diplegic cerebral palsy. Yonsei Med J 42:180, 2001.
14. Self, BP, Greenwald, R, and Pflaster, DS: A biomechanical analysis of medial unloading brace for osteoarthritis in the knee. Arthrit Care Res 13:191, 2000.
15. Gok, H, et al: Effects of ankle-foot orthoses on hemiparetic gait. Clin Rehab 17:137, 2003.
16. White, H, et al: Clinically prescribed orthoses demonstrate an increase in the velocity of gait in children with cerebral palsy: A retrospective study. Dev Med Child Neurol 44:227, 2002.
17. McCulloch, M, et al: The effect of foot orthotics and gait velocity on lower limb kinematics and temporal events. J Orthop Sports Phys Ther 17:2, 1993.
18. Eng, JJ, and Pierrynowski, MR: The effect of soft foot orthotics on three-dimensional lower limb kinematics and kinetics during walking and running. Phys Ther 74:836, 1994.
19. Radka, SA, et al: A comparison of gait with solid, dynamic and no ankle-foot orthoses in children with spastic cerebral palsy. Phys Ther 77:395, 1997.
20. Granata, KP, Abel, MF, and Damiano, DL: Joint angular velocity in spastic gait and the influence of muscle-tendon lengthening. J Bone Joint Surg [Am] 82:174, 2000.
21. Damiano, DL, et al: Effects of quadriceps muscle strengthening on crouch gait in children with spastic diplegia. Phys Ther 75:658, 1995.
22. Van Swearingen, JM, et al: The Modified Gait Abnormality Rating Scale for recognizing the risk of recurrent falls in community-dwelling elderly adults. Phys Ther 76:994, 1996.
23. Shumway-Cook, A, et al: Predicting the probability for falls in community-dwelling older adults. Phys Ther 77:812, 1997.
24. Wall, JC, and Scarbrough, J: Use of a multimemory stopwatch to measure temporal gait parameters. J Orthop Sports Phys Ther 25:277, 1997.
25. Sutherland, DH: The evolution of clinical gait analysis. Part 11 kinematics. Gait Posture 16:159, 2002.
26. Craik, RL, and Otis, CA: Gait assessment in the clinic: Issues and approaches. In Rothstein, JM (ed): Measurement in Physical Therapy. Churchill Livingstone, London, 1985, p 169.
27. Dumholdt, E: Physical Therapy Research, ed 2. WB Saunders, Philadelphia, 2000.
28. Strube, MJ, and DeLitto, A: Reliability and measurement theory. In Craik, R, and Oatis, C (eds): Gait Analysis: Theory and Application. Mosby-Yearbook, St. Louis, 1995, p 88.
29. Perry, J: Gait Analysis: Normal and Pathological Function. Slack, Thorofare, NJ, 1992.
30. Pathokinesiology Service and Physical Therapy Department: Observational Gait Analysis Handbook. Los Amigos Research and Education Institute, Inc, Downey, CA, 2001.
31. Southerland, CC: Gait evaluation. In Valmassy, RL (ed): Clinical Biomechanics of the Lower Extremities. Mosby-Yearbook, St. Louis, 1996, p 149.
32. Bernhardt, J, et al: Accuracy of observational kinematic assessment of upper-limb movements. Phys Ther 78:3, 1998.
33. Russell, DJ, et al: Training users in the gross motor function measure: Methodological and practical issues. Phys Ther 74:630, 1994.
34. Eastlack, ME, et al: Interrater reliability of videotaped observational gait-analysis assessments. Phys Ther 71:465, 1991.
35. Krebs, DE: Interpretation standards in locomotor studies. In Craik, R, and Oatis, C (eds): Gait Analysis: Theory and Application. Mosby-Yearbook, St. Louis, 1995, p 334.
36. McGinley, JL, et al: Accuracy and reliability of observational gait analysis data: Judgment of push-off in gait after stroke. Phys Ther 83:146, 2003.
37. Stuberg, WA, et al: Comparison of a clinical gait analysis method using videography and temporal-distance measures with 16-mm cinematography. Phys Ther 68:1221, 1988.
38. Levangie, P, and Norkin, C: Joint Structure and Function: A Comprehensive Analysis, ed 3. FA Davis, Philadelphia, 2001.
39. Nelson, AJ: Functional ambulation profile. Phys Ther 54:1059, 1974.
40. Harada, N, et al: Screening for balance and mobility impairment in elderly individuals living in residential care facilities. Phys Ther 75:462, 1995.
41. Wolf SL, Catlin, PA, and Gage, K: Establishing the reliability and validity of measurements of walking using the Emory Functional Ambulation Profile. Phys Ther 79:1122, 1999.
42. Shields, RK, et al: Reliability, validity and responsiveness of functional tests in patients with total joint replacement. Phys Ther 75:169, 1995.
43. The Guide for Uniform Data System for Medical Rehabilitation (Including the FIM™ Instrument), Version 5.1. University of Buffalo Foundation Activities, Inc, Amherst, New York, 1997.
44. Santa Clara Valley Medical Center (2004). The Center for Outcome Measurements in Brain Injury (COMBI). http://www.tbims.org/combi (August 23, 2004).
45. Ottenbacher, KJ, et al: Interrater agreement and stability of the functional independence measure for children (WeeFIM): Use in children with developmental disabilities. Arch Phys Med Rehabil 78:1309, 1997.
46. Woolacott, MA, and Tang, PF: Balance control during walking in the older adult: Research and its implications. Phys Ther 77:646, 1997.
47. Di Fabio, RP, and Seay, R: Use of the "Fast Evaluation of Mobility, Balance and Fear" in elderly community dwellers: Validity and reliability. Phys Ther 77:904, 1997.
48. Morton, T: Uniform data system for rehab begins: First tool measures dependence level. Progress Report, American Physical Therapy Association, Alexandria, VA, 1986.
49. Wolfson, AM, Doctor, JN, and Burns, SP: Clinical judgments of functional outcomes: How bias and perceived accuracy affect rating. Arch Phys Med Rehabil 81:1567, 2000.
50. Hobart, JC, et al: Evidence-based measurement: Which disability scale for neurologic rehabilitation? Neurology 57:639, 2001.
51. Linn, RT, et al: Does the Functional Assessment Measure (FAM) extend the Functional Independence Measure (FIM™) Instrument? A Rasch analysis of stroke inpatients. J Outcome Measure 3:339, 1999.
52. Woolacott, MA, and Tang, PF: Balance control during walking in the older adult: Research and its implications. Phys Ther 77:646, 1997.

53. Robinett, CS, and Von Dran, MA: Functional ambulation velocity and distance requirements in rural and urban communities: A clinical report. Phys Ther 63:1371, 1988.
54. Walsh, M, et al: Physical impairments and functional limitations: A comparison of individuals 1 year after total knee arthroplasty with control subjects. Phys Ther 78:248, 1998.
55. Winter, DA, et al: Biomechanical walking pattern changes in the fit and healthy elderly. Phys Ther 70:340, 1990.
56. Blanke, DJ, and Hageman, PA: Comparison of gait of young men and elderly men. Phys Ther 69:144, 1989.
57. Bohannon, RW, et al: Walking speed: Reference values and correlates for older adults. J Orthop Sports Phys Ther 77:86, 1996.
58. Ostrosky, JM, et al: A comparison of gait characteristics in young and old subjects. Phys Ther 74:637, 1994.
59. Todd, FN, et al: Variations in the gait of normal children: A graph applicable to the documentation of abnormalities. J Bone Joint Surg 71A:196, 1989.
60. Murray, M, et al: Walking patterns in normal men. J Bone Joint Surg 46A:335, 1964.
61. Murray, M, et al: Walking patterns of normal women. Arch Phys Med Rehabil 51:637, 1970.
62. Spyropoulos, P, et al: Biomechanical gait analysis in obese men. Arch Phys Med Rehabil 72:1065, 1991.
63. Hills, AP, and Parker, AW: Gait characteristics of obese children. Arch Phys Med Rehabil 72:403, 1991.
64. McGibbon, CA, and Krebs, DE: Discriminating age and disability effects in locomotion: Neuromuscular adaptations in musculoskeletal pathology. J Appl Physiol 96:149, 2004.
65. Connelly, DM, and Vandervoort, AA: Effects of detraining on knee extensor strength and functional mobility in a group of elderly women. J Orthop Sports Phys Ther 26:340, 1997.
66. Sutherland, DH, et al: The development of mature gait. J Bone Joint Surg 61A:336, 1980.
67. Schenkman, M, et al: Reliability of impairment and physical performance measures for persons with Parkinson's disease. Phys Ther 77:19, 1997.
68. Mossberg, KA: Reliability of a timed walk test in persons with acquired brain injury. Am J Phys Med Rehabil 82:385, 2003.
69. Shumway-Cook, A, and Woollacott, WJ: Motor Control Theory and Practical Applications, ed 2. Williams & Wilkins, Baltimore, 2001.
70. Robinson, JL, and Smidt, GL: Quantitative gait evaluation in the clinic. Phys Ther 61:351, 1981.
71. Coleman, KL, et al: Step activity monitor: Long-term continuous recording of ambulatory function. J Rehab Res Dev 36:1, 1999.
72. Moe-Nilssen, R: Test-retest reliability of trunk accelerometry during standing and walking. Arch Phys Med Rehabil 79:1377, 1998.
73. Henriksen, M, et al: Test-retest reliability of trunk accelerometric gait analysis. Gait Posture 19:288, 2004.
74. Menz, HB, Lordm SR, and Fitzpatrick, RC: Acceleration patterns of the head and pelvis when walking on level and irregular surfaces. Gait Posture 18:35, 2003.
75. Tong, K, and Granat, MH: A practical gait analysis system using gyroscopes. Med Eng Phys 21:87, 1999.
76. Bowen, A, et al: Dual-task effects of talking while walking on velocity and balance following a stroke. Age Aging 30:319, 2001.
77. Pomeroy, VM, et al: Reliability of measurement of temporo-spatial parameters of gait after stroke using Gait Mat II. Clin Rehabil 18:222, 2004.
78. Wolf, SL, and Binder-Macleod, SA: Use of the Krusen limb load monitor to quantify temporal and loading measurements of gait. Phys Ther 62:976, 1982.
79. Powers, CM, et al: The influence of lower-extremity muscle force on gait characteristics in individuals with below-knee amputations secondary to vascular disease. Phys Ther 76:369, 1996.
80. Morris, ME, et al: Changes in gait and fatigue from morning to afternoon in people with multiple sclerosis. J Neurol Neurosurg Psychiatry 72:361, 2002.
81. Powers, CM, et al: The effect of patellar taping on stride characteristics and joint motion in subjects with patello-femoral pain. J Orthop Sports Phys Ther 26:286, 1997.
82. Powers, CM, et al: Are patellofemoral pain and quadriceps femoris muscle torque associated with locomotor function? Phys Ther 77:1063, 1997.
83. O'Shea, S, Morris, ME, and Iansek, R: Dual task interference during gait in people with Parkinson's disease: Effects of motor versus cognitive secondary tasks. Phys Ther 82:888, 2002.
84. Evans, MD, Goldie, PA, and Hill, KD: Systematic and random error in repeated measurements of temporal and distance parameters of gait after stroke. Arch Phys Med Rehabil 78:725, 1997.
85. Huitema, BB, Hof, AL, and Postema, K: Ultrasonic motion analysis system: Measurement of temporal and spatial gait parameters. J Biomech 35:837, 2002.
86. Kim, CM, and Eng, JJ: Magnitude and pattern of 3D kinematic and kinetic gait profiles in persons with stroke: Relationship to walking speed. Gait Posture 20:140, 2004.
87. Neptune, RR, Zajac, FE, and Kautz, SA: Muscle force redistributes segmental power for body progression during walking. Gait Posture 19:194, 2004.
88. Schwartz, MH, Novacheck, TF, and Trost, J: A tool for quantifying hip flexor function during gait. Gait Posture 12:122, 2000.
89. Maurer, BT, et al: Quantitative identification of ankle equinus with applications for treatment assessment. Gait Posture 3:19, 1993.
90. Thomas, SS, et al: Stair locomotion in children with spastic hemiplegia: The impact of three different ankle foot orthosis (AFOs) configurations. Gait Posture 16:180, 2002.
91. Tiexeira-Salmela, LF, et al: Effects of muscle strengthening and physical conditioning training on temporal, kinematic and kinetic variables during gait in chronic stroke. J Rehabil Med 33:53, 2001.
92. Schwartz, MH, et al: Comprehensive treatment of ambulatory children with cerebral palsy: An outcome assessment. J Pediatr Orthop 24:45, 2004.
93. Brinkmann, JR, and Perry, J: Rate and range of knee motion during ambulation in healthy and arthritic subjects. Phys Ther 65:7, 1985.
94. Hinmann, JE, et al: Age-related changes in speed of walking. Med Sci Sports Exerc 20:1611, 1988.
95. Hageman, PA, and Blanke, DJ: Comparison of gait of young women and elderly women. Phys Ther 66:1382, 1986.
96. Cho, SH, Park, JM, and Kwon, OY: Gender differences in three dimensional gait analysis data form 98 healthy Korean adults. Clin Biomech 19:145, 2004.
97. Sutherland, DH, et al: Clinical use of prediction regions for motion analysis. Dev Med Child Neurol 38:773, 1996.
98. Kaufman, KR: Future directions in gait analysis. Retrieved November 30, 2004 from http://www.vard.org/mono/gait/kaufman.htm
99. Romei, M, et al: Use of the normalcy index for the evaluation of gait pathology. Gait Posture 19:85, 2004.
100. Mulroy, S, et al: Use of cluster analysis for gait pattern classification of patients in the early and late recovery phases following strike. Gait Posture 18:114, 2003.
101. Randolph, AL: Reliability of measurements of pressure applied to the foot during walking by a computerized insole sensor system. Arch Phys Med Rehabil 81:573, 2000.
102. Birke, J, et al: The effectiveness of a modified wedge shoe in reducing pressure at the area of previous great toe ulceration in individuals with diabetes mellitus. Wounds 16:109, 2004.
103. Mueller, MJ: Use of an in-shoe pressure measurement system in the management of patients with neuropathic ulcers or metatarsalgia. J Orthop Sports Phys Ther 21:328, 1995.
104. Armstrong, DG, et al: Peak foot pressures influence the healing time of diabetic foot ulcers treated with total contact casts. J Rehab Res Dev 35:1, 1998.
105. Wertsch, JJ, et al: A portable insole plantar measurement system. J Rehab Res Dev 29:13, 1992.
106. Warren, GL, Maker, RM, and Higbie, EJ: Temporal patterns of plantar pressure and lower-leg muscle activity during walking: Effect of speed. Gait Posture 19:91, 2004.
107. Waters, RL, et al: Comparable energy expenditure after arthrodesis of the hip and ankle. J Bone Joint Surg 70A:1032, 1988.
108. Marsolais, MD, and Edwards, BG: Energy costs of walking and standing with functional neuromuscular stimulation and long leg braces. Arch Phys Med Rehabil 69:243, 1988.
109. Herbert, LM, et al: A comparison of oxygen consumption during walking between children with and without below-knee amputations. Phys Ther 74:943, 1994.
110. Davies, MJ, and Dalsky, GP: Economy of mobility in older adults. J Orthop Sports Phys Ther 26:69, 1997.

111. Torburn, L, et al: Energy expenditure during ambulation in dysvascular and traumatic below-knee amputees: A comparison of five prosthetic feet. J Rehabil Res Dev 32:111, 1995.
112. Ebbling, CJ, et al: Lower extremity mechanics and energy cost of walking in high-heeled shoes. J Orthop Sports Phys Ther 19:190, 1994.
113. Olgiati, R, et al: Increased energy cost of walking in multiple sclerosis: Effect of spasticity, ataxia, and weakness. Arch Phys Med Rehabil 69:846, 1988.
114. Olney, SJ, Monga, TN, and Costiganm PA: Mechanical energy of walking of stroke patients. Arch Phys Med Rehabil 67:92, 1986.
115. McGibbon, CA, Krebs, DE, and Puniello, MS: Mechanical energy analysis identifies compensatory strategies in disabled elders' gait. J Biomech 34:481, 2001.
116. MacGregor, J: The Objective Measurement of Physical Performance with Long-Term Ambulatory Physiological Surveillance Equipment (LAPSE). Proc 3rd Int Symp on Ambulatory Monitoring, London, 29–39, 1979.
117. Boyd, R, et al: High- or low-technology measurements of energy expenditure in clinical gait analysis? Dev Med Child Neurol 41:676, 1999.
118. Bowen, TR, et al: Variability of energy-consumption measures in children with cerebral palsy. J Pediatr Orthop 18:738, 1998.
119. Ijzerman, MJ, et al: Validity and reproducibility of crutch force and heart rate measurements to assess energy expenditure of paraplegic gait. Arch Phys Med Rehabil 80:1017, 1999.
120. Ijzerman, MJ, and Nene, AV: Feasibility of the physiological cost index as an outcome measure for the assessment of energy expenditure during walking. Arch Phys Med Rehabil 83:1777, 2002.
121. Nene, AV: Physiological cost index of walking in able-bodied adolescents and adults. Clin Rehabil 7:319, 1993.
122. Stein, RB, et al: Improved efficiency with a wheelchair propelled by the legs using voluntary activity or electric stimulation. Arch Phys Med Rehabil 82:1198, 2001.
123. Cross, J, and Tyson, SF: The effect of a slider shoe on hemiplegic gait. Clin Rehabil 17:817, 2003.
124. Stallard, J, and Major, RE: The influence of orthosis stiffness on paraplegic ambulation and its implications for functional electrical stimulation (FES) walking systems. Prosthet Orthot Int 19:108, 1995.
125. Hood, VL, et al: A new method of using heart rate to represent energy expenditure: The Total Heart Beat Index. Arch Phys Med Rehabil 83:1266, 2002.
126. Titianova, EB, et al: Gait characteristics and functional ambulation profile in patient with chronic unilateral stroke. Am J Phys Med Rehabil 82:778, 2003.
127. Baer, HR, and Wolf, SL: Modified Emory Functional Ambulation Profile: An outcome measure for rehabilitation for post stroke gait dysfunction. Stroke 32:973, 2001.
128. Hawley, CA, et al: Use of functional assessment measure (FIM + FAM) in head injury rehabilitation: A psychometric analysis. J Neurol Neurosurg Psychiatry 67:749, 1999.
129. Donaghy, S, and Wass, PJ: Interrater reliability of the Functional Assessment Measure in a brain injury rehabilitation program. Arch Phys Med Rehabil 79(10):1231, 1998.
130. Resnick, B, et al: Measurement of activity in older adults: Reliability and validity of the Step Activity Monitor. J Nurs Meas 9:275, 2001.
131. Brandes, M, and Rosenbaum, D: Correlations between the Step Activity Monitor and the DynaPort ADFL-Monitor. Clin Biomech 19:91, 2004.
132. Hartsell, H, et al: Accuracy of a custom-designed activity monitor: Implications for diabetic foot ulcer healing. J Rehabil Res Dev 39:395, 2002.
133. Maluf, KS, and Mueller, MJ: Comparison of physical activity and cumulative plantar tissue stress among subjects with and without diabetes mellitus and a history of recurrent plantar ulcers. Clin Biomech 18:567, 2003.
134. Aminian, K, et al: Spatio-temporal parameters of gait measured by an ambulatory system using miniature gryoscopes. J Biomech 35:689, 2002.
135. Bliney, B, Morris, M, and Webster, K: Concurrent validity of the GAITRite walkway system for quantification of the spatial and temporal parameters of gait. Gait Posture 17:68, 2003.
136. McDonough, AL, et al: The validity and reliability of the GAITRite System's measurements: A preliminary evaluation. Arch Phys Med Rehabil 82:419, 2001.
137. Titianova, AEB, and Tarka, IM: Asymmetry in walking performance and postural sway in patients with chronic unilateral cerebral infarction. J Rehabil Res 32:236, 1995.
138. Nelson, AJ, et al: The validity of the GaitRite and Functional Ambulation Performance scoring system in the analysis of Parkinson gait. NeuroRehabil 17:255, 2002.
139. Van Uden, CJT, and Besser, MP: Test-retest reliability of temporal and spatial gait characteristics measured with an instrumented walkway system (GAITRite ^{R}). BMC Musculoskel Dis 5:13, 2004.
140. Menz, HB, et al: Reliability of the GAITRite walkway system for quantification of temporo-spatial parameters of gait in young and older people. Gait Posture 20:25,2004.
141. Besser, M, Anton, N, and Quaile, S: Criterion validity of the Ariel Performance Analysis System (APAS) for the calculation of joint angles using APAS and GaitLab software. Proceedings of the 20th Annual Meeting of the American Society of Biomechanics, Atlanta, Georgia, 1996. Retrieved November 30, 2004, from http://asb-biomech.org/onlineabs/abstracts96/besser.html.
142. Wilson, DJ, et al: Accuracy of reconstructed angular estimates obtained with the Ariel Performance Analysis System. Phys Ther 77:1741, 1997.

Appendix A: Blank Sample Recording Form for Observational Gait Analysis

Patient's name ______________________ Age ________ Sex ________ Height ________ Weight ________
Diagnosis ______________________
Footwear ______________________ Assistive devices ______________________
Date ______________________ Therapist ______________________

DIRECTIONS: Place a check in the space opposite the deviation if the deviation is observed.

		Stance										Swing							
Body Segment	**Deviation**	**HS**		**FF**		**MST**		**HO**		**TO**		**ACC**		**MSW**		**DEC**		**Possible Cause**	**Analysis**
Ankle and foot	None	R	L	R	L	R	L	R	L	R	L	R	L	R	L	R	L		
Observations in the sagittal plane	Foot flat																		
	Foot slap																		
	Heel off																		
	No heel off																		
	Excessive plantarflexion																		
	Excessive dorsiflexion																		
	Toe drag																		
	Toe clawing																		
	Contralateral vaulting																		
Observations in the frontal plane	Varus																		
	Valgus																		
Knee	None																		
Observations in the sagittal plane	Excessive flexion																		
	Limited flexion																		
	No flexion																		
	Hyperextension																		
	Genu recurvatum																		
	Diminished extension																		

Body Segment	Deviation	HS	Stance FF	MST	HO	TO	ACC	Swing MSW	DEC	Possible Cause	Analysis
Observations in the frontal plane	Varum										
	Valgum										
Hip	None										
Observations in the sagittal plane	Excessive flexion										
	Limited flexion										
	No flexion										
	Diminished extension										
Observations in the frontal plane	Abduction										
	Adduction										
	External rotation										
	Internal rotation										
	Circumduction										
	Hiking										
Pelvis	None										
Observations in the sagittal plane	Anterior tilt										
	Posterior tilt										
	Increased backward rotation										
	Increased forward rotation										
	Limited backward rotation										
	Limited forward rotation Drops on contralateral side										

(*continued*)

Appendix A: Blank Sample Recording Form for Observational Gait Analysis (continued)

Body Segment	Deviation	HS	Stance FF	MST	HO	TO	ACC	Swing MSW	DEC	Possible Cause	Analysis
Trunk	None										
Observations in the frontal plane	Backward rotation										
	Lateral lean										
	Forward rotation										
	Backward lean										
	Forward lean										

Appendix B: Completed Sample Recording Form for Observational Gait Analysis

Patient's name Edna Smith Age 65 Sex F Height 5'3" Weight 160 lbs.
Diagnosis Post total Hip Arthroplasty—Peripheral Neuropathy—Diabetes
Footwear Shoes Assistive devices NONE
Date 5/6/98 Therapist Norkin

DIRECTIONS: Place a check in the space opposite the deviation if the deviation is observed.

Body Segment	Deviation	HS		Stance FF		MST		HO		TO		ACC		Swing MSW		DEC		Possible Cause	Analysis
Ankle and foot	None	R	L	R	L	R	L	R	L	R	L	R	L	R	L	R	L	Weakness dorsiflexors	
Observations in the sagittal plane	Foot flat	✔																	
	Foot slap																		
	Heel off																		
	No heel off																		
	Excessive plantarflexion			✔		✔						✔		✔		✔		Weakness dorsiflexors	
	Excessive dorsiflexion																		
	Toe drag											✔		✔				Weakness dorsiflexors	
	Toe clawing																		
	Contralateral vaulting																		
Observations in the frontal plane	Varus																		
	Valgus																		
Knee	None																		
Observations in the sagittal plane	Excessive flexion																		
	Limited flexion																		
	No flexion																		
	Hyperextension																		
	Genu recurvatum																		
	Diminished extension																		

(continued)

Appendix B: Completed Sample Recording Form for Observational Gait Analysis (continued)

Body Segment	Deviation	HS	Stance FF	MST	HO	TO	ACC	Swing MSW	DEC	Possible Cause	Analysis
Observations in the frontal plane	Varum										
	Valgum										
Hip	None										
Observations in the sagittal plane	Excessive flexion										
	Limited flexion										
	No flexion										
	Diminished extension										
Observations in the frontal plane	Abduction										
	Adduction			✓						Drop of pelvis	
	External rotation										
	Internal rotation										
	Circumduction										
	Hiking										
Pelvis	None										
Observations in the sagittal plane	Anterior tilt										
	Posterior tilt										
	Increased backward rotation										
	Increased forward rotation										
	Limited backward rotation										

Body Segment	Deviation	Stance HS	FF	MST	HO	TO	ACC	Swing MSW	DEC	Possible Cause	Analysis
	Limited forward rotation										
	Drops on contralateral side	TO THE LEFT	✔	✔	✔					Weakness Right hip abductors	
Trunk	None										
Observations in the frontal plane	Backward rotation										
	Lateral lean										
	Forward rotation									Weakness	Compensation to counteract
	Backward lean	✔	✔	✔						Hip extensors	Flexion moment
	Forward lean										

Appendix C: Manufacturer Contact Information for Motion Analysis Equipment

Advanced Medical Technology, Inc (AMTI)
176 Waltham Street
Watertown, MA 02172-4800
Web site: http://www.amtiweb.com

Ariel Performance Analysis System
Ariel Dynamics
Galicante St.
Trabuco Canyon, CA 92679
Web site: http://www.arielnet.com

ELITE Motion Analysis System
Bioengineering Technology Systems (BTS)
BTS North America
35 Tillinghast Trace
Newnan, GA 30265
Web site: http://www.bts.it

EMED Pedar-in Shoe
Novel Electronics, Inc
964 Grand Ave
St. Paul, MN 55105
Web site: http://www.novel.de

FAM
Santa Clara Valley Medical Center
751 S. Bascom Ave, Box 70
San Jose, CA 95128

Flock of Birds
Ascension Technology Corporation
P.O. Box 527
Burlington, VT 05402
Web site: http://www.ascension-tech.com

Force Plates
Kistler Instrument Corporation
75 John Glenn Dr.
Amherst, NY 14228
Web site: http://www.kistler.com

F-Scan In-Shoe Pressure Measurement System
Tekscan, Inc
307 W. First St.
South Boston, MA 02127-1309
Web site: http://www.tekscan.com

Functional Independence Measure (FIM™)
Uniform Data System for Medical Rehabilitation,
UB Foundation Activities, Inc
Amherst, NY 14228

GAITMAT II™
EQ, Inc
P.O. Box 16
Chalfont, PA 18914-0016
Web site: http://www.gaitmat.com

GAITRite®
CIR Systems, Inc
790 Bloomfield Ave Suite 10
P.O. Box 4402
Clifton, NJ 07012
Web site: http://www.gaitrite.com

Gaitway
Kistler Instrument Corporation
75 John Glenn Dr.
Amherst, NY 14228
Web site: http://www.kistler.com

Mat-Scan
Tekscan, Inc
307 W. First St.
South Boston
MA 02127-1309
Web site: http://www.tekscan.com

Optotrak Motion Analysis System
Northern Digital, Inc
13 Randall Dr.
Waterloo, Ontario, Canada N2V1C5
Web site: http://www.ndigital.com

OrthoTrak
Motion Analysis Corporation
3617 Westwind Blvd
Santa Rosa, CA 95403
Web site: http://www.motionanalysis.com

Peak Motus
Peak Performance Technologies, Inc
7388 S. Revere Parkway
Suite 901
Centennial, CO 80112
Web site: http://www.peakperform.com

Selspot
Selcom, Inc
21654 Melrose
Southfield, MI 48075
(248) 355-5900

Step Watch Activity Monitor 3™ (SAM)
Cyma Corporation
8515 35th Ave, NE, Suite C
Seattle, WA 98115-3675
Web site: http://www.cymatech.com

Stride Analyzer
B and L Engineering
3002 Dow Ave, Suite 416
Tustin, CA 92780
Web site: http://www.bleng.com

Vicon Motion Analysis System
Vicon Motion Systems, Inc
9 Spectrum Pointe Dr.
Lake Forest, CA 92630
Web site: http://www.vicon.com

WeeFIM®
Uniform Data System for Medical Rehabilitation, a Division of UB Foundation Activities, Inc
Amherst, NY 14228

Appendix D: Simple Tabulated Output from the Stride Analyzer System

YOUR DEPARTMENT'S NAME
YOUR INSTITUTION'S NAME
STRIDE ANALYZER REPORT—WALKING

NAME:	JOHN SMITH	RUN:	JS01
I.D. NUMBER:	1234	STRIDES:	4
DATE:	05/13/93	DISTANCE (M):	6.00
AGE:	29	TEST CONDITIONS:	
SEX:	M	WALK	
DIAGNOSIS:	Sprained Right Ankle		

STRIDE CHARACTERISTICS	ACTUAL	%NORMAL
VELOCITY (M/MIN):	60.3	74.0
CADENCE (STEP/MIN):	100.4	92.7
STRIDE LENGTH (M):	1.201	79.8
GAIT CYCLE (SEC):	1.20	106.8

SINGLE LIMB SUPPORT	-R-	-L-
(SEC):	0.429	0.418
(%NORMAL):	86.4	84.2
(%GC):	35.9	35.0
SWING (%GC):	33.5	34.5
STANCE (%GC):	66.5	65.5
DOUBLE SUPPORT		
INITIAL (%GC):	15.2	15.4
TERMINAL (%GC):	15.4	15.2
TOTAL (%GC):	30.6	30.6

LEFT FOOT (stance = 65.5% GC)

HEEL	– Normal contact at 0.0% GC (0.0% Stance) Delayed cessation at 50.6% GC (77.2% Stance)
5TH METATARSAL	– Premature contact at 3.8% GC (5.7% Stance) Delayed cessation at 63.3% GC (96.6% Stance)
1ST METATARSAL	– Normal contact at 22.4% GC (34.2% Stance) Delayed cessation at 63.9% GC (97.5% Stance)
TOE	– Normal contact at 33.7% GC (51.4% Stance) Delayed cessation at 65.5% GC (100.0% Stance)

RIGHT FOOT (stance = 66.5% GC)

HEEL	– Normal contact at 0.0% GC (0.0% Stance) Delayed cessation at 50.8% GC (76.4% Stance)
5TH METATARSAL	– Premature contact at 4.0% GC (6.0% Stance) Delayed cessation at 64.8% GC (97.5% Stance)
1ST METATARSAL	– Normal contact at 19.6% GC (29.4% Stance) Delayed cessation at 63.8% GC (96.0% Stance)
TOE	– Normal contact at 38.1% GC (57.3% Stance) Delayed cessation at 65.2% GC (98.1% Stance)

From Craik, RL, and Oatis, CA,[26, p 133] with permission.

CHAPTER

11

LEARNING OBJECTIVES

1. Discuss the concepts of health status, impairment, functional limitation, and disability.
2. Define functional activity, and discuss the purposes and components of a functional examination.
3. Select activities and roles appropriate to an individual's particular characteristics and condition to guide examination of functional status and activity level.
4. Compare and contrast characteristics of various formal tests of function, including physical function tests and multidimensional functional assessment instruments.
5. Identify factors to be considered in the selection of formal instruments for testing function.
6. Compare and contrast various scoring methods used in functional instruments.
7. Discuss the issues of reliability and validity as they relate to functional instruments.
8. Using the case study example, apply clinical decision making skills in evaluating data from the examination of functional status.

Examination of Functional Status and Activity Level

Andrew A. Guccione, DPT, PhD, FAPTA
David A. Scalzitti, PT, MS, OCS

OUTLINE

The ultimate objective of any rehabilitation program is to return the individual to a lifestyle that is as close to the premorbid level of function as possible or, alternatively, to maximize the current potential for function and maintain it. For an otherwise healthy patient with a fractured arm, this may be a reasonably simple process: improving range of motion and strength will reestablish skills in dressing and feeding. However, considering the patient with a stroke as an example, the task is much more complex because the problems are much more extensive, complicated, and interwoven. The two cases, however, are broadly similar. In both instances, the therapist begins by describing the patient's problem in functional terms obtained from the patient history, performing a systems review and detailed examination using selected tests and measures, evaluating the data, establishing a diagnosis and prognosis, implementing interventions to reduce or to eliminate the problems identified, and documenting the progress of the patient toward the desired functional outcome.[1]

Every individual values the ability to live independently. Functional activities encompass all those tasks, activities, and roles that identify a person as an independent adult or as a child progressing toward adult independence. These activities require the integration of both cognitive and affective abilities with motor skills. Functional activity is a patient-referenced concept and is dependent on what the individual self-identifies as essential to support physical and psychological well-being as well as to create a personal sense of meaningful living. Function is not totally individualistic, however; there are certain categories of activities that are common to everyone. Eating, sleeping, elimination, and hygiene are major components of survival and protection common to all animals. Particular to humans are the evolutionary advancements of bipedal locomotion and complex hand activities, which permit independence in the personal environment. Work and recreation are functional activities in a social context.

This chapter presents a conceptual framework for examining functional status and introduces the reader to terminology used in the field. It presents an overview of the purposes of functional status examination and the range and rigor of formal test instruments currently available to clinicians and researchers. Considerations in test selection and principles of administration are also presented.

A Conceptual Framework

Chronically ill and disabled persons represent a large segment of the population in the United States. Approximately 34 million individuals suffer from physical or mental impairments that limit their capacity to perform some daily functional activity.[2] Traditionally, these individuals have been categorized or classified according to their medical diseases or conditions. Medical procedures such as physical examination and laboratory tests are the primary tools to delineate the problems created by disease. Strict focus on a biomedical model, with its emphasis on the characteristics of *disease* (etiology, pathology, and clinical manifestations), may contribute to reducing patients to the medical labeling of these individuals; for example, referring to people as amputees, paraplegics, arthritics, or strokess rather than as individuals with these conditions. This model virtually ignores the equally important psychological, social, and behavioral dimensions of the **illness**, which accompanies the disease. Illness refers to the personal behaviors that emerge when the reality of having a disease is internalized and experienced by an individual. Factors related to illness often play a key role in determining the success or failure of rehabilitation efforts well beyond the nature of the medical condition that prompted a patient's referral to physical therapy. In helping the individual with a disease, physical therapists come to understand each person's illness as well.

A broad conceptual framework is necessary to fully understand the concept of health and its relationship to functional disability. Terms such as well-being, health-related quality of life, and functional status are often used interchangeably to describe health status. The most global definition of **health** has been provided by the World Health Organization (WHO), which defined health as "a state of complete physical, mental, and social well-being, and not merely the absence of diseases and infirmity."[3, p 459] Although such global definitions are useful as philosophical statements, they lack the precision necessary for a clinician or researcher.

Nagi has been particularly influential in developing a model found throughout the American literature that explicates health status and the relationship among the various terms used to describe health status.[4–8] This model, used in this chapter to capture the concept of health status and the processes by which an individual becomes disabled, begins with the pathology or disease process that mobilizes the body's defenses and response mechanisms. Physical signs and symptoms set the individual's clinical presentation apart as abnormal and indicate the body's attempts to cope with this attack on its normal functioning. **Physical signs** are the directly observable or measurable changes in an individual's organs or systems. **Symptoms** are the more subjective reactions to the changes experienced by the individual. Thus the individual demonstrates an elevated blood pressure (a physical sign) and reports feeling dizzy (a symptom). Many medical conditions are, in fact, not labels for a single pathological entity, but clusters of signs and symptoms that designate a syndrome. Two common examples of "diseases" that are really syndromes are congestive heart failure (CHF) and acquired immune deficiency syndrome (AIDS). Although the definition of disease presented above implies an active condition, many of the physical signs and symptoms that are important to physical therapy examination and treatment are not associated with active or ongoing medical conditions. For example, a resolved myocardial infarction is a fixed lesion with great importance for physical therapists, but is not an active disease process in itself (Fig. 11.1).

Impairments, as described within Nagi's model, evolve as the natural consequence of pathology or disease and are defined as any alteration or deviation from normal in anatomical, physiological, or psychological structures or functions.[6–8] The partial or complete loss of a limb or an organ, or any disturbance in body part, organ, or system function are examples of impairments. Physical therapists are concerned primarily with impairments of the musculoskeletal, neuromuscular, cardiopulmonary, and integumentary systems; for example, loss of range of motion, strength, endurance, or scar formation. Impairments may be temporary or permanent and represent an overt manifestation of the disease or pathological state. Some impairments are themselves sequelae of other impairments. For example, a patient with a swollen and stiff joint may eventually develop weakness in the muscles surrounding the joint. Therefore, impaired muscle strength would be an **indirect (secondary) impairment** resulting from impaired joint mobility, rather than a specific disease or pathological process.[9,10]

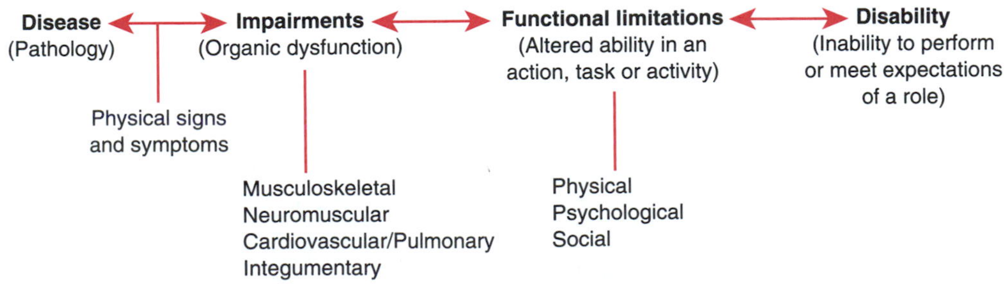

Figure 11.1 Schematic representation of Nagi's model of the process of disablement.

A **functional limitation** is the inability of an individual to perform an action or activity in the way it is done by most people, usually as the result of an impairment.[6–8] Accurate judgment about the relationship between impairments and functional limitations is at the heart of all physical therapist examination, evaluation, and intervention.[1,5] Three main categories of function have been delineated: physical function, psychological function, and social function. **Physical function** refers to those sensory-motor skills necessary for the performance of usual daily activities. Getting out of bed, walking, and climbing stairs are examples of physical functional activities. Physical therapists are traditionally most involved with this category of functional status examination and intervention. These sensory–motor skills underlie the tasks of daily self-care such as feeding, dressing, hygiene, and physical mobility that are known as **basic activities of daily living (BADL)**. Advanced skills that are considered vital to an individual's independent living in the community are termed **instrumental activities of daily living (IADL)**. These include a wide range of high-level tasks and activities such as managing personal affairs, cooking and shopping, home chores, and driving. The ability to work, including the "work" associated with normal childhood development, may be investigated as an aspect of physical function. Participation in community and recreational activities are no less important than work to maintain quality of life and also fall under the examination of physical function. Examination of recreational activities, however, is not limited to sports. A number of physically demanding activities, such as dancing and gardening, require a relatively high degree of balance, flexibility, and strength. Even sedentary activities, such as stamp collecting or playing chess, require a certain degree of physical ability in the hand and upper extremity and therefore may be meaningful measures of function and activity levels for some patients.

Psychological function has two components: mental and affective. **Mental function** refers to the intellectual or cognitive abilities of an individual. Factors such as initiative, attention, concentration, memory, problem solving, or judgment are important components of normal mental function. **Affective function** refers to the affective skills and coping strategies needed to deal with the everyday "hassles" as well as the more traumatic and stressful events each person encounters over the course of a lifetime. Factors such as self-esteem, attitude toward body image, anxiety, depression, and the ability to cope with change are examples of affective functions. Finally, **social function** refers to an individual's performance of social roles and obligations. Categories of roles and activities relevant to determining an individual's social function include social activity, including participation in recreational activities and clubs; social interaction, such as telephoning or visiting relatives or friends; and social roles created and sustained through interpersonal relationships specific to one's personal life and occupation.

When an individual is limited in a number of functional activities and unable to engage in critical social roles (e.g., worker, student, spouse), this person may be regarded as disabled as conceptualized within the Nagi model.[6–8] **Disability** is characterized by discordance between the actual performance of an individual in a particular role and the expectations of the community regarding what is "normal" for an adult. Thus, disability is a term that takes its meaning from the community in which the individual lives and the criteria for "normal" within that social group. Many factors can influence the connections among disease, impairment, and function, not the least of which will be the individual's personal response. Patients with the same disease and the same impairments may not always have the same functional limitations. Furthermore, although an individual may perform functional activities differently than is "normal," this person may successfully accomplish expected social roles and escape the label of being "disabled." Physical therapists most often think of "normal" adulthood in terms of independence in self-care activities, competence and autonomy in decision making, and productivity. In some cultural subgroups, social expectations may be quite different, particularly if the individual has certain impairments or functional limitations. Physical therapists should account for the effects of culture and social expectations in determining what is "normal" function for an individual, especially when the therapist and the patient do not share the same social or cultural backgrounds.

In 1976 the WHO initially adopted the International Classification of Impairments, Disability, and Handicaps (ICIDH)[4] with the goal of promoting the use of consistent terminology and to provide a framework for discourse among health professionals by standardizing four key terms: disease, impairment, disability, and handicap. The original ICIDH framework had a similar intent to the Nagi model to describe the consequences of disease.[11] The ICIDH underwent extensive revision, beginning in 1993. Draft revisions of the ICIDH-2, as it was known at the time, that were circulated for review internationally in 1997 and 1999 continued using the term "impairment," but abandoned the terms disability and handicap in favor of the terms *activity limitation* and *participation restriction*, respectively.[12] These proposed changes in ICIDH terminology, if they had been adopted as originally presented when the revision began, would have put the revised ICIDH closer to the notions of functional limitation and disability used in the Nagi model and greatly reduced the overall differences between the two sets of concepts.

The conceptual orientation of the ICIDH also was changed during the revision process. Instead of orienting toward the consequences of disease, the underlying framework was directed toward describing the components of health.[11] This re-direction in conceptual focus altered the operationalization of the terms activity and participation when the revision, now known as the International Classification of Functioning, Health and Disability (but abbreviated as the ICF), was adopted in 2001. As in the Nagi model, the ICF recognizes that activity limitations (the ICF analog to functional limitations in the Nagi model) occur when an individual experiences difficulties in performing actions, tasks, or activities. Similarly, an individual experiences participation restrictions in specific life situations, not unlike the Nagi conceptualization of disability in which a person experiences limitations in a particular sociocultural context. Thus, within the Nagi model, a functional limitation contributes to disability if that particular task or activity is a component of the role expectation.[6] The ICF takes a completely different approach to understanding activity limitations and restricted participation because of its concerns to be a classification system for coding as well as a conceptual model of health and functioning. The ICF operationalized activity and participation with the same lists of actions, tasks, and activities, but distinguished between the two concepts by appealing to the differences between a person's capacity in a standardized environment with and without human or mechanical assistance and a person's performance in that individual's actual environment with or without assistance.

The ICF approach to distinguishing between activity and participation has met with mixed enthusiasm, and further refinement in the years ahead appears likely. Much of the success of this conceptual approach will depend on the strength of its utility as a classification system for clinical practice and research. The classification scheme for coding may be particularly intriguing for physical therapists in its delineation of actions, tasks, and activities in an implicit hierarchy of functioning. Within this hierarchy, actions (e.g., rolling, bending, sitting, standing, lifting and reaching) are constituents of tasks and activities (e.g., bathing, dressing, and grooming). Tests and measures of actions are particularly relevant to physical therapist practice as they capture the complex integration of systems that permits an individual to maintain a posture, transition to other postures, or sustain safe and efficient movement.

Nagi's model never had a term to cover the concept of handicap, a term which is rarely used nowadays owing to its negative connotations. *Handicap* was a term that described the social disadvantage of disability as a function of a society's response to needs of people with different abilities.[6] In some instances, even a person who is functioning independently could still be handicapped by the social stigma of some impairments or the environmental barriers confronted when using an assistive device such as a wheelchair. Within this context, the concept of handicap is more generally expressed in less negative terminology by recognizing environmental factors that may be physical or social. The ICF, and further refinements of the Nagi model such as the Institute of Medicine's enabling-disabling process (Fig. 11.2),[13] emphasize the interaction between the person and the environment as critical to understanding functioning

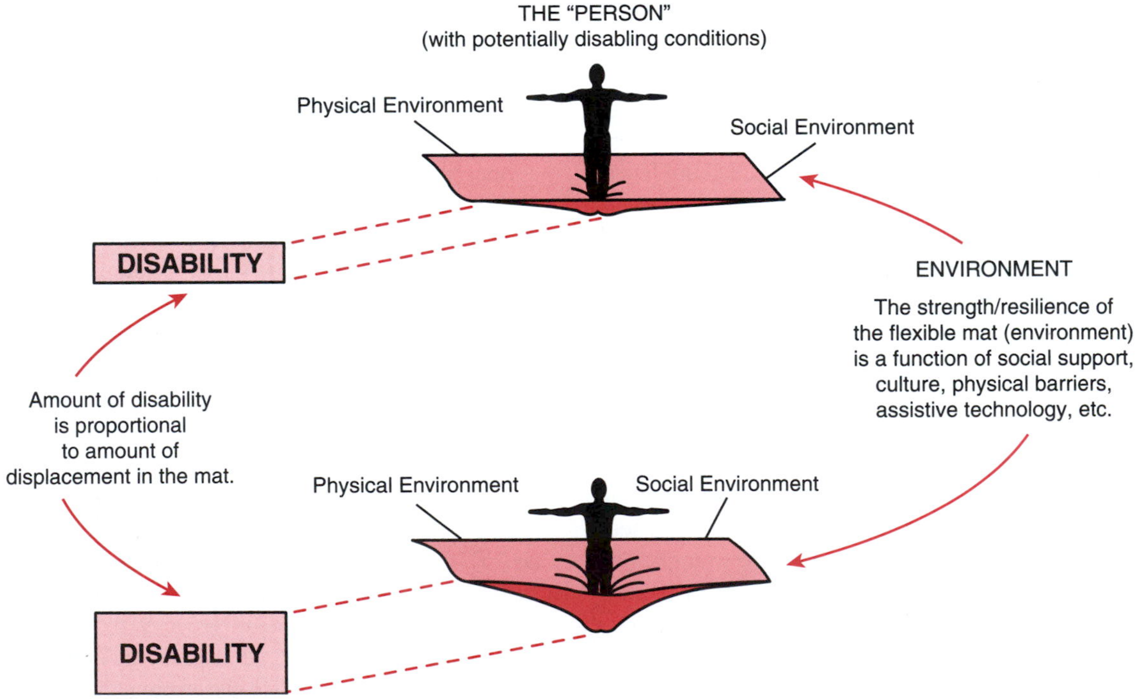

Figure 11.2 The Institute of Medicine model of the enabling-disabling process. Disability is a function of the interaction between the person and the environment. The amount of displacement represents the amount of disability that is experienced by the individual. Displacement is a function of the strength of the physical and social environments that support an individual and the magnitude of the potentially disabling condition. (From Brandt, EN, Jr, and Pope AM (eds): Enabling America: Assessing the Role of Rehabilitation Science and Engineering. National Academy Press, Washington DC, 1997, p 9, with permission.)

and disability. Physical therapists can help change discriminatory social attitudes and environmental restrictions such as architectural barriers that stigmatize individuals and restrict participation in all aspects of society.

Although deficits in behavioral or motor skills or limitations in function may typically exist in certain disease categories, the exact empirical relationship between a particular set of impairments and a specific functional disability is not yet known.[14] The cause-and-effect relationship between an impairment and a functional limitation is most often inferred in the clinic from empirical evidence. For example, physical therapists may assume that the reason a patient cannot transfer independently is causally linked to the fact that the individual has lost enough lower extremity range of motion at the hip (e.g., hip flexion contractures) to prevent balancing in a fully upright posture. The return of function following remediation of the impairment of joint mobility is then considered clinical evidence of a causal relationship between the impairment and the functional limitation. For data to be clinically useful, functional assessment must be linked to the other tests and measures which are used by a physical therapist to examine a patient.

Examination of Function

Purpose of Examination of Functional Status

Analysis of function focuses on the identification of pertinent **functional activities** and measurement of an individual's ability to successfully engage in them. In essence, functional testing measures how a person does certain tasks or fulfills certain roles in the various dimensions of living described above. Application of selected functional tests and measures yield data that can be used as (1) baseline information for setting function-oriented goals and outcomes of intervention; (2) indicators of a patient's initial abilities and progression toward more complex functional levels; (3) criteria for placement decisions, for example, the need for inpatient rehabilitation, extended care, or community services; (4) manifestations of an individual's level of safety in performing a particular task and the risk of injury with continued performance; and (5) evidence of the effectiveness of a specific intervention (medical, surgical, or rehabilitative) on function.

General Considerations

Physical therapists possess a unique body of knowledge related to the identification, remediation, and prevention of movement dysfunction. Thus, they have traditionally been involved in the examination of physical function. Other members of the rehabilitation team, including the occupational therapist, nurse, rehabilitation counselor, and recreational therapist, are also typically involved in administering and interpreting functional tests. Some formal instruments were designed to be completed collectively by the team. Other tests are compiled in separate sections by specific health professionals and housed together in the patient's chart. Where teams exist, physical therapists are typically responsible for the testing of **functional mobility skills (FMS)**, that is, bed mobility, transfers, and locomotion (wheelchair mobility, ambulation, negotiation of stairs and graded elevations, walking for longer distances in the community). A typical ADL or IADL battery may be administered by a physical therapist alone or cooperatively with other health professionals. When overlap among team members exists, for example, the performance of toilet transfers, the data may be collected by the physical therapist, an occupational therapist, or a nurse. In these instances, testing should be coordinated to reduce duplication and unnecessary patient stress. In noninstitutional settings or where there is no team, the physical therapist is often responsible for determining all aspects of physical function.

Testing Perspectives

Function tests can utilize two highly divergent perspectives on what is to be tested or measured by the physical therapist. It is extremely important that the therapist determine in advance whether data are needed to describe the *habitual level* of a patient's ability to do certain tasks and activities, or to identify the patient's *capacity* to perform certain tasks and activities, whether the patient habitually performs up to that level or not, or even performs them at all.

These divergent viewpoints directly affect what types of tests and measures should be chosen and what parameters of measurement are appropriate to yield data useful to making clinical judgments. Most importantly, physical therapists must consider the differences between capacity for function and habitual function in determining the prognosis for rehabilitation and estimating the likelihood of the success of an intervention. Patients accept a therapist's recommendations regarding the anticipated goals of treatment only if there is the perceived need and motivation to function habitually at the highest level of ability. Understanding the difference between what a person actually does or would be willing to do and what that person potentially could do is an essential component of designing realistic, and achievable, functional goals. For example, even though a person might have the capacity to climb stairs, there may not be any willingness to do so. Ultimately, physical therapists must abide by each patient's own decision regarding which tasks and activities will be incorporated into a daily routine and what is a meaningful level of function, regardless of the therapist's professional opinion.

Irrespective of the particular instrument used, there are several basic considerations to be kept in mind. The setting chosen must be conducive to the type of testing and free of distractions. Instructions should be precise and unambiguous. Testing may be biased by fatigue. If a patient performs best in the morning but tires by afternoon, an accurate determination of functional ability must consider the variation in the patient's performance. Therapists should be aware of patients whose energy fluctuates during the day, and interpret the data accordingly. In general, information from functional tests should always be interpreted in the context provided by other data generated during the initial examination (e.g., tests and measures of joint integrity and mobility, motor function, muscle performance, and sensory integrity). Retesting should occur at regular intervals during treatment to document progress and at discharge from the episode of care.

Types of Instruments

Performance-Based Tests

A **performance-based test** may be administered by a therapist who observes the patient during the performance of an activity. Generally speaking, the therapist who chooses a performance-based test is searching for an indication of what a patient can do under a specific set of circumstances, which may or may not be similar to the natural environment in which the patient functions. If a performance-based test is chosen with the intention of making inferences about how the patient will perform at home, then the conditions and setting should be as similar as possible to the actual environment in which the patient usually performs the tasks and activities. A performance-based approach may be used either to describe the patient's current level of function or to identify the maximum level of function possible.

During the administration of the test, each task is presented and the patient is asked to perform it. For example, to examine current level of function in wheelchair mobility, a patient would receive this instruction, "Push your wheelchair over to that red chair and stop." To determine the patient's maximum level of function in this activity, the instruction might specify a particular manner of performance: "Push your wheelchair over to that red chair *as quickly as you can* and stop." Understanding the difference between these two commands, even though both are observation-based performance of wheelchair mobility, is essential to sound clinical decision making. Data from the first example identify only what the patient can do under specific circumstances, but does not support the inference that the patient will be able to wheel across a busy intersection in the short time span allotted to a typical pedestrian walkway. The form of the instruction determines whether an inference can be made about the patient's maximal level of function in formulating the goals for intervention and the plan of care.

In either case, a patient is given no additional instructions or assistance unless he or she is unable or unsure of how to perform. Then only as much direction or assistance as is needed is given. Appropriate safety precautions should be taken during the session so that the patient does not attempt tasks that are potentially dangerous.

There are a number of tests of impairments that are sometimes also referred to as functional performance measures, including the 6-Minute Walk Test,[15] the Physical Performance and Mobility Examination,[16] the Functional Reach Test,[17,18] the Get Up and Go Test,[19] the Timed Up and Go Test,[20] and the Physical Performance Battery.[21] A performance instrument of this sort typically measures either a complex integration of impairments, the performance of actions, or a combination a both by direct observation. Overall, the tests do provide some insight into the individual's capabilities to maintain a posture, transition to other postures, or sustain safe and efficient movement. The data from such a test, gathered under controlled conditions, characterize a person's performance limitations as a result of impairments, and may purport to predict the success or failure of an individual in performing goal-directed tasks or activities under natural conditions, using a score that summates the combined impacts of impairments throughout and across systems on movement dysfunction. Each of these tests can contribute to an understanding of a person's function, but they do not examine a functional limitation in a particular BADL or IADL. Although these tests employ the method of direct observation of performance, they most often do not measure the task or activity as it might be accomplished in the "real" world of the patient, which is also influenced by motivation and habit.

Self-Reports

In contrast to the method of direct observation, useful data on how a person functions may also be gathered by *self-report,* in which the patient is asked directly either by the therapist or a trained interviewer (*interviewer report*) or through the use of a *self-administered report* instrument. The critical issue in the ability of a self-report to capture function correctly and completely lies in providing clearly worded questions without language bias, concise directions on completing the questions, and a format that encourages accurate reporting of answers to all questions. Self-report is a valid method of determining function, and may be preferable to performance-based methods in some circumstances.[22] Self-reports should be designed so that questions are asked in a standard format and answers are recorded as specified by the predetermined choices. Long paper-and-pencil tests may be difficult for those with upper extremity disability.

Clinical personnel who will act as interviewers must be trained to administer a questionnaire and should practice until they have reached a high degree of agreement with expert examiners of the same cases. Periodic retraining may be necessary if interviewers do not have frequent practice administering the instrument. The interview should be scheduled with the patient in advance and conducted in an environment conducive to complete concentration. Interviews may be conducted by phone or in person, but the mode of administration should be kept consistent if comparisons of the data are to be made. Ad lib prompting by the interviewer or caregivers for answers is discouraged because these intrusions into the patient's self report tend to bias results. If the patient has had help in filling out a form or responding to questions, this should be noted. Similarly, if the data have been provided by a spouse, family member, or caregiver, this should be documented as well.

The distinction in perspectives on function that was discussed regarding performance-based measures of function also holds for self-reports. It is extremely important to distinguish between questions that indicate a person's habitual performance (e.g., "*Do* you cook your own meals?") and those that identify a person's perceived capacity to perform a task (e.g., "If you had to, *could* you cook your own meals?").

The time frame reference of self-reporting is also a relevant consideration. A therapist should decide in advance if the relevant "window" on a person's functional level is the past 24 hours, last week, last month, or the previous year. One can easily imagine how the same person might respond differently regarding the same functional activity depending on frame of reference. Instruments that examine only short-term objectives may not relate well to the long-term objectives of a rehabilitation program.

Instrument Parameters and Formats

Performance-based and self-report instruments grade performance on a number of different criteria in a variety of formats. There is no one parameter or format that is perfect for every type of clinical encounter or research need. It is particularly important that documentation of a patient's progress not be blunted by *floor*" or *ceiling* effects of various descriptors. For example, if a therapist wishes to measure changes in function among generally well elderly patients and the most advanced functional activity on an instrument measures "independent ambulation on level surfaces," there would be no room to demonstrate either progression or decline except around ambulation on level surfaces. Similarly, a patient who was severely debilitated might improve in transfers from needing the maximum assistance of two persons to maximum assistance of one. If the instrument only measures change from "maximum assistance" to "moderate assistance," this patient's real improvement will not be recorded.

Descriptive Parameters

Therapists should use descriptive terms that are well defined and unambiguous. Meanings of descriptive terms should be clear to all others using the medical record. Box 11.1 provides a sample set of acceptable terms and definitions. Additional terms used to qualify function include *dependence* and *difficulty*. Most often, the term *independent* refers to the complete absence of a need for human or mechanical assistance to accomplish a task, but some scoring systems consider reliance on devices and aids as a modified form of independence when used without the help of another person. The use of equipment during the performance of a functional task should be explicitly noted; for example, independent in ambulation with axillary crutches or independent in dressing with adapted clothing and a long-handled shoe horn.

Difficulty is a hybrid term that suggests an activity poses an extra burden for the patient, regardless of dependence level. It is unclear whether it is a measure of overall perceptual-motor skill, coordination, endurance, efficiency, or a combination of measures. Difficulty can be measured in two ways. One approach assumes that difficulty is likely to be present and quantifies the degree of difficulty that the individual experiences while performing the activity (e.g., "How much difficulty do you have while doing household chores? None, some, or a great deal?"). The other approach quantifies the frequency that the difficulty is encountered (e.g., "How often do you have difficulty putting on your shoes? Never, sometimes, very often, or always?").

Often it is helpful to qualify a person's performance by linking observations with nonspecific indicators of impairments such as the energy consumption required to complete the functional task and the degree to which patients must exert themselves to engage in the activity. Simple measurements of a patient's physiological response to activity generally include heart rate, respiratory rate, and blood pressure, both at rest (baseline measurements) and during the most stressful elements of the functional task. For example, "heart rate increased to 100 beats per minute with independent ambulation on stairs; no increase in respiratory rate." In addition, the patient's perceived fatigue, perception of exertion, and overt signs of physiological stress, such as shortness of breath, also should be noted. These notations may assist the therapist in a quick identification of some obvious impairments that limit function, which should be followed by more specific tests and measures of impairment.

Additional descriptors frequently used to qualify functional performance further include (1) pain, (2) fluctuations according to the time of day, (3) medication level, and (4) environmental influences. Any factors that modify a patient's function should be carefully noted and considered by the physical therapist evaluating examination data.

Quantitative Parameters

The time it takes to complete a series of functional activities is often used to enhance a therapist's quantification of function when a given speed of performance is required or an improvement in performance speed is expected. A common example of timed functional skills is found in pre- and post-medication performance of individuals with Parkinson's disease who are placed on L-dopa therapy. Examples of activities that may be timed include (1) walking a set distance; (2) writing one's signature; (3) donning an article of clothing; and (4) crossing a street during the time of a "Walk" light. Scores of timed tests should not be taken as

Box 11.1 Functional Examination and Impairment Terminology

DEFINITIONS

1. **Independent:** patient is able consistently to perform skill safety with no one present.
2. **Supervision:** patient requires someone within arm's reach as a precaution; low probability of patient having a problem requiring assistance.
3. **Close guarding:** person assisting is positioned as if to assist, with hands raised but not touching patient; full attention on patient; fair probability of patient requiring assistance.
4. **Contact guarding:** therapist is positioned as with close guarding, with hands on patient but not giving any assistance; high probability of patient requiring assistance.
5. **Minimum assistance:** patient is able to complete majority of the activity without assistance.
6. **Moderate assistance:** patient is able to complete part of the activity without assistance.
7. **Maximum assistance:** patient is unable to assist in any part of the activity.

DESCRIPTIVE TERMINOLOGY

A. Bed mobility
   1. Independent—no cuing[a] is given
   2. Supervision
   3. Minimum assistance
   4. Moderate assistance
   5. Maximum assistance

   (2–5: may require cues)

B. Transfers, Ambulation
   1. Independent—no cuing is given
   2. Supervision
   3. Close guarding
   4. Contact guarding
   5. Minimum assistance
   6. Moderate assistance
   7. Maximum assistance

   (2–7: may require cues)

C. Functional Balance Grades

1. Normal	Patient able to maintain steady balance without support (static). Accepts maximal challenge and can shift weight easily and within full range in all directions (dynamic).
2. Good	Patient able to maintain balance without support, limited postural sway (static). Accepts moderate challenge; able to maintain balance while picking object off floor (dynamic).
3. Fair	Patient able to maintain balance with handhold support; may require occassional minimal assistance (static). Accepts minimal challenge; able to maintain balance while turning head/trunk (dynamic).
4. Poor	Patient requires handhold and moderate to maximal assistance to maintain posture (static). Unable to accept challenge or move without loss of balance (dynamic).
5. No balance	

[a]Types of cues: verbal, visual, or tactile. In some instances (e.g., a person with a memory deficit, short attention, learning disability, visual loss), a decrease in the number of cues may represent treatment progress, even though the level of dependence remains the same. Interim progress notes can denote these changes by citing frequencies (e.g., 2 out of 3 tries) or an arbitrarily defined rank order scale (e.g., always/occasionally/rarely).

absolute, but rather as one dimension of performance. Although the ability to complete a particular activity in a specified period of time does provide one kind of important data on a patient's overall ability, it may not always be correct to conclude that what is being measured as "quicker" can be interpreted as "better." For example, the patient may get dressed quickly (within seconds), but do so with poorly coordinated movements and a haphazard outcome. When the task is slowed down, the movements may become more coordinated, with a more satisfactory functional outcome, even though the time taken to do the task increases. Similarly, certain medical conditions that affect energy expenditure may require that the patient properly pace a functional activity to complete it successfully. Thus, time scores alone do not always yield the complete functional picture. When interpreted in light of other aspects of the patient's clinical presentation, they do provide an added dimension to the evaluation of data collected during a functional examination.

Response Formats

Nominal Measures

One of the simplest formats in functional tests uses a **nominal** level of measurement by presenting a **checklist** of various functional tasks on which the patient is simply scored as able to do/not able to do, independent/dependent, completed/incomplete, or the like. The results are not particularly descriptive of the exact nature of an individual's limitations and usually require further examination prior to interpretation.

Ordinal Measures

A few tests use descriptive scales that describe a range of performance or the degree to which a person can perform the task. Most commonly, the scales are **ordinal or rank-order scales** (e.g., "no difficulty," "some difficulty," or "unable to do"; or "always," "sometimes," "rarely," or "never"). Scales may be graded in ascending or descending order. The primary drawback in using such a system to score function is that these grades do not define categories that are separated by equal intervals. For example, it is not possible to tell whether the patient who went from maximal assistance to moderate assistance changed as much as a patient who also went one level between moderate assistance and minimal assistance.

Summary or Additive Measures

Summary or **additive measures** grade a specific series of skills, award points for part or full performance, and sum the subscores as a proportion of the total possible points, such as 60/100 or 6/24 and so forth. One example, which is well known to physical therapists, is the Barthel Index (Table 11.1).[23] Some formal, standardized instruments for testing function summarize detailed information about a complex area of function into an overall index score. Use of these instruments facilitates the interpretation of complex data and enables the clinician to perform cross-disease, cross-program, and cross-population comparisons of function. Caution must be exercised in considering only summated scores, however, because potentially important individual differences in functional ability can be masked.[24] A patient who is limited in only a few of the many tasks covered on a functional test will most likely score well, despite what could be substantial limitations in discrete functional activities that are pertinent to the physical therapist's anticipated goals of treatment. Similarly, two patients with the same numeric score might be quite different in their functional deficits, having gained (or lost) their points on different activities. Although these measures yield a "hard number," which is regarded statistically as an interval level of measurement, the degree to which "points" are truly equal intervals apart should be carefully scrutinized.

Visual Analog Scales

Visual or linear analog scales attempt to represent measurement quantities in terms of a straight line placed horizontally or vertically on paper (Fig. 11.3). The endpoints of the line are labeled with descriptive or numeric terms to anchor the extremes of the scale and provide a frame of reference for any point in the continuum between them. Some scales will also use descriptors or numeric intervals

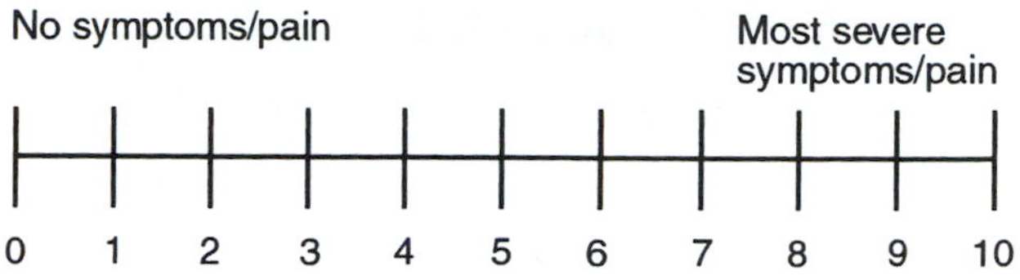

Figure 11.3 A visual analog scale for measuring pain or other symptoms. The patient is instructed to mark the line at the point that corresponds to the degree of pain or severity of symptoms that are experienced.

between the endpoints to assist the individual in grading responses. Commonly the entire visual analog line is 10 centimeters (cm) long, but distances of 15 and 20 cm are also used. The patient is asked to bisect the line at a point representing self-reported position on the scale. The patient's score is then obtained by measuring from the zero mark to the mark bisecting the scale.

Video Recordings

With ever-increasing application of technology to clinical data collection, new tools are available to clinicians and researchers for recording changes in function. Although more costly than traditional methods, videotaping or filming can be a valuable adjunct to functional testing. Visual recordings are appropriate methods for examining and validating the effectiveness of new interventions or treatment approaches. They are also useful to patients in displaying the quality of their movement patterns and in depicting the true extent of their limitation. Video recordings are valuable tools for training staff to score tasks reliably by reaching agreement on observed performance.

Interpreting Test Results

Clearly, the single most important consideration in examining functional status is using the test results correctly to establish and revise the anticipated goals and expected outcomes of intervention and the plan of care. The therapist should carefully delineate the contributing factors that result in the functional deficit. When diminished ability is evident, the therapist must attempt to ascertain the cause of the problem. Some important questions to ask include:

1. What are the normal movements necessary to perform the task?
2. Which impairments inhibit performance or completion of the task? For example, do factors such as poor motor planning and execution, decreased strength, decreased range of motion, or altered joint integrity impede function? Does fatigue hamper functional ability?
3. Are the patient's functional deficits the result of impaired communication, perception, vision, hearing, or cognition?

Table 11.1 Barthel Index[a]

Patient's Name ______________________	Date ____________ Initial ____________
FEEDING 10 = Independent. Able to apply any necessary device. Feeds in reasonable time. 5 = Needs help (e.g., for cutting).	______________
BATHING 5 = Independent	______________
PERSONAL TOILET 5 = Independently washes face, combs hair, brushes teeth, shaves (manages plug if electric).	______________
DRESSING 10 = Independent. Ties shoes, fastens fasteners, applies braces. 5 = Needs help, but does at least half of work in reasonable time.	______________
BOWELS 10 = No accidents. Able to use enema or suppository, if needed. 5 = Occasional accidents or needs help with enema or suppository.	______________
BLADDER 10 = No accidents. Able to care for collecting device if used. 5 = Occasional accidents or needs help with device.	______________ ______________
TOILET TRANSFERS 10 = Independent with toilet or bedpan. Handles clothes, wipes, flushes, or cleans pan. 5 = Needs help for balance, handling clothes or toilet paper.	______________
TRANSFERS—CHAIR AND BED 15 = Independent, including locking of wheelchair, lifting footrests. 10 = Minimum assistance or supervision. 5 = Able to sit, but needs maximum assistance to transfer.	______________
AMBULATION 15 = Independent for 50 yards. May use assistive devices, except for rolling walker. 10 = With help, 50 yards. 5 = Independent with wheelchair for 50 yards if unable to walk.	______________
STAIR CLIMBING 10 = Independent. May use assistive devices. 5 = Needs help or supervision.	______________ ______________
	Totals ______________

[a]A score of zero (0) is given in any category in which the patient does not achieve the stated criterion.

From Mahoney, F, and Barthel, D,[23, pp 62–65] with permission.

Examples of the kinds of questions a therapist must pose to assess function and integrate findings into a comprehensive treatment program are found in the case vignettes that follow:

Case A	Case B
36-year-old male construction worker	72-year-old female homemaker
dx: traumatic right transtibial amputation; post fracture left femur	dx: CVA with right hemiplegia with global aphasia
Partial Examination Findings	
Motor Control and Muscle Performance	
Decreased in all extremities following prolonged immobilization	Flaccid paralysis right extremities
Functional Limitations	
Unable to transfer from bed to wheelchair	Unable to transfer from bed to wheelchair

Although the functional disability in each case is in fact identical, the contributing factors, goals and outcomes, and the interventions would be markedly different. In case A, the patient's inability to transfer can reasonably be attributed to decreased strength. When ameliorated, it is likely that the patient will go on to achieve an outcome of independent ambulation with a prosthesis. The patient in case B has factors that cannot be addressed solely through physical therapy. In addition, it may be difficult to determine whether it is the paralysis or the aphasia that compromises efforts to assess and improve function. Although a similar goal of independence in wheelchair mobility and transfers may be proposed, reexamination throughout the episode of care may demonstrate that functional deficits persist, despite improvement in motor function. In that case, the impairments in comprehension and language function may be the more important factors contributing to functional limitation. Thus, the design of rehabilitation programs is based on the impairments that presumably underlie the functional deficits. If remediation of the impairment does not solve the functional problem, the therapist needs to reexamine the initial clinical impression by looking for other potentially causative factors.

Some functional tasks may need to be analyzed more precisely. Activities can be broken down into subordinate parts, or subroutines. A **subordinate part** is defined as an element of movement without which the task cannot proceed safely or efficiently. For example, bed mobility includes the following subordinate parts: (1) scooting in bed (changing position for comfort or skin care and getting to the edge), (2) rolling onto the side, (3) lowering the legs, (4) sitting up, and (5) balancing at the edge of the bed. A functional loss of independent bed mobility may result from an inability to perform any or all of these subroutines. These are not only checkpoints for examining patients, but they also later represent the anticipated goals of various interventions. The more involved the patient, the slower the learner, or complex the task, the more the functional task may need to be broken down into subordinate parts.

Determining the Quality of Instruments

Within the rehabilitation setting, many tools have been developed primarily for in-house use and may have spread from facility to facility as staff members have moved. In most instances, the instruments underwent many modifications and the original sources have been lost. Other tests have been designed more rigidly and tested in clinical trials, examining the instrument's psychometric properties and providing documentation of its **reliability** and **validity** in the literature. If the reliability and validity of an instrument are not established, little faith can be put in the results obtained or in the conclusions drawn from the results. A poorly constructed instrument can produce data that are questionable, if not worthless. In light of the fact that the viability of physical therapy as a reimbursable service rests on the demonstration of functional outcomes, the importance of these concepts to functional testing becomes clear. Some of the more recently developed instruments have undergone extensive testing of their measurement properties. In accordance with the American Physical Therapy Association's Standards of Measurement, physical therapists should use only those instruments whose reliability and validity are known.[25] Although no instrument will have perfect reliability or validity, therapists must be able to gauge the certainty of their data and the appropriate scope of inferences drawn from the data.

Reliability

A reliable instrument measures a phenomenon dependably, time after time, accurately, predictably, and without variation. If a functional test is not reliable, the patient's initial baseline status or the true effect of treatment can be concealed. An instrument with acceptable *test–retest reliability* is stable and will not indicate change when none has occurred. Tests performed by the same therapist of the same performance should be highly correlated (*intrarater reliability*). Instruments should also have strong *interrater reliability*, or agreement among multiple observers of the same event. If a particular patient is examined by several therapists in the course of treatment, or reexamined over time to determine long-term change, the reliability of the functional tool must be known.

A flaw in the clinical use of most types of standardized tests and measures is the tendency to disregard interrater reliability. To use functional tests with maximum accuracy, (1) scoring criteria must be defined clearly and must be mutually exclusive; (2) criteria must be strictly applied to each clinical situation; and (3) all therapists in a facility must be retrained periodically in the use of the instrument to ensure similarity.

Validity

Validity is a multifaceted concept and established in many different ways. Questions regarding an instrument's validity attempt to determine (1) whether an instrument designed to measure function truly does just that; (2) what the appropriate applications of the instrument are; and (3) how the data should be interpreted. First, the valid instrument should, on the face of it, appear to measure what it purports to measure (*face validity*).[26] Another critical dimension is whether the assessment instrument measures all the important or specified dimensions of function (*content validity*). If there were a **gold standard** (an unimpeachable measure of a phenomenon, such as a laboratory test with normative values), then a new instrument could be tested against the results of this standard (*criterion-related validity*). Such a gold standard does not exist for functional instruments. New functional measurement tools can, however, be compared to existing ones that are accepted measures of the same functional activities. The degree to which the two instruments agree helps to establish *concurrent validity*. Concurrent validity can also be demonstrated by showing that an instrument corresponds appropriately to measures of other phenomena. This method is particularly relevant for self-report instruments. The concurrent validity of some self-report instruments has been determined by comparison with clinician ratings and other clinical findings; for example, a person's level of function as indicated by an instrument correlates directly with clinician's ratings of improvement and inversely with the patient's reports of pain. There is also the *predictive validity* of a test or measure, which indicates the likelihood of a subsequent phenomenon or event (e.g., return to work) on the basis of a prior phenomenon (e.g., a baseline measure of function). Finally, the degree to which an instrument measures abstract concepts such as physical mobility or social interaction can be established over time (*construct validity*). Construct validation, using a variety of statistical procedures, is a never-ending process as our understanding of the construct is further refined as instruments are developed to measure it.

Other Factors

In addition to reliability and validity, a measure of functional status should be (1) sufficiently sensitive to reflect meaningful changes in patient status and (2) concise enough to be clinically useful.

Considerations in Selection of Instruments

A large number of instruments have been developed to assess and to classify functional ability. Given the plethora of instruments that currently exist, it is quite reasonable to ask how these instruments compare with one another. It is important to remember that no instrument is perfect for all patients or all situations. No instrument can measure all the items potentially relevant to a particular individual and provide the perfect composite picture. For example, one instrument may provide an extensive measure of activities of daily living (ADL), but not deal with psychological or social dimensions of function. Another instrument may investigate social functioning while omitting some ADL tasks. Many items overlap from instrument to instrument. For example, a question on the ability to ambulate is a common item found in most physical function instruments. Although instruments may cover the same kind of activity, the questions posed about the performance of the same activity may be quite different. For example, one instrument may investigate the degree of difficulty and of human assistance required to "dress yourself, including handling of closures, buttons, zippers, snaps." Another may ask, "How much help do you need in getting dressed?" As discussed, differences also may exist in the time frames sampled in the various instruments.

Critical questions to ask, therefore, in selecting an instrument include:

1. What are the domains or categories that the assessment instrument focuses on?
2. How adequately does the instrument measure the domain or domains being sampled?
3. What areas of physical function are included? Does the instrument measure ADL? IADL? Functional mobility skills?
4. What aspect of function is being measured? Is the level of dependence–independence considered? What is the length of time required to complete the functional task? Degree of difficulty? Influence of pain?
5. What is the time frame sampled in the instrument?
6. What is the mode of administration?
7. What type of scoring system is used?
8. Are multiple instruments necessary to provide a more complete picture of functional status?

Extrapolating items from a variety of instruments may provide the kind of data desired but should be considered with extreme caution inasmuch as this process changes reliability or validity of the measurements. Factors such as the theoretic orientation of the user, the purpose for using the instrument, and the relevance of particular functional items to certain patient populations all enter into the decision-making process. In the final analysis, the choice of instrument may be dictated by practical considerations. For example, self-report instruments, which rely on information from the patient, are limited in use to mentally competent individuals. Time and resources for administration also may influence test selection. In any case, there are many suitable instruments available for assessing functional status, some of which are quite commonly used by clinicians as well as researchers.

Selected Instruments Assessing Physical Function

Barthel Index

The *Barthel Index* was developed by a physical therapist about 40 years ago.[23] Although not as commonly used today as some other instruments, this assessment tool represents one of the earliest contributions to the functional status literature and identifies physical therapists' long-standing inclusion of functional mobility and ADL measurement within their scope of practice. The Barthel Index specifically measures the degree of assistance required by an individual on 10 items of mobility and self-care ADL (see Table 11.1). Levels of measurement are limited to either complete independence or needing assistance. Each performance item is scored on an ordinal scale with a specified number of points assigned to each level or ranking. Variable weightings were established by the developers of the Barthel Index for each item based on clinical judgment or other implicit criteria. An individual who uses human assistance in eating, for example, would receive 5 points; independence in eating would receive a score of 10 points. A single global score, ranging from 0 to 100, is calculated from the sum of all weighted individual item scores, so that a 0 equals complete dependence for all 10 activities, and 100 equals complete independence in all 10 activities. The Barthel Index has been used widely to monitor functional changes in individuals receiving inpatient rehabilitation, particularly in predicting the functional outcomes associated with stroke.[27,28] Although its psychometric properties have never been fully examined, the Barthel Index has demonstrated strong interrater reliability (0.95) and test–retest reliability (0.89) as well as high correlations (0.74 to 0.80) with other measures of physical disability.[29]

Katz Index of Activities of Daily Living

The *Katz Index of ADL* focuses on patient performance and the degree of assistance required in six categories of basic ADL: bathing, dressing, toileting, transferring, continence, and feeding (Table 11.2).[30,31] Using both direct observation and patient self-report over a 2-week period, the examiner scores 1 point for each activity that is performed without human help. A score of 0 is given if the activity is performed with human assistance or is not performed. Activity scores are combined to form a cumulative scale in letter grades (A through G) in order of increasing dependency. An individual's global letter score indicates an exact pattern of responses to the list of items. A score of B in the Katz Index, for example, means that the individual is independent in performing all but one of the six basic ADL categories. On the other hand, a score of D means that the individual is independent in all but bathing, dressing, and one additional function. The combination of categorical deficits in the Katz Index reflects a particular theoretical orientation. The developers of the Katz Index assumed a developmental and hierarchical organization of function in constructing their instrument. This organizational model is based on the empirically noted integration of neurological and locomotor responses seen in children. One version of the scale demonstrated agreement ratios of 0.68 and 0.98 between different professional raters. Test–retest reliability of respondent self-reports produced intraclass correlation coefficients ranging from 0.61 to 0.78.[32]

The Katz Index, originally developed for use with institutionalized patients, has been adapted for use in community-based populations.[33] A major disadvantage of using the Katz Index in rehabilitation settings is its failure to include an item on ambulation. The predictive validity of the instrument for long-term survival also has been reported.[31]

Summary of Physical Function Tests

Neither of the single physical functional assessment instruments presented in the preceding paragraphs covers all areas of physical function (Table 11.3). Even items that appear to measure the same function may, depending on how the item is worded, be concerned with a different aspect of performance.[34] Therefore, one of these instruments may be chosen to match the specific needs of the clinician for a brief, unidimensional functional measure, but only if the likely functional limitations of the clinical population served are described by the items on the instrument.

Multidimensional Functional Assessment Instruments

The previous discussion of functional instruments that describe only one dimension of health status highlights a clinician's need to understand a patient's health status in all its domains. Further instrument development in the last 20 years has resulted in the emergence of multidimensional health status instruments to measure the spectrum of health status domains more comprehensively. Most concentrate on two or three dimensions of a patient's function, and record little about a person's disease or impairments. Therefore, to some small degree the term *health status* frequently used to describe these instruments is a misnomer, inasmuch as these instruments actually measure multiple dimensions of function as they contribute to a person's health and not "health" in, and of, itself. Similarly, these instruments are also sometimes referred to as measuring *health-related quality of life*. Without bringing in the patient's perspective on personal meaningfulness to the individual, the gold standard quality of life, such terminology may overstate the value of these instruments. However, used in conjunction with traditional clinical methods of examining signs and

Table 11.2 **The Katz Index of ADL**

Name ______________ Day of examination ______________

For each area of functioning listed below, check description that applies. (The word "assistance" means supervision, direction, or personal assistance.)

Bathing—either sponge bath, tub bath, or shower.		
☐ Receives no assistance (gets in and out of tub by self if tub is usual means of bathing).	☐ Receives assistance in bathing only one part of the body (such as back or a leg).	☐ Receives assistance in bathing more than one part of the body (or not bathed).
Dressing—gets clothes from closets and drawers—including underclothes, outer garments and using fasteners (including braces if worn).		
☐ Gets clothes and gets completely dressed without assistance.	☐ Gets clothes and gets dressed without assistance except for assistance in tying shoes.	☐ Receives assistance in getting clothes or in getting dressed, or stays partly or completely undressed.
Toileting—going to the "toilet room" for bowel and urine elimination, cleaning self after elimination, and arranging clothes.		
☐ Goes to "toilet room," cleans self, and arranges clothes without assistance (may use object for support such as cane, walker, or wheelchair and may manage night bedpan or commode, emptying same in morning).	☐ Receives assistance in going to "toilet room" or in cleansing self or in arranging clothes after elimination or in use of night bedpan or commode.	☐ Doesn't go to room termed "toilet" for the elimination process.
Transfer		
☐ Moves in and out of bed as well as in and out of chair without assistance (may be using object for support such as cane or walker).	☐ Moves in and out of bed or chair with assistance.	☐ Doesn't get out of bed.
Continence		
☐ Controls urination and bowel movement completely by self.	☐ Has occasional "accidents."	☐ Supervision helps keep urine or bowel control; catheter is used, or is incontinent.
Feeding		
☐ Feeds self without assistance.	☐ Feeds self except for getting assistance in cutting meat or buttering bread.	☐ Receives assistance in feeding or is fed partly or completely by using tubes or intravenous fluids.

The Index of Independence in Activities of Daily Living is based on an evaluation of the functional independence or dependence of patients in bathing, dressing, going to toilet, transferring, continence, and feeding. Specific definitions of functional independence and dependence appear below the index.

A—Independent in feeding, continence, transferring, going to toilet, dressing, and bathing.
B—Independent in all but one of these functions.
C—Independent in all but bathing and one additional function.
D—Independent in all but bathing, dressing, and one additional function.
E—Independent in all but bathing, dressing, going to toilet, and one additional function.
F—Independent in all but bathing, dressing, going to toilet, transferring, and one additional function.
G—Dependent in all six functions.
Other—Dependent in at least two functions, but not classifiable as C, D, E, or F.

Independence means without supervision, direction, or active personal assistance, except as specifically noted below. This is based on actual status and not on ability. A patient who refuses to perform a function is considered as not performing the function, even though he is deemed able.

(*continued*)

Table 11.2 The Katz Index of ADL (continued)

Bathing (sponge, shower, or tub)
Independent: assistance only in bathing a single part (as back or disabled extremity) or bathes self completely

Dependent: assistance in bathing more than one part of body; assistance in getting in or out of tub or does not bathe self

Dressing
Independent: gets clothes from closets and drawers; puts on clothes, outer garments, braces; manages fasteners; act of tying shoes is excluded

Dependent: does not dress self or remains partly undressed

Going to toilet
Independent: gets to toilet; gets on and off toilet; arranges clothes; cleans organs of excretion (may manage own bedpan used at night only and may or may not be using mechanical supports)

Dependent: uses bedpan or commode or receives assistance in getting to and using toilet

Transfer
Independent: moves in and out of bed independently and moves in and out of chair independently (may or may not be using mechanical supports)

Dependent: assistance in moving in or out of bed and/or chair; does not perform one or more transfers

Continence
Independent: urination and defecation entirely self-controlled

Dependent: partial or total incontinence in urination or defecation; partial or total control by enemas, catheters, or regulated use of urinals and/or bedpans

Feeding
Independent: gets food from plate or its equivalent into mouth (precutting of meat and preparation of food, as buttering bread, are excluded from evaluation)

Dependent: assistance in act of feeding (see above); does not eat at all or parenteral feeding

From Katz, S, et al.[31, p 20] with permission.

symptoms, multidimensional functional status instruments can add an important comprehensive view of a patient's function to the overall health status. In this respect they add a crucial, and previously missing, component in evaluating the health of individuals. A few of these instruments representative of the current "state of the art" are discussed below.

The Functional Independence Measure

The *Functional Independence Measure (FIM)*[35,36] is an 18-item measure of physical, psychological, and social function that is part of the Uniform Data System for Medical Rehabilitation (UDS_{MR}).[37] The UDS_{MR} collects data from participating rehabilitation facilities and issues summary reports of the records that have been entered into the UDS_{MR} database. The FIM uses the level of assistance an individual needs to grade functional status from total independence to total assistance (Fig. 11.4). A person may be regarded as independent if a device is used, but this is recorded separately from "complete" independence. The instrument lists six self-care activities: feeding, grooming, bathing, upper body dressing, lower body dressing, and toileting. Bowel and bladder control, aspects of which some may consider as impairments rather than function, are categorized separately. Functional mobility is tested through three items on transfers. Under the category of locomotion, walking and using a wheelchair are listed equivalently, while stairs are considered separately. The FIM also includes two items on communication and three on social cognition.

The FIM measures what the individual does, not what that person could do under certain circumstances. The interrater reliability of the FIM has been established at an acceptable level of psychometric performance (intraclass correlation coefficients ranging from 0.86 to 0.88).[36] The face and content validity of the FIM as well as its ability to capture change in a patient's level of function have also been determined. Any clinical worker can administer the FIM after appropriate training in using the response set for each item.

For persons with stroke, the motor scale of the FIM has been shown to have high concurrent validity with the Barthel Index ($ICC \geq 0.83$).[38] Gosman-Hedstrom and

Table 11.3 Items Covered in Selected Physical Function Instruments

	Barthel	Katz
Mobility		
Transfers	+	+
Ambulation	+	–
Inclines/stairs	+	–
ADL		
Bathing	+	+
Grooming	+	–
Dressing	+	+
Feeding	+	+
Toileting	+	+

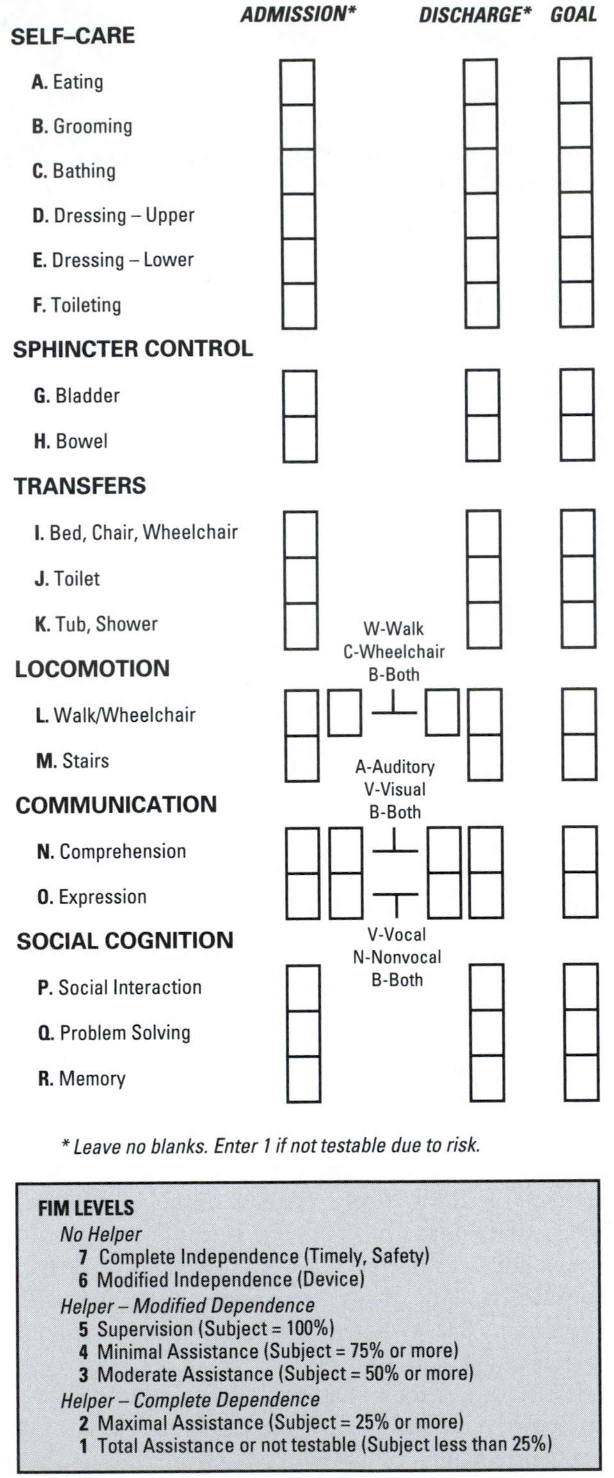
ADMISSION* DISCHARGE* GOAL

SELF-CARE
A. Eating
B. Grooming
C. Bathing
D. Dressing – Upper
E. Dressing – Lower
F. Toileting

SPHINCTER CONTROL
G. Bladder
H. Bowel

TRANSFERS
I. Bed, Chair, Wheelchair
J. Toilet
K. Tub, Shower

LOCOMOTION
W-Walk
C-Wheelchair
B-Both
L. Walk/Wheelchair
M. Stairs

COMMUNICATION
A-Auditory
V-Visual
B-Both
N. Comprehension
O. Expression
V-Vocal
N-Nonvocal
B-Both

SOCIAL COGNITION
P. Social Interaction
Q. Problem Solving
R. Memory

* Leave no blanks. Enter 1 if not testable due to risk.

FIM LEVELS
No Helper
7 Complete Independence (Timely, Safety)
6 Modified Independence (Device)
Helper – Modified Dependence
5 Supervision (Subject = 100%)
4 Minimal Assistance (Subject = 75% or more)
3 Moderate Assistance (Subject = 50% or more)
Helper – Complete Dependence
2 Maximal Assistance (Subject = 25% or more)
1 Total Assistance or not testable (Subject less than 25%)

Figure 11.4 The Functional Independence Measure (FIMJ) instrument scores function using a seven-point scale based on percentage(s) of active participation from patient. (From the Uniform Data System for Medical Rehabilitation, a division of UB Foundation Activities, Inc [$UDS_{MR}{}^{SM}$]. Guide for the Uniform Data Set for Medical Rehabilitation [including the FIM™ instrument], Version 5.1. Buffalo, NY 14214: State University of New York at Buffalo; 1997, with permission.)

Svensson have shown strong construct validity between items on the Barthel and items on the FIM that measure functional limitations.[39] Rasch analysis has been applied to the scale scores of the FIM which are ordinal measures, in order to create interval scale measurements.[40] In addition, the *WeeFIM*, an 18-item instrument based on the FIM, has been developed for use for children between the ages of 6 months and 18 years.[41]

The Sickness Impact Profile

The *Sickness Impact Profile (SIP)* was developed to address the need for an instrument that was precise enough to detect meaningful changes in perceived function.[42–47] Intended for use across types and severities of illness, it is designed to detect small impacts of illness. The SIP contains 136 items in 12 categories of activities. These include sleep and rest, eating, work, home management, recreation, ambulatory mobility, body care and movement, social interaction, alertness, emotional behavior, and communication. A sample SIP measure of affective functioning specific to emotional behavior is presented in Table 11.4. The entire test can be either self-administered or administered by an interview in

Table 11.4 Sickness Impact Profile (SIP): Affective Function

Please respond to (check) *only* those statements that you are *sure* describe you today and are related to your state of health.

1. I say how bad or useless I am; for example, that I am a burden on others. ______
2. I laugh or cry suddenly. ______
3. I often moan and groan in pain or discomfort. ______
4. I have attempted suicide. ______
5. I act nervous or restless. ______
6. I keep rubbing or holding areas of my body that hurt or are uncomfortable. ______
7. I act irritable and impatient with myself; for example, talk badly about myself, swear at myself, blame myself for things that happen. ______
8. I talk about the future in a hopeless way. ______
9. I get sudden frights. ______

CHECK HERE WHEN YOU HAVE READ ALL STATEMENTS ON THIS PAGE ☐

Reprinted by permission of Marilyn Bergner, PhD.[43]

20 to 30 minutes. SIP scores are percentage ratings based on the ratio of the summed scale scores to the summed values of all SIP items. Higher scores indicate greater dysfunction.

The SIP test–retest reliability coefficients range from 0.75 to 0.92 for the overall score and from 0.45 to 0.60 for items checked.[44] Validity has been determined using subjective self-report, clinician measurement, and subjects' scores on other instruments. Correlations relevant to establishing multiple forms of validity range from a low of 0.35 to a high of 0.84.[43] The SIP has been used as a measure of function in many studies including describing the physical and psychosocial functions of individuals in an outpatient setting in relation to the duration of disease[48] and the efficacy of using transcutaneous electrical nerve stimulation (TENS) with low back pain patients.[49] There are, however, some concerns regarding its use and suitability in certain kinds of studies. In examining disability, SIP focuses only on whether a person selects statements that are very broad about the inability to perform activities; for example, "I do not maintain balance"; "I kneel, stoop, or bend down only by holding on to something"; "I am very clumsy in body movements." It neglects the range of performance in between, with some potential loss of precision. The SIP also combines many functional activities into a single item, which may also reduce its discriminatory ability, such as "I have difficulty doing handwork; for example, turning faucets, using kitchen gadgets, sewing, carpentry." A few investigators have noted that the SIP may be more sensitive to detecting deterioration of status than to improvement, which may diminish its suitability as an instrument for monitoring the progress of rehabilitation for individuals over time.[50]

The Outcome and Assessment Information Set

The *Outcome and Assessment Information Set (OASIS)* was designed to ensure the collection of pertinent data on the adult patient in the home care setting that would allow home health agencies to assess the quality of care by measuring the outcomes of care.[51,52] During the years of its initial development, use of the OASIS by home health agencies had been voluntary. However, as of January 1, 1999, home health agencies were mandated to use the OASIS as a *Condition of Participation in the Medicare program* by the Health Care Financing Administration. Developed over a 10-year period, the current version of OASIS, known as OASIS-B, contains 79 core items covering sociodemographic characteristics, environmental factors, social support, health status, and functional status. OASIS is not designed to be a comprehensive examination of a patient, or an "add-on" measurement. OASIS items are meant to be integrated into the clinical record to highlight various aspects of a patient's status that identify particular needs for care upon admission to the home health service, at follow-up every 60 days, and at discharge. The OASIS was intended to be a discipline-neutral record, administered by any health professional including physical therapists. Created as part of a research program to develop outcomes measures applicable to home health, the OASIS has been field-tested through demonstration projects and refined by a panel of experts. Reliability testing is ongoing.

Ease of administration increases with familiarity with the instrument. Unlike most other instruments, the response sets that accompany each item are specifically matched to the item. Some response sets have only two possible descriptions of behavior, whereas others have as many as nine possible descriptions of behavior. Therefore, the user must be familiar with the possible response set to each item, and anticipate that comfort level in using this instrument will increase over a learning curve. The ADL/IADL section is composed of 14 different items (Table 11.5) including grooming, dressing the upper body, dressing the lower body, bathing, toileting, transfers, ambulation/locomotion, feeding, meal preparation, transportation, laundry, housekeeping, shopping, and the ability to use the telephone. The format of the instrument in this section allows recording of both prior and current functional status on each of the items.

The SF-36

The *SF-36* contains 36 items based on questions used in the RAND Health Insurance Study. These 36 items were culled from the 113 questions used by RAND in the Medical Outcomes Study (MOS) to explore the relationship between physician practice styles and patient outcomes.[53] Thus, it was named the SF-36, because it was a short form of the MOS instrument with only 36 questions. The MOS provided important data on the functional status of adults with specific chronic conditions[54] and the well-being of patients experiencing depression compared to subjects with a chronic medical condition.[55] The SF-36 demonstrated high reliability and validity (correlation coefficients ranging from 0.81 to 0.88).[56–59] Normative data for these self-report items have been collected.[60]

All but one of the 36 questions of the SF-36 are used to form eight different scales: physical function, social function, role function, mental health, energy/fatigue, pain, and general health perceptions. The last question considers self-perceived change in health during the past year. Items are scored on nominal (yes/no) or ordinal scales. Each possible response to an item on a scale is assigned a number of points. The total points for all items within a scale are then added and transformed mathematically to yield a percentage score, with 100 percent representing optimal health. Sample items on physical function and role function are presented in Table 11.6. The SF-36 has been used in a number of studies that describe the health status and physical functioning of patients with a variety of impairments receiving physical therapy services.[61–66]

Table 11.5 Outcome and Assessment Information Set (Oasis): ADL/IADLs

(M0640) Grooming: Ability to tend to personal hygiene needs (i.e., washing face and hands, hair care, shaving or make up, teeth or denture care, fingernail care).

Prior	*Current*	
☐	☐	0—Able to groom self unaided, with or without the use of assistive devices or adapted methods.
☐	☐	1—Grooming utensils must be placed within reach before able to complete grooming activities.
☐	☐	2—Someone must assist the patient to groom self.
☐	☐	3—Patient depends entirely upon someone else for grooming needs.
☐		UK—Unknown

(M0650) Ability to Dress *Upper* Body (with or without dressing aids) including undergarments, pullovers, front-opening shirts and blouses, managing zippers, buttons, and snaps:

Prior	*Current*	
☐	☐	0—Able to get clothes out of closets and drawers, put them on and remove them from the upper body without assistance.
☐	☐	1—Able to dress upper body without assistance if clothing is laid out or handed to the patient.
☐	☐	2—Someone must help the patient put on upper body clothing.
☐	☐	3—Patient depends entirely upon another person to dress the upper body.
☐		UK—Unknown

(M0660) Ability to Dress *Lower* Body (with or without dressing aids) including undergarments, slacks, socks or nylons, shoes:

Prior	*Current*	
☐	☐	0—Able to obtain, put on, and remove clothing and shoes without assistance.
☐	☐	1—Able to dress lower body without assistance if clothing and shoes are laid out or handed to the patient.
☐	☐	2—Someone must help the patient put on undergarments, slacks, socks or nylons, and shoes.
☐	☐	3—Patient depends entirely upon another person to dress lower body.
☐		UK—Unknown

(M0670) Bathing: Ability to wash entire body. ***Excludes*** **grooming (washing face and hands only).**

Prior	*Current*	
☐	☐	0—Able to bathe self in *shower or tub* independently.
☐	☐	1—With the use of devices, is able to bathe self in shower or tub independently.
☐	☐	2—Able to bathe in shower or tub with the assistance of another person: (a) for intermittent supervision or encouragement or reminders, *OR* (b) to get in and out of the shower or tub, *OR* (c) for washing difficult to reach areas.
☐	☐	3—Participates in bathing self in shower or tub, *but* requires presence of another person throughout the bath for assistance or supervision.
☐	☐	4—*Unable* to use the shower or tub and is bathed in *bed or bedside chair.*
☐	☐	5—Unable to effectively participate in bathing and is totally bathed by another person.
☐		UK—Unknown

(M0680) Toileting: Ability to get to and from the toilet or bedside commode.

Prior	*Current*	
☐	☐	0—Able to get to and from the toilet independently with or without a device.
☐	☐	1—When reminded, assisted, or supervised by another person, able to get to and from the toilet.
☐	☐	2—*Unable* to get to and from the toilet but is able to use a bedside commode (with or without assistance).

(*continued*)

Table 11.5 Outcome and Assessment Information Set (Oasis): ADL/IADLs (continued)

☐	☐	3—*Unable* to get to and from the toilet or bedside commode but is able to use a bedpan/urinal independently.
☐	☐	4—Is totally dependent in toileting.
☐		UK—Unknown

(M0690) Transferring: Ability to move from bed to chair, on and off toilet or commode, into and out of tub or shower, and ability to turn and position self in bed if patient is bedfast.

Prior	*Current*	
☐	☐	0—Able to independently transfer.
☐	☐	1—Transfers with minimal human assistance or with use of an assistive device.
☐	☐	2—*Unable* to transfer self but is able to bear weight and pivot during the transfer process.
☐	☐	3—Unable to transfer self and is *unable* to bear weight or pivot when transferred by another person.
☐	☐	4—Bedfast, unable to transfer but is able to turn and position self in bed.
☐	☐	5—Bedfast, unable to transfer and is *unable* to turn and position self.
☐		UK—Unknown

(M0700) Ambulation/Locomotion: Ability to *SAFELY* walk, once in a standing position, or use a wheelchair, once in a seated position, on a variety of surfaces.

Prior	*Current*	
☐	☐	0—Able to independently walk on even and uneven surfaces and climb stairs with or without railings (i.e., needs no human assistance or assistive device).
☐	☐	1—Requires use of a device (e.g., cane, walker) to walk alone *or* requires human supervision or assistance to negotiate stairs or steps or uneven surfaces.
☐	☐	2—Able to walk only with the supervision or assistance of another person at all times.
☐	☐	3—Chairfast, *unable* to ambulate but is able to wheel self independently.
☐	☐	4—Chairfast, unable to ambulate and is *unable* to wheel self.
☐	☐	5—Bedfast, unable to ambulate or be up in a chair.
☐		UK—Unknown

(M0710) Feeding or Eating: Ability to feed self meals and snacks. **Note: This refers only to the process of *eating, chewing,* and *swallowing, not preparing* the food to be eaten.**

Prior	*Current*	
☐	☐	0—Able to independently feed self.
☐	☐	1—Able to feed self independently but requires: (a) meal set-up; *OR* (b) intermittent assistance or supervision from another person; *OR* (c) a liquid, pureed or ground meat diet.
☐	☐	2—*Unable* to feed self and must be assisted or supervised throughout the meal/snack.
☐	☐	3—Able to take in nutrients orally *and* receives supplemental nutrients through a nasogastric tube or gastrostomy.
☐	☐	4—*Unable* to take in nutrients orally and is fed nutrients through a nasogastric tube or gastrostomy.
☐	☐	5—Unable to take in nutrients orally or by tube feeding.
☐		UK—Unknown

(M0720) Planning and Preparing Light Meals (e.g., cereal, sandwich) or reheat delivered meals:

Prior	*Current*	
☐	☐	0—(a) Able to independently plan and prepare all light meals for self or reheat delivered meals; *OR* (b) Is physically, cognitively, and mentally able to prepare light meals on a regular basis but has not routinely performed light meal preparation in the past (i.e., prior to this home care admission).
☐	☐	1—*Unable* to prepare light meals on a regular basis due to physical, cognitive, or mental limitations.
☐	☐	2—Unable to prepare any light meals or reheat any delivered meals.
☐		UK—Unknown

(continued)

Table 11.5 Outcome and Assessment Information Set (Oasis): ADL/IADLs (continued)

(M0730) Transportation: Physical and mental ability to *safely* use a car, taxi, or public transportation (bus, train, subway).

Prior	Current	
☐	☐	0—Able to independently drive a regular or adapted car; *OR* uses a regular or handicap-accessible public bus.
☐	☐	1—Able to ride in a car only when driven by another person; *OR* able to use a bus or handicap van only when assisted or accompanied by another person.
☐	☐	2—*Unable* to ride in a car, taxi, bus, or van, and requires transportation by ambulance.
☐		UK—Unknown

(M0740) Laundry: Ability to do own laundry—to carry laundry to and from washing machine, to use washer and dryer, to wash small items by hand.

Prior	Current	
☐	☐	0—(a) Able to independently take care of all laundry tasks; *OR* (b) Physically, cognitively, and mentally able to do laundry and access facilities, *but* has not routinely performed laundry tasks in the past (i.e., prior to this home care admission).
☐	☐	1—Able to do only light laundry, such as minor hand wash or light washer loads. Due to physical, cognitive, or mental limitations, needs assistance with heavy laundry such as carrying large loads of laundry.
☐	☐	2—*Unable* to do any laundry due to physical limitation or needs continual supervision and assistance due to cognitive or mental limitation.
☐		UK—Unknown

(M0750) Housekeeping: Ability to safely and effectively perform light housekeeping and heavier cleaning tasks.

Prior	Current	
☐	☐	0—(a) Able to independently perform all housekeeping tasks; *OR* (b) Physically, cognitively, and mentally able to perform *all* housekeeping tasks but has not routinely participated in housekeeping tasks in the past (i.e., prior to this home care admission).
☐	☐	1—Able to perform only *light* housekeeping (e.g., dusting, wiping kitchen counters) tasks independently.
☐	☐	2—Able to perform housekeeping tasks with intermittent assistance or supervision from another person.
☐	☐	3—*Unable* to consistently perform any housekeeping tasks unless assisted by another person throughout the process.
☐	☐	4—Unable to effectively participate in any housekeeping tasks.
☐		UK—Unknown

(M0760) Shopping: Ability to plan for, select, and purchase items in a store and to carry them home or arrange delivery.

Prior	Current	
☐	☐	0—(a) Able to plan for shopping needs and independently perform shopping tasks, including carrying packages; *OR* (b) Physically, cognitively, and mentally able to take care of shopping, but has not done shopping in the past (i.e., prior to this home care admission).
☐	☐	1—Able to go shopping, but needs some assistance: (a) By self is able to do only light shopping and carry small packages, but needs someone to do occasional major shopping; *OR* (b) *Unable* to go shopping alone, but can go with someone to assist.
☐	☐	2—*Unable* to go shopping, but is able to identify items needed, place orders, and arrange home delivery.
☐	☐	3—Needs someone to do all shopping and errands.
☐		UK—Unknown

(*continued*)

Table 11.5 Outcome and Assessment Information Set (Oasis): ADL/IADLs (continued)

(M0770) Ability to Use Telephone: Ability to answer the phone, dial numbers, and *effectively* use the telephone to communicate.

Prior	*Current*	
☐	☐	0—Able to dial numbers and answer calls appropriately and as desired.
☐	☐	1—Able to use a specially adapted telephone (i.e., large numbers on the dial, teletype phone for the deaf) and call essential numbers.
☐	☐	2—Able to answer the telephone and carry on a normal conversation but has difficulty with placing calls.
☐	☐	3—Able to answer the telephone only some of the time or is able to carry on only a limited conversation.
☐	☐	4—*Unable* to answer the telephone at all but can listen if assisted with equipment.
☐	☐	5—Totally unable to use the telephone.
☐	☐	NA—Patient does not have a telephone.
☐		UK—Unknown

From OASIS-B, Center for Health Services and Policy Research, Denver, CO, 1997, with permission.

Recently, a shortened version has been developed that uses a subset of items from the SF-36.[67] This version, known as SF-12, includes items from each of the eight concepts represented in the SF-36 and allows for the calculation of physical and mental subscale scores. An advantage to using fewer questions is less time is required to complete the survey. This, however, may be at the expense of having a less precise score that may not be as sensitive to change for an individual patient.[68] The development of the SF-36 stands as the premier example of a complete and published exploration of the psychometric properties of an instrument as an essential part of its development, and a testament to the responsibility of its creators in verifying the quality of the SF-36 as a scientific tool (see Evidence Summary Box 11.2).

Summary of Multidimensional Functional Instruments

For the purposes of illustration, four multidimensional instruments have been presented. Choice of a multidimensional instrument carries the same caveats mentioned for

Table 11.6 The SF-36: Physical and Role Function

The following questions are about activities you might do during a typical day. Does *your health* limit you in these activities? If so, how much? (Mark one box on each line.)	Yes, limited a lot	Yes limited a little	No, not limited at all
a. *Vigorous activities*, such as running, lifting heavy objects, participating in strenuous sports	1 ☐	2 ☐	3 ☐
b. *Moderate activities*, such as moving a table, pushing a vacuum cleaner, bowling, or playing golf	1 ☐	2 ☐	3 ☐
c. Lifting or carrying groceries	1 ☐	2 ☐	3 ☐
d. Climbing *several* flights of stairs	1 ☐	2 ☐	3 ☐
e. Climbing *one* flight of stairs	1 ☐	2 ☐	3 ☐
f. Bending, kneeling, or stooping	1 ☐	2 ☐	3 ☐
g. Walking *more than a mile*	1 ☐	2 ☐	3 ☐
h. Walking *several blocks*	1 ☐	2 ☐	3 ☐
i. Walking *one block*	1 ☐	2 ☐	3 ☐
j. Bathing or dressing yourself	1 ☐	2 ☐	3 ☐

During the *past 4 weeks*, have you had any of the following problems with your work or other regular daily activities *as a result of your physical health*? (Mark one box on each line.)	Yes	No
a. Cut down the *amount of time* you spent on work or other activities	1 ☐	2 ☐
b. *Accomplished less* than you would like	1 ☐	2 ☐
c. Were limited in the *kind* of work or other activities	1 ☐	2 ☐
d. Had *difficulty* performing the work or other activities (for example, it took extra effort)	1 ☐	2 ☐

From Ware, J, et al.[67]

Evidence Summary Box 11.2

Reliability and Validity of the SF-36

Study	Study Design	Sample	Setting	Reliability	Validity	Comments
Stewart, AL, et al,[54] 1989	Cross-sectional	9,385 persons 18 years and older who had visited a physician	Ambulatory care	Internal consistency of scale scores .67 to .88	Not addressed	Used MOS SF-20
Stewart, AL, et al,[56] 1988	Cross-sectional	11,186 English-speaking persons 18 years and older who had visited a physician	Ambulatory care in three large cities	Internal consistency of scale scores .81 to .88	Used internal consistency as a validity measure; also compared good and poor health samples to discriminate; also correlated to sociodemographic factors.	Used MOS SF-20
McHorney, CA, et al,[59] 1994	Cross-sectional and longitudinal	3,445 English-speaking persons 18 years and older with chronic medical and psychiatric conditions	Ambulatory care in three large cities	Internal consistency reliability of scale scores .78 to .93	Item discriminant validity from .09–.58 to .20–.62	SF-36
Ware, J, et al,[67] 1996	Longitudinal	$n = 2{,}333$, including adults with chronic conditions	Participants in the National Survey of Functional Health Status and the Medical Outcomes Study	2-week test–retest .89 for physical component score and .76 for mental component score, in the general US population	Discriminant validity of SF-12 similar to SF-36 in groups of patients known to differ in physical and mental conditions.	Article on construction of SF-12
Riddle, DL, et al,[68] 2001	Longitudinal	101 consecutive patients with low back pain	Three physical therapy clinics in the Richmond, VA area	Not addressed	SF-36 completed before initial examination and at time of discharge. SF-12 items extracted from SF-36. No significant differences were found for the comparison of change scores between the physical component score of the SF-36 and SF-12.	
King, JT, et al,[69] 2002	Cross-sectional	88 persons with cervical spondylotic myelopathy	Outpatient neurosurgery clinic	Internal consistency reliability (Cronbach's alpha) of scale scores .79 to .92	Construct validity was demonstrated using myelopathy scales constructed by Nurick, Cooper, and Harsh as well as a Western modification of the scale developed by the Japanese Orthopedic Association.	

Evidence Summary Box 11.2

Reliability and Validity of the SF-36 (Continued)

Study	Study Design	Sample	Setting	Reliability	Validity	Comments
Kosinski, M, et al,[70] 1999a	Cross-sectional	1,016 persons with osteoarthritis or rheumatoid arthritis	Outpatient or inpatient setting	Internal consistency reliability of baseline scale scores .75 to .91	Not addressed	
Kosinski, M, et al,[70] 1999b	Longitudinal	1,016 persons with osteoarthritis or rheumatoid arthritis	Outpatient or inpatient setting	Not addressed	SF-36 administered before treatment and 2 weeks after treatment. Discriminant validity was demonstrated in groups of patients with clinical measures of arthritis severity and across patients who improved with treatment.	
Hagen, S, et al,[71] 2002	Prospective, observational	153 persons recruited within 1 month of a recent stroke. SF-36 administered at 1, 3 and 6 months	24 general practices in Scotland	Internal consistency of scale scores >.7 at all time points except for Vitality at 1 month = .68 and General Health at 3 months = .66	Construct validity examined with Barthel Index, Canadian Neurological Scale and Mini-Mental State Examination. Strongest correlations were between Barthel Index and Physical Functioning and Social Functioning subscales.	
Findler, M, et al,[72] 2001	Cross-sectional	597 participants of whom 326 had a traumatic brain injury (TBI) who were at least 1 year post injury	Residents of New York State	Internal consistency of scale scores for individuals with TBI .79 to .92	Compared with Beck Depression Inventory, TIRR Symptom Checklist and Health Problems List. Significant correlations were found between the SF-36 scales and the other measures.	
Yip, JY, et al,[73] 2001	Cross-sectional	32 persons 60 years of age and older and their proxy respondents	Community dwelling older adults recruited from senior housing programs, assisted living facilities and senior centers	Correlations for scale scores of respondents and their proxies .31 to .84	Not addressed	

(continued)

Evidence Summary Box 11.2

Reliability and Validity of the SF-36 (Continued)

Study	Study Design	Sample	Setting	Reliability	Validity	Comments
Andersen, EM, et al,[74] 1999	Longitudinal	128 nursing home residents with scores of 17 or more on the Mini-Mental State Examination and at least 3 months residence	Nursing home	1 week test-retest for scales from .55 to .82 (ICC)	Convergent validity of physical health scales with activities of daily living index from −0.37 to −.0.43. Mental health scales correlated with Geriatric Depression Scale (−0.63 to −0.71). No SF-36 scales correlated strongly with the Mini-Mental State Examination.	
Hobart, JC, et al,[75] 2002	Cross-sectional	126 males and 51 females with stroke at time of admission; mean age 62 years	Three hospitals in Indianapolis	Not addressed	Limited discriminant validity in this sample of persons with stroke due to floor and ceiling effects. Assumptions for generating 5 of the 8 scales and for the 2 summary scores not satisfied.	

instruments examining physical function.[76] No instrument measures all potentially relevant items. Table 11.7 presents a comparison of items covered. In the physical function area, questions on the ability to ambulate are the only items these instruments have in common. Aspects of physical function not covered in any of these instruments include bed mobility and dexterity. The FIM and the OASIS include more BADL items than either the SIP or the SF-36. The SIP and the SF-36 investigate work performance, whereas the FIM and the OASIS do not. This is not surprising, given that the FIM was originally developed as a tool for the inpatient rehabilitation setting and the OASIS was expressly designed for home health agencies, both generally serving older patients. In contrast, the development of the SIP and SF-36 was focused on younger adult populations in ambulatory care. Anxiety and depression are addressed as areas of psychological function in the SIP, the SF-36, and the OASIS, but not in the FIM. The OASIS does not explore social function, while the other three instruments do. Finally, only the SF-36 records general health perceptions.

Summary

This chapter has presented a conceptual framework for understanding health status and examination of functional status. The traditional medical model with its narrow focus on disease and its symptoms fails to consider the broader social, psychological, and behavioral dimensions of illness. All these factors have an impact on an individual's function. Examination of functional status, therefore, must be viewed as a broad, multidimensional process. Three main categories of function have been delineated—physical, psychological, and social. Instrumentation has been presented that addresses the physical dimension of function, the area of examination that physical therapists are traditionally most involved with, as well as other dimensions. Finally, specific aspects of functional examination have been discussed, including purpose, selection of instruments, aspects of test administration, interpretation of test results, and determination of instrument quality.

Table 11.7 Items Covered in Selected Multidimensional Functional Assessment Instruments

	FIM	SIP	SF-36	OASIS
Symptoms	–	+	+	+
Physical function				
Transfers	+	–	–	+
Ambulation	+	+	+	+
ADL				
Bathing	+	+	+	+
Grooming	+	–	–	+
Dressing	+	–	+	+
Feeding	+	–	–	+
Toileting	+	–	–	+
IADL				
Indoor home chores	–	+	+	+
Outdoor home chores/shopping	–	+	+	+
Community travel/ drive car	–	+	+	+
Work/school	–	+	+	–
Affective function				
Communication	+	+	–	+
Cognition	+	+	–	+
Anxiety	–	+	+	+
Depression	–	+	+	+
Social function				
Interaction	+	+	+	–
Activity/leisure	–	+	+	–
General health perceptions	–	–	+	–

Questions for Review

1. How do functional status and measurement of function relate to health status?
2. Your rehabilitation facility uses the FIM. How can reliability be ensured so that the results can be used with confidence in both treatment planning and research?
3. What criteria can be used in the selection of a functional instrument?
4. Discuss the uses, advantages, and disadvantages of performance-based instruments, interviewer reports, and self-administered reports.
5. Explain how environment, fatigue, and other related issues affect measurement of function. Suggest ways to control these factors in the clinic.
6. Identify the major types of scoring systems used in functional instruments. What are some common errors in interpretation of testing results?
7. Review Tables 11.1 through 11.7. Hypothesize a caseload in a particular setting and indicate how and when you could use each of these instruments with the proposed population. Describe the advantages and disadvantages of each. Imagine that you are looking to follow the progress of these same patients to another setting. Which instruments would you choose?
8. Using one of the instruments, develop a set of results and use them to identify treatment goals and outcomes and to formulate a plan of care.
9. For each of the following, identify particular physical tasks relevant to that individual's functional status.
   - a 22-year-old female file clerk
   - a 31-year-old male physical therapist assistant
   - a 39-year-old female homemaker with children
   - a 45-year-old male construction worker
   - a 56-year-old female school teacher
   - a 65-year-old male journalist
10. Discuss the relationship among disease, impairment, functional limitations, and disability.

Case Study

A 78-year-old woman with a diagnosis of osteoarthritis was admitted for a right total hip replacement. The patient reported a long-standing history of discomfort. She described the hip pain as radiating posteriorly to the buttock and low back and exacerbated by weightbearing and stair climbing. Over the past 12 months she has experienced a very marked increase in pain and stiffness. Radiographic findings demonstrated degenerative changes of both the acetabulum and femoral head consistent with osteoarthritis. The surgical intervention replaced the right femoral head and neck with a metallic prosthesis and the acetabulum was resurfaced with a plastic cup. Past medical history is unremarkable.

SOCIAL HISTORY

The patient is a retired manager of a small accounting firm that she and her husband established. Her husband is deceased. She has three grown children who all live in neighboring communities. Prior to the functional limitations imposed by the hip pain, the patient had been independent in all ADL and IADL. She also volunteered her accounting services 1 day per week to a local charity that provides meals to homebound individuals. She was a regular participant in family outings, enjoyed going to the theater, concerts, and special museum events, and was an active member of the community historical preservation society. Recently, these activities had to be curtailed owing to the increased hip discomfort. She essentially had no activities outside the home for 3 months prior to admission and used a walker to minimize weight bearing and reduce pain. She also required the assistance of a home care aide 4 hours a day two times per week (primarily for shopping, errands, and some household management tasks). She expressed considerable distress at being unable to take a bath and having to rely on the assistance of another person for some basic care activities. She had been using aspirin for its analgesic and anti-inflammatory effects. However, the pain experienced in recent months was not alleviated by the aspirin and other conservative measures. She has been instructed to use local applications of heat, periodic rest intervals, and gentle range of motion exercises. The patient has extensive medical insurance coverage and is without financial concerns.

POSTSURGICAL RIGHT HIP PRECAUTIONS

No hip flexion beyond 90°.
Avoid crossing one leg or ankle over the other.
Avoid internal rotation of right lower extremity.

REVIEW OF SYSTEMS

Communication, Affect, Cognition, Learning Style: Fully communicative and oriented × 3. Cooperative and motivated. Hearing intact. Wears corrective lens; experiences "night blindness," which she describes as seeing poorly in dim light and her eyes take several seconds longer than normal to adjust from brightness to dimness.

Cardiopulmonary: HR = 84; BP = 130/78; RR = 16; No appreciable increases with activity.

Integumentary: Surgical wound healing well; staples removed.

Strength: Upper extremity gross ROM is WNL. Gross strength generally good to normal, except hands. Left hip, knee, and ankle at least good on break test. Partial weightbearing on right lower extremity.

Joint Integrity and Mobility: Patient reports some sporadic episodes of wrist and finger stiffness upon awakening in the morning and after periods of immobility. Crepitus noted in right knee. Heberden's nodes noted at the DIP and PIP joints of the left index finger.

Range of Motion: Right knee and ankle within functional limits; right hip not tested.

Muscle Performance: Grip strength is reduced bilaterally (4–15).

Pain: Patient denies pain in wrist or fingers, or right hip.

Gait, Locomotion, and Balance: The patient is ambulating on level surfaces with supervision using bilateral standard aluminum axillary crutches with partial weightbearing on the right lower extremity. Stair climbing also requires minimal assistance. It is anticipated the patient will be independent with ambulation on level surfaces at time of discharge from the hospital.

Functional Status: Impaired bed mobility (modified independence device), sit-to-stand, transfers (minimum assistance).

Home Environment: The patient lives alone in a fifth-floor apartment in a building with an elevator. The living space is a one-bedroom apartment on a single level.

Patient Goals: The patient is extremely motivated to once again be an independent manager of her personal care and household management needs. The prosthetic replacement has successfully relieved much of the pain experienced in the hip prior to surgery (most of her current discomfort is described as minor and associated with the surgical incision). She would also like to return to her family, volunteer, social, and leisure activities. She is very determined to discontinue the home care assistance as soon as possible.

GUIDING QUESTIONS

1. Based on the findings of the initial examination, discuss the links between the patient's impairments, functional limitations, and disability as presented in the Nagi model of the process of disablement.

2. Identify the specific ADL and IADL skills that would need to be examined to return this patient to the highest level of function and achieve the patient's goals for rehabilitation. Discuss the appropriateness of the instruments presented in this chapter for measuring her function and documenting the outcomes of patient management.

References

1. American Physical Therapy Association: The Guide to Physical Therapist Practice, ed 2. Phys Ther 81:9, 2001.
2. Schiller, JS, Adams, PF, and Nelson, ZC: Summary health statistics for the U.S. population: National Health Interview Survey, 2003. Vital Health Stat 10. Apr (224):1, 2005.
3. World Health Organization (WHO): The First Ten Years of the World Health Organization. World Health Organization, Geneva, 1958.
4. World Health Organization (WHO): International Classification of Impairments, Disabilities, and Handicaps. World Health Organization, Geneva, 1980.
5. Guccione, AA: Physical therapy diagnosis and the relationship between impairments and function. Phys Ther 71:499, 1991.
6. Nagi, S: Disability concepts revisited. In Pope, AM, and Tarlov, AR (eds): Disability in America: Toward a National Agenda for Prevention. National Academy Press, Washington, DC, 1991, p 309.
7. Nagi, S: Disability and Rehabilitation. Ohio State University Press, Columbus, 1969.
8. Nagi, S: Some conceptual issues in disability and rehabilitation. In Sussman, M: Sociology and Rehabilitation, Ohio State University Press, Columbus, 1965, p 100.
9. Schenkman, M, and Butler, RB: A model for multisystem evaluation, interpretation, and treatment of individuals with neurologic dysfunction. Phys Ther 69:538, 1989.
10. Schenkman, M, and Butler, RB: A model for multisystem evaluation and treatment of individual's with Parkinson's disease. Phys Ther 69:932, 1989.
11. World Health Organization (WHO): International Classification of Functioning, Disability and Health. World Health Organization, Geneva, 2001.
12. ICIDH-2: International Classification of Impairments, Activities and Participation. A Manual of Dimensions of Disablement and Functioning. Beta-1 draft for field trials. World Health Organization, Geneva, 1997.
13. Brandt, EN, Jr, and Pope, AM (eds): Enabling America: Assessing the Role of Rehabilitation Science and Engineering. National Academy Press, Washington, DC, 1997.
14. Jette, AM, and Keysor, JJ: Disability models: Implications for arthritis exercise and physical activity interventions. Arthrit Rheum 49:114, 2003.
15. Guyatt, GH, et al: The 6-minute walk: A new measure of exercise capacity in patients with chronic heart failure. Can Med Assoc J 132:923, 1985.
16. Winograd, CH, et al: Development of a physical performance and mobility examination. J Am Geriatr Soc 42:743, 1994.
17. Duncan, PW, et al: Functional reach: A new clinical measure of balance. J Gerontol 45:192, 1990.
18. Duncan, PW, et al: Functional reach: Predictive validity in a sample of elderly male veterans. J Gerontol 47:93, 1992.
19. Mathias, S, et al: Balance in elderly patients: The "Get Up and Go" test. Arch Phys Med Rehabil 67:387, 1986.
20. Podsiadlo, D, and Richardson, S: The timed "Up and Go": A test of basic functional mobility for frail elderly persons. J Am Geriatr Soc 39:142, 1991.
21. Guralnik, JM, et al: A short physical performance battery assessing lower extremity function: Association with self-reported disability and prediction of mortality and nursing home admission. J Gerontol 49:85, 1994.
22. Tager, IB, et al: Reliability of physical performance and self-reported functional measures in an older population. J Gerontol 53:295, 1998.
23. Mahoney, F, and Barthel, D: Functional evaluation: The Barthel Index. Md Med J 14:61, 1965.
24. Guccione, AA, et al: Defining arthritis and measuring functional status in elders: Methodological issues in the study of disease and disability. Am J Public Health 80:949, 1990.
25. Standards for Tests and Measurements in Physical Therapy Practice. Phys Ther 71:589, 1991.
26. Portney, LG, and Watkins, MP: Foundations of Clinical Research: Applications to Practice, ed 2. Prentice-Hall Health, Upper Saddle River, NJ, 2000.
27. Granger, CV, et al: The Stroke Rehabilitation Outcome Study—Part I: General Description. Arch Phys Med Rehabil 69:506, 1988.
28. Granger, CV, et al: The Stroke Rehabilitation Outcome Study: Part II. Relative merits of the total Barthel Index score and a four-item subscore in predicting patient outcomes. Arch Phys Med Rehabil 70:100, 1989.
29. Granger, C, et al: Outcome of Comprehensive Medical Rehabilitation: Measurement by Pulses Profile and the Barthel Index. Arch Phys Med Rehabil 60:145, 1979.
30. Katz, S, et al: Studies of illness in the aged. The Index of ADL: A standardized measure of biological and psychosocial function. JAMA 185:914, 1963.
31. Katz, S, et al: Progress in the development of the Index of ADL. Gerontologist 10:20, 1970.
32. Liang, M, and Jette, A: Measuring functional ability in chronic arthritis. Arthritis Rheum 24:80, 1981.
33. Branch, L, et al: A prospective study of functional status among community elders. Am J Public Health 74:266, 1984.
34. Guccione, AA, and Jette, AM: Assessing limitations in physical function in patients with arthritis. Arthrit Care Res 1:170, 1988.
35. Granger, CV, et al: Advances in functional assessment for medical rehabilitation. Top Geriatr Rehabil 1:59, 1986.
36. Granger, CV, et al: Functional assessment scales: A study of persons with multiple sclerosis. Arch Phys Med Rehabil 71:870, 1990.
37. Guide for the Uniform Data Set for Medical Rehabilitation (Adult FIM), Version 4.0. Buffalo, Uniform Data System for Medical Rehabilitation, UB Foundation Activities, Inc, 1993.
38. Hsueh, IP, et al: Comparison of the psychometric characteristics of the functional independence measure, 5 item Barthel index, and 10 item Barthel index in patients with stroke. J Neurol Neurosurg Psychiatry 73:188, 2002.
39. Gosman-Hedstrom, G, and Svensson, E. Parallel reliability of the functional independence measure and the Barthel ADL index. Disabil Rehabil 22:702, 2000.
40. Heinemann, AW, et al: Relationships between impairment and physical disability as measured by the functional independence measure. Arch Phys Med Rehabil 74:566, 1993.
41. Ottenbacher, KJ, et al: Measuring developmental and functional status in children with disabilities. Dev Med Child Neurol 41:186, 1999.
42. Gilson, B, et al: The Sickness Impact Profile: Development of an outcome measure of health care. Am J Public Health 65:1304, 1975.
43. Bergner, M, et al: The Sickness Impact Profile: Validation of a health status measure. Med Care 14:57, 1976.
44. Pollard, W, et al: The Sickness Profile: Reliability of a health status measure. Med Care 14:146, 1976.
45. Carter, W, et al: Validation of an interval scaling: The Sickness Impact Profile. Health Serv Res 11:516, 1976.
46. Bergner, M, et al: The Sickness Impact Profile: Development and final revision of a health status measure. Med Care 19:787, 1981.
47. Deyo, R, et al: Measuring functional outcomes in a chronic disease: A comparison of traditional scales and a self-administered health status questionnaire in patients with rheumatoid arthritis. Med Care 21:180, 1983.

48. Deyo, R, et al: Physical and psychosocial function in rheumatoid arthritis. Clinical use of a self-administered health status instrument. Arch Intern Med 142:870, 1982.
49. Deyo, R, et al: A controlled trial of transcutaneous electrical stimulation (TENS) and exercise for chronic low back pain. N Engl J Med 322:1627, 1990.
50. MacKenzie, C, et al: Can the Sickness Impact Profile measure change: An example of scale assessment. J Chron Dis 39:429, 1986.
51. Krisler, KS, et al: OASIS Basics: Beginning to Use the Outcome and Assessment Information Set. Center for Health Services and Policy Research, Denver, 1997.
52. Shaughnessy, PW, and Crisler, KS: Outcome-based Quality Improvement. A Manual for Home Care Agencies on How to Use Outcomes. National Association for Home Care, Washington, DC, 1995.
53. Tarlov, AR, et al: The Medical Outcomes Study: An application of methods for monitoring the results of medical care. JAMA 262:925, 1989.
54. Stewart, AL, et al: Functional status and well-being of patients with chronic conditions: Results from the Medical Outcomes Study. JAMA 262:907, 1989.
55. Wells, KB, et al: The functioning and well-being of depressed patients: Results from the Medical Outcomes Study. JAMA 262:914, 1989.
56. Stewart, AL, et al: The MOS short general health survey: Reliability and validity in a patient population. Med Care 26:724, 1988.
57. Ware, JE, and Sherbourne, CD: The MOS 36-item short form health survey (SF-36): I. Conceptual framework and item selection. Med Care 30:473, 1992.
58. McHorney, CA, et al: The MOS 36-item short form health survey (SF-36): II. Psychometric and clinical tests of validity in measuring physical and mental health constructs. Med Care 31:247, 1993.
59. McHorney, CA, et al: The MOS 36-item short form health survey (SF-36): III. Tests of data quality, scaling assumptions, and reliability across diverse patient groups. Med Care 32:40, 1994.
60. Ware, JE, et al: SF-36 Health Survey: Manual and Intepretation Guide. Boston, The Health Institute, New England Medical Center, 1993.
61. Mossberg, KA, and McFarland, C: Initial health status of patients at outpatient physical therapy clinics. Phys Ther 75:1043, 1995.
62. Jette, DU, and Downing, J: Health status of individuals entering a cardiac rehabilitation program as measured by the Medical Outcomes Study 36-item short form survey (SF-36). Phys Ther 74:521, 1994.
63. Jette, DU, and Downing, J: The relationship of cardiovascular and psychological impairments to the health status of patients enrolled in cardiac rehabilitation programs. Phys Ther 76:130, 1996.
64. Jette, DU, and Jette, AM: Physical therapy and health outcomes in patients with spinal impairments. Phys Ther 76:930, 1996.
65. Jette, DU, and Jette, AM: Physical therapy and health outcomes in patients with knee impairments. Phys Ther 76:1178, 1996.
66. Jette, DU, et al: The disablement process in patients with pulmonary disease. Phys Ther 77:385, 1997.
67. Ware, J, Kosinski, M, and Keller, SD: A 12-Item Short-Form Health Survey: construction of scales and preliminary tests of reliability and validity. Med Care 34:220, 1996.
68. Riddle, DL, Lee, KT, and Stratford, PW: Use of SF-36 and SF-12 health status measures: a quantitative comparison for groups versus individual patients. Med Care 39:867, 2001.
69. King, JT, and Roberts, MS: Validity and reliability of the Short Form-36 in cervical spondylotic myelopathy. Spine 97:180, 2002.
70. Kosinski, M, et al: The SF-36 health survey as a generic outcome measure in clinical trials of patients with osteoarthritis and rheumatoid arthritis: tests of data quality, scaling assumptions and score reliability. Med Care 37:MS10, 1999.
71. Hagan, S, et al: Psychometric properties of the SF-36 in the early post-stroke phase. J Adv Nurs 44(5):461, 2003.
72. Findler, M, et al: The reliability and validity of the SF-36 health survey questionnaire for use with individuals with traumatic brain injury. Brain In 15(8):715, 2001.
73. Yip, JY, et al: Comparison of older adult subject and proxy responses on the SF-36 health-related quality of life instrument. Aging Ment Health 5(2):136, 2001.
74. Andresen, EM, et al: Limitations of the SF-36 in a sample of nursing home residents. Age Aging: 28:562, 1999.
75. Hobart, JC, et al: Quality of life measurement after stroke: uses and abuses of SF-36. Stroke 33:1348, 2002.
76. Guccione, AA, and Jette, AM: Multidimensional assessment of functional limitations in patients with arthritis. Arthrit Care Res 3:44, 1990.

Supplemental Readings

Dittmar, S, and Bresham, G: Functional Assessment and Outcome Measures for the Rehabilitation Health Professional. Aspen, Gaithersburg, MD, 1997.

Finch E, et al: Physical Rehabilitation Outcome Measures: A Guide to Enhanced Clinical Decision Making, ed 2. Lippincott Williams & Wilkins, Baltimore, 2002.

Hazuda, HP, et al: Development and validation of a performance-based measure of upper extremity functional limitation. Aging Clin Exp Res 17(5):394, 2005.

McDowell, I, and Newell, C: Measuring Health: A Guide to Rating Scales and Questionnaires, ed 2. Oxford University Press, New York, 1996.

Nickel, MK, et al: Changes in instrumental activities of daily living disability after treatment of depressive symptoms I elderly women with chronic musculoskeletal pain: A double-blind, placebo-controlled trial. Aging Clin Exp Res 17(4): 293, 2005.

Peel, C, et al: Assessing mobility in older adults: The UAB Study of Aging Life-Space Assessment. Phys Ther 85(10):1008, 2005.

Shaver, JC, and Allan, DE: Care-receiver and caregiver assessments of functioning: Are there gender differences? Can J Aging 24(2):139, 2005.

Vittengl, JR, et al: Comparative validity of seven scoring systems for the instrumental activities of daily living scale in rural elders. Aging Ment Health 10(1):40, 2006.

CHAPTER

12

LEARNING OBJECTIVES

1. Identify the roles and responsibilities of the physical therapist in examination of the physical environment.
2. Understand the importance of environmental accessibility in optimizing patient function.
3. Identify common home, work place, and community environmental barriers that impact patient function.
4. Identify the tests and measures, tools used for gathering data, and data generated during examination of environmental, home, and work barriers.
5. Describe examination instruments used to measure environmental impact on patient function.
6. Identify strategies to improve patient function through environmental modifications.
7. Describe the scope of adaptive equipment and assistive technology options available for individuals with functional limitations and disability.
8. Recognize the importance of an examination of the environment within the context of a comprehensive plan of care.

Examination of the Environment

Thomas J. Schmitz, PT, PhD

OUTLINE

The *physical environment* in which an individual functions consists of a variety of both built and natural objects. Built objects refer to buildings and structures created by humans; natural objects include other humans as well as geographical objects such as vegetation, mountains, rivers, uneven terrain, and so forth.[1] The environment encompasses a substantial range of components that impact human function and includes the individual's home, neighborhood, community, and method(s) of transportation, in addition to the individual's educational, workplace, entertainment, commercial, and natural settings.[2]

Environmental barriers are defined as physical impediments that prevent individuals from functioning optimally in their surroundings, and include safety hazards, access problems, and home or workplace design difficulties.[3] **Accessibility** is the degree to which an environment affords use of its resources with respect to an individual's level of function. **Accessible design** typically refers to structures that meet prescribed standards for accessibility. In the United States, these standards are available from the American National Standards Institute (Accessible and Usable Buildings and Facilities, ICC/ANSI A117.1-1998),[4] the Fair Housing Amendments Act of 1988, and the Uniform Federal Accessibility Standards (UFAS). Requirements for public and commercial buildings are regulated by the accessibility guidelines of the Americans with Disabilities Act (ADA).[5]

Universal design (also called *life-span design*) refers to "the design of products and environments to be usable by all people, to the greatest extent possible, without the need for adaptation or specialized design."[6, p 1] This design concept emphasizes social inclusion by creating environments that are useable by a wide range of individuals of different ages, stature, sizes, and abilities as well as addresses the changing needs of human beings across the life span. Although universal design is both accessible and free of barriers, it is not the same as bringing existing buildings or structures into compliance with the ADA Standards for Accessible Design[5] or other building codes or laws. Applying such standards to existing structures often results in important but selective accessibility. In contrast, universal design is applied from the *inception* of a building plan. Ostroff[7] argues there is confusion about the importance of incorporating universal design principles into architectural plans versus creating new structures and then approaching the task of eliminating of environmental barriers: "We see the poor design and the problems created by this confusion, especially in thoughtless new designs that end up looking like retrofits. Ramps added in new construction are a good example, where none would have been needed if the architects had considered the needs of all users as fundamental in the earliest stages of the programming process, rather than a technical requirement to be added at the end of the design process."[7, p 1.5]

Incorporated into initial planning, universal design principles are essentially "invisible" as compared to adaptations made to existing structures. They apply to all features and spaces of a dwelling. Several examples of universal design elements include stepless entrances, wide hallways and doorways, level transitions between rooms (no doorway thresholds), use of nonslip floors, lever door handles, rocker light switches, single-handle sink faucets, and no-step shower access. Reinforced walls capable of supporting handrails or grab bars and large closets aligned from floor to floor suitable for housing a residential elevator are examples of universal design elements intended to meet the future needs of residents.[8–10]

The seven Principles of Universal Design developed at The Center for Universal Design (North Carolina State University) are presented in Appendix A. Although universal design originated in response to the need for environmental access for individuals with functional limitations and disability, many of its design elements proved useful and have been embraced by the general public. Riley[8] provides a fitting example of this trend, "Think for a moment of the automatic garage door, which originated out of necessity for a client whose disability prevented him from lifting a heavy door. Now a staple of living for nearly all of us so-called "able-bodied" people as well as those with disabilities, it is but one of many examples of how Universal Design has raised the bar for home design of all kind."[8, p XII]

Reflective of the importance of **environmental accessibility**, an internationally recognized *wheelchair symbol* identifies buildings accessible to individuals with a disability. The Rehabilitation Act of 1973 (Sections 503 and 504) requires that all organizations receiving federal funding provide accessible programs and activities. The Americans with Disability Act (1990) expanded accessibility to the private sector to improve employment opportunities as well as environmental access to retail businesses, cultural events, movie theaters, restaurants, travel, and so forth. Other access symbols identify the availability of assistive listening devices, telephones with inter-active text capabilities (TTY), which allow the user to communicate using a keyboard and visual display, volume-controlled telephones, availability of sign language interpretation, and so forth. The 12 Disability Access Symbols are presented in Figure 12.1. These symbols are prominently displayed to identify and make public the availability of accessible services (Fig. 12.2).

Purpose

A primary outcome of rehabilitation intervention is for the patient to be fully functional in a former environment and lifestyle. To achieve this outcome, continuity of accessibility must exist within the individual's environmental context. With full accessibility as a goal, examination of the environment must address the patient–environment relationship relative to accessibility, safety, usability, and function. The purposes of an environmental examination are multiple and serve to:

1. Determine the degree of patient safety and level of function in the physical environment.
2. Identify design barriers that may impact usability or compromise performance of customary tasks or activities.
3. Make realistic recommendations regarding environmental accessibility and accommodations to the patient, support network (family, friends, caregivers, significant others, coworkers, professional colleagues, neighbors), employer, government agencies or other potential funding sources, and third-party payers.
4. Determine the need for **adaptive equipment** or assistive technology to support and promote function.
5. Assist in preparing the patient and support network for the patient's return to a former environment and to help determine whether further services may be required (i.e., outpatient treatment, home care services, and so forth).

Examination Strategies

Physical therapists use a variety of tests and measures to examine physical impediments (e.g., safety hazards, access problems, design barriers) impacting the patient–environment relationship. The data generated are used to suggest modifications to the environment, guide recommendations for adaptive equipment, assistive technology, and/or propose alternative approaches to performing a task or activity (e.g., improve safety, conserve energy) to promote optimum function. The *Guide to Physical Therapist Practice*[3] includes examination of environmental, home, and work (job/school/play) barriers among the list of 24 categories of tests and measures that may be used by physical therapists. Table 12.1 presents an overview of examination components including the types of tests and

	**Symbol for Accessibility** The wheelchair symbol should only be used to indicate access for individuals with limited mobility including wheelchair users. For example, the symbol is used to indicate an accessible entrance, bathroom or that a phone is lowered for wheelchair users. Remember that a ramped entrance is not completely accessible if there are no curb cuts, and an elevator is not accessible if it can only be reached via steps.
	**Access (Other Than Print or Braille) for Individuals Who Are Blind or Have Low Vision** This symbol may be used to indicate access for people who are blind or have low vision, including: a guided tour, a path to a nature trail or a scent garden in a park; and a tactile tour or a museum exhibition that may be touched.
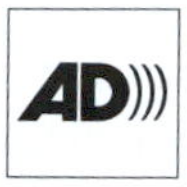	**Audio Description** A service for persons who are blind or have low vision that makes the performing arts, visual arts, television, video, and film more accessible. Description of visual elements is provided by a trained Audio Describer through the Secondary Audio Program (SAP) of televisions and monitors equipped with stereo sound. An adapter for non-stereo TVs is available through the American Foundation for the Blind, (800) 829-0500. For live Audio Description, a trained Audio Describer offers live commentary or narration (via headphones and a small transmitter) consisting of concise, objective descriptions of visual elements (e.g., a theater performance or a visual arts exhibition).
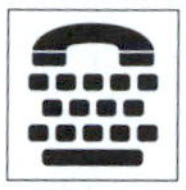	**Telephone Typewriter (TTY)** This device is also known as a text telephone (TT), or telecommunications device for the deaf (TDD). TTY indicates a device used with the telephone for communication with and between deaf, hard of hearing, speech impaired and/or hearing persons.
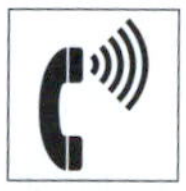	**Volume Control Telephone** This symbol indicates the location of telephones that have handsets with amplified sound and/or adjustable volume controls.
	**Assistive Listening Systems** These systems transmit amplified sound via hearing aids, headsets or other devices. They include infrared, loop and FM systems. Portable systems may be available from the same audiovisual equipment suppliers that service conferences and meetings.
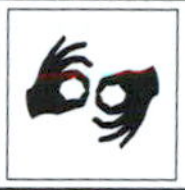	**Sign Language Interpretation** The symbol indicates that Sign Language Interpretation is provided for a lecture, tour, film, performance, conference or other program.
Large Print	**Accessible Print (18 pt. or Larger)** The symbol for large print is "Large Print" printed in 18 pt. or larger text. In addition to indicating that large print versions of books, pamphlets, museum guides and theater programs are available, you may use the symbol on conference or membership forms to indicate that print materials may be provided in large print. Sans serif or modified serif print with good contrast is important, and special attention should be paid to letter and word spacing.
	**The Information Symbol** The most valuable commodity of today's society is information; to a person with a disability it is essential. For example, the symbol may be used on signage or on a floor plan to indicate the location of the information or security desk, where there is more specific information or materials concerning access accommodations and services such as "LARGE PRINT" materials, audio cassette recordings of materials, or sign interpreted tours.
CC	**Closed Captioning (CC)** This symbol indicates a choice for whether or not to display captions for a television program or videotape. TV sets that have a built-in or a separate decoder are equipped to display dialogue for programs that are captioned when selected by the viewer. The Television Decoder Circuitry Act of 1990 requires TV sets (with screens 13" or larger) to have built-in decoders as of July, 1993. Also, videos that are part of exhibitions may be closed captioned using the symbol with instruction to press a button for captioning.
OC	**Opened Captioning (OC)** This symbol indicates that captions, which translate dialogue and other sounds in print, are always displayed on the videotape, movie or television program. Open Captioning is preferred by many including deaf and hard-of-hearing individuals, and people whose second language is English. In addition, it is helpful in teaching children how to read and in keeping sound levels to a minimum in museums and restaurants.
Braille	**Braille Symbol** This symbol indicates that printed material is available in Braille, including exhibition labeling, publications, and signage.

The Disability Access Symbols were produced by the Graphic Artists Guild Foundation with support and technical assistance from the Office for Special Constituencies, National Endowment for the Arts. Special thanks to the National Endowment for the Arts. Graphic design assistance by the Society of Environmental Graphic Design. Consultant: Jacqueline Ann Clipsham, with permission.

Figure 12.1 Disability access symbols.

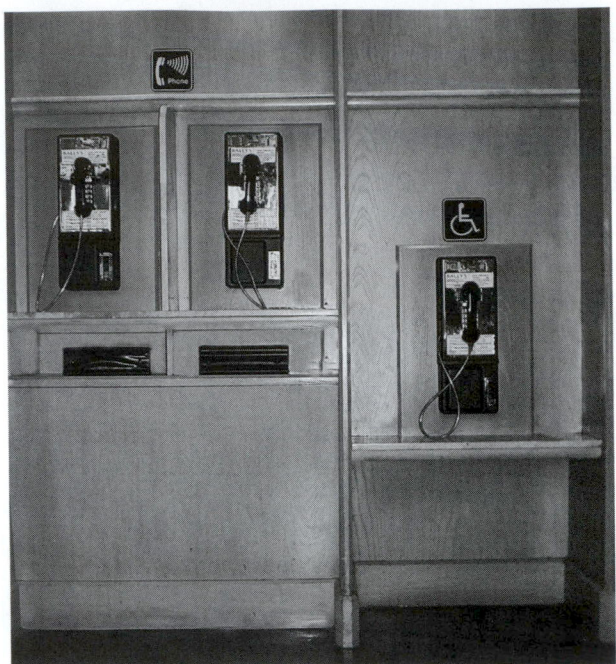

Figure 12.2 Availability of accessible services. Shopping mall telephones display the symbol for volume control telephones (*left*) and the wheelchair symbol of accessibility (*right*).

measures used, tools used for gathering data, and types of data generated.

Depending on the nature of the patient's functional limitation or disability, data collection tools used for examination of the environmental may include (1) *interviews,* (2) *self-reports (checklists, questionnaires)* and *performance-based measures (observation) of function,* (3) *measures of environmental impact on function,* (4) *visual depictions (photographs, videotapes)* and *dimensions of physical space (structural specifications),* and (5) *on-site visits.* A combination of two or more of these strategies may be warranted to generate all needed data. The current era of cost containment has placed restrictions on time and travel allocations for on-site visits. In such situations, several data collection alternatives (e.g., interview, self-report, and performance-based measures; and use of photographs and/or diagrams [with dimensions] of the physical space) can be implemented to achieve the goals of the environmental examination.

Sanford et al[11] reported on a novel cost-effective alternative approach to the in-home examination. The authors compared data from an actual on-site home examination with those obtained from remote video-conferencing technology. The data suggest that videoconferencing has the potential for enabling therapists to examine the patient's environment regardless of distance or location. The data from the remote examination identified 51 of the 59 problems (86.4 percent) documented from the on-site visit and 54 of the 60 quantitative measures (90 percent) obtained from the on-site visit.[11]

Interview

Exploration of the environment is typically initiated by interviewing the patient and support network members. If

Table 12.1 Environmental, Home, and Work (Job/School/Play) Barriers: Types of Tests and Measures Used, Tools Used for Gathering Data, and Types of Data Generated.

Environmental, home, and work (job/school/play) barriers are the physical impediments that keep patients/clients from functioning optimally in their surroundings. The physical therapist uses the results of tests and measures to identify any of a variety of possible impediments, including safety hazards (e.g., throw rugs, slippery surfaces), access problems (e.g., narrow doors, thresholds, high steps, absence of power doors and elevators), and home or office design barriers (e.g., excessive distances to negotiate, multistory environments, sinks, bathrooms, counters, placement of controls or switches). The physical therapist also uses the results to suggest modification to the environment (e.g., grab bars in the shower, ramps, raised toilet seats, increased lighting) that will also allow the patient/client to improve functioning in the home, workplace, and other settings.

Tests and Measures	Tools Used for Gathering Data	Data Generated
Tests and measures may include those that characterize or quantify: • Current and potential barriers (e.g., checklists, interviews, observations, questionnaires) • Physical space and environment (e.g., compliance standards, observations, photographic assessments, questionnaires, structural specifications, technology-assisted assessments, videographic assessments)	Tools for gathering data include: • Cameras and photographs • Checklists • Interviews • Observations • Questionnaires • Structural specifications • Technology-assisted analysis systems • Video cameras and videotapes	Data are used in providing documentation and may include: • Descriptions of: – barriers – environment • Documentation and description of compliance with regulatory standards • Observations of environment • Quantifications of physical space

From American Physical Therapy Association,[3, p 68] with permission.

the patient's functional limitations or disability impact only isolated tasks or activities or if accessibility issues involve limited environmental barriers, an interview may be all that is needed to determine the physical impediments and provide suggestions and guidelines for improving performance and resolving access problems. In the presence of more formidable functional limitations or disability, the interview may be the first of several strategies used to collect data about the patient's environment. The interview can be used to establish the general characteristics of the environment (number of levels, stairs, railings, and so forth), identify any special problems previously encountered by the patient, alert the therapist to potential safety hazards, and determine the need for further tests and measures to obtain essential information. The interview process also provides the therapist an opportunity to gain knowledge of support network characteristics including (1) attitude toward the patient; (2) the extent of their desire to have the patient return to his or her environment; (3) their caregiving goals and capabilities[1]; and (4) attitude toward rehabilitation team members, which may influence receptivity to suggested environmental modifications.

Self-Report and Performance-Based Measures of Function

Self-reports involve asking the patient to provide information about the ability to perform certain tasks and activities in specific environments. Administration can be either in a paper-and-pencil format or by way of an interview conducted by the therapist. An inherent shortcoming of self-report instruments is that an individual may overestimate performance capabilities or underestimate the impact of environmental barriers. Accuracy of reporting can be improved by requesting the patient (1) focus the performance information on a recent time interval (e.g., *within* the previous week) and (2) distinguish between actual performance of an activity (e.g., *daily* use of shower for bathing) versus perceived ability in the absence of consistent execution of the task.

Performance-based measures address classification of functional abilities and identification of functional limitations. They are administered by the therapist who observes patient performance of the activity. A variety of instruments are available that include quantitative scoring systems. Examples include the *Functional Reach Test*,[12] *Get Up and Go Test*,[13] the *Short Physical Performance Battery* (SPPB),[14] the *Functional Independence Measure* [FIM],[15] timed walking tests,[16–21] and the *Berg Balance Test*.[22,23] The therapist interprets the data by comparison to normative performance. The measures yield important information about the impact of impairments on function and help predict patient performance within his or her natural environment. The reader is referred to Chapter 11 for additional information on both self-reports and performance-based measures.

Measures of Environmental Impact on Function

The environment directly impacts the ability to perform tasks and activities that support physical, social, and psychological well-being. Environmental factors can either *constrain* or *promote* patients' abilities to perform customary actions within their social/cultural contexts. A variety of instruments have been developed that address the impact of environmental determinants on function. Examples of these instruments include:

- The *Physical Activity Resource Assessment (PARA)*.[24] Based on the close link between aspects of the physical environment and physical activity levels, this instrument was designed to examine and document the available resources that promote activity within a neighborhood or community environment. The PARA is used to examine the type, quantity, accessibility, quality, and features of physical activity resources within a patient's environment.
- *Home and Community Environment (HACE)* instrument.[25] The HACE is a self-report instrument used to identify features of the patient's home or community that may impact level of function. The environmental domains examined include home and community mobility, basic mobility and communication devices, transportation factors, and attitudes.
- *Safety Assessment of Function and the Environment for Rehabilitation (SAFER)* tool.[26] A comprehensive functional and environmental examination tool designed for use with the elderly. It includes 15 areas of concern: living situation, mobility, kitchen, eating, household management, fire hazards, dressing, grooming, bathroom, medication, communication, recreation, general items, wandering, and memory aids. Each category is examined within the content of the home environment and the functional capabilities of the patient.
- *Usability in My Home (UIMH)*.[27–30] This self-report instrument examines features of the home environment that either constrain or promote activity performance (see Appendix B). It addresses aspects of both basic (BADL) and instrumental activities of daily living (IADL) and consists of 23 items, 16 of which are scored on a scale of 1 to 7 (1 representing the most negative response; 7 the most positive response). In addition, the instrument includes 7 open-ended questions (6 for description of specific usability problems and 1 for expressing additional opinions). Usability is conceptually defined as the extent to which a patient's needs and preferences can be met within the home. The UIMH includes a personal, environmental, and activity component.
- *Housing Enabler*.[27,29] This instrument is administered using a combination of interview and observation and is

designed to examine home accessibility. It includes three steps: (1) determination of functional limitations (13 items) and dependence on mobility devices (2 items); (2) examination of environmental barriers (188 items) including indoor and outdoor accessibility, entrances, and communication features; and (3) calculation of an accessibility score (higher scores reflect greater accessibility problems).

- *Environmental Analysis of Mobility Questionnaire (EAMQ).*[31,32] The EAMQ is a self-report instrument that examines the impact of the environment on community mobility. It includes 24 characteristics of the environment grouped into 8 dimensions. Each characteristic includes both an encounter question ("How often do you?") and an avoidance question ("How often do you avoid?"). A five-item ordinal scale is used to document frequency of encounter and avoidance responses (never, rarely, sometimes, often, always).[32, p 394] Encounter and avoidance scores are averaged to generate a *summary environmental score* and a *summary avoidance score.*
- *Craig Handicap Assessment and Reporting Technique (CHART).*[33] This instrument was developed to document an individual's functioning within his or her societal context. It examines level of involvement within six domains of function: physical independence, cognitive independence, mobility, occupation, social integration, and economic self-sufficiency. Each area is scored based on 100 points (600 points maximum) with greater levels of participation receiving higher scores. The CHART-SF[34] is a 20-item shortened version of the CHART.
- *Craig Hospital Inventory of Environmental Factors (CHIEF).*[35,36] This inventory rates frequency and impact of 25 environmental barriers defined as any impediments that prevent functioning within the home and community. In addition to physical and architectural barriers, the instrument includes social, attitudinal, and policy barriers; response items carry numeric values. The CHIEF (see Appendix C) gathers information about the frequency of encounters with each barrier (daily = 4, weekly = 3, monthly = 2, less than monthly = 1, never = 0) and the magnitude of the problem (big problem = 2 or little problem = 1). Scores are calculated by multiplying the frequency of occurrence by the magnitude of the problem to provide an *impact score.* Higher scores indicate greater impact of environmental barriers. A CHIEF short form (CHIEF-SF) contains 12 items from the original inventory.
- *ADL Staircase.*[37–42] Based on the original Katz ADL-Index,[39] the ADL-Staircase (see Appendix D) is an index of four instrumental activities (cleaning, shopping, transportation and cooking)[37,38] combined with six personal daily life activities (bathing, dressing, going to the toilet, transfer, continence, and feeding).[39] The ability to perform each activity is scored using a three-point scale: *independence, partly dependent,* and *dependent.* Dependence means that assistance from another person is required. The ratings can then be dichotomized into *independence* or *dependence,* and arranged into one conditional ordered scale of ADL-steps 0 to 9/10. ADL-step 0 means independent in all activities, and ADL-step 9/10 dependent in all activities. When continence is included there are 10 steps and when it is excluded there are 9 steps. The responses from the ADL-Staircase have an ordered structure which means that statistical methods for ordinal data should be used in analysis as well as in reliability studies (Ulla Sonn, personal communication, October 11, 2005). The reliability and validity of the instrument have been established.[37–42]
- *Environmental Functional Independence Measure (Enviro-FIM™).*[43] This instrument is derived from the widely used 18-item Functional Independence Measure (FIM™) that addresses aspects of physical, psychological, and social function[44] (see Chapter 11). "The principal distinction between the two measures is that the Enviro-FIM™ instrument expands the FIM™ instrument's 7-point rating scale to an 11-point scale. This change gives the Enviro-FIM™ instrument sensitivity to the physical environment's role in the disablement process by adding four additional levels of function and organizing the resulting eleven level[s] of function scores into four categories"[43, p 2] (see Appendix E). The scores range from 0 to 10. A score of 10 indicates *independence,* scores of 6 to 9 denote *modified independence* with each score representing a specific qualifying parameter of performance (e.g., a score of 6 indicates personal safety is compromised; a score of 8 identifies the need for an assistive device), scores of 3 to 5 indicate *modified dependence* (e.g., supervision or physical assistance is required), and 0 to 2 designate *dependence* (e.g., maximal assistance or unable to complete activity). Enviro-FIM™ function scores are guided by starting at the top of a decision tree and working down through the various question branches (see Appendix F).
- *Functional Performance Measure (FPM™).*[45] This instrument is comprised of two scales: Level of Effort Scale (LES™) and Level of Assistance Scale (LAS™). The FPM™ is used to identify needed environmental adaptations required to improve performance. The design of the instrument separates patient *effort* from the amount of *assistance* required from caregivers. The LES™ includes eight levels of effort expended during activity performance; none, blocked, declined, impossible, maximum, moderate, and minimal (see Appendix G). Scores are influenced by factors such as performance time required, safety, frequency of complaints, and frequency of interruptions in task performance. Similar to the Enviro-FIM™, assignment of scores is guided by

working through a decision tree (see Appendix H). The LAS™ also includes eight categories used for coding the level of assistance required during task performance (see Appendix I) and a decision tree to guide score determination (see Appendix J). Scores are influenced by whether assistance provided is only incidental to performance, merely facilitates performance, or constitutes direct performance of the task.

- *Environmental Utility Measure (EUM™)*[46] is comprised of two identically formatted companion measures: the *Difficulty Rating Scale* (DRS™) and the *Acceptability Rating Scale* (ARS™). The EUM is a 7-point bipolar rating scale adapted from an earlier published and tested 15-point sequential judgment scale.[47] It examines the patient's perceptions of the comparative ease or *difficulty* of task performance (that may or may not be consistent with the observer's rating) as well as the *acceptability* of performing within a selected environmental context. After performance of an activity, the DRS™ is administered in a two-step process: (1) following completion of an activity, the patient initially characterizes performance as: *difficult, moderate,* or *easy* using a simplified version of the scale; (2) the patient is then asked to position the initial characterization on the relevant subsection of the 7-point scale (Appendix K). The ARS™ examines the *perceived level of acceptability* of the physical environment for activity performance within the context of individual functional limitations or disability. Administration also uses a two-step process: (1) following completion of an activity, the patient initially characterizes the environment as: *unacceptable, moderate,* or *acceptable*; (2) the patient then refines perceptions by characterizing the environment on the appropriate subsection of the 7-point scale (Appendix L).

Visual Depictions and Dimensions of Physical Space

The therapist may request support network members provide visual depictions (e.g., photographs, videotapes, diagrams, floor plans) and physical dimensions (structural specifications obtained with a tape measure) of the environment in which the patient is expected to function. If visuals are unavailable, an inexpensive disposable camera works well for this purpose.

Suggestions for modifications can be made from the visual representations and measured dimensions of the patient's environment. Such environmental information will allow the therapist to simulate aspects of the patient's surroundings (prior to discharge) for practicing tasks while directing attention to maximizing safety and function. This will also assist the therapist to determine the need for adaptive equipment.

On-Site Visit

On-site visits require that rehabilitation team members together with the patient travel to the physical location where the patient will be required to function. A major advantage of the on-site visit is that it allows observation of performance in the actual environment in which the activities must be accomplished. On-site visits are often useful in reducing patient, support network, and/or employer apprehension concerning the patient's ability to function within the environment. The on-site visit also provides an important opportunity for the therapist to identify safety hazards and make recommendations regarding altering, coping with, or adapting specific environmental barriers. During the visit, patient activity should be interspersed with adequate rest intervals to ensure fatigue is not a mitigating factor.

Whichever examination strategy or combination of strategies are applied, the scope and breadth of the information gathered will be enhanced by involvement of members of the patient's support network. Because it is usually not feasible for the therapist to examine all aspects of the patient's total environment, involvement of other individuals can be instrumental in ensuring that the goal of maximum accessibility is met. This is particularly important for determination of general community access. The therapist can direct and guide an investigation of access to community recreational, educational, and commercial facilities as well as availability of public transportation. The therapist can also provide guidance in the essential role of exploring funding sources for needed environmental modifications (potential funding sources are addressed later in this chapter).

Home Visit

Prior to an on-site visit to the patient's home, occupational and physical therapy treatment sessions should be scheduled that will include participation from support group members. These visits serve several functions. They provide an opportunity to become familiar with the patient's capabilities and functional limitations. They give the support network members time to learn safe methods (e.g., proper body mechanics, guarding techniques) for assisting with ambulation, transfers, exercise, and functional activities. During these treatment session visits the occupational and physical therapists will have an opportunity to provide instruction in the use of assistive devices, adaptive equipment, and assistive technology. The time spent in education of family and caregivers is often pivotal in facilitating the patient's reclamation to the home, community, and/or work (job/school/play) environments.

CLINICAL NOTE: Although sometimes restricted by reimbursement issues, when feasible, a day or weekend patient visit to his or her home should be encouraged and arranged prior to the on-site visit. During such a visit, problems not previously anticipated by the therapist or support network may be uncovered. Emphasis can then be placed on initial development of a plan to solve these problems prior to the on-site visit and the patient's actual return to the environment.

Preceding the on-site visit, information should be gathered about several important areas that will influence both the preparation for and the types of suggestions made during the visit. This information includes:

- Detailed information about present level of function (e.g., communication skills, bed mobility, transfers, gait, and so forth); data should be gathered from all involved disciplines (occupational therapist, physical therapist, speech-language pathologist, and so forth).
- Knowledge of physical assistance or verbal cueing required for activity performance.
- Characteristics and dimensions of adaptive devices (e.g., raised toilet seat, environmental controls) and assistive devices (e.g., canes, crutches, long-handled reachers).
- Information about predicted level of optimum function or improvement (anticipated outcomes).
- Nature of the functional limitations or disability (i.e., static or progressive).
- Insurance coverage, financial resources, and availability of potential funding sources (in terms of capacity to modify environment or obtain needed adaptive and assistive devices or assistive technology).
- Knowledge of the patient's future plans (household management, family care, employment outside the home, school, vocational training, and so forth).
- Knowledge of whether the house or apartment is owned or rented; the type and ownership of the home can impact or preclude the type of modifications the patient may require. However, it should be noted that the Fair Housing Act requires landlords to allow individuals with disabilities to make reasonable access modifications to both personal living space as well as common space such as entryways.
- Information about the relative permanence of the dwelling; if the patient plans to move in the near future, it will influence the type of modifications recommended (e.g., installing permanent ramps vs removable ones, or paving a gravel driveway).

This information can be obtained from a variety of sources including the patient, rehabilitation team conferences, patient/family and caregiver conferences or interviews, medical record documentation from all disciplines involved, and social service interviews. Once this information is gathered, decisions can be made concerning what adaptive or assistive devices will be needed and the appropriate team members to accompany the patient on the visit.

Ideally, given their complementary expertise and skills, both the physical and occupational therapist accompany the patient on the home visit. They assume shared responsibility for examining the patient–environment interface. Depending on the specific needs of the patient and/or support network members, a speech-language pathologist, social worker, or nurse also may be among the rehabilitation team members visiting the home. For purposes of organization and structure, home visits are often divided into two global elements: (1) accessibility of the dwelling's *exterior* and (2) examination of the home's *interior*. An inexpensive disposable camera is useful for providing images of architectural barriers to accompany letters of justification for needed modifications. A tape measure and home visit examination form are also important tools during the visit. Many rehabilitation departments develop their own home survey forms to meet the particular needs of their patient population. The forms (or checklists) help to organize the visit and are useful in directing attention to all necessary details. A sample is provided in Appendix M. This form can be expanded or modified, depending on the specific needs of the individual or patient population. Some caution must be used in interpreting data from home survey forms that have not been standardization or examined for reliability.

On arrival at the home for the on-site visit, the patient may need to rest for a short while before beginning the home examination. This is an important consideration, because patients may become very excited or emotional when returning to a cherished home environment after a lengthy absence. This may be true even if a day or weekend visit occurred prior to the formal home visit.

One method of gathering data about the interior of the home is to begin with the patient in bed as though it were morning. Simulation of all daily tasks and activities, including dressing, grooming, bathroom activities, and preparation of meals can ensue. The patient should attempt to perform all transfer, exercise, locomotion, self-care, and homemaking activities as independently as possible. This will provide an additional opportunity to teach the family members and caregivers how and when to assist the patient.

Patient–Home Environment Relationship: Overview of Access, Usability, and Safety

Data from an examination of the environment are used to evaluate the need for specific access, usability, and safety interventions. Corcoran and Gitlin[1] identify five major areas of environmental intervention strategies. These include (1) *assistive* or *adaptive devices* such as grab bars, reachers, adapted eating utensils (e.g., rocker knife), canes, or walkers; (2) *safety devices* such as lighting, smoke detectors, or sensing devices; (3) *structural alterations,* which include widening doors, installing railings or ramps, or removing a doorway threshold; (4) *modification* or *altered location of environmental objects* such as disabling a stove, placing locks on doors, use of extension levers on door handles, removing throw rugs, or moving furniture; and (5) *task modification* such as use of visual, auditory, or other sensory cuing, work simplification, and energy conservation or joint preservation techniques.

The following sections offer suggestions for examination and modification of the home and workplace environment. The information presented is neither exhaustive nor inclusive of the needs of every patient. The environmental considerations are intended to direct attention to some of the more common access, usability, and safety concerns.

Exterior Accessibility

Route of Entry

1. If there is more than one entry to the dwelling, the most accessible should be selected (closest to driveway, most level walking surface, fewest stairs, available handrails, and so forth).
2. Ideally, the driveway should be a smooth, level surface with easy access to the home. Walking surfaces to the entrance should be carefully examined. Cracked and uneven surfaces should be repaired or an alternate route selected.
3. The entrance should be level, well-lighted, and provide adequate cover from adverse weather conditions. Package shelves near the entrance are useful for freeing hands to unlock and/or open doors.
4. The height, number, and condition of stairs should be noted. Ideally, steps should not be greater than 7 in. (180 mm) high with a minimum depth of 11 in. (280 mm).[4] *Nosings,* also referred to as "lips," are the 1/2 in. (13 mm) curved overhangs on the front edge of stairs. These overhangs are often problematic because they can cause a patient's toe to "catch" and prevent smooth transition to the next step. Nosings should be removed or reduced, if possible. Nosing can be minimized by installing small wood bevels under the overhangs that taper down toward the lower step and provide a smoother contour (Fig. 12.3 [top]). The steps also should have a nonslip surface to improve traction. This can be accomplished by adding abrasive strips to improve traction (Fig. 12.3 [bottom]).
5. Handrails should be installed, if needed. In general, handrail height should measure between a minimum of 34 in. (865 mm) and a maximum of 38 in. (965 mm) high. This range in handrail height allows for modifications to accommodate needs of particularly tall or short individuals. At least one handrail should extend a minimum of 12 in. (305 mm) beyond the foot and top of the stairs. Outside cross-sectional diameter of circular handrails should be between a minimum of 1.25 in. (32 mm) and a maximum of 2 in. (51 mm). If mounted adjacent to a wall, clearance between the handrail and wall should be a minimum of 1.50 in. (38 mm).[4]
6. Installation of a ramp requires adequate space. Large ramps are typically constructed of wood or concrete; smaller ramps can be made from aluminum or fiberglass. The minimum **ramp grade** (incline or slope) for a wheelchair ramp is that for every inch of threshold height there is a corresponding 12 in. (305 mm) of ramp length (a running slope of 1:12).[4] Outdoor ramps exposed to inclement weather such as snow or ice formation require a more gradual running slope of approximately 1:20. Ramps should be a minimum of 36 in. (915 mm) wide, with a nonslip surface. The overall rise of any ramp should be no greater than 30 in. (760 mm). Handrails also should be included on the ramp with a minimum height of 34 in. (865 mm) and a maximum height of 38 in. (965 mm) and extend 12 in. (305 mm) beyond the top and bottom of the ramp (Fig. 12.4).[4] Small commercially available ramps can be used for traversing curbs and small step heights.

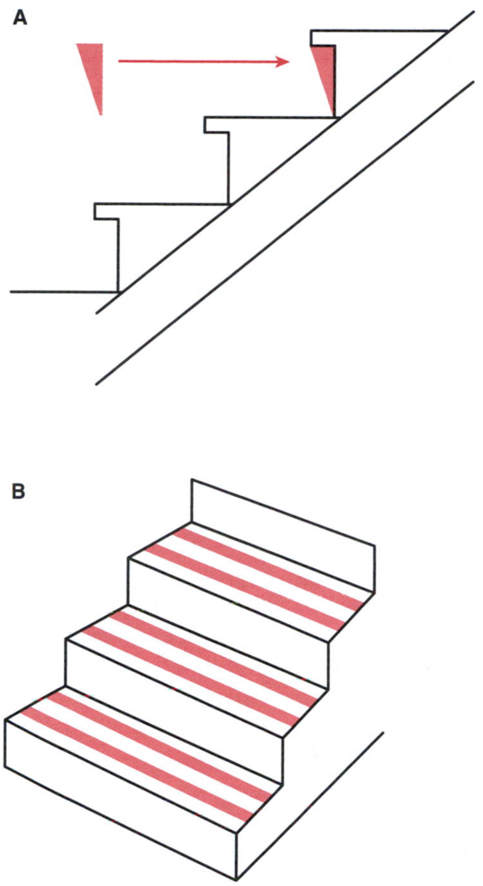

Figure 12.3 (*A*) Wood bevels placed under nosings minimize the danger of "toe-catching" during transition to the next step. (*B*) Abrasive strips improve traction and depth perception.

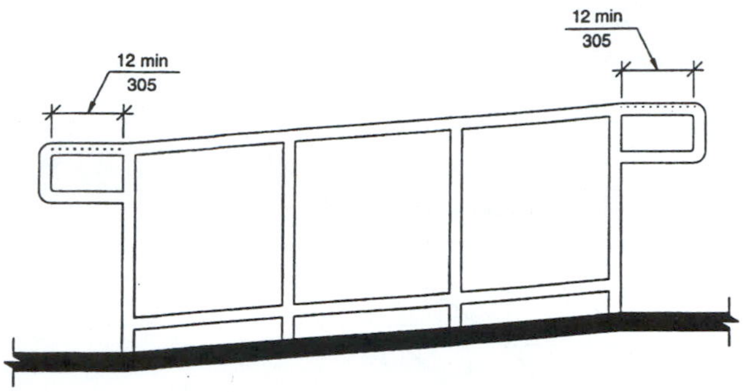

Figure 12.4 Handrail extensions should run a minimum of 12 in. (305 mm) beyond the top and bottom edge of ramp. (From American National Standards Institute, Inc,[4, p 37] with permission.)

7. *Vertical platform lifts* and *stairway inclined lifts* are commercially available and may be a consideration when inadequate space is available for a ramp. Vertical platform lifts travel approximately 8 feet (243.84 cm) straight up and down. Both open and enclosed models are available. Platform lifts are often installed adjacent to stairs with an upper landing. The lift (approximately 30 × 40 in. [76 × 102 cm]) brings the wheelchair user from the ground level to the landing level to access the entrance to the home (these lifts can be used indoors as well). Stairway inclined lifts are installed directly onto existing stairways and are typically used indoors. The stairway lifts are mounted on runners that traverse the length of the stairs and slightly beyond. Many models allow the platform to fold up against an adjacent wall to allow free stair access for other members of the home. Residential elevators are another more costly option; they require construction of an enclosed shaft.

Entrance

1. For individuals using a wheelchair, the entrance should have a platform large enough to allow the patient to rest and to prepare for entry. This platform area is particularly important when a ramp is in use. It provides for safe transit from the inclined surface to the level surface. If an individual using a wheelchair is required to open a door that swings out, this area should be at least 5 × 5 feet (153 × 153 cm). If the door swings away from the patient, a space at least 3 feet (91.5 cm) deep and 5 feet (153 cm) wide is required.
2. The door locks should be accessible to the patient. The height of the locks should be determined as well as the amount of force required to turn the key. Alternative lock systems (e.g., voice- or card-activated, remote control locks, keypad electronic security systems, and push-button padlocks) may be an important consideration for some patients. Particular attention should be directed toward ensuring that the locking mechanism on the door is sufficiently illuminated.
3. The door handle should be turned easily by the patient. Rubber doorknob covers (that stretch over a round doorknob will provide a textured grip) or lever-type handles (Fig. 12.5) are often easier to use for patients with limited grip strength (screw fastened, slip-on levers are also available that convert a round doorknob to lever-type handle).
4. The door should open and close in a direction that is functional for the patient. A long canvas "door strap" may be attached to the outside of the door (or around door handle) to help an individual using a wheelchair close the door when leaving.
5. Remote control automatic door openers are available that attach to existing doors that can open, close, and lock the door; some are equipped with customized "stay-open" features to accommodate the time required to enter or exit. These devices can be activated by a hand-held remote control or a touch pad.
6. Installation of an intercom system allows the patient to see and/or hear who is at the door. Some allow remote control opening of a door from any location in the home.
7. If there is a raised threshold in the doorway, it should be removed. If removal is not possible, the threshold should be lowered to no greater than 1/2 in. (13 mm) in height, with beveled edges.[4] If needed, weather-stripping the door will help prevent drafts.
8. The doorway width should be measured. Generally, 32 to 34 in. (815 to 865 mm) is an acceptable doorway width to accommodate most wheelchairs.
9. If the door is weighted to aid in closing, the pressure should not exceed 8 pounds to be functional for the patient.

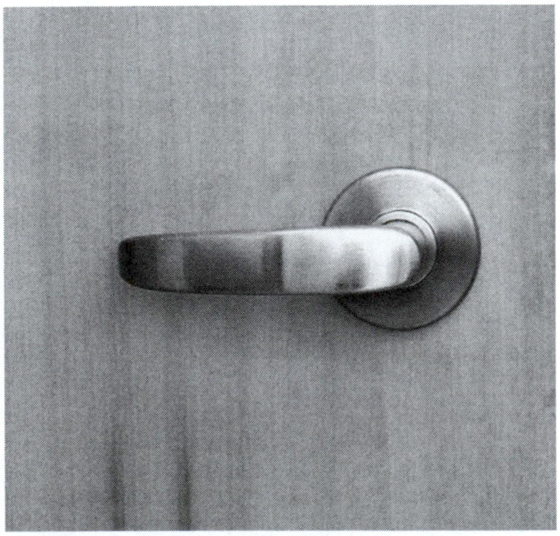

Figure 12.5 Lever-style door handle (a frequent universal design element) is particularly useful for individuals with limited grip strength as they can be activated with other body parts (e.g., fisted hand, forearm, elbow).

10. A kick plate (metal guard) may be added to doors frequently entered by individuals using a wheelchair or ambulatory assistive devices. The kick plate should measure 12 in. (305 mm) in height from the bottom of the door.

General Considerations: Interior Accessibility

Furniture Arrangement and Features

1. Sufficient room should be made available for maneuvering a wheelchair or ambulating with an assistive device. An initial step is to move as much furniture as possible against the walls to increase clearance and stability (i.e., prevent sliding of furniture during movement transitions). Further stability can be achieved by placing rubber suction cups under the legs of sofas and chairs. Access to furniture should not be obstructed by items such as coffee tables, foot stools, or telephone or electrical wires.
2. Clear passage must be allowed from one room to the next.
3. Typically, overstuffed sofas and chairs do not provide the needed support for movement transitions (e.g., sit-to-stand). Although generally not the case, living room chairs should have double arm rests, a firm seating surface, and an upright back. Sometimes a suitable chair can be found in a different location within the home and moved to the living room. Another option is to modify the current furniture by placing a fitted wooden board under the seat cushion and behind the seat back (if removable). If a new chair is to be purchased, recommended features of the chair should be provided to the patient, family member, and/or caregiver (e.g., the height of the seat should allow the knees to flex approximately 90° with the feet flat on the floor, a firm cushioned seat, a firm cushioned back that provides adequate upright support, and double arm rests).
4. Use of any unstable furniture such as rocking chairs should be discouraged for most patients. Use of leather furniture should also be avoided as it can hinder movement. Chairs that provide mechanized elevation of the back of the seat are commercially available but should be used with caution. It may be difficult for a patient to stabilize the feet as the seat is elevating. This causes the feet (and pelvis) to slide forward resulting in a fall.

Electrical Controls

1. Unrestricted access should be provided to wall switches, and electrical outlets. Power strips (surge protectors) can be used to increase the number of outlets as well as improve access. Outlets may need to be raised and wall switches lowered. For individuals using a wheelchair, use of pull cord extensions may allow control of some high electrical switches.
2. Some patients may benefit from replacement of standard toggle electric switches (e.g., overhead fixtures) with rocker switches that require less fine motor skill to activate. Rocker switches are available with lighted surfaces and with occupancy sensor devices that automatically turn on or off upon entering or leaving the room. Light-switch plates come in a variety of colors and will be easier to see if they contrast with the existing wall color. For example, in rooms with light colored walls (white, off-white, beige), darker electrical outlet and light-switch plates can be selected. A ground fault circuit interrupter (GFCI) should be installed in wet locations such as bathrooms to prevent against electrical shock. A GFCI outlet acts as a monitor for current imbalance between the hot and neutral wires and breaks the circuit if that situation occurs (e.g., faulty appliances, worn cords, or appliance contact with water) (Fig. 12.6).

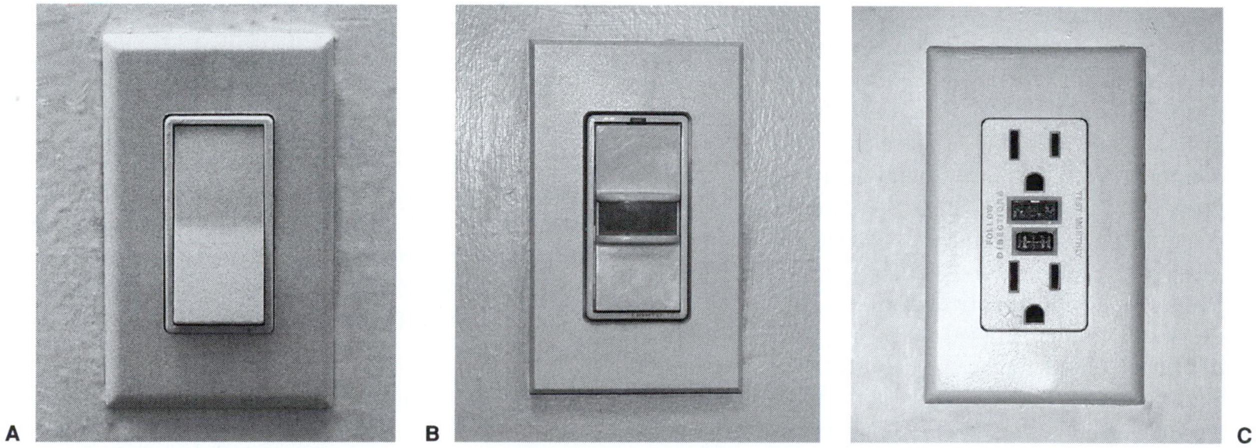

Figure 12.6 Electrical switches. (*A*) Rocker switch (available with lighted surface). (*B*) Rocker switch with light sensor that turns on or off upon entering or leaving the room. (*C*) Ground fault circuit interrupter (GFCI) for use in wet locations to prevent electrical shock.

3. For some patients, vision may be enhanced by use of higher wattage bulbs, fluorescent lighting, full-spectrum bulbs, or high-intensity halogen lamps. Use of long-life light bulbs reduces the frequency of required bulb changes.
4. Inexpensive, programmable electrical timers can be used to regularly turn lights on and off throughout the day and night.
5. Inexpensive night-lights with motion sensors can be placed in strategic locations to provide additional illumination.
6. Touch pad dimmer switches can be used to activate lamps with small control knobs. The dimmer module is plugged into a wall outlet and the lamp attached to the module. The lamp can be turn "on" or "off" or level of brightness changed by touching the pad. Voice activated dimmers are also available.
7. Inexpensive remote control units can be used in any room of the home to control lights or small appliances. The simplest designs of these remote control units send signals through existing wires (receiver modules are plugged into existing outlets and appliances are plugged into the receiver and controlled by a hand-held remote); others are wireless and utilize radio signals. Receiver modules can also be wired directly into the electrical system of the dwelling. Remote control units are available with large-print buttons and numbers.

Floors

1. Floors should be nonslip and level. All floor coverings should be glued or tacked to the floor. This will prevent bunching or rippling under wheelchair use. When carpeting is used, a dense, low pile, low-level loop generally provides for easiest movement of a wheelchair or ambulatory assistive device. Industrial-style or "in-door out-door" carpeting typically meet these requirements.
2. Floors should be examined for uneven or unlevel areas. This may be particularly problematic with older wooden floors. Optimally, these areas should be repaired or replaced. If restoration is not possible, several other solutions might be recommended: (1) establish a path of movement for the patient that eliminates use of the problematic area; (2) place a piece of furniture over the offending area; or (3) place brightly colored tape along the borders of the area to continually remind the patient to avoid this area of the potential danger.
3. Scatter rugs should be removed; larger area rugs can be secured with a good quality carpet tape. Use of nonskid waxes should be encouraged.
4. If flooring is to be replaced, matte finishes should be recommended to reduce glare. Patients with visual impairments will benefit from a contrasting colored border along the perimeter of the room to help mark the boundaries of the space. Wide-colored tape can also be used effectively.

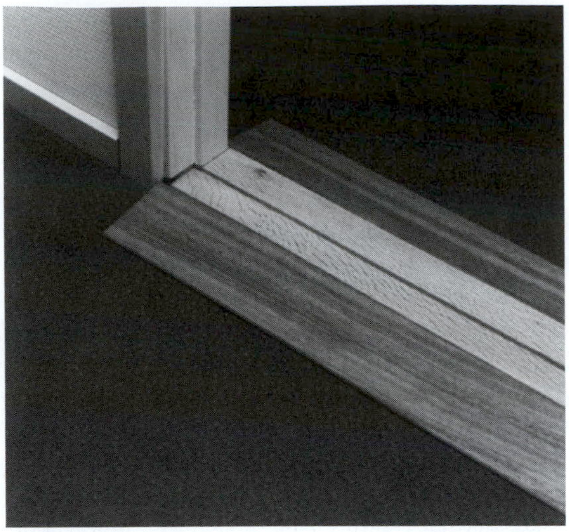

Figure 12.7 Common materials used for threshold ramps are wood (shown) and aluminum with a lacquered non-slip surface. They can be used between rooms if the floor surface height changes slightly. (Courtesy of Guldmann, Inc, Tampa, FL 33634.)

Doors

1. Raised thresholds should be removed to provide a flush, level surface. If structural elements prevent removal, threshold ramps ("transition wedges") can be easily installed (Fig. 12.7).
2. Doorways may need to be widened (if less than 32 in. [815 mm] wide) to allow clearance for a wheelchair or assistive device. Doors may have to be removed, reversed (e.g., to open outward for easier exit, especially in the case of an emergency), or replaced with folding doors, or a door of lighter weight. Several other options are available to increase door clearance. These options include:
   - Installation of pocket doors, which slide into the adjacent wall when not in use; some sliding doors allow installation on the outside of the door frame and wall to minimize structural changes.
   - Removal of the wood strips on the inside of a door frame will add approximately 3/4 to 1 in. (19 to 25.4 mm) of clearance.
   - Use of *offset* hinges (also called *swing-clear* hinges), which swing the open door clear of the frame provide approximately 2 additional in. (51 mm) of space.
   - Removal of the door with installation of a curtain (inexpensive spring-loaded curtain rods and a fabric or plastic shower curtain can be used).
3. As mentioned in regard to exterior doors, handles inside the home should also be examined. Rubber doorknob covers or lever-type handles may be important considerations. Knurled (roughened) surface door handles are used on interiors of buildings and dwellings when frequented by persons with visual impairments. These

abrasive, knurled surfaces provide tactile clues that the door leads to a hazardous area and alerts the individual to danger. (Note: Brightly colored roughened areas are also used on flooring to indicate potential danger; for example, the edge of a train or subway platform.)

Windows

1. To reduce glare, window films can be installed; frosted films are effective at diffusing light without appreciably reducing ambient light.
2. Heavy draperies or shades can also be used with the added benefit of absorbing internal background noise to improve hearing and conversation.
3. Remote control systems for closing or opening window coverings either partially or fully are commercially available.
4. Although not frequently seen in older dwellings, casement windows provide several important features for individuals using a wheelchair or for patients with limited upper extremity function. Casement windows open using a crank-style handle and can be locked with a single lever locking mechanism located near the bottom of the window. Automatic openers can be installed on these windows.

Stairs

1. All indoor stairwells should have handrails and should be well-lighted. Ideally, handrails should extend a minimum of 12 in. (305 mm) past the top and bottom of the stairs for added safety.[4] Battery-operated touch switch lamps are a practical supplement where electrical light sources are unavailable. Inexpensive track lighting provides multiple adjustable lamps and requires only a single electrical source. Lighting should be bright with glare and reflection minimized. Motion detection lights that automatically turn on when the patient approaches the stairs (or other area of the home) can also be an important safety consideration.
2. Stairs should be free of clutter. Rather than climbing the stairs to move a single item to the next level, patients sometimes "store" or collect items on the stairs. This creates several safety hazards: (1) initially bending over to pick-up the items prior to stair climbing can alter postural stability; (2) negotiating stairs holding several objects can impair balance and limit use of the handrail; and (3) other household members may not see the item(s), precipitating a fall. As an alternative, a canvas bag or "stair basket" with handles (that can be held in one hand) can be placed near the stairs to collect the items until the patient is ready to move to another floor level.
3. For individuals with decreased visual acuity or age-related visual changes, adhesive light reflective *tactile warning strips* provide contrasting textures on the surface of the top and bottom stair(s) to alert them that the end of the stairwell is near. They can also be used on each step to identify its edge. Circular bands of tape also can be placed at the top and bottom of the handrail for the same purpose. Tactile warning strips placed on the floor can also be used to signal a change in level of the walking surface or entrance to another area or room of the dwelling.
4. Many patients with visual impairment will benefit also from bright, contrasting color tape on the border of each stair. Warm colors (reds, oranges, and yellows) are generally easier to see than cool colors (blues, greens, and violets).
5. For patients unable to negotiate stairs who require access to the second floor of a dwelling, a motorized stairlift may be an option (Fig. 12.8). These battery-powered units are available with a variety of options such as swing-away arms for wheelchair transfers, adjustable seat width (22.5 to 25.5 in. [572 mm to 648 mm]), and wireless call/send controls. Outdoor models are also available as well as units to accommodate curves or turns in the stairwell. Although a more costly alternative, residential elevators are also commercially available. If possible, these elevators are typically installed in stacked closet space to minimize construction to the dwelling.

Heating Units

1. All radiators, heating vents, and hot water pipes should be appropriately screened off or insulated with pipe covers to prevent burns, especially for patients who have sensory impairments. Adaptations may be required to

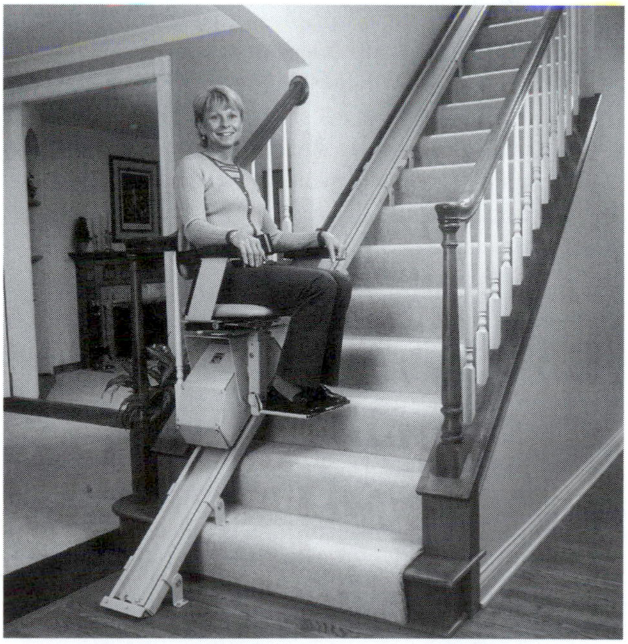

Figure 12.8 Battery-powered stairlift. (Courtesy of Bruno Independent Living Aids, Inc, Oconomowoc, WI 53066.)

allow patient access to heat controls (e.g., remote control thermostat control, use of reachers or enlarged, extended, or adapted handles on heat control valves).
2. The heating source should be clear of combustible material and clutter. Use of space heaters should be discouraged.
3. Smoke alarms and carbon monoxide detectors should be in the home and checked regularly by pressing the test button. Some newer models allow testing the unit using a flashlight.

Specific Considerations: Interior Accessibility

Bedroom Area

1. The bed should be stationary and positioned to provide ample space for transfers. Stability may be improved by placing the bed against a wall or in the corner of the room (except when the patient plans to make the bed). Additional stability may be achieved by placing rubber suction cups under each leg.
2. The height of the sleeping surface must be considered to facilitate transfer activities. The height of the bed can be raised by use of wooden blocks with routed depressions to hold each leg (blocks may be used to raise the height of chairs, as well). The use of an extra-thick mattress or box spring can also provide additional height to the bed. The bed height can be lowered by using commercially available reduced-height box springs.
3. The mattress should be carefully examined. It should provide a firm, comfortable surface. If the mattress is in relatively good condition, a firm bed board inserted between the mattress and box spring may suffice to improve the sleeping surface adequately. If the mattress is badly worn, a new one should be suggested.
4. A bedside table or cabinet should be available; it can be used to hold a lamp, telephone (preferably cordless with a memory dial for frequently used numbers or emergency phone numbers), necessary medications, and call bell if assistance is needed from a caregiver.
5. The closet clothes bar may require lowering to provide wheelchair accessibility. The bar should be lowered to 52 in. (132 cm) from the floor. Wall hooks also may be a useful addition to the closet area and should be placed between 40 in. (101.6 cm) and 56 in. (142.2 cm) from the floor. Shelves also can be installed at various levels in the closet (Fig. 12.9). The highest shelf should not exceed 45 in. (115.5 cm). Clothing and grooming articles frequently used by the patient should be placed in the most easily accessible bureau drawer. Free-standing modular storage units are also commercially available in a variety of dimensions. These units typically provide clothes bar, shelves, and drawers that can be adjusted to meet the needs of the user. Figure 12.10 illustrates the basic components and dimensions of an accessible bedroom.

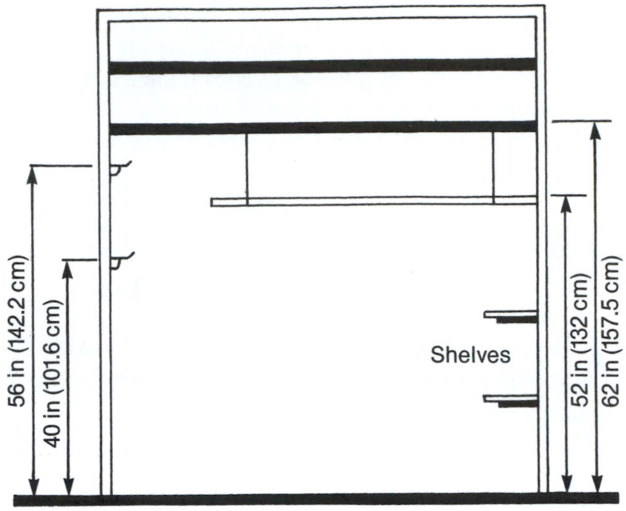

Figure 12.9 Closet modifications to provide accessibility for an individual using a wheelchair. Values denoted in inches and centimeters. (From Cotler, SR, and DeGraff, AH: Architectural Accessibility for the Disabled of College Campuses. New York State University Construction Fund, Albany, 1976, p 57, with permission.)

Bathroom

1. If the doorframe prohibits passage of a wheelchair, the patient may transfer at the door to a chair with casters attached. As mentioned above, several other solutions are available to address the problem of narrow door frames (see Interior Accessibility: General Considerations, Doors).
2. An elevated toilet seat can be used to facilitate transfers. Some models allow the height to be custom adjusted while others provide a fixed height elevation. They are also available with grab bars. Power-lift toilet seats with grab bars are designed to assist the patient to standing (elevation initiated from the posterior aspect of the seat). As with other types of mechanized seat elevators, they should be used with caution as it may be difficult to stabilize the feet as the seat is elevating. For new construction, a wall-mounted toilet seat may be recommended that can be placed at the optimum height for the user and provide more floor space for transfer positioning.
3. Grab bars securely fastened to a reinforced wall will assist in both toilet and tub transfers. Grab bars should have a circular cross section diameter of 1.25 in. (32 mm) minimum and 2 in. (51 mm) maximum and be knurled. For use in toilet transfers, the bars should be mounted horizontally 33 to 36 in. (840 to 915 mm) from the floor. The length of the grab bars should be between 42 and 54 in. (1065 and 1370 mm) on the side wall and between 24 and 36 in. (610 and 915 mm) on the back wall (Fig. 12.11). Ideally, two grab bars are secured horizontally to the back wall for use in tub transfers. One is placed 33 to 36 in. (840 to 915 mm) from the floor of the tub and

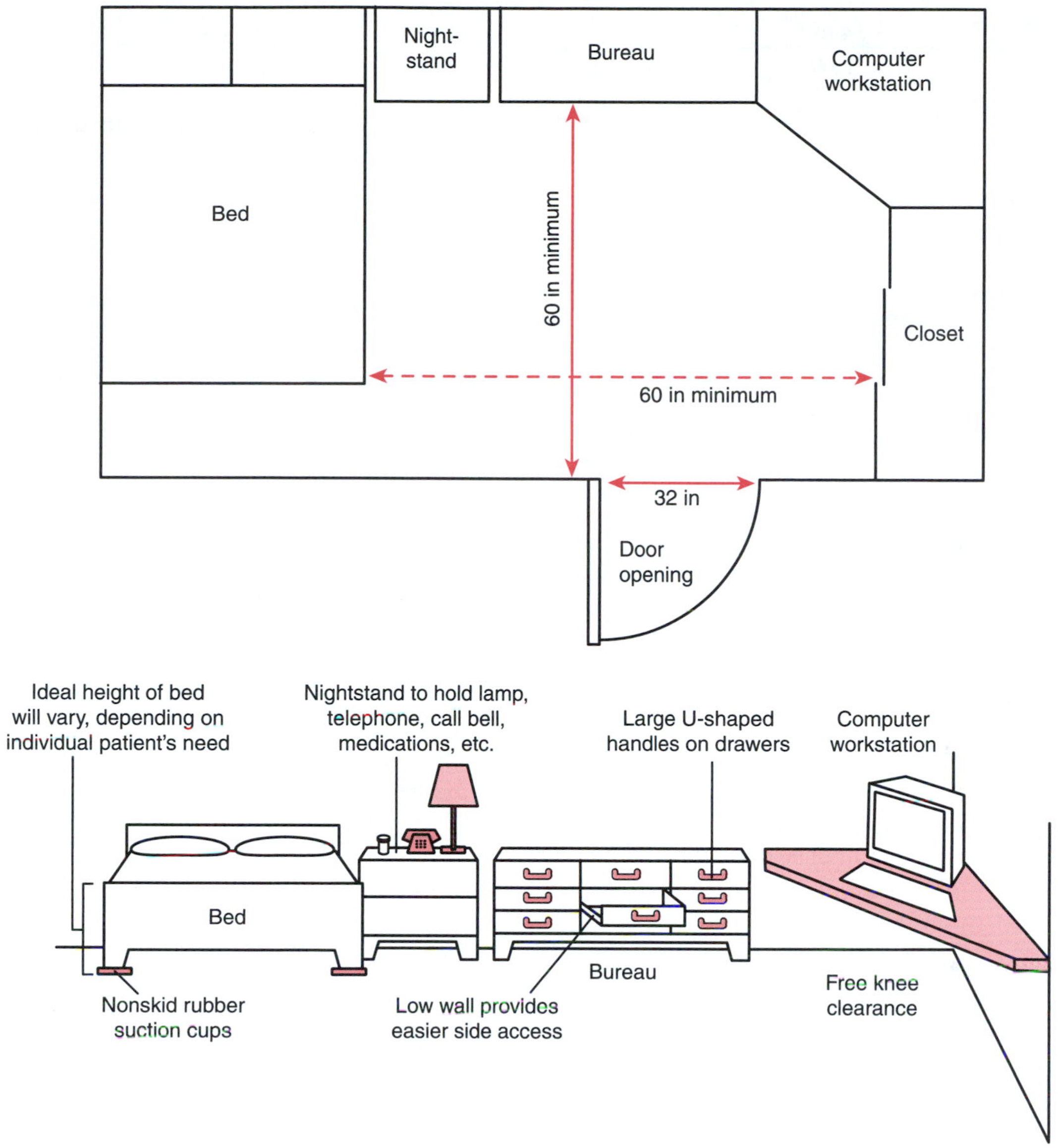

Figure 12.10 Sample dimensions and features of an accessible bedroom.

the second 9 in. (230 mm) above the rim of the bathtub. Grab bars may also be mounted horizontally at the foot-end wall of the bathtub (recommended length is 24 in. [610 mm] with placement at the front edge of the bathtub) and at the head-end wall of the bathtub (recommended length is 12 in. [305 mm] with placement at the front edge of the bathtub) (Fig. 12.12). Knurled surfaces are typically used on grab bars to improve grasp and prevent slipping.

4. A tub transfer bench (tub seat) may be recommended for bathing. Many types of commercially produced benches are available. In selecting a tub transfer bench (tub seat), function and safety are primary considerations. The bench should provide a wide base of support (some are designed with suction feet; and some provide height adjustment), a back rest, and an appropriate seating surface to facilitate transfers in and out of the tub (Fig. 12.13A and B). Tub transfer benches with relatively long seating surfaces are typically positioned with two legs in the tub and two legs on the floor adjacent to the tub. Smaller benches are available that require all four legs be placed inside the bathtub.
5. In shower stall areas, a collapsible seat may be permanently attached to the wall (Fig. 12.14). When not in use it folds flat against the wall, allowing easy shower access from a standing position as well.
6. Nonskid adhesive strips may be placed on the floor of the tub or shower area.
7. Additional bathroom considerations may include a handspray attachment to the bathtub or shower faucet

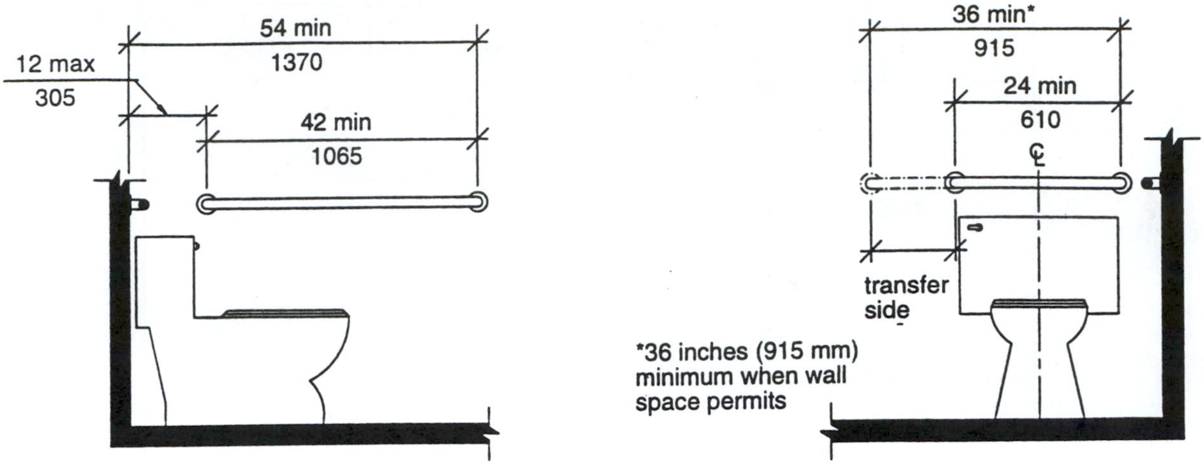

Figure 12.11 Location and dimensions of bathroom grab bars on the side wall (*left*) and rear wall (*right*). Values denoted in inches and millimeters. The bars should be mounted horizontally 33 in. (840 mm) to 36 in. (915 mm) from the floor. (From American National Standards Institute, Inc,[4, p 41] with permission.)

(see Fig. 12.12), antiscald valves to prevent water temperature from rising above a preset limit (also called *scald-guard valves* or *high temperature stops*), water volume-control mechanisms (to prevent a sudden surge of water with resultant change in temperature), enlarged faucet handles on the tub or sink (single-lever system faucets are optimal owing to their ease of use), motion-sensor faucets, a spray attachment at the sink (allows washing hair without entering the bathtub or shower), a towel rack and small shelf for toiletry articles, and a call bell within easy reach of the patient.

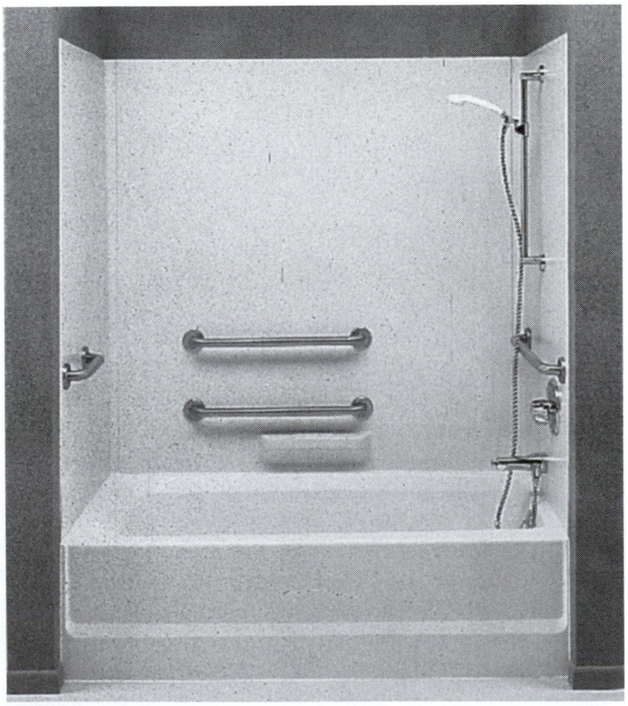

Figure 12.12 Bathtub with grab bars secured to back, foot-end, and head-end walls. The handspray faucet attachment facilitates control of water flow direction from a sitting position. (Courtesy of The Swan Corporation, St. Louis, MO 63101.)

CLINICAL NOTE: To prevent injury in the presence of sensory impairments, patient, family, and caregiver education should include using a thermometer to test water temperature prior to bathing.

8. Ideally, sinks should provide clear knee space below and any exposed hot water pipes should be insulated to prevent burns (Fig. 12.15). In new construction, shallow sinks may be installed to increase knee clearance with faucets placed on the side for easier access. Storage space lost from beneath the sink can be partially compensated for by an under-the-sink roll-out cabinet that can be easily moved for wheelchair access. An enlarged mirror over the sink with the top tilted away from the wall facilitates use from a sitting position (Fig. 12.16). Forward tilting mirrors are also available with adjustable hinges for alternating placement against and away from the wall. Hinged-wall, gooseneck, or accordion fold-up mirrors (with one side magnified) are also helpful for close work.

Figure 12.17 illustrates the minimum space requirements of a wheelchair-accessible bathroom.

Kitchen

1. The height of countertops (work space) should be appropriate for the individual. When using a wheelchair, the armrests should be able to fit under the working surface. The ideal height of counter surfaces should

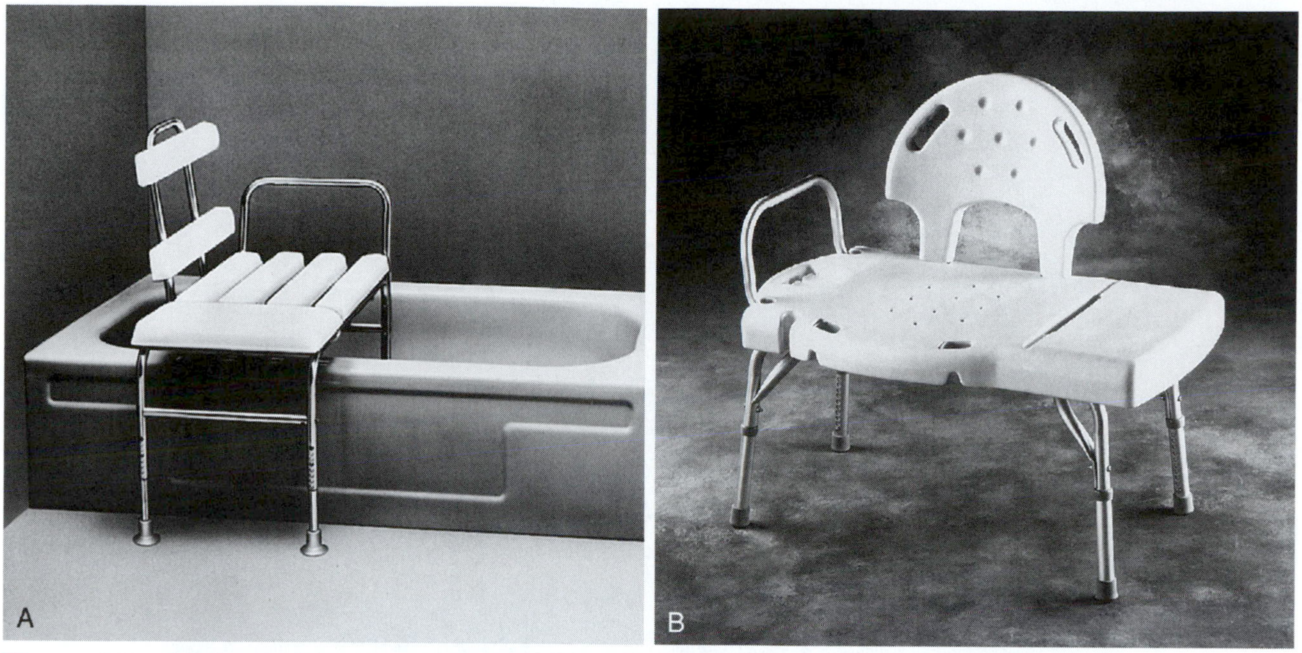

Figure 12.13 Two tub transfer bench designs each providing a wide base of support, a secure back rest, and a long seating surface to facilitate transfers. (Courtesy of Lumex, Inc., Bay Shore, NY 11706.)

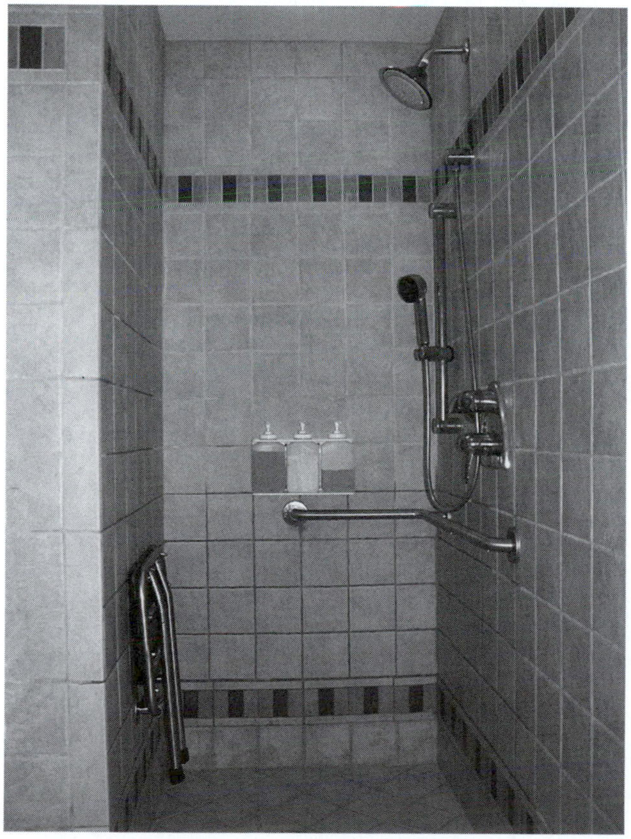

Figure 12.14 Shower stall with collapsible shower seat, grab bars, and handspray attachment.

be no greater than 31 in. (794 mm) from the floor with a knee clearance of 27.5 to 30 in. (705 to 769 mm). Counter space should provide a depth of at least 24 in. (615 mm). All surfaces should be smooth to facilitate sliding of heavy items from one area to another. Slide-out counter spaces are useful in providing an over-the-lap working surface. A section of base cabinetry can be removed to provide a seated countertop workspace. For patients who are ambulatory, stools (preferably with back and footrests) may be placed strategically at the main work area(s). For patients with visual impairments, placing colored tape along the border of the countertop that contrasts sharply with the color of the counter surface will help identify boundaries of the workspace. Under-the-counter cabinets with glide-out height-adjustable shelves improve access to storage areas (Fig. 12.18).

2. Improved function and safety may be provided by a sink equipped with large blade-type handles or a single-lever style faucet, scald-guard valves, or electronic sensors that allow hands-free operation by automatically turning water off and on. A spray-hose fixture allows filling heavy pots without needing to lift them from a sink. Pressure-balanced valves can be used to equalize hot and cold water; other faucets allow preprogramming desired water temperature. Hot water dispensers are helpful for preparing coffee or tea and instant soups or cereals minimizing the need for using the stove. Shallow sinks 5 to 6 in. (128 to

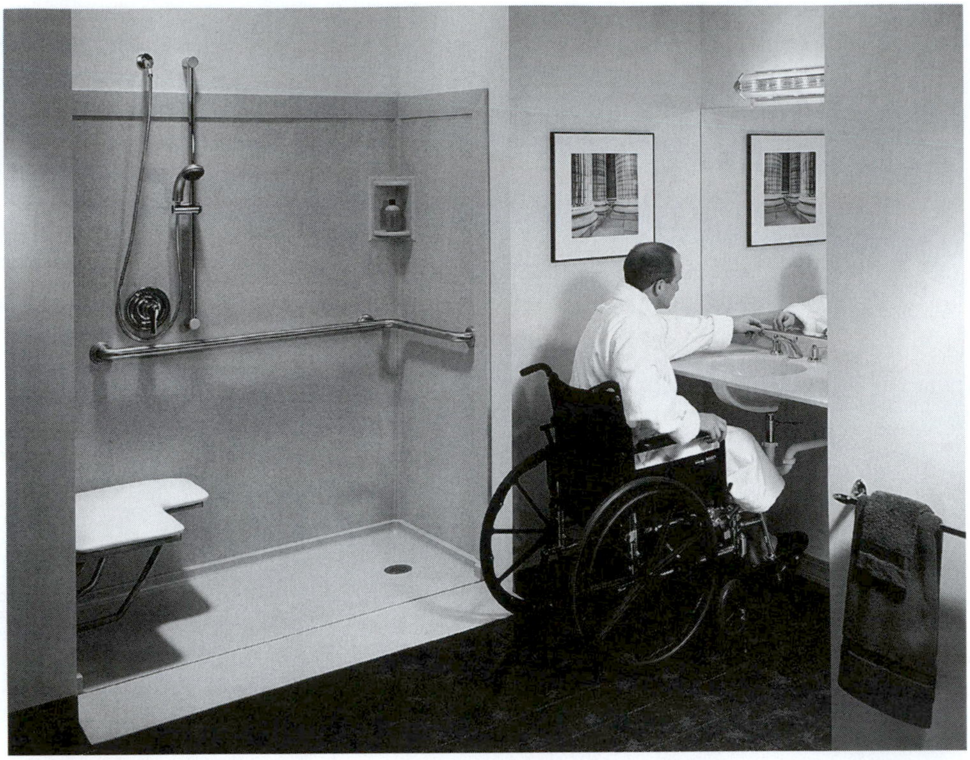

Figure 12.15 Accessible bathroom with knee clearance below sink and insulated piping. The shower entrance includes a small ramp to accommodate a difference in floor surface heights. Note that the shower handspray is held by a vertical slide-bar (to change height) allowing for a seated shower. Alternately, the handspray can be hand-held to direct water flow to specific areas. (Courtesy of The Swan Corporation, St. Louis, MO 63101.)

153 mm) deep will improve knee clearance below. Providing sink access to an individual using a wheelchair may require removal of under-the-sink cabinets. As in the bathroom, hot water pipes under the kitchen sink should be insulated to prevent burns. Motorized adjustable sinks (Fig. 12.19) are designed to be mounted against a wall between two stationary cabinets with free space beneath. By activating the control switch, the sink height can be adjusted for the individual user whether seated in a wheelchair or standing.

3. A small cart with casters may be helpful to improve ease of movement of articles from refrigerator to counter and other such activities.
4. The height of tables also should be checked and the tables may have to be raised or lowered.
5. Equipment and food storage areas should be selected with optimum energy conservation in mind. All frequently used articles should be within easy reach, and unnecessary items should be eliminated. Additional storage space may be achieved by installation of open shelving or use of pegboards for pots and pans. If shelving is added, adjustable shelves are preferable and should be placed 16 in. (410 mm) above the countertop.[48] Electronically powered storage cabinets are also available that automatically lower for counter-top access (Fig. 12.20).
6. Electric stoves are generally preferable to open-flame gas burners. For optimum safety, controls should be located on the front or side border of the stove to eliminate the need for reaching across the burners. Burners that are placed beside each other provide a safer arrangement than those placed one behind the other. A heat-resistant burn-proof counter surface adjacent to the burners will facilitate movement of hot items once cooking is completed. Smooth, ceramic cooktop surfaces also reduce the amount of lifting required while cooking (Fig. 12.21). If cooktops provide knee clearance beneath, exposed or potential contact surfaces must be insulated. Electromagnetic stoves are also available that heat food without flames or heating elements.[49]
7. For patients with visual impairments, large-print label-making devices and large-print stencil overlays can be used to enlarge appliance control indicators and dials (e.g., on/off or temperature indicators on thermostats,

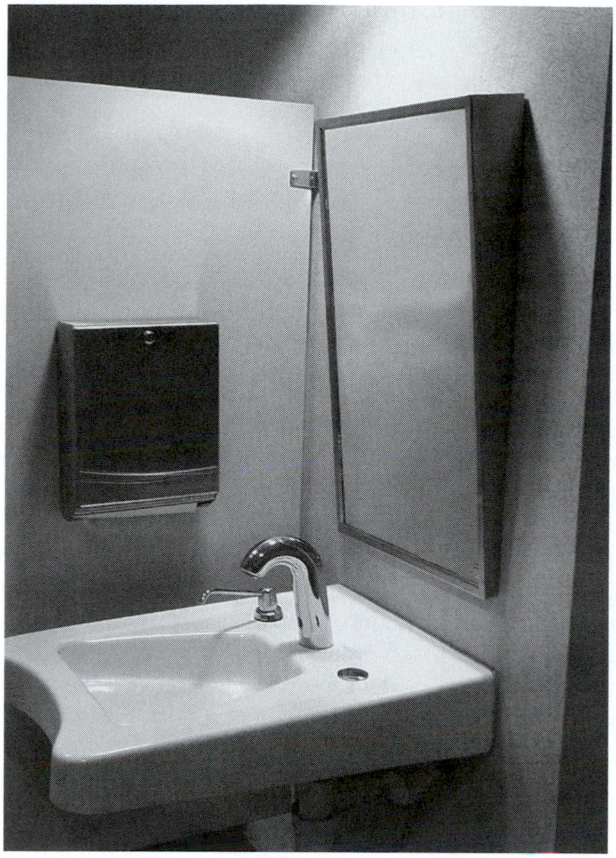

Figure 12.16 Over-sink mirror with top tilted away from wall to allow use from a seated position.

microwaves, stoves, and ovens). Timers, wall clocks, and telephones with large-print numbers are also available.[49]

8. Wall-mounted ovens (separate from the stove) should be placed 30 to 34 in. (76 to 102 cm) from the floor with a side-opening door. These cooking units are generally more easily accessible than a single, low-level combined oven and burner unit. Oven units should be self-cleaning.
9. For many individuals, a countertop microwave oven is essential for food preparation.
10. Dishwashers should be elevated 6 in. (152 mm), be front-loading, with pull-out shelves and front-mounted controls. Elevated (6 in. [152 mm]) side-by-side clothes washers and dryers should also be front-loading with front-mounted controls.
11. Access to the refrigerator will be enhanced by use of a side-by-side (refrigerator-freezer) model.
12. A standard or remote control smoke detector and one or more, easily accessible, portable fire extinguishers should be available. It is generally recommended that fire extinguishers be mounted in open view near an exit and away from cooking appliances. For patients with hearing impairments, the smoke detector can be attached to a signaling system that activates both an audible and strobe light response to visually warn of danger. These signaling systems also can be used to activate flashing lights in response to a doorbell, knock on the door, telephone ring, or burglar alarm.

Figure 12.22 presents sample features of a kitchen designed for an individual using a wheelchair.

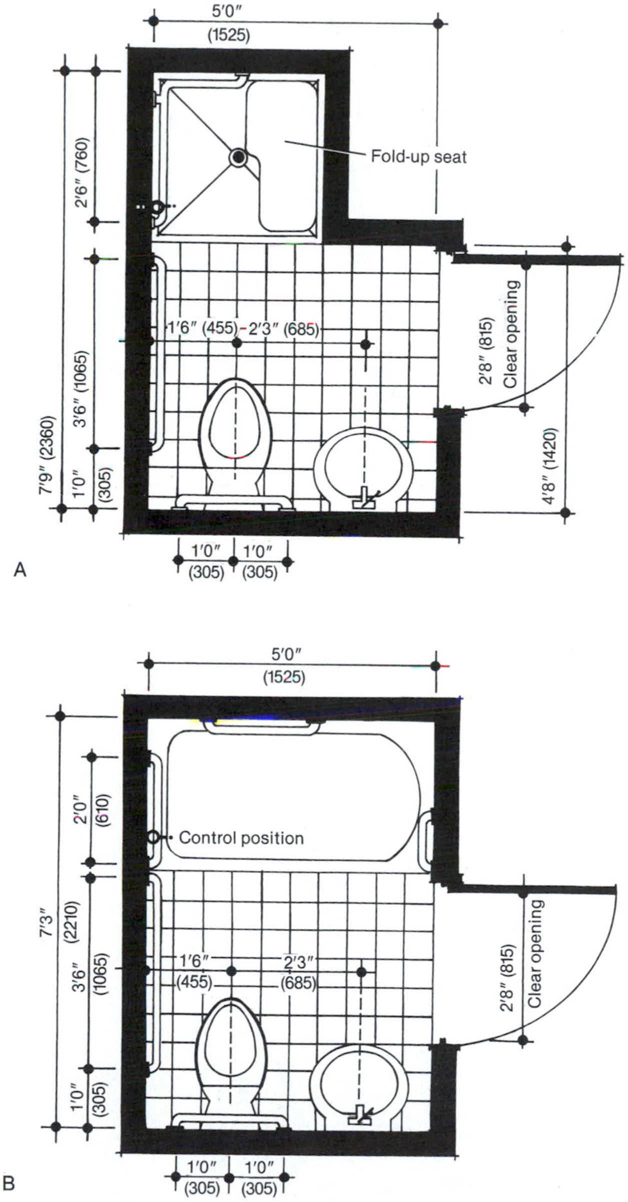

Figure 12.17 Minimum space requirements of a residential bathroom with (*A*) a shower stall and (*B*) a bathtub. The dotted line indicates lengths of wall that require reinforcement to receive grab bars or supports. (From Nixon, V: Spinal Cord Injury: A Guide to Functional Outcomes in Physical Therapy Management. Aspen Systems Corporation, Rockville, MD, p 186, with permission.)

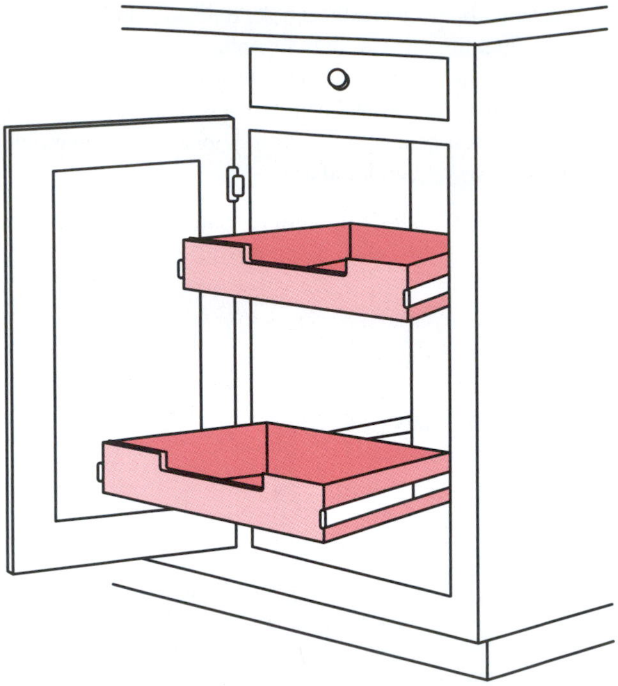

Figure 12.18 Glide-out under cabinet shelves improve access to storage areas.

CLINICAL NOTE: Although important for many patients, an examination of the home environment is often essential for older adults with specific areas of the home presenting greater hazards than others. Gitlin and co-workers[50] addressed the types of difficulties older adults experience in their home. Data were collected from 296 participants (mean age 73.24 years) using interviews, self-reports, clinical assessment, and direct observation of the home environment. The researchers focused on nine areas of the homes: bathroom, kitchen, bedrooms, entry to home, dining/living/family room, outdoor spaces, common rooms, stairs, and the area from street to house. The areas where subjects encountered the greatest environmental difficulties were: bathrooms (88 percent), kitchens (76 percent), bedrooms (61 percent), and entryways (58 percent).

Adaptive Equipment

A large variety of **adaptive equipment** is commercially available to increase independence, speed, skill, and efficiency in performing activities of daily living (ADL). Adaptive equipment is available to assist performance in such areas as bathing, personal care, dressing, meal preparation, and general household tasks. Typically, adaptive equipment is a component of a *compensatory training approach* that focuses on achieving the highest level of function possible by using remaining abilities. This approach involves considering alternate ways to accomplish a task, use of intact segments to compensate for those lost, use of energy conservation and joint preservation techniques, and adapting the environment to optimize performance.

Table 12.2 presents suggestions for adaptive equipment to improve function in several areas of ADL. The table is organized around adaptive equipment recommendations and compensatory strategies for four impairments including (1) one upper extremity or body side involvement, (2) reduced upper extremity range of motion and strength, (3) incoordination of upper extremities, and (4) mobility limitations without upper extremity involvement. The table also identifies common medical diagnoses associated with each impairment together with the rationale for the suggested compensatory strategies.[51]

A

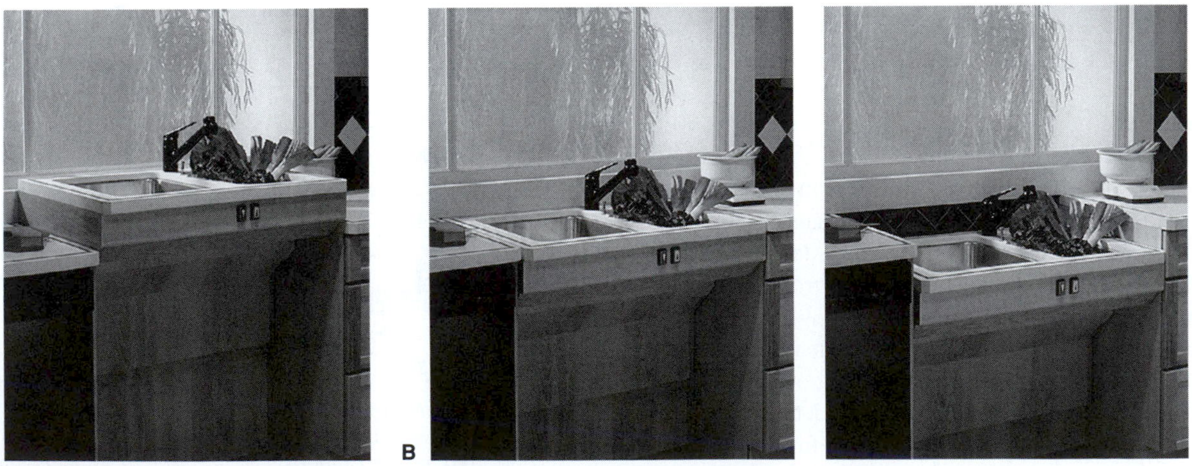

B C

Figure 12.19 A motorized adjustable height sink can be raised or lowered for comfortable use from either a seated or standing position. Height-adjustment controls are located on the anterior panel of the sink ([*A*] high, [*B*] middle, and [*C*] low positions). (Courtesy of General Electric, Fairfield, CT 06431.)

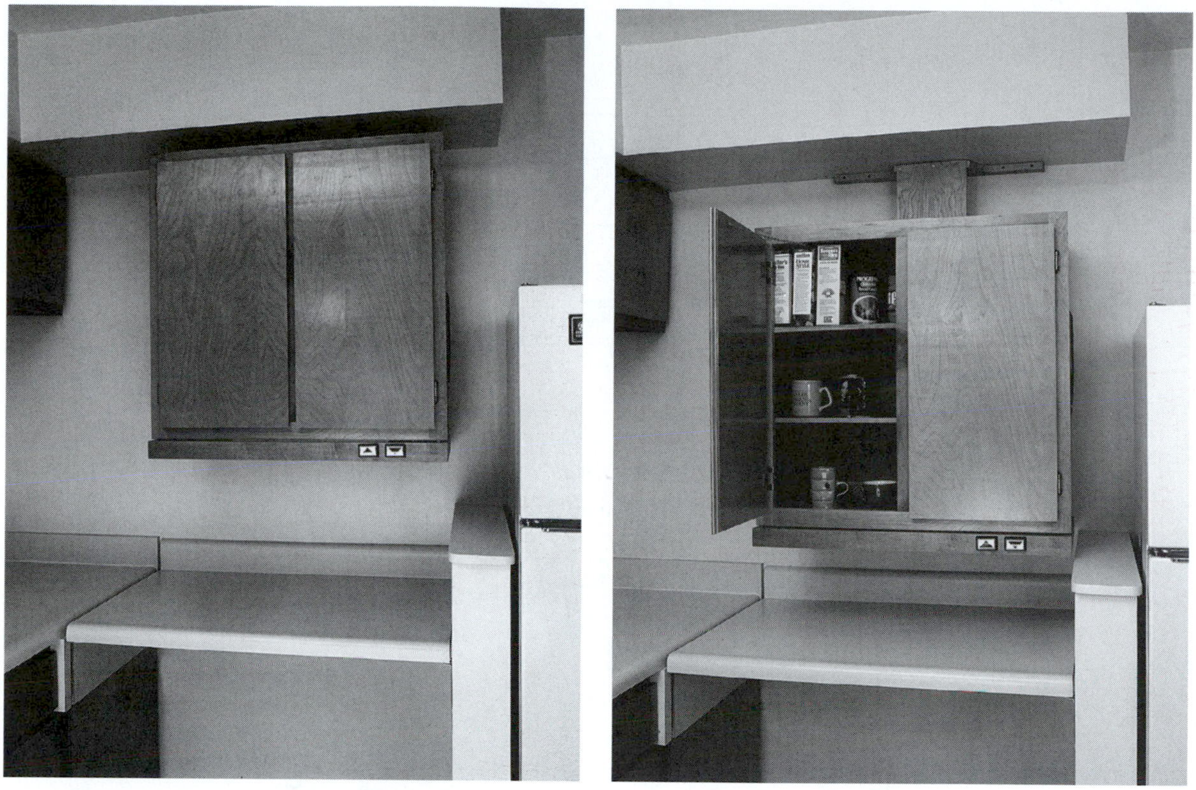

A B

Figure 12.20 Motorized storage cabinets that can be lowered from the resting position to allow counter-top access. Height-adjustment controls ([*A*] high and [*B*] low) are located on the right anterior panel of the cabinet. (Courtesy of AD-AS, Boise, ID 83709.)

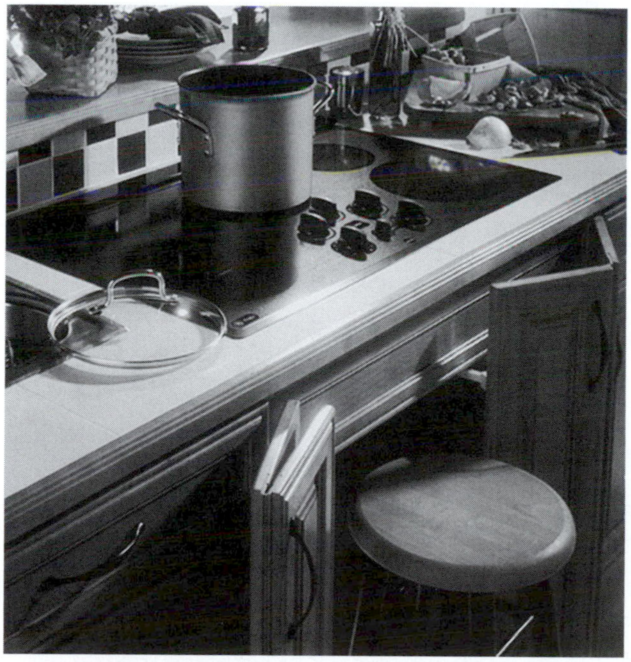

Figure 12.21 Cooktop with front-mounted controls and smooth surface that allows sliding (rather than lifting) from burner to heat-resistant countertop. Knee clearance beneath is accessed by folding doors. (Courtesy of General Electric, Fairfield, CT 06431.)

Assistive Technology

In the Technology-Related Assistance for Individuals with Disabilities Act of 1988, assistive technology is defined as "any item, piece of equipment, or product system, whether acquired commercially off the shelf, modified, or customized, that is used to increase, maintain, or improve functional capabilities of individuals with disabilities."[52] Assistive technologies can be simple mechanical or mobility devices but the term usually denotes some type of electronic, computer (e.g., hardware, software, peripherals), or microprocessor-based (prosthetic knee control) device.

Assistive technologies (ATs) enable individuals with disabilities to perform daily activities by compensating for lost or impaired function. They promote greater independence and typically improve quality of life by assisting in such areas as communication, education, environmental accessibility, and work or recreation activities. Three important considerations in determining the need for ATs include (1) the individual's available function, (2) the nature of the tasks or activities that will be performed, and (3) the environmental context in which it will be used.

An enormous variety of ATs are commercially available. Ideally, the evaluation and prescription for specific items is accomplished by an interdisciplinary team that includes the

(text continues on page 426)

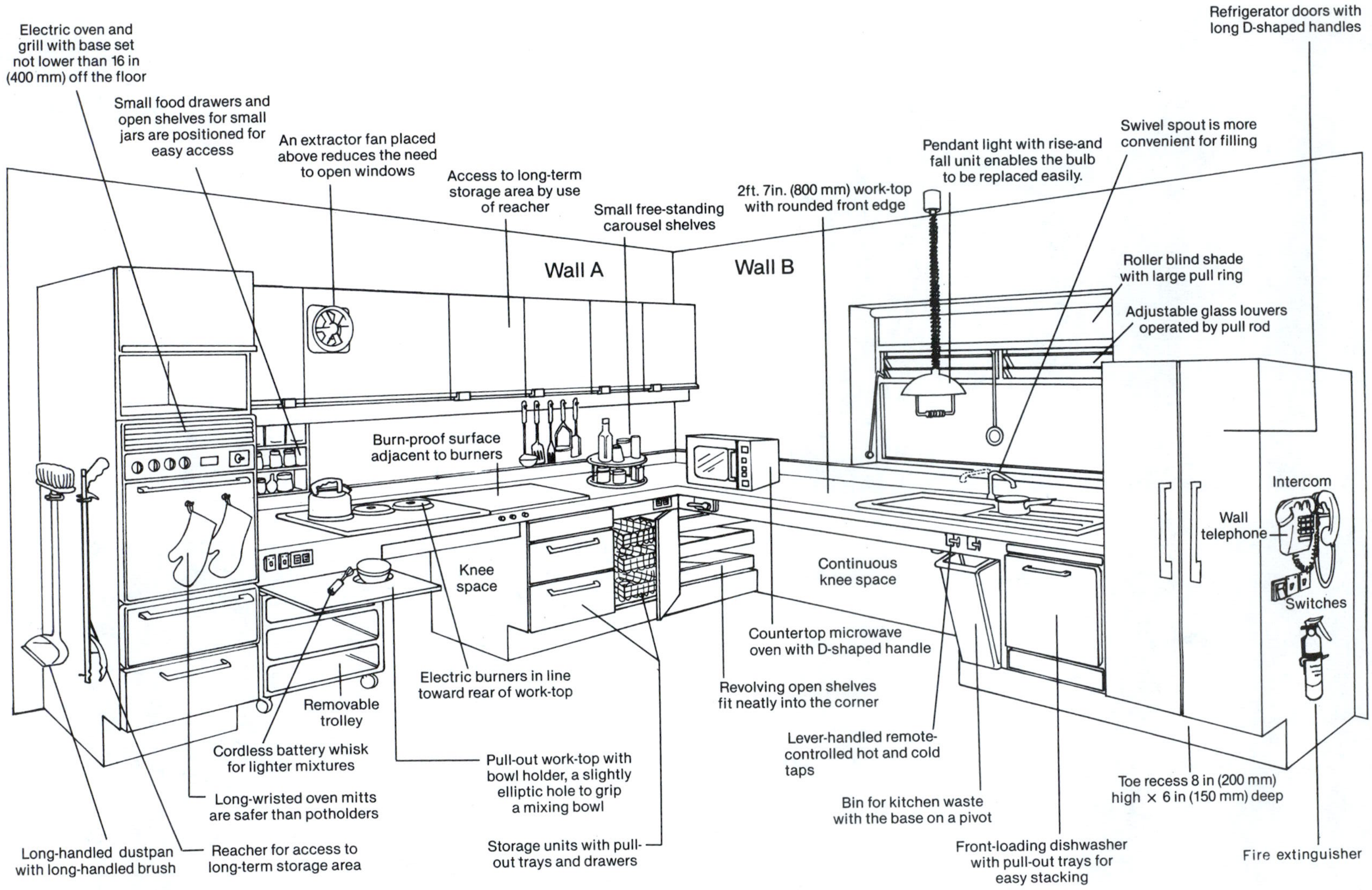

Figure 12.22 Sample features of a kitchen area that provides access for an individual using a wheelchair. (Adapted from Conran, T: The Kitchen Book, Mitchell Beazley, London, 1977, p 118, with permission.)

Table 12.2 **Adaptive Equipment and Compensatory Strategies for Selected Areas of ADL**

Impairment
One upper extremity or body side involvement.

Common Medical Diagnoses Associated with Impairment
Hemiplegia (cerebrovascular accident [CVA] or brain injury), unilateral trauma or amputation, temporary conditions such as burns and peripheral neuropathy.

Rationale for Using Compensatory Strategies
To allow for safe, one-handed performance: to stabilize objects for task completion; with hemiplegia, to compensate for loss of balance and mobility.

ADL Area	Adaptive Equipment	Adaptive Techniques
Meal preparation and cleanup	To stabilize objects, consider use of: • Adapted cutting board with stainless steel or aluminum nails for cutting or peeling. Raised corners on the board can stabilize bread to spread ingredients or make a sandwich. • Suction devices to stabilize bowls or dishes during food preparation. • Pot stabilizer. To allow for safe, one-handed performance: • Adapted jar openers. • Electric appliances such as food processor and hand mixer save time and energy. *Note:* patient safety and judgment need to be considered when electrical appliances are recommended. • Rocker knife. • Battery-operated whisk to mix food. To compensate for decreased standing tolerance and mobility, consider use of: • Utility cart to transport objects. • If cooking is done at wheelchair level or seated, use angled mirror over the stove to watch food on the stove. For cleanup, consider use of: • Hand-held spray for rinsing dishes. • Rubber mat at bottom of sink to reduce breakage. • Suction-type brush to clean glassware.	If balance is affected, it is recommended that the task be done in a seated position. • Pots and pans can be slid across counters, rather than lifted. • To open a jar, place it in a drawer, then lean against it to stabilize it before opening. • Scissors can be used to open plastic bags. • Milk cartons can be opened by using a fork. • An egg can be cracked by holding it in the palm of the hand, hitting the egg against the edge of the bowl, and separating the egg shell with the index and middle fingers. For clean-up: • Soak and air-dry dishes for easier clean-up.
Clothing management (laundry, ironing, clothing repair)	• Laundry can be transported to and from washer and dryer using a wheeled cart.	
Housecleaning	• Long-reach duster. • Long-handled dustpan and brush. • Self-wringing mop.	• Incorporate energy conservation by making bed completely at each corner before progressing to the next corner. • No-wax floors are easier to care for. • If balance problems are present, some floor care can be managed from a seated position.

(*continued*)

Table 12.2 Adaptive Equipment and Compensatory Strategies for Selected Areas of ADL (continued)

Impairment
Reduced upper-extremity range of motion and strength.

Common Medical Diagnoses Associated with Impairment
Spinal cord injury, burns, arthritis, upper-extremity amputation, multiple sclerosis, amyotrophic lateral sclerosis, orthopedic and other traumatic injuries.

Rationale for Using Compensatory Strategies
To compensate for lack of reach or hand grip; to compensate for lack of strength or tolerance for prolonged activity; to allow gravity to assist; to compensate for decreased balance.

ADL Area	Adaptive Equipment	Adaptive Techniques
Meal preparation and cleanup	Consider the use of: • Adapted jar opener. • Built-up handles on utensils. • Universal cuff to hold utensils to compensate for reduced grip. • Long-handled reacher to obtain lightweight objects from overhead or low places. • Wheeled cart to transport objects. • Adapted cutting board. • Loop handles can be added to utensils to substitute for reduced grasp. • If using a walker, a walker basket can help transport objects. For marketing: • Marketing by phone or computer is recommended (objects may be out of reach in store).	• Joint protective measures (rheumatoid arthritis). • Position electrical appliances within easy reach to conserve energy. • Also to conserve energy, work in a seated position. • Consider convenience foods to minimize food preparation. • Tenodesis action (wrist extension and finger flexion; wrist flexion and finger extension) can be used to pick up lightweight objects. • Use a fork to open milk cartons. • Use lightweight pots, pans, and utensils.
Housecleaning	• Long-handled reacher allows objects to be picked up from the floor. • Long-handled sponge to clean bath tub. • Self-wringing mop. • Use lightweight tools such as sponge mops and brooms for floor care.	• Use aerosol cleaners to dissolve dirt before cleaning surfaces. • When making the bed, do not tuck sheets in.
Laundry	• If patient is ambulatory, the preference is for a top-loading washer to avoid the need to bend. • Push-button controls on the washer and dryer are easier to use than knobs. If knobs are present, they may need to be adapted. • If patient chooses to iron, set iron at a low temperature setting. An asbestos pad can be placed at the end of the ironing board to eliminate the need to stand iron up after each ironing stroke.	• Use premeasured packages of soap or bleach to avoid handling large containers. It may be more economical to buy larger containers and have someone else measure soap or bleach into single packets. • Place hangers near dryer to hang permanent press items as they come out of the dryer. Remain seated to do ironing.

(continued)

Table 12.2 Adaptive Equipment and Compensatory Strategies for Selected Areas of ADL (continued)

Impairment
Incoordination of upper extremities.

Common Medical Diagnoses Associated with Impairment
Brain injury, cerebral palsy, CVA, multiple sclerosis, tumors, other neurological conditions.

Rationale for Using Compensatory Strategies
To stabilize proximal portion of limbs; to reduce movements distally by using weight; to stabilize objects for task completion; to provide an environment in which patient is safe and proficient; to avoid breakage or accidents with sharp utensils or hot food or equipment.

ADL Area	Adaptive Equipment	Adaptive Techniques
Meal preparation and cleanup	• Use pots and casseroles with double handles to provide greater stability. • Weighted wrist cuffs may reduce tremors. • Use adapted cutting board to stabilize food while cutting. • A serrated knife is less likely to slip than a straight-edged knife. • Free-standing appliances, electric skillet, microwave oven, and countertop mixer are safer than transferring objects out of oven or using hand-held mixer. • Use a milk carton holder with handles to pour milk. • A stove with front controls is preferred to eliminate reaching over hot pots to the back of the stove. • A wheeled cart that is weighted for transporting food. • Place a rubber mat or sponge cloth at the bottom of the sink to cushion fall of dishes.	• During food preparation such as cutting and peeling, stabilize arms proximally to reduce tremors. • Start the stove after the food has been placed on the burner. • Sliding food and dishes over a counter is preferable to lifting. • To avoid breakage, soak dishes, rinse with hand sprayer and drip dry; minimize dish handling.
Housecleaning	• Heavier work tools are useful. A dust mitt is easier to handle than gripping a duster. • Fitted sheets on a bed are recommended.	• Eliminate or store excess household decorations to reduce dusting.

(continued)

Table 12.2 Adaptive Equipment and Compensatory Strategies for Selected Areas of ADL (continued)

Impairment
Mobility limitations without upper extremity involvement.

Common Medical Diagnoses Associated with Impairment
Paraplegia, osteoarthritis, lower-extremity amputation, burns, leg and knee fractures.

Rationale for Using Compensatory Strategies
Mobility may be provided by a wheelchair. Wheelchair accessibility includes consideration of work heights, maneuverability, and access to storage, equipment, and supplies.
Other types of mobility devices (walker, crutches) may require increased endurance.

ADL Area	Adaptive Equipment	Adaptive Techniques
Meal preparation and cleanup	• Transport items using a wheelchair laptray. The laptray can be used as a work surface to protect lap from hot pans. • Stove controls should be in the front. • Use an angled mirror to see the contents of pots.	• Place frequently used items on easy-to-reach shelves, above and below counter-top level.
Laundry	• Use front-loading washer and dryer.	
Housekeeping	• Use self-propelled lightweight vacuums.	

Adapted from Culler,[51, p 371] with permission.

patient, family member(s) and/or caregiver(s), physical and occupational therapists, speech-language pathologist, and a rehabilitation engineer. Depending on the needs of the patient, other contributors may include a special education teacher, seating specialist, rehabilitation technology supplier, augmentative communication specialist, and medical social worker or funding specialist. Box 12.1 provides an overview of the general categories of ATs.

Environmental control units (ECUs) are an important example of how ATs can enhance function and improve independence. ECUs are electronic interfaces that allow the user to control a variety of appliances and devices (e.g., telephones, bed controls, various components of an entertainment unit, room temperature and lighting, open and close curtains, open doors). These devices combine operation of all appliances into a central control panel, providing increased independence for individuals with severe disability.

The three main components of an ECU include (1) the input device, (2) the control unit, and (3) the appliance. The *input device* controls the ECU using whatever voluntary movement the individual has available (e.g., joystick, control panel, keypad, keyboard [ECU computer software programs are available], a series of switches, touch pads and screens, light pen, optical pointers, and voice, mouthstick, and eye control). The *control unit* is the central processor that translates the input signal to an output signal to regulate the target appliance. The *appliance* can be virtually any device that can be controlled electronically.

Examination of the Workplace

An investigation of the workplace is an important component of a comprehensive examination of the environment. It is used to explore the *worker–job–environment relationship* and to determine the feasibility of returning to a former job or if reasonable accommodations will provide the needed support to resume work. The tests and measures used by physical therapists to examine the workplace fall into two broad categories: (1) *ergonomics,* which is the application of scientific and engineering principles to the worker–job–environment relationship to improve safety, efficiency, and quality of movement;[3] and (2) *body mechanics,* which is the interaction of muscles and joints in response to forces placed on or generated by the body.[3] Within the context of these two examination categories, Table 12.3 presents the tests and measures used by physical therapists together with the tools for gathering data, and the types of data generated.

Information Gathering

Job Analysis Interview

An initial component of the examination is a preliminary *job analysis interview.* The purpose of the interview is to gather information about (1) the functional requirements

Box 12.1 Categories of Assistive Technology

Aids for Daily Living: Aids or devices that enhance performance of ADL and level of independence in such activities as eating, meal preparation, dressing, personal hygiene, bathing, or household management. *Examples*: Grab bars, ramps, stair lifts, lowered counters, bathtub seats, adapted doorknobs, and alternative doorbells.

Augmentative Communication: Devices used to enhance personal expressive and receptive communication. *Examples*: Augmentative communication devices (electronic), bookholders, communication boards, electric page turners, headwands, mouthsticks, light pointers, reading machines, personal voice amplification, signal systems, and telephone adaptations.

Computer Applications: Hardware, software, and devices to enhance computer access. *Examples*: Modified, chording, expanded or alternate keyboards; voice recognition systems; alternate work stations (electrically powered height and tilt adjustments); Braille translation software (conversion from print and Braille); Braille printers; access aids (head-control sticks, light pointers, eye gaze input); alternative switches (minimal pressure, voice activated) and cursor (mouse) control; voice synthesizers, large print software that allows user to alter background and text colors; magnification screens, touch screens, on-screen keyboard, screen reader; keyguards, forearm supports; text-to-speech software; optical character recognition (OCR) system that scans written text to a computer and read by a speech synthesis/screen review system; and robotic wheelchair mounting to support a laptop computer.

Environmental Control Systems: Electronic systems that enhances ability to control various devices. *Examples*: Electronic control of appliances, lights, doors, and security systems in the home.

Hearing Technology: Devices designed to enhance receptive communication (assistive listening devices). *Examples*: Closed captioning, FM amplification systems (isolate and amplify a sound source), hearing aids, infrared amplification systems, personal amplification systems, TDDs/TTYs, television amplifiers, telephone adaptations, and visual and tactile alerting systems

Mobility Technology: Devices designed to provide an alternative means for walking or moving within the environment. *Examples*: Manual or powered wheelchairs; powered scooters; vehicle modification (driving adaptations, hand controls, wheelchair lifts); stair lifts; bus lifts; kneeling buses; and ambulatory assistive devices.

Seating and Positioning: Wheelchair (or other seating system) interventions to improve postural alignment, stability, head control and reduce skin pressure. *Examples*: Custom-molded seating surface, control blocks, pressure-relieving seat cushions, head and neck supports, adductor cushions, abductor pommel, lumbar supports, torso supports, and pelvic and foot positioners.

Vision Technology: Devices designed to enhance interaction with the environment for individuals with visual impairments. *Examples*: Talking devices (clocks, watches, calculators, thermometers, scales, hand-held spell checkers, dictionaries, and thesauruses), magnifiers, speech output devices, large-print screens, mini pocket tape recorders, voice-activated daily planners, large-button phone, large print books, magazines, and newspapers, closed circuit television to magnify documents, audio books, and books on disc (can be loaded onto a computer and read to user with a voice synthesizer).

of the job based on a review of duties and responsibilities and (2) the characteristics of the physical space in which the individual is required to work (job analysis will continue during the on-site visit). Interview questions are developed based on the type of employment (e.g., assembly work, food service tasks, motor vehicle operation, manual material handling, factory work). During the interview, the patient/client should be encouraged to provide detailed information about responsibilities and tasks performed while on duty (e.g., duration of performance, weight and distance of items lifted, carried or pulled, body positions used and so forth). A sample of suggested job analysis interview questions appropriate for a clerical position is presented in Table 12.4.

A **job analysis** provides the basis for accommodating individuals with disabilities. It typically includes a job function statement that identifies the overall purpose as well as a description of (1) the essential functions of a job and relative time spent on each; (2) the physical environment in which the essential functions are performed (e.g., indoors, outdoors, temperature fluctuations, noise levels); (3) the physical requirements (e.g., lifting, push/pull activities, bending, reaching); (4) the skills needed (cognitive processes, language, writing, or computer skills); and (5) the social context of the job (level of supervision, independent, contact with the public).

Job analyses provide a description of the job (not the potential employee). Generally, the analysis is preformed when a job is created to guide hiring of individuals with disabilities. (A sample job analysis form is presented in Appendix N.) The physical therapist may also be called on to analyze a patient/client's current job following the onset of disability to make recommendations for reasonable accommodations.

Functional Capacity Evaluation (FCE)

Typically, the most effective means of examining the patient/client–work environment interface is an on-site visit. However, a variety of standardized functional capacity evaluation (FCE) instruments are commercially available that

Table 12.3 Ergonomics and Body Mechanics: Tests and Measures, Tools Used for Gathering Data, and Data Generated.

Ergonomics is the relationship among the worker; the work that is done; the actions, tasks, or activities inherent in that work (job/school/play); and the environment in which the work (job/school/play) is performed. Ergonomics uses scientific and engineering principles to improve safety, efficiency, and quality of movement involved in work (job/school/play). Body mechanics are the interrelationships of the muscles and joints as they maintain or adjust posture in response to forces placed on or generated by the body. The physical therapist uses these tests and measures in examining both the worker and the work (job/school/play) environment and in determining the potential for trauma or repetitive stress injuries from inappropriate workplace design. These tests and measures may be conducted after a work injury or as a preventative step. The physical therapist may conduct tests and measures as part of work hardening or work conditioning programs and may use the results of tests and measures to develop such programs.

Tests and Measures	Tools Used for Gathering Data	Data Generated
Tests and measures may include those that characterize or quantify: Ergonomics • Dexterity and coordination during work (job/school/play) (e.g., hand function tests, impairment rating scales, manipulative ability tests) • Functional capacity and performance during work actions, tasks, or activities (e.g., accelerometry, dynamometry, electroneuromyography, endurance tests, force platform tests, goniometry, interviews, observations, photographic assessments, physical capacity tests, postural loading analyses, technology-assisted assessments, videographic assessments, work analyses) • Safety in work environments (e.g., hazard identification checklists, job severity indexes, lifting standards, risk assessment scales, standards for exposure limits) • Specific work conditions or activities (e.g., handling checklists, job simulations, lifting models, preemployment screenings, task analysis checklists, workstation checklists) • Tools, devices, equipment, and workstations related to work actions, tasks, or activities (e.g., observations, tool analysis checklists, vibration assessments) Body mechanics • Body mechanics during self-care, home management, work, community, or leisure actions, tasks, or activities (e.g., activities of daily living [ADL] and instrumental activities of daily living [IADL] scales, observations, photographic assessments, technology-assisted assessments, videographic assessments)	Tools for gathering data include: • Accelerometers • Cameras and photographs • Checklists for exposure standards, hazards, lifting standards • Dynamometers • Electroneuromyographs • Environmental tests • Force platforms • Functional capacity evaluations • Goniometers • Hand function tests • Indexes • Interviews • Muscle tests • Observations • Physical capacity and endurance tests • Postural loading tests • Questionnaires • Scales • Screenings • Technology-assisted analysis systems • Video cameras and videotapes • Work analyses	Data are used in providing documentation and may include: Ergonomics • Characterizations of efficiency and effectiveness of use of tools, devices, and workstations • Characterizations of environmental hazards, health risks, and safety risks • Descriptions of tools, devices, equipment, and workstations • Descriptions and quantification of: – abnormal movement patterns associated with work actions, tasks, or activities – dexterity and coordination – functional capacity – repetition and work/rest cycle in work actions, tasks or activities – work actions, tasks, or activities • Presence or absence of actual, potential, or repetitive trauma in the work environment Body Mechanics • Characterizations of abnormal or unsafe body mechanics • Descriptions and quantifications of limitations in self-care, home management, work, community, and leisure actions, tasks, or activities

From American Physical Therapy Association,[3, pp 70–71] with permission.

Table 12.4 Suggested Interview Questions Appropriate for a Clerical Position. Interview Questions Are Used to Gather General Data About Functional Requirements of the Job and the Physical Space In Which the Individual is Required to Work.

1.	Y N	Do you frequently lift more than 35 pounds?
2.	Y N	Are you required to lift objects from below knee level or above shoulder level on an occasional or frequent basis?
3.	Y N	When you lift, do you reach across other objects or at arms' length in order to accomplish the lift?
4.	Y N	Do you frequently reach for objects above shoulder level during the day?
5.	Y N	Do you sit for more than 4 hours per day?
6.	Y N	Does your job require you to maintain one position or posture for 30 to 60 minutes or longer at one time? If yes, what posture is it?________
7.	Y N	Are repetitive exertions required on a regular basis (e.g., typing)?
8.	Y N	Does your job require frequent motions of the fingers, wrists, elbows, or shoulders? (If yes, circle all that apply.)
9.	Y N	Do you feel that your desk height is at a comfortable level?
10.	Y N	a) Is your chair comfortable for you?
	Y N	b) Do you feel that it fits you properly?
	Y N	c) Do you know how to adjust your chair?
11.	Y N	Is there ample space for your to perform your job?
12.	Y N	Does your job involve frequent bending, twisting, or jerking movements?

From Hunter,[60, p 68] with permission.

can be used to gather preliminary data prior to an on-site visit. Depending on the job task requirements, the FCE may be all that is needed to determine ability to return to a previous job or to assume alternative job placement. The FCE provides a series of objective tests and measures designed to identify both work-related capabilities as well as functional limitations. Measurement parameters typically include endurance, ROM (flexibility), strength, force generation, posture, coordination, manual dexterity, and consistency of performance.[53–56]

The FCE is used to measure performance in specific components of work-related tasks. The specificity of the job will dictate the functional movements required. FCE instrument capabilities are then selected based on these requirements in order to examine the specific group of skills that comprise the employment tasks (e.g., lifting, stooping, trunk rotation, reaching). An example of a FCE instrument is the *ER Functional Testing System* (Baltimore Therapeutic Equipment [BTE] Co., Hanover, MD 21076-3105). This computer-integrated system (Fig. 12.23) allows replication of physical task demands using either standardized testing protocols or customized physical tests. A variety of tasks can be simulated including, but not limited to: lifting (Fig. 12.24), crouching, sitting, stoop-to-stand, and kneeling tolerance, overhead reaching, pushing (Fig. 12.25), carrying capacity, and pulling (Fig. 12.26). Other examples of physical work capacity instruments include the *Joule Functional Capacity Evaluation System* (Valpar International Corporation, Tucson, AZ 85703-5767), the *Physical Work Performance Evaluation (PWPE)* (Ergo Science, Inc, Birmingham, AL 35223), and the *Isernhagen Work Systems Functional Capacity Evaluation* (WorkWell Systems, Inc, Aliso, CA 92656).

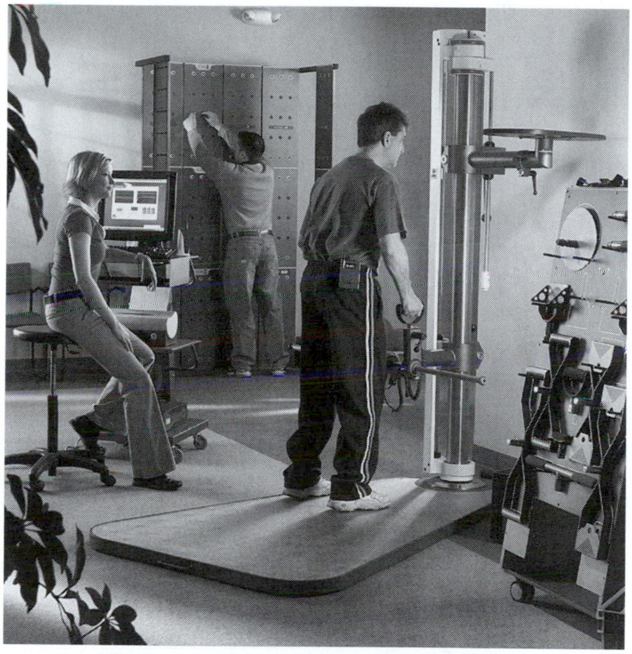

Figure 12.23 Functional Capacity Evaluation System. (Courtesy of BTE Technologies, Hanover, MD 21076.)

Software programs allow comparison of FCE data with normative values such as strength and ROM. Data can also be compared against the *demand minimum functional capacities (DMFC)* contained in the Dictionary of Occupational Titles (DOT)[57] which is a US government publication that defines physical demands of jobs in the United States.[58] Data from the FCE assist the physical therapist with:

- Predicting the individual's work capacity and ability to safely return to work.

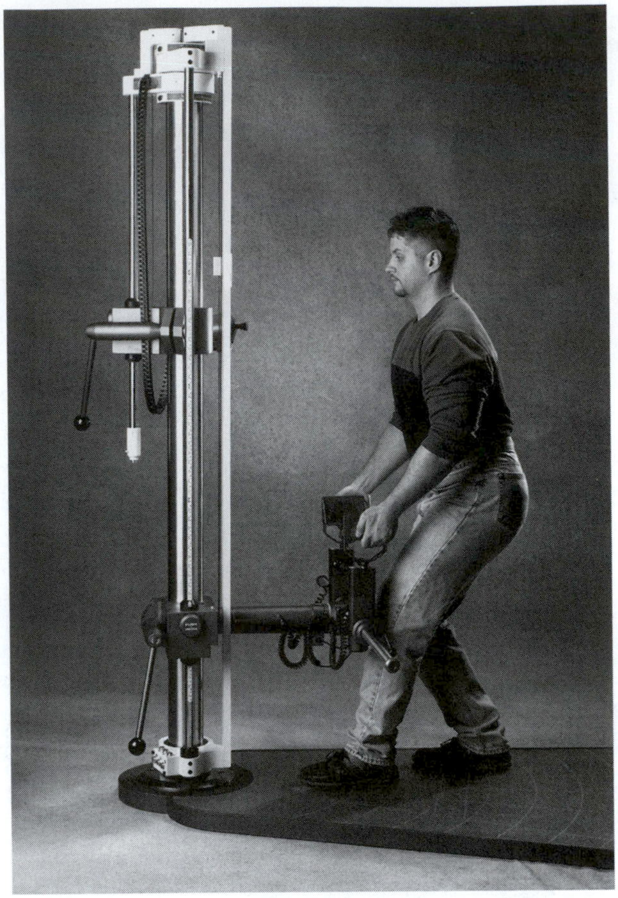

Figure 12.24 Dynamic lifting task. (Courtesy of BTE Technologies, Hanover, MD 21076.)

- Identifying parameters of the physical environment needed to optimize function and prevent further injury (reasonable accommodations).
- Identifying extent of functional limitations (e.g., compensation process).
- Matching abilities to appropriate job placement.
- Projecting potential benefits of a work hardening program.

Work Hardening

The term work hardening refers to treatment interventions aimed at improving worker capabilities and function. "*Work hardening* is a highly structured, goal-oriented, individualized intervention program designed to return the patient/client to work. Work hardening programs, which are multidisciplinary in nature, use real or simulated work activities designed to restore physical, behavioral, and vocational functions. Work hardening addresses the issues of productivity, safety, physical tolerances, and worker behaviors."[59, p 2] Work hardening programs typically involve progressive function-based exercise programs established from an analysis of work-related activities with careful attention to ergonomic and body mechanic principles. The anticipated goals and expected outcomes of work hardening programs are based on specific job requirements. Elements of the program may include (1) interventions to develop joint integrity and mobility, improve motor function, muscle performance (i.e., strength, power, endurance), ROM, and cardiovascular/pulmonary status; (2) guided practice and instruction in simulated work activities; (3) education (e.g., body mechanics, safety and injury prevention); and (4) promotion of self-management strategies.[59]

Work hardening products (Fig. 12.27) are commercially available that allow the therapist to progressively challenge the patient using simulated work activities such as lifting tasks using objects of different shapes and weight (Fig. 12.28A) to and from different heights, assembly tasks (Fig. 12.28B), sorting tasks, shoveling, pushing and pulling activities, use of table top- and wall-mounted work stations, and so forth.

On-Site Visit

Intervention in the workplace is an expanding area of interest within physical therapy.[60–73] The on-site visit to the workplace typically includes (1) further refinement of the job analysis by observation of the patient/client performing work tasks within the environment in which they must be accomplished and (2) application of ergonomic principles to identify the immediate or predicted risks of musculoskeletal injury for an individual worker. Data from the on-site visit will allow the therapist to establish a *plan for risk reduction* that provides recommendations to eliminate the potential for injury, and a *plan to optimize function* that may include suggestions for fitting the job to the patient/client's anatomical and physiological characteristics in a way that enhances efficiency and performance within the work environment.[61,62]

When examining level of function during an on-site visit to the work environment, the principles of energy conservation, ergonomics, body mechanics, and anthropometrics are of prime importance in prevention of injury and maximizing the worker's efficiency and comfort. Capabilities should be weighed against the physical demands of the work environment, and the therapist, using knowledge of adaptive equipment and applied biomechanics, may suggest changes appropriate to the situation.

Many of the areas examined, recommendations, and adaptive strategies employed in the home will be used in the work environment as well. Several considerations specific to the work setting are described below.

External Accessibility

A parking space should be available within a short distance of the building if the patient/client plans to drive to and from work. For wheelchair users, parking spaces should be a minimum of 96 in. (2440 mm) wide, with an adjacent access aisle 60 in. (1525 mm) wide (Fig. 12.29).[4] The location should be clearly marked as a reserved parking area.

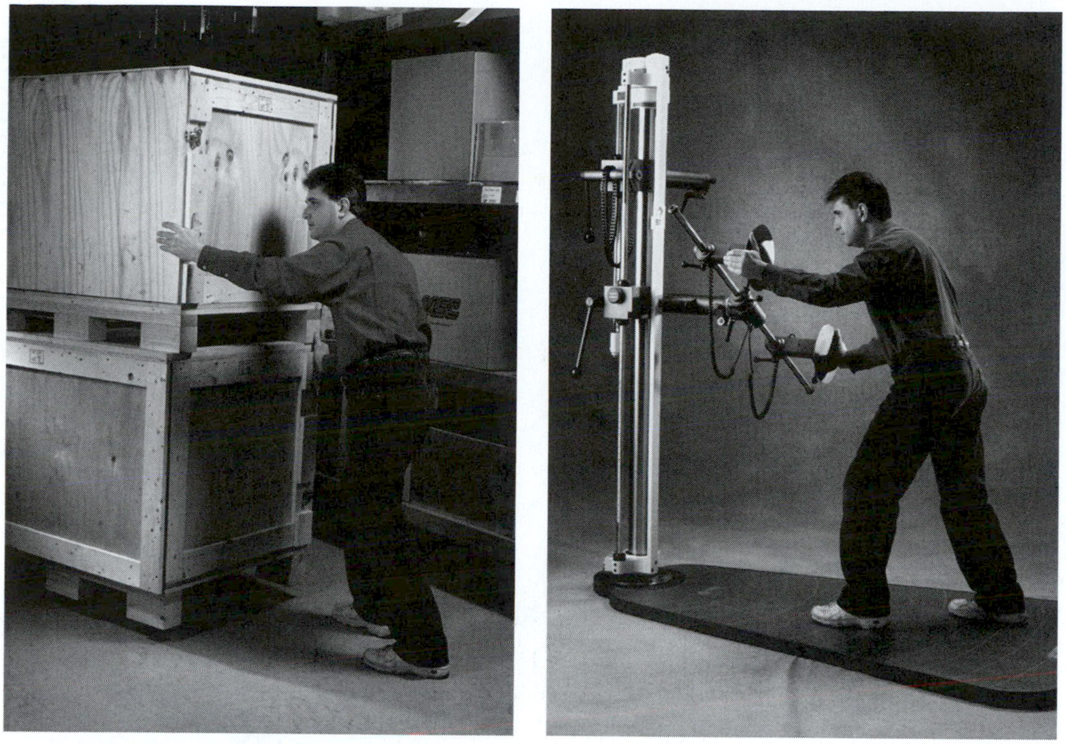

A B

Figure 12.25 Comparison of (*A*) actual and (*B*) simulated pushing activity. (Courtesy of BTE Technologies, Hanover, MD 21076.)

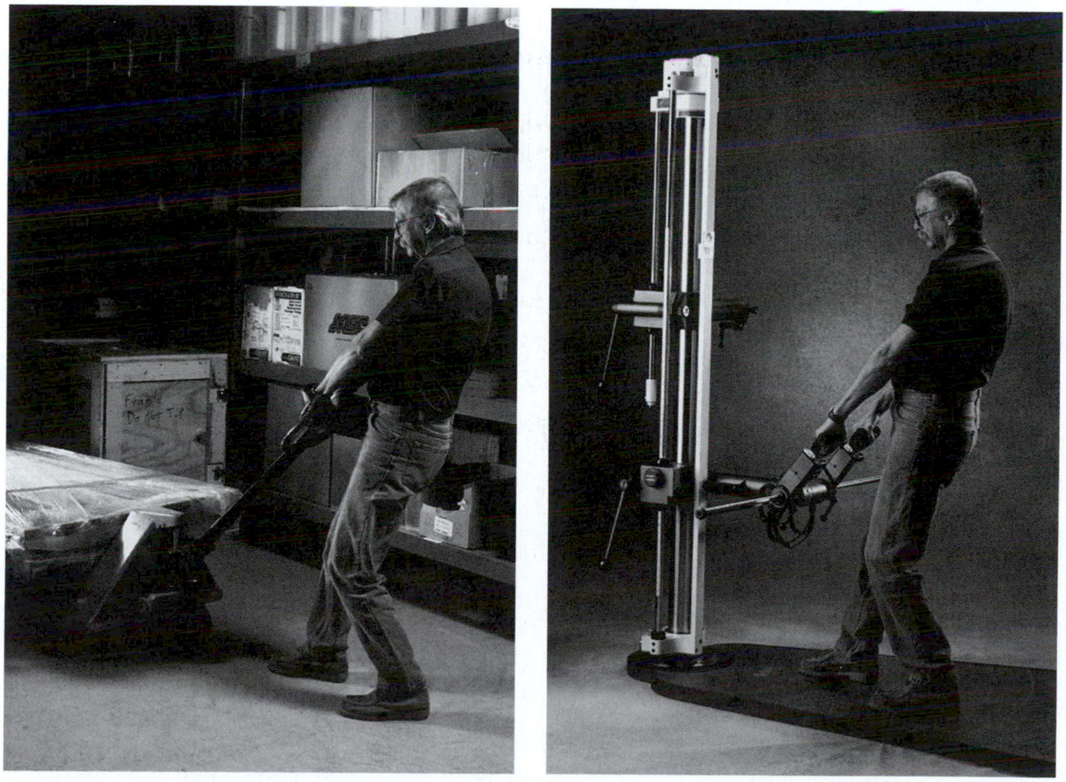

A B

Figure 12.26 Comparison of (*A*) actual and (*B*) simulated pulling activity. (Courtesy of BTE Technologies, Hanover, MD 21076.)

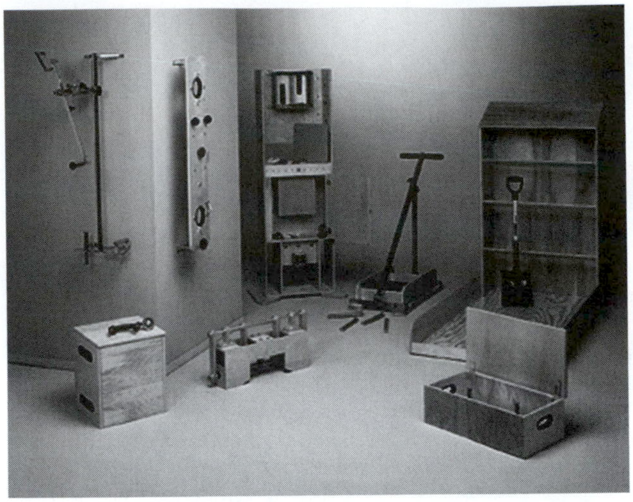

Figure 12.27 Work hardening equipment allows development of progressive therapeutic exercise (conditioning) programs based on simulation of a variety of tasks and assembly activities using sound ergonomic and body mechanic principles. (Courtesy of Bailey Mfg Co, Lodi, OH 44254.)

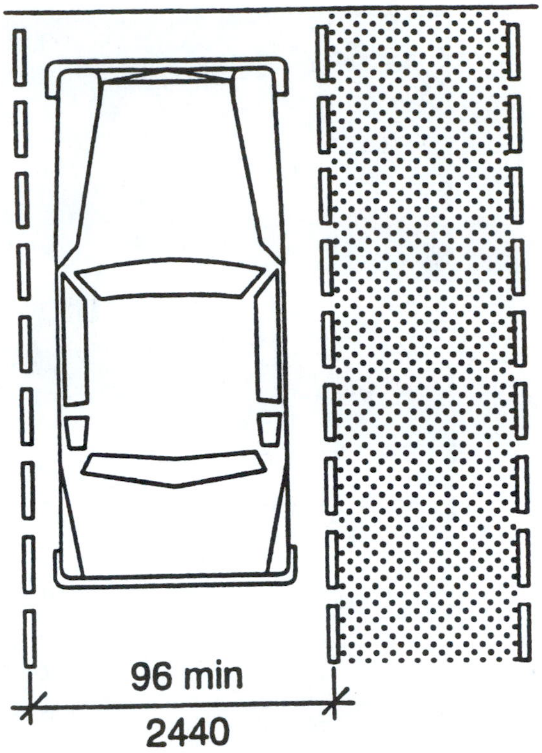

Figure 12.29 Vehicle parking spaces should be a minimum of 96 in. (2440 mm) wide, with an adjacent access aisle 60 in. (1525 mm) wide. Values denoted in inches and millimeters. (From American National Standards Institute, Inc,[4, p 33] with permission.)

External accessibility of the building should be addressed using guidelines similar to those presented for home exteriors.

Internal Accessibility

Initially, the component requirements of the work task are identified. The complexity of some tasks or the needed interface with the work environment may render the analysis of such tasks prior to the on-site visit inappropriate. This will include determination of mobility requirements (movement within and outside the primary work area), as well as determination of demands or skill required in each of the following areas: muscle performance including strength, power, and endurance (trunk, upper vs lower extremities), ROM, posture, manual dexterity, eye-hand coordination, vision, hearing, and communication.

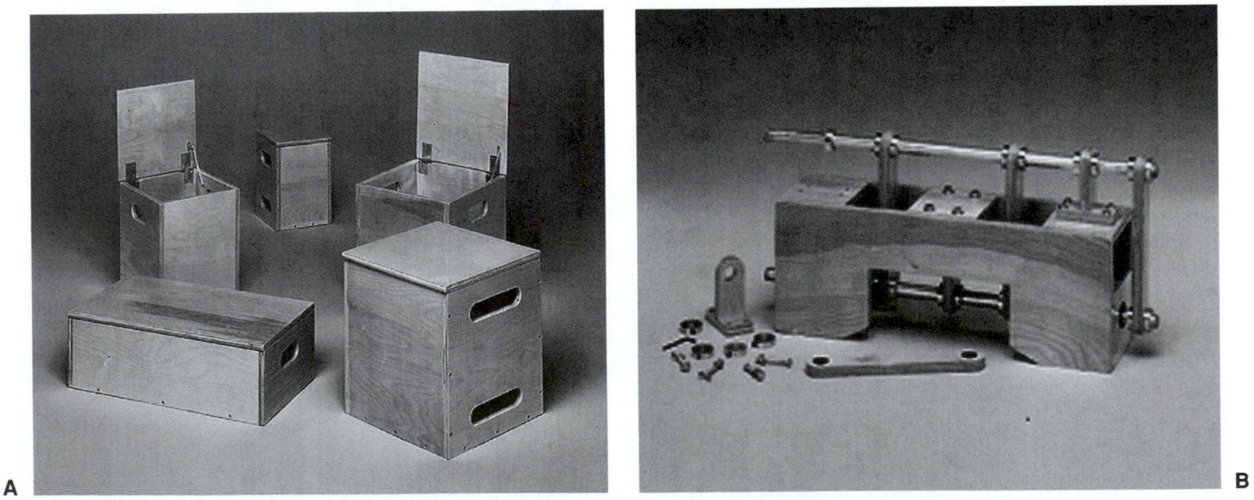

Figure 12.28 (*A*) Series of boxes of different shapes, sizes, and weights (progressively added) for lifting activities. (*B*) Table top unit includes bolts, washers, and nuts used for either manual or tool (e.g., use of a wrench) assembly. (Courtesy of Bailey Mfg Co, Lodi, OH 44254.)

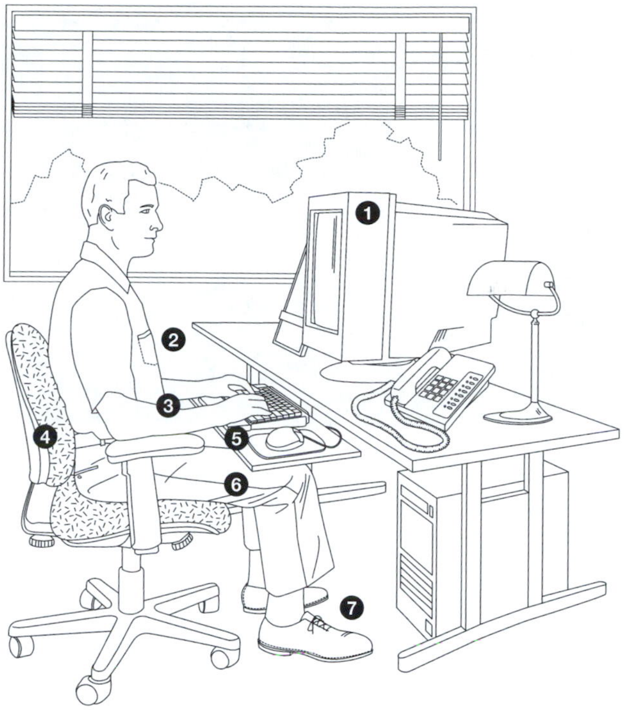

Figure 12.30 Overview of positioning recommendations for computer workstations: (1) monitor screen top slightly below eye level; (2) body centered in from of the monitor and keyboard; (3) forearms level or tilted-up slightly; (4) lower back supported by chair; (5) wrists free while typing; (6) thighs horizontal; and (7) feet resting flat on the floor. (From Workplace Ergonomics Reference Guide,[74, p 2] with permission.)

The immediate work area should be carefully examined. This includes lighting; temperature; seating surface (if other than a wheelchair); the height and size of the workstation (some patients may benefit from a variable height or tilting work surface); and exposure to noise, vibration, or fumes. Access to supplies, materials, or equipment should be considered with respect to the patient's vertical and horizontal reaching capabilities. Access to public telephones, drinking fountains, and bathrooms should also be addressed.

Owing to the prevalence of computer workstations in many employment settings, therapists may be called on to make recommendations to optimize efficiency and reduce the potential for trauma or repetitive stress injury from poorly designed work areas. Although individual patient parameters may require variations, the foundational principles for positioning at a computer workstation include screen slightly below eye level, body centered directly in front of monitor and keyboard, forearms level or tilted slightly upward, wrists free while typing, lower back well-supported, thighs horizontal on seating surface, and feet resting flat on the floor (Fig. 12.30).[74]

During examination of workstations for individuals using a wheelchair, functional sitting reach is an important

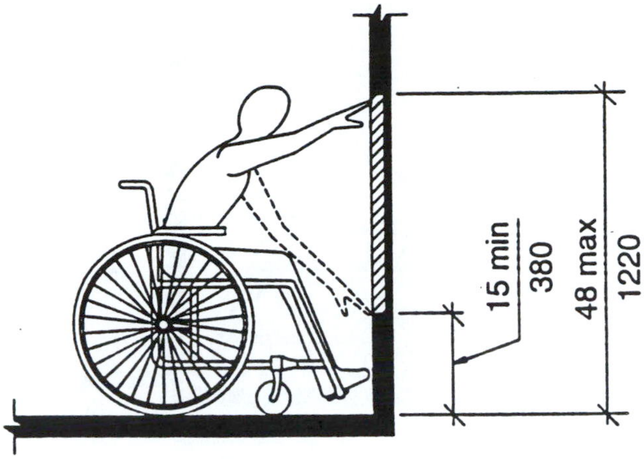

Figure 12.31 Unobstructed high forward reach is a maximum of 48 in. (1220 mm) from the floor and the low forward reach is a minimum of 15 in. (380 mm) from the floor. Values denoted in inches and millimeters. (From American National Standards Institute, Inc,[4, p 11] with permission.)

consideration. From an upright wheelchair sitting position, the unobstructed high forward reach is a maximum of 48 in. (1220 mm) from the floor and the low forward reach is a minimum of 15 in. (380 mm) from the floor (Fig. 12.31). When the high forward reach is over a work surface of not greater than 20 in. (510 mm), the maximum reach distance is 48 in. (1220 mm) from the floor (Fig. 12.32A). Progressively deeper work surfaces will alter the forward reach accordingly. For example, a work surface depth between 20 and 25 in. allows a maximum forward reach of not greater than 44 in. (1120 mm) from the floor (Fig. 12.32B).[4] For individuals with good trunk control, reaching capacity will be increased.

A variety of building survey forms have been developed to facilitate the on-site examination of the workplace. These forms assist with attending to all necessary details during the visit. A sample of such a form is provided in Appendix O.

Community Access

To attain the goal of full accessibility, the viability of community resources, services, and facilities must be investigated. As mentioned, when direct involvement by the therapist is not possible, this may best be accomplished by providing the support network members with guidelines for exploring access to local facilities.

Another important consideration is to refer the patient, family, and/or caregivers to community organizations such as the Arthritis Foundation, National Easter Seal Society, Multiple Sclerosis Society, the Mayor's Office, Chamber of Commerce, or the Veterans Administration. These groups can provide information on services available to individuals

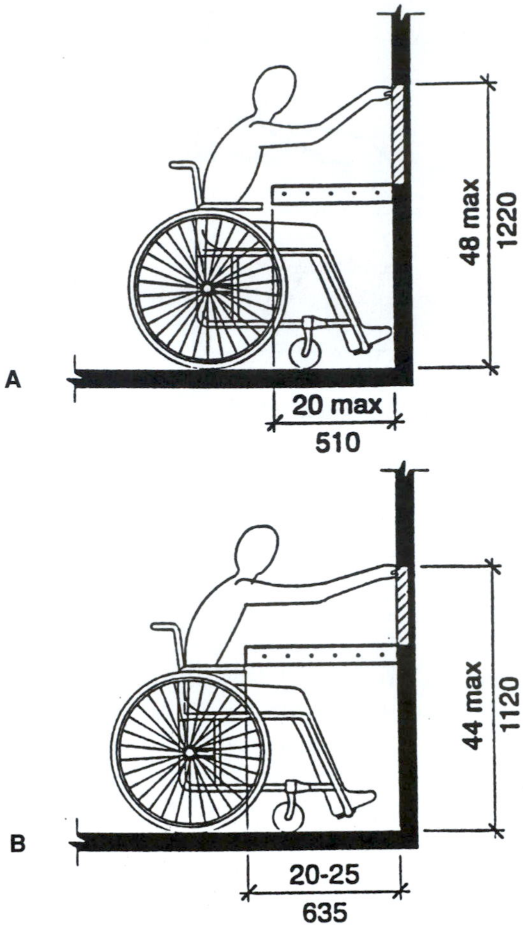

Figure 12.32 (*A*) High forward reach over a 20-in. (510 mm) deep work surface is a maximum of 48 in. (1220 mm) from the floor. (*B*) A work surface depth of 20 to 25 in. (510 to 635 mm) allows a maximum forward reach of not greater than 44 in. (1120 mm) from the floor. Values denoted in inches and millimeters. (From American National Standards Institute, Inc,[4, p 11] with permission.)

with a disability who reside in the community. Individuals who are returning to school should be encouraged to contact the campus student services office, which addresses the needs of students with disabilities. Information will be offered on housing, special services, and general campus resources.

Transportation

Currently the availability of accessible public transportation varies considerably among geographical areas. As such, careful exploration by the patient, family, and/or caregivers will be needed to determine what resources are obtainable in specific locales. Many communities provide at least part-time service of partially or completely accessible buses. These include the so-called kneeling buses equipped with a hydraulic unit that lowers

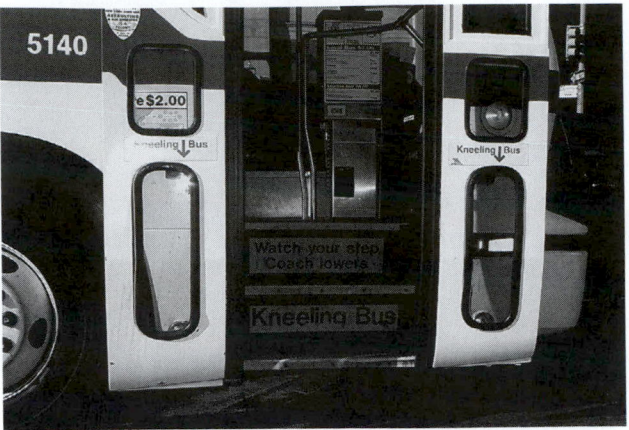

Figure 12.33 A kneeling bus lowers the steps to within 3 to 6 in. of the curb. Buses designed to kneel typically display a sign (Kneeling ↓ Bus) either on or next to the door.

the entrance to curb level for easier boarding (Fig. 12.33). Many buses are now designed with hydraulic lifts to allow direct entry by an individual using a wheelchair (Fig. 12.34).

Not all public transportation systems in the United States allow use by individuals who are nonambulatory or by those with limited ambulatory capacity. However, many urban transit systems are gradually making accommodations for individuals with mobility impairments (e.g., installation of elevators, alternatives to turnstile entrances, identified space for wheelchair riders). In many areas where public transportation is unavailable, door-to-door accessible van transportation is provided to residents with disabilities. Again, availability of such services may be limited in some rural locations.

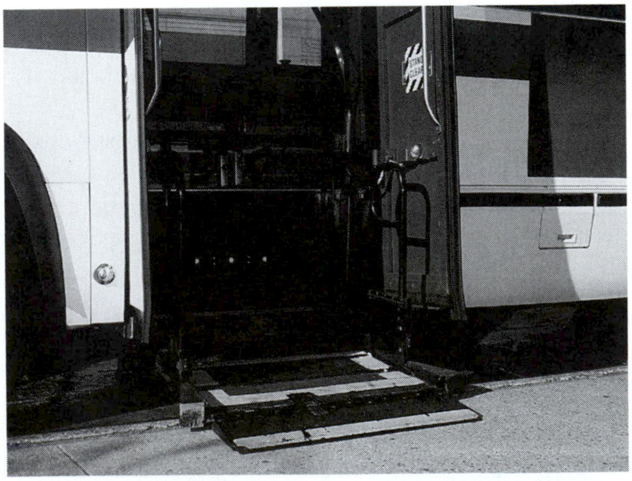

Figure 12.34 Bus lifts are able to accommodate wheelchairs and motorized scooters. The international wheelchair symbol for accessibility is typically displayed on the doors of the bus.

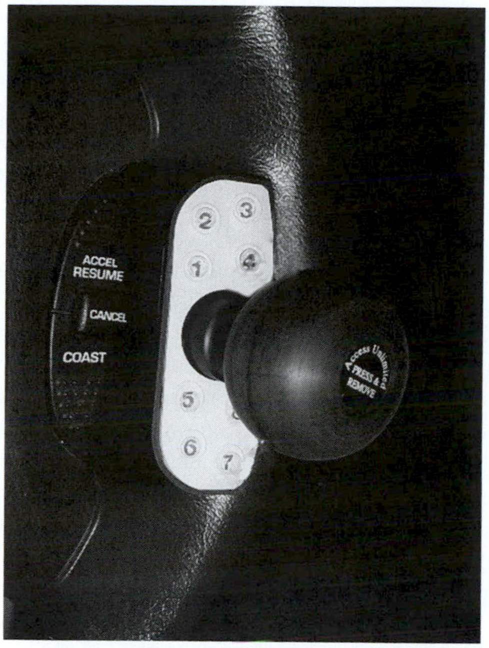

Figure 12.35 A steering wheel-mounted control pad can be used to control multiple vehicle controls such as windshield wipers, turn indicators, and high/low beams. (Courtesy of Access Unlimited, Binghamton, NY 13903.)

Some patients will want to master driving an adapted automobile or van. This, of course, will improve opportunities for community travel significantly. Motor vehicle adaptations are selected based on the physical capabilities of the individual. Common adaptive equipment includes hand controls to operate the brakes and the accelerator; steering wheel attachments, such as knobs or universal cuffs, for individuals with limited grip strength (Fig. 12.35); lifting units to assist with placement of the wheelchair into the vehicle; and, for patients with tetraplegia or high-level paraplegia, self-contained lifting platforms for entry to a van while remaining seated in a wheelchair. Driver training programs are offered by some rehabilitation centers.

For patients whose capacity for long-distance ambulation is limited and/or whose endurance is low, community-going electric "scooters" (Fig. 12.36) may be a practical alternative for travel within a reasonable proximity of the home.

Access to Community Facilities

Several considerations incorporated into examination of the workplace warrant attention for general community access, as well. Briefly stated, area facilities used by the patient should be explored for the availability of appropriate parking areas; beveled curbs; external and internal structural accessibility of buildings; and availability of accessible public telephones, drinking fountains, bathrooms, and restaurants. Theaters, auditoriums, and lecture halls must be considered with respect to accessible seating areas. Many such public presentation spaces are now designed with an accessible isle leading to open floor space interspersed within a row of standard seats to accommodate a wheelchair. This allows the individual using a wheelchair the option of either sitting next to a person who is ambulatory or someone using a wheelchair. Locations of emergency exits should also be noted for all facilities. In addition to these general considerations, stores and shopping areas should also be inspected for access to merchandise (especially for individuals using a wheelchair), appropriate aisle widths, and adequate space at checkout counters.

Another useful source of information on community access is the guidebook offered by many larger cities (funded as a community service by local businesses). These books provide information on accessibility of local cultural, civic, and religious institutions; government offices; theaters; hotels; restaurants; shopping areas; transportation; and social and recreational facilities. These publications usually can be obtained from the city's chamber of commerce, the mayor's office, or the office of tourism. Combined use of such guides and phoning ahead for details

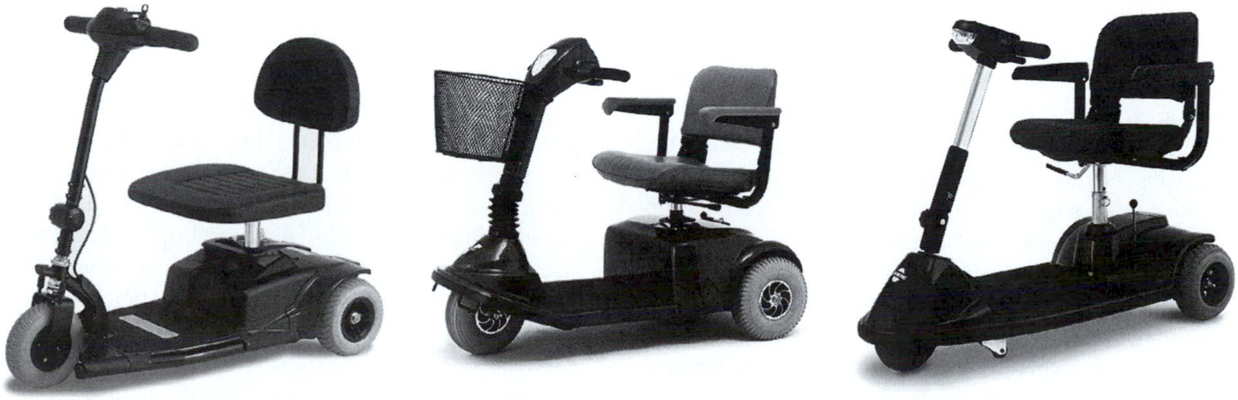

Figure 12.36 Examples of motorized scooters suitable for outdoor travel. (Courtesy of Pride Mobility Products, Corp, Exeter, PA 18643.)

of accessibility will facilitate travel both within and outside the local community.

Documentation

Once examination of the environment is complete, a final collaborative report is prepared that includes information from each participating team member. This report consists of information obtained from the home and, if applicable, the workplace or school setting. Information should also be included about the measures taken to explore general community accessibility.

Documentation of the on-site visit should incorporate a completed home or building survey form. Additional information that should be provided includes (1) a description of the methods used to assist the patient in ambulation or functional activities, (2) identification of the type and quantity of adaptive equipment required (including source and cost), (3) AT recommendations, and (4) suggested environmental modifications with precise specifications.

Documentation related to community access should include verification of the patient's knowledge of available community resources. The sources of this information, as well as whether the therapist was directly or indirectly involved in the community investigation, should be reported.

The completed report is then included as part of the patient's medical record. Copies of the report are typically submitted to the patient's support network, the physician, third-party payer(s) or other potential funding sources, and any community-based health care or social service agencies that will be providing care.

Funding for Environmental Modifications

The patient and support network may require assistance in locating appropriate financial resources to achieve environmental accessibility. Typically, the social worker within the patient care facility will provide direction in this area. Information on resource organizations can also be obtained from the National Council on Disabilities. Potential sources of funding include private medical insurance companies, home equity or other types of bank loans, Veterans Administration, the Division of Vocational Rehabilitation (DVR), the Worker's Compensation Commission, and local chapters of national groups (e.g., Kiwanis International, Veterans of Foreign Wars, Masons/Shriners Lodges, and Lions International) or diagnosis-specific organizations (e.g., National Stroke Association, National Multiple Sclerosis Society, National Parkinson Foundation).

An important consideration is that not all patients will have current housing that is amenable to modification (e.g., an individual who previously lived in a third-floor walk-up apartment and now uses a wheelchair). In such instances, the local Housing and Urban Development (HUD) Office will be an important resource. This office can provide a listing of accessible housing within the community. Because there are often waiting lists for such dwellings, early application is warranted.

Finally, creative funding for specific items (such as specialized adaptive equipment not covered by other resources) may be available through private organizations or foundations. Considerable time, research, and perseverance may be required in locating a receptive organization. General suggestions the patient, family, and/or caregiver(s) might consider in seeking assistance include contacting local businesses or corporate giving offices, civic or service clubs, churches or synagogues, labor unions, Jaycees, and the Knights of Columbus.

Legislation

Much attention has been focused on the importance of environmental accessibility. Through legislation and a variety of private organizations, significant strides have been made in this area. In 1990 the *Americans with Disabilities Act (ADA)* was signed into law. This legislation is among the most comprehensive of the civil rights laws enacted for individuals with disabilities. It guarantees civil rights protection and equal opportunity in the areas of government services, employment, public transportation, privately owned transportation available to the public, telephone service, and public accommodations.[75] This law requires that all "public places of accommodation" be made accessible to people with a disability unless it imposes "undue hardship" to the establishment. This law specifies that reasonable accommodations be made by restaurants, movie theaters, hotels, professional offices, retail stores, and so forth.

With respect to an individual, disability is defined in the ADA as "a physical or mental impairment that substantially limits one or more major life activities of such an individual; a record of such impairment; or being regarded as having such impairment."[75, p 4] Undue hardship includes excessive direct cost of adapting the environment, limited resources of the establishment, or situations where these changes would fundamentally alter the nature or daily operation of a business. Connolly[76] suggests that the cost of changes cannot be used as a defense during litigation unless the financial burden would threaten the very existence of the business. The ADA also provides a federal tax credit incentive for measures taken by businesses to comply with this law.

The *Fair Housing Act*, as amended in 1988, prohibits discrimination in housing on the basis of race, color, religion, gender, disability, familial status, and national origin. The act includes private housing, state and local government housing, as well as any housing that receives federal financial support. It requires landlords to allow individuals with disabilities to make reasonable, access-related modifications to their living space, as well as common areas of the building. However, the landlord is not required to pay for these modifications. The Fair Housing Act also provides accessible construction standards for multifamily housing units built for first occupancy after March, 1991.

The *Rehabilitation Act of 1973* provided that access must be established in all federally funded buildings and transportation facilities constructed after 1968. The law prohibits discrimination in federal employment, stipulates accessibility within federal buildings, and established the Architectural Transportation Barriers and Compliance Board. Because many federally funded institutions provided low compliance with the 1973 Rehabilitation Act, an amendment was passed in 1978. The Comprehensive Rehabilitation Services Amendments (P.L. 95-602) of 1978 strengthened the enforcement of the original 1973 Rehabilitation Act. The Architectural and Transportation Barriers Compliance Board is the governing body responsible for enforcing this legislation.

The *Architectural Barrier Act of 1968* (P.L. 90-480) provided that certain buildings that were financed by federal funds be designed and constructed "to insure that physically handicapped persons will have ready access to, and use of, such buildings."[77, p 719] Another important item of legislation related to environmental accessibility is the Public Buildings Act of 1983, which functioned to establish public building policies for the federal government. This act (section 307) provided several amendments to the Architectural Barrier Act of 1968 to further strengthen and delineate the importance of accessibility. The term *fully accessible* in this act was defined as "the absence or elimination of physical and communications barriers to the ingress, egress, movement within, and use of a building by handicapped persons and the incorporation of such equipment as is necessary to provide such ingress, egress, movement, and use and, in a building of historic, architectural, or cultural significance, the elimination of such barriers and the incorporation of such equipment in such a manner as to be compatible with the significant architectural features of the building to the maximum extent possible."[78, p 373]

Despite the recent gains made in architectural accessibility, barriers continue to exist. Inasmuch as most public transportation systems were built before 1968, accessibility is not required by law. However, the ADA indicates that all concerns that offer public transit along a fixed route must also provide buses that are accessible to individuals with disabilities, including access by wheelchairs. Other areas that continue to be problematic include revolving doors, the design of many supermarkets and shopping areas (barriers imposed by checkout areas and items displayed on high shelves), lack of available parking spaces, multiple levels of stairs at the entrance to some buildings, and the design of some theaters and auditoriums that do not have specifically designated areas for individuals using a wheelchair.

The ADA homepage (http://www.ada.gov) provides a rich resource for information related to accessibility, planning of new construction, guidelines for modification of existing facilities, and answers to frequently asked questions about federal accessibility requirements. An ADA information line (800.514.0301 [voice] 800.514.0383 [TDD]), provides technical assistance on accessibility standards and a 24-hour automated service for ordering ADA material. Also available is the ADA video gallery and an ADA Technical Assistance CD-ROM that includes regulations, design standards, and technical assistance.

Although increasing numbers of buildings are being designed to provide accessibility, this area warrants further involvement from therapists. Physical therapists can be effective advocates and are equipped to provide a leadership role in compliance with existing and new laws. They have important knowledge and skills to enable them to provide valuable input into the initial planning and/or modification of barrier-free designs.

Summary

Examination of the environment is an important factor in facilitating the patient's transition to the home, work, and community. The rehabilitation team uses the data to determine the level of patient access, safety, and function within the environment. The information is also used to determine the need for additional treatment interventions, ATs, environmental modifications, outpatient services, and adaptive equipment. In addition, the examination assists in preparing the patient, family, caregivers, and/or work colleagues and employer for the individual's return to a given setting.

This chapter has presented a sample approach to examination of the environment. Common environmental features that typically warrant consideration have been highlighted. Inasmuch as a return to a former environment is often a primary goal of rehabilitation, early consideration of these issues is warranted. Collaboration among team members, the patient, family, and/or caregivers will ensure an optimum and highly individualized patient–environment interface.

Questions for Review

1. Identify the roles and responsibilities of the physical therapist in examination of the physical environment.
2. Discuss examples of the tests and measures; tools used for gathering data; and data generated during examination of environmental, home, and work barriers.
3. In lieu of an on-site visit to a patient's home, discuss alternative approaches to gathering information about the patient's environment.
4. Develop a list of information you would need to acquire prior to an actual on-site visit to a patient's home environment.
5. Provide examples of how the principles of universal design can be incorporated into new construction.
6. What specific aspects of the *exterior* of a patient's home should be examined during an on-site visit? Your response should address the route to the entrance and actual entrance to the home.
7. What specific aspects of the *interior* of a patient's home should be examined during an on-site visit? Your response should address furniture arrangement, floor surfaces, doors, stairs, and considerations specific to the bedroom, bathroom, and kitchen areas of the dwelling.
8. Discuss how a job analysis can promote accommodating individuals with disabilities within the work environment.
9. What civil rights of individuals with disabilities are protected by the 1990 Americans with Disabilities Act?
10. Describe the information that should be included in documentation of an on-site environmental examination.

Case Study

A 78-year-old woman with a diagnosis of osteoarthritis was admitted for a right total hip replacement. The patient reported a long-standing history of discomfort. She described the hip pain as radiating posteriorly to the buttock and low back and was exacerbated by weight-bearing and stair climbing. Over the past 12 months she has experienced a very marked increase in pain and stiffness. Radiographic findings demonstrated degenerative changes of both the acetabulum and femoral head consistent with osteoarthritis. The surgical intervention replaced the right femoral head and neck with a metallic prosthesis and the acetabulum was resurfaced with a plastic cup. Past medical history is unremarkable.

SOCIAL HISTORY

The patient is a retired manager of a small accounting firm that she and her husband established. Her husband is deceased. She has three grown children who all live in neighboring communities. Prior to the functional limitations imposed by the hip pain, the patient had been independent in all BADL and IADL. She also volunteered her accounting services one day per week to a local charity which provides meals to homebound individuals, she was a regular participant in family outings, enjoyed going to the theater, concerts, and special museum events, and was an active member of the community historical preservation society. Recently, these activities had to be curtailed owing to the increased hip discomfort.

She essentially had no activities outside the home for 3 months prior to admission and used a walker to minimize weightbearing and reduce pain. She also required the assistance of a home care aide 4 hours a day two times per week (primarily for shopping, errands, and some household management tasks). She expressed considerable distress at being unable to take a bath and having to rely on the assistance of another person for some basic care activities. She had been using aspirin for its analgesic and anti-inflammatory effects. However, the pain experienced in recent months was not alleviated by the aspirin and other conservative measures she has been instructed to use (e.g., local applications of heat, periodic rest intervals, and gentle ROM exercises). The patient has medical insurance coverage and is without financial concerns.

REVIEW OF SYSTEMS

Cognitive function: Intact.

Vision: Wears corrective lens; experiences night blindness, which she describes as seeing poorly in dim light and her eyes take several seconds longer than normal to adjust from brightness to dimness.

Hearing: Intact.

Strength:

Upper extremities

Generally within functional limits; patient reports some sporadic episodes of wrist and finger stiffness on awakening in the morning and after periods of immobility. Grip strength is reduced bilaterally (MMT of finger flexors = G–). Heberden's nodes noted at the DIP and PIP joints of the left index finger. Patient denies pain in wrist or fingers.

Lower extremities

Left: within functional limits.

Right: within functional limits (hip motions not tested owing to surgical intervention); crepitus noted in right knee.

Weightbearing status on right lower extremity: partial weightbearing

Range of Motion:
Within functional limits (with the exception of the right hip, which was not tested)

Postsurgical Right Hip Precautions:
No hip flexion beyond 90°.
Avoid crossing one leg or ankle over the other.
Avoid internal rotation of right lower extremity.

Coordination: Within normal limits.
Sensation: Intact.
Gait:
The patient is ambulating on level surfaces with supervision using bilateral standard aluminum axillary crutches with partial weightbearing on the right lower extremity. Stair climbing also requires minimal assistance. It is anticipated the patient will be independent with household ambulation on level surfaces at time of discharge from the hospital.

PATIENT GOALS

The patient is extremely motivated to be independent in her personal care and household management. The prosthetic replacement has successfully relieved much of the pain experienced in the hip prior to surgery (most of her current discomfort is described as "minor" and associated with the surgical incision). She would also like to return to her family, volunteer, social, and leisure activities. She is very determined to discontinue the home care assistance as soon as possible.

HOME ENVIRONMENT

The patient lives alone in a fifth floor apartment in a building with an elevator. The living space is a one-bedroom apartment on a single level. At your request, one of the patient's children has provided dimensions of door frames and height of sleeping and seating surfaces together with several photographs of each room of the patient's home. The physical dimensions and photographs indicate the following:

- Bedroom: two small area rugs, a nightstand with an alarm clock, a bureau, a wooden platform bed with a sleeping surface 1 1/2 feet from the floor, and a ceiling lamp fixture controlled by a switch adjacent to the door.
- Bathroom: an area rug, standard toilet and sink, bathtub does not include a shower, a doorway entrance 30 in. wide.
- Kitchen: polished linoleum floors, adequate counter space, and a dining table in the center of the room.
- Living room: overstuffed upholstered furniture with low seating surfaces, a large carpet that appears to ripple in several areas, a centered coffee table, a telephone with an extra-long extension wire placed on the coffee table, a manual control television, two end tables and a bookcase.
- Hallway (between rooms): poorly lit with a long, narrow area rug.

GUIDING QUESTIONS

With general knowledge of the patient's living space, what environmental modifications, adaptive equipment, or additional instruction would you suggest or provide to optimize safety and function in each of the following areas of the home?

1. Bedroom
2. Bathroom
3. Kitchen
4. Living room
5. Hallway

References

1. Corcoran, M, and Gitlin, L: The role of the physical environment in occupational performance. In Christiansen, CH, and Baum, CM (eds): Occupational Therapy Enabling Function and Well-Being, ed 2. Slack, Thorofare, NJ, 1997, p 336.
2. Lawton, MP, et al: Assessing environments for older people with chronic illness. J Ment Health Aging 3:83, 1997.
3. American Physical Therapy Association: Guide to physical therapist practice, ed 2. Phys Ther 81:1, 2001.
4. American National Standards Institute, Inc: American National Standard: Accessible and Usable Buildings and Facilities (ICC/ANSI A117.1-1998). International Code Council, Inc, Falls Church, VA, 1998.
5. ADA Standards for Accessible Design (28 CFR Part 36). US Department of Justice, Revised, July 1, 1994. Retrieved September 15, 2005 from http://www.usdoj.gov/crt/ada/stdspdf.htm
6. Mace, R: About Universal Design: What Is Universal Design? NC State University, The Center for Universal Design, an initiative of the College of Design, 1997, p 1. Retrieved September 15, 2005 from http://www.design.ncsu.edu/cud/index.html.
7. Ostroff, E: Universal design: The new paradigm. In Preiser, W, and Ostroff, E (eds): Universal Design Handbook. McGraw-Hill, New York, 2001, p 1.3.
8. Riley, CA: High-Access Home: Design and Decoration for Barrier-Free Living. Rizzoli International Publications, New York, 1999.
9. Mace, RL: Universal design in housing. Asst Technol 10(1):21, 1998.
10. Levine, D (ed): Universal Design: New York. The City of New York, Mayor's Office for People with Disabilities. Center for the Inclusive Design and Environmental Access, University of Buffalo, The State University of New York, 2003.
11. Sanford, JA, et al: Using telerehabilitation to identify home modification needs. Assist Technol 16(1):43, 2004.
12. Duncan, PW, et al: Functional reach: Predictive validity in a sample of elderly male veterans. J Gerontol 47(3):M93, 1992.
13. Mathias, S, Nayak, US, and Isaacs, B: Balance in elderly patients: The "Get Up and Go" test. Arch Phys Med Rehabil 67(6):387, 1986.

14. Guralnik, JM, et al: A short physical performance battery assessing lower extremity function: Association with self-reported disability and prediction of mortality and nursing home admission. J Gerontol 49(2):M85, 1994.
15. Keith, RA, et al: The functional independence measure: A new tool for rehabilitation. Adv Clin Rehabil 1:6, 1987.
16. Brooks, D, et al: Reliability of the two-minute walk test in individuals with transtibial amputation. Arch Phys Med Rehabil 83(11): 1562, 2002.
17. Hamilton, DM, and Haennel, RG: Validity and reliability of the 6-minute walk test in a cardiac rehabilitation population. J Cardiopulm Rehabil 20(3):156, 2000.
18. ATS Committee on Proficiency Standards for Clinical Pulmonary Function Laboratories: ATS statement: Guidelines for the six-minute walk test. Am J Respir Crit Care Med 166(1):111, 2002.
19. Kervio, G, Carre, F, and Ville, NS: Reliability and intensity of the six-minute walk test in healthy elderly subjects. Med Sci Sports Exerc 35(1):169, 2003.
20. Solway, S, et al: A qualitative systematic overview of the measurement properties of functional walk tests used in the cardiorespiratory domain. Chest 119(1): 256, 2001.
21. Gibbons, WJ, et al: Reference values for a multiple repetition 6-minute walk test in healthy adults older than 20 years. J Cardiopulm Rehabil 21(2):87, 2001.
22. Berg, KO, et al: Measuring balance in the elderly: Validation of an instrument. Can J Public Health 83(Suppl 2):S7,1992.
23. Steffen, TM, Hacker, TA, and Mollinger, L: Age- and gender-related test performance in community-dwelling elderly people: Six-Minute Walk Test, Berg Balance Scale, Timed Up & Go Test, and gait speeds. Phys Ther 82(2):128, 2002.
24. Lee, RE, et al: The Physical Activity Resource Assessment (PARA) instrument: Evaluating features, amenities and incivilities of physical activity resources in urban neighborhoods. Int J Behav Nutr Phys Act 2(1):13, 2005.
25. Keysor, J, Jette A, and Haley, S: Development of the home and community environment (HACE) instrument. J Rehabil Med 37(1):37, 2005.
26. Oliver, R, et al: Development of the Safety Assessment of Function and the Environment for Rehabilitation (SAFER) tool. Can J Occup Ther 60(2):78, 1993.
27. Fänge, A, and Iwarsson, S: Changes in accessibility and usability in housing: An exploration of the housing adaptation process. Occup Ther Int 12(1):44, 2005.
28. Fänge, A, and Iwarsson, S: Changes in ADL dependence and aspects of usability following housing adaptation—a longitudinal perspective. Am J Occup Ther 59(3):296, 2005.
29. Fänge, A, and Iwarsson, S: Accessibility and usability in housing: Construct validity and implications for research and practice. Disabil Rehabil 25(23):1316, 2003.
30. Fänge, A, and Iwarsson, S: Physical housing environment: Development of a self-assessment instrument. Can J Occup Ther 66(5):250, 1999.
31. Shumway-Cook, A, et al: Assessing environmentally determined mobility disability: Self-report versus observed community mobility. J Am Geriatr Soc 53(4):700, 2005.
32. Shumway-Cook, A, et al: Environmental components of mobility disability in community-living older persons. J Am Geriatr Soc 51(3):393, 2003.
33. Whiteneck, GG, et al: Quantifying handicap: A new measure of long-term rehabilitation outcomes. Arch Phys Med Rehabil 73(6):519, 1992.
34. Whiteneck, G, et al: Environmental factors and their role in participation and life satisfaction after spinal cord injury. Arch Phys Med Rehabil 85(11):1793, 2004.
35. Whiteneck, GG, Gerhart, KA, and Cusick, CP: Identifying environmental factors that influence the outcomes of people with traumatic brain injury. J Head Trauma Rehabil 19(3):191, 2004.
36. Whiteneck, GG, et al: Quantifying environmental factors: A measure of physical, attitudinal, service, productivity, and policy barriers. Arch Phys Med Rehabil 85(8):1324, 2004.
37. Åsberg, KH, and Sonn, U: The cumulative structure of personal and instrumental ADL in the elderly: A study of elderly people in a health service district. Scand J Rehab Med 21(4):171, 1989.
38. Sonn, U, and Åsberg, KH: Assessment of activities of daily living: A study of a population of 76-year-olds in Gothenburg, Sweden. Scand J Rehab Med 23(4):193, 1991.
39. Katz, S, et al: Studies of illness of the aged. The Index of ADL: A standardized measure of biological and psychosocial function. JAMA (Sept 21)185:914, 1963.
40. Sonn, U, Grimby, G, and Svanborg, A: Activities of daily living studied longitudinally between 70 and 76 years of age. Disabil Rehabil 18(2):91, 1996.
41. Sonn, U: Longitudinal studies of dependence in daily life activities among elderly persons. Scand J Rehab Med 34:1 (Suppl 34), 1996.
42. Sonn, U, and Svensson, E: Measures of individual and group changes in ordered categorical data: Application to the ADL Staircase. Scand J Rehabil Med 29(4):233, 1997.
43. Danford, GS, and Steinfeld, E: User's Guide for the Environmental Functional Independence Measure (Enviro-FIM™). Center for Inclusive Design and Environmental Access, School of Architecture and Planning, State University of New York at Buffalo, Buffalo, NY 14214, 2001.
44. Granger, CV, et al: Advances in functional assessment for rehabilitation. Top Geriatr Rehabil 1:59, 1986.
45. Danford, GS, and Steinfeld, E: User's Guide for the Functional Performance Measure (FPM™): Level of Effort Scale (LES™) and Level of Assistance Scale (LAS™). Center for Inclusive Design and Environmental Access, School of Architecture and Planning, State University of New York at Buffalo, Buffalo, NY, 14214, 2001.
46. Danford, GS, and Steinfeld, E: User's Guide for the Environmental Utility Measure (EUM™): Difficulty Rating Scale (DRS™) and Acceptability Rating Scale (ARS™). Center for Inclusive Design and Environmental Access, School of Architecture and Planning, State University of New York at Buffalo, Buffalo, NY, 14214, 2001.
47. Pitrella, F, and Kappler, W: Identification and Evaluation of Scale Design Principles in the Development of the Extended Range Sequential Judgment Scale. Research Institute for Human Engineering, Wachtberg, Germany, 1988.
48. Building Design Requirements for the Physically Handicapped, Revised Edition. Eastern Paralyzed Veterans Association, New York, undated.
49. Beaver, KA, and Mann, WC: Overview of technology for low vision. Am J Occup Ther 49:913, 1995.
50. Gitlin, LN, et al: Factors associated with home environmental problems among community-living older people. Disabil Rehabil 23(17):777, 2001.
51. Culler, KH: Treatment for work and productive activities: Home and family management. In Neistadt, ME, and Crepeau, EB (eds): Willard & Spackman's Occupational Therapy, ed 9. Lippincott-Raven, Philadelphia, 1998, p 369.
52. Technology-Related Assistance for Individuals with Disabilities Act of 1988 as Amended in 1994 (Public Laws 100-407 and 103-218). Retrieved October 7, 2005 from http://www.resna.org/taproject/library/laws/techact94.htm.
53. Hart, DL, Isernhagen, SJ, and Matheson, LN: Guidelines for functional capacity evaluation of people with medical conditions. J Orthop Sports Phys Ther 18(6):682, 1993.
54. Gibson, L, and Strong, J: A conceptual framework of functional capacity evaluation for occupational therapy in work rehabilitation. Austral Occup Ther J 50(2):64, 2003.
55. Kibg, PM, Tuckwell, N, and Barrett, TE: A critical review of functional capacity evaluations. Phys Ther 78(8):852, 1998.
56. Gross, DP, and Battié, MC: Factors influencing results of functional capacity evaluations in workers' compensation claimants with low back pain. Phys Ther 85(4):315, 2005.
57. Fishbain, DA, et al: Measuring residual functional capacity in chronic low back pain patients based on the Dictionary of Occupational Titles. Spine 19(8):872, 1994.
58. United States Department of Labor: Dictionary of Occupational Titles, ed 4, Revised 1991. Retrieved October 15, 2005 from http://www.oalj.dol.gov/libdot.html
59. American Physical Therapy Association Board of Directors: Occupational Health Physical Therapy Guidelines: Work Conditioning and Work Hardening Programs. BoD 03-01-17-58 (Program 32). Retrieved October 8, 2005 from http://www.apta.org/AM/PrinterTemplate.cfm?Section=Home&CONTENTID=15628&TEMPLATE=/CM/ContentDisplay.cfm.

60. Hunter, S: Using CQI to improve worker's health. PT Magazine of Physical Therapy 3(11):64, 1995.
61. Owens, TR, Hoffman, GL, and Kumar, S: An ergonomic perspective on accommodation in accessibility for people with disability. Disabil Rehabil 18(8):402, 1996.
62. Alpert, J: The physical therapist's role in job analysis and onsite education. Orthop Phys Ther Pract 5:8, 1993.
63. Helm-Williams, P: Industrial rehabilitation: Developing guidelines. PT Magazine of Physical Therapy 1(3):65, 1993.
64. Wynn, KE: A continuum of care to treat the injured worker. PT Magazine of Physical Therapy 2(1):52, 1994.
65. Hebert, LA: OSHA ergonomics guidelines and the PT consultant. PT Magazine of Physical Therapy 3(7):54, 1995.
66. Wynn, KE: Setting corporate trends with on-site PT. PT Magazine of Physical Therapy 4(7):66, 1996.
67. Lawrence, LP: Practicing where industry lives. PT Magazine of Physical Therapy 6(3):28, 1998.
68. Cohn, R: Direct contracting: Is it for you? PT Magazine of Physical Therapy 7(5):22, 1999.
69. Davolt, S: Carving their niches: One-of-a-kind practitioners. PT Magazine of Physical Therapy 6(11):34, 1998.
70. Woods, EN: Forming partnerships with employers. PT Magazine of Physical Therapy 2(1): 56, 1994.
71. Dininny, P: Keeping industry's "athletes" on the job. PT Magazine of Physical Therapy 2(1):48, 1994.
72. Lechner, D, et al: The work-injured population. In Boissonnault, WG (ed): Primary Care for the Physical Therapist: Examination and Triage. Elsevier Saunders, St. Louis, 2005, p 271.
73. Ries, E: Working solutions: PTs and ergonomics. PT Magazine of Physical Therapy 12(9):38, 2004.
74. Workplace Ergonomics Reference Guide: A Publication of the Computer/Electronic Accommodations Program, US Department of Defense. Retrieved October 14, 2005 from http://cap.tricare.osd.mil/acc_sol/Ergonomics.cfm (www.tricare.osd.mil/cap)
75. The Americans with Disabilities Act of 1990 (As Amended): Public Law 101-336.
76. Connolly, JB: Understanding the ADA. Clinical Management 12(2): 40, 1992.
77. Architectural Barriers Act, Public Law 90-480, 1968.
78. Public Buildings Act, 98th Congress, 1st session, 1983.

Supplemental Readings

Agree, EM, Freedman, VA, and Sengupta, M: Factors influencing the use of mobility technology in community-based long-term care. J Aging Health 16(2):267, 2004.

Agree, EM, and Freedman, VA: A comparison of assistive technology and personal care in alleviating disability and unmet need. Gerontologist 43(3):335, 2003.

Cook, AM, and Hussey, SM: Assistive Technologies: Principles and Practice, ed 2. Mosby, St. Louis, 2002.

Fänge, A, and Iwarsson, S: Accessibility and usability in housing: Construct validity and implications for research and practice. Disabil Rehabil 25(23):1316, 2003.

Gitlin, LN: Conducting research on home environments: Lessons learned and new directions. Gerontologist 43(5):628, 2003.

Gitlin, LN, et al: Effects of the home environmental skill-building program on the caregiver-care recipient dyad: 6-month outcomes from the Philadelphia REACH initiative. Gerontologist 43(4):532, 2003.

Iwarsson, S: A long-term perspective on person-environment fit and ADL dependence among older Swedish adults. Gerontologist, 45(3):327, 2005.

Iwarsson, S, and Ståhl, A: Accessibility, usability, and universal design—Positioning and definition of concepts describing person-environment relationships. Disabil Rehabil 25(2):57, 2003.

Jensen, G, Iwarsson, S, and Ståhl, A: Theoretical understanding and methodological challenges in accessibility assessments, focusing the environmental component: An example from travel chains in urban public bus transport. Disabil Rehabil 24(5):231, 2002.

Knecht, B: Accessibility regulations and a universal design philosophy inspire the design process. Archit Rec 1:145, 2004.

Mann, WC, et al: Effectiveness of assistive technology and environmental interventions in maintaining independence and reducing home care costs for the frail elderly: A randomized controlled trial. Arch Fam Med 8(3):210, 1999.

McClain, L: Shopping center wheelchair accessibility: Ongoing advocacy to implement the Americans with Disabilities Act of 1990. Public Health Nurs 17(3):178, 2000.

Preiser, W, and Ostroff, E (eds): Universal Design Handbook. McGraw-Hill, New York, 2001.

Newman, S: The living conditions of elderly Americans. Gerontologist 43(1):99, 2003.

Sandler, LA, and Blanck, P: The quest to make accessibility a corporate article of faith at Microsoft: Case study of corporate culture and human resource dimensions. Behav Sci Law 23(1):39, 2005.

Sanford, JA, and Butterfield, T: Using remote assessment to provide home modification services to underserved elders. Gerontologist 45(3):389, 2005.

Schur, L, Kruse, D, and Blanck, P: Corporate culture and the employment of persons with disabilities. Behav Sci Law 23(1):3, 2005.

Shumway-Cook, A, et al: Environmental demands associated with community mobility in older adults with and without mobility disability. Phys Ther 82(7):670, 2002.

Sonn, U: Longitudinal studies of dependence in daily life activities among elderly persons: Methodological development, use of assistive devices and relation to impairments and functional limitations. Scand J Rehabil Med (Suppl) 34:1, 1996.

Spataro, SE: Diversity in context: How organizational culture shapes reactions to workers with disabilities and others who are demographically different. Behav Sci Law 23(1):21, 2005.

Steinfeld, E, and Danford, GS (eds): Enabling Environments. Measuring the Impact of Environment on Disability and Rehabilitation. Kluwer Academic Plenum, New York, 1999.

Thapar, N, et al: A pilot study of functional access to public buildings and facilities for persons with impairments. Disabil Rehabil 26(5):280, 2004.

Ward, AC, and Baker, PM: Strategies for workplace integration. Behav Sci Law 23(1):143, 2005.

Wooten, LP, and James, EH: Challenges of organizational learning: Perpetuation of discrimination against employees with disabilities. Behav Sci Law 23(1):123, 2005.

Appendix A

THE PRINCIPLES OF UNIVERSAL DESIGN

1. EQUITABLE USE

The design is useful and marketable to people with diverse abilities.

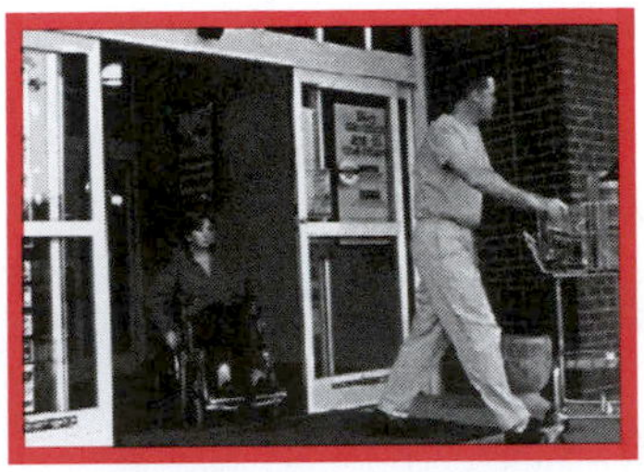

GUIDELINES

1a. Provide the same means of use for all users: identical whenever possible; equivalent when not.

1b. Avoid segregating or stigmatizing any users.

1c. Make provisions for privacy, security, and safety equally available to all users.

1d. Make the design appealing to all users.

EXAMPLES

- Power doors with sensors at entrances that are convenient for all users.
- Integrated, dispersed, and adaptable seating in assembly areas such as sports arenas and theaters.

2. FLEXIBILITY IN USE

The design accommodates a wide range of individual preferences and abilities.

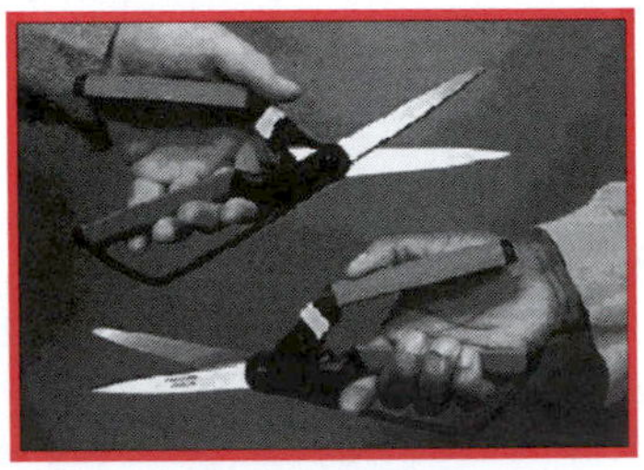

GUIDELINES

2a. Provide choice in methods of use.

2b. Accommodate right- or left- handed access and use.

2c. Facilitate the user's accuracy and precision.

2d. Provide adaptability to the user's pace.

EXAMPLES

- Scissors designed for right- or left- handed users.
- An automated teller machine (ATM) that has visual, tactile, and audible feedback, a tapered card opening and a palm rest.

3. SIMPLE AND INTUITIVE USE

Use of the design is easy to understand regardless of the user's experience, knowledge, language skills, or current concentration level.

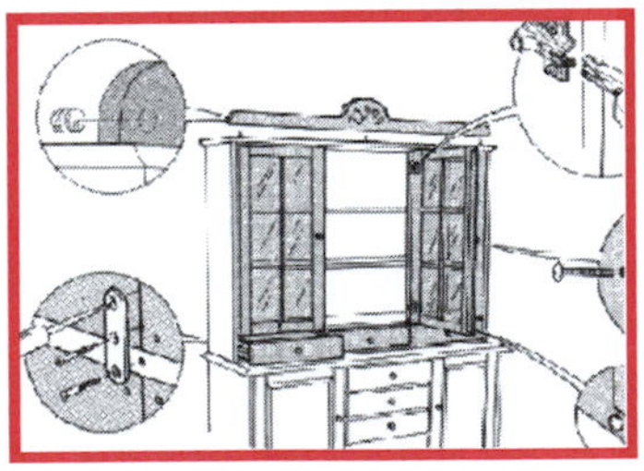

GUIDELINES

3a. Eliminate unnecessary complexity.

3b. Be consistent with user expectations and intuition.

3c. Accommodate a wide range of literacy and language skills.

3d. Arrange information consistent with its importance.

3e. Provide effective prompting and feedback during and after task completion.

EXAMPLES

- A moving sidewalk or escalator in a public space.
- An instruction manual with drawings and no text.

4. PERCEPTIBLE INFORMATION

The design communicates necessary information effectively to the user, regardless of ambient conditions or the user's sensory abilities.

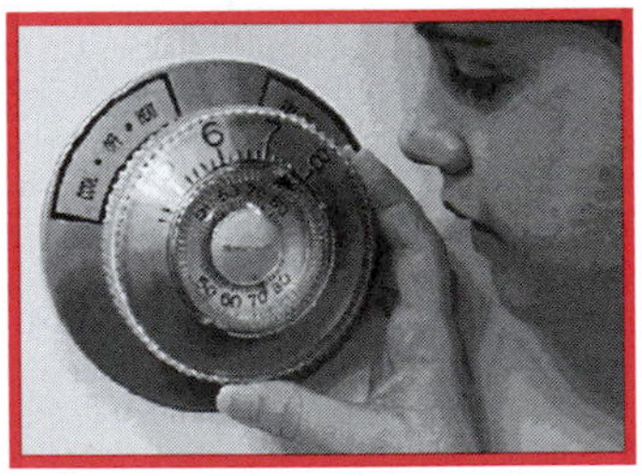

GUIDELINES

4a. Use different modes (pictorial, verbal, tactile) for redundant presentation of essential information.

4b. Maximize "legibility" of essential information.

4c. Differentiate elements in ways that can be described (i.e., make it easy to give instructions or directions).

4d. Provide compatibility with a variety of techniques or devices used by people with sensory limitations.

EXAMPLES

- Tactile, visual, and audible cues and instructions on a thermostat.
- Redundant cueing (e.g., voice communications and signage) in airports, train stations, and subway cars.

THE PRINCIPLES OF UNIVERSAL DESIGN

5. TOLERANCE FOR ERROR

The design minimizes hazards and the adverse consequences of accidental or intended actions.

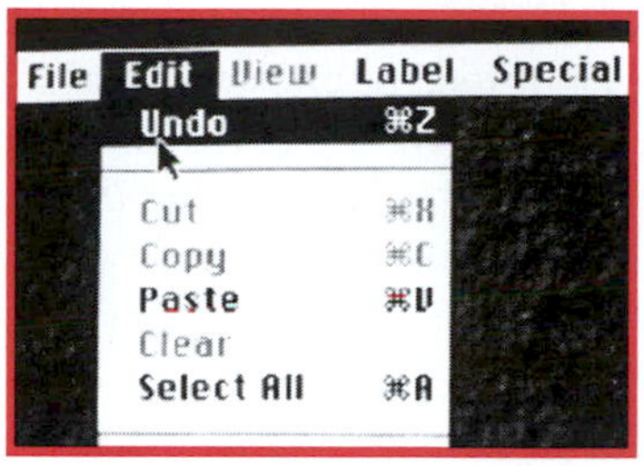

GUIDELINES

- **5a.** Arrange elements to minimize hazards and errors: most used elements, most accessible; hazardous elements eliminated, isolated, or shielded.
- **5b.** Provide warnings of hazards and errors.
- **5c.** Provide fail safe features.
- **5d.** Discourage unconscious action in tasks that require vigilance.

EXAMPLES

- A double-cut car key easily inserted into a recessed keyhole in either of two ways.
- An "undo" feature in computer software that allows the user to correct mistakes without penalty.

6. LOW PHYSICAL EFFORT

The design can be used efficiently and comfortably and with a minimum of fatigue.

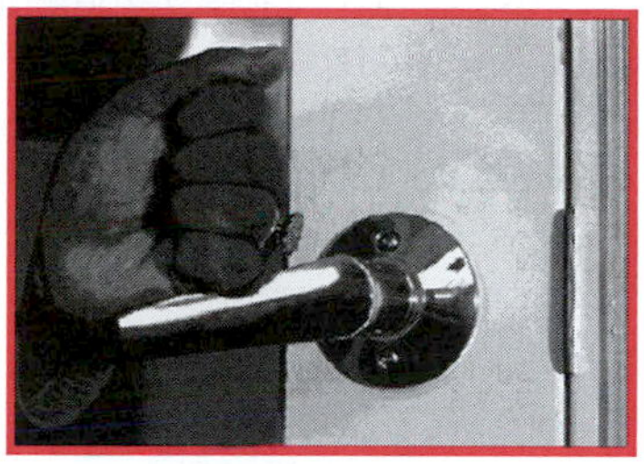

GUIDELINES

- **6a.** Allow user to maintain a neutral body position.
- **6b.** Use reasonable operating forces.
- **6c.** Minimize repetitive actions.
- **6d.** Minimize sustained physical effort.

EXAMPLES

- Lever or loop handles on doors and faucets.
- Touch lamps operated without a switch.

7. SIZE AND SPACE FOR APPROACH AND USE

Appropriate size and space is provided for approach, reach, manipulation, and use regardless of user's body size, posture, or mobility.

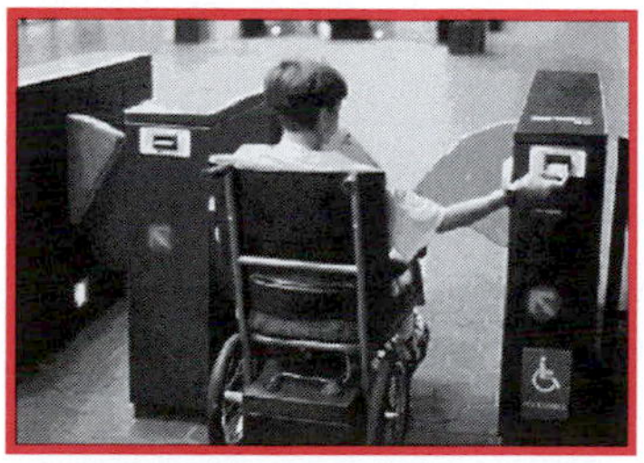

GUIDELINES

- **7a.** Provide a clear line of sight to important elements for any seated or standing user.
- **7b.** Make reach to all components comfortable for any seated or standing user.
- **7c.** Accommodate variations in hand and grip size.
- **7d.** Provide adequate space for the use of assistive devices or personal assistance.

EXAMPLES

- Controls on the front and clear floor space around appliances, mailboxes, dumpsters, and other elements.
- Wide gates at subway stations that accommodate all users.

THE PRINCIPLES WERE COMPLIED BY ADVOCATES OF UNIVERSAL DESIGN, IN ALPHABETICAL ORDER:

Bettye Rose Connell, Mike Jones, Ron Mace, Jim Mueller, Abir Mullick, Elaine Ostroff, Jon Sanford, Ed Steinfeld, Molly Story, and Gregg Vanderheiden.

NOTE:

The Principles of Universal Design are not intended to constitute all criteria for good design, only universally usable design. Certainly, other factors are important, such as aesthetics, cost, safety, gender and cultural appropriateness, and these aspects must also be taken into consideration when designing.

Appendix B: Usability in My Home–A Self-Report Instrument

Directions: The questionnaire consists of two parts, with a number of questions about the design of the *physical housing environment* in which you live. You are asked to answer the questions by assessing how you feel that the design and form of the physical housing environment suits you, your needs, and your wishes.

By physical housing environment is meant here your home, the car park, garage, or parking space that you use if you have a car, your own letterbox, the dustbin/refuse storage place, the storage space, and the shared laundry, if there is one. This includes all the routes along which you move on the site to and from these places. It also includes a balcony, patio, and garden where applicable.

The questions are very general, and the aim is to capture your immediate perception of how the physical housing environment suits you.

For each question there are seven response alternatives in the form of the numbers 1 to 7. The number 1 stands for what is the worst and lowest alternative for you, while 7 stands for the best and highest alternative. The numbers 2 to 6 describe the positions that lie between the best and the worst alternatives. The number 4 is the neutral point on the scale, neither good nor bad. Put a circle round the alternative that agrees best with your perception.

Example: If you are so dissatisfied with your physical housing environment that it could not, in your opinion, be worse for you, then circle the number 1. If you are so satisfied with the design of your physical housing environment that it could not, in your opinion, be better, then circle the number 7. You use the numbers 2 to 7 to describe how close to the best or worst alternative you find the features of your housing environment.

There now follow a number of questions about how well you feel that the design of your physical housing environment suits your needs and wishes. Some questions concern security, social interaction, etc., while others concern how the design of the housing environment makes it easy or difficult to do the everyday tasks you wish and need to perform.

Draw a circle round the number that you think agrees best with your own perception.

(From Fänge, A. [2002]. Usability in My Home: Manual and Instrument Form. Division of Occupational Therapy, Lund University, Sweden. © Agneta Fänge, 2002, with permission.)

1. In relation to how you normally manage your personal hygiene, dressing, visiting the toilet, or how you eat; to what extent is the housing environment suitably designed? (*If you do not manage any of these at all, cross out the whole question.*)

1 2 3 4 5 6 7

Not at all suitable — Very suitable

2. In relation to how you normally manage your cooking/heating of food or preparation of snacks; to what extent is the housing environment suitably designed? (*If you do not manage any of these at all, cross out the whole question.*)

1 2 3 4 5 6 7

Not at all suitable — Very suitable

3. In relation to how you normally manage your washing up, cleaning, care of flowers; to what extent is the housing environment suitably designed? (*If you do not manage any of these at all, cross out the whole question.*)

1 2 3 4 5 6 7

Not at all suitable — Very suitable

4. In relation to how you normally manage your washing, ironing, or repair of clothes; to what extent is the housing environment suitably designed? (*If you do not manage any of these at all, cross out the whole question.*)

1 2 3 4 5 6 7

Not at all suitable — Very suitable

5. How secure do you feel in your housing environment?

1 2 3 4 5 6 7

Not at all secure — Completely secure

6. To what extent does the design of the housing environment allow you to be by yourself when you so wish?

1 2 3 4 5 6 7

Not at all — As much as I want to

7. To what extent does the design of the housing environment allow you to socialize with the friends and acquaintances you want to meet?

1	2	3	4	5	6	7
Not at all				As much as I want to		

8. To what extent does the design of the housing environment allow you to do hobbies/leisure pursuits and relax?

1	2	3	4	5	6	7
Not at all				As much as I want to		

9. If your health should change, to what extent would it be possible for you to make simple changes to your housing environment (e.g., to use a different parking place, to use a different toilet, to rearrange the furniture, to use a different room as a bedroom, etc.)?

1	2	3	4	5	6	7
Not at all				As much as I need to		

There now follow a number of questions about how usable you feel that your housing environment is. First you make an overall assessment (question 10). This is followed by a number of more detailed questions about usability in different parts of the housing environment. State the problems you perceive and make an assessment of how accessible each part of the housing environment is, with regard to the problems you have stated (questions 11 to 22). If you do not feel that there are any special problems, please say so. Do not forget to assess each part of the physical housing environment, even if you have not stated any specific problem.

10. How usable do you feel that your housing environment is in general?

1	2	3	4	5	6	7
Not at all usable					Fully usable	

11. What problems do you perceive in the physical environment just outside your home (e.g., paths and pavements, car park/garage/carport, the design of the refuse storage place, the placing of your letterbox, etc.)?

____

____

12. In view of the above problems in question 11, how usable do you feel that the environment outside your home is?

1	2	3	4	5	6	7
Not at all usable					Fully usable	

13. What problems do you find in the design of the entrance to your home (e.g. heavy doors, narrow stairs, ramps, cramped lift, poor lighting, etc.)?

____

____

14. In view of the above problems in question 13, how usable do you feel that the entrance to your home is?

1	2	3	4	5	6	7
Not at all usable					Fully usable	

15. What problems do you find in the design of the secondary spaces in your home (e.g., store rooms, attic/basement, refuse storage place, laundry [if any], and the routes you have to follow indoors to reach these places)?

____

____

16. In view of the above problems in question 15, how usable do you feel that the secondary spaces in your home are?

1	2	3	4	5	6	7
Not at all usable					Fully usable	

17. What problems do you have in reading and understanding markings and signs outside the building or at the entrance? (For example, are lift buttons fully visible and easy to use? Are the signs at the waste sorting station clear and easy to understand? Are the markings in staircases easy to see?) (*The questions should only be answered by people living in apartments. If you live in your own house, omit this question and question 18.*)

____

____

18. In view of the above problems in question 17, to what extent would you say that the markings and signs outside the building and at the entrance can be read and understood?

1	2	3	4	5	6	7
Not at all					Perfectly easily	

19. What problems do you find in the design of your balcony, patio, or garden? (*If you do not have any balcony, patio, or garden, please say so. You may then omit question 20.*)

____

____

20. In view of the above problems in question 19, how usable do you feel that the balcony, patio, or garden are?

1 2 3 4 5 6 7

Not at all usable Fully usable

21. What problems do you find in the design of the interior of your home?

____

____

22. In view of the above problems in question 21, how usable do you feel that the interior of your home is?

1 2 3 4 5 6 7

Not at all usable Fully usable

To conclude, there is a general question which allows you to express your wishes and needs.

23. If you were able to wish for anything at all concerning your home and your housing environment, what would you wish for?

____

____

____

____

____

____

____

____

Appendix C

Craig Hospital Inventory of Environmental Factors

From Craig Hospital, Research Department, 3425 S. Clarkson Street, Englewood, CO, 80110, with permission.

Being an active, productive member of society includes participating in such things as working, going to school, taking care of your home, and being involved with family and friends in social, recreational and civic activities in the community. Many factors can help or improve a person's participation in these activities while other factors can act as barriers and limit participation. First of all, do you think you have had the same opportunities as other people to participate in and take advantage of:

Education	_____ yes	_____ no
Employment	_____ yes	_____ no
Recreation/leisure	_____ yes	_____ no

First, please tell me how often each of the following has been a barrier to your own participation in the activities that matter to you. Think about the past year, and tell me whether each item on the list below has been a problem **daily, weekly, monthly, less than monthly, or never.** If the item occurs, then answer the question as to how big a problem the item is with regard to your participation in the activities that matter to you.

(Note: if a question asks specifically about **school or work** and you neither work nor attend school, check not applicable)

	Daily	Weekly	Monthly	Less than monthly	Never	Not applicable	Big problem	Little problem
1. In the past 12 months, how often has the availability of transportation been a problem for you?	○	○	○	○	○			
When this problem occurs has it been a big problem or a little problem?							○	○
2. In the past 12 months, how often has the design and layout of your home made it difficult to do what you want or need to do?	○	○	○	○	○			
When this problem occurs has it been a big problem or a little problem?							○	○
3. In the past 12 months, how often has the design and layout of buildings and places you use at school or work made it difficult to do what you want or need to do?	○	○	○	○	○	○		
When this problem occurs has it been a big problem or a little problem?							○	○
4. In the past 12 months, how often has the design and layout of buildings and places you use in your community made it difficult to do what you want or need to do?	○	○	○	○	○			
When this problem occurs has it been a big problem or a little problem?							○	○
5. In the past 12 months, how often has the natural environment - temperature, terrain, climate - made it difficult to do what you want or need to do?	○	○	○	○	○			
When this problem occurs has it been a big problem or a little problem?							○	○
6. In the past 12 months, how often have other aspects of your surroundings - lighting, noise, crowds, etc. - made it difficult to do what you want or need to do?	○	○	○	○	○			
When this problem occurs has it been a big problem or a little problem?							○	○
7. In the past 12 months, how often has the information you wanted or needed not been available in a format you can use or understand?	○	○	○	○	○			
When this problem occurs has it been a big problem or a little problem?							○	○
8. In the past 12 months, how often has the availability of the education and training you needed been a problem for you?	○	○	○	○	○			
When this problem occurs has it been a big problem or a little problem?							○	○
9. In the past 12 months, how often has the availability of health care services and medical care been a problem for you?	○	○	○	○	○			
When this problem occurs has it been a big problem or a little problem?							○	○
10. In the past 12 months, how often has the lack of personal equipment or special adapted devices been a problem for you? Examples might include hearing aids, eyeglasses or wheelchairs.	○	○	○	○	○			
When this problem occurs has it been a big problem or a little problem?							○	○

	Daily	Weekly	Monthly	Less than monthly	Never	Not applicable	Big problem	Little problem
11. In the past 12 months, how often has the lack of computer technology been a problem for you?	O	O	O	O	O			
When this problem occurs has it been a big problem or a little problem?							O	O
12. In the past 12 months, how often did you need someone else's help in your home and could not get it easily?	O	O	O	O	O			
When this problem occurs has it been a big problem or a little problem?							O	O
13. In the past 12 months, how often did you need someone else's help at school or work and could not get it easily?	O	O	O	O	O	O		
When this problem occurs has it been a big problem or a little problem?							O	O
14. In the past 12 months, how often did you need someone else's help in your community and could not get it easily?	O	O	O	O	O			
When this problem occurs has it been a big problem or a little problem?							O	O
15. In the past 12 months, how often have other people's attitudes toward you been a problem at home?	O	O	O	O	O			
When this problem occurs has it been a big problem or a little problem?							O	O
16. In the past 12 months, how often have other people's attitudes toward you been a problem at school or work?	O	O	O	O	O	O		
When this problem occurs has it been a big problem or a little problem?							O	O
17. In the past 12 months, how often have other people's attitudes toward you been a problem in the community?	O	O	O	O	O			
When this problem occurs has it been a big problem or a little problem?							O	O
18. In the past 12 months, how often has a lack of support and encouragement from others in your home been a problem?	O	O	O	O	O			
When this problem occurs has it been a big problem or a little problem?							O	O
19. In the past 12 months, how often has a lack of support and encouragement from others at school or work been a problem?	O	O	O	O	O	O		
When this problem occurs has it been a big problem or a little problem?							O	O
20. In the past 12 months, how often has a lack of support and encouragement from others in your community been a problem?	O	O	O	O	O			
When this problem occurs has it been a big problem or a little problem?							O	O
21. In the past 12 months, how often did you experience prejudice or discrimination?	O	O	O	O	O			
When this problem occurs has it been a big problem or a little problem?							O	O
22. In the past 12 months, how often has the lack of programs and services in the community been a problem?	O	O	O	O	O			
When this problem occurs has it been a big problem or a little problem?							O	O
23. In the past 12 months, how often did the policies and rules of businesses and organizations make problems for you?	O	O	O	O	O			
When this problem occurs has it been a big problem or a little problem?							O	O
24. In the past 12 months, how often did education and employment programs and policies make it difficult to do what you want or need to do?	O	O	O	O	O	O		
When this problem occurs has it been a big problem or a little problem?							O	O
25. In the past 12 months, how often did government programs and policies make it difficult to do what you want or need to do?	O	O	O	O	O			
When this problem occurs has it been a big problem or a little problem?							O	O

THE ADL-STAIRCASE

Note: In this instrument, the term **personal activities of daily living (P-ADL)** is synonymous with **basic activities of daily living (BADL).**

DEFINITIONS

Cleaning: ***performs house cleaning, vacuum cleaning, washing floors***

Independent: Performs the activity when necessary.
Partly dependent: Gets assistance in taking the carpets outdoors or assistance very seldom.
Dependent: Does not perform the activity or gets assistance with some part of the activity regularly.

Shopping: ***gets to the store, manages stairs and other obstacles, takes out groceries, pays for them and carries them home***

Independent: Performs the activity when necessary.
Partly dependent: Performs the activity but together with another person.
Dependent: Does not perform the activity or needs assistance with some part of the activity.

Transportation: ***gets to the stop for public transportation, get on and goes by bus, tram, or train***

Independent: Performs the activity when needed.
Partly dependent: Performs the activity but together with another person.
Dependent: Does not perform the activity.

Cooking: ***gets to the kitchen, prepares the food, manage the stove***

Independent: Performs the activity when needed.
Partly dependent: Does not prepare dinner-food or only heating up prepared food.
Dependent: Does not perform the activity.

Bathing: ***means sponge bath, tub bath, or shower***

Independent: Receives no assistance (gets in and out of tub by self if tub is usual means of bathing).
Partly dependent: Receives assistance in bathing only one part of the body (such as back or leg).
Dependent: Receives assistance in bathing more than one part of the body (or does not bathe self).

Dressing: ***means getting all needed clothing from closets and drawers and getting dressed, includes using fasteners, and putting on brace if worn***

Independent: Gets clothes and gets completely dressed without assistance.
Partly dependent: Gets clothes and gets dressed without assistance except for help with tying shoes.
Dependent: Receives assistance in getting clothes or in getting dressed, or stays partly or incompletely dressed.

Toileting: ***means going to the "toilet room" for bowel and urine elimination, cleaning self after elimination, and arranging clothes***

Independent: Goes to the "toilet room," clean self and arrange clothes without assistance. (May use support object such as cane, walker, or wheelchair, and may manage a night bedpan or commode, emptying it in the morning.)
Partly dependent: Receives assistance in going to the "toilet room" or in cleaning self or in arranging clothes after elimination, or using the night bedpan or commode.
Dependent: Does not go to the "toilet room" for elimination.

Transfer: ***means moving in and out of bed and in and out of chair***

Independent: Moves in and out of bed and out of chair without assistance. (May use support object such as cane or walker.)
Partly dependent: Moves in and out of bed or chair with assistance.
Dependent: Does not get out of bed.

Continence: ***means function of controlling elimination from the bladder and bowel***

Independent: Controls urination and bowel movement completely by self.
Partly dependent: Has occasional "accidents."
Dependent: Supervision helps keep urine or bowel control, or catheter is used, or is incontinent.

Feeding: ***means the basic process of getting food from plate or equivalent into the mouth***

Independent: Feeds self without assistance.
Partly dependent: Feeds self except for getting assistance in cutting meat or buttering bread.
Dependent: Receives assistance in feeding or is fed partly or completely through tubes or with intravenous fluids.

THE ADL-STAIRCASE

Definitions of personal (P -) and instrumental (I -) ADL according to a cumulative scale of conditional ADL-steps (the ADL Staircase)

ADL-Steps in I and P-ADL

Step 0	Independent in all activities
Step 1	Dependent on one activity
Step 2	Dependent on cleaning and one more activity
Step 3	Dependent on cleaning, shopping, and one more activity
Step 4	Dependent on cleaning, shopping, transportation, and one more activity
Step 5	Dependent in all I-ADLs and one P-ADL
Step 6	Dependent in all I-ADLs, bathing, and one more P-ADL
Step 7	Dependent in all I-ADLs, bathing, dressing, and one more P-ADL
Step 8	Dependent in all I-ADLs, bathing, dressing, going to the toilet, and one more P-ADL
Step 9	Dependent in all activities
"Others"	Dependent in two or more activities but not classifiable as above

If the item continence is included, the definitions of the last two steps will be as follows:

Step 9	Dependent in all I-ADLs, bathing, dressing, going to the toilet, transfer, and one more P-ADL
Step 10	Dependent in all activities

ADL-step 0
ADL-step 1 Cleaning
ADL-step 2 Shopping
ADL-step 3 Transportation
ADL-step 4 Cooking
ADL-step 5 Bathing
ADL-step 6 Dressing
ADL-step 7 Toileting
ADL-step 8 Transfer
ADL-step 9 Continence
ADL-step 10 Feeding

Appendix E: The Enviro-FIM™ Instrument's Eleven Levels of Function and Their Associated Scores

Independent

The person receives no help with any of the behavioral components involved in the activity.

10 **No Assistance**—The person completes the activity without taking an inappropriate amount of time, without using an assistive device(s) or aid(s), without changing (or causing someone else to change) the environmental context, and without risking personal safety or well-being.

Modified Independent

The person receives no help with any of the behavioral components involved in the activity. The person completes the activity independently but either takes an inappropriate amount of time, uses an assistive device(s) or aid(s), changes (or causes some one else to change) the environmental context or risks personal safety or well-being.

9 **Additional time**—The person completes the activity independently and safely but takes an inappropriate amount of time. At least one of the following is true: the person hesitates, makes repeated attempts, takes at least one period of rest or simply takes at least double the amount of time normally required to complete the activity.

8 **Assistive device**—The person completes the activity independently and safely by using an assistive device(s) or aid(s). The person may or may not take an inappropriate amount of time.

7 **Modified environment**—The person completes the activity independently and safely after changing (or causing some one else to change) the environmental context. The person may or may not take an inappropriate amount of time and may or may not use an assistive device(s) or aid(s).

6 **Safety considerations**—Either the person completes the activity independently with some risk to personal safety or well-being or the actions of another person present indicate that something about the activity poses a hazard. The person may or may not take an inappropriate amount of time, may or may not use an assistive device(s) or aid(s) and may or may not change (or cause some one else to change) the environmental context.

(From Danford and Steinfeld,[43, p 3] with permission)

Modified Dependent

The person requires and receives help in the form of either supervision or physical assistance with at least one of the behavioral components involved in the activity. The person nevertheless contributes at least half (50% to 100%) of the total effort expended to complete the activity.

5 **Supervision or setup**—The person requires and receives help that only involves supervision (e.g., standing by, cueing, coaxing, setting up needed items or applying orthoses)—i.e., no physical contact with a helper occurs during completion of the activity. The person contributes all (100%) of the effort expended to complete the activity.

4 **Minimal contact assistance**—The person requires and receives assistance that involves physical contact with a helper during completion of the activity. The person contributes nearly all (75–99%) of the effort expended to complete the activity.

3 **Moderate assistance**—The person requires and receives help that involves physical contact with a helper during completion of the activity. The person still contributes most (50–74%) of the effort expended to complete the activity.

Dependent

The person requires and receives help in the form of physical assistance with at least one of the behavioral components involved in the activity. Either the person contributes less than half (0–49%) of the effort expended to complete the activity or the activity is not completed.

2 **Maximal assistance**—The person contributes some (25–49%) of the effort expended to complete the activity.

1 **Total assistance**— The person contributes little or none (0–24%) of the effort expended to complete the activity.

0 **Activity not completed**—The person either is unable to complete the activity even with total assistance or declines to perform the activity.

Appendix F: The Enviro-FIM™ instrument's decision tree.

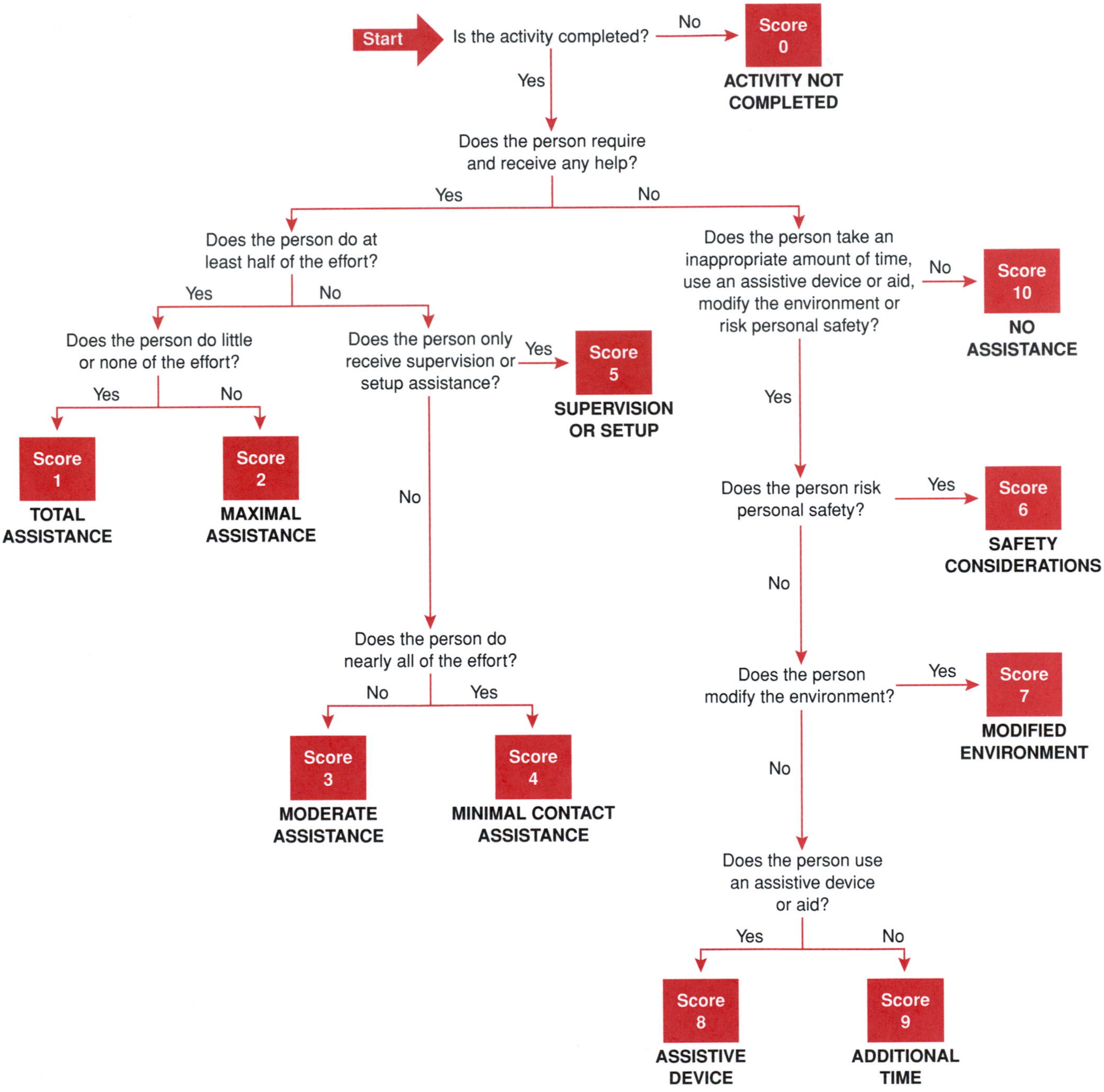

Start
Is the activity completed?
No
Score 0
ACTIVITY NOT COMPLETED
Yes
Does the person require and receive any help?
Yes
No
Does the person do at least half of the effort?
Yes
No
Does the person do little or none of the effort?
Yes
No
Score 1
TOTAL ASSISTANCE
Score 2
MAXIMAL ASSISTANCE
Does the person only receive supervision or setup assistance?
Yes
Score 5
SUPERVISION OR SETUP
No
Does the person do nearly all of the effort?
No
Yes
Score 3
MODERATE ASSISTANCE
Score 4
MINIMAL CONTACT ASSISTANCE
Does the person take an inappropriate amount of time, use an assistive device or aid, modify the environment or risk personal safety?
No
Score 10
NO ASSISTANCE
Yes
Does the person risk personal safety?
Yes
Score 6
SAFETY CONSIDERATIONS
No
Does the person modify the environment?
Yes
Score 7
MODIFIED ENVIRONMENT
No
Does the person use an assistive device or aid?
Yes
No
Score 8
ASSISTIVE DEVICE
Score 9
ADDITIONAL TIME

(From Danford and Steinfeld,[43, p 5] with permission)

Appendix G: The Functional Performance Measure's LES™ Eight Levels of Effort and Their Defining Characteristics

Level X—Unknown: Performance of the task is not observable.

Level 0—None: No effort is expended either because task performance is not required for completion of the activity in the observed situation or because the task is self-performing.

Level 6—Blocked: The person's ability to perform the task is thwarted either because characteristics of the observed situation make attempting the task futile or because the activity was aborted before the task could be attempted.

Level 5—Declined: The opportunity to perform the task is declined.

Level 4—Impossible: The task is not completed successfully or the task is completed successfully only after someone else performs the task on the person's behalf.

Level 3—Maximum: At least one of the following is true: the person performs the task successfully only after more than one attempt; successful task performance takes much more than the amount of time (i.e., at least double) that would be typical for a member of the general population functioning under similar circumstances; the person offers frequent or lengthy complaint (verbal or nonverbal) as an expression of frustration, inconvenience or anxiety during task performance; or there is frequent or lengthy interruption in the continuity of task performance.

Level 2—Moderate: At least one of the following is true: successful task performance takes only a little more than the amount of time (i.e., less than double) that would be typical for a member of the general population functioning under similar circumstances; the person offers only infrequent or brief complaint (verbal or nonverbal) as an expression of frustration, aggravation, inconvenience or anxiety during task performance; or there is only infrequent or brief interruption in the continuity of task performance.

Level 1—Minimum: All of the following are true: successful task performance takes no more time than would be typical for a member of the general population functioning under similar circumstances; the person offers no complaint as an expression of frustration, aggravation, inconvenience or anxiety during task performance; and there is no interruption in the continuity of task performance.

(From Danford and Steinfeld,[45, p 3] with permission)

Appendix H: The Functional Performance Measure's LES™ Decision Tree

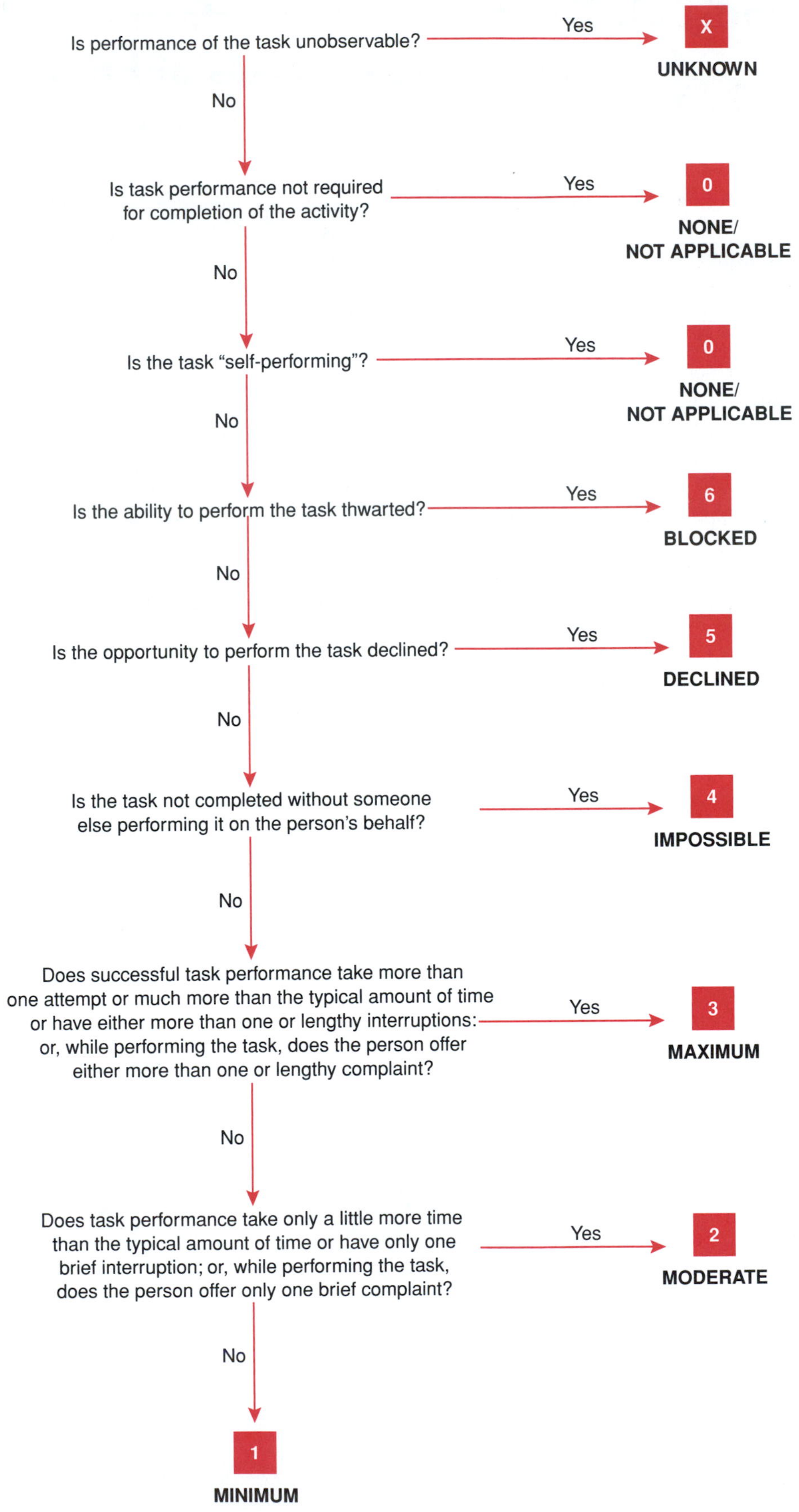
Is performance of the task unobservable?
Yes
X
UNKNOWN
No
Is task performance not required for completion of the activity?
Yes
0
NONE/ NOT APPLICABLE
No
Is the task "self-performing"?
Yes
0
NONE/ NOT APPLICABLE
No
Is the ability to perform the task thwarted?
Yes
6
BLOCKED
No
Is the opportunity to perform the task declined?
Yes
5
DECLINED
No
Is the task not completed without someone else performing it on the person's behalf?
Yes
4
IMPOSSIBLE
No
Does successful task performance take more than one attempt or much more than the typical amount of time or have either more than one or lengthy interruptions: or, while performing the task, does the person offer either more than one or lengthy complaint?
Yes
3
MAXIMUM
No
Does task performance take only a little more time than the typical amount of time or have only one brief interruption; or, while performing the task, does the person offer only one brief complaint?
Yes
2
MODERATE
No
1
MINIMUM

(From Danford and Steinfeld,[45, p 8] with permission)

Appendix I: The Functional Performance Measure's LAS™ Eight Levels of Assistance and Their Defining Characteristics

Level X—Unknown: Assistance with task performance is not observable.

Level 0—None: No assistance is provided because task performance is not required for completion of the activity in the observed situation, because the task is self-performing, or because the person performing the task requires no assistance.

Level 6—Blocked: The ability to provide assistance is thwarted either because characteristics of the observed situation make assisting the task performance futile or because the activity was aborted before assistance with task performance could be attempted.

Level 5—Declined: The opportunity to provide assistance is refused.

Level 4—Impossible: The task is not completed successfully even though assistance is provided that involves an attempt to perform the task on the person's behalf.

Level 3—Maximum: The assistance provided effectively constitutes direct performance of the task on behalf of the person performing the activity.

Level 2—Moderate: The assistance provided merely facilitates performance of the task by the person performing the activity.

Level 1—Minimum: The assistance provided is only incidental to performance of the task by the person performing the activity.

(From Danford and Steinfeld,[45, p 13] with permission)

Appendix J: The Functional Performance Measure's LAS™ Decision Tree

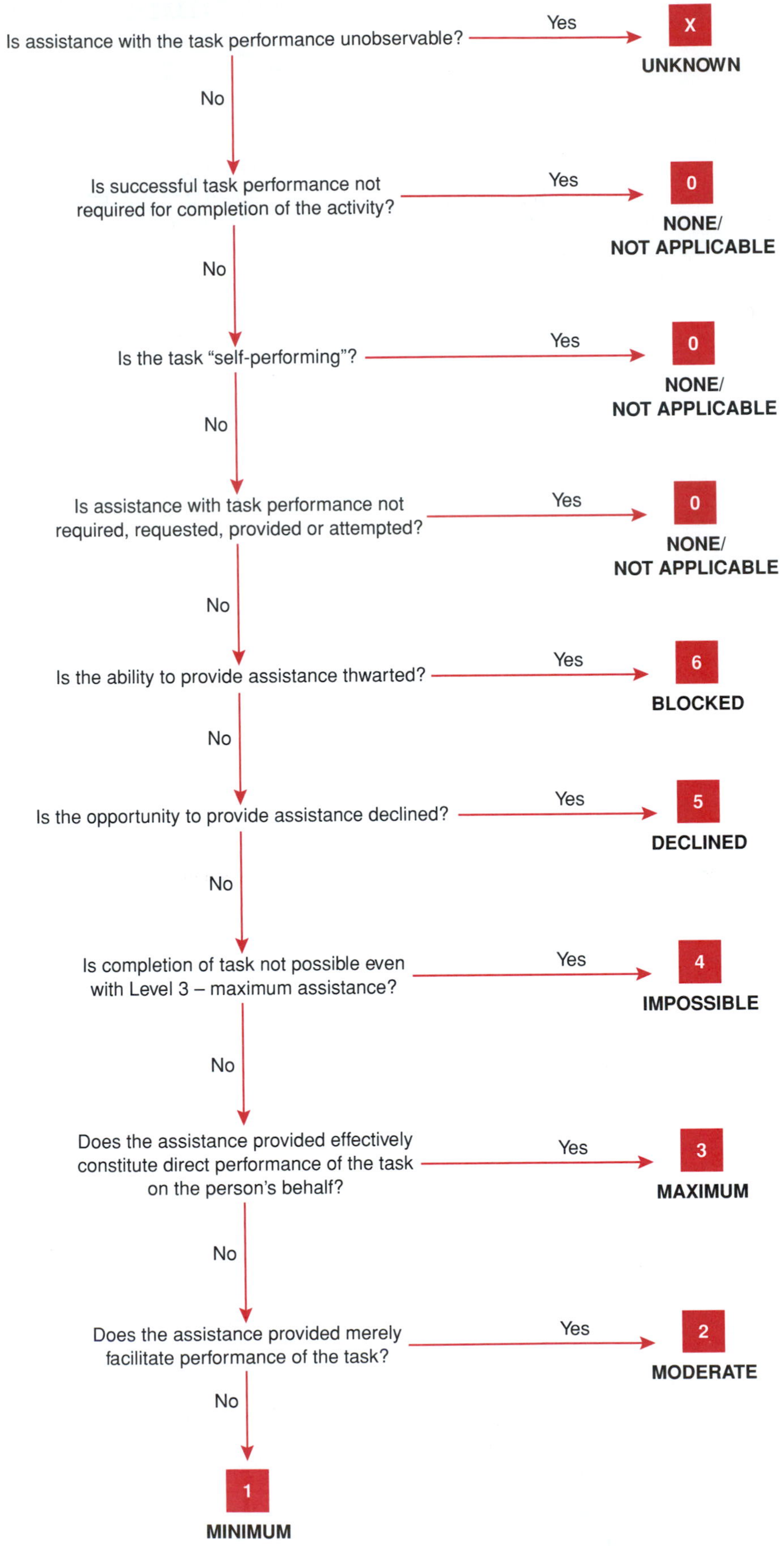
Is assistance with the task performance unobservable?
Yes
X
UNKNOWN
No
Is successful task performance not required for completion of the activity?
Yes
0
NONE/ NOT APPLICABLE
No
Is the task "self-performing"?
Yes
0
NONE/ NOT APPLICABLE
No
Is assistance with task performance not required, requested, provided or attempted?
Yes
0
NONE/ NOT APPLICABLE
No
Is the ability to provide assistance thwarted?
Yes
6
BLOCKED
No
Is the opportunity to provide assistance declined?
Yes
5
DECLINED
No
Is completion of task not possible even with Level 3 – maximum assistance?
Yes
4
IMPOSSIBLE
No
Does the assistance provided effectively constitute direct performance of the task on the person's behalf?
Yes
3
MAXIMUM
No
Does the assistance provided merely facilitate performance of the task?
Yes
2
MODERATE
No
1
MINIMUM

(From Danford and Steinfeld,[45,p 17] with permission)

Appendix K: The Environmental Utility Measure's Difficulty Rating Scale (DRS™)

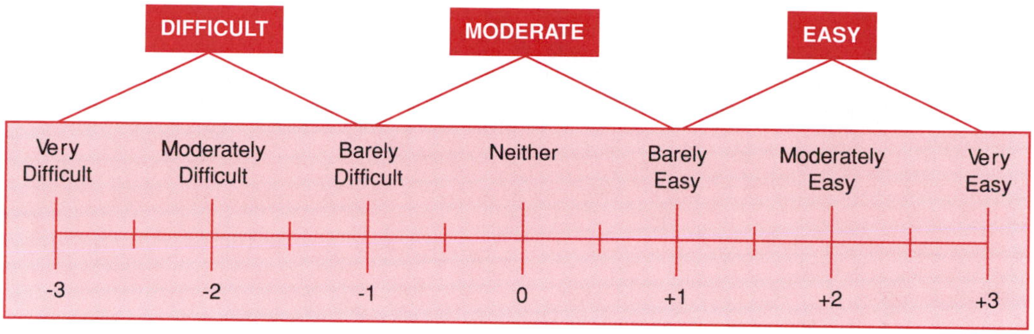

Administration

Step 1: Using a simplified version to the DRS™ rating scale (below) the patient is asked if the functional task just completed seemed ***difficult, moderate,*** or ***easy***.

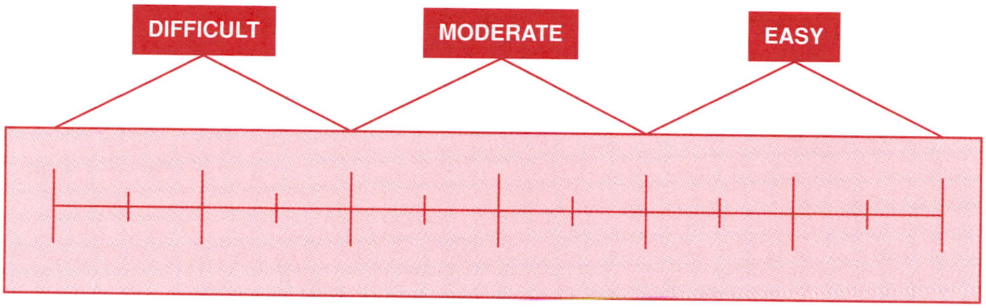

Step 2: Based on the response to Step 1, the appropriate subscale is selected. In this example, the task was perceived as ***difficult***. The patient is then presented with the Difficult Subscale (below) and asked to point to the position that identifies "how difficult?" Three choices are labeled (***very difficult* [-3]**, ***moderately difficult* [-2]**, and ***barely difficult* [-1]**), with two choices between the three anchor points: -2.5 and -1.5.

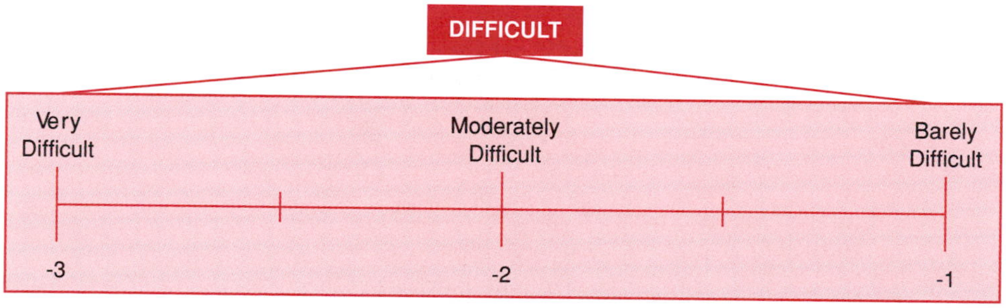

Additional Subscales:

The Moderate Subscale ("how moderate?") responses and scores include:
***Barely Difficult* (-1)**, ***Neither* (0)**, and ***Barely Easy* (+1)** with two anchor choices: -.5 and +.5.

The Easy Subscale ("how easy?") responses and scores include: ***Barely Easy* (+1)**, ***Moderately Easy* (+2)**, and ***Very Easy* (+2.5)** with two anchor choices: +1.5 and +2.5.

Appendix L: The Environmental Utility Measure's Acceptability Rating Scale (ARS™)

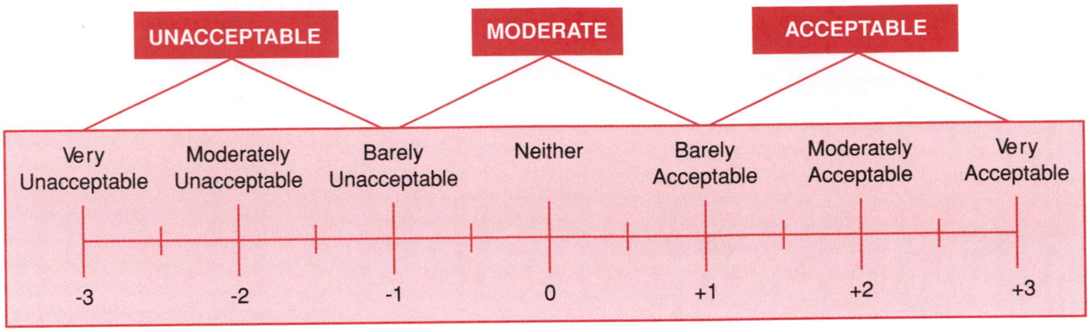

Administration

Step 1: Using a simplified version of the ARS™ rating scale (below) the patient indicates the acceptability of a functional task using three options: ***unacceptable***, ***moderate***, or ***acceptable***.

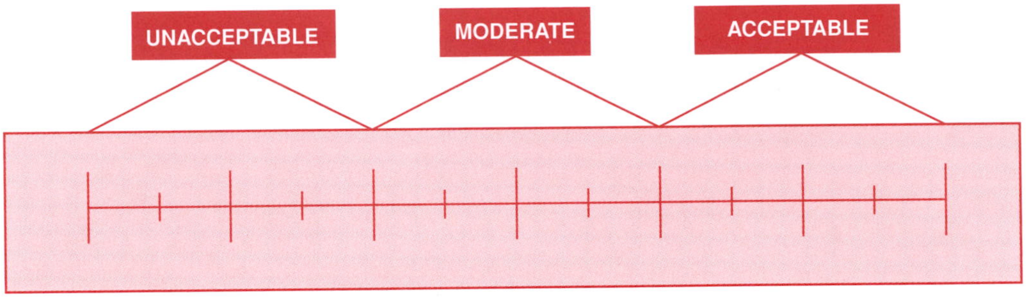

Step 2: Based on the response to Step 1, the appropriate subscale is selected. In this example, the usability rating was ***unacceptable***. The patient is then presented with the Unacceptable Subscale (below) and asked to point to the position that identifies, "how unacceptable?" Three choices are labeled ***very unacceptable* [-3]**, ***moderately unacceptable* [-2]**, and ***barely unacceptable* [-1]**, with two choices between the three anchor points: -2.5 and -1.5.

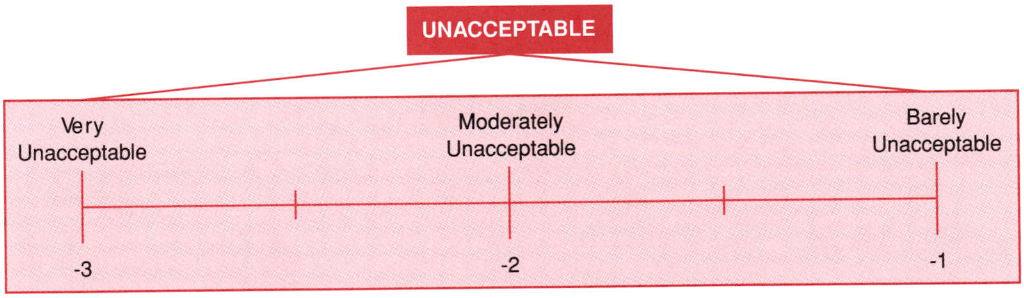

Additional Subscales:

Moderate Subscale: ***Barely Unacceptable* (-1)**, ***Neither* (0)**, and ***Barely Acceptable* (+1)**, and two anchor choices: -.5 and +.5.

Acceptable Subscale: ***Barely Acceptable* (+1)**, ***Moderately Acceptable* (+2)**, and ***Very Acceptable* (+3)**, and two anchor choices: +1.5 and +2.5.

(From Danford and Steinfeld,[46, p 7] with permission)

Appendix M: Home Survey Form

Type of Home

_______ Apartment
Is elevator available? _______
What floor does patient live on? _______
_______ Single family home.
_______ Two or more floors.
_______ Does patient live on only one floor, or use all floors of home?
_______ Basement. Does patient have or use basement area?

Entrances to Building or Home

Location

Front Back Side (Circle one)
Which entrance is used most frequently or easily? _______
Can patient get to entrance? _______

Stairs

Does patient manage outside stairs? _______
Width of stairway _______
Number of steps _______ Height of steps _______
Railing present as you go up? R _______ L _______
Both _______
Is ramp available for wheelchair? _______

Door

Can patient unlock, open, close, lock door? (Circle for yes)
If doorsill is present, give height _______ and material _______
Width of doorway _______
Can patient enter _______ leave _______ via door?

Hallway

Width of hallway _______
Are any objects obstructing the way? _______

Approach to Apartment or Living Area

(Omit if not applicable)
Obstructions? _______
____

Steps

Width of stairway _______
Number of steps _______ Height of steps _______
Railing present as you go up? R _______ L _______
Both _______
Is ramp available? _______

Door

Can patient unlock, open, close, lock door? (Circle one)
Doorsill? Give height _______ material _______
Width of doorway _______
Can patient enter _______ leave _______ via door?

Elevator

Is elevator present? _______ Does it land flush with floor? _______
Width of door opening _______
Height of control buttons _______
Can patient use elevator alone? _______

Inside Home

Note width of hallways and of door entrances.
Note presence of doorsills and height.
Note if patient must climb stairs to reach room.
Can patient move from one part of the house to another?
Hallways _______
Bedroom _______
Bathroom _______
Kitchen _______
Livingroom _______
Others _______
Can patient move safely?
Loose rugs _______
Electrical cords _______
Faulty floors _______
Highly waxed floors _______
Sharp-edged furniture _______
Note areas of particular danger for patient.
Hot water pipes _______
Radiators _______

Bedroom

Is light switch accessible? _______
Can patient open and close windows? _______

Bed

Height _______ Width _______
Both sides of bed accessible? _______ headboard present? _______ footboard? _______
Is bed on wheels? _______ Is it stable? _______
Can patient transfer from wheelchair to bed? _______ and bed to wheelchair? _______
Is night table within patient's reach from bed _______ Is telephone on it? _______

Clothing

Is patient's clothing located in bedroom? _______
Can patient get clothes from dresser? _______ closet? _______ elsewhere? _______

Bathroom

Does patient use wheelchair _______ walker _______ in bathroom?
Does wheelchair _______ walker _______ fit into bathroom?

Light switch accessible? ______ Can patient open and close window? ______
What material are bathroom walls made of? ______
If tile, how many inches does tile extend from the floor beside the toilet? ______
How many inches does tile extend from the top of the rim of the bathtub? ______
Does patient use toilet? ______
Can patient transfer independently to and from toilet? ______
Does wheelchair wheel directly to toilet for transfers? ______
What is height of toilet seat from floor? ______
Are there bars or sturdy supports near toilet? ______
Is there room for grab bars? ______
Can patient use sink? ______ What is height of sink? ______
Is patient able to reach and turn off faucets? ______
Is there knee space beneath sink? ______
Is patient able to reach necessary articles? ______ mirror? ______ electrical outlet? ______

Bathing
Does patient take tub bath? ______ shower? ______ sponge bath? ______
If using tub, can patient safely transfer without assistance? ______
Bars or sturdy supports present beside tub? ______
Is equipment necessary? (tub seat, handspray attachment, tub rail, no-skid strips, grab rails, other ______)
Can patient manage faucets and drain plug? ______
Height of tub from floor to rim ______
Is tub built-in ______ or on legs? ______
Width of tub from the inside ______
If uses separate shower stall, can patient transfer independently and manage faucets? ______
If patient takes sponge bath, describe method. ______
______
______

Living Room Area
Light switch accessible? ______ Can patient open and close window? ______
Can furniture be rearranged to allow manipulation of wheelchair? ______
Can patient transfer from wheelchair to and from sturdy chair? ______
Height of chair ______
Can patient transfer from wheelchair to and from sofa? ______
Height of sofa ______
Can ambulatory patient transfer to and from chair or sofa? ______
Can patient manage television and radio? ______

Dining Room
Light switch accessible? ______
Is patient able to use table? ______ Height of table ______

Kitchen
What is the table height? ______ Can wheelchair fit under? ______
Can patient open refrigerator door and take food? ______
Can patient open freezer door and take food? ______
Sink
Can patient be seated at sink? ______
Can patient reach faucets? ______ Turn them on and off? ______
Can patient reach bottom of basin? ______
Shelves and cabinets
Can patient open and close? ______
Can patient reach dishes, pots, eating utensils, and food? ______
Comments: ______
______
______

Transport
Can patient carry items from one part of kitchen to another? ______
Stove
Can patient reach and manipulate controls? ______
Manage oven door? ______
Place food in oven and remove? ______
Manage broiler door? ______
Put food in and remove? ______
Other Appliances
Can patient reach and turn on appliances? ______
Can patient use outlets? ______
Counter space: Is there enough for storage and work area? ______
Diagram (include stove, refrigerator, microwave, sink, table, counters, others if applicable)

Laundry
If patient has no facilities, how will laundry be managed?
Location of facilities in home or apartment and description of facilities present:
Can patient reach laundry area? ______
Can patient use washing machine and dryer? ______
Load and empty? ______
Manage doors and controls? ______
Can patient use sink? ______
What is height of sink? ______
Able to reach and turn on faucets? ______
Knee space beneath sink? ______
Able to reach necessary articles? ______
Is laundry cart available? ______
Can patient hang clothing on line? ______

Ironing board ______
Location: ______
Is it kept open? ______
If not kept open, can patient set up and take down ironing board? ______
Can patient reach outlet? ______

Cleaning

Can patient remove mop, broom, vacuum, pail from storage? ______
Use equipment? (mop, broom, vacuum and so forth) ______

Emergency

Location of telephone in house: ______
Could patient use fire escape or back door in a hurry if alone? ______
Does patient have numbers for neighbors, police, fire and physician? ______

Other

Will patient be responsible for child care? ______
If so, give number of children ______ and ages: ______
Will patient do own shopping? ______
Is family member or friend available? ______
Is delivery service available? ______
Does family have automobile? ______
Is family member or friend available to help with lawn care, changing high light bulbs, and so forth? ______
______
______

Guidelines for Completing Essential and Marginal Job Function Analysis Form

Purpose and Use

- It qualifies a position, describing the purposes and needs within the respective department.
- It is a comprehensive job description describing both the tasks performed and the physical and cognitive needs of the job.
- It maximizes interview information to determine the candidate's ability to perform the Essential Functions.
- It identifies performance evaluation criteria.
- It is required for all job accommodation requests when a health condition necessitates ADA modification/accommodation.
- It must accompany all new positions that need to be advertised and a reclassification request if the position is currently vacant and needs to be advertised.

Help Table

Department: The department where the position is performed.

Position/Job Code Title: Merit classification or professional and scientific classification.

Job Code: University of Iowa Job Code (EX: GB11, PC67).

Incumbent: Name of person currently in position or "vacant."

Position Number: HRIS assigned 8–digit position number (EX: 00000755).

Requisition Number: For advertising, match Requisition Number to Functional Analysis.

Position Summary: Basic purpose of job and rationale for existence.

Function Statements: Action outcome statements, starting with a verb, either essential (primary) or marginal (secondary) to the position, identified by percentange of time performed to add up to 100%.

Essential Function: Functions defined by the frequency with which they are performed, the amount of time it takes to perform them, how the job is impacted if not performed by this position, or whether these functions could be assigned to another position.

Marginal Function: Function that needs to be performed only infrequently, with usually minimal consequence to the mission of the job if performed by another person.

Position Context Variables: Needed for the performance of essential functions. Check "YES" even if only one variable applies at this time.

Comments: Add anything not already covered that is needed to perform the essential functions of the job, or to further explain context variables.

Cognitive Processes: Level of training needed to perform the essential functions of the position, split between high school level training and post high school college/technical training. Check "YES" even if only one variable applies at this time.

Bilingual Requirements: Foreign languages used in the performance of the position.

Degree of Push–Pull Activity: Designate all forms of push–pull on the job to add up to a total of 100% for performance of the essential functions.

Physical Requirements: Movements that <u>CANNOT</u> be performed concurrently and reflect the essential functions on pages 1 and 2.

Physical Requirements: Movement that <u>CAN</u> be performed concurrently to reflect the essential functions of the job.

Vision Clarity: With corrected vision to perform the essential functions.

Equipment, Tools, Electronic Devices and Software: Equipment, tools, electronic devices, and software operated to perform the essential functions.

Physical Surroundings and Hazards: Applicable to all areas where essential functions of a position are performed (e.g., office, job site, lab, hospital, kitchen, and so forth).

Comments: Any that pertain to the physical surroundings or possible hazards involved in the performance of the essential functions of the position.

Vehicle Driven: Only if needed to perform the essential functions (out-of-town work, delivery, and so forth).

Locations: All job sites where essential functions are performed.

Day/Hour Schedule: The work shift or shifts if rotating.

Name and Title of Supervisor: Name of person to whom this incumbent reports.

Person Completing this Form: Incumbent or supervisor (print or type).

Signature of Incumbent: Signature of person currently in position. If "vacant" or "new," leave blank.

THE UNIVERSITY OF IOWA
University Human Resources
Faculty and Staff Disability Services
121 University Services Building, Ste20
Iowa City, Iowa 52242-1911

ESSENTIAL AND MARGINAL JOB FUNCTION ANALYSIS

Tab field-to-field to enter data (or click with mouse). Press the F1 key at any field to see a description of that field.

Department: ____________________ **Position Title:** ________________ **Job Code:** ____________________

Incumbent: ____________________ **Position #:** ____________________ **Requisition #:** ________________

POSITION SUMMARY:

Provide a position summary. If you need more space, please attach a separate sheet. A position summary consists of concise, qualitative statements crystallizing the basic purpose of the job and rationale for its existence.

FUNCTION STATEMENTS:

A job function statement should focus on the purpose, the result to be accomplished, and the productivity required rather than the manner in which the function is performed. Begin each statement with a verb. Each statement is to contain one action that produces the desired outcome. Identify whether the functions are essential or marginal (primary or secondary) to the position.

Provide the projected percent of time to be devoted to each job function during a typical time period.

Essential (Primary) Functions	%	Marginal (Secondary) Functions	%
1.	0.00	1.	0.00
2.	0.00	2.	0.00
3.	0.00	3.	0.00
4.	0.00	4.	0.00
5.	0.00	5.	0.00
6.	0.00	6.	0.00
7.	0.00	7.	0.00
8.	0.00	8.	0.00
9.	0.00	9.	0.00
10.	0.00	10.	0.00
11.	0.00	11.	0.00
12.	0.00	12.	0.00
13.	0.00	13.	0.00
14.	0.00	14.	0.00
Essential Column Total**	0.00%	Marginal Column Total**	0.00%

**Essential and Marginal Column Totals must total 100%.

JOB FUNCTION ANALYSIS Page 2

POSTION CONTEXT VARIABLES:

Indicate the responsibilities and aptitudes required to perform the essential/primary functions for this position.

Yes	No	Place an "X" in the appropriate box (or click box with mouse to use as toggle).
❑	❑	Work with frustrating situations: Job objectives are hindered by events beyond the employee's control.
❑	❑	Advise: Counsel others based on legal, financial, scientific, technical, or other specialized areas; recommend, guide caution.
❑	❑	Coordinate: Negotiate, monitor and organize activities of others to achieve objectives, but without direct authority.
❑	❑	Instruct: Teach others, formally or informally.
❑	❑	Group activities: Participate in activities requiring interpersonal skills and cooperation with others.
❑	❑	Work under time pressure: Rush or urgent time lines.
❑	❑	Work on an irregular schedule: Unscheduled overtime, called in to work, unanticipated changes in work pace.
❑	❑	Work with numerous distractions: Telephone calls, visitors, coworkers.
❑	❑	Handle multiple assignments, conflicting demands or priorities.
❑	❑	Concentration: Maintain attention to detail over extended period of time, continually aware of variations in changing situations.
❑	❑	Reaction or response: Quick reaction/immediate response to emergencies of severe consequences.
❑	❑	Research and analysis: Fact-finding, interpretation, investigation in preparing reports or evaluations.
❑	❑	Accountability and consequence of error: Responsible for money, equipment, or personnel. Severe consequences to department, University, or coworkers if work objectives are not met.
❑	❑	Work independence: Work is performed independently or with minimal on-site supervision.
❑	❑	Supervise: Recruit, screen, hire, assign and/or review work, train and/or evaluate other employees.
❑	❑	Confidentiality: Work with confidential information, materials, records.

Comments:

COGNITIVE PROCESSES:

Indicate cognitive abilities required to complete the essential functions.

Yes	No	Type an "X" in the appropriate box (or click box with mouse to use as toggle).
❑	❑	Inspect products, objects, or materials.
❑	❑	Analyze information or data.
❑	❑	Plan sequence of operations or actions.
❑	❑	Make decisions of moderate to substantial effects, with variety of alternatives and moderate to substantial consequences.
❑	❑	Use logic to define problems, collect information, establish facts, draw valid conclusions, interpret information, deal with abstract variables.
❑	❑	Perform basic counting, addition, and subtraction of numbers.
❑	❑	Perform calculations using algebra, geometry, and statistics.
		Comprehend written communication:
❑	❑	a. Basic instructions, safety rules, office memoranda at high school graduate level.
❑	❑	b. Technical or professional materials, financial or legal reports at post secondary level.
		Compose written communication:
❑	❑	a. Compose letters or memos using standard business English at high school graduate level.
❑	❑	b. Compose and edit report or technical, professional material at post secondary level.
		Verbal comprehension:
❑	❑	a. Comprehend simple verbal sentences and instructions at high school graduate level.
❑	❑	b. Comprehend technical and complex information at post-secondary level.
		Verbal communication:
❑	❑	a. Converse in Standard English at high school graduate level.
❑	❑	b. Converse using complex technical or professional English at post secondary level.

Foreign Language Requirements:

Comments:

JOB FUNCTION ANALYSIS Page 3

DEGREE OF PUSH/PULL ACTIVITY:

Indicate the percent of time that pushing and pulling activities are performed. The total should equal 100%.

		N/A	<25%	25-49%	50-74%	>75%
SEDENTARY	Exert up to 10 lbs. of force occasionally* and/or a minute amount frequently**	❑	❑	❑	❑	❑
LIGHT	Exert up to 20 lbs. of force occasionally* and/or up to 10 lbs. of force frequently**	❑	❑	❑	❑	❑
MEDIUM	Exert 20-50 lbs. of force occasionally* and/or 10-15 lbs. of force frequently**	❑	❑	❑	❑	❑
HEAVY	Exert 50-100 lbs. of force occasionally* and/or 25-50 lbs. of force frequently**	❑	❑	❑	❑	❑
VERY HEAVY	Exert 100 lbs. of force occasionally* and/or 50 lbs. of force frequently**	❑	❑	❑	❑	❑

***Occasionally: activity or conditions exist up to 1/3 of the time**

****Frequently: activity or conditions exist from 1/3 to 2/3 of the time**

PHYSICAL REQUIREMENTS:

Indicate the percent of time the following are performed.

The following activities cannot be performed concurrently, so the total should equal 100%.

		N/A	<25%	25-49%	50-74%	>75%
KNEEL	To bend legs at the knee, come to rest on knees	❑	❑	❑	❑	❑
CROUCH	To bend the body down and forward, bending the legs and spine	❑	❑	❑	❑	❑
CRAWL	Move on the hands, knees and feet	❑	❑	❑	❑	❑
CLIMB	Ascend/descend ladders, stairs, ramps	❑	❑	❑	❑	❑
SIT	For up to two hours at a time	❑	❑	❑	❑	❑
STAND	**For up to two hours at a time**	❑	❑	❑	❑	❑
WALK	**Move about on foot**	❑	❑	❑	❑	❑

The following can be performed concurrently, so the amounts need not be totaled.

		N/A	<25%	25-49%	50-74%	>75%
LIFT	To raise or lower an object >10 lbs. from one level to another	❑	❑	❑	❑	❑
LIFT	To raise or lower an object >25 lbs. from one level to another	❑	❑	❑	❑	❑
CARRY	To transport an object	❑	❑	❑	❑	❑
PUSH	To press with steady force, thrust objects forward, downward, outward	❑	❑	❑	❑	❑
PULL	To drag or tug objects	❑	❑	❑	❑	❑
BEND	To bend downward and forward by bending the spine at the waist	❑	❑	❑	❑	❑
BALANCE	Exceeding ordinary body equilibrium	❑	❑	❑	❑	❑
REACH	Extend hands and arms, in any direction	❑	❑	❑	❑	❑
HANDLE	Seize, hold, turn with hands	❑	❑	❑	❑	❑
FINGER	Pinch, type, activity with fingers	❑	❑	❑	❑	❑
REP MOT[1]	Repetitious movements of arms, hands, wrists, etc.	❑	❑	❑	❑	❑
TALK	Express or exchange ideas verbally	❑	❑	❑	❑	❑
HEAR	Perceiving sound by ear	❑	❑	❑	❑	❑
SEE***	Obtain impressions through the eye	❑	❑	❑	❑	❑

*****Check all that apply:**
❑ vision clarity greater than 20 inches
❑ vision clarity less than 20 inches
❑ ability to distinguish color

[1] Repetitive motion

JOB FUNCTION ANALYSIS Page 4

EQUIPMENT, TOOLS, ELECTRONIC AND COMMUNICATION DEVICES, AND SOFTWARE:

List the items the employee will use to perform the essential/primary functions.

1.		4.	
2.		5.	
3.		6.	

PHYSICAL SURROUNDINGS AND HAZARDS:

Indicate which statements are applicable.

❑ Spends approximately 80% or more of time indoors.
❑ Spends approximately 80% or more of time outdoors.
❑ Activities occur inside or outside in approximately equal amounts.

❑ Temperatures may be below 32 degrees for more than one hour at a time.
❑ Temperatures may be above 100 degrees for more than one hour at a time.

❑ Noise is sufficient to cause the employee to shout in order to be heard.
❑ Exposure to vibrating movements to the extremities or entire body.
❑ Risk of bodily injury due to proximity to moving mechanical parts, electrical current, animals, etc.
❑ Conditions that affect the respiratory system or the skin, i.e., fumes, odors, air particles.

GENERAL INFORMATION:

Comments: ______

Must a vehicle be driven to perform the essential/primary functions? ❑ YES ❑ NO

Location(s) where work is performed: ______________________________

Day/Hour schedule: ______________________________

Name/phone of Supervisor to whom this position reports: ______________________________

Title of Supervisor: ______________________________

Name of person completing form: ______________________________ Date ______________

Signature of incumbent:* ______________________________ Date ______________

***Signature of person currently in position. If "vacant" or "new," leave blank.**

If you are requesting the establishment of a new Merit position or reclassification of existing Merit position, submit this form to: Compensation and Classification, 121-11 USB.

All merit requisitions must have an EFMA on file In the hiring department before the requisition will be processed.

It is recommended all P & S requisitions have an EFMA on file in the hiring department at the time of advertising.

Comments: ______

Appendix O: Building Survey Form

Name of building: ______________________ Date of survey: ______________________

Location: ______________________ Surveyor: ______________________

	Yes	No
Parking Area		
1. Are accessible parking spaces with adjacent access aisle to accommodate a wheelchair available?	____	____
2. Are curb cutouts available and appropriately labeled?	____	____
3. Are parking spaces easily accessible to walkway without requiring negotiating behind parked cars?	____	____
Entrances to Building		
1. Is at least one major entrance available for use by an individual using a wheelchair?	____	____
2. Does the entrance provide access to a level where elevators are available?	____	____
Elevators		
1. Is a passenger elevator available?	____	____
2. Does the elevator reach all levels of the building?	____	____
3. Are control buttons (both inside and outside of the elevator) no more than 48 in (122 cm) from the floor?	____	____
4. Are control buttons raised and easy to push?	____	____
5. Is an emergency telephone accessible?	____	____
Public Telephones		
1. Are an appropriate number of phones available and accessible to individuals using a wheelchair?	____	____
2. Are they dial or pushbutton?	____	____
3. Is the height of the dial mechanism no more than 44 in (112 cm) from the floor?	____	____
4. Is a receiver volume control available?	____	____

	Yes	No
Floor Surfaces		
1. Are surfaces nonslip?	____	____
2. If carpeting is present, is it tightly woven and securely glued to floor (to prevent rippling under wheelchair)?	____	____
Rest Rooms		
1. Is there an adequate number of accessible rest rooms available?	____	____
2. Is there at least 48 in (122 cm) between inside wall and partitions enclosing toilet?	____	____
3. Is entrance to cubicle at least 48 in (122 cm) wide?	____	____
4. Are grab bars present and securely mounted?	____	____
5. Is height of seat not more than 17.5 in (44.5 cm)?	____	____
6. Is toilet paper holder within easy reach?	____	____
7. Is adequate turning space (6 ft × 6 ft [183 cm × 183 cm]) available in main area of rest room?	____	____
8. Is there adequate space for clearance of knees under sink?	____	____
9. Are drain and hot-water pipes covered or shielded to avoid burns?	____	____
10. Are faucet handles large (blade-type) and accessible?	____	____
Water Fountains		
1. Is the fountain height appropriate for use by someone in a wheelchair?	____	____
2. Are controls pushbutton or blade-type?	____	____
3. Is a foot control available?	____	____
4. Is adequate space (at least 3 ft [92 cm]) provided near fountain to permit wheelchair mobility?	____	____

From Cotler, SR, and DeGraff, AH: Architectural Accessibility for the Disabled of College Campuses. New York State Univ. Construction Fund, Albany, 1976.

S E C T I O N   T H R E E

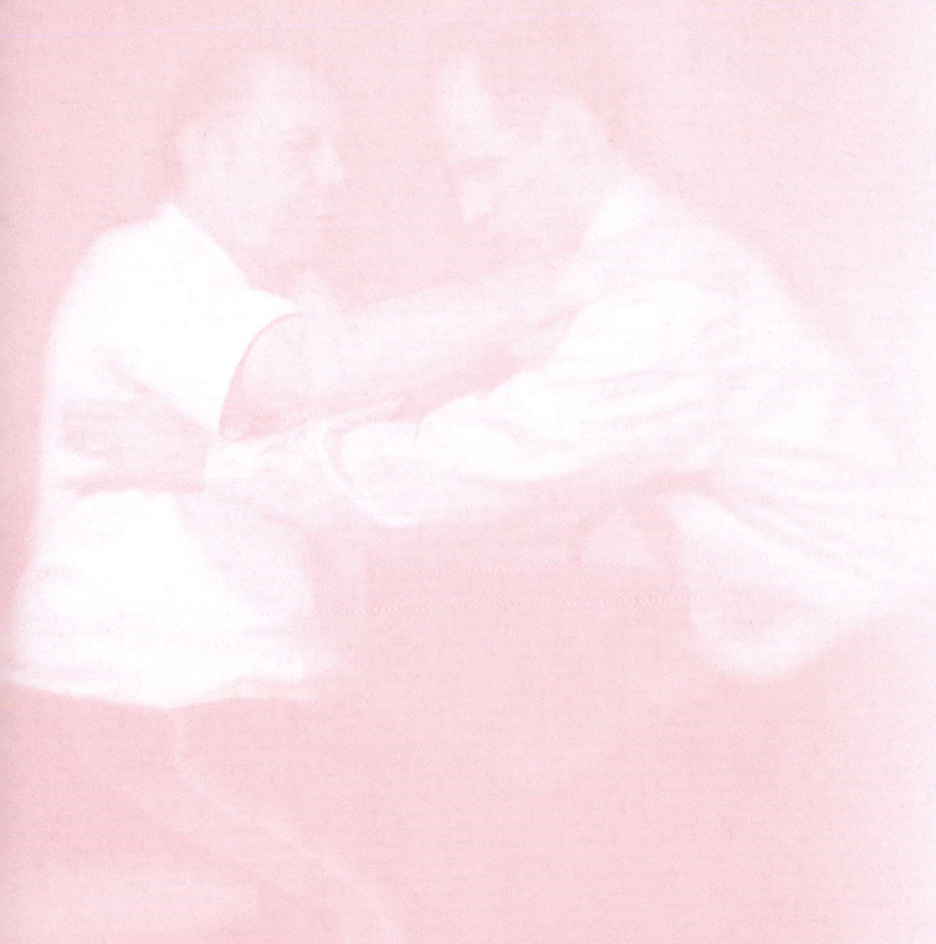

Intervention Strategies for Rehabilitation

CHAPTER

13

LEARNING OBJECTIVES

1. Describe a model for clinical decision making that incorporates components of normal motor control and motor learning.
2. Identify factors critical to motor control and describe intervention strategies designed to optimize the acquisition of motor control.
3. Identify key factors in recovery of function and describe intervention strategies designed to optimize recovery.
4. Identify factors critical to motor learning and describe intervention strategies designed to optimize learning.
5. Differentiate among the following: functional training, neurofacilitation training, and compensatory training.
6. Analyze and interpret patient data, formulate anticipated goals and expected outcomes, and develop a plan of care that presents an integrated approach to treatment when presented with a clinical case study.

Strategies to Improve Motor Function

Susan B. O'Sullivan, PT, EdD

OUTLINE

Developing strategies to improve motor function (motor control, motor recovery, and motor learning) requires a thorough understanding of the neural processes involved in producing movement and learning, and the pathologies that may affect the central nervous system (CNS). In addition, knowledge of recovery processes following CNS insult is essential. Treatment models based on theories of motor control, recovery, and learning allow the therapist to organize thinking and approach clinical decision making in a coherent manner. Patients with disorders of motor function frequently demonstrate a wide variety of impairments, functional limitations, and disabilities. Careful examination of sensorimotor and learning behaviors and the environmental contexts in which they occur provides an appropriate base for planning. Different intervention strategies and techniques have been developed by physical therapists to address disorders of motor function. An optimal plan of care (POC) must address the individual needs of the patient, maintain a focus on minimizing or eliminating functional limitations and physical disabilities, and enhance overall quality of life.

Motor Control

Motor control has been defined as "an area of study dealing with the understanding of the neural, physical, and behavioral aspects of movement."[1, p 465] Information processing of human motor behavior occurs in stages (Fig. 13.1). The initial stage is *stimulus identification.* Relevant stimuli concerning current body state and environmental context are selected and identified. Meaning is attached based on past sensorimotor experiences. Perceptual and cognitive processes including memory, attention, motivation, and emotional control all play an integral role in ensuring the ease and accuracy of information processing during this stage. Selection of relevant sensory input is sensitive to the clarity and intensity of the stimuli received. Thus, stronger and crisper stimuli result in enhanced attentional mechanisms and information processing. Processing is also influenced by stimulus pattern complexity. Complicated, novel patterns of stimuli prolong stimulus identification. An intrinsic knowledge of movement (e.g., position of limb,

Within the CNS

Stimulus ➤	Stimulus Identification	Response Selection	Response Programming	➤ Movement output
	sensing perceiving memory contact	interpreting planning deciding	translating structuring initiating R	
	sensitive to s clarity s intensity s pattern complexity	sensitive to nu. of alternatives S-R compatability	sensitive to R complexity R duration R-R compatability	

Nu = number, CNS = central nervous system, S = stimulus, R = response

Figure 13.1 Model of information-processing stages of movement control.

length of limb, distance to goal, and so forth) is a critical characteristic of motor behavior. In the *response selection stage* the plan for movement is developed.

A **motor plan** is defined as an idea or plan for purposeful movement that is made up of component motor programs. A general rather than detailed response is selected; that is, a prototype of the final movement. Decision making during this stage is sensitive to the number of different movement alternatives possible and the overall compatibility between the stimulus and response. The more natural the association between stimulus and response, the easier the decision making. For example, in a well-learned movement like crossing at a street light, an individual easily responds to the green light by moving forward. If a crossing guard signals the individual to move forward even though the light is red, the individual is likely to be more hesitant in responding.

The final stage is termed *response programming*. Neural control centers translate and change the idea for movement into muscular actions defined by a motor program. A **motor program** is defined as "an abstract representation that, when initiated, results in the production of a coordinated movement sequence."[1, p 466] The structuring of motor programs includes attention to specific parameters such as synergistic component parts, force, direction, timing, duration, and extent of movement. Parametric specification is based on the constraints of the individual, the task, and the environment. Information processing during this stage is sensitive to the complexity of the desired movement and duration. Thus, complex and lengthier movement sequences increase the duration of processing during this stage. Programming can also be affected by response–response compatibility. This is the compatibility for dual movement tasks that either occur simultaneously (e.g., bouncing a ball while walking) or when choices are required (e.g., one paired movement response must occur before another). During response execution (movement output), muscles are selected against an appropriate background of postural control. **Feedforward**, the sending of signals in advance of movement to ready the system, allows for anticipatory adjustments in postural activity. **Feedback**, response-produced information received during or after the movement, is used to monitor output for corrective actions. Although this simplified model gives the appearance that the information flow is linear, actual processing by the CNS is both serial and parallel. Thus, both single and multiple pathways are engaged to process information.[1] Figure 13.2 provides a schematic depiction of the major directions of information flow within the CNS during voluntary movement.

Theories of Motor Control

A theory is the orderly explanation of observations. Different theories of motor control have been developed over time, and reflect current understanding and interpretation of nervous system function. Because theories provide an important framework for clinical practice, a brief overview is warranted. The reader is also referred to the excellent works of Schmidt[1] and Shumway-Cook and Woollacott[2] for further review and study.

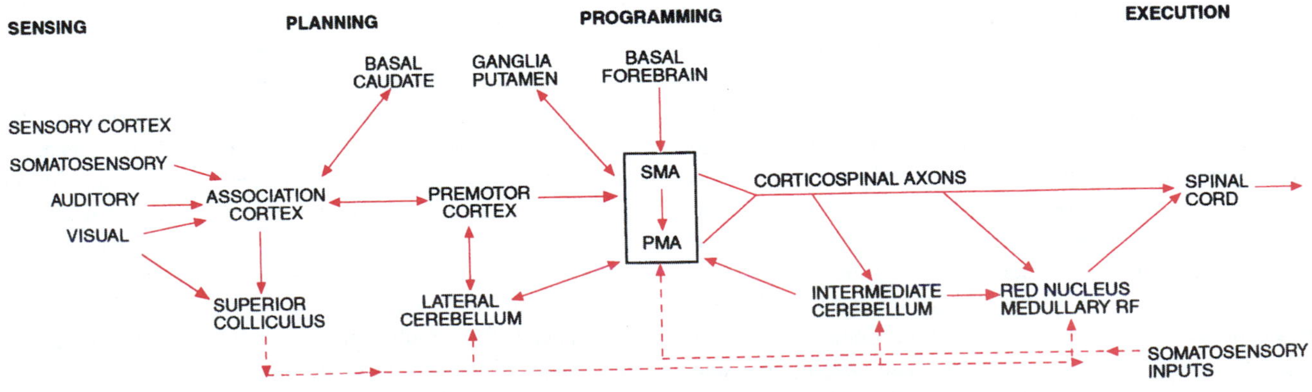

Figure 13.2 Major directions of information flow during a voluntary movement to and from the primary motor areas (PMA) and supplementary motor areas (SMA), only some of the connections of the superior colliculus are shown. RF = reticular formation. (From Brooks,[5, p 199] with permission.)

An early theory of motor control, *reflex theory,* was established by Sherrington.[3] His research on sensory receptors led to the view that movement was the result of a stimulus–response sequence of events or **reflex** based. Complex movements were nothing more than the coupling or chaining together of a number of reflexes to produce the final outcome. Thus, sensation assumed a primary role in the initiation and production of movement. Limitations in reflex theory abound. It fails to consider that voluntary movements can be activated in the absence of a sensory stimulus. It also fails to consider that some movements occur so fast as to not allow use of available feedback. Finally, it does not consider the infinite variability that allows for different movements in response to the same stimulus.[2]

Hierarchical theory dates back to the work of Hughlings Jackson.[4] This theory is based on the assumption that the CNS is organized into three primary levels of control: high, middle, and low centers. Control was viewed as proceeding in a descending direction from higher to lower centers, a "top-down" progression. Reflex theory integrated with hierarchical theory presents the view that reflexes are components of the lower centers that became integrated during normal maturation and development as higher centers assumed control. Conversely, reflexes reemerge in control of movement when higher centers become damaged. A more current interpretation of this model proposes a theory of *flexible hierarchies.*[5] Within this modification, the command hierarchies have been more fully elaborated. The association cortex operates as the highest level (elaborating perceptions and planning strategies), while the sensorimotor cortex in association with portions of the basal ganglia, brainstem, and cerebellum function as the middle level (converting strategies into motor programs and commands). The spinal cord functions at the lowest level, translating commands into muscle actions resulting in the execution of movement. Modern hierarchical theory proposes that the three levels do not operate in a rigid, top-down order as originally described but rather as a flexible system in which each level can exert control on the others. Shifts in control are dependent on the demands and complexity of the task with the higher centers always assuming control whenever the task demands are high.

Systems theory, proposed by Bernstein,[6] is based on the view that motor control is the result of the cooperative actions of many interacting systems, working to accommodate the demands of the specific task. Both internal factors (joint stiffness, inertia, movement-dependent forces) and external factors (gravity) must be taken into consideration in the planning of movements. It assumes a shifting locus of neural control, referred to as a *distributed model of control.* Thus, large areas of the CNS may be engaged for complex motor tasks while relatively few centers are engaged for more discrete movements. This type of multilevel control allows for the control of a number of separate independent dimensions of movement, termed *degrees of freedom.* The executive level is freed from the responsibility of control for simple movements or the demands of having to control many degrees of freedom at one time. *Coordinative structures* are used to simplify control, and to initiate coordinated patterns or synergies to produce movements. The use of *synergies* for the control of locomotion (central pattern generators) and posture (postural synergies) is well documented.[7]

Motor Programming Theory

Motor programs allow for movements to occur in the absence of sensation (deafferentation) or in situations in which limitations in speed of processing feedback negate control (rapid movements). Motor programs also free the nervous system from conscious decisions about movement, reducing the problem of multiple degrees of freedom. Motor programs can be run off virtually without the influence of peripheral feedback or error detection processes, termed an **open-loop control system** (Fig. 13.3). This is in contrast to a **closed-loop control system** (Fig. 13.4), which employs feedback and a reference for correctness to compute error and initiate subsequent corrections. Feedback and closed-loop processes play a critical role in the learning of new motor skills (response selection) and in the shaping and correction of ongoing movements (response execution). Feedback is also essential for the ongoing maintenance of body posture and balance.

The complexity of human movement negates any simplistic model of movement control. An *intermittent control hypothesis* described by Schmidt[1] proposes a blending of both open-loop and closed-loop processes, in

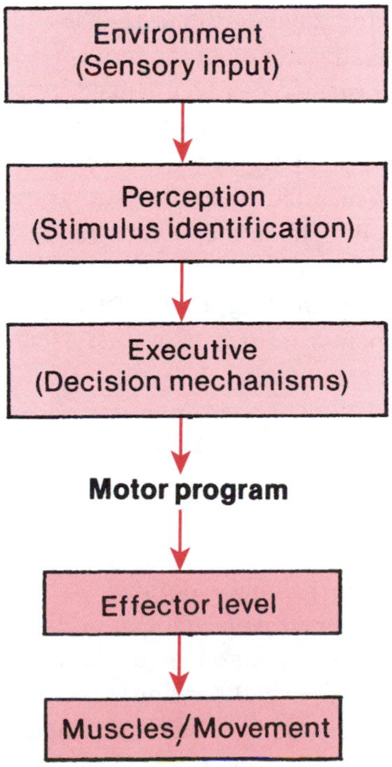

Figure 13.3 Open-loop control system.

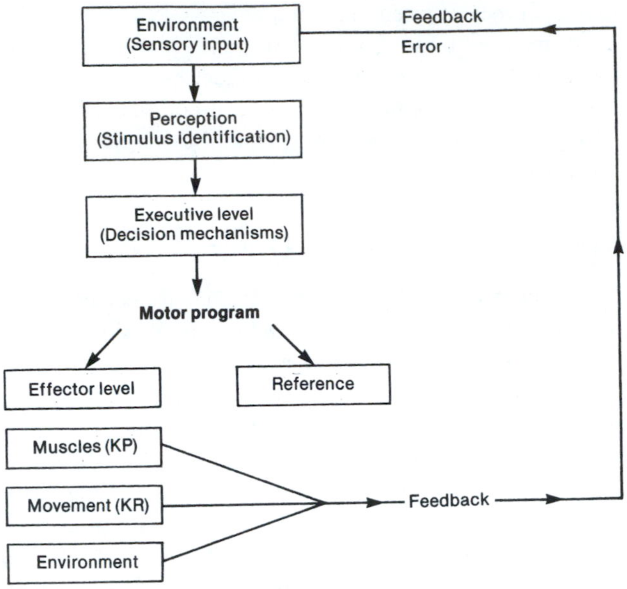

Figure 13.4 Closed-loop control system. KP = knowledge of performance, KR = knowledge of results.

which both operate in concert as part of the larger system. Motor programs provide the generalized code for motor events **(schema)**, while feedback is used to refine and perfect movements. Either may assume a dominant role, depending on the task at hand. Both may operate within a given movement but at different times and with different functions. Generalized motor programs include both invariant characteristics and parameters. *Invariant characteristics* are the unique features of the stored code: relative force, relative timing, and order of components. *Parameters* are the changeable features that ensure flexibility of motor programs and variations in movements from one performance to the next. These include overall force and overall duration of the movement. For example, walking performance can be changed by speeding up or slowing down (changes in overall duration) while the basic order of stepping cycle and relative timing of the components (invariant characteristics) are maintained.[8] Patients with deficits in motor function may demonstrate impairments in voluntary movements (impaired motor planning or programming) or the corrective actions (feedback adjustments) needed to initially learn and coordinate movements.

Motor Learning

Motor learning has been defined as "a set of internal processes associated with practice or experience leading to relatively permanent changes in the capability for skilled behavior."[1, p 466] Learning a motor skill is a complex process that requires spatial, temporal, and hierarchical organization of the CNS. Changes in the CNS are not directly observable but rather are inferred from changes in motor behavior. Improvements in **performance** result from practice or experience and are a frequently used measure of learning. For example, with practice an individual is able to develop appropriate sequencing of movement components with improved timing and reduced effort and concentration. Performance, however, is not always an accurate reflection of learning. It is possible to practice enough to temporarily improve performance but not retain the learning. Conversely, factors such as fatigue, anxiety, poor motivation, or medications may cause performance to deteriorate while learning may still occur. Because performance can be affected by a number of factors, it can be reasonably defined as a "temporary change in motor behavior seen during practice sessions."[2, p 24] **Retention** provides a better measure of learning. Retention refers to the ability of the learner to demonstrate the skill over time and after a period of no practice **(retention interval)**. Performance after a retention interval may decrease slightly, but should return to original performance levels within relatively few practice trials. For example, riding a bike is a well-learned skill that is generally retained even though an individual may not have ridden for years. The ability to apply a learned skill to the learning of other similar tasks, termed **generalizability**, is another important measure of learning. Individuals who learn to transfer from wheelchair to platform mat can apply that learning to other types of transfers (e.g., wheelchair to car, wheelchair to tub). The time and effort required to organize and learn these new types of transfers is reduced. Finally, learning can be measured by **resistance to contextual change**. This is the adaptability required to perform a motor task in altered environmental situations. Thus, an individual who has learned a skill (e.g., walking with a cane on indoor level surfaces) should be able to apply that learning to new and variable situations (e.g., walking outdoors, walking on a busy sidewalk). Motor learning is the direct result of practice and is highly dependent on sensory information and feedback processes. The relative importance of the different types of sensory information varies according to task and to the phase of learning. Individual differences exist **(motor capacity)** and may influence both the rate and degree of learning possible. Impairments in learning are common for the patient with CNS dysfunction.

Theories of Motor Learning

Adams[9] developed a theory of motor learning based on closed-loop control (closed-loop theory). He postulated that sensory feedback from ongoing movement is compared with stored memory of the intended movement (perceptual trace) to provide the CNS with a **reference of correctness** and error detection. Memory traces are then used to produce an appropriate action and to evaluate outcomes. The stronger the perceptual trace developed through practice, the greater the capability of the learner to use closed-loop processes for learning movements. Adams concentrated on examining slow, linear-positioning responses. This theory does not adequately explain learning under conditions of rapid movements (open-loop control processes). It also does not explain learning that can occur in the absence of sensory feedback (deafferentation studies).

Schema theory, proposed by Schmidt,[10] is based on the concepts that slow movements are feedback-based while rapid movements are program-based. He proposed that schema were used for storage into memory. Schema is defined as "a rule, concept, or relationship formed on the basis of experience."[1, p 467] Schema can include such things as initial conditions (body position, weight of objects, and so forth), relationships between parameters of movement, environmental outcomes, and sensory consequences of movement. *Recall schema* are used to select and define the initial movement conditions while *recognition schema* are used to evaluate movement responses based on expected sensory consequences. Clinically, this theory supports the concept that practicing a variety of movement outcomes would improve learning through the development of expanded rules or schema. It also provides a plausible explanation for the learning of novel and open skills performed in a variable and changing environment.

Stages of Motor Learning

The process of motor learning has been described by Fitts and Posner[11] as occurring in relatively distinct stages, termed cognitive, associated, and autonomous. These stages provide a useful framework for describing the learning process and for organizing training strategies. Table 13.1 provides a summary.

Cognitive Stage

During the initial **cognitive stage** of learning, the major task at hand is to develop an overall understanding of the skill, termed the *cognitive map* or cognitive plan. This decision making phase of *"what to do"* requires a high level of cognitive processing as the learner performs successive approximations of the task, discarding strategies that are not successful and retaining those that are. The resulting trial-and-error practice initially yields uneven performance with frequent errors. Processing of sensory cues and perceptual–motor organization eventually leads to the selection of a motor strategy that proves reasonably successful. Because the learner progresses from an initially disorganized and often clumsy pattern to more organized movements, improvements in performance can be readily observed during this acquisition phase. The learner relies heavily on vision to guide early learning and movement. A stable environment free from distractors optimizes learning during this initial stage.

Associative Stage

During the middle or **associative stage** of learning, refinement of the motor strategy is achieved through continued practice. Spatial and temporal aspects become organized as the movement develops into a coordinated pattern. As performance improves, there is greater consistency and fewer errors and extraneous movements. The learner is now concentrating on "how to do" the movement rather than on what to do. Proprioceptive cues become increasingly important, while dependence on visual cues decreases. The learning process takes varying lengths of time depending on a number of factors. The nature of the task, prior experience and motivation of the learner, available feedback, and organization of practice can all influence acquisition of learning.

Autonomous Stage

The final or **autonomous stage** of learning is characterized by motor performance that after considerable practice is largely automatic. There is only a minimal level of cognitive monitoring, with motor programs so refined they can almost "run themselves." The spatial and temporal components of movement are becoming highly organized, and the learner is capable of coordinated motor patterns. The learner is now free to concentrate on other aspects, such as *"how to succeed"* at a competitive sport. Movements are largely error-free with little interference from environmental distractions. Thus the learner can perform equally well in a stable, predictable environment (termed **closed motor skills**) or in a changing, unpredictable environment (termed **open motor skills**).

Strategies to Enhance Motor Learning

Motor learning involves a significant amount of practice and feedback, with a high level of information processing related to control, error detection, and correction. Motor learning can be facilitated through the use of effective training strategies (summarized in Table 13.1).

Strategy Development

The overall goal during the early cognitive stage of learning is to facilitate task understanding and organize early practice. The learner's knowledge of the skill and any existing problems must be ascertained. The therapist should highlight the purpose of the skill in a functionally relevant context. The task should seem important, desirable, and realistic to learn. The therapist should demonstrate the task exactly as it should be done (i.e., coordinated action with smooth timing and ideal performance speed). This helps the learner develop an internal cognitive map or *reference of correctness*. Attention should be directed to the desired outcome and critical task elements. The therapist should point out similarities to other learned tasks so that subroutines that are part of other motor programs can be retrieved from memory. Features of the environment critical to performance should also be highlighted.

Table 13.1 Characteristics of Motor Learning Stages and Training Strategies

Cognitive Stage Characteristics	Training Strategies
The learner develops an understanding of task; **cognitive mapping** assesses abilities, task demands; identifies stimuli, contacts memory; selects response; performs initial approximations of task; structures motor program; modifies initial responses "*What to do*" decision	Highlight purpose of task in functionally relevant terms. Demonstrate ideal performance of task to establish a **reference of correctness**. Have patient verbalize task components and requirements. Point out similarities to other learned tasks. Direct attention to critical task elements. Select appropriate feedback. • Emphasize intact sensory systems, intrinsic feedback systems. • Carefully pair extrinsic feedback with intrinsic feedback. • High dependence on vision: have patient watch movement. • **Knowledge of Performance** (KP): focus on errors as they become consistent; do not cue on large number of random errors. • **Knowledge of Results** (KR): focus on success of movement outcome. Ask learner to evaluate performance, outcomes; identify problems, solutions. Use reinforcements (praise) for correct performance, continuing motivation. Organize feedback schedule. • Feedback after every trial improves performance during early learning. • Variable feedback (summed, fading, bandwidth designs) increases depth of cognitive processing, improves retention; may decrease performance initially. Organize initial practice. • Stress controlled movement to minimize errors. • Provide adequate rest periods (distributed practice) if task is complex, long, or energy costly or if learner fatigues easily, has short attention, or poor concentration. • Use manual guidance to assist as appropriate. • Break complex tasks down into component parts, teach both parts and integrated whole. • Utilize bilateral transfer as appropriate. • Use blocked (repeated) practice of same task to improve performance. • Use variable practice (serial or random practice order) of related skills to increase depth of cognitive processing and retention; may decrease performance initially. • Use mental practice to improve performance and learning, reduce anxiety. Assess, modify arousal levels as appropriate. • High or low arousal impairs performance and learning. • Avoid stressors, mental fatigue. Structure environment. • Reduce extraneous environmental stimuli, distractors to ensure attention, concentration. • Emphasize closed skills initially gradually progressing to open skills.
Associated Stage Characteristics	**Training Strategies**
The learner practices movements, refines motor program: spatial and temporal organization; decreases errors, extraneous movements Dependence on visual feedback decreases, increases for use of proprioceptive feedback; cognitive monitoring decreases "*How to do*" decision	Select appropriate feedback. • Continue to provide KP; intervene when errors become consistent. • Emphasize proprioceptive feedback, "feel of movement" to assist in establishing an internal reference of correctness. • Continue to provide KR; stress relevance of functional outcomes. • Assist learner to improve self-evaluation, decision making skills. • Facilitation techniques, guided movements may be counterproductive during this stage of learning.

Table 13.1 **Characteristics of Motor Learning Stages and Training Strategies (continued)**

	Organize feedback schedule. • Continue to provide feedback for continuing motivation; encourage patient to self-assess achievements. • Avoid excessive augmented feedback. • Focus on use of variable feedback (summed, fading, bandwidth) designs to improve retention. Organize practice. • Encourage consistency of performance. • Focus on variable practice order (serial or random) of related skills to improve retention. Structure environment. • Progress toward open, changing environment. • Prepare the learner for home, community, work environments.
Autonomous Stage Characteristics	**Training Strategies**
The learner practices movements, continues to refine motor responses, spatial and temporal highly organized, movements are largely error-free, minimal level of cognitive monitoring "*How to succeed*" decision	Assess need for conscious attention, automaticity of movements. Select appropriate feedback. • Learner demonstrates appropriate self-evaluation, decision making skills. • Provide occasional feedback (KP, KR) when errors evident. Organize practice. • Stress consistency of performance in variable environments, variations of tasks (open skills). • High levels of practice (massed practice) are appropriate. Structure environment. • Vary environments to challenge learner. • Ready the learner for home, community, work environments. Focus on competitive aspects of skills as appropriate, e.g., wheelchair sports.

Highly skilled individuals who have been successfully discharged from rehabilitation can be expert models. Their success in returning to the "real world" will also have a positive effect in motivating patients new to rehabilitation. For example, it is very difficult for a therapist with full use of muscles to accurately demonstrate appropriate transfer skills to an individual with C6 complete tetraplegia. A former patient with a similar level injury can accurately demonstrate how the skill should be performed. Demonstration has also been shown to be effective in producing learning even with unskilled patient models. In this situation, the learner/patient benefits from the cognitive processing and problem solving used while watching the unskilled model attempt to correct errors and arrive at the desired movement.[12] Demonstrations can be live or videotaped. Developing a video library of demonstrations of skilled former patients is a useful strategy to ensure availability of effective models.

During initial practice, the therapist should give clear and concise verbal instructions and not overload the patient with excessive or wordy commands. It is important to reinforce correct performance and intervene when movement errors become consistent or when safety is an issue. The therapist should *not* attempt to correct all the numerous errors that characterize this stage but rather allow for some trial-and-error learning. Feedback, particularly visual feedback, is important during early learning. The learner should be directed to watch the movements closely. The learner's initial performance trials can also be recorded for later viewing and analysis.

Guidance

Guidance involves physically assisting the learner during the task. It is effective during early learning in improving performance of an unfamiliar skill by preventing or limiting errors. The therapist's hands can effectively substitute for missing elements, holding part of a limb stable while constraining unwanted movements and guiding the patient toward correct performance.[13] It also allows the learner to experience the tactile and kinesthetic inputs inherent in task performance, that is, to learn the "sensations of movement."[14] The supportive use of hands can allay fears and instill confidence while ensuring safety. The key to success in using guided movements is to intersperse active practice with guided movements, providing only as much assistance as needed and removing assistance as soon as possible. As manual guidance is reduced, verbal guidance can be increased. Overuse of guided movements is likely to result in dependence on the therapist for assistance, thus becoming a "crutch." Guidance is most effective for slow postural responses (positioning tasks) and less effective during rapid or ballistic tasks.[1] Once guidance is removed, studies have shown that performance gains are not well maintained on retention tests.[15]

Active Decision Making

As learning progresses, the patient should be actively involved in self-monitoring, analysis, and self-correction of movements. The therapist can prompt the patient in early decision making by posing key questions. Specifically, the patient can be asked:

- What is the intended outcome of movement?
- What problems were present during the movement?
- What do you need to do to correct the problems in order to achieve a successful outcome?
- For complex movements, what are the components or steps of the task?
- How should the components be sequenced?

The therapist should confirm the accuracy of the patient's responses. If movement errors are consistent, the patient's efforts can be redirected. For example, if the patient consistently falls to the right while standing, questions can be more directed (In what direction did you fall? What do you need to do to correct this problem?). The therapist can also use augmented cues (i.e., tapping or light resistance) to assist the patient in correcting postural responses. The development of decision-making skills is critical in ensuring continued learning.

Strategy Refinement

During the associated and autonomous phases of learning, the patient continues to refine movement strategies with high levels of practice. Random errors decrease. As consistent errors are identified, solutions are generated. The focus is on refinement of skills and movement consistency in varied environments. This will ensure an overall range of movement patterns that are adaptable and match the changing demands of open environments. The patient's attention should be now focused on proprioceptive feedback, the "feel of the movement." Thus, the patient is directed to attend to the sensations intrinsic to the movement itself and to associate those sensations with the motor actions. Guided movements and facilitation techniques are counterproductive at this stage because they maintain dependence on the therapist and detract from active control. During late-stage learning, the use of distracters such as ongoing conversation or dual task training (e.g., ball skills during standing and walking) can yield important evidence of a developing level of autonomous control. It is important to remember that many patients undergoing active rehabilitation do not reach the final stage of learning. For example, in patients with traumatic brain injury, performance may reach consistent levels within structured environments, while safe, consistent performance in more open environments is not possible.

Feedback

The vast body of motor learning and therapeutic literature stresses the critical role of feedback in promoting motor learning. Feedback can be either **intrinsic**, occurring as a natural result of the movement, or provided by **extrinsic, augmented** sensory cues not typically received in the task. Proprioceptive, visual, vestibular, and cutaneous signals are examples of types of intrinsic feedback, while visual, auditory, or tactile cues are forms of extrinsic feedback (e.g., verbal cues, manual cues, biofeedback devices—EMG, pressure-sensing devices—forceplates, foot pad). During therapy, both intrinsic and extrinsic feedback can be manipulated to enhance motor learning. *Concurrent feedback* is given during task performance while *terminal feedback* is given at the end of task performance. Augmented feedback about the end result or overall outcome of the movement is termed **knowledge of results (KR)**. Augmented feedback about the nature or quality of the movement pattern produced is termed **knowledge of performance (KP)**.[1, p 465] The relative importance of KP and KR varies according to the skill being learned and the availability of feedback from intrinsic sources.[16–20] For example, tracking tasks are highly dependent on intrinsic visual and kinesthetic feedback (KP) while KR has less influence on the accuracy of the movements. In other tasks (e.g., transfers) KR provides the key information about how to shape the overall movements for the next attempt while KP may not be as useful. Performance cues (KP) should focus on key task elements that lead to a successful final outcome. Clinical decisions about feedback include:

- What type of feedback should be employed (mode)?
- How much feedback should be used (intensity)?
- When should feedback be given (scheduling)?

Choices about type of feedback involve the selection of which intrinsic sensory systems to highlight, what type of augmented feedback to use, and how to pair extrinsic feedback to intrinsic feedback. The selection of sensory systems depends on specific examination findings of sensory integrity. The sensory systems selected must provide accurate and usable information. If an intrinsic sensory system is impaired and provides distorted or incomplete information (e.g., impaired proprioception with diabetic neuropathy) then use of alternate sensory systems (vision) should be emphasized. Supplemental augmented feedback can be used to enhance learning. Decisions are also based on stage of learning. Early in learning, visual feedback is easily brought to conscious attention and therefore is important. Less consciously accessible sensory information such as proprioception is more useful during the middle and end stages of learning.

Decisions about frequency and scheduling of feedback (when and how much) must be reached. Frequent feedback (e.g., given after every trial) quickly guides the learner to the correct performance but slows retention. Conversely, feedback that is varied (not given after every trial) slows initial acquisition of the skill while improving performance on a retention test.[21–25] This is most likely due to the increased depth of cognitive processing that accompanies the variable presentation of feedback. Varied feedback schedules include (1) *summed feedback,* feedback given after a set number of trials (e.g., after every other trial or every third trial); (2) *faded feedback,* feedback given at first after every trial and then less frequently (e.g., after every second trial, progressing to every fifth trial); and (3) *bandwidth feedback,* feedback given only when performance is outside a given error range. *Delayed feedback,* feedback given after a brief time delay (e.g., a 3-second delay), can also be beneficial in allowing the learner a brief time for introspection and self-assessment.[26] In contrast, the therapist who bombards the patient immediately after task completion with excessive augmented verbal feedback may preclude active information processing by the learner. The patient's own decision-making skills are minimized, while the therapist's verbal skills dominate. Winstein[27] points out that this may well explain why many studies on the effectiveness of therapeutic approaches cite minimal carryover and limited retention of newly acquired motor skills. A feedback delay interval that is prolonged or filled with practice of other movements results in interference that may decrease learning. Finally, the withdrawal of augmented feedback should be gradual and carefully paired with the patient's efforts to correctly utilize intrinsic feedback systems.

Practice

The second major influence on motor learning is **practice**. In general, the more the practice, the greater the learning. The therapist's role is to ensure that the patient practices the desired movements. Practice of incorrect movement patterns can lead to a negative learning situation in which "faulty habits and postures" must be unlearned before the correct movements can be mastered. The organization of practice will depend on several factors, including the patient's motivation, attention span, concentration, endurance, and the type of task. An additional factor is the frequency of allowable therapy sessions, which is often dependent on hospital scheduling and availability of services and payment. For outpatients, practice at home is highly dependent on motivation, family support, and suitable environment.

Clinical decisions about practice include:

- How should practice periods and rest periods be spaced (distribution of practice)?
- What tasks and task variations should be practiced (variability of practice)?
- How should the tasks be sequenced (practice order)?
- How should the environment be structured (closed vs open)?

Massed versus Distributed Practice

Massed practice refers to a sequence of practice and rest times in which the rest time is much less than the practice time.[1, p 465] Fatigue, decreased performance, and risk of injury are factors that must be considered when using massed practice. **Distributed practice** refers to spaced practice intervals in which the practice time is equal to or less than the rest time.[1, p 463] Although learning occurs with both, distributed practice results in the most learning per training time although the total training time is increased.[1] It is the preferred mode for many patients undergoing active rehabilitation who demonstrate limited performance capabilities and endurance. With adequate rest periods, performance can be improved without the interfering effects of fatigue or increasing safety issues. Distributed practice is also of benefit if motivation is low or if the learner has a short attention span, poor concentration, or motor planning deficits (e.g., dyspraxia). Distributed practice should also be considered if the task itself is complex, long, or has a high energy cost. Massed practice can be considered when motivation and skill levels are high and when the patient has adequate endurance, attention, and concentration. For example, the patient with spinal cord injury in the final stages of rehabilitation may spend long practice sessions acquiring the wheelchair skills needed for community access.

Blocked versus Random Practice

Blocked practice refers to a practice sequence organized around one task performed repeatedly, uninterrupted by practice of any other task.[1, p 462] **Random practice** refers to a practice sequence in which a variety of tasks are ordered randomly across trials.[1, p 466] While both allow for motor skill acquisition, random practice has been shown to have superior long-term effects in terms of retention.[28–30] For example, a variety of different transfers (e.g., bed to wheelchair, wheelchair to toilet, wheelchair to tub transfer seat) can be practiced all within the same training session. Although skilled performance of individual tasks may be initially delayed, improved retention of transfer skills can be expected. The constant challenge of varying the task demands provides high *contextual interference* and increases the depth of cognitive processing through retrieval practice from memory stores. The acquired skills can then be applied more easily to other task variations or environments. Constant practice will result in superior initial performance because of low contextual interference and may be required in certain situations (e.g., the patient with traumatic brain who requires a high degree of structure and consistency for learning).

Practice Order

Practice order refers to the sequence in which tasks are practiced. *Blocked order* refers to the repeated practice of a task or group of tasks in order (three trials of task 1, three trials of task 2, three trials of task 3: 111222333). *Serial order* refers to a predictable and repeating order (practice of multiple tasks in the following order: 123123123). *Random order* refers to a nonrepeating and nonpredictable order (123321312). Although skill acquisition can be achieved with all three, differences have been found. Blocked order produces improved early acquisition of skills (performance) while serial and random order produce better retention and generalizability of skills. This is again due to contextual interference and increased depth of cognitive processing.[31,32] The key element here is the degree to which the learner is actively involved in memory retrieval. For example, a treatment session can be organized to include practice of a number of different tasks (e.g., forward-, backward- and side-stepping and stairclimbing). Random ordering of the tasks may initially delay acquisition of the desired stepping movements but over the long term will result in improved retention and generalizability.

Mental Practice

Mental practice is a practice strategy in which performance of the motor task is imagined or visualized without overt physical practice.[1, p 465] Beneficial effects result from the cognitive rehearsal of task elements. It is theorized that underlying motor programs for movement are activated but with sub-threshold motor activity.[1] Brain mapping techniques have also revealed activation of similar brain areas during imagined movements as those activated during actual movement.[33,34] Mental practice has consistently been found to facilitate the acquisition of motor skills.[35–38] It should be considered for patients who fatigue easily and are unable to sustain physical practice. Mental practice is also effective in alleviating anxiety associated with initial practice by previewing the upcoming movement experience. Mental practice when combined with physical practice has been shown to increase the accuracy and efficiency of movements at significantly faster rates than physical practice alone.[39] When using mental practice, it is important to make sure the patient understands the task and is actively rehearsing the correct movements. This can be ensured by having the patient verbalize aloud the steps being rehearsed. It is generally contraindicated in patients with profound cognitive, communication, and/or perceptual deficits.

Part versus Whole Practice

Complex motor skills can be broken down into component parts for practice. The component parts are practiced before practice of the whole task is attempted. For example, during initial wheelchair transfer training the transfer steps are practiced in isolation before practicing the whole transfer (e.g., locking the brakes, lifting the foot pedals, moving forward in the chair, standing up, pivoting, and sitting down). It is important to identify the key steps through accurate task analysis and to sequence them in the required order. It is also important to practice the integrated whole in conjunction with the parts practice so that the learner develops the whole idea for the required task (i.e., cognitive map). Delaying practice of the integrated whole can interfere with transfer effects and learning.[1] Part–whole practice is most effective with discrete or serial motor tasks that have highly independent parts. Part–whole practice is not as effective for continuous movement tasks (e.g., walking) or for complex tasks with highly integrated parts. Both require a high degree of coordination with spatial and temporal sequencing of elements. For these tasks, practice of the integrated whole will result in superior learning.

Transfer of Learning

Transfer of learning refers to the gain (or loss) in the capability of task performance as a result of practice or experience on some other task.[1, p 436] Learning can be promoted through practice using contralateral extremities, termed **bilateral transfer**. For example, a patient with stroke first practices the desired movement pattern using the more normal (unaffected) extremity. This initial practice enhances formation or recall of the necessary motor program, which can then be applied to the opposite, involved extremity. This method cannot, however, substitute for lack of movement potential of the affected extremities (e.g., a flaccid limb on the hemiplegic side). Transfer effects are optimal with similarity of the tasks (e.g., identical components and actions) and environments.[40] For example, optimal transfer can be expected with practice of an upper extremity flexion pattern first on one side, then with an identical pattern on the other side.

Practice of *lead-up activities* is commonly used in physical therapy. Lead-ups are simpler task versions of a required complex task. The subtasks are practiced, typically in easier postures with significantly reduced degrees of freedom. Anxiety is also reduced and safety is ensured. Thus initial upright postural control can be practiced in kneeling, half-kneeling, or plantigrade before standing. The patient develops the required hip extension/abduction stabilization control required for upright stance but without the demands of the standing position or fear of falling. The more closely the lead-ups (subskills) resemble the final task, the better the transfer.

Closed versus Open Environments

Altering the environmental context is an important consideration in structuring practice sessions. Early learning benefits from practice in a stable or predictable, *closed environment.* As learning progresses the environment should be varied, and incorporate more variable features consistent with real world, *open environments.* Practicing walking only within the physical therapy clinic might lead to successful performance in that setting (context-specific learning) but does little to prepare the patient for ambulation at home or in the community. The therapist should begin to gradually modify the environment as soon as performance becomes consistent. It is important to remember that some patients (e.g., a patient with traumatic brain injury and limited recovery) may never be able to function in anything but a highly structured environment.

Functional Skills

The development of functional skills is a continuously evolving process that proceeds throughout the lifespan. Foundational skills are learned in infancy and childhood with the emergence of specific markers of developmental maturation.[41–44] These skills are often referred to as *developmental motor skills* although they remain *essential functional skills* throughout the lifespan. Examples include rolling, supine-to-sit or sit-to-stand, maintaining stability or moving in progressively more challenging antigravity postures (i.e., sitting, kneeling, standing), upper extremity manipulation, and locomotion. Essential functional skills can be grouped into four broad categories of motor skills: mobility, static postural control (stability), dynamic postural control (controlled mobility), and skill. See Table 13.2 for a description of these categories together with examples of activities/postures and impairments. These activities and postures are a focus of functional training during rehabilitation. Careful attention to the demands of the postures can effectively address the degrees of freedom problem in controlling body segments. For example, the prone-on-elbows posture focuses on development of shoulder, upper trunk, and head control while eliminating all demands for movement control in the lower body. Because the center of mass (COM) is low and the base of support (BOS) wide it is inherently safe. Kneeling and half-kneeling postures can be used to improve trunk and hip control without the demands for control of the knee and ankle. As with prone-on-elbows posture, the low COM and wide BOS reduce the likelihood of falls and injury. Table 13.3 presents a list of developmental postures and possible treatment benefits. It is clear that considerable variability exists in the development and refinement of these motor skills in both children and adults and a specific sequence for acquisition of skills cannot be applied.

Age-related factors result in modification and adaptation of functional skills in adults.[45–48] All stages of information processing are affected by aging.[49] Sensory losses (decline in receptor sensitivity, recognition, and sensory encoding) affect stimulus identification. Response selection and programming are also affected by CNS changes.[50] An age-related slowing of movements is well documented with increases noted in both reaction and movement times.[51] Coordination changes result from changes in motor unit size with deficits particularly noticeable in fine motor control. Older adults are also more sensitive to complexity of movement.[52,53] The principle of *speed–accuracy tradeoff* typically applies as adults age, that is, the accuracy of a movement is decreased as its speed is increased. To accommodate for this change, older adults typically move slower, especially when accuracy is required. Decreasing levels of cardiovascular fitness and strength and increased weight commonly associated with a sedentary lifestyle can also affect the performance of motor skills.[54] Finally, older adults often experience multiple disease pathologies that affect their ability to move and learn.[55] For example, an older adult may alter the method used to roll over and sit up secondary to an increase in body weight, a decrease in overall strength and fitness, or an emerging pathology such as Parkinson's disease.

Table 13.2 Motor Skills

Categories	Characteristics	Examples	Impairments
Mobility	Ability to move from one position to another	Rolling; supine-to-sit; sit-to-stand; transfers	Failure to initiate or sustain movements through the range; poorly controlled movements
Static postural control (stability, static equilibrium, or static balance)	Ability to maintain postural stability and orientation with the COM over the BOS with the body not in motion	Holding in antigravity postures: prone-on-elbows, quadruped, sitting, kneeling, half-kneeling, plantigrade, or standing	Failure to maintain a steady body position; excessive postural sway; wide BOS; high guard position or handhold; loss of balance
Dynamic postural control (controlled mobility, dynamic equilibrium, or dynamic balance)	Ability to maintain postural stability and orientation with the COM over the BOS while parts of the body are in motion	Weight shifting and reaching in any of the above postures	Failure to control posture during weight shifting or reaching tasks; loss of balance
Skill	Ability to consistently perform coordinated movement sequences for the purposes of investigation and interaction with the physical and social environment	Upper extremity reach and manipulation Bipedal ambulation	Poorly coordinated movements; lack of precision, control, consistency, and economy of effort

BOS = base of support; COM = center of mass.

Table 13.3 Neurodevelopment Postures and Potential Treatment Benefits

Posture	Treatment Benefits
1. Prone-on-elbows	• Improve upper trunk, UE, and neck/head control • Weightbearing through shoulders, elbows flexed • Increase extensor ROM at hip extensors • Improve head/neck and shoulder stabilizers strength • Wide BOS, low COG
2. Quadruped	• Improve upper trunk, lower trunk, LE, UE, and neck/head control • Weightbearing through hips and shoulders and extended UEs • Improve hip, shoulder, and elbow stabilizers strength • Decrease extensor tone at knees by prolonged weightbearing • Decrease flexor tone at elbows, wrists, and hands by prolonged weightbearing • Increase extensor ROM at elbows, wrists and fingers • Wide BOS, low COG
3. Bridging	• Improve lower trunk and LE control • Increase hip stabilizers strength • Weightbearing through feet and ankles • Lead-up activity for bed mobility, sit-to-stand • Wide BOS, low height of COM
4. Sitting	• Improve upper trunk, lower trunk, LE, and head/neck control • Weightbearing in upright, antigravity position; can include weightbearing through extended UEs • Functional posture, important for reaching and ADL skills • Improve balance reactions • Medium BOS, medium height of COM
5. Kneeling and half-kneeling	• Improve head/neck, upper trunk, lower trunk, and LE control • Weightbearing through hips in upright, antigravity position • Decrease extensor tone at knees by prolonged weightbearing • Increase hip and trunk stabilizers strength • Improve balance reactions • Weightbearing through ankle in half-kneeling • Narrow BOS, intermediate height of COM (kneeling) • Wide BOS, intermediate height of COM (half-kneeling)
6. Modified plantigrade	• Improve head/neck, upper trunk, lower trunk, and UE and LE control • Weightbearing through extended UEs and LEs, upright antigravity position • Improve balance reactions • Functional posture, lead-up for standing, stepping and reaching • Decrease tone in elbow, wrist, and finger flexors by prolonged weightbearing • Increase extensor ROM at wrists and fingers • Wide BOS, high COM
7. Standing	• Improve head/neck, upper trunk, lower trunk, and LE control • Weightbearing through extended LEs, full upright, antigravity position • Improve balance reactions • Functional posture, important for ADL skills; lead-up for gait • Narrow BOS, high COM

BOS = base of support; COM = center of mass; LE = lower extremity; ROM = range of motion; UE = upper extremity;

Recovery

Recovery is the "re-acquisition of movement skills lost through injury."[2, p 23] In complete recovery the performance of the reacquired skills is identical in every way to preinjury performance. It is far more likely that the individual with CNS insult will demonstrate recovery using preinjury skills that are modified in some way. **Compensation** is defined as "behavioral substitution, that is, alternative behavioral strategies are adopted to complete a task."[2, p 38] For example, the patient recovering from stroke learns to dress independently using the nonaffected upper extremity; the patient with a complete T1 level spinal cord injury is taught to roll using upper extremities and momentum.

Immediately after insult, a cascade of events occurs, producing a prolonged but reversible depression of neuronal activity. Changes at a cellular level occur in the immediate area of damaged brain tissue. Disruption of the blood–brain barrier results in edema, with an accumulation of intracellular fluid and leakage of blood cells, proteins, and other toxic substances that disrupt nerve function. There is a release of neurotransmitters, glutamate, and calcium that activate enzymes associated with neuron death and neuronal degeneration. Free radical damage from toxic particles of oxygen and iron also are associated with cell death. *Denervation supersensitivity,* defined as postsynaptic neuronal hypersensitivity, results in decreased synaptic efficiency. Changes also occur in areas remote from the injured brain. Blood flow changes suggestive of depressed neural activity have been found to exist on both sides of the brain and in both cortical and subcortical structures, areas that are remote from the injured site.[56] *Injury-related cortical reorganization* is evidenced by a reduction in motor cortex excitability of the involved areas, a decrease in the cortical representation area of paretic muscles, and impairment of motor function.[57–60]

Brain injury was for a long time thought to be permanent with little potential for brain repair and recovery. This is now viewed as incorrect and can represent a dangerous *self-fulfilling prophecy* when applied to the individual who suffers from such injuries. **Neuroplasticity** (plasticity) has been defined as "the ability of the brain to change and repair itself."[56, p 134] Mechanisms of neuroplasticity include neuroanatomical, neurochemical, and neuroreceptive changes. Anatomical changes include nerve growth (*neural regeneration*). Trophic molecules (*nerve growth factors*) have been shown to play a key role in growth and repair processes. Nerve cells also change their interactions with each other, with physiological changes occurring at the level of the synapses. *Regenerative synaptogenesis* refers to sprouting of the injured axons to innervate (reclaim) previously innervated synapses. *Reactive synaptogenesis (collateral sprouting)* refers to the reclaiming of synaptic sites of the injured axon by dendritic fibers from neighboring axons. Neurotransmitter release and receptor sensitivity are improved (*synaptic plasticity*). Changes in synaptic strength, *long-term potentiation (LTP),* firm up neuronal connections and serve as a basis for all memory and learning. It is important to remember that these neuroplastic changes may be adaptive (functional) or maladaptive (nonfunctional). Neural regeneration, repair, and reorganization is a topic of intense ongoing research. For excellent reviews, the reader is referred to the work of Stein, Brailowsky, and Will[56] and Ploughman.[61]

Recovery can be categorized into two main types: (1) *spontaneous recovery* resulting from repair processes occurring immediately after the insult and (2) **function-induced recovery**, the neural reorganization that occurs as a result of increased use of involved body segments in behaviorally relevant tasks. Initial spontaneous recovery is influenced by the return to function of undamaged parts of the brain with the resolution of temporary blocking factors (i.e., shock, edema, decreased blood flow, decreased glucose utilization). This process has been termed *diaschisis* and takes place over a relatively short time frame, typically 3 to 4 weeks. For example, the patient with cerebral edema following stroke is likely to demonstrate early worsening of clinical signs as edema develops followed by spontaneous improvement within a few weeks as the edema resolves.

Function-Induced Recovery

Function-induced recovery (*use-dependent cortical reorganization*) refers to the ability of the nervous system to modify itself in response to changes in activity and the environment. It is important to remember that the brain is organized with parallel and distributed circuits that provide multiple inputs to many areas and overlapping function. Different and underutilized areas of the brain (e.g., cortical supplementary and association areas) can take over the functions of damaged tissue, a process that has been called *vicariance.* Another possibility is that the CNS has backup or fail-safe systems (parallel cortical maps) that become operational when the primary system breaks down. The unmasking of new, redundant neuron pathways permits cortical map reorganization and maintenance of function. Whole different areas of the brain are also capable of becoming reprogrammed, a process termed *substitution.* An example of substitution is the increased sensitivity of the hands as a sensory information system for the person who becomes blind. In this example, the changes in sensory strategy lead to structural reorganization within the brain. Newer techniques in brain mapping have led to better understanding of these processes. These include (1) positron emission tomography (PET) scanning used to measure regional cerebral blood flow (rCBF), (2) focal transcranial magnetic stimulation (TMS) used to measure responses in motor cortical regions to focal magnetic field stimulation, and (3) functional magnetic resonance imaging (fMRI) used to measure small changes in blood flow during brain activation.[57–59] Recovery is a complex and dynamic process, and likely involves all of the above processes.

There is an accumulating body of research on **constraint-induced movement therapy** (*CI therapy* or *forced-use therapy*) in patients following stroke that has demonstrated significant and large improvements of upper extremity (UE) function.[62–71] Treatment-induced cortical reorganization has been demonstrated in studies using TMS[64] and fMRI.[65] Box 13.1 presents a summary of evidence from selected research in this area. Two factors are critical to the successful outcomes achieved in these studies. The first is the concentrated and repetitive practice of the involved UE. Training was intensive (averaging 6 hours/day) and focused on practice of common functional tasks. All subjects started with some voluntary movement (wrist and finger extension) in their affected limb. Second, movement was restricted in the sound UE through the use of mitts or splints and slings for up to 90 percent of waking hours. Behavioral shaping techniques (operant conditioning) were used in which the patients were rewarded for improvement with verbal reinforcement but not blamed (punished) for failure. The tasks were selected and tailored to address the specific motor deficits of the patient and ordered to allow for improving movement control and appropriate rest intervals.

Locomotor training using partial body weight support (BWS), a treadmill (TM), and manually assisted limb movements has also been shown to promote function-induced recovery.[72–75] As in CI therapy, practice is intense and task-specific. The limbs are maximally loaded to tolerance while movements are coordinated to stimulate actual walking. Compensatory strategies are minimized or eliminated. Training is progressed by decreasing the amount of loading (body weight support) and assistance and moving toward overground and community ambulation. See discussion in Chapter 14 and Evidence Summary Boxes in Chapters 18 and 23.

Effect of the Environment on Recovery of Function

Beneficial effects on brain function (increased cortical depth, brain weight, dendritic branching, and enzyme activity) have been demonstrated in rodents exposed to enriched environments.[76–79] The enriched environments consisted of manipulative toys for play, and structures for climbing, running, or swinging. In contrast, intact rodents raised in impoverished or small cage environments did not demonstrate the same level of brain development. When lesions were induced in rodents, exposure to enriched environments and activity prior to surgical insult had a protective effect with greater sparing of function and improved recovery.[80,81] Lesioned rodents exposed post-surgery to enriched environments also demonstrated improved recovery and performance when compared to impoverished, rodents.[82–84] Finally, socialization influenced outcomes. Rats housed in social groups in enriched environments demonstrated superior recovery over isolated rats.[85] Animal studies have also revealed that there may exist an optimal time period for such exposure. When rats with brain lesions less than 7 days were given intensive training, additional neuronal injury was demonstrated. These findings suggest that during the early post-lesion period, the damaged brain may be vulnerable to the stress imposed by intense training with additional injury.[86]

In humans, an unfamiliar and unpredictable hospital or rehabilitation environment may contribute to depression, disorientation, and decline of function. This same environment may be overly structured and protective to the point that it contributes to learned helplessness and disuse.[87] Carr and Shepherd argue that poor recovery after stroke may be partially explained by the impoverished and nonchallenging environments that many individuals recovering from stroke are exposed to.[88–89] While there are few environmental studies, there is evidence that patients recovering from stroke who were treated on an acute stroke unit demonstrated better recovery and functional outcomes than patients who received a comparable amount of physical therapy while on a general medical unit.[90–92] As Carr and Shepherd[93] point out, an important consideration is the amount of "down time" patients typically experience while in rehabilitation. Upwards of 30 to 40 percent of the day can be spent in passive pursuits while time in therapy is limited (e.g., for patients receiving stroke rehabilitation, only 93 minutes/day were spent in physical therapy and occupational therapy).[94–96] During nontherapy time, there is often little attention to self-directed practice, thereby further limiting the potential for optimal recovery of function.

Framework for Intervention

Different neurorehabilitation approaches and therapeutic techniques have evolved for patients with disorders of motor function. Historically many practical treatment ideas have evolved from empirical knowledge and clinical practice. Theory has been applied to explain the success of these interventions and to organize them into a coherent treatment philosophy. Recent emphasis on *evidence-based practice* has resulted in increased efforts to validate therapeutic interventions through research. Figure 13.5 presents a framework of current neurorehabilitation intervention strategies.

Functional Training

Evidence from research on function-induced recovery has led to **functional/task-oriented training**.[62–75] Central to this approach is the idea that specific task-oriented training with extensive practice is essential to reacquiring skill and

(text continues on page 488)

Evidence Summary Box 13.1
Constraint-Induced Movement Therapy

Reference	Subjects	Design/ Intervention	Duration	Results	Comments
Levy, CE, et al[65] 2001	2 patients, post-stroke (3–4 months); post-rehab, with moderate motor deficit; convenience sample. IC: 20°, voluntary wrist ext. and 10° finger ext	Nonrandomized cohort design; CI training of affected UE with restrictive mitt worn on nonaffected hand; behavioral shaping techniques; Pre- and posttreatment testing using: WMFT MAL fMRI	6 hours/day, 5 days/week for 2 weeks	Significant and large improvement in motor function and performance time. fMRI : ↑ motor cortex activity near lesion site; ↑ bilateral hemisphere activation	Small N, no controls; Findings support use of CI to reverse deficits and prevent learning nonuse; fMRI is a useful tool to monitor recovery and treatment effects.
Liepert, J, et al[64] 2000	13 patients, post-stroke (>6 months); post-rehab, with moderate motor deficit; convenience sample; IC: 20°, voluntary wrist ext. and 10° finger ext; no balance or cognitive problems	Nonrandomized cohort design; CI training of affected UE with restrictive hand splint and sling worn on nonaffected UE during 90% of waking hours; behavioral shaping techniques; Pre- and posttreatment testing using: MAL TMS	6 hours/day, 4 days/week for 2 weeks	Significant and large improvement in motor functions; Significant enlargement of cortical motor ouput area in the affected hemisphere; Treatment gains maintained up to 6 months post-treatment.	Small N, no controls; Supports CI therapy as a powerful treatment for improving UE function post-stroke; significant brain changes seen with short time course.
Dromerick, A, Edwards, D; and Hahn, M[66] 2000	20 patients, post-stroke within 14 days of ischemic stroke, with moderate motor deficit and in active rehab; screening tools for inclusion: NIHSS MAS IC: acute stroke, preserved cognitive function, presence of UE protective response	Single randomized clinical trial; Treatment group: CI training of affected UE with restrictive hand mitt worn on nonaffected UE at least 6 hours/day; Control group: traditional OT treatment; behavioral shaping techniques. Pre- and posttreatment testing using: ARA	2 hours/day, 5 days/week for 2 weeks	Mean total ARA score was significantly higher in treatment group ($r = 0.66$); No difference in disability measure (BI).	Small *N*, with controls; Supports CI therapy as a powerful treatment for improving UE function post-stroke; Lower treatment intensities than other studies; BI not a sensitive measure of UE changes; Average age of control group was 10 years greater than treatment group; No long-term follow-up.

(*continued*)

Evidence Summary Box 13.1

Constraint-Induced Movement Therapy (continued)

Reference	Subjects	Design/ Intervention	Duration	Results	Comments
Blanton, S, and Wolf, S[67] 1999	Single patient 4 months post-stroke; post-rehab, with moderate motor deficit; Screening tools for inclusion: MAL MMSE IC: 10°, voluntary wrist ext. and finger ext; no balance or cognitive problems	Single case report design; CI training of affected UE with restrictive mitten worn on nonaffected UE during waking hours; behavioral shaping techniques; Pre- and posttreatment, 3 months follow-up testing using: WMFT MAL	6 hours/day 5 days/week for 2 weeks	Significant improvement of motor abilities and timed abilities on WMFT; ↑ self-report use of UE on MAS; Treatment gains maintained 3 months posttreatment.	Small *N*, no controls; Supports CI therapy as a powerful treatment for improving UE function post-stroke; May reverse effects of learned non-use.
Miltner, W, et al[68] 1999	15 patients, post-stroke, post-rehab. with moderate motor deficit (mean time = 5.1 years); Convenience sample; Screening tools for inclusion: EMG, EEG, MRI, TMS, Cognitive battery IC: 20°, voluntary wrist ext, 10° finger ext; no balance or cognitive problems	Nonrandomized cohort design; CI training of affected UE with restrictive hand splint and sling worn on nonaffected UE during 90% of waking hours; behavioral shaping techniques; Pre and post-treatment testing using: WMFT MAL	7 hours/day, 4 days/week for 12 days	Significant and very large improvement on motor tests (MAL, WMFT); Gains maintained 6 months post-treatment	Small *N*, no controls; Supports CI therapy as a powerful treatment for improving UE function post-stroke; Mean chronicity of 5.1 years discounts effects of spontaneous recovery or prior therapy.
Kunkel, A, et al[69] 1999	5 patients, post-stroke, post-rehab with moderate motor deficit (time post-stroke = 3–15 yrs); convenience sample. Screening tools for inclusion: MRI Cognitive battery IC: 20°, voluntary wrist ext, 10° finger ext; no cognitive problems	Nonrandomized cohort design; CI training of affected UE with restrictive hand splint and sling worn on nonaffected UE during 90% of waking hours; behavioral shaping techniques; Pre- and posttreatment testing using: WMFT MAL AMAT AAUT	6 hours/day 5 days/week for 2 weeks	Significant and large improvement in performance times (AMAT, WMFT); quality of movement (AMAT, WMFT, MAL); and use of UE in real world (AAUT); Gains maintained 3 mo. post-treatment	Small *N*, no controls; Supports CI therapy as a powerful treatment for improving UE function post-stroke; More than 100% in active use of UE.

Evidence Summary Box 13.1

Constraint-Induced Movement Therapy (continued)

Reference	Subjects	Design/ Intervention	Duration	Results	Comments
Van der Lee, J, et al[70] 1999	66 patients, post-stroke (median time = 3 years) with moderate motor deficit; Screening tools for inclusion: ARA IC: at least 1 year post-stroke; 20° voluntary wrist ext, 10° finger ext; no cognitive or balance problems	Single randomized clinical trial; Treatment group: CI training of affected UE with restrictive splint/sling worn on nonaffected UE; Control group: traditional PT treatment according to NDT method (bimanual training); behavioral shaping techniques; Pre- and posttreatment testing using: ARA RAP FMA (UE motor subtest) MAL	6 hours/day, 5 days/week for 2 weeks	Small and significant improvement in motor performance (dexterity measured by ARA) and use of UE (MAL); Gains in ARA maintained 1 yr. post-treatment	Larger *N* than other studies; Supports CI therapy as a treatment for improving UE function post-stroke; Benefits found in those patients with sensory disorders; Both RAP and FMA failed to reveal any differences suggesting inadequate responsiveness of instruments to chronic stroke.
Taub, E, et al[71] 1993	9 patients, post-stroke with moderate motor deficit (median post-stroke time = 4.1 years); Screening tools for inclusion: Cognitive tests IC: at least 1 year post-stroke; 20° voluntary wrist ext, 10° finger ext; no cognitive or balance problems	Single randomized clinical trial Treatment group: CI training of affected UE with restrictive splint/sling worn on nonaffected UE 90% of waking hours Control group: Received training strategies to focus attention on using affected UE; traditional PT (PROM) behavioral shaping techniques Pre- and posttreatment testing using: WMFT MAT	7 hours/day, 5 days/week for 2 weeks	Significant and large improvement in motor performance (performance time, quality of movement on WMFT) and use of UE (MAT); Gains maintained during 2-year follow-up.	Small *N*; Supports CI therapy as a treatment for improving UE function post-stroke; Long follow-up period Attention training of control group reduces likelihood improvement due to attention/placebo factors.

↑ = increased; AAUT = Actual Amount of Use Test (includes 21 items of self-report of arm use); AMAT = Arm Motor Ability Test (includes 13 complex tasks); ARA = Action Research Arm Test (includes 19 items of UE strength, dexterity, and coordination); BI = Barthel Index (measure of basic ADL and disability); CI = Constraint-Induced Movement Therapy: intensive, supervised task-specific practice of affected upper extremity (UE) with restriction of non-affected UE; EEG = electroencephalography; EMG = electromyography; Ext = extension; fMRI = functional magnetic resonance imaging; FMA = Fugl-Meyer Assessment Scale (stroke-specific instrument with upper extremity motor section); IC = inclusion criteria; MAL = Motor Activity Log (structured interview that identifies performance on 30 daily activities); MAS = Motor Assessment Scale (stroke-specific instrument); MMSE = Mini-Mental State Exam (Folstein); N = number of subjects; NDT = Neurodevelopmental Treatment; NIHSS = National Institutes of Health Stroke Scale (stroke-specific instrument); OT = occupational therapy; RAP = Rehabilitation Activities Profile (based on ICIDH, semistructured interview that assesses disabilities and handicaps and consists of 21 items in 5 domains); Rehab = rehabilitation; TMS = focal transcranial magnetic stimulation; WMFT = Wolf Motor Function Test, an UE functional test that includes 14 timed activities and 2 strength tests.

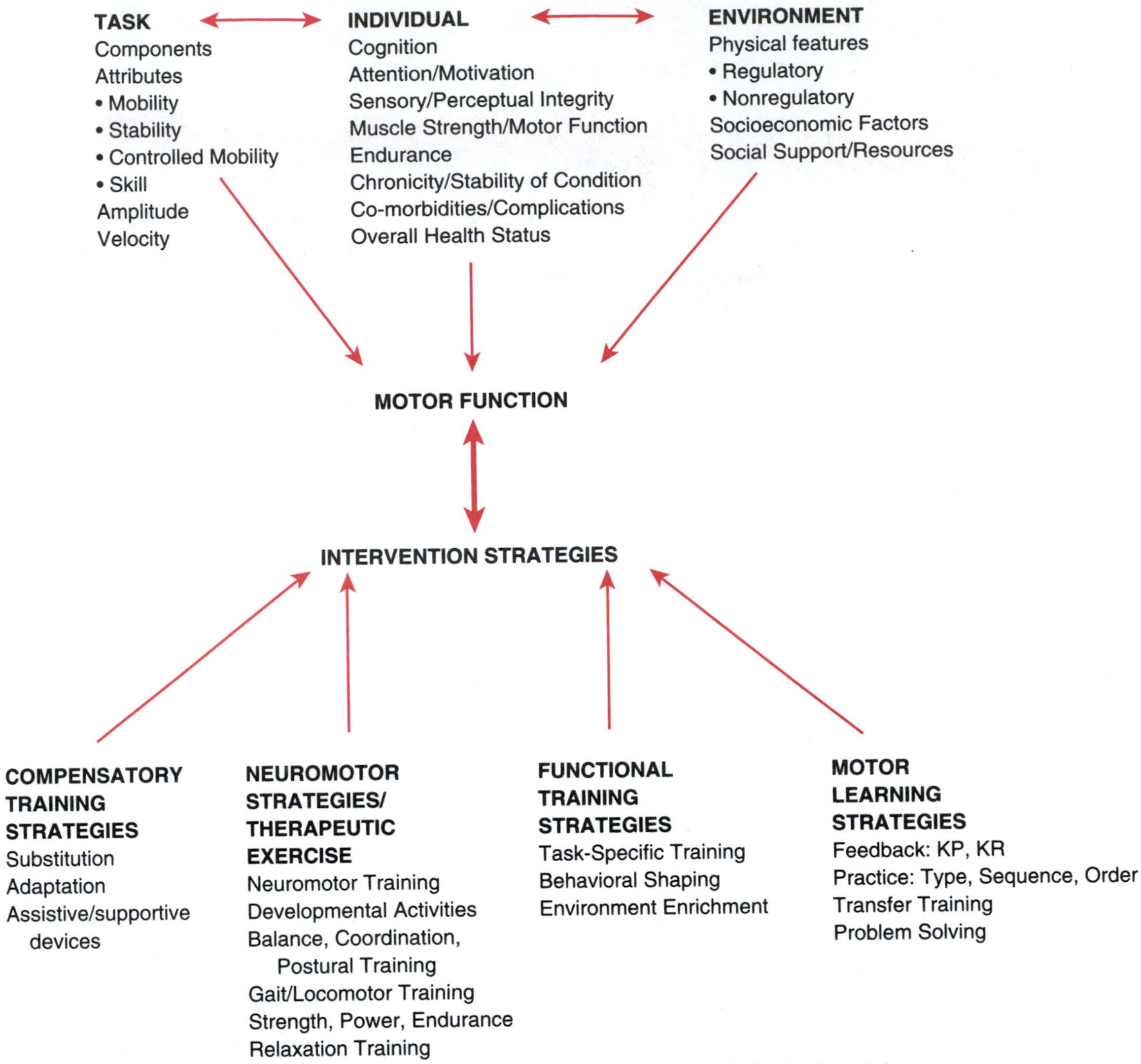

Figure 13.5 Motor function emerges from interaction among the task, the individual, and the environment. Deficits in motor function can be improved using *Neuromotor, Functional/Task Oriented, Motor Learning,* and/or *Compensatory* intervention strategies.

enhancing recovery. Theoretically, the interacting systems of the CNS are viewed as organized around essential functional tasks. Thus, an understanding of tasks, the essential elements within each task, and the context or environment in which tasks occur is key to structuring appropriate training (see Chapter 8, Box 8.1). Tasks important for daily function (e.g., grasp and release, standing and walking) are emphasized. Involved segments are targeted for training (i.e., constraint-induced movement therapy). Level of difficulty is varied and initial tasks are selected to ensure patient motivation and success. Motor learning strategies are used to enhance function, including **behavioral shaping techniques** that use reinforcement and reward to promote skill development. This approach represents a shift away from a traditional neurotherapeutic focus that utilizes extensive hands-on therapy (e.g., facilitated movements). While initial movements can be assisted or guided, active movements are the overall goal. The therapist serves as coach, providing appropriate feedback and encouraging the patient. Task-oriented training effectively counteracts the effects of immobility and the development of indirect impairments such as muscle weakness or loss of flexibility. It also prevents *learned nonuse* of the involved segments while stimulating CNS recovery. Box 13.2 presents a summary of task-oriented training strategies to promote function-induced recovery.

Task-oriented training is not an appropriate for every patient. Its selection is dependent on the degree of recovery and severity of motor deficits. Animal studies have suggested that early overemphasis on use-dependent training may increase the vulnerability of the brain to additional damage.[85] Patients who are not able to participate in task-oriented training include those who lack voluntary control or cognitive function. For example, a patient with traumatic brain injury who is in the early recovery stages has limited

Box 13.2 Task-Oriented Training Strategies to Promote Function-Induced Recovery

Focus on early training as soon as possible after brain damage to utilize specific windows of opportunity and avoid learned nonuse.

Consider the individual's past history, health status, age, and experience in designing appropriate, interesting and stimulating activities.

Involve the patient in goal-setting and decision making, thereby enhancing motivation and promoting active commitment to recovery.

Structure practice utilizing task-related training activities.

- Select tasks important for independent function; include tasks that are important to the patient.
- Identify the patient's abilities/strengths and level of recovery/learning; choose tasks that have potential for patient success.
- Target active movements involving the affected extremities; constrain or limit compensatory strategies.
- Utilize repetition and extensive (massed) practice.
- Include both supervised and unsupervised practice using an activity log.
- Assist (guide) the patient to successfully carry out initial movements as needed.
- Provide augmented verbal feedback and verbal reward for small improvements in task performance.
- Provide modeling of task performance as needed.
- Promote practice of variable behaviors to facilitate adaptation of skills.

Structure context-specific practice.

- Promote initial practice in a supportive environment, free of distractors.
- Progress to variable practice in real-world environments.

Maintain focus on role as *training coach* while minimizing hands-on therapy.

Continue to monitor recovery closely and document progress using valid and reliable functional outcome measures.

Be cautious about timetables and predictions as recovery may take longer than expected.

potential to succeed with this type of intensive training. Similarly, patients with stroke who experience profound upper extremity paralysis would not be eligible for constraint-induced (CI) UE training. One of the consistent exclusion criteria for CI therapy has been inability to perform voluntary wrist and finger extension of the involved hand. Thus threshold abilities to perform the basic components of the task need to be identified. Careful analysis of underlying impairments with a focus on intervention (e.g., strength, ROM) complements task-oriented training. For example, during locomotor training using BWS and a TM system, patients are guided in their stepping and pelvic motions into an efficient motor pattern. Patients need to demonstrate essential prerequisites of basic head and trunk stability during upright positioning in order to be considered appropriate candidates for this type of training.

Neuromotor Development Training

Neuromotor development training includes developmental activities training, motor training, movement pattern training, and neuromuscular education or reeducation. Neuromuscular/sensory stimulation techniques and therapeutic exercises are used to alter sensorimotor impairments and promote functional movements. The affected body segments are targeted for training while compensatory movements by intact segments are not allowed. A hands-on approach is used to stimulate, guide, or assist movements for correct performance.

Gordon[97] points out the dominant treatment philosophy at the time these approaches were developed was one of muscular reeducation (e.g., Kenny method), which could not be easily adapted to patients with CNS disorders. As therapists sought to develop more appropriate approaches for this group of patients, these approaches evolved. A central concept was the use of sensory inputs to modify the CNS and stimulate motor output. These approaches evolved in a time when hierarchical theory of motor control was the prevailing motor control theory during the 1950s and 1960s. Thus the goal of treatment was initially viewed as assisting the higher centers of the CNS in regaining control of motor function. Acquisition of function was viewed as modeling the acquisition of movement patterns seen in normal development. Thus a common base was developmental activities training (e.g., prone-on-elbows, quadruped, sitting). Following remediation of impairments (e.g., reduction of tone and abnormal reflexes) treatment progressed to functional movement patterns. Modifications in these approaches have emerged from the changing scientific evidence and theories of motor control. Currently there is a much greater emphasis on functional training. Motor learning strategies have always been a strong component. Two of the most popular approaches in current use are *Neurodevelopmental Treatment (NDT)* and *Proprioceptive Neuromuscular Facilitation (PNF).*

These approaches are not appropriate for every patient. Patients who demonstrate sufficient recovery and consistent voluntary movement would not benefit from neuromuscular stimulation and an intensive hands-on approach. Rather these patients are candidates for active task-oriented training. Interventions organized around a behavioral goal provide a better vehicle for promoting continuing functional recovery and long-term retention than interventions that target remediation of a impairments (e.g., spasticity). Also, continued use of interventions (e.g., guided movement) may result in the patient becoming dependent on the therapist, a phenomenon appropriately labeled the "my therapist syndrome." For example, a therapist who is covering for another therapist hears the patient remark that he or she is not helping correctly. It has to be done the way "my therapist" does it. This patient is demonstrating an overreliance on the therapist for movement. In summary, these techniques can provide important choices for treatment. They can help the patient bridge the gap between absent or severely disordered movements and active movements. Once the patient develops independent voluntary control of movement, these treatment approaches are generally counterproductive.

Neurodevelopmental Treatment (NDT)

Neurodevelopmental treatment (NDT) is a treatment approach developed in the late 1940s and early 1950s by Dr. Karel Bobath, an English physician, and Berta Bobath, a physiotherapist.[14,98] Their work focused on patients with neurological dysfunction (cerebral palsy and stroke). The essential problems of these patient groups were identified as a release of abnormal tone (spasticity) and abnormal postural reflexes (primitive spinal cord and brainstem reflexes) from higher center CNS control with resulting loss of the normal postural reflex mechanism (righting, equilibrium, protective extension reactions) and normal movements. The role of sensory feedback was viewed as critical in inhibiting abnormal reactions and facilitating more normal movement patterns.

Current NDT has realigned itself with newer theories of motor control (systems theory and a distributed model of CNS control).[99] Many different factors are recognized as contributing to loss of motor function in patients with neurological dysfunction including the full spectrum of sensory and motor deficits (weakness, limited ROM, impaired tone and coordination). Emphasis is on the use of both feedback and feedforward mechanisms to support postural control. Postural control is viewed as the foundation for all skill learning. Normal development in children and normal movement patterns in all patients are stressed. The patient learns to control posture and movement through a sequence of progressively more challenging postures and activities. NDT uses physical *handling techniques* and *key points of control* (e.g., shoulders, pelvis, hands, and feet) directed at supporting body segments and assisting the patient in achieving active control. Sensory stimulation (facilitation and inhibition via primarily proprioceptive, and tactile inputs) is used during treatment. Postural alignment and stability are facilitated while excessive tone and abnormal movements are inhibited. For example, in the patient with stroke, abnormal obligatory synergy movements are restricted while out-of-synergy movements are facilitated. Activities are selected that are functionally relevant and varied in terms of difficulty and environmental context. Compensatory training strategies (use of the less involved segments) are avoided. Carryover is promoted through a strong emphasis on patient, family, and caregiver education. NDT is taught today in recognized training courses. Appendix A presents an overview of NDT principles and techniques.

Proprioceptive Neuromuscular Facilitation (PNF)

Motor function can be improved using *Proprioceptive Neuromuscular Facilitation (PNF),* an approach initially developed by Dr. Herman Kabat and Maggie Knott (a physical therapist).[100] Synergistic patterns of movement were identified as components of normal movement. A developmental emphasis was added later by Voss to include practice of various different activities (rolling, prone-on-elbows, quadruped, kneeling, half-kneeling, modified plantigrade, standing, and gait). Extremity patterns of movement are rotational and diagonal in nature (labeled Diagonal 1 [D1] and Diagonal 2 [D2]) rather than straight plane movements. Coordination within and between patterns is stressed. For example, the technique of slow reversals is used to establish smooth linkages between agonist and antagonist actions during reversing patterns. Patterns can be unilateral or bilateral and combined with various trunk patterns and postures. A number of different facilitation techniques, largely proprioceptive, are utilized to facilitate movement (e.g., stretch, resistance, traction, approximation, and so forth). Precise manual contacts are used to provide important directional cues and enhance the function of underlying muscles. PNF also incorporates a number of important motor learning strategies (e.g., practice, repetition, visual guidance of movement, verbal commands, and so forth). It is directed at improving functional performance and coordinated patterns of movement and has been used effectively to treat patients with both neuromuscular or musculoskeletal deficits.[101] PNF is taught today in recognized training courses. Appendix B presents an overview of PNF principles and techniques.

Neuromuscular/Sensory Stimulation Techniques

A number of therapeutic techniques can be used to facilitate, activate, or inhibit muscle contraction. These have been collectively called facilitation techniques, although this term is a misnomer, because they also include techniques used for inhibition. The term **facilitation** refers to the enhanced capacity to initiate a movement response through increased neuronal activity and altered synaptic potential. An applied stimulus may lower the synaptic threshold of the alpha motor neuron but may not be sufficient to produce an observable movement response. **Activation** on the other hand refers to the actual production of a movement response and implies reaching a critical threshold level for neuronal firing. **Inhibition** refers to the decreased capacity to initiate a movement response through altered synaptic potential. The synaptic threshold is raised, making it more difficult for the neuron to fire and produce movement. The combination of spinal inputs and supraspinal inputs acting on the alpha motor neuron (final common pathway) will determine whether a muscle response is facilitated, activated, or inhibited.

Several general guidelines are important. First, facilitative techniques can be additive. That is, several inputs applied simultaneously, such as quick stretch, resistance, and verbal commands commonly combined in PNF patterns, produce the desired motor response, whereas use of a single stimulus may not. This demonstrates the property of spatial summation within the CNS. Repeated application of the same stimulus (e.g., repeated quick stretches) may also produce the desired motor response owing to temporal summation within the CNS, whereas a single stimulus does not. Thus, stretch is used repeatedly to ensure that the patient with a weak muscle is able to move from the lengthened to the shortened range. The response to stimulation or inhibition is unique to each patient and dependent on a number of different factors, including level of intactness of the CNS, arousal, and the specific level of activity of the motoneurons in question. For example, a patient who is depressed and hypoactive may require large amounts of stimulation to achieve the desired response. Stimulation is generally contraindicated for the patient with hyperactivity while inhibition/relaxation techniques are of benefit. The intensity, duration, and frequency of simulation need to be adjusted to meet individual patient needs. Unpredicted responses can result from inappropriate application of techniques. For example, stretch applied to a spastic muscle may increase spasticity and negatively impact voluntary movement. Facilitation techniques are not appropriate for patients who demonstrate adequate voluntary control; they should be viewed primarily as a bridge to voluntary movement control. Appendix C presents an overview of neuromuscular/sensory stimulation techniques.

Compensatory Training

The focus of *compensatory training* is early resumption of functional skills using the uninvolved or less involved segments for function. For example, the patient with hemiplegia is taught to dress using the less-affected upper extremity; the patient with paraplegia regains functional mobility and wheelchair independence using the upper extremities. Central to this approach is the concept of substitution. The patient is made aware of movement deficiencies (cognitive awareness is developed). Changes are then made in the patient's overall approach to functional tasks. Alternate ways to accomplish the task are suggested, simplified, and adopted. The patient practices and relearns the task using the new pattern. The patient then practices the new pattern in the environment in which the function is expected to occur. Energy conservation techniques are incorporated to ensure the patient can successfully complete all daily tasks. A second central tenet of this approach is modification of the task and environment **(adaptation)** to facilitate relearning of skills, ease of movement, and optimal performance. For example, the patient with unilateral neglect is assisted in dressing by color coding of the shoes (red tape on the left shoe, yellow tape on the right shoe). The wheelchair brake toggle is extended and color coded to allow the easy identification by the patient.

One of the major criticisms of this approach is the focus on uninvolved segments may suppress recovery for certain patients and contribute to learned nonuse of impaired segments.[102] For example, the patient with stroke fails to learn to use the involved extremities. Compensatory training can also lead to development of *splinter skills,* which are skills acquired in a manner inconsistent with skills the individual already possesses. Splinter skills cannot be easily generalized to other task variations or to other environments.

A compensatory training approach may be the only realistic approach possible when recovery is limited or the patient presents with significant impairments and functional limitations with little or no expectation for additional recovery. Examples include the patient with complete spinal cord injury or the patient recovering from stroke with severe sensorimotor deficits and extensive co-morbidities (e.g., severe cardiac and respiratory compromise or memory deficits associated with Alzheimer's disease). The latter is severely limited in the ability to actively participate in rehabilitation and to relearn motor skills.

Integrating Approaches

An understanding of how the brain regulates movement is essential to making sound clinical decisions in selecting interventions. Therapists must be cautious not to develop a "disciple-like" adherence to one approach. Therapists who become certified in, and a proponent of, a particular approach must be particularly cautious about overreliance on a single group of treatment interventions. The diversity of problems experienced by patients with disordered motor function negates the idea that any one approach could be successful for all patients. As patients recover, their abilities and needs change. Therapists must be attuned to the patient's changing status and recognize anticipated goals and expected outcomes may change. A variety of interventions is likely to be the most effective approach in meeting the diverse needs of patients. A common base for all intervention is training to improve functional skills and motor learning. Interventions also need to promote adaptability of skills for function in real-world environments. In selecting interventions, the therapist must consider those that have the greatest chance of success. The choice of interventions must also take into consideration other factors, including ability to deliver care, cost-effectiveness in terms of length of stay and number of allotted physical therapy visits, age of the patient and number of co-morbidities, social support, and potential discharge placement. Examples of

Box 13.3 Examples of General Goals and Outcomes for Patients with Disorders of Motor Function

Impact of pathology/pathophysiology is reduced.
- Risk of recurrence of condition is reduced.
- Risk of secondary impairment is reduced.
- Intensity of care is decreased.

Impact on impairments is reduced.
- Alertness, attention, and memory are improved.
- Joint integrity and mobility are improved
- Sensory awareness and discrimination are improved.
- Motor control is improved.
- Coordination is improved.
- Muscle performance (strength, power, and endurance) is improved.
- Postural control and balance improved.
- Gait and locomotion are improved.
- Endurance is increased.

Ability to perform physical actions, tasks, or activities is improved.
- Functional independence in activities of daily living (ADL) and instrumental activities of daily living (IADL) is increased.
- Level of supervision for task performance is decreased.
- Tolerance of positions and activities is increased.
- Flexibility for varied tasks and environments is improved.
- Motor learning skills are improved.
- Decision making is improved.
- Safety of patient/client, family, and caregivers is improved.

Disability associated with acute or chronic illness is reduced.
- Ability to assume/resume self-care, home management, work (job/school/play), community, and leisure roles is improved.

Health status is improved.
- Sense of well-being is increased.
- Insight, self-confidence, and self-image are improved.
- Health, wellness, and fitness are improved.

Satisfaction, access, availability, and services are acceptable to patient/client.

Patient/client, family, and caregiver knowledge and awareness of the diagnosis, prognosis, anticipated goals/expected outcomes, and interventions are increased.

Adapted from *Guide to Physical Therapist Practice*[103]

general goals and outcomes for improving motor function adapted from the *Guide to Physical Therapist Practice*[103] are presented in Box 13.3. These can serve as a basis for developing specific anticipated goals and expected outcomes for an individual patient.

Intervention Strategies to Improve Motor Control

Strength, Power, and Endurance Training

Muscle performance is defined as "the capacity of a muscle or group of muscles to generate forces."[103, p 688] **Muscle strength** is the "muscle force exerted by a muscle or a group of muscles to overcome a resistance under a specific set of circumstances."[103, p 688] **Muscle power** is "the work produced per unit of time or the product of strength and speed."[103, p 688] **Muscle endurance** is "the ability to sustain forces repeatedly or to generate forces over a period of time."[103, p 688] Muscle performance is regulated by a number of factors, including motor unit recruitment, motoneuron firing patterns, muscle length and tension, muscle fiber composition, fuel storage and delivery, speed and type of contraction, and movement arm.[104] Techniques that optimize these factors while addressing the specific demands of the task and environment will yield maximum functional outcomes. Improved sense of well-being and confidence are also important outcomes.

Patients undergoing neurorehabilitation commonly present with disruption of motoneurons from central pathways, the direct result of upper motor neuron lesions. Weakness or paralysis can affect one side of the body (hemiparesis, hemiplegia), both lower limbs (paraparesis, paraplegia), all four limbs (tetraparesis, tetraplegia), or a single limb or segments of a limb. As recovery progresses, the status of muscle strength and performance may change (e.g., the patient recovering from incomplete spinal cord injury). In addition, prolonged periods of disuse and immobility result in diminished neural activity, atrophy, and weakness. Older adults typically demonstrate a preferential loss of type II fibers. It is also important to recognize that the patient may have been inactive prior to insult or injury resulting in preexisting deconditioning.

Muscle Strengthening

Strength training produces a number of neuromuscular changes. There is an increase in the production of maximal force due to changes in neural drive (increased motor unit recruitment, increased rate, and synchronization of firing rate) and changes in muscle (hypertrophy of muscle fibers, improved metabolic/enzymatic adaptations, increased size and number of myofibrils, muscle fiber type adaptation with conversion of type IIB to type IIA). Connective tissue tensile strength and bone mineral density are increased. Body composition is improved in terms of body mass ratio of fat to lean. Reaction time, functional performance, and sense of well-being are also improved. The effectiveness of a strengthening program is dependent on achieving an adequate training stimulus. For strength and power training, an *exercise prescription* should include the following elements: *mode* of exercise (type of muscle contraction, application of resistance, arc of movement), *intensity* (exercise load or level of resistance), *frequency* (number of repetitions and sets; number of exercises per set), *rest interval* (recuperation time between sets and exercise sessions), and *duration* (total time of resistance training). Additional determinants include use of *correct alignment* and *stabilization* and consideration of replication of *functional demands*.[105]

Basic principles of effective strengthening programs include overload, specificity, cross training, and reversibility.[106] The loads placed on muscle must be greater than those normally incurred **(overload principle)**. Application of a progressive resistance sequence that achieves 80 percent maximum voluntary strength is a generally accepted criteria for effective strengthening. Free weights, pulley systems, elastic resistance bands, mechanical resistance machines, isokinetic dynamometers, and manual resistance all provide sources of external load on muscle. Training effects are specific to the mode of exercise stress imposed on the exercising muscles **(specificity principle)**. Thus, the training effects from an isometric protocol are specific to the exercising muscle and the point in the range that the muscle is holding. Effects do not carry over to improved dynamic performance (concentric or eccentric contractions). Nor will exercise training of the upper extremities transfer to improved lower extremity performance. **Cross training** refers to a training program that includes a variety of training elements (e.g., isometric, concentric, eccentric, and endurance). Cross training is used to place broadest possible demands on the neuromuscular system and overcome the effects of specificity. **Reversibility principle** refers to the failure to sustain the benefits of strength training if muscles are not regularly used in a maintenance program of resistance or functional exercises. Detraining effects include a reduction in muscle performance, decreased neural recruitment, and muscle fiber atrophy.[107]

Strength training methods have been well described and documented.[105,108] Selection of a particular training sequence must be based on the specific needs of the patient and the potential benefits of a particular method. For example, isometric training will result in gains in static strength without added joint motion. This may be important during early rehabilitation when pain is a factor or when postural stability is the focus of treatment. Dynamic exercise (concentric and eccentric) allows for joint movement and excursion of a body segment and is essential to develop the strength, power, and endurance required for functional mobility skills.

Patients with deficits in motor function may demonstrate deficits in muscle activation. Early training should focus on isometric and eccentric contractions because muscle tension is better maintained than with concentric contractions. This is due primarily to the improved peripheral reflex support of contraction as opposed to the spindle unloading that occurs as the muscle moves into the shortened range of a concentric contraction. The patient is initially asked to actively hold at midrange where the greatest tension can be generated. The patient is then asked to slowly lower the limb (an eccentric contraction) and hold (an isometric contraction). Once control is achieved in both of these types of contractions, concentric contractions can be attempted. For isotonic contractions prestretching the muscle by starting the contraction in the lengthened range optimizes tension development through increased use of viscoelastic forces *(length–tension relationship)* and peripheral reflex support. Weak muscles can be initially lightly resisted (*tracking resistance*) to facilitate contraction through proprioceptive loading of the muscle spindle. Control of velocity is also important to ensure efficiency of initial movement attempts. During concentric contractions, total tension decreases as velocity increases. Thus, patients may be able to generate a contraction at slow speeds but not at high speeds. For example, the patient with stroke who demonstrates limited control should be instructed to begin with slow and controlled movements. As movements become more efficient, they can be progressed to faster speeds.

Open-chain exercises involve the distal segment of the limb moving in space without simultaneous motions at adjacent joints. Muscle activation occurs predominately in the prime mover(s) crossing the moving joint. Resistance is applied to the distal moving segment, typically in non-weightbearing positions. *Closed-chain exercises* involve motions in which the distal part is fixed (foot or hand) while the proximal segments are moving (e.g., weight shifting in standing, bilateral short-arc squats). They are performed in weightbearing postures and involve simultaneous actions of synergistic muscles at multiple joints. The added joint approximation and stimulation of joint and muscle proprioceptors enhances neuromuscular control and joint stabilization (co-contraction). A limitation of closed chain exercise is the substitution of other agonist muscles for specific muscle weakness. In comparison, open-chain exercises can be used to isolate contraction of a muscle or muscle group and enhance specific training.[105] *Pylometric training* involves quick powerful movements with pre-stretching of the muscle for improved neuromuscular responses (using stretch-shortening principles). For example, when performing a vertical jump, slightly lowering the body in a partial squat first provides increased stretch on the quadriceps and heelcords and enhances the push-off. Plyometric exercise drills are used during the advanced stages of rehabilitation to prepare individuals for explosive movements required for certain sports.[108]

Gains in strength can be obtained through progressive resistive exercises (PRE) using free weights or fixed mechanical resistance machines. A major disadvantage of PRE is that the weight selected is determined by the amount that can be lifted by the muscle at the weakest point of the range. Isokinetic training devices offer the advantage of providing accommodating resistance throughout the range. Muscle performance is therefore not limited to the weakest part of the range. The amount of force generated is recorded, providing an important objective measure of performance. Different isokinetic protocols using concentric and eccentric contractions have been developed. The speed of movement can be predetermined. This is an important consideration for training the patient who demonstrates neuromuscular impairments in timing and velocity control. For example, the patient recovering from stroke may be unable to generate the acceleration and deceleration forces needed during the different phases of gait. This results in delayed sequencing of muscle components and a general slowing of gait. Isokinetic training that focuses on the timing of these various components can improve gait function. Carryover to improved functional performance with any of these resistance training methods is not assured.[109] Additional functional training is necessary to ensure effective transference of strength and timing parameters to functional skills (specificity principle).

Manually resisted patterns of movement (PNF patterns) offer the advantage of functionally based, synergistic movements. Patterns of motion are spiral and diagonal in nature as opposed to straight planes of motion. The therapist can accommodate to the patient's specific level of weakness by providing repetitive graded resistance throughout the range and by adding additional facilitation as needed to improve or maintain performance. Effective verbal commands improve the magnitude of muscle contraction. Stretch is applied in the lengthened range to assist in the initiation of contraction and throughout the range as needed to sustain contraction. Approximation is applied to assist extensor patterns while traction is applied to assist flexor patterns. Specific PNF techniques (e.g., slow reversal, repeated contractions, and so forth) are described in Appendix B. Elastic resistance bands or pulley weights can also be used to provide resistance in PNF patterns.

Strength gains can be achieved through functional training that uses task-related practice.[110,111] Resistance is provided by gravity and body weight and is applied simultaneously to multiple moving segments. It can be supplemented with manual resistance of the therapist, weights, elastic resistance bands, or resistance of water during pool therapy. Activities can be selected that focus on specific body segments and progressed to involve increasingly larger segments of the body. This serves to increase the level of difficulty and the degrees of freedom that must be controlled during the movement. Benefits of functional training include improved coordination of muscles, improved postural control and balance, and improved muscle extensibility and flexibility. Functional training helps the patient develop control of synergistic muscle groups acting in multiple axes and planes of movements. It also fosters the control of varying types and combinations of muscle contractions (concentric, eccentric, isometric) that are used interchangeably during normal movement. This is a very different focus from the straight planes of motion and isolated movements commonly employed during PRE and isokinetic training. Intrinsic sensory input (somatosensory, vestibular, visual) is maximized during functional training.

Combining strength training protocols with task-specific practice is an effective strategy to maximize transfer gains to functional skills. For example, strengthening of weak lower limb extensor muscles can be first achieved using an isokinetic machine that targets both eccentric and concentric contractions of the quadriceps. This training can effectively be followed up with repetitive practice of functional activities also demanding similar extensor control (e.g., partial squats, sit-to-stand transfers, and stair climbing). The important consideration here is to match the strength training protocol to the requirements of the functional task in terms of range of motion achieved and type, magnitude, and speed of contraction.[109]

Endurance Training

Muscle endurance can be improved with exercise using dynamic contractions of large muscle groups repeated over time. Effects of endurance training are both central (cardiovascular) and peripheral (muscular). Peripheral adaptations include improved oxygen delivery to the exercising muscles, improved metabolic exchange, an increase in the number and size of mitochondria, increased myoglobin, and improved enzymatic activity. Essential components of an exercise prescription include the following interdependent elements: frequency, intensity, time or duration, and type or exercise mode (the *FITT equation*) along with progression of physical activity.[112] Training modes and equipment include walking and jogging (overground, treadmill, pool), cycling (ergometers), stepping (steps), or swimming (pools).

Patients with deficits in motor function may demonstrate poor muscular endurance and fatigue. **Fatigue** is defined as the inability to contract muscle repeatedly over time. Thus exercise cannot be sustained and exercise tolerance is reduced. The onset of fatigue is variable from patient to patient. Although many different factors may play a role, among the most important are the type and intensity of exercise. With the onset of fatigue, patients will demonstrate a decrement in force production progressing to total exhaustion (a ceiling effect). Fatigue can arise from neuromuscular disease affecting three primary sites: (1) the CNS (central fatigue), (2) the peripheral nerves or neuromuscular junction, or (3) the muscle itself.[113] Examples of conditions that can produce debilitating fatigue include multiple sclerosis, Guillain-Barré syndrome, chronic fatigue syndrome, and post-polio syndrome. The real danger of exercise training with these patients is the risk of injury and **overwork weakness**, defined as a prolonged decrease in absolute strength and endurance as a result of excessive activity.[114] For example, following an exercise session a patient with post-polio syndrome may demonstrate prolonged weakness and fatigue that does not recover with rest. If exercise is exhaustive, the patient may be unable to get out of bed the next day or perform normal ADL. Even a simple conditioning program should be carefully monitored and progressed slowly to avoid overexertion and injury.[115–117] In general, moderate intensities of exercises in the range of 60 to 70 percent of maximal oxygen consumption or "somewhat hard" Ratings of Perceived Exertion are recommended while high intensities are contraindicated. A frequency of 3 days/week or alternate days is ideal using a discontinuous protocol that carefully balances exercise with rest.[118,119] Energy conservation, activity pacing, stress management, and lifestyle modification are essential components of the educational program.

Flexibility Exercises

Joint range of motion (ROM) and muscle flexibility must be adequate to allow for normal functional excursions of muscle and biomechanical alignment. Prolonged periods of disuse and immobility can lead to changes in muscle and joint function, postural alignment, and a host of indirect impairments (e.g., muscle tightness, atrophy, fibrosis, contracture, joint ankylosis, postural deformity). Older adults demonstrate age-related changes affecting joint flexibility. These include increased viscosity of synovial fluid, stiffening of the joint capsule and ligaments, and calcification of articular cartilage.[120] Early intervention is critical in maintaining joint motion, tissue extensibility, physical ability, and function. Additional benefits include improved circulation and tissue nutrition to the limbs and pain inhibition.

Techniques include ROM exercises, muscular stretching, and joint mobilization. The use of a preliminary therapeutic heat modality (e.g., hot pack or ultrasound) increases muscle temperature and elasticity, and collagen extensibility.[121,122] A warm-up period of exercise can also be used. For example, calisthenics or low-resistance cycling will gradually increase tissue temperatures and elasticity, thereby enhancing the safety of stretching. Cold modalities can be used to cool muscles and decrease muscle spasm and physiological splinting.[123] Patients with spasticity may benefit from preliminary prolonged icing and relaxation techniques (e.g., rhythmic rotation, cognitive relaxation). Icing can also be added following stretching, if necessary, to reduce tissue inflammation.

ROM Exercises

Range of motion is "the arc through which movement occurs at a joint or a series of joints."[103, p 690] ROM can be *active (AROM)*, performed and controlled entirely by the voluntary muscular efforts of the patient), *active-assisted (AAROM*, requiring some degree of external assistance for voluntary efforts) or *passive (PROM)*, performed solely by therapist or caregiver). The *Guide to Physical Therapist Practice* classifies the first two as therapeutic exercise while passive ROM is classified as manual therapy.[103] PROM is typically used when active movement is not possible (e.g., due to pain, paralysis, or unresponsiveness). AROM and AAROM have additional benefits of improving circulation, decreasing atrophy, and improving motor function. Progression should be to AROM exercises whenever possible as they are an important component of the home exercise program (HEP). ROM exercises are performed through the patient's full available range. The limb should be well supported with stable positioning of the patient to prevent joint trauma. The movements should be slow and rhythmic and within the patient's tolerance. Excess force and pain are contraindicated. This is especially important when working with the patient at risk for osteoporosis and heterotopic ossifications. External force during PROM or AAROM can also be applied mechanically (e.g., continuous passive motion machine, pulleys).

ROM exercises can be administered in anatomic planes of motion or in diagonal patterns of motion (PNF patterns). The latter may be more efficient as ROM can be administered throughout a limb, combining motions at more than one joint. ROM can also be achieved during functional training activities (e.g., shoulder ROM is achieved during weight shifting in quadruped or plantigrade positions). An added benefit may be the patient's lack of attention to joint motion during the activity with less protective splinting. Functional activity training should follow ROM exercises. The adage "use it or lose it" holds true for maintaining the benefits of both strengthening and ROM exercises.

Stretching Techniques

Stretching involves the application of manual or mechanical force to elongate (lengthen) structures that have adaptively shortened and are hypomobile.[105] The term *static stretching* refers to a method of stretching in which the muscle is slowly elongated to tolerance and the end position (greatest tolerated length) is held at least 20 to 30 seconds or longer depending upon the patient's tolerance. The use of slow, prolonged stretch minimizes muscle spindle activation and reflex contraction of the muscle being stretched. Maintaining the position at maximal end range results in the firing of the Golgi tendon organs (GTOs) with resulting inhibition of the muscle being stretched through mechanisms of autogenic inhibition. The combined neurophysiological effects result in improved muscle elongation. Additional benefits of static stretching using low loads include less danger of soft tissue tearing, less muscle soreness, and decreased energy requirements.[124–127] Low-load, long duration mechanical stretching can be applied for 30 minutes up to several hours using mechanical pulleys and weights or specialized orthotic devices. Prolonged positioning on a tilt table with wedges and straps can also be used to effectively to improve lower extremity range.[128,129]

Ballistic stretching involves the use of a high-load, short-duration, intermittent stretch. For example, bouncing movements of the body during sitting toe touch can be used to increase range in young, healthy individuals as part of a conditioning program. They can be appropriate as part of an advanced training program for high-velocity sports, particularly when used in conjunction with static stretching.[130] Ballistic stretching is generally contraindicated for the elderly, the chronically ill, or for patients undergoing active rehabilitation with neuromuscular impairments. It involves high-velocity, high-intensity movements that are not easily controlled. In addition, activation of muscle stretch receptors (muscle spindle Ia endings) results in reflex contraction and limits muscle elongation. Also in chronic contractures, connective tissue is more brittle and tears easily. Thus it is associated with high rates of microtrauma and injury.[105]

Facilitated stretching refers to the use of neuromuscular inhibition techniques to relax (inhibit) and elongate muscles when used in conjunction with stretching. PNF facilitated stretching techniques include Hold-Relax (HR), Contract-Relax (CR), and Active Contraction (AC)[100] (see Appendix B). The limb is actively moved to the lengthened, range-limited position. The patient is then instructed to perform a maximal isometric contraction of the tight muscles in the antagonist pattern. The prestretch contraction results in muscle inhibition from activation of the GTO (autogenic inhibition). This is followed by voluntary relaxation. The limb can then be passively moved into the elongated position (HR) or can be actively moved into the elongated position (Hold-Relax with Active Contraction, HRAC). The CR technique utilizes strong, small range isotonic contraction of the restricting muscles (antagonists) with emphasis on the rotators followed by an isometric hold. Movement into the newly gained range of the agonist pattern is active, not passive (CR with Active Contraction, CRAC). AC produces additional reciprocal inhibition effects (i.e., agonist contraction further inhibits the tight muscle via muscle spindle activity). Although these techniques were originally meant to be applied while using PNF patterns, clinicians have also used them in anatomical planes of motion. Research has demonstrated the effectiveness and superiority of facilitated stretching techniques over static and ballistic stretching techniques.[131–136] An additional benefit is that patients frequently report less discomfort with the application of facilitated stretching techniques as compared to other stretching methods. Because the inhibitory mechanisms affect primarily muscle and depend on voluntary contraction, these techniques are not effective with very weak or paralyzed muscles or range limitation associated with substantial connective tissue changes (chronic contracture).

Frequency of stretching (number of sessions per day or per week) varies according to underlying cause, the chronicity and severity of contracture, the patient's age and level of tissue integrity and healing, and medical management (use of corticosteroids).[105] Optimally multiple sessions per week (i.e., two to five sessions/week) are balanced with adequate rest in between to minimize tissue soreness. Exercises should be followed by active functional movements that maximize the mobility gained. Patients and/or their families/caregivers should be taught stretching exercises (i.e., self-stretching) as part of the HEP to maintain carryover outside of the clinic setting.

Strategies to Manage Tone

Tonal abnormalities are one of a number of features that can affect motor function. **Muscle tone** refers to firmness of the tissue and is the resistance to passive elongation or stretch. It is a function of both mechanical–elastic properties of muscle and neural drive. The term **postural tone** refers to the overall level of tension in the body musculature necessary to maintain body posture against gravity. Changes in tone can vary from higher than normal tone (hypertonia) to lower than normal tone (hypotonia) or fluctuating tone (dystonia). See Chapter 8 for a complete discussion of tonal abnormalities and examination procedures.

Patients with upper motor neuron (UMN) syndrome may exhibit spasticity. **Spasticity** is defined as velocity-dependent hypertonia and hyperactive tendon reflexes (increased deep tendon reflexes, DTRs). Additional *positive signs* associated with UMN syndrome include clonus, spasms, mass reflex responses (exaggerated cutaneous and autonomic reflexes, flexor reflex afferents [FRAs]), and pathological reflexes (e.g., Babinski, Hoffman). *Negative signs* include muscle weakness, slowness of muscle activation, abnormal motor unit recruitment, dyssynergic patterns or obligatory synergies, and loss of coordination and dexterity. Functionally the patient demonstrates poor volitional control of movements and limitations in functional skills. The limbs are typically held in fixed, abnormal postures with antigravity muscles primarily affected. For example, the upper extremity typically assumes an abnormal flexor posture while the lower extremity assumes an abnormal extensor posture. If left untreated, spasticity can lead to the development of secondary impairments such as contracture, postural asymmetries, and deformity. In contrast, the patient with hypotonia typically demonstrates loss of tone with weak or paralyzed muscles, joint instability, and deformity. Following neurological insult, tone varies relative to recovery stage. For example, the patient with a new or recent stroke or spinal cord injury will present with initial flaccidity during the stage of cerebral or spinal shock while the same patient in the post-acute stage will often demonstrate emerging spasticity. Asymmetries of tone between limbs, between the two sides of the body, or between limbs and the trunk are common. Asymmetries may also occur within a limb from muscle to muscle. For example, the proximal muscles are spastic while the distal hand muscles are flaccid.

Strategies for Managing Hypertonia

A number of interventions can be used to manage spasticity. These include prolonged icing, prolonged stretch, inhibitory pressure, and neutral warmth. See Appendix C for a complete description of these techniques. Rhythmic rotation (RRo) is a highly effective exercise technique that can be used to reduce hypertonicity and increase range (see Appendix B). Precise handling of a spastic limb is important. The therapist should use constant, firm manual contacts positioned over nonspastic areas to avoid directly stimulating spastic muscles. To maintain soft tissue range, limbs are slowly moved out of the spastic pattern. Positioning out of the spastic pattern is effective in sustaining the inhibition and range achieved. For example, the patient with stroke is positioned in sitting. Rhythmic rotation is used to move the affected upper limb out of a flexed, adducted position into weightbearing with the elbow extended, hand open, and wrist and fingers extended. Weight shifting during sitting can then be used to maintain inhibition and range. Johnstone[137] advocates the use of inflatable pressure splints to decrease hypertonicity and maintain limbs in optimal tone-reducing positions during functional training. For example, an inflatable pressure cuff is applied to maintain the upper limb in an extended position during weightbearing activities in sitting. At best, inhibitory techniques can be expected to produce a temporary reduction in tone, with results lasting 20 to 30 minutes or up to a few hours. They do not permanently alter tone. Thus, these techniques must be viewed as preparatory techniques to enhance ROM, stretching, and functional movement training and not as the primary focus of treatment. For example, ROM exercise for the patient with severe lower extremity spasticity resulting from multiple sclerosis will likely be ineffective without first applying a tone-reducing technique. Relaxation can be obtained through RRo with both lower extremities positioned on a ball (patient supine with the hips and knees flexed to 90°) and gently rocked side-to-side. Once relaxation occurs, the therapist can then effectively range the limbs to ensure adequate length of muscle and joint position. Resting splints can then be applied to maintain the muscles in an elongated state with positioning of the ankle in a neutral position.

Exercise training is key to lasting improvement in tone and motor function. The following guidelines can be used:

- Primary focus should be on first activating contraction of antagonist muscles (muscles opposite the spastic muscles) to provide inhibition and lengthen spastic muscles.
- Assistance (RRo, active assistive or guided movements) can be used initially as needed but withdrawn as soon as active movements are possible.
- Reciprocal actions are then attempted. Agonist (spastic muscle) contractions are initiated first in small ranges (short arcs) progressing to larger arcs of movement. Smooth, reciprocal movements are practiced.
- Highly stressful and effortful activities should be minimized during early training as they may reinforce (heighten) tone and activate abnormal associated reactions.
- Important functional skills are targeted for training. For example, the patient practices reciprocal reaching, sit-to-stand movements, stepping, or walking.
- Isokinetic exercises are effective in improving function in patients with spasticity.[138–141]
- Strength training can be used and is helpful in improving motor function in patients with spasticity.[142–145]
- Aerobic conditioning can be implemented and is beneficial in improving motor function in patients with spasticity.[146–148]
- Patients and their family or caregivers should be educated about the need to maintain length of spastic muscles. Daily ROM exercises are stressed as well as effective use of stretching, positioning, and splinting techniques.

Serial Casting

Serial casts combined with stretching are effective in reducing hypertonicity, improving range, and reducing deformity.[149–161] *Serial casting* is used when traditional techniques fail and the patient is at risk for development of contractures and deformity, or demonstrates ineffective movement patterns or severe limitations in hygiene and skin care. Inhibitory and ROM techniques are first used to move the limb into its fully lengthened range. Nerve blocks can also be used to improve range prior to casting. The cast is then applied while the limb is held at the end of available range. The sustained position produces relaxation of the spastic muscles, thought to be the result of GTO autogenic inhibition and adaptation of stretch receptors.[162] Neutral warmth and continuous even pressure may also be contributing factors. Inhibitory casting has been found to promote changes in muscle or tendon length and sarcomere distribution.[163] The casts are typically changed every 5 to 7 days (serial application) to gradually increase available range. Poor casting techniques include lack of end-range positioning of the limb, loose-fitting cast, or insufficient padding. Faulty technique may result in a lack of improvement or even increased tone, skin breakdown especially on bony prominences, or nerve compression. An overly restrictive cast can result in decreased circulation and peripheral edema. Highly agitated patients may potentially injure themselves and demonstrate increased risk of skin breakdown and cast breakage. Patients with cognitive or communication impairments should be monitored closely because they will be unable to indicate pain or discomfort and potential skin breakdown. Casting is contraindicated in patients with severe heterotropic ossification; muscle rigidity; skin conditions such as open wounds, blisters, or abrasions; impaired circulation and edema; uncontrolled hypertension; unstable intracranial pressure; pathological inflammatory conditions such as arthritis or gout; or in individuals at risk for compartment syndrome or nerve impingement. Application to individuals with long-standing contractures (longer than 6 to 12 months) is also contraindicated.[164,165]

Adjustable orthoses have also been used to provide passive, sustained stretch with the added benefits of easy removal for hygiene and observation. These devices use a rotating adjustable dial attached to metal rods and a flexible acrylic thermoplastic base.[166,167] The required adjustments are easier and less time consuming than fabricating an entirely new serial cast. Dynamic orthoses, primarily used on elbow or knee flexion contractures, use a spring-loaded or hydraulic mechanism to provide nearly constant pressure.[168,169] Reported outcomes of studies using these devices include reduction of contractures with minimal complications.

Modalities

Neuromuscular electrical stimulation (NMES) has been used to reduce spasticity and improve motor function.[170] Applications to the tibialis anterior muscle or to the common peroneal nerve have been shown to reduce spasticity in the plantarflexor muscles and ankle clonus.[171–173] Electrical stimulation of forearm muscles has been shown to reduce flexor tone and posturing of the hand.[174,175] Spinal cord stimulators have been utilized to reduce severe flexor and extensor spasms, with variable results.[170] Transcutaneous electrical nerve stimulation (TENS) has been used to improve motor function and reduce tone in patients with UMN syndrome.[176,177] Finally, EMG biofeedback has been used to relax spastic muscles by monitoring muscle activity of during slow, passive stretch. Patients are encouraged to decrease EMG activity during passive or active stretch. Conversely, antagonists to the spastic muscles have also been monitored, with patients encouraged to increase EMG activity and muscle contraction.[178–180]

Strategies for Managing Hypotonia

Intervention techniques to increase tone for patients with hypotonia (flaccidity) can include quick stretch, tapping, resistance, approximation, and positioning (see Appendix C). Patients typically also demonstrate weakness and at times it is difficult to differentiate between the two states. Strengthening exercises that do not overload the weak, hypotonic muscles are indicated. Postural instability is a common problem. Interventions should be designed to improve postural stability in functional positions (see following section on postural stability training). Supportive and protective devices may be necessary to prevent injury to limbs and postural asymmetries (e.g., a Swedish knee cage can be used to prevent hyperextension). NMES can also be used to activate hypotonic muscles, improve strength, and generate movement in paralyzed limbs while preventing disuse atrophy. It is important to focus the patient's attention on the desired movement and verbally cue the patient's movement attempts at volitional contraction. Without such cueing and movement attempts, carryover to volitional control is not possible. Electrical stimulation should ideally be coupled with functional training activities to optimize outcomes.

Postural Control Training

Postural control (balance) is the ability to maintain the body in equilibrium or to control the body's position in space for stability and orientation. **Postural orientation** is the ability to maintain normal alignment relationships between the various body segments and between the body and environment. **Postural stability control** (static equilibrium, static balance, or stability) is the ability to maintain stability and orientation with the center of mass (COM) over the base of support (BOS) with the body at rest (no motion). **Dynamic postural control** (dynamic equilibrium, dynamic balance, or controlled mobility) is the ability to maintain stability and orientation with the COM over the BOS while parts of the body are in motion (see Table 13.2).[2] An intervention program to improve postural control must be based on an accurate evaluation of data obtained during examination of deficits (see Chapter 8). Training activities can be used to:

- Improve static postural control, biomechanical alignment, and symmetrical weight distribution.
- Improve dynamic postural control including musculoskeletal responses necessary for movement and balance.
- Improve adaptation of balance skills for varying task and environmental conditions.
- Improve sensory function including sensory integration and sensory compensation.
- Improve safety awareness and compensatory strategies for effective fall prevention.

Strategies to Improve Static Postural Control

Patients who demonstrate impairments in static postural control are unable to maintain or hold a steady position for a number of reasons, including decreased strength, tonal imbalances (hypotonia, spasticity), impaired voluntary control and hypermobility (ataxia, athetosis), sensory hypersensitivity (tactile-avoidance reactions), or increased anxiety or arousal (high sympathetic state). Instability is associated with excessive postural sway, wide BOS, a high guard hand position or handhold, and loss of balance.

The therapist can select any of a number of weight bearing (antigravity) postures to develop stability control (see Table 13. 3). Postures are selected on the basis of (1) patient safety and level of control and (2) variety in terms of functional tasks. It is important to remember that some activities may cause the patient distress initially. The patient will feel threatened when placed in situations where he or she is in jeopardy of losing balance. The therapist should ensure patient confidence by providing a clear explanation of what is going to happen, and what is expected of the patient in terms that are easy to understand. Support may be given initially to reduce fear if using a new posture, but should be withdrawn as soon as possible to allow focus on active control. The therapist varies the level of activities, selecting activities that both provide success as well as appropriately challenge the patient.

In sitting or standing, the patient is instructed to "hold steady" while sitting or standing tall and maintaining a visual focus on a forward target. Progression is to holding for longer and longer durations. Neuromuscular/sensory stimulation techniques that can be used to enhance stabilizing muscle contractions include quick stretch, tapping, resistance, approximation, manual contacts, and verbal cues (see Appendix C). For the patient unable to actively stabilize the body, the therapist can begin with resisted isometric contractions of antagonist postural muscle groups using the technique of Rhythmic Stabilization (RS) (see Appendix B). For example, the patient with severe instability following traumatic brain injury who is unable to sit independently may need to practice holding first in the side-lying position during application of RS. The therapist can then progress training through postures that demand increasing amounts of upright (antigravity) postural control—prone-on-elbows to quadruped and finally sitting. In each position the therapist carefully provides matching resistance using RS. If an imbalance exists, the stabilizing activity can be followed by a strengthening activity for the weak muscles.[101] As the trunk becomes more stable, the patient is expected to assume active control in stabilizing in the posture. For a patient with hyperkinetic disorders (e.g., ataxia, athetosis), the PNF technique of Stabilizing Reversals (Slow Reversals) is appropriate (see Appendix B). Alternating isotonic contractions are used, allowing only very small range movements. Progression is toward decreasing range (decrements of range) until finally the patient is asked to stabilize and hold steady in the posture.

Additional strategies to improve stability include the use of elastic resistance bands or weights to enhance *proprioceptive loading* and contraction of stabilizing muscles. For example, in the prone-on-elbows position, bands can be placed around the forearms. The patient is instructed to push out against the band and maintain the forearms apart against the resistance. This selectively loads and facilitates contraction of the shoulder stabilizers (abductors and rotator cuff muscles). In bridging, kneeling, or standing, elastic resistance bands can be placed around the thighs. The patient is instructed to maintain the thighs apart against the resistance of the bands. This selectively loads and facilitates contraction of the hip stabilizers (abductors, extensors), improving stability control at the hips.

The therapist can have the patient stabilize while sitting on a therapy ball (also known as Swiss or stability ball). Gentle bouncing provides joint approximation through the vertebral joints, facilitating extensors and an upright posture. For patients requiring more assistance, sitting control can first be practiced on a compliant surface (foam, wobble board, or Dynadisc™) placed on a platform mat or sitting on a ball with a ball holder underneath the therapy ball. Task difficulty can be increased by reducing the BOS (feet apart to feet together to single limb support).

Aquatic therapy can also be used to enhance proprioceptive loading. The water provides a degree of unweighting and resistance to movement. This can be quite effective in reducing hyperkinetic movements and enhancing postural stability. For example, a patient recovering from traumatic brain injury who demonstrates significant ataxia may be able to sit or stand in the pool with minimal assistance while these same activities outside the pool are not possible.

To improve standing control, the patient is directed to practice neuromuscular *fixed-support strategies* that occur at the ankle and hip joints. Feedback is provided to assist the patient in recruiting the correct pattern. To recruit *ankle strategies,* the patient practices small-range, slow-velocity shifts. Attention is directed to the action of ankle muscles to move the body (COM) over the fixed feet (BOS). Standing on a wobble board or foam roller with the flat side down progressing to flat side up are effective activities to recruit ankle strategies. The patient is also directed to practice tasks that normally recruit *hip strategies.* These are recruited with larger shifts in the COM, that approach the limits of stability (LOS), and/or faster body sway motions and are characterized by early activation of proximal hip and trunk muscles. Hip flexion and extension responses are generated during anterior–posterior (AP) displacements and lateral hip motions are generated during lateral displacements. Patients can be instructed to move their upper body forward and backward while standing on a foam roller. Tandem standing or tandem standing on a foam roller can be used to recruit lateral hip strategies.

Anticipatory postural adjustments should also be practiced, because predictive control must be operational for functional balance. The patient is provided with advance information about the upcoming demands of the task. For example, "I want you to catch this 5-pound weighted ball while maintaining your sitting position. The prior knowledge serves as an important source of information in initiating the correct postural pattern. To promote generalizabilty, practice should occur in a variety of environments. For example, training can progress from a closed or fixed environment to a more variable environment such as the physical therapy gym. Balance training must ultimately be context specific to real-life settings of home or community to ensure functional carryover.

Strategies to Improve Dynamic Postural Control

Patients who demonstrate impairments in dynamic postural control are unable to control postural stability and orientation while moving segments of the body. A number of impairments may be contributing factors, including tonal imbalances (spasticity, rigidity, hypotonia), ROM restrictions, impaired voluntary control and hypermobility (ataxia, athetosis), impaired reciprocal actions of the antagonists (cerebellar dysfunction), or impaired proximal stabilization. Clinically, the patient demonstrates difficulty weight shifting from side-to-side, forward–backward, or diagonally. Difficulties are also apparent in moving one or more limbs while maintaining a posture (sometimes referred to as *static-dynamic control*). For example, one limb is freed for movement (reaching or stepping) while the patient maintains the sitting or standing posture. Or from the quadruped position the patient is asked to lift one arm or leg or to lift the opposite arm and leg. These added movements increase the demand for stabilization control because the overall BOS is reduced and the COM must shift over the remaining support segments before the dynamic limb movement can be successful.

The therapist can select any of a number of weightbearing (antigravity) postures to develop dynamic postural control. Practice begins with movements emphasizing smooth directional changes that engage antagonist actions (e.g., weight shifts). As control improves, the movements are gradually expanded through an increasing range (increments of range). Dynamic movements can be facilitated using quick stretch, tapping, light tracking resistance, manual contacts, and dynamic verbal commands (see Appendix C). Although active movement is the goal, assistance may be required during initial movement attempts for both the dynamic movements as well as the stabilizing body segments. Specific task-oriented training (e.g., reaching, stepping) are more motivating, especially if the task is important to the patient.

PNF extremity patterns can be used to increase the level of difficulty. For example, in sitting the patient is asked to move the dynamic limbs in a chop/reverse chop pattern while maintaining a stable posture. The patient's full attention is focused on performing the pattern and not on the stabilizing postural components. This ability to redirect cognitive attention is an important measure of developing postural control as intact postural control functions largely on an automatic and unconscious level. Specific PNF techniques appropriate for assisting patients include Dynamic Reversals (Slow Reversals), Repeated Contractions, Rhythmic Initiation, and Combination of Isotonics (Agonist Reversals) (see Appendix B). For example, in bridging the patient's movements are resisted in assuming the bridge posture (isotonic contractions) and during movement from the bridge position to hooklying (eccentric contractions) using the Combination of Isotonics technique. This activity is an important lead-up for other functional activities that require similar combinations including sit-to-stand transitions, moving from kneeling to heel sitting, and ascending–descending stairs.

Therapy ball activities are effective in developing dynamic stability control. For example, the patient sits on a ball and gently moves the ball side-to-side, forward–backward, or in a combination (pelvic clock motions). Or the patient sits on the ball while performing voluntary movements of the arms or legs (alternate leg or arm raises). Progression is from unilateral to bilateral and finally to reciprocal limb movements (e.g., Mexican hat dance). Voluntary trunk motions can be practiced while sitting on the ball (e.g., head and trunk rotations or forward/backward leans).[181] Resistance can be introduced by using elastic resistance bands or weight cuffs on the ankles or wrists. Difficulty can also be increased by adding a second task (*dual task training*) such as catching and throwing a weighted ball, balloon volleyball, or kicking a ball. Group activities can be introduced when patients can safely perform each of the activities individually.[182]

To improve standing control, the patient is directed to practice neuromuscular *stepping strategies*. The traditional view holds that stepping strategies occur when the COM exceeds the LOS.[183–185] Perturbation is used to provide the COM displacement. Stepping movements are accompanied by early activation of hip abductors and ankle co-contraction for medial–lateral stability during single-limb support.[186] Maki and McIlroy[187] investigated the role of limb movements in maintaining upright stance, specifically compensatory stepping and grasping movements of the upper limbs, which they termed *change-in-support strategies* (as opposed to the fixed-support strategies at the ankle and hip). These investigators found that both stepping and arm movements were very common reactions to loss of balance. Moreover they were initiated well before the COM reached the LOS, contradicting the traditional view that they are strategies of last resort. They also found that stepping may actually be a preferred strategy to using a hip strategy. The direction and magnitude of change-in-support strategies were found to vary according to the magnitude and direction of the perturbation. For example, stepping may occur forward or backward in response to anterior or posterior displacements. Lateral displacements typically resulted in cross-stepping pattern (seen in 87 percent of lateral stepping responses) as opposed to straight side-stepping. Lateral destabilization with its increased demands for lateral weight transfer is particularly problematic for a large portion of older adults who experience falls. Arm reactions in response to whole-body instability were also found to be prevalent with activation of shoulder muscles occurring in 85 percent of destabilizing trials. Increased understanding of the range and variability of postural strategies for balance negates any simplistic view of balance based on a developmental perspective of reflex control (i.e., righting and equilibrium reactions). Overall, the organization of balance strategies must be viewed as flexible, not rigid, involving multiple body segments. In that context, patterns will vary according to a number of different factors including initial conditions, perturbation characteristics, learning, and intention.[188] Training should therefore include practice of voluntary stepping movements in all directions (i.e., anterior, posterior, or lateral side steps). Elastic resistance bands positioned around the pelvis can be used to improve the strength of stepping responses. Manual perturbations of increasing force can also be used to elicit stepping responses.[182]

Postural Awareness Training

Faulty postures such as forward head, kyphosis, lordosis, excessive hip and knee flexion, or pelvic asymmetries can result in decreased postural stability, inaccurate kinesthetic awareness of true vertical, and pain. Although mild deficits may not affect balance control, deficits that significantly alter the COM position can impair balance.[189] Patients are typically unable to self-correct faulty postures. Physical therapy interventions should focus first on improving specific musculoskeletal impairments (e.g., limited ROM, weakness). For example, active exercises to improve standing balance can include standing heel-cord stretches, heel-rises, toe-offs, partial wall squats, chair-rises, side-kicks, back-kicks, and marching in place using touch-down support of the hands as needed (sometimes referred to as the "kitchen sink exercises"). Postural reeducation begins with demonstration of the correct posture. Verbal cues should focus on control of essential postural elements, that is, stable (neutral) pelvis, axial extension (e.g., sit or stand tall), and normal alignment (e.g., head erect, shoulders back, weight evenly distributed under both hips [sitting] or feet [standing]). Patients can benefit from tactile cues during initial practice (manual or surface-related). For example, patients can stand with the back positioned against a wall or patients with a lateral lean (e.g., post-stroke patients with pusher syndrome) can sit with their side positioned against the seated therapist or a wall. Corner standing or standing between two plinths can be effective for patients with significant COM distortion. Mirrors provide important visual cues regarding vertical position but are generally contraindicated for the patient with visuospatial perceptual deficits. Application of correct postures to real-life functional situations is important to ensure carryover and lasting change.

Center-of-Mass Control Training

The therapist should focus on obtaining symmetrical, balanced weightbearing. Patients may present with specific directional instabilities, such as weightbearing more on one side than the other. For example, after a stroke the patient typically keeps weight centered toward the sound side. Practice should focus on redirecting the patient into a centered position by moving toward the affected side, both in sitting and standing positions. Limits of stability (LOS) should be explored. For example, in sitting or standing, the patient is instructed to slowly sway forward–backward and side-to-side. The outer point at which the COM is still maintained within the BOS is termed the LOS. Loss of balance occurs when the LOS have been exceeded, for example, when the COM extends beyond the BOS. Practice of volitional body sway is important to assist the patient in developing accurate perceptual awareness of stability limits, an important component of an overall CNS internal model of postural control. Because LOS change with different tasks, a variety of functional activities should be practiced in different environmental settings.

Posturography Feedback

Balance training using augmented visual feedback has become increasingly popular in treating the elderly and other patients at risk for falls. Research reports substantiate its effectiveness in improving balance.[190–196] Force-platform devices are used to measure forces and provide center of pressure (COP) biofeedback or *posturography feedback.* COP displacement is associated with movement of the COM or postural sway. While COP excursion always exceeds COM sway, this relationship is close during ankle motions (ankle strategies) when the body moves like a pendulum over the feet. However, when a hip strategy is used (upper body motion focused at the hips) the COP:COM relationship becomes distorted and does not accurately reflect sway.[197,198] A computer analyzes the data and provides relevant biofeedback concerning sway path and COP position on a visual monitor. Some units also provide auditory feedback.

Posturography training can be used to shape sway movements to enhance symmetry and steadiness. The patient can be instructed to increase or decrease sway movements or move the COP cursor on the computer screen to achieve a designated range or to match a designated target. It is an effective training mode for patients who demonstrate problems in force generation. For example, the patient with decreased force generation (hypometria) as typically demonstrated by individuals with Parkinson's disease is directed toward achieving larger and faster sway movements during posturography training. The patient with too much force (hypermetria), as typically demonstrated by the individual with cerebellar ataxia, is directed toward decreasing sway movements progressing to holding a stable, centered posture.[194,195] It is important to remember that balance retraining using posturography biofeedback does not automatically transfer to functional skills like gait. Winstein[199,200] found that a reduction in standing balance asymmetry did not result in a concomitant reduction in asymmetrical limb movement patterns associated with hemiparetic locomotion. Given the specificity of training principle, this is not a surprising finding. Finally, a set of bathroom scales or limb load monitors can provide a low tech, low cost form of biofeedback weight information to assist patients in achieving symmetrical weightbearing.[201,202]

Strategies to Improve Safety

Prevention of falls for the patient with balance deficiency is an important goal of therapy. Lifestyle counseling is important to help recognize potentially dangerous situations and reduce the likelihood of falls. For example, high-risk activities likely to result in falls include turning, sit-to-stand transfers, reaching and bending over, and stair climbing. Patients should also be discouraged from clearly hazardous activities such as climbing on step stools, ladders, and chairs, or walking on slippery or icy surfaces. The education plan should stress the harmful effects of a sedentary lifestyle. Patients should be encouraged to maintain an active lifestyle, including a program of regular exercise and walking. Medications should be reviewed and those medications linked to increased risk of falls (e.g., medications that result in postural hypotension) should be addressed. A consult with the physician for medication review may be indicated.

Compensatory training strategies should be utilized. The patient should be instructed in how to maintain an adequate BOS at all times. For example, the patient should widen BOS when turning or sitting down. If a force is expected, the patient should be instructed to widen the BOS in the direction of the expected force (e.g., leaning into the wind). If greater stability is needed, instruction should be provided in how to lower the COM (e.g., crouching down to reduce the likelihood of a fall). Greater stability can also be achieved if friction is increased between the body and the support surface. The patient should therefore be instructed to wear shoes with low heels and rubber-soles for better gripping (e.g., athletic shoes). Assistive devices should be used assist to balance when necessary. Consideration should always be given to using the least restrictive device (LRD) while at the same time ensuring safety. Light touch-down support using a vertical or slant cane (used by individuals who are blind) has been shown to improve balance.[203] A fall prevention program must also address environmental factors that contribute to falls. See Box 13.4 for recommendations for reducing falls in the home environment (see also Chapter 12).

Sensory Training

Several general concepts are important to an understanding of the role of sensation in movement. Sensation allows one to interact with the environment, guiding the selection of movement responses. Sensory inputs are used to modify movements and shape motor programs through feedback for corrective actions. Variability and adaptability of movements to environmental change are made possible by the information processing of sensory inputs. Finally, sensory inputs are used to prevent or minimize injury. Interaction of sensory and motor systems occurs throughout the CNS. Much of the sensory information received is not consciously perceived. Spinal-level interactions are largely reflexive in nature, whereas supraspinal centers modulate more complex levels of sensorimotor behavior. Conscious perception and interpretation of sensory information occurs at the highest level, the cortex.

The various types of sensory receptors demonstrate differential sensitivity. Each receptor is highly sensitive to a preferential stimulus while being relatively insensitive to other stimuli at normal intensities. Use of appropriate intensities of sensory stimulation is important to ensure that the desired receptors are stimulated. Excess stimulation can activate unwanted sensory receptors and produce undesired responses, including generalized arousal and sympathetic fight-or-flight reactions. Another special characteristic of sensory receptors is their adaptation to stimuli over time. Generally, they can be divided into two categories, slow- and fast-adapting receptors. In treatment, fast-adapting, phasic receptors such as touch receptors are generally more effective in initiating dynamic movements, whereas slow-adapting, tonic receptors such as joint receptors, Golgi tendon organs, and muscle spindles are used more in monitoring and regulating postural responses. Velocity of movement is also a consideration. At slow velocities, afferent stimuli can contribute to movement responses, while at high velocities there is insufficient time to allow for afferent information to effect motor control (open skills). Certain body segments such as the face, palms of the hands, and soles of the feet demonstrate both high concentrations of tactile receptors and increased representation in the sensory cortex. These areas are highly responsive to stimulation and are closely linked to both protective and exploratory functions.

Damage to the CNS can produce impairments in sensory function. Alterations in tactile, proprioceptive, visual,

Box 13.4 Fall Prevention Strategies: Modifying the Home Environment

- Adequate lighting is essential. Both low light and glare can be hazardous, particularly for the elderly. Glare can be reduced with translucent shades or curtains.
- Light switches should be positioned at the entrance to a room and fully accessible. Timers can ensure that lights come on routinely at dusk. Clapper devices can be used to enable the patient to turn on lights from across the room. Nightlights typically used in bathrooms or hallways do not provide enough light to ensure adequate balance.
- Carpets with loose edges should be tacked down. Scatter or throw rugs should be removed.
- Furniture that obstructs walkways should be removed or repositioned.
- Chairs should be of adequate height and firmness to assist in sit-to-stand transfers. Chairs with armrests and elevated seat heights may be required. Motorized chairs that elevate the patient into standing may be hazardous for (1) some patients who are unable to initiate active balance responses in a timely manner during initial standing and (2) those with impaired LE strength unable to maintain firm foot contact with the floor as the chair rises.
- Stairs are the site of many falls. Ensure adequate lighting. Contrast tape using bright warm colors (red, orange, or yellow) can be used to highlight steps. Handrails are important for safety on stairs and, if not present, may need to be installed.
- Grab bars or rails reduce the incidence of falls in the bathroom. Nonskid mats or strips in the bathtub along with a tub or shower seat can also improve safety. Toilet seats can be elevated to facilitate independent use.

or vestibular systems can affect a patient's ability to move and learn new activities. Deafferentation in animals and in humans is associated with nonuse of a limb, although gross movements are possible under forced situations. Learning of new movements through corrective actions is impaired. The therapist must focus on forced training of sensory-deficient limbs even though the patient may have little interest in moving the limb. The movements obtained should not be expected to be normal, however, because significant deficits have been noted in fine motor control in deafferentated limbs. Following damage to the CNS, sensory inputs may be reduced or distorted. Perceptions are therefore impaired. Sensory training strategies can be used to sharpen and heighten perceptions and assist in reorganizing the CNS.

Training Strategies for Sensory Loss

Sensory stimulation refers to the structured presentation of stimuli to improve (1) alertness, attention, and arousal; (2) sensory discrimination; or (3) initiation of muscle activity and improvement of movement control. Effects are immediate and specific to the current state of the nervous system. See Appendix C for a complete discussion of these techniques. The techniques are important elements of the neurofacilitation approaches.[98–100] Behaviors are modified using techniques to increase or decrease attention and arousal. Movements are elicited and modified through the use of specific stimuli (e.g., stretching, tapping). The effects do not carry over to subsequent movement attempts. Because the movements rely on augmented inputs, their greatest use is to assist the patient with absent or severely disordered voluntary control (e.g., a patient who sustained a stroke and who is unable to consistently initiate muscle contractions). Once a desired motor response is obtained, focus should shift to active movements that utilize naturally occurring intrinsic sensory information. Thus, sensory stimulation techniques may be an effective *bridge* to assist early attempts at movement but should be withdrawn as soon as possible. Repeated use of sensory stimulation long after it is necessary can result in movements that become stimulus dependent, and can further limit the patient's ability to regain voluntary control.

Sensory integration training refers to "the use of enhanced, controlled sensory stimulation in the context of a meaningful, self-directed activity in order to elicit adaptive behavior"[204, p 23] Varied sensory stimuli are presented (tactile, vestibular-proprioceptive, and visual) in order to engage higher brain centers for central processing of sensory information (see Appendix C). The overall goals are to (1) improve sensory discrimination: identification of specific stimuli (e.g., shapes, weights, texture, numbers written on skin), intensities, and localization of stimuli and (2) improve perception: selection, attention, and response to sensory inputs with appropriate use of information to generate specific motor responses. The key elements are multimodal presentation of various different stimuli combined with functional task training. Focus is also on postural training activities with progression to more difficult adaptive motor responses.

Sensory reeducation has been used successfully to improve sensory function in patients with peripheral nerve damage.[205] Patients with stroke-related impairments have also shown benefits from specific sensory training programs.[206–208] Components of these programs consist of having the patient practice sensory identification tasks (numbers, letters drawn on the hand or arm), discrimination tasks (detecting size, weight and texture of objects placed in the hand), and passive-assisted drawing using a pencil. The tasks are alternated between both affected and unaffected hands. Each training session starts and ends with a sensory task the patient could successfully master. The training group showed a positive and significant improvement in sensory function.[208] An important feature of this study was that the subjects were at least 2 years post-stroke, providing strong evidence that the effects were due to training and not recovery. Continued practice with functionally relevant tasks is necessary to maintain the positive effects of any sensory training program. Important considerations for the therapist include having the patient concentrate on the relevant sensory cues, structuring the environment for optimal success, and providing verbal and visual cues. Yekatiel and Guttman[208] suggest that sensory retraining should be considered as a regular component of rehabilitation programs along with motor training following stroke.

Sensory Training Strategies for Balance

An important focus of balance training is utilization and integration of appropriate sensory systems. Normally three sources of inputs are utilized to maintain balance: somatosensory inputs (proprioceptive and tactile inputs from the feet and ankles), visual inputs, and vestibular inputs.[209] Careful examination can identify the patient's use of inputs to maintain balance (e.g., *Clinical Test for Sensory Interaction and Balance* [CTSIB]). See Chapter 8 for a discussion of this test. Training is directed to using varying sensory conditions to challenge the patient. For example, patients who demonstrate a high degree of dependence on vision can practice balance tasks with eyes open and eyes closed, in reduced lighting, or in situations of inaccurate vision (petroleum-coated lenses or prism glasses). Altering the visual inputs allows the patient to shift focus and reliance to other sensory inputs, in this case to intact somatosensory and vestibular inputs. Patients can practice varying somatosensory inputs by standing and walking on different surfaces, from flat surfaces (floor) to compliant surfaces (low to high carpet pile), to dense foam. A patient who is barefoot or wearing thin-soled shoes is better able to attend to sensation from the feet than if wearing thick-soled shoes. Challenges to the vestibular system can be introduced by reducing both visual and somatosensory inputs through sensory conflict situations. For example, the patient practices standing on dense foam with the eyes closed. The patient can also be directed to walk on foam with eyes closed, a condition that requires maximum use of vestibular inputs. Patients should also practice varying environmental influences such as walking outside, progressing from relatively smooth terrain (sidewalks) to uneven terrain to moving surfaces (escalator, elevator). Repetition and practice are important factors in assisting CNS adaptation.

Patients with significant sensory loss will require assistance in shifting toward the intact systems to monitor and adjust balance using *compensatory training strategies*. For example, the patient with proprioceptive losses will need to learn to shift focus onto the visual system for functional mobility and balance. Thus, the patient with bilateral amputations learns to rely heavily on visual inputs for control in standing and walking. If deficits exist in more than one of the major sensory systems, compensatory shifts are generally inadequate and balance deficits will be pronounced.[2] Thus, the patient with diabetic neuropathy and retinopathy will be at high risk for loss of balance and falls. Compensatory training with an assistive device is indicated. Other patients must be encouraged to ignore distorted information (e.g., impaired proprioception accompanying stroke) in favor of more accurate sensory information (e.g., vision). Augmented feedback can assist in training (e.g., verbal commands, light-touch finger contact, biofeedback cane with auditory signals, limb load monitor).

Gait and Locomotion Training

Substantial rehabilitation efforts are directed toward improving gait to restore or improve a patient's functional mobility and independence. Walking is frequently the number one goal of patients who "want to walk" above all other considerations. Ability to ambulate independently is often a significant factor in determining discharge placements (e.g., return to home or extended care facility). The alternate to walking is locomotion using a wheelchair. To establish a realistic plan of care, the physical therapist must accurately analyze the patient's walking ability. Comprehensive gait analysis including gait variables and common gait deviations is discussed in Chapter 10. The functional demands of the patient's home, community, or work environment must be considered in planning successful interventions and in predicting a patient's future status.

Gait is a complex skill that requires integrated function of many interacting systems. Basic requirements for walking include (1) establishment of a rhythmic stepping pattern, (2) body support and propulsion in the intended direction, (3) dynamic postural control, and (4) ability to adapt to changing task and environmental demands.[210] Multiple muscle groups are active in alternating synergistic patterns. Stabilizing muscles contribute to stability of the stance limb and trunk during weight acceptance and single limb support. Other muscles contribute to limb advancement of the dynamic limb during the swing phase. The pattern is then reversed as the gait cycle progresses. As the speed of walking increases, the requirements for timing and control increase. Older adults can be expected to have reduced walking speed, shorter strides, shorter steps, increased time in double support, and decreased time in swing phase than young adults.[53]

Interventions must first be directed at improving function of individual gait components. For example, attention is directed first at improving ROM and strength of weak muscles such as hip abductors or knee extensors. Emphasis can then shift to improving synergistic control of muscles and flexibility through functional training activities. Important *lead-up* or *preambulation activities* that improve strength, range, and control necessary for gait include bridging, sit-to-stand transfers, and static and dynamic postural control activities in kneeling, half-kneeling, modified plantigrade, and standing. Finally, stepping first in modified plantigrade and then in standing are important lead-up activities. See Chapter 14 for a detailed discussion on locomotor training.

Task-Specific Training

Walking is typically practiced first under supportive conditions using parallel bars or assistive devices (e.g., walker, cane, crutches). The goal is early mobilization of the patient out-of-bed or out-of-chair is to prevent further indirect impairments (e.g., weakness, decreased endurance, loss of mobility, and so forth). Gait is typically slow and deliberate with a great deal of conscious effort. Therapists often assist required gait elements, including the weight shift, stabilization of the stance limb, or advancement of the dynamic limb. These compensatory strategies are effective in promoting early ambulation but do little to promote the balance and dynamic control needed for independent gait.

Once out of the parallel bars close stand-by guarding may be necessary. In general, a hands-off approach is recommended as soon as possible. Initially, the patient can use light touch-down (fingertip) support walking next to a treatment table or wall to maintain balance. Progression is then to walking away from the wall with no touch-down support. The therapist can verbally cue the patient to maintain the pace and symmetry of gait.

A variety of walking patterns should be practiced, including forwards, backwards, and sidewards. Side-stepping and crossed-stepping can be practiced first holding on to the outside of the parallel bars or to an oval bar progressing to no support. The PNF activity of *braiding* is a skill-level gait activity that involves alternating side-steps with cross-steps. One limb steps out to the side while the other limb alternates between stepping up and across in front of the other leg (in a D1 flexion pattern) or back and around the other leg (in a D2 extension pattern). Alternating the patterns results in improved pelvic/lower trunk rotation and LE control. Locomotion can also be resisted using the PNF technique of Resisted Progression (RP). Manual contacts placed on the pelvis first lightly stretch and then resist motion. Improved timing and control of pelvic rotation is the goal. Resistance can also be provided using elastic resistance bands wrapped around the pelvis. The therapist walks near the patient, holding the ends of the resistance bands. Speed elements can be controlled using a metronome or brisk marching music. This is an important consideration for the patient with Parkinson's disease who responds well to rhythmic auditory cues (see Evidence Summary Box in Chapter 21).

Walking should be practiced on varying surfaces, from smooth surfaces to uneven terrain outside. Varying the BOS can challenge walking. The patient is instructed to walk first using a normal BOS to narrow BOS to finally semitandem or tandem walking. Having the patient walk with eyes open progressing to eyes closed can vary visual inputs. Having the patient walk while moving the head right and left or up and down can vary vestibular inputs. Walking with directional changes and abrupt starts and stops should be practiced. For example, the patient is asked to make an abrupt start and stop on command and to turn on command. Initially turns are wide progressing to more narrow turns; partial turns (90° turns) are progressed to full turns (180° turns). Attention can be varied by having the patient practice walking with while performing a second task (dual-task training). For example, the patient walks and carries an object or bounces a ball. Talking to the patient while walking can also divert attention (Walkie-Talkie Test). Walking through an obstacle course around and over objects can also be used to challenge control. Patients can be asked to stop and perform a task (march in place on a foam cushion) before proceeding on to the next obstacle.[182]

Climbing stairs is an important functional skill. For many patients, it may mean the difference between going home or going to an alternative living environment. Important lead-up activities for stair climbing include sit-to-stand transfers, standing weight shifting and stepping activities. Step-up and step-down exercises can be practiced using varying step heights from low (4 in. [10 cm]) to high (8 in. [20.3 cm]). The patient initially is instructed to step-up and step-down in the same direction and progressed to stepping up and down in different directions (up and over the step). Practice can begin in the parallel bars or next to a treatment table or wall for light touch-down support. Stair climbing is then practiced, first with limited stairs and progressing to a full flight of stairs. Consideration is given to the number of stairs required in the patient's home. Initial upper extremity support on handrails may be used to compensate for any instability the patient may experience. However, pulling forward with the hand during ascent or pushing during descent masks active control of trunk and lower extremity muscles. As soon as possible stair climbing should be practiced without upper extremity support. Practice on ramps may also be necessary for some patients. For patients with knee extension instability, ramps pose an increased challenge during descent while knee stabilization is enhanced during ascent.

Locomotor Training Using Body Weight Support Treadmill Training (BWSTT)

Locomotor training using partial BWS, a TM, and manually assisted limb movements has already been discussed in a previous section in this chapter as well as in Chapters 14, 18, and 23. There is no underestimating the importance this type of training has had in influencing recovery of gait. Evidence supports its efficacy as a training strategy for diverse groups of patients with deficits in motor function. Studies comparing traditional physical therapy approaches to gait with BWSTT have shown significant improvements in gait speed for the BWSTT group. Once treatment is stopped, the differences between the two groups become less apparent.[72,211,212]

Summary

This chapter outlined a conceptual framework for rehabilitation of the patient with deficits in motor function based on normal processes of motor control, motor learning, and recovery. Clinical decision making is based on a thorough examination of the patient's deficits in terms of impairments, functional limitations, and disability. The unique problems of each patient require that the therapist also recognize a number of interrelated factors, including individual needs, motivation, goals, concerns, and potential for independent function. Given the tremendous variability of patients with deficits in motor function, it is unrealistic to expect that any one intervention can be successful with all patients. Interventions must be carefully chosen to improve function and to minimize injury, future impairments, or disability. The effective use of motor learning strategies can dramatically improve treatment outcomes. Carefully planned and structured education empowers the patient. Patient skills in self-evaluation, problem solving, and decision making are promoted to foster independence. If patient independence is not possible because of the complexity of deficits and limitations in recovery, education of family, friends, and caregivers assumes paramount importance.

Questions for Review

1. Differentiate between the terms *motor control* and *motor learning*. How can impairments in motor control be distinguished from those of motor learning?
2. Describe how information is processed within the CNS to arrive at an appropriate plan for movement. What is the difference between a motor program and a motor plan?
3. Differentiate between the three stages of motor learning. How should training strategies differ during each stage?
4. Discuss motor learning training strategies designed to improve retention and generalizability. How do they differ from strategies that optimize performance?
5. Define neuroplasticity. What are the different theories proposed to explain recovery of function?
6. Define functional/task-specific training. Give three examples of interventions based on this approach.
7. Define the neurofacilitation approaches of NDT and PNF. How do they differ from each other? From compensatory training strategies? Give three examples of interventions of each.
8. Define compensatory training. Identify three interventions that can be considered compensatory training strategies.

Case Study

HISTORY

The patient is a 36-year-old man who sustained a traumatic brain injury following a motorcycle accident. On admission to a local hospital, the patient was found to have a left frontal laceration with an underlying linear skull fracture. CT scan revealed edema, a right basal ganglia contusion, and a left frontal contusion. The patient was comatose on admission. His acute hospital course was complicated by increased intracranial pressure and severe spasticity which required casts and splints. A gastric tube was inserted.

The patient's neurological status did not substantially improve at the acute hospital. He was transferred to a rehabilitation hospital 4 weeks post-injury for intensive rehabilitation. He had a brief readmission to the acute hospital during his sixth week post injury for stabilization of acute hypothermia and hypothyroidism. He was then returned to the rehabilitation facility for continued intensive rehabilitation. His medications consisted of Tegretol (200 mg po qid), multivitamins, and Colace.

PART I: PHYSICAL THERAPY EXAMINATION FINDINGS (INITIAL ADMISSION TO REHAB, 4 WEEKS POST-INJURY)

Cognition: The patient is semicomatose and unresponsive. He inconsistently responds to a command to "look at me" with eye opening and to "lift up your leg" with movement of the right leg only. Otherwise there is no response to auditory or visual stimulation.

Language–Communication: Unable to examine.

Social: Married with no children. Wife is a registered nurse and very supportive of her husband.

Vital Signs: Heart rate 60 bpm; blood pressure 122/70 mm Hg; respiratory rate 14 breaths per minute; O_2 sat level is 92.

Sensation: Localizes to pinprick with withdrawal.

Passive Range of Motion:
- RUE is limited in elbow ROM (0 to 70°); LUE elbow ROM is (10 to 100°).
- Both lower extremities (BLEs) are within normal limits except for ankle dorsiflexion 0 to 5° on R and 0 to 10° on L.

Motor Function

Tone: (Modified Ashworth Scale grades [M-AS]) Severe flexor tone and spasms of the trunk that result in the patient moving in bed from a supine to a left sidelying, curled-up (fetal) position, M-AS = 4

- Right upper extremity (RUE) extensor tone, M-AS = 3
- Right lower extremity (RLE) extensor tone, M-AS = 3
- LUE flexor tone, M-AS = 3
- LLE extensor tone, M-AS = 2

Reflexes:
- Frequent asymmetrical tonic neck reflex posturing with head rotated to the right
- Flexor withdrawal reflexes bilaterally in response to pain (delayed on the left with decreased intensity of response)
- Positive support reflex on the left
- Hyperactive deep tendon reflexes throughout
- At times the patient displays decorticate posturing with mass patterning. The lower extremities scissor at times, especially when upper body flexor tone increases

Voluntary Movements:
- The patient is agitated with restless movements and is frequently diaphoretic.
- No head or trunk control, dependent sitting
- Movement of RUE is spontaneous, purposeful at times, and out-of-synergy.

- Movement of the RLE is spontaneous, nonpurposeful, and out-of-synergy.
- LUE no active movement
- LLE movement is spontaneous, nonpurposeful, with abnormal obligatory synergy.

Coordination: Unable to assess; unresponsive.

Skin: Multiple healed lacerations on the knees and calves and pressure sores bilaterally on the lateral malleoli and calcanei from bivalve positioning splints.

Bladder and Bowel: Incontinent of bowel and bladder, and has external catheter in place.

Functional Activities: Dependent in all activities

PART I (QUESTIONS 1–3)

1. Identify and prioritize the clinical problems presented in this case in terms of direct and indirect impairments, and functional limitations based on initial admission data.
2. Identify the goals and outcomes of physical therapy intervention for this patient at this point in his recovery (initial admission).
3. Identify treatment interventions appropriate for this patient at this point in his recovery (initial admission).

PART II: REEXAMINATION 6 MONTHS POST-INJURY

Cognition:
- **Orientation:** The patient is alert, oriented × 3.
- **Memory:** Memory is impaired; shows limited carryover for relearned tasks such as self-care; past memories show more depth and detail than short-term memory.
- **Attention:** Attention span is reduced; he requires repetition and structure to complete activities.
- **Insight:** He demonstrates little insight into disability or safety awareness.

Behavior:

He is functioning at Rancho Levels of Cognitive Functioning (RLOCF) Level VI Confused-Appropriate. He shows some limited goal-directed behavior but is dependent on external direction. He shows some carryover for new learning but at a significantly decreased rate. Becomes easily frustrated and responds with disinhibited behaviors (name calling and swearing).

Language–Communication: The patient is dysarthric; speech is usually intelligible but difficult to understand and delayed in onset. Auditory comprehension is good.

Vital signs: WNL
Skin: Lacerations are healed.

Sensation:
- **Vision and hearing** are within normal limits.
- **LUE:** Absent sensation
- **LLE:** Impaired sensation, decreased proprioception.
- **RUE and RLE:** Intact

Range of Motion:
- **RUE:** elbow ROM 0 to 90°; LUE: elbow ROM 5 to 110°
- **BLEs:** Within normal limits except for ankle dorsiflexion bilaterally of 0 to 15°

Motor Function
- **Tone:** (modified Ashworth Scale grades, M-AS)
  Trunk: Tone in the trunk is within normal limits except for occasional flexor spasms
  RUE and RLE: Extensor tone, M-AS = 1
  LUE: Flexor tone, M-AS = 2
  LLE: Extensor tone, M-AS = 1

- **Reflexes:** Exhibits strong associated reactions in the LUE and increased flexor posturing with stressful activities.

- **Voluntary Movements:**
  RUE and RLE: Demonstrates purposeful, full, isolated motions through available ROM against gravity. Strength is grossly F+ in the RUE and RLE.
  LUE: No voluntary movement
  LLE: Movement is purposeful and in abnormal synergy; strength is grossly F.
  Head and Trunk: Movement is functional and strength is grossly F.

- **Coordination:**
  Exhibits moderate to severe ataxia in the head, trunk, and extremities.
  Demonstrates moderate impairment in finger-to-nose and toe-tapping test.

- **Balance:**
  Sitting:
  Static: Poor; requires handhold support and moderate assistance; demonstrates sacral siting with posterior tilt of the pelvis
  Dynamic: Poor; unable to accept challenge or move without loss of balance

Standing:
Static: Poor, requires maximal assist of two persons to stand in the parallel bars
Dynamic: Unable

Functional Activities:
- **Bed mobility:** Rolls to right and left with supervision (S)
- **Supine-to-sit:** Mod dependence, requires Min A to close S
- **Transfers:** Mod A × 1 in stand-pivot transfers

- **Wheelchair Locomotion:** Maneuvers power wheelchair with close S for safety
- **Gait:** Unable

PART II (QUESTIONS 4–6)

4. Identify and prioritize this patient's problems in terms of direct and indirect impairments, and functional limitations (6 months post-injury).
5. Identify the goals and outcomes of physical therapy intervention for this patient at this point in his recovery (6 months post-injury).
6. Identify treatment interventions appropriate for this patient at this point in his recovery (6 months post-injury).

References

1. Schmidt, R, and Lee, T: Motor Control and Learning, ed. 4. Human Kinetics, Champaign, IL, 2005.
2. Shumway-Cook, A, and Woollacott, M: Motor Control Theory and Practical Applications, ed 2. Lippincott Williams & Wilkins, Baltimore, 2001.
3. Sherrington, C. The Integrative Action of the Nervous System, ed 2. Yale University Press, New Haven, CT, 1947.
4. Taylor, J (ed): Selected Writings of John Hughlings Jackson. Basic Books, New York, 1958.
5. Brooks, V: The Neural Basis of Motor Control. Oxford University Press, New York, 1986.
6. Bernstein, N: The Coordination and Regulation of Movements. Pergamon Press, Oxford, 1967.
7. Kelso, JA: Dynamic Patterns: The Self-Organization of Brain and Behavior. MIT Press, Cambridge, MA, 1995.
8. Magill, R: Motor Learning Concepts and Applications, ed 4. Brown & Benchmark, Madison, WI, 1993.
9. Adams, J: A closed-loop theory of motor learning. J Motor Behav 3:111, 1971.
10. Schmidt, R: A schema theory of discrete motor skill learning. Psychol Rev 82:225, 1975.
11. Fitts, P, and Posner, M: Human Performance. Brooks/Cole, Belmont, CA, 1967.
12. Lee, T, and Swanson, L: What is repeated in a repetition? Effects of practice conditions on motor skill acquisition. Phys Ther 71:150, 1991.
13. Davies, P: Starting Again—Early Rehabilitation after Traumatic Brain Injury or Other Severe Brain Lesion. Springer-Verlag, New York, 1994.
14. Bobath, B: Adult Hemiplegia: Evaluation and Treatment, ed 2. Heinemann, London, 1978.
15. Singer, R, and Pease, D: A comparison of discovery learning and guided instructional strategies on motor skill learning, retention, and transfer. Res Q 47:788, 1976.
16. Salmoni, A, et al: Knowledge of results and motor learning: A review and critical appraisal. Psychol Bull 95:355, 1984.
17. Lee, T, et al: On the role of knowledge of results in motor learning: Exploring the guidance hypothesis. J Mot Behav 22:191, 1990.
18. Bilodeau, EA, et al: Some effects of introducing and withdrawing knowledge of results early and late in practice. J Exp Psychol 58:142, 1959.
19. Magill, R: Augmented feedback in motor skill acquisition. In Singer, RN, Hausenblas, HA, and Janell, CM (eds). Hanbook of Sport Psychology, ed 2, Wiley, New York, 2001, p 86.
20. Winstein, C, et al: Learning a partial-weight-bearing skill: Effectiveness of two forms of feedback. Phys Ther 76:985, 1996.
21. Bilodeau, E, and Bilodeau, I: Variable frequency knowledge of results and the learning of a simple skill. J Exp Psychol 55:379, 1958.
22. Ho, L, and Shea, J: Effects of relative frequency of knowledge of results on retention of a motor skill. Percept Mot Skills 46:859, 1978.
23. Sherwood, D: Effect of bandwidth knowledge of results on movement consistency. Percept Mot Skills 66:535, 1988.
24. Winstein, C, and Schmidt, R: Reduced frequency of knowledge of results enhances motor skill learning. J Exp Psychol Learn Mem Cogn 16:677, 1990.
25. Lavery, J: Retention of simple motor skills as a function of type of knowledge of results. Can J Psych 16:300, 1962.
26. Swinnen, S, et al: Information feedback for skill acquisition: Instantaneous knowledge of results degrades learning. J Exp Psychol Learn Mem Cogn 16:706, 1990.
27. Winstein, C: Knowledge of results and motor learning: Implications for physical therapy. Phys Ther 71:140, 1991.
28. Shea, J, and Morgan, R: Contextual interference effects on the acquisition, retention, and transfer of a motor skill. J Exp Psychol: Hum Learn 5:179, 1979.
29. Wulf, G, and Schmidt, R: Variability in practice facilitation in retention and transfer through schema formation or context effects? J Mot Behav 20:133, 1988.
30. Wulf, G, and Schmidt, R: Variability of practice and implicit motor learning. J Exp Psychol: Learn, Mem, Cogn 23:987, 1997.
31. Lee, T, Wulf, G, and Schmidt, R: Contextual interference in motor learning: Dissociated effects due to the nature of task variations. Q J Exp Psychol 44A:627, 1992.
32. Lee, T, and Magill, R: The locus of contextual interference in motor skill acquisition. J Exp Psychol Learn Mem Cogn 9:730, 1983.
33. Jeannerod, M: Neural simulation of action: A unifying mechanism for motor cognition. Neuroimage 14:103, 2001.
34. Jeannerod, M, and Frak, V: Mental imaging of motor activity in humans. Curr Opin Neurobiol 9:735, 1999.
35. Feltz, D, and Landers, D: The effects of mental practice on motor skill learning and performance: A meta-analysis. J Sports Psychol 5:25, 1983.
36. Richardson, A: Mental practice: A review and discussion (Part 1). Res Q 38:95, 1967.
37. Richardson, A: Mental practice: A review and discussion (Part 2). Res Q 38:263, 1967.
38. Warner, L, and McNeill, M: Mental imagery and its potential for physical therapy. Phys Ther 68:516, 1988.
39. Maring, J: Effects of mental practice on rate of skill acquisition. Phys Ther 70:165, 1990.
40. Lee, TD: Transfer-appropriate processing: A framework for conceptualizing practice effects in motor learning. In: Meijer O and Roth K (eds). Complex Movement Behavior: The Motor-Action Controversy. North Holland, Amsterdam, 1988, p 201.
41. Bayley, N: The development of motor abilities during the first three years. Monogr Soc Res Child Dev 1 (1, serial no 1), 1935.
42. Gesell, A, and Amatruda, C: Developmental Diagnosis. Harper, New York, 1941.
43. McGraw, M: The Neuromuscular Maturation of the Human Infant. Hafner, New York, 1945.
44. Keogh, J, and Sugden, D: Movement Skill Development. Macmillan, New York, 1985.
45. VanSant, A: Life span development in functional tasks. Phys Ther 70:788, 1990.
46. VanSant, A: Rising from a supine position to erect stance: Description of adult movement and a developmental hypothesis. Phys Ther 69:185, 1988.
47. Woollacott, M, and Shumway-Cook, A: Changes in posture control across the life span: A systems approach. Phys Ther 70:799, 1990.
48. Woollacott, M, and Shumway-Cook, A (eds): Development of Posture and Gait Across the Life span. University of South Carolina Press, Columbia, 1989.
49. Light, K: Information processing for motor performance in aging adults. Phys Ther 70:821, 1990.

50. Schlendorf, S: Effects of aging and exercise on the adult central nervous system: A literature review. Neurology Report (now JNPT) 15:24, 1991.
51. Salthouse, T, and Somberg, B: Isolating the age deficit in speeded performance. J Gerontol 37:59, 1982.
52. Light, K, and Spirduso, W: Effects of adult aging on the movement complexity factor of response programming. J Gerontol 45:107, 1990.
53. Spirduso, W: Physical fitness, aging, and psychomotor speed: A review. J Gerontol 35:850, 1980.
54. Shephard, R: Physical Activity and Aging, ed 2. Aspen, Rockville, MD, 1987.
55. Morris, J, and McManus, D: The neurology of aging: Normal versus pathologic change. Geriatrics 46:47, 1991.
56. Stein, D, Failowsky, B, and Will, B: Brain Repair. Oxford University Press, New York, 1995.
57. Cicinelli, P, Traversa, R, and Rossini, P: Post-stroke reorganization of brain motor output to the hand: A 2–4 month follow-up with focal magnetic transcranial stimulation. Electroenceph Clin Neurophysiol 105:438, 1997.
58. Traversa, R, et al: Mapping of motor cortical reorganization after stroke. Stroke 28:110, 1997.
59. Pohl, P, and Richards, L: Changes in brain activity with motor learning in humans. Neurology Report (now JNPT) 22:79, 1998.
60. van Praag, H, Kemperman, G, and Gage, F: Running increases cell proliferation and neurogenesis in adult mouse dentate gyrus. Nat Neurosci 2:266, 1999.
61. Ploughman, M: A review of brain neuroplasticity and implications for the physiotherapeutic management of stroke. Physiother Can, Summer: 164, 2002.
62. Liepert, J, et al: Motor cortex plasticity during constraint-induced movement therapy in stroke patients. Neurosci Lett 250:5, 1998.
63. Liepert, J, et al: Training-induced changes of motor cortex representations in stroke patients. Acta Neurol Scand 101:321, 2000.
64. Liepert, J, et al: Treatment-induced cortical reorganization after stroke in humans. Stroke 31:1210, 2000.
65. Levy, C, et al: Functional MRI evidence of cortical reorganization in upper-limb stroke hemiplegia treated with constraint-induced movement therapy. Am J Phys Med Rehabil 80:4, 2001.
66. Domerick, A, Edwards, D, and Hahn, M: Does the application of constrain-induced movement therapy during acute rehabilitation reduce arm impairment after ischemic stroke? Stroke 31:2984, 2000.
67. Blanton, S, and Wolf, S: Case Report: An application of upper-extremity constraint-induced movement therapy in a patient with sub-acute stroke. Phys Ther 79:847, 1999.
68. Miltner, W, et al: Effects of constraint-induced movement therapy on patients with chronic motor deficits after stroke: A replication. Stroke 30:586, 1999.
69. Kunkel, A, et al: Constraint-induced movement therapy for motor recovery in chronic stroke patients. Arch Phys Med Rehabil 80:624, 1999.
70. Van der Lee, J, et al: Forced use of the upper extremity in chronic stroke patients: Results from a single-blind randomized clinical trial. Stroke 30:2369, 1999.
71. Taub, E, et al: Technique to improve chronic motor deficit after stroke. Arch Phys Med Rehabil 74:347, 1993.
72. Richards, C, et al: Task-specific physical therapy for optimization of gait recovery in acute stroke patients. Arch Phys Med Rehabil 74:612, 1993.
73. Visitin, M, et al: A new approach to retrain gait in stroke patients through body weight support and treadmill stimulation. Stroke 29:1122, 1998.
74. Visintin, M, and Barbeau, H: The effects of body weight support on the locomotor pattern of spastic paretic patients. Can J Neurol Sci 16:315, 1989.
75. Field-Fote, E: Spinal cord control of movement: Implications for locomotor rehabilitation following spinal cord injury. Phys Ther 80:477, 2000.
76. Kempermann, G, Kuhn, H, and Gage, F: More hippocampal neurons in adult mice living in an enriched environment. Nature 386:493, 1997.
77. Comery, T, et al: Increased density of multiple-head dendritic spines on medium-sized spiny neurons of the striatum of rats reared in a complex environment. Neurobiol Learn Mem 66:93, 1996.
78. Rosenzweig, M, and Bennet, E: Effects of differential environments on brain weights and enzyme activities in gerbils, rats, and mice. Dev Psycholbiol 2:87, 1969.
79. Smith, R, Parts, T, and Lynch, G: A comparison of the role of the motor cortex in recovery from cerebellar damage in young and adult rats. Behav Biol 12:77, 1974.
80. Held, J, Gordon, J, and Gentile, A: Environmental influences on locomotor recovery following cortical lesions in rats. Behav Neurosci 99:678, 1985.
81. Held, J: Environmental enrichment enhances sparing and recovery of function following brain damage. NeuroReport 22:74, 1998.
82. Ohlsson, A, and Johansson, B: Environment influences functional outcome of cerebral infarction in rats. Stroke 26:644, 1995.
83. Johansson, B, and Ohlsson, A: Environment, social interaction and physical activity as determinants of functional outcome after cerebral infarction in the rat. Exp Neurol 139:322, 1996.
84. Kozlowski, D, James, D, and Schallert, T: Use-dependent exaggeration of neuronal injury after unilateral sensorimotor cortex lesions. J Neurosci 16:4776, 1996.
85. Humm, J, et al: Use-dependent exaggeration of brain injury: Is glutamate involved? Exp Neurol 157:349, 1999.
86. Humm, J, et al: Use-dependent exacerbation of brain damage occurs during an early post-lesion vulnerable period. Brain Res 783:286, 1988.
87. Lawton, P: Therapeutic environments for the aged. In Canter, S and Canter, D (eds): Designing Therapeutic Environments. A review of Research. New York, John Wiley, p 233.
88. Carr, J, and Shepherd, R: A Motor Relearning Programme for Stroke, ed 2. Aspen, Rockville, MD, 1987.
89. Carr, J, and Shepherd, R: A motor learning model for rehabilitation. In Carr, J and Shephard, R (eds): Movement Science. Foundations for Physical Therapy in Rehabilitation. Aspen, Rockville MD, p 31.
90. Karla, L: The influence of stroke unit rehabilitation on functional recovery following stroke. Stroke 25:821, 1994.
91. Indredavik, B, et al: Stroke unit treatment. Long term effects. Stroke 28:1861, 1997.
92. Langhorne, P, and Duncan, P: Does the organization of post acute stroke care really matter? Stroke 32:268, 2001.
93. Carr, J, and Shepherd, R: Neurological Rehabilitation: Optimizing Motor Performance. Butterworth Heinemann, Oxford, 1998.
94. Lincoln, N, et al: Behavioural mapping of patients on a stroke unit. Int Disabil Studies 11:149, 1989.
95. Tinson, D: How stroke patients spend their days. Int Disabil Stud 11:45, 1989.
96. Mackey, F, et al: Stroke rehabilitation: Are highly structured units more conducive to physical activity than less structured units? Arch Phys Med Rehabil 77:1066, 1996.
97. Gordon, J: Assumptions underlying physical therapy intervention: Theoretical and historical perspectives. In Carr, J, and Shepherd, R (eds): Movement Science Foundations for Physical Therapy Rehabilitation. Aspen, Rockville, MD, 2000, p 1.
98. Bobath, B: The treatment of neuromuscular disorders by improving patterns of coordination. Physiotherapy 55:1, 1969.
99. Howle, J: Neuro-Developmental Treatment Approach. Neuro-Developmental Treatment Association, Laguna Beach CA, 2002.
100. Voss, D, et al: Proprioceptive Neuromuscular Facilitation, ed 3. Harper & Row, Philadelphia, 1985.
101. Adler, S, Beckers, D, and Buck, M: PNF in Practice, ed 2. Springer-Verlag, New York, 2003.
102. Taub, E: Movement in nonhuman primates deprived of somatosensory feedback. Exerc Sports Sci Rev 4:335, 1976.
103. American Physical Therapy Association: Guide to physical therapist practice. Phys Ther 81:1, 2001.
104. Smidt, G, and Rogers, M: Factors contributing to the regulation and clinical assessment of muscular strength. Phys Ther 62:1283, 1982.
105. Kisner, C, and Colby, L: Therapeutic Exercise Foundations and Techniques, ed 4. FA Davis, Philadelphia, 2002.
106. Enoka, R: Chronic adaptations. In Enoka R (ed): Neuromechanical Basis of Kinesiology, ed 3. Human Kinetics, Champaign, IL, 2002.
107. Harris, B, and Watkins, M: Adaptations to strength conditions. In Frontera, W, Dawson, D, and Slovik, D (eds): Exercise in Rehabilitation Medicine. Human Kinetics, Champaign, IL, 1999. p 71.

108. Bandy, W, and Sanders, B: Therapeutic Exercise—Techniques for Intervention. Lippincott Williams & Wilkins, Philadelphia, 2001.
109. Eng, J: Strength training in individuals with stroke. Physiother Can 56:189, 2004.
110. O'Sullivan, S, and Schmitz, T: Physical Rehabilitation Laboratory Manual: Focus on Functional Training. FA Davis, Philadelphia, 1999.
111. Hall, C, and Brody, L: Therapeutic Exercise—Moving Toward Function, ed 2. Lippincott Williams & Wilkins, Philadelphia, 2005.
112. American College of Sports Medicine: ACSM's Guidelines for Exercise Testing and Prescription, ed 6. Lippincott Williams & Wilkins, Philadelphia, 2000.
113. Curtis, C, and Weir, J: Overview of exercise responses in healthy and impaired states. Neurology Report (now JNPT) 20:13, 1996.
114. Bennett, R, and Knowlton, G: Overwork weakness in partially denervated skeletal muscle. Clin Orthop 12:22, 1958.
115. Dean, E: Effect of modified aerobic training on movement energetics in polio survivors. Orthopedics 14:1253, 1991.
116. Fillyaw, M, et al: The effects of long-term non-fatiguing resistance exercise in subjects with post-polio syndrome. Orthopedics 14:1252, 1991.
117. Aitkens, S, et al: Moderate resistance exercise program: Its effects in slowly progressive neuromuscular disease. Arch Phys Med Rehabil 74:711, 1993.
118. American College of Sports Medicine: ACSM's Exercise Management for Persons with Chronic Diseases and Disabilities. Human Kinetics, Champaign, IL, 1997.
119. American College of Sports Medicine: ACSM's Resources for Clinical Exercise Physiology. Lippincott Williams & Wilkins, Philadelphia, 2002.
120. Spirduso,W: Physical Dimensions of Aging. Human Kinetics, Champaign, IL, 1995.
121. Lentell, G, et al: The use of thermal agents to influence the effectiveness of a low-load prolonged stretch. J Orthop Sports Phys Ther 16:200, 1992.
122. Wessling, K, et al: Effects of static stretch versus static stretch and ultrasound combined on triceps surae muscle extensibility in healthy women. Phys Ther 67:674, 1987.
123. Cornelius, W, and Jackson, A: The effects of cryotherapy and PNF techniques on hip extensor flexibility. J Athl Train 19:183, 1984.
124. Kottke, F, et al: The rationale for prolonged stretching of shortened connective tissue. Arch Phys Med Rehabil 47: 345, 1982.
125. Anderson, B, and Burke, E: Scientific, medical, and practical aspects of stretching. Clin Sports Med 10:63, 1991.
126. Bandy, W, and Irion, J: The effects of time on static stretch on the flexibility of the hamstring muscles. Phys Ther 74:845, 1994.
127. Gajdosik, R: Effects of static stretching on the maximal length and resistance to passive stretch of short hamstring muscles. J Orthop Sports Phys Ther 13:126, 1991.
128. Bohannon, R, and Larkin, P: Passive ankle dorsiflexion increases in patients after a regimen of tilt table: Wedge board standing. Phys Ther 65:1676, 1985.
129. Light, K, et al: Low-load prolonged stretch vs. high-load brief stretch in treating knee contractures. Phys Ther 64:330, 1984.
130. Zachazewski, J: Flexiblity for sports. In: Sanders, B (ed): Sports Physical Therapy. Appleton & Lange, Norwalk, CT, 1990, p 201.
131. Sady, S, et al: Flexibility training: Ballistic, static or proprioceptive neuromuscular facilitation. Arch Phys Med Rehabil 63:261, 1982.
132. Markos, P: Ipsilateral and contralateral effects of proprioceptive neuromuscular facilitation techniques on hip motion and electromyographic activity. Phys Ther 59:1366, 1979.
133. Etnyre, B, and Abraham, L: Gains in range of ankle dorsiflexion using three popular stretching techniques. Am J Phys Med 65:189, 1986.
134. Etnyre, B, and Lee, E: Chronic and acute flexibility of men and women using three different stretching techniques. Res Q 59:222, 1988.
135. Cornelius, W, et al: The effects of cold application and modified PNF stretching techniques on hip flexibility in college males. Res Q Exerc Sport 63:311, 1992.
136. Osternig, L, et al: Differential response to proprioceptive neuromuscular facilitation (PNF) stretch technique. Med Sci Sports Exerc 22:106, 1990.
137. Johnstone, M: Restoration of Normal Movement After Stroke. Churchill Livingstone, New York, 1995.
138. Giuliani, C: The relationship of spasticity to movement and consideration for therapeutic interventions. Neurol Report (now JNPT) 21: 78, 1997.
139. Light, K, and Giuliane, C: Effect of isokinetic exercise effort on arm coordination of spastic hemiparetic subjects. Neurology Report (now JNPT) 16:19, 1992.
140. Giuliani, C, Light, K, and Rose, D: The effects of isokinetic exercise program in gait patterns of patients with hemiparesis. Neurology Report (now JNPT) 4:23, 1993.
141. Brown, D, and Kautz, S: Increased workload enhances force output during pedaling exercise in persons with poststroke hemiplegia. Stroke 29:598, 1998.
142. Damiano, D, and Abel, M: Functional outcomes of strength training in spastic cerebral palsy. Arch Phys Med Rehabil 79:119, 1998.
143. Damino, D, Vaughan, C, and Abel, M: Muscle response to heavy resistance exercise in children with spastic cerebral palsy. Dev Med Child Neurol 38:731, 1995.
144. Miller, G, Light, K, and Kellog, R: Comparison of isometric force control measures in spastic muscle of post-stroke individuals before and after graded resistive exercise. Neurol Report 20:92, 1996.
145. Hall, C, and Light, K: Heavy restrictive exercise effect on reciprocal movement coordination of closed-head injured subjects with spasticity. Neurology Report (now JNPT) 14:19, 1990.
146. Hunter, M, Tomberlin, J, and Kuna, S: Progressive exercise testing in closed head-injuried subjects comparison of exercise apparatus in assessment of a physical conditioning program. Phys Ther 70:363, 1990.
147. Jankowski, LW, and Sullivan, SJ: Aerobic and neuromuscular training: Effect on the capacity efficiency and fatigability of patients with traumatic brain injuries. Arch Phys Med Rehab 71(7):500, 1990.
148. Potempa, K, et al: Physiologic outcomes of aerobic exercise training in hemiparetic stroke patients. Stroke 26:101, 1995.
149. Booth, B, Doyle M, and Montgomery J: Serial casting for the management of spasticity in the head-injuried adult. Phys Ther 63:1960, 1983.
150. Barnard, P, et al: Reduction of hypertonicity by early casting in a comatose head-injured individual: A case report. Phys Ther 64:1540, 1984.
151. Booth, BJ, et al: Serial casting for the management of spasticity in the head-injured adult. Phys Ther 63:1960, 1983.
152. Lehmkuhl, L, et al: Multimodality treatment of joint contractures in patients with severe brain injury: Cost, effectiveness, and integration of therapies in the application of serial/inhibitive cases. J Head Trauma Rehabil 5:23, 1990.
153. Hill, J: The effects of casting on upper extremity motor disorders after brain injury. Am J Occup Ther 48:219, 1994.
154. Moseley, A: The effect of casting combined with stretching on passive ankle dorsiflexion in adults with traumatic head injuries. Phys Ther 77:240, 1997.
155. Singer, B, et al: Evaluation of serial casting to correct equinovarus deformity of the ankle after acquired brain injury in adults. Arch Phys Med Rehabil 84:483, 2003.
156. Bronski, B: Serial casting for the neurological patient. American Physical Therapy Association, Physical Disabilities Special Interest Section Newsletter 18:4, 1995.
157. Zablotny, C, et al: Serial casting: Clinical applications for the adult head-injured patient. J Head Trauma Rehabil 2:46, 1987.
158. Sullivan T, et al: Serial casting to prevent equinus in acute traumatic head injury. Physiother Can 40:346, 1988.
159. Singer, B, Singer, K, and Allison, G: Serial plastering to correct equinovarus deformity of the ankle following acquired brain injury in adults: Review and clinical applications. Disabil Rehabil 23:829, 2001.
160. Kent, H, et al: Case control study of lower extremity serial casting in adult patients with head injury. Physiother Can 42:189, 1990.
161. Rothstein, J, et al: The effect of casting combined with stretching on passive ankle dorsiflexion in adults with traumatic head injuries. Phys Ther 77:248, 1997.
162. Gracies, J: Pathophysiology of impaiment in patients with spasticity and the use of stretch as a treatment for spastic hypertonia. Phys Med Rehabil Clin North Am 12:747, 2001
163. Tabary, J, et al: Physiological and structural changes in the cat's soleus muscle due to immobilization at different lengths by plaster casts. J Physiol 224:231, 1972.

164. Feldman, P: Upper extremity casting and splinting. In Glenn, M, and Whyte, J (eds): The Practical Management of Spasticity in Children and Adults. Lea & Febiger, Philadelphia, 1990.
165. Giorgetti, M: Serial and inhibitory casting: Implications for acute care physical therapy management. Neurology Report (now JNPT) 17:18, 1993.
166. Collins, K, et al: Customized adjustable orthosis: Their use in spasticity. Arch Phys Med Rehabil 66:397, 1985.
167. Grissom, S, and Blanton, S: Treatment of upper motoneuron plantarflexion contractures by using an adjustable ankle-foot orthosis. Arch Phys Med Rehabil 82:270, 2001.
168. Hepburn, GR: Case studies: Contracture and stiff joint management with Dynasplint. J Orthop Sports Phys Ther 8:498, 1987.
169. MacKay-Lyons, M: Low-load, prolonged stretch in treatment of elbow flexion contractures, secondary to head trauma: A case report. Phys Ther 69:292, 1988.
170. Stefanovska, A, et al: Effects of electrical stimulation on spasticity. Crit Rev Phys Rehabil Med 3:59, 1991.
171. Sieb, T, et al: The quantitative measurement of spasticity: Effect of cutaneous electrical stimulation. Arch Phys Med Rehabil 75:746, 1994.
172. Levin, M, and Hui-Chan, C: Relief of hemiparetic spasticity by TENS is associated with improvement in reflex and voluntary motor functions. Electroencephalogr Clin Neurophysiol 85:131, 1992.
173. Carmick, J: Managing equines in children with cerebral palsy: Electrical stimulation to strengthen the triceps surae muscle. Dev Med Child Neurol 37:965, 1995.
174. Cauraugh, J, et al: Chronic motor dysfunction after stroke: Recovering wrist and finger extension by electromyography-triggered neuromuscular stimulation. Stroke 31:1360, 2000.
175. Kraft, G, Fitts, S, and Hammond, M: Techniques to improve function of the arm and hand in chronic hemiplegia. Arch Phys Med Rehabil 73:220, 1992.
176. Hui-Chan, C, and Levin, M: Stretch reflex latencies in spastic hemiparetic subjects are prolonged after transcutaneous electrical nerve stimulation. Can J Neurol Sci 20:97, 1993.
177. Belanger, AY: Neuromuscular electrostimulation in physiotherapy: A critical appraisal of controversial issues. Physiother Theo Pract 7:83, 1991.
178. Barton, L: Uses of surface EMG for neuromuscular evaluation and training in patients with neurological impairments. Biofeedback Newsmagazine of the AAPB 24:12, 1996.
179. Colborne, G, et al: Feedback of triceps surac EMG in gait of children with cerebral palsy: A controlled study. Arch Phys Med Rehabil 75:40, 1994.
180. Glanz, M, et al: Biofeedback therapy in post-stroke rehabilitation: A meta-analysis of the randomized controlled trials. Arch Phys Med Rehabil 76:508, 1995.
181. Creager, C: Therapeutic Exercises using the Swiss Ball. Executive Physical Therapy, Boulder, CO, 1994.
182. Rose, D: Fall Proof – A Comprehensive Balance and Mobility Training Program. Human Kinetics, Champaign, IL, 2003.
183. Nashner, L: Fixed patterns of rapid postural responses among leg muscles during stance. Exp Brain Res 30:13, 1977.
184. Nashner, L: Adapting reflexes controlling the human posture. Exp Brain Res 26:59, 1976.
185. Horak, F, and Nashner, L: Central programming of postural movements: Adaptation to altered support surface configurations. J Neurophysiol 55:1369, 1986.
186. McIlroy, W, and Maki, B: Adaptive changes to compensatory stepping responses. Gait Posture 3:43, 1995.
187. Maki, B, and McIlroy, W: The role of limb movements in maintaining upright stance: The “change-in-support” strategy. Phys Ther 77:488, 1997.
188. Horak, F, et al: Postural perturbations: New insight for treatment of balance disorders. Phys Ther 77:517, 1997.
189. Damis, C, et al: Relationship between standing posture and stability. Phys Ther 78:502, 1998.
190. Wannstedt, F, and Herman, R: Use of augmented sensory feedback to achieve symmetrical standing. Phys Ther 58:553, 1978.
191. Hocherman, S, et al: Platform training and postural stability in hemiplegia. Arch Phys Med Rehabil 65:588, 1984.
192. Shumway-Cook, A, Anson, D, and Haller, S: Postural sway biofeedback: Its effect on reestablishing stance stability in hemiplegic patients. Arch Phys Med Rehabil 69:395, 1988.
193. Hammon, R, et al: Training effects during repeated therapy sessions of balance training using visual feedback. Arch Phys Med Rehabil 73:738, 1992.
194. Moore, S, and Woollacott, M: The use of biofeedback devices to improve postural stability. Phys Ther Practice 2:1, 1993.
195. Nichols, D: Balance retraining after stroke using force platform biofeedback. Phys Ther 77:553, 1997.
196. Kasser, S, Rose, D, and Clark, S: Balance training for adults with multiple sclerosis: Multiple case studies. Neurol Report (now JNPT) 23:5, 1999.
197. Nashner, L, and McCollum, G: The organization of human postural movements: A formal basis and experimental synthesis. Behav Brain Sci 8:135, 1985.
198. Benda, B, et al: Biomechanical relationship between center of gravity and center of pressure during standing. IEEE Trans Rehab Eng 2:3, 1994.
199. Winstein, C, et al: Standing balance training: Effect on balance and locomotion in hemiparetic adults. Arch Phys Med Rehabil 70:755, 1989.
200. Winstein, C: Balance retraining: Does it transfer? In Duncan, P (ed): Balance. American Physical Therapy Association, Alexandria, VA, 1990, p 95.
201. Gapsis, J, et al: Limb load monitor: Evaluation of a sensory feedback device for controlling weight-bearing. Arch Phys Med Rehabil 63:38, 1982.
202. Gauthier-Gagnon, C, et al: Augmented sensory feedback in the early training of standing balance of below-knee amputees. Physiother Can 38:137, 1986.
203. Jeka, J: Light touch contact as a balance aid. Phys Ther 77:476, 1997.
204. Bundy, AC, Lane, SJ, and Murray, EA: Sensory Integration: Theory and Practice, ed 2. FA Davis, Philadelphia, 2002.
205. Wynn Parry, C, and Salter, M: Sensory re-education after median nerve lesions. The Hand 8:250, 1976.
206. Goldman, H: Improvement of double simultaneous stimulation perception in hemiplegic patients. Arch Phys Med Rehabil 47:681, 1966.
207. Weinberg, S, et al: Training sensory awareness and spatial organization in people with right brain damage. Arch Phys Med Rehabil 60:491, 1979.
208. Yekatiel, M, and Guttman, E: A controlled trial of the retraining of the sensory function of the hand in stroke patients. J Neurol Neurosurg Psychiatry 56:241, 1993.
209. Nashner, L: Sensory, neuromuscular, and biomechanical contributions to human balance. In Duncan, P (ed): Balance. American Physical Therapy Association, Alexandria, VA, 1990, p 5.
210. Forssberg, H: Spinal locomotor functions and descending control. In Sjolund, G and Bjorklund, A (eds) Brain Stem Control of Spinal Mechanisms. Elsevier Biomedical Press, New York, 1982, p 103.
211. Harburn, K, et al: An overhead harness and trolley system for balance and ambulation assessment and training. Arch Phys Med Rehabil 74:220, 1993.
212. Hesse, S, Konrad, M, and Uhlenbroch, D: Treadmill walking with partial body weight support versus floor walking in hemiparetic subjects. Arch Phys Med Rehabil 80:421, 1999.

Supplemental Readings

Carr, J, and Shephard, R: Neurological Rehabilitation Optimizing Motor Performance. Butterworth-Heinemann, Woburn, MA, 1998.

Frontera, W, Dawson, D, and Slovik, D (eds): Exercise in Rehabilitation Medicine. Human Kinetics, Champaign, IL, 1999.

Schmidt, R, and Lee, T: Motor Control and Learning, ed 4. Human Kinetics, Champaign, IL, 2005.

Shumway-Cook, A, and Woollacott, M: Motor Control Theory and Practical Applications, ed 2. Lippincott Williams & Wilkins, Philadelphia, 2001.

Appendix A: Neurodevelopmental Treatment Approach (NDT)[98,99]

I. NDT Basic Principles

- NDT is based on an ongoing analysis of sensorimotor function and carefully planned interventions designed to improve function. Principles of motor control, motor learning, and motor development guide the planning process.
- Therapy focuses on the client's strengths and competencies while at the same time addressing impairments, functional limitations, and disabilities. Negative signs (weakness, impaired postural control, and paucity of movement) are equally important to address in treatment as positive signs (spasticity, hyperactive reflexes).
- The POC is developed in partnership with the patient, family, and interdisciplinary team.
- Treatment focuses on the relationship between sensory input and motor output.
- Therapeutic handling is the primary NDT intervention strategy. Facilitatory and/or inhibitory inputs are provided to influence the quality of motor responses.
- Training is focused on specific task goals and functional skills. The task and/or environment is modified as needed to enhance function.
- Active participation by the patient is a goal and an expectation of treatment.
- A major role of the therapist is assisting in an accurate analysis of motor problems and development of effective solutions.
- Motor learning principles are adhered to in the therapeutic setting, including verbal reinforcement, repetition, facilitation of error awareness (trial and error learning), an environment conducive to learning, engaging the patient/client/family and ensuring motivation.
- Direct teaching of the patient/client/family/caregiver to ensure carryover of functional activities in the home and community setting is an important component.

II. NDT Intervention Strategies and Techniques

Therapeutic Handling: Therapeutic handling is used to influence the quality of the motor response and is carefully matched to the patient's abilities to use sensory information and adapt movements. It includes neuromuscular facilitation, inhibition, or frequently a combination of the two. Manual contacts are used to:

- "Direct, regulate, and organize tactile, proprioceptive and vestibular input,
- Direct the client's initiation of movement more efficiently and with more effective muscle synergies,
- Support or change alignment of the body in relation to the BOS and with respect to the force of gravity prior to and during movement sequences,
- Decrease the amount of force the client uses to stabilize body segments,
- Guide or redirect the direction, force, speed, and timing of muscle activation for successful task completion,
- Either constrain or increase the flexibility in the degrees of freedom needed to stabilize or move body segments in a functional activity,
- Dense the response of the client to sensory input and the movement outcome and provide nonverbal feedback for reference of correction,
- Recognize when the client can become independent of the therapist's assistance and take over control of posture and movement, and
- Direct the client's attention to meaningful aspects of the motor task."[99, p 259]

Key Points of Control: Key points are parts of the body the therapist chooses as optimal to control (inhibit or facilitate) postures and movement. *Proximal key points* include the shoulders and pelvis and are used to influence proximal segments and trunk. *Distal key points* upper and lower extremities (typically the hands and feet).

Key points of control are also used to provide inhibition of abnormal tone and postures. Examples include:

- Head and trunk flexion decreases shoulder retraction, trunk and limb extension (key points of control: head and trunk).
- Humeral external rotation and flexion to 90 degrees decreases flexion tone of the upper extremity (key point of control: humerus).
- Thumb abduction and extension with forearm supination decreases flexion tone of the wrist and fingers (key point of control: the thumb).
- Femoral external rotation and abduction decreases extensor/adductor tone of the lower extremity (key point of control: hip).

Facilitation: Components of posture and movement that are essential for successful functional task performance are facilitated through therapeutic handling and key points.

Inhibition: Components of posture and movement that are atypical and prevent development of desired motor patterns are inhibited. While originally this term referred strictly to the reduction of tone and abnormal reflexes, in current NDT practice it refers to reduction of any underlying impairment that interferes with functional performance. It can be used to:

- "Prevent or redirect those components of a movement that are unnecessary and interfere with intentional, coordinated movement,
- Constrain the degrees of freedom, to decrease the amount of force the client uses to stabilize posture,
- Balance antagonistic muscle groups, or
- Reduce spasticity or excessive muscle stiffness that interferes with moving specific segments of the body."[99, p 261]

Appendix B: Proprioceptive Neuromuscular Facilitation (PNF)[100,101]

I. PNF Basic Procedures for Facilitation

Patterns of Motion: Normal motor activity occurs in synergistic and functional patterns of movement. PNF patterns are "spiral and diagonal" in character and combine motion in all three planes (flexion/extension, abduction/adduction, and transverse rotation). They closely resemble patterns used in normal functional activity and sports.

Extremity patterns are named for the action occurring at the proximal joint or by the diagonal (antagonist pairs of patterns make up the diagonal).

Upper Extremity (UE) Diagonal 1 = Flexion, Adduction, External Rotation (D1 Flexion) and Extension, Abduction, Internal Rotation (D1 Extension)

UE Diagonal 2 = Flexion, Abduction, External Rotation (D2 Flexion) and Extension, Adduction, Internal Rotation (D2 Extension)

Lower Extremity (LE) Diagonal 1 = Flexion, Adduction, External Rotation (D1 Flexion) and Extension, Adduction, Internal Rotation (D1 Extension)

LE Diagonal 2 = Flexion, Abduction, Internal Rotation (D2 Flexion) and Extension, Adduction, External Rotation (D2 Extension)

Patterns are varied by changing the action of the intermediate joint (i.e., elbow or knee) or by changing the position of the patient (i.e., supine, sitting, standing). Patterns can be unilateral or bilateral (i.e., symmetrical, asymmetrical, or reciprocal).

Trunk patterns include chop and lift patterns, bilateral lower extremity (LE) patterns, scapula and pelvis patterns, and head/neck patterns.

Timing: Normal timing ensures smooth, coordinated movement. In PNF patterns normal timing is from distal to proximal. Distal segments (hand/wrist or foot/ankle) move first followed closely by more proximal components. Rotation occurs throughout the pattern, from beginning to end.

Timing for Emphasis (TE): Maximum resistance is used to elicit a strong contraction and allow overflow to occur from strong to weak components within a synergistic pattern; the strong muscles are resisted isometrically ("locking in") while motion is allowed in the weaker muscles.
Indications: Weakness and/or incoordination

Resistance: Resistance facilitates muscle contraction and motor control. Both intrafusal and extrafusal muscle fibers contract, resulting in recruitment of motor units and improved strength of contraction. Resistance is applied manually and functionally through the use of gravity to all types of contractions (isotonic—concentric and eccentric; isometric).

- **Tracking or Light Resistance** applied to weak muscles is facilitatory and is usually applied in combination with light stretch.
- **Maximal Resistance** (the greatest amount of resistance tolerated by the patient) is used to generate maximal effort and adjusted to ensure smooth, coordinated movement; maximal resistance varies according to the individual patient.

Indications: Facilitate weak muscles to contract; enhance kinesthetic awareness of motion; increase strength; increase motor control and motor learning.

Overflow or Irradiation: Refers to the spread of muscle response from stronger muscles in a synergistic pattern to weaker muscles; maximal resistance is the main mechanism for securing overflow or irradiation. Stronger patterns can also be used to reinforce weaker patterns through mechanisms of overflow or irradiation from one extremity to the other, or extremity to trunk.
Indications: Enhance synergistic actions of muscles, increase strength.

Manual Contacts (MC): Precise manual contacts (grip) are used to provide pressure to tactile and pressure receptors overlying muscles to facilitate contraction and guide direction of movements; pressure is applied opposite to the direction of the desired motion.
Indications: Enhance contraction and synergistic patterns.

Positioning: Muscle positioning at optimal range of function allows for optimal responses of muscles (*length–tension relationship*). The greatest muscle tension is generated in mid-ranges with weak contractile force (*active insufficiency*) occurring in the shortened ranges.

The lengthened range provides optimal stretch for muscle spindle support of contraction while the shortened range with muscle spindle unloading provides the least amount of muscle spindle support for contraction.
Indications: Enhance weak contraction.

Therapist Position and Body Mechanics: Therapist is positioned directly *in line* with the desired motion (facing the direction of the movement) in order to optimize the direction of resistance that is applied.

Indications: Enhance therapist's control of the patient's movements; reduce therapist fatigue through effective use of body weight and position.

Verbal Commands (VCs): Verbal commands allow for the use of well-timed words and appropriate vocal volume to direct the patient's movements.

- *Preparatory commands* ready the patient for movement (what to do) and need to be clear and concise. They are optimally accompanied by demonstration and/or guided movement.
- *Action commands* guide the patient through the movement (when and how to move). Strong, dynamic action commands are used when maximal stimulation of movement is the goal; soft action commands are used when relaxation is the goal. Timing is critical to coordinate the patient's actions with the therapist's VCs, resistance, and MCs.
- *Corrective commands* provide augmented feedback to help the patient modify movements.

Indications: Verbal stimulation to enhance strength of muscle contraction and guide the synergistic actions in patterns of movement; verbal corrections provide augmented feedback to enhance motor learning.

Vision: Vision is used to guide the patient's movements, enhance muscle contractions, and synergistic patterns of movement.

Indications: Enhance initial motor control and motor learning.

Stretch (STR): The elongated position/lengthened range and the stretch reflex are used to facilitate muscle contraction. All muscles in the pattern are elongated to optimize the effects of stretch. Commands for voluntary movement are always synchronized with stretch to enhance the response.

- *Repeated stretch* can be applied throughout the range to reinforce contraction in weak muscles that are fading out.

Indications: Enhance strength of muscle contraction and synergistic patterns of movement.

Approximation (AP): Approximation (compressing the joint surfaces) is used to facilitate extensor/stabilizing muscle contraction and stability; can be applied manually, functionally through the use of gravity acting on body during upright positions, or mechanically using weights or weighted vests or belts. Approximation is applied manually during upright, weightbearing positions and in PNF extensor patterns.

Indications: Weakness, inability of extensor muscle to function in weightbearing for stabilization control

Traction (TR): A distraction force (separating the joint surfaces) is used to facilitate muscle contraction and motion, especially in flexion patterns or pulling motions; force is applied manually during PNF. Gentle distraction is also useful in reducing joint pain.

Indications: Weakness, inability of flexor muscles to function in mobilizing or antigravity patterns

II. PNF Techniques

Reversal of Antagonists: A group of techniques that allow for agonist contraction followed by antagonist contraction without pause or relaxation.

- **Dynamic Reversals (Slow Reversals):** Utilizes isotonic contractions of first agonists, then antagonists performed against resistance. Contraction of stronger pattern is selected first with progression to the weaker pattern. The limb is moved through full ROM.

Indications: Impaired strength and coordination between agonist and antagonist, limitations in ROM, fatigue

- **Stabilizing Reversals:** Utilizes alternating isotonic contractions of first agonists, then antagonists against resistance, allowing only very limited ROM.

Indications: Impaired strength, stability and balance, coordination

- **Rhythmic Stabilization (RS):** Utilizes alternating isometric contractions of first agonists, then antagonists against resistance; no motion is allowed.

Indications: Impaired strength and coordination, limitations in ROM; impaired stabilization control and balance

Repeated Contractions, RC (Repeated Stretch): Repeated isotonic contractions from the lengthened range, induced by quick stretches and enhanced by resistance; performed through the range or part of range at a point of weakness. Technique is repeated (i.e., three or four stretches) during one pattern or until contraction weakens.

Indications: Impaired strength, initiation of movement, fatigue, and limitations in active ROM

Combination of Isotonics (Agonist Reversals, AR): Resisted concentric, contraction of agonist muscles moving through the range is followed by a stabilizing contraction (holding in the position) and then eccentric, lengthening contraction, moving slowing back to the start position; there is no relaxation between the types of contractions. Typically used in antigravity activities/assumption of postures (i.e., bridging, sit-to-stand transitions).

Indications: Weak postural muscles, inability to eccentrically control body weight during movement transitions, poor dynamic postural control

Rhythmic Initiation (RI): Voluntary relaxation followed by passive movements progressing to active-assisted and active-resisted movements to finally active movements. Verbal commands are used to set the speed and rhythm of the movements. Light tracking resistance is used during the resistive phase to facilitate movement.

Indications: Inability to relax, hypertonicity (spasticity, rigidity); difficulty initiating movement; motor planning deficits (apraxia or dyspraxia); motor learning deficits; communication deficits (aphasia)

Contract-Relax (CR): A relaxation technique usually performed at a point of limited ROM in the agonist pattern. Strong, small range isotonic contraction of the restricting muscles (antagonists) with emphasis on the rotators is followed by an isometric hold. The contraction is held for 5 to 8 seconds and is then followed by voluntary relaxation and movement into the new range of the agonist pattern. Movement can be passive but active contraction is preferred.

- **Contract-relax-active-contraction (CRAC):** Active contraction into the newly gained range serves to maintain the inhibitory effects through reciprocal inhibition.

Indications: Limitations in ROM

Hold-Relax (HR): A relaxation technique usually performed in a position of comfort and below a level that causes pain. Strong isometric contraction of the restricting muscles (antagonists) is resisted, followed by voluntary relaxation, and passive movement into the newly gained range of the agonist pattern.

- **Hold-Relax-Active Contraction (HRAC):** Similar to HR except movement into the newly gained range of the agonist pattern is active, not passive. Active contraction serves to maintain the inhibitory effects through reciprocal inhibition.

Indications: Limitations in PROM with pain

Replication (Hold-Relax Active Motion, HRA): The patient is positioned in the shortened range/end position of a movement and is asked to hold. The isometric contraction is resisted followed by voluntary relaxation and passive movement into the lengthened range. The patient is then instructed to move back into the end position; stretch and resistance are applied to facilitate the isotonic contraction. For each repetition, increasing ROM is desired.

Indications: Marked weakness; inability to sustain a contraction in the shortened range

Resisted Progression (RP): Stretch, approximation, and tracking resistance is applied manually to facilitate pelvic motion and progression during locomotion; the level of resistance is light so as to not disrupt the patient's momentum, coordination, and velocity. RP can also be applied using elastic band resistance.

Indications: Impaired timing and control of lower trunk/ pelvic segments during locomotion, impaired endurance

Rhythmic Rotation (RRo): Relaxation is achieved with slow, repeated rotation of a limb at a point where limitation is noticed. As muscles relax the limb is slowly and gently moved into the range. As a new tension is felt, RRo is repeated. The patient can use active movements (voluntary effort) for RRo or the therapist can perform RRo passively. Voluntary relaxation when possible is important.

Indications: Relaxation of excess tension in muscles (hypertonia) combined with PROM of the range-limiting muscles

Appendix C: Neuromuscular/Sensory Stimulation Techniques

The term **neuromuscular technique** refers to the facilitation or inhibition of muscle contraction or motor responses. The term **sensory stimulation** refers to the structured presentation of stimuli to improve (1) alertness, attention, and arousal; (2) sensory discrimination; or (3) initiation of muscle activity and improvement of movement control. Effects are immediate and specific to the current state of the nervous system. Additional practice using relevant inputs and feedback is necessary for meaningful and lasting functional change to occur. Variable perceptions exist among individuals; may see decreased sensitivity in some older adults and with some neurological conditions.

I. Proprioceptive Facilitation Techniques

1. Quick Stretch

Stimulus: Brief stretch applied to a muscle.
Activates muscle spindles (facilitates Ia endings); sensitive to velocity and length changes. Has both segmental (spinal cord) and suprasegmental (CNS higher centers) effects.

Response: Stretch reflex: facilitates or enhances agonist muscle contraction; phasic.

Additional peripheral reflex effects: inhibits antagonists, facilitates synergists (*reciprocal innervation effects*). Influences perception of effort.

Techniques: Quick stretch; more effective when applied in the lengthened range (e.g., PNF patterns); tapping over muscle belly or tendon

Comments: A low-threshold response, relatively short-lived; can add resistance to maintain contraction.

Adverse Effects: May increase spasticity when applied to spastic muscles.

2. Prolonged Stretch

Stimulus: Slow, maintained stretch, applied at maximum available lengthened range
Activates muscle spindles (higher threshold response, primarily IIs), Golgi tendon organs (Ib endings); sensitive to length changes; has both segmental (spinal cord) and suprasegmental (CNS higher centers) effects.

Response: Inhibits or dampens muscle contraction and tone due largely to peripheral reflex effects (*stretch-protection reflex*).

Techniques: Positioning; inhibitory splinting, casting; mechanical low-load weights using traction

Comments: Higher threshold response; may be more effective in extensor muscles than flexors due to the added effects of II inhibition. To maintain inhibitory effects, follow with activation of antagonist muscles (*reciprocal inhibition effects*).

3. Resistance

Stimulus: A force exerted to muscle
Activates muscle spindles (Ia and II endings) and golgi tendon organs (Ib endings); sensitive to velocity and length changes. Has both segmental (spinal cord) and suprasegmental (CNS higher centers) effects.

Response: Facilitates or enhances muscle contraction due to: (1) peripheral reflex effects: muscle spindle effects via reciprocal innervation (facilitates agonist, inhibits antagonists, facilitates synergists); Golgi tendon effects via autogenic inhibition: dampens or smooths out the force of contraction and (2) suprasegmental effects: recruits both alpha and gamma motoneurons, additional motor units. Hypertrophies extrafusal muscle fibers; enhances kinesthetic awareness.

Techniques: Manual resistance, carefully graded for optimal muscle function.
Use of body weight and gravity using upright positions.
Mechanical resistance: use of weights, cuffs or vests.
Isokinetic resistance: resistance is applied to a muscle contracting at a constant rate.

Comments: *Tracking (light manual) resistance* is used to facilitate and accommodate to very weak muscles.
With weak hypotonic muscles, eccentric and isometric contractions are used before concentric (enhances muscle spindle support of contraction with less spindle unloading). Maximal resistance may produce overflow from strong to weak muscles within the same muscle pattern (synergy) or to contralateral extremities.

Adverse Effects: Too much resistance can easily overpower weak, hypotonic muscles and prevent voluntary movement, encouraging substitution. May possibly increase spasticity in spastic muscles.

4. Joint Approximation

Stimulus: Compression of joint surfaces
Activates joint receptors, primarily static, type I receptors. Has both segmental (spinal cord) and suprasegmental (CNS higher centers) effects.

Response: Facilitates postural extensors and stabilizing responses (co-contraction); enhances joint awareness

Techniques: Manual joint compression
Mechanical using weighted harness, vest, or belt
Elastic tubing with compression of joints during movement
Bouncing while sitting on a Swiss ball
Comments: Used in PNF extensor extremity patterns, pushing actions.
Approximation applied to top of shoulders or pelvis in upright weightbearing positions facilities postural extensors and stability (e.g., sitting, kneeling, or standing).
Adverse Effects: Contraindicated with inflamed joints.

5. Joint Traction

Stimulus: Traction of joint surfaces
Activates joint receptors, possibly phasic, type II. Has both segmental (spinal cord) and suprasegmental (CNS higher centers) effects.
Response: Facilitates joint motion; enhances joint awareness
Techniques: Manual distraction
Mechanical: wrist or ankle cuffs
Comments: Used in PNF flexor extremity patterns, pulling actions.
Joint mobilization uses slow, sustained traction to improve mobility, relieve muscle spasm, and reduce pain.
Adverse Effects: Contraindicated in hypermobile or unstable joints.

6. Inhibitory Pressure

Stimulus: Deep, maintained pressure applied across the longitudinal axis of tendons; prolonged positioning in extreme lengthened range
Activates muscle receptors (Golgi tendon organs) and tactile receptors (pacinian corpuscles). Has both segmental (spinal cord) and suprasegmental (CNS higher centers) effects.
Response: Inhibition, dampens muscle tone.
Techniques: Firm, maintained pressure applied manually or with positioning.
Pressure from prolonged weightbearing on knees (e.g., quadruped or kneeling) dampens extensor tone.
Pressure from prolonged weightbearing on extended arm, wrist, and fingers dampens flexor tone (e.g., sitting, modified plantigrade).
Pressure over calcaneus dampens plantarflexor tone.
Tactile pressure over acupressure points relieves pain and dampens muscle tone.

Mechanical: firm objects (cones) in hand, inhibitory splints or casts (e.g., wrist, lower leg).
Comments: Inhibitory effects can be enhanced by combination with other relaxation techniques (e.g., deep breathing techniques, soothing environment)
Adverse Effects: Sustained positioning may dampen muscle contraction enough to affect functional performance (e.g., difficulty walking after prolonged kneeling).

II. Exteroceptive Stimulation Techniques

1. Manual Contacts

Stimulus: Firm, deep pressure of the hands in contact with the body
Activates tactile receptors and muscle proprioceptors (somatosensation).
Has both segmental (spinal cord) and suprasegmental (CNS higher centers) effects.
Response: Can facilitate contraction in muscle directly under the hands.
Provide sensory awareness, directional cues to movement.
Provide security and support to unstable body segments.
Comments: Can be used with or without resistance.
Adverse Effects: *Contraindicated* over spastic muscles, and open wounds.

2. Light Touch

Stimulus: A brief, light contact to skin
Activates fast adapting tactile receptors
Has both segmental (spinal cord) and suprasegmental (CNS higher centers) effects.
Potential for interaction with autonomic nervous system, sympathetic division
Response: Protection and alerting responses: protective withdrawal (flexion and adduction) of stimulated extremity withdrawing away from the stimulus; can also see contralateral extension in the lower extremity
Increased arousal
Discriminative responses: identification of touch stimuli, spatial discrimination
Techniques: Brief, light stroke of the fingertips
Brief swipe with ice cube
Light pinch or squeezing or pressure to nail bed
Applied to areas of high tactile receptor density (hands, feet, lips) that are more sensitive to stimulation
Comments: Low threshold response, accommodates rapidly.
Effective in initially mobilizing patients with low response levels (e.g., the patient with traumatic brain injury who is minimally responsive)
Can apply tracking resistance to maintain contraction.
Adverse Effects: Overstimulation may produce sympathetic arousal (rebound effects) with undesirable *fight-or-flight responses.*
Contraindicated for patients with generalized arousal or autonomic instability (e.g., the patient with traumatic brain injury who is agitated and combative).
Brief icing should be used with caution on face, forehead, midline back because of risk of adverse sympathetic and arousal effects.

3. Maintained Touch

Stimulus: Deep, maintained touch/pressure
Activates tactile receptors. Has both segmental (spinal cord) and suprasegmental (CNS higher centers) effects.

Potential for interaction with autonomic nervous system, parasympathetics

Response: Calming effect, generalized inhibition, decreased fight/flight responses; desensitizes skin.

Techniques: Firm manual contacts

Firm pressure to midline abdomen, back, lips, palms, and/or soles of feet

Firm rubbing midline back

Comments: Useful for patients with agitation and high arousal (e.g., the patient with traumatic brain injury)

Useful for patients with hypersensitivity (e.g., the patient with peripheral nerve injury and paresthesias or the patient with tactile defensiveness).

Can be used in combination with other maintained stimuli and sensory discrimination training. Brief touch stimuli should be avoided.

4. Slow Stroking

Stimulus: Slow stroking, applied to paravertebral spinal region

Activates tactile receptors. Has both segmental (spinal cord) and suprasegmental (CNS higher centers) effects.

Potential for interaction with autonomic nervous system, parasympathetics

Response: Calming effect, generalized inhibition, decreased fight-or-flight responses

Techniques: The patient is placed in a supported position such as prone, or sitting head and arms supported and resting forward on a table top.

A flat hand is used to apply firm, alternating strokes in a downward direction over the paravertebral region for approximately 3 to 5 minutes.

Comments: Useful with patients who demonstrate high arousal, increased sympathetic (fight-or-flight) responses.

Can combine with other relaxation techniques (e.g., deep breathing exercises, quiet environment).

Patients with large amounts of body hair may be less responsive to calming effects; hair follicle stimulation may be irritating.

5. Neutral Warmth

Stimulus: Retention of body heat

Activates tactile and thermoreceptors. Has both segmental (spinal cord) and suprasegmental (CNS higher centers) effects.

Potential for interaction with autonomic nervous system, primarily parasympathetics

Response: Generalized inhibition of tone; warming produces a calming effect, relaxation, and reduction of pain

Techniques: Wrapping body or body parts: ace wraps, towel wraps

Application of snug fitting clothing (gloves, socks, tights)

Air splints

Tepid baths

Duration variable depending on patient response

Comments: Useful for patients with high arousal, or increased sympathetic activity; spasticity.

Adverse Effects: Overheating should be avoided, may produce rebound effects (increased arousal or tone).

6. Prolonged Icing

Stimulus: Cold applications

Activates thermoreceptors. Has both segmental (spinal cord) and suprasegmental (CNS higher centers) effects.

Potential for interaction with autonomic nervous system, sympathetics

Response: Decreases neural and muscle spindle firing.

Provides inhibition of muscle tone and painful muscle spasm.

Decreases metabolic rate of tissues.

Techniques: Immersion in cold water, ice chips,

Ice towel wraps or ice packs

Ice massage

Cooling suit

Duration variable depending on patient response

Comments: Monitor effects carefully.

Adverse Effects: Can produce sympathetic nervous system arousal, protective withdrawal responses, fight-or-flight responses.

Contraindicated in patients with sensory deficits, generalized arousal, autonomic instability, and vascular problems.

III. Vestibular Stimulation Techniques

1. Slow Vestibular Stimulation

Stimulus: Low-intensity, slow and rhythmic vestibular stimulation

Activates primarily otolith organs (tonic receptors); lesser effects on semicircular canals (phasic receptors) with inputs via CN VIII (vestibulocochlear) to CNS higher centers and spinal cord; potential for interaction with autonomic nervous system, primarily parasympathetics

Response: Generalized relaxation: inhibition or dampening of tone and motor output (vestibulospinal reflexes); decreased arousal, fight/flight responses

Techniques: Passive, manually assisted or active motions: slow, repetitive rolling or rocking movements, e.g., sidelying rolling, sitting rocking,

Mechanical: use of a rocking chair or bed, therapy ball or bolster, equilibrium board, hammock, swing; wheelchair ride

Comments: Useful with patients who are hypertonic, hyperactive, or who demonstrate high arousal, or tactile defensiveness (e.g., the patient with traumatic brain injury who is combative)

Can be combined with other relaxation techniques (e.g., deep breathing, cognitive/imagery techniques, quiet environment).

2. Vestibular Stimulation

Stimulus: Vestibular stimulation via head and body movements

Activates semicircular canals (phasic receptors that detect rotational acceleration and deceleration), otolith organs (tonic receptors that detect head position with respect to gravity and linear acceleration) with inputs via CN VIII (vestibulocochlear) to CNS higher centers (vestibular nucleus, spinal cord, reticular formation, superior colliculus, cerebellum).
Vestibulospinal and vestibuloocular reflexes
Potential for interaction with autonomic nervous system

Response: Postural and tonal adjustments
Head and eye movements
Improvement of retinal image stability (vestibuloocular reflex), decreased post-rotatory nystagmus
Improvement of motor coordination
Generalized arousal and consciousness

Techniques: Change of position or movement
Fast spinning and linear movements with acceleration and deceleration components heightens alertness and motor responses (e.g., spinning in a chair, mesh net or hammock; prone on a scooter board).
Equipment: equilibrium boards, wobble boards, therapy ball, dynamic posturography

Comments: Useful with:
Hypotonic patients (e.g., an individual with Down syndrome)
Patients with sensory integrative dysfunction (e.g., a child with hyperactivity)
Patients with coordination problems (e.g., stroke, cerebral palsy)
Helpful in overcoming the effects of akinesia or bradykinesia (e.g., a patient with Parkinson's disease)

Adverse Effects: Prolonged effects may include behavioral changes, seizures, and sleep disturbances.
Contraindicated for patients with recurrent seizures or who are intolerant to sensory stimulation.

IV. Augmented Visual Stimulation Techniques

Stimuli: Visual objects: pen light, brightly colored blocks, familiar objects, photo card
Visual backgrounds: checkerboard background, moving surround screen
Videotapes
Visual biofeedback
Activates photoreceptors (rods and cones) with inputs via CN II (optic) to CNS higher centers (lateral geniculate nucleus, primary visual cortex in the occipital lobe, association areas)

Response: Visual discrimination: conscious awareness and recognition of objects; visual tracking
Alerting, orienting responses: startle response to an unexpected visual stimulus
Visual proprioception: processes information about body in space and spatial relationships.
Contributes to control motor responses: active movements, postural/tonal adjustments.
Can contribute to relaxation response.
Potential for emotional responses (limbic system)

Techniques: Structured application of visual stimuli: presentation of visual objects: vary colors, size, distance, and orientation
Moving visual targets
Computer programs for visual–perceptual training
Environmental: altered lighting:
Soft lights and cool colors for promotion of relaxation (e.g., the patient with traumatic brain injury and confused/agitated response levels)
Bright lights, bright colors, and repetitive even patterns for generalized stimulation of consciousness, attention, and alertness (e.g., a patient with traumatic brain injury with decreased response levels)
Visual biofeedback can be used to aid movement control, strength of muscle contraction, or muscle relaxation.

Comments: Visual scanning activities are important for patients with hemianopsia and unilateral spatial inattention.
Elimination of extraneous visual stimuli and visual distractors using a quiet or closed environment may be necessary to ensure patient attention and visual perception (e.g., for the patient with traumatic brain injury in the confused recovery stages).
Utilize gradual reintroduction of distracting visual stimuli in a variable or open environment as recovery permits.

Adverse Effects: Avoid sensory overload, irritating stimuli that may cause agitation.
Altered or decreased visual perception occurs with busy, open clinic environments; visual distractors or sudden, unexpected visual stimuli disrupt motor performance.

V. Augmented Auditory Stimulation Techniques

Stimuli: Verbal commands (VCs)
Variable sounds: rattle, cluster bells
Metronome
Audiotapes: familiar music or voices
Auditory biofeedback
Activates cochlear receptors via CN VIII (vestibulocochlear) to CNS higher centers (cochlear nucleus, reticular formation, inferior colliculus, and medial geniculate body)

Response: Auditory discrimination: conscious awareness and recognition of sounds, auditory tracking responses
Alerting, orienting responses: startle response to a loud noise
Motor responses: active movement responses, postural/tonal adjustments
Relaxation responses
Emotional responses (limbic system)

Techniques: Structured application of auditory stimuli: presentation of varying auditory sounds.
With VCs: consideration of pitch, tone, and level, volume/intensity is important; adaptation occurs with constant volume.
Relaxing, soft, familiar music aids relaxation and reduction of tone.
Rhythmic auditory stimulation and brisk music aids movement initiation and the development of timing and rhythm of a movement sequence (e.g., marching music for patients with Parkinson's disease).
Music aids socialization; useful in group classes.
Auditory biofeedback can be used to aid movement control, strength of muscle contraction, or muscle relaxation.

Comments: Precise, dynamic VCs are an important element of PNF.
Positive emotional effects occur with VCs that are motivating and encouraging.
Elimination of extraneous noise and auditory distractors using a quiet or closed environment may be necessary to ensure patient attention and auditory perception (e.g., for the patient with traumatic brain injury in the confused recovery stages).
Utilize gradual reintroduction of distracting auditory stimuli in a variable or open environment as recovery permits.

Adverse Effects: Avoid sensory overload, irritating stimuli that may cause agitation.
Negative emotional effects occur with VCs that express anger and frustration.
Altered or decreased auditory perception occurs with busy, open clinic environments; auditory distractors or sudden loud noises disrupt motor performance.

VI. Augmented Olfactory Stimulation Techniques

Stimuli: Varying odors that stimulate the sense of smell
Pleasant odors: vanilla, perfume, favorite foods
Stimulant odors: ammonia, vinegar
Activates nasal olfactory receptors (fast adapting) to CN I (olfactory) to temporal and frontal lobes without synapsing in thalamus, higher centers.
Limbic system: Emotional responses

Response: Relaxation responses with pleasant, familiar odors:
Pleasure, positive mood
Reduction of tone and hyperkinetic movements

Alerting, orienting, arousal responses with noxious odors:
Alertness, arousal (e.g., after fainting)
In the minimally conscious patient (e.g., traumatic brain injury): alertness, arousal, withdrawal responses
Motor responses: active movement responses, postural/ tonal adjustments

Techniques: Structured application of stimuli: presentation of varying scents.

Comments: Consider patient's premorbid interests and likes as well as odors in the external environment and scents you may be wearing.

Adverse Effects: Avoid sensory overload; irritating stimuli that cause agitation.
Adverse fight/flight or emotional responses can occur.
Contraindicated in patients with hypersensitivity.

VII. Gustatory Stimulation Techniques

Stimuli: Taste stimuli
Activates taste receptors on posterior tongue to CN IX (glossopharyngeal); anterior and sides of tongue to CN X (vagus) and CN VII (facial) to higher centers (temporal lobe)

Response: Recognition of tastes; fast adapting

Techniques: Structured application of stimuli: presentation of varying tastes.
Feeding is a multisensory experience including taste, smell, pressure, texture, and temperature.

Comments: Various foods evoke emotional contexts.

Adverse Effects: Dysphagia management requires careful control of food inputs (e.g., taste, texture, size).

VIII. Sensory Integration Training

Stimuli: Multimodal: varied sensory stimuli are presented in the context of meaningful activities (tactile, vestibular-proprioceptive, and visual).
Activates sensory receptors and higher brain centers: engages central processing areas of sensory information.

Response: Improved sensory discrimination: identification of specific stimuli (e.g., shapes, weights, texture, numbers written on skin), intensities, and improved ability to localize stimuli
Improve perception: selection, attention, and response to sensory inputs with appropriate use of information to generate specific motor responses

Techniques: Multimodal, presentation of various different stimuli is combined with functional task training.
Tactile: deep touch-pressure activities (e.g., stroking or rubbing the skin, use of a vibrator, manipulation and identification of objects, drawing letters on skin, learning to read Braille); one-handed and two-handed (bimanual) activities
Vestibular–proprioceptive: activities designed to stimulate a variety of movement experiences (e.g., linear and accelerated movements, resisted movements, gasping and moving objects, throwing objects, therapy ball or wobble board activities) Emphasis is on functional tasks, interlimb control.
Visual: visual cues, tracking tasks
Focus is on postural training activities with progression to more difficult adaptive motor responses.

Comments: Sensory organization training is an important component of balance training: activities focus on isolating, suppressing, and combining different inputs under varying conditions.

Used for patients with sensory integrative dysfunction who have a poor ability to discriminate touch, movement, force, or information about their bodies. May underlie disorders of bilateral integration, sequencing, and dyspraxia.

Some patients present with decreased discrimination abilities and intense craving for certain types of sensory inputs (e.g., the hyperactive child with frequent outbursts)

Maintain optimal concentration and attention: provide frequent rests and change of task.

Reduce environmental distractors; combine with relaxation techniques.

Adverse Effects: Sensory overload may produce prolonged after-effects (e.g., pupil dilation, changes in respiratory rate, flushing or pallor, nausea, sleep disturbance).

CHAPTER

14

LEARNING OBJECTIVES

1. Discuss the major elements of physical therapy intervention for patients with gait impairments.
2. Formulate general goals of an exercise program designed to prepare a patient for locomotor training.
3. Describe the characteristic features and focus of control of each posture included in the preparatory exercise program.
4. Contrast and compare the advantages and limitations of using parallel bars for locomotor training.
5. Explain the rationale for each component of the indoor overground sequence.
6. Describe the rationale for locomotor training using body weight support and a motorized treadmill.
7. Describe the guidelines for selection and measurement of canes, crutches, and walkers.
8. Identify the common gait patterns and guarding technique used with assistive devices.
9. Describe strategies for varying task and environmental demands during locomotor training.
10. Using the case study example, apply clinical decision-making skills within the context of locomotor training.

Locomotor Training

Thomas J. Schmitz, PT, PhD

OUTLINE

Walking is the final and highest level of motor control (skill). It represents a foundational component of independent human function that supports and enhances effective interaction with the environment. It is also a functional skill commonly impaired by pathology or injury. Independent ambulation is an expected outcome for many patients who seek physical therapy intervention.

The major requirements for successful walking include:

- Support of body mass by the lower extremities (LEs)
- Production of locomotor rhythm
- Dynamic balance control of the moving body
- Propulsion of the body in the intended direction
- Adaptability of locomotor responses to changing task and environmental demands

The examination of gait presented in Chapter 10 includes identification of gait deviations that impair or prevent ambulation as well as their possible causes. Evaluation of gait analysis data allows the therapist to develop an appropriate plan of care (POC) to address locomotor impairments and typically includes a program of preparatory exercises and locomotor training. The general goal of intervention is to provide the patient with a method of locomotion that allows maximum independence and safety at a reasonable energy cost.

Interventions for impairments that restrict or prevent ambulation are applicable to a broad spectrum of patients/clients seen by physical therapists. The *Guide to Physical Therapist Practice*[1] includes elements of gait and locomotor training as an intervention category within each of the four preferred practice patterns. The continuum of procedural interventions for this category include developmental activities training; gait training; implement and device training; standardized, programmatic, complementary exercise approaches; and wheelchair training.[1] (Wheelchair training is addressed in Chapter 33.)

This chapter presents a general discussion of preparatory exercises and locomotor training strategies that can be modified to meet the needs of an individual patient. Several factors will be of major influence in determining the extent and type of training activities required to achieve the desired expected outcomes. These factors include the

Box 14.1 Locomotor Training: Major Elements of Physical Therapy Intervention

A. Preparation for Locomotor Training
Instruction and training in:

- Bridging
- Quadruped
- Sitting
- Sit-to-stand
- Kneeling and half-kneeling
- Modified plantigrade
- Standing

B. Parallel Bar Progression
Instruction and training in:

- Moving from sitting to standing and reverse
- Standing balance and limits of stability (LOS) training
- Stepping, side-stepping, cross-stepping
- Use of appropriate gait pattern, forward progression, and turning
- Moving from sitting to standing, and reverse, with assistive device[a]
- Standing balance and weight shifting activities with assistive device[a]
- Use of assistive device (with appropriate gait pattern) for forward progression and turning[a]

C. Indoor Overground Progression
Instruction and training in:

- Walking forward and backward
- Resisted progression
- Side-stepping and cross-stepping
- Braiding
- Stair climbing
- Falling techniques (generally included for individuals who are active ambulators; particularly important for individuals who require long-term use of an assistive device)

D. Outdoor Overground Progression
Instruction and training in:

- Opening doors and passing through thresholds that lead outdoors
- Curb climbing; negotiating ramps, stairs, and sloped surfaces
- Walking on even and uneven surfaces
- Walking within imposed timing requirements (e.g., crossing at a stoplight)
- Use of open community environments; outside doors and thresholds
- Entering/exiting transportation vehicles
- Use of elevators, revolving doors

E. Locomotor Training Using Body Weight Support and a Motorized Treadmill
Instruction and training in:

- Walking on treadmill using body weight support (BWS) progressing to no BWS
- Production of locomotor rhythm: slow speed progressing to faster speeds
- Forward propulsion of the body
- Dynamic balance control of the moving body
- Reciprocal stepping patterns: assisted movements (pelvis and LE) to unassisted
- Strategies to improve speed, symmetry, and endurance

F. Indoor Overground Progression Using Body Weight Support
Instruction and training in:

- Indoor walking on level surfaces with body weight support (BWS) progressing to no BWS
- Use of assistive device (if indicated) for ambulation on level surfaces
- Elevation activities: step-ups
- Opening doors and passing through doorways

[a]Owing to limited space, use of the parallel bars may not be possible. However, when adjustable-width bars are available, they provide added security for preliminary use of the assistive device. An alternative approach would be to begin use of the device outside and next to standard parallel bars or oval-shaped parallel bars.

patient's goals for ambulation; information obtained from the gait analysis and subsequent evaluation of these data; and the diagnosis, prognosis, and weightbearing status. For example, the progression of locomotor training activities indicated for an otherwise healthy individual with a non-weightbearing tibial fracture would be very different from those developed for a patient with paraplegia or stroke.

The major elements of physical therapy intervention that comprise locomotor training are outlined in Box 14.1. It should be noted that the entire sequence of intervention will not be indicated for each patient. Depending on individual patient need, multiple segments may be accomplished concurrently, a more rapid progression may be used, or portions may be completely omitted.

Preparatory Exercises for Locomotor Training

Preparatory exercises ready a patient for assuming the upright position and typically involve a large component of mat work. Many of these preparatory activities are based on a developmental framework and progress from initial activities with a large base of support (BOS) and a low center of mass (COM) through later activities that have a smaller BOS and high COM. The techniques utilized within each posture of the preparatory exercises are sequenced and progress from (1) *mobility,* which incorporates initiation of movement techniques, including *assist to position* in which the therapist manually assists the patient to achieve a given posture; to (2) *stability,* characterized by the ability to maintain a posture against gravity; to (3) *dynamic stability,* which is the ability to maintain postural control during weight shifting and movement; and finally to (4) *skill,* which is the highest level, characterized by discrete motor control superimposed on proximal stability. The techniques used within each posture typically progress from assisted or guided movement to active movement to resisted movement to independent movement.

These preparatory mat exercises or lead-up activities (the term *lead-up* implies that the activities are preparatory for or "lead up" to ambulation) have important functional carryover to other daily activities as well, such as relieving pressure, dressing, and bed mobility. Many forms of exercise provide important components of an overall program of preparatory exercises (e.g., progressive resistive exercises, endurance and cardiovascular training, and mobility, flexibility, and coordination exercises).

Depending on level of patient involvement, the development of specific anticipated goals for a preparatory exercise program, is based on the following general goals:

1. Improve strength, power, and endurance.
2. Increase or maintain range of motion (ROM).
3. Improve motor function (motor control and motor learning).
4. Enhance sensory integration.
5. Instruct the patient in handling and moving the affected extremity or extremities.
6. Develop postural stability in sitting and standing.
7. Develop dynamic stability as evidenced by the ability to move within and between postures.
8. Improve trunk and pelvic control.
9. Develop functional balance responses.

A general outline of suggested preparatory mat exercises follows. The activities should be ordered from easiest to most difficult. Total mastery of one activity is not necessary before moving to the next higher level. Sequences may be planned in such a way that multiple postures may be overlapped and used in an exercise program concurrently. With adult patients it is common to work on several levels of activities concurrently. The specific activities and techniques selected, as well as the sequence, will be determined by the anticipated goals established with the individual patient. Chapter 13 should be consulted for descriptions of the individual techniques and additional treatment suggestions. The preparatory mat sequence that follows uses a number of activities and postures, including bridging, quadruped, sitting, kneeling and half-kneeling, modified plantigrade, and, finally, standing.

Bridging, Pelvic Elevation

Bridging allows weightbearing through the feet and is an important precursor to assuming the kneeling position and in developing sit-to-stand control. For this activity the patient is in a hooklying position (supine with hips and knees flexed and feet flat on the mat) and elevates the pelvis off the mat (Fig. 14.1). The BOS is thus reduced and the COM is raised. This activity is particularly useful for facilitating pelvic motions and strengthening the low back and hip extensors in preparation for the stance phase of gait. In addition, bridging has several important functional implications, including bed mobility, use of a bedpan, pressure relief, LE dressing, movement from sit-to-stand, and stair climbing. Specific pelvic motions (e.g., pelvic forward motion, rotation, and lateral shift) required during gait also can be initiated and practiced in this position. Several suggestions that can be used as a progression within this posture follow.

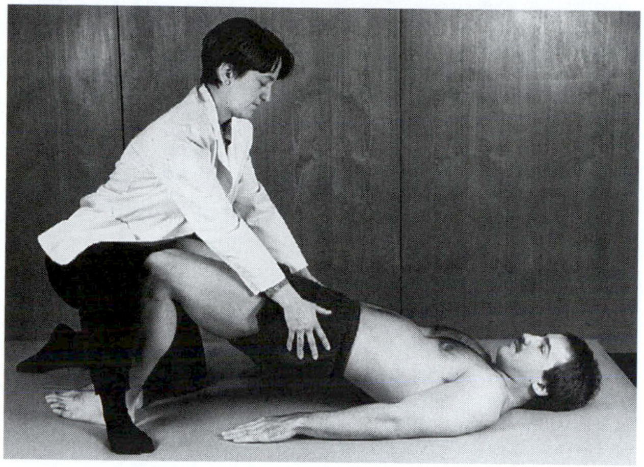

Figure 14.1 Bridging, pelvis elevation. Manual contacts at the pelvis can be used to assist or to resist pelvic elevation.

1. Initial activities will involve assisted assumption and assisted maintenance of the position. Manual contacts (MCs) to assist to position are at the pelvis. Assistance during early bridging activities also can be provided by having the patient abduct the upper extremities (UEs) on the mat to provide a larger BOS.
2. The ability to maintain, or to hold, the posture can be facilitated by use of isometric contractions. The technique of stabilizing reversals (alternating isometrics) can be used to promote stability.
3. Independent maintenance of the posture should be practiced with a progressive decrease in the BOS provided by the UEs (i.e., moving arms closer to body or to the arms-crossed position).
4. The technique of dynamic reversals (slow reversal and slow reversal-hold) can be used to facilitate pelvic rotation and lateral shifting.
5. Strengthening can be accomplished during bridging by application of resistance with MCs at the anterior superior iliac spines. Resistance also can be applied diagonally (greater emphasis of resistance to one side) to facilitate pelvic rotation and/or to increase ROM selectively on one side.

6. Bridging can be used to facilitate hip abduction and adduction. This can be accomplished either symmetrically (resistance applied against the same motion in each extremity) or asymmetrically (resistance applied against opposing motions) by use of alternating isometrics with manual contacts at the knees. Theraband® tubing can be placed around the patient's distal thighs to increase contraction of the hip abductor muscles (gluteus medius) and to increase proprioceptive loading.
7. Resisted (e.g., using agonist reversal) and unassisted movement into and out of the posture.
8. Several modifications to bridging can be made to make the activity more demanding by altering the BOS. These modifications include (a) performing the activity with support from only one LE in preparation for weight acceptance during the stance phase of gait; (b) decreasing the angle of hip and knee flexion (i.e., moving the feet distally); and (c) performing the activity with the upper trunk supported on a therapy ball (walk-out position).

Quadruped Posture

This all-fours (hands and knees) posture further decreases the BOS and raises the COM with weightbearing through multiple joints. The *quadruped* position allows weightbearing through the hips and is particularly useful for promoting control of the lower trunk and hips. For patients with spasticity, this posture can be used to provide inhibitory pressure to the quadriceps and long finger flexors (using an open hand position) to diminish tone.

Assumption of the quadruped position can be achieved from two positions. If the patient is able to sit, the patient may be guided into sidesitting by rotating the trunk to allow weightbearing on the hands with the elbows extended. The therapist then guides the lower trunk into the quadruped position, with MCs on the pelvis to assist movement of the pelvis up and over the knees.

The quadruped position also may be assumed from a prone-on-elbows position. Using this approach the therapist straddles the patient's LEs with one foot placed parallel to each thigh. With the therapist's hips and knees bent, he or she then lifts and guides the pelvis over the knees as the patient "walks" backward on elbows. Once the pelvis is positioned over the knees, the patient extends elbows or is assisted into weightbearing on hands with full elbow extension. Several suggested techniques and activities that can be incorporated into the quadruped position follow.

1. Initial activities involve assisted assumption and assisted maintenance of the position. If these activities are difficult, a therapy ball can first be used to support the patient's trunk during the movement transition from sidesitting to the quadruped position and then during maintenance of the position. The ball can be placed centrally under the trunk or moved toward the upper or LEs, depending on the area of impaired strength. Additional arm support for the patient with stroke can be achieved with the use of an airsplint.
2. Stabilizing reversals (alternating isometrics) will facilitate co-contraction of shoulder, hip, and trunk musculature. Manual application of approximation force can be used to facilitate co-contraction of shoulder and/or hip stabilizing muscles.
3. Weight shifting can be used in a forward, backward, and side-to-side direction to increase weightbearing over two extremities simultaneously to improve dynamic stability.
4. Rocking through increments of range (forward, backward, side-to-side, and diagonally) will facilitate balance and proprioceptive responses as well as increase ROM at the proximal weightbearing joints.
5. Static-dynamic activities, such as freeing one or more extremities from a weightbearing position, may be used in the quadruped position. A progression is frequently made from unweighting one UE to unweighting one LE to unweighting opposite upper and LEs simultaneously. This activity will provide greater joint approximation forces on the supporting extremities and increase dynamic holding of postural muscles (Fig. 14.2).
6. Unassisted movement into and out of the quadruped posture can be practiced.
7. Movement within the quadruped position (creeping) has several important implications for ambulation. This activity requires trunk counterrotation, an important prerequisite for ambulation. Creeping can also be used to improve strength (resisted progression), facilitate dynamic balance reactions, and improve coordination and timing. Movement within the quadruped position is also an important training activity to assist patients who fall in assuming a standing position from the floor (e.g., after a fall a patient can creep to a chair or sofa prior to again assuming an upright posture).

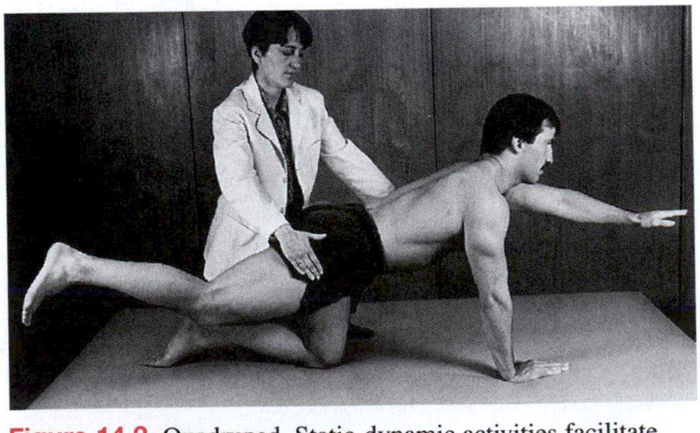

Figure 14.2 Quadruped. Static-dynamic activities facilitate dynamic holding of postural muscles by increasing weightbearing demands on the static limbs.

Sitting

Sitting can be used effectively to promote static and dynamic postural control, reactive and anticipatory balance control, vertical midline orientation and postural alignment, as well as weightbearing through the UEs. In addition, improved stability of the head and neck can be achieved in this position. Two types of sitting are often incorporated into a mat program:

- *Short sitting.* In this position the patient's hips and knees are flexed with the feet flat on the floor (small BOS and intermediate COM).
- *Long sitting.* In this position the hips are flexed and the knees are extended on the supporting surface. The long sitting position provides a large BOS.

CLINICAL NOTE: A factor that warrants consideration in selection of a sitting posture is the ROM required to assume the position. The long sitting position will be difficult for some patients owing to limited ROM in the low back and/or hamstrings. Hamstring tightness in the long sitting position will result in alterations in pelvic position, causing the patient to sit back on the ischia (referred to as sacral sitting).

The BOS in sitting may be altered by changing the positions of UE and LE support. UE support may be placed posterior to the pelvis (large BOS), lateral to the pelvis (small BOS), or anterior to the pelvis (intermediate BOS). LE support can vary from both feet down to legs crossed and one foot down. Several suggestions that can be incorporated into a progression of activities used in sitting follow.

1. Initial activities include assisted assumption (supine-to-sit transitions) and assisted maintenance of the position. Focus is placed on holding (static postural control) with UE weightbearing on the mat; light approximation force may be applied at the shoulder to facilitate activity of stabilizing shoulder muscles. The head, pelvis, and trunk should be in a vertical midline position. A mirror may be used to improve awareness of symmetrical sitting posture. For patients with spasticity, sitting with extended arm support with the hand open and flat on the mat will provide inhibitory input to the long finger flexors to dampen tone.
2. Weight shifting may be practiced in all directions (forward, backward, side-to-side, and diagonally). Typically this will begin with bilateral UE support, progressing to unilateral, and then no support. Weight shifting can also be effectively practiced with the UEs supported on a therapy ball placed directly in front of the patient. Exploration of limits of stability (LOS) should be addressed by practicing extremes of reach without losing balance and return to the starting position. Active reaching in all directions follows.
3. Sitting balancing may be practiced by completely eliminating UE support. The UEs may be held across the chest (cradle position) or altered by movement into shoulder flexion, abduction, and so forth while maintaining trunk balance. Further challenges may be imposed by movement of the trunk (forward, backward, and side-to-side) without UE support; a progression can be made to application of light tracking resistance to trunk movements. Balance may be manually challenged at the trunk (perturbations) or by active movements of the LEs (e.g., crossing the legs). Changing the sitting surface can also increase the challenge (e.g., sitting on a disc or wobble board). Additional practice strategies include engaging the patient in balloon tapping, throwing and catching a ball to and from various directions, or involvement in functional activities such as putting on a pair of socks, tying shoes, and so forth.
4. A variety of PNF techniques can be used in sitting to challenge postural control and stability and to promote diagonal and rotational movements. Examples include UE D1F, D1E, D2F, D2E, Chop/Reverse Chop, and Lift/Reverse Lift.
5. Foot placement can be altered by starting with feet flat on the floor, then to no floor contact (raised seating surface).
6. A progression can be made to sitting on a moveable surface such as a rocker or equilibrium board, roller, or small therapy ball.
7. Sitting push-ups are an important preparatory activity for transfers and locomotor training with assistive devices as well as for proficient positional changes. This activity is accomplished by placing arms at sides, extending the elbows, and depressing the shoulders to lift the buttock from the mat. The activity can be accomplished initially with bearing weight on the base of the hands (or a fisted hand to eliminate excessive stretch on the wrist and finger flexors) placed directly on the mat or using push-up blocks with graded increments in height. A modification of the sitting push-up is placement of both hands on one side of the body in a long sitting position (sidesitting). The patient then pushes down on both UEs to lift the buttocks off the mat. This facilitates lower trunk rotation needed for gait as well as movement transitions from sitting to quadruped positions.
8. Movement within this posture (scooting) has direct functional carryover to transfers, ambulation, and positional changes, and can be practiced in both long- and short-sitting. This activity involves shifting weight onto one hip and then moving the opposite hip forward using a pelvic thrust. The therapist may initially assist by supporting the moving limb with MCs at the feet/ankle (long sitting) or distal thigh (short sitting).

Sit-to-Stand

Movement transitions from sit-to-stand should emphasize symmetrical weightbearing as well as coordination and timing of motor response. Initially, the patient shifts weight forward by using momentum and actively flexing the trunk forward (mass flexion pattern). The feet are placed back partially under the supporting surface to engage the dorsiflexors in forward rotation.

1. Forward weight shifts can be promoted by instructing the patient to focus on a visual target at eye level directly in front and use of appropriate verbal cues from the therapist ("rock your shoulders forward, continue rocking, and come to standing").
2. The patient's UEs can be used effectively to facilitate the weight transfer required of this movement transition by using a forward reaching movement or clasped together in a prayer position and swung forward (momentum). With the therapist positioned directly in front of the patient, active-assistive transitions can be accomplished by placing the patient's UEs (shoulders flexed, elbows extended, and hands clasped together) on one of the therapist's shoulders. Alternately, the patient's UEs can be extended against the therapist's sides (lower trunk). The therapist uses MCs on the patient's upper trunk to promote forward weight shift. Active-assistive transitions can also be practiced with a low table placed in front of the patient. With hands placed on the table, the patient practices partial stand-ups with the hands weightbearing on the table (sit-to-plantigrade). A large therapy ball can also be used to promote weight transfer. With the ball directly in front of the patient, his or her hands are placed on the ball being stabilized by the therapist. The therapist coordinates forward movement of the ball with the forward weight shift.
3. The height of the sitting surface can also be varied. This may be particularly important for patients with hip and knee extensor weakness that limits vertical movement into the upright position. The required extensor force can be decreased by raising the seat height. A gradual progression is then made to lower seat heights.
4. Agonist reversals can be incorporated to strengthen hip and knee extensors both during the *standing up* and *sitting down* phases of the movement. Modified wall squats can also be used to strengthen these muscle groups.
5. Once the patient is upright, lower trunk rotation can be promoted by active lateral shifts of the pelvis to one side and then sitting down next to the original start position. The position of the feet is then adjusted.
6. Self-initiated functional balance tasks such as reaching, bending, and turning can also be utilized. These can be practiced first on a stable sitting surface with progression to an unstable surface (e.g., sitting on a therapy ball) to further promote dynamic balance control.

CLINICAL NOTE: Sit-to-stand activities should be selected carefully based on anticipated goals for the individual patient. Another training strategy is for the patient to "push off" with both hands on a support surface (usually the chair armrests) to move from sit-to-stand. This involves having the patient scoot to the front of the chair, position the feet well under the seating surface, lean forward, and push up into vertical standing using UE support. This is a compensatory training strategy that effectively assists the patient with the movement transition. However, some caution is warranted in selecting this approach. It is typically not effective in developing the forward weight transfer critical for some patients (e.g., stroke). Early and focused use of this strategy may limit dynamic weight shifting ability as well as subsequently restrict the patient to use of only those seating surfaces that provide a "push off" option (i.e., armrests).

Kneeling and Half-Kneeling

The kneeling position further decreases the BOS and raises the COM. It provides weightbearing at the hips simulating the demands of upright standing alignment. This position is particularly useful for establishing lower trunk and pelvic control and further promoting upright balance control. The position also facilitates the LE pattern (initiated during bridging) of combined hip extension with knee flexion necessary for ambulation. In addition, kneeling can be used to provide inhibition to the quadriceps muscle and thus to dampen tone in patients with spasticity. Reduction of extensor tone may be an important preparatory activity to standing and walking for some patients.

It is usually easiest to assist the patient into a kneeling position from a quadruped position. From quadruped, the patient moves or "walks" the hands backward until the knees further flex and the pelvis drops toward the heels. The patient will be "sitting" on the heels. From this position the patient may be assisted to kneeling by using the UEs to climb stall bars (wall ladder) while the therapist guides the pelvis. Another method is for the therapist to assume a heel-sitting position directly in front of the patient. The patient's UEs are supported on the therapist's shoulders while the therapist manually guides the pelvis. Several suggested techniques and activities that can be utilized during kneeling follow.

1. Initial activities concentrate on assisted assumption and assisted maintenance of the position. Stabilizing reversals (alternating isometrics) also can be used to promote stability in this position. MCs are at the pelvis, shoulders, or both shoulders and pelvis. Light approximation force may be applied at the hips to facilitate stabilizing activity of hip muscles. UE weightbearing with hands placed on a chair or therapy ball can also be used for initial stability.
2. The PNF technique of slow reversal or slow reversal-hold is effective in facilitating pelvic forward motion, lateral shifting, and rotation.
3. Eccentric hip control can be facilitated by agonist reversals. This technique uses a smooth reversal between concentric and eccentric contractions. With MCs at the pelvis,

the hips are moved into increments of flexion with a return to extension. The excursion of movement is gradually increased. This technique also improves ability to move from heel-sitting to the kneeling or side-sitting to kneeling position.

4. Transfer of weight from one knee to the other will promote stability on the supporting limb.
5. Balancing activities may be practiced, progressing from support with one UE to balancing without UE support. The patient's balance also may be challenged in this position by kneeling on discs or foam rollers. Throwing and catching a ball from various directions also can be used as a component of these balance activities.
6. Unassisted assumption of the posture can be facilitated by use of reverse chop or lift trunk patterns.
7. Hip hiking and forward progression, or "kneel walking," while the UEs are supported on the therapist's shoulders can be included in this position. A resisted progression can be used to facilitate forward movement. A progression is then made to a resisted progression with the UEs unsupported.

In half-kneeling (Fig. 14.3) the COM is the same as in kneeling; however, the BOS is widened. Greater demands are now placed on the posterior weightbearing limb in preparation for weight acceptance during the stance phase of gait. Weight on the forward limb is now borne through the foot. This position allows facilitation of hip extension, lateral pelvic control, and ankle movements as well as increasing proprioceptive input through the foot. The following techniques and activities are appropriate for use in the half-kneeling position.

1. Initial activities will include assisted assumption and assisted maintenance of the posture.
2. Rhythmic stabilization or alternating isometrics may be used in this position to improve stability. Several combinations of manual contacts may be used: shoulder and pelvis, shoulder and anterior knee, and pelvis and anterior knee.
3. Anterior–posterior diagonal weight shifting in this position will facilitate ROM of the hip, knee, and is particularly effective in mobilizing foot and ankle musculature (see Fig. 14.3).
4. Resistance may be introduced with manual contacts at the pelvis during weight shifting (e.g., slow reversal or slow reversal-hold)
5. Practice in assuming the posture (moving from kneeling to half-kneeling) is an important prerequisite to accomplishing movement transitions from the floor to upright standing (e.g., after a fall).

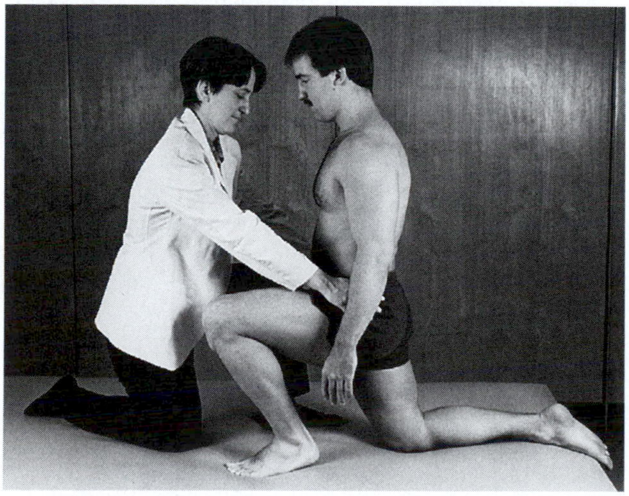

Figure 14.3 Half-kneeling. Anterior weight shifting onto forward limb.

Modified Plantigrade

Modified plantigrade (Fig. 14.4) is an early weightbearing posture that can be used in preparation for erect standing and walking. In this position there is a large BOS and high COM. This posture inherently promotes stability because weightbearing demands are placed on all four extremities and the forward position of the COM creates an extension moment, enhancing knee extension. Modified plantigrade is an important precursor to walking inasmuch as it superimposes close to full weightbearing on an advanced LE pattern. This pattern, required during gait, combines hip flexion with knee extension and ankle dorsiflexion.

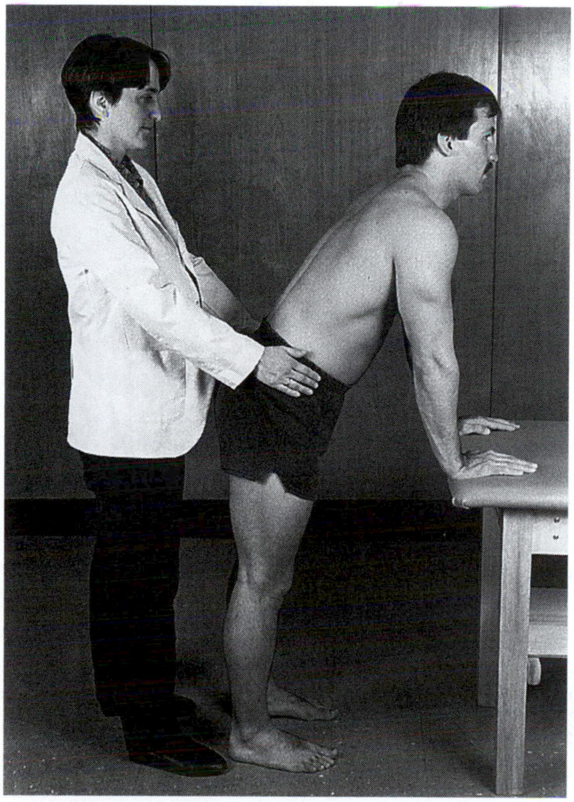

Figure 14.4 Modified plantigrade.

Initial assist-to-position activities are usually easiest from a sitting position. The patient is seated directly in front of a treatment table or other stable surface of appropriate height. A guarding belt may be warranted during early transitions from sitting to plantigrade positions. The patient is asked (or assisted) to scoot forward in the chair. The feet should be well under the seating surface (COM over the BOS), and the hands placed forward on the support surface. The patient shifts weight forward and moves into the modified plantigrade posture. The therapist provides the needed level of assistance by use of the guarding belt and/or MCs. Several suggested activities and techniques that can be used in this posture follow.

1. Initial activities involve assisted assumption and assisted maintenance of the posture.
2. The patient is asked to hold in the modified plantigrade position. Stability can be enhanced by use of manual approximation force at both the shoulders and the pelvis. Stabilizing reversals (alternating isometrics) also can be used to promote stability in this position. MCs are at the pelvis, shoulders, or both shoulders and pelvis.
3. ROM can be increased and dynamic stability further enhanced by rocking through increments of range. Rocking can be used in multiple directions (e.g., forward, backward, diagonally) and is effective in increasing weightbearing over one or more extremities. Guided weight shifting is effectively accomplished by the therapist standing behind the patient with MCs at the pelvis.
4. A progression can be made to static-dynamic activities. Freeing one UE (e.g., reaching in different directions) or one LE (e.g., stepping forward–backward, side-stepping) will place increased demands on the three remaining weightbearing limbs and promote dynamic stability. Body weight is then shifted over the dynamic limb while the static limb remains stationary. This will facilitate pelvic motion and lateral shifting. Rotation of the lower trunk also can be emphasized during static-dynamic LE activities.

Standing

Initially, the patient should be allowed time to become acclimated to the upright posture. During initial standing, the therapist should be alert to complaints of nausea or lightheadedness, which may indicate an onset of *orthostatic (postural) hypotension* caused by a drop in blood pressure. These symptoms typically disappear as tolerance to the upright posture improves. However, if the patient has been confined to bed and/or a wheelchair for a prolonged period, these symptoms may be severe. In these situations a gradual progression of tilt-table activities and careful monitoring of vital signs (see Chapter 4) may be warranted prior to standing. Use of compressive stockings or wraps and an abdominal support or binder will further minimize these effects.

In erect standing the BOS is small with a high COM, requiring maximum balance control. Standing activities can be initiated in the parallel bars (described in the next section). For many patients these activities can be more effectively initiated outside but next to standard parallel bars, next to an oval parallel bar, appropriate height treatment table or other supporting surface such as a wall.

CLINICAL NOTE: Some patients may demonstrate sufficient stability to maintain a standing posture prior to being able to assume the position independently.

It should be noted that achieving a specific level of motor control within an individual posture of the preparatory exercise sequence *does not guarantee translation of gains to standing*. Subcomponents (e.g., hip stability in quadruped) do not translate into standing function without context-specific practice. Motor learning relies on sensory information and feedback provided by practice and experience to shape specific functions. Components of the lead-up activities must be incorporated in upright standing to ensure transfer of subcomponents into a functional whole. The amount of practice required and the rate of learning vary among patients. The following activities and techniques can be used in the standing position.

1. Initial activities involve assisted assumption (see earlier *sit-to-stand* section) and assisted maintenance of the position. With the feet positioned parallel and equal weight distributed on both LEs, holding the posture is practiced. The ability to maintain the posture can be promoted by stability techniques such as stabilizing reversals (alternating isometrics) with manual contacts at the pelvis, scapula, or both scapula and pelvis. With the LEs in a symmetrical stance position, Theraband® tubing can be placed around the thighs to increase proprioceptive loading and pelvic stabilization by the hip abductors.
2. Limits of stability (LOS) training involves determining how far the patient's COM can be displaced while balance is maintained. Without altering the BOS, early exploration of LOS can be accomplished using guided anterior-posterior weight shifts forward and backward; and lateral weight shifting from side-to-side; MCs on the pelvis. Additional support may be provided by placement of the patient's hands on the support surface or the therapist's shoulders (bilateral support progressing to single-hand support); as stability improves, UE support should be eliminated. A platform biofeedback device can be used to enhance limits of stability training as well as centered stance with weight borne equally on both LEs.
3. Dynamic stability activities of the trunk can be practiced in standing using weight shifting with the feet symmetrical or in stride. Anterior–posterior, lateral, and rotational movements of the trunk can be emphasized. A platform biofeedback device can be used to enhance weight shift training (e.g., the patient with stroke is encouraged to shift weight toward the more affected side).

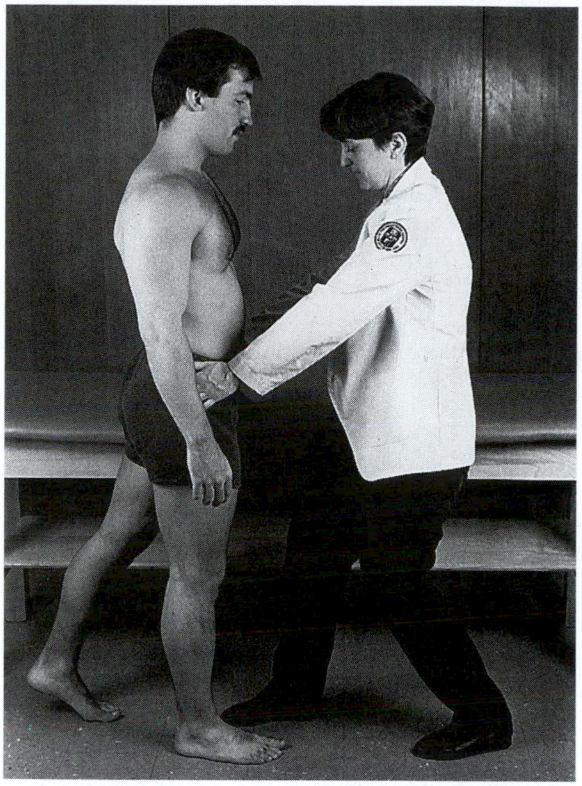

Figure 14.5 Stepping (static-dynamic activity) will promote weight acceptance on the advancing dynamic limb, forward pelvic rotation, and lateral shift of the pelvis.

4. Stepping will promote weight acceptance by advancing the dynamic limb forward and moving body weight over the advanced limb. MCs at the pelvis during stepping are particularly effective in promoting forward rotation and lateral shift of the pelvis (Fig. 14.5). The patient steps forward with one leg, shifts weight anteriorly, and returns to the starting position (normal BOS). This is alternated with stepping backward with one leg, shifting the weight posteriorly, and returning to the starting position. Light tracking resistance can be applied with MCs at the pelvis (e.g., slow reversals). Practice includes stepping forward, backward, forward and backward diagonal shifts, and forward and lateral step-ups. UE movements can also be superimposed on these activities to promote trunk rotation (e.g., reciprocal arm swing) needed for gait.

This section presented a series of activities and exercises designed to prepare the patient for locomotor training. Table 14.1 summarizes the incremental *focus of control* of these activities progressing from more proximal elements (lower trunk, pelvis) using a large BOS and low COM to more distal segments (knee, ankle) that incorporate a small BOS and high COM. The preparatory activities and exercises will require careful and appropriate sequencing to meet individual patient needs. In conjunction with these preparatory activities, patients may also benefit from a concurrent program of strengthening, flexibility, and coordination exercises; transfer training with emphasis on sit-to-stand transitions; and balance training focusing on both static and dynamic control. Figure 14.6 presents a summary overview of preparatory activities and concurrent interventions for locomotor training. For a more detailed description of preparatory therapeutic exercise interventions for locomotor training the reader is referred to *Physical Rehabilitation Laboratory Manual: Focus on Functional Training*.[2]

Table 14.1 Focus of Control: Preparatory Activities for Locomotor Training

Preparatory Activity	Focus of Control
Bridging	Lower trunk Hips/pelvis Lower extremities
Quadruped	Trunk Proximal and intermediate upper extremities Proximal lower extremities
Sitting	Upper trunk Pelvis Proximal and intermediate upper extremities
Kneeling/half-kneeling	Trunk Pelvis Proximal and distal lower extremities (knee and ankle) Reciprocal control of lower extremities
Modified plantigrade	Trunk Upper extremities Proximal, intermediate, and distal control of lower extremities
Standing	Trunk Lower extremities

Locomotor Training Strategies

The discussion of locomotion training strategies is divided into the following sections: (1) parallel bar progression, (2) indoor overground progression, (3) outdoor overground progression, (4) locomotor training using body weight support and a motorized treadmill, (5) overground training using body weight support, and (6) locomotor training with assistive devices.

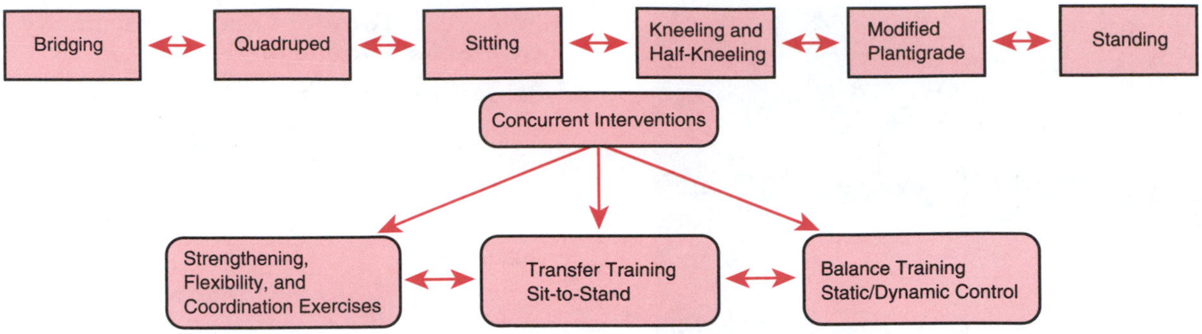

Figure 14.6 Overview of preparatory activities and concurrent interventions for locomotor training.

The following section addresses the parallel bar progression. Parallel bars have a time-honored tradition in conventional locomotor training. They provide a reasonably safe and stable environment to become acclimated to upright standing; and allow early walking practice on a relatively normal indoor floor surface for short distances. They also permit the UEs to assist in maintaining an erect posture, static/dynamic balance control, and to partially or fully unweight a LE. As a high level of stability is provided by UE support, there is less demand imposed for balance control and the highly coordinated movements required of normal locomotor rhythm. Prolonged parallel bar training promotes compensatory practice and learning of skills that often transfer poorly to independent overground walking and use of an assistive device. Owing to the increased weight borne by the UEs, a forward head and trunk posture (limiting hip extension ROM and loading) is imposed and practiced. Locomotor speed, symmetry, and rhythm (timing) are typically diminished and appropriate dynamic balance mechanisms cannot be effectively promoted. In addition, the amount of body weight relief cannot be easily monitored.

In recent years, the availability of partial body weight support (BWS) training devices has diminished the routine use of parallel bars in many facilities. BWS training can be used in conjunction with treadmill training (TT) or used on overground surfaces and involves the patient donning a harness attached to a frame that supports him or her in an upright vertical posture. Treadmill training using BWS is addressed later in this chapter.

Parallel Bar Progression

Prior to standing, two important preliminary activities include fitting the patient with a guarding belt and adjusting the parallel bars. The initial adjustment of the parallel bars is an estimate based on the patient's height. Ideally the bars should be adjusted to allow 20 to 30° of elbow flexion and come to about the level of the greater trochanter. Considering individual variations in body proportions and arm length, the elbow measurement is usually most accurate. Once the patient is standing, the height of the bars can be checked. If adjustments are required, the patient should be returned to a sitting position.

Prior to beginning locomotor training in the parallel bars, wheelchair positioning and use of a guarding belt are important considerations. The patient's wheelchair should be positioned at the end of the parallel bars. The brakes should be locked, the footrests placed in an upright position, and the patient's feet on the floor well under the seating surface (COM over the BOS). The guarding belt should be fastened securely around the patient's waist. Guarding belts provide several critical functions. They increase the therapist's effectiveness in controlling or preventing potential loss of balance; they improve patient safety; they facilitate the therapist's use of proper body mechanics in untoward circumstances; and finally, they are an important consideration regarding issues of liability. The safety implications of the guarding belt should be explained to the patient carefully.

Locomotor training in the parallel bars is initiated with patient instruction and demonstration. First, the entire progression should be presented before breaking it into sequential component parts. This will include instruction and demonstration in how to assume a standing position in the parallel bars, guarding techniques to be used by the therapist, the components of initial standing balance activities, gait pattern to be used, how to turn in the parallel bars, and how to return to a sitting position. Demonstrating these activities by assuming the role of the patient during verbal explanations will facilitate learning. Each component of the parallel bar progression should then be reviewed prior to the patient's actual performance of the activity. A sequence of activities for use in the parallel bars follows.

Assuming the Standing Position

To prepare for standing, the patient should be instructed to move forward in the chair. The therapist is positioned directly in front of the patient. A method of guarding should be selected that does not interfere with the patient's use of the UEs while moving to standing. Having moved forward in the chair with the supporting foot or feet on the floor well under the seating surface, the patient should be instructed to come to a standing position by leaning or rocking forward and pushing down on the armrests of the wheelchair with verbal cueing from the therapist ("rock your shoulders forward, continue rocking, push down on the armrests, and come to standing"). The patient should not be allowed to stand by pulling up on the parallel bars as this approach has little functional carry-over. As the patient nears an erect posture, the hands should be released from the armrests one at a time and placed on the parallel bars. The patient's COM should be guided over the BOS to promote a stable standing posture.

Training Activities

During initial parallel bar activities, the therapist usually stands inside the bars facing the patient or outside the bars on the patient's weaker side. In guarding the patient from inside the bars, one hand should grasp the guarding belt anteriorly, and the opposite hand should be in front of, but not touching, the patient's shoulder. From outside the bars one hand should grasp the belt posteriorly with the opposite hand in front of, but not touching, the patient's shoulder. This method of guarding provides effective hand placement for an immediate response should the patient lose his or her balance. It also eliminates the patient's feeling of being "held back" or "pushed forward," which may occur with manual contacts at the shoulders. The following initial activities in the parallel bars can be modified relative to the patient's weightbearing status and the specific requirements (e.g., use of a prosthesis or orthosis). Guarding techniques are maintained by the therapist during these activities.

1. Standing, holding, acclimation to upright position; feet in symmetrical stance position, equal weight on both LEs; hands supported on parallel bars.
2. LOS training (weight shifts; alteration in hand placement on parallel bars).
   a. Lateral weight shift from side-to-side without altering the BOS; hand placement on the parallel bars is not altered.
   b. Anterior–posterior weight shifting forward and backward without altering the BOS; hand placement on the parallel bars is not altered.
   c. Anterior–posterior hand placement and weight shift; patient moves hands forward on bars and shifts weight anteriorly; alternated with posterior hand placement, and weight is shifted backward.
   d. Single-hand support; patient balances with support from only one hand on the parallel bars; hands are alternated. A progression of this activity involves gradual changes in position of the freed hand and UE. For example, moving the freed hand several inches above the bar and gradually progress to alternate positions such as shoulder flexion, abduction, crossing the midline, and so forth. A progression can be made to balancing with both hands freed from the bars.
3. Stepping forward and backward. Patient steps forward with one LE, anterior weight shift, and then returns foot to starting position (normal BOS); alternated with stepping backward with one LE, posterior weight shift, with return of foot to starting position. Light tracking resistance can be applied with MCs at the pelvis to promote rotation.
4. Side-stepping and cross-stepping. Patient turns 90° from a forward-facing position and places both hands on one parallel bar; weight shifted over support limb and dynamic limb side-steps. Progression made to cross-stepping; weight shifted over support limb and dynamic limb alternately placed anteriorly and posteriorly across or behind the stance limb.
5. Forward progression. Ambulation in the parallel bars using selected gait pattern and appropriate weightbearing (e.g., partial, full).

CLINICAL NOTE: The patient should be instructed to push down rather than to pull on the parallel bars while ambulating, inasmuch as this is the motion that eventually will be required with an assistive device. This will be easier if the patient is instructed to use a loose or open grip on the bars rather than a tight grip; the loose or open grip facilitates correct use of the parallel bars and, ultimately, the assistive device.

6. Turning. Once the desired distance in the parallel bars has been reached, the patient should be instructed to turn toward the stronger side. For example, with a non-weightbearing left LE, the turn should be toward the right. The patient should be instructed to turn by stepping in a small circle and not to pivot on a single extremity. This technique will carry over to ambulation outside the bars, when pivoting will always be discouraged because of the potential loss of balance by movement on a small BOS. Guarding can be accomplished two ways. The therapist can remain in front of the patient, maintain the same hand positions, and turn with the patient. This will keep the therapist positioned in front of the patient. A second method is not to turn with the patient but, rather, to guard from behind on the return trip. In this method hand placements will change during the turn. Hand placement is changed gradually by first placing both hands on the guarding belt as the patient initiates the turn. One hand then remains on the posterior aspect of the belt and the freed hand is placed anterior to, but not touching, the shoulder on the patient's weaker side for the return trip toward the chair. Although both techniques are acceptable, the latter is probably more practical, considering the limited space available in the parallel bars.
7. Return to seated position. When reaching the chair the patient should again turn as described above. Once completely turned, patients are typically instructed to continue backing up until they feel the seat of the chair on the back of their legs (this will require substitution with visual or auditory clues for patients with impaired sensation). At this point the patient releases the stronger hand from the parallel bar and reaches back for the wheelchair armrest.

Once this hand has securely grasped the armrest, the patient should be instructed to bend forward slightly, release the opposite hand from the parallel bar and place it on the other armrest. Keeping the head and trunk forward, the patient gently returns to a seated position.

Indoor Overground Progression

The sequence of activities in the standing indoor overground progression typically includes walking forward and backward, resisted progression, side-stepping and cross-stepping, and stair climbing. MCs are used to guide and assist control of pelvic movement. Verbal cueing is used to promote normal timing and locomotor rhythm. UE support may initially be required (e.g., hands on therapist's shoulders). MCs, verbal cueing, and UE support are progressively decreased and then eliminated.

1. Walking forward and backward. This activity can begin with standing, stepping in place with emphasis on diagonal weight shifts forward and backward onto stance limb; and pelvic rotation in combination with advancing the swing limb. During forward progression, MCs at the pelvis can be used to guide movements and facilitate missing components. During backward progression, MCs can be placed posteriorly over the gluteal region to promote hip extension as weight is accepted onto the stance limb. This activity combines hip extension with knee flexion and is particularly useful for patients with hemiplegia with synergy influence in the LEs.
2. Resisted progression. Walking forward and backward is initiated actively and progressed to application of resistance through MCs at the pelvis. During forward progression, the therapist may be standing or sitting on a rolling stool with bilateral MCs on the pelvis. Light tracking resistance is used initially to promote timing of pelvic movements. Approximation can be used to enhance stability of the stance limb and light phasic stretch can be used to facilitate pelvic rotation on the swing limb. Resistance can also be applied using Theraband® around the pelvis and held from behind by the therapist. Wands held simultaneously by the patient and therapist can be used to promote reciprocal UE movements and provide the patient some stability.
3. Side-stepping and cross-stepping. Side-stepping involves abduction of the leading dynamic limb with foot placement followed by movement of the remaining limb to a parallel position with the first (symmetrical stance). Emphasis should be placed on keeping the pelvis level. Cross-stepping involves side-stepping and then crossing the remaining limb up and over the other limb. Movements can be guided and facilitated with MCs at the pelvis. A progression can then be made to application of resistance (resisted progression) with MCs at the pelvis and thigh.
4. Braiding. This activity involves a crossed and side-step progression with one limb advancing alternately anteriorly and posteriorly across the other while the second limb sidesteps. It incorporates lower trunk rotation as well as crossing the midline. This is a challenging activity and may require support from the therapist standing in front of the patient (forearms supinated, patient's hands lightly touching therapist's hands) or by use of a modified plantigrade position with UEs lightly supported on treatment table. A resisted progression may be incorporated with MCs on the lateral pelvis for sideward movement, the anterior pelvis during forward limb crossing, and the posterior pelvis during backward limb crossing.
5. Step-ups. To practice stepping up, a portable step can be placed directly in front of the patient. The patient weight shifts laterally toward the support limb and places the dynamic limb on the step. The limb is then returned to the original stance position. Verbal cues and manual guidance is provided as needed. The height of the step can be varied to increase or decrease the difficulty of the activity. For example, a 4-in. (10 cm) step can be used initially with a gradual progression to a standard 7-in. (17.5-cm) step. A progression is made to a step-over-step pattern on stairs. Early activities will require support from a railing. An erect trunk posture should be maintained and "pulling" on the railing should be avoided.

Additional indoor overground practice activities may be included:

- Walking with head turns on verbal command such as *look right, look left, look up,* or *look down*
- Increasing speed and rhythm of gait by using pacing cues to vary speed such as *walk slow* and *walk fast*
- Use of a metronome or marching music to increase speed and improve rhythm
- Progress to longer distances with decreased number of rest intervals to improve duration of walking
- Practice dual-task walking (e.g., walk and talk; walk and catch/throw a ball)
- Practice walking on varied indoor surfaces such as tile, wood flooring, and carpeting

Box 14.2 presents strategies for varying task demands during locomotor training. It provides practice activities for enhancing specific (missing) components of gait that can be incorporated into the indoor overground progression.

Outdoor Overground Progression

Activities on outdoor surfaces are among the final components of locomotor training. They must be specifically examined to determine their appropriateness for an individual patient.

1. Curbs. A useful lead-up activity to curb climbing is provided by a series of interlocking portable steps arranged in increments of height. For additional security they can be placed next to a treatment table, wall or other support

Box 14.2 Strategies for Varying Task Demands During Locomotor Training

Upright Postural Alignment
- Practice walking upright.
- Long poles can be used to increase upright alignment and reduce forward head and trunk lean (common with use of an assistive device such as a walker).

Foot Placement/Toe Clearance
- Practice heel-toe floor contact; tactile cues can be provided to dorsal foot by tapping over pretibial muscles.
- Practice high step marching in place (high steppage).
- Practice foot placement during walking using foot markers on floor or floor grid for promoting even steps, or increasing step length or step width.
- Practice walking with altered base of support (BOS); progressing from wide (8 to 12 in. apart) to narrow (2 in. apart) to tandem (heel-to-toe).
- Practice walking on a 3-in. wide line taped to floor; half-foam roller.

Single and Double Limb Support
- Practice controlled lateral and diagonal weight shifts.
- Combine diagonal weight shifts with pelvic rotation movements and stepping forward and backward.

Forward Progression and Push-Off
- Practice push-ups (toe rises) in stance; progress to toe-walking.
- Practice heel-rises in stance; progress to heel-walking.
- Practice forceful push-off on command during walking.
- Practice walking against resistance using resisted progression; walking against Theraband® positioned around pelvis.

Trunk Counterrotation and Arm Swing
- Practice walking with exaggerated arm swings.
- Practice walking with long poles; therapist is behind and holds one end of poles; patient is in front and holds other end of poles.

Stepping
- Practice stepping onto and off varied surfaces (e.g., foam pad, half foam roller, Dyna Disc®).

Stopping and Starting
- Practice abrupt stops and starts on command.
- Practice turns on command progressing from a quarter turn to half turn to full turn.
- Practice forward, backward, sidewards, and crossed steps.
- Practice step-ups and step-downs forward and sideways; vary step height, progressing from low (4-in.) to high (8-in.).

surface. A progression can be made from a 3- or 4-in. (7.62-cm or 10.16-cm) increment to a 7-in. (17.78-cm) curb height.

2. Ramps and slopes. Ramps and other slopping surfaces can be negotiated in several ways. If the incline is very gradual, it may be sufficient simply to instruct the patient to use smaller steps. For steeper inclines the patient should be instructed to use smaller steps and to traverse the ramp (use a diagonal, zigzag pattern) for both ascending and descending. Practice should include inclines of varying height. Walking up an inclined surface is associated with decreased speed, cadence, and step length.
3. Terrain variations. Outdoor walking presents a variety of terrains that require adaptation of locomotor skills. Practice should include uneven surfaces such as sidewalks, grassy surfaces, parking lots, and so forth.
4. Timing requirements. Several outdoor walking settings impose precise time restrictions (coincident timing) on movement. Walking should be practiced within these time constraints and can include crossing at a stoplight, stepping on and off a moving walkway, walking onto an elevator, and walking through a revolving door.
5. Open environment. Walking should be practiced in a variable open community environment such as a shopping mall, community center, grocery store, or other patient-specific location. As learning is task and environment specific, walking should be practiced in all environments normally used by the patient.

Additional outdoor overground practice activities include:

- Exit and entrance through outside doors and thresholds
- Outdoor stair climbing (e.g., cement stairs)
- Entering and exiting public or private transportation
- Variations in visual conditions (e.g., full to reduced lighting)

Locomotor Training Using Body Weight Support and a Motorized Treadmill

Considerable recent attention has been focused on the impact of partially supporting body weight during locomotor training.[3–27] Locomotor training using BWS and a motorized treadmill (TM) involves having the patient don a trunk harness with adjustable straps that attach to an overhead suspension system. The harness and its attachments support the desired amount of weight required for the individual patient. The wheeled base with locking casters is positioned over a treadmill (Fig. 14.7). The lift function brings the patient to upright standing (Fig. 14.8) and the straps allow adjustment to promote a symmetrical standing posture. The system can also accommodate limited weightbearing requirements on a single LE (e.g., partial weightbearing).

The concept of body weight support (BWS) locomotor training in humans was first introduced by Finch and Barbeau.[16] The rationale for its use is supported by animal studies of cats with thoracic spinal cord lesions that regained hind limb stepping patterns when supported by a harness over a moving treadmill.[28–30] These findings suggest the spinal cord is capable of reciprocal locomotor patterns produced by

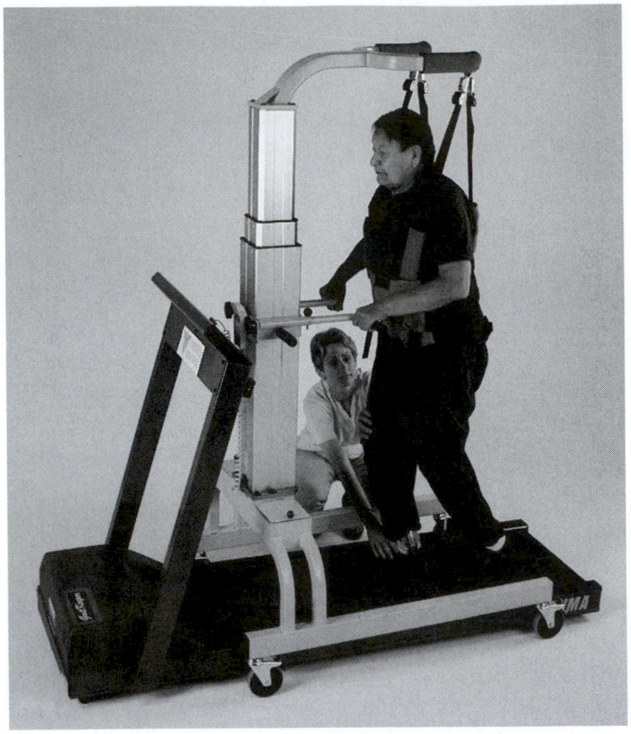

Figure 14.7 Locomotor training using partial body weight support and a motorized treadmill provides a safe patient environment, promotes an upright posture, and allows the therapist to manually guide limb movements. (Courtesy of Mobility Research, Tempe, AZ 85281.)

central pattern generators (CPGs) at the spinal cord level in the absence of supraspinal input.[15] CPGs are also influenced by sensory input allowing motor output modification based on environmental demands.[10]

A key element of locomotor training using BWS and a TM is facilitation of automatic walking movements within the context of intensive, task-specific training (whole-task practice). With body weight supported, the TM speed provides a rhythmic input. Manually guided movements are used to enhance the rhythmicity of the gait pattern. This continues until the patient is able to participate in generating the reciprocal stepping patterns before a progression is introduced.[14] Thus, training can occur well before development of the prerequisite skills required of more traditional gait training strategies.

Conventional gait training approaches are often delayed by the time required to practice component elements such as balance, weight-shifting, coordination, or sit-to-stand transitions (parts-to-whole practice). Early use of parallel bars and assistive devices can promote compensatory patterns (e.g., forward displacement of upper body, compensatory asymmetry, dependence on UE support to substitute for impaired LE function) that are undesirable and difficult to change as intervention progresses.[3] In addition, these activities can place such overwhelming demands on the patient and therapist to ensure adequate static/dynamic balance control that only limited locomotor training can actually occur (preventing optimum use of treatment time for skilled intervention by the therapist).[3]

Sufficient evidence has accumulated to suggest that locomotor training using BWS and a TM may become a mainstay intervention for some patient groups. The efficacy has largely been examined with patients having neurological involvement, most notably patients with stroke and spinal cord injury (SCI). Many of these studies compare more conventional gait training approaches to locomotor training strategies using BWS and a TM; improvements are typically noted in the later group, although this is not exclusively the case (Evidence Summary Box 14.3). For patients with stroke, increased stance time has been documented[7] as well as improvements in gait symmetry[17]

(text continues on page 540)

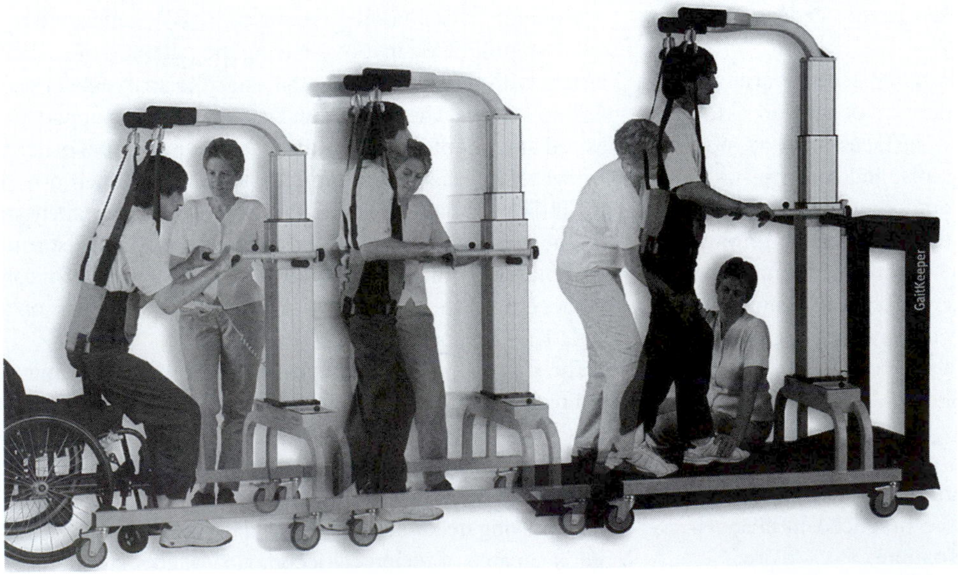

Figure 14.8 Body weight support system lifting a patient to upright in preparation for locomotor training. (Courtesy of Mobility Research, Tempe, AZ 85281.)

Evidence Summary Box 14.3
Locomotor Training

Reference	Purpose	Subjects/ Design	Results	Conclusions/ Comments
Brown, TH, et al[3] 2005	To determine whether locomotor training using body weight support and a motorized treadmill (BWSTT) is more effective than conventional over-ground gait training (COGT) in the chronic traumatic brain injury (TBI) population.	Randomized control trial. Twenty participants (14 men, 6 women) in post-acute phase of rehabilitation for TBI, randomly placed in 2 groups (BWSTT or COGT). Pre-testing/post-testing consisted of the TUG test, the FAC, the FR, and collection of gait parameters. All subjects walked a total of 15 minutes during a 30-minute session, resting when needed and received 30 minutes of therapeutic exercise. COGT group: walking on level surfaces with assistance/device deemed appropriate. BWSTT: treadmill walking with 30% unweighting, decreasing by 10% when subjects were able to achieve 10 consecutive heel strikes. Speed was increased as tolerated.	Both groups significantly narrowed step width. BWSTT group showed an increase in step length asymmetry, while COGT group showed a decrease. No significant improvement in FR, FAC, or TUG test for either group, nor was there a difference between groups. While these results were not statistically significant, the results showed a trend toward improvement.	Since these subjects sustained their injuries between 7 and 23 years prior, improvement could be attributed to the treatment provided during the study. Significant decrease in step width can be seen as an improvement in balance. These results do not support the hypothesis that BWSTT would lead to greater improvements in gait than COGT. Two limiting factors: not a long enough time frame, trunk control was not practiced while trying to maintain maximal comfortable speed.
Field-Fote, EC[4] 2001	To examine the effect of an intervention combining body weight support (BWS), functional electrical stimulation (FES), and treadmill training, on overground walking speed (OGWS), treadmill walking speed (TWS), distance, and lower extremity motor scores (LEMS) in patients with chronic incomplete SCI.	Pre-test/post-test comparison. 19 subjects (13 men, 6 women, mean age 31.7). All subjects had ASIA class C injuries. Test measures included: OGWS without BWS or FES (2-minute timed walk on an 80-ft oblong track) with needed devices at their chosen comfortable pace, treadmill walking with BWS (up to 30%) and FES for optimal gait, and strength examination in the LE using the LEMS. Intervention included: 36-session program of BWS and FES-assisted (common peroneal nerve in the weaker limb) treadmill walking. Subjects were allotted a 1.5-hour block of time and choose their walk/rest periods. Time and distance were recorded. No attempts were made to decrease BWS or FES.	6 subjects needed manual assistance to advance weaker leg initially, only 2 subjects post-intervention. Mean OGWS and TWS increased significantly. All but 2 subjects significantly increased their treadmill distance per session. LEMS scores significantly increased over the course of training. A moderate correlation was found between pre-training OGWS and LEMS scores. Four participants were available for follow-up at 2 months to 1 year. 3 subjects demonstrated that OGWS was as good as or better than their final evaluation. The other individual had undergone surgery, and had a prolonged period without ambulation.	All subjects had a SCI of at least 1 year's duration, thus improvements can be attributed to the training in the study. There is little evidence in this study's results to suggest that a change in OGWS correlates with a change in TWS. That LEMS scores correlate with improved function is debatable. None of the subjects approached normal values for OGWS. The lack of a control/comparison group in this study allows for the possibility that other interventions may have given the same results. Overall, this study suggests that BWS/FES treadmill training may have a positive effect on functional measures in patients with chronic incomplete SCI.

(*continued*)

Evidence Summary Box 14.3

Locomotor Training (continued)

Reference	Purpose	Subjects/ Design	Results	Conclusions/ Comments
Colby, SM, et al[5] 1999	To determine: (1) the muscular activity and cardiovascular response of a normal population during locomotor training using body weight support and a motorized treadmill (BWSTT); (2) if lower extremity (LE) muscular activity changes with BWS; and (3) if muscle activation can be preserved while decreasing loads on healing tissues, conserving energy, and reducing pain.	10 healthy recreational athletes, mean age 28.9 years. Electrodes were placed over the following muscle groups on the dominant side: vastus lateralis, vastus medialis obliquus, rectus femoris, biceps femoris, semimembrinosus and semitendinosus, and the medial gastrocnemus. Subjects walked on a treadmill at 1.34 m/s. O_2 consumption and HR were recorded during the last minute of a 5-minute exercise period. BWS was changed from 0% (FWB) to 20% to 40%.	Average EMG activity did not change significantly for any muscle groups when FWB was compared to 20% BWS ambulation. Average EMG activity decreased significantly in 40% BWS when compared to FWB in the quadriceps, but not in the hamstrings and gastrocnemius. O_2 consumption decreased significantly from FWB to 20% BWS and from FWB to 40% ambulation. HR did not change significantly for any conditions.	Findings suggest that muscle activation can be preserved while possibly decreasing load and pain at the knee. However, this does not mean the muscles around the knee are being strengthened. Overall, this study supports use of BWSTT as a method of providing functional exercise which does not compromise most muscle activity about the knee and lowers the energy cost.
Miller, EW, et al[6] 2002	To determine: (1) the feasibility and patient tolerance for using a BWS system for overground ambulation; and (2) to measure the function of patients with chronic stroke prior to and following BWSTT and BWS overground training.	Pretest posttest comparison. Two participants: one 87-year-old woman 10 years post-stroke (Participant A), one 93-year-old woman 14 years post-stroke (Participant B). Prior to and after training, participants were given the following tests: Berg Balance Scale, 10-m timed walk test, and the gait section of the Tinetti Test of Balance and Mobility. Templates of footprints were taken, step length was measured, and gait observation was noted. BWS training occurred 2–3 times per week over a 6 to 7-week period. Each session included 4 bouts of ambulation (first 3 on treadmill, the last being overground) separated by a 5-minute rest interval. Each bout was limited by patient tolerance. BWS started at 40% and progressed to 20% and 0%; treadmill speed progressed from 0.5 mph to 0.75 mph to 1.0 mph. Speed of overground training was determined by patient comfort.	Participant A – Showed improvements in Berg Balance Scale scores (26/56–40/56), Tinetti Gait and Balance Assessment, and 10-m walk speed (0.35 m/s–0.65 m/s). Her right and left step lengths improved by 35% and 41%. Gait symmetry improved as indicated by observation, however bilateral trunk sway during single-leg stance remained. Self-reports and family reports of her gait illustrated positive changes. Participant B—Minimal improvements in gait and balance were evident. The greatest improvement was a 22% increase in her 10-m walk time. Her step length for each LE improved by 35% and 25%.	While participant B showed less improvement than participant A, both showed positive signs after receiving BWS treatment. Participant B had occasional days of agitation and confusion that may have contributed to her limited improvements. Participant A displayed more motivation to improve than did Participant B. Participant B had bilateral foot deformities that may have contributed as well. For both subjects, BWS ambulation training was both feasible and well-tolerated.

Evidence Summary Box 14.3

Locomotor Training (continued)

Reference	Purpose	Subjects/ Design	Results	Conclusions/ Comments
Hesse, S, et al[7] 1999	To compare the gait of subjects with hemiplegia during locomotor training using body weight support and a motorized treadmill (BWSTT) and overground walking.	18 subjects with hemiplegia; mean age 59.9 years. Mean time since onset was 5.7 months. TM walking was done with FWB, 15%, and 30% BWS. Velocity was kept constant during all trials and was self-selected by each subject. Floor walking occurred at a self-selected velocity on a 15-m walkway at a mean velocity of .33 m/s. Gait analysis was done for all conditions. Velocity, cadence, and cycle, stance, swing and double support durations were recorded (average of 10 cycles). GRF at heel and toe off and EMG activity for anterior tibialis, medial gastrocnemius, biceps femoris, vastus lateralis, gluteus medius, and erector spinae on the affected side and for the anterior tibialis and medial gastroc on the nonaffected side were recorded.	Single-leg stance time of affected limb increased with increased BWS and was longer for TM walking than ground walking. Subjects walked more symmetrically on TM than on the floor. GRF decreased more prominantly on the affected limb with increased BWS. Mean activity levels of the gastrocnemius and vastus lateralis were less during TM walking. There was decreased clonus activity in the gastrocnemius before and after initial contact and decreased co-contraction with antagonistic muscles at the lower leg with treadmill walking. Mean velocity and cadence were significantly increased for ground walking, however stride length did not change.	Training of stance on the affected limb is considered highly relevant for restoring gait. Increasing stance time may promote balance, weightbearing, and strength in paretic limbs. Decreases in co-contraction may lead to more efficient movement patterns. BWS training should not be used in excess or for a prolonged period of time due to the significant decrease in the activation of weightbearing muscles (gastrocnemius and vastus lateralis).
Protas, EJ, et al[8] 2001	To determine if locomotor training using body weight support and a motorized treadmill (BWSTT) will improve gait (speed, endurance, walking status, assistive device use, orthotic use) and reduce the oxygen costs of walking.	Repeated measures pilot study. 3 men with chronic, incomplete, thoracic SCIs. Three scales to examine gait: (1) Garrett scale of walking; (2) assistive device usage scale; (3) orthotic device usage scale. Gait speed measured using a timed 5-m walk; endurance by the distance walked in a 5-minute period. O_2 consumption, minute ventilation, and respiratory exchange ratio were measured. Neurological and muscle testing were performed, together with bilateral EMG recordings of the quadriceps, hip abductors, tibialis anterior, triceps surae, paraspinal, and abdominal muscles. BWSTT for 1 hour/day, 5 days/week, for 12 weeks. A total of 20 minutes of walking was targeted for each session. BWS began at 40%, treadmill speed began at .16 kmph. BWS and speed gradually progressed. Overground walking was attempted after 3 weeks of training.	Walking speed, endurance, and energy expenditure improved significantly for all subjects after 12 weeks of training. All subjects improved or maintained their ambulation status and use of assistive device; however these changes were not statistically significant. Muscle strength tended to increase, but these changes also were not significant. Subjects 2 and 3 displayed a distribution of motor control in the LE that shifted toward values seen in healthy subjects.	Subjects walked faster, farther, and with more efficiency after training. The measures for assistive device usage, orthotic device usage, and muscle strength test were not sensitive enough to detect small changes. Small group size limits conclusiveness of study.

Evidence Summary Box prepared by Stephen A. Caronia.

ASIA = American Spinal Injury Association; FAC = functional ambulation category; FR = functional reach; FWB = full body weight; GRF = ground reaction force; HR = heart rate; SCI = spinal cord injury; TM = treadmill; TUG = Timed Up and Go.

speed,[17,20,31] endurance,[31] and distance[20,31] parameters. Similar findings including improvements in speed[8,18,19,21] and endurance[8,19] have been documented for patients with SCI. In patients with Parkinson's disease, Miyai et al[32] found an increase in ambulation speed and stride length following locomotor training using BWS and a TM. For further discussion on this topic as well as additional clinical trial examples, see sections on locomotor training using BWS and a TM and Evidence Summary Boxes in Chapters 18 and 23.

Evidence suggests that sensory input such as appropriately timed manually assisted limb movements can promote function-induced recovery.[15,18] Within a task-specific and safe patient environment, locomotor training using BWS and a TM allows the therapist access to hips, pelvis, and LEs to manually assist, guide, or adjust locomotor rhythm, limb placement, weight shifts, and symmetry. Movements are coordinated to simulate normal gait; upright posture and balance is maintained, and speed of walking is controlled. Kosak and Reding[10] emphasize the role of sensory input during locomotor training using BWS and a TM by stating, "Stride and cadence vary with treadmill speed, indicating local sensory feedback to a lumbosacral gait pattern-generator. The intensity and timing of sensory feedback from pressure receptors in the sole of the foot and joint proprioceptors from the ankle, knee, and hip are thought to provide facilitory and inhibitory effects on flexor-extensor motor neuron pools in the spinal cord at appropriate time during the gait cycle (p 14)."

Descriptions by Shepherd and Carr[9] and Seif-Naraghi and Herman[14] provide an apt summary of the advantages of locomotor training using BWS and a TM as follows:

- Inter- and intralimb timing can be practiced before limbs are capable of fully supporting body weight.[9]
- Gait training can be initiated earlier within an episode of care.[14]
- Specific elements of the gait cycle (e.g., midstance limb loading; swing phase unweighting and stepping) can be trained within a dynamic task-specific strategy.[14]
- Limb loading can be varied based on ability to support weight.[9]
- Gait deviations may be addressed early using greater BWS and low TM velocities.[14]
- Owing to forced stepping movements, "learned non-use" may be prevented by focusing attention on both involved and uninvolved limbs.[9]
- Opportunity to practice walking is provided without undue fear of falling.[9]
- Dynamic balance training can be enhanced by decreasing BWS and increasing TM speed.[14]
- Compensatory strategies (e.g., upper limb support) to compensate for lower limb impairment are reduced.[9]
- Peripheral sensory input is enhanced to promote muscle activation.[14]
- Constant speed of the TM provides rhythmic input that reinforces a coordinated reciprocal gait pattern.[14]
- Hip extension is facilitated.[14]

As reciprocal patterns emerge and improve, training is progressed. This is accomplished by increasing *TM speed,* and decreasing the *amount of BWS,* and *manual guidance.* For example, training may be initiated at very low speeds (e.g., 0.25 mph) with minimal or no weightbearing and constant manual guidance, and progressed until walking speeds of approximately 1.0 mph are achieved with 100% weightbearing and no manual input.[14]

Intensity of treatment is required to attain a training effect. Recommendations are between 30 and 60 minutes (divided into two or three bouts with intervening rest intervals), five times per week. However, with severe involvement, training sessions may be as short as 3 minutes with 5-minute rest intervals.[14]

Overground Locomotor Training Using Body Weight Support

The task-oriented approach to locomotor training using BWS is continued by progressing to overground walking. Unlocking the casters and moving the BWS system away from the treadmill creates a mobile, safe, and efficient environment for continuing the controlled reduction in body weight support to overground surfaces.

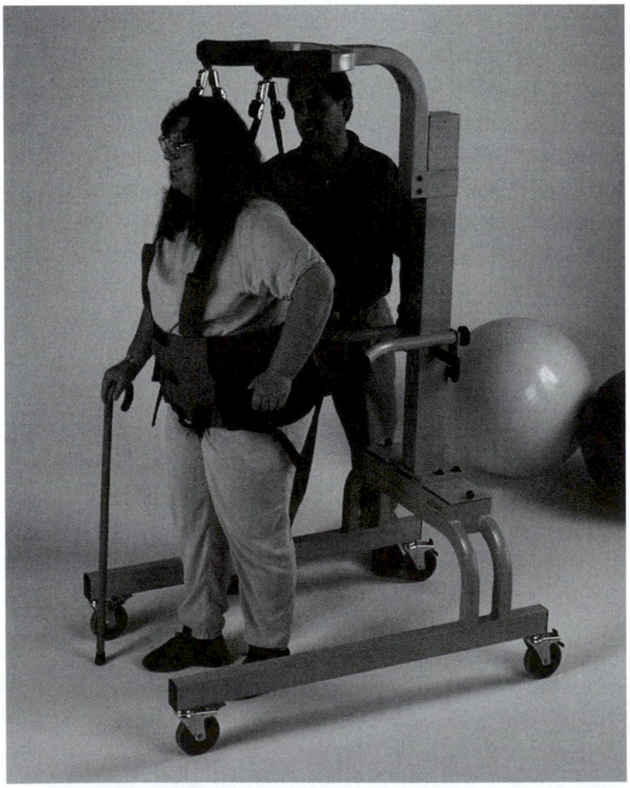

Figure 14.9 Body weight support overground locomotor training using a cane. (Courtesy of Mobility Research, Tempe, AZ 85281.)

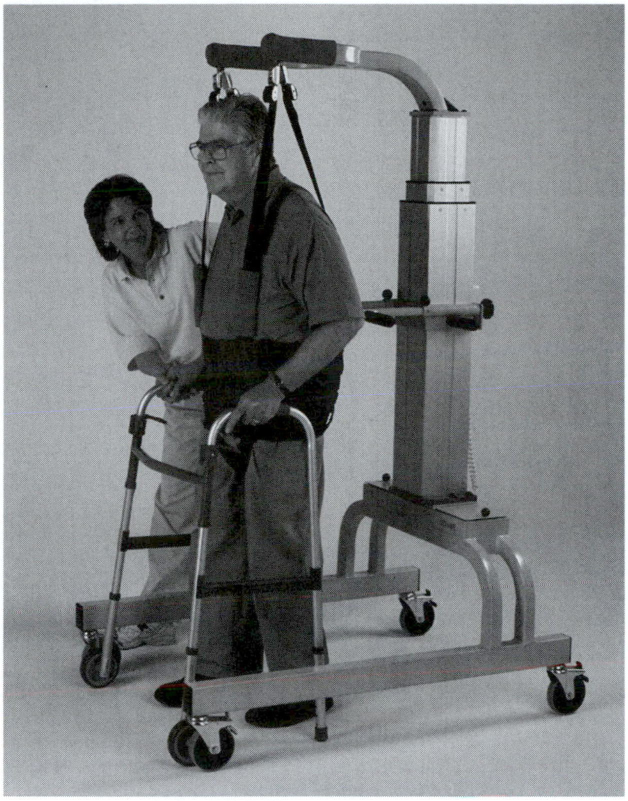

Figure 14.10 Body weight support overground locomotor training using a walker. (Courtesy of Mobility Research, Tempe, AZ 85281.)

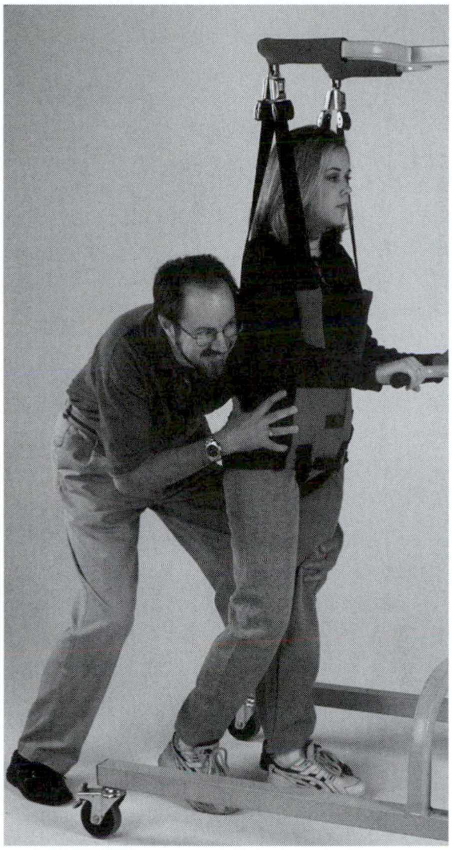

Figure 14.11 Body weight support overground locomotor training without an assistive device. Hand placements allow the patient to move and steer the unit during forward progression. (Courtesy of Mobility Research, Tempe, AZ 85281.)

During initial overground training, verbal cueing and manual guidance is continued as needed. Gait speeds will typically be slower on overground surfaces with elimination of the rhythmic steady-state input provided by the TM. Ambulatory assistive devices such as a cane (Fig. 14.9) or a walker (Fig. 14.10) can be incorporated into overground training. The BWS device is manually moved to keep pace with the patient's forward progression. For use without an assistive device, the patient can move and steer the unit with the UEs prior to progressing to an assistive device or hands-free reciprocal arm movements (Fig 14.11).

Some BWS devices are designed specifically for overground use (Fig. 14.12). These units are relatively lightweight (20 lbs), have swiveling wheels to allow turning in small areas, can fit over a wheelchair or toilet, provide adjustable support and are available in wide and heavy duty designs. They support body weight during standing and walking as well as sit-to-stand transitions. As these devices have a reasonably small turning radius of 20 in. (50.8 cm), they are suitable for the home setting for patients requiring long-term use. Disadvantages of these units are that the amount of body weight supported cannot be precisely determined and the design of the sidebars prevents unsupported reciprocal arm swing.

Assistive Devices

There are three major categories of ambulatory assistive devices: *canes, crutches,* and *walkers.* Each has several modifications to the basic design, many of which were developed to meet the needs of a specific patient problem or diagnostic group. Assistive devices are prescribed for a variety of reasons, including problems of balance, pain, fatigue, weakness, joint instability, excessive skeletal loading, and cosmesis. Another primary function of assistive devices is to eliminate weightbearing fully or partially from a LE. This unloading occurs by transmission of force from the UEs to the floor by downward pressure on the assistive device.

Canes

Most canes used in current clinical practice are constructed of lightweight aluminum. The function of a cane is to *widen the BOS* and *improve balance.*[33] Canes are not intended for use with restricted weightbearing gaits (such as non- or **partial-weightbearing**). Patients are typically instructed to hold a cane in the hand *opposite the affected extremity.* This positioning of the cane most closely approximates a normal reciprocal gait pattern

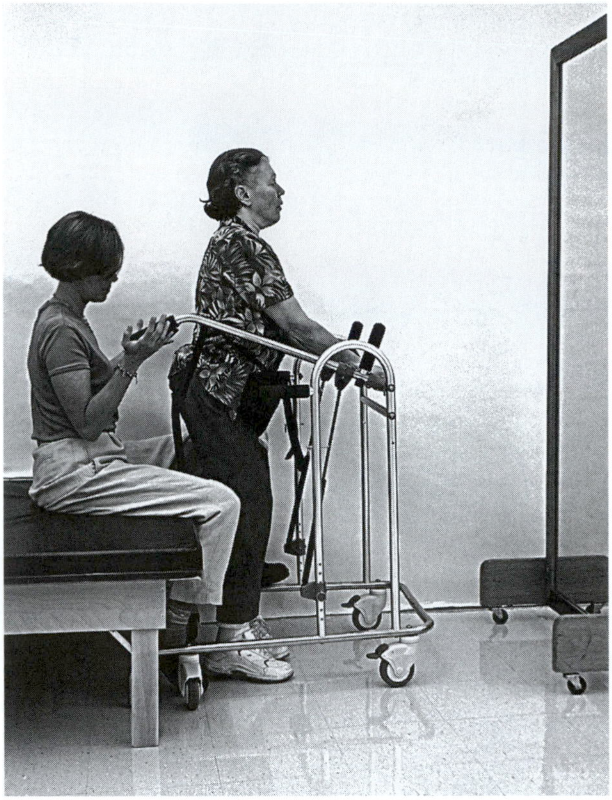

Figure 14.12 Body weight support system designed specifically for overground use. The patient depicted is practicing sit-to-stand transitions and standing using a mirror for postural alignment feedback.

with the opposite arm and leg moving together. It also widens the BOS with less lateral shifting of the COM than when the cane is held on the ipsilateral side.

Contralateral positioning of the cane is particularly important in reducing forces created by the abductor muscles acting at the hip.[34] During normal gait, the hip abductors of the stance extremity contract to counteract the gravitational moment at the pelvis on the contralateral side during swing. This prevents tilting of the pelvis on the contralateral side but results in a compressive force acting at the stance hip. Use of a cane in the UE opposite the affected hip will reduce these forces. The floor (ground) reaction force created by the downward pressure of body weight on the cane counterbalances the gravitational movement at the affected hip.[35] Thus, the need for tension in the abductor muscles is reduced, with a subsequent decrease in joint compressive forces.

Several components of floor reaction forces that create joint compression at the hip can be reduced by use of a cane. Ely and Smidt[36] found that contralateral use of a cane decreased the vertical and posterior components of the floor reaction force produced by the affected foot. They noted that the reductions in vertical floor reaction peaks were probably due to a shifting of body weight toward the cane, which was a contributing factor in reducing contact force at the affected hip. Neumann[34] found that contralateral use of a cane reduced

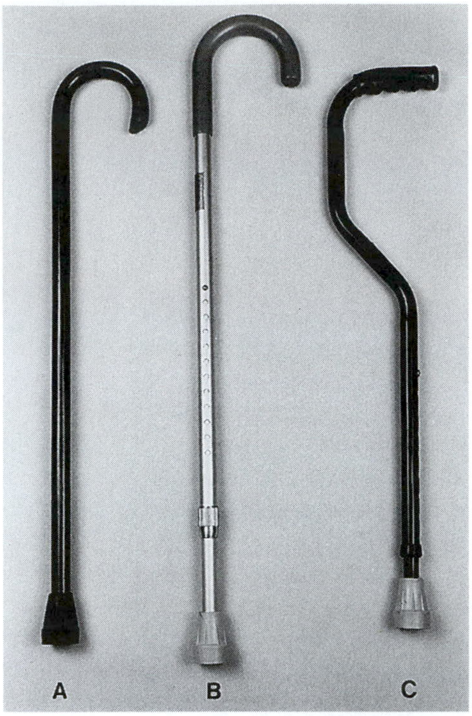

Figure 14.13 Shown here are (*A*) standard wooden cane, (*B*) standard adjustable aluminum cane, and (*C*) adjustable offset cane.

the average hip abductor muscle EMG activity to 31 percent below that generated when not using a cane.

Research suggests that use of a cane is an effective method of reducing forces acting at the hip.[34,36] This concept is particularly important for activities such as stair climbing, when the forces generated at the hip are significantly increased.[35] Clearly, use of a cane has important implications for hip involvement such as joint replacements or degenerative joint disease.

In addition to altering the forces on the affected extremity, canes are selected on the basis of their ability to improve gait by providing increased dynamic stability and improving balance. This is achieved by the increased BOS provided by the additional point(s) of floor contact. The level of stability provided by canes is on a continuum. The greatest stability is provided by the broad-based canes and the least by a standard cane. The following section presents several of the more common types of canes in clinical use and identifies their advantages and disadvantages.

Standard Cane

This assistive device also is referred to as a regular or conventional cane (Fig. 14.13A). It is made of aluminum, wood or plastic and has a half circle ("crook") handle. The distal rubber tip is at least 1 in. in diameter or larger.

Advantages. This cane is inexpensive and fits easily on stairs or other surfaces where space is limited.

Disadvantages. The standard cane is not adjustable and must be cut to fit the patient. Its point of support is anterior to the hand, not directly beneath it.

Standard Adjustable Aluminum Cane

This assistive device (Fig. 14.13B) has the same basic design as the regular or standard cane. It is made of aluminum tubing and has a half-circle handle with a molded plastic covering. The telescoping design of this cane enables the height to be adjusted using a push-button mechanism. Variations in available height range differ slightly with manufacturers. However, they are generally adjustable within the range of approximately 27 to 38.5 in. (68 to 98 cm). The distal rubber tip is at least 1 in. in diameter or larger. (*Note:* Most adjustable aluminum assistive devices use a push-button mechanism to alter height; some include a reinforcing cuff that is tightened by a thumbscrew or a rotation sleeve.)

Advantages. This cane is quickly adjustable, facilitating ease of determining appropriate height. It is lightweight and fits easily on stairs.

Disadvantages. The point of support is anterior to the hand, not directly beneath it. This cane is more costly than a standard cane.

Adjustable Aluminum Offset Cane

The proximal component of the body (shaft) of this cane is offset anteriorly creating a *straight* (or *offset*) handle. It is made of aluminum tubing with a plastic or rubber molded grip-shaped handle (Fig. 14.13C). The telescoping design allows the height to be adjusted from approximately 27 to 38.5 in. (68 to 98 cm) by a push-button mechanism. The diameter of the distal rubber tip is at least 1 in.

Advantages. The design of this cane allows pressure to be borne over the center of the cane for greater stability. This cane also is quickly adjusted, lightweight, and fits easily on stairs.

Disadvantages. This cane is more costly than standard or adjustable aluminum canes.

Quad (Quadruped or Four-Prong Cane)

This assistive device is constructed of aluminum and aluminum tubing and is available in a variety of designs depending on the manufacturer. Both large-based quad canes (LBQC) and small-based quad canes (SBQC) are commercially available (Figs. 14.14 and 14.15). The characteristic feature of these canes is that they provide a broad base with four points of floor contact. Each point (leg) is covered with a rubber tip. The legs closest to the patient's body are generally shorter and may be angled to allow foot clearance. On many designs the proximal portion of the cane is offset anteriorly. The handpiece is usually one of a variety of contoured plastic grips. A telescoping design allows for height adjustments. Quad canes are generally adjustable from approximately 28 to 38 in. (71 to 91 cm).

Advantages. This cane provides a broad-based support. Bases are available in several different sizes. This cane is also easily adjustable.

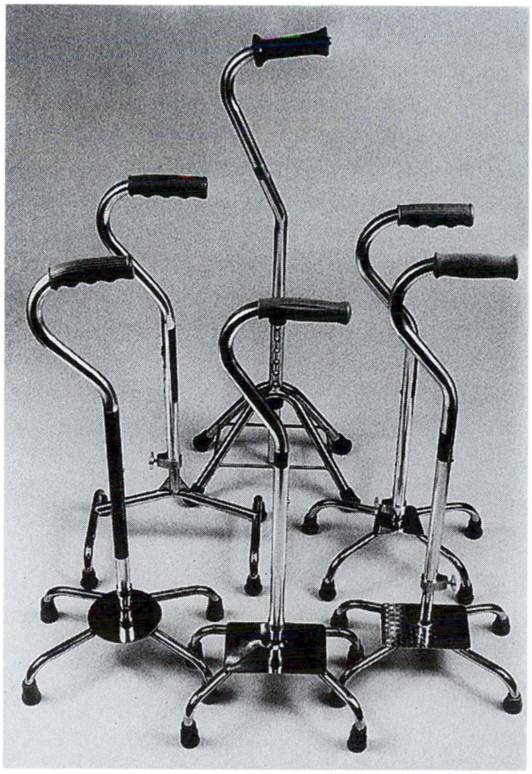

Figure 14.14 Shown here are a variety of large-based quadruped canes.

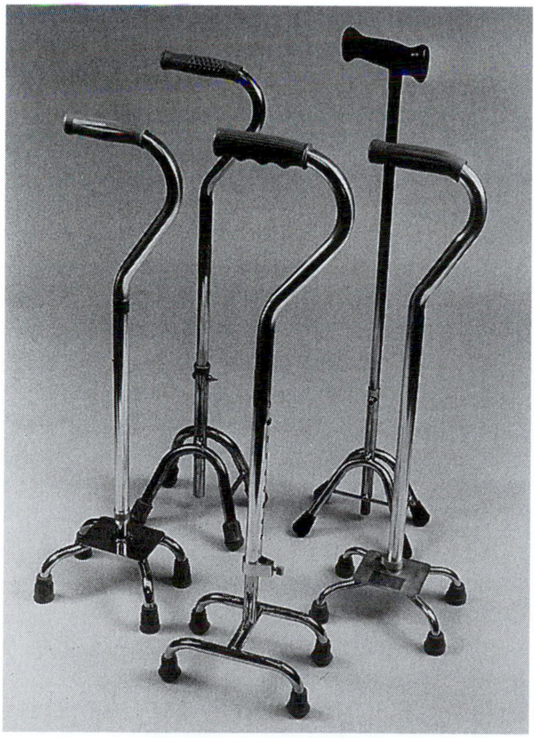

Figure 14.15 A variety of small-based quadruped canes.

Disadvantages. Depending on the specific design of the cane, the pressure exerted by the patient's hand may not be centered over the cane and may result in patient complaints of instability. As a result of the broad BOS, some quad canes may not be practical for use on stairs. Another disadvantage of broad-based canes is that they warrant use of a slower gait pattern. If a faster forward progression is used, the cane often "rocks" from rear legs to front legs, which decreases effectiveness of the cane. Patients should be instructed to place all four legs of the cane on the floor simultaneously to obtain maximum stability.

Walk Cane

The walk cane also is constructed of aluminum and aluminum tubing (Fig. 14.16). It provides a very broad base with four points of floor contact. Each point (leg) is covered with a rubber tip. The legs farther from the patient's body are angled to maintain floor contact and to improve stability. The handgrip is molded plastic around the uppermost segment of aluminum tubing. Walk canes fold flat and are adjustable in height from approximately 29 to 37 in. (73 to 94 cm).

Advantages. Walk canes provide very broad-based support and are more stable than a quad cane. These canes also fold flat for travel or storage.

Disadvantages. As with the quad canes, the specific design of a walk cane or handgrip placement may not allow pressure to be centered over the cane. Walk canes cannot be used on most stairs. They require use of a slow forward progression and are generally more costly than quad canes.

Rolling Cane

Constructed of aluminum and aluminum tubing (Fig. 14.17), this cane provides a wide wheeled base allowing uninterrupted forward progression. It includes contoured handholds, easy height adjustment from 28 to 37 in. (71 to 94 cm), and a pressure-sensitive brake built into the handle engaged using pressure from the base of the hand.

Advantages. The wheeled base allows weight to be continuously applied as the need to lift and place the cane forward is eliminated. This also provides for a faster forward progression. The second and third handles placed between the uprights can assist in rising to standing (brake engaged).

Disadvantages. This cane is more costly than standard quadruped canes, and requires sufficient UE and grip strength to engage the braking mechanism. This cane is not suitable for patients displaying a propulsive gait pattern (e.g., Parkinson's disease).

Hand Grips

A general consideration relevant to all canes is the nature of the handgrip. There are a variety of styles and sizes

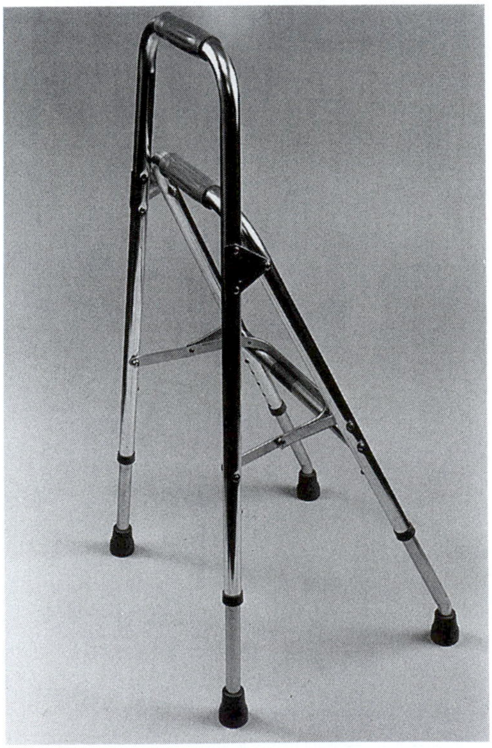

Figure 14.16 Walk cane.

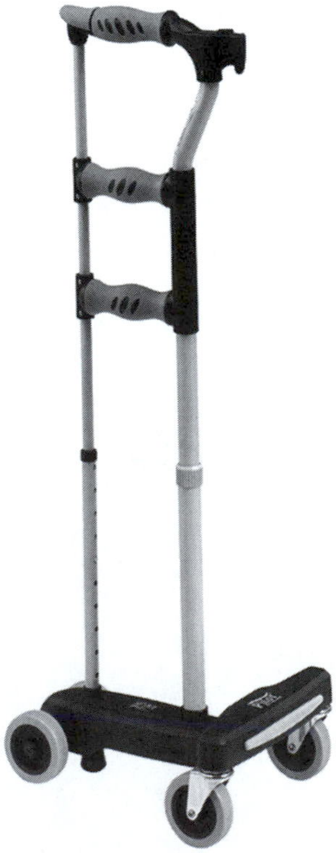

Figure 14.17 Rolling cane. (Courtesy of Full Life Products, LLC, Moorestown, NJ 08057.)

available. The type of handgrip should be judged and selected primarily on the basis of patient comfort and on the grip's ability to provide adequate surface area to allow effective transfer of weight from the UE to the floor. The more common types of handgrips are (1) the *crook* handle, (2) the *straight* (or *offset*) handle, (3) the *shovel* handle, and (4) the *pistol* handle, which conforms to the patient's hand. It is useful to have several handgrip styles available for examination and trial with individual patients.

Measuring Canes

In measuring cane height, the cane (or center of a broad-based cane) is placed approximately 6 in. from the lateral border of the toes. Two landmarks typically are used during measurement: the *greater trochanter* and the *angle at the elbow.* The top of the cane should come to approximately the level of the greater trochanter, and the elbow should be flexed to about 20 to 30°. Because of individual variations in body proportion and limb lengths, the degree of flexion at the elbow is generally considered the more important indicator of correct cane height.

This elbow flexion serves two important functions. It allows the arm to shorten or to lengthen during different phases of gait, and it provides a shock-absorption mechanism. Finally, as with all assistive devices, the height of the cane should be considered with regard to patient comfort and the cane's effectiveness in accomplishing its intended purpose.

Gait Pattern for Use of Canes

As discussed, the cane should be held in the UE opposite the affected limb. For ambulation on level surfaces, the cane and the involved extremity are advanced simultaneously (Fig. 14.18). The cane should remain relatively close to the body and should not be placed ahead of the toe of the involved extremity. These are important considerations, because placing the cane too far forward or to the side will cause lateral and/or forward bending, with a resultant decrease in dynamic stability.

When bilateral involvement exists, a decision must be made as to which side of the body the cane will be held. This question is most effectively resolved by a problem-solving approach with input from both the patient and therapist. Questions to be considered include:

1. On which side is the cane most comfortable?
2. Is one placement superior in terms of improving balance and/or ambulatory endurance?
3. If gait deviations exist, is one position more effective in improving the overall gait pattern?
4. Is safety influenced by cane placement (e.g., during transfers, stair climbing, or ambulation on outdoor surfaces)?
5. Is there a difference in grip strength between hands?
6. Are two canes needed for stability?

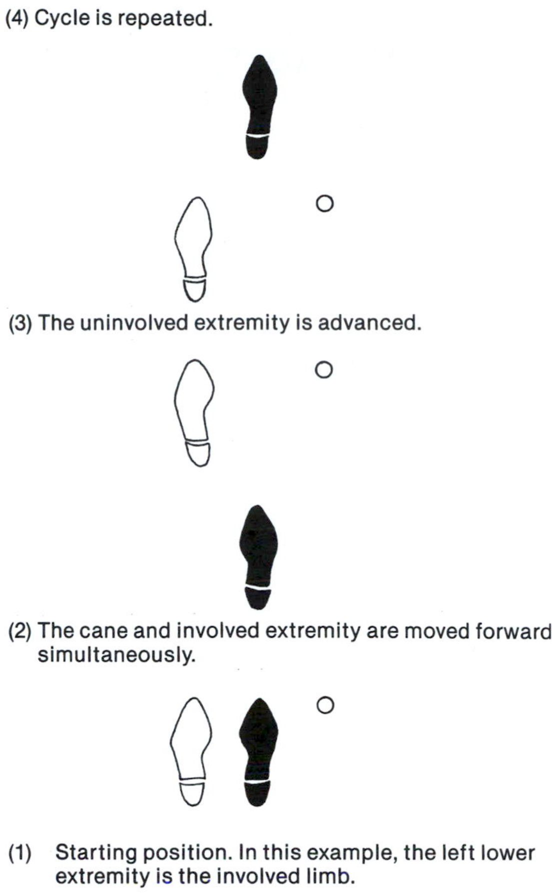

(4) Cycle is repeated.
(3) The uninvolved extremity is advanced.
(2) The cane and involved extremity are moved forward simultaneously.
(1) Starting position. In this example, the left lower extremity is the involved limb.

Figure 14.18 Gait pattern for use of cane.

Consideration of these questions will generally provide sufficient information to determine the most effective cane placement and use when bilateral involvement exists.

Crutches

Crutches are used most frequently to improve balance and to either relieve weightbearing fully or partially on a LE. They are typically used bilaterally, and function to increase the BOS, to improve lateral stability, and to allow the UEs to transfer body weight to the floor. This transfer of weight through the UEs permits functional ambulation while maintaining a restricted weightbearing status. There are two basic designs of crutches in frequent clinical use: *axillary* and *forearm* crutches.

Axillary Crutches

These assistive devices also are referred to as regular or standard crutches (Fig. 14.19A). They are made of lightweight wood or aluminum. Their design includes an axillary bar, a handpiece, and double uprights joined distally by a single leg covered with a rubber suction tip (which should have a diameter of 1.5 to 3 in.). The single leg allows for height variations. Height adjustments for wooden crutches are accomplished by altering the placement of screws and wing bolts in predrilled holes. The design of most aluminum crutches

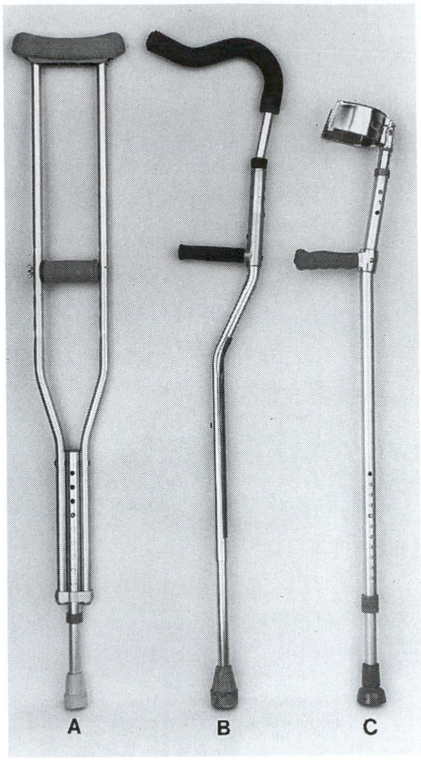

Figure 14.19 (*A*) Axillary crutch, (*B*) ortho crutch, and a (*C*) forearm crutch.

incorporates a push-button pin mechanism for height adjustments similar to those found on aluminum canes. Some aluminum crutches also have patient height markers adjacent to the notches to assist in adjustment. The height of the handgrips for wooden and some aluminum crutches is adjusted by placement of screws and wing bolts in predrilled holes. The handgrip height on some aluminum crutches is adjusted using a push-button mechanism with a reinforcing clip-lock (Fig. 14.20). Both the overall height of the crutch as well as the height of the handgrip typically adjust in 1-in. increments. Axillary crutches are generally adjustable in adult sizes from approximately 48 to 60 in. (122 to 153 cm), with children's and extra-long sizes available.

A modification to this basic design is the ortho crutch (Fig. 14.19B). This type of axillary crutch is made of aluminum. Its design includes a single upright, an axillary bar covered with sponge-rubber padding, and a handgrip covered with molded plastic. The crutch adjusts both proximally (to alter elbow angle) and distally (to alter height of crutch). Adjustments are made using a push-button mechanism. The distal end of the crutch is covered with a rubber suction tip.

Advantages. Axillary crutches improve balance and lateral stability, and provide for functional ambulation with restricted weightbearing. They are easily adjusted, inexpensive when made of wood, and can be used for stair climbing.

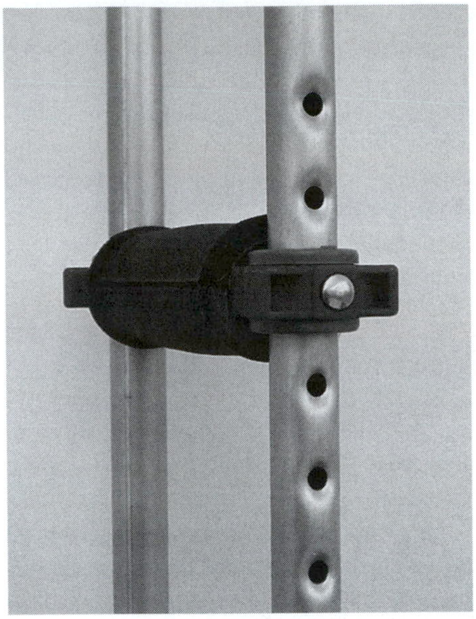

Figure 14.20 Push-button handgrip adjustment with reinforcing clip-lock.

Disadvantages. Because of the tripod stance required to use crutches and the resultant large BOS, crutches are awkward in small areas. For the same reason, the safety of the user may be compromised when ambulating in crowded areas. Another disadvantage is the tendency of some patients to lean on the axillary bar. This causes pressure at the radial groove (spiral groove) of the humerus, creating a situation of potential damage to the radial nerve as well as to adjacent vascular structures in the axilla.

Platform Attachments

These attachments (Fig. 14.21) are also referred to as *forearm rests* or *troughs*. Although they are described here, they also are used with walkers. Their function is to allow transfer of body weight through the forearm to the assistive device. A platform attachment is used when weightbearing is contraindicated through the wrist and hand (e.g., arthritis, Colles fracture). The forearm piece is usually padded, has a dowel or handgrip, and has Velcro® straps to maintain the position of the forearm. Platform crutches are also commercially available.

Forearm Crutches

These assistive devices are also known as *Lofstrand* and *Canadian* crutches (Fig. 14.19C). They are constructed of aluminum. Their design includes a single upright, a forearm cuff, and a handgrip. This crutch adjusts both proximally to alter position of the forearm cuff and distally to alter the height of the crutch. Adjustments are made using a push-button mechanism. The available heights of forearm crutches are indicated from handgrip to floor and are generally adjustable in adult sizes from 29 to 35 in. (74 to 89 cm), with children's and extra-long sizes available. The

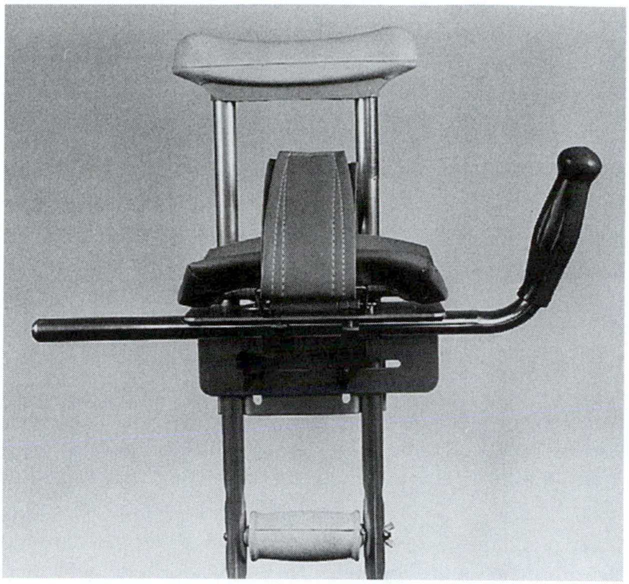

Figure 14.21 Platform attachment to axillary crutch.

distal end of the crutch is covered with a rubber suction tip. The forearm cuffs are available with either a medial or anterior opening. The cuffs are made of metal and can be obtained with a plastic coating.

Advantages. The forearm cuff allows use of hands without the crutches becoming disengaged. They are easily adjusted and allow functional stair climbing activities. Many patients feel they are more cosmetic and they fit more easily into an automobile owing to the overall decreased height. They are also the most functional type of crutch for stair climbing activities for individuals wearing bilateral knee-ankle-foot orthoses (KAFOs).

Disadvantages. Forearm crutches provide less lateral support owing to the absence of an axillary bar. The cuffs may be difficult to remove.

Measuring Crutches

Axillary Crutches

Several methods are available for measuring axillary crutches. The most common use a standing or a supine position. Measurement from standing is most accurate and is the preferred approach.

Standing. From a supported standing position, crutches should be measured from a point approximately 2 in. below the axilla. The width of two fingers is often used to approximate this distance. During measurement, the distal end of the crutch should be resting at a point 2 in. lateral and 6 in. anterior to the foot. A general estimate of crutch height can be obtained prior to standing by subtracting 16 in. from the patient's height. With the shoulders relaxed, the handpiece should be adjusted to provide 20 to 30° of elbow flexion.

Supine. From this position the measurement is taken from the anterior axillary fold to a surface point (mat or treatment table) 6 to 8 in. (5 to 7.5 cm) from the lateral border of the heel.

Forearm Crutches

Standing is the position of choice for measuring forearm crutches. From a supported standing position, the distal end of the crutch should be positioned at a point 2 in. lateral and 6 in. anterior to the foot. With the shoulders relaxed the height should then be adjusted to provide 20 to 30° of elbow flexion. The forearm cuff is adjusted separately. Cuff placement should be on the proximal third of the forearm, approximately 1 to 1.5 in. (2.5 to 3.8 cm) below the elbow.

Gait Patterns for Use of Crutches

Gait patterns are selected on the basis of the patient's balance, coordination, muscle function, and weightbearing status. The gait patterns differ significantly in their energy requirements, BOS, and the speed with which they can be executed.

Prior to initiating instruction in gait patterns, several important points should be emphasized to the patient:

1. During axillary crutch use, body weight should always be borne on the hands and not on the axillary bar. This will prevent pressure on both the vascular and nervous structures located in the axillary region.
2. Balance will be optimal by always maintaining a wide (tripod) BOS. Even when in a resting stance, the patient should be instructed to keep the crutches at least 4 in. (10 cm) to the front and to the side of each foot. The foot should not be allowed to achieve parallel alignment with the crutches. This will jeopardize anterior–posterior stability by decreasing the BOS.
3. When using standard crutches, the axillary bars should be held close to the chest wall to provide improved lateral stability.
4. The patient should also be cautioned about the importance of holding the head up and maintaining good postural alignment during ambulation.
5. Turning should be accomplished by stepping in a small circle rather than pivoting.

Three-Point Gait

In this type of gait three points of support contact the floor. It is used when a non-weightbearing status is required on one LE. Body weight is borne on the crutches instead of on the affected LE. The sequence of this gait pattern is illustrated in Figure 14.22.

Partial Weightbearing Gait

This gait is a modification of the three-point pattern. During forward progression of the involved extremity, weight is

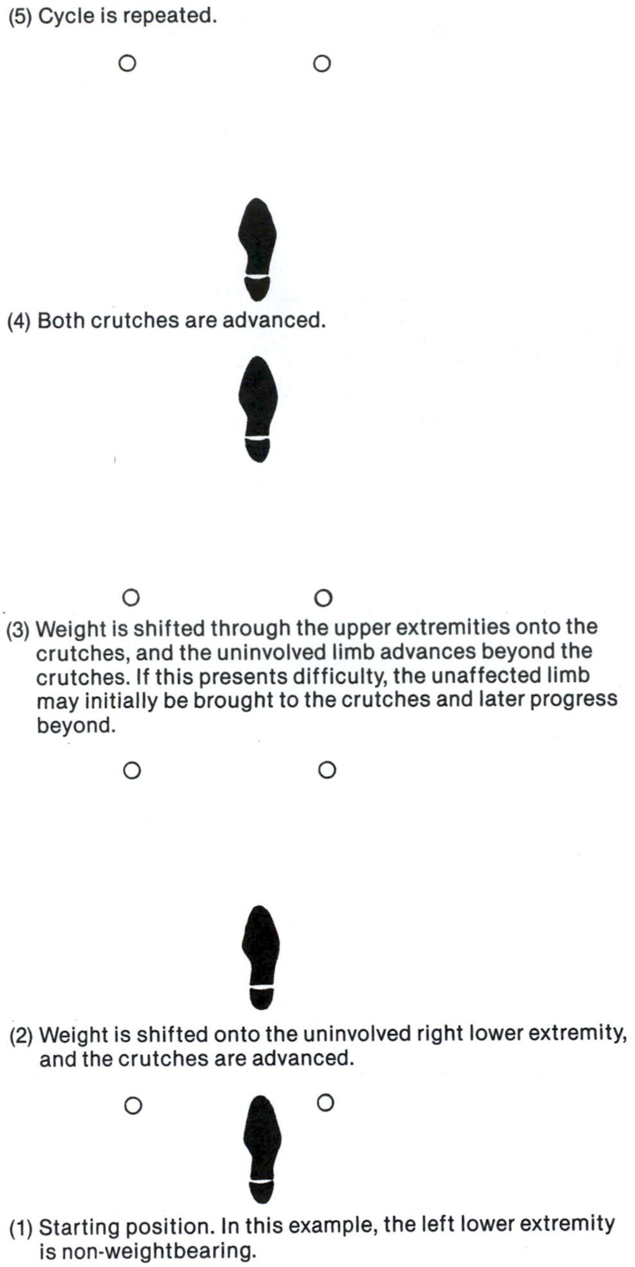

(5) Cycle is repeated.
(4) Both crutches are advanced.
(3) Weight is shifted through the upper extremities onto the crutches, and the uninvolved limb advances beyond the crutches. If this presents difficulty, the unaffected limb may initially be brought to the crutches and later progress beyond.
(2) Weight is shifted onto the uninvolved right lower extremity, and the crutches are advanced.
(1) Starting position. In this example, the left lower extremity is non-weightbearing.

Figure 14.22 Three-point gait pattern.

borne partially on both crutches and on the affected extremity (Fig. 14.23). During instruction in the partial weightbearing gait, emphasis should be placed on use of a normal heel–toe progression on the affected extremity. Often the term partial weightbearing is interpreted by the patient as meaning that only the toes or ball of the foot should contact the floor. Use of this positioning over a period of days or weeks will lead to heel cord tightness. Limb load monitors are often a useful adjunct to partial weightbearing gait training and are described later in this chapter. These devices provide auditory feedback to the patient regarding the amount of weight borne on an extremity.

Four-Point Gait

This pattern provides a slow, stable gait as three points of floor contact are maintained. Weight is borne on both LEs and typically is used with bilateral involvement due to poor balance, incoordination, or muscle weakness. In this gait pattern one crutch is advanced and then the opposite LE is advanced. For example, the left crutch is moved forward, then the right LE, followed by the right crutch and then the left LE (Fig. 14.24).

Two-Point Gait

This gait pattern is similar to the four-point gait. However, it is less stable because only two points of floor contact are maintained. Thus, use of this gait requires better balance. The two-point pattern more closely simulates normal gait, inasmuch as the opposite lower and UE move together (Fig. 14.25).

Two additional, less commonly used crutch gaits are the swing-to and swing-through patterns. These gaits are often used when there is bilateral LE involvement, such as in SCI. The swing-to gait involves forward movement of both crutches simultaneously, and the LEs "swing to" the

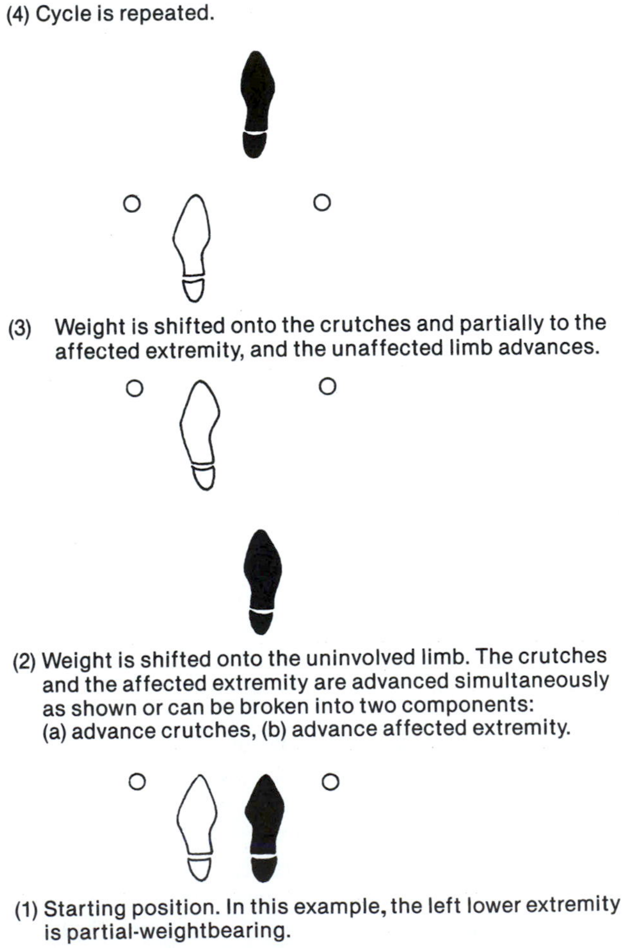

(4) Cycle is repeated.
(3) Weight is shifted onto the crutches and partially to the affected extremity, and the unaffected limb advances.
(2) Weight is shifted onto the uninvolved limb. The crutches and the affected extremity are advanced simultaneously as shown or can be broken into two components: (a) advance crutches, (b) advance affected extremity.
(1) Starting position. In this example, the left lower extremity is partial-weightbearing.

Figure 14.23 Partial weightbearing gait; modification of the three-point gait pattern.

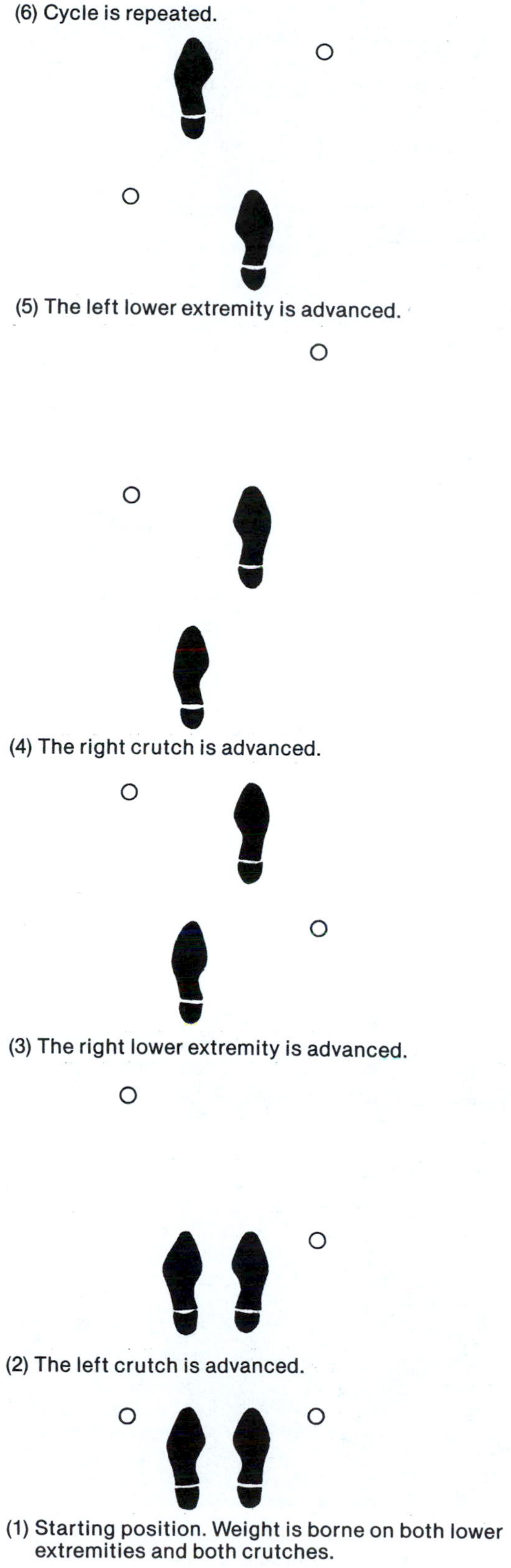
(6) Cycle is repeated.
(5) The left lower extremity is advanced.
(4) The right crutch is advanced.
(3) The right lower extremity is advanced.
(2) The left crutch is advanced.
(1) Starting position. Weight is borne on both lower extremities and both crutches.

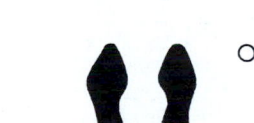

Figure 14.24 Four-point gait pattern.

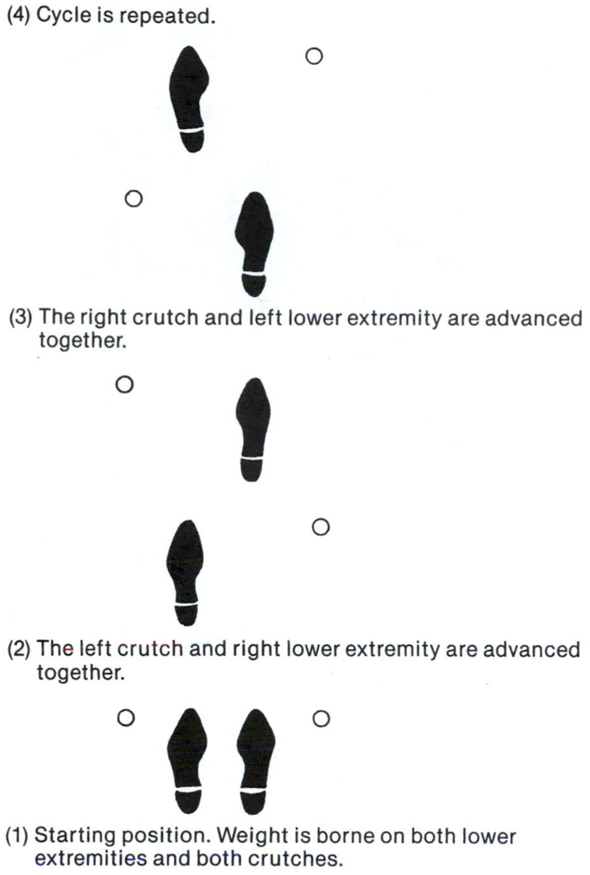
(4) Cycle is repeated.
(3) The right crutch and left lower extremity are advanced together.
(2) The left crutch and right lower extremity are advanced together.
(1) Starting position. Weight is borne on both lower extremities and both crutches.

Figure 14.25 Two-point gait pattern.

crutches. In the swing-through gait, the crutches are moved forward together, but the LEs are swung beyond the crutches. Both these crutch patterns are discussed in greater detail in Chapter 23.

Walkers

Walkers are used to improve balance and relieve weight-bearing either fully or partially on a LE. Of the three categories of ambulatory assistive devices, walkers afford the greatest stability. They provide a wide BOS, improve anterior and lateral stability, and allow the UEs to transfer body weight to the floor.

Walkers are typically made of tubular aluminum with molded vinyl handgrips and rubber tips. They are adjustable in adult sizes from approximately 32 to 37 in. (81 to 92 cm), with children's, youth, and tall sizes available. Several design variations and modifications to the standard design are available and are described below.

Glides

Glides are small, plastic attachments placed on the posterior legs of walkers typically in combination with wheels on the front legs (Fig. 14.26). They promote a smooth forward progression without having to lift and place the walker with each step. They are typically made of high-density plastic in an inverted mushroom-shape. Other common

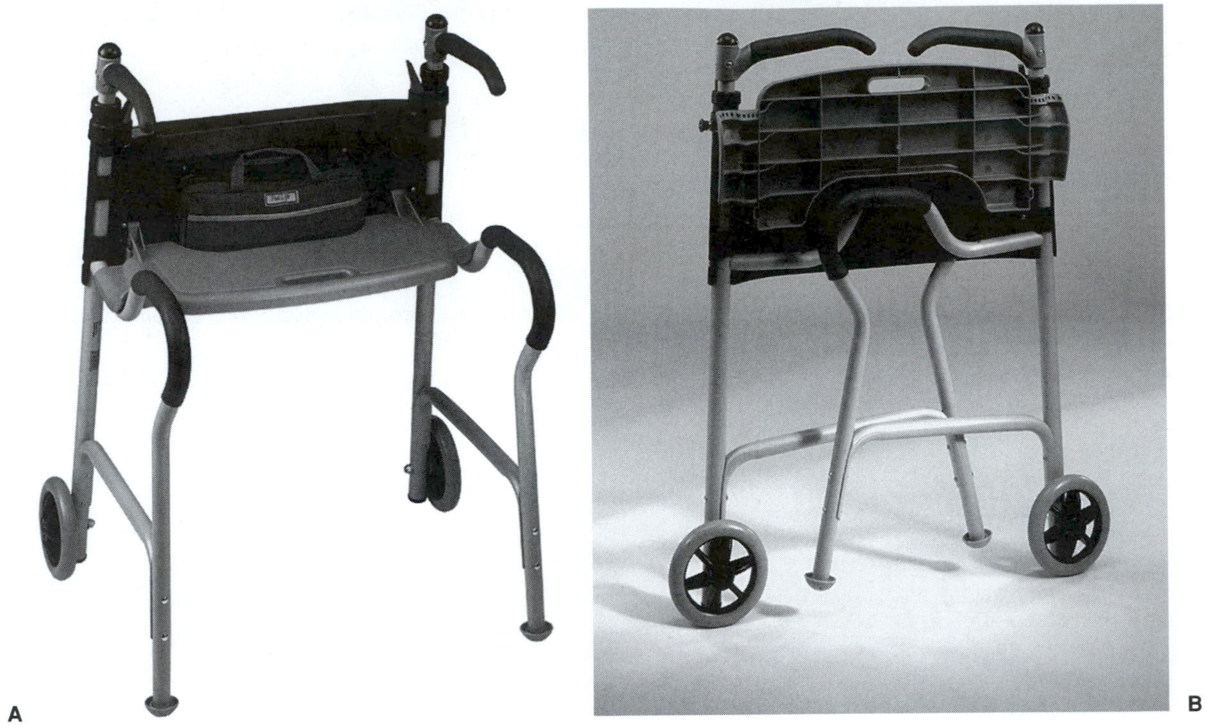

Figure 14.26 Walker in (*A*) open, and (*B*) folded position. This walker has several unique features including: plastic posterior glides, a built-in seat with a molded back bar to support the user during rest intervals (the seat flips up for folding), large front wheels (6 in.) to improve ease of use on multiple terrains, a second set of handles set at approximately the seat level to assist sit-to-stand transitions in the absence of chair armrests or for movement on and off a toilet, and a removable walker pouch for storing personal items. Height of handles adjust using a collar and pin mechanism that eliminates having to turn the walker over to change the height. (Courtesy of Full Life Products, LLC, Moorestown, NJ 08057.)

glide designs include a 1-in. diameter "disk" with a central stem that slides into the tubular leg and is tightened into place with a screwdriver; and a fitted cap that is placed directly onto the walker leg (in the same manner the rubber tip is attached). Another style of glide incorporates a tennis ball within a fixed housing (Fig. 14.27).

Folding Mechanism

Folding walkers are particularly useful for patients who travel. These walkers can be easily collapsed to fit in an automobile or other storage space (see Fig. 14.26A).

Handgrips (Handles)

Enlarged and molded handgrips are available, and may be useful for some patients with arthritis. Some walkers offer a second set of handles to assist with sit-to-stand transitions (see Fig 14.25A).

Platform Attachments

This adaptation is used when weightbearing is contraindicated through the wrist and hand (described in crutch section).

Wheel Attachments

This adaptation to walkers (often called *rollators* or *rolling* walkers) includes the addition of wheels (either to the two front wheels only or to all four wheels). The addition

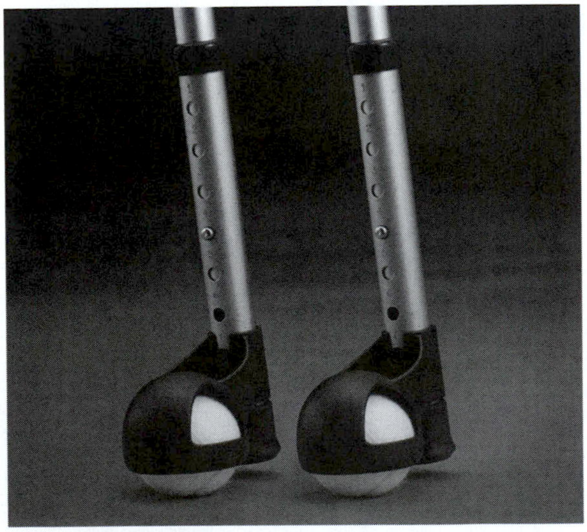

Figure 14.27 The design of these walker glides incorporates a tennis ball within a fixed housing, a spring-loaded brake for intermittent braking during walking, and brake lock-out clips used to deactivate the braking feature for uninterrupted forward motion. The tennis ball can be manually rotated to unworn areas or completely removed to "snap-in" a replacement. (Courtesy of Invacare Corp, Elyria, OH 44036.)

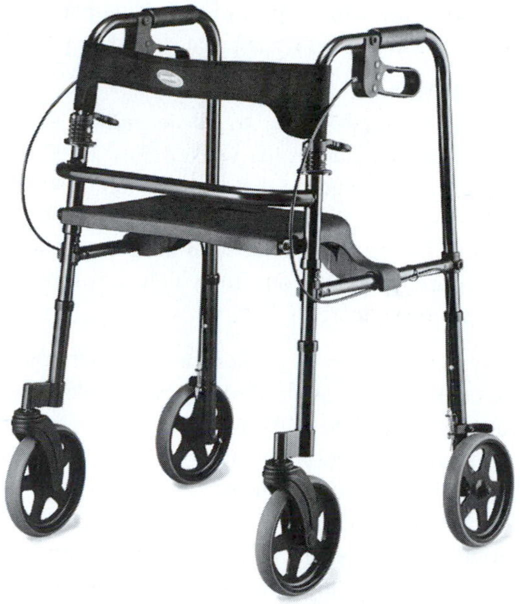

Figure 14.28 The front wheels of this walker swivel freely in all directions. Handbrakes allow locking the rear wheels. (Courtesy of Invacare Corp, Elyria, OH 44036.)

of wheels frequently allows functional ambulation for patients who are unable to lift and to move a conventional walker (e.g., frail elderly). *Swivel wheels* turn freely in a complete circle (Fig. 14.28). *Fixed wheels* rotate around a central axis (Fig. 14.29). Wheels are generally available in 3-, 5-, and 6-in. diameters. Eight-inch diameter wheels are also available and can be used to add height for tall users.

Braking Mechanism

A braking system is an essential feature of walkers designed with wheels. Walkers with four wheels frequently include handbrakes that lock the rear wheels (see Fig. 14.28). Posterior pressure brakes are effective when wheels are placed only on the front walker legs.

Tripod Rollators

Three-wheel rollators incorporate a tripod design (Fig 14.30). A major advantage of this device is ease of maneuverability and turning. Height adjustments are made at the handles; the unit folds for storage and travel.

Storage Attachments

The ability to transport items is an important consideration for many patients and is often essential for those needing frequent access to medications, a cordless or cellular phone, remote control devices, or appointment books. A variety of sizes and styles of attachable baskets and pouches are available (Fig. 14.31; also see Fig 14.25A).

Seating Surface

A variety of walker seat designs are available that fold out of the way when not in use (see Fig. 14.25A and 14.29B). The structural design of many walkers also includes a contoured back support. Seats are an important consideration for individuals with limited endurance (i.e., post-polio syndrome) as well as for community ambulators who require periodic rest intervals. Walker seats should be carefully examined for

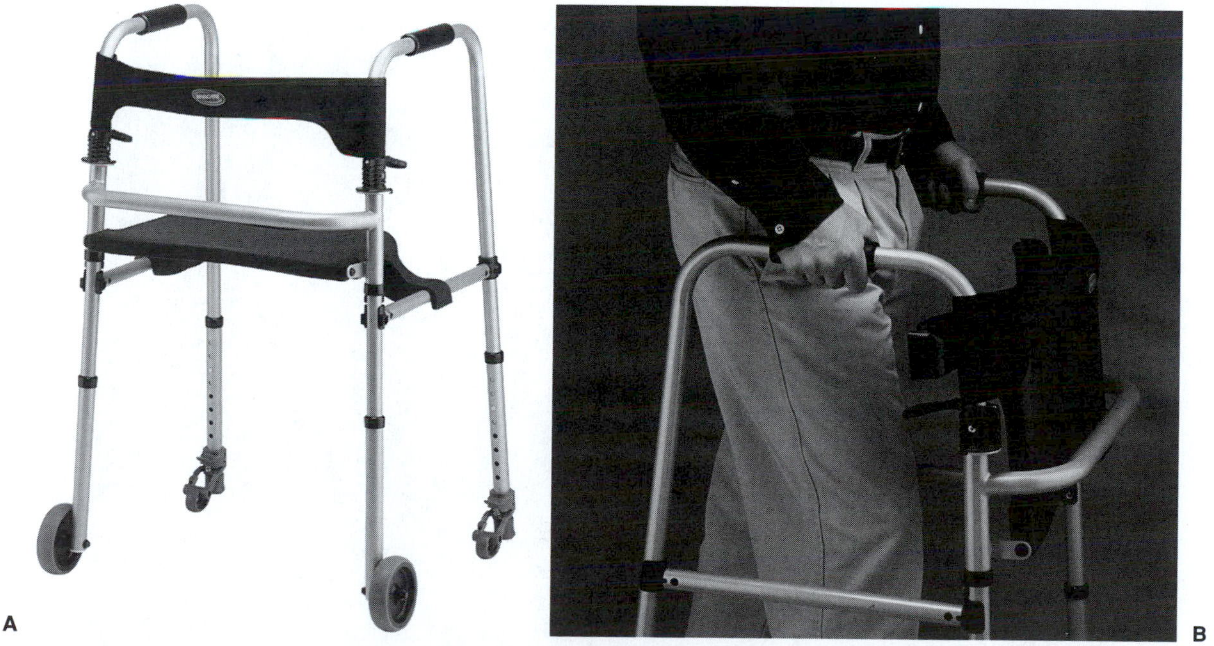

Figure 14.29 Walker seat (*A*) positioned for use, and (*B*) flipped-up for ambulation. The 5-in. fixed front wheels of this walker rotate around a single axis. Features of this walker include rear spring-loaded brakes, a flexible backrest for sitting, a dual-paddle folding mechanism, and adjustable seat-to-floor height. (Courtesy of Invacare Corp, Elyria, OH 44036.)

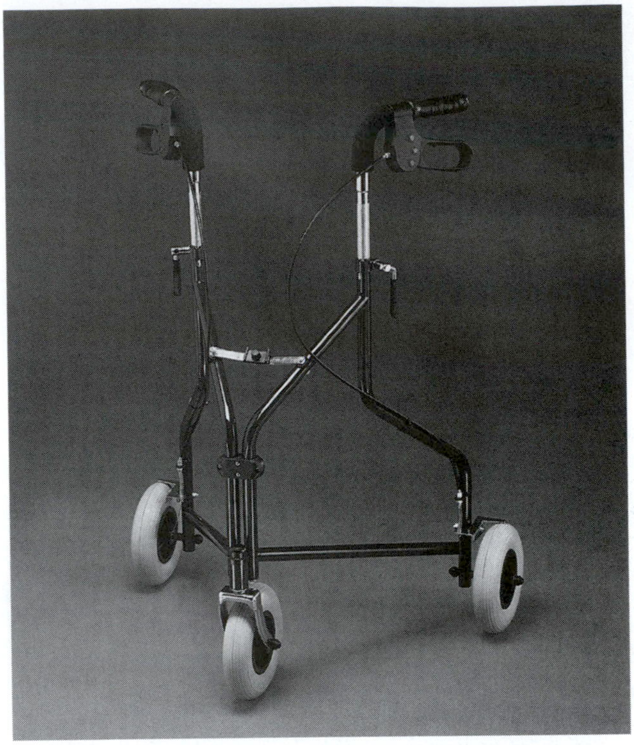

Figure 14.30 Three-wheel rollator with handbrakes and polyurethane tires to improve performance on a variety of terrains. (Courtesy of Invacare Corp, Elyria, OH 44036.)

stability and safety with respect to individual patient needs. Patient practice in use the walker seat should be provided.

Reciprocal Walkers

These walkers are designed to allow unilateral forward progression of one side of the walker (Fig. 14.32). A disadvantage of this design is that some inherent stability of the walker is lost. However, they are useful for patients incapable of lifting the walker with both hands and moving it forward (in situations in which a rolling walker might be contraindicated).

Advantages. Conventional walkers provide four points of floor contact with a wide BOS. They provide a high level of stability. They also provide a sense of security for patients fearful of ambulation. They are relatively lightweight and easily adjusted.

Disadvantages. Walkers tend to be cumbersome, are awkward in confined areas, and are difficult to maneuver through doorways and into cars. They eliminate normal arm swing and cannot be used safely on stairs.

Measuring Walkers

The height of a walker is measured in the same way as that of a cane. The handgrip or handle of the walker should come to approximately the greater trochanter and allow for 20 to 30° of elbow flexion.

Gait Patterns: Conventional Walkers

Prior to initiating instruction in gait patterns using a conventional walker (4 points of floor contact without wheel

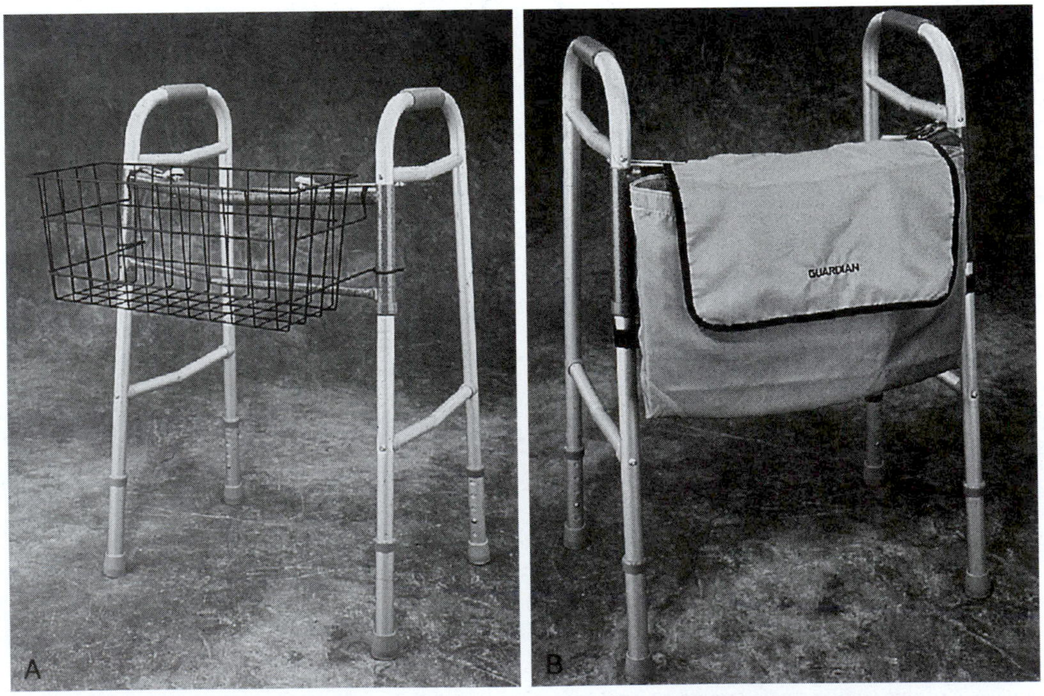

Figure 14.31 Walker basket (*left*) and walker pouch (*right*). (Courtesy of Sunrise Medical, Longmont, CO 80503.)

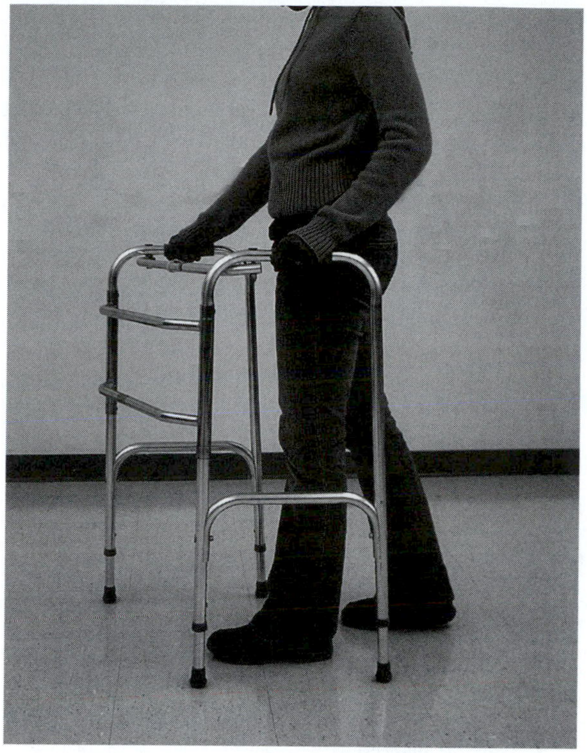

Figure 14.32 Reciprocal walkers allow unilateral movement of one side of the walker while the opposite side remains stationary.

attachments), several points related to use of the walker should be emphasized with the patient:

- The walker should be picked up and placed down on all four legs simultaneously to achieve maximum stability. Rocking from the back to front legs should be avoided because it decreases the effectiveness and safety of the assistive device.
- The patient should be encouraged to hold the head up and to maintain good postural alignment; forward flexion of the trunk, neck, and head should be avoided.
- The patient should be cautioned not to step too close to the front crossbar. This will decrease the overall BOS and may result in a fall.

There are three types of gait patterns used with conventional walkers. These are the full, partial, and non-weightbearing gaits (rolling devices are not recommended for patients with altered weightbearing status). The sequence for each pattern follows.

Full Weightbearing Gait

1. The walker is picked up and moved forward about an arm's length.
2. The first LE is moved forward.
3. The second LE is moved forward past the first.
4. The cycle is repeated.

Partial Weightbearing Gait

1. The walker is picked up and moved forward about an arm's length.
2. The involved LE is moved forward, and body weight is transferred partially onto this limb and partially through the UEs to the walker.
3. The uninvolved LE is moved forward past the involved limb.
4. The cycle is repeated.

Non-Weightbearing Gait

1. The walker is picked up and moved forward about an arm's length.
2. Weight is then transferred through the UEs to the walker. The involved limb is held anterior to the patient's body but does not make contact with the floor.
3. The uninvolved limb is moved forward.
4. The cycle is repeated.

Note: Rolling walkers generally allow use of a reciprocal gait pattern as the walker can be rolled forward while walking. As the need to lift the walker forward following each step is eliminated, a smoother forward progression can be achieved.

Locomotor Training Using Assistive Devices

Level Surfaces

Several important preparatory activities should precede locomotor training on level surfaces with the assistive device. These activities may be completed in the parallel bars for added security. However, if the width of the bars is not adjustable, the BOS of the assistive device may make movement within the bars difficult and unsafe. An alternative is to move the patient outside but next to the parallel bars (or oval bar) or near a treatment table or wall. These preparatory activities include:

1. Instruction in assuming the standing and seated positions with use of the assistive device. These techniques are outlined in Box 14.4 for each category of assistive device.
2. Standing balance activities with the assistive device (similar to those using the parallel bars, described earlier).
3. Instruction in use of assistive device (with selected gait pattern) for forward progression and turning.

As mentioned, demonstrating these activities by assuming the role of the patient during verbal explanations is an effective teaching approach. Following the demonstration, manual contacts, verbal cuing, and explanations can be used again to guide performance of the activity. **Mental practice** (mental rehearsal of a task) is another important strategy to assist in the learning and performance of motor tasks.[37–46] The literature suggests that mental practice

Box 14.4 **Assuming Standing and Seated Positions with Assistive Devices**

I. Cane

A. *Coming to standing*
- Patient moves forward in chair.
- Cane is positioned on uninvolved side (broad-based cane) or leaned against armrest (standard cane).
- Patient leans forward and pushes down with both hands on armrests, comes to a standing position, and then grasps cane. With use of a standard cane, the cane may be grasped loosely with fingers prior to standing and the base of the hand used for pushing down on armrests.

B. *Return to sitting*
- As the patient approaches the chair, the patient turns in a small circle toward the uninvolved side.
- The patient backs up until the chair can be felt against the patient's legs.
- The patient then reaches for the armrest with the free hand, releases the cane (broad-based), and reaches for the opposite armrest. A standard cane is leaned against the chair as the patient grasps the armrest.

II. Crutches

A. *Coming to standing*
- The patient moves forward in the chair.
- Crutches are placed together in a vertical position on the affected side.
- One hand is placed on the handpieces of the crutches; one on the armrest of the chair.
- The patient leans forward and pushes to a standing position.
- Once balance is gained, one crutch is cautiously placed under the axilla on the unaffected side.
- The second crutch is then carefully placed under the axilla on the affected side.
- A tripod stance is assumed.

B. *Return to sitting*
- As the patient approaches the chair, the patient turns in a small circle toward the uninvolved side.
- The patient backs up until the chair can be felt against the patient's legs.
- Both crutches are placed in a vertical position (out from under axilla) on the *affected* side.
- One hand is placed on the handpieces of the crutches; one on the armrest of the chair.
- The patient lowers to the chair in a controlled manner.

Note: See Chapter 23 for alternative methods using bilateral knee ankle orthoses.

III. Walker

A. *Coming to standing*
- The patient moves forward in the chair.
- The walker is positioned directly in front of the chair.
- The patient leans forward and pushes down on armrests to come to standing.
- Once in a standing position, the patient reaches for the walker, one hand at a time.

B. *Return to sitting*
- As the patient approaches the chair, the patient turns in a small circle toward the stronger side.
- The patient backs up until the chair can be felt against the patient's legs.
- The patient then reaches for one armrest at a time.
- The patient lowers to the chair in a controlled manner.

facilitates acquisition of a motor skill as well as improves retention. The physiological basis for mental practice remains in question. However, it has been suggested that mental rehearsal may be functionally similar to motor preparation.[37] Kohl and Roenker[40] propose that imagined movements and actual performance are closely related and may partially share a common physiological substrate. Mental practice is generally considered most effective when combined with physical practice.

Following these preliminary instructions, gait training using the assistive device can be begun on level surfaces. The following guarding technique (Fig. 14.33) should be used.

1. The therapist stands posterior and lateral to the patient's weaker side.
2. A wide BOS should be maintained with the therapist's leading LE following the assistive device. The therapist's opposite LE should be externally rotated and follow the patient's weaker LE.
3. One of the therapist's hands is placed posteriorly on the guarding belt and the other anterior to, but *not touching*, the patient's shoulder on the weaker side.

Should the patient's balance be lost during training, the hand guarding at the shoulder should make contact. Frequently, the support provided by the therapist's hands at the shoulder and on the guarding belt will be enough to allow the patient to regain balance. If the balance loss is severe, the therapist should move in toward the patient so that the body and guarding hands can be used to provide stabilization. The patient should be allowed to regain balance while "leaning" against the therapist. If balance is not recovered and it is apparent the patient must be moved to the floor, further attempts should not be made to hold the patient up because this is likely to result in injury to the patient and/or the therapist. In this situation, the therapist should continue to brace the patient against the body to break the fall and to protect the head and move with the patient to a sitting position on the floor. It is also important to talk to the patient ("Help me lower you to the floor") so that the patient does not continue to struggle to regain balance.

Gait training activities on level surfaces should include instruction and practice in passage through doorways, elevators, and over thresholds. When using crutches, doorways are most easily approached from a diagonal. A hand

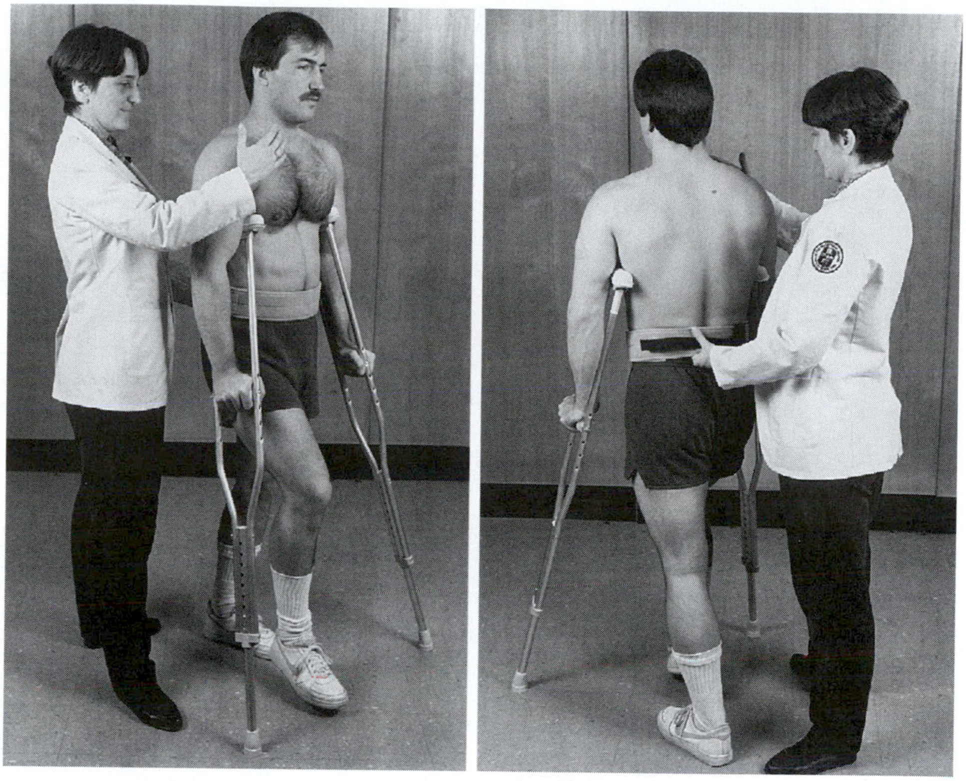

Figure 14.33 Anterior (*left*) and posterior (*right*) views of guarding technique for level surfaces, demonstrated with use of crutches. The same positioning is used with canes and walkers.

must be freed to open the door and one crutch must be placed in a position to hold it open. The patient then gradually proceeds through the doorway, using the crutch to open the door wider if necessary.

Because many patients using a walker or cane may have balance problems, careful examination will determine the safest methods for passage through doorways. A patient using a conventional walker with sufficient balance may be able to use a technique similar to that described above.

Stair Climbing

Several general guidelines should be relayed to the patient during instruction in stair climbing. First, if a railing is available it should always be used. This is true even if it requires placing an assistive device in the hand in which it is not normally used. For stair climbing with axillary crutches using a railing, both crutches are placed together under one arm. Second, the patient should be cautioned that the stronger LE always leads going up the stairs, and the weaker or involved limb always leads coming down (*"up with the good and down with the bad"*).

The progressions of stair climbing techniques are presented in Box 14.5. The following guarding technique should be used by the therapist during stair climbing.

Ascending Stairs (Fig. 14.34)

1. The therapist is positioned posterior and lateral on the affected side behind the patient.

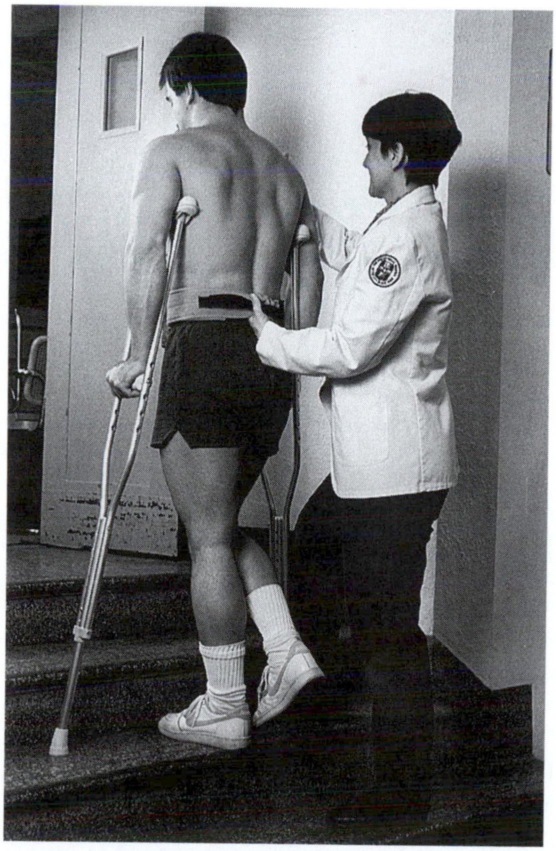

Figure 14.34 Guarding technique for ascending stairs.

Box 14.5 Stair-Climbing Techniques[a]

I. Cane

A. *Ascending*

1. The unaffected lower extremity leads up.
2. The cane and affected lower extremity follow.

B. *Descending*

1. The affected lower extremity and cane lead down.
2. The unaffected lower extremity follows.

II. Crutches: Three-Point Gait (non-weight-bearing gait)

A. *Ascending*

1. The patient is positioned close to the foot of the stairs. The involved lower extremity is held back to prevent "catching" on the lip of the stairs.
2. The patient pushes down firmly on both handpieces of the crutches and leads up with the unaffected lower extremity.
3. The crutches are brought up to the stair that the unaffected lower extremity is now on.

B. *Descending*

1. The patient stands close to the edge of the stair so that the toes protrude slightly over the top. The involved lower extremity is held forward over the lower stair.
2. Both crutches are moved down *together* to the *front* half of the next step.
3. The patient pushes down firmly on both handpieces and lowers the unaffected lower extremity to the step that the crutches are now on.

III. Crutches: Partial Weight-Bearing Gait

A. *Ascending*

1. The patient is positioned close to the foot of the stairs.
2. The patient pushes down on both handpieces of the crutches and distributes weight partially on the crutches and partially on the affected lower extremity while the unaffected lower extremity leads up.
3. The involved lower extremity and crutches are then brought up together.

B. *Descending*

1. The patient stands close to the edge of the stair so that the toes protrude slightly over top of the stair.
2. Both crutches are moved down *together* to the *front* half of the next step. The affected lower extremity is then lowered (depending on patient skill, these may be combined). *Note:* When crutches are not in floor contact, greater weight must be shifted to the uninvolved lower extremity to maintain a partial weight-bearing status.
3. The uninvolved lower extremity is lowered to the step the crutches are now on.

IV. Crutches: Two- And Four-Point Gait

A. *Ascending*

1. The patient is positioned close to the foot of the stairs.
2. The right lower extremity is moved up and then the left lower extremity.
3. The right crutch is moved up and then the left crutch is moved up (patients with adequate balance may find it easier to move the crutches up together).

B. *Descending*

1. The patient stands close to the edge of the stair.
2. The right crutch is moved down and then the left (may be combined).
3. The right lower extremity is moved down and then the left.

[a] The sequences presented here describe stair-climbing techniques without the use of a railing. When a secure railing is available, the patient should be instructed to use it always.

2. A wide BOS should be maintained with each foot on a different stair.
3. A step should be taken only when the patient is not moving.
4. One hand is placed posteriorly on the guarding belt and one is anterior to, but not touching, the shoulder on the weaker side.

Descending Stairs (Fig. 14.35)

1. The therapist is positioned anterior and lateral on the affected side in front of the patient.
2. A wide BOS should be maintained with each foot on a different stair.
3. A step should be taken only when the patient is not moving.
4. One hand is placed anteriorly on the guarding belt and one is anterior to, but not touching, the shoulder on the weaker side.

Should the patient's balance be lost during stair climbing, the following procedure should be followed. First, contact should be made with the hand guarding at the shoulder. Next, the therapist should move toward the patient to help brace the patient (the patient should never be pulled toward the therapist on stairs) or leaned toward the wall of the stairwell (if available). Finally, if needed, the therapist can move with the patient to sit the patient down on the stairs. Remember to inform the patient of your intentions ("I'm going to sit you down").

Note: As described under the section on *Outdoor Overground Progression,* locomotor training using assistive devices should also include outdoor training and practice with curbs, ramps, and slopes; uneven terrains; timed activities (e.g., crossing at a stoplight); and negotiating open community environments as well as outside doors and thresholds, and public or private transportation.

Adjunct Training Devices

Limb Load Monitors

A limb load monitor is a form of biofeedback used clinically as an adjunct intervention during gait training. The limb load monitor incorporates a strain gauge attached to the sole or

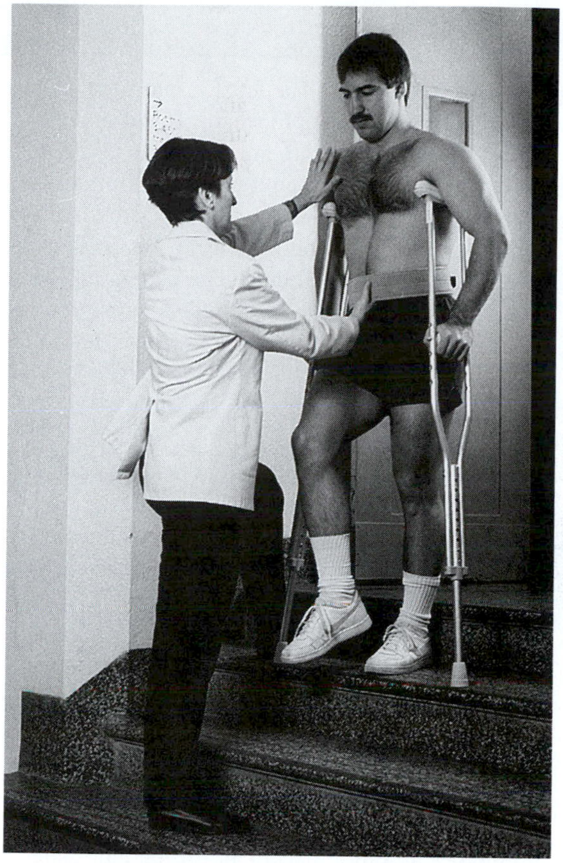

Figure 14.35 Guarding technique for descending stairs.

heel of the shoe. When a force or pressure is applied, the strain gauge is deformed and an auditory signal provides feedback to the wearer. As pressure increases, the signal becomes louder or more rapid. This feedback provides information about the amount of weightbearing on a limb. Limb load monitors can also be used to reinforce the correctness or timing of a movement. For example, an audible noise or buzzer sounding when the heel makes contact with the floor can provide immediate feedback on foot placement. Similar devices can also be attached to a cane (often referred to as a *biofeedback cane*). The principle of operation is the same and incorporates a strain gauge. Auditory signals provide the patient with information on placement as well as pressure applied to the cane.

Summary

Recovery of independent locomotion is an important goal for many patients seeking physical therapy intervention. It is a functional skill that directly impacts performance of expected roles within the patient's social, cultural, and physical environment. A general framework of preparatory exercises and locomotor training strategies has been presented that can be modified to meet the needs of an individual patient. Through a process of careful examination and communication with the patient, family, and/or caregivers, the appropriate preparatory activities and specific training strategies can be identified.

Questions for Review

1. What factors influence the extent and type of locomotor training activities required to achieve desired outcomes for an individual patient?
2. What are the major elements of physical therapy intervention for patients with gait impairments?
3. List the general goals of a program of therapeutic exercise designed to prepare a patient for locomotor training.
4. What are the characteristic features and focus of control of each posture (bridging, sitting, kneeling, half-kneeling, modified plantigrade, and standing) included in the preparatory exercise program leading up to locomotor training?
5. Contrast and compare the advantages and limitations of using parallel bars for locomotor training.
6. Explain the rationale for each component of the indoor overground locomotor training sequence.
7. Describe the rationale and procedure for locomotor training using body weight support and a motorized treadmill.
8. Contrast and compare the advantages and disadvantages of each category of ambulatory assistive device: canes, crutches, and walkers.
9. Describe the guidelines for selection and measurement of canes, crutches, and walkers.
10. Describe the sequence for instructing a patient to rise from and return to a sitting position with a cane, crutches, and a walker.
11. Describe therapist positioning and hand placement for guarding the patient on level surfaces and stairs.
12. Describe the sequence for the following crutch gaits: four-point, two-point, three-point, and partial weight-bearing.
13. Identify the common gait patterns and guarding technique used with canes and walkers.
14. Describe strategies for varying task and environmental demands during locomotor training.

Case Study

The patient is a 26-year-old male who was involved in a motorcycle accident 3 days ago. He sustained closed transverse fractures of the left tibia and fibula secondary to angulatory forces acting on the limb during the accident. Disruption of the periosteum and surrounding soft tissue was evident. The mid-shaft fractures were reduced and a long leg cast applied with the knee flexed to 30° (to help control rotation at the fracture site). The cast is to remain in place for 4 weeks with progression to a below-knee patellar tendon weight-bearing cast.

A Colles fracture of the right wrist was also sustained as the patient attempted to break his fall landing on an open hand with the forearm pronated. The main transverse fracture line is at the flared out distal metaphysis of the radius with avulsion of the ulnar styloid. The fracture was reduced and a cast applied to the wrist and forearm. The thumb and fingers were left free. A series of repeat radiographs are planned at 2-week intervals to ensure satisfactory alignment is maintained. The plan is to progress to functional fracture bracing of the right wrist within 4 weeks.

Past Medical History: Unremarkable.

Social History: The patient lives with his mother, stepfather, and two younger siblings. He has a bachelor's degree in engineering, is employed by a large automotive manufacturer, and is working part-time toward a master's degree. He plans to be married in 6 months. The patient is an avid sportsman with particular interests in sailing, archery, and skiing.

REVIEW OF SYSTEMS

Vision:	Intact
Respiration:	14/minute
Hearing:	Intact
Coordination:	Intact
Blood pressure:	124/80
Sensation:	Intact
Pulse:	60/minute
Cognition:	Intact

Weightbearing status: Non-weightbearing left LE; no weight is to be borne on the right wrist.

ROM examination: The left LE and right wrist and fingers not tested owing to fractures. ROM for all other joints is within normal limits (WNL).

Manual muscle testing: The left LE and right wrist and fingers not tested owing to fractures. All other strength values are within normal limits (WNL).

Plan: The patient is to remain hospitalized for another 48 hours for observation and physical therapy intervention. He will then be followed as an out-patient through the orthopedic clinic. The patient has been referred for gait training activities. Assume you have selected axillary crutches as the assistive device for this patient.

GUIDING QUESTIONS

1. What advantages would selection of the axillary crutches have for this patient?
2. Would you recommend any special attachments to the axillary crutches? If yes, give the rationale for your selection.
3. What type of gait pattern would you select for this patient? Provide a rationale for your selection.
4. As you plan the parallel bar progression for this patient, you decide to provide a verbal description of the gait pattern while you concurrently demonstrate proper use of the crutches. Identify how you would *verbally describe* the sequencing of crutches and foot placement for the gait pattern selected.
5. Prior to initiating instruction in use of the axillary crutches, what general guidelines for their use would you emphasize with the patient?
6. Are there any special considerations or modifications you would need to make to the parallel bar progression for this patient? Describe an appropriate sequence and progression of parallel bar activities.
7. Describe the appropriate therapist positioning and hand placements for guarding the patient during gait training on level surfaces.
8. Describe the sequence of crutch and foot placement for ascending and descending stairs using both crutches (for this response, assume a railing is unavailable).
9. Describe the appropriate therapist positioning and hand placements for guarding the patient while ascending and descending stairs.
10. What basic outdoor activities would you include during gait training for this patient?

References

1. American Physical Therapy Association: Guide to physical therapist practice, ed 2. Phys Ther 81:1, 2001.
2. O'Sullivan, SB, and Schmitz, TJ: Physical Rehabilitation Laboratory Manual: Focus on Functional Training. FA Davis, Philadelphia, 1999.
3. Brown, TH, et al: Body weight-supported treadmill training versus conventional gait training for people with chronic traumatic brain injury. J Head Trauma Rehabil 20(5):402, 2005.
4. Field-Fote, EC: Combined use of body weight support, functional electric stimulation, and treadmill training to improve walking ability in individuals with chronic incomplete spinal cord injury. Arch Phys Med Rehabil 82(6):818, 2001.
5. Colby, SM, Kirkendall, DT, and Bruzga, RF: Electromyographic analysis and energy expenditure of harness supported treadmill walking: Implications for knee rehabilitation. Gait Posture 10(3):200, 1999.
6. Miller, EW, Quinn, ME, and Seddon, PG: Body weight support treadmill and overground ambulation training for two patients with chronic disability secondary to stroke. Phys Ther 82(1):53, 2002.
7. Hesse, S, Konrad, M, and Uhlenbrock, D: Treadmill walking with partial body weight support versus floor walking in hemiparetic subjects. Arch Phys Med Rehabil 80(4):421, 1999.
8. Protas, EJ, et al: Supported treadmill ambulation training after spinal cord injury: A pilot study. Arch Phys Med Rehabil 82(6):825, 2001.
9. Shepherd, R, and Carr, J: Treadmill walking in neurorehabiliation. Neurorehabil Neural Repair 13(3):171, 1999.
10. Kosak, MC, and Reding, MJ. Comparison of partial body weight-supported treadmill gait training versus aggressive bracing assisted walking post stroke. Neurorehabil Neural Repair 14(1):13, 2000.
11. Dobkin, BH: An overview of treadmill locomotor training with partial body weight support: A Neurophysiologically sound approach whose time has come for randomized clinical trials. Neurorehabil Neural Repair 13(3):157, 1999.
12. Barbeau, H, Fung, J, and Visintin: New approach to retrain gait in stroke and spinal cord injured subjects. Neurorehabil Neural Repair 13(3):177, 1999.
13. Barbeau, H, et al: Walking after spinal cord injury: Evaluation, treatment, and functional recovery. Arch Phys Med Rehabil 80(2):225, 1999.
14. Seif-Naraghi, AH, and Herman, RM: A novel method for locomotion training. J Head Trauma Rehabil 14(2):146, 1999.
15. Field-Fote, EC: Spinal cord control of movement: Implications for locomotor rehabilitation following spinal cord injury. Phys Ther 80(5):477, 2000.
16. Finch, L, and Barbeau, H: Hemiplegic gait: New treatment strategies. Physiother Can 38(1):36, 1986.
17. Pillar, T, Dickstein, R, and Smolinski, Z: Walking reeducation with partial relief of body weight in rehabilitation of patients with locomotor disabilities. J Rehabil Res Dev 28(4):47, 1991.
18. Visintin, M, and Barbeau, H: The effects of body weight support on the locomotor pattern of spastic paretic patients. Can J Neurol Sci 16:315, 1989.
19. Wernig, A, et al: Laufband therapy based on 'rules of spinal locomotion' is effective in spinal cord injured persons. Eur J Neurosci 7(4):823, 1995.
20. Malouin, F, et al: Use of an intensive task-oriented gait training program in a series of patients with acute cerebrovascular accidents. Phys Ther 72(11):781, 1992.
21. Gardner, MB, et al: Partial body weight support with treadmill locomotion to improve gait after incomplete spinal cord injury: A single-subject experimental design. Phys Ther 78(4):361, 1998.
22. Schindl, MR, et al: Treadmill training with partial body weight support in nonambulatory patients with cerebral palsy. Arch Phys Med Rehabil 81(3):301, 2000.
23. Miller, EW: Body weight supported treadmill and overground training in a patient post cerebrovascular accident. NeuroRehabilitation 16(3):155, 2001.
24. Trueblood, PR: Partial body weight treadmill training in persons with chronic stroke. NeuroRehabilitation 16(3):141, 2001.
25. da Cunha Filho, IT, et al: Gait outcomes after acute stroke rehabilitation with supported treadmill ambulation training: A randomized controlled pilot study. Arch Phys Med Rehabil 83(9):1258, 2002.
26. Ada, L, et al: A treadmill and overground walking program improves walking in persons residing in the community after stroke: A placebo-controlled, randomized trial. Arch Phys Med Rehabil 84(10):1486, 2003.
27. Sullivan, K, Knowlton, B, and Dobkin, B: Step training with body weight support: Effect of treadmill speed and practice paradigms on poststroke locomotor recovery. Arch Phys Med Rehabil 83(5):683, 2002.
28. Barbeau, H, and Rossignol, S: Recovery of locomotion after chronic spinalization in the adult cat. Brain Res 26:84, 1987.
29. Lovely, RG, et al: Effects of training on the recovery of full-weight-bearing stepping in the adult spinal cat. Exp Neurol 92(2):421, 1986.
30. de Leon, RD, et al: Locomotor capacity attributable to step training versus spontaneous recovery after spinalization in adult cats. J Neurophysiol 79(3):1329, 1998.
31. Visintin, M, et al: A new approach to retrain gait in stroke patients through body weight support and treadmill stimulation. Stroke 29(6):1122, 1998.
32. Miyai, I, et al: Long-term effect of body weight-supported treadmill training in Parkinson's disease: A randomized controlled trial. Arch Phys Med Rehabil 83(10):1370, 2000.
33. Holden, MK, et al: Clinical gait assessment in the neurologically impaired. Reliability and meaningfulness. Phys Ther 64(1):35, 1984.
34. Russell, DJ, et al: The gross motor function measure: A means to evaluate the effects of physical therapy. Dev Med Child Neurol 31(3):341, 1989.
35. Milczarek, JJ, et al: Standard and four-footed canes: Their effect on the standing balance of patients with hemiparesis. Arch Phys Med Rehabil 74(3):281, 1993.
36. Neumann, DA: Hip abductor muscle activity as subjects with hip prostheses walk with different methods of using a cane. Phys Ther 78(5):490, 1998.
37. Levangie, PK, and Norkin, CC: Joint Structure and Function: A Comprehensive Analysis, ed 4. FA Davis, Philadelphia, 2005.
38. Ely, DD, and Smidt, GL: Effect of cane on variables of gait for patients with hip disorders. Phys Ther 57(5):507, 1977.
39. Stephan, KM, et al: Functional anatomy of the mental representation of upper extremity movements in healthy subjects. J Neurophysiol 73(1):373, 1995.
40. Kohl, RM, and Roenker, DL: Behavioral evidence for shared mechanisms between actual and imaged motor responses. J Hum Mov Stud 17:173, 1989.
41. Overdorf, V, et al: Mental and physical practice schedules in acquisition and retention of novel timing skills. Percept Mot Skills 99(1):51, 2004.
42. Liu, KP, et al: Mental imagery for relearning of people after brain injury. Brain Inj 18(11):1163, 2004.
43. Davis, FD, and Yi, MY: Improving computer skill training: Behavior modeling, symbolic mental rehearsal, and the role of knowledge structures. J Appl Psychol 89(3):509, 2004.
44. Yoo, E, Park, E, and Chung, B: Mental practice effect on line-tracing accuracy in persons with hemiparetic stroke: A preliminary study. Arch Phys Med Rehabil 82(9):1213, 2001.
45. Hall, JC: Imagery practice and the development of surgical skills. Am J Surg 184(5):465, 2002.
46. Yaguez, L, et al: A mental route to motor learning: Improving trajectorial kinematics through imagery training. Behav Brain Res 90(1):95, 1998.

Supplemental Readings

Behrman, AK, et al: Locomotor training progression and outcomes after incomplete spinal cord injury. Phys Ther 85(12):1356, 2005.

Brown, DA, Nagpal, S, and Chi, S: Limb-loaded cycling program for locomotor intervention following stroke. Phys Ther 85(2):159, 2005.

Cavanaugh, JT, et al: Comparison of head- and body-velocity trajectories during locomotion among healthy and vestibulopathic subjects. J Rehabil Res Dev 42(2):191, 2005.

Chen, G, et al: Gait deviations associated with post-stroke hemiparesis: Improvement during treadmill walking using weight support, speed, support stiffness, and handrail hold. Gait Posture 22(1):57, 2005.

Gerin-Lajoie, M, Richards, CL, and McFadyen, BJ: The negotiation of stationary and moving obstructions during walking: Anticipatory locomotor adaptations and preservation of personal space. Motor Control 9(3):242, 2005.

Hesse, S: Recovery of gait and other motor functions after stroke: Novel physical and pharmacological treatment strategies. Restor Neurol Neurosci 22(3–5):359, 2004.

Hornby, TG, Zemon, DH, and Campbell, D: Robotic-assisted, body-weight-supported treadmill training in individuals following motor incomplete spinal cord injury. Phys Ther 85(1):52, 2005.

Reisman, DS, Block, HJ, and Bastian, AJ: Interlimb coordination during locomotion: What can be adapted and stored? J Neurophysiol 94(4):2403, 2005.

White, SC, and Lifeso, RM: Altering asymmetric limb loading after hip arthroplasty using real-time dynamic feedback when walking. Arch Phys Med Rehabil 86(10):1958, 2005.

Wirz, M, et al: Effectiveness of automated locomotor training in patients with chronic incomplete spinal cord injury: A multicenter trial. Arch Phys Med Rehabil 86(4):672, 2005.

CHAPTER

15

LEARNING OBJECTIVES

1. Define the disease processes (including definition, etiology, pathophysiology, clinical presentation, and clinical course) of chronic obstructive pulmonary disease, asthma, cystic fibrosis, and restrictive lung disease.
2. Describe examination procedures (including patient interview, vital signs, observation, inspection, palpation, auscultation, and laboratory tests) for a patient with pulmonary disease.
3. Identify the anticipated goals and expected outcomes of pulmonary rehabilitation.
4. Describe the rehabilitative management of a patient with chronic pulmonary dysfunction.
5. Value the therapist's role in the management of a patient with chronic pulmonary dysfunction.
6. Analyze and interpret patient data, formulate realistic goals and outcomes, and develop a plan of care when presented with a clinical case study.

Chronic Pulmonary Dysfunction

Julie Ann Starr, PT, MS, CCS

OUTLINE

Pulmonary rehabilitation is a multidisciplinary program of care for patients with chronic respiratory impairment that is individually tailored and designed to optimize physical and social performance and autonomy.[1] Years ago, patients with chronic pulmonary disease were given a standard prescription for rest and avoidance of exercise.[2] The stress imposed by exercise was considered deleterious to people with pulmonary disorders. A pivotal study by Pierce et al. (1964) provided the impetus to change direction in the treatment of pulmonary dysfunction.[3] Exercise training effects of decreased heart rate, respiratory rate, minute ventilation, oxygen consumption, and carbon dioxide production at submaximal exercise levels was documented in their subjects with chronic obstructive pulmonary disease (COPD). Increased maximal aerobic capacity was also documented.[3] Reconditioning of patients with pulmonary disease was found to be possible!

COPD, asthma, and cystic fibrosis are the most common chronic obstructive lung diseases for which pulmonary rehabilitation is rendered. Patients with restrictive lung disease have also demonstrated improvement in functional abilities following pulmonary rehabilitation.[4] Rehabilitation for patients with chronic lung disease is now a well-established and widely accepted means of optimizing function.[5]

In this chapter, the most common chronic pulmonary diseases are discussed, as well as the physical therapy examination and treatment of patients with chronic pulmonary disease. A brief review of ventilation and respiration is warranted for a better understanding of the disease pathologies, and for understanding the rationale of the physical therapy procedures. The supplemental readings list at the end of this chapter contains references for a more thorough review of respiratory physiology.

Respiratory Physiology

Air is inspired through the nose or mouth, through all of the conducting airways until it reaches the distal respiratory unit, which contains the respiratory bronchiole, alveolar ducts, alveolar sacs, and the alveoli (Fig. 15.1).

The movement of air through the conducting airways is termed *ventilation.* At full inspiration, the lungs contain their maximum amount of gas. This volume of air is called *total lung capacity (TLC),* which can be divided into four separate volumes of air: (1) tidal volume, (2) inspiratory reserve volume, (3) expiratory reserve volume, and (4) residual volume. Combinations of two or more of these

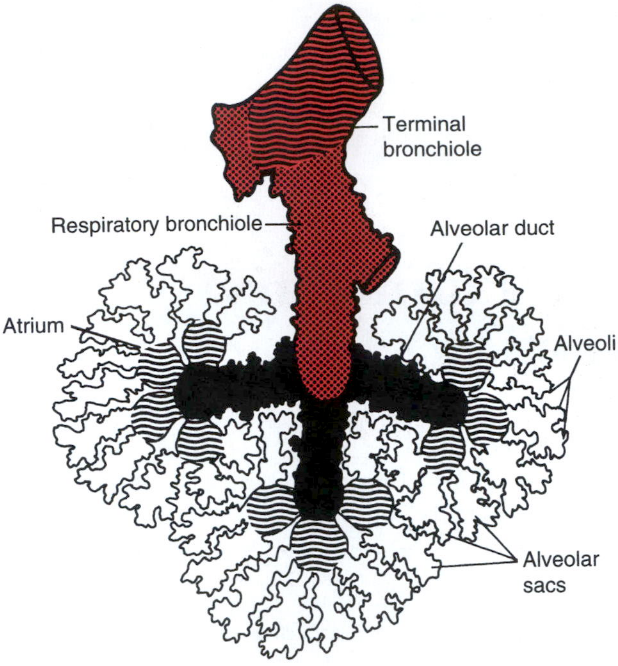

Figure 15.1 Anatomy of the distal conducting airway, the terminal bronchiole and the respiratory unit, the respiratory bronchiole, alveolar ducts, aveolar sacs, and alveoli. (From Brannon, FJ, et al: Cardiopulmonary Rehabilitation: Basic Theory and Application, ed 2. FA Davis, Philadelphia, 1993, p 43, with permission.)

lung volumes are termed capacities. Figure 15.2 illustrates the relationship of lung volumes and capacities.

The amount of air inspired and expired during normal resting ventilation is termed *tidal volume (TV)*. As this tidal volume of air enters the respiratory system, it travels through the conducting airways to reach the respiratory units. Tidal volume is about 500 mL/breath for a young, healthy, white male. The amount of inspired air that actually reaches the distal respiratory unit and takes part in gas exchange is about 350 mL of the 500 mL total. The remaining 150 mL of the inhaled tidal breath remains in the conducting airways and does not take part in gas exchange. When only a tidal breath occupies the lungs, there is "room" for additional air that can be further inhaled. This volume in excess of that used in tidal breathing is the *inspiratory reserve volume (IRV)*. Aptly named, it is the volume of air that can be inspired when needed, but is usually kept in reserve. There is a quantity of air that can potentially be exhaled beyond the end of a tidal exhalation. Although it is kept in reserve, the volume of air that can be exhaled in excess of tidal breathing is called the *expiratory reserve volume (ERV)*. The lungs are not completely emptied of air even after maximally exhaling the expiratory reserve volume. The volume of air remaining within the lungs when ERV has been exhaled is called the *residual volume (RV)*.

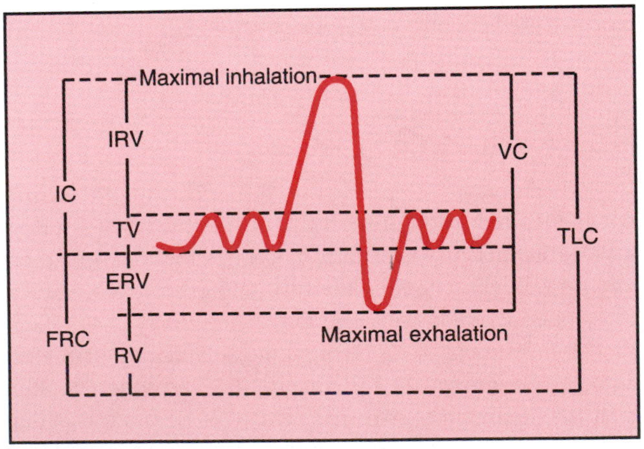

Figure 15.2 Lung volumes and capacities. ERV = expiratory reserve volume; FRC = functional residual capacity; IC = inspiratory capacity; IRV = inspiratory reserve volume; RV = residual volume; TLC = total lung capacity; TV = tidal volume; VC = vital capacity.

The sum of two or more volumes is referred to as a capacity. Tidal volume plus the inspiratory reserve volume is known as the *inspiratory capacity (IC)*. This refers to the volume of air that can be inspired beginning from a tidal exhalation. The combination of residual volume and expiratory reserve volume is the *functional residual capacity (FRC)*. Functional residual capacity is the volume of air that remains in the lungs at the end of a tidal exhalation. The sum of inspiratory reserve volume, tidal volume, and expiratory reserve volume is called the *vital capacity (VC)*. It is the total volume of air within the lungs that is under volitional control. The common method of measuring VC is to achieve maximal inspiration, then forcibly exhale all of the air into a measuring device as hard and as fast as possible until ERV has been exhausted. Because this is a forced expiratory maneuver, it is termed the forced vital capacity (FVC). As stated earlier, all volumes together equal total lung capacity;

$$TV + IRV + ERV + RV = TLC.$$

Flow rate measures the volume of gas moved in a period of time. Expiratory flow rates, therefore, are measurements of exhaled gas volume divided by the amount of time required for the volume to be exhaled. Flow rates reflect the ease with which the lungs can be ventilated and are related to the elasticity of the lung parenchyma. An important airflow measurement is the volume of air that can be forcefully exhaled during the first second of a forced vital capacity maneuver. This is called the *forced expiratory volume* in 1 second *(FEV_1)*. This flow rate is thought to reflect the status of the airways of the lungs. In healthy individuals, FEV_1 is 70 percent or more of the total FVC (FEV_1/FVC > 70%).[6] Inspiratory flow rates can also be determined by measuring the amount of air inspired and the amount of time necessary for the inhalation.

Maximum inspiratory pressure (PI_{max}) reflects the greatest static inspiratory effort that can be generated from residual volume. It is measured as a pressure in millimeters of mercury or cubic centimeters of water and reflects the strength of the muscles of inspiration. *Maximal sustained inspiratory pressure* (SIP_{max}) is a test of inspiratory muscle endurance. The patient is initially challenged with –6 cm H_2O pressure resistance. Gradually the resistance is increased –2 cm H_2O every 2 minutes until the patient can no longer achieve adequate ventilation flow levels.[7] The maximal pressure is defined as the highest level that the patient could tolerate during the testing procedure.

Lung volumes, capacities, flow rates, and mechanics depend on the size and configuration of the thorax. Therefore, height, gender, and race influence static and dynamic lung measurements. Any alteration in the properties of the lungs or chest wall due to the aging process or a disease process will change the lung volumes, capacities, flow rates, or mechanics.

Respiration is a term used to describe the gas exchange within the body. This should not be confused with ventilation, which describes only the movement of air. External respiration is the exchange of gas that occurs at the alveolar capillary membrane between atmospheric air and the pulmonary capillaries. Internal respiration takes place at the tissue capillary level between the tissues and the surrounding capillaries. The following discussion traces the course of gas exchange, specifically that of oxygen and carbon dioxide, during both external and internal respiration.

For external respiration to take place, there must first be an inhalation of air from the environment, through the conducting airways, and into the respiratory bronchioles and alveoli. Oxygen diffuses through the walls of the respiratory unit, through the interstitial space, and through the pulmonary capillary wall. Most of the oxygen (98.5 percent) then travels through the blood plasma into red blood cells where it occupies one of the gas-carrying sites of hemoglobin. A small portion of dissolved oxygen (1.5 percent) is carried in the plasma.

The oxygenated blood returns to the left side of the heart via the pulmonary veins; from there it travels through the aorta, and then through a network of connecting arteries, arterioles, and capillaries, until its destination, the tissue, is reached. Internal respiration begins when the arterial blood reaches the tissue level. Oxygen diffuses from the gas-carrying sites of hemoglobin, out of the red blood cell, out of the capillary, through the cell membranes, and into the mitochondria of the working cells. Again, this process occurs through diffusion.

Carbon dioxide (CO_2), which is produced at the tissue level as a by-product of metabolism, diffuses out of the working cells and into the capillaries. Carbon dioxide is transported through the venous system into the right side of the heart. Once the carbon dioxide makes its way to the pulmonary capillary, it diffuses out through the capillary membrane, through the interstitial space, and into the alveoli, where it is finally exhaled into the atmosphere.

When the cycle of external and internal respiration has occurred, oxygen has been extracted from the environment and provided to the body tissues meanwhile, carbon dioxide has been removed from the body and released into the external environment. Of course, this system is dependent upon an intact cardiovascular system to pump the blood through the lungs, deliver it to the working cells, and then return it back to the lungs, all in a timely fashion.

Chronic Lung Diseases

Chronic Obstructive Pulmonary Disease

Chronic obstructive pulmonary disease (COPD) is the most common chronic pulmonary disorder, afflicting 14 million adults in the United States and is a leading cause of morbidity.[8] It is the fourth leading cause of death worldwide with a mortality rate that continues to rise.[6]

The 2001 Global Initiative for Chronic Obstructive Lung Disease (GOLD) was a collaborative work of the United States Heart, Lung, and Blood Institute and the World Health Organization (WHO) that set out to increase world-wide awareness of COPD and decrease morbidity and mortality from the disease.[6] According to GOLD, COPD is defined as a "disease state characterized by airflow limitation that is not fully reversible. The airflow limitation is usually both progressive and associated with an abnormal inflammatory response of the lungs to noxious particles or gases."[6, p 6] Disease severity is based on both clinical symptoms and measurements of airflow limitation. See Table 15.1 for the classification of severity of COPD.

Risk Factors

Risk factors for the development of COPD contain both host factors and environmental factors. Host factors that would make a person more susceptible to the development of COPD would include hyperreactivity of the airways, overall lung growth, and genetics. One well known genetic cause of COPD is an alpha-1 antitrypsin deficiency.[9] Recent studies have also investigated inflammatory mediated genes that may influence the development of the disease.[10]

Environmental factors that contribute to the development of COPD include primary and secondary tobacco smoke as well as occupational exposures, and indoor and outdoor pollutants.[6] Cigarette smoking is the major environmental causal agent in the development of COPD.[6] There is a relationship between the amount and duration of cigarette smoking and the severity of the lung disease, although significant individual variation does exist.[5] It is perplexing that not all smokers develop airway inflammation and that not all persons with airway inflammation go on to develop clinically significant COPD. It would appear that the development of COPD results from a combination of host and environmental factors.

Table 15.1 The GOLD Classification System for Severity of Chronic Obstructive Pulmonary Disease

Stage	Characteristics
0: At Risk	• Normal spirometry • Chronic symptoms (cough, sputum production)
I: Mild COPD	• $FEV_1/FVC < 70\%$ • $FEV_1 \geq 80\%$ predicted • With or without chronic symptoms (cough, sputum production)
II: Moderate COPD	• $FEV_1/FVC < 70\%$ • $50\% \leq FEV_1 < 80\%$ predicted • With or without chronic symptoms (cough, sputum production)
III: Severe COPD	• $FEV_1/FVC < 70\%$ • $30\% \leq FEV_1 < 50\%$ predicted • With or without chronic symptoms (cough, sputum production)
IV: Very Severe COPD	• $FEV_1/FVC < 70\%$ • $FEV_1 < 30\%$ predicted or $FEV_1 < 50\%$ predicted plus chronic respiratory failure

Classification based on postbronchodilator FEV_1.

FEV_1 = forced expiratory volume in 1 second; FVC = forced vital capacity; respiratory failure = arterial partial pressure of oxygen (Pa_{O_2}) < 8.0 kPa (60 mm Hg) with or without arterial partial pressure of CO_2 (Pa_{CO_2}) > 6.7 kPa (50 mm Hg) while breathing air at sea level.

Reprinted with permission, NILBI/WHO Global Initiative for Chronic Obstructive Lung Disease (GOLD) workshop summary.[6]

Pathophysiology

COPD is a combination of airway narrowing, parenchymal destruction, and pulmonary vascular thickening. These changes are related to chronic airway inflammation and are most pronounced in the peripheral airways. In addition, there are imbalances of proteinases/antiproteinases and oxidants/antioxidants in patients with COPD.[6] Chronic inflammation, characterized by an increase in neutrophils, macrophages, and T lymphocytes, damages the endothelial lining of the airways. Airway damage results in airway repair, leading to airway remodeling. These airway changes appear to be most pronounced in the smaller peripheral airways.[6] The glands and goblet cells within the bronchial walls hypertrophy producing excessive secretions, which either partially or completely obstruct the airways. Decreases in ciliary function and alterations in physiochemical characteristics of bronchial secretions also impair airway clearance and contribute to airway obstruction. Damaged and inflamed mucosa shows an increased sensitivity of irritant receptors within the bronchial walls, which in turn cause bronchial *hyperreactivity.*

During inspiration, the lungs and the airways are pulled open, increasing the diameter of the lumen. During exhalation, as the thorax returns to its resting position, the airways decrease in size. In COPD, the airways are pulled open wide by thoracic expansion, allowing air to enter. During exhalation, the airway narrowing from inflammation, remodeling and excessive secretions, causes premature airway closure, trapping air in the distal airways and airspaces. This air trapping is called *hyperinflation,* which is defined as an abnormal increase in the amount of air within the lung tissue.

The most common parenchymal changes found in COPD are dilatation and destruction of the respiratory bronchioles, which is thought to be due to an imbalance of proteinases and antiproteinases in the lung.[6] This change in pulmonary tissue results in loss of the normal elastic recoil properties of the lungs. The pulmonary vasculature is also altered early in the development of COPD. There are endothelial changes that result in thickening of the vessel wall. In advanced stages of the disease, there is destruction of the pulmonary capillary bed.[6]

Ventilation in the alveoli and *perfusion* in the capillary membrane are no longer matched. This results in *hypoxemia,* a condition in which a decreased amount of oxygen is carried by the blood to the tissues. As the disease progresses and more areas of the lung become involved, hypoxemia will worsen and *hypercapnea,* a condition in which there is an increased amount of carbon dioxide within the arterial blood, will develop. Increased pulmonary vascular resistance secondary to capillary wall damage and destruction and reflex vasoconstriction in the presence of hypoxemia and hypercapnea results in right ventricular hypertrophy, termed *cor pulmonale. Polycythemia,* an increase in the amount of circulating red blood cells, is another complication of advanced COPD.

Clinical Presentation

Patients with COPD will present with symptoms of chronic cough, expectoration, and exertional dyspnea. The

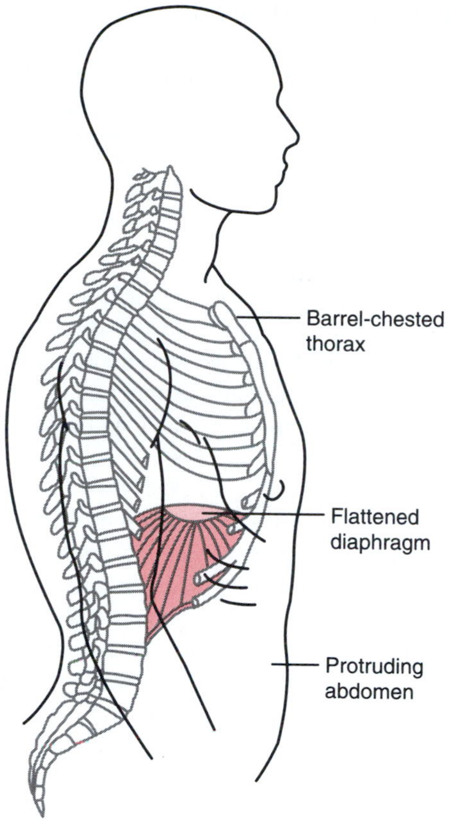

Figure 15.3 Changes in the configuration of the thorax with chronic obstructive pulmonary disease.

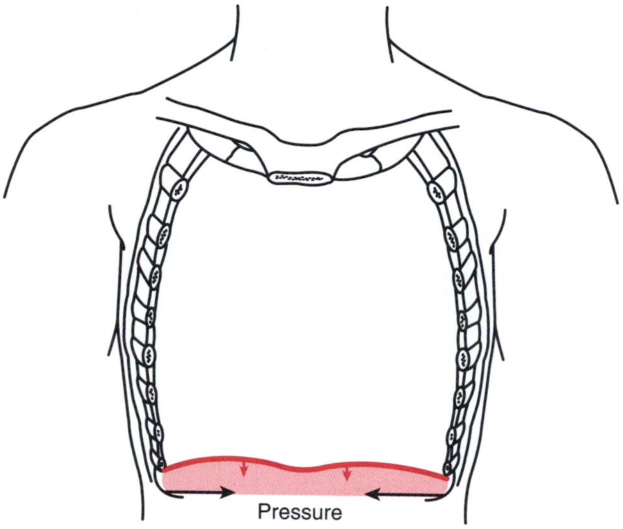

Figure 15.4 Alteration in alignment of fibers of the diaphragm due to hyperinflation. (From Levangie, P, and Norkin, C: Joint Structure and Function, ed 4, 2005, p 204, with permission.)

intensity of each symptom varies from patient to patient. Cough and expectoration appear slowly and insidiously. Dyspnea is first evidenced during exertion. As the disease progresses, symptoms worsen. Dyspnea occurs at progressively lower activity levels. Severely involved patients may appear dyspneic even at rest.

On physical examination, the thorax appears enlarged owing to loss of lung elastic recoil. The anterior–posterior (AP) diameter of the chest increases and a dorsal kyphosis is noted. These anatomical changes give the patient a barrel-chest appearance (Fig. 15.3).

The resting position of the thorax is in a more inspiratory mode, there is a decreased available range of motion, i.e., decreased thoracic excursion. There are changes in the alignment of fibers of the diaphragm with hyperinflation. The diaphragm becomes flatter, or less domed. The angle of pull of these fibers changes as the disease progresses, altering the biomechanics of the thorax. In severe disease, the diaphragm fiber alignment may be horizontal, resulting in an inward motion of the lower ribs during inhalation (Fig. 15.4).

Breath sounds and heart sounds may be distant and difficult to hear. Partially obstructed bronchi and bronchioles may result in expiratory wheezing. Crackles may also be present. Hypertrophy of accessory muscles of ventilation, pursed-lip breathing, cyanosis, and digital clubbing may all be present in the advanced stages of COPD. (See the section on Examination for clarification of terms.)

Significant and progressive airway limitation is reflected in altered pulmonary function tests. Lung volumes and capacities, especially residual volume and functional residual capacity, are increased from the normal value due to air trapping. Figure 15.5 shows the changes in lung volumes and capacities that occur in obstructive pulmonary disease.

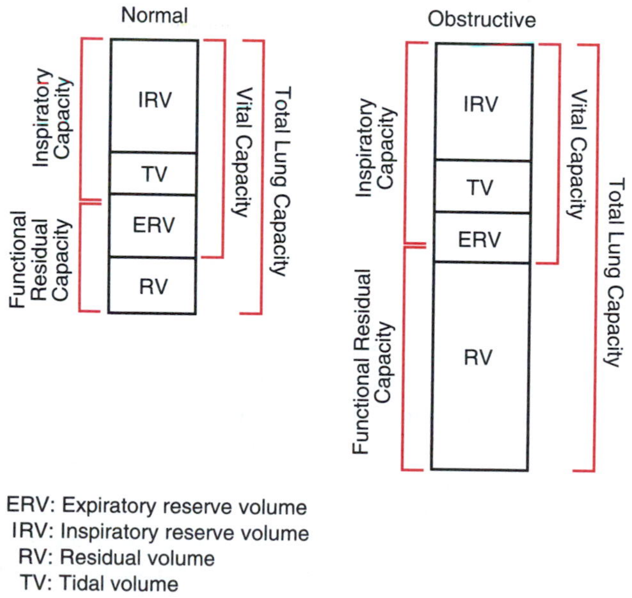

Figure 15.5 Lung volumes of a healthy pulmonary system compared with the lung volumes found in obstructive disease. (Adapted from Rothstein, J, Roy, S, and Wolf, S: The Rehabilitation Specialist's Handbook. FA Davis, Philadelphia, 2005, p 428, with permission.)

Expiratory flow rates, especially FEV_1, are decreased. The ratio of FEV_1 to FVC is also decreased (<70 percent). These changes in pulmonary function do not show a major reversibility in response to pharmacological agents.

Arterial blood gas analyses may reflect hypoxemia in the early stages of COPD. Hypercapnea appears as the disease progresses. With disease progression, chest radiographs show several characteristic findings. These include depressed and flattened diaphragm; alteration in pulmonary vascular markings; hyperinflation of the thorax, evidenced by an increased AP diameter of the chest; and an increase in the size of the retrosternal airspace, hyperlucency, elongation of the heart, and right ventricular hypertrophy.

Course and Prognosis

The clinical course of COPD has an insidious onset with a disease progression that can run for many years. Early identification of those individuals at risk for the development of COPD has been elusive. While smoking is the most prevalent risk factor for the development of disease, only a percentage of smokers develop clinically significant lung disease. Therefore, a smoking history in and of itself is not predictive for the development of COPD. Certain pulmonary function tests, for example, mid-maximal expiratory flow rate, once thought to be indicative of potential disease, also lack predictive value. Stage 0 COPD of the GOLD guidelines (clinical complaints of cough and sputum production without pulmonary function test abnormality) is currently proposed as a way to identify the population at risk for the development of COPD.[6] Some patients may demonstrate these clinical findings for many years before developing signs and symptoms of airway limitation. However, recent research has not proven stage 0 to be a predictor of future disease.[11,12] Once COPD is established, expiratory flow rates measured during stable periods are good indicators of the progression of COPD. The patient's age, severity of airway obstruction as measured by FEV_1 and level of dyspnea are correlates of mortality.[6,13,14]

Asthma

Asthma is a common chronic pulmonary disease, affecting approximately 14.9 million persons.[15] The disease is characterized by episodic periods of reversible airway narrowing in the presence of aeroallergens, irritants, or exercise. Airway narrowing is due to inflammation, smooth muscle, *bronchospasm,* and increased airway secretions.[16] These attacks improve either spontaneously or with medical intervention and are interspersed with intervals that are symptom free.

Diagnosis

The diagnosis of asthma is clinically based on a history of episodic wheezing, shortness of breath, tightness in the chest and/or coughing which may be worse at night in the absence of any other obvious cause. The forced expiratory volume in one second (FEV_1) during exacerbations will be less than 80 percent of the predicted value. With the use of a rescue drug (inhaled short-acting $beta_2$ agonist), an improvement of at least 12 percent in FEV_1 should be demonstrated.[17]

Etiology

There is an association between asthma and allergy. Airway hyperreactivity, genetic predisposition, indoor and outdoor environmental irritants, infections, and active airway inflammation has been implicated in the development of asthma.[17,18] Symptoms of asthma may begin at any age.

Pathophysiology

The major physiological manifestation of asthma is widespread narrowing of the airways in response to a trigger, such as a cold environment or other irritants, infections, or cigarette smoke. The airway narrowing occurs as a result of eosinophilic inflammation of the bronchial mucosa, bronchospasm, and increased bronchial secretions. The narrowed airways increase the resistance to airflow and cause air trapping, leading to hyperinflation. These narrowed airways provide an abnormal distribution of ventilation to the alveoli. Even during periods of remission, some degree of airway inflammation is present.

Clinical Presentation

The clinical symptoms of asthma are cough, dyspnea, and wheezing during quiet or forced exhalation. During an acute exacerbation, the chest is usually held in an expanded position, indicating that hyperinflation of the lungs has occurred. Accessory muscles of ventilation are used for breathing. Intercostal, supraclavicular, and substernal *retractions* may be present on inspiration. Wheezing may occur during expiration and crackles may be present. With severe airway obstruction, breath sounds may markedly decrease owing to poor air movement and wheezing may be present not only throughout inhalation, but may also become present on inspiration.

Chest radiographs taken during an asthmatic exacerbation usually indicate hyperinflation, as evidenced by an increase in the AP diameter of the chest and hyperlucency of the lung fields. Less commonly, chest radiographs may reveal areas of infiltrate or **atelectasis** from the bronchial obstruction. Normal chest radiographs can be seen between asthmatic exacerbations.

The most consistent change during an exacerbation of asthma is decreased expiratory flow rates (FEV_1). Residual volume and functional residual capacity are increased because of air trapping at the expense of vital capacity and inspiratory reserve volume, which are reduced. The reversibility of these pulmonary function test abnormalities is characteristic of asthma. During remission, the patient with asthma may have normal or near-normal values.

The most common arterial blood gas finding during an asthmatic exacerbation is mild to moderate hypoxemia. Usually some degree of hypocapnia is present secondary to hyperventilation. With severe attacks, hypoxemia may be more pronounced and with further clinical deterioration, hypercapnia occurs, indicating the patient is exhausted and respiratory failure may follow.

Clinical Course

By the time adulthood is reached, many children with asthma no longer have symptoms of the disease.[19,20] When the onset of symptoms begins later in life, the clinical course is usually more progressive, showing changes in pulmonary function tests even during periods of remission. Airway remodeling in response to the chronic eosinophilic airway inflammation is thought to be responsible for the progressive nature of the disease.

Cystic Fibrosis

Cystic fibrosis (CF) affects the excretory glands of the body. Secretions made by these glands are thicker, more viscous and can affect a number of systems of the body: pulmonary, pancreatic, hepatic, sinus, and reproductive. Dysfunction of the pulmonary system is the most common cause of morbidity and mortality in patients with CF. Thickened pulmonary secretions will narrow or obstruct airways leading to hyperinflation, infection, and tissue destruction. Other presentations may occur due to the affect of the disease on other organ systems such as failure to thrive, diabetes, sinusitis, biliary disorders, and infertility.

Etiology

CF is a genetic pulmonary disease transmitted by an autosomal recessive trait. The incidence of disease in children is approximately 1 in 2,500 live births.[21] Caucasians make up 94.6 percent of all cases of CF in the United States. CF is less common in the Hispanic (white and black) population (6.4 percent) and is rare in the African-American population (3.7 percent).[21] The CF gene (cystic fibrosis transmembrane regulator or CFTR) has been identified on the long arm of chromosome 7. The CFTR functions as a chloride channel in epithelial cells. More than 1,000 mutations of this gene have been described and grouped into six different classes. The most common defect is class 2: defective processing.[22]

Pathophysiology

Chronic pulmonary disease in CF is related to the abnormally viscous mucus secreted by the tracheobronchial tree. The function of the mucociliary transport system is impaired by the altered secretions, resulting in airway obstruction and hyperinflation. Exaggerated and sustained neutrophilic airway inflammation in response to infection is also a feature of this disease.[23] Partial or complete obstruction of the airways reduces ventilation to the alveolar units. Ventilation and perfusion within the lungs are uneven. Fibrotic changes are ultimately found in the lung parenchyma.

Diagnosis

The diagnosis of CF may be suspected in patients who present with a positive family history of the disease, with recurrent respiratory infections from *Staphylococcus aureus* and *Pseudomonas aeruginosa,* or with a diagnosis of malnutrition and/or failure to thrive. A chloride concentration of 60 mEq/L found in the sweat of children is a positive test for the diagnosis of CF. Genotyping for the most common CFTR mutations can also be done.

Clinical Presentation

The clinical presentation of CF can be related to any number of involved systems. Failure to thrive due to gastrointestinal dysfunction, diabetes due to pancreatic dysfunction or frequent respiratory infections are all possible presentations of the disease. The severity of the disease, while quite variable, has been linked to the classification of the CFTR mutation.[22]

With pulmonary involvement, a patient presents with thick bronchial secretions that may be difficult to clear. With advancing disease, the chest wall will become "barreled" with an increased AP diameter and an increased dorsal kyphosis. Hyperinflation causes a decrease in thoracic excursion. Breath sounds may be decreased with adventitious sounds of crackles and wheezes. Hypertrophy of accessory muscles of ventilation, pursed-lip breathing, cyanosis, and digital clubbing may all be present.

Pulmonary function studies show obstructive impairments including decreased FEV_1, decreased FVC, increased residual volume, and increased FRC. The abnormal ventilation–perfusion relationship within the lungs results in hypoxemia and hypercapnia, as shown by arterial blood gas analysis. As the disease progresses, destruction of the alveolar capillary network causes pulmonary hypertension and cor pulmonale. In advanced disease, chest radiographs show diffuse hyperinflation, increased lung marking, and atelectasis.

Course and Prognosis

Although some patients die in infancy and early childhood, the majority of patients currently survive into adulthood. Life expectancy continues to increase owing to advances in early diagnosis and improved medical management. The predicted survival age of patients with CF was 31.6 years in 2002, a remarkable improvement from 1955, when few children made it to school age.[21] Respiratory failure is the most frequent cause of death in patients with CF. Therefore, treatment of the pulmonary dysfunction including removal of the abnormal secretions and prompt treatment of pulmonary infections, is key to the management of CF. Gastrointestinal dysfunction from CF can be aided by proper diet, vitamin supplements, and replacement of pancreatic enzymes. Aerobic fitness is a strong correlate with 8-year survival.[24] Nutritional status is also a powerful predictor of prognosis.[25]

Restrictive Lung Disease

Restrictive lung disease is a grouping of diseases with differing etiologies that result in a difficulty in expanding the lungs and a reduction in lung volume. This restriction can come from diseases of the alveolar parenchyma and/or the pleura, changes in the chest wall or an alteration in the neuromuscular apparatus of the thorax. For the purpose of this discussion, those diseases most likely to be encountered in a pulmonary rehabilitation setting—restrictive diseases of the lung parenchyma and pleura—will be presented.

Etiology

This group of disorders has a variety of causes. Numerous agents, such as radiation therapy, inorganic dust, inhalation of noxious gases, oxygen toxicity, and asbestos exposure can cause damage to the pulmonary parenchyma and pleura and result in restrictive pulmonary disease. The most common restrictive lung disease is *idiopathic pulmonary fibrosis (IPF)*. The etiology of IPF is not known; however, there is an immunological reaction in some cases.

Pathophysiology

The particular changes occurring within the lung tissue (parenchyma) and pleura depend on the etiological factors of restrictive disease. Parenchymal changes often begin with chronic inflammation and a thickening of the alveoli and interstitium. As the disease progresses, distal airspaces become fibrosed, making them more resistant to expansion (i.e., less distensible). Consequently, lung volumes are reduced. A reduced pulmonary vascular bed eventually leads to hypoxemia and cor pulmonale. *Asbestosis* (asbestos- induced pulmonary fibrosis) is a type of restrictive lung disease that shows both parenchymal fibrosis and pleura involvement in the form of pleural plaques. These changes may be due to injury or inflammatory reactions that ultimately lead to parenchymal and pleural fibrosis.

Clinical Presentation

Dyspnea is the classic symptom of restrictive lung diseases. A nonproductive cough is often encountered; weakness and early fatigue are also common. Signs of restrictive lung disease include rapid, shallow breathing; limited chest expansion; crackles, especially over the lower lung fields; digital clubbing; and cyanosis.[26]

In the early stages of parenchymal restrictive disease, the chest radiograph reveals fine interstitial markings defined as a ground glass appearance, honeycombing, visible intralobular bronchioles, and fibrotic consolidations. Reduction in lung volumes can be seen serially on chest radiographs. Radiographic evidence of pleural involvement, when present, can also be seen.

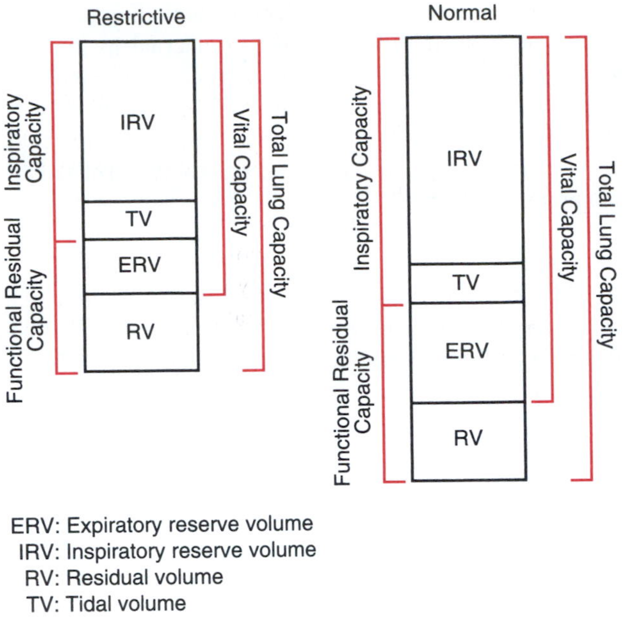

Figure 15.6 Lung volumes of a healthy pulmonary system compared with the lung volumes found in restrictive disease. (Adapted from Rothstein, J, Roy, S, and Wolf, S: The Rehabilitation Specialist's Handbook. FA Davis, Philadelphia, 2005, p 428, with permission.)

Pulmonary function tests reveal a reduction in VC, FRC, and TLC. Residual volume may be normal or near normal, and expiratory flow rates remain near normal. Figure 15.6 shows the changes in lung volumes and capacities that occur in restrictive pulmonary disease.

Arterial blood studies show varying degrees of hypoxemia and hypocapnea. Hypoxemia at rest is usually exacerbated by exercise. Exercise may significantly lower oxygenation, even for patients with normal oxygenation at rest.

Course and Prognosis

Restrictive pulmonary disease may have a slow onset but is chronic and progressive in nature. Survival depends on the type of restrictive disease, the etiological factors, and the treatment. Almost 50 percent of patients with IPF die within 5 years of diagnosis.[26] Chest radiographs are insensitive indicators of the extent of the disease. Hypercapnea is an ominous sign, indicating the terminal stage of pulmonary fibrosis.

Medical Management

Medical management of chronic pulmonary disease includes smoking cessation, pharmacological agents, and the use supplemental oxygen. The following discussion provides a brief description of these medical interventions.

Smoking Cessation

Smoking is the major causal agent in the development of COPD, as well as a contributing cause to many other disease processes. Smoking cessation is the most important intervention for improving the outcomes of patients with COPD.[27] Smoking increases the annual rate of decline of lung function as measured by FEV_1 from –25 ml/year in a non-smoker to –40 ml/year in a smoker.[28] Smoking cessation shows an initial small recovery (2 percent) in FEV_1, but more importantly, the annual rate of decline of lung function was approximately half the rate of continuing smokers.[29] Therefore, special focus on the benefits of being a nonsmoker and intervention for successful smoking cessation should be included in the medical management of patients with pulmonary disease.

There are many types of smoking cessation programs, such as education, behavior modification, "cold turkey," diversion therapy, aversion therapy, nicotine gum, or nicotine patch. Advice from a clinician, counseling, and behavior therapies can increase the success of a patient's intent to quit smoking. Nicotine replacement therapy either by patch, gum, or spray may improve cessation rates even further.[5] In the Lung Health Study, a comprehensive treatment approach including physician recommendation, group participation with a health educator, behavior modification, nicotine replacement therapy, and the use of inhalers had an impressive 59 percent cessation rate among participants who were followed at 4 months. A 22 percent cessation rate among participants was found at the end of 5 years.[30,31] While this amount of intervention may not be possible for most patients, it appears that any and all attempts to encourage smoking cessation are worthwhile. The regional offices of the American Lung Association and the American Cancer Society are good resources for local smoking cessation programs.

Pharmacological Management

Pharmacological agents provide relief from the symptoms of chronic lung disease and improvement in the health and functional status of individuals with lung disease. Each different pulmonary diagnosis and the severity of that disease will require a tailored plan of care. Table 15.2 shows the recommended treatments according to the severity of COPD as described by the GOLD standards.[6]

It is not unusual for patients to be on a combination of drugs for the management of their pulmonary disease. These drugs can affect exercise performance, heart rate, and blood pressure, both at rest and with exercise. This

Table 15.2 Suggested Pharmacological Management Based on the GOLD Classification of Severity of Lung Disease.

Old	0: At Risk	I: Mild	II: Moderate		III: Severe
			IIA	IIB	
New	**0: At Risk**	**I: Mild**	**II: Moderate**	**III: Severe**	**IV: Very Severe**
Characteristics	• Chronic symptoms • Exposure to risk factors • Normal spirometry	• $FEV_1/FVC < 70\%$ • $FEV_1 \geq 80\%$ • With or without symptoms	• $FEV_1/FVC < 70\%$ • $50\% \leq FEV_1 < 80\%$ • With or without symptoms	• $FEV_1/FVC < 70\%$ • $30\% \leq FEV_1 < 50\%$ • With or without symptoms	• $FEV_1/FVC < 70\%$ • $FEV_1 < 30\%$ or $FEV_1 < 50\%$ predicted plus chronic respiratory failure
	Avoidance of risk factor(s); influenza vaccination				
		Add short-acting bronchodilator when needed			
			Add regular treatment with one or more long-acting bronchodilators *Add* rehabilitation		
				Add inhaled glucocorticosteroids if repeated exacerbations	
					Add long-term oxygen if chronic respiratory failure *Consider* surgical treatments

Reprinted with permission, NILBI/WHO Global Initiative for Chronic Obstructive Lung Disease (GOLD) workshop summary.[6]

Table 15.3 Common Drugs Used in the Medical Management of Patients with Chronic Pulmonary Disease

	Drug	Trade Name	Action	Adverse Reactions
Maintenance	Anticholinergic	Atrovent	Bronchodilation	Throat irritation Drying of tracheal secretions Tachycardia Palpitations
	Long-acting Beta$_2$ agonist	Serevent	Bronchodilation	Tachycardia Palpitations GI distress Nervousness Tremor Headache Dizziness
	Steroids	Flovent Prednisone	Reduces the inflammatory response	Increase BP Sodium retention (edema) Muscle wasting Osteoporosis GI irritation Atherosclerosis Hypercholesterolemia Increased susceptibility to infection
	Cromolyn sodium	Intal	Prevents the inflammatory response	Throat irritation Cough Bronchospasm
	Leukotriene receptor antagonist	Singulair	Blocks allergic reaction (blocking leukotrienes)	GI distress Sore throat Upper respiratory tract infection Dizziness Headache Nasal congestion
Rescue	Short-acting Beta$_2$ agonist	Albuterol Ventolin	Bronchodilation	Tachycardia Palpitations GI distress Nervousness Tremor Headache Dizziness

discussion will provide information on both maintenance drugs and rescue drugs used in the care of patients with pulmonary disease. Table 15.3 provides basic information on the pharmacological management of lung disease.

Maintenance Drugs

This category of drugs is used to reduce or minimize pulmonary symptoms throughout the day. These drugs tend to be taken on a regular schedule to keep symptoms at bay. Anticholinergics, long acting beta$_2$ agonists, steroids, cromolyn sodium, and leukotriene antagonists are commonly prescribed drugs for patients with chronic pulmonary disease. Theophylline, while an effective drug for the treatment of chronic pulmonary diseases, is less frequently prescribed as there are safer medications available for the maintenance of chronic pulmonary disease. Routes of administration of maintenance drugs are usually inhalation or ingestion. When inhalation is effective, it is the advisable route of administration as it limits systemic side effects of these drugs.

Inhaled anticholinergics are a commonly prescribed drug classification for patients with COPD.[32] Their action is to promote airway smooth muscle relaxation, thus promoting bronchodilation. Inhaled long-acting beta agonists are also used to block smooth muscle constriction in patients with chronic pulmonary disease, thereby promoting bronchodilation. Steroids, either inhaled or systemic, are the mainstay of medical management of the chronic eosinophilic inflammation of asthma.[16] Steroids do not appear to have the same potent affect in the management of COPD. Therefore, inhaled steroids are used as a complement to bronchodilators. Inhaled cromolyn sodium is used to prevent the inflammatory response by stabilizing the mast cell within the alveolar units. Used prior to exposure of a known trigger for bronchoconstriction, cromolyn sodium can prevent airway narrowing before it can begin. It is therefore helpful in patients with predictable bronchoconstriction, such as exercise induced bronchospasm. Leukotriene antagonists are systemic drugs that reduce airway inflammation and relax airway smooth muscle. Again, all of these maintenance drugs are used for the long-term management of chronic lung disease. They are tailored to the severity of disease, the patient's symptoms, and response to the medication.

Rescue Drugs

Rescue drugs are used for a more immediate relief of breakthrough symptoms. Inhaled short-acting $beta_2$ agonists are used for this purpose. Patients are advised to use their prescribed inhaled short acting $beta_2$ agonist on an as needed basis, rather than a schedule. If a patient reports the frequent use of a rescue drug, it is indicative of a flaw in the maintenance regimen or a change in the patient's pulmonary status. Short acting $beta_2$ agonists can be used prior to the onset of activity to enhance exercise performance.[33]

Although the mechanism of action of each bronchodilator is different, there may be an increase in resting heart rate and blood pressure with their use. Employing the Karvonen formula for exercise intensity acknowledges the elevated resting heart rate and an appropriate target heart rate can be calculated. Other common side effects of bronchodilators include nervousness, tremor, anxiety, and nausea. The side effects of systemic steroids, including osteoporosis, myopathies, and muscle wasting, may require modifications to an exercise program such as muscle strengthening and low-impact exercise.

Antibiotics

Pulmonary infections are frequent in patients with chronic pulmonary disease. They can be devastating to the patient and cause major setbacks in pulmonary rehabilitation efforts. The early signs of an infection are often noted by some change in the patient's baseline status (i.e., a change in exercise ability, dyspnea, color or amount of sputum, or an increase in the use of rescue inhalers). Antibiotics are used to interfere with the growth and proliferation of bacteria. The action of these drugs is either bacteriostatic or bactericidal. There are many categories of antibiotics (e.g., penicillins, cephalosporins, tetracyclines) that are effective on different organisms. It is important to identify the infecting organism in order to prescribe the appropriate antibiotic. The Alliance for the Prudent Use of Antibiotics (APUA) encourages the use of antibiotics for only diagnosed bacterial infections to reduce antibiotic resistant strains of bacteria.[34]

Supplemental Oxygen

The use of supplemental oxygen has been shown to prolong the survival of patients with COPD whose resting Pa_{O_2} is lower than 60 mm Hg.[35] An absolute indication for use of long-term oxygen therapy is an arterial partial pressure of oxygen (Pa_{O_2}) of 55 mm Hg or less, which correlates with an Sa_{O_2} of 88 percent or less.[36] If a patient is limited in the ability to exercise due to dyspnea, then supplemental oxygen may be warranted.[37] Patients with nonhypoxemic COPD may be able to more rapidly increase their exercise capacity using supplemental oxygen.[38] The amount of oxygen used should be titrated individually to maintain an Sa_{O_2} of at least 90 percent, if possible.[39] There are various delivery methods available: continuous flow, pulsed flow, and reservoir are among the most common.

Surgical Management

There are few surgical options for the patient with pulmonary disease. Lung volume reduction surgery (LVRS) is a surgical technique that removes nonfunctional, overdistended lung tissue, in order to restore the normal biomechanics of the thorax. Patients with heterogeneous emphysema have areas of their lungs that are relatively nonfunctional along with functional lung tissue. The surgical procedure removes approximately 20 to 35 percent of the most diseased lung tissue, relieving the more normal tissue of its burden. The purpose of the surgical procedure is to decrease residual volume and functional residual capacity (i.e., decrease hyperinflation). This allows for a more normal resting position of the diaphragm with a possible increase in diaphragmatic excursion and more normal chest wall excursion and lung mechanics.[40] Postoperative results show variable improvements in exercise capacity, lung function, quality of life, and gas exchange in patients with moderate disease.[41] Patients with severe lung disease ($FEV_1 \leq$ to 20 percent of predicted) do not appear to benefit from this intervention. This group of patients showed both a high mortality rate and only slight improvement in functional abilities and quality of life scores.[42,43] A preoperative pulmonary rehabilitation program is advocated at many centers. Patients who participated in pulmonary rehabilitation prior to LVRS demonstrated shorter hospital stays and fewer days on mechanical ventilation.[44] Lung transplantation for end-stage pulmonary disease has an overall survival rate of

60 to 65 percent at 2 years and approximately 40 percent at 5 years.[45] The goals of lung transplantation are to restore normal lung function, restore normal exercise capacity, and prolong life.[46] People awaiting a lung transplant may include patients with emphysema, cystic fibrosis, idiopathic pulmonary fibrosis, and pulmonary hypertension. The number of patients awaiting lung transplantation continues to grow, far exceeding the number of organs available for transplantation. The average wait for a organ transplant is approximately 2.9 years, making transplantation a reality for only a small number of individuals.[47]

Physical Therapy Management

Chronic pulmonary disease and its associated dysfunction have a slow yet progressive course. The person with pulmonary dysfunction often avoids activities that result in the uncomfortable sensation of dyspnea. A slow but steady decrease in these patients' functional activities follows, resulting in a progressive aerobic deconditioning. It is not uncommon for someone with pulmonary disease to have lost many functional abilities before ever seeking medical help. The intended outcome of pulmonary rehabilitation is to interrupt this downward spiraling of physical ability, improve functional capacity, and improve quality of life.

Goals and Outcomes

The *Guide for Physical Therapist Practice* provides a general framework for physical therapy intervention for patients with impaired ventilation, respiration, and aerobic capacity and endurance associated with ventilatory pump dysfunction (Practice Pattern 6F).[48] The development of specific anticipated goals and expected outcomes for the individual patient with pulmonary impairment is based on the following general goals:

- Increased understanding of patient and family of disease process, expectations, goals, and outcomes.
- Increased cardiovascular endurance.
- Increased strength, power, and endurance of peripheral muscles.
- Improved performance of physical tasks, both basic activities of daily living and instrumental activities of daily living.
- Increased strength, power, and endurance of ventilatory muscles.
- Improved independence in airway clearance.
- Decreased work of breathing.
- Improved decision making ability regarding the use of health care resources.
- Enhanced self-management of symptoms and self-management of pulmonary disease.

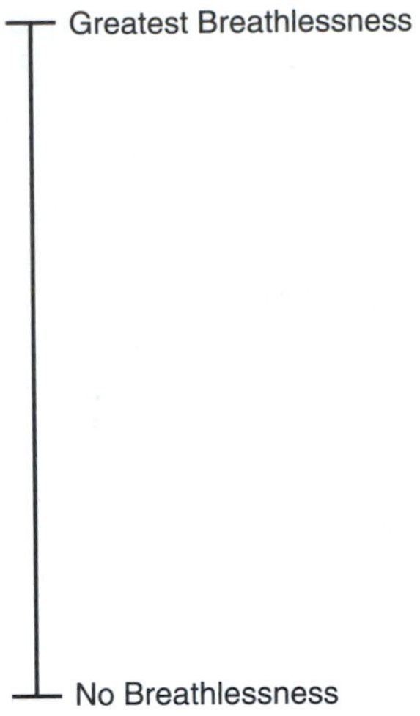

Figure 15.7 The visual analogue scale is an empty vertical line with end caps labeled "Greatest Breathlessness" and "No Breathlessness." The patient is asked to mark the point on the line that reflects his level of breathlessness. (From Mahler, D, et al.,[49] p 215, with permission.)

Examination

The examination of a patient's pulmonary status has several purposes: (1) to evaluate the appropriateness of the patient's participation in a pulmonary rehabilitation program; (2) to determine the therapeutic measures most appropriate for the participant's treatment program; (3) to monitor the participant's physiological response to exercise; and (4) to appropriately progress the participant's treatment program over time.

Patient History

A patient interview should begin with the chief complaint, the patient's perception of why pulmonary rehabilitation is being sought. Commonly, the chief complaint is often shortness of breath and/or loss of function. Quantifying dyspnea at the beginning and the end of a rehabilitation program and during periods of exacerbation can be accomplished through a visual analog scale (Fig. 15.7) or the *Baseline Dyspnea Index* (Table 15.4).[49,50] Quality of life measures such as the *SF36* or the *Chronic Respiratory Questionnaire* may also be helpful in determining the patient's baseline health-related quality of life.[51,52] A medical history contains pertinent pulmonary symptoms specific to that patient: cough, sputum production, wheezing, and shortness of breath. Occupational, social, medication, and family histories should also be recorded.

Tests and Measures

Vital Signs

Temperature and resting blood pressure, heart rate, and respiratory rate should be determined and recorded (see

Table 15.4 Baseline Dyspnea Index

Functional Impairment			Magnitude of Effort		
______	Grade 4:	*No Impairment.* Able to carry out usual activities and occupation without shortness of breath.	______	Grade 4:	*Extraordinary.* Becomes short of breath only with the greatest imaginable effort. No shortness of breath with ordinary effort.
______	Grade 3:	*Slight Impairment.* Distinct impairment in at least one activity but no activities completely abandoned. Reduction in activity at work *or* in usual activities that seems slight or not clearly caused by shortness of breath.	______	Grade 3:	*Major.* Becomes short of breath with effort distinctly submaximal. Tasks performed without pause unless the task requires extraordinary effort that may be performed with pauses.
______	Grade 2:	*Moderate Impairment.* Patient has changed jobs *and/or* has abandoned at least one usual activity due to shortness of breath.	______	Grade 2:	*Moderate.* Becomes short of breath with moderate effort. Tasks performed with occasional pauses and require more time to complete than the average person.
______	Grade 1:	*Severe Impairment.* Patient unable to work *or* has given up most or all customary activities due to shortness of breath.	______	Grade 1:	*Light.* Becomes short of breath with little effort. Tasks performed with little effort or more difficult tasks with frequent pauses and requiring 50–100% longer to complete than the average person might require.
______	Grade 0:	*Very Severe Impairment.* Unable to work *and* has given up most or all customary activities due to shortness of breath.	______	Grade 0:	*No Effort.* Becomes short of breath at rest, while sitting, or lying down.
______	W:	*Amount Uncertain.* Patient is impaired owing to shortness of breath, but amount cannot be specified. Details are not sufficient to allow impairment to be categorized.	______	W:	*Amount Uncertain.* Patient has limited exertional capacity due to shortness of breath, but amount cannot be specified. Details are not sufficient to allow impairment to be categorized.
______	X:	*Unknown.* Information unavailable regarding impairment.	______	X:	*Unknown.* Information unavailable regarding limitation of effort.
______	Y:	*Impaired for Reasons Other than Shortness of Breath.* For example, musculoskeletal problem or chest pain.	______	Y:	*Impaired for Reasons Other than Shortness of Breath.* For example, musculoskeletal problem or chest pain.
Magnitude of Task					
______	Grade 4:	*Extraordinary.* Becomes short of breath only with extraordinary activity, such as carrying very heavy loads on the level, lighter loads uphill, or running. No shortness of breath with ordinary tasks.			
______	Grade 3:	*Major.* Becomes short of breath only with such major activities as walking up a steep hill, climbing more than three flights of stairs, or carrying a moderate load on the level.			
______	Grade 2:	*Moderate.* Becomes short of breath with moderate or average tasks, such as walking up a gradual hill, climbing less than three flights of stairs, or carrying a light load on the level.			
______	Grade 1:	*Light.* Becomes short of breath with light activities, such as walking on the level, washing, standing, or shopping.			
______	Grade 0:	*No Task.* Becomes short of breath at rest, while sitting, or lying down.			
______	W:	*Amount Uncertain.* Patient has limited exertional capacity due to shortness of breath, but amount cannot be specified. Details are not sufficient to allow impairment to be categorized.			
______	X:	*Unknown.* Information unavailable regarding limitation of magnitude of task.			
______	Y:	*Impaired for Reasons Other than Shortness of Breath.* For example, musculoskeletal problem or chest pain.			

From Mahler, D, et al.,[49] p 399, with permission.

Chapter 4). An individual's height should be measured as there is a direct relationship between height and lung volume. Weight should be measured on a standard scale and each subsequent measure should be performed on the same scale.

Observation, Inspection, and Palpation

By observing the neck and shoulders of a patient with pulmonary disease, the use of accessory muscles of ventilation can be observed. A normal configuration of the thorax reveals a ratio of AP to lateral diameter of 2:1. Destruction of the lung parenchyma results in an increase in the AP diameter and a reduction of this ratio (up to 1:1). During inhalation and exhalation both sides of the thorax should move symmetrically.

Cyanosis is a bluish discoloration of the skin that can be observed periorally, periorbitally, and in nail beds; it indicates acute hypoxemia. An indicator of more chronic hypoxemia is digital clubbing of the fingers and toes. In *clubbing*, there is an increase in the angle created by the distal phalanx and the point where the nail exits from the digit. The tip of the distal phalanx becomes bulbous (Fig 15.8).

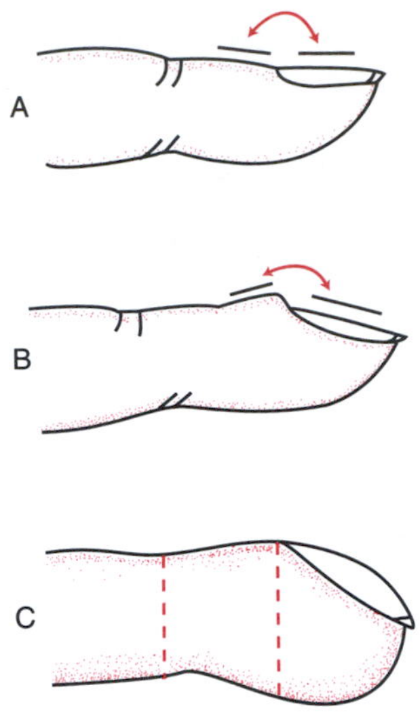

Figure 15.8 Digital clubbing is a sign of chronic tissue hypoxia. (From Effgen, S: Pediatric Physical Therapy, FA Davis, Philadelphia, 2004, p 307, with permission.)

Auscultation of the Lungs

Auscultation involves listening over the chest wall as gas enters and exits the lungs. To perform auscultation of the lungs, a stethoscope is placed firmly on the patient's thorax anteriorly, laterally, and posteriorly. The patient is asked to inspire fully through an open mouth, then to exhale quietly. Inhalation and the beginning of exhalation normally produce a soft rustling sound. The end of exhalation is normally silent. This characteristic of a normal breath sound is termed *vesicular.* When a louder, more hollow and echoing sound occupies a larger portion of the ventilatory cycle, the breath sounds are referred to as *bronchial.* When the breath sounds are very quiet and barely audible, they are termed *decreased.* These three terms—vesicular, bronchial, and decreased—allow the listener to describe the intensity of the breath sound.[53]

In addition to the normal and abnormal intensity of the breath sound, there may be additional sounds and vibrations heard during auscultation. These are called *adventitious breath sounds*. These sounds are superimposed on the previously described intensity of the breath sound. According to the American College of Chest Physicians and the American Thoracic Society, there are two types of adventitious sounds: crackles and wheezes.[54] *Crackles*, historically termed rales, sound like the rustling of cellophane. *Wheezes* are more musical in nature. A decrease in the size of the lumen of the airway will create a wheezing sound, much as stretching the neck of an inflated balloon narrows the passageway through which air must escape and produces a whistling sound.

Measurement of Strength

Patients with pulmonary disease may show peripheral and/or ventilatory muscle weakness due to deconditioning, malnutrition, chronic hypoxemia, and hypercapnea or steroid use.[55] Peripheral and ventilatory muscle weakness can contribute to exercise limitations and an inability to perform activities of daily living.[56] Therefore, measurement of peripheral muscle strength and maximal inspiratory pressure should be assessed to determine the need for strength training during rehabilitation.

Laboratory Tests

Various laboratory studies may be performed to examine patients with pulmonary disease. These include radiology, pulmonary function tests (PFTs), graded exercise tests (GXT), arterial blood gas (ABG) analysis, oxygen saturation measurements (Sao_2), and electocardiograms.

Exercise Testing in Patients with Pulmonary Disease

A determination of functional capacity is part of the examination of a patient with pulmonary disease. A *graded exercise test* (GXT, exercise tolerance test) can provide the objective information to (1) document a patient's symptomatology and physical impairment; (2) prescribe safe exercise; (3) document changes in oxygenation during exercise and determine the need for supplemental oxygen; and (4) identify any changes in pulmonary function during exercise intervention.

There are a number of testing methods available to determine the maximal oxygen consumption and functional abilities of patients with pulmonary disease. A GXT protocol, usually utilizing a treadmill or cycle ergometer, gradually increases exercise intensity in order to stress the patient with pulmonary dysfunction to the point of limitation. Vital signs are monitored throughout the test to ensure safety. The ECG, continuously recorded during exercise, records the exercise heart rate and electrical activity of the cardiac conduction system. Blood pressure measurements

Table 15.5 Exercise Testing Protocols Used for the Patient with Pulmonary Disease

Test	Author	Protocol
Walk Test (6- or 12-minute)	American Thoracic Society/ American College of Chest Physicians[57]	Ambulate (walk) as far as possible in the allotted time
10-M Shuttle Test	Revill[59]	Walking between two markers, 10 m apart, at increasing walking velocities, which are synchronized to an auditory signal or metronome
Cycle tests	Jones[60]	Begin at 100 kpm, increase 100 kpm every minute
	Berman[61]	Begin at 100 kpm, increase 100 kpm every minute, or 50 kpm if FEV_1 is <1 L/s
Treadmill tests	Bruce[62]	Begin at 1.7 mph, 10% treadmill grade; increase both speed and grade every 3 min
	Naughton[63]	Begin at 1.2 mph 0% grade; increase speed and 3% grade every 2 min
	Balke-Ware and Ware[64]	Begin at constant speed of 3.3 mph, increase grade 3.5% every min

recorded at 1- to 3-minute intervals during exercise and during recovery from the test, provide information on the hemodynamic status of the patient. ABGs measured during exercise provide the best method for determining arterial oxygenation and the adequacy of alveolar ventilation, though the invasive nature of this test limits its use. Arterial oxygen saturation monitoring provides less information, but the noninvasive nature of the test makes its use more widespread. A number of these protocols are outlined in Table 15.5.[57–64]

The symptom-limited GXT requires the patient to continue the exercise protocol until symptoms dictate cessation. Criteria for stopping a pulmonary exercise test are presented in Box 15.1.

The *10-Meter Shuttle Test (10-m Shuttle)* is a walking protocol that uses a recorded audio signal to dictate incremental walking speeds on a level 10-meter field. The results of the 10-m Shuttle have a positive correlation with $\dot{V}O_2$.[59] The *12- or 6-Minute Walk Test* asks a patient to cover as much distance as possible in the time frame given. The 12- and 6-Minute Walk Tests have been shown to be a good predictor of functional abilities.[58] Both the 10-m Shuttle and the timed walk tests are easy to administer and the ready availability of the required equipment make them good tools for pre- and post-exercise measurements. Refer to the section on exercise testing in Chapter 16 for more information on exercise protocols.

Determination of functional capacity using by an exercise test allows for appropriate vocational counseling and provides the necessary documentation for addressing disability.[65] The need for supplemental oxygen is indicated if a patient becomes hypoxemic during the exercise test session. A decrease in the Pa_{O_2} of less than 55 mm Hg, corresponding to an Sa_{O_2} of 88 percent or less, are

Box 15.1 Graded Exercise Test Termination Criteria

1. Maximal shortness of breath
2. A fall in Pa_{O_2} of greater than 20 mm Hg or a Pa_{O_2} less than 55 mm Hg
3. A rise in Pa_{CO_2} of greater than 10 mm Hg or greater than 65 mm Hg
4. Cardiac ischemia or arrhythmias
5. Symptoms of fatigue
6. Increase in diastolic blood pressure readings of 20 mm Hg, systolic hypertension greater than 250 mm Hg, decrease in blood pressure with increasing workloads
7. Leg pain
8. Total fatigue
9. Signs of insufficient cardiac output
10. Reaching a ventilatory maximum

From Brannon, F, et al: Cardiopulmonary Rehabilitation: Basic Theory and Application. FA Davis, Philadelphia, 1998, p 300, with permission.

indications of a need for oxygen supplementation during exercise.[39,66]

PFTs performed prior to and following an exercise test document the effects of exercise on lung function. A reduction of 15 percent in FEV_1 is an indication of a positive pulmonary test.[66] Finally, a prescription for exercise that will safely promote cardiopulmonary fitness can be developed based on the GXT. This is the topic of the next section.

Exercise Prescription

Exercise prescription incorporates four variables that together provide an individually tailored exercise formula designed to produce an increase in functional capacity. These variables are mode, intensity, duration, and frequency.

Mode

Any type of sustained **aerobic exercise** is recommended for pulmonary rehabilitation. Lower extremity (LE) activities, including walking, jogging, rowing, cycling, and swimming, are recommended to improve exercise tolerance. Upper extremity (UE) aerobic exercise, arm ergometry, or free weights should also be included. The combination of UE and LE training in a rehabilitation program results in improved functional status compared to either exercise alone.[67] Many programs utilize a circuit approach to train different muscle groups and maintain the participant's interest.

Intensity

Three parameters used to prescribe exercise intensity are oxygen consumption, heart rate, and a *Rating of Perceived Exertion/Shortness of Breath*. Below is a discussion of each means of prescribing exercise intensity.

Exercise Intensity as a Percent of $\dot{V}O_{2MAX}$

A GXT reports functional capacity in terms of $\dot{V}O_{2max}$. Exercise intensity can be prescribed using 60 to 75 percent of the maximum $\dot{V}O_2$ achieved on a GXT. Patients with severe pulmonary disease may not tolerate long periods of activity at this level. Lowering exercise intensity may not be the answer to this situation as lesser to no training effects have been found by using lower percentages of $\dot{V}O_2$.[68] Rather, exercise will be tolerated and a training effect achieved when short bursts of activity at up to 60 to 80 and even up to 95 percent of $\dot{V}O_{2max}$ are interspersed with rest periods.[69,70]

Exercise Intensity as a Percent of Heart Rate Reserve

While using a percentage of $\dot{V}O_2$ may be the most accurate method of prescribing exercise from a graded exercise test, it does not give the clinician a means to monitor exercise intensity during the performance of the exercise session. Exercising heart rate is a commonly used parameter for prescribing exercise intensity. The *target heart rate range (THRR)* defines safety guidelines for exercise intensity during the treatment session. The **target heart rate (THR)** for a specific patient defines the most appropriate heart rate within the prescribed target heart rate range to ensure endurance training.

A common method to determine the THRR and the THR for patient populations is the **heart rate reserve method** or *Karvonen's formula*.[64] The heart rate reserve is the difference between the resting heart rate (HR_{rest}) in the seated position and the maximal heart rate (HR_{max}) achieved on a GXT. To calculate the THRR, percentages of the heart rate reserve are added to the resting heart rate. The equation for determining the THRR is:

$$THRR = [(HR_{max} - HR_{rest}) \times 0.40 \text{ and } 0.85] + HR_{rest}$$

For example, on a GXT a patient achieved a maximal heart rate of 165 beats per minute (b/min). Resting heart rate was 85 beats/min. The heart rate reserve is calculated to be 165 − 85 = 80 beats/min; 40 percent of 80 beats/min[32] + resting heart rate[85] = 117 beats/min; 85 percent of 80 beats/min[68] + resting heart rate[85] = 153 beats/min. Thus, for this patient, a THRR of 117 to 153 beats/min has been calculated.

Determining the appropriate THR (i.e., where in this wide range of 117 to 153 beats/min to exercise) requires careful consideration of individual abilities and functional limitations. Correlating the THR with a percent of $\dot{V}O_{2max}$ from the exercise test will help determine the most appropriate exercise intensity. Patients with mild to moderate pulmonary disease do not usually have a pulmonary limitation to exercise, therefore, a maximal cardiovascular exercise test is likely to have been performed. For these patients, the THR is often calculated using a minimum of 50 percent and a maximum of 60 to 70 percent of the heart rate reserve. In the above example, a THR of 120 to 136 beats/min would ensure cardiovascular training. Patients with severe pulmonary impairment will likely approach their ventilatory maximum before their cardiovascular maximum is reached; that is, their maximal exercise heart rate may be lower than their cardiovascular heart rate maximum owing to pulmonary constraints. For these patients, exercise intensities that approach their maximum ventilatory limits or the upper end of the THRR, 70 to 85 percent of heart rate reserve, can be used.[71] In the example, this would be a THR of 136 to 148 beats/minute. It should be emphasized that exercise intensity should be prescribed with an upper and lower heart rate limit, not a single number.

Exercise Intensity by Rating Perceived Exertion

Using heart rate parameters for the prescription of exercise intensity does not directly address the cause of physical limitation in patients with low ventilatory reserves. Rating of perceived exertion (i.e., the Borg RPE scales®) provide important information about how the patient feels or perceives the intensity of exercise, i.e., how heavy or strenuous the exercise feels to the patient. The perceptions are based on the strain and fatigue of exercising muscles (peripheral factors) and feelings of breathlessness or aches in the chest (central factors).[72] The Borg CR10 scale uses scores that range from 0 (nothing at all) to 10 (extremely strong, maximum perception) (Table 15.6). RPE is a valid and reliable indicator of an individual's exercise tolerance and is highly correlated with HR and VO_2. Perceived shortness of breath (dyspnea) has been examined using a similar rating scale and shown to correlate with VO_2[73] (Table 15.7). Ratings between 3 (moderate shortness of breath) and 6 (between severe and very severe shortness of breath) define the range within which patients with pulmonary dysfunction generally exercise. A rating of 3 corresponds to approximately 50 percent of VO_{2max}. A rating of 6 corresponds to approximately 85 percent of VO_{2max}.[66]

The prescription for exercise intensity should incorporate symptoms of shortness of breath and perceived exertion, rather than being based solely on THR, fixed work levels, or $\dot{V}O_2$. Clinicians often prefer to prescribe exercise by utilizing a combination of prescription by THR and RPE or perceived shortness of breath parameters.

Table 15.6 Rating of Perceived Exertion: The Borg CR10 Scale

The Borg CR10 Scale®		
0	Nothing at all	"No P"
0.3		
0.5	Extremely weak	Just noticeable
1	Very weak	
1.5		
2	Weak	Light
2.5		
3	Moderate	
4		
5	Strong	Heavy
6		
7	Very strong	
8		
9		
10	Extremely strong	"Max P"
11		
•	Absolute maximum	Highest possible

For correct usage of the scale, the exact design and instructions given in Borg's folders must be followed. See Borg, G., 1998, Borg's Perceived Exertion and Pain Scales. Human Kinetics, Champaign, IL or www.borgproducts.com. With permission.

Table 15.7 Rating of Perceived Shortness of Breath

Scale	Perceived Shortness of Breath
0	Nothing at all
0.5	Very, very slight (just noticeable)
1	Very slight
2	Slight
3	Moderate
4	Somewhat severe
5	Severe
6	
7	Very severe
8	
9	Very, very severe (almost maximal)
10	Maximal

Duration

Exercising within the THR for at least 20 to 30 minutes is recommended. The duration of the training session varies according to patient tolerance, with some participants not being able to maintain continuous exercise for 20 to 30 minutes. Frequent rest periods can be interspersed with exercise to accomplish a total of 20 to 30 minutes of discontinuous exercise.

Frequency

The frequency of exercise refers to the number of sessions performed on a weekly basis during the exercise training period. The frequency of exercise is often dependent on the intensity that can be achieved and the duration that can be maintained. If 20 to 30 minutes of continuous aerobic exercise can be accomplished within the THR, then three to five evenly spaced workouts per week are recommended. More frequent exercise sessions are recommended for patients with lower functional abilities. One to two daily sessions are advisable for patients with very low functional work capacities.

Pulmonary Rehabilitation

Aerobic Training

The aerobic training portion of a pulmonary rehabilitation session includes the following components: check-in, warm-up, aerobic exercise, and cool-down periods. The check-in period is a time to take vital signs, including resting heart rate, respiratory rate, and blood pressure; auscultation of the lungs, and weight. It is also the time to discuss with patients their medication schedule, any problems they have encountered, and any changes that need to be noted and addressed by a member of the pulmonary rehabilitation team. If the patient was found to have a decrease in FEV_1 of 10 percent or more on the GXT, a prescribed inhaler should be used at this time. If a patient was found to have a significant decrease in oxygenation with exercise, the supplemental oxygen should be readied at this time.

Prior to the aerobic period of exercise, the participant performs stretching exercises to help prevent musculoskeletal injuries. Stretching exercises should be performed during exhalation to prevent a Valsalva maneuver, which would worsen a participant's pulmonary capabilities. Patients often use accessory muscles of ventilation during the exercise program; therefore, the neck and upper extremities should be incorporated into the stretching program. The warm-up component is a time to slowly increase the HR and BP to ready the cardiovascular system for aerobic exercise. This is usually accomplished by performing the same mode of exercise that will be used in the aerobic portion of the program but at a lower intensity, with an emphasis on controlled breathing. For example, cycling with no resistance could be used as a warm-up activity for a patient with a biking program. The warm-up portion of the program lasts between 5 and 15 minutes.

The aerobic portion of the exercise session consists of a mode or modes of aerobic activity at the appropriate intensity to maintain the THR of the exercise prescription for the advised duration. This portion of the program lasts for at least 20 minutes. The participant can be monitored by using a rating of perceived shortness of breath, perceived exertion, heart rate values, respiratory rate, and oximetry. The aerobic training period should be followed immediately by a cool-down period. This consists of 5 to 15 minutes of low-level aerobic activities that slowly return the cardiovascular system to near pre-exercise levels. Again, there is an emphasis on controlled breathing. Finally, stretching exercises are repeated to maintain joint and muscle integrity and to help prevent injury.

Strength Training

Strength of both upper and lower extremities will increase with appropriate training.[56] Strength training can use similar modes of exercise as the endurance training with a change to higher resistance and lower repetitions (i.e., increase the grade of treadmill, increase resistance on stationary cycle or arm ergometer), or weight training of the involved muscle groups can be prescribed. Participants should be encouraged to refrain from using the Valsalva maneuver during training as this may impair ventilatory exchange and effect exercise performance.

Exercise Progression

Modifications in the duration and intensity of the exercise session should be made as an individual physiologically adapts to exercise. Exercise progression is appropriate when the individual perceives the intensity of the exercise session to be easier or when the same exercise intensity is performed with a lesser degree of shortness of breath and lower heart rate.

Exercise progression should first be directed toward increasing the duration of exercise by extending the amount of time spent in continuous aerobic activity and decreasing the amount of time spent in rest periods. The goal of duration progression is to achieve at least 20 minutes of continuous aerobic activity without the need for a rest. When 20 minutes of activity can be accomplished, then an increase in exercise intensity can be proposed. Frequency should be adjusted as necessary, based on duration and intensity.

A patient's age, functional ability, symptoms, and severity of disease must be considered prior to any change in the exercise prescription. When considerable change in a participant's ability has occurred, it is advisable to perform a new GXT. The new exercise prescription will allow for a safe and comfortable progression of exercise under controlled guidance.

Program Duration

Improved exercise tolerance can occur during an inpatient hospital admission, as an outpatient, or with a program of home-based care.[1] Because of the limited length of stays for many hospital admissions, most increases in functional capacity occur during an outpatient or home program. Generally, conditioning exercises are conducted up to three times per week over a course of 6 to 8 weeks. At the end of the rehabilitation program, both quality of life measurements and functional abilities should be reexamined. An exit exercise test may be performed to assess the exercise prescription for continuation of care. Although GXTs may provide a wealth of clinical information, a 6- or 12-Minute Walk Test or the 10-m Shuttle, with their ease of administration, makes them a valuable pre- and post-pulmonary rehabilitation program measures.

Home Exercise Programs

A home exercise program (HEP) begins while the participant is still enrolled in an outpatient pulmonary rehabilitation program. When the team deems it feasible (based on exercise and laboratory data), the participant can be assigned exercise activities to be done at home. The patient returns to the outpatient clinic with an exercise log containing the heart rate, RPEs, exercise parameters, and any problems that may have occurred during the home program. The team analyzes the data and adjusts the home program if necessary. Progression of the patient to a home program and to independent exercise is an important goal of the rehabilitation program.

An unfortunate reality is that patients with pulmonary dysfunction often have respiratory setbacks from exacerbations of their disease. Continued contact and encouragement in the form of periodic evaluation are essential to maintain the new level of physical activity. However, reimbursement for such care can be difficult to obtain. Patients are encouraged to join community-based groups that facilitate compliance with their medical and exercise regimens.

Multispecialty Team

A diversity of health professionals is essential to meet the medical, physical, social, and psychological needs of the patient with pulmonary disease. The team may include a nurse, physician, physical therapist, occupational therapist, nutritionist, pharmacist, respiratory care practitioner, exercise physiologist, psychologist, and most importantly, the patient and the patient's family and caregivers.

Although aerobic exercise training is integral to pulmonary rehabilitation, patients require additional services and information to optimize their exercise capability and to improve quality of life. The following section addresses other elements of a pulmonary rehabilitation program: patient education, secretion removal techniques, ventilatory muscle training, and pacing. Smoking cessation should also be considered as a component of pulmonary rehabilitation. Please see section on smoking cessation in the medical management section of this chapter.

Patient Education

The concept of self-management is promoted in the educational sessions of a pulmonary rehabilitation program. By using both individual and group sessions for education, the benefits of both types of interaction can be attained. Participants are given individual, one-on-one time to identify their own needs and address issues that are particular to themselves. Benefits from group discussions include support from peers regarding the patient's feelings or needs, learning from others' experiences and questions, and the socialization only a group can provide. Key components of a patient education program are presented in Box 15.2.

Education makes it possible for patients to assume the responsibility for their own wellness. A patient will carry out the required activities to produce the desired outcome only if the patient knows what to do, how to do it, and also wants to do it. This theory of self-efficacy for the patient with pulmonary disease begins with a daily routine that includes self-assessment, adherence to a medication schedule, performance of airway clearance techniques, activities of daily living with pacing, and a home exercise program.

Self-assessment is used to recognize the first sign of an exacerbation of the disease (increased dyspnea, decreased exercise tolerance, change in sputum color or consistency, pedal edema, or any other significant change from baseline). An exacerbation protocol is devised for each patient that includes a set of standard instructions consistent with the participant's disease and abilities. These behaviors may include the use of airway clearance techniques, pacing techniques, a change in the exercise prescription, as well as a call to the primary care physician for a review of symptoms and pharmacological management.

Box 15.2 Education Topics

Anatomy and physiology of respiratory disease
Airway clearance techniques
Nutritional guidelines
Energy-saving techniques
Stress management and relaxation
Benefits of being smoke free
Impact of environmental factors on COPD
Pharmacology/use of MDIs
Oxygen delivery systems
Psychosocial aspects of COPD
Diagnostic techniques
Management of COPD
Community resources
Exercise: Effects, contraindications, adherence

COPD = chronic obstructive pulmonary disease; MDIs = metered dose inhalers.

Individuals can be taught to manage their lung disease through an educational program that addresses the needs of individuals with pulmonary disorders. Compared to education alone, education as part of a comprehensive pulmonary rehabilitation program produced significantly improved exercise abilities, decreased dyspnea, and greater self-efficacy.[74] Once the patient has progressed through pulmonary rehabilitation, access to new information and continued support is possible through community support groups (e.g., the Better Breathing Club, sponsored by the American Lung Association).

Secretion Removal Techniques

Secretion retention can interfere with ventilation and the diffusion of oxygen and carbon dioxide in some patients with pulmonary disease. Patients with secretion retention may improve their performance on an exercise regimen if proper secretion removal techniques have been performed prior to the exercise session. The preferred practice pattern from the *Guide to Physical Therapist Practice* for these individuals would be 6C-1: Impaired ventilation, respiration and aerobic capacity associated with airway clearance dysfunction.[48] An individualized program of secretion removal techniques directed to the areas of involvement can optimize ventilation and therefore gas exchange capabilities. Secretion removal techniques include dependent programs that rely on a caregiver (postural drainage, percussion, and shaking) or independent programs such as the *Active Cycle of Breathing Technique* (ACBT), airway oscillation devices, or *Positive Expiratory Pressure* (PEP) devices.

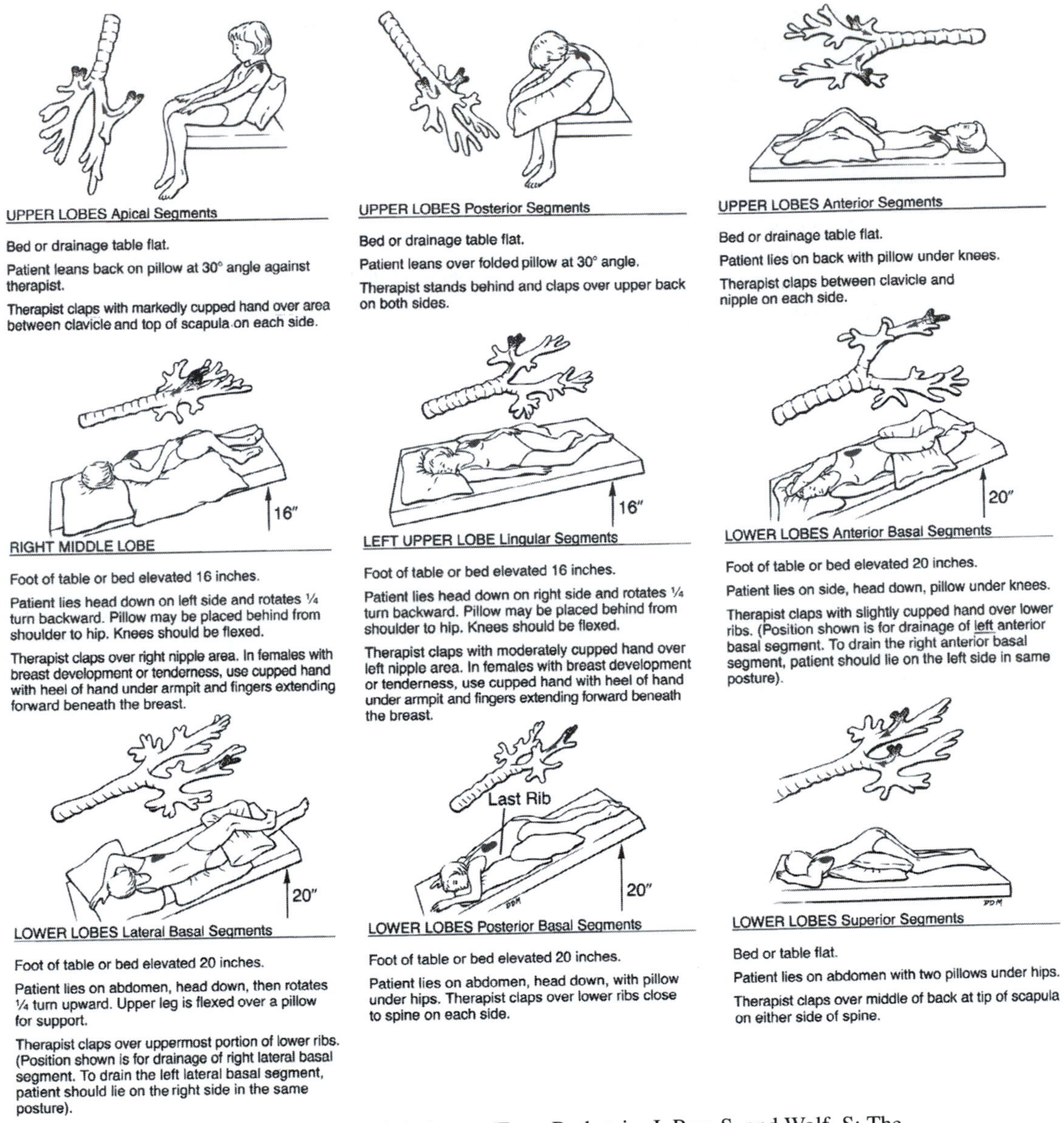
UPPER LOBES Apical Segments
Bed or drainage table flat.
Patient leans back on pillow at 30° angle against therapist.
Therapist claps with markedly cupped hand over area between clavicle and top of scapula on each side.
UPPER LOBES Posterior Segments
Bed or drainage table flat.
Patient leans over folded pillow at 30° angle.
Therapist stands behind and claps over upper back on both sides.
UPPER LOBES Anterior Segments
Bed or drainage table flat.
Patient lies on back with pillow under knees.
Therapist claps between clavicle and nipple on each side.
16″
RIGHT MIDDLE LOBE
Foot of table or bed elevated 16 inches.
Patient lies head down on left side and rotates ¼ turn backward. Pillow may be placed behind from shoulder to hip. Knees should be flexed.
Therapist claps over right nipple area. In females with breast development or tenderness, use cupped hand with heel of hand under armpit and fingers extending forward beneath the breast.
16″
LEFT UPPER LOBE Lingular Segments
Foot of table or bed elevated 16 inches.
Patient lies head down on right side and rotates ¼ turn backward. Pillow may be placed behind from shoulder to hip. Knees should be flexed.
Therapist claps with moderately cupped hand over left nipple area. In females with breast development or tenderness, use cupped hand with heel of hand under armpit and fingers extending forward beneath the breast.
20″
LOWER LOBES Anterior Basal Segments
Foot of table or bed elevated 20 inches.
Patient lies on side, head down, pillow under knees.
Therapist claps with slightly cupped hand over lower ribs. (Position shown is for drainage of left anterior basal segment. To drain the right anterior basal segment, patient should lie on the left side in same posture).
20″
LOWER LOBES Lateral Basal Segments
Foot of table or bed elevated 20 inches.
Patient lies on abdomen, head down, then rotates ¼ turn upward. Upper leg is flexed over a pillow for support.
Therapist claps over uppermost portion of lower ribs. (Position shown is for drainage of right lateral basal segment. To drain the left lateral basal segment, patient should lie on the right side in the same posture).
Last Rib
20″
LOWER LOBES Posterior Basal Segments
Foot of table or bed elevated 20 inches.
Patient lies on abdomen, head down, with pillow under hips. Therapist claps over lower ribs close to spine on each side.
LOWER LOBES Superior Segments
Bed or table flat.
Patient lies on abdomen with two pillows under hips.
Therapist claps over middle of back at tip of scapula on either side of spine.

Figure 15.9 Positions used for postural drainage. (From Rothstein, J, Roy, S, and Wolf, S: The Rehabilitation Specialist's Handbook, ed 3. FA Davis, Philadelphia, 2005, p 444, with permission.)

Postural Drainage

Positioning a patient so that the bronchus of the involved lung segment is perpendicular to the ground is the basis for **postural drainage.** Using gravity, these positions assist the mucociliary transport system in removing excessive secretions from the tracheobronchial tree. Standard postural drainage positions are presented in Figure 15.9. Although these postural drainage positions are optimal for gravity drainage of specific lung segments, they may not be realistic for some patients. Modification of these standard positions may prevent any untoward effects yet still enhance secretion removal. Box 15.3 lists precautions that should be considered prior to instituting postural drainage with patients enrolled in an outpatient pulmonary rehabilitation program. These are not absolute contraindications, but relative precautions. The

Box 15.3 Precautions for Postural Drainage

Precautions for the use of the *Trendelenburg* position
- Circulatory: congestive heart failure, hypertension
- Pulmonary: pulmonary edema, shortness of breath made worse with Trendelenberg position (head of bed lower than foot)
- Abdominal: obesity, abdominal distention, hiatal hernia, nausea, recent food consumption

Precautions for the use of the side-lying position
- Vascular: axillofemoral bypass graft
- Musculoskeletal: arthritis, recent rib fracture, shoulder bursitis, or tendonitis, any conditioning that would make appropriate postural drainage positioning uncomfortable

list is not meant to be inclusive; however, it does provide the reader with a range of dysfunction that should be considered prior to instituting postural drainage.

Percussion

Percussion is a force rhythmically applied with the therapist's cupped hands to the patient's chest wall. The percussion technique is applied to a specific area on the thorax that corresponds to an underlying involved lung segment. The technique is typically administered for 3 to 5 minutes over each involved lung segment. Percussion is thought to release the pulmonary secretions from the wall of the airways and into the lumen of the airway. By coupling percussion with the appropriate postural drainage position for a specific lung segment, the probability of secretion removal is enhanced. Because percussion is a force directed to the thorax, there are precautions that need to be considered prior to its use. These precautions are outlined in Box 15.4. The list is again by no means inclusive. It does provide some general guidelines that deserve consideration when percussion is part of the therapeutic regimen. It should be noted also that some modification of this technique can be made to enhance patient tolerance.

Shaking

Following a deep inhalation, a bouncing maneuver is applied to the rib cage throughout the expiratory phase of breathing. This **shaking** is applied to a specific area on the thorax that corresponds to the underlying involved lung segment. Five to seven trials of shaking are appropriate to hasten the removal of secretions via the mucociliary transport system. Shaking is commonly used following percussion in the appropriate postural drainage position. Because this technique consists of a force applied to the thorax, the same considerations are needed as in the application of percussion.

Airway Clearance

Once the secretions have been mobilized with postural drainage, percussion, and shaking or vibration, the task of removing the secretions from the airways is undertaken using an airway clearance technique. *Coughing* is the most common and easiest means of clearing the airway. High intrathoracic pressures, such as those generated during coughing, can force the closing of small airways in some patients. By trapping air behind the closed airway, the forced expulsion of air during a cough becomes ineffective in clearing secretions.

Box 15.4 Precautions for the Use of Percussion and Shaking

Circulatory: hemoptysis, coagulation disorders (increased partial thromboplastin time, [PTT] or prothrombin time [PT], platelet count below 50,000)
Musculoskeletal: fractured ribs, frail chest, degenerative bone disease

Huffing is another method of airway clearance that is useful for patients with COPD. A huff uses many of the same steps of coughing, without creating the high intrathoracic pressures. The patient is asked to take a deep breath and rapidly contract the abdominal muscles and forcefully saying "HA HA HA." This allows a forced expiration through a stabilized open airway and makes secretion removal more effective.[75]

Active Cycle of Breathing Techniques

Active Cycle of Breathing Techniques (ACBT) is an independent breathing exercise program that includes a breathing control phase, thoracic expansion exercises, and the forced expiratory technique to clear secretions from the airways. ACBT begins with a few minutes of the breathing control phase, defined as relaxed, diaphragmatic, tidal volume breathing. Three to four thoracic expansion exercises, defined as deep inhalations with a 3-second hold followed by a passive exhalation are performed next. A return to the breathing control phase follows. Depending on the patient's needs, this breathing control phase can last for seconds to minutes. If the patient feels that there are secretions ready to be moved upward, then the forced expiratory technique completes the cycle. If secretions are not ready to be moved, the patient returns to thoracic expansion exercises followed by another period of breathing control for rest and evaluation of status. The forced expiratory technique, defined as one or two huffs from tidal volume down to low lung volumes, is used to expel secretions from the airways rather than a cough. The forced expiratory technique is followed by a rest period of breathing control. Using ACBT, secretions are milked from smaller to larger airways. Once the secretions have moved into the larger airways, huffs or coughs from mid or high lung volumes remove the secretions. This independent technique has been demonstrated to be as effective as postural drainage, percussion, and shaking.[76]

Oral Airway Oscillation Devices

Airway oscillation devices, for example, the flutter or the acapella (Fig. 15.10), alter the exhaled airflow throughout the airways. The patient inhales a breath, approximately 3/4 of his or her vital capacity, and holds it for two or three seconds. During active exhalation through the device, the exhaled air causes an intermittent backward air pressure that jars the airways. The usual procedure is to exhale 5 to 10 of these breaths through the device, followed by two large exhaled volumes through the device and finally a huff or cough to clear mobilized secretions. This routine is repeated until all secretions are cleared from the lungs. An airway oscillation device has been shown to help in the removal of secretions from airways.[77,78]

Positive Expiratory Pressure

The positive expiratory pressure (PEP) uses a mask or mouthpiece with a valve to regulate expiratory resistance (Fig. 15.11). Inhalation through the mask or mouthpiece at tidal volume is unresisted. Active exhalation is against a

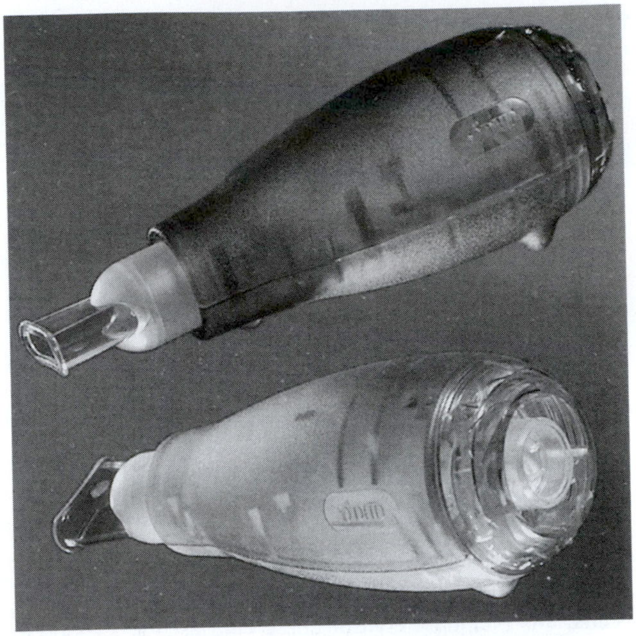

Figure 15.10 The acapella device used for an independent program of secretion removal. (Courtesy of DHD Healthcare, Wampsville, NY 13163.)

positive expiratory pressure. Low pressure PEP uses a resistance that will measure 10 to 20 cm H_2O during mid exhalation. After approximately 10 breaths, the mask is removed and the patient huffs to clear secretions. After a brief rest period, the routine is repeated until all secretions have been cleared from the airways. For patients with unstable airways, high-pressure PEP of 50 to 120 cm H_2O can be used. High pressure PEP requires that the resistance be individually set at the point where the patient is able to exhale a larger FVC with the device in place than

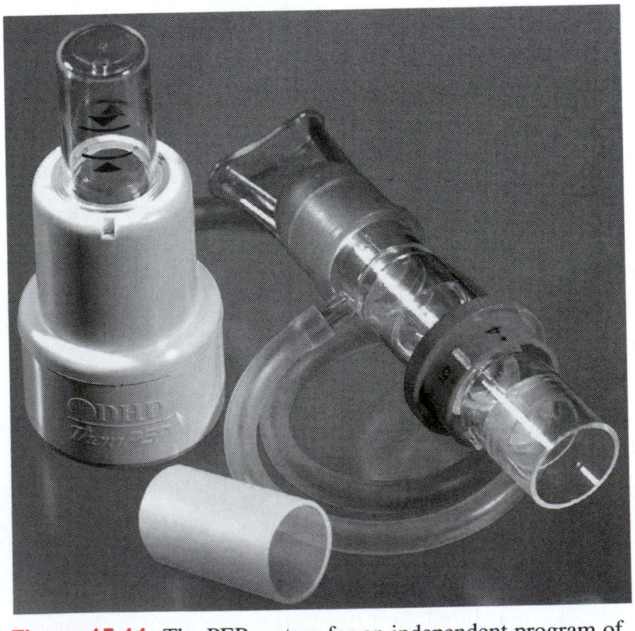

Figure 15.11 The PEP system for an independent program of secretion removal. DHD Healthcare, Wampsville, NY. (Courtesy of DHD Healthcare, Wampsville, NY 13163.)

without. PEP has been shown to be equally effective to postural drainage, percussion, and shaking.[79,80]

Ventilatory Muscle Training

The inability to sufficiently increase ventilation and the sensation of breathlessness may be limiting factors in the performance of functional activities and exercise in patients with pulmonary dysfunction. Ventilatory muscle training devices provide resistance to the inspiratory phase, the expiratory phase, or both phases of ventilation in order to improve strength and endurance of the muscles of ventilation (Fig. 15.12).

Many research studies have demonstrated the ability to increase ventilatory muscle strength and endurance using these loading devices, especially in the presence of known respiratory muscle weakness.[81–87] Ventilatory muscles trainers have also been studied for their ability to alter the perception of dyspnea. While results varied, a number of studies have demonstrated an improvement in the sensation of dyspnea with inspiratory muscle training.[82–84,86] Most importantly, the question is whether training the muscles of ventilation translates into a clinically significant functional improvement. Statistically significant changes in 6-Minute Walk Test and Shuttle Walk Test have been demonstrated.[83,84,87] However, these changes do not always translate into a clinically significant improvement. For example, a change of greater than 54 m needs to be realized on a 6-Minute Walk Test in order to be clinically significant.[88] Although Weiner et al[83] found a statistically significant increase in distance on the 6-Minute Walk Test, the increase was less than 54 m in two of the three treatment groups. The meta-analysis by Lotters[81] states that the ability to affect functional improvement by the use of ventilatory muscle training is yet to be determined. Weiner et al[83] present information that suggests ventilatory muscle training may have different effects based on the patient's severity of lung disease. In patients with severe disease and documented inspiratory muscle weakness, training improved their ventilatory muscle function. However, in patients with

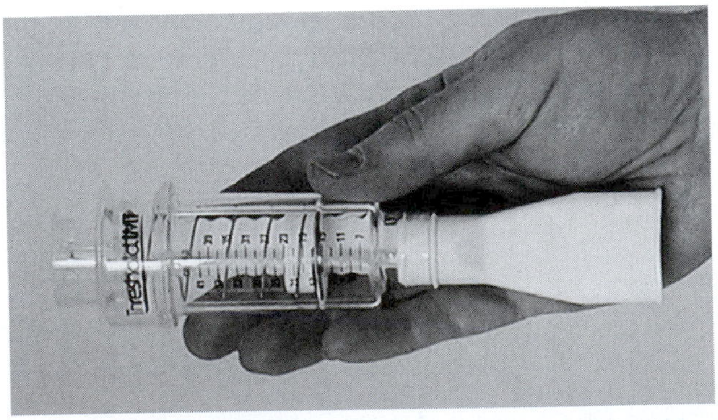

Figure 15.12 A threshold inspiratory muscle trainer for the use in improving strength and endurance of the muscles of inspiration. (Courtesy of Fitness Mart®, [Country Technology, Inc], Gays Mills, WI 54631.)

Evidence Summary Box 15.5
Ventilatory Muscle Testing

Design	Subjects	Methods	Duration	Results	Comments
Larson, JL, et al[82] 1999	53 patients with moderate to severe COPD	Pretest, posttest, randomly assigned to 3 treatment, +1 control groups Treatment 1: IMT Treatment 2: Cycle training Treatment 3: Cycle and IMT Control: education	Cycle: Intensity of 50% of peak work rate on GXT, 20 min/day, 5 days/week, 4 months IMT: 5 days a week 30 min/day at 30% of MIP	Significant increase in MIP with IMT posttraining No change in MEP post training Significant increases in peak work rate and peak oxgen uptake in the cycle and cycle + IMT group post training Significant decreased perception of dyspnea with CET and CET with IMT post training	4 people dropped out of the study, from the CET + IMT group, because of difficulty with training. Addition of IMT did not enhance training effect IMT alone did not reduce exercise induced dyspnea Home-based program
Weiner, P, et al[83] 2003	32 patients with COPD, FEV_1 < 50% predicted FEV_1/FVC < 70%	Pretest, posttest, randomly assigned to 3 treatment + 1 control groups SIMT group: high load IMT and low load EMT SEMT group: High load EMT and low load IMT SEMT and SIMT group: high load IMT and EMT Control group: low load IMT and EMT	1 hour/day (1/2 hour of IMT and ½ hour of EMT), 6 days/week for 3 months. High load was ramped up to 60% of max by the end of first month. Low load was 7 cm H_2O pressure.	Groups that trained inspiratory muscles showed a significant increase in PI_{max} Groups that trained expiratory muscles showed a significant increase in PE_{max} Significant increase in 6 min walk test in treatment groups Significant change in dyspnea scores in only the SIMT and SEMT + SIMT group Significant change in perception of dyspnea in only the SIMT and SEMT + SIMT group	Small sample size of only 8 participants per group Increases in 6-min walk test were statistically significant but the SEMT and the SEMT + SIMT did not reach clinical significance for improvement in that test (>54 m)
Riera, HS, et al[84] 2001	20 patients with severe COPD FEV_1 <50%	Pretest, posttest, randomly assigned to 2 groups Treatment group: IMT at 60% of SIP_{max} Control group: zero resistance through flowmeter	Treatment and control groups: 15 minutes of training on device, 2 × /day, 6 days/week for 6 months	Significant increase in SIP_{max} and PI_{max} post training Significant increase in SWT distance post training Significant decrease in dyspnea post training Significant improvement in CRQ scores (quality of life) No significant change in $\dot{V}O_{2\,max}$, VE_{max}, or W_{max} No significant change in Borg Scores	Home based program Training was at 60% of Sustatined Inspiratory pressure that is approximately 30% of PI_{max}. Device controlled inhalation and exhalation time via visual feedback

(continued)

Evidence Summary Box 15.5

Ventilatory Muscle Testing (Continued)

Design	Subjects	Methods	Duration	Results	Comments
DeJong, W, et al[85] 2001	16 patients with CF. FEV_1 = 70% predicted	Pretest, posttest, assigned to two groups Treatment: IMT at 40% PI_{max} Control: minimal pressure load of 10% PI_{max}	Threshold trainer 20 min/day, 5 days/week for 6 weeks % PI_{max} was ramped from 20% to 40% by week 3	Significant change in inspiratory muscle endurance post-training No significant change in inspiratory muscle strength post training No significant changes in exercise capacity post training No significant change in subjective findings of fatigue or dyspnea	Mean Inspiratory pressure in each group was 100% predicted Mean inspiratory muscle endurance was 50% of PI_{max}
Scherer, TA, et al[86] 2000	30 patients with COPD $FEV_1 < 70\%$ $FEV_1/FVC < 70\%$ <15% improvement in FEV_1 with bronchodilation	Pretest, posttest, Randomly assigned to two groups Treatment: respiratory muscle endurance training Control: Use of incentive spirometry	Twice daily, 15 minutes per session, 5 days per week for 8 weeks. Training apparatus was set at frequency of 60% MVV and tidal volume of 50–60% VC	Significant increase in respiratory muscle endurance post training Significant increases in PE_{max}, 6 min walk test, VO_2 peak and physical components of SF12 post training No change in PI_{max} or mental component of the SF12 post training No change in dyspnea index nor treadmill endurance post training	Training apparatus was not a threshold nor resistance trainer, but a device that used a fixed TV and frequency rather than resistance to provide the endurance training.

EMT = Expiratory muscle training; GXT = Graded Exercise Test; IMT = inspiratory muscle training; MIP = maximal inspiratory pressure; MVV = maximal voluntary ventilation; PE_{max} = maximal expiratory pressure; PI_{max} = maximal inspiratory pressure; SIP_{max} = maximal sustained inspiratory pressure.

mild to moderate disease, training did not significantly improve muscle function. Also, in patients with mild and moderate lung disease, improvements in dyspnea were documented while patients with severe disease did not show an alteration in their perception of dyspnea with training. Finally, there is a suggestion that the use of ventilatory muscle training may increase hyperinflation in patients with severe pulmonary disease, making this treatment potentially harmful.[87] Use of this intervention should be made individually, based on the type of disease, the severity of disease, motivation of the participant and the progress made with the ventilatory muscle training program. Current research on this intervention is presented in the Evidence Summary Box (Box 15.5).

Pursed-Lip Breathing and Pacing

Pursed-lip breathing, when used by patients with COPD, has been shown to decrease respiratory rate and increase tidal volume.[66] Pursed-lip breathing may delay or prevent airway collapse, allowing for better gas exchange. Most patients demonstrate this behavior during periods of dyspnea and rarely need to be taught the technique.

Activity pacing refers to the performance of an activity within the limits or boundaries of that patient's breathing capacity. Often, this means that an activity that usually causes dyspnea needs to be broken down into component parts such that each component can be performed at a rate that does not exceed breathing abilities. By breaking activities down into component parts and interspersing rest periods between each component, the total activity can be completed without dyspnea or undo fatigue. Pacing can and should be part of every activity that would otherwise cause dyspnea. Pacing should be used when performing activities of daily living, ambulation, stair climbing, and other daily tasks. Pacing is not a technique to be used during the aerobic portion of a pulmonary rehabilitation program. During exercise, some shortness of breath should and will occur.

Summary

Pulmonary rehabilitation programs are a well established treatment for patients with chronic pulmonary disease. Components of these programs typically include exercise testing and training, secretion removal instruction, education, and psychosocial support. Increases in exercise tolerance have been documented and maintained in follow-up studies. Pulmonary rehabilitation results in an increase in aerobic capacity, an increase in skeletal muscle strength, an improvement in the symptom of dyspnea both during exercise and activities of daily living and an increase in the perception of health related quality of life. Gains made in pulmonary rehabilitation programs can make the difference between a lifestyle of dependence and one of independence. Physical therapists have the important role of evaluating patients, determining their potential, and through exercise prescription and exercise programs, ensuring that rehabilitation goals are realized.

Questions for Review

1. How does the clinical presentation of obstructive disease differ from the clinical presentation of restrictive disease?
2. Explain how altered airway structure leads to airflow limitation.
3. What would be the expected breath sounds of a patient with COPD? With asthma during an exacerbation? (Remember to describe intensity as well as adventitious sounds.)
4. Identify the tests and measures required to determine the extent of pulmonary disease.
5. What are the pulmonary end points to a symptom-limited graded exercise test?
6. How does exercise prescription differ for a patient with mild pulmonary disease and the patient with severe pulmonary disease?
7. How do you know when to progress a patient's exercise program? What is the nature of that progression? When is another exercise test warranted?
8. How would you explain stair climbing that utilizes the principles of activity pacing to a patient with pulmonary disease? How would you combat the patient's assumption that it would take longer to climb stairs with pacing than without?
9. Design a secretion removal treatment plan for a patient with CF that can be carried out independently prior to coming to pulmonary rehabilitation.
10. What evidence is presented in the current literature regarding the benefits of pulmonary rehabilitation?

Case Study: Patient with COPD

A 67-year-old white female was admitted to the hospital with a diagnosis of acute bacterial pneumonia. She was treated with mechanical ventilation for 5 days, steroids, antibiotics, and bronchodilators. After the acute care hospital stay of 7 days, the patient was transferred to a rehabilitation facility for 7 days. She is now referred to outpatient physical therapy.

PAST MEDICAL HISTORY

COPD, pneumonia 4 times over the past 2 years, s/p lumpectomy of right breast 8 years ago, smoking history of 45 *pack/years,* quit on day of admission to hospital for acute bacterial pneumonia.

MEDICATIONS

2 L/min of pulsed oxygen, Atrovent 4 puffs qid, albuterol PRN, prednisone 5 mg/day.

OCCUPATION

Secretary, works 32 hours/week. Presently on medical leave.

SOCIAL AND ENVIRONMENTAL

Lives with husband in own home. Ramp to front door, six stairs within the home.

OBJECTIVE FINDINGS

Interview

Mental Status: awake, alert, talks in three- to four-word sentences. Adequate historian. Chief complaint: shortness of breath limiting function. Patient is able to walk 150 ft before needing to rest to catch her breath. No complaints of increased secretions. Baseline dyspnea index: functional impairment, grade 1; magnitude of task, grade 1; magnitude of effort, grade 1. Patient's desired functional outcome is to be oxygen free and able to care for grandchildren without shortness of breath.

Vital Signs

HR 72, BP 96/74, Sao_2 at rest 86% on RA, 98% on 2 L/min pulsed O_2 on 1 pulse/breath, RR 34, Temp 98.5° F.

Observation, Inspection, Palpation

Thin, frail-looking female wearing nasal cannula. Kyphosis noted. Patient uses posture of forward sitting with arms supported to enhance ventilatory accessory muscle use. Increased AP diameter of thorax, accessory muscle use at rest. Labored, symmetrical breathing pattern. No venous distention, no edema, no cyanosis, minimal clubbing evident.

Auscultation

Decreased breath sounds throughout both lung fields, especially at bases. End expiratory wheezes at left lateral base.

Strength

Bilateral lower extremity manual muscle testing: hip flexion 4/5, knee extension 3/5, plantar flexion 4/5, dorsiflexion, 4/5. Bilateral upper extremity elevation, abduction, elbow flexion, wrist flexion and extension, 4/5. Patient unable to lie flat or prone for further testing. Tested in alternate positions, other muscle groups able to move against gravity with near maximal resistance. Maximal inspiratory effort (PI_{max}): 52 mm Hg. SIP_{max} 26 mm Hg.

Functional Independence Measurements (FIM scores)

Ambulation: 6 (modified independence—slow gait with pacing necessary). Stairs: 6 (modified independence: requires pacing and railing). RPE of 6 (The Borg CR-10 Scale) with one flight of stairs. Patient is dependent in shopping, house cleaning, and laundry.

Exercise Test Data

Patient performed a 7-min, staged (3 min/stage) exercise test using a modified protocol. Treadmill speed was held constant at 2 mph, grade increased from 0% (stage 1) to 2% (stage 2) to 3% (stage 3). ECG was within normal limits. HR_{rest} was 84 beats/min, HR_{max} 121 beats/min. On 2 L pulsed O_2, Sao_2 resting 98%, 93% at max exercise, 90%during the first minute of cool down, returned to baseline within 4 min of recovery. Rate of perceived shortness of breath at max exercise was 7 (1–10 scale) . Exercise was terminated due to patient request. There was no change in pulmonary function tests post-exercise. 6-Minute Walk Test: 200 m on pulsed O_2

Laboratory Test Data

Pulmonary	FEV_1	1.107 L/sec (45% predicted)
Function Tests:	FVC	1.78 L (64% predicted)
	FEV_1/FVC	62%

GUIDING QUESTIONS

1. What are the patient's impairments and functional limitations?
2. Identify anticipated treatment goals.
3. Identify anticipated functional outcomes of physical therapy.
4. Formulate a physical therapy plan of care for week 1. Patient will be seen 3 times/week for this first week of therapy.

References

1. American Thoracic Society: Pulmonary Rehabilitation—1999. Am J Respir Crit Care Med 159:1666, 1999.
2. Hughes, R, and Davison, R: Limitation of exercise reconditioning in COLD. Chest 83:241, 1983.
3. Pierce, A, et al: Responses to exercise training in patients with emphysema. Arch Intern Med 114:28, 1964.
4. Foster, S, and Thomas, H: Pulmonary rehabilitation in lung disease other than chronic obstructive pulmonary disease. Am Rev Respir Dis 141:601, 1990.
5. Morgan, MD, and Britton, JR: Chronic obstructive pulmonary disease 8: Non-pharmacological management of COPD. Thorax 58:453, 2003.

6. Pauwels, R, et al: Global strategy for the diagnosis, management, and prevention of chronic obstructive pulmonary disease. NHLBI/WHO global initiative for chronic obstructive lung disease (GOLD) workshop summary. Am J Respir Crit Care Med 163:1256, 2001.
7. Martyn, JB, et al: Measurement of inspiratory muscle performance with incremental threshold loading. Am Rev Respir Dis 135:919, 1987.
8. Celli, B: The importance of spirometry in COPD and asthma. Chest 117:15S, 2000.
9. Laurell, CB, and Eriksson, S: The electrophoretic alpha-1 globulin pattern of serum in alpha-1 antitrypsin deficiency. Scand J Clin Lab Invest 15:132, 1963.
10. Chen, Y: Genetics and pulmonary medicine. 10: Genetic epidemiology of pulmonary function. Thorax 54:818, 1999.
11. Vestbo, J, and Lange, P: Can GOLD stage 0 provide information of prognostic value in Chronic Obstructive Pulmonary Disease? Am J Respir Crit Care Med 166:329, 2002.
12. Kohler, D, et al: Usefulness of GOLD classification of COPD severity. Thorax 58:825, 2003.
13. Nishimura, K, et al: Dyspnea is a better predictor of 5 year survival than airway obstruction in patients with COPD. Chest 121:1434, 2002.
14. Anthonisen, NR, et al: Prognosis in chronic obstructive pulmonary disease. Am Rev Respir Dis 133:14, 1986.
15. National Heart, Lung, and Blood Institute: Asthma Fact Sheet; Asthma Statistics, 1999. Retrieved February 12, 2006 from http://www.nhlbi.nih.gov/health/prof/lung/asthma/asthstat.pdf
16. DeKorte, CJ: Current and emerging therapies for the management of chronic inflammation in asthma. Am J Health Syst Pharm 60:1949, 2003.
17. National Asthma education and prevention program. Guidelines for the diagnosis and management of asthma. NIH publication 97–4051, 1997.
18. Sibbaid, B, et al: Genetic factors in childhood asthma. Thorax 35:671, 1980.
19. Weinberger, M: Clinical patterns and natural history of asthma. J Pediatr 142:515, 2003.
20. Panhuysen, CI, et al: Adult patients may outgrow their asthma. Am J Respir Crit Care Med 155:1267, 1997.
21. Cystic Fibrosis Foundation Patient Registry 2002. Annual Report, Bethesda, MD, 2002.
22. McKone, EF, et al: Effect of genotype on phenotype and mortality in cystic fibrosis: A retrospective cohort study. Lancet 361:1671, 2003.
23. Ratjen, F, and Doring, G: Cystic fibrosis. Lancet 361:681, 2003.
24. Kerem, E, et al: Prediction of mortality in patients with cystic fibrosis. N Engl J Med 326:1187, 1992.
25. Durie, PR, and Pencharz, PB: Cystic fibrosis nutrition. Br Med Bull 48:823, 1992.
26. Sharma, O: Editorial review: Idiopathic pulmonary fibrosis. Curr Opin Pulm Med 2:343, 1996.
27. Sin, DD, et al: Contemporary management of chronic obstructive pulmonary disease: Scientific review. JAMA, 290:2301, 2003.
28. Kerstjens, HA, et al: Decline of FEV_1 by age and smoking status: Facts, figures and fallacies. Thorax 52:820, 1997.
29. Scanlon, PD, et al: Smoking cessation and lung function in mild to moderate chronic obstructive pulmonary disease. The Lung Health Study. Am J Respir Crit Care Med 161:381, 2000.
30. O'Hara, P, et al: Design and results of the initial intervention program for the Lung Health Study. The Lung Health Study Research Group. Preventive Medicine. 22(3):304, 1993.
31. Anthonisen, NR, et al: Effects of smoking intervention and the use of an inhaled anticholinergic bronchodilator on the rate of decline of FEV_1: The Lung Health Study. JAMA 272:1497, 1994.
32. Tiep, B: Disease management of COPD with pulmonary rehabilitation. Chest 112:1630, 1997.
33. Belman, M, et al: Inhaled bronchodilators reduce dynamic hyperinflation during exercise in patients with chronic obstructive pulmonary disease. Am J Respir Crit Care Med 153:967, 1996.
34. Alliance for the Prudent Use of Antibiotics (APUA): When and How to Take Antibiotics. Retrieved February 2, 2006 from http://www.tufts.edu/med/apua/Patients/How2Take.html
35. Nocturnal Oxygen Therapy Trial Group: Continuous or nocturnal oxygen therapy in hypoxemic chronic obstructive lung disease: A clinical trial. Ann Intern Med 93(3):391, 1980.
36. Man, SF, et al: Contemporary management of chronic obstructive pulmonary disease: Clinical applications. JAMA 290:2313, 2003.
37. Garrod R, et al: Supplemental oxygen during pulmonary rehabilitation in patients with COPD with exercise hypoxaemia. Thorax 55:539, 2000.
38. Emtner, M: Benefits of supplemental oxygen in exercise training in nonhypoxemic chronic obstructive pulmonary disease patients. Am JRespir Crit Care Med 168:1034, 2003.
39. British Thoracic Society: Standards of care subcommittee on pulmonary rehabilitation. Thorax 56 (11):827, 2001.
40. Bendett, J, and Albert, R: Surgical options for patients with advanced emphysema. Clin Chest Med 18:577, 1997.
41. Criner, GJ, et al: Prospective randomized trial comparing bilateral lung volume reduction surgery to pulmonary rehabilitation in severe chronic obstructive pulmonary disease. Am J Respir Crit Care Med 160:2018, 1999.
42. National Emphysema Treatment Trial Research Group: Patients at high risk of death after lung volume reduction surgery. N Engl J Med 345:1075, 2001.
43. National Emphysema Treatment Trial Research Group: A Randomized trail comparing lung-volume reduction surgery with medical therapy for severe emphysema. N Engl J Med 348:2059, 2003.
44. Szekely, LA, et al: Preoperative predictors of operative morbidity and mortality in COPD patients undergoing bilateral lung volume reduction surgery. Chest 111(3):550, 1997.
45. American Thoracic Society: International guidelines for the selection of lung transplant candidates. Am J Respir Crit Care Med 158:335, 1998.
46. Kesten, S: Pulmonary rehabilitation and surgery for end stage lung disease. Clin Chest Med 18:173, 1997.
47. Organ Procurement and Transplantation Network and the Scientific Registry of Transplant Receipients (OPT/SRTR): 2003. Retrieved February 12, 2006 from http://www.optn.org/AR 2003/default.htm
48. American Physical Therapy Association: Guide to Physical Therapist Practice, ed 2. Phys Ther 81:1, 2001.
49. Mahler D, et al: The impact of dyspnea and physiologic function in general health status in patients with chronic obstructive pulmonary disease. Chest 102:395, 1992.
50. Mahler, D: Dyspnea: Diagnosis and management. Clin Chest Med 8:215, 1987.
51. Guyatt, GH, et al: A measure of quality of life for clinical trials in chronic lung disease. Thorax 42:73, 1987.
52. Brazier, JE, et al: Validating the SF-36 health survey questionnaire: New outcome measure for primary care. Br Med J 305:160, 1992.
53. Murphy, R: Auscultation of the lung: Past lessons, future possibilities. Thorax 36:99, 1981.
54. American College of Chest Physicians and American Thoracic Society: ACCP-ATS joint committee on pulmonary nomenclature: Pulmonary terms and symbols: A report of the ACCP-ATS joint committee on pulmonary nomenclature. Chest 67:583, 1975.
55. Casaburi, R: Skeletal muscle function in COPD. Chest 117:267S, 2000.
56. American Thoracic Society/European Respiratory Society: Skeletal muscle dysfunction in chronic obstructive pulmonary disease. Am J Respir Crit Care Med 159:S1, 1999.
57. American Thoracic Society/American College of Chest Physicians: ATS/ACCP statement on cardiopulmonary exercise testing: Am J Respir Crit Care Med 167:211, 2003.
58. Steele, B: Timed walking test of exercise capacity in chronic cardiopulmonary illness. J Cardiopulmonary Rehabil 16:25, 1996.
59. Revill, SM, et al: The endurance shuttle walk: A new field test for the assessment of endurance capacity in chronic obstructive pulmonary disease. Thorax 54:213, 1999.
60. Jones, N: Exercise testing in pulmonary evaluation: Rationale, methods and the normal respiratory response to exercise. N Engl J Med 293:541, 1975.
61. Berman, L, and Sutton, J: Exercise for the pulmonary patient. J Cardiopulm Rehabil 6:55, 1986.
62. Bruce, RA, et al: Maximal oxygen intake and nomographic assessment of functional aerobic impairment in cardiovascular disease. Am Heart J 85:546, 1973.
63. Naughton, J, et al: Modified work capacity studies in individuals with and without coronary artery disease. J Sports Med 4:208, 1964.
64. Balke, B, and Ware, R: An experimental study of physical fitness of air force personnel. US Armed Forces Med J 10:675, 1959.

65. American Thoracic Society: Evaluation of impairment secondary to respiratory disease. Am Rev Respir Dis 126:945, 1982.
66. American College of Sports Medicine: Guidelines for Exercise Testing and Prescription, ed 5. Lea & Febiger, Philadelphia, 1995.
67. Lake, F, et al: Upper limb and lower limb exercise training in patients with chronic airflow obstruction. Chest 97:1077, 1990.
68. Normandin, EA, et al: An evaluation of two approaches to exercise conditioning in pulmonary rehabilitation. Chest 121:1085, 2002.
69. Maltais, F, et al: Skeletal muscle adaptation to endurance training in patients with chronic obstructive pulmonary disease. Am J Respir Crit Care Med 154:442, 1996.
70. Maltais, F, et al: Intensity of training and physiologic adaptation in patients with chronic obstructive pulmonary disease. Am J Respir Crit Care Med 155:555, 1997.
71. Punzal, P, et al: Maximum intensity exercise training in patients with chronic obstructive pulmonary disease. Chest 100:618, 1991.
72. Borg, G: Borg's Perceived Exertion and Pain Scales. Human Kinetics, Champaign, IL, 1998.
73. Horowitz, MB, et al: Dyspnea ratings for prescribing exercise intensity in patients with COPD. Chest 109: 1169, 1996.
74. Ries, A, et al: Effects of pulmonary rehabilitation of physiologic and psychosocial outcomes in patients with chronic obstructive pulmonary disease. Ann Intern Med 122:823, 1995.
75. Hietpas, B, et al: Huff coughing and airway patency. Respir Care 24:710, 1979.
76. Wilson, GE, et al: A comparison of traditional chest physiotherapy with the active cycle of breathing in patients with chronic suppurative lung disease. Eur Respir J 8(Suppl 19), 171S, 1995.
77. Konstan, MH, et al: Efficacy of the flutter device for airway mucus clearance in patients with cystic fibrosis. J Pediatr, 124, 689, 1994.
78. Gondor, M, et al: Comparison of flutter device and chest physical therapy in the treatment of cystic fibrosis during pulmonary exacerbation. Pediatr Pulmonol, 28, 255, 1999.
79. Van Asperen, PP, et al: Comparison of a positive expiratory pressure (PEP) mask with postural drainage in patients with cystic fibrosis. Austral Paediatr J 23:283, 1987.
80. Steen, HJ, et al: Evaluation of the PEP mask in cystic fibrosis. Acta Paediatr Scand 80(1):51, 1991.
81. Lotters, F, et al: Effects of controlled inspiratory muscle training in patients with COPD: A meta-analysis. Eur Respir J 20:570, 2002.
82. Larson JL, et al: Cycle ergometer and inspiratory muscle training in chronic obstructive pulmonary disease. Am J Respir Crit Care Med 160:500, 1999.
83. Weiner, P, et al: Comparison of specific expiratory, inspiratory, and combined muscle training programs in COPD. Chest 124:1357, 2003.
84. Riera, HS, et al: Inspiratory muscle training in patients with COPD: Effect on dyspnea, exercise performance and quality of life. Chest 120:748, 2001.
85. de Jong, W, et al: Inspiratory muscle training in patients with cystic fibrosis. Respir Med 95:31, 2001.
86. Scherer, TA, et al: Respiratory muscle endurance training in chronic obstructive pulmonary disease: Impact on exercise capacity, dyspnea, and quality of life. Am J Respir Crit Care Med 162: 1709, 2000.
87. American Thoracic Society: ATS Statement: Guidelines for 6 minute walk test. Am J Respir Crit Care Med 166:111, 2002.

Supplemental Readings

American College of Chest Physicians/American Association of Cardiovascular and Pulmonary Rehabilitation: Evidence Based Guidelines. Chest 112:1363, 1997.
American College of Sports Medicine. Guidelines for Exercise Testing and Prescription, ed 6. Lippincott, Williams & Wilkins, Philadelphia, 2000.
American Thoracic Society/American College of Chest Physicians: ATS/ACCP Statement on Cardiopulmonary Exercise Testing: Am J Respir Crit Care Med 167:211, 2003.
Goodman, C, Boissonnault, W, and Fuller, K: Pathology: Implications for the Physical Therapist, ed 2. WB Saunders, Philadelphia, 2003.
Pauwels, R, et al: Global strategy for the diagnosis, management, and prevention of chronic obstructive pulmonary disease. NHLBI/WHO global initiative for chronic obstructive lung disease (GOLD) workshop summary. Am J Respir Crit Care Med 163:1256, 2001.
Man, SF, et al: Contemporary management of chronic obstructive pulmonary disease: Clinical applications. JAMA 290:2313, 2003.
Ratjen, F, and Doring, G: Cystic fibrosis. Lancet 361:681, 2003.

CHAPTER

16

LEARNING OBJECTIVES

1. Describe the etiology, pathophysiology, symptomatology, and sequelae of coronary heart disease.
2. Describe the etiology, pathophysiology, symptomatology, and sequelae of congestive heart failure.
3. Identify and describe the examination procedures used to evaluate patients with heart disease and establish a diagnosis and plan of care.
4. Describe the role of the physical therapist in assisting the patient in recovery from heart disease in terms of interventions, patient-related instruction, coordination, communication, and documentation.
5. Identify and describe strategies of intervention during various phases of cardiac rehabilitation.
6. Analyze and interpret patient data, formulate realistic anticipated goals and expected outcomes, and develop a plan of care when presented with a clinical case study.

Heart Disease

Kate Grimes, DPT, MS, CCS

OUTLINE

The term heart disease includes a variety of clinical diagnoses, including myocardial infarction (MI) or heart attack, angina, heart failure, arrhythmias, sudden death, and valvular dysfunction.[1] The most prevalent type of heart disease is disease of the coronary arteries, also known as **coronary artery disease (CAD)**, coronary heart disease (CHD), or ischemic heart disease. The World Health Organization identifies coronary heart disease as either an acute or chronic cardiac disability resulting from a reduction (or arrest) of blood supply to the myocardium with associated coronary arterial disease.[2]

Epidemiology

In the United States, heart disease is the leading cause of death for males, females, whites, blacks, Asians, American Indians, and Hispanics.[3] Since 1900, cardiovascular disease has been the number one cause of mortality every year except 1918 (influenza pandemic).[3] An estimated 13.7 million people have CHD in the United States; in 2004, the estimated incidence of new coronary events in the United States was 700,000, and for recurrent attacks, 500,000.[3] Atherosclerosis is the most common cause of CHD; besides its fatty deposits within the coronary arteries, atherosclerosis also affects moderate and large size arteries such as carotid and femoral arteries. Therefore, if heart and blood vessel disease were looked at together, an estimated 70 million Americans would have one or more forms of cardiovascular (i.e., heart or blood vessel) disease.[3] Cardiovascular disease is the leading cause of death in the United States today. It accounts for nearly 1 million deaths each year, or approximately 43 percent of all deaths.

Cardiovascular Disease

The pathophysiological conditions that underlie cardiovascular disease are atherosclerosis, altered myocardial muscle mechanics, valvular dysfunction, arrhythmias, and hypertension. Atherosclerosis is a disease in which lipid-laden plaque (lesions) is formed within the intimal layer of the blood vessel wall of moderate and large size arteries; over time the plaque may extend into the lumen causing a decreased lumenal diameter. Atherosclerosis is also a primary contributor to cerebrovascular disease (stroke) and peripheral vascular disease (PVD).

Alteration in myocardial muscle mechanics involving the systolic and/or diastolic properties of the myocardium results in an impairment of left ventricular (LV) functioning. Heart failure is a clinical diagnosis that results from impaired LV functioning and is referred to as **congestive heart failure (CHF)** when it is accompanied by signs and symptoms of edema (i.e., congestion). There are many causes of heart failure, including myocardial scarring and remodeling as a result of an MI, cardiomyopathy from various causes, or impairment in valvular function, especially the mitral and aortic valves.

Arrhythmias are caused by a disturbance in the electrical activity of the heart, resulting in impaired electrical impulse formation or conduction. Arrhythmias may present as benign or malignant (i.e., life threatening). Examples of malignant arrhythmias are sustained ventricular tachycardia (v-tach) and ventricular fibrillation (v-fib). An example of a common benign arrhythmia in the elderly population would be atrial fibrillation (a-fib) with a controlled ventricular response.

Hypertension is "the most prevalent cardiovascular disease in the United States and one of the most powerful contributors to cardiovascular morbidity and mortality." (4 p.8) The Joint National Committee (JNC VII) that evaluates and makes recommendations for hypertension management defines three stages of hypertension: prehypertension, stage 1, and stage 2. (5) (Table 16.1)

Table 16.1 Stages of Hypertension as Defined by JNC VII[5]

Hypertension is defined by either systolic or diastolic elevation. A BP of 110/90 is Stage 1 diastolic hypertension; a BP of 160/60 is Stage 3 systolic hypertension.

Stages of Hypertension	Systolic Blood Pressure (mm Hg)	Diastolic Blood Pressure (mm Hg)
Prehypertension	120–130	80–89
Stage 1	130–140	90–100
Stage 2	140–160	100–110
Stage 3	>160	>110

Normal: 119/79 or below.

The clinical presentations of cardiovascular disease are diverse and depend on the source of the impairment: perfusion of coronary arteries, contractility of LV myocardium, or alteration of electrical activity. Common signs and symptoms associated with heart disease are chest pressure, dyspnea, fatigue, syncope, and palpitations. However, although these clinical manifestations are strongly associated with heart disease, they are not exclusive for heart disease. Therefore, taking a thorough patient history and performing an appropriate examination and evaluation are crucial to establishing the physical therapy diagnosis, goals, outcomes, and plan of care.

It is also important to consider that there is no direct objective measurement of functional limitations based solely upon the cardiac diagnosis and pathology. Individuals with seemingly similar cardiac pathology may experience different functional limitations. Functional limitations experienced by the patient who has a diagnosis of CAD or heart failure may vary widely and are influenced by many factors other than the amount of intact, perfused myocardium, or the functioning of the LV (LV function). In response to cardiac impairments, neurohormonal and cardiovascular compensatory mechanisms are activated that allow cardiac functioning to continue for a while before the patient becomes symptomatic or there is a significant change in function. Functional limitations are therefore influenced by the amount of compensation as well as the pharmacological management.

The clinical significance of heart disease is determined by the impact of the disease on cardiac output (CO). The majority of diseases primarily affect the LV (i.e., ischemia, infarction, cardiomyopathy, heart failure). When the right ventricle (RV) is involved, it will be documented within the medical record based on findings from diagnostic testing, such as the EKG, echocardiogram, or cardiac catheterization.

Patients with CAD, including MI, ischemia, and revascularization procedures (e.g., coronary artery bypass graft [CABG] and angioplasty), as well as patients with cardiomyopathy, arrhythmias, and hypertension, are all included under Practice Pattern 6D in the Guide to Physical Therapist Practice.[6] This pattern is entitled, "Impaired Aerobic Capacity/Endurance Associated with Cardiovascular Pump Dysfunction or Failure." The reader is referred to this source for general guidance in planning examination and intervention strategies with this population.

Cardiac Anatomy and Physiology

Surface Anatomy

The heart lies within the left thoracic cavity. The base of the heart is located superiorly, approximately between the second and third rib; the apex is located inferiorly, approximately at the level of the 5th rib. In this position, the heart is rotated in the sagittal plane so that the RV is positioned anterior to the LV and tipped, bringing the apex closer to the chest wall. In the posterior–anterior (PA) view of a chest x-ray (CxR), the RV occupies a significant portion of the frontal plane. The right atrium (RA) is generally located in the area of the second intercostal spaces and the *angle of Louis.* When one palpates the sternum, the angle of Louis is the "bump" that demarcates the manubrium from the body of the sternum. The second intercostal spaces are lateral and slightly below the angle of Louis. The second intercostal spaces are an important auscultatory landmark; the right space is known as the aortic area, the left as the pulmonic area. The apex of the normal heart is in the fifth intercostal space at the mid-clavicular line. In a healthy heart, this area, known as the *point of maximal impulse (PMI),* is where the contraction of the LV is most pronounced. The clinical reference point for the filling pressures of the heart is measured from the angle of Louis. For example, when it is documented that the jugular vein is distended by 4 in (10 cm), it means 4 in (10 cm) above the angle of Louis.

Muscle and Connective Tissue Structures

The major tissue structures of the heart are composed of muscle, connective tissue, blood vessels, and nerves. The wall of the LV consists of muscle (the myocardium) sandwiched between two connective tissue layers: the endocardium on the inner surface and the epicardium, which forms the outer surface. The endocardium is in contact with the blood that fills the ventricles, while the epicardium is in contact with the pericardial fluid. The endocardium not only serves as a lining for the inner surface of the chambers, but also contributes to the formation of the valves. The valves are composed of dense connective tissue. The epicardium lines the outer surface of the heart and forms the visceral layer of the pericardial sac. The pericardium surrounds and cushions the heart; its two layers are the outer parietal layer and the inner visceral layer (the epicardium). Between these two layers is pericardial fluid, which serves as a lubricant allowing the two surfaces to slide past one another. The status of the pericardium primarily influences the diastolic behavior of the heart, specifically compliance. A decrease in compliance of the pericardium may limit ventricular filling. Connective tissue is also found within the walls of blood vessels. It is important to note that any disease that affects the connective tissue in other areas of the body may also affect any of the connective tissue structures located within the cardiovascular system, endocardium, epicardium, valves, pericardium, and blood vessels.

Coronary Arteries

The coronary arteries originate in the sinus of Valsalva located in the wall of the aorta near the aortic valve. The right coronary originates from the area near the right aortic leaflet, the left coronary from the area near the left aortic leaflet. When the aortic valve is open during systole, the origins of the coronary arteries are located behind the aortic leaflets within the wall; when the aortic valve is closed during diastole, the openings of the coronaries are clearly exposed, allowing them to be easily perfused. The coronary arteries therefore receive the majority of their blood flow during diastole, unlike the other arteries of the body that are perfused during systole. The left coronary artery begins as the left main (LM) and then branches into the left anterior descending (LAD) and the circumflex (CX). The LAD may have further divisions, known as diagonal branches, that come off of the primary LAD. The LAD and its diagonal branches primarily supply the anterior and apical surfaces of the LV, as well as portions of the interventricular septum. The circumflex may also have branches, known as marginal branches. The circumflex and its marginal branches supply the lateral and part of the inferior surfaces of the LV and portions of the left atrium (LA). The right coronary artery (RCA) supplies the RA, most of the RV, part of the inferior wall of the LV, portions of the interventricular septum, and the conduction system. The posterior descending artery (PDA) is most commonly a branch of the RCA and perfuses the posterior heart (Fig. 16.1). If the RCA does not perfuse the posterior heart, the circumflex will supply this area.

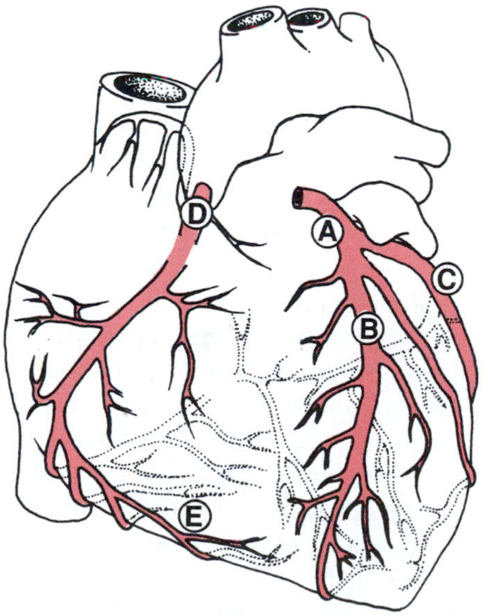

Figure 16.1 Coronary circulation. (A) left main (LM); (B) left anterior descending (LAD); (C) left circumflex (CX) (D) right coronary (RCA); (E) posterior descending (PDA). The branches of the LAD are known as diagonals; the branches of the Circ are known as marginals.

When the PDA comes from the RCA, the anatomy is referred to as being right dominant; if the PDA comes from the circumflex, the anatomy is referred to as being left dominant. For physical therapists, there is no clinical importance to whether the anatomy of the myocardium is either left or right dominant.

The inner diameter (i.e., the opening) of the arteries through which the blood flows is the lumen. The size of the lumen is critical for adequate blood flow. A significant narrowing of the lumen, such as that which occurs with a fixed atherosclerotic lesion of CAD, will decrease the available blood supply to the myocardium. Lumen size may also be altered by the smooth muscle within the walls of the arteries, as smooth muscle regulates vasomotor tone of the coronary arteries. Vasodilation will increase lumen diameter as a result of relaxation of smooth muscle, and vasoconstriction will decrease lumenal diameter as a result of smooth muscle contraction. The responsiveness of arterial smooth muscle is also influenced by the integrity of the endothelium, the lining of the coronary artery that is in direct contact with the lumen. The endothelium has a number of normal functions and "plays the central role in controlling the biology of the vessel wall."[7, p 1265] Some of these important functions are anti-inflammatory actions, growth inhibition, anti-thrombotic activity, as well as its influence on vasodilation. Endothelial cells release *endothelial derived relaxing factor (EDRF),* which facilitates vascular smooth muscle relaxation. Nitric oxide (NO) is the most prevalent EDRF. An injury to endothelium can result in impaired NO release and a decrease in vasodilatation.[8] NO release is influenced by many factors including acetylcholine, norepinephrine, serotonin, ADP, bradykinin, and histamine.[8]

The etiology of the clinical condition known as **coronary spasm**, in which smooth muscle contraction within the walls of the artery results in narrowing of the coronary artery, is not clearly understood. Coronary spasm occurs in arteries that have endothelial injury (e.g., atherosclerosis), as well as in those arteries that appear to be normal but exhibit hyperreactivity to a variety of vasoconstrictor stimuli, such as serotonin and ergonovine, and loss of endothelium dependent relaxing factor.[9]

The role of the arterioles of the coronary arteries is to regulate blood flow through the capillary beds to provide adequate oxygen for aerobic metabolism. Arteriolar tone is influenced by a variety of factors, such as sympathetic nervous system neurotransmitters, hormones, and autoregulation. The greatest influence on coronary artery arteriolar tone is autoregulation. Autoregulation provides a mechanism for a quick and direct response to a change in local metabolism or blood flow alterations and can thereby be more specific and faster responding than sympathetic neurotransmission or blood-borne catecholamines. In the normal healthy heart, autoregulation provides an almost immediate response of the arterioles to vasodilate in response to local metabolic changes such as a decrease in oxygen, an increase in carbon dioxide, or an increase in hydrogen ions. In this way, the heart is able to quickly and adequately provide for its aerobic energy needs. In diseased arteries, autoregulation will respond to a decrease in perfusion pressure due to decreased arterial blood flow by vasodilating the arterioles. Autoregulation provides a mechanism to maintain adequate capillary bed filling of the diseased arteries by influencing local arteriolar vasodilation. In this case, it is important to remember that autoregulation is a local not systemic effect; it influences the arterioles of the diseased vessels only.

Cardiac Cycle

The cardiac cycle consists of two interrelated phases: systole, the contraction phase, and diastole, the filling phase. (*Note:* systole and diastole occur within both the right and left ventricles; because the essential functioning of the heart is primarily dependent upon LV function, only the LV will be referenced). During diastole, the LV is filled with blood from the LA via an open mitral valve. The first two thirds of the filling is passive; during the last one third the atria contract and push the blood into the LV. This contraction is known as the *atrial kick*. After the atrial kick, diastole ends and the mitral valve closes. Systole begins with both the mitral and aortic valves closed. An initial isovolumetric contraction, similar to an isometric contraction of striated muscle, increases the pressure within the LV, and the aortic valve opens. The LV then undergoes a concentric contraction, causing the stroke volume (SV) to be ejected. After the SV is ejected, the aortic valve closes and systole is over. The cardiac cycle is defined by the presence of normal heart sounds, S_1 and S_2. Heart sounds are associated with valvular closings; S_1 is associated with mitral valve closure, and S_2 is associated with aortic valve closure. Systole occurs between S_1 and S_2, and diastole occurs between S_2 and S_1 (Fig. 16.2).

Hemodynamics

Blood enters the heart via the superior and inferior vena cava into the RA. Blood moves forward from the RA

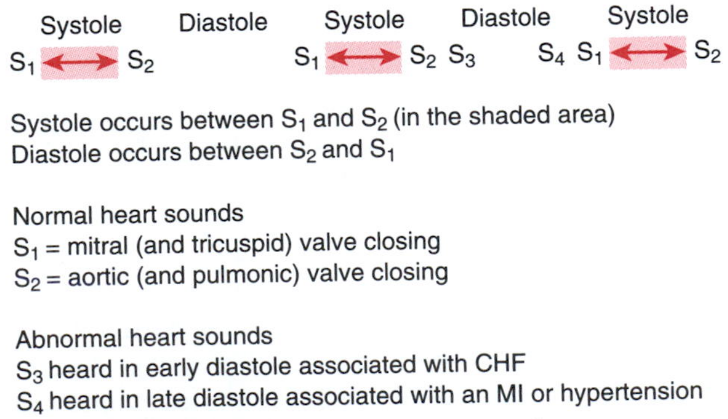

Systole
Diastole
Systole
Diastole
Systole
S1 S2
S1 S2 S3
S4 S1 S2
Systole occurs between S1 and S2 (in the shaded area)
Diastole occurs between S2 and S1
Normal heart sounds
S1 = mitral (and tricuspid) valve closing
S2 = aortic (and pulmonic) valve closing
Abnormal heart sounds
S3 heard in early diastole associated with CHF
S4 heard in late diastole associated with an MI or hypertension

Figure 16.2 Heart sounds of the cardiac cycle.

through the tricuspid valve to the RV, through the pulmonic valve to the pulmonary artery (PA) and pulmonary capillaries. The capillaries perfuse the alveoli, and the alveolar capillary membrane is the site of gas exchange. Newly oxygenated blood within the pulmonary veins (PV) travels to the LA, and passes through the mitral valve into the LV. Blood within the LV travels down to the apex, where it is squeezed in a wringing motion during systole and moved from the apex to the LV outflow tract and finally out through the aortic valve to the aorta.

Blood volume in any chamber or vessel generates a pressure; the normal pressure recordings for the cardiovascular system are presented in Table 16.2. Because of the relationship of blood volumes and pressures, direct determination of blood volumes within the heart may be done by invasive monitoring of the intravascular or chamber pressures. In a *right heart catheterization,* a catheter with pressure-sensitive recording ability is inserted into the internal jugular or subclavian vein and progressed antegrade through the right heart. Common measurements taken with a right heart catheterization are RA pressure, PA pressure, and *pulmonary capillary wedge pressure (PCWP).* The PCWP is an indirect measure of the *left ventricular end diastolic pressure (LVEDP),* one of the most sensitive measures of LV function. An advantage of a right heart catheterization is the ability to monitor filling pressures not only on the right side, but also, by estimation, of left heart pressures without the need for the more difficult and risky LV catheterization. Invasive monitoring can also be done by a left heart catheterization by placing a catheter into the femoral or radial artery and advancing it retrograde to the flow of blood through the aorta, across the aortic valve, and into the LV where LVEDP can be directly monitored. The LV catheter lies within a high-pressure system (the left heart and aorta), and therefore can stay in place for only a short period of time (e.g., an hour) because of the difficulties associated with cannulating a high-pressure system. In contrast, the right heart catheter, which lies within a relatively low-pressure system (the right heart), provides continuous monitoring of pressures and can be kept in place for days.

Table 16.2 Hemodynamic Variables

Right Heart Catheterization	Normal Ranges
Central venous pressure (CVP)	0–8 mm Hg
Right atrial (mean)	0–8 mm Hg
Pulmonary artery (PA)	Systolic 20–25 mm Hg Diastolic 6–12 mm Hg Mean 9–19 mm Hg
Pulmonary capillary wedge Pressure (PCWP)	6–12 mm Hg
Left Heart Catheterization	**Normal Ranges**
Left ventricular end diastolic pressure	5–12 mm Hg
Left ventricular peak systolic pressure	90–140 mm Hg
Systemic arterial pressure	Systolic 110–120 mm Hg Diastolic 70–80 mm Hg Mean 82–102 mm Hg
Cardiac output (CO)	4–5 L/min
Cardiac index (CO ÷ body surface area)	2.5–3.5 L/min
Stroke volume	55–100 ml/beat
Systemic vascular Resistance	800–1200 dynes/sec/cm^{-5}

Adapted from Braunwald, E, Zipes, D, and Libby, R (eds): Heart Disease: A Textbook of Cardiovascular Medicine, ed 6. Saunders, Philadelphia 1997, p 188; and Parrillo, JE: Current Therapy in Critical Care Medicine. BC Decker Inc, 1987, p 36.

Neurohormonal Influences

The autonomic nervous system (ANS) influences the heart and blood vessels through direct neural and indirect neurohormonal mechanisms. The heart has dual direct innervation from the sympathetic and parasympathetic nervous systems.[10] The sympathetic receptors of the heart are primarily beta-adrenergic receptors[11] and are located on the sinus node and within the myocardium. Stimulation of the receptors by the neurotransmitter norepinephrine (noradrenaline) increases the overall activity of the heart by increasing the heart rate (*chronotropy*) and force of contraction (*inotropy*), and also results in coronary artery dilatation.[12] Sympathetic stimulation of the alpha-adrenergic receptors on peripheral blood vessels will result in vasoconstriction and an increase in *peripheral vascular resistance (PVR).*

The sympathetic nervous system may also stimulate the adrenal cortex to secrete the catecholamine epinephrine. This blood-borne hormone will have sympathetic effects that at times may even be more long lasting and potent than direct sympathetic activation. Epinephrine is released as part of the normal exercise response, especially when exercise is continued beyond a few minutes. The increase in HR and contractility noted with exercise is in part due to this hormonal influence. Many cardiovascular drugs either enhance or suppress sympathetic functioning. Those that mimic the action of the sympathetic nervous system are known as *sympathomimetics;* those that suppress sympathetic functioning are known as *sympatholytics*. Frequently used sympathomimetics are dopamine, epinephrine, and atropine, which are commonly used in critical care settings. Dopamine and epinephrine increase CO, while atropine increases HR in the presence of critical *bradycardia.*

Frequently used sympatholytics are the category of drugs known as beta-blockers (beta-adrenergic antagonists) that suppress beta-adrenergic activity. They are commonly used as part of an anti-ischemic drug regimen and for the medical management of hypertension.

The normal parasympathetic influence via the vagus nerve has a primary impact on the resting heart, influencing resting HR substantially more than the sympathetic nervous system. Parasympathetic stimulation results in a depression of HR, decreased force of atrial contraction, and decreased speed of conduction through the A–V node. Vagal fiber innervation of ventricular myocardium is relatively small; therefore the effect on LV function is minimal.[11] During exercise, the effects of the sympathetic nervous system and catecholamine release significantly override any effect from the parasympathetic system. The impact of direct parasympathetic influence on peripheral blood vessels is limited to a vasodilatory effect on the bowel, bladder, and genitals.

The catecholamine role in myocardial functioning during exercise is especially crucial for the patient who has lost direct sympathetic activation to the heart. For a patient who has undergone a heart transplant, the heart is essentially denervated; the sympathetic and parasympathetic fibers to the heart are excised. Sympathetic influence on the denervated heart is therefore solely dependent on catecholamine stimulation of the beta-adrenergic myocardial receptors to increase HR and contractility.

Blood Pressure

Systemic arterial blood pressure (BP) is a product of CO and PVR. The influences on BP are multifactorial[13] (Fig. 16.3). Factors that influence CO include venous pressure, HR, and LV contractility. Factors that influence peripheral vascular resistance include arteriolar tone, vasoconstriction, and to a lesser extent, blood viscosity. The central nervous system (CNS) regulatory site for BP control is the vasomotor center primarily located within the medulla. The vasomotor center mediates sympathetic and vagal inputs and is influenced by neural impulses arising in the baroreceptors, chemoreceptors, hypothalamus, cerebral cortex, and skin. [(14)] The *baroreceptor reflex* is activated by either pressure or stretch receptors located within the internal carotid (carotid sinus) and aortic arch. They are more responsive to constantly changing pressure than to sustained constant pressure. Therefore, they play a key role in the short-term adjustment of BP that was altered abruptly and not in long-term BP control.[12] These receptors respond to an increase in arterial pressure by facilitating a compensatory decrease in CO and PVR. Activation of the baroreceptor reflex by an increase in arterial pressure results in a decrease in sympathetic activation of the heart, arterioles, and veins, and an increase in parasympathetic activation. Conversely, a decrease in arterial pressure will decrease firing of the arterial baroreceptors, resulting in an increase in sympathetic activation of the heart, veins, and arterioles, and a decrease in parasympathetic activity of the heart. The increase in sympathetic and decrease in parasympathetic activity will result in an increase in CO and PVR, thereby increasing systemic BP (Fig. 16.3). Patients at risk for hypotension include those who have lost blood volume with a subsequent decrease in CO and those who may have an alteration in peripheral nerve responsiveness (e.g., diabetic neuropathy, spinal cord injury).

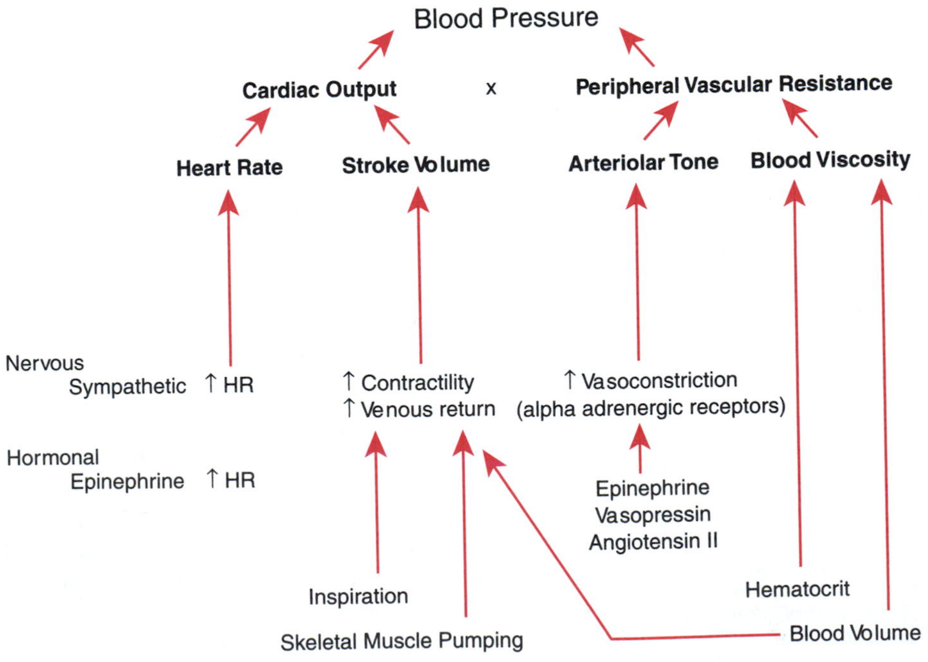

Figure 16.3 Factors that influence blood pressure. Some of the major influences on blood pressure include hormones, nerves, respiration, muscle pumping, blood viscosity, and blood volume. (Adapted from Vander, AJ, Sherman, JH, and Luciano, DS: Human Physiology, McGraw-Hill, New York, 1990.)

Systolic and diastolic measures are the most common clinical measures of BP. However, the *mean arterial pressure (MAP)* is an important measure to use in the critical care setting (i.e. ICU) when the goal is to keep MAP > 60 mm Hg. The MAP is the arterial pressure within the large arteries over time (the cardiac cycle) and is dependent upon mean blood flow and arterial compliance.[13] It may be approximated by taking the sum of the systolic pressure (SBP) and twice the diastolic pressure (DBP) and dividing by 3 (e.g., SBP + 2 DBP ÷ 3); a BP of 90/60 will therefore have a MAP of 70 mm Hg.

Cardiac Output

The goal of the heart is to provide adequate cardiac output (CO) and, therefore, aerobic energy for the body's metabolic demands. Because the energy demands of the body are constantly changing, the heart's CO must also be able to adapt to the changing systemic energy demands, as well as to its own myocardial oxygen needs. Influencing CO are three key physiological principles: (1) adequate oxygen supply to the myocardium by the coronary arteries; (2) contractility of the myocardium through its properties of diastole and systole; and (3) formation and conduction of an electrical impulse from the sinus node to the ventricles.

CO is defined as amount of blood that leaves the ventricles per minute, expressed in L/min; normal CO is 4 to 6 L/min. It is influenced by HR (expressed as beats per minute [bpm]) and stroke volume (expressed as ml/min). **Stroke volume (SV)** is the amount of blood that is ejected with each myocardial contraction and is influenced by three factors: (1) *preload,* the amount of blood in the ventricle at the end of diastole (also known as left ventricular end diastolic volume, LVEDV); (2) *contractility,* the ability of the ventricle to contract; and (3) *afterload,* the force the LV must generate during systole to overcome aortic pressure and open the aortic valve. Afterload may also be described as the "load . . . against which the LV contracts during left ventricular ejection."[15, p 378] In general, stroke volume will increase with an increase in preload or contractility and will decrease with an increase in afterload. Normally about 55 to 75 percent of the preload is ejected as the SV. The **ejection fraction (EF)** demonstrates this relationship between SV and LVEDV such that EF = SV ÷ LVEDV, normal EF is approximately 55 to 75 percent; (67 ± 8 percent[16]). EF is widely used clinically as an index of contractility.[17]

Clinically, especially in critical care settings, the concept of **cardiac index (CI)** is often preferred to CO. CI expresses the CO in relationship to the surface area of the body (BSA) expressed in meters such that CI = CO/ BSA. Normal CO range is 4 to 5 L/min; normal CI range is 2.5 to 3.5 L/min/m^2. CI provides a more complete determination of the adequacy of an individual's CO than CO alone. For example, in comparing a 6-ft tall individual and a 5-ft tall individual each with a CO of 3 L/min, the 5-ft tall person will have a higher CI and therefore better tissue perfusion because there is less body surface area requiring the 3 L of CO. Determination of BSA and CI is often done using nomograms based upon the Geigy scientific tables.[18]

Myocardial Oxygen Supply and Demand

Myocardial oxygen supply and myocardial oxygen demand must be in balance. *Myocardial oxygen supply* depends on the delivery of oxygenated blood through the coronary arteries, the oxygen carrying capacity of arterial blood, and the ability of the myocardial cells to extract oxygen from the arterial blood. *Myocardial oxygen demand ($M\dot{V}O_2$)*, the energy cost to the myocardium, is dependent upon many factors.[19] Clinically, however, $M\dot{V}O_2$ is calculated by the product of HR and systolic blood pressure (SBP), known as the *rate pressure product (RPP)* or double product.[20] Any activity that increases HR and/or BP will increase $M\dot{V}O_2$. Therefore, any increase in systemic oxygen demand (e.g., exercise) will increase the energy cost of the heart and $M\dot{V}O_2$.

The myocardium is routinely very efficient at extracting oxygen from its blood supply. Therefore, during times of increased energy demand, very little increase in extraction can occur. The primary mechanism for increasing myocardial oxygen supply during times of increased demand is by an increase in *coronary blood flow (CBF)*.[11] In general, there is a linear relationship between CBF and $M\dot{V}O_2$. During exercise, CBF may increase five times above resting level in response to the increased demand. Unlike skeletal muscle, which has the capability of both aerobic and anaerobic metabolism, the heart muscle (myocardium) is essentially dependent on aerobic metabolism and has very limited anaerobic capacity.

Pathophysiology

The prime reason for a decrease in myocardial oxygen supply is the presence of atherosclerosis. Atherosclerosis is a progressive inflammatory disease of primarily large and medium sized arteries, whose lesions will become more complex if the inflammatory process is not abated. The etiology of atherosclerosis is hypothesized as an inflammatory reaction in response to an injury[21] that caused endothelial dysfunction or even perhaps denudation.[22] The lesion initially forms within the intima and contains elements of the inflammatory response such as macrophages, lymphocytes, and platelets as well as fibroproliferative response cells such as fibroblasts, foam cells, connective tissue, calcium, and lipids. In response to the injury, smooth muscle cells migrate from the media into the intima of the arterial wall. In an advanced, complicated lesion, it may contain necrotic tissue covered by a fibrous cap. The causes of endothelial dysfunction are varied and again not clearly understood. Proposed possible causes include elevated and modified low-density lipoprotein (LDL) levels, elevated

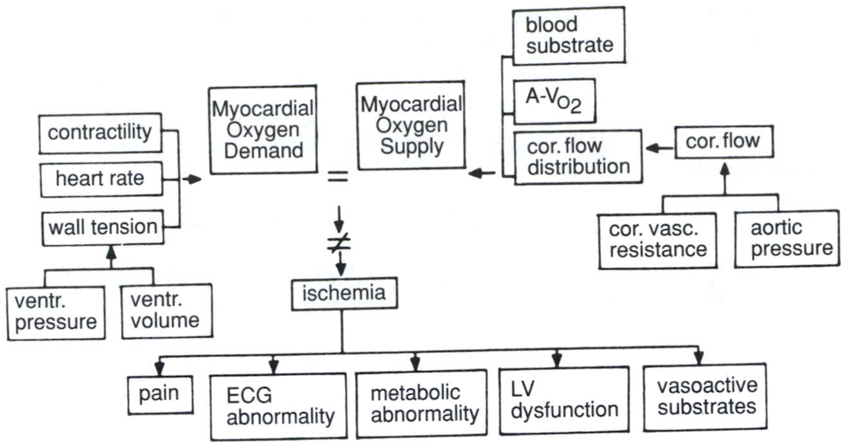

Figure 16.4 Myocardial oxygen supply and demand ($M\dot{V}O_2$) relationship. Myocardial oxygen supply and demand are influenced by many factors; demand is strongly influenced by contractility, heart rate and wall tension; supply is primarily influenced by coronary blood flow. (Adapted from Ellestad M: Stress Testing Principles and Practice, ed 2. FA Davis, Philadelphia, 1980, p 24, with permission.)

plasma homocysteine, and the presence of free radicals in response to hypertension, cigarette smoking, diabetes mellitus, genetic abnormalities, and infectious microorganisms such as herpes viruses or *Chlamydia pneumonia*.[22] Passive exposure to cigarette smoking is also associated with loss of endothelium-dependent vasodilation. As compared to premenopausal women, postmenopausal women exhibit impaired endothelial vasomotor function.[23] The presence of atherosclerosis itself appears to result in a dysfunction of the endothelium, resulting in, among other things, decreased vasodilation capacity. The cause of this is not completely understood, but may be attributed to the production of oxygen-free radicals. Alexander noted "excessive production of oxygen radicals may be a general metabolic feature of atherosclerotic arteries that may explain, in part, the abnormal vasomotor control and tendency toward vasospasm."[7, p 1265] A potent endothelial vasodilator is EDRF, a form of which is nitric oxide (NO). NO facilitates vascular smooth muscle relaxation; atherosclerosis, however, may interfere with the availability of NO and therefore result in a decreased vasodilatory capacity of the coronary arteries.

When a patient's oxygen supply is inadequate to meet the oxygen demand, a condition known as **ischemia** occurs (Fig. 16.4). Clinical diagnoses of **ischemia** or myocardial infarction (MI) are due to an imbalance between myocardial oxygen supply and demand.

Contractility

Throughout the cardiac cycle, diastole and systole place different demands on the ventricles. During diastole, the ventricles must be compliant, able to stretch to accommodate the blood entering the ventricles (preload). During systole, the ventricles must be able to contract adequately to eject the SV. The principle of Starling's length–tension relationship is applicable to the myocardium and the relationship between the properties of diastole and systole. During diastole as muscle length increases (e.g., the ventricular chamber size increases) the ability of the myocardium to develop force is increased, up to a point. Beyond a certain length, however, force development is impaired owing to the inadequate alignment of actin and myosin (Fig. 16.5).

Pathophysiology

Contractility occurs during systole; a decrease in contractility results in systolic dysfunction. Common reasons for systolic dysfunction are loss of myocardial contractile proteins, such as that which occurs with a MI, or diminished contractility from inadequate coupling of actin and myosin, such as that which occurs with an enlarged, dilated LV. LV dilation is a common compensatory mechanism that occurs in response to LV injury.[24] LV dilation may occur in

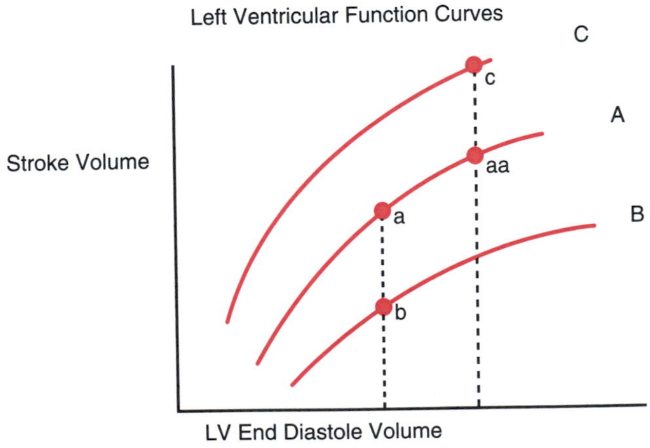

Figure 16.5. Left ventricular (LV) function curves. (*A*) With normal LV function, as the left ventricular volume increases, stroke volume will also increase. (*B*) With LV function impairment, the curve will shift to the right, and for any given length, stroke volume is decreased compared to normal (point *b* has a deceased SV compared to point *a*). (*C*) When normal LV function experiences an increase in sympathetic activity, the curve will shift to the left and SV will increase (note that point *c* is greater than point *aa*).

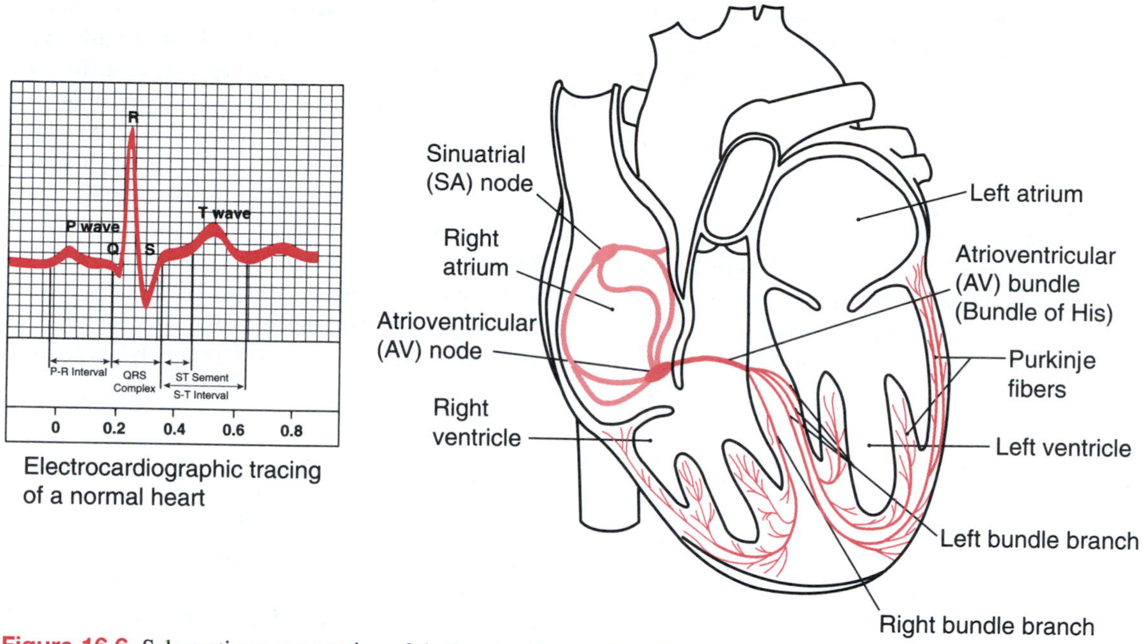

Figure 16.6 Schematic representation of the heart and normal cardiac electrical activity. The EKG is the body surface manifestation of the depolarization and repolarization waves of the heart. The P wave is generated by atrial depolarization, the QRS by ventricular muscle depolarization, and the T wave by ventricular repolarization. The PR interval is a measure of conduction time from atrium to ventricle, and the QRS duration indicates the time required for all of the ventricular cells to be activated. The QT interval reflects the duration of the ventricular action potential. (Adapted from Taber's Cyclopedic Medical Dictionary, ed 18. FA Davis, Philadelphia, PA, 1997, p 852, with permission.)

response to a variety of stimuli, such as myocardial injury from a large MI; alcoholic, bacterial, or viral cardiomyopathy; valvular heart disease; or certain types of chemotherapy.

If the diastolic properties of the ventricle are impaired, myocardial function will also be impaired. Decreased LV filling occurs whenever the LV is limited in its ability to stretch adequately to accommodate preload. Examples of impaired diastolic function include inflamed pericardium (e.g., pericarditis), thickening and stiffening of myocardium due to hypertension, pericardial effusions, scar tissue, and connective tissue changes associated with diabetes.

Electrical Conduction

Contraction depends on an intact electrical conduction system that results in depolarization of the myocardium and timely repolarization. In *normal sinus rhythm (NSR)* the impulse begins in the sinus node, travels through the atria, the A–V node, bundle of His, Purkinje fibers, septum, and ventricles.

Electrical conduction can be viewed via the electrocardiogram (EKG) complex (Fig. 16.6). Each component of the complex reflects a certain phase of conduction: P wave, sinus node and atrial depolarization; PR segment, conduction through AV node; QRS complex, ventricular depolarization; ST segment, initiation of ventricular repolarization; and T wave, completion of ventricular repolarization.[25,26] Each EKG complex represents one cardiac cycle, one heartbeat. In a series of EKG complexes representing sinus rhythm, each QRS complex should be preceded by a P wave and the QRS complexes should be equally spaced apart, indicating a regular rhythm.

Pathophysiology

A HR greater than 100 bpm is known as *tachycardia;* a HR less than 60 bpm is known as *bradycardia.* Exercise commonly results in a tachycardia as part of the normal response to the increased systemic oxygen demand ($\dot{V}O_2$). Volume loss, such as that with surgery or dehydration, may result in a *compensatory tachycardia* to maintain CO in the presence of a reduced SV (remember CO $=$ HR $\times$ SV). Bradycardia at rest is commonly seen in people with good aerobic capacities as a result of regular endurance exercise; however, their HR will appropriately increase in response to the increased $\dot{V}O_2$ of exercise. Patients may have bradycardia because of impaired conduction, a sick sinus node, or certain medications (e.g., beta-blockers). If HR does not increase appropriately when $\dot{V}O_2$ is increased, CO will decrease. Inadequate CO may produce a variety of clinical signs and symptoms as a result of inadequate tissue or organ perfusion such as lightheadedness, alteration in mental status, and angina. Insufficient HR response in the presence of increased $\dot{V}O_2$ is known as *chronotropic incompetence*.

A rhythm is either regular or irregular. A regular rhythm indicates a consistent relationship between each QRS complex as measured by the R-to-R interval between EKG complexes. An irregular rhythm indicates an inconsistent relationship between each QRS complex. There are many different types arrhythmias and conduction delays. The most common are the atrial arrhythmias of atrial fibrillation (a-fib), paroxysmal atrial tachycardia (PAT),supraventricular tachycardia (SVT), and the ventricular arrhythmias of bigeminy, trigeminy, v-tach, and ventricular fibrillation (v-fib). The severity of any arrhythmia is determined by its impact on CO. Because the ventricular arrhythmias are more likely to cause a decrease in CO, particularly if prolonged, they usually have a more detrimental effect on cardiac functioning than atrial arrhythmias.

Exercise Response

Normal Exercise Response

An increase in $\dot{V}O_2$ occurs with an increase in external workload (i.e., mph, kpm,). There is a direct, almost linear relationship between HR and external workload (Fig. 16.7). Therefore, if the physical therapy intervention requires an increase in systemic oxygen consumption expressed as either an increase in MET levels, kcal, L/O_2, or ml O_2 per kg of body weight per minute, then HR should also increase. Although some cardiac medications, particularly the *beta-blockers,* which suppress the sympathetic nervous system's effect on the heart, will limit the actual amount of increase, HR should rise nonetheless. Failure of the HR to increase with increasing workloads (chronotropic incompetence) should be of concern for the physical therapist. Other physiological parameters should be quickly examined, such as BP, respiratory rate, skin color, and temperature as well as the patient's level of cognition and perceived exertion. An adverse response in any of these parameters is an indication of the patient's inability to hemodynamically respond to the given amount of work.

BP should be taken before and immediately after exercise with the patient in the same position (i.e., supine, sitting, standing) and from the same arm each time. Ideally, BP should be taken during exercise to determine the actual hemodynamic response to the increased workload. However, depending on the type of exercise modality, this is often technically difficult. If HR and BP are both to be taken following exercise, HR should be taken first. Whenever possible, a more accurate examination of BP and HR response to exercise is obtained if these measurements can be taken during exercise. As with HR, a linear increase in systolic pressure is expected with increasing levels of work (Fig. 16.7). Hellerstein et al[27] reported that for each 10 percent increment of maximal HR, systolic BP increased 12 to 15 mm Hg. Naughton and Haider[28] interpreted an increase in systolic BP in excess of 12 mm Hg/MET as a hypertensive exercise response and an increase below 5 mm Hg as a hypotensive exercise response. Diastolic pressure exhibits limited changes with exercise; it may not change, or either increase or decrease by 10 mm Hg.

As systemic oxygen requirements increase, the depth and rate of respirations will normally increase from rest (i.e., tidal volume).

Inappropriate Exercise Response

The American College of Sports Medicine has identified signs and symptoms of excessive effort (Box 16.1). Obviously, if a patient experiences any of these symptoms, the activity should be stopped and the patient stabilized. It is also important to inform patients that some responses may be delayed for as long as several hours after exercise. Observation of the patient throughout the physical therapy intervention provides a mechanism for ongoing examination. By paying attention to any subtle changes in the patient's facial expression, skin color, tone of voice, or thought processing that may indicate activity intolerance, the physical therapist may quickly respond and modify the intervention after critically evaluating the patient status.

Besides the patient's subjective complaint of fatigue or discomfort, there are other responses that should terminate an exercise session. These abnormal responses include (1) failure of the systolic pressure to rise as exercise

Box 16.1 Signs and Symptoms of Excessive Effort

- Persistent dyspnea
- Dizziness or confusion
- Pain
- Severe leg claudication
- Excessive fatigue
- Pallor, cold sweat
- Ataxia
- Pulmonary rales

Responses that may be delayed for as long as several hours include:

- Prolonged fatigue
- Insomnia
- Sudden weight gain owing to fluid retention

From American Colleges of Sports Medicine: Guidelines for Exercise Testing and Training, ed 4. Lea & Febiger, Philadelphia, 1991, with permission.

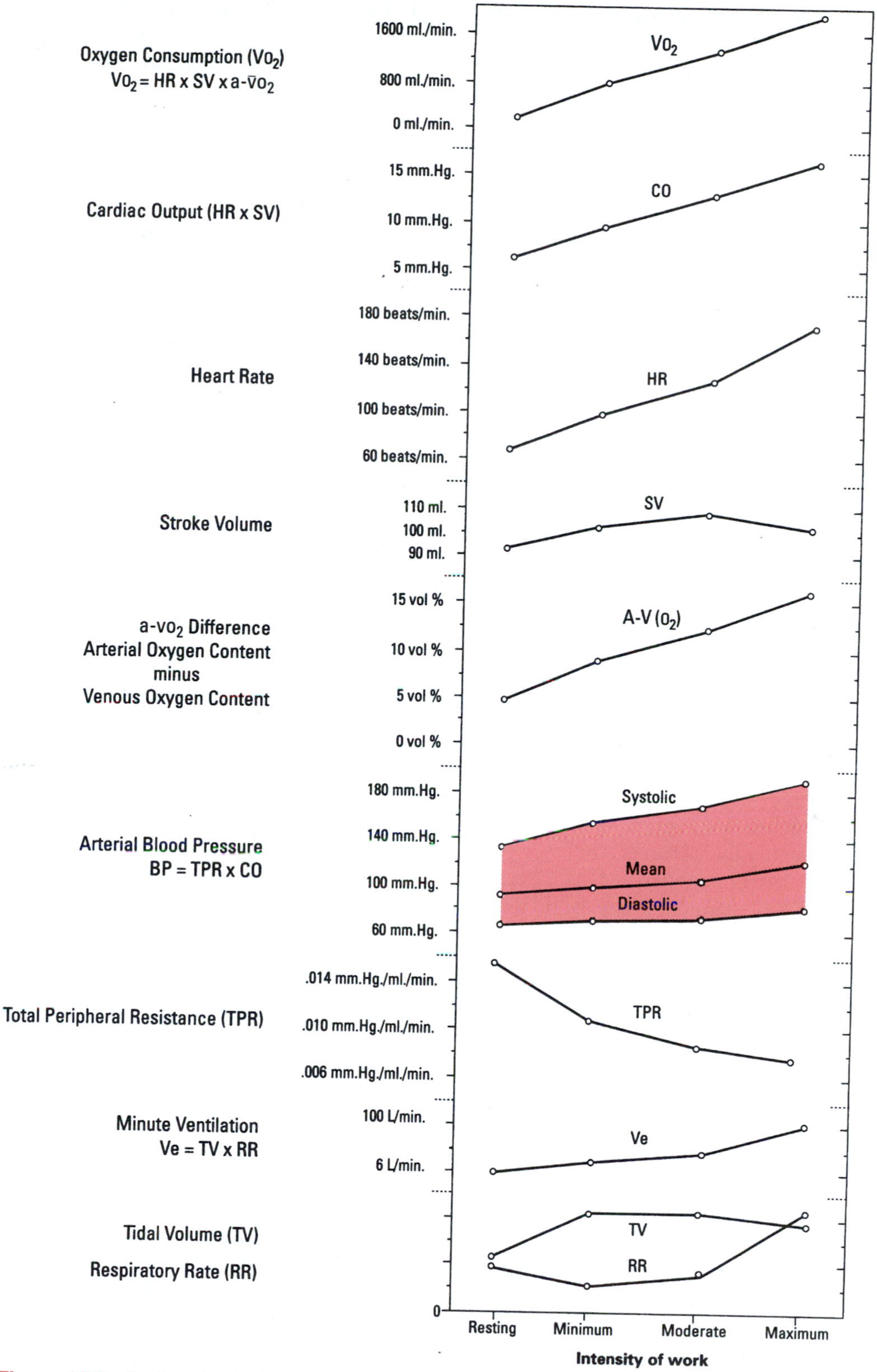

Figure 16.7. Cardiopulmonary response to acute aerobic exercise. (Adapted from Berne, RM and Levy, MN: Cardiovascular Physiology, ed 5. CV Mosby, St. Louis, 1986, p 237; Zadai, CC: Clinics in Physical Therapy, Pulmonary Management in Physical Therapy, Churchill Livingstone, New York, 1992, p 27; and McArdle WD et al: Essentials of Exercise Physiology, Lea & Febiger, Philadelphia, 1994, p 230.)

continues; (2) a hypertensive BP response, including a systolic pressure of greater than 200 mm Hg and/or a diastolic pressure greater than 110 mm Hg; or (3) a progressive fall in systolic pressure of 10 to 15 mm Hg.[29] In addition, a significant change in cardiac rhythm detected either by palpation or by EKG monitoring warrants termination.

Cardiovascular Examination

The physical therapist must determine how cardiac impairment has impacted cardiac function in order to plan safe and appropriate exercise interventions. $\dot{V}O_2$ is directly related to CO; an increase in $\dot{V}O_2$, such as that with exercise, will result in an increase demand for CO. Therefore, anything that limits CO will limit the amount of systemic energy that the patient has available. Depending on the practice site of physical therapy, the availability of patient information will be varied. Before planning an intervention for any cardiac patient, in addition to questions concerning medical history, medications, and review of systems, the following questions need to be answered:

- What is the patient's cardiac diagnosis and history (e.g., ischemia, noncomplicated MI, complicated MI, CHF)?
- Does the patient presently have ischemia? If so, how does the angina present?
- What is the result of the latest exercise tolerance test (ETT) in order to identify the ischemic RPP?
- What is the patient's baseline rhythm and rate? (Identify any ectopy and the EKG interpretation of the rhythm.)
- What is the BP? Is it the same in both arms? What is it sitting and standing?
- If the patient has been revascularized, what vessels were involved and what is the status of the other vessels?
- Does the patient continue to have ischemia after the revascualarization?

The patient history is critical in directing the appropriate questions.

Medical Record Review

Review of the medical record is helpful in understanding the patient's status and in planning physical therapy interventions. The medical record of a patient with cardiovascular impairments may at times be so overwhelming and time-consuming that a brief initial interview can be helpful in providing and in sorting out the information. Depending on the type of setting (e.g., inpatient, outpatient, acute, rehabilitation), the specific contents of the medical record may vary. The acute inpatient record is generally the most thorough regarding medical/surgical interventions. Items important to note include the following:

1. Medical problems, past medical history, physician's examination
2. Medications including type, dosage, and schedule
3. Laboratory tests
   - Blood tests for specific cardiac enzymes that may indicate an MI has occurred, such as a positive CK-MB or troponin level.
   - Electrolytes, especially potassium (K), if ventricular arrhythmias are present, and albumin if CHF is present.
   - Complete blood count (CBC), which may indicate the presence of anemia via the hemoglobin and hematocrit values and also the status of kidney and liver function.
   - Presence of CAD risk factors, such as elevated lipid values (e.g., total cholesterol, low-density lipoproteins [LDL], triglyceride), and elevated blood sugars (glucose).
   - Arterial blood gases (ABGs)
4. Results of any diagnostic studies or interventions: CxR, EKGs, ETT, cardiac catheterization, surgical reports, hemodynamic monitors (e.g., pressure readings from central line and/ or arterial line)
5. Nursing and other health care provider notes

The medical record contains information regarding what has happened to the patient, as well as the status of the patient within the last 24 hours or since the last health care provider intervention. It often is not sufficiently up-to-date to give the immediate status. The use of flow charts, which record vital signs, temperature, oxygenation requirements, and volume status, provide more up-to-date patient data and may therefore provide invaluable information for the physical therapist, especially when working with the more medically challenged patient.

Patient Interview

The formal patient interview should follow the medical record review. A determination of overall cognition (e.g., orientation, memory, learning needs, comprehension) should be made. Information regarding the patient's lifestyle, previous level of functioning, recreational interests, work requirements, and goals is important in establishing the intervention. Data should also be obtained about the patient's response to health and illness, coping status, support systems, and knowledge of heart disease. It is important to note that not all the information from the interview needs to be obtained on the first session. During subsequent sessions, the patient may begin to feel better and less anxious and may therefore be able to communicate more easily. Patient education can often be woven into the interview process, either subtly or overtly. The patient should describe, in his or her own words, the quality and location of the symptom for which medical attention is being sought. It is common for physical therapists to ask a patient about pain; for patients with cardiac disease, one should be cautious about assuming that the patient's symptom is pain. Many patients will not use pain as their qualifier, but instead describe their symptoms as pressure, heaviness, shortness of breath (dyspnea), aching, heartburn, or general malaise, to identify a few. Knowing the symptom presentation for each individual will make patient education and activity progression easier. It is also important to identify any consistent precipitating factors and alleviators as well as duration and frequency of symptoms.

The interview also helps to establish rapport and trust between therapist and patient, creating an environment for mutual goal setting and facilitating easier compliance with the overall rehabilitation program. Patients who are recovering from an MI or from surgery need to have an understanding of time frames for healing and convalescence. Education for family members and significant others is also crucial for patient compliance and understanding.

Vital Signs

The physical therapist will take and monitor vital signs (see Chapter 4) at rest and with activity, auscultate the heart (and lungs), as well as perform a general inspection of the patient. An overview of the pertinent components is presented.

HR and Rhythm

In taking an initial HR, either by palpation or auscultation, it is important to count for a full minute. When examining the patient's response to an activity and no arrhythmia is present, an immediate post-exercise HR can be taken for 10 seconds. Always note if the rhythm is regular or irregular and report it as such. Unless there is EKG monitoring, it is impossible to identify a specific rhythm by palpation or auscultation alone. Note that there is a normal respiratory variation in HR; inspiration results in an increase in HR, exhalation in a slowing down of HR. Obviously, since the patient is going to be both inhaling and exhaling throughout the counting, do not identify the rhythm as irregular.

Respiratory Rate, Rhythm, and Shortness of Breath

As with the heart, both rate and rhythm of respirations should be noted, as well as the breathing pattern and use of accessory muscles. Patients with cardiac impairments frequently complain of shortness of breath *(dyspnea)* and report that it is anxiety provoking. The patient needs to seek immediate medical care if dyspnea occurs at rest. Frequently, dyspnea is associated with activity and is known as *dyspnea on exertion (DOE)*. It is important for the physical therapist to document and understand the amount and types of activity that provoke DOE. Patients may also describe a type of dyspnea that awakens them from sleep but is relieved when they assume an upright posture. This is known as *paroxysmal nocturnal dyspnea (PND)* and is associated with LV failure. It is also important to ask the patient how many pillows are needed to feel comfortable breathing while sleeping. Patients with LV failure frequently use more than one pillow to sleep; by elevating the trunk, venous return is slightly delayed and the work of the LV is temporarily decreased. This is recorded as *two pillow orthopnea* (or whatever number of pillows are needed). *Orthopnea* refers to the dyspnea that is influenced by the effect of gravity on increased venous return (e.g., occurs in the supine but not in the upright position). In heart failure, orthopnea may be exacerbated by the shift of blood volume from the periphery to the pulmonary circulation.[30] Some patients may experience dyspnea as their anginal equivalent; that is, they do not have the typical chest discomfort often associated with ischemia but instead experience shortness of breath. Treatment should be immediate and follow the guidelines for ischemia.

Blood Pressure

Arterial BP is a product of CO and PVR (BP = CO × PVR). An increase in either of these factors will increase BP, and a decrease in either may decrease blood pressure. BP is normally slightly higher in supine than in either sitting or standing because of the increase in venous return in the gravity-minimized position. This increase in venous return contributes to an increase in CO. In the upright position, gravity will delay venous return and there will be a transient, brief, asymptomatic decrease in BP until peripheral muscle contractions and sympathetic venoconstriction are able to increase venous return and sympathetic arteriolar vasoconstriction increases PVR. Although difficult to substantiate, clinical observation indicates that BP usually normalizes within seconds to a minute of standing.

Orthostatic Hypotension

Orthostatic (postural) hypotension is the sudden prolonged drop in BP that accompanies a position change from lying to either sitting or standing. Common symptoms include lightheadedness, dizziness, and loss of balance.[31] A drop of systolic blood pressure of more than 20 mm Hg between measurements (lying versus sitting versus standing) is unacceptable; a standing BP less than 100 mm Hg systolic may be abnormal. Both situations require further clinical examination and intervention.[31] If the patient has any of the above symptoms with position change, she or he should be managed as if there was an orthostatic response, even if BP is only minimally decreased. Patients at risk for orthostatic changes are those who have been on prolonged bed rest, who may be volume depleted, who may have PVD or muscle atrophy, or who may be taking vasodilators or antihypertensive medications.

Interventions used to decrease the occurrence of postural hypotension involve a slow, stepwise progression from supine to sit, gradually elevating the head of the bed to allow physiological adaptation to occur. When sitting on the side of the bed, the feet should be supported and the patient encouraged to take deep breaths and perform ankle pumps, all of which facilitate venous return. Use of support stockings or ace wraps to increase venous return may also be indicated for some patients.

Observation, Inspection, and Palpation

The patient's skin color should be inspected. *Cyanosis,* a bluish color of the skin, nail beds, and possibly lips and tongue, may be present when arterial oxygen saturation is 85 percent or less.[32] *Pallor,* the absence of a pink, rosy color, may indicate a decrease in CO. *Diaphoresis* (excess sweating, cool clammy skin) should also be noted because it may indicate excessive effort or inadequate cardiovascular response. Cold fingertips may be due to compensatory vasoconstriction in response to a decreased CO or from the suppressed beta-sympathetic response of some beta-blockers.

Palpation includes monitoring the femoral, dorsalis pedis, and posterior tibialis pulses, which are compared bilaterally and documented as bounding (4+), normal (3+), weak (2+), thready (1+), or absent (0). A diminished pulse may be due to a decrease in CO or a local arterial occlusion.

The extremities are inspected for the presence of edema; patients with LV failure may have an increase in peripheral edema owing to the increase in hydrostatic intravascular pressure associated with increased pressure from the LV transmitted retrograde through the heart to venous system. Edema is examined for its level of *pitting* (indentation) when moderate pressure is applied. Bilateral peripheral edema may be a result of CHF. Edema of one leg, however, is usually associated with local factors within the same leg such as varicose veins, lymphedema, or thrombophlebitis.[32] The patient with chronic CHF who has a weight gain owing to sodium and water retention may notice edema of the ankles and lower legs during the day (due to an increase in hydrostatic pressure) that diminishes during the night.

Auscultation

Invaluable information as to the status of the heart is obtained from *auscultation* (listening) of the heart sounds. Normal heart sounds are identified as S_1 (lub), which occurs at the time of the closure of the mitral (and tricuspid) valve and marks the beginning of systole and S_2 (dub), which occurs at the time of aortic (and pulmonic) valve closure and marks the end of systole (see Fig. 16.2).

Abnormal Heart Sounds

Murmurs are abnormal heart sounds commonly the result of valvular disorders due to the changes in blood flow around and through the altered valve.[33] A *systolic murmur* will present as audible turbulence between S_1 and S_2, and a *diastolic murmur* as turbulence between S_2 and S_1. A *stenotic* valve has impaired opening, and a regurgitant valve has impaired closing. A valve may be both stenotic and regurgitant.

Other abnormal sounds are S_3 and S_4. S_3, also known as a *ventricular gallop,* occurs after S_2 and is clinically associated with LV failure. S_4, also known as an *atrial gallop,* occurs before S_1 and is clinically associated with an MI or chronic hypertension. The abnormal heart sounds are therefore "bookending" the normal heart sounds such that they would be ordered as: S_4, S_1, S_2, S_3.

Another type of auscultatory finding is the *pericardial friction rub.* These friction sounds are high pitched with a leathery and scratchy quality, although they may vary in intensity from hour-to-hour or day-to-day, or may even transiently disappear.[34] The pericardial rub has been described as similar to the squeaking sound of rubbed leather.[35] This rub results from an inflammation of the pericardial sac, either with or without excessive fluid. Pericardial disease may result from many causes such as trauma, infections, tumors, collagen diseases, anticoagulants, and MI. Post-MI pericarditis is known as *Dressler's syndrome.*[36] An example of documentation for heart sounds would be: *Cor: RRR Ø m, g, r,* which would be interpreted as *Heart: regular rate and rhythm without murmurs, gallops, or rubs.*

Auscultating the lungs is an important component of the cardiac physical examination. Patients who have LV failure often have the adventitious sounds of *crackles.* Crackles may also appear as a result of atelectasis; in that case, deep breathing with an inspiratory hold and coughing may correct this impairment. A patient with decreased breath sounds or consolidations may have a decrease in the oxygen content of his or her blood; a decrease in oxygenation may result in an increase in myocardial work and aggravate a preexisting cardiac impairment.

Auscultation is used to determine the presence of an abnormal sound known as a *bruit,* which is associated with a narrowing within an artery. It is heard most commonly in the carotid and femoral arteries and indicates the probable presence of atherosclerotic disease. Auscultation of the heart borders is also done to examine size. The location of the apex and point of maximal impulse (PMI) is noted; if the LV has increased in size, as frequently occurs with patients in LV failure, the PMI will be displaced laterally toward the axilla.

Additional examination details may be found in many medical and nursing texts for physical assessments.[37–39]

Tests and Measures

A number of clinical tests and measures are used to examine myocardial function. A few of the more commonly used are described below.

Electrocardiogram (EKG, ECG)

The EKG (also referred to as ECG) is used to examine HR, rhythm, conduction delays, and coronary perfusion.

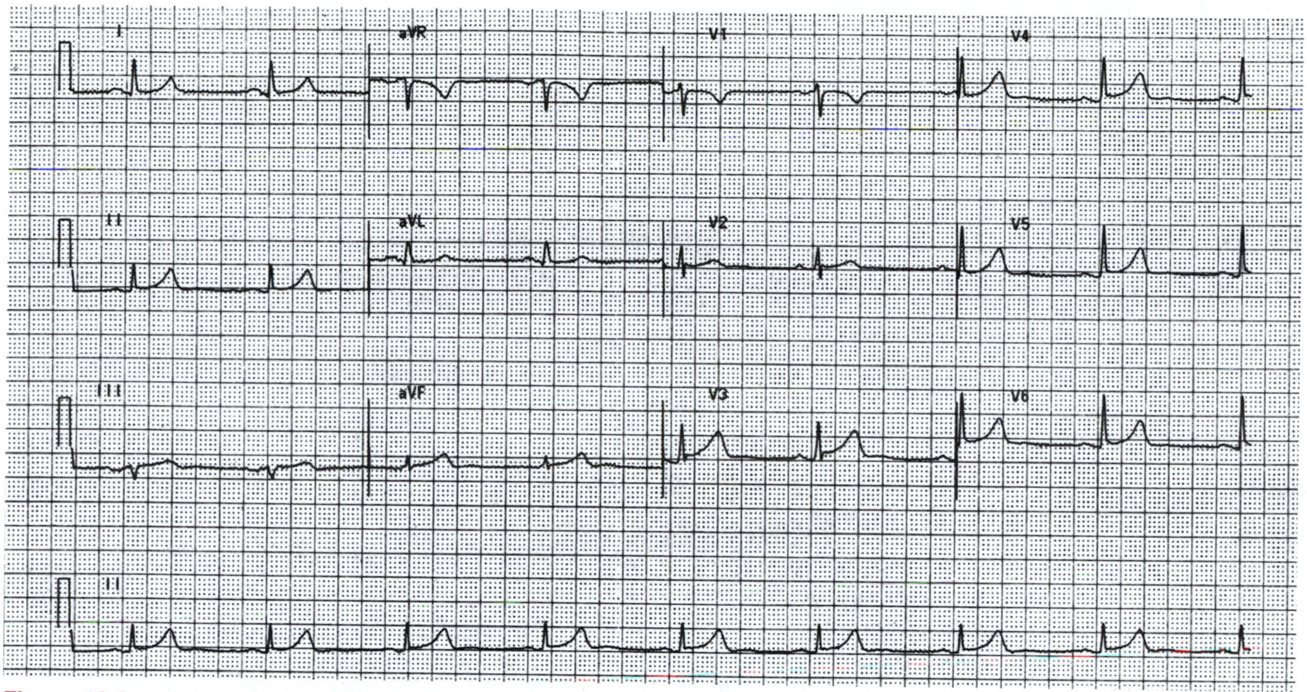

Figure 16.8 Normal 12 lead EKG from 50-year-old woman; slight ST elevation is insignificant. Twelve leads are presented; at the bottom of the page is a rhythm strip from Lead II. Heart rate from the rhythm strip is approximately 52 (there are 5.8 large boxes between complex 3 and 4; therefore 300/5.8 = 52).

Two of the most common types of EKG are the single lead and the 12-lead (Fig. 16.8). In the single lead, only one area of the heart (e.g., anterior, lateral, inferior) may be viewed at a time. This area may be changed, however, by altering the location of the electrodes. In the 12-lead, 12 areas may be viewed almost simultaneously. The single lead is sensitive to rate and rhythm changes and is commonly used for monitoring patients during ambulation and activity. Monitoring is accomplished either via telemetry (radio transmission), allowing the patient freedom to move around when wearing this portable device, or by hardwire, where the patient is attached to the monitor by a cable approximately 15 ft long, therefore limiting mobility. A variation of the single lead is the 3-lead, which is usually hardwire and is used for monitoring in an inpatient setting. It can be worn continuously throughout an entire treatment session or throughout the entire hospitalization.

The 12-lead EKG is sensitive to changes in perfusion as well as rate, rhythm, and conduction. Each coronary artery is represented by a cluster of leads that, although not absolutely correlated with each individual's anatomy, gives a general schema for myocardial perfusion. For example, changes in the perfusion of the RCA affects the inferior part of the heart and are generally displayed in leads II, III, AVF; left coronary perfusion of the anterior, anterior–lateral, and anterior–septal parts of the heart are displayed by various combinations of the other leads (Table 16.3). Unlike the single-lead system, the 12-lead does not provide continuous monitoring (except during an **exercise tolerance test [ETT]**). Two common uses for the 12-lead are the resting EKG taken with the patient quietly supine and the ETT. Twelve-lead EKGs are invaluable in identifying perfusion impairments in the coronary arteries and in assisting with arrhythmia detection. During the ETT, the EKG is continuously monitored to determine the presence of ischemia or arrhythmias with each increase in workload.

EKG interpretation is an important component of the evaluation process. For a more thorough understanding of EKGs and for guided practice, there are several excellent texts available on EKG interpretation.[40–42]

Table 16.3 Electrocardiographic Lead Changes Associated with Anterior, Lateral, Inferior, and Posterior Transmural Infarctions

Infarction Site[a]	ECG Changes
1. Anterior infarction:	Q or QS in V1 to V4
2. Lateral infarction:	Q or QS in lead I, aVL
3. Inferior infarction:	Q or QS in leads II, III, aVF
4. Posterior infarction:	Large R waves in V1–V3 ST depression V1, V2, or V3

[a]Standard 12-lead electrocardiogram: leads I to III, aVR, aVL, and aVF are limb leads; V1 to V6 are chest leads.

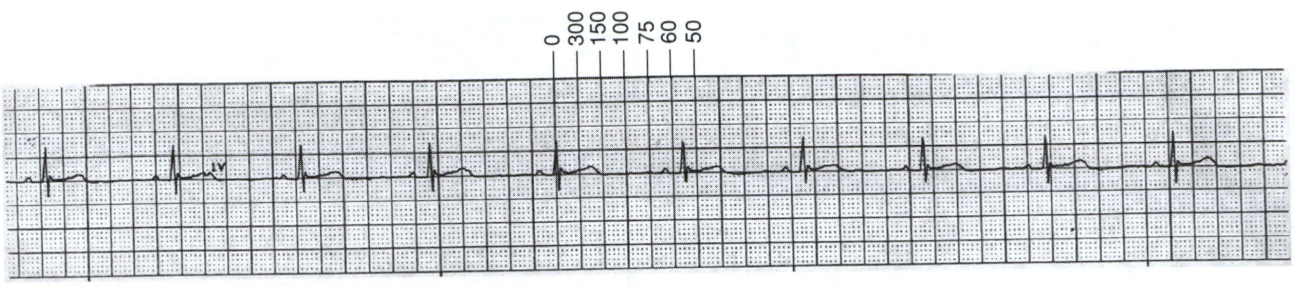

Figure 16.9 Calculation of a heart rate from a rhythm strip. Begin with the fifth complex (which falls on a large black line) and count each large black line to the right of this complex in the order of 300, 150, 100, 75, 60, 50. The sixth complex falls between two large lines (i.e., 50 and 60). There are five small lines between each large line. Between 50 and 60 there are 10 beats, therefore each small line in this case would be two beats. The heart rate would be 60 − 4 = 56. An alternate method would be to count the number of complexes in a 6-second strip and multiply by 10.

Rate

The EKG graph paper consists of a series of small boxes (represented by light black lines) and large boxes (represented by heavy black lines). Each large box is made up of five small boxes. The horizontal axis represents time; when the EKG paper is moving at the usual speed of 25 mm/sec, five large boxes constitutes one second. Knowing that time is on the x-axis, there are many ways to calculate a HR from the EKG graph paper. An easy way to calculate a minute rate is to count the number of complexes in 6 seconds (i.e., 30 large boxes) and multiply by 10. Often the EKG paper will have 3-second intervals premarked. An alternative approach is to identify an R wave from one EKG complex that is close to or on a heavy black line (i.e., a large box), and then assign each of the following heavy black lines (large boxes) a number in the following order: 300, 150, 100, 75, 60, 50, 40. The heavy line closest to the next R wave will provide an approximation of HR (Fig. 16.9). Finally, dividing 300 by the number of large boxes between two R waves will also indicate the HR. If the rate is regular, any of the preceding strategies will work. If the rate is irregular, however, the complexes will need to be counted over a long time frame, a minimum of a 6-second strip should be used.

ST Segment

The clinical usefulness of the ST segment is to identify the presence of impaired coronary perfusion, either ischemia or injury. The J point, the point where the S wave turns into the ST segment, is the point of reference for interpreting the ST segment. On the EKG paper, if the ST segment is depressed (one or two small boxes) at two small boxes beyond the J point, then ischemia is likely present. Ischemia is transient, and when myocardial supply and demand are rebalanced, the ST segment will return to baseline. Unlike the ST depression of ischemia, a transmural myocardial injury (i.e., infarction) presents as ST segment elevation (Fig. 16.10). A nontransmural myocardial injury, however, presents as ST depression and is usually accompanied by laboratory values (e.g., CK-MB, troponin) that indicate infarction has occurred.

Left Heart Catheterization/Coronary Angiogram

Left heart cardiac catheterization or *cath,* as it is commonly referred to, involves insertion of a catheter into a major artery (often the femoral or radial artery) and advancing it retrograde through the aorta until it reaches the LV. The catheter may then proceed into the LV and is used to measure hemodynamic pressures during systole and diastole and to examine LV function. The ejection fraction (EF) is a clinically useful measure of systolic LV function. The EF is the relationship between the SV and the LVEDV (EF = SV/LVEDV). Normal EF is 55 to 75 percent, meaning that with each contraction 55 to 75 percent of the volume of blood that was in the LV at the end of diastole has been ejected into the aorta during systole. In systolic dysfunction, a general rule of thumb is that the lower the EF, the more impaired the LV function. The *angiogram* component involves injecting a radiopaque dye into the ostium of each coronary artery, observing blood flow through each of the arteries to determine the presence of lesions or blood flow obstructions. Depending on the information desired, the patient's status, and the planned interventions, a cardiac cath procedure may last from 1 to 3 hours.

Echocardiogram

With ultrasound technology, the echocardiogram is used to examine wall motion integrity, valvular status, wall thickness, chamber size, and LV function. The EF may also be calculated using the data obtained from the echocardiogram. An echocardiogram may accompany a stress test and is known as a *stress echo*. The purpose of a stress echo is to compare LV function and wall motion between rest and exercise when an increased $\dot{V}O_2$ results in an increased $M\dot{V}O_2$. A

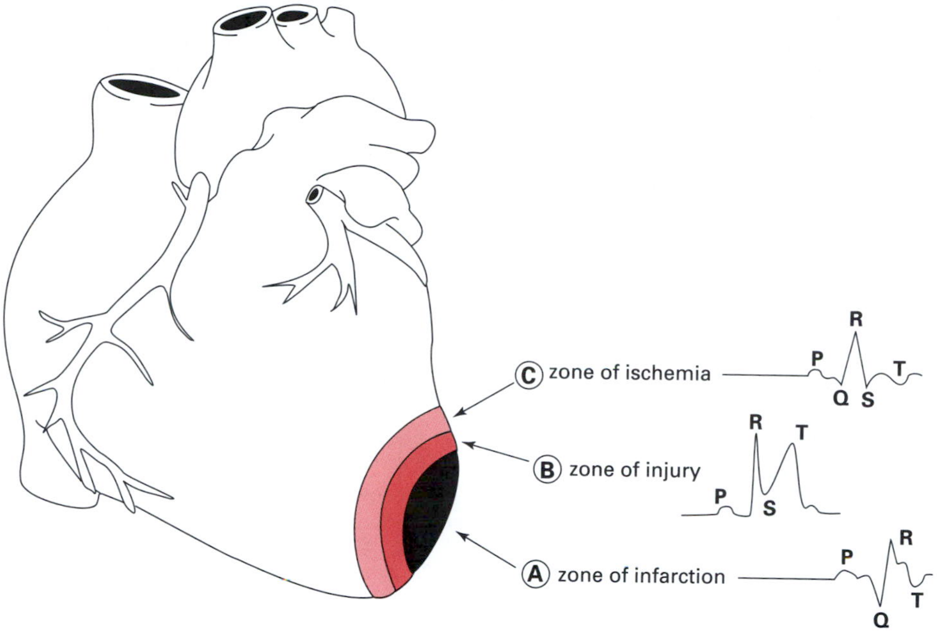

Figure 16.10 EKG following an MI. (*A*) *Zone of infarction*: when infarction occurs through the full thickness of the myocardium (transmural) an abnormal Q wave usually appears. (*B*) *Zone of injury*: ST elevation occurs in the area of injury. (*C*) *Zone of ischemia*: ST depression and/or T wave inversion occurs in an area of decreased perfusion (ischemia).

positive stress echo indicates a worsening of LV function as activity increases; a negative stress echo indicates that the LV has adequately adapted to the increase in energy demand.

Invasive Monitors

When is it not feasible to perform a left heart catheterization to examine LV function, or if continuous monitoring of myocardial function is desired, a catheter may be inserted through the vessels entering the right side of the heart to record the following pressures: central venous pressure (CVP), PA pressure, and pulmonary capillary wedge pressures (PCWP). This catheter is referred to as a central line. A common type of central line for hemodynamic monitoring is the Swan-Ganz catheter. Because the cardiovascular system is a closed loop and the LV depends on the integrity of the RV to function appropriately, recording right-sided pressures gives an indirect indication of the status of the LV. By comparing the actual readings from the patient to the expected norm, a failing LV may be identified by elevated pressures, while lowered pressures may identify a volume-depleted LV. Patients in intensive care settings are frequently invasively monitored to determine minute-to-minute hemodynamic changes over extended periods of time. If the patient is relatively hemodynamically stable, physical therapy intervention may be appropriate. Activity is limited, however, to bed or possibly chair activity.

Exercise Tolerance Tests

To examine the ability of the cardiovascular system to accommodate to increasing $\dot{V}O_2$, an exercise tolerance test (ETT, stress test or graded exercise test) is useful. The patient exercises through stages of increasing workloads, expressed in units of oxygen. Oxygen cost may be expressed in L/min, ml O_2 / kg /min, kcal, or **metabolic equivalents (METs)**; a MET represents the basic systemic oxygen requirement at rest, roughly 3.5 ml O_2/kg/min. The clinical usefulness of METs is that an activity can be expressed in comparison to resting energy cost. For example, the first stage of the Bruce protocol requires roughly 5 METs of energy (i.e., it requires five times the energy expended at rest). The most common modalities used in exercise testing of patients with cardiac impairments are the treadmill, bicycle, and arm ergometer (Fig. 16.11). In the earlier years of exercise testing for examination of CAD, the step test was routinely used; however, it has for the most part been replaced by the other modalities. The step test is useful for fitness screening in the relatively healthy population and in exercise training for both the cardiac and noncardiac populations.

Knowledge of systemic energy requirements is important in prescribing exercise and activity guidelines, as well as in exercising testing for patients with cardiac impairments. Many charts are available that express systemic energy requirements using a variety of oxygen equivalents (Table 16.4).

The two major goals of exercising testing are to detect the presence of ischemia and to determine the functional aerobic capacity of the individual. The patient is monitored with a 12-lead EKG throughout the test and recovery; information regarding perfusion, rhythm, or conduction changes is therefore immediately available. In addition to the EKG, other diagnostic tools may be used, most commonly the echocardiogram and nuclear imaging. The stress

(text continues on page 608)

FUNCTIONAL CLASS	CLINICAL STATUS	O2 COST ml/kg/min	METS	STEP TEST	BICYCLE ERGOMETER	TREADMILL PROTOCOLS													
						Bruce		Cornell		Balke-Ware	ACIP		mACIP		Naughton			Ware	
				Nagle Balke Naughton; 2 min stages 30 steps min; Step height increased 4 cm q 2 min	1 watt= 6kpds; For 70 kg body weight	3-min stages		2-min stages		% grad at 3.3 mph; 1-min stages	2-min stages First 2 stages 1 min				2-min stages			2-min stages	
				Height (cm)	KPDS	MPH	%GR	MPH	%GR		MPH	%GR	MPH	%GR	%GR 2 MPH	%GR 3 MPH	%GR 3.4 MPH	MPH	%GR
						5.5	20												
						5.0	18	5.0	18	26, 25, 24						32.5	26		
Normal and I	Healthy dependent on age, activity	56.0	16							23						30	24		
		52.5	15					4.6	17	22, 21	3.4	24	3.4	24		27.5	22		
		49.0	14		1500					20	3.1	24	3.1	24		25	20		
		45.5	13		1350	4.2	16	4.2	16	19, 18						22.5	18		
		42.0	12	40						17, 16	3	21	2.7	24		20	16		
		38.5	11	36	1200			3.8	15	15, 14	3	17.5	2.3	24		17.5	14	3.4	14.0
	sedentary healthy	35.0	10	32	1050	3.4	14			13, 12						15	12	3.0	15.0
		31.5	9	28						11									
	Limited	28.0	8	24	900			3.0	13	10, 9	3	14	2	24		12.5	10	3.0	12.5
		24.5	7	20	750	2.5	12	2.5	12	8, 7	3	10.5	2	18.9	17.5	10	8	3.0	10.0
II	Symptomatic	21.0	6	16	600			2.1	11	6, 5					14	7.5	6	3.0	7.5
		17.5	5	12	450	1.7	10	1.7	10	4, 3, 2	3.0	7.0	2	13.5	10.5	5	4	2.0	10.5
III		14.0	4	8	300	1.7	5	1.7	5	1	3.0	3.0	2	7	7	2.5	2	2.0	7.0
		10.5	3	4	150						2.5	2.0	2	3.5	3.5	0		2.0	3.5
		7.0	2			1.7	0	1.7	0		2.0	0	2	0	0			1.5	0
IV		3.5	1															1.0	0

Figure 16.11 Estimated oxygen requirements for step, bicycle, and treadmill. The standard Bruce protocol begins at 1.7 mph and 10 percent grade (roughly 5 METs). Oxygen requirements increase with progressive increases in workload for all modalities. (Adapted from Fletcher, GF et al[81] p 156).

Table 16.4 Metabolic Equivalent (MET) Chart

Intensity (70-kg Person)	Endurance Promoting	Occupational	Recreational
1½–2 METs 4–7 mL/kg/min 2–2½ kcal/min	Too low in energy level	Desk work, driving auto, electric calculating machine operation, light housework, polishing furniture, washing clothes	Standing, strolling (1 mph), flying, motorcycling, playing cards, sewing, knitting
2–3 METs 7–11 mL/kg/min 2½–4 kcal/min	Too low in energy level unless capacity is very low	Auto repair, radio and television repair, janitorial work, bartending, riding lawn mower, light wood-working	Level walking (2 mph), level bicycling (5 mph), billiards, bowling, skeet shooting,shuffleboard, powerboat driving, golfing with power cart, canoeing, horseback riding at a walk
3–4 METs 11–14 mL/kg/min 4–5 kcal/min	Yes, if continuous and if target heart rate is reached	Brick laying, plastering, wheelbarrow (100-lb load), machine assembly, welding (moderate load), cleaning windows, mopping floors, vacuuming, pushing light power mower	Walking (3 mph), bicycling (6 mph), horseshoe pitching, volleyball (6-person, non-competitive), golfing (pulling bag cart), archery, sailing (handling small boat), fly fishing (standing in waders), Horseback riding (trotting), badminton (social doubles)
4–5 METs 14–18 mL/kg/min	Recreational activities promote endurance; occupational activities must be continuous, lasting longer than 2 min	Painting, masonry, paperhanging, light carpentry, scrubbing floors, raking leaves, hoeing	Walking (3½ mph), bicycling (8 mph), table tennis, golfing (carrying clubs), dancing (foxtrot), badminton (singles), tennis (doubles), many calisthenics, ballet
5–6 METs 18–21 mL/kg/min	Yes	Digging garden, shoveling light earth	Walking (4 mph), bicycling (10 mph), canoeing (4 mph), horseback riding (posting to trotting), stream fishing (walking in light current in waders), ice or roller skating (9 mph)
6–7 METs 21–25 mL/kg/min 7–8 kcal/min	Yes	Shoveling 10 times/min (4½ kg or 10 lb), splitting wood, snow shoveling, hand lawn mowing	Walking (5 mph), bicycling (11 mph), competitive badminton, tennis (singles), folk and square dancing, light downhill skiing, ski touring (2½ mph), water skiing, swimming (20 yards/min)
7–8 METs 25–28 mL/kg/min 8–10 kcal/min	Yes	Digging ditches, carrying 36 kg or 80 lb, sawing hardwood	Jogging (5 mph), bicycling (12 mph), horseback riding (gallop), vigorous downhill skiing, basketball, mountain climbing, ice hockey, canoeing (5 mph), touch football, paddleball
8–9 METs 28-32 mL/kg/min 10–11 kcal/min	Yes	Shoveling 10 times/min (5½ kg or 14 lb)	Running (5½ mph), bicycling (13 mph), ski touring (4 mph), squash (social), handball (social), fencing, basketball (vigorous), swimming (30 yards/min), rope skipping
10+ METs 32+ mL/kg/min 11+ kcal/min	yes	Shoveling 10 times/min (7½ kg or 16 lb)	Running (6 mph = 10 METs, 7 mph = 11½ METs, 8 mph = 13½ METs, 9 mph = 15 METs, 10 mph = 17 METs), ski touring (5+ mph), handball (competitive), squash (competitive), swimming (greater than 40 yards/min)

From Fox, SM, et al: Physical activity and cardiovascular health: 3. The exercise prescription: Frequency and type of activity. Mod Con Cardiovasc Dis 41:26, 1972, with permission.

echo examines wall motion abnormalities that may or may not be present at rest, but may become more pronounced with increasing workloads. Nuclear imaging (e.g., thallium sestamibi) compares coronary perfusion between rest and exercise. If there is no decrease in perfusion with increasing workloads, the test is negative; if there is a decrease, the test is considered positive.

Stress tests are interpreted as either positive (+) or negative (−). A *positive ETT* indicates that there is a point at which the myocardial oxygen supply is inadequate to meet the myocardial oxygen demand, and the test is therefore positive for ischemia. A *negative ETT* indicates that at every tested physiological workload there is a balanced oxygen supply and demand. Patients are often confused regarding this grading system; it is helpful to reassure them that in this case, a negative test is in fact good. Stress tests are not unlike other diagnostic tools; however, they are not 100 percent specific and sensitive in identifying the presence of ischemia. A *false-negative ETT* is one that is interpreted as negative but the patient in fact has ischemia. Conversely, a *false-positive ETT* is one that is interpreted as positive but the patient does not have ischemia. Although relatively safe for a vast majority of patients, there are certain contraindications to exercise testing that should be noted (Box 16.2).

When a patient is unable to perform an exercise test because of limitations such as musculoskeletal or neurological impairments, a pharmacological stress test such as a *persantine thallium* test is often recommended. Persantine, when given intravenously, decreases coronary vascular resistance by causing arterioles to vasodilate, and therefore increases the blood flow through the capillary beds. If an artery is atherosclerotic, its arteriole may have gradually dilated over time in an attempt to increase capillary blood flow by means of pressure autoregulation. Therefore, when persantine is given, the diseased arteries may have a limitation in the amount of further arteriolar dilation that can occur. In comparison to the nondiseased arteries, there will be a relative decrease in blood flow through the capillary beds of the diseased arteries. Imaging studies will thus detect a relative decrease in blood flow to the area of the myocardium that is perfused by the diseased artery compared to that perfused by a nondiseased artery. Adenosine, which is a coronary and peripheral vasodilator (as well as an antiarrhythmic), has similar effects as persantine and may be used instead.[43]

Box 16.2 Contraindications to Exercise Testing

Absolute contraindications

- A recent significant change in the resting ECG suggesting infarction or other acute cardiac event
- Recent complicated myocardial infarction (unless patient is stable and pain free)
- Unstable angina
- Uncontrolled ventricular arrhythmia
- Uncontrolled atrial arrhythmia that compromises cardiac function
- Third-degree AV heart block without pacemaker
- Acute congestive heart failure
- Severe aortic stenosis
- Suspected or known dissecting aneurysm
- Active or suspected myocarditis or pericarditis
- Thrombophlebitis or intracardiac thrombi
- Recent systemic or pulmonary embolus
- Acute infections
- Significant emotional distress (psychosis)

Relative contraindications

- Resting diastolic blood pressure >115 mm Hg or resting systolic blood pressure >200 mm Hg
- Moderate valvular heart disease
- Known electrolyte abnormalities (hypokalemia, hypomagnesemia)
- Fixed-rate pacemaker (rarely used)
- Frequent or complex ventricular ectopy
- Ventricular aneurysm
- Uncontrolled metabolic disease (e.g., diabetes, thyrotoxicosis, or myxedema)
- Chronic infectious disease (e.g., mononucleosis, hepatitis, AIDS)
- Neuromuscular, musculoskeletal, or rheumatoid disorders that are exacerbated by exercise
- Advanced or complicated pregnancy

From the American College of Sports Medicine, Guidelines for Exercise Testing and Prescription, ed 5. Williams & Wilkins, Baltimore, 1995, p 42, with permission.

Pathophysiology and Physical Therapy Intervention

Simply stated, the heart is a muscular pump whose primary function is to provide adequate cardiac output for the body's metabolic needs. The pathophysiology of the heart, for the most part, can be viewed as a failure of any of the three interrelated factors that influence pump functioning: (1) the oxygen supply to the heart, (2) the contractility of the ventricles, or (3) the electrical impulse initiation or conduction. Clinically, an imbalance of myocardial oxygen supply and demand is the hallmark of CAD, inadequate myocardial oxygen supply to meet the metabolic oxygen demands of the myocardium. A decrease in myocardial contractility impairs the systolic functioning of the myocardium; a decrease in the compliancy of the myocardium impairs the diastolic functioning of the myocardium. Heart failure may result from either impairment in systolic or diastolic functioning. An alteration in either the initiation of the electrical impulse or in its conduction pathways is the basis for many arrhythmias. Because the work of the LV is really the powerhouse of the entire heart, and its energy requirements are significantly greater than the energy requirements of the RV, most clinical problems result from an impairment of the LV (e.g., inadequate LV perfusion via the coronary arteries, or inadequate LV contractility). Impaired RV functioning can occur in combination with LV dysfunction, as in *biventricular failure*. Impaired RV function seen separately, is seen in either cor pulmonale, which is right-sided failure owing to pulmonary abnormalities, or right-sided valvular disorders (tricuspid, pulmonic). Clinically, however, LV failure is much more common than RV failure.

Coronary Artery Disease

The primary impairment in CAD is an imbalance of myocardial oxygen supply to meet the $M\dot{V}O_2$. The decrease in supply is due to a narrowing of the lumen of the coronary artery, usually due to a fixed atherosclerotic lesion. The lesion results from an initial endothelial injury that causes changes within the intima of the blood vessel and progresses to lumenal narrowing. The cause of the initial injury is not well understood, but risk factors have been identified that are associated with an increased risk for the formation of an atherosclerotic lesion. The earliest identified risk factors by epidemiological studies such as The Framingham Heart Study included smoking, high cholesterol, hypertension, diabetes, emotional stress, and family history.[44–46] In recent years, obesity, sedentary lifestyle, and elevated blood homocysteine and fibrinogen levels have also been identified as possible contributors.[47]

Premenopausal women appear to have added protection from atherosclerosis. Initial clinical manifestation of coronary disease is delayed an average of 10 years for woman compared to men; the incidence of MIs presents as much as two decades later.[48] Starting at age 75, the prevalence of cardiovascular disease among women is greater than that for men.[3] The use of hormone replacement therapy (HRT) in postmenopausal women has been a topic of much discussion. In 1997, Hennekens reviewed 31 observational studies and estimated that there was a 44 percent reduction in coronary heart disease among postmenopausal women receiving estrogen replacement.[49] However, published studies in 1998 and 2002 resulted in suppressing the routine use of HRT due to the risk of hormone sensitive cancers outweighing any questionable cardiovascular benefit.[50,51] In 1998, the Heart and Estrogen Replacement Study (HERS) reported no beneficial effect of HRT on women with documented CAD[52]; in 2002, The Women's Health Initiative (WHI) reported similar findings from its study of healthy postmenopausal women without documented CAD.[53] Therefore, at this time, the use of HRT as either a primary or secondary prevention strategy for CAD is not clinically accepted.[54,55]

Clinical Manifestations

Patients may have occlusions within their coronary arteries and not have symptoms; in general, symptoms of CAD are not experienced until the lumen is at least 70 percent occluded. There are, therefore, many patients who are unaware of their subacute occlusions. It is imperative that an individual's risk factors are known and interventions and monitoring adjusted accordingly.

The clinical conditions resulting from CAD are due to inadequate myocardial oxygen supply to meet the $M\dot{V}O_2$. The most common clinical presentations of CAD are ischemia, infarction, or arrhythmias. It has been estimated, however, that as many as 50 percent of patients with CAD present with *sudden death* (cardiac arrest) as their first symptom. Ventricular fibrillation is the arrhythmia most commonly associated with sudden death.[56]

Ischemia

Ischemia is a temporary deficiency in oxygenated blood flow to tissues, and is due to arterial disease. Ischemia is a temporary condition; when the balance of myocardial oxygen supply and demand is reestablished, ischemia will be reversed. Recall that the factors that influence myocardial demand are HR and systolic BP (the RPP). When ischemia is present, reducing the RPP by stopping the aggravating activity and decreasing the $\dot{V}O_2$ may correct the myocardial oxygen imbalance because as systemic O_2 demand decreases so too will HR and SBP. A blockage of 70 percent or more of the coronary artery reduces blood flow enough to cause ischemia. This blockage is most commonly due to the presence of an atherosclerotic lesion. A less common cause of coronary narrowing is spasm of the smooth muscle within the walls of the vessels.

As a result of myocardial ischemia, the patient will feel the symptom of **angina**. The classical presentation of angina is substernal chest pressure accompanied by the *Levine sign* (the patient clenching his or her fist over the sternum). The Levine sign has a high diagnostic accuracy for ischemia.[57] For some patients, angina does not present in the classic way but rather may present as a pain or heaviness in the shoulder, jaw, arm, elbow, or upper back between scapulae. Angina may radiate from the chest to the arm or up to the throat, or it may present as indigestion or even shortness of breath. The patient is often asked to rank his or her discomfort on a scale of 1 to 10, with 10 being the most pain/discomfort ever experienced. The term *stable angina* is used when angina occurs at a predictable RPP and is alleviated by decreasing the RPP, commonly by stopping the activity and resting and the possible use of nitroglycerin (NTG; TNG). In stable angina, the patient often describes the sensation as an intensity less than 5/10, which improves to 0/10 when the oxygen supply is able to balance the demand. It is important to remember that any report of angina requires intervention; the clinician cannot ignore the symptoms even when the patient describes the sensation as light (1 to 2/10). The pathophysiology of an *unstable angina*, sometimes referred to as preinfarction angina, does not occur at a predictable RPP. It typically occurs at rest without any obvious precipitating factors or with minimal exertion, and therefore does not necessarily respond to a decrease in RPP. Unstable angina usually warrants immediate medical intervention, as the patient is at impending risk for further complications such as a MI or a lethal arrhythmia (v-tach, v-fib).

Ischemic myocardium demonstrates both systolic and diastolic dysfunctions. During the time of ischemia, there is a marked depression in contractility and an increase in myocardial stiffness (decreased compliance) in the affected area. Reversal of these myocardial dysfunctions will occur if the myocardial oxygen supply is reestablished after a short interruption. The longer the ischemic period, the longer it will take for normal contractility and relaxation to occur; [58] the patient is then at risk for irreversible damage such as MI (heart attack).

Infarction

Individual myocardial cells may differ in their tolerance for ischemia; however, irreversible changes start to appear 20 minutes to 2 hours from the onset of myocardial ischemia[58] The actual process of an infarction evolves over a period of hours. Angina commonly precedes an MI, but the intensity of the symptoms is dramatically increased. Patients frequently describe their discomfort as a 10 out of 10 on the pain scale. Infarction is irreversible. Whereas ischemia is due to a partial blockage of the coronary artery, an infarction results from complete occlusion of the vessel. This occlusion commonly results from a rupture of a vulnerable plaque with resultant formation of a thrombus. The type of plaque, more so than the size, will influence the risk of rupture. Lipid rich and soft plaques are more vulnerable to rupture than collagen-rich and hard plaque. Angiographically large plaque lesions are not necessarily more susceptible to rupture than smaller lesions. Because atherosclerosis begins within the walls of the artery, many vulnerable plaques are invisible via angiogram[59] or appear smaller than their actual size. Although not as common as plaque rupture, coronary occlusion can occur as a result of coronary spasm, coronary emboli, congenital anomalies, and a wide variety of inflammatory diseases.[59] The actual cause of plaque rupture is not clearly understood; however, as a result of the rupture, a thrombus is formed. There may be several mechanisms for thrombosis formation, such as mechanical obstruction of the lumen, release of tissue thromboplastin and the initiation of the clotting cascade, and platelet plug formation from the contact of platelets and exposed collagen.[60] Only lesions that occlude the lumen by 70 percent or more can cause ischemia, but smaller lesions can and do cause MIs. It is important to remember that the size of the initial lesions does not determine whether or not an MI can occur; a small plaque lesion of 30 percent as well as a larger lesion of 80 percent may rupture and subsequently form a thrombus that occludes the remainder of the lumen. The majority of MIs occur as a result of initial plaque lesions that are less than 60 percent, which are not hemodynamically significant to cause ischemia.[61] The effects on the ventricle as a result of the infarction often extend beyond the acute infarction period; these long-term effects occur primarily in ventricles that have sustained a moderate to large MI. As the ventricle heals, a process of *remodeling* occurs as a result of the presence of the infarcted tissue and subsequent dilation. Over time, this reengineering process produces an alteration in ventricular size, shape, and function. Thus, the resultant ventricle often operates at an increased myocardial energy cost due to its inefficient muscle mechanics.

Often pictured as three concentric circles (although not absolutely histologically correct), the area of infarction would be at the center of the circle surrounded first by an area of injury and then an outside area of ischemia (see Fig. 16.8).

MIs are identified by EKG findings, such as *Q wave* or *non-Q wave,* whether or not the ST segment was elevated or not at the time of intervention, the MI location (anterior, inferior, lateral, septal or posterior), and the resulting EF. A Q wave MI is identified by the presence of an abnormal Q wave on the EKG. A Q wave MI was formerly known as a *transmural MI* because it was believed to involve the full thickness of the ventricular wall. A non-Q wave MI was formerly known as a *nontransmural or subendocardial MI* because it involved the endocardium. However, it is possible that a Q wave may be absent from a transmural MI, so the newer classification was chosen. Anatomical classifications for MIs are based upon the surfaces of the LV, not the anatomic heart; an anterior MI involves the anterior surface of the LV, an inferior MI involves the inferior surface of the LV (the diaphragmatic region), a lateral MI involves the lateral surface of the LV (also may be referred to the free wall of the LV for the lateral wall is not adjacent to another structure), a septal MI involves the septum, and a posterior MI involves the LV posterior wall. If the MI involves the RV, it will be referred to as a RV infarct; because the RV and the inferior wall of the LV are commonly perfused by the RCA, it is possible to have an inferior MI with RV involvement. An EF of less than 35 percent is considered a large MI with significant systolic dysfunction and with the potential for LV failure (recall that a normal EF is approximately 55 to 75 percent). An MI that initially presents with an elevated ST segment on the EKG (*STEMI*: ST elevation MI) may be an indication for emergent thrombolytic therapy or revascularization.[62]

Although most MIs heal initially without incident, complications may occur. The major complications following an MI are recurrence of ischemia, LV failure, and ventricular arrhythmias. Therefore, when a patient is said to have had a *complicated MI*, either ischemia, LV failure, or significant ventricular arrhythmias have developed in the acute post MI period. Ischemia post MI is important to document because it indicates that there may be vulnerable myocardium with a reduced oxygen supply that may go on to infarct and thereby potentially enlarging the MI. The ultimate complication would be **cardiogenic shock** with inadequate CO and arterial blood pressure to perfuse the major organs as a result of severe LV failure. This may necessitate extraordinary medical interventions such as the *intra-aortic balloon pump (IABP)*.[63] The IABP facilitates CO, decreases $M\dot{V}O_2$, and increases coronary artery perfusion. The IABP is a balloon catheter placed within the aorta that inflates during diastole thereby increasing coronary artery perfusion and deflates during systole thereby decreasing afterload. The IABP may be used in other conditions besides post-MI cardiogenic instability, for example, patients with hemodynamic decompensation who are awaiting heart transplantation, patients with unstable angina and malignant arrhythmias (such as v-tach and v-fib), or post-cardiac surgical patients with severe hemodynamic instability.[63]

Once a MI has occurred, the wound healing process begins. In general, the stability of the wound is established within the first 4 to 6 weeks. During this time, the patient may engage in low-level activity, but aerobic training intensity should generally be avoided. After 4 to 6 weeks, it is common for the patient to undergo a symptom-limited maximal exercise tolerance test (ETT). The treadmill is the most common modality for exercise testing, and a variety of protocols may be followed. The bicycle may also be used.

Most patients will have a negative ETT at this time, indicating that there is no apparent ischemic myocardium at the workload achieved. A positive ETT means that ischemia is present at a certain workload. The physician will report at what HR and BP the ischemia occurred (the ischemic RPP), as well as the time during the test it occurred. As a result of a positive test, the physician may suggest altering the patient's medications to provide more anti-ischemic benefits or suggest a cardiac catheterization to determine the feasibility of a revascularization procedure such as *coronary artery bypass grafting (CABG)* or *angioplasty (PTCA)*. (see following section). After the ETT, patients may undergo an aerobic and strength-training program for the next 2 to 4 months, followed by a maintenance program. Cardiac rehabilitation and maintenance programs include not just exercise but education and support for the suggested behavioral changes and the patient's individual pharmacological management.

Diagnostic Tests and Medical Management

The classic diagnostic tool for examining a patient's complaint of suspected angina is the 12-lead EKG. If ischemia is present, the ST segment will be depressed, and the T wave may also be inverted (flipped) in those leads corresponding to the coronary perfusion pattern of the involved artery. Ischemic changes will be present only while the ischemia is present; when the ischemia has resolved, the EKG will return to normal. If a transmural MI is present, a series of changes will occur; the ST will initially elevate, indicating an area of injury, and a pathological Q wave will emerge within hours of the MI (see Fig. 16.10). A non-transmural (non-Q wave) MI will not have a Q wave, and the EKG will exhibit ST depression in the leads corresponding to the involved artery with decreased perfusion.

If the patient presents to the emergency room with the symptom of angina that is supported by EKG (e.g., ST depression), the physiological goal is to decrease $M\dot{V}O_2$ and/or increase myocardial oxygen supply. The patient is given supplemental oxygen by nasal cannula and administered the medication nitroglycerin (NTG). Nitroglycerin is a potent vasodilator of arteries and veins; it will (1) decrease myocardial work (i.e., energy requirements of the heart) by decreasing BP (afterload) and venous return (preload) and (2) increase coronary blood supply by dilating coronary arteries. The impact of coronary artery dilation is minimal compared to the other effects. Patients not responsive to these and other interventions are at risk for a MI. They may, therefore, be candidates for an emergent cardiac catheterization to locate and identify the critical lesion and be considered for a revascularization procedure to decrease the atherosclerotic lesion, such as *percutaneous transluminal coronary angioplasty (PTCA) with stent,* rotational *atherectomy* of the lesion, laser surgery, or CABG.

If the patient's EKG is consistent with a pattern of injury, ST elevation, a *thrombolytic agent* such as streptokinase or tissue plasminogen activase (TPA) may be given. The effect of the thrombolytics is to lyse the new active thrombus being formed within the coronary artery. This reduction in thrombus size will help to restore at least partial blood flow to the myocardium and either avert an MI or reduce its potential size.

Two of the most common methods for determining whether a patient has had an MI are EKG findings and blood work; specific to the latter is the presence of elevated levels of *CK-MB*, an isoenzyme released with intracellular myocardial damage. Unlike in an MI, there are no definitive blood tests that indicate the presence of ischemia or injury. Other markers that may be used to diagnose an acute MI are the proteins *troponin I, troponin T,* and myoglobin. Alexander and colleagues[64] note that total CK-MB, troponin I, and troponin T have a high sensitivity for the diagnosis of an MI. CK-MB and myoglobin may be the most sensitive biomarkers for patients presenting for emergent medical intervention within 6 to 10 hours of the onset of an MI.[64] For patients presenting after 10 hours, troponin biomarkers are preferred over CK-MB because of their increased sensitivity.[64] CK is found in many tissues besides the myocardium, especially striated muscle, brain, and liver. Injury to these areas will elevate total CK. To differentiate the type of tissue injured, use of CK-MB will isolate the source to the myocardium. Troponin levels should not be elevated in the setting of striated muscle trauma.

Once the diagnosis of an MI has been reached (i.e., the patient is "ruled in" for an MI), the goal of medical management is to keep the patient hemodynamically stable and optimize the wound healing of the myocardium. Usually after an uneventful 24 hours of bed rest, the patient may gradually begin to increase his or her activity, ideally under the supervision of a physical therapist.

Revascularization

PTCA uses a balloon on the tip of a catheter that is inserted into either the femoral or radial artery and advanced retrograde along the aorta to the openings of the coronary arteries. The catheter is inserted into the coronary artery and at the site of the lesion the balloon is inflated to compress the plaque against the wall of the coronary artery, thereby increasing the lumenal area. A wire like cage (stent) is placed over the compressed area to help it stay in place. The cage is commonly coated with a drug (e.g., the drug eluting stent) to prevent endothelial cell proliferation, which may occur in response to endothelial trauma and the presence of a foreign object placed within the coronary artery.

CABG uses a donor vessel to bypass the involved lesion and establish an alternate blood supply. The donor vessel may be the radial artery of the nondominant hand, the saphenous vein, or the internal mammary artery. The patient's harvested saphenous vein or radial artery must be completely detached from both its proximal and distal insertions; the graph is sutured proximally into the aorta and distally into the involved artery beyond the occlusion. The internal mammary artery maintains its native proximal attachment while the distal segment is reattached below the area of occlusion. Bypass surgery techniques are constantly changing; traditionally, the full sternum was cut and retracted, but newer minimally invasive techniques have emerged that involve less sternal cutting and some techniques involve no sternal cutting at all, but access the heart via the intercostal space. Most CABG procedures involve placing the patient on an artificial heart–lung machine (bypass pump), which maintains the oxygenation and circulation of the blood while the heart is stopped during the surgical procedure. As a result of the bypass pump, patients may have additional fluid weight gain following surgery, may feel fatigued, and some patients may have transient atrial fibrillation and cognitive changes.

Pharmacological Management

Cardiovascular pharmacological agents are critical in the medical management of patients with CAD. There are a variety of drugs designed to reestablish the balance of myocardial supply and demand, with new drugs being added all the time. The major anti-ischemic categories are beta-blockers, calcium channel blockers, and nitrates. *Beta-blockers* decrease beta sympathetic activity on the heart, resulting in a decrease in HR and contractility and therefore energy demand ($M\dot{V}O_2$). *Calcium channel blockers* reduce blood pressure and therefore decrease the work of the heart. Calcium channel blockers are also somewhat unique in preventing coronary smooth muscle spasm and thereby may increase myocardial blood supply. *Nitrates,* one of the oldest categories of drugs, are potent vasodilators that decrease preload and afterload, and therefore decrease myocardial work, as well as dilate coronary arteries. *Afterload reducers,* particularly those that affect the renin–angiotensin–aldosterone system such as *ACE inhibitors* (angiotensin converting enzyme inhibitor) and *ARBs (angiotensin receptor blocker)* are frequently used to counteract the adverse effects of ventricular remodeling that occurs following MIs (see CHF section).

There are many excellent resources for further study of pharmacological management for heart disease, including Ciccone,[65] Malone,[66] Kupersmith,[67] and Grimes and Cohen.[68] Therapists working with patients who have CAD must be familiar with these medications and their side effects, especially their effect on exercise response. The effect of some of the more widely used cardiac drugs on HR, BP, and EKG findings are presented in Table 16.5.

Physical Therapy Intervention for Patients with Coronary Artery Disease

According to the APTA *Guide to Physical Therapist Practice,* the preferred practice pattern for management of patients with cardiovascular disease is Pattern 6-D. The development of specific anticipated goals and expected outcomes for the individual with CAD is based on the following general goals of physical therapy intervention.[6]

1. Aerobic capacity is increased.
2. Ability to perform physical tasks related to self-care, home management, community and work integration or reintegration, and leisure activities is increased.
3. Physiological response to increased oxygen demand is improved.
4. Strength, power, and endurance are increased.
5. Symptoms associated with increased oxygen demand are decreased.
6. Ability to recognize a recurrence is increased, and intervention is sought in a timely manner.
7. Risk of recurrence is reduced.
8. Behaviors that foster healthy habits, wellness, and prevention are acquired.
9. Decision making is enhanced regarding health of patient and the use of health care resources by patient/client, family, significant others, and caregivers.

Physical therapists treat not only patients who have a primary diagnosis of heart disease, but also, and perhaps more commonly, patients with multiple medical diagnoses, only one of which is cardiac. Physical therapy intervention during the traditional acute cardiac rehabilitation phase involves following the patient while recovering from his or her cardiac event, such as an MI, providing hemodynamic monitoring of progressive activity, discharge guidelines, education, and information regarding outpatient referral. It may include outpatient management as well, ideally in a multidisciplinary setting including nursing and nutrition. Patients with cardiac histories commonly have physical therapy needs at other points throughout their lives. For example, the patient with a previous MI might require ambulation training as a result of a fractured hip, an outpatient knee rehabilitation program following a skiing injury, tennis elbow intervention, prosthetic

Table 16.5 Effects of Medications on Heart Rate, Blood Pressure, ECG, and Exercise Capacity

Medications	Heart Rate	Blood Pressure	ECG	Exercise Capacity
I. Beta blockers (including labetalol)	↓* (R and E)	↓ (R and E)	↓ HR* (R) ↓ ischemia† (E)	↑ in patients with angina; ↓ or ⟷ in patients without angina
II. Nitrates	↑ (R) ↑ or ⟷ (E)	↓ (R) ↓ or ⟷ (E)	↑ HR (R) ↑ or ⟷ HR (E) ↓ ischemia† (E)	↑ in patients with angina; ⟷ in patients without angina; or ⟷ in patients with congestive heart failure (CHF)
III. Calcium channel blockers				↑ in patients with angina; ⟷ in patients without angina
Felodipine, Isradipine, Nicardipine, Nifedipine	↑ or ⟷ (R and E)	↓ (R and E)	↑ or ⟷ HR (R and E) ↓ ischemia (E)	
Bepridil, Diltiazem, Verapamil	↓ (R and E)		↓ HR (R and E) ↓ ischemia† (E)	
IV. Digitalis	↓ in patients w/atrial fibrillation and possibly CHF Not significantly altered in patients w/sinus rhythm	⟷	May produce nonspecific ST-T wave changes (R) May produce ST segment depression (E)	Improved only in patients with atrial fibrillation or in patients with CHF
V. Diuretics	⟷	⟷ or ↓ (R and E)	⟷ (R) May cause PVCs and "false possitive" test results if hypokalemia occurs. May cause PVCs if hypomagnesemia occurs (E)	⟷ except possibly in patients with CHF
VI. Vasodilators, nonadrenergic	↑ or ⟷ (R and E)	↓ (R and E)	↑ or ⟷ HR (R and E)	⟷ except ↑ or ⟷ in patients with CHF
ACE inhibitors	⟷	↓ (R and E)	⟷	⟷ except ↑ or ⟷ in patients with CHF
Alpha-adrenergic blockers	⟷	↓ (R and E)	⟷	⟷
VII. Nicotine	↑ or ⟷ (R and E)	↑ (R and E)	↑ or ⟷ HR May provoke ischemia, arrhythmias (R and E)	⟷ except ↓ or ⟷ in patients with angina

Adapted from American College of Sports Medicine: Guidelines for Exercise Testing and Prescription, ed 5. Williams & Wilkins, Baltimore, 1995, pp 246, 247, 251, with permission.

Key: ↑ = increase; ⟷ = no effect; ↓ = decrease.

*Beta-blockers with ISA lower resting HR only slightly.

†May prevent or delay myocardial ischemia.

R = rest; E = exercise.

ambulation training, or intervention following a cerebrovascular accident (CVA). If the physical therapist understands the pathophysiology of the cardiac condition, and the energy demands that are being placed on the patient, then the therapist will be able to adjust the plan of care accordingly.

It is important to remember that a patient with known CAD may not have symptomatic ischemia, either because the lesions are not of significant size to interfere with blood flow, or the anti-ischemic medications are able to keep the patient's physiological response to activity below his or her ischemic threshold. Following a noncomplicated MI, ischemia should not occur in the area perfused by the involved artery because infarcted tissue cannot become ischemic. However, if there is disease in other arteries, then ischemia can occur in any noninfarcted tissue that has a compromised blood supply. A physical therapist working with patients with significant CAD must be aware that their basic cardiac impairment is an imbalance of myocardial oxygen supply and demand, and any increase in systemic oxygen consumption will increase myocardial oxygen consumption. A past medical history of CAD does not mean that the disease occurred in the past and is no longer present; once a person has been diagnosed with CAD they have the potential for atherosclerosis progression at any later point in time. Even in patients with lesions that are less than 70 percent there is the possibility of plaque rupture. Although the precipitating factors for plaque rupture are not clearly understood, the plaque with increased levels of oxidized LDLs is thought to be unstable with a greater potential for rupture.[69] It is important to note that plaque rupture may occur with lesions of any size, not just those that are greater than 70 percent. [61,70] Therefore, it is prudent for the physical therapist to know the status of all the coronary arteries, not just those that were revascularized or have a greater than 70 percent lesion.

The degree of a patient's risk for increased morbidity and mortality is based on a number of factors. The American Association of Cardiovascular and Pulmonary Rehabilitation (AACVPR) and the American College of Physicians provide a framework for stratifying cardiac patients (Table 16.6).

Exercise Prescription

The Clinical Practice Guidelines for Cardiac Rehabilitation were established after extensive and critical review of published scientific literature.[71] These guidelines support the beneficial effect of exercise training on exercise tolerance for patients with heart disease. The most consistent benefit appeared to occur with exercise training at least three times per week for 12 or more weeks' duration. The duration of aerobic exercise training sessions varied from 20 to 40 minutes at an intensity approximating 70 to 85 percent of the baseline maximal exercise test HR. Exercise prescriptions are based on frequency, intensity, time (duration), and type (mode), the FITT equation. Activity should be gradually progressive in a logical stepwise fashion of increasing energy costs (i.e., METs, kilocalories) with appropriate HR and BP monitoring.

Although exercise is highly recommended for the patient with heart disease, there are conditions in which exercise is unwise. The American Association of Cardiovascular and Pulmonary Rehabilitation (AACVPR) established guidelines for evaluating a patient's appropriateness for exercise participation. They recommend that patients with the following conditions be excluded from exercise training: unstable angina, symptomatic heart failure, uncontrolled arrhythmias, moderate to severe aortic stenosis, uncontrolled diabetes, acute systemic illness or fever, uncontrolled tachycardia (HR $>$ 100 bpm), resting systolic BP $\geq$ 200 mm Hg, resting diastolic blood pressure $\geq$ 110 mm Hg, thrombophlebitis, as well as other conditions.[72] The patient should be evaluated once these conditions have been corrected and, when appropriate, begin (or resume) the exercise program. Recognizing that cardiac disease is a dynamic process, and that the patient who was stable and able to participate in physical therapy last week may not be stable this week is a critical concept. The importance of a patient-specific examination and evaluation prior to each session will allow the physical therapist to critically plan the appropriate intervention.

Exercise Intensity

Intensity may be prescribed by either HR or by subjective report, a *rating of perceived exertion (RPE)*. Subjective ratings of intensity of exertion have been used to quantify effort during exercise. The original **Rating of Perceived Exertion scale (The Borg RPE Scale)**, developed by Borg, has been used extensively[73] (Table 16.7). It consists of numbers ranging from 6 to 20, which patients use to rate their perceptions of how hard they are working. Descriptive words accompany the numbers, such as hard or very hard. Commonly, patients are asked to limit their exertion to between fairly light and somewhat hard. Borg also developed a category-ratio scale of 0-10 (Chapter 15, Table 15.6). Both local symptoms, such as muscle aches, cramps, pain, or fatigue, and central symptoms, such as feelings of fatigue or breathlessness, contribute to the overall feelings of work performance. High correlation of RPE ratings with HR and aerobic power has been found in normal individuals and in patients with cardiac disease.

A common aerobic exercise prescription based on HR is 70 to 85 percent of HR_{max}. However, the more deconditioned patient may be aerobically trained at as low as 50 to 60 percent of HR_{max}. Any patient who has documented CAD should have a medically supervised ETT before beginning an aerobic exercise program. Without an ETT, it is impossible to assume what the maximum HR would be for a patient with cardiac disease. The EKG monitoring during the ETT is useful in the detection of exercise-induced ischemia. If there are no ETT data available, it is unwise to prescribe an exercise based on HRs. Cautious progression of activity is warranted, along with use of RPE and knowledge of adverse signs and symptoms for exercise intolerance. An easy tool for self-monitoring is for the patient to be able to talk without becoming breathless while exercising. This provides a fair indication that the patient is appropriately exercising below his or her maximal oxygen capacity.

Exercise Frequency

Exercise is commonly prescribed three to five times per week. The patient should not experience increased fatigue

Table 16.6 Risk Stratification Criteria for Cardiac Patients by the American College of Physicians (ACP), and American Association of Cardiovascular and Pulmonary Rehabilitation (AACVPR)

ACP	AACVPR
Low Risk	
Uncomplicated MI or CABG	Uncomplicated MI, CABG, angioplasty, or atherectomy
Functional capacity ≥8 METs 3 weeks after clinical event	Functional capacity ≥6 METs 3 or more weeks after clinical event
No ischemia, left ventricular dysfunction or complex arrhythmias	No resting or exercise-induced myocardial ischemia manifested as angina and/or ST segment displacement No resting or exercise-induced complex arrhythmias
Asymptomatic at rest with exercise capacity adequate for most vocational and recreational activities	No significant left ventricular dysfunction (EF ≥ 50%)
Intermediate (Moderate) Risk	
Functional capacity <8 METs 3 weeks after clinical event	Functional capacity <5–6 METs 3 or more weeks after clinical event
Shock or CHF during recent MI (<6 months)	Mild to moderately depressed left ventricular function (EF 31–49%)
Failure to comply with exercise prescription Inability to self-monitor heart rate	Failure to comply with exercise prescription
Exercise-induced ST-segment depression <2 mm	Exercise-induced ST-segment depression of 1–2 mm or reversible ischemic defects (echocardiography or nuclear radiography)
High Risk	
Severely depressed LV function (EF <30%)	Severely depressed LV function (EF ≤30%)
Resting complex ventricular arrhythmias (low grade IV or V)	Complex ventricular arrythmias at rest or appearing or increasing with exercise
PVCs appearing or increasing with exercise	
Exertional hypotension (≥15 mm Hg decrease in systolic pressure during exercise)	Decrease in systolic blood pressure of >15 mm Hg during exercise or failure to rise consistent with exercise workloads
Recent MI (<6 months) complicated by serious ventricular arrhythmias	MI complicated by CHF, cardiogenic shock, and/or complex-ventricular arrhythmias
Exercise-induced ST-segment depression >2 mm	Patients with severe CAD and marked (>2 mm) exercise-induced ST-segment depression
Survivor of cardiac arrest	Survivor of cardiac arrest

From American College Sports Medicine: Guidelines For Exercise Testing, ed 5. Williams & Wilkins, Baltimore, 1995, pp 20, 21, with permission.

CABG = coronary artery bypass graft; MET = metabolic equivalent; EF = ejection fraction; CHF = congestive heart failure; LV = left ventricular; PVC = premature ventricular contraction.

as a result of exercise. If fatigue does occur, then the frequency and/or intensity of exercise should be decreased. Patients who choose to exercise daily must watch for signs and symptoms of fatigue and overexertion, recognizing that fatigue may not just occur during the activity, but be delayed until later in the day or the next day.

Exercise Duration (Time)

The goal of 30 to 40 minutes of aerobic exercise with an additional 5 to 10 minutes of warmup and an adequate cool-down is appropriate. If this amount of activity is uncomfortable for the patient, whatever amount he or she can do comfortably without adverse symptoms is appropriate.

Table 16.7 Rating of Perceived Exertion: The Borg RPE Scale

The Borg RPE Scale
6 No exertion at all
7
8 Extremely light
9 Very light
10
11 Light
12
13 Somewhat hard
14
15 Hard (heavy)
16
17 Very hard
18
19 Extremely hard
20 Maximal exertion

For correct usage of the scale(s) the exact design and instructions given in Borg's folders must be followed. See Borg, G., 1998, Borg's Perceived Exertion and Pain Scales. Champaign, IL: Human Kinetics, 1998, or www.borgproducts.com.

Patients who are deconditioned may require interval work, brief rests every 5 minutes during their early training. Adequate warmup is crucial for all patients but especially for patients with CAD. By gradually increasing the $M\dot{V}O_2$ and allowing the coronary arteries time to vasodilate, a balanced myocardial supply and demand may be possible with subsequent activity.

Mode of Exercise (Type)

The variety of exercise equipment has expanded in the last 20 years. The good news is that the patient has the opportunity to experience a variety of equipment including treadmills, stair climbers, bicycles, rowers, cross-country ski simulators, reclining bicycles, steppers, arm ergometers, and others. Patients frequently ask which is the best equipment; the one that they enjoy and the one that they will use is by far the best for them.

If a patient becomes symptomatic with angina during a physical therapy intervention, the immediate goal is to decrease $M\dot{V}O_2$; the activity should be immediately stopped. The patient should sit or, if possible, lie down on a bed or plinth. The physical therapist should take the patient's HR and blood pressure as soon as possible to determine the $M\dot{V}O_2$ at which the patient became ischemic, the ischemic threshold. If the patient is in an inpatient facility, help should be sought immediately to ensure that facility guidelines are quickly initiated. Such guidelines may include supplemental oxygen, a 12-lead EKG, administration of NTG, and other anti-ischemic medications. If the patient is in an outpatient setting and has his or her own NTG (which the patient should be carrying at all times), the patient should take it and follow the prescribed guidelines. NTG should produce a tingling or burning sensation if it is effective; failure of the NTG to produce these may indicate that the NTG is outdated. Patients are generally instructed to take one NTG sublingually (under the tongue), although some patients use an NTG spray. Wait 5 minutes and repeat administration if the symptoms are not completely gone. A third NTG may also be taken after waiting another 5 minutes. Patients are frequently told that if the symptoms have not resolved completely after three doses of NTG they should come to the emergency room for further management. If the patient is in an outpatient setting without his or her own NTG and has symptoms that do not resolve after a few minutes of rest, then the facility guidelines to activate advanced care for the patient should begin quickly. If the patient's symptoms escalate, even after the first NTG, emergency care needs to be initiated immediately. If the patient is climbing stairs, the patient should stop, take a few easy deep breaths, and then descend when the symptoms have abated and walk slowly to the first available support. However, if the patient's symptoms are quickly accelerating despite stopping the activity and taking deep breaths, the patient should be assisted to a position of comfort and further medical assistance sought immediately. The therapist should present a calm demeanor, reassuring the patient that this situation can be handled efficiently and easily (which it can).

Physical therapists must be sensitized to the fact that not all chest pain is necessarily cardiac in origin; there are many differential diagnoses including visceral (Fig. 16.12) and musculoskeletal that may mimic cardiac pain. They must therefore be able to differentiate musculoskeletal from cardiac pain, which at times may be difficult. Listening to the patient's subjective report of his or her symptoms, identifying pertinent risk factors, and performing screening tests to clear the musculoskeletal system are all indicated. Generally, cardiac pain is associated with an increase in myocardial demand, that is, an increase in HR and BP, and therefore is often associated with activity. When the intensity of the activity decreases, the symptoms should resolve or decrease. Breathing patterns, body positions, or range of motion generally do not affect the pain of cardiac origin. The absolute measure of ischemia is the EKG; the ST segment will depress or the T wave will invert with ischemia and remain as such as long as ischemia is occurring.

Cardiac Rehabilitation: Myocardial Infarction

Although it is common today to take cardiac rehabilitation for granted, it really was not that long ago that treatment

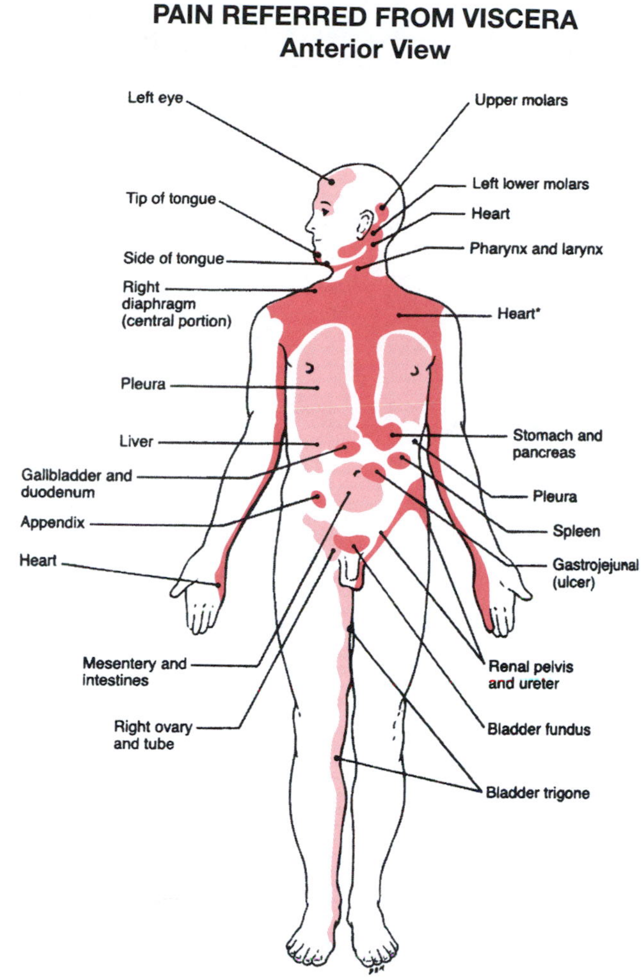

Figure 16.12 Pain referred from viscera. The pain of coronary insufficiency can involve any aspect of the anterior chest: interscapular, retrosternal, shoulders, arms, and epigastric area. Another site for myocardial ischemia is jaw discomfort. Also note the varieties of differential diagnosis that may present in the same locations as myocardial ischemic pain. (From Rothstein, J et al: The Rehabilitation Specialist's Handbook, ed 2. FA Davis, Philadelphia, 1998, p 484, with permission).

for patients with MI included weeks of prolonged bed rest. In the pivotal 1952 study by Levine and Lown,[74] chair rest and low-level activity was found to be more beneficial than the traditional 8 weeks of bed rest. Today, the patient with a noncomplicated MI may be hospitalized for as few as 3 to 5 days.

Cardiac rehabilitation (cardiac rehab) is multidisciplinary and may include the physician, nurse, physical and occupational therapists, exercise physiologist, nutritionist, and social service caseworker. Cardiac rehab begins in the hospital and extends indefinitely into the maintenance phase. The inpatient component is referred to as *Phase I.* Outpatient phases include *Phase II,* the exercise training period, and *Phase III,* the maintenance period. The AACVPR describes Phase II as occurring immediately after discharge, requiring intensive monitoring and supervision including EKG monitoring and intensive risk factor interventions.[75] Aerobic and strength training may begin based upon the results of the ETT, which is usually done at approximately 4 weeks. In Phase III, the patient has stabilized and requires EKG monitoring only if signs and symptoms necessitate; endurance training and risk factor modification continue. Ideally, Phase II is initiated within 2 weeks of hospital discharge. It is important to note that these phases are not absolutes and the timelines and activities of these phases may vary according to managed care models, contracts with reimbursement plans, and treatment protocol designs. Owing to insurance coverage, some patients do not enter into a formal cardiac rehab program until after their symptom-limited maximum ETT at 4 to 6 weeks post-MI.

Inpatient/Phase 1

The length of hospital stay for a patient with an MI has changed dramatically in the last decade and is commonly 3 to 5 days for an *uncomplicated MI* (no post-MI angina, malignant arrhythmias, or heart failure), compared to at least three to four times that duration in the early 1980s. Inpatient cardiac rehab uses a team approach based on activity progression, patient education, and hemodynamic and EKG monitoring, together with medical and pharmacological management. The role of the physical therapist is to monitor activity tolerance, prepare for discharge, educate the patient to recognize adverse symptoms with activity, support risk factor modification techniques, provide emotional support, and collaborate with other team members.

Vital sign monitoring occurs before and after and, if possible, during activity. The intensity of the activity is considered to be low level, perceived exertion for the patient should be comparable to the "fairly light range" of the Borg RPE Scale (see Table 16.7). For an increase of one to two METs, a HR increase of 10 to 20 bpm is appropriate, if beta-blockers or other HR suppressers are not used; however, the absence of beta blockade in Phase I is uncommon. If a beta-blocker is used, there is no standardization as to the degree of HR suppression; subjective ratings of perceived exertion and objective observation of patient effort become increasingly important. A patient on beta-blockers who has a HR increase of 20 bpm during low-level inpatient activity would be considered inadequately medicated, unless the activity level was considerably higher than appropriate. A decrease in HR or BP during activity for any patient, regardless of medications, should be evaluated for the presence of an arrhythmia. Following the physical therapy intervention, the patient's tolerance of activity and hemodynamic stability should be documented.

There are a variety of inpatient cardiac rehab programs, frequently progressive based upon levels of increasing energy costs (e.g., MET levels). Each facility will establish their own levels and criteria for activity progression and education; an example of an inpatient program is shown in Table 16.8. Following are some general comments and recommendations about the various levels. It is important to note that activity progression occurs along a continuum

Table 16.8 Inpatient Cardiac Rehabilitation Program

CCU–Essentially Bedrest
Level 1 1–1.5 METs Evaluation and patient education Arms supported for meals and ADLs Bed exercises and dangle with feet supported (if CPKs have peaked and patient has no complications) Education Introduction to inpatient cardiac rehab and role of physical therapy Education Monitored progression of activity Home exercise/activity guidelines/outpatient cardiac rehab
Sitting–Limited Room Ambulation
Level 2 1.5–2 METs Sitting 15–30 min, 2–4 times/day Leg exercises Commode privileges Reclining upright chair Limited ADL Electric razor Limited supervised room ambulation for small uncomplicated MI Education Identification of CAD risk factors Concept of "healing interval" and need to pace activities
Room–Limited Hall Ambulation
Level 3 2–2.5 METs Room or hall ambulation up to 5 min as tolerated 3–4 times/day Standing leg exercises optional[a] Sit on side of bed or in bathroom to wash (per discration nurse/PT) Manual shave Bathroom privileges Independent or assisted ambulation in room or hall as advised by PT Education Size of infarct and how it relates to the need for gradual resumption of activities Impact of exercise on reducing the patient's risk factors Teach use of Borg's Scale for Rating of Perceived Exertion and appropriate parameters with activity
Progressive Hall Ambulation
Level 4 2.5–3 METs Hall ambulation 5–7 min as tolerated 3–4 times/day Standing trunk exercises optional[a] Independent or assisted ambulation in hall as advised by PT Education Teach pulse taking and appropriate parameters with activity Reinforce benefits of outpatient cardiac rehabilitation
Progressive Hall Ambulation
Level 5 3–4 METs Hall ambulation 8–10 min as tolerated Arm exercises optional[a] Standing shower Independent hall ambulation as advised by PT Education Written home exercise/activity guidelines reviewed Patient given written information on outpatient cardiac rehab

(continued)

Table 16.8 Inpatient Cardiac Rehabilitation Program (continued)

Stair Climbing
Level 6 4–5 METs Progressive hall ambulation as tolerated Full flight of stairs (or as required at home) up and down one step at a time[b] Education Answer patient's questions Check for understanding of activity guidelines
Patient Outcome–No Evidence of Hemodynamic Compromise with Activity Progression (All Levels)
No systolic drop in BP >10 mm Hg or increase >30 mm Hg No HR increase >12 if beta blocked, or no HR increase >20 if not beta blocked No complaints of dizziness, lightheadedness, or angina Perceived exertion <13/20
Hemodynamic Monitoring
Level 1 HR and BP before and after supine bed exercises Orthostatic signs supine and dangling at bedside Level 2 Orthostatic signs (supine, sit, and stand) before exercises and transfer HR and BP after leg exercises/transfer to chair HR and BP after return to bed Levels 3–6 HR and BP in sitting and standing prior to activity HR and BP immediately following activity HR and BP 5 min after activity

From Rehabilitation Services Department, Newton Wellesley Hospital, Newton, MA, with permission.

[a]Optional exercises are at the discretion of the physical therapist (PT) and may be used to establish the patient's CV response in the room, prior to moving on to more challenging hallway ambulation; or in those patients who require general strengthening exercises.

[b]Stair climbing activities should take place after the ETT if the scheduling of the ETT permits. Otherwise patients may, at the discretion and supervision of the PT, climb stairs on the day prior to the ETT.

and is not done in a rigid format. Although a patient must demonstrate the ability to sit at the bedside with appropriate hemodynamic response before ambulating in the hallway, the patient's individual response and medical history will dictate how quickly he or she is able to progress. A patient may progress through more than one level within any treatment session.

Level 1. The patient is in the intensive care unit (ICU) and is stable; generally physical therapy intervention does not begin until after the first 24 hours from admission or until the patient has been stable for 24 hours. Physical therapy intervention should begin after the blood work has indicated the MI is completed. CK and troponin (both I and T) levels are monitored. For both CK and Troponin levels, reliable diagnostic sensitivity (greater than 90 percent) is reached within 12 to 16 hours of the onset of symptoms.[76] CK peak levels occur between 14 and 36 hours, with a return to normal level after 48 to 72 hours; troponin peaks at 24 to 36 hours, with a return to normal levels within 10 to 12 days.[76] Commonly, three sets of CPK levels collected 8 hours apart are collected. Because CK is released very quickly into the bloodstream with cellular damage, it is typical for the first and second CK levels to show a progressive increase and the third set to be less than the second (i.e., the CK peak has occurred, and the values are now trending downward). Because CK may be released with cellular damage to areas other than to the myocardium, specific myocardial isoenzymes known as CK-MB are monitored.

Appropriate activity for the patient in the ICU during the first 24 hours is to move comfortably within the bed, perform ankle pumps, deep breathing exercises, commode use (if hemodynamically stable), and perform limited personal care.

Level 2. Once the patient has been hemodynamically stable for 24 hours he or she may progress OOB (out of bed). The therapist should also be alert to signs of orthostatic hypotension when the patient changes position from supine to sitting on the side of the bed. The patient's feet should be supported on a stool to assist venous return if they are not able to touch the floor. The patient walks to a bedside chair. The patient sits in an upright chair for up to 30 minutes a few times a day. There is a real temptation for many health care providers to have the patient "do" something while seated, such as washing, eating, or visiting with family. It is probably wise to just let the patient sit for the first time, without being encumbered with other tasks. The therapist is thus better able to evaluate the patient's response to being upright. If the patient has had a large MI or requires a slow progression to upright posture, then the use of a reclining chair is a way to gradually assume the upright position. The patient performs LE exercises such as ankle pumps, knee extensions, or marching in place. Vital signs are monitored for hemodynamic stability and appropriate activity response. The importance of healing time, pacing activities, and creating a healthful environment are components of a comprehensive patient education program.

Level 3. Patients are instructed to gradually increase their ambulation. One approach is to educate patients to judge their ambulation in terms of time instead of distance. Time is a more reproducible measurement, while distance may be difficult to judge (e.g., "I want you to walk for 2 minutes" vs "I want you to walk 200 ft"). It also allows for an easier transition to the home exercise program, which is commonly based on length of time. For documentation purposes, it is most effective to document the distance covered in the time period whenever possible (e.g., Patient ambulated 500 ft in 6 minutes with a RPE of 10/20). Information regarding CAD risk factors allows patients to begin to take responsibility for their choices about activity and lifestyle. However, for some patients this may be too early in their recovery, and they are unable to focus on what is being said. Giving patients written information is a good way to provide education and yet give patients the choice when to read it. Use of the Borg RPE scale assists the patient in monitoring of activity intensity.

Levels 4 Through 6. Patients gradually increase the frequency and time of their walks at a comfortable and leisurely pace. The goal is to progress walks from 2 minutes, to 5 minutes, to 10 minutes with appropriate hemodynamic response. Stairs may be climbed foot over foot with a planned rest half way or so, or one foot at a time, depending on the status of the patient. Patients are often hesitant to move, especially in stretching their arms overhead; therefore performing a variety of trunk, arm, and standing leg exercises for a few repetitions each often allays the fear and helps the patient feel more comfortable moving.

Patients need to be made aware of the fatigue that often accompanies seemingly innocuous activities (e.g., showering) and plan their rests accordingly. Visitors are often a hidden energy cost; patients are often very excited and reassured to have visitors, but the fatigue that follows is sometimes very disconcerting. Helping the patient understand the concept of energy and the cost of not just physical but emotional and mental activities is invaluable. Comparing energy costs to money may help the patient to pace activity. Patients are told that they have a dollar's worth of energy and everything they do is going to cost them some part of that dollar; however, they can never spend more than 50 or 60 cents at one time. Every time they rest, it is like going to the ATM for a quick refill. In this way, patients become knowledgeable about the expendability of energy and yet are given the responsibility to spend (and save) as they choose.

Documentation

There are many ways to document physical therapy examination and intervention. In this patient population, appropriate documentation would include:

1. Objective activity data, including time period and distance ambulated, type of sitting and standing exercises, and stair climbing (number of steps); number and duration of rests
2. Patient's vital sign response to each activity including a statement that addresses patient performance with respect to vital signs (e.g., Patient ambulated 6 minutes covering 500 ft and climbed 10 steps foot over foot using handrail with adaptive VS response without signs or symptoms of hemodynamic compromise).
3. Education provided and response of patient, family, and caregivers.

Home Exercise Program (HEP)

Two of the more important concepts for a patient to understand at the time of discharge are symptom recognition and appropriate activity guidelines. It is crucial that the patient be aware of, and recognize, cardiac symptoms and understand the action to take if they occur.

Physical therapists establish activity guidelines during the first 4 to 6 weeks post-MI while the myocardium is healing. During this healing phase, physical activity involves a gradual increase in ambulation time, with a goal of 20 to 30 minutes of ambulation one to two times per day at 4 to 6 weeks post-MI. Patients are encouraged to walk comfortably, dress appropriately, and to try to exercise in ambient temperature at indoor malls if weather is not appropriate (i.e., below 40°F including wind chill factor, over 80°F, or excessive humidity and poor air quality). Some patients are very sensitive to environmental factors and should exercise only in ambient conditions or indoors. For some patients, home exercise equipment is affordable and may be a reasonable alternative to outdoor exercise. For safety reasons, the patient should be monitored on similar equipment before independently beginning to exercise at home. This is not the time for a patient to try a new type of exercise modality but to stay with what is familiar. Walking appears to be the exercise of choice owing to its ease and familiarity.

The patient's days will be a combination of rest and low-level activity including ambulation and LE and UE mobility. The patient should be encouraged to try and change positions or activity every 1 to 2 hours. For example, it is generally not a good idea for the patient to be up all morning and then rest all afternoon. It is invaluable to have patients verbally outline what their days will include once they are discharged. This affords an opportunity to better understand the interests of the patient and make specific suggestions, as well as provide an opportunity to determine the patient's understanding of activity guidelines and energy conservation techniques.

Outpatient Phase II

Patients commonly undergo a symptom-limited maximal stress test (ETT) at 4 to 6 weeks post-MI. Based on the results of the tests, either positive (+) for ischemia or negative (−) for ischemia, an exercise prescription is prescribed. For a (−) ETT, a common exercise prescription would be 70 to 85 percent of the peak achieved on the test (i.e., HR_{max}); however an equally effective alternative would be 65 to 80 percent of HR_{max}. Understanding that a negative test does not mean the patient is disease free and that vulnerable plaques may exist, a conservative prescription may be a wiser choice.

Positive Exercise Tolerance Test

If a patient has had a *positive ETT,* the exercise prescription becomes relatively simple: during aerobic training, it is important to keep $M\dot{V}O_2$ below the patient's ischemic $M\dot{V}O_2$. Remember that a clinical measure of $M\dot{V}O_2$ is the product of HR and SBP, known as the rate pressure product (RPP = HR × SBP). The importance of considering the ischemic threshold is the recognition that BP will vary during use of different pieces of exercise equipment owing in part to the differences in muscle recruitment. If there is a difference in BP for a given HR, then there will be a difference in the $M\dot{V}O_2$ to the patient. For example, if a patient has a HR of 100 bpm and a BP of 140/80 mm Hg while exercising on the treadmill, and a HR of 100 bpm and a BP of 160/80 mm Hg while exercising on the stationary bicycle, the bicycle is costing the myocardium more energy than the treadmill, even though HR is the same. Depending on the patient's ischemic threshold, it is possible that angina may occur on the bicycle but not on the treadmill. A good safety tip is to not exceed 90 percent of the ischemic RPP. The remainder of the exercise prescription may follow the common guidelines for aerobic training in regard to frequency, intensity, and duration for patients with cardiac involvement.

Strength Training

The inclusion of strength training in a cardiac rehab program is a relatively recent addition to the traditional cardiac rehabilitation program.[77] Initial concern was that resistance work would inordinately increase $M\dot{V}O_2$ and ventricular arrhythmias and therefore be detrimental. A publication by Beniamini et al[78] gives excellent insight into this area. The AACVPR's thorough review of the literature on this topic concluded, "resistance exercise has been shown to be a safe and effective method for improving strength and cardiovascular endurance, modifying risk factors and enhancing self efficacy in low-risk cardiac patients."[75] Resistance training may begin with the use of elastic bands, and light hand weights (one to three pounds) and progress to a load that allows 12 to 15 repetitions comfortably.[79] AACVPR guidelines further state that resistance training should not begin until the patient has been in a cardiac rehab program for at least 3 weeks and is at least 5 weeks post-MI or 8 weeks post-CABG.[79] Some guidelines for resistance training include (1) exercising large muscle groups before small, (2) stressing exhalation with exertion, (3) avoiding sustained tight grip, (4) focusing on RPE 11-13, (5) using slow controlled movements, and (6) stopping exercise with any warning of concerning or uncomfortable signs or symptoms.[79] The American Heart Association, American College of Sports Medicine, and the AACVPR all advocate the importance of muscular fitness for the patient with cardiac impairment and support the inclusion of resistance training into the patient's exercise program.[75,79–81]

Revascularization

It is important to review the surgical and catheterization reports to determine which vessels were revascularized, and which vessels have less than 70 percent lesions and were therefore not revascularized. Just because a vessel is not a candidate for revascularization does not mean that it cannot be problematic at a later date, either by rupturing or continuing to demonstrate progressive atherosclerosis. It would be short sighted for a clinician to believe that a patient who has had a revascularization procedure cannot become ischemic.

Percutaneous Transluminal Coronary Angioplasty (PTCA)

There are at present no strict guidelines for when a patient may resume aerobic training following an angioplasty. Conventional wisdom, however, favors waiting approximately 2 weeks to allow the inflammatory process resulting from the intervention an appropriate time to subside. The new exercise prescription should be based on the results of the post-angioplasty ETT, not the pre-angioplasty ETT, which was more than likely positive. Patients may continue to ambulate at a low intensity and comfortable pace during the first 1 to 2 weeks following the PTCA, but should avoid the moderate to higher intensities associated with aerobic training.

Coronary Artery Bypass Graft

For patients who have had bypass surgery (e.g., CABG), recovery is somewhat slower than that for PTCA owing to the complexity of the surgical procedure and the incisional healing. The number and location of incisions depend on the surgeon's technique (i.e., either a full sternal cut, partial sternal cut, or intercostal approach). The donor graph site may require additional incisions: a leg incision if saphenous vein is used, a nondominant arm incision if radial artery is used, or no additional incision if grafted with the internal mammary artery. Physical therapy intervention should address any soft tissue impairments that may be affected by the incision to maintain appropriate flexibility and postures, with an awareness that patients often indicate soreness and/or discomfort around the donor site. If a sternal wound is present, appropriate posture, scapula retraction, and functional shoulder movements should be encouraged. Proprioceptive Neuromuscular Facilitation (PNF) upper extremity (UE) diagonal patterns often work well, as do the traditional cardinal plane ROM exercises. Patients should be reminded that only a few repetitions at a time throughout the day are better tolerated than more intensive reps (5 to 10) 1 to 2 times per day; the latter regimen often results in incisional soreness. Some surgeons choose to limit UE flexibility exercises during the 4 to 6 weeks following surgery while the sternum is healing; however, it is unclear as to the rationale for the limitation. A professional collegial relationship with the surgical team to discuss surgical techniques and mobility concerns will ensure the best outcome for the patient. To avoid sternal discomfort, all patients will benefit from splinting the incision with a hand or pillow when laughing, coughing, or sneezing. Patients should be instructed to avoid lifting, pushing, and pulling objects until 4 to 6 weeks post-surgery when the sternum is well healed. Patients will also appreciate information regarding energy conservation and rest periods. Even though the functioning of the heart is perhaps the best it has been in quite some time, the effects of major surgery on energy level and mobility must be emphasized. The impact of fatigue on the patient's sense of well being may be profound, and it is important that patients understand the need for rest as well as ambulation. Early ambulation and mobility beginning the first day post surgery will assist in the patient's physical and emotional recovery.

During the initial weeks following cardiac surgery, the early in-hospital limitations following cardiac surgery have perhaps more to do with the surgical procedure and altered mobility and less to do with the heart itself, which is theoretically healthier than it was before surgery. Postoperative fatigue may be due to a combination of factors, including anesthesia, blood loss, initial weight gain due to cardiopulmonary bypass machine, common arrhythmias such as atrial fibrillation, and the energy cost of healing. As with the post-MI recovery period, when the surgical patient returns home it is a good idea to break the day into many subunits including rest, leisure activity, and perhaps visiting with friends by phone or in person. Developing a schedule but keeping it flexible helps the patient exert some control over the day and energy level.

The patient is encouraged to gradually increase walking, with a goal of 30 minutes of ambulation 1 to 2 times per day at 4 to 6 weeks post-surgery. If the patient is walking in the neighborhood, suggest that the initial walks be back and forth in front of the house rather than around the block. In this way, if the patient overestimates his or her energy level, the close proximity of home will provide a welcomed rest and prevent overexertion. Many patients ambitiously begin their walk only to find themselves suddenly fatigued and further from home than they would like. Continuing exercises for posture, UE and trunk mobility, and sternal protection are also important components of the home exercise program.

Once a patient's incisions have healed (approximately 6 weeks), and his or her blood counts including hematocrit and hemoglobin are in acceptable ranges, cardiac rehabilitation may begin. The patient may have a maximal ETT and begin aerobic and strength training according to the general guidelines.

Heart Failure

With the marked improvement in anti-ischemic medications, increased knowledge and management of CAD risk factors, availability of sophisticated monitoring, and revascularization techniques, more patients are living longer with coronary disease than similar patients 20 or 30 years ago. New technology and medications continually improve the understanding and management of CAD; however, an undesired effect of long-term CAD may be the increased prevalence of heart failure, also known as **congestive heart failure (CHF)**. For the year 2004, the estimated direct and indirect cost of CHF in the United States was projected to be $28.8 billion.[3] Coronary disease may well be the most common etiology of CHF.[82] According to the Heart Disease and Stroke Statistics—2004 Update, the prevalence of CHF in the United States in 2001 was 5 million Americans, 2.5 million males and 2.5 million females.[3] Although disease prevalence is similar between males and females, female mortality exceeded that of males within the same time period, 33.0 thousand versus 19.8 thousand; female deaths accounted for 62½ percent of all deaths due to CHF, male deaths 37½ percent.[3] Heart failure has surpassed MI as the leading cause of cardiac deaths in the United States. Heart failure is also the most frequent cardiac diagnosis for hospital admissions and readmissions.[3] In 1998, it was reported that once signs of overt failure appear, approximately 50 percent of patients would die within 5 years, despite medical management.[4] As understanding of the disease process improves along with new drug combinations, these statistics may improve.

Types of Heart Failure

Although the term heart failure most commonly refers to LV failure, heart failure may include both right and left ventricles or be limited to the RV alone. As a result of LV failure, increased pressure gradients may occur not only in the LV but may continue in a retrograde fashion to include the RV as well. When left and right heart failure coexist, *biventricular* failure is present. Right heart failure may occur independently of left heart failure with pulmonary disease such as chronic obstructive pulmonary disease (COPD), in which chronically elevated PA pressures result in RV failure; this is referred to as cor pulmonale (Table 16.9).

LV failure is also identified as primarily a systolic or diastolic dysfunction, depending upon whether the impairment is primarily one of ventricular contractility (systolic dysfunction) or ventricular relaxation and/or filling (diastolic dysfunction).[83] The clinical presentation of systolic dysfunction relates to inadequate CO with resultant signs and symptoms of hypoperfusion (e.g., fatigue, weakness,

Table 16.9 Example of Hemodynamic Pressures Associated with Heart Failure

An increase in PA and/or PCWP pressures is associated with LV failure; an increase in CVP is associated with RV failure; and an increase in CVP, PA, and PCWP pressures is associated with biventricular failure.

Pressure (Norms)	LV Failure	RV Failure	Biventricular Failure
CVP (0–8 mm Hg)	6 mm Hg	12 mm Hg	12 mm Hg
PA (9–19) mm Hg	22 mm Hg	16 mm Hg	22 mm Hg
PCWP (6–12) mm Hg	18 mm Hg	10 mm Hg	18 mm Hg

and reduced exercise tolerance).[83] Diastolic dysfunction presents with elevated filling pressures and decreased ventricular capacity. Systolic dysfunction has characteristics of decreased contractility and resultant decrease in EF. Diastolic dysfunction has characteristics of decreased compliance and a normal or increased EF.

There are three common classifications of *cardiomyopathies:* dilated, hypertrophic, and restrictive.[84] CAD is the prime cause of *dilated cardiomyopathy,* resulting in LV failure and systolic dysfunction; myocarditis and alcohol abuse are causes as well. *Hypertrophic cardiomyopathy* presents as diastolic dysfunction with an increased ventricular mass; chronic hypertension and aortic stenosis are examples of hypertrophic cardiomyopathy. *Restrictive cardiomyopathy* also presents as diastolic dysfunction due to the presence of excessively rigid ventricular walls, resulting in a decrease in compliance.[84,85] The connective tissue changes of the heart associated with diabetes are an example of a restrictive cardiomyopathy. The EF of patients with ischemic or dilated cardiomyopathies (systolic dysfunction) is decreased from normal, usually by more than 70 percent; patients with hypertrophic or restrictive cardiomyopathies (diastolic dysfunctions) may have a normal or even above normal EF. Because of the decreased LVEDV, diastolic dysfunction may present with a "normal" EF (EF = SV/ LVEDV). In this case, however, it is important to remember that an EF in the normal range of approximately 55 to 75 percent does not mean normal LV function. For example, a patient without heart disease may have a LVEDV of 100 ml and a SV of 60 ml and would therefore have a normal EF of 60 percent; a patient with systolic dysfunction may have a LVEDV of 100 ml and a SV of 30 ml and would have an EF of 30 percent, while a patient with diastolic dysfunction might have a LVEDV of 65 ml and a SV 50 ml for an EF of 77 percent. Although either systolic or diastolic dysfunction may be the initial presentation early in the disease process,[85] as the disease progresses, components of both dysfunctions may coexist.[83] Besides coronary disease, alcohol, viral or bacterial infections, chronic hypertension, and valvular dysfunction, cardiomyopathy may also result from an unknown (idiopathic) cause. It is important to note that cardiomyopathy may occur at any age and is not an exclusive disease of the elderly.

A common classification system, Class I, II, II, IV, for heart failure has been established by the New York Heart Association based upon the patient's subjective report of functional activity limitations based upon their "ordinary physical activity."[86] Grading using this classification is based on the individual physician's judgment from listening to the patient. It is not presently based upon any formal objective measurements (Table 16.10).

Pathophysiology of Congestive Heart Failure

Heart failure results from a complex series of events involving neurohormonal and mechanical factors in response to an initial myocardial injury. When the myocardium has received significant injury (e.g., as a result of a large MI or multiple MIs), compensatory mechanisms are activated with the goal of maintaining adequate CO. The compensatory mechanisms include: (1) increased sympathetic tone (increased HR, myocardial contractility, and peripheral vascular vasoconstriction); (2) ventricular remodeling (myocardial dilation and hypertrophy); (3) activation of the renin angiotensin system (increased sodium and water reabsorption by action of aldosterone and peripheral vasoconstriction by action of angiotensin II); and (4) redistribution of blood flow away from periphery toward central circulation. Actions of the these mechanisms result in an increase in CO from sympathetic effects on HR and contractility, an alteration of the length–tension relationship due to the enlarged LV from ventricular remodeling resulting in an increased LVEDV, and an increase in plasma volume, increasing LVEDV, from the aldosterone effect. For a while, compensatory mechanisms are able to provide adequate cardiac functioning and the patient remains asymptomatic (Fig. 16.13).

The body can maintain the compensatory mechanisms only for a limited time, the energy cost of the compensatory mechanisms will eventually become too much for the impaired ventricle; the patient will become symptomatic. The increase in LVEDV contributes to a rise in LV pressure. The increased pressure is transmitted retrograde toward the LA and the pulmonary veins. This increase in hydrostatic pressure in the pulmonary veins causes fluid to move out of the veins and into the interstitial space of the lung, resulting in **pulmonary edema**. This increased pressure may continue from the pulmonary veins and capillaries and extend into the pulmonary artery, right heart, and the peripheral venous system. The increase in hydrostatic pressure in the peripheral veins will result in peripheral edema. Sympathetic nervous system activation in heart failure results in tachycardia and blood flow redistribution. As a result of decreased contractility, SV decreases and, in

Table 16.10 Functional Classifications of Patients with Diseases of the Heart

Functional	Continuous–Intermittent Permissible Work Loads	Maximum
Class I	4.0–6.0 cal/min Patients with cardiac disease but without resulting limitations of physical activity. Ordinary physical activity does not cause undue fatigue, palpitation, dyspnea, or anginal pain.	6.5 METs
Class II	3.0–4.0 cal/min Patients with cardiac disease resulting in slight limitation of physical activity. They are comfortable at rest. Ordinary physical activity results in fatigue, palpitation, dyspnea, or anginal pain.	4.5 METs
Class III	2.0–3.0 cal/min Patients with cardiac disease resulting in marked limitation of physical activity. They are comfortable at rest. Less than ordinary physical activity causes fatigue, palpitation, dyspnea, or anginal pain.	3.0 METs
Class IV	1.0–2.0 cal/min Patients with cardiac disease resulting in inability to carry on any physical activity without discomfort. Symptoms of cardiac insufficiency or of the anginal syndrome may be present even at rest. If any physical activity is undertaken, discomfort is increased.	1.5 METs

Four-level classification system based on functional limitations.
Reprinted by permission of the American Heart Association, New York.

an attempt to maintain CO, there is a compensatory increase in HR. A resting tachycardia, therefore, may not be an unusual finding, especially for patients in Class III or IV heart failure. Blood flow redistribution occurs in response to a depressed CO. In an effort to maintain perfusion to the central circulation and major organs, peripheral vasoconstriction occurs, redistributing blood to the central circulation. The renin–angiotensin–aldosterone system is activated by a decrease in renal artery perfusion as a result of the decrease in CO. This decrease in kidney function as a result of heart failure is known as *prerenal failure,* meaning the mechanism for renal failure occurred in the organ preceding the kidneys (i.e., the heart). In response to the perceived inadequate volume, the renin-angiotensin system stimulation and activation of aldosterone results in retention of salt and water. In reality, however, there is not too little blood volume, but rather an inappropriate allocation of volume (within the heart or venous system), resulting in a decrease in arterial blood flow. Sodium and water retention contributes to the formation of pulmonary edema (and its associated shortness of breath) and peripheral edema.[87] Activation of renin–angiotensin, especially owing to the contribution of angiotensin, also causes peripheral vasoconstriction. Vasoconstriction redistributes blood to the central circulation and, by increased PVR, may contribute to an increase in BP and, therefore, peripheral perfusion pressure.

Clinical Manifestations of Congestive Heart Failure

The clinical presentation of the patient with CHF depends not only on the amount of LV failure, but also on the status of compensatory mechanisms and drug therapy. Over time, the energy cost of the compensatory mechanisms proves to be too much for the impaired myocardium. The patient presents with CHF signs and symptoms, and now moves from being asymptomatic to symptomatic. Although the terminology may be somewhat confusing, it is important to appreciate that when a patient is referred to as being in *compensated heart failure,* the patient's congestive symptoms can be relieved by medical therapy.[82] A patient who is noncompensated is showing signs and symptoms of congestion and requires medical and pharmacologic readjustment.

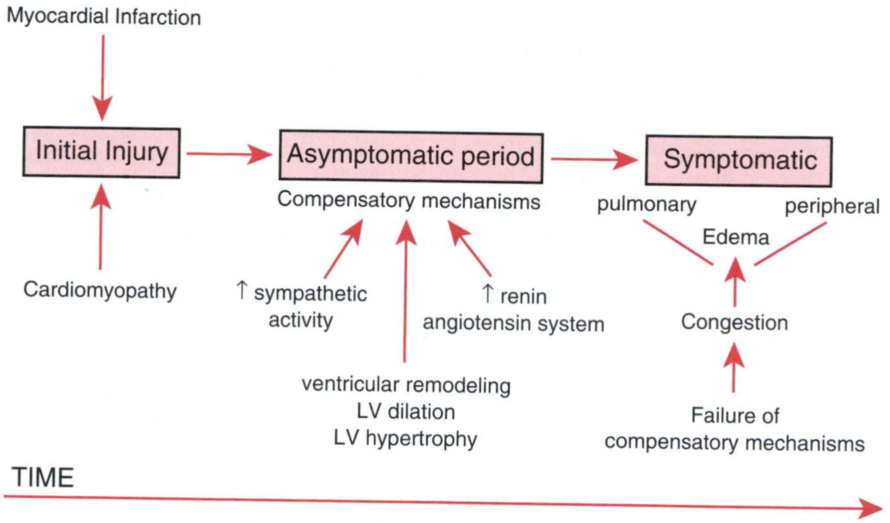

Figure 16.13 Development of congestive heart failure. An initial injury to the LV causes activation of compensatory mechanisms in order to maintain adequate LV function. When the patient is adequately compensated there are no symptoms of congestion (i.e., edema). The failure of the compensatory mechanisms results in signs and symptoms of congestion (e.g., pulmonary and peripheral congestion).

Common signs and symptoms of CHF include fatigue, dyspnea, edema (pulmonary and peripheral), fluid weight gain, presence of an S_3 heart sound, and renal dysfunction. Pulmonary edema may be evident by chest X-ray film, and auscultation of adventitious sounds (e.g., crackles). Peripheral edema may be evident in gravity dependent lower extremities by the presence of indentations in the skin when pressure is applied, i.e., **pitting edema**. Pitting edema due to CHF is usually bilateral and may extend from the foot to the pretibial area.[88,89] Documentation should include not only the amount of pitting, but also the area covered.

The usual abnormal heart sound associated with CHF is the presence of an S_3, probably resulting from altered LV compliance. Heart murmurs, especially that of mitral regurgitation, may also be present owing to the effect of the enlarged LV pulling on the mitral valve. Dyspnea, either positional (orthopnea, paroxysmal nocturnal) or exertional, is frequently associated with pulmonary edema. Dyspnea may also result from the increased energy cost of activity as a result of decreased peripheral endurance and peripheral muscle changes. Weight gain and peripheral edema are among the signs of systemic volume overload. Increased arterial resistance results in an increase in afterload and therefore in $M\dot{V}O_2$. The increased resistance may result from a combination of factors, including (1) increased sympathetic adrenergic stimulation; (2) decreased vasodilation of vascular smooth muscle as a result of a decrease in the availability of the endothelium-derived relaxant factor nitric oxide; (3) an increase in the endothelial-derived smooth muscle vasoconstrictor, endothelin-1; (4) an increase in vascular stiffness as a result of salt and water retention; and (5) the presence of the powerful peripheral vasoconstrictors angiotensin II and vasopressin.[87]

One of the common complaints of patients with CHF that affects their activity tolerance is early onset of muscle fatigue. The cause of their muscle fatigue may be multifactorial, including a decrease in peripheral blood flow, changes within the peripheral vascular beds, peripheral vasoconstriction, atrophy of muscle fibers, or increased utilization of anaerobic metabolism.[90,91] The contribution of intracellular mechanisms to muscle fatigue has been studied. Examples of these intracellular mechanisms include an alteration in the control of calcium release and reuptake[92] and myocyte apoptosis.[93] In addition to peripheral muscle functioning in patients with heart failure, exercise studies have also investigated various other factors, including oxygen uptake kinetics, neurohormonal parameters, and endothelial function that may influence the exercise response.[94–96] Although there are many potential reasons for the fatigue associated with CHF (especially Class III and IV), a recently identified contributor is obstructive sleep apnea. Sleep apnea may be treated in this patient population with the use of continuous positive airway pressure (CPAP) worn while sleeping.[97,98]

CHF is not just a disease of the heart; it is complex and systemic. Although the precipitating cause is LV dysfunction, the sequelae of the disease process involves far more than the LV, including the kidneys, peripheral vascular system, skeletal muscle, and neurohormonal influences.[87]

Pharmacological Management of CHF

With the advent of new medications in the management of CHF, such as combined alpha and beta-blockers, ACE inhibitors, and vasodilators, the symptoms of volume overload are more effectively managed.[99,100] The principles of drug management with CHF are quite simple: increase contractility and relieve congestion. Drugs that increase contractility are known as *positive inotropes;* the common oral drug in this category is digoxin. Diuretics decrease preload, thereby decreasing LVEDV. Patients are often on a sliding scale dosage of diuretics depending on the amount of fluid weight gain; they are instructed to weigh themselves daily and adjust diuretics accordingly. Afterload reducers, particularly those that block the effects of the renin–angiotensin system (e.g., ACE inhibitors, known as ACE inhibitors or angiotensin receptor blockers known as ARBs), are often a critical component of drug management in this population. By blocking salt and water retention through aldosterone suppression, preload is decreased, by blocking vasoconstriction through angiotensin II suppression, afterload is reduced. The increase in sympathetic activity that accompanies heart failure causes an increase in $M\dot{V}O_2$ (from beta-receptor stimulation), peripheral vasoconstriction, and resultant reduction in peripheral blood flow (from alpha-receptor stimulation). Drugs that combine both beta-receptor blockade and alpha-receptor blockade minimize these affects; beta-blockade will result in a decrease in $M\dot{V}O_2$, and alpha-blockade will result in decreased afterload due to suppression of the vasoconstriction associated with alpha activation. A relatively new approach to CHF management is the use of a potent vasodilator, sildenafil (trade name Viagra), which is being investigated in this patient population with the goal of decreasing pulmonary artery pressures (PA) and therefore LV and RV work.[101]

Mechanical and Surgical Support

For the symptomatic patient in Class III/IV, there are dramatic surgical options that may improve function, such as heart transplant, left ventricular devices (LVAD) and myoplasty. It is beyond the scope of this chapter to discuss in detail the complexity of each of these procedures. Heart transplantation involves replacing the patient's heart with a donor heart. The donor heart will be denervated; therefore, it will not have any direct sympathetic or parasympathetic connection and will be dependent on the intrinsic pacemaker of the SA node and hormonal stimulation to increase HR. The patient with a heart transplant requires careful pharmacological management. Immune suppressing drugs are used to prevent the body from rejecting the organ, as well as for careful control of infection. The LVAD is a temporary pump that is inserted into the patient to perform the work of the LV or to augment the function of the failing heart. The patient is connected to an external energy source but also has the option of wearing a battery pack that allows freedom of movement for hours, in which the patient can go shopping, to the movies, etc. Myoplasty is a surgical procedure in which an enlarged LV undergoes a size reduction by removing dilated, scarred myocardium that is ineffective in contributing to contractility.

A new class of pacemaker, the biventricular pacer, is being used for the more involved CHF population with an intraventricular conduction delay (e.g., left bundle branch block on the EKG). This pacer coordinates the contraction of the right and left ventricles and in doing so provides a more effective LV contraction and increased CO.[102]

Physical Therapy Intervention for Patients with CHF

According to the APTA *Guide to Physical Therapist Practice,* the management of CHF is included under the category of Impaired Aerobic Capacity and Endurance Associated with Cardiovascular Pump Dysfunction or Failure, Pattern 6-D. The development of specific anticipated goals and expected outcomes for the patient with CHF is based on the following general goals:

1. Physiological response to increased oxygen demand is improved.
2. Self-management of symptoms is improved.
3. Ability to perform physical tasks is increased.
4. Behaviors that foster healthy habits, wellness, and prevention are acquired.
5. Disability associated with acute or chronic illness is reduced.
6. Risk of secondary impairments is reduced.
7. Awareness and use of community resources is improved.
8. Performance of and independence in ADL is increased.

Exercise Prescription

Exercise programs for patients with CHF are relatively recent. Patients whose cardiac status was once thought to be too fragile to participate in organized exercise are now not only participating, but exercise is recommended as an integral component of their medical management.[103–106] Studies have shown that patients with heart failure can exercise safely and regular exercise may improve functional status, quality of life, exercise capacity and decrease symptoms.[107–113] (See Evidence Summary Box 16.3.)

The safety and importance of strength training and peripheral adaptations have also been studied.[114,115] Using a multidisciplinary approach that includes a thorough physical examination before each exercise session with a review of symptoms and medications, low-level exercise may begin if the patient is hemodynamically stable. CHF is a multisystem disease that affects not just the heart but peripheral muscle and arteries as well. Studies have demonstrated muscle fiber atrophy of skeletal and respiratory muscle, as well as an alteration in arterial vasodilation capacity. Exercise has been shown to limit some of these adverse changes; therefore, an exercise program should consider not only systemic conditioning, but also peripheral endurance training, low-level resistance training, and respiratory muscle training.[116–118] Oxygen saturation via pulse oximetry is a valuable tool in monitoring adequate tissue oxygenation. Patients may

Evidence Summary Box 16.3

Studies Investigating the Effect of Exercise on Patients with CHF.

Reference	Subjects	Design	Intervention	Duration	Results	Comments
Wielenga, RP, et al[107] 1999	*N* = 80 Characteristics: Male: Age: 40–75 ± 56.6 ± 8.3 years); Class II–III; EF: < 40%; (26.5 ± 9) $\dot{V}o_2$ < 20 ml O_2/kg/min	RCT Location: outpatient clinic	Intensity: RHR + (60% of HRmax RHR); Frequency: 3×/week; Duration: 3 10-min endurance sessions separated by 5 min of rest	12 weeks	Exercise time ↑ 24% in trained group, NSD in control; 10% ↑ $\dot{V}o_2$ max; ↑ anaerobic threshold; ↑ QOL; no training related adverse effects	Short duration interval training shown to be safe and effective in men
Dubach, D, et al[108] 1997	*N* = 25 Characteristics: Class II–III; previous MI but no previous dx of CHF Age: 56 ± 5 EF: 31.5 ± 6.7	RCT Location: patients in residence	Intensity: 70–80% HR max; > 70% peak $\dot{V}o_2$ Frequency: daily; 4×/week Modality/duration: walk/ daily 1 hour bid Cycle/45 min × 4 weeks	8 weeks	↑ CO ↑ A-V O_2 ↓ PCWP ↑ $\dot{V}o_2$ by 29%	High-frequency and intensity training improved exercise capacity without worsening myocardial function
Piepoli, M[109] 1998	*N* = 134 Characteristics: Class I–III; Age: 60.5 ± 8.6 years[44–77]; EF: 25.0 ± 8.9%[9–43]	RCT Location: home-based and clinic	Intensity: 70–80% of peak HR Modality: cycle and calisthenics (Canadian Air Force XBX for Women) Frequency: 4–5 days week Duration: 20 min	16 weeks (6–16) Majority at 8 weeks	↑ 13% $\dot{V}o_2$ max ↑ 17% exercise ↑ BP with peak exercise; ↓ noradrenaline, aldosterone, rennin, ANP, and adrenaline Cycle plus calisthenics had > benefits than cycling alone home + clinic (vs. home alone) had > benefits	Improvement in both M and F; ischemic pts showed less improvement than nonischemic in $\dot{V}o_2$ max; greater gains in pts who participated for 16 weeks than 6 weeks; 6-week training duration may be too short
Coats, AJS, et al[110] 1992	*N* = 19 Characteristics: Class II–III; ischemic cardiomyopathy Age: 61.8 ± 1.5 years EF: 19.6 + 2.3%; $\dot{V}o_2$ peak: 12.5–13.3 ml/min/kg	Controlled crossover trial Location: home-based with activity restriction	Intensity: 80% of HR_{max} Modality: Cycle Frequency: 5×/week Duration: 20 min	16 weeks 8 weeks training, 8 weeks restricted activity	Improved submax Exercise response with training delayed anaerobic threshold during exercise, occurring at a higher $\dot{V}o_2$; improved autonomic function	Neuroendocrine function demonstrated an ↑ in parasympathetic activity and ↓ sympathetic

(continued)

Evidence Summary Box 16.3

Studies Investigating the Effect of Exercise on Patients with CHF (Continued)

Reference	Subjects	Design	Intervention	Duration	Results	Comments
Giannuzzi, PG, et al[111] 1997	*N* = 80 (76 M, 4 F); Post-MI; EF: 34.4% ± 4.5	Multicenter, RCT; Location: home + clinic	Intensity: 80% HR_{max} Modality: cycle, walk Frequency: 3×/week Duration: 30-min cycle; > 30-min walk	6 months 2 months supervised then F/U at home with q 2 clinic visit and exercise prescription changed as needed	→ LV volume and dilation in exercise group however signif ↑ in control; ↑ in exercise group but not in control; ↑ QOL in exercise group	Improve global and regional (LV) function over time in patients with ↓ EF following MI
Willenheimer, R, et al[112] 1998	*N* = 54 Characteristics: Male and female Age: < 75 years; EF: 36% ± 11.5	RCT Location: outpatient clinic	Intensity: 80% of $\dot{V}O_2$ max Modality: cycle Frequency: 2–3×/week Duration: interval training; 90-s exercise, 30-s rest Increase in duration from 15 min 2×/week to 45 min 3×/week from week 7–16	4 months	↑ Max exercise capacity ↑ $\dot{V}O_2$ max in M ischemic etiology; not in F ↑ QOL → submax performance	Men and women differ in their response to exercise training Included ischemic CHF and non-ischemic patients
McKelvie, RS, et al[113] 2002	*N* = 181 80% M; 20% F Characteristics: Class I–III; Age: 66.1 + .99 ex group EF: 27.7% + .9 in ex group $\dot{V}O_2$: 14 ml/kg	RCT, single blind comparing 3 months of supervised training followed by 9 months of home based	Intensity: HR 60–70% of HR_{max} Resistance training: 40% 1RM increasing to 60% Modality: cycle, TM, arm ergometer Frequency: 3×/week: clinic 2×/week, home 1×/week Duration: 30 min aerobic Resistance: 3 sets per ex session; arm curls, knee ext, leg press	12 months	↑ 6MWT performance at 3 and 12 months for both ex and control group and 12 months ex and control; ↑ $\dot{V}O_2$ by 10% post 3 months; NSD 12 months ↑ strg at 3 months, none at 12 months → QOL → LV function	Adherence to exercise decreased with home-based exercise Patients required close supervision programs to ensure compliance with exercise training

CHF = Congestive heart failure; CO = cardiac output; EF = ejection fraction; F = female; HR = heart rate; LV = left ventricle; M = male; MI = myocardial infarction; 6MWT = 6-Minute Walk Test; N = number; PCWP = pulmonary capillary wedge pressure; QOL = quality of life; RCT = randomized control trial; RM = resistance maximum; $\dot{V}O_2$ = oxygen consumption per unit time.

desaturate if their CO is inadequate or if pulmonary gas exchange is decreased owing to pulmonary congestion. At times pulse oximetry may be difficult to obtain via finger probe due to the effect of peripheral vasoconstriction as a result of blood flow redistribution directed away from the periphery toward the central circulation. Regardless of the reason, it is prudent to stop and reexamine the intensity of the activity as well as determine the need for supplemental oxygen. Patient examination should include vital sign monitoring, auscultation, observation, and recording of RPE.

A recommendation for an exercise prescription is to keep intensity low and duration gradually increasing as the patient tolerates. Because of the decrease in diastolic filling time and the potential alteration in cardiac function at higher HRs, keeping the exercise HR below 115 bpm is prudent. However, as a result of drug management with beta-blockade, many patients may find that their HR increases only approximately 10 to 20 bpm above resting for an adequate work out intensity. RPE is a valuable tool within this population and should be kept to a rating of fairly light. In the normal heart, an increase in HR is accompanied by an increase in inotropy. In the failing heart, an increase in HR may actually result in a decrease in force; this is known as the *negative treppe effect*.[87] Duration of exercise depends on the physiological response of the patient. A compensated Class III patient may be able to complete 20 continuous minutes of low-level sustained activity such as treadmill walking or recumbent cycle ergometry. Another patient may require an intermittent schedule with planned rests after every minute of exercise. Light calisthenics in the sitting position are often a good initial exercise for the most compromised of patients. Besides low intensity and long duration, the exercise prescription should include a prolonged warmup and cool-down period and avoidance of isometrics.[119] Inclusion of light resistance work has shown to be safe in this population.[120] Modalities for resistance training may include elastic bands for mild upper and lower extremity resistance work or light weights. A patient's hemodynamic status may change quickly with activity; therefore, it is prudent to be prepared for signs/symptoms of exertional hypotension, chronotropic incompetence, and significant dysrhythmias.[119]

Functional examination of this population may be done with the *6-minute walk test (6MWT)*. Patients are asked to walk as far as they can in 6 minutes, taking as many rests as needed during this time.[119,121,122] One study reported that in patients with heart failure, the oxygen consumption ($\dot{V}O_2$) measured at the end of a standardized 6MWT was on average only 15 percent less than the peak $\dot{V}O_2$ attained on an ETT.[123] Quality of life questionnaires such as the Minnesota Living with Heart Failure Questionnaire are valuable for tracking patients' responses over time. The reader is referred to the following Web site for additional information on this questionnaire: http://www.mlhfq.org.

Conduction Abnormalities

Ectopic Beats

A beat that originates from a site other than the sinus node is known as an ectopic beat. The common ectopic beats are atrial *(premature atrial contractions [PACs])* and ventricular *(premature ventricular contractions [PVCs])*. PVCs may occur either by themselves or in groups such as couplets (two PVCs) or triplets (three PVCs), or alternating with sinus beats such as bigeminy (every other beat a PVC) or trigeminy (every third beat a PVC). There may also be a premature junctional beat from the A-V node, but at times this is difficult to differentiate from the atrial beat, so they are commonly referred to as ectopic *supraventricular beats,* occurring above the ventricles in either the atria or A-V node. The presence of ectopic beats results in an irregular rhythm. Usually, ectopic beats are transient, and their severity depends on their impact on CO. It is certainly common to have a few PVCs even in a normal heart. Many people may have ectopic beats during times of stress or with stimulants such as nicotine and caffeine. Even though this may be a common response in a normal heart, it is important to educate patients with myocardial impairments who may have ectopic beats or irregular rhythms to avoid these aggravators. An increase in ectopy is undesired. It is unwise for any patient with cardiac disease to engage in exercise following recent cigarette smoking. Although the specific time frame that a patient may be at risk for increased ectopy is not clearly known, a good rule of thumb may be abstinence of smoking for at last 2 hours either before or after exercise.

Conduction

Changes in the length of the PR interval, the width of the QRS complex, and the length of the QT interval are some of the EKG measurements indicative of conduction abnormalities.

Conduction delays through the A-V node are classified as first-, second-, or third-degree A-V block. *First-degree heart block* occurs when the conduction time through the A-V node is prolonged; therefore, the EKG will have an increased length of the PR interval. There are two categories of *second-degree heart block:* Mobitz type I and Mobitz type II; each is hallmarked by the presence of dropped beats. Mobitz I, also known as *Wenckebach,* presents with a gradual increase in PR length in the preceding beats and then an eventual dropped beat; Mobitz II has normal PR intervals in all the beats preceding the dropped beat. In *third-degree heart block,* a mismatch of atrial and ventricular conduction exists, so there is no consistency between the atrial contraction and the ventricular contraction (i.e., no relationship between P waves and QRS complex on the EKG).

Conduction delays through the bundle of His are known as either right bundle branch block (RBBB) or left bundle branch block (LBBB). Bundle branch blocks are not true arrhythmias because there is no change in the actual rhythm, just in the timing of conduction through the bundle of His. The heart is still depolarized from the same pacemaker; only the route of activation is changed. Bundle branch blocks present on the EKG as a distortion of the QRS complex with an increase duration (i.e., widening). The presence of a LBBB on the EKG is usually permanent and indicates a pathological condition. RBBB may occur from a variety of reasons; it may be a permanent change due to underlying disease, or it may be benign. RBBB can also occur transiently. LBBB usually indicates the presence of more significant disease than RBBB.

Physical Therapy Intervention for Patients with Arrhythmias

Atrial Fibrillation (Fig. 16.14A)

A-fib is the classic irregular rhythm, characterized by a varied number of nonsinus originating P waves (known as flutter waves) for each QRS complex. Patients may exhibit this rhythm continuously as their baseline rhythm. Physical therapy intervention may be appropriate for patients in a-fib who have a good ventricular response at rest, with appropriate hemodynamic and HR increase with exercise. A good rule of thumb is to avoid physical therapy interventions and seek medical consultation if the patient's resting HR is greater than 115 bpm, if the patient appears uncomfortable, or if there is an inadequate hemodynamic response. Because this rhythm is irregular, it is important to monitor the HR for a full minute.

Premature Atrial Contraction (PAC) (Fig. 16.14B)

A PAC is an ectopic beat that originates in the atria and may present as an irregular rhythm. Usually, PACs will not compromise CO, and physical therapy intervention may be appropriate if accompanied by adequate hemodynamic and an appropriate ventricular response. A run of PACs occurring at a fast rate (100 to 200 bpm) is known as *paroxysmal atrial tachycardia (PAT)*. A common cause of PAT is digoxin toxicity. It may be difficult to distinguish a PAC from a premature junctional contraction (PJC), an ectopic beat that originates in the A-V node. A run of either PACs or PJCs at a rate of 150 to 250 bpm is known as supraventricular tachycardia (SVT) (Fig. 16.14C). In some cases, it may be difficult to distinguish PAT from SVT; SVT usually responds to a carotid massage whereas PAT does not. No physical therapist should ever initially instruct a patient in the use of a carotid massage or perform a carotid massage because adverse rhythm changes may occur with its use; a physician must first carefully screen patients during EKG monitoring. No physical therapy intervention should occur during an episode of SVT or PAT. These rhythms usually last for a short time (minutes, not hours), and activity may usually be resumed after the patient has been examined, the patient is comfortable, and the etiology determined and corrected, if possible.

Premature Ventricular Contraction (PVC) (Fig. 16.14D)

PVC is an ectopic beat that originates in the ventricle and may present as an irregular rhythm. Usually, single PVCs will not compromise CO if less than 7 per minute. Therefore, physical therapy intervention may be appropriate if accompanied by an adequate hemodynamic response. If PVCs increase with activity, the activity should be stopped and the patient examined for possible myocardial ischemia. PVCs that come from different ectopic sites within the ventricle are known as multifocal PVCs. They are more serious than unifocal PVCs, and, therefore, the patient should be medically evaluated before beginning or continuing an activity.

Ventricular Bigeminy (Fig. 16.14E) and Ventricular Trigeminy (Fig. 16.14F)

In ventricular bigeminy, every other beat is a PVC; in trigeminy, every third beat is a PVC. These rhythms occur transiently or episodically, and many patients have frequent bursts of these rhythms. Altered LV function and ischemia are two of the more common causes; therefore, medical management is directed toward improved LV function and perfusion whenever possible, as well as arrhythmia control. Physical therapy intervention is conservative at best and depends on the hemodynamic stability of the patient. If ectopy increases with activity, then activity should be immediately stopped.

Ventricular Couplets (Fig. 16.14G) and Ventricular Triplets

When two PVCs occur together, it is known as a couplet; when three PVCs occur together, it is known as a triplet. Couplets and triplets are important in that they suggest a higher level of ventricular irritability than bigeminy or trigeminy. In general, activity should be stopped for anyone who has a couplet or triplet, and the patient should be examined for myocardial ischemia. Activity should not continue until the patient has received medical clearance.

Ventricular Tachycardia (Fig. 16.14H)

A run of four or more PVCs in a row is known as v-tach. V-tach may be either sustained or nonsustained. *Sustained v-tach,* by definition, occurs at a HR of at least 100 bpm and lasts for at least 30 seconds.[124] The patient may or may not have a palpable pulse and, if present, the pulse will be weak. Because of the severe decrease in CO and rapid hemodynamic deterioration associated with this rhythm, the presence of sustained v-tach is considered an emergency situation. Medical intervention must be initiated as soon as possible. No physical therapy intervention is appropriate, except assisting the patient in stabilization, initiating CPR when indicated, and activating the advanced

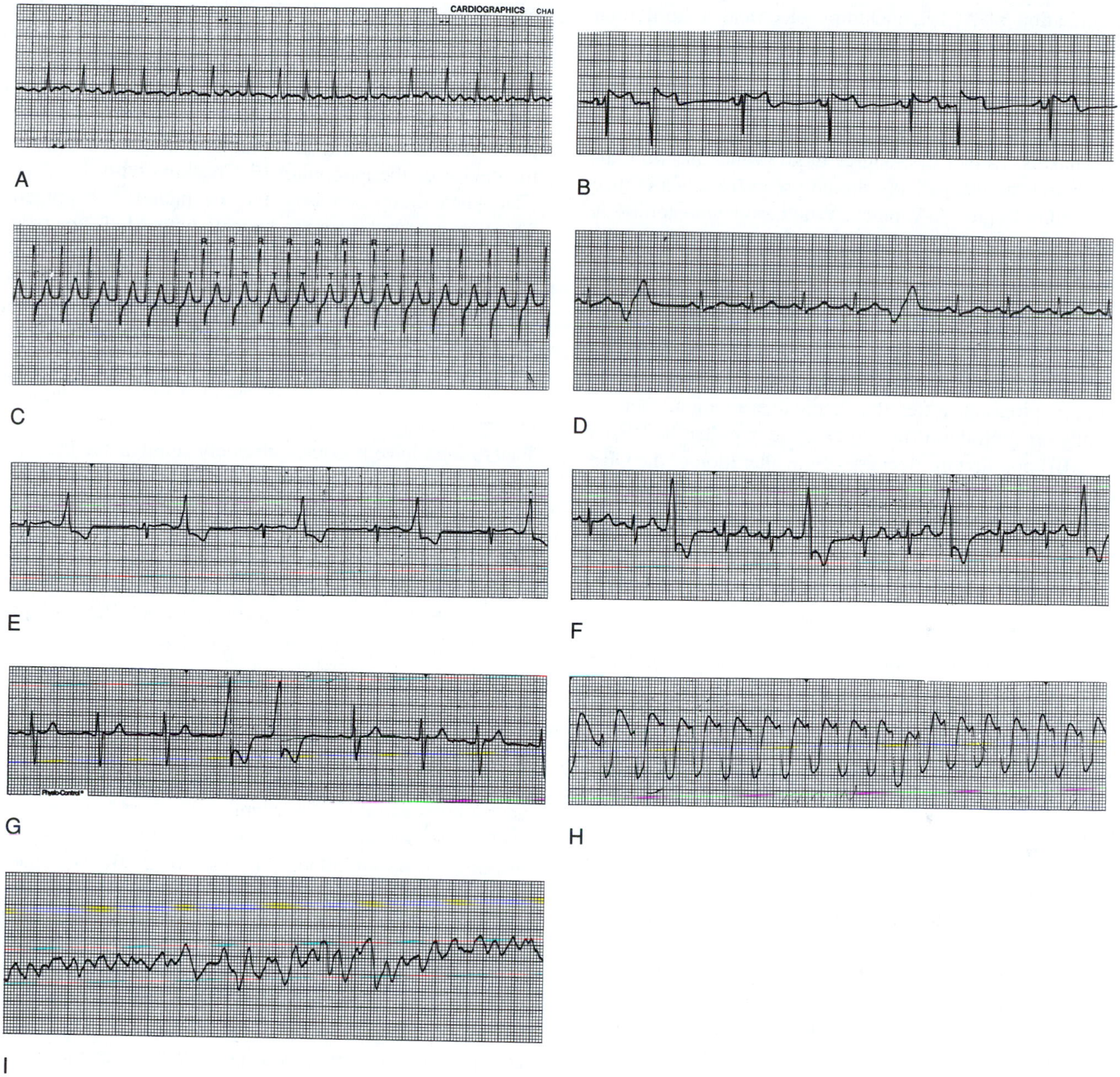

Figure 16.14 Examples of ectopy and arrhythmias. (*A*) Atrial fibrillation. (*B*) Atrial premature beat, also known as premature atrial contraction (PAC) (note third complex). (*C*) Supraventricular tachycardia (SVT). (*D*) Premature ventricular contraction (PVC) (note third complex). (*E*) Bigeminy (note second, fourth, and sixth complexes are PVCs). (*F*) Trigeminy (note second, fifth, and eighth complexes are PVCs). (*G*) Couplets (note fourth and fifth complexes are PVCs). (*H*) Ventricular tachycardia (v-tach). (*I*) Ventribular fibrillation (v-fib) (v-tach deteriorates into v-fib). (From Brown, K, and Jacobson, S: Mastering Dysrhythmias: A Problem-Solving Guide, FA Davis, Philadelphia, 1988, p 30, with permission).

cardiac life support (ACLS) system. V-tach may deteriorate quickly into ventricular fibrillation.

Nonsustained V-Tach occurs either in groups of three to five PVCs known as *salvos,* or a run of six or more PVCs lasting for up to 30 seconds.[124] Nonsustained v-tach is considered a high-risk indicator for potentially lethal arrhythmias. Because the rhythm is nonsustained, the decrease in CO may not be sufficient to cause symptoms. However, until the etiology of the arrhythmia is identified and the rhythm controlled, physical therapy intervention is generally inappropriate.

Ventricular Fibrillation (Fig. 16.14I)

When the ventricles do not contract but instead fibrillate, there is ineffective CO. The patient will expire if this rhythm is not altered immediately; the treatment of choice is activation of ACLS, including electrical defibrillation and medication.

Conduction Abnormalities

Patients with third-degree A-V block are candidates for pacemakers. Unlike first-degree block, which has no limitations to exercise, patients should not exercise while they are in third-degree A-V block. Whether or not exercise is permitted with second-degree A-V block depends on the etiology and subsequent hemodynamic response; the attending physician should clear this patient population before beginning any exercise.

The presence of a new bundle branch block should be medically evaluated before beginning or progressing an exercise program. After the medical evaluation, there is usually no contraindication to exercise in either the RBBB or LBBB population. Because of the alteration of the QRS complex and as a result the ST segment, the sensitivity of the EKG in detecting ischemia via ST depression is lost in the patient with LBBB.

Special Exercise Considerations

For a brief overview of areas for consideration when designing an exercise prescription for patients following a CABG, valvular surgery, PTCA, pacemaker, automatic *implantable cardioverter defibrillator (AICD),* or heart transplant,[125–130] and for those patients with a diagnosis of silent ischemia or severe LV dysfunction, refer to Table 16.11.[126]

Heart Transplant

Patients who have undergone a heart transplant may present with the following: (1) calf cramps (occurring in approximately 15 percent of patients) owing to the immunosuppressive drug cyclosporine; (2) decreased lower extremity strength; (3) obesity owing to long-term corticosteroid use; (4) increased risk of fracture owing to osteoporosis associated with long-term, high-dose corticosteroids; and (5) an increased probability of developing atherosclerosis in the coronary arteries of the donor heart after the first year post surgery.[127] Because the heart is denervated, HR alone provides a limited measure of exercise intensity. Therefore, BP and perceived exertion should be included in the routine data collection.

Automatic Implantable Cardioverter-Defibrillator (AICD)

AICD (ICD) are placed in patients who have life-threatening ventricular arrhythmias (v-tach, v-fib). The AICD is programmed to deliver an electric shock if it detects a HR higher than its programmed HR limit. Therefore, it is important for the physical therapist to know this limit and avoid an exercise intensity that may inadvertently activate the device.[128] In addition to knowing the HR settings for the patient with a pacemaker, there are other considerations. ST segment changes on the EKG may be common and are not specific for ischemia; therefore, other diagnostic studies must be done. In addition, UE aerobic or strengthening exercises should be avoided initially after placement of the pacer to avoid inadvertently dislodging the device or the lead wires.[128] Checking with the physician when these exercises may be included is prudent. There may be a danger for patients with AICDs or pacemakers from electromagnetic signals such as anti-theft devices, either causing the AICD to discharge or causing pacers to slow down or speed up. It may be no problem for patients to walk through these devices but lingering within a few feet could be dangerous.[129]

Pacemaker

Pacemakers have become extremely sophisticated in their capabilities and are no longer used just for the patient with bradycardia. Other indications for pacemaker use include the following; (1) symptomatic second- or third- degree A-V conduction block, either acquired or as a complication post MI; (2) bifasicular or trifasicular second-degree A-V block; (3) sinus node dysfunction; and (4) recurrent syncope due to hypersensitive carotid sinus reflex or neurocardiac syndrome.[136] Pacemakers have rate and rhythm sensitivity as well as the ability to override certain arrhythmias. Pacemakers may also be combined with AICD capabilities. Pacemakers are coded by either a three- or five-category system according to which chamber (atria or ventricle) is sensed, what chamber is paced (atria or ventricle), and whether the electrical stimulus will trigger a response or be inhibited.[130] (Table 16.12) Because pacemakers may fail to work properly, whenever VS response and HR appear abnormal during rest or activity, EKG monitoring is helpful to determine if the pacer is working properly.

As stated previously, patients with Class III CHF and left bundle branch block may be candidates for a specialized pacemaker known as a biventricular pacemaker, the purpose of which is to synchronize LV contractility to provide a more effective CO. The biventricular pacer does not influence HR or rhythm.

Education for Patients with Heart Disease

For patients with heart disease, patient and family education develops along a continuum, depending on the patient's baseline status and readiness to attend to the information. The physical therapist, along with other members of the health care team, must to determine the patient's and family's ability to understand the information and, when needed, to recommend home care personnel for supervision and safety. Appropriate discharge or ongoing outpatient topics to be addressed include the following:

Table 16.11 Special Considerations for Early Rehabilitation

Classification	Key Factors	Exercise Prescription
CABG or valvular surgery	• Incisional discomfort • Infectious processes • Anemia	• RPE of 11–14 • Range of motion for trunk and upper extremities • Muscular strength and endurance for upper extremities
PTCA (or similar procedure), MI, or angina	• Intravascular inflammation post procedure • Signs or symptoms of continued ischemia • Anxiety • Symptom denial • New ischemia (signs or symptoms) • Resting (unstable) angina	• HR criteria if below ECG signs of ischemia • Limited by symptoms • RPE
Silent ischemia	• Associated signs (e.g., shortness-of-breath, nausea, general malaise) • Sudden decrease in exercise capacity • Sudden changes in overall condition or "sense of well-being" (prodromal symptoms)	• RPE preferred for monitoring
Severe LV dysfunction and CHF	• Significant weight gain (>4 lb) over short duration (1–2 days) • Decreased (or failure to increase) SBP during exercise • Resting or abnormal exercise shortness-of-breath	• RPE • SBP response to exertion • Symptoms
Pacemakers or AICDs	• Pacemaker type and method of function • Symptoms similar to pacemaker insertion • AICD threshold discharge rate • Ectopy or ventricular tachycardia	• RPE • HR (if available from postinsertion GXT) • HR and intensity threshold for exercise-induced ventricular tachycardia • Ventricular ectopy pattern(s)
Heart transplant	• Delayed and attenuated exercise HR response • Elevated resting HR • Signs of rejection • Infection • Medication side effects	• RPE • Signs and symptoms

Adapted from American College of Sports Medicine: Guidelines for Exercise. Testing and Training, ed 5, Williams & Wilkins, Baltimore, 1995, p 191, with permission.

Table 16.12 Pacemaker Classification System

Chamber Paced	Chamber Sensed	Response	Rate Responsive Pacing
O = none	O = none	O = none	R = rate responsive
A = atria	A = atria	I = inhibit	
V = ventricle	V = ventricle	T = trigger	
D = dual chamber	D = dual chamber	D = capacity to both inhibit and trigger	

Pacemakers are commonly identified by a three-letter code as displayed in the first three columns. Pacemakers may also have the capacity to respond to physiologic stimuli to increase rate (column 4) and to override atrial tachycardia. A fifth column for antitachycardiac function, is rarely used due to the increased sophistication of the newer implantable defibrillators/pacemakers which renders this function unnecessary. Example: VVI pacer will provide an electrical impulse to the ventricle if it senses that there is no ventricular activity within an appropriate time frame. If there is intrinsic ventricular electrical activity, the pacemaker will be inhibited.

Activity Guidelines

Patients (and family) need to be able to understand specific activity guidelines, which include planned exercise sessions as well as leisure time and rests.

Self-Monitoring

Patients may monitor the intensity of their activity in a variety of ways; two of the more common ways are palpating a pulse and RPE. Because many older patients have decreased sensitivity in their palpation skills, the use of RPE may be easier and more reliable. Those patients that are able to take a pulse or choose to invest in a HR monitor may prefer to use those methods. Self-monitoring not only involves HR or RPE, but awareness of other symptoms or signs that may suggest exercise intolerance, such as lightheadedness, mental confusion, dyspnea, and inability to carry on a brief conversation while performing an activity. Patients with CHF commonly use the dyspnea scale and the Borg RPE scale.

Symptom Recognition and Response

Being able to recognize their specific cardiac symptoms and to know how to respond is a key component in patient education. Patients should have written information regarding the action they should take when symptoms occur, for example, when to call their physician or go to the hospital. Angina is the most common symptom associated with coronary heart disease, while weight gain (2 pounds over 1 to 2 days), dyspnea, LE edema, and increased pillows for sleep are common signs and symptoms for CHF.

Nutrition

Patients commonly meet with a nutritionist to discuss their usual dietary habits and to make recommendations when needed for a more heart-healthy diet. Most commonly, patients with coronary heart disease are instructed to reduce fat intake; patients with CHF are instructed to monitor salt and fluid intake.

Medications

Patients receive written information regarding the desired action of their medications, potential side effects, dosage, and timing of medications. Patients should also know which nonprescription drugs such as cold, sinus, allergy, or anti-inflammatory medications they should avoid because of possible interactions with prescription drugs. Patients should also be encouraged to disclose all herbal remedies and supplements that they may be taking.

Lifestyle Issues

Many factors influence whether a patient will return to work after a cardiac event. Many patients with CAD return to work if they were employed before their event; patients with CHF are, in general, an older population when compared to patients with CAD and therefore may have already retired.

Resumption of sexual activity may be an uncomfortable discussion for some patients. There may be many issues of concern for the patient (e.g., fear, anxiety, performance concerns, lack of libido). Patients and their partners are encouraged to verbalize their concerns to each other and to seek appropriate information from their health care team. Some medications (e.g., beta-blockers) may blunt the sexual response, and it is important that patients communicate this with their physician. Often, another medication or category of medication may be better tolerated. When patients feel ready for sex, their energy level throughout the day is satisfying for them and they are able to walk outdoors and climb stairs comfortably, they are probably ready for sexual activity. It may be helpful for patients to remember that sexual activity is not unlike other physical activity with respect to energy cost, and therefore planning, pacing, and warmup are powerful contributors for a more comfortable outcome. In some cases, the physician may recommend taking a prophylactic nitroglycerin prior to sexual activity.

Psychological/Social Issues

Cardiac disease may not only create new emotional issues but also enhance some that might have existed before the cardiac event. Reassure patients that many of these issues are normal sequelae of their event. Encourage them to seek guidance and counseling in whatever arena they feel appropriate (health care, counseling, religion).

Many studies have addressed the relationship of emotional depression following CABG.[131–133] Although depression is reported to exist, there is difficulty in objectively measuring the direct impact of CABG on subsequent depression. Some of the difficulty arises in the use of depression scales (Beck or CES-D), grading criteria, the presurgical emotional status, and gender. Burg et al reported two studies in 2003 in which 89 men were followed preoperatively and up to 2 years following surgery.[131,132] They found that presurgical depression was an independent predictor of postoperative prolonged surgical pain and failure to return to previous activity. In the study by Blumenthal et al, 817 patients were studied preoperatively, up to a mean of 5.2 years postoperatively. They reported that the patients with moderate to severe depression at baseline (preoperatively) that persisted postoperatively had an increased death rate compared to the nondepressed.[133] Ai et al reported that the presence of preoperative co-morbidities strongly influenced whether depression existed.[134] McKhann et al, in their study of 124 patients, concluded that the majority of patients depressed after surgery were in fact depressed prior to surgery.[135] Pirraglia et al reported on 237 patients and noted that 43 percent were classified as depressed preoperatively and only 23 percent postoperatively. Factors that influenced post surgical scores were length of ICU stay and the amount of reported social support.[136] The decrease in postoperative depression compared to preoperatively was supported by Lindquist et al in 2003; they studied more than 650 men and women and found less anxiety and depression following surgery than preoperatively.[137] Of interest, they also noted that women's report of QOL was lower than men's up to one year following surgery. Westin et al also reported a gender difference in CABG outcomes in regard to depression and QOL measures. In their study of more than 300 patients, women scored lower on the QOL and higher on depression scale than men at 1 month and 1 year following CABG, compared to men.[138] Phillips et al reported women to be at greater risk for both cognitive difficulties and anxiety than men at 1-year postop CABG than men.[139] The physical therapist needs to be aware that depression may exist following surgery and, as a member of the health care team, assist in directing appropriate care and support for the patient.

Heart Failure Education

As listed in Box 16.4, the US Department of Health & Human Services Clinical Practice Guidelines for Patients with CHF[140] suggests additional topics for patient and family education for patients with LV dysfunction.

Box 16.4 Suggested Topics for Patient, Family, and Caregiver Education and Counseling

General counseling
Explanation of heart failure and the reason for symptoms
Cause or probable cause of heart failure
Expected symptoms
Symptoms of worsening heart failure
What to do if symptoms worsen
Self-monitoring with daily weights
Explanation of treatment/care plan
Clarification of patient's responsibilities
Importance of cessation of tobacco use
Role of family members or other caregivers in the treatment/care plan
Availability and value of qualified local support group
Importance of obtaining vaccinations against influenza and pneumococcal disease

Prognosis
Life expectancy
Advance directives
Advice for family members in the event of sudden death

Activity recommendations
Recreation, leisure, and work activity
Exercise
Sex, sexual difficulties, and coping strategies

Dietary recommendations
Sodium restriction
Avoidance of excessive fluid intake
Fluid restriction (if required)
Alcohol restriction

Medications
Effects of medications on quality of life and survival
Dosing
Likely side effects and what to do if they occur
Coping mechanisms for complicated medical regimens
Availability of lower cost medications or financial assistance

Importance of compliance with the treatment care plan

From Clinical Practice Guidelines, Number 11, Heart Failure: Evaluation and Care of Patients With Left-Ventricular Systolic Dysfunction, AHCPR Publication No. 94-0612, p 42, with permission.

Primary Prevention of Coronary Artery Disease

Patients who do not have documented CAD but who have identifiable risk factors should be encouraged to adopt lifestyle behaviors that can modify their risk factors. Health education and primary prevention programs through individualized education and exercise guidelines attempt to modify an individual's risk factors and thereby prevent CAD.

Patients are instructed in appropriate dietary guidelines including low fat, adequate fiber, minerals and vitamins, and decreased salt, particularly if the patient has high BP. Besides lowering total dietary fat, patients are instructed to decrease their percentage of saturated fats and avoid trans fatty acids. Elevated levels of the amino acid homocysteine appear to increase the risk of arterial endothelial disease. Folic acid, a B vitamin, lowers homocysteine levels. If weight loss is needed, patients are encouraged to see a nutritionist to design a sensible eating plan. Patients are encouraged to gradually increase their endurance activity, such as walking toward a goal of 30 to 40 minutes (not including warmup and cool-down) four times a week. The American College of Sports Medicine and the American Heart Association recommend that anyone over the age of 40 with two or more risk factors should have an ETT before beginning an aerobic or strengthening exercise program. The purpose of the ETT is to identify the presence of any latent ischemia.

If no ischemia is present, a typical aerobic exercise prescription might be:

- Intensity: 70 to 85 percent of HR_{max} as the aerobic training zone
- Duration: 30 to 40 minutes in the aerobic training zone; appropriate warmup of 5 to 10 minutes, and cool-down
- Frequency: three to four times per week.

Maximum HR may be estimated by subtracting the person's age from 220; this, however, is not an exact science for any individual and cannot be accurate if the person is on any cardiac medications, such as beta-blockers, that may decrease the maximum HR. Supplemental resistance work is also encouraged at moderate intensities, with initial monitoring of HR and BP.

Modification of the other CAD risk factors is also key to the success of any primary prevention intervention. Patients are encouraged to identify risk factors and to seek resources to assist in modifying them. There are many community-based smoking cessation programs or medically supervised programs that a patient might explore. Stress management programs are also varied and can be adapted to the individual's needs. Proper and consistent use of any medications that might be used in controlling risk factors, such as antihypertensives, antihypercholesterolemias, blood glucose lowering agents (hypoglycemics), and anti-anxiety or antidepressants, is crucial to the success of any program.

Hypertension, as the most prevalent cardiovascular disease in the United States, is one of the most powerful contributors to cardiovascular morbidity and mortality.[4] The Joint National Committee on Detection, Evaluation and Treatment of High Blood Pressure recommends a multifactorial approach and suggests that lifestyle modifications including weight reduction, physical activity and moderation of dietary sodium are recommended as either definitive or adjunctive therapy for hypertension.[141]

Summary

Physical activity is important for all individuals and is especially beneficial for those individuals already diagnosed with CAD,[71,72] are at risk for the development of CAD,[142] or who are diagnosed with CHF.[143] Individuals with heart disease should understand that a consistent exercise program is part of the management for their disease and is as necessary as their medications. Having heart disease means that the person needs to understand the parameters in which he or she may safely participate in activity either recreationally or as a prescribed exercise. The role of the physical therapist is to provide a safe exercise prescription for all patients.

During the time of illness, the effects of decreased activity can be devastating (Box 16.5). A paradox exists, however, in that the less activity that is done, the less activity can be done as a result of a decreased work capacity. Therefore, the relative energy cost of all activity increases, and the heart actually works harder for any given task. Not encouraging the patient to resume activity when he or she is medically stable is a disservice. As physical therapists, our role is clear: to understand the pathophysiology of the disease process, to accurately examine the patient, and to establish a safe plan of care. The ultimate goal is to improve the patient's physiological response to activity and, in doing so, decrease the work of the cardiovascular system.

Box 16.5 Deconditioning Effects of Prolonged Bedrest

A decrease in physical work capacity
An increase in the heart rate response to effort
A decrease in adaptability to change in posture, which is manifested primarily as orthostatic hypotension
A decrease in the circulation blood volume (with plasma volume decreasing to a greater extent than red cell mass)
A decrease in lung volume and vital capacity
A decrease in serum protein concentration
A negative nitrogen and calcium balance
A decrease in the contractile strength of the body musculature

From Wenger, N: Coronary Care: Rehabilitation after Myocardial Infarction. American Heart Association, New York, 1973, with permission.

Questions for Review

1. Discuss the role of the endothelium in atherosclerosis.
2. Describe the evolutionary process of an MI, addressing plaque formation, plaque rupture, thrombus formation, and the role of TPA.
3. Compare pertinent findings in the medical record: ECG, physical examination, heart sounds, lung sounds, peripheral pulses, blood work, presenting clinical symptoms, and so forth, between ischemia, infarction, and CHF.
4. Discuss the physical therapy management if a patient has angina during a treatment session.
5. Design a HEP for a patient who has a positive ETT.
6. Discuss the compensatory mechanisms associated with LV failure
7. Discuss the difference between compensated and noncompensated CHF.
8. Design a HEP for a patient with Class II CHF.
9. Identify the various potential presentations of angina. Discuss how you would instruct your patient in symptom recognition.
10. What is the usual clinical course following a non-complicated MI? What is a complicated MI?
11. Discuss the HEP for a patient being discharged from the hospital 5 days post CABG.
12. Identify and discuss the components of CO. (a) How does a patient respond to an increase in $\dot{V}O_2$? (b) What symptoms/signs may your patient present when there is a decrease in CO?
13. Discuss factors regulating BP. Discuss what actions you may take and why if your patient becomes hypotensive.

Case Study

A 58-year-old man presents to the local emergency room with chief complaint of SOB and difficulty sleeping last night; patient had to sit up all night to make symptoms even a little better. Patient came to ER because he was unable to get ready for work owing to increased SOB. Patient reports that he has felt SOB off and on for a couple of months, usually associated with physical activity; symptoms, however, usually resolved with rest. Today's episode was the first related to sleeping.

PAST MEDICAL HISTORY

Coronary artery disease: Anterior MI 4 years ago
Hypercholesterolemia
Peripheral vascular disease

MEDICATIONS

Digoxin, captopril, furosemide (Lasix), diltiazem, simvastatin (Zocor)

FAMILY/SOCIAL

Patient works full-time as an engineer; travels 3 to 4 days per month.

Married, lives with his wife in a two-story home on a 2-acre lot; three college-aged children.

Patient is an avid golfer; enjoys gardening and landscaping.

Present illness

PHYSICAL EXAM

Heart sounds: S_1, S_2 normal; S_3 present, no S_4; 2/6 systolic murmur
Lung sounds: Crackles 1/3 way
Rhythm/rate: Irregular, 140 bpm
Blood pressure: 100/60 mm Hg
Respiratory rate: 26 breaths/minute
SaO_2: 90%
JVD: 5 cm
Echocardiogram: Akinetic apex, akinetic distal septum and anterior wall; dilated atria and LV, Chest X-ray: Unavailable.

LABORATORY DATA

Enzyme pending; CBC WNL except BUN and creatinine slightly elevated.

Patient remained in the hospital for 2 days while medications were adjusted. During this time patient underwent further testing, including an ETT.

RESULTS OF ETT

Bruce protocol: 4 minutes; estimated $\dot{V}_2$ max; 20 ml O_2/kg/min (approximately 6 METs); Max VS: 130 bpm HR; 120/60 mm Hg BP
ECG: (−) negative for ischemia, chest pain
Reason for stopping: absolute exhaustion.
Exam immediately post-ETT: (+) S_3
Physical and occupational therapy were requested to assist with exercise guidelines and discharge planning.

PATIENT'S GOALS

Return to work.
Resume hiking.
Begin to prepare his garden for spring planting within the next 5 weeks.

PHYSICAL THERAPY INTERVENTION

Exercise tolerance via low level exercises sitting and standing, as well as 5-minute walk.

Vital Signs

Sitting (rest): HR 90 bpm; BP 110/60 mm Hg
Sitting exercises: HR 108 bpm; BP 110/60 mm Hg
Standing (rest): HR 110 bpm; BP 108/60 mm Hg
Standing exercise: HR 116 bpm: BP 110/60 mm Hg
5-minute walk: 1000 ft; HR 120 bpm; BP 116/60 mm Hg

HOME INSTRUCTIONS

Meetings planned with patient and his family to discuss discharge guidelines over the next 4 to 8 weeks.

FOLLOW-UP

Patient returns to his PCP 3 months after discharge. Echocardiogram is unchanged with EF 30%. Patient states that he has been following discharge guidelines.

Vital Signs

HR 100 bpm; BP 116/70 mm Hg (resting).
Patient states that he feels great and just wants to get on with his life.

GUIDING QUESTIONS

1. What is a reasonable presenting diagnosis? Identify each piece of information (and how you interpreted it) that you used to make this diagnosis.
2. Explain the pathophysiology of the patient's presenting symptoms. Discuss the significance of his HR and rhythm in relation to his symptoms
3. If the patient's symptoms and signs worsened, and he was admitted to the CCU,
   a. What do you think his Swan-Ganz reading could reasonably look like?
   b. What would you expect these signs/ symptoms would be that would bring the patient to the CCU?
   c. What might be a reasonable cause of his signs/symptoms worsening?
   d. What other drugs/interventions might be given in the CCU?
4. What rhythm do you think the patient is in and why? What do you think might be a reason that he is in this rhythm?
5. What do you think the CxR would look like and why?
6. What is your interpretation of the patient's vital sign response to PT intervention? What is your plan for your next session?
7. What exercise prescription would you recommend for the patient at home (modality, intensity, duration, frequency)?

References

1. Adams, PF, and Marano, MA: Current Estimates from the National Health Survey, United States 1994. Vital and Health Statistics. Vol. DHHS pub no (PHS) 96-1521: US Government Printing Office, Washington, DC, 1995.
2. World Health Organization (WHO): MONICA Manual revised edition, Cardiovascular Diseases Unit. WHO MONICA Project. Geneva, Switzerland, 1990.
3. American Heart Association (AHA): Heart Disease and Stroke Statistics 2005 Update. AHA, Dallas, TX. Retrieved December 17, 2005 from www.americanheart.org.
4. Thom, TJ, et al: Incidence, prevalence and mortality of cardiovascular disease in the United States. In Fuster, V, Alexander, RW, and O'Rourke, R (eds): Hurst's The Heart, ed 10. McGraw-Hill, New York, 2001, p 3.
5. US Department of Health and Human Services: The Seventh Report of the Joint National Committee on Prevention, Detection, Evaluation, and Treatment of High Blood Pressure. National Institute of Health, National Heart, Lung, and Blood Institute. NIH Publication; 2003. No. 03-5233.
6. American Physical Therapy Association: Guide to Physical Therapist Practice, ed 2. Phys Ther 81(1):471, 2001.
7. Alexander, RW: Coronary ischemic syndromes: Relationship to the biology of atherosclerosis. In Schlant, RC, Alexander, RW, and Fuster, V (eds): Hurst's The Heart, ed 9. McGraw-Hill, New York, 1998, p 1263.
8. Maseri, A, et al: Coronary blood flow and myocardial ischemia. In Fuster, V, Alexander, RW, and O'Rourke, R, (eds): Hurst's The Heart, ed 10. McGraw-Hill, New York, 2001, p 1109.
9. Griendling, KK, et al: Biology of vessel wall. In Fuster V, Alexander RW, O'Rourke, R, (eds): Hurst's The Heart, ed 11. Mc-Graw Hill, New York, 2004, p 135.
10. Berne, RM, and Levy, MN: Cardiovascular Physiology, ed 8. CV Mosby, St. Louis, 2001, p 85.
11. Lewinter, M, and Osol, G: Normal physiology of the cardiovascular system. In Fuster, V, Alexander, RW, and O'Rourke, R, (eds): Hurst's The Heart, ed 10. McGraw-Hill, New York, 1994, p 63.
12. Berne, RM, and Levy, MN: Cardiovascular Physiology, ed 8. CV Mosby, St. Louis, 2001, p 227.
13. Berne, RM, and Levy, MN: Cardiovascular Physiology, ed 8. CV Mosby, St. Louis, 2001, p 135.
14. Berne, RM, and Levy, MN: Cardiovascular Physiology, ed 8. CV Mosby, St. Louis, 2001, p 175.
15. Opie, L: Mechanisms of cardiac contraction and relaxation. In Braunwald, E, Zipes, D, and Libby, R (eds): Heart Disease: A Textbook of Cardiovascular Medicine, ed 6. WB Saunders, Philadelphia, 1997, p 443.
16. Braunwald, E: Normal and abnormal myocardial function, assessment of cardiac function. In Kasper, D, et al: Harrison's Principles of Internal Medicine, ed 16. McGraw-Hill, New York, 2001, p 1309.
17. Berne, RM, and Levy, MN: In Cardiovascular Physiology, ed 8. CV Mosby, St. Louis, 2001, p 55.
18. Lentner, C (ed): Geigy Scientific Tables, ed 8. Ciba Geigy, Basel, Switzerland, 1981.
19. Alpert, JS: Myocardial ischemia. In Physiology of the Cardiovascular System. Little, Brown, Boston, 1984, p 19.
20. Fletcher, GF, and Schlant, RC: The exercise test. In Schlant, RC, and Alexander, RW (eds): Hurst's The Heart, ed 8. McGraw-Hill, New York, 1994, p 423.
21. Ross, R: The pathogenesis of atherosclerosis: A perspective for the 1990's. Nature 362:801, 1993.
22. Ross, R: Atherosclerosis: An inflammatory disease. N Engl J Med 340:115, 1998.
23. Charo, S, et al: Endothelial dysfunction and coronary risk reduction. J Cardiopulm Rehabil 18:60, 1998.

24. Schoen, FJ: The Heart. In Cotran, RS, Kumar, V, and Collins (eds): Robbins Pathologic Basis of Disease, ed 6. WB Saunders, Philadelphia, 1999, p 543.
25. Phillips, RE, and Feeney, MK: The Cardiac Rhythms, ed 3. WB Saunders, Philadelphia, 1990, p 44.
26. Hillegass, EA: Electrocardiography. In Hillegass, EA, and Sadowsky, HS (eds): Essentials of Cardiopulmonary Physical Therapy, ed 2. WB Saunders, Philadelphia, 2001, p 380.
27. Hellerstein, HK, et al: Principles of exercise prescription. In Naughton, JP (ed): Exercise Testing and Exercise Training in Coronary Heart Disease. Academic, New York, 1973, p 147.
28. Naughton, J, and Haider, R: Methods of exercise testing. In Naughton, JP, and Hellerstein, HK (eds): Exercise Testing and Exercise Training in Coronary Heart Disease. Academic, New York, 1973, p 80.
29. American College of Sports Medicine. Exercise Prescription for Cardiac Patients. In ACSM's Guidelines for Exercise Testing and Prescription. Lippincott Williams & Wilkins, Philadelphia, 2000, p 165.
30. Alexander, RW: Dyspnea and fatigue. In Schlant, RC, and Alexander, RW (eds): Hurst's The Heart, ed 8. McGraw-Hill, New York, 1994, p 469.
31. Perry, AG, and Potter, PA: Vital Signs and Clinical Assessment. Clinical Nursing Skills and Techniques. CV Mosby, St. Louis, 1998, p 269.
32. Hurst, JW, and Morris, DC: The history: Symptoms and past events related to cardiovascular disease. In Schlant, RC, and Alexander, RW (eds): Hurst's The Heart, ed 8. McGraw-Hill, New York, 1994, p 205.
33. Guyton, AC, and Hall, JE: Textbook of Medical Physiology, ed 9. WB Saunders, Philadelphia, 1996, p 275.
34. O'Rourke, RA, Siverman, M, and Shaver, J: History, physical examination and cardiac auscultation. In Fuster, V, Alexander RW, and O'Rourke RA (eds): Hurst's The Heart, ed 11. McGraw-Hill, New York, 2004, p 217.
35. Collin, V: Contribution to diseases of the heart and pericardium: I. Historical Introduction. Bull NY Med Coll 18:1, 1955.
36. Holt, B: Diseases of the pericardium. In Fuster, V, Alexander, RW, and O'Rourke R (eds): Hurst's The Heart, ed 10. McGraw-Hill, New York, 2001, p 2061.
37. Bickley, L: Bates' Guide to Physical Examination and History Taking, ed 9. Lippincott Williams & Wilkins, Philadelphia, 2005.
38. Seidel, HM, et al: Mosby's Guide to Physical Examination. CV Mosby, St. Louis, 1995.
39. Jarvis, C: Physical Examination and Health Assessment. WB Saunders, Philadelphia, 2004.
40. Thaler, MS: The Only EKG Book You'll Ever Need. Lippincott, Philadelphia, 1998.
41. Golderberger, A, and Golderberger, E: Clinical Electrocardiography: A Simplified Approach. CV Mosby, St. Louis, 1981.
42. Dubin, D: Rapid Interpretation of EKGs. Cover, Tampa, 1974.
43. McGuinness, ME, and Talbert, RL: Cardiovascular Testing. In Dipiro, J (ed): Pharmacotherapy: A Pathophysiologic Approach. McGraw-Hill, New York, 2002, p 123.
44. Kannel, WB, et al: Factors of risk in the development of coronary heart disease—six-year follow-up experience. The Framingham Study. Ann Intern Med 55:33, 1961.
45. Kannel, WB, Castelli, WP, and Gordon, T: Cholesterol in the prediction of atherosclerotic disease. New perspectives based on the Framingham study. Ann Intern Med 90(1):85, 1979.
46. Wilson, PW: Established risk factors and coronary artery disease, the Framingham Study. Am J Hypertens 7(7 pt2):7S, 1994.
47. Grundy, SM, et al: Assessment of cardiovascular risk by use of multiple-risk-factor assessment equations: A statement for health care professionals from the American Heart Association and the American College of Cardiology. Circulation 100(13):1481, 1999.
48. Wenger, NK: Coronary heart disease in women: Evolving knowledge in dramatically changing clinical care. In Julian, DG, and Wenger, NK (eds): Women and Heart Disease. Mosby, CV St. Louis, 1997, p 20.
49. Hennekens, CH: Coronary disease: Risk intervention. In Julian, DG, and Wenger, NK (eds): Women and Heart Disease. CV Mosby, St. Louis, 1997, p 44.
50. US Preventative Services Task Force: Postmenopausal hormone replacement therapy for primary prevention of chronic conditions: Recommendations and rationale.Ann Intern Med 37(10):148, 2002.
51. Haas, JS, et al: Changes in the use of postmenopausal hormone therapy after the publication of clinical trial results. Ann Intern Med 140(3):184, 2004.
52. Hulley, S, et al: Randomized trial of estrogen plus progestin for secondary prevention of coronary heart disease in postmenopausal women. Heart and Estrogen/progestin Replacement Study (HERS) Research Group. JAMA 280:605, 1998.
53. Ressouw, JE, et al: Risks and benefits of estrogen plus progestin in healthy postmenopausal women: Principal results from the Women's Health Initiative randomized controlled trial. JAMA 288:321, 2002.
54. Herrington, DM, et al: The Estrogen Replacement and Atherosclerosis (ERA) study: Study design and baseline characteristics of the cohort. Control Clin Trials 21:257, 2000.
55. Deady, J: Clinical monograph: Hormone replacement therapy. J Manag Care Pharm Jan-Feb 10(1):33, 2004.
56. Pinto, D, and Josephson, M: Sudden cardiac death. The mechanisms, predictors and prevention of sudden cardiac death. In Fuster, V, Alexander RW, and O'Rourke RA (eds): Hurst's The Heart, ed 11. McGraw-Hill, New York, 2004, p 1051.
57. Schlant, RC, and Alexander, RW: Diagnosis and management of patients with chronic ischemic heart disease. In Alexander, RW, et al (eds): Hurst's The Heart, ed 9. McGraw-Hill, New York, 1998, p 1275.
58. Alpert, JS: Myocardial ischemia. In Physiology of the Cardiovascular System, Little, Brown, Boston, 1984, p 35.
59. Antman, EM, and Braunwald, E: Acute myocardial infarction. In Kasper, D, et al (eds): Harrison's Principles of Internal Medicine, ed 15. McGraw Hill, New York, 2001, p 1386.
60. Factor, SM, and Bache, RJ: Pathophysiology of myocardial ischemia. In Alexander, RW, et al (eds): Hurst's The Heart, ed 9. McGraw-Hill, New York, 1998, p 1241.
61. Falk, E: Atherogenesis and its determinants. In Fuster, V, Alexander, RW, and O'Rourke, R. (eds): Hurst's The Heart, ed 10. McGraw Hill, New York, 2001, 1065.
62. Antman, E, et al: ACC/AHA Guidelines for the management of patients with ST-elevation myocardial infarction-executive summary: A report of the American College of Cardiology/American Heart Association Task Force on Practice Guidelines. Circulation 110(5):588, 2004.
63. Richenbacher, WE, and Pierce, WS: Treatment of heart failure: Assisted circulation. In Braunwald, E (ed): Heart Disease: A Textbook of Cardiovascular Medicine, ed 6. WB Saunders, Philadelphia, 2001, p 600.
64. Alexander, RW, et al: ST-Segment elevation myocardial infarction: Clinical presentation, diagnostic evaluation and medical management. In Fuster, V, Alexander, RW, and O'Rourke,R (eds): Hurst's The Heart, ed 11. McGraw-Hill, New York, 2004, 1277.
65. Ciccone, C: Pharmacology in Rehabilitation, ed 3. FA Davis, Philadelphia, 2002.
66. Malone, T: Physical and Occupational Therapy: Drug Implications for Practice. Lippincott, Philadelphia, 1989.
67. Kupersmith, J: Antiarrhythmic Drugs. The Pharmacologic Management of Heart Disease. Williams & Wilkins, Baltimore, 1997.
68. Grimes, K, and Cohen, M: Cardiac pharmacology. In Hillegass, E, and Sadowsky, HSS (eds): Essentials of Cardiopulmonary Physical Therapy, ed 2. WB Saunders, Philadelphia, 2001, p 536.
69. Maehara, A, et al: Morphologic and angiographic features of coronary plaque rupture detected by intravascular ultrasound. J Am Coll Cardiol 40(5):904, 2002.
70. Cheng, JWM: Recognition, pathophysiology and management of acute myocardial infarction. Am JHealth Syst Pharm 58(18): 1709, 2001.
71. US Department of Health and Human Services: Effects of Cardiac Rehabilitation Exercise Training. Clinical Practice Guidelines, Cardiac Rehabilitation, AHCPR No. 17 publication No. 96-0672, October 1995.
72. American Association of Cardiovascular and Pulmonary Rehabilitation. Program Components, Risk Stratification,

Monitoring. In Guidelines for Cardiac Rehabilitation Programs, AACVPR, ed 2. Human Kinetics, Champaign, IL, 1995, p 7.
73. Borg, G: Borg's Perceived Exertion and Pain Scales. Human Kinetics, Champaign, IL, 1998.
74. Levine, SA, and Lown, B: Armchair treatment of acute coronary thrombosis. JAMA 1948:1356, 1952.
75. American Association of Cardiovascular and Pulmonary Rehabilitation. Phases of Cardiac Rehabilitation. In Guidelines for Cardiac Rehabilitation Programs. Human Kinetics, Champaign, IL, 1995, p 49.
76. American Association of Cardiovascular and Pulmonary Rehabilitation patient Education, Psychological Issues and Outcomes. In Guidelines for Cardiac Rehabilitation Programs, AACVPR ed 2. Human Kinetics, Champaign, IL, 1995, p 57.
77. McCartney, N: Role of resistance training in heart disease. Med Sci Sports Exerc S396, 1998.
78. Beniamini, Y, et al: Effects of high intensity strength training on quality of life parameters in cardiac rehabilitation patients. Am J Cardiol 841, 1997.
79. American Association of Cardiovascular and Pulmonary Rehabilitation: Graded exercise testing, exercise prescription, and resistance training. In Guidelines for Cardiac Rehabilitation Programs, AACVPR, ed 2. Human Kinetics, Champaign, IL, 1995, p 27.
80. American College of Sports Medicine: General principles of exercise prescription. In ACSM's Guidelines for Exercise Testing and Prescription, ed 6. Lippincott Williams & Wilkins, Philadelphia, 2000, p 137.
81. Fletcher, GF, et al: Exercise standards for testing and training: A statement for healthcare professionals from the American Heart Association. Circulation 104(14):1694, 2001.
82. Kannel, WB: Epidemiological aspects of heart failure. Cardiol Clin 7:1, 1989
83. Braunwald, E: Heart Failure. In Kapser, D, et al (eds): Harrison's Principles of Internal Medicine, ed 15. McGraw-Hill, New York, 2001, p 309.
84. Cahalin, LP: Cardiac muscle dysfunction. In Hillegass, E, Sadowsky, HSS (eds): Essentials of Cardiopulmonary Physical Therapy. WB Saunders, Philadelphia, 1995, p 106.
85. Wynne, J, and Braunwald, E: The cardiomyopathies and myocarditides. In Braunwald, E, Zipes, D, and Libby, R (eds): Heart Disease: A Textbook of Cardiovascular Medicine, ed 6. WB Saunders, Philadelphia, 1997, p 1404.
86. The Criteria Committee of the New York Heart Association: Nomenclature and Criteria for Diagnosis of Diseases of the Heart and Great Vessels, ed 9. Little, Brown, Boston, 1994, p 253.
87. Schlant, RC, and Sonnenblick, EH: Pathophysiology of heart failure. In Alexander, RW, Schlant, RC, Fuster, V (eds): Hurst's The Heart, ed 9. McGraw-Hill, New York, 1998, p 687.
88. Bickley, L: Peripheral vascular system. In Bickley, L (ed): Bates' Guide to Physical Examination and History Taking, ed 8. Lippincott, Philadelphia, 2003, p 441.
89. Jarvis, C: Physical Examination and Health Assessment, ed 3. WB Saunders, Philadelphia, 2004.
90. Atsumi, H, et al: Cardiac sympathetic nervous disintegrity is related to exercise intolerance in patients with chronic heart failure. Nucl Med Commun 19:451, 1998.
91. Linjiing, X, et al: Effect of heart failure on muscle capillary geometry: Implications for O_2 exchange. Med Sci Sports Exerc 30:1230, 1998.
92. Lunde, PK, et al: Skeletal muscle fatigue in normal subjects and heart failure patients: Is there a common mechanism? Acta Physiol Scand 162:215, 1998.
93. Vescovo, G, et al: Apoptosis in the skeletal muscle of patients with heart failure: Investigation of clinical and biochemical changes. Heart 84(4):431, 2000.
94. Rocca, HPBL, et al: Oxygen uptake kinetics during low level exercise in patients with heart failure: Relation to neurohormones, peak oxygen consumption, and clinical findings. Heart 81:121, 1999.
95. Bank, AJ: Effects of short-term forearm exercise training on resistance vessel endothelial function in normal subjects and patients with heart failure. J Card Fail 4:193, 1998.
96. Genth-Zotz, S, et al: Changes of neurohumoral parameters and endothelin-1 in response to exercise in patients with mild to moderate congestive heart failure. Int J Cardiol 30:137, 1998.
97. Yan, AT, Bradley, TD, and Liu, PP: The role of continuous positive airway pressure in the treatment of congestive heart failure. Chest 120(5):167, 2001.
98. Mansfield, DR, et al: Controlled trial of continuous positive airway pressure in obstructive sleep apnea and heart failure. Am J Respir Crit Care Med 169(3):361, 2004.
99. Avezum, A, et al: Beta-blocker therapy for congestive heart failure: A systemic overview and critical appraisal of the published trials. Can J Cardiol 14:1045, 1998.
100. Cleland, JG, et al: Beta-blockers for chronic heart failure: From prejudice to enlightenment. J Cardiovasc Pharmacol 32:S36, 1998.
101. Aleddini, J, et al: Sildenafil and assessment of pulmonary arterial reactivity in heart failure. Congest Heart Fail 993:176, 2003.
102. Salukhe, TV, Dimopoulos, K, and Francis, D: Cardiac resynchronization may reduce all-cause mortality: Meta analysis of preliminary COMPANION data with CONTAK-CD, InSync ICD, MIRACLE and MUSTIC. Int J Cardiol 93(2-3):101, 2004.
103. Rossi, P: Physical training in patients with congestive heart failure. Chest 101(5 Suppl):350S, 1992.
104. Afzal, A, et al: Exercise training in heart failure. Prog Cardiovasc Dis 41:175, 1998.
105. Piepoli, MF, et al: Exercise training meta-analysis of trials in patients with chronic heart failure (exTraMATCH). Br Med J 328(7433):189, 2004.
106. Kokkinos, PF, et al: Chronic heart failure and exercise. Am Heart J 140(1):21, 2000.
107. Wielenga, RP: Safety and effects of physical training in chronic heart failure: Results of the chronic heart failure and graded exercise study (CHANGE). Eur Heart J 20:872, 1999.
108. Dubach, D, et al: Hemodynamic response to training in CHF. JACC 29(7):1591, 1997.
109. Piepoli, M: Experience from controlled trials of physical training in chronic heart failure. Eur Heart J 19:466, 1998.
110. Coats, A, et al: Controlled trial of physical training in chronic heart failure: Exercise performance, hemodynamics, ventilation and autonomic function. Circulation 85:2119, 1992.
111. Giannuzzi, P, et al: Attenuation of unfavorable remodeling by exercise training in postinfarction patients with left ventricular dysfunction: Results of the exercise in left ventricular dysfunction (ELVD) trial. Circulation 96:790, 1997.
112. Willenheimer, R, et al: Exercise training in heart failure improves quality of life and exercise capacity. Eur Heart J 774, 1998.
113. McKelvie, RS, et al: Effects of exercise training in patients with heart failure: The Exercise Rehabilitation Trial (EXERT). Am Heart J 144:23, 2002.
114. Hambrecht, R, et al: Effects of exercise training on left ventricular function and peripheral resistance in patients with chronic heart failure: A randomized trial. JAMA 283(23):3095, 2000.
115. Tyni-Lenne, R, et al: Improved quality of life in chronic heart failure patients following local endurance training with leg muscles. J Card Fail 2:111, 1996.
116. Johnson, PH, et al: A randomized controlled trial of inspiratory muscle training in stable chronic heart failure. Eur Heart J 19:1249, 1998.
117. Balady, GJ: Exercise training in the treatment of heart failure: What is achieved and how? Ann Med 30(Suppl 1):61, 1998.
118. Cahalin, LP: Heart Failure. Phys Ther 76:516, 1996.
119. Myers, JN: Congestive heart failure. In ACSM's Exercise Management for Persons with Chronic Disease and Disabilities. Human Kinetics, Champaign, IL, 1997, p 48.
120. McKelvie, RS, et al: Comparison of hemodynamic responses to cycling and resistance exercises in congestive heart failure secondary to ischemic cardiomyopathy. Am J Cardiol 76:977, 1995.
121. Schaufelberger, SM, and Swedberg, K: Is six-minute walk test of value in congestive heart failure? Am Heart J 136:371, 1998.
122. Cahalin, L: The six-minute walk test predicts peak oxygen uptake and survival in patients with advanced heart failure. Chest 110:325, 1996.
123. Faggiano, P, et al: Assessment of oxygen uptake during the six-minute walking test in patients with heart failure: Preliminary experience with a portable device. Am Heart J 134:203, 1997.
124. Myerburg, RJ, et al: Recognition, clinical assessment, and management of arrhythmias and conduction disturbances. In Fuster, V, Alexander, RW, and O'Rourke, R (eds): Hurst's The Heart, ed 10. McGraw-Hill, New York, 2001, p 797.

125. Braith, RW: Exercise training in patients with CHF and heart transplant recipients. Med Sci Sports Exerc 30(Suppl 10), 1998.
126. American College of Sports Medicine: Exercise prescription for cardiac patients. In ACSM's Guide For Exercise Testing and Prescription, ed 6. Williams & Wilkins, Baltimore, 2000, p 165.
127. Keteyian, SJ, and Brawner, C: Cardiac transpantation. In American College of Sports Medicine: ACSM's Exercise Management for Persons with Chronic Diseases and Disabilities. Human Kinetics, Champaign, IL, 1997, p 54.
128. West, M, Johnson, T, and Roberts, SO: Pacemakers and implantable cardioverter Defibrillators. In American College of Sports Medicine: ACSM's Exercise Management for Persons with Chronic Diseases and Disabilities. Human Kinetics, Champaign, IL, 1997, p 37.
129. Harvard Heart Letter: Hazards for patients with cardiac pacemakers and defibrillators. Harvard Heart Lett 19:6, 1999.
130. Mitrani, RD, et al: Cardiac pacemakers. In Fuster, V, Alexander, RW, and O'Rourke, RA (eds): Hurst's The Heart, ed 10. McGraw-Hill, New York, 2001, p 963.
131. Burg, MM, et al: Presurgical depression predicts medical morbidity 6 months after coronary artery bypass graft surgery. Psychosom Med 65(1):111, 2003.
132. Burg, MM, et al: Depressive symptoms and mortality two years after coronary artery bypass graft surgery (CABG) in men. Psychosom Med 65(4):508, 2003.
133. Blumenthal, JA, et al: Depression as a risk factor for mortality after coronary artery bypass surgery. Lancet 362(9384):604, 2003.
134. Ai, AL, et al: Psychological recovery from coronary artery bypass graft surgery: The use of complementary therapies. J Altern Complement Med 3(4):343, 1997.
135. McKhann, GM, et al: Depression and cognitive decline after coronary artery bypass grafting. Lancet 349(9061):1282, 1997.
136. Pirraglia, PA, et al: Depressive symptomatology in coronary artery bypass graft surgery patients. Int J Geriatr Psychiatry 14(8):668, 1999.
137. Lindquist, R, et al: Comparison of health-related quality-of-life outcomes of men and women after coronary artery bypass surgery through 1 year: Findings from the POST CABG Biobehavioral Study. Am Heart J 146(6):935, 2003.
138. Westin, L, et al: Differences in quality of life in men and women with ischemic heart disease: A prospective controlled study. Scand Cardiovasc J 33(3):160, 1999.
139. Phillips, BB, et al: Female gender is associated with impaired quality of life 1 year after coronary artery bypass surgery. Psychosom Med 65(6):944, 2003.
140. US Department of Health and Human Services: Clinical Practice Guideline, Number 11, Heart Failure: Management of Patients with Left Ventricular Systolic Dysfunction. AHCPR Publication No. 94-0613, 1994.
141. National High Blood Pressure Education Program: The Seventh Report of The Joint National Committee on Detection, Evaluation, and Treatment of High Blood Pressure, NHLBI Obesity Education Initiative. US Government Printing Office, Washington, DC, 2003.
142. Miller, T, et al: Exercise and its role in the prevention and rehabilitation of cardiovascular disease. Ann Behav Med 19:220, 1997.
143. Pina, IL, et al: Exercise and heart failure: A statement from the American Heart Association on exercise, rehabilitation, and prevention. Circulation 107(8):1210, 2003.

Supplemental Readings

American College of Sports Medicine: ACSM's Exercise Management for Persons with Chronic Diseases and Disabilities. Human Kinetics, Champaign, IL, 1997.

American College of Sports Medicine: ACSM's Guidelines for Exercise Testing and Prescription, ed 6. Lippincott, Williams & Wilkins, Baltimore, 2000.

Astrand, PO, et al: Textbook of Work Physiology, Physiological Bases of Exercise, ed 4. Human Kinetics, Champaign, IL, 2003.

Braunwald, E, et al (eds): Braunwald's Heart Disease: A Textbook of Cardiovascular Medicine, ed 6. WB Saunders, Philadelphia, 2001.

Braunwald, E, and Goldman, L: Primary Cardiology, ed 2. WB Saunders, Philadelphia, 2003.

DeTurk, WE, and Cahalin, LP: Cardiovascular and Pulmonary Physical Therapy: An Evidence-Based Approach. McGraw-Hill, New York, 2004.

Hillegass, EA, and Sadowsky, HS: Essentials of Cardiopulmonary Physical Therapy. WB Saunders, Philadelphia, 2001.

CHAPTER

17

LEARNING OBJECTIVES

1. Understand the anatomy, physiology, and pathophysiology of the vascular, lymphatic, and integumentary systems.
2. Describe wound physiology as it relates to normal and abnormal wound healing.
3. Recognize the characteristics and risk factors of common disorders of the vascular, lymphatic, and integumentary systems.
4. Identify the components of a comprehensive examination of a patient with a disorder related to the vascular, lymphatic, and/or integumentary systems.
5. Analyze and integrate wound examination data to complete the physical therapy evaluation.
6. Describe the rationale for skin and wound care treatment with particular attention to moist wound healing, arterial wound hydration, venous wound compression, lymphedema treatment, pressure ulcer prevention, and foot care for the patient with diabetes.
7. Design an appropriate plan of care for an individual with a vascular, lymphatic, and/or integumentary disorder.
8. Collaborate with other disciplines to determine a realistic and comprehensive plan of care.

Vascular, Lymphatic, and Integumentary Disorders

Deborah Graffis Kelly, PT, MSEd

OUTLINE

Patients and clients with disorders of the vascular, lymphatic, and integumentary systems have complex needs. Interest in the function of these essential systems has grown as options for improved intervention have expanded significantly. This chapter provides foundational material on which to build sound clinical decisions. While interrelated, the systems discussed have unique characteristics and functions. This chapter facilitates understanding of the separate systems and then illustrates how the systems are intricately and essentially related. Chapter 27 in this text covers burn wounds and is complementary and supplemental to the information in this chapter.

Anatomy and Physiology of the Vascular, Lymphatic, and Integumentary Systems

In the microscopic world of circulation, blood and lymph vessels permeate most tissues, carrying oxygen and nutrients while removing carbon dioxide and wastes. Not all vessels involved are the "large tubes" so often associated with the circulatory system. Capillaries are woven throughout most of the tissues of the body, around muscle fibers, through connective tissues, and below the basement membrane of the epithelium.[1] Arteries and veins are too large and too thick to allow diffusion between the bloodstream and surrounding tissues. Thus, a delicate network of blood and lymph capillaries controls all chemical and gaseous exchange between blood, interstitial fluid, and lymph.[1] In the normal system, homeostatic mechanisms adjust blood flow across the capillary walls to meet the needs of peripheral tissues. Every year, new information is uncovered that further elucidates the complexities of the circulatory system and how it interacts with the other systems of the body. It is important to have a clear understanding of the delicate vessels that carry blood to the peripheral tissues and the normal processes that occur there to gain insight into the disorders discussed later in the chapter.

Vascular

Arterial

Arteries carry rich, oxygenated blood away from the heart, branching off into sections with smaller diameters called **arterioles**, leading ultimately to capillaries. Arteries have three-layered walls that give them strength and elasticity. The walls of arteries are generally thicker than those of veins because they have to bear strong blood flow pressures generated by the heart. Arteries are strong and durable, able to keep their cylindrical shape when stretched. The movement of blood through arteries is dependent on heart function. Arteries have the ability to change in diameter when the volume of blood passing through them changes. They can also change in diameter when the sympathetic division of the autonomic nervous system (ANS) is triggered, either contracting (*vasoconstriction*), or relaxing (*vasodilation*). Because they have contractile abilities, arteries do not need valves to effect blood flow. These terms will be important when the chapter discussion turns to peripheral vascular disease and capillary blood flow.

Venous

Veins return oxygen depleted blood from tissues and organs to the heart. At the beginning of the venous system, superficial blood capillaries empty into *venules* that carry blood toward medium-sized veins (about the size of muscular arteries). Superficial veins run above the fascia of the muscles. Deep veins run below the fascia. Perforating veins run between the superficial and the deep, penetrating the fascia to connect the superficial and deep vessels. Veins also have three-layered walls but they do not need to be as muscular or elastic as arteries because the blood pressure in veins is lower than in arteries. Venous walls are so thin that they do not hold their shape well under stress, collapsing or tearing when stretched. As blood moves through the outermost regions of the body (the peripheral vascular system) from the arteries to the veins, blood pressures decrease. The blood pressure in the medium-sized veins is so low that it cannot oppose the force of gravity without structural assistance.[1] In the limbs, medium-sized veins contain *valves* that project from the inner walls of the veins, pointing in the direction of blood flow. Under normal conditions, the valves allow blood to flow in one direction, preventing backflow of blood. When the valves are working normally, any movement that compresses or pulls on a vein will push blood toward the heart. Skeletal muscle contraction will squeeze blood toward the heart. When the walls of veins weaken, or are enlarged, the valves cannot function properly and blood pools in the veins. Eventually the veins become distended, leading to *varicose veins*. If a valve or valves do not close properly, this leads to a condition known as *venous reflux*.

Lymphatic

Although parallel, and working in concert with the venous system, the lymphatic system is separate and unique. Because of its many roles and diffuse locations throughout the body, anatomists place discussion of the lymphatic system with the immune system, the circulatory system, and the integumentary system. The two primary functions of the lymphatic system are to protect the body from infection and disease via the immune response and to facilitate movement of fluid back and forth between the bloodstream and the interstitial fluid, removing excess fluid, blood waste, and protein molecules in the process of fluid exchange. *Lymphatics* are located in all portions of the body except the central nervous system and cornea.[2] The lymphatic system includes lymph vessels (superficial, intermediate, and deep, also referred to as lymphatics); lymph fluid; and lymph tissues and organs (lymph nodes, tonsils, spleen, thymus, and the thoracic duct).

Lymph fluid is first absorbed at the capillary level, then channeled through small vessels called *precollectors,* and finally picked up by the larger, valved vessels called *collectors*. The collectors have contractile, smooth muscle, and valves. Lymphatics are even thinner and more likely to collapse under pressure than veins.[2–4] Lymph moves throughout the body by a number of mechanisms. Superficially, lymph fluid is moved by the process of diffusion and filtration. Below the dermis, intrinsic contractions drive lymph propulsion in the deeper collectors. The force to generate a lymph vessel contraction does not come from the heart but from *lymphangions,* small pump-like segments within the larger lymph vessels. The human body is wonderfully equipped to provide a variety of stimuli that have an impact on lymphangion contraction:[4–8]

- Parasympathetic, sympathetic, and sensory *nerve stimulation*
- *Contraction of muscles* adjacent to a vessel
- *Pulsation of arteries* adjacent to a lymph vessel (even precapillary arterioles have pulsation)
- Abdominal and thoracic cavity pressure changes that occur during *breathing*
- *Volume changes* within each lymphangion (internal receptors respond to tension and trigger a contraction)
- *Mild mechanical stimulation* of dermal tissue increases the frequency of lymphangion contractions

Excess lymph fluid is transported through the thoracic duct and emptied into the venous angles at the left and right jugular vein trunks. Under normal conditions, lymph flow is not adversely affected by gravity. Under abnormal conditions, the lymphatic system may exhibit excess lymph pooling related to gravity, especially in the lower extremities (LEs).

Integumentary

Also referred to as an organ, this system is the most often seen and touched by a physical therapist of all the body systems. The integumentary system has a functional relationship to many other body systems. The health of the integumentary system is dependent on the normal functions of the arterial, venous, and lymphatic capillaries (dermal circulation). A thorough review of the functions of the skin illustrates the importance of even a small area of damage to this organ. The discussion on skin anatomy, with diagrams, in Chapter 27 will supplement this overview. The *epidermis* is avascular and water-resistant. It provides protection from infection, abrasion, and chemicals and assists with heat regulation, retention, and dissipation. Melanocytes determine skin color and provide protection from ultraviolet radiation. The epidermis regenerates rapidly. The *dermis* is 20 to 30 times thicker than epidermis. It contains blood vessels and lymphatics; hair follicles; sweat glands, and sebaceous glands; nerves and nerve endings; and collagen, elastin, and ground substance that provide structure, strength, flexibility, and elasticity. The nails are located in dermis but project through the epidermis to the surface of the skin. The *hypodermis* (also referred to as the *subcutaneous* layer) is not part of the integument but is important in stabilizing skin over skeletal muscles and organs. It consists of loose connective tissue and fat cells and provides insulation and protection to underlying structures.

CLINICAL NOTE: Subcutaneous fat and fascia (firm and adherent) should not be confused with yellow slough (soft and stringy) in a deep wound.

As a result of injury, some or all of the components of the integument are impaired, resulting in sequelae such as edema, decreased lubrication, and loss of elasticity and tensile strength.

Wound Physiology

Normal Wound Healing

In the human body, an elegant sequence of events takes place to ensure that when injury occurs, wounds will heal. Within the endogenous fluids of the body, every cell and chemical mediator is programmed and ready to act when needed. When conditions are normal, the body is equipped to heal itself.

Phases of Healing

The classic model of overlapping phases of wound healing describes a process that is continuous, its phases not distinct. The model is used in this chapter to draw attention to the normal process and to provide guidelines for what can be expected in normal healing. The number of days to complete each phase will vary owing to factors such as age, size of wound, comorbidities, continued trauma, nutrition, blood flow, medications, stress, and infection. The process of repair is the same for all wounds but the sequence will be much quicker in more shallow wounds with less tissue loss. In all stages of healing, wounded tissues are striving to achieve homeostasis. Italicized words below stress important concepts.

- *Inflammation* (Phase I)
  - The *normal* immune system reaction to injury
  - *The* central activity in wound healing
  - Temporary repair initiated by coagulation (clotting factors, platelets) and *short term decreased* blood flow
  - *Necrosis* occurs after cells have been injured or destroyed.
  - The spread of pathogens is slowed: debris and bacteria are attacked by a host of cells. If the wound is acute, some periwound edema, erythema, and drainage can be expected.[9] If fluid accumulates at the injury site it is called *pus*.
  - Oxygen is delivered via *increased* blood flow to keep the phagocytic cells alive and functioning.
  - Permanent repair is facilitated by creating a clean wound, *setting the stage* for the next phase of healing; signals are generated that re-epithelialization can begin.
  - Time frame: day of injury to approximately day 10.
  - *Rate* of inflammatory process is affected by blood supply, available nutrients, and the extrinsic environment.
  - If this phase is interrupted or delayed, *chronic inflammation can result,* lasting from months to years (see Abnormal Wound Healing and the Chronic Wound)
- *Proliferation* (Phase II)
  - *New tissue* fills in the wound as fibroblasts secrete collagen.
  - Skin integrity is restored by re-epithelialization and/or contraction (see discussion below).
  - Angiogenesis occurs: new blood vessel growth from endothelial cells, fragile capillary buds grow into the wound bed; new reddish, slightly bumpy tissue is called granulation tissue.
  - Epithelial cells differentiate into type I collagen. *Collagen synthesis* occurs but the resulting new scar tissue is fragile and must be protected; trauma during this phase may return the wound to the inflammatory process.
  - Time frame: day 3 of injury to approximately day 20.
  - *Rate* of proliferation is affected by blood supply, available nutrients, and the extrinsic environment.
  - If this phase is interrupted or delayed, the result may be a chronic wound.
- *Maturation/remodeling* (Phase III)
  - Maturation begins while granulation tissue is forming during the prior (proliferative) phase.
  - Epithelial cells continue to differentiate into type I collagen.
  - New skin has *tensile strength* that is 15 percent of normal. Scar tissue is rebuilding but at best reaches 80 percent of original tensile strength.
  - Underlying granulation tissue is replaced by *less vascular* tissue.

- In deep wounds, dermal appendages are rarely repaired (hair follicles, sebaceous and sweat glands, nerves) but instead are replaced by *fibrous tissue*.
- Over time the scar tissue matures, changing from red to pink to white and from raised and rigid to flat and flexible.
- Time frame: approximately day 9 of injury up to 2 years.
- *Rate* is affected by blood supply, available nutrients, and the extrinsic environment.

The Role of Oxygen in Wound Healing

Oxygen reaches the wound bed through blood flow to the area. The need for oxygen to sustain life is apparent, not only at the systemic level, but also at the cellular level of human physiology. Most cells in the wound environment have an enzyme that converts oxygen to a form that allows the cell to support wound healing.[10] Wound contraction, collagen deposition, angiogenesis, and granulation are examples of wound healing steps supported by oxygen. Oxygen even has an antibiotic effect allowing tissues to resist pathogens.[11] Wound tissue oxygenation is a sensitive indicator for the risk of postoperative infection.[12,13] Wound perfusion may be limited for a variety of reasons. The presence of edema and necrotic tissue makes it more difficult for oxygen to reach the wound. Since compression can reduce edema and débridement can reduce the presence of necrotic tissue, these procedural interventions are important components of most wound care. Unless contraindicated owing to arterial disease, compression and débridement will decrease the obstruction to wound oxygenation. Peripheral vasoconstriction can also limit wound perfusion. Problems with vasoconstriction cannot always be improved readily. Interventions that will increase wound perfusion and are appropriate for all individuals include keeping the wound area warm, avoiding smoking, hydrating the individual, and controlling pain and anxiety. Several clinical studies have shown that keeping patients warm and giving them supplemental oxygen decreases the rate of infection and shortens hospital stay.[14,15] Improvement of oxygen levels in wound tissue alone may trigger wound healing. Adequate oxygen levels will also enhance the effectiveness of growth factors and a host of other cells that require oxygenation to maintain their function. The delivery of exogenous oxygen will be discussed later in the chapter under intervention. The nutritional status of the individual as discussed below, will also have an impact on oxygenation since hemoglobin, iron, vitamin B_{12}, and folic acid are needed to enable red blood cells to carry oxygen to healing tissues.

The Role of Moisture in Wound Healing

In the past, the goal of wound care was to create and maintain a dry wound, packed with dry dressings, dried by heat lamps, and exposed to the air. Modern wound management is based on the concept of creating and maintaining a moist wound environment to facilitate wound healing. More than 50 years ago, research confirmed that a dry wound creates an environment that is hostile to wound healing. A dry wound allows the formation of wound scab and eschar which inhibit migration of epithelial cells, provide food for pathogens, and affect blood flow to the wound bed.

A dry wound also allows cooling of the wound surface; without a protective barrier, the surface temperature of the wound is decreased and healing is slowed. Adhesion of gauze or other dry dressings to the wound bed causes trauma upon removal. Bacteria enter a dry wound more readily because of the lack of a protective barrier. As the wound dries, fluid loss occurs. The rich endogenous fluids that are lost contain the elements necessary for timely wound healing. Patient discomfort is increased.

Wound management experts agree that adequate wound hydration is the most important external factor responsible for optimal wound healing.[16–19] Wounds are typically covered with an occlusive or semiocclusive dressing. This type of dressing is also called a moisture retentive dressing because the dressing retains fluids on the wound bed. There are many types and styles of dressings that will facilitate a moist environment. See the section on Dressings for further discussion. Maintaining a moist wound with an occlusive dressing will hold endogenous fluids on the wound, preserving the cells needed for healing and keeping them in contact with the wound bed. It also softens wound scab and eschar; under the right conditions, the body's own enzymes will dissolve the eschar in a process called **autolytic débridement**. Occlusive dressings maintain appropriate wound surface temperature to prevent delays in healing, protect the wound surface from trauma and from bacteria and other contaminants. Wound cleansing is facilitated during autolytic débridement and further breakdown of skin in the periwound area is prevented.

Patient comfort is increased. Basic principles of moist wound healing include covering the wound with a barrier (occlusive dressing) that preserves adequate wound hydration; limiting fluid loss from the wound surface while the dressing is in place; allowing gaseous exchange; maintaining periwound integrity; controlling heavy exudates; and removing the dressing when exudate begins to leak out from edges of dressing.

It has long been believed that occlusive dressings should not be applied over infected wounds because trapped bacteria could fulminate. Studies are now producing evidence that the opposite may be true.[20–24] Since endogenous fluids have bacteria fighting chemical elements, evidence of colonized bacteria in the wound does not automatically preclude the use of occlusive dressings. Specially selected dressings such as hydrocolloids are a good choice in this situation. With the use of a systemic antibiotic and a close watch for signs of change in the patient's symptoms, clinicians may be able to utilize occlusive or moisture-retentive dressings over many types of wounds that are infected.[25] The use of this dressing technique may broaden if the evidence continues to build in strength.

Despite half a century of research to support the concepts of moist wound healing, there are still practitioners who ignore the evidence and utilize outdated methods of wound management. Clinicians must strive to educate patients, families, and all members of the wound care team about appropriate wound care concepts.

The Role of Nutrition in Wound Healing

It is well established that nutritional status can have a significant impact on wound healing. Literature abounds with information about important nutritional issues such as the role of specific nutrients in wound healing, how poor nutritional status can delay wound healing, the use of special pharmacological interventions, and appropriate routes for nutritional support (enteral versus parenteral).[26–34]

In response to this information, nutrition and metabolic support of acutely and chronically ill patients is emerging as an important branch of medicine. Nutrients that must be present for a wound to heal include iron, vitamin B_{12} and folic acid (essential so that red blood cells can deliver oxygen to tissues), vitamin C and zinc (essential for tissue repair), vitamin A (essential to stimulate collagen cross-linking), and arginine (enhances healing and immune function).[35,36] High protein intake provides the amino acids required to build new tissue. Protein and calorie needs will vary depending on the size of the wound and the medical condition of the patient.

As a part of the wound care team, a physical therapist will make contributions to the plans for nutritional support of the patient. Clinicians will collect data through chart review, observation, history taking, and the use of dietary examination methods.[37]

Wound Characteristics

The characteristics of wounds may be defined as dry, wet, or granulating. Wounds can also be defined by their etiology such as diabetic, vascular, or traumatic. Wound characteristics describe the physical appearance of the wound but often provide the clues to the etiology, phase of healing, and likelihood of closure. Wound characteristics can provide valuable information needed to make sound clinical judgments about treatment. For example, the location of the wound may prompt the clinician to select a particular dressing, change patient positioning, or prescribe orthotic footwear. When wound characteristics are described in documentation, they can indicate progress (or failure to progress) toward closure and healing. Wound characteristics should be identified during the initial examination and then monitored at least weekly during the wound healing phase. Depending on the etiology and chronicity of the wound, some characteristics may not be evident upon initial examination but could appear at a later date as complications of the wound healing process. The following are characteristics that should be tracked and documented throughout the phases of wound healing:

- *Location*: where on the body
- *Size*: depth, width, and length
- *Shape*: irregular versus distinct
- *Edges*: condition and shape of wound edges, evidence of premature healing
- *Tunneling, undermining, sinus tracts*: presence and depth
- *Base*: characteristics of the wound base compared to sides and edges
    - Necrosis, eschar, slough: amount, color, texture, adherence to wound bed
    - Exudate: amount, color, odor
    - Granulation tissue: presence or absence, amount, location
    - Epithelialization: presence or absence, premature or on schedule
    - Exposed structures: color and condition of bone, tendon, ligament
- *Periwound area*: edema, induration, maceration
- *Pain*: although not a visible characteristic, it is measurable and significant to the intervention
- *Quantity of bacteria*: amount present in a wound. This is referred to as the *bio-burden.*

The quantitative biopsy is the gold standard for obtaining a wound culture but it is not used universally owing to cost, lack of lab facilities, and potential pain for the patient.[10] A swab culture is often used as an alternative but it is limited to detecting surface contamination, not tissue infection. Some literature supports swab culture, when used appropriately, as an adjunct in the management of chronic wounds.[38] Clinical intuition is also important in determining if infection is probable.

The examination will include data about the characteristics that have been gathered using methods such as observation, palpation, measurement, photography, and tracing. A clinician who is new to the wound care team should remember that these are skills that take practice.

Wound Closure

Primary Intention

Healing by primary intention occurs when a surgeon closes a wound by bringing the edges together. Approximating the edges can occur through the use of sutures, staples, glue, skin grafts, or skin flaps. (See skin grafting in Chapter 27.) Wounds closed by primary intention still pass through the phases of wound healing but on a smaller scale. A wound closed by primary intention that later opens up again owing to maceration or infection has opened by the process of *dehiscence* (Fig. 17.1). Following

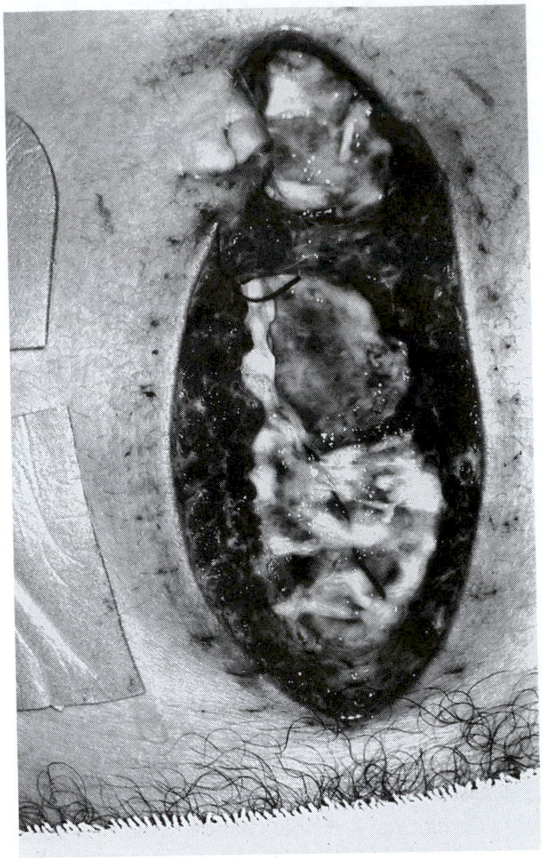

Figure 17.1 Wound dehiscence following appendectomy.

dehiscence, a wound is almost always allowed to close by secondary intention.

Secondary Intention

Healing by secondary intention occurs when a wound is left to heal on its own. Wound healing by secondary intention will close by contraction, re-epithelialization, or a combination of both. Deeper wounds heal by replacing injured tissue with scar tissue as collagen fills the wound bed.

During the process of contraction, existing tissue migrates, pulling the wound edges toward the center of the wound. No new tissue is formed by this process. New tissue may be forming in the wound simultaneously but not via contraction. Growth factors trigger myofibroblasts to pull the wound edges inward. Myofibroblasts can be influenced positively or negatively by physiological factors such as the amount of oxygen and nutrients available, and by mechanical factors such as external compression and the shape of the wound. Even though contraction is a normal occurrence in certain types of wound healing, if it is too rapid, it can cause disfiguring scars and impaired tissue function. Since there is centripetal movement of the entire thickness of the surrounding skin, tissue elongation may not keep up with the pace of contraction, causing significant functional and cosmetic deformity. Clinicians often intervene by applying special types of pressure to the tissues to slow the deforming forces of contraction. (See the section on scar management under Intervention.)

As noted in the phases of normal wound healing, chemical mediators send signals for reepithelialization to begin in Phase I or the inflammatory phase. Actual repair begins in Phase II when tissue is formed to cover the wound. Growth factors stimulate specialized epithelial cells, *keratinocytes,* to begin to migrate from the edges of the wound toward the center. In partial-thickness wounds in which the dermal appendages have not been destroyed, the cells will also migrate from the hair follicles, sebaceous glands, and sweat glands. In smaller, more shallow wounds this process may be triggered to begin as early as 12 hours after wounding. In larger wounds, it may be 10 days or longer before the cells begin to migrate. In a chronic wound there are many reasons why this process is not triggered or is interrupted. (See discussion under Abnormal Wound Healing and the Chronic Wound.) Re-epithelialization stops by *contact inhibition.*

When epithelial cells meet at the center of the wound, migration ends and cells will stop dividing. This is referred to as *contact inhibition.* At the time of contact inhibition and/or full re-epithelialization, wound *closure* has occurred. Wound *healing,* however, may continue for several years. A significant amount of treatment intervention is still required to support the wound successfully from "closed" to "healed" status.

Factors affecting closure by secondary intention include:

- *Wound shape*: linear wounds (surgical) contract most rapidly, circular wounds (pressure ulcers) contract most slowly.[39]
- *Wound depth*: all things equal, the more shallow the wound, the quicker the closure.[40–42]
  - *Superficial* (loss of the epidermis): closes by re-epithelialization.
  - *Partial-thickness* (loss of the epidermis and dermis): closes primarily by re-epithelialization with minimal contraction.
  - *Full-thickness* (loss of all layers of the epidermis, dermis, and deeper structures): closes by contraction and scar formation; however, epithelial cells will migrate from the wound edges to assist in wound closure if the environment is homeostatic.
- *Wound location*: areas with least pressure, most perfusion (face) will close more rapidly than areas with most pressure, least perfusion (sacrum, heel).
- *Wound etiology*: least traumatic (surgery) will close more rapidly than most traumatic (pressure ulcer, burn).

As deeper wounds heal, the wound is filled but the repair process does not replace lost muscle, fat or dermis with those same types of tissue. The wound is filled with granulation or scar tissue made up primarily of collagen. Because the original tissue is not replaced with more of the same, a wound that is closed, and finally healed, does not return to its prewounded state. This concept becomes particularly important when understanding the position on reverse staging of pressure ulcers as described in the section on Tests and Measurements. It is also important to understand this concept when planning protection, positioning, patient education, foot wear, and exercise programs for individuals with all types of wounds whether they are acute, closed, healed, or chronic wounds.

Tertiary Intention

Also called *delayed primary*, this occurs when a wound is allowed to heal by secondary intention and then is closed by primary intention as the final treatment. The delay in primary closure is usually owing to the presence of infection, or waiting for granulation tissue to form.

Abnormal Wound Healing and the Chronic Wound

When the sequence of events that leads to normal wound healing does not occur, a chronic wound results. The characteristics and causes of chronic wounds vary owing to the diverse nature of the individuals with wounds, their medical histories, and the etiology of the wound. Even if the chronic wound moves through the classic phases of wound healing, it does so in an abnormal manner. Vital actions and reactions necessary for wound healing are interrupted, stunted, or absent in the chronic wound.

While the characteristics of abnormal wound healing may be varied, concepts can be used to illustrate the failure of a wound to pass through phases of wound healing in a timely manner. The following discussion focuses on the results of interruption to the classic phases of wound healing:

- Inflammation: if there is inadequate blood flow and oxygen supply to support cellular life and activity, cells may not initiate the repair sequence. Debris and bacteria build up, pathogens spread more rapidly. Bio-burden is measured as greater than 10^5 organisms/g of tissue, the classic definition of infection.
  - Clinical signs: increase in amount of drainage, change in color or odor, lingering swelling, eschar/necrosis from the ischemic conditions, periwound maceration, chronic inflammation, tunneling, undermining, and infection may develop if the host's immune system is unable to resist the impact of the bacterial load.
- Proliferation: if collagen synthesis is delayed, skin integrity will be poor. If angiogenesis is delayed, myofibroblasts will be too few to initiate wound contraction. The need for oxygen and nutrients will be very high and without them, available cells will be unable to reproduce rapidly, resulting in delayed epithelialization.
  - Clinical signs: keratinocytes do not migrate because the wound bed is not moist, healthy, clean, and granulating. Epithelial cells may attempt to migrate from the wound edges but without a wound bed that is ready, they will build up at the wound edge and may migrate over the edge, forming a lip that curls under. Granulation tissue is either absent, pale, or delayed; new tissue is weak and breaks down or bleeds easily; tunneling, eschar, and periwound maceration may be evident. Necrosis, if it has not been removed, will delay angiogenesis. Changes in drainage color, amount, odor, or lingering swelling, may signal a return to the inflammation stage.
- Remodeling: if the synthesis and lysis of collagen is out of balance, weakened tissue will break down too easily or hypertrophic scarring will build up too rapidly.
  - Clinical signs: newly formed skin breaks down with little provocation, scar tissue builds up within the outline of the original wound (hypertrophic), or beyond the margins of the original wound (keloid).

Infection in Wound Healing

Wound infection is a significant problem for any individual. Bio-burden has a greater impact on wound healing than most underlying medical conditions.[9,43] Infection may turn life-threatening if the patient is elderly or critically ill. Regardless of the condition of the individual, wound infection is detrimental to wound closure and healing time.

- Effects of infection
  - Inefficient cellular activity, decreased collagen metabolism, chemical mediators absent or dilute, cells absent or confused by lack of instructions from chemical mediators and presence of other cells. When the bio-burden is greater than 10^5 organisms/g of tissue, epithelialization may not occur.[38]
  - Decreased oxygen in the wound bed, need to supply enough oxygen to support the regeneration of tissue and to assist in the prevention of infection
  - Increased rate of cell necrosis
  - Overall decline of body systems contributes to strain on the specialized cells
  - Risk of wound sepsis, osteomyelitis, gangrene
- Signs of potential infection
  - Change in wound drainage: amount, color, odor
  - Swelling
  - Periwound redness or warmth (less obvious with darker skin)
  - Increase in pain or tenderness
  - Change in the quality of granulation tissue or failure to produce good quality tissue (may be pale, soft, easily broken down)
  - No measurable wound contraction within 2 to 4 weeks
  - Tissue culture/punch biopsy results of greater than 10^5 organisms/g of tissue
  - Fever, nausea, fatigue, loss of appetite

Clinicians should use a structured approach to identify clinical infection. Careful identification of infection may help to avoid the risk of overuse of antibiotics.[44]

Factors Contributing to Abnormal Wound Healing

The factors or triggers that may contribute to abnormal wound healing are varied but can be placed into broad categories for better understanding. Most abnormal wound healing will be influenced by factors from all the categories. Treatment intervention that addresses factors from one category and not others will be incomplete.

Intrinsic Factors

Intrinsic or internal factors are conditions within the body that may contribute to abnormal healing. These factors relate primarily to the wound and periwound areas, and include hypoxemia owing to inadequate blood flow and oxygen supply and aging skin. Decreased moisture content, brittle quality, delayed renewal time affects the stratum corneum. *Rete pegs,* undulations between contact layers of the epidermis and dermis, become less functional with increased risk of sheering.

Changes in the dermis include a decrease in elasticity, collagen, and mast cell production, along with a decrease in the vascularity and number of pain receptors. Available fat in the subcutaneous layer begins to resorb after age 70, leading to a decrease in protection against pressure and sheering. Finally, underlying disease will impact acute and chronic wound healing. The more common conditions known to impact healing are diabetes, cancer, circulatory insufficiencies, human immunodeficiency virus infection, and connective tissue diseases.

Extrinsic Factors

Extrinsic or environmental factors are those influences that come from outside the body. The medical professionals caring for the person with a wound may be able to moderate the impact of extrinsic factors on the wound environment. These include the effects of radiation therapy or chemotherapy; incontinence; medication, smoking, recreational drugs, and alcohol (all slow or eliminate cellular reactions needed for healing); dehydration and malnutrition (both slow the delivery of oxygen to wound tissues); bio-burden/infection (healing is slowed by pathogens, necrotic tissue, granulomas); and stress (negative effects of stress can lead to impaired healing).[41,45–50]

Iatrogenic Factors

Iatrogenic refers to any injury or illness that occurs as the result of medical care. Theoretically, these items are under the control of the medical professionals who care for the patient and are therefore, preventable. Poor wound management occurs with frequent disruption of wound through inappropriate cleansing, use of inappropriate dressings and dressing techniques, cytotoxic topical agents that lead to inefficient cellular activity, and lack of moisture resulting in delayed or absent migration of keratinocytes. Infection is caused by cross-contamination, improper use of gloves and other protective devices, inadequate use of sterile and clean technique, lack of proper handwashing, lack of adherence to universal precautions, and inadequate clean or sterile technique.

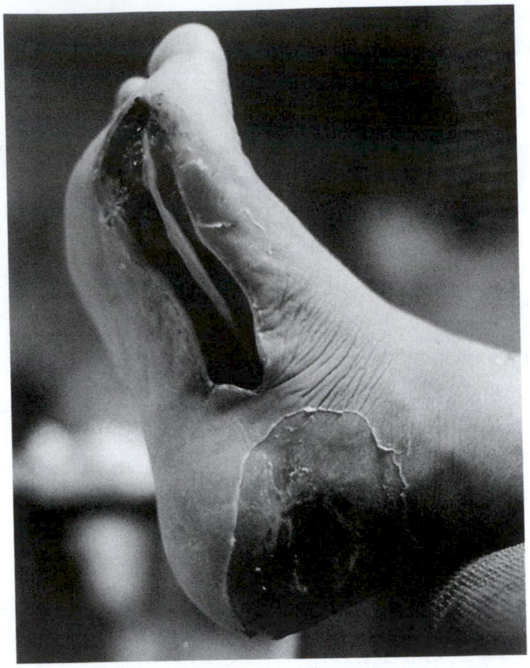

Figure 17.2 Chronic wound.

Sheer injuries (skin tears) can occur during transfers and repositioning. Ischemia results from unrelieved pressure owing to inadequate turning schedules or absent or inadequate *pressure relieving devices (PRDs).* In general, the larger the wound and more traumatic the cause, the more likely a delay in healing time.

Complications of Chronicity

A chronic wound creates a complex and serious health problem for an individual (Fig. 17.2). Chronic wounds may lead to complications including any or all of the following: impairments of body function and structures, restrictions in activities and participation, need for assisted living or home care, decreased quality of life perceptions, depression, infection, malnutrition and weight loss, protein depletion, tissue fibrosis, loss of limb, and death. Every year over 5 million Americans are treated for chronic wounds at a cost of billions of dollars, making this type of wound one of the most costly challenges in health care.[51] A chronic wound fails to heal because of an underlying pathology and will not heal until the cause is corrected or improved. The clinician must determine the factors contributing to abnormal wound healing and then develop an appropriate plan of care (POC) to overcome or address the obstacles.

Vascular, Lymphatic, and Integumentary Disorders

Arterial Insufficiency and Ulceration

Arterial insufficiency refers to a lack of adequate blood flow to a region or regions of the body. Many different disorders may arise from arterial insufficiency and can be classified by a variety of descriptors. For the purposes of this chapter, references will be to arterial insufficiency owing to organic disruption of blood flow to the extremities or to **peripheral vascular disease (PVD)**. PVD is a general term used to describe any disorder that interferes with arterial or venous blood flow of the extremities. Factors that lead to PVD owing to arterial insufficiency include smoking, cardiac disease, diabetes, hypertension, renal disease, and elevated cholesterol and triglycerides. Obesity and a sedentary lifestyle are related contributors in the cycle of disease and vessel obstruction. The damage caused by these factors is reflected in structural changes in the walls of the arteries, causing abnormal blood flow. The following is a brief overview of these disorders:

- Arteriosclerosis: thickening, hardening, loss of elasticity of arterial walls
- **Atherosclerosis:** the most common form of arteriosclerosis, associated with damage to the endothelial lining of the vessels and the formation of lipid deposits, eventually leading to plaque formation.
- **Arteriosclerosis obliterans:** a peripheral manifestation of atherosclerosis characterized by intermittent claudication, rest pain, trophic changes. This is the arterial disease most likely to lead to ulceration.[52] Known risk factors for development of the disease are smoking, diabetes mellitus, hypertension, hyperlipidemia, and hyperhomocysteinemia.
- Thromboangiitis obliterans (Buerger's disease): inflammation leads to arterial occlusion and tissue ischemia, especially in young men who smoke.
- **Raynaud's disease:** a functional vasomotor disease of small arteries and arterioles, not likely to cause ischemic necrosis
- Ulceration: a peripheral sign of a long-standing disease process; by definition, arterial ulcers are associated with arterial insufficiency.

Between 10 and 25 percent of LE ulcers are caused by arterial disease.[53] The incidence of arterial disease and LE ulceration is significantly lower than that for venous disease and ulceration; however, arterial wounds more frequently lead to loss of limb and death.

Clinical Presentation

- Most frequently located on the LEs: lateral malleoli, dorsum of feet, toes.
- When wounds are present on an ischemic limb, atherosclerotic occlusion of the peripheral vasculature is almost always present.
- The majority of patients with arterial insufficiency also have diabetes.
- Trophic changes are present and include abnormal nail growth, decreased leg and foot hair, dry skin.
- Skin is cool upon palpation.
- Wounds are painful and patient may also describe pain in the legs and/or feet (see discussion below about intermittent claudication).
- Wound base is necrotic and pale, lacking **granulation tissue**.
- Skin around the wound may be black, *gangrenous*, mummified (dry gangrene).
- Other signs of arterial insufficiency will be evident: decreased pulses, **pallor** on elevation, and *rubor* when dependent.

History

Painful cramping or aching of the LEs during walking is the most common complaint in patients with chronic arterial occlusion of the LEs. The pain is caused by *intermittent claudication* that occurs when exercising muscles are not receiving the blood perfusion needed for normal function. Patients should be examined for other signs of arterial insufficiency if intermittent claudication is occurring. Rest pain that develops at night, awakens the patient, or requires analgesics for relief is considered more severe than claudication. The individual with vascular dysfunction may also be diabetic. Diabetes will contribute to slower healing times and difficulty fighting infection. A wound in a distal, ischemic area is not likely to heal unless the vascular supply is enhanced or restored. Individuals with arterial disease and diabetes are more likely to have hypertension, may have previous bypass grafts or amputations of the toes, pain on ambulation or rest, pain with elevation, cold hands and feet, and color changes of fingers and toes. Owing to the long latency period between injury to the arterial circulation and clinical appearance of disorders, healthcare providers, families, caregivers, and patients must join forces with education, prevention, and vigilance.

Tests and Measurements

One of the most important tests to perform or have performed for individuals with arterial disease is the **Ankle-Brachial Index (ABI)**. The ABI is a test designed to examine the vascular system. Results provide useful information about the potential loss of perfusion in the LE. Refer to Arterial Perfusion in the section on Tests and Measurements under Patient Management.

Intervention

If an ulceration is present, treatment should enhance chemical and gaseous homeostasis in the wound bed, facilitate superficial blood flow to target tissues, and educate patients about the importance of facilitating blood

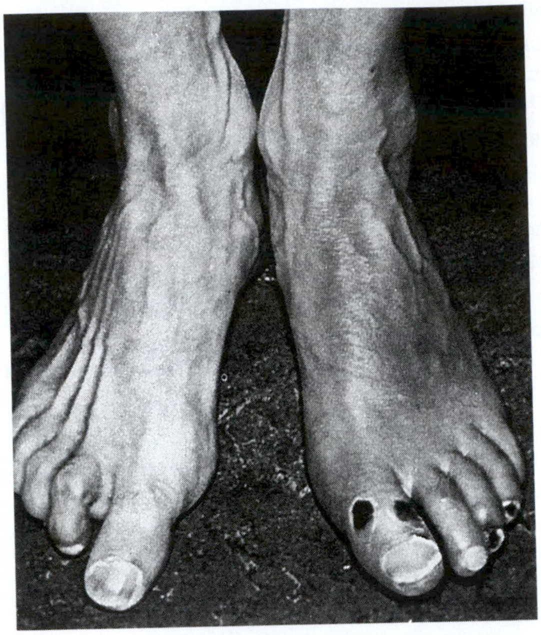

Figure 17.3 Clinical presentation of arterial insufficiency.

flow to the extremities. Treatment will include appropriate wound care as well as important adjuncts to wound care (see Intervention under Patient Management). Results of the ABI will guide the therapist and referring practitioner in the appropriate use of compression. In a diagnosis of mixed arterial and venous disease the condition that is more severe should be treated first. If the arterial condition is worse, compression may be inappropriate even when edema is present. A nonhealing wound on an ischemic limb can lead to gangrene, amputation, further amputation and/or loss of life (Fig. 17.3). In the most severe cases, conditions are inhospitable to wound closure. Necrotic tissue should not be débrided, since the tissue will not be replaced. Skin grafts do not adhere to the virtually lifeless wound bed. Antibiotics cannot reach the wound systemically and topical agents are too superficial to stop infection. At this point, vascular surgery may be an option for some individuals. A bypass graft is used to restore arterial circulation to the ischemic tissue. For others, living with a chronic nonhealing wound or coming to terms with amputation are the only options. Most experts agree that the single most important intervention in peripheral vascular disease is prevention of smoking. The second most important intervention is exercise for weight control, improvement of collateral circulation and lipid profiles, and management of hypertension. A physical therapist plays a crucial role in wound care for arterial wounds and should address patient education and exercise in the intervention plan.

Venous Insufficiency and Ulceration

Venous insufficiency refers to inadequate drainage of venous blood from a body part, usually resulting in edema

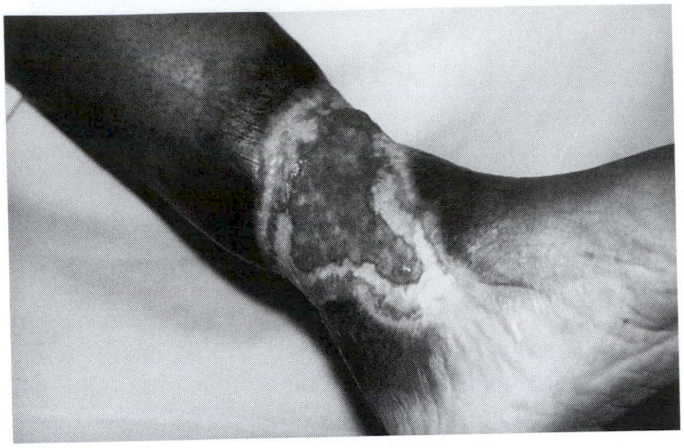

Figure 17.4 Venous insufficiency with leg ulcer.

and/or skin abnormalities and ulcerations. **Chronic venous insufficiency** (CVI) refers to venous insufficiency that persists over a long period of time. The majority of individuals with peripheral vascular disease are diagnosed with CVI. CVI is the most common cause of leg ulcers.[54] In current literature, venous insufficiency is synonymous with venous hypertension, defining the beginning of a chain of pathophysiological events that often end in ulceration. Some authors still use the term *venous stasis ulcer* although it has been shown that blood stasis (blood pooling) is not the cause of these wounds.[55] While it is clear that ulcerations are the result of inadequate venous circulation, the mechanism by which this happens is not clear. Attention is currently focused on the contribution to skin breakdown made by dysfunction of circulating white blood cells (WBCs), endothelial cell dysfunction, fibrin deposition, edema, and lymphatic congestion.[56,57]

The incidence of venous ulceration is much higher than that of arterial ulceration (Fig. 17.4). In fact, 80 percent of all leg ulcers are caused by venous disease[53] The higher incidence is not clearly understood even though years of clinical and laboratory research have been devoted to understanding venous disease. The path from CVI to ulceration can take many turns. Aging, lack of exercise, obesity, pregnancy, long hours of standing or sitting, and heredity will predispose an individual to venous hypertension and subsequent CVI. Predictors for ulceration include the factors just listed as well as: history of deep vein thrombosis (DVT), number of pregnancies for women, family history of ulceration, and history of vigorous activity in the presence of other risk factors.[58]

Clinical Presentation

- Swelling of unilateral or bilateral LEs relieved in the early stages by elevation
- Complaints of itching, fatigue, aching, heaviness in involved limb(s)
- Skin changes including **hemosiderin staining** and lipodermatosclerosis

- *Fibrosis* of the dermis
- Increase in skin temperature of lower legs
- Wounds
  - Most frequently located on the LEs: proximal to medial malleolus although can occur anywhere (arterial wounds may also occur at this location)
  - Not significantly painful; usually complaints of minor dull leg pain are relieved with elevation.
  - Granulation tissue is usually present in the wound bed.
  - Tissue is *wet* from a typically large amount of draining *exudate*.
- Signs and symptoms of lymphedema may be present (chronic inflammation and fluid overload can trigger the onset of lymphedema).

History

Because the incidence of CVI increases with age, clinicians should be suspicious of the disease in older patients. The slow development of venous disease and ulceration usually implies a history of lingering swelling, slow healing, repeated infection, and frequent recurrence of skin breakdown. Once ulceration occurs, venous wounds can exist for years. This progression of symptoms frequently leads to a mechanical overload of the lymphatic system and subsequent development of lymphedema. If the individual is older than age 50, it is likely there are comorbidities such as diabetes, hypertension, congestive heart failure, or history of DVT. Owing to the long latency period between injury to the venous circulation and clinical manifestations, health care providers, patients, families, and caregivers must join forces using the tools of education, prevention, and vigilance.

Tests and Measurements

One of the most important tasks during the examination process is to rule out an arterial component to the venous pathology. If there is arterial insufficiency, healing will be impaired and compression may be contraindicated.[53,59,60] Skin temperature of the lower leg may be elevated. This sign can imply a worsening or impending complication of CVI.[61] Existing edema may decrease with elevation unless it occurs in the advanced stages of disease or in combination with lymphedema. With venous disease, pitting edema may occur in the periwound area, the foot and ankle, or anywhere on the body. Advanced edema and lymphedema are generally unaffected by elevation and require compression as part of treatment. With the exception of mixed arterial and venous disease, the vascular exam results for venous insufficiency will show strong distal pulses and a normal ABI.

Intervention

The most important therapeutic measure for prevention and treatment of venous leg ulcers is *compression therapy*. Even though edema is a natural characteristic of the first phase of wound healing, excessive edema can delay wound healing by slowing perfusion of tissues and facilitating the growth of bacteria.[16] Along with compression and appropriate wound care, treatment will include exercise to increase mobility, and positioning to support and enhance venous blood flow.[54] Compression therapy is essential for timely healing if arterial disease has been ruled out. As mentioned earlier, in a diagnosis of mixed arterial and venous disease, the more severe pathology is treated first. Significant arterial disease will most likely preclude the use of compression. For the individual with a diagnosis of venous disease or mixed (mild) arterial/venous disease, a combination of therapeutic measures will accelerate results.[62] These include compression bandaging and garments, gait training, *manual lymphatic drainage (MLD)*, and exercise including range of motion (ROM). Wound care should avoid whirlpool use owing to the risks of dependent positioning, cross-contamination, cytotoxic additives, and unnecessary costs.

In some cases, surgical correction of venous abnormalities is indicated.

Lymphedema

Lymphedema is a chronic disorder characterized by an abnormal accumulation of lymph fluid in the tissues of one or more body regions.[2,63] The accumulation of fluid can be caused by a number of events but is most often owing to a mechanical insufficiency of the lymphatic system. Some lymphatic components are not functioning sufficiently to manage the lymph fluid present in the body region. Lymphedema can be classified as *primary* or *secondary* lymphedema. *Primary lymphedema* (Fig. 17.5) is caused by a condition that is congenital or hereditary. With primary lymphedema, lymph node or lymph vessel formation is abnormal. The most common abnormality is *hypoplasia,* a

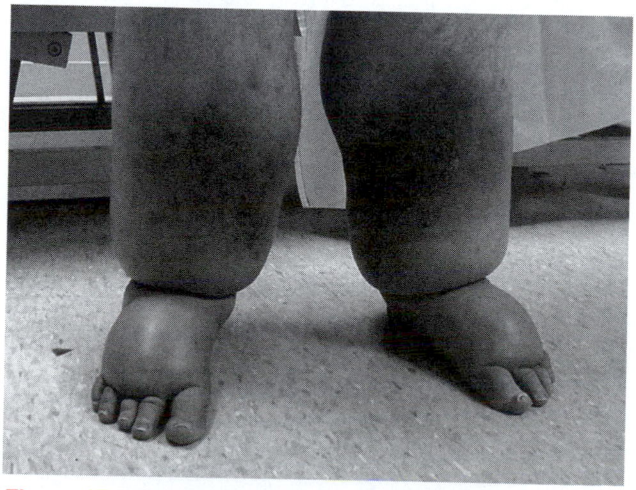

Figure 17.5 Primary lymphedema of bilateral LEs.

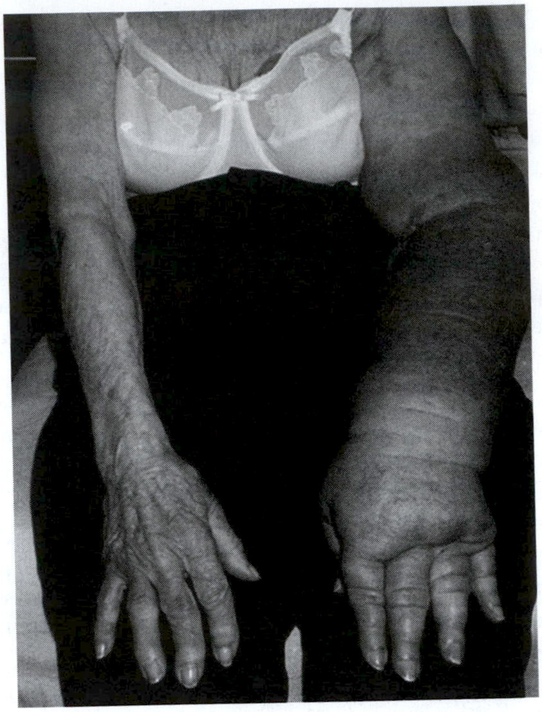

Figure 17.6 Secondary lymphedema of unilateral UE.

condition in which there are fewer lymphatic vessels and they are smaller than normal. One of the more common forms of primary lymphedema appears in *Milroy's disease*. *Secondary lymphedema* (Fig. 17.6) is caused by injury to one or more components of the lymphatic system: some portion of the lymphatic system has been blocked, dissected, fibrosed or otherwise damaged or altered.

Secondary lymphedema is more prevalent than primary. In developed countries, the most common cause of secondary lymphedema is surgery and/or radiation therapy as part of breast cancer treatment. The rise in incidence of other types of cancer and the subsequent treatments for those cancers has lead to an increase in reports of lymphedema following treatment for cancer of the prostate, bladder, uterus, ovaries, and skin. Cancer is not the only causative factor for lymphedema. It is common for an individual with CVI to develop lymphedema, triggered by longstanding fluid overload in the LEs. Secondary lymphedema can also be triggered by the complications of paralysis, disuse in chronic regional pain syndrome, or trauma to regional lymph nodes following liposuction, pelvic fracture, hernia repair, and other surgical interventions where lymph nodes or lymph vessels are located.[64–66] Collection of data on the incidence of noncancer–related secondary lymphedema is limited by the lack of specific education related to lymphedema among health care professionals and by a lack of clinical suspicion when examining individuals with a history of swelling. In the tropical and subtropical regions of the world, secondary lymphedema is most often caused by *filariasis*. In filariasis, nematode worm larvae live a full life cycle in the lymphatic vessels, causing inflammation and blocked lymphatic vessels.

Clinical Presentation

- Swelling distal to or adjacent to the area where lymph system function has been impaired
- Swelling usually not relieved by elevation
- Pitting edema in the early stages of disease, nonpitting edema in later stages, as fibrotic changes occur
- Feelings of fatigue, heaviness, pressure, or tightness in the affected region
- Numbness and tingling
- Discomfort varying from mild to intense
- Fibrotic changes of the dermis
- Dermal abnormalities such as *cysts, fistulas, lymphorrhea, papillomas, hyperkeratosis*
- Increased susceptibility to infection, at first local to the affected region but often becoming systemic
- Loss of mobility and ROM
- Impaired wound healing

History

A patient history consistent with lymphatic system damage or deformity will be pivotal in the diagnosis of lymphedema. A patient's history might include cancer, cancer treatment, radiation therapy, lymph node disruption, CVI, trauma, surgery, or (in primary lymphedema) onset of swelling at birth or puberty. There may be a long latency period between injury to the lymphatics and clinical manifestations; thus health care providers and patients must adhere to prevention guidelines and be suspicious of any signs and symptoms that might suggest lymphedema. Chronic inflammation of a body region may eventually lead to lymphedema. Lymphedema can develop within a few weeks of insult or as long as 30 years later.

Tests and Measurements

The diagnosis of lymphedema can be made without the use of special tests for most individuals. A patient history consistent with lymph system damage or deformity, a systems review, differential diagnosis, inspection, and palpation of the integument and girth measurements are adequate for accurate diagnosis in most cases. Unique findings might include *Stemmer's sign,* skin texture changes, skin folds, fibrosis, increase in girth, *papules,* lymph leakage, and *elephantiasis. Severity* is determined by a collection of data including presence of fibrotic tissue changes (brawny, woody, and/or lobular); number of episodes of cellulitis; condition of the superficial integument of the lymphedematous limb (papules, leakage, fungus, venous wounds); circumference or volume differences between involved and uninvolved limbs; and quality of life issues (sleep, mobility, activities of daily living [ADLs], relationships).

Intervention

A physical therapist should be cautious about the application of pressure to an edematous or lymphedematous body part. Although compression is an essential intervention, pressures that are too high will occlude superficial lymph capillaries and prevent the initial step of fluid absorption needed to control edema and lymphedema.[4]

Current intervention for the patient/client with lymphedema requires attention to detail and a level of expertise not often provided in entry-level professional educational programs. Practitioners are best served by gaining additional education to better prepare them to treat these patients. The current recommended course of care is a two-phase program of *Complete Decongestive Therapy (CDT)*. Phase I (intensive) includes skin care, MLD, lymphedema bandaging, exercise, and compression garment at the *end* of Phase I. Phase II (self-management) includes skin care, compression garment during the day, exercise, lymphedema bandaging at night, MLD as needed. Appendix A provides Web sites for training programs or other information on CDT, trained therapists, and patient education related to the treatment of lymphedema.

As with many progressive, chronic disorders, the effectiveness of treatment is significantly improved by early intervention. Accurate and early diagnosis occurs when health care professionals are sensitized to the signs and symptoms and carefully evaluate the examination data. In the POC, the number and frequency of treatments should not be determined by lymphedema staging or by circumferential differences between limbs (although the severity of the condition is not determined by these data alone). Some individuals with lymphedema may present with more involved signs and symptoms than the measurements imply.

Pressure Ulcers

A *pressure ulcer* is a wound caused by unrelieved pressure to the dermis and underlying vascular structures, usually between bone and support surfaces. When pressure is not relieved in time, the damage is of such magnitude that the tissues cannot repair and recover on their own. As deeper vessels are occluded, decreased blood flow leads to cell death, tissue necrosis, and finally a visible wound. The superficial dermis can tolerate *ischemia* for 2 to 8 hours before breakdown occurs. Deeper muscle, connective, and fat tissues tolerate pressures for 2 hours or less. Thus, there may be significant damage to underlying tissues while the epidermis and dermis remain intact. The clinical implications of this phenomenon are discussed below and in the section on Tests and Measurements. Readers can gain greater understanding about depth of damage to the integument by referring to Chapter 27 in this text to view cross-sections of skin, illustrating which components of the skin are lost at descending levels of damage.

Pressure ulcers occur most frequently among individuals who are immobilized for long periods of time. While pressure ulcers can occur at any age during prolonged periods of immobility, they are more likely to occur on individuals who are hospitalized, elderly, incontinent, and/or underweight and among individuals of all ages following spinal cord injury (SCI).[44,67–69] Up to 25 percent of hospital-acquired pressure ulcers may originate during surgery.[70] According to Reed et al, the presence of low albumin levels, confusion, and a *Do Not Resuscitate (DNR)* order are also pressure ulcer risk factors.[71] Pressure ulcers increase the risk of death for elderly individuals whether at home or in a hospital or long-term care setting.[72] The incidence of chronic wounds, including pressure ulcers, is increasing as the population ages.

Clinical Presentation

The severity of pressure ulceration can be estimated by observing clinical signs. A progression from least tissue damage to most severe damage is presented.

- The first clinical sign of pressure ulceration is *blanchable erythema* along with increased skin temperature. If pressure is relieved, tissues may recover in 24 hours. If pressure is unrelieved, nonblanchable erythema occurs.
- Progression to superficial abrasion, blister, or a shallow crater indicates involvement of the dermis.
- When full-thickness skin loss is apparent, the ulcer appears as a deep crater. Bleeding is minimal, and tissues are *indurated* and warm. **Eschar** formation marks the full-thickness skin loss. Tunneling or undermining is often present (see staging system described in Table 17.2).
- The majority of all pressure ulcers develop over six primary bony areas (Fig. 17.7): sacrum (Fig. 17.8), coccyx, greater trochanter, ischial tuberosity, calcaneus (heel), and lateral malleolus.

History

If an individual has a history of a period of immobility followed by the discovery of a warm, red, spot over a bony prominence, a pressure ulcer can usually be confirmed. If the spot is unnaturally soft to the touch, sometimes referred to as "boggy," this is enough evidence to suspect that damage is deeper than the epidermis.

Tests and Measurements

During examination, along with general wound characteristics, pressure ulcers are classified by grading or staging systems that describe the degree of tissue damage observed. It is important to also use an examination tool to measure an individual's risk of developing a pressure ulcer before a pressure ulcer exists. These measures can also be used to prevent recurrence after wound healing.

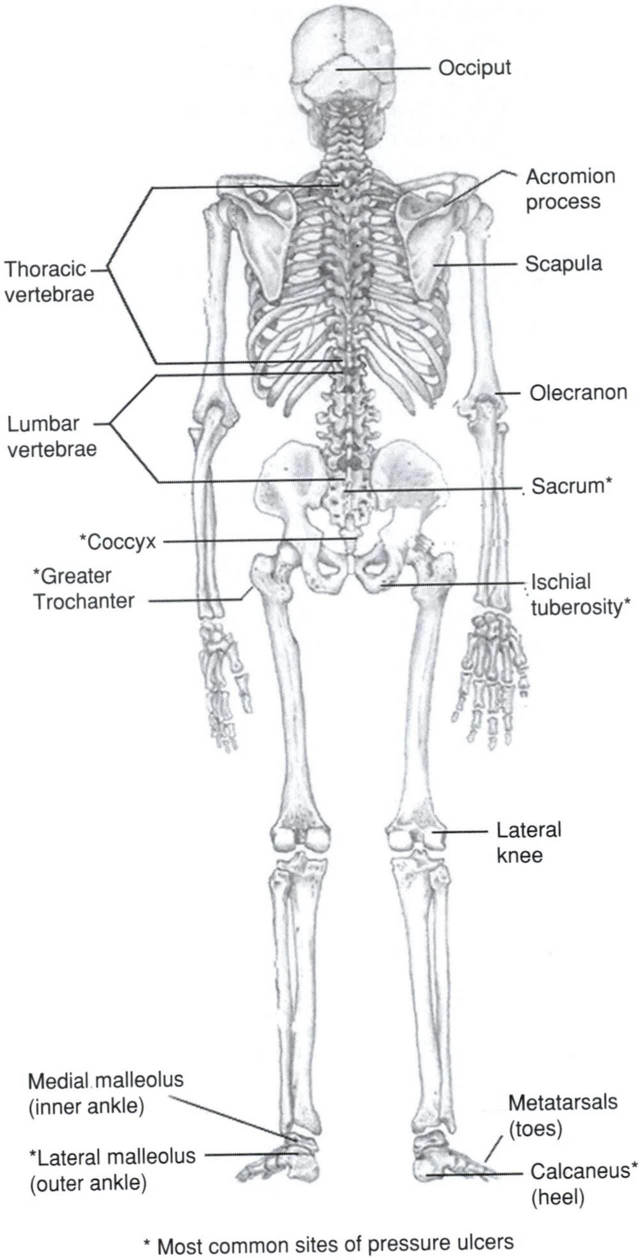

Figure 17.7 Pressure points of bony prominences.

Intervention

A physical therapist treats integumentary disorders that involve the epidermis, the dermis, hypodermis or below into exposed bone, tendon, muscle, and organs. For healing to occur, intervention for disorders of the integument must facilitate local and regional homeostasis of the vascular and lymphatic systems. In addition to appropriate wound care, it is imperative that the underlying cause of pressure be addressed. Wounds will not heal and remain closed unless the reduction of pressure and prevention of future breakdown are top priorities in the intervention plan. Pressure management is accomplished with the use of PRDs, *pressure mapping* to determine pressure loads,

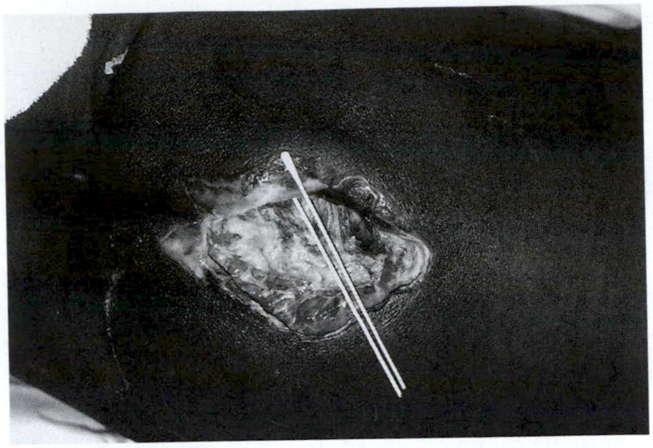

Figure 17.8 Sacral pressure ulcer. (From Kloth, LC, and McCulloch, JM,[137] Plate 31, with permission.)

positioning/turning schedules, and *education* of the patient, family and caregivers. Other factors that contribute to ulceration or risk of ulceration such as shear, friction, mobility, sensation, moisture, nutrition, age, and underlying medical condition should also be addressed. With appropriate wound care, control of pressure, and attention to risk factors, a wound should progress through the phases of wound healing, showing signs of improvement in a matter of weeks. Partial-thickness wounds typically take 1 to 2 weeks, while clean full-thickness wounds can take 2 to 4 weeks.[40,73–76]

Neuropathy

Neuropathy can be defined as any disease of nerves and can include peripheral nerves, cranial nerves, and/or autonomic nerves. Neuropathy exists in many disease processes; however, the most common disease process seen with neuropathy is diabetes. For most chronic diseases, including diabetes, the effects of neuropathy are peripheral. The etiology of diabetic neuropathy is not well understood but thought to be related to high levels of glucose in the blood over a long period of time. *Diabetic neuropathy* is a generic term for any diabetes mellitus-related disorder of the peripheral or autonomic nervous systems or the cranial nerves. The majority of symptoms from diabetic neuropathy will be located in the LE with foot insensitivity and subsequent ulceration being the most common (Fig. 17.9).

Between 5 and 12 percent of LE leg ulcerations are caused by the complications of diabetes.[53] In addition, many individuals with diabetes have coexisting arterial disease because the conditions are not mutually exclusive. While this percent is lower than venous and arterial wounds in general, the underlying diabetic condition creates a difficult environment in which to close a wound. The incidence of neuropathic LE wounds is likely to grow as the population ages and the incidence of diabetes continues to escalate. According to the U.S. Department of Health and Human Services (HHS), someone in America is diagnosed with diabetes every 25 seconds.[77] Almost half of all

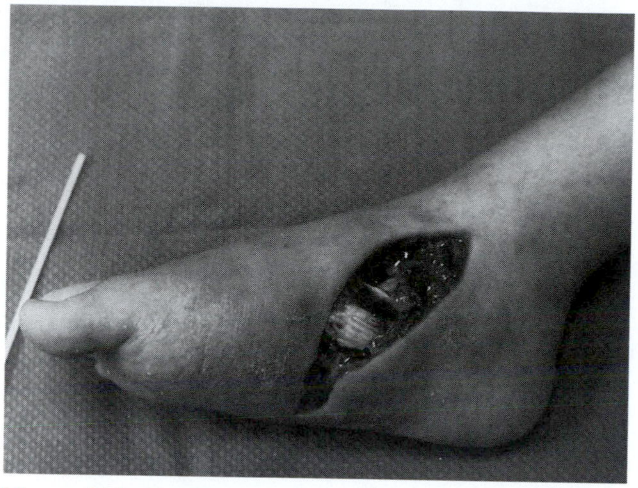

Figure 17.9 Chronic wound as a result of diabetic neuropathy.

adults now are at risk for the disease.[78] Based on information from the Centers for Disease Control and Prevention (CDC) diabetes affects more than 18 million people of all ages in the United States. This figure represents 6.3 percent of the population. About 60 to 70 percent of people with diabetes have mild to severe forms of neuropathy and more than 60 percent of the nontraumatic lower-limb amputations that are performed in the United States occur among people with diabetes.[79] At least half of the amputations were preceded by a foot ulcer, many of which could have been prevented by appropriate team management. If current trends prevail, the impact of diabetic neuropathy on future wound care needs will continue to expand.

Clinical Presentation

- Ulceration usually located on the weightbearing surfaces of the foot
- Usually anesthetic, round, over bony prominences but can be located anywhere
- Sensory neuropathy, if present:
  - Patient unable to sense pain and pressure
  - Risk of skin breakdown without patient awareness
  - Mechanical, repetitive stresses are most common causative factors of wounds.
- Motor neuropathy, if present:
  - Loss of intrinsic muscles
  - Hammer-toe, claw-toe deformities adding to risk of breakdown owing to poor weight distribution and rubbing
  - Foot drop
- Autonomic neuropathy, if present:
  - Decreased or absent sweat and oil production leading to dry, inelastic skin
  - Increased susceptibility to skin breakdown and injury
  - Propensity for heavy callus formation
- Dysvascular symptoms, if present:
  - Usually arterial disorders but can be complicated by reduced cardiac function from autonomic causes
  - Ischemia
  - Impaired healing time (also present owing to diabetes)
  - Impaired transport of oxygen, antibiotics, and nutrients needed for healing

History

A history of diabetes is sufficient to warrant investigation of diabetic neuropathy. If the individual has had diabetes for a number of years or has had trouble regulating insulin levels even for a few years, the presence of diabetic neuropathy is very likely. When an ulceration is visible, the history will include specific details about the wound in addition to information about other symptoms.

Tests and Measurements

During the examination, every patient with diabetes should be checked, using monofilaments, for the presence of protective sensation in the LEs. This should be part of a systems review for patients with diabetes even when diabetes is not the primary diagnosis. Data on skin temperature of the LEs should also be recorded during the examination. Information about blood glucose levels should be obtained as part of the examination and must be considered for safe development of the POC.

Intervention

Physical therapists are in an ideal position to provide education and comprehensive foot care intervention for the diabetic population. According to a recent National Diabetes Fact Sheet, comprehensive foot care programs can reduce amputation rates by 45 to 85 percent.[79] In addition to appropriate wound care, and maintenance of acceptable blood glucose levels, intervention must include some method of decreasing weightbearing stresses. Options for off-loading include crutches or walker, changes in gait patterns, walking casts or splints, and specialized footwear. It would not be unusual to utilize all of the off-loading options over the course of treatment for a foot ulceration. Intervention must include a comprehensive program including elements of wound care, foot care, education, PRDs, orthotics, exercise, and modalities. Every effort should be made by clinicians and patients alike to improve or retain skin integrity of the foot. Refer to Appendix B for patient education information on foot care. In addition to other medical complications of diabetes, altered circulation to the foot can complicate symptoms from diabetic neuropathy. Intervention should address the worst problem first but with lower expectations for healing when vascular disorders coexist with neuropathy.

The five most common disorders of the vascular, lymphatic, and integumentary systems have been discussed. Disorders caused by surgery, trauma, malignancy, hematologic disease, connective tissue disease, and thermal injury *will* impact the systems discussed in this chapter. Owing to space restrictions, however, they will not be discussed at this time. Interested readers should seek one of the texts mentioned in the reference list to supplement information presented here. Examination and treatment of other disorders would utilize the same tests and measurements and treatment interventions discussed in this chapter based on the patient's unique characteristics.

Patient Management

Examination

History

A thorough history will include seeking information on systems beyond the local affected area. As noted in Chapter 1 of this text, physical therapy examinations for all disorders begin with gathering data from the patient, family, and other involved individuals. For the disorders discussed in this chapter, information needed from the history will be similar. Many of the disorders discussed in this chapter have a slow or insidious onset, making history taking challenging but important. Refer to Chapter 1 to review the type of data that may be generated from taking a thorough history.

Systems Review

It might be tempting to skip a systems review before using other tests and measurements in the examination process to save time. This step, however, is of utmost importance as physical therapists move toward greater autonomy. Results may alert the physical therapist to problems that may require referral to another practitioner. A systems review is particularly important here because the disorders discussed in this chapter are the result of dysfunction in other systems of the body. For example, diabetes may lead to wounds of the feet, breast cancer surgery may lead to lymphedema, heart disease may lead to arterial wounds of the legs, and paralysis may lead to pressure ulcers. A comprehensive approach to observing and examining the patient will set the stage for the investigation and data collection that follows.

Tests and Measurements

Owing to the close relationship among disorders of the vascular, lymphatic, and integumentary systems, the importance of differential diagnosis, and the likelihood of a patient or client presenting with more than one disorder, a physical therapist will make use of a wide variety of available tests and measurements during the examination. The tests and measurements discussed in this chapter are described in the order in which they are presented in the *Guide to Physical Therapist Practice*.[80] A review of the test and measurement categories themselves should serve as a reminder of the responsibility of the examining therapist to document thoroughly. For purposes of space, only the most essential categories have been addressed. An annotated version of selected tests and measurements has been included to assist the reader in greater understanding of the tests and the conditions under examination.

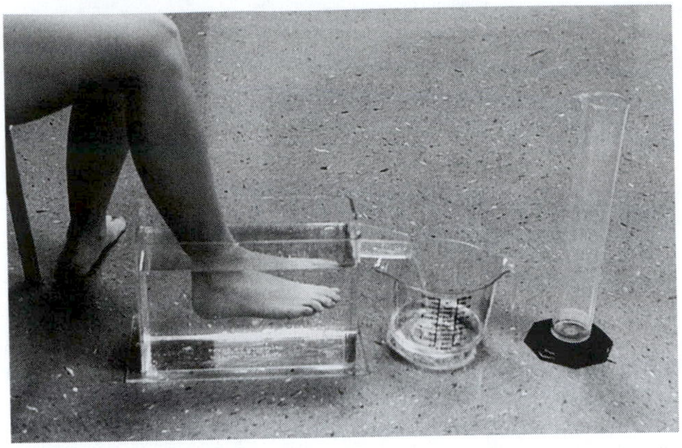

Figure 17.10 Volumetric examination for edema.

Aerobic Capacity/Endurance

Aerobic capacity during functional activities will be important to measure since activity will be encouraged as part of long-term management of the majority of the disorders in this chapter. In addition to information obtained during the systems review (i.e., blood pressure, respiratory rate, heart rate), the gathering of additional data will depend on the individual patient. This might include the use of angina, claudication and dyspnea scales, pulmonary function tests, and ECG. A determination of heart rhythm sounds, and breath and voice sounds may also be required.

Anthropometric Characteristics

Height and Weight. Data on height and weight are necessary to address and track normal weight values especially for the patient with a disorder that results in abnormal fluid retention such as diabetes, edema, lymphedema, venous disease, or underlying cardiopulmonary disease.

Volumetric Measurement. Volumetrics are performed utilizing special containers that hold water, and a graduated cylinder for water collection (Fig. 17.10). This method is accurate for measuring changes in body dimensions; however, it is time consuming, awkward and may be inappropriate for open wounds owing to cross-contamination risks.

Girth Measurement. Girth is recorded using a tape measure to determine circumferential body dimensions (Fig. 17.11). Ideally, a tape measure specially designed to measure girth should be used. While bony landmarks are sometimes used as reference points in taking girth measurements, the standard among experts who treat edema is to use consistent centimeter intervals instead. For example, in measuring the LE, circumferential measurements are taken every 3 cm, starting with 3 cm from the floor or weightbearing surface to the groin. Some clinicians choose intervals of 4, 6, or 10 cm. The smaller the interval, the better the representation of body dimensions. Special measuring boards can be obtained for measuring the LE or a well-placed clipboard can be utilized to establish the beginning measurement. Girth measurements should not be utilized alone

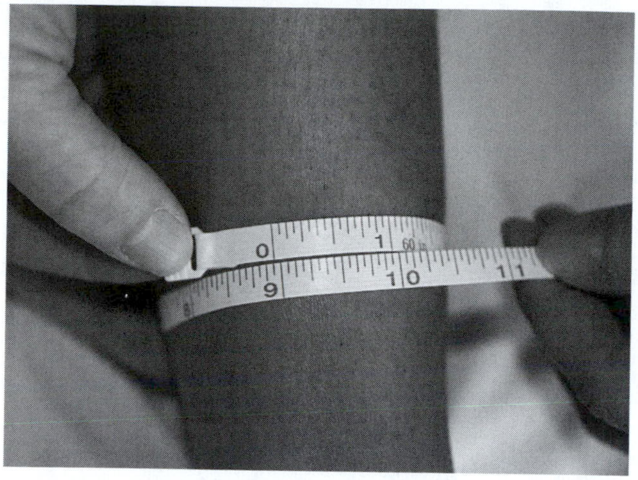

Figure 17.11 Tape measure examination for girth measurement.

to determine severity, frequency of visits, or duration of the episode of care. Advanced fibrotic changes can occur to the dermis and underlying connective tissue without significant increase in girth of a limb.[2,65]

Additional Tools. Data on anthropometric measurements may be collected using *tonometry* or *bioelectrical impedance*. Although not a standardized procedure, soft-tissue tonometry uses a device that measures tissue tension at the surface of the skin. The greater the tension reading, the less pliable the skin, implying the presence of fluid and/or tissue fibrosis. Data from tonometry can be useful for subclinical evidence of edema, lymphedema, and fibrotic changes before they are visible or palpable. Bioelectrical impedance analysis provides accurate measurements to help predict the onset of lymphedema, often many months before a clinical diagnosis is possible. The technique involves passing a very small amount of AC current through the limb to be tested and measuring the impedance to its flow at various frequencies. This technique is much more sensitive than limb volume measurements in detecting changes in the extracellular fluid volume. In studies thus far the false-negative rate has been zero.[81–83]

Staging or Grading of Lymphedema. In an effort to categorize levels of severity, some professionals use staging or grading systems for edema and lymphedema in addition to one or more of the measurement techniques above.[2] Grading or staging of edema and lymphedema is not universally utilized by health professionals and should be accompanied by objective information in the examination results. One of the more frequently used systems by Foldi et al[63] is:

- Subclinical: patient begins to feel "heaviness" in limb, fibrotic changes and fluid accumulation occur before visible swelling or pitting; approximately 50 percent of patients with minimal edema report a feeling of heaviness or fullness in the extremity.[84]
- Stage I, reversible lymphedema: accumulation of protein-rich fluid, elevation reduces swelling; pits on pressure.
- Stage II, spontaneously irreversible lymphedema: proteins stimulate fibroblast formation, connective and scar tissues proliferate; minimal pitting even with moderate swelling.
- Stage III, lymphostatic elephantiasis: hardening of dermal tissues, papillomas of the skin, appearance of skin is elephant-like.

Palpation/Pitting Scale. Palpation of soft tissues must be a regular part of vascular, lymphatic, and integumentary examinations. There is no universal pitting scale currently used by healthcare professionals. Some scales are based on how deep an indentation is left after applying fingertip pressure. Other scales are based on how severe the examiner believes the pitting to be. The following scale, most commonly used by physical therapists and physicians, gives a numerical grade to the pitting based on how long it remains after fingertip pressure is applied:

1+	Indentation is barely detectable
2+	Slight indentation visible when skin is depressed, returns to normal in 15 seconds
3+	Deeper indentation occurs when pressed and returns to normal within 30 seconds
4+	Indentation lasts for more than 30 seconds

If using a pitting scale during an examination, it is wise to document an explanation of the grades or scoring system utilized. Pedal edema may be attributed to chronic wounds, inflammation, infection, cellulitis, diabetes, liver disease, renal disease, CVI, lymphedema, phlebo-lymphedema, congestive heart failure (CHF), or trauma.

Arousal, Attention, and Cognition

After recording screening results during the history and systems review, the physical therapist will decide whether there is a clinical indication for tests and measurements in this category. It is important for the therapist to understand the patient's level of motivation, orientation, attention, and ability to process instructions. Many of the disorders in this chapter, such as diabetic neuropathy, chronic venous insufficiency and lymphedema, require life-long adherence to the self-care component of the treatment in order to retain the gains made during intervention. Most of this information can be obtained through interviews and observations. Additional tools would include cognitive and behavior scales, safety checklists, and learning profiles.

Assistive and Adaptive Devices

It is very likely that patients with vascular, lymphatic, or integumentary disorders will need assistive devices during the intervention and self-care phases of management. Data will most often be obtained by observation. Pressure-sensing devices offer objective data and will be discussed under Tests and Measurements for Integumentary Integrity.

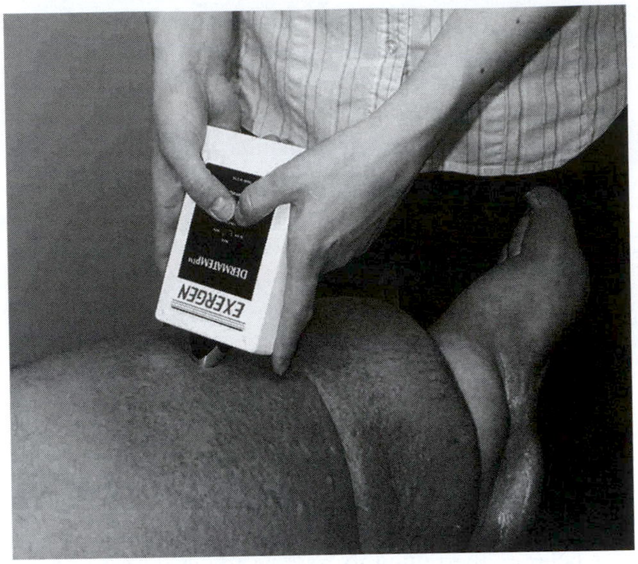

Figure 17.12 Skin temperature examination using a skin thermometer.

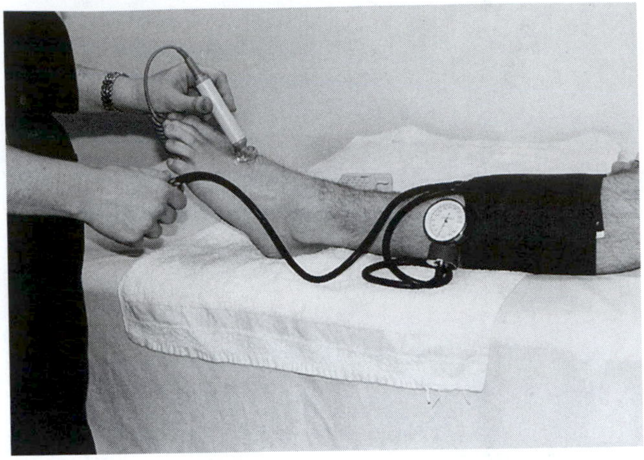

Figure 17.13 ABI test.

Circulation

Collecting data about the movement of blood and lymph through the arterial, venous, and lymphatic systems is interrelated with the tests and measurements for integumentary integrity. Tests and measurements for skin changes that may occur with impairment of the circulation are discussed under the section on Integumentary Integrity. The presence or risk of pathology of the circulatory systems can be detected in many cases by skilled observation and palpation (e.g., temperature and pulses).

Temperature. Temperature can be examined by palpation. Objective data should also be collected and quantified using a *radiometer* or a *thermistor* as superficial skin temperature changes are often indicative of pathology (Fig. 17.12). A decrease in skin temperature can indicate poor arterial perfusion. An increase can indicate infection or active disease processes such as a *Charcot joint*. An increase can also indicate a worsening or impending complication of CVI.[61]

Arterial Perfusion. The therapist collects data to determine whether adequate blood flow is reaching distal tissues. If blood flow is adequate, the oxygen supply will be adequate. Some noninvasive tests and measurements are designed to determine *blood flow* and *skin perfusion,* while others address *oxygen levels* in the tissues. Pulses should be palpated initially to provide information about possible vascular system involvement. The examination should include palpation of the following arteries: brachial and radial, femoral, popliteal, dorsalis pedis, and posterior tibialis. The following scale, commonly used by physical therapists and physicians, gives a numerical grade to the pulses quality:

0 = *No pulse*
1+ = *Weak* pulse, difficult to palpate
2+ = Palpable but not normal, *diminished*
3+ = *Normal,* easy to palpate
4+ = *Bounding,* very strong, may imply the possibility of an aneurysm or other pathological condition.

Auscultation by stethoscope of major pulse points may identify a *bruit*. If turbulent blood flow is heard, the patient may have partial blockage of the artery. Barriers to effective pulse taking include scar tissue, edema, fibrosis, and tissue induration.

Doppler ultrasound is considered an essential component of the vascular examination.[52,55,85,86] The examiner uses a hand-held probe to direct a sound wave into the vessel to be tested. The sound wave is reflected by red blood cells moving in the vessel. The sound wave signal is changed into audible sound that is transmitted from a small, hand-held unit. The ABI is the most frequently performed test using Doppler ultrasound. A blood pressure cuff is inflated to occlude blood flow temporarily then deflated as the examiner listens for the return of flow. This is performed on the upper extremity (UE) at the brachial artery and on the LE at the posterior tibial and the dorsalis pedis arteries (Fig. 17.13). The ABI is a ratio of the LE pressure divided by the UE pressure. Table 17.1 presents the ranges of ABI values and potential vascular indications. Obtaining

Table 17.1 Ankle-Brachial Indices with Corresponding Indications

ABI Ranges	Possible Indication
>1.2	Falsely elevated, arterial disease, diabetes
1.19–0.95	Normal
0.94–0.75	Mild arterial disease, + intermittent claudication
0.74–0.50	Moderate arterial disease, + rest pain
<0.50	Severe arterial disease

an ABI will provide useful information about the arterial system since the ABI is an indicator of loss of perfusion in the LE. Results will guide the therapist in decisions about the use of compression and débridement, and will help to predict the likelihood of wound closure. When the examiner cannot occlude blood flow with the blood pressure cuff, calculations may show a falsely elevated ABI. Arteriosclerosis or calcified vessels (from diabetes) can make it difficult for the cuff to compress enough to get an accurate ABI. The target arteries would be documented as *noncompressible vessels*. Test options when the vessels are noncompressible include taking toe pressures with a special cuff, proceeding with transcutaneous oxygen testing (see below) or recommending referral for vascular laboratory workup.

Trophic Changes. *Trophic changes* occur in the skin of the LEs when circulation is impaired by poor arterial blood flow. Observation is the most accurate way to note changes. Trophic changes include dry, shiny skin (pale in Caucasians), decreased or absent leg hair, and thick toenails. It should be noted that these signs are also a predictable part of aging but not to the same degree as can be seen with trophic changes. The presence of changes indicates the need for other tests of circulation.

Pain. When related to circulation, a thorough pain history may be all that is necessary to suggest the possibility of arterial disease. Reports of pain indicate the need for further tests and measurements of the vascular system. Pain as the result of intermittent claudication (IC) is described earlier in this chapter. Rest pain that develops at night, awakens the patient, or requires analgesics for relief is considered more severe than IC. Pain can be measured for severity on a Visual Analog Scale. The degree of impairment from IC is often measured in terms of how far an individual can walk before experiencing acute leg pain or fatigue. IC can be classified objectively with a rating scale to indicate severity based on distance walked before onset of pain. The *Walking Impairment Questionnaire (WIQ)* is a disease-specific questionnaire commonly used to examine claudication. It does not, however, measure the impact of claudication on quality of life (QoL).[87,88] The most extensively researched disease specific QoL questionnaire for IC is the *Claudication Scale (CLAU-S)*.[87,89,90]

Special Tests. There are many other noninvasive and invasive tests used to detect, examine, diagnose, or confirm arterial disease and dysfunction. Appendix C presents a brief description of special tests for arterial and venous function including *Rubor of Dependency, Air Plethysmography (APG), Transcutaneous Oxygen ($TcPO_2$)* measurement, and *Skin Perfusion Pressure (SPP)* measurement. Although some of the tests are useful for predicting healing of ulcers and amputation wounds, they may not be readily reimbursed when performed by a physical therapist. The APG, $TcPO_2$, and SPP, are used primarily for research purposes because they are time consuming to perform.

Venous Patency. Venous disease and dysfunction can be detected with a wide range of tests and measurements. The amount of time available for examination as well as reimbursement issues may impact decisions about which tests to utilize. Refer to Appendix C for a brief description of *Venous Filling Time, Percussion Test,* and the *Trendelenburg Test*. Owing to inconsistencies in interpretation and administration, the *Homans' Test,* or Homans' sign (pain in the calf when the foot is passively dorsiflexed) should not be relied upon to detect a deep vein thrombosis (DVT). A physician should be contacted and a Doppler study utilized if an individual exhibits two of the following signs: change in skin temperature, change in skin color (darker), pain in the calf (experienced by approximately half of patients), or swelling.

Lymph Vessel Integrity. Patient history and clinical findings are utilized most often to make a diagnosis of lymphedema. Most invasive tests have lost popularity because of the risk of triggering the onset of lymphedema or an exacerbation of existing lymphedema owing to the irritation caused by dye and/or needle puncture. When invasive tests are indicated, the most common test procedure is *lymphoscintigraphy*. This test, using dye and a special camera and computer, can visualize many lymphatic system functions.[2,91]

Gait, Locomotion, and Balance

The importance of movement to impact blood and lymphatic flow, and to facilitate the overall return to function for most individuals, will validate the use of tests and measurements to document patient abilities in this area. During the initial examination, gathering data through observation, gait analysis, and postural control tests is usually adequate. The examination results may indicate the need for additional tests such as inventories, or batteries of tests to further document safety (fall risk) or equipment needs.

Integumentary Integrity

Collection of data about skin and subcutaneous tissues is interrelated with the tests and measurements for circulation and cutaneous sensation.

Observation and Palpation. Characteristics of the skin are noted almost entirely by observation and palpation. A comparison between involved and normal integument is made with careful attention to color, moisture, texture, firmness, temperature, elasticity, symmetry, and shape. In the presence of a wound, the wound tissue, the periwound area, and the wound exudates should all be observed and data recorded regarding the observations. The location of a wound, presence of edema and lymphedema can be documented using a *body diagram*.

Trophic Changes. Because they are an important part of many disorders involving the integument, trophic changes are mentioned again under this section. As in the section on circulation, observation is an important approach to noting changes. Characteristics to consider include the predictable signs of aging.

Fibrosis. Palpation is the best way to detect fibrotic changes of the skin. Tissues will feel thickened, firm, and unyielding or immobile. Testing for the presence or absence of the *Stemmer's sign* is an objective measurement that can be added to the examination for lymphedema. When the dorsal skin folds of the toes or fingers are resistant to lifting or cannot be lifted at all, the Stemmer's sign is said to be "present." The clinician must be cautious, however, as a negative or "absent" skin fold test does not rule out lymphedema.

Coloration. Skin color will vary based on the underlying disease. Observation is the best way to note comparisons between normal tissues and those under examination. The most abnormal color changes include red, purple, and brown. Color changes may indicate a chronic condition such as hemosiderin staining or an acute situation such as redness associated with DVT. If color changes are intermittent they may signal a disease such as **Raynaud's**.

Temperature. Temperature is most often examined by palpation but data can be objectively collected and quantified using a radiometer or a thermistor. A decrease in superficial skin temperature changes may indicate poor arterial perfusion. An increase may indicate infection or active disease processes such as Charcot joint disease. Maintenance of normal skin temperatures is essential for good wound healing.

Wound Size and Depth. There are a number of tools as well as scales available for gathering data about wounds, edema, lymphedema, and other aspects of integumentary integrity. Wounds not classified with staging or grading can be described based on the depth of tissue damage. The descriptions used for depth of burn injury, *superficial, partial,* and *full thickness,* can also be used to describe wound depth in other types of wounds. Objective measures included in documentation are vital for communication about the patient. A calibrated grid, photographs, tracings, graphs, and specifically designed forms are most commonly used to document wound size and depth.

Staging. Pressure ulcers are typically classified using a *staging* or *grading* system that gives information about the severity of the wound based on depth of tissue destruction. Both the National Pressure Ulcer Advisory Panel (NPUAP) and the Agency for Health Care Research and Quality (AHRQ) support the use of the universal, four-stage classification system described in Table 17.2.[92,93] Despite some standardization and acceptance by some government agencies, staging of pressure ulcers is controversial among wound management experts because it is often misused and even more often misleading. The misuse most often occurs because the staging system describes only the depth of tissue destruction and not other characteristics of the wound that need to be considered. Treatment plans should not be based solely on the staging system. Staging can be misleading in that tissue damage may be deeper than what appears on the surface, wounds cannot be staged when necrotic tissue is present and darker skin does not always show the reddened alterations indicating stage I. The staging descriptions are intended for use with pressure ulcers but are often used inaccurately to describe the severity of other wound types.

Table 17.2 Pressure Ulcer Staging Criteria

Pressure Ulcer Stage	Definition
Stage I	An observable pressure-related alteration of intact skin whose indicators, as compared with the adjacent or opposite area on the body, may include changes in one or more of the following: skin temperature (warmth or coolness), tissue consistency (firm or boggy feel), and/or sensation (pain, itching). The ulcer appears as a defined area of persistent redness in lightly pigmented skin, whereas, in darker skin tones, the ulcer may appear with persistent red, blue, or purple hues.
Stage II	Partial-thickness skin loss involving epidermis or dermis, or both. The ulcer is superficial and presents clinically as an abrasion, blister, or shallow crater.
Stage III	Full-thickness skin loss involving damage or necrosis of subcutaneous tissue, which may extend down to but not through underlying fascia. The ulcer presents clinically as a deep crater, with or without undermining of adjacent tissue.
Stage IV	Full-thickness skin loss with extensive destruction, tissue necrosis, or damage to muscle bone or supporting structures (such as tendon, joint capsule).

The NPUAP position on staging: Staging should not be used in reverse order (also called back-staging or down-staging). The staging system is not a measure of healing. A stage IV ulcer is always a stage IV. If it is healed, it would be referred to as a healed stage IV, not a stage 0.

The NPUAP has developed and validated the *Pressure Ulcer Scale for Healing* tool (PUSH tool).[94] This tool documents pressure ulcer healing.

Wound Healing Tools. A variety of wound healing tools can be utilized to document wound status and wound healing.[42] Since there is no single wound characteristic that can be used alone to monitor healing or predict outcomes, it is best to use a tool that includes multiple characteristics as measures of wound healing. The three tools with the most well-established reliability and validity are the *Sussman Wound Healing Tool (SWHT)*,[42] the *Pressure Ulcer Scale for Healing (PUSH)*[42,94] and the *Pressure Sore Status Tool (PSST)*.[42] The PUSH tool is presented in Appendix D. The *Wagner Ulcer Grade Classification* system is a tool designed for examination of the diabetic foot when neuropathy and ischemia are present.[95]

Risk Factor Assessment. Although all individuals can be subjected to the same intensities of pressure for similar amounts of time, they all will not develop pressure ulcers. As a result, factors related to individual risk, susceptibility or tolerance capacity should be determined. Data can be very helpful in planning cost effective intervention strategies. As discussed earlier in the chapter, there are many factors that put some people more at risk for developing pressure ulcers such as poor peripheral circulation, diabetes, nutritional status, mobility, and continence issues to name a few. To objectify and standardize risk assessment, a number of reliable tools have been validated by research:

- *Norton Risk Assessment Scale*: original risk assessment instrument scores individuals on physical condition, mental condition, activity, mobility, and incontinence.[96]
- *Gosnell Scale-Pressure Sore Risk Assessment*: refinement of Norton's scale includes changes to the following scoring categories: nutrition, mental condition, activity, mobility, continence, skin appearance, medication, diet, and fluid balance.[97]
- *Braden Scale for Predicting Pressure Sore Risk*: the six scoring categories of this instrument include sensory perception, moisture, activity, mobility, nutrition, and friction/shear.[98,99]

Muscle Performance

Muscle strength screening during the systems review and specific manual muscle testing is often included during examination of the individual with a disorder of the vascular, lymphatic, or integumentary system. Functional muscle strength identified during an examination of functional mobility skills and activities of daily living (ADL) is also important. Lack of strength and immobility go hand in hand, often leading to problems such as pressure ulcers, CVI, increased LE edema and lymphedema, varicosities, and poor control of diabetic sequelae.

Orthotic, Protective, and Supportive Devices

An examination of the need for devices if not currently in use and an evaluation of the appropriateness and fit of those already in use is indicated. For the individual with impaired sensation of the feet, *extra depth* shoes may be indicated. Existing shoes should be checked periodically for fit and wear. A referral to another professional for protective footwear may be needed. Compression garments and bandaging, considered *supportive devices,* must be checked periodically for fit and function to ensure they retain their effectiveness. Garments and bandages will be essential intervention choices for most individuals with edema and lymphedema. In the later stages, a patient's need for devices may provide a way to quantify the remediation of impairments or functional limitations imposed by the symptoms of the disorder.

Pain

Owing to the high incidence of comorbidity in patients with disorders of the vascular, lymphatic, and integumentary systems, the measurement of pain may also assist in making a differential diagnosis. The presence or absence of pain, its location and intensity, its effect on sleep, and other quality of life factors (QoL), should be measured (see Chapter 28). Pain scales, drawings, and maps are effective for documentation.

Posture

Indications for examination of posture include pain, heavy limbs, scar tissue, poor body image (e.g., following cancer treatment), obesity, and decreased sensation. Data can be obtained with the combined use of a posture grid, tape measure, observation, and palpation.

ROM

The need for adequate ROM cannot be underestimated. Following ROM screening during the systems review, specific ROM measurements are often indicated, especially with persons for whom movement is an essential part of symptom management. Examples are numerous but include ankle ROM for the person with CVI, shoulder ROM following breast cancer surgery, or knee ROM in the individual with lymphedema of the LE. A universal goniometer and a tape measure are the minimum tools required to obtain objective ROM data.

Self-Care and Home Management

Functional limitations and disability are common. Examination, education, and training that allow the patient to safely perform self-care and home management activities are of great importance in planning and implementing the self-management phase. Descriptions and quantifications are needed for documentation and goal setting. Examination tools should include functional measures of both basic (BADL) and instrumental (IADL) activities of daily living (discussed in Chapter 11) as well as fall risk scales.

Sensation

Information from the history and systems review may indicate the need for a detailed examination of sensory function. Therapists should not rely on history alone as an indication for sensory testing, however, because many individuals are unaware of their deficits until tested. Sensory tests are particularly important when symptoms are long-standing, or include complaints of numbness, tingling, or burning. Patients who should routinely be tested are those who may receive LE compression treatments, and all individuals who have a diagnosis of peripheral neuropathy, diabetes, and/or arterial disease. In addition to observation and palpation, initial tests should include testing for protective sensation using filaments such as the *Semmes Weinstein monofilaments*. The filaments are supplied in varying sizes and are each mounted on a handle. The filament is applied to the skin until it bends. The patient is asked to report, with eyes closed, whether the filament is touching the body part. Each monofilament supplies a specific amount of force when it is placed on the test area and gently bent. The monofilaments are available in a large set but most testing can be accomplished using a few filaments. An individual has *normal sensation* when the 4.17 monofilament (1 *g* of force) can be felt. An individual has *protective sensation* intact when the 5.07 filament (10 *g* of force) can be felt (Fig. 17.14). With loss of protective sensation, the individual cannot sense trauma to the foot, often leading to foot ulceration. For the individual who has lost protective sensation, the use of special protective footwear is indicated. Lack of sensation, especially protective sensation can be a characteristic of longstanding diabetes. Decreased sensation may signal a disorder such as **scleroderma**. To test for sharp/dull sensation, vibratory sensation, pressure and other sensations, tools for gathering data include a pressure scale, tuning fork, and/or aesthesiometer. For more information, the reader is referred to Chapter 5.

Ventilation and Respiration

Tests and measures should be used to determine if the patient has adequate ventilation and respiration to meet normal oxygen demands. The presence of pathology might be indicated from a predictable source such as breath sounds or the color of nailbeds. Pathology could also be indicated by a less predictable sign, such as swelling around the ankles. Initial data may be gathered by examining arterial blood gases, observing the work of breathing, or utilizing a spirometer. Additional appropriate tests include the airway clearance test and use of a pulse oximeter.

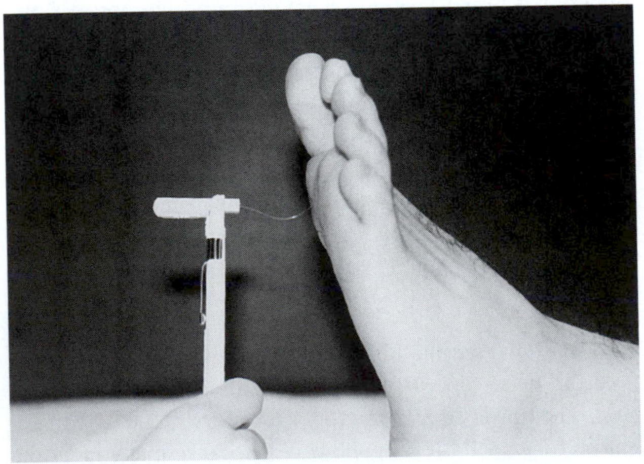

Figure 17.14 Use of Semmes-Weinstein monofilament.

Evaluation, Diagnosis, Prognosis

Once the examination is complete, the physical therapist evaluates the data and determines the diagnosis and prognosis. As presented in Chapter 1 and outlined in *the Guide to Physical Therapist Practice*,[80] the physical therapist needs to consider a number of factors including clinical findings, overall physical function and health status, social support, multisystem involvement and comorbid conditions, and chronicity, severity, and stability of the condition.

The next step is the design and implementation of the plan of care (POC) including procedural interventions.

Intervention

Physical therapist intervention for disorders of the vascular, lymphatic, and/or integumentary systems should include a variety of techniques to address the problems identified during the examination. It is common for patients with disorders in these systems to present with multiple factors contributing to the primary diagnosis. The intervention plan should reflect a holistic view of the patient. For example, an individual with signs and symptoms of venous disease may also present with poor ankle ROM, a LE wound, and lymphedema. The wound must be cleansed and dressed but the limb should also receive compression for optimum healing. Ankle ROM must be improved since ambulation will enhance calf pump function. Another example of the need to view patients holistically would be an individual with signs and symptoms of arterial disease who also presents with decreased LE strength, diabetes, and peripheral neuropathy. Exercise is important for this person but it must be carefully coordinated to address arterial health, diabetes management, and skin protection.

Coordination, Communication, Documentation

In keeping with practice standards, the physical therapist coordinates intervention efforts to ensure the patient receives the highest quality of care. Critical to this goal is open communication among the wound care team, patient, family, and caregivers. The wound care team includes a physician, nurse, physical therapist, occupational therapist, dietitian, and social worker. Referrals to other health care professionals (e.g., podiatrist) who can support the patient can also be made. Meticulous documentation will have a significant impact on issues such as continuity of care, receiving adequate number of visits for procedures, and a stronger working relationship with referring practitioners. The use of photographs, special forms for data collection, and body graphs are very effective tools to enhance communication and documentation. Appendix E provides an example of an examination form that might be utilized to document data collected for a patient with a wound.

Patient/Client-Related Instruction

Disorders of the vascular, lymphatic, and integumentary systems represent major health events for patients and their families and require life-long management strategies. Patients and families often react with anger, despair, or at least confusion when learning about a condition that may be permanent. The value of patient and family education cannot be underestimated. Patient education will be the key to preparing individuals to manage their symptoms, prevent recurrence, and remain vigilant about their condition. Information should be provided that is appropriate to the patient/family/caregiver's educational level with provisions for follow-up and repetition. Motivation strategies are important to ensure adherence to self-management. For many chronic disorders, high-quality patient education has been shown to result in positive changes in health behaviors, QoL perceptions, and adherence to home programs. Instruction for the patient should include resources, education materials, and a home program.

- Resources
  - Community services and support groups related to the patient's diagnosis
  - Counseling services, as needed, especially for assistance with QoL issues
  - Internet sites (refer to Appendix F for Internet Resources)
  - Family member participation in care
- Education materials
  - Instructional materials, multimedia tools
  - Self-management strategies
  - Available resources include *Wound Care* by Sussman[100] or *Living Well with Lymphedema* by Ehrlich.[101]
- Home program
  - Skin and/or wound care; prevention practices; scar management
  - Compression garment or bandage wear and care
  - Exercise
  - Edema control
  - Pressure relieving devices
  - Foot care for patients with diabetes (refer to Appendix B for a foot care guide).

Outpatient or home therapy may be required for some patients. Follow-up visits at regularly scheduled intervals may be the best way to facilitate adherence to the home program and to prevent recurrence or exacerbation of symptoms.

Procedural Interventions

This section has been organized in the order in which a physical therapist would provide patient care. Within each section, information has been organized from most invasive/least selective to least invasive/most selective. In developing the POC, a physical therapist should select interventions that are least invasive/most selective, always trying to create an environment that is conducive to healing. The ultimate goal should be to optimize the body's opportunity to heal. Despite tremendous gains in the management of vascular, lymphatic, and integumentary disorders, there are still an alarming number of practitioners using outdated and often harmful methods to treat these disorders. Overused agents such as povidone-iodine, wet-to-dry dressings, whirlpool, and compression pumps have been replaced for at least a decade with more advanced, biocompatible, and cost-effective methods of treatment. The use of inappropriate agents can delay healing and may cause harm. Supporting literature abounds for the clinician seeking evidence-based practice. Elements of skin and wound care that are often overlooked or underestimated for their impact include pressure relieving devices (PRDs), positioning, exercise, patient education, compression, and orthotics.

Cleansing

Wound cleansing is differentiated from wound débridement that follows in the next section. The wound cleansing method should be selected based on its ability to support or return a wound bed to homeostasis. Chemical and mechanical trauma should be minimized even in the presence of infection. A decision to cleanse should be made carefully, as many wounds do not need to be cleansed at every dressing change.

Whirlpool

Since whirlpool can be classified as a means of cleansing and mechanical débridement, it is discussed in both categories of intervention. Despite at least a decade of investigation, with little evidence to support its use, whirlpool is still used for both nonselective mechanical débridement and for wound cleansing. However, many clinicians involved in wound care have decreased their use of whirlpool significantly with the evolution of wound care and subsequent publication of the Agency for Health Care Research and Quality (AHRQ) guidelines. Standards have changed with the increased knowledge of the microenvironment in the wound bed and a greater understanding of the chemical mediators necessary for homeostasis.

The historical rationale for use of whirlpool was based on its use in deodorization, skin and wound cleansing, mechanical nonselective débridement, wound decontamination and infection control, and softening adherent necrotic tissue in preparation for débridement. There is little evidence to support whirlpool as the *optimal* method for achieving these. If using whirlpool for an infected wound, the AHRQ recommends that whirlpool be discontinued when the ulcer is clean. First issued in 1994, the guidelines are considered to still be current.[93] It includes more than 300 references; bibliographic sources and updates that can be easily obtained.[102]

Evidence-based rationale for changes in the use of whirlpool is based on a number of factors.[3,103–105] There is risk of contamination from waterborne pathogens to clean wounds and of patient cross-contamination. The dependent position can initiate or increase venous congestion and extremity edema. There is loss of endogenous fluids from the wound bed and heat loss affecting core body temperature and/or the local wound area. Even mild changes in core body temperature (hypothermia) have negative effects on cells important to wound healing. Mechanical disruption of granulation tissue, epithelial cells, and new skin grafts occurs, primarily from the use of agitation. Whirlpool saturates wound tissue and surrounding skin creating the potential for maceration and skin breakdown and temporarily inactivates normal skin defenses through immersion. Thus there is the potential to prolong inflammation and delay wound healing. Whirlpool can also increase heart and respiratory rates. Finally, the use of whirlpool is labor intensive and costly in terms of use of water, utilities, linen, and staff.

Based on current standards of care and guidance from the literature cited earlier, it may be possible to justify the use of whirlpool in the following situations. Wounds that need intensive cleansing that cannot be accomplished with other methods might benefit from whirlpool. Minimal agitation of water is recommended with only small body areas treated for short amounts of time (5 to 10 minutes) to limit the negative effects of temperature and pressure changes. Unless infection is confirmed with tissue culture, cytotoxic agents in the water should be avoided (e.g., povidone-iodine, chlorine). Wounds that need softening of loosely adherent tissue before sharp, enzymatic or autolytic débridement might benefit from whirlpool when other tissue softening methods are not appropriate. (Note: there is little to no reimbursement for the use of whirlpool to soften tissue before débridement). Wounds that would benefit from stimulation of peripheral circulation might benefit from whirlpool. Neutral warmth or normothermia (normal body temperature 98.6°F [37°C]) is recommended.

Pulsatile Lavage with Suction

Pulsatile lavage with suction (*PLWS*, also referred to as *forceful irrigation*) is a method of wound irrigation combined with suction (Fig. 17.15).[106] Pulsed irrigation and simultaneous suction removes the irrigation fluid, wound exudates, and loose debris. In use for over twenty years, this wound cleansing and débridement method has several advantages over whirlpool cleansing.[107] It uses less water, less staff support, less treatment time, and requires less clean up time. PLWS can be performed bedside and in the home. (Note: family or visitors are not allowed in the room during the procedure owing to aerosolization of microorganisms.)[108] It collects wound exudates and debris efficiently and delivers topical antibiotics, antiseptics, and antibacterial solutions efficiently. PLWS speeds healing by rapid removal of contaminants and treats tunneling wounds and undermining wounds using special cannula tips. Risk of periwound maceration and cross-contamination is eliminated with use of disposable equipment.

While the advantages are clear, there are disadvantages to using PLWS. These include risk of overuse especially with clean, granulating wounds and risk of trauma to newly formed tissue from plastic tips, pulsed irrigant, and/or suction. Treatment may be painful to the patient.

PLWS use should be limited to experienced therapists who are well versed in anatomy especially when irrigating tracts, undermining, exposed bone, tendon, blood vessels, cavity linings, grafts, or flaps. All staff involved in treatment must wear disposable personal protective equipment (PPE).

Compared to other irrigation options, disposable, single-use equipment contributes to landfill burden. There is increased cost (labor, PPE, equipment).

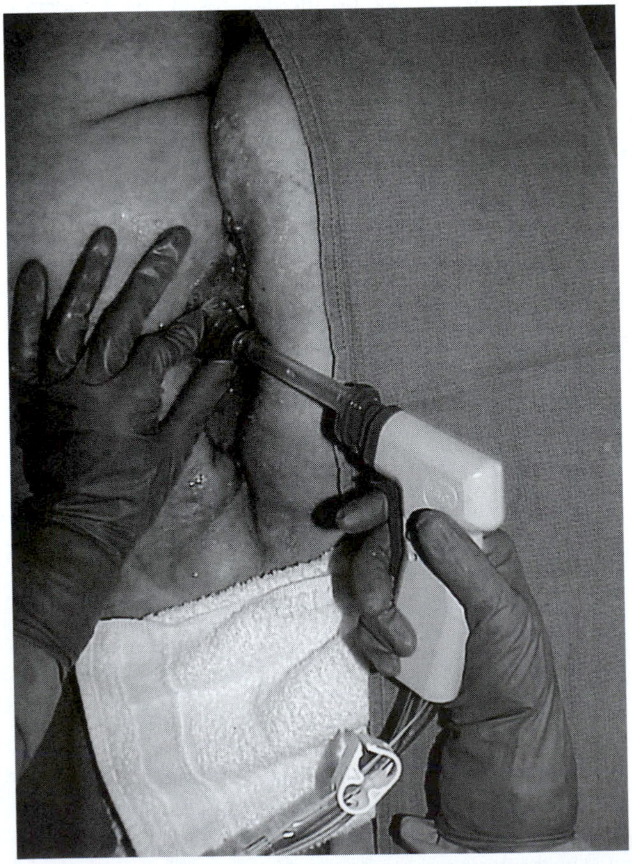

Figure 17.15 Physical therapist's fingers mold PLWS shield to sacral wound surface. (From Kloth, LC, and McCulloch, JM,[137] p 221, with permission.)

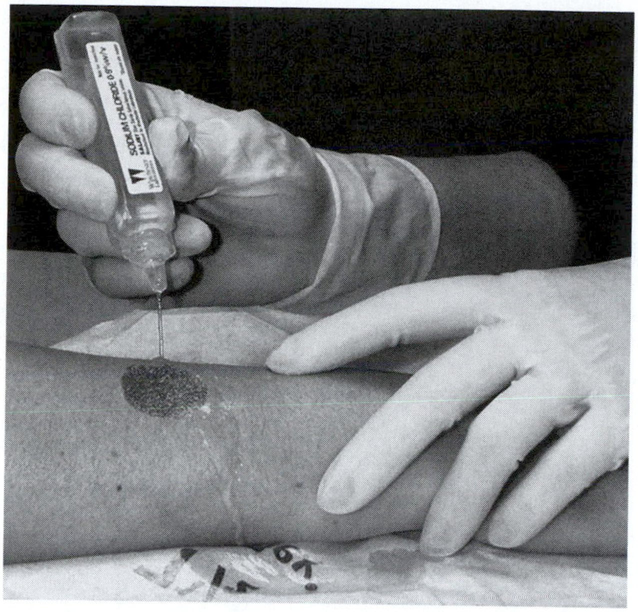

Figure 17.16 Wound cleansing with nonforceful irrigation.

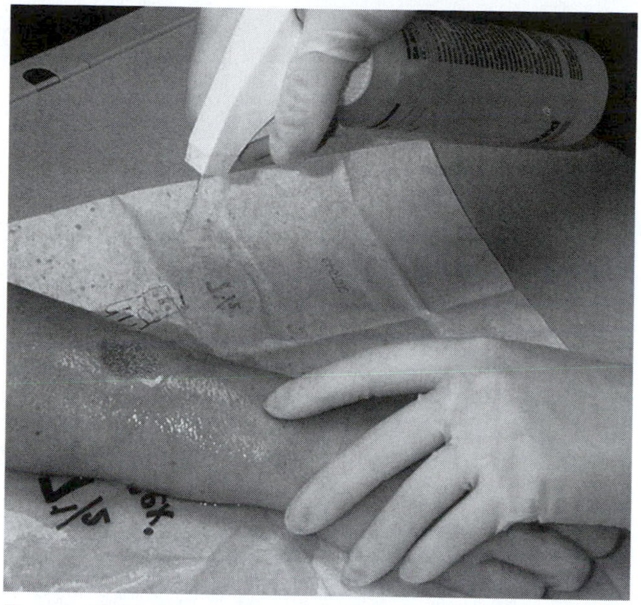

Figure 17.17 Wound cleansing with a spray cleanser.

Nonforceful Irrigation

As soon as possible, wound cleansing should be accomplished with minimal pressure or force on the wound bed by nonforceful irrigation. This can be accomplished by pouring a solution over a wound, or using a bulb syringe, or other device designed to deliver an irrigant to the wound (Fig. 17.16). There are several products that package saline specifically for wound cleansing: Blairex® Wound Wash Saline manufactured by Blairex Laboratories, Inc, Columbus, IN 47201 and Saljet®, single-dose sterile saline manufactured by Winchester Laboratories, LLC, St. Charles, IL 60174. Several manufacturers produce a spray container that delivers saline or a surfactant at very gentle pressures (Fig. 17.17). Infected wounds can also be effectively cleaned with nonforceful irrigation. Wounds with necrotic tissue or debris, however, may respond best to a few sessions of a more forceful type of cleansing. For wounds that are clean, with new tissue growth, cleansing should be done only to remove excess endogenous fluids or residue left by dressing products.

Débridement

Débridement is defined as the removal of foreign material and dead or damaged tissue. Removal of devitalized or infected tissue is an important intervention to prevent or control bacterial growth, encourage normal cellular activity in the wound bed, and enhance the rate of tissue repair. *Nonselective débridement* removes all tissue both necrotic and living. Methods in this category may be quick but are often painful and frequently cause damage to nearby healthy tissue. *Selective débridement* removes necrotic tissue in a controlled method. Selective methods are more comfortable and gentle to the wound bed but may remove tissue more slowly. When choosing a method of débridement, clinicians must consider not only the wound status but also the physiological, emotional, and financial status of the patient. Modern wound management experts avoid débridement techniques that cause the wound to bleed owing to the highly damaging effects to the wound tissues.

Nonselective Débridement

Wet-to-Dry Dressings. A wet-to-dry (WTD) dressing consists of wet gauze applied to the wound bed and allowed to dry on the wound. Removal of the dry dressing débrides the wound, pulling away any cellular material that has adhered to the gauze. This method of débridement removes necrotic tissue as well as rich endogenous fluids, fibrin, and other cells critical to wound healing. It is also frequently uncomfortable for the patient, often causing bleeding and trauma to the wound bed. Wound management experts agree with a multidisciplinary panel: "One of the most routinely and inappropriately used forms of nonselective mechanical débridement is the wet-to-dry dressing."[34, p 28] Once believed to be less costly than other dressing options, it has been shown that WTD dressings are actually more costly than advanced dressings. Research addressing the negative impact of WTD dressings on wounds is summarized in Evidence Summary Box 17.1 As WTD dressings can be classified as a tool for mechanical débridement and/or a primary wound dressing, they have been discussed in both categories.

Surgical

Surgical débridement provides rapid results when treating life-threatening necrosis, large wounds, tunneling wounds, and necrotic or infected bone. Wide excision, removing viable and nonviable tissue, is usually done in the operating

Evidence Summary Box 17.1

Outcome Studies Using Wet-to-Dry (WTD) Dressings as Part of Wound Care

Reference	Subjects	Design/Intervention	Duration	Results	Comments
Ovington, LG[109] 2001	N/A	Systematic review	N/A	WTD dressings have been standard procedure for wound care although research indicates gauze dressings are not optimal for the patient, the clinician, or the health care system.	Gauze dressings do not support optimal healing and are more labor intensive than advanced dressings. This article provides clinicians with the rationale and evidence to collaborate with physicians in choosing cost-effective products to achieve positive patient outcomes.
Lawrence, JC, Lilly, HA, and Kidson, A[111] 1994	Simulated wounds: 7 subjects, 14 dressing changes IC: colonized burn wounds	Experimental	Two dressing changes per wound	Removing dry or damp gauze from a wound released significant numbers of organisms into the air. Significantly fewer organisms were released when removing an occlusive dressing. Significant numbers of bacteria were still in the air as long as 30 minutes after removal of gauze dressings.	Wounds are often undressed in open areas, sometimes with other patients nearby. Some health care practitioners do not wear masks when undressing a wound. There is an appreciable cross-contamination hazard from removing dry or damp gauze dressings without protection to all individuals in the room.
Svensjo, T, et al[17] 1997	3 porcine animals with a total of 70 wounds IC: Female, Yorkshire pigs, 3 months, 30–40 kg	Experimental	16 days	12 days after wounding 0% of dry, 20% of moist and 86% of wet treated wounds were re-epithelialized.	The basic mechanisms of skin wound repair: granulation tissue formation, re-epithelialization, and contraction were influenced by moisture level. Dry wounds heal more slowly.
Lim, JK, et al[112] 1999	10 subjects with 10 wounds and 10 control areas IC: full-thickness skin ulcers	Experimental	6 hours, with fluid assay every 30 minutes	With evaporation allowed by gauze dressings, test fluids became hypertonic.	Evaporation and saturation are difficult to control with gauze dressings. Fluids under a dressing remain isotonic until the gauze becomes completely saturated (which occurs prematurely in a heavily exudating wound) or until the gauze dries out as is often allowed on purpose. To remain isotonic, gauze dressings must be changed frequently.
Mosher, BA, et al[113] 1999	9 specialists IC: multidiscipline, independent clinical experts in geriatric care, familiar with 4 débridement models	Nonexperimental: computer modeling and decision analysis/therapy with each of 4 débridement methods	1 month	The likelihood of achieving a clean wound bed was 70% with collagenase, 57% for fibrinolysin, 50% for autolysis, and 30% for WTD dressings. Cost for treatment was highest with WTD and lowest with collagenase.	WTD dressings are often used as a débridement technique. They are not as effective as other options, their use leads more often to infection and they are costly to the health-care system.

Rodeheaver, G, et al[34] 1994	Roundtable of 7 IC: multi-discipline, experts in wound care	Report of expert community	N/A	A multidisciplinary panel of experts convened to discuss wound care with a special emphasis on 4 types of débridement: mechanical (WTD), surgical, chemical, and enzymatic.	WTD is one of the most routinely but inappropriately used forms of non-selective mechanical débridement. The disadvantages are numerous: bleeding, pain, removal of granulation tissue, desiccation (drying) and cost.
Kohr, R[114] 2001	1 (Case Study) IC: wound that had failed to heal	Moist wound environment applied to wound that had failed to heal with WTD for 21 days.	10 days	Switch from WTD to moist-wound-healing (MWH):10 days to significant wound healing.	The temperature in the wound was optimized, autolytic débridement promoted. Cost comparison issues between WTD and MWH also well illustrated in the article.
Eriksson, E, et al[18] 1996	1 (Case Study) IC: chronic wound, failure to heal	Moist wound environment applied to infected wound that had failed to heal with WTD for 7 years.	10 weeks. Follow-up at 24 months.	Significant changes in 2 weeks. Wound closed at 10 weeks. Remained closed at 24 months.	The wound was bathed in endogenous (its own) fluids continuously, eliminating the discomfort, wound bed disruption, dessication, and risk of infection associated with frequent WTD dressing changes.
Colwell, JC, Foreman, MD, and Trotter, JP[115] 1993	70 patients with 97 pressure ulcers IC: noninfected stage II or stage III pressure ulcers	Prospective, randomized, controlled study	15 months	22% of ulcers receiving hydrocolloid therapy healed as compared to 2% receiving moist gauze therapy.	There is an overwhelming difference in healing between gauze and advanced dressings. The per diem cost of the moist gauze dressing was $12.26; the per diem cost of the hydrocolloid dressing was $3.55.
Capasso VA, and Munro, BH[116] 2003	50 adult patients with wounds, IC: 25-WTD dressings, 25-amorphous hydrogel dressings	Nonexperimental, retrospective chart review	4 biweekly data collection points	The overall cost of wound care was significantly higher for patients in the normal saline group, with a higher number and cost of home nursing visits.	Demonstrating the value and cost effectiveness of hydrogel dressings should enhance therapeutic decision making and guide treatment decisions.

[a]See also Lawrence,[110] 1992.

IC = inclusion criteria; WTD = wet to dry.

room with anesthesia. Laser débridement, another form of surgical débridement, may be appropriate when an individual is not a candidate for operating room procedures. Surgical débridement is not within the scope of practice of a physical therapist.

Pulsatile Lavage with Suction

PLWS will provide nonselective débridement while cleansing a wound. Refer to the detailed discussion of PLWS in the previous section on Cleansing.

Whirlpool

Whirlpool can be utilized for mechanical débridement through its feature of water agitation. It can also be used to soften necrotic tissue in preparation for sharp, enzymatic, or autolytic débridement. There are, however, often better methods of preparing tissue for débridement than whirlpool. See discussion in the previous section on Cleansing.

Selective Débridement

Sharp. *Sharp débridement* is defined as the removal of dead or necrotic tissue or foreign material from and around a wound using sterile instruments such as a scalpel, scissors, and/or forceps (Fig. 17.18). Considered the *gold standard* of methods for removal of necrotic tissue, sharp débridement is a minor, tissue sparing procedure that is performed bedside or in a procedure room. In the vast majority of states in the United States, it is within the scope of practice for a physical therapist to perform sharp débridement. It is incumbent on the therapist to be aware of his or her own practice act regarding regulations. In the June 2000 American Physical Therapy Association position statement, sharp débridement should be performed exclusively by physical therapists, not other personnel. Additional information can be found in the *Guide to Physical Therapist Practice*.[80] A physical therapist should not débride except in the presence of necrotic tissue.

Even though sharp débridement is effective for all types of necrotic tissue, there are situations where this form of débridement is not appropriate. It is contraindicated for vascular wounds with limited blood flow and eschar serving as a cap for a chronic open wound. Without adequate perfusion, there is little hope of wound closure. It is not appropriate for wounds with tunneling (the wound bed cannot be seen) or areas affected by dry gangrene. Patients with low platelet counts, on anticoagulants, or with other conditions that inhibit clotting are not suitable candidates. It is also contraindicated for pressure ulcers on the heels covered with dry eschar (Note: Some experts maintain that in this scenario, eschar provides protection as long as there is no infection present; others maintain that eschar must be removed because it inhibits epithelial cell growth.)

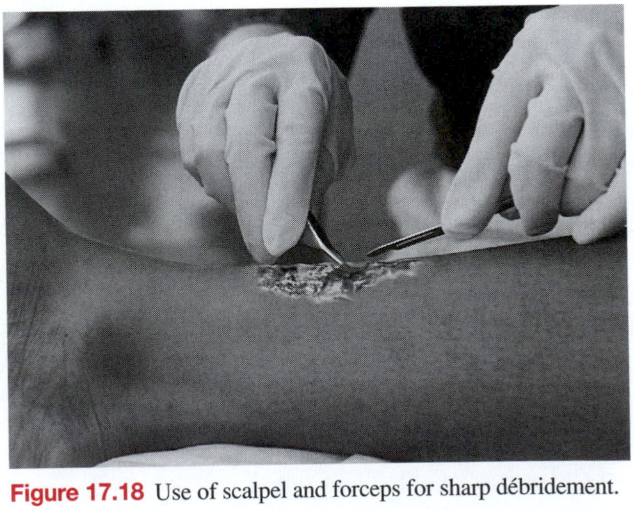

Figure 17.18 Use of scalpel and forceps for sharp débridement.

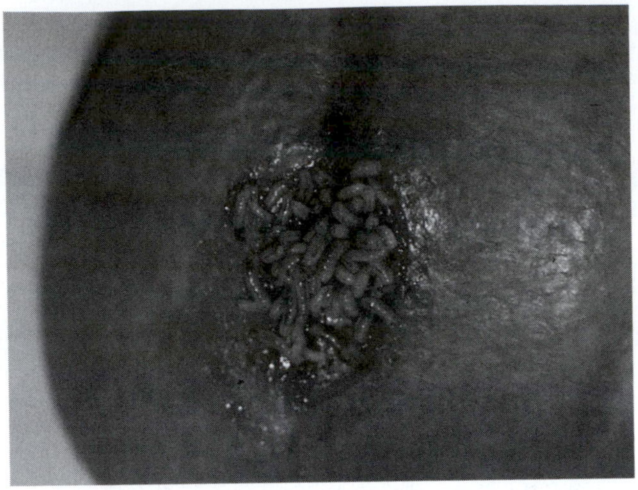

Figure 17.19 Maggot therapy for a cavity wound. (Courtesy of the Biosurgical Research Unit, Surgical Materials Testing Laboratory, Bridgend, UK.)

Chemical or Enzymatic. This type of selective débridement includes the application of a topical agent containing enzymes that act by dissolving necrotic tissue. A referral for treatment and a prescription for the enzyme agent from a referring practitioner are currently required in most regions of North America. There are several types and brands of enzymatic agents, each designed to affect a certain type of necrotic tissue. Advantages for this type of treatment are that débridement is selective, patient discomfort is minimal, and application procedures are simple. Disadvantages include the potential development of dermatitis of the intact periwound skin, frequent dressing changes disrupting the wound bed, and eschar which may have to be cross-hatched with a scalpel so that the enzyme can penetrate the wound.

Biosurgery. Biosurgery as a form of selective débridement is also referred to as *maggot débridement therapy (MDT),* or maggot or larval therapy (Fig 17.19). While it has been in use in the western world for over 150 years, its popularity declined with the advent of antibiotics. Biosurgery is now generating new interest owing to the rise of multiresistant bacteria such as methicillin-resistant *Staphylococcus aureus*. Sterile, newly hatched larvae are placed on chronic wounds and held in place with dressings for 2 to 5 days before removal. Biosurgery has been shown to remove devitalized tissue, decrease the risk of infection and improve wound healing without side effects in a wide variety of wound types. Biosurgery is recommended for osteomyelitis and deep wound infections that remain unresponsive to more conventional antibiotic and surgical therapy. Although moist wound healing is compatible with biosurgery, a very wet wound environment has an adverse effect on larval survival. Certain types of moisture-retentive wound dressings are more compatible with larval survival than others.[117–124]

Autolytic. *Autolytic débridement* uses the endogenous enzymes on the wound bed to digest devitalized tissue and promote granulation tissue formation. In practice, the body's natural fluids are held in contact with the wound base with a moisture retentive dressing for 3 to 7 days. By increasing the moisture content of slough and necrotic tissue with the body's own enzyme-rich fluids, autolytic activity is facilitated. While this method is the least invasive/ most selective as well as inexpensive, painless, and biocompatible, each patient is examined to determine if this type of débridement is best for the existing wound. The type of moisture retentive dressing selected to promote autolytic débridement will be based on the health of the periwound tissues and the level of fungal or bacterial loads. As described and referenced in the discussion on moist wound healing, the presence of infection does not rule out the use of occlusive dressings.

Topical Agents

Current standards for chronic wound care have decreased the use of topical agents even in the presence of infection. In the literature these agents may be referred to as *antiseptics, disinfectants,* and/or *antimicrobials.* Other topical agent categories include *antibiotics* and *analgesics.* When discussing the use of topical agents with a physician, always evaluate cytotoxicity, biocompatibility, safety, and efficacy. Even under Direct Access, in most states physical therapists are not permitted to prescribe medications, even over-the-counter products, for wound care. Guidelines reveal that almost all man-made products are cytotoxic to white blood cells even when diluted.[93] Many agents once thought to be safe are now known to be unsafe to healing tissue, causing adverse reactions at any concentration. Many agents once thought to be effective as antibacterial or decontaminating agents are now known to be ineffective. When striving for wound bed homeostasis, preserving cellular life in endogenous fluids is almost always more desirable than destroying it with additives. Many physicians and wound management experts use the following adage to guide in the decision-making process: "It is desirable never to put anything in the wound that cannot be tolerated comfortably in the conjunctival sac."[16, p 179]

Antiseptics

Povidone-Iodine. The combination of iodine plus a polymer provides bactericidal effects. One commonly known product name is Betadine (Purdue Frederick Co, Stamford, CT 06901). Used indiscriminately for many years on acute and chronic wounds, it is now recommended mainly for wounds infected with *Staphylococcus aureus.* The AHRQ guidelines published in 1994 state: "Do not clean ulcer wounds with skin cleansers or antiseptic agents (e.g., povidone-iodine, iodophor, sodium hypochlorite solution [Dakin's solution], hydrogen peroxide, acetic acid)."[93, p 15] Although the guidelines address pressure ulcers, the wound healing evidence is applicable to all wound treatments. This evidence implies that the use of povidone-iodine as well as other antiseptics is inconsistent with practice standards. In rare instances when such agents are recommended by a physician and are indeed appropriate, clinicians should document sound reasoning behind the use of these products because they will be held accountable to these published and respected guidelines. The literature does not support clinically or legally adequate reasons to use povidone-iodine for managing wounds.[125] In addition, the Food and Drug Administration (FDA) has not approved the use of povidone-iodine solution or povidone-iodine surgical scrub solution for wounds.[126] Its use is contraindicated for the noninfected wound.[93]

Hypochlorite Solutions: Dakin's (Bleach and Boric Acid), Sodium Hypochlorite (Household Bleach). Sodium hypochlorite is cytotoxic even at very dilute concentrations. It damages **fibroblasts** and endothelial cells and causes cellular damage to granulation tissue. It is irritating to the skin and can initiate severe reactions in some individuals. It is used in the management of wounds with purulent exudates. Treatment should be discontinued when the wound is clean. Its use is contraindicated for the noninfected wound.[93]

Acetic Acid Solution. Acetic acid is traditionally used to inhibit bacterial infections however, the solution has been found to be more damaging to fibroblasts than to bacteria.[127] A common form of acetic acid is found in vinegar. It is corrosive and cytotoxic at any dilution. Most recently, it has been utilized to manage contamination by *Pseudomonas aeruginosa.* Its use is contraindicated for the noninfected wound.[93]

Oxidizing Agents: Hydrogen Peroxide Solution. When this solution comes in contact with tissue, there is a release of oxygen and temporary antimicrobial activity. Its bubbling action is used for nonselective débridement to loosen small debris. It is cytotoxic unless diluted to a very weak concentration. It is contraindicated in wounds that are noninfected, tunneling, or granulating.[93]

Antibacterials

This section includes a sample of commonly utilized topical antimicrobials, antibiotics, and antibacterials. These topical agents are each effective against a variety of bacteria and are selected by the physician based on the species cultured for an individual patient. All of them share risk of similar side effects such as burning, itching, contact dermatitis, and/or allergic sensitivity. There is little evidence in the literature to show levels of cytotoxicity in these topical agents. Examples include:

- Bacitracin/Baciguent: associated with allergic reactions.
- Neosporin/neomycin sulfate: causes greatest incidence of allergic reactions.
- Silvadene/silver sulfadiazine: primarily for thermal injuries, silver is selectively toxic to bacteria but may inactivate topical proteolytic enzymes.[128]
- Furacin/nitrofurazone: cytotoxic in animal studies.[129]
- Sulfamylon/mafenide acetate: diffuses easily through eschar, primarily for thermal injuries.
- Bactroban/mupirocin ointment: currently effective against all species of staphylococcus.
- Gentamicin/Geramycin: currently effective against all species of staphylococcus and streptococcus.

Owing to the paucity of information on cytotoxicity, the risk of side effects and the growing incidence of antibiotic-resistant bacteria, use of these products for chronic wounds should be considered carefully and is usually contraindicated for the noninfected wound.

Creams and Ointments (Over-the-Counter). Some antibacterial ointments and creams such as are Bacitracin and Neosporin can be purchased without a prescription. These are minimally bacteriostatic owing to their dilution. Once they lose their antibacterial strength, the ointments may trap bacteria and encourage bacterial growth from surface contamination. If ointments or creams are used, the wound should be cleansed regularly to remove potential contamination, however, frequent cleansing may disrupt the healing process. These preparations provide moisture (albeit expensive) to a dry wound but they may create a greasy wound bed, making early epithelial cell migration difficult. A more biocompatible ointment that will provide moisture to a healing wound is Aquaphor (Beiersdorf-Jobst, Charlotte, NC 28209).

Analgesics

The use of topical anesthetics to control wound pain is controversial in the literature. Conflicting reports and the lack of substantial research have led to concerns about the impact of anesthetics on the wound bed. This issue is further complicated by the broad profile of patients with wounds, their etiologies and comorbidities. The more common agents used topically are lidocaine and EMLA (eutectic mixture of local anesthetics) cream, which is a mixture of lidocaine and prilocaine (AstraZeneca, Wilmington, DE 19803). Amitriptyline, a tricyclic antidepressant, has local anesthetic properties and has shown promise as an option for treating wound pain.[130] While topical anesthetics may be under scrutiny for their effects, vasoconstriction in particular, there is a need for more investigation since pain is a major issue for most patients with wounds.

Growth Factors

Endogenous growth factors normally abound in the fluids of a wound. In some chronic wounds where the normal timetable for healing has been delayed or stopped, and growth factors in the wound bed are decreased or absent, they can be added topically. Increasing strength of evidence supports the practice of adding growth factors to a wound to facilitate healing. The application of exogenous growth factors in conjunction with good wound care increases wound healing outcomes.[131–136] Growth factors can be isolated from an individual's own tissue, added to a liquid formula and reapplied to the wound. An example of an autologous growth factor product with a name familiar to many clinicians is Procuren (Curative Health Services, Hauppauge, NY 11788). Recombinant DNA technology has resulted in other products such as becaplermin gel, trade name Regranex® Gel (Ortho-McNeil Pharmaceutical, Inc, Raritan, NJ 08869). Reimbursement for application of growth factors varies and should be checked before use. For example, becaplermin gel is FDA approved for the treatment of LE diabetic neuropathic ulcers that extend into the subcutaneous tissue or beyond but currently not approved for the treatment of pressure, venous, or other nondiabetic-related wounds.

Topical Agents and Acute Wounds

The use of antiseptics and antibiotics to reduce bacterial levels in acute, traumatic wounds follows a different rationale from that of chronic wounds. For wounds resulting from trauma or thermal injury, the risk for contamination is high. It is accepted practice to utilize cytotoxic products such as povidone-iodine or Silvadene in the *early* management of acute traumatic wounds. The goal is to discontinue use of cytotoxic agents as soon as the wounds are clean and able to produce and support endogenous fluids.

Mechanical Modalities

Procedures for use of modalities vary based on unique patient characteristics and individual patient response. A useful place to begin is with protocols recommended in comprehensive wound management texts such as *Wound Healing: Alternatives in Management* by Kloth and McCulloch[137] and *Wound Care* by Sussman and Bates-Jensen.[138] Owing to the ever-changing rules of reimbursement, it is prudent to check current reimbursement and documentation guidelines when billing for these services.

Ultrasound

Therapeutic ultrasound (US) application for wound management differs from its use as a modality to treat pain. US stimulates cell activity, accelerating processes such as inflammation. Once thought to target only the sluggish wound in the inflammatory stage, evidence now demonstrates that the effects can be seen throughout all wound healing phases. Basic science evidence and clinical research have established that skin repair and wound contraction can be accelerated, collagen secretion can be stimulated, and elastin properties affected to strengthen scar tissue. Standard

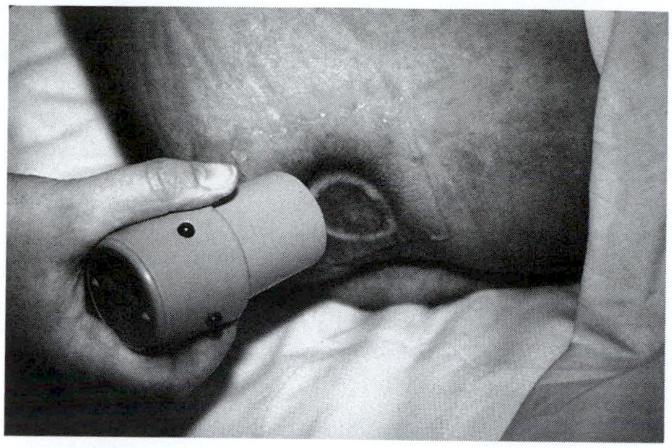

Figure 17.20 Application of ultrasound to wound and periwound tissues with hydrogel sheet coupling. (From Kloth, LC, and McCulloch, JM,[137] Plate 15, with permission.)

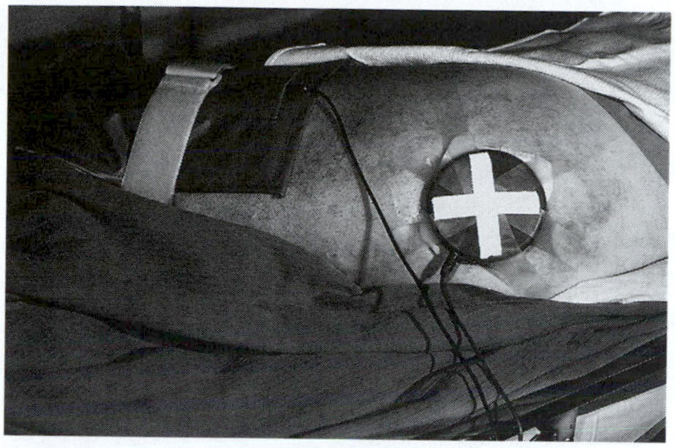

Figure 17.21 Electrical stimulation direct [one electrode (+) on wound] electrode placement method. (From Kloth, LC, and McCulloch, JM,[137] Plate 48, with permission.)

procedure for the treatment is to cover the wound with a sheet of hydrogel, or an application of amorphous hydrogel. US is then delivered with a hand-held applicator (Fig. 17.20). Another option for treatment is to apply US transmission gel to the periwound area and treat from this region in addition to or instead of the wound bed.[139–144]

Electrical Stimulation

The use of electrical stimulation (ES) to treat chronic, and more recently, acute wounds is well documented. ES is recommended to eliminate bacterial load, promote granulation, decrease inflammation, reduce edema, reduce wound-related pain, and augment blood flow. Human skin, wounds, and the cells that facilitate wound healing all have measurable electrical currents.[145] ES affects various types of cells and their activities by supporting, altering, or providing electrical currents to accelerate wound healing. A clear understanding of medical electricity will assist the clinician in applying an appropriate ES treatment. The available literature is diverse and instructive.[146–153] There are a variety of options for treatment setup depending on the goals of treatment, the type of wound, and the condition of the patient. Standard equipment for the direct method of application will include an ES unit, treatment and nontreatment electrodes, and a substance such as saline soaked gauze or a hydrogel dressing applied to the wound bed or cavity to enhance electrical conductivity under the treatment electrode (Fig. 17.21). For the indirect method, electrodes straddle the wound and interface with the periwound skin using gel electrodes. Clinical decisions related to voltage, electrode placement, dosage, and other variables must be made on a case-by-case basis. Information about treatment protocols, strength of evidence, and guidelines for treatment can be found in detailed wound care texts.[154,155]

Thermal and Nonthermal Diathermy

Pulsed short wave diathermy (PSWD), continuous shortwave diathermy (CSWD), and pulsed radiofrequency stimulation (PRFS) have been used successfully to treat chronic open wounds, facilitating progress from one phase of wound healing to the next. These diathermy treatments utilize radio waves to provide thermal and nonthermal effects respectively. All transmit radiation from an applicator head to the target tissues. PSWD heats superficial and deep tissues. CSWD heats deep muscle and joint tissues. PRFS can influence tissue at the cellular level. Wound sites treated with diathermy have demonstrated increased fibroblast proliferation, collagen formation, tissue perfusion, and metabolic rate. While the number of clinical studies is smaller than that of other modalities, the evidence is mounting for the role diathermy plays in wound healing. The clinical use of these modalities has increased since the publication of a number of studies regarding the nonthermal effects of pulsed diathermy and the production of smaller treatment units for clinical use.[156–158] Equipment needed for treatment includes a diathermy unit/electronic console, and one or two applicator heads. Treatment is usually delivered without touching the skin. Wounds should be carefully prepared before treatment according to guidelines. With newer units such as the Provant unit pictured in Figure 17.22, the pad can be placed over wound dressings, compression gar-

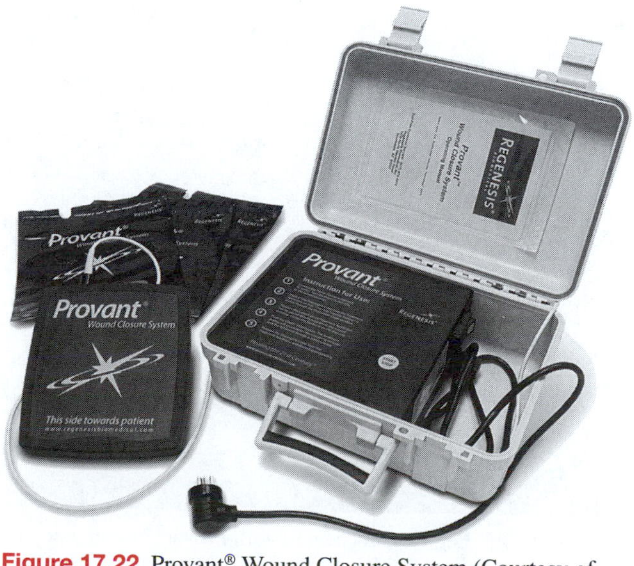

Figure 17.22 Provant® Wound Closure System (Courtesy of Regenesis® Biomedical Inc., Scottsdale, AZ 85257.)

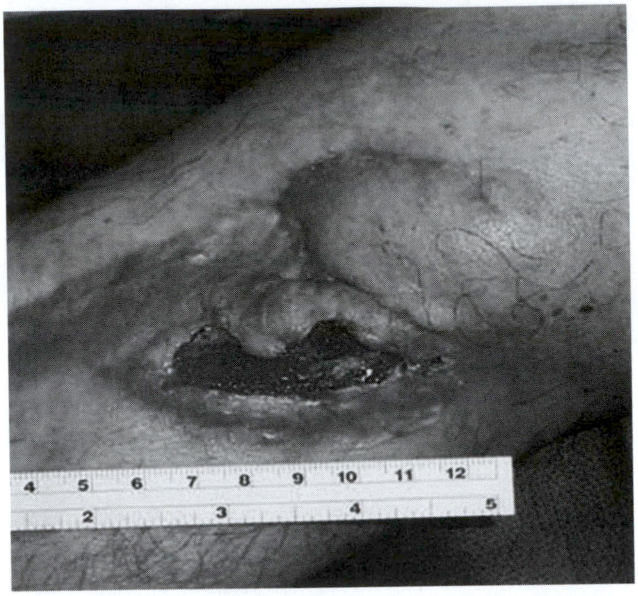

Figure 17.23 Wound being treated with Provant® radiofrequency stimulus. (Courtesy of Regenesis® Biomedical Inc, Scottsdale, AZ 85257.)

ments, and casts. Because the effects of heat may continue after the treatment, patients should be observed carefully and protocol guidelines should be followed closely. Figure 17.23 presents a wound currently under treatment with the Provant unit; Figure 17.24 depicts the Provant treatment pad in place over a leg wound.

Ultraviolet Radiation

Ultraviolet radiation (UV) energy is a form of radiation between X-ray and visible light on the electromagnetic spectrum.[159] UV wavelengths have been divided into wavelengths and bands. The three bands most useful for their effects on human skin are UVA, UVB, and UVC. UV has cutaneous and bactericidal effects that include increased blood flow, enhanced granulation tissue formation, destruction of bacteria, stimulation of vitamin D production, and thickening of the stratum corneum. The effects of UV radiation on antibiotic-resistant bacteria make it a useful tool in wound care.[160–163] UVC in particular has been found effective in the treatment of methicillin-resistant *Staphylococcus aureus* (MRSA).[164] The treatment is typically delivered to a clean wound with dressings removed, using a UVB or UVC lamp (Fig. 17.25). Treatment distance and dosage, frequency, and subsequent clinical outcomes will vary based on the goals of the treatment and the status of the wound. The varied physiological effects make this treatment appropriate for a variety of skin diseases as well as acute and chronic wounds.[139,165,166]

Hyperbaric Oxygen Therapy

Hyperbaric oxygen therapy (HBO) delivers 100 percent oxygen to an individual resting inside a sealed chamber. The oxygen is delivered at a pressure greater than the atmosphere. This *systemic* treatment increases the amount of oxygen available for cell metabolism, improving oxygen delivery to hypoxic tissue. Systemic HBO is, however, associated with risks related to oxygen toxicity. The literature demonstrates positive responses to this treatment when used as an adjunct to other forms of wound care but few controlled, randomized trials have been completed.[139,167–171] Chambers to deliver *topical* oxygen have been available for at least a decade. Discussion among investigators comparing the effects of systemic versus topical oxygen is ongoing. In some studies, topical oxygen is also referred to as *topical hyperbaric oxygen (THBO)*, and *O_2 therapy*.[12,172,174] Instead of the full body chamber used for HBO, THBO is delivered in a localized

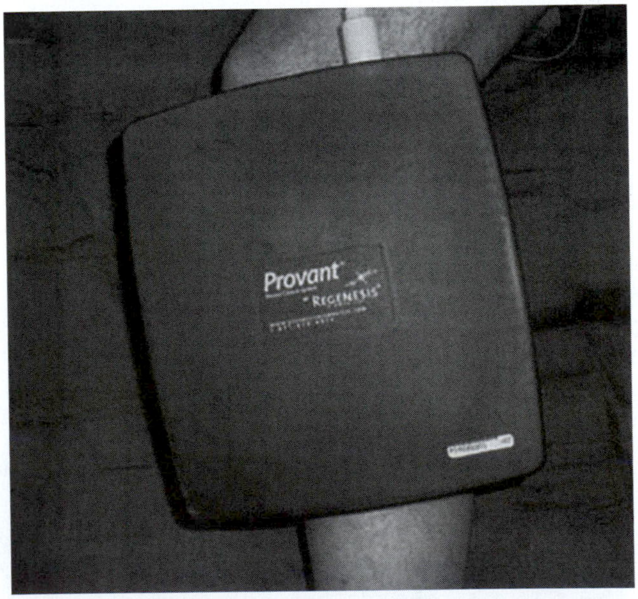

Figure 17.24 Leg wound covered with Provant® treatment pad. (Courtesy of Regenesis® Biomedical Inc, Scottsdale, AZ 85257.)

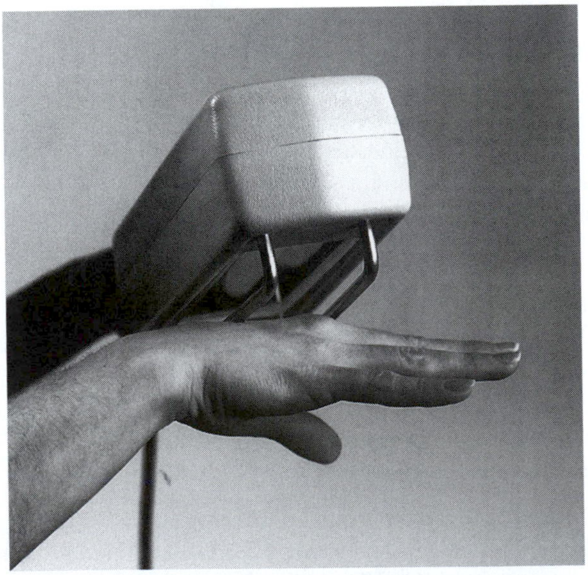

Figure 17.25 Application of ultraviolet light treatment using Dermawand™. (Courtesy of National Biological Corporation, Twinsburg, OH 44087.)

limb chamber. Using THBO, oxygen is delivered directly to the surface of a wound through a portable unit large enough to enclose a limb or the sacral area.[12,172] THBO has been combined with electrical stimulation and also with cold laser for the treatment of pressure ulcers and neuropathic foot wounds.[173,174] Topical O_2 therapy has enhanced the effects of growth factors in investigations within the last few years.[10] Renewed interest by investigators has lead to more refined protocols and improved strength of evidence in the field. If investigations continue to provide positive results, the use of topical O_2 in wound care could result in more cost-effective and efficient care, fewer risks and applicability to a wider population as compared to systemic O_2.

Thermotherapy (Radiant Heat)

The process of warming wounds to promote healing is an important part of wound care intervention. Owing to their location, the type of treatment used and/or the loss of skin protection, most wounds are *hypothermic* (below core body temperature). It is not surprising that wounds heal more efficiently if they are *normothermic* (normal body temperature).[70,175] While reaching normothermia can be accomplished in a number of ways, the Warm-Up Wound Therapy System™ (Arizant, Inc, Eden Prairie, MN 55344) may be the most efficient way to deliver warmth to chronic wounds (Fig. 17.26). Controlled, moist heat is delivered through a noncontact, semiocclusive dressing. A small warming card is placed into a special sleeve on top of the sterile wound cover so that radiant warmth can be delivered to the wound bed. The card warms to 100.4°F (38°C). An additional dressing is not needed since the wound cover edges are absorbent and the top is clear for viewing the wound. The wound cover can be utilized just as semiocclusive dressings are used for moist wound healing and can be left in place for up to 72 hours or until the absorbent edge of the cover becomes saturated.[139,175–179] Although formerly marketed in North America and still being used here, availability is now limited. These devices, however, are successfully utilized and marketed in Europe.

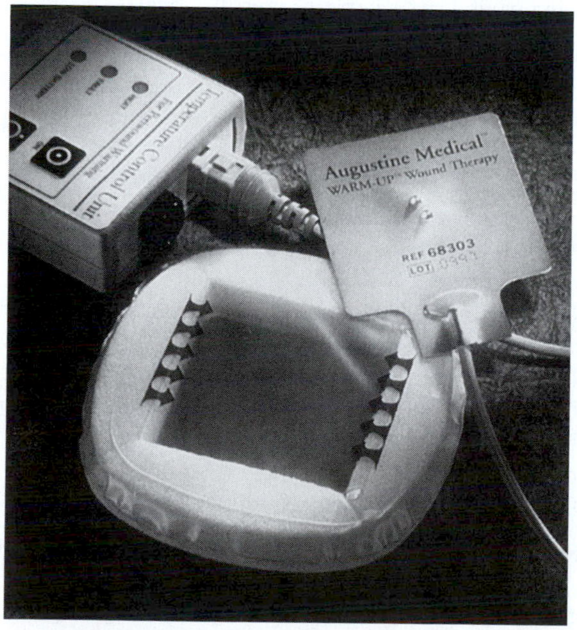

Figure 17.26 Warm-Up™ radiant heating unit. (Courtesy of Arizant Inc, Eden Prairie, MN 55344.)

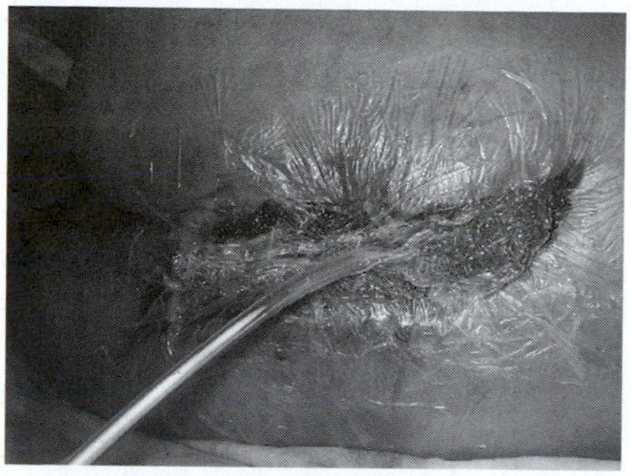

Figure 17.27 A stage IV sacral pressure ulcer with reticulated foam dressing, tubing, and polyurethane sheet covering the entire wound to maintain the vacuum during treatment with vacuum assisted closure. (From Kloth, LC, and McCulloch, JM,[137] Plate 14, with permission.)

Negative Pressure Wound Therapy

Negative pressure wound therapy (NPWT) is used as an adjunct to wound healing to facilitate wound closure in acute surgical wounds as well as with more challenging, slow-to-heal wounds. *Vacuum-assisted closure* or *VAC®* is the name of the device used to provide the negative pressure treatment (Kinetic Concepts, Inc, San Antonio, TX 78230). An open cell foam dressing is placed in the wound and a suction tube is connected from the foam to a portable pump. An airtight seal is created over the foam and the suction tube with a clear, occlusive film (Fig. 17.27). A controlled amount of negative (subatmospheric) pressure is applied through the foam to the entire wound bed. Typically, for the first few days (48 hours) the negative pressure is applied continuously via the portable pump system. After a significant amount of excess wound fluid has been withdrawn, the pump is programmed to apply pressure intermittently. The foam dressing is changed every 12 hours (infected wounds) to 48 hours or longer (clean wounds). The strength of evidence is mounting as basic research explores the effects of this treatment. NPWT has been shown, in some studies, to enhance granulation tissue formation, promote wound edge approximation, remove edema from wounds, and improve oxygen levels in the wound.[180–184] One claim that is still under investigation is the ability of the VAC to remove bacteria from the wound bed. According to Weed et al, the use of the VAC may actually increase the bacterial bio-burden but this fact did not negate the beneficial effects of the treatment in their study.[43] Although this type of therapy must be ordered by a physician, many are unaware of this intervention and would be responsive to an appropriate recommendation by the therapist. In different environments, administration of the technique may be performed by therapists, nurses, or other clinical staff.

Cold Laser Therapy

Cold laser is also referred to in the literature as low-level cold laser, low-level infrared laser, or monochromatic infrared photo energy (MIRE). Low-energy laser treatment uses light in the infrared spectrum. This therapy has been promoted for augmenting wound healing[185] and reversing the symptoms of peripheral neuropathy in individuals with diabetes.[186,187] It is thought that the effects of laser increase circulation and reduce pain by increasing the release of nitric oxide into the microcirculation. While supportive, peer-reviewed literature is modest at this point, published studies citing success with this treatment are mounting.[188–191] Owing to the perceived lack of adequate evidence, some third party payers do not cover treatment except when used as a heat modality. This may soon change as the strength of evidence increases. The most well known product on the market is called Anodyne Therapy System (Fig. 17.28). (Anodyne Therapy, LLC, Tampa, FL 33626). Figure 17.29 depicts use of a special foot pad to deliver infrared photo energy.

Dressings

The type of wound dressings selected for a wound may have a profound effect on healing time. There are hundreds of choices for the discerning clinician. Information on indications, contraindications, and expected outcomes can be obtained from individual vendors listed in Appendix G, as well as from texts devoted entirely to wound care.[154,155] This chapter includes introductory information

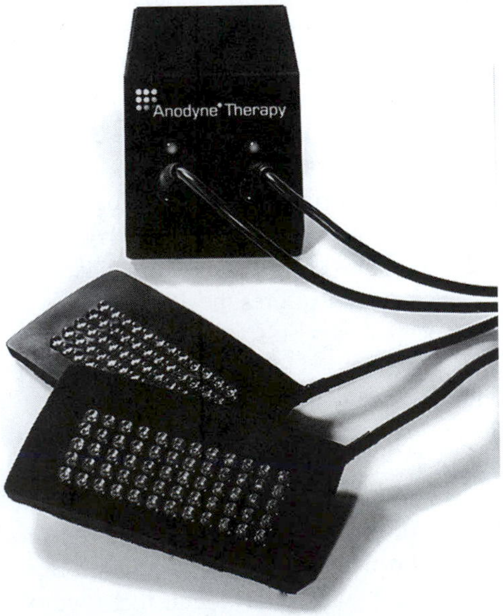

Figure 17.28 Anodyne® System Home Unit with two pads. (Courtesy of Anodyne Therapy, LLC, Tampa, FL 33626.)

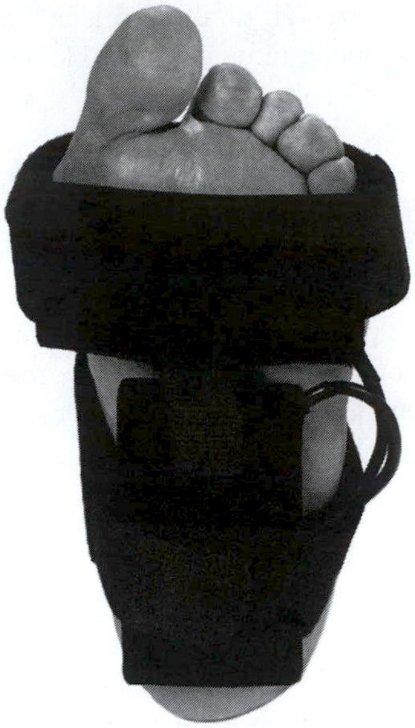

Figure 17.29 Application of infrared photo energy to the foot using an Anodyne® Therapy foot pad. (Courtesy of Anodyne Therapy, LLC, Tampa, FL 33626.)

necessary to make clinical decisions about dressings: the characteristics of the dressing categories and the effects of the dressings on the wound bed. Refer to Appendix H for a listing of dressings categorized by treatment goal (purpose) or type of wound (indication).

Choosing appropriate dressings should be directed by the characteristics of the wound and periwound tissues, not by what is available in the supply closet. A product that preserves wound hydration and limits fluid loss is usually ideal. In addition to following the principles of moist wound healing in most dressing selections, the following wound characteristics must be considered:

- Infection: absent or present; prevent or treat
- Necrosis: remove or not; autolytic or mechanical
- Drainage: dry, adequate or excessive; restore, retain or remove
- Granulation tissue: present or absent; protect, facilitate or slow down formation
- Epithelialization: present or absent; facilitate or slow down formation
- Periwound area: intact, at risk or macerated; protect or treat
- Incontinence: present or absent; protect or monitor
- Cavities and tunneling: present or absent; fill or prevent
- Friction: present, some risk, significant risk; cushion, protect or prevent
- Odor: minimal or need reduction; ignore or add odor reducing dressings

The dressing that is applied directly to the wound is referred to as the *primary* dressing. The dressing that is applied over the primary dressing is referred to as the *secondary* dressing. Some advanced dressings serve as the

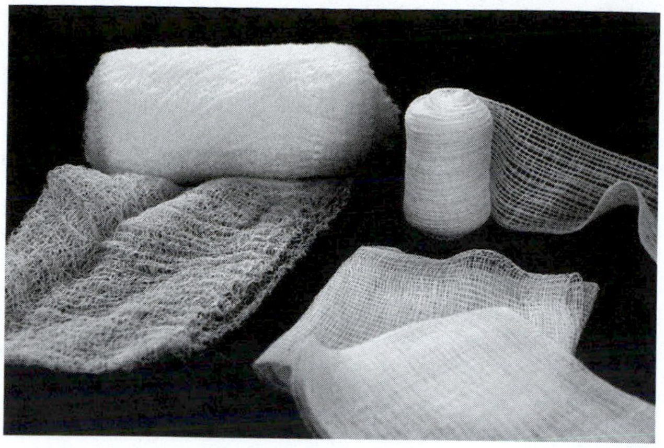

Figure 17.30 Samples of gauze dressings.

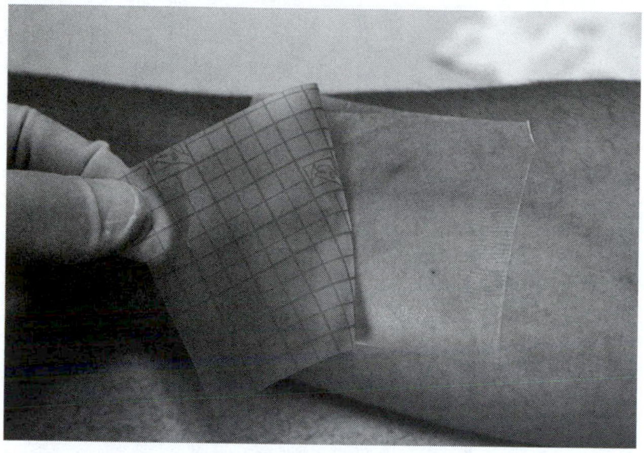

Figure 17.31 Application of a film dressing.

primary and secondary, including adhesive and absorptive qualities in the same dressing.

Gauze/Fiber

Gauze dressings (Fig. 17.30) are considered by many wound management experts to be outside the description of modern wound dressings. Used and misused for decades, there are more reasons not to use gauze than there are indications for use. As a primary dressing, gauze leaves contaminating fibers in the wound, contributes to desiccation, is permeable to bacteria, can be adherent to the wound, releases excessive amounts of bacteria into the air upon removal, and causes pain upon removal if it adheres to the wound surface. Once thought to be cost effective, it has been shown in more than one study, to be more costly than other dressing choices. (See Evidence Summary Box 17.1.) Gauze ribbon can be used to maintain an opening for drainage in a tunneling wound. It can also be used successfully to gently support a cavity wound but should not be used to aggressively pack any shape of wound. It was once thought that cavity wounds should be packed very full but it has since been established that granulation tissue and epithelial cells do not survive well with aggressive gauze packing. The additional pressure from a tightly packed wound will impede the flow of oxygen and nutrients to the granulating wound bed. Gauze can be an effective secondary dressing, especially if the dressings will be changed frequently or if exudate is heavy. Gauze 4 × 4s and a roll of gauze are typically used to create a WTD dressing. Because WTD dressings can be classified as a tool for mechanical débridement or as a primary wound dressing, they are discussed in both categories.

Impregnated Gauze

Designed to be less adherent, this category includes products made of tightly meshed synthetic fibers or woven products such as cellulose acetate. Fiber materials are impregnated with a petroleum emulsion such as Vaseline®, intended to prevent the gauze from sticking to the wound surface. Used as a primary dressing this choice is minimally absorptive, provides minimal protection, does not enhance a moist environment, and may create a greasy wound bed.

Transparent Films

Films are made of a transparent membrane with an acrylic adhesive layer (Fig. 17.31). Transparent films do not allow bacteria or moisture into the wound. Currently, few films have absorptive qualities and cannot be used on highly exuding wounds. They facilitate a moist wound environment, trapping endogenous fluids in the wound bed to assist with autolytic débridement, wound bed homeostasis, and *angiogenesis*. Films assist in protecting skin from the effects of shearing, friction, and the contaminating effects of incontinence. Removal, however, can cause skin tears especially with frail or aging skin.

Foam

Foams are highly absorbent pads, sheets, or packing of polyurethane available in many sizes with many features (Fig. 17.32). They are available with or without adhesive backing so that they can be used as a primary and/or a secondary dressing. They are highly absorptive but also help to create an occlusive environment for moist wound

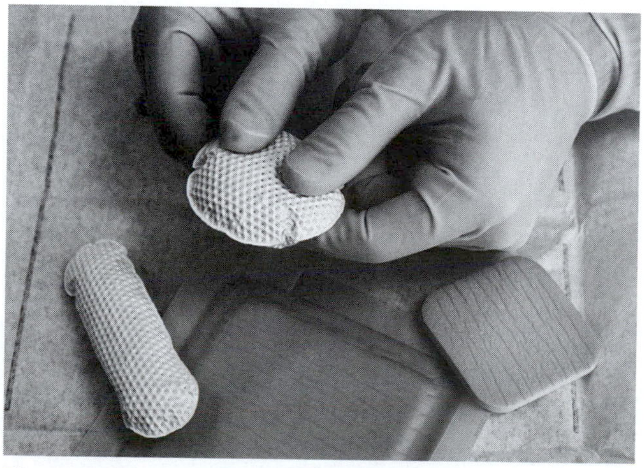

Figure 17.32 Samples of foam dressings.

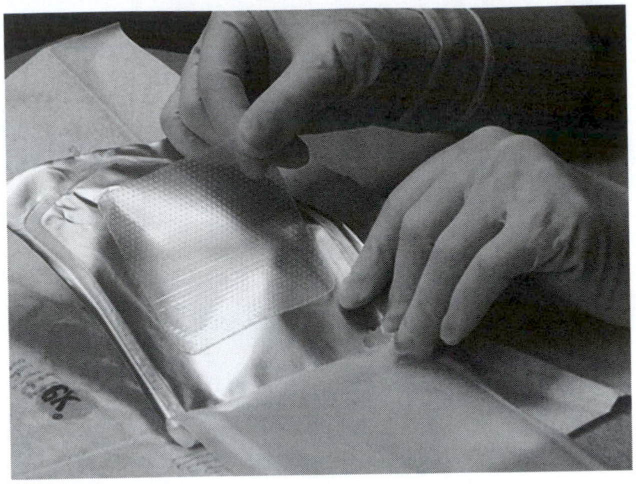

Figure 17.33 Sample of a hydrogel sheet dressing.

healing. They should not be used alone on a dry wound but could serve as a secondary dressing if the primary dressing was a gel product.

Hydrogels

Hydrogels are categorized as *amorphous,* referring to a liquid-like gel or as *sheets,* consisting of a thin, flexible sheet of polymer containing at least 90 percent water (Fig. 17.33). Both types are used to increase moisture in a dry wound bed, soften necrotic tissue and support autolytic débridement. Both have some absorptive qualities and will swell slightly until they are saturated. The amorphous gel (Fig. 17.34) must be contained in the wound with a secondary dressing. The flexible sheets usually require a secondary dressing but are available through some vendors with tape attached to the borders. Patient response is usually very positive to the soothing sensation of the hydrogel application.

Hydrocolloids

Considered the most occlusive of the moisture-retentive dressings, hydrocolloids are also available in less occlusive or semipermeable styles as well. As with foams, these

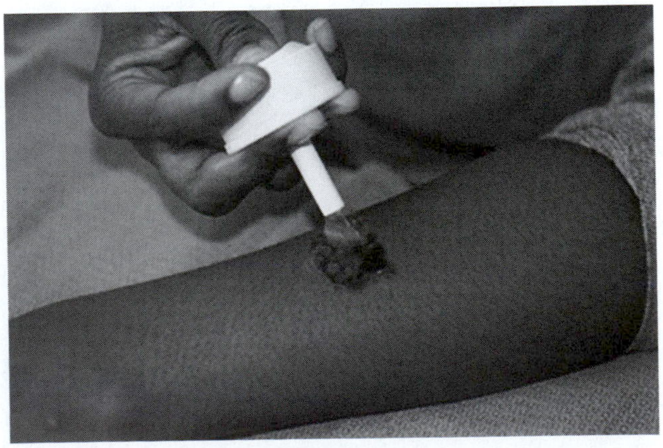

Figure 17.34 Application of a gel dressing.

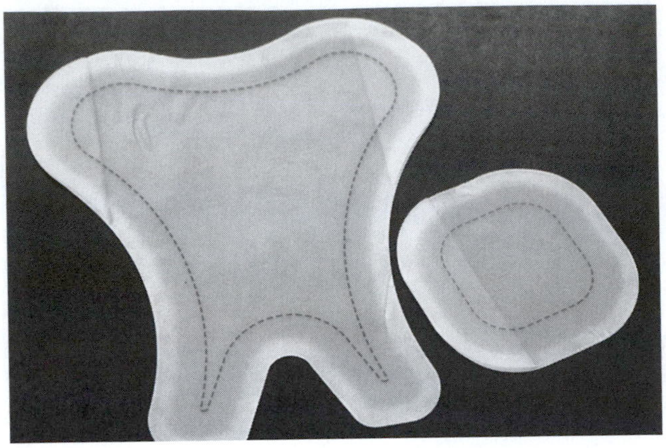

Figure 17.35 Samples of hydrocolloid dressings.

dressings come in a variety of styles and shapes including pastes, granules, powder, and sheets. They typically consist of an absorbent colloidal material combined with a film or foam backing (Fig. 17.35). They work best on mild to moderate exudating wounds. When wound exudates combine with the colloidal polymer, a soft, gelatinous, often yellow, and malodorous mass is formed. Patients, families, caregivers, and other health care providers must be informed about this harmless reaction so that infection is not assumed. Hydrocolloids have been used successfully as occlusive dressings over infected wounds without fulmination of existing bacteria.

Alginates

This dressing category is also known as *calcium alginate* because the dressings are manufactured using the calcium salts of alginic acid derived from marine algae and kelp (seaweed). The raw material is woven and then converted into flat sheets, ropes, or ribbon shapes (Fig. 17.36). Alginates absorb 20 to 30 times their own weight, are gentle to apply and remove, and biocompatible with the wound bed. A chemical reaction between the dressing and wound

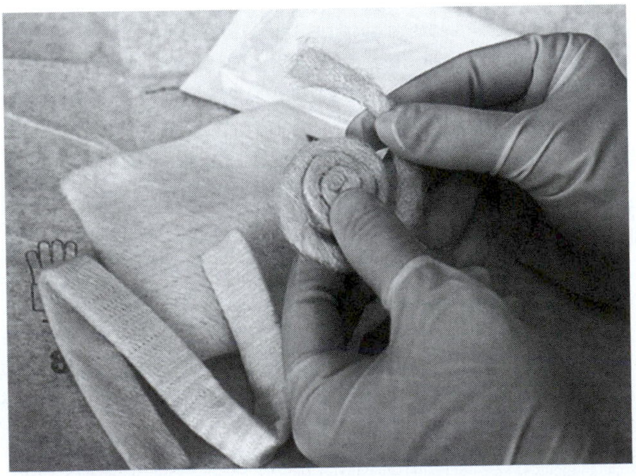

Figure 17.36 Samples of alginate dressings.

Table 17.3 Examples of Skin Substitutes

Product Name Manufacturer	Source of Skin Cells/ Product Ingredient	Type of Wound
Apligraftneonatal Novartis Pharma AG	Male foreskin	Venous leg ulcers
Dermagraft Smith & Nephew	Neonatal male foreskin	Chronic diabetic foot ulcers
Integracollagen Johnson & Johnson	Matrix with silicon layer	Dermal regeneration for treatment of severe burns
Transcyteneonatal Smith & Nephew	Fibroblast cells plus porcine dermal collagen	Full-thickness and partial-thickness burns
Oasis Cook Medical	Porcine-based product	Classified as an exotic dressing, not skin substitute, diabetic foot ulcers
Biobrane II Bertek Pharmaceuticals	Porcine-based product silicon bonded to nylon	Partial-thickness burn wounds

exudate creates a gel substance that helps to maintain a moist wound environment while absorbing excess exudates. Because they are permeable, alginates do not provide a barrier against bacteria. Conversely, this characteristic makes them an effective choice when an infected wound cannot be covered with an occlusive dressing. Most alginates currently require a secondary dressing to hold them in place. Several manufacturers are combining alginates with other products, such as hydrocolloids, to maximize their effectiveness. There is growing interest in the use of silver in advanced dressings to combine the antimicrobial action of silver with the absorptive qualities of alginates. An example of this type of dressing is SILVERCEL® (Johnson & Johnson Wound Management, ETHICON, Inc, Somerville, NJ 08876).

Skin Substitutes

Considered by some to be topical applications and by others to be dressings, human skin equivalents, and bioengineered tissues are finding their place in the wound care arena. Created using a variety of techniques and substances, living skin applications resemble skin structure and function and may include epidermal and dermal layers. Skin substitutes are of human origin or bioengineered tissue. They are useful as temporary coverage, providing skin protection for the wound bed. Some have been shown to stimulate endogenous cell activity. Most are marketed to use on wounds that have not responded to conventional therapy or for burn care. Selected examples of product names, their source of skin cells, and the type of wound they are used to treat are found in Table 17.3.

Innovative Dressings

New products are entering the market yearly as research and development continue to grow and expand in the area of wound care. Too many to mention all, categories include options such as polysaccharide dressings, absorptive fillers, hydrophilic fiber, composite dressings, collagen, and biological products. Examples of products gaining attention are:

- Hydroactive dressings are designed to have a selective absorptive capacity. They have the combined positive characteristics of foam and gel dressings. Their properties allow growth factors and other peptides to survive on the wound bed. Aquacel® (ConvaTec, Princeton, NJ 08543) is a spun Hydrofiber® dressing that readily absorbs moisture (Fig. 17.37). Aquacel® Ag adds ionic silver to the absorbent dressing.
- Flexible film dressings made with chitin, a natural material found in the extracellular macromolecules of the body.[192]
- Hyalofill-F® (ConvaTec, Princeton, NJ 08543) is a hyaluronic acid derivative dressing that is applied directly to the wound. First used most on neuropathic foot ulcers, it has been used successfully in a clinical trial for venous leg ulcers.[193]

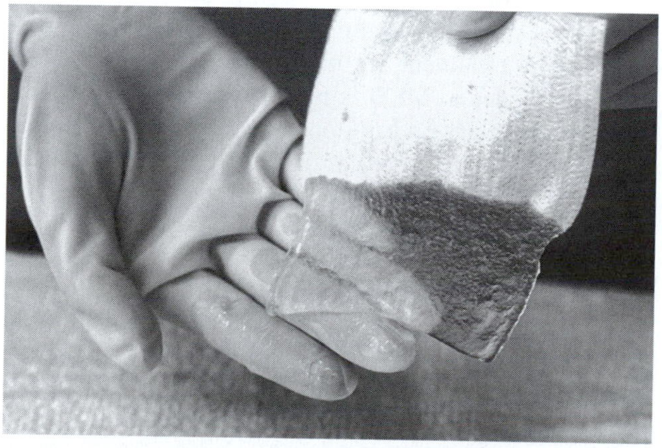

Figure 17.37 Sample of AQUACEL®, a Hydrofiber® dressing simulating the change in consistency from dry to gel as wound drainage is absorbed.

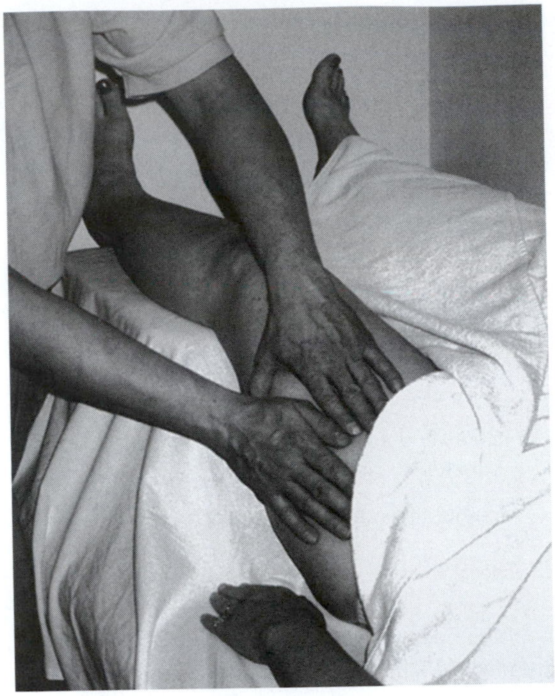

Figure 17.38 Manual lymphatic drainage to the LE. (Courtesy of Klose Training & Consulting, LLC, Red Bank, NJ 07701.)

Manual Lymphatic Drainage

Manual lymph drainage (MLD) is a specialized manual therapy technique that affects primarily superficial lymphatic circulation. It is considered to be one of the five elements of an effective treatment intervention for lymphedema and many types of edema. MLD will increase the frequency of lymphangion contractions, improve lymph transport capacity, redirect lymph flow toward collateral vessels, anastomoses, and uninvolved lymph regions and mobilize excess lymph fluid that has overwhelmed a body segment or region. The techniques of MLD are gentle and specific, requiring specialized education to be performed accurately (Fig. 17.38). Appendix A provides contact information for training facilities that provide specialized education in MLD and CDT. The benefits of this treatment are not limited to the population with lymphedema. MLD is used successfully for edema from sports injury and postoperative swelling. It is contraindicated for treating cardiac and pulmonary related edema.[2,194–196]

Compression Therapy

Controlling edema or lymphedema is critical to all types of healing. Edema not only inhibits wound healing by affecting perfusion of tissues, but also inactivates the ability of the skin to manage bacteria.[197] Unless there are red flags, compression should be part of every treatment for individuals with lymphedema, edema, and CVI. Compression therapy should be introduced as soon as clinical signs of swelling or fibrosis appear. When leg wounds are present, compression is essential for timely wound healing. For the individual with mixed arterial and venous disease, an ABI test is indicated to provide information about the safety of using compression on the LE. A greater understanding of how the lymphatic system functions has created a paradigm shift in the way intervention for all types of swelling is planned and delivered. Aggressive compression techniques were once used to "milk" the fluid out of a limb. It is now understood that deep pressure and mechanical "milking" techniques are counterproductive and harmful to the superficial capillary network that filters lymph and interstitial fluids.[4]

Elevation

Although elevation is not compression therapy, it is used as means of controlling some types of swelling and is often a precursor to compression. Mild, acute swelling of the extremities may be relieved temporarily with elevation. Active ROM exercises (e.g., ankle pumps) can be used to facilitate blood flow. Patients should be educated about how to elevate safely, paying attention to positioning so that optimal venous and lymphatic circulation is facilitated. Elevation should be viewed as a temporary or complementary measure while other means of controlling swelling are employed.

Unna's Boot

Compression for the LE with a venous wound can be applied using zinc paste impregnated gauze or Unna's boot (Fig. 17.39). Examples of conveniently packaged products are: Medicopaste (Graham-Field Inc, Bay Shore, NY 11706), Unna-Flex (Bristol-Myers Squibb, Princeton, NJ 08540), and Gelo-cast (BSN-JOBST, Charlotte, NC 28209). There is little information in the literature to support the topical application of zinc for wound healing. The success of this treatment application is most likely owing

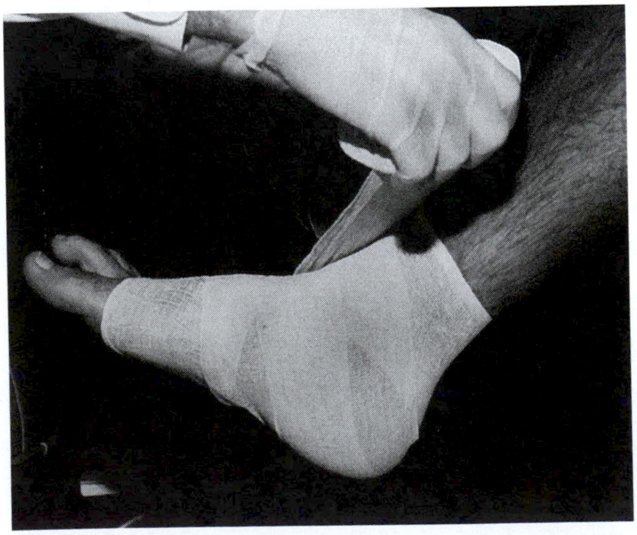

Figure 17.39 Unna's boot application.

to the compression. It is an inexpensive means of covering a wound, providing compression and supporting the calf pump to empty venous blood from the LE. Unna's boot is not appropriate for arterial or mixed arterial/venous ulcers. There may be more comfortable and efficient methods for treating venous wounds than with an Unna's boot.[198]

Four-Layer Bandage System

Four-layer bandage systems have been associated with excellent leg ulcer closure. They include a wound covering with modest absorptive qualities, and several layers of compression. The bandage system has been shown to be comfortable and cost-effective.[199] An example of a well known system is Profore (Fig. 17.40) (Smith & Nephew, Inc, Largo, FL 33773). For the appropriate patient, four-layer bandage systems can be left in place for up to a week.

Long-Stretch and Short-Stretch Bandages

Both long- and short-stretch bandages are utilized to control edema and supply therapeutic levels of compression to support the venous and lymphatic systems. Long-stretch bandages such as Ace® bandages provide a *high resting pressure,* which means that they continue to constrict when the wearer is resting. Owing to their extensibility or stretchiness, they do not provide significant *working pressure,* the ability to resist muscle contraction during activity. Long stretch bandages are readily available and require little training to apply. Short-stretch bandages such as Comprilan® and Rosidal® provide *low resting pressure* and *high working pressure* (Fig. 17.41). They are less extensible or stretchy, providing a more rigid shell when applied to a limb. This feature makes short stretch bandages more appropriate for treating edema and lymphedema. Higher working pressures increase the efficiency of the muscle pump during activity while lower resting pressures make the bandages more tolerable to wear. Short-stretch bandages require special training to apply. The number of layers of bandage, the age and condition of the bandages, the tension on the bandage when it is applied, and the skill of the clinician will all influence the amount of working and resting pressure delivered to the limb.

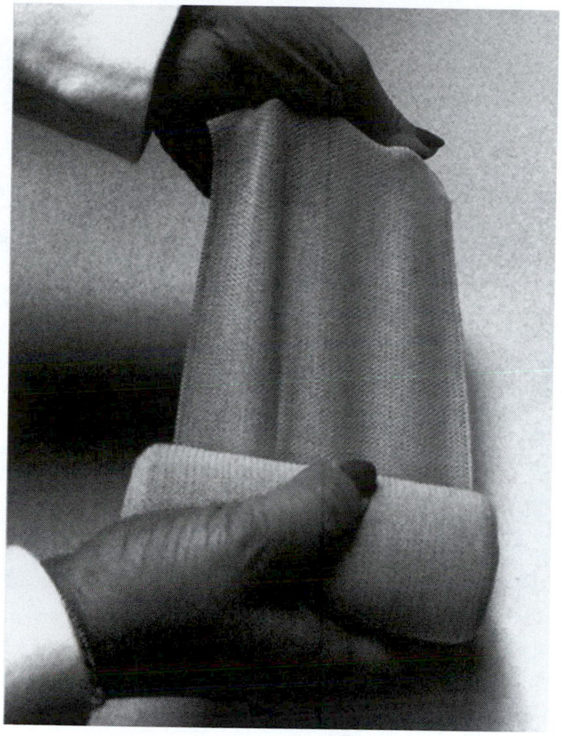

Figure 17.41 Sample of short stretch bandage.

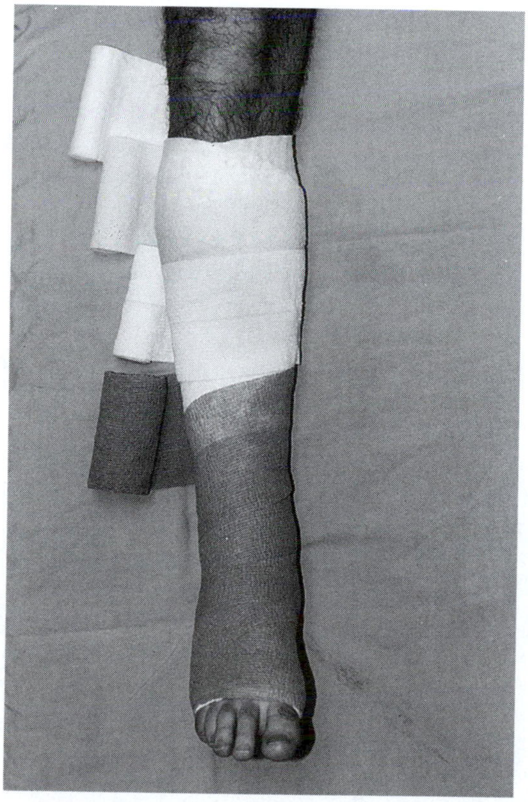

Figure 17.40 Profore™ is a four layer bandage system consisting of a cotton, crepe, and two compression layers (top to bottom).

Lymphedema Bandaging

This highly specialized form of bandaging utilizes multiple layers of unique padding materials and short stretch bandages to create a supportive structure for edematous and lymphedematous body segments. Lymphedema bandaging provides support for tissues that have lost elasticity, facilitates a mild increase in tissue pressure, assisting lymph vessels to empty, prevents refilling of the interstitium between MLD treatments, improves the efficiency of the muscle pump during activity and provides localized pressure where indicated to soften fibrotic tissue.

Bandaging protocols include techniques for applying compression to the head and neck, fingers, and hands

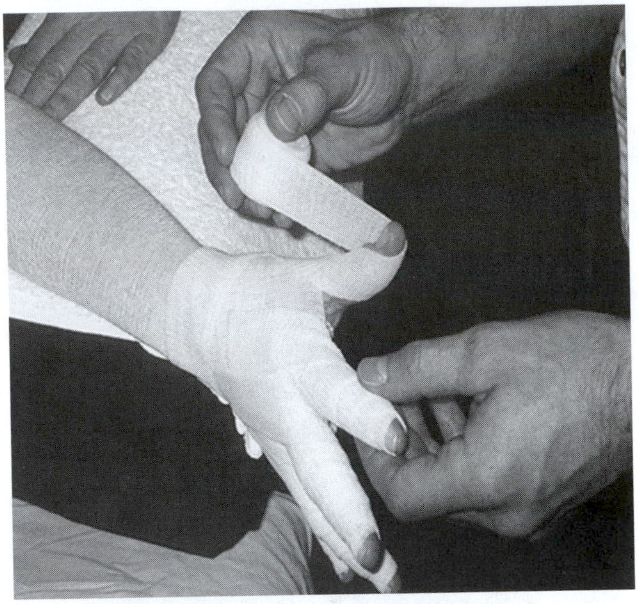

Figure 17.42 Application of lymphedema bandaging to fingers and hand. (Courtesy of Klose Training & Consulting, LLC, Red Bank, NJ 07701.)

(Fig. 17.42), UE (Fig. 17.43), and LE (Fig. 17.44). The chest, abdomen, genital area, and back can also receive specialized support from compression products. As with MLD, the benefits of this treatment are not limited to the population with lymphedema. When compression is indicated, standard or modified lymphedema bandaging can be beneficial to the population with edema (e.g., postoperative, CVI, venous ulcers, orthopedic injury).[195,196, 200–205]

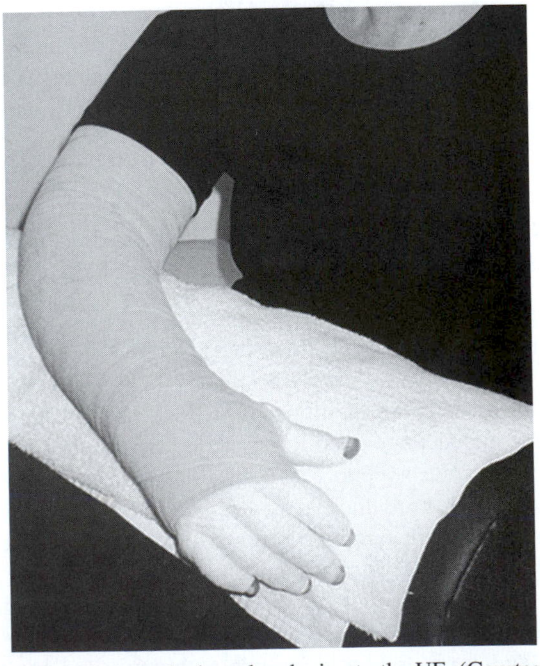

Figure 17.43 Lymphedema bandaging to the UE. (Courtesy of Klose Training & Consulting, LLC, Red Bank, NJ 07701.)

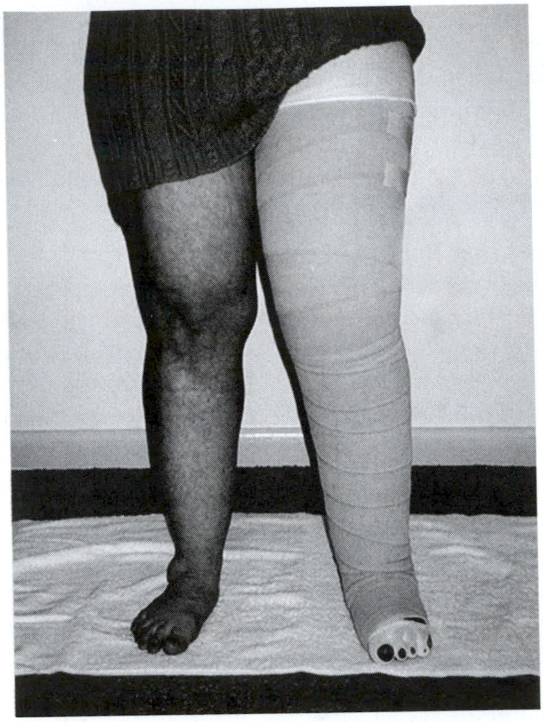

Figure 17.44 Lymphedema bandaging to the LE. (Courtesy of Klose Training & Consulting, LLC, Red Bank, NJ 07701.)

Compression Garments

Compression garments are utilized by many patient/client populations (Fig. 17.45). Originally designed to assist venous blood flow in the LEs, they are now specifically designed to manage burn and surgical scars, provide support to venous circulation, and to prevent reaccumulation of fluid in the lymph-edematous limb. There are a variety of design styles and fabrics, custom and off-the-shelf, garments to meet the unique needs of different populations. When appropriately selected and fitted by a trained professional and worn correctly by a prepared patient, the garments serve an essential role in managing chronic, life-long conditions such as CVI and lymphedema (Fig. 17.46).[205] Garments should not be used as a treatment to remove excess fluids

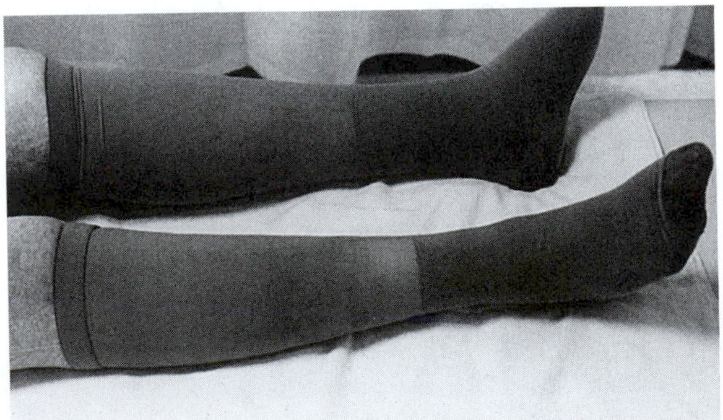

Figure 17.45 Patient wearing custom fitted compression garments.

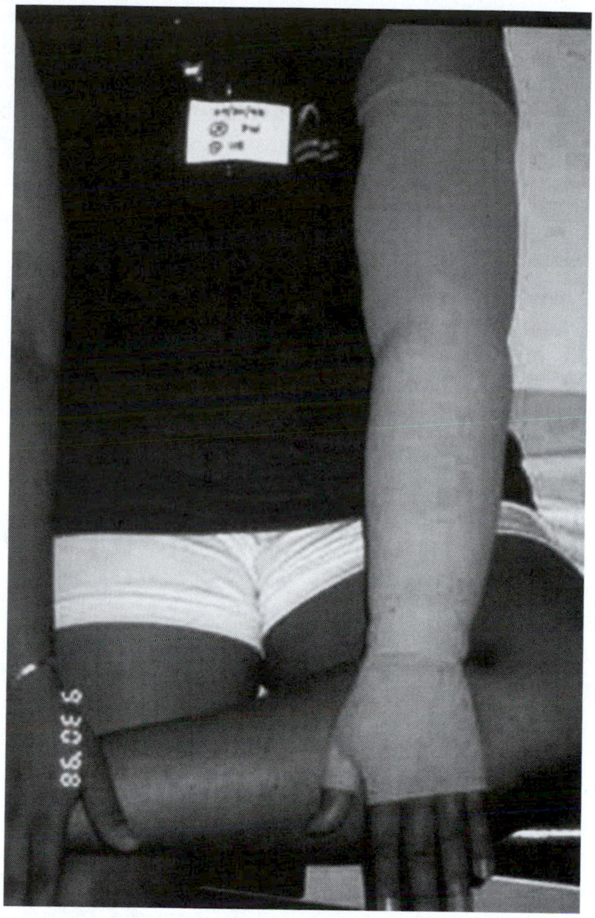

Figure 17.46 Patient wearing custom fitted compression garment after reduction of swelling from lymphedema.

from an extremity. Applied to an extremity that has not been adequately evacuated, the garments will be uncomfortable and may worsen the patient's symptoms.[84,206–208] Currently manufacturers are participating in clinical research supporting the use of silver in compression garments. Juzo® Silver (Juzo®, Cuyahoga Falls, OH 44223) adds permanently bonded silver to the textile fiber of LE garments to inhibit bacterial growth and reduce odor.

Another option for some individuals is a quilted garment that can provide compression and easy donning and doffing (Fig. 17.47). This option may be useful for a person who is unable to apply a more fitted support garment independently or whose skin is compromised or fragile. These specialized garments can be made to support venous circulation or lymphatic drainage by altering the style and the stitching channels. For added compression, they can be used with additional support wraps over them. If appropriate, shoes can be worn while in this type compression. An example of a specialized garment in this category is the ADVI (JoviPak®, Tri-D Corporation, Kent, WA 98032).

Compression treatment should be customized to the characteristics of each individual. To assist in clinical decision making, the following is a summary of general guidelines for compression bandaging and garments for edema and lymphedema:

- Arterial wounds: No compression or very light compression with close involvement of the referring practitioner. Long-stretch bandaging or off-the-shelf low compression garment (12 to 25 mm Hg) can be used. Edema will not be great and will evacuate quickly.
- Venous wounds: Compression is an essential component of treatment for wound healing and support of the venous system. Short-stretch bandaging with high working pressure and low resting pressure will facilitate the effects of calf pump during activity. High pressure of 40 mm Hg at the ankle has been suggested.[203]
- Neuropathic wounds: Compression is contingent on blood flow. Fifteen percent of these patients also have an arterial component to their disease and must have ABI checked before compression is applied. If no arterial involvement, compress with short-stretch wrap.
- Lymphedema: Short-stretch compression wrap until limb reduction goal reached then moderate to high compression garments at 20 to 30 mm Hg to 30 to 40 mm Hg depending on location and severity of swelling as well as ability of the patient to don and doff garments.
- Edema: Case studies and reports from the field establish that the compression treatment for lymphedema also works well for edema.[204] Short-stretch compression bandage is worn 23 hours/day, graduating to daytime only, decreasing as edema resolves.

Relative contraindications for compression should be evaluated including history of deep vein thrombosis, acute local infection, congestive heart failure, cor pulmonale, and acute dermatitis.

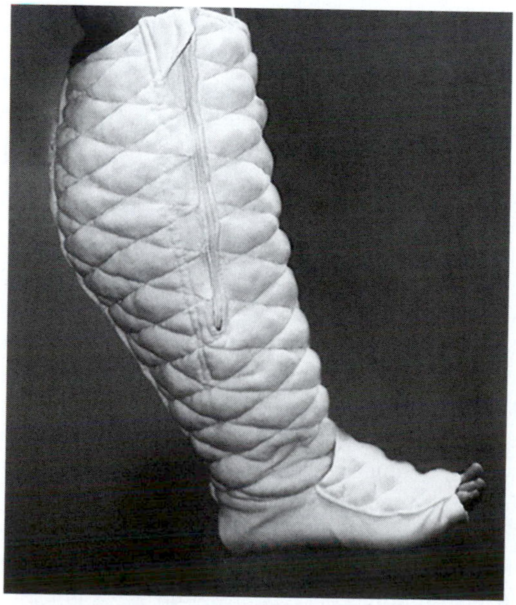

Figure 17.47 JoviPak® Quilted channel compression garment.

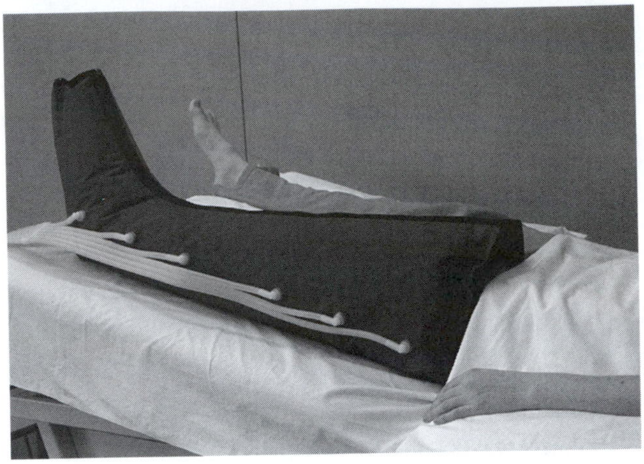

Figure 17.48 Intermittent pneumatic compression pump.

Pneumatic Pump

Until the 1990s, intermittent pneumatic compression (IPC) was one of the few clinical interventions utilized to treat swelling (Fig. 17.48). Since then, new information about the physiology of edema and lymphedema as well as lymphatic system function, has limited its value in treating some edema and most lymphedema. Intermittent compression pumps can facilitate venous return and may be an important adjunct to other forms of compression for the individual with a venous disorder.[3,209] A review of the evidence provided only modest support for the use of ICP for the treatment of venous leg ulcers.[210] Many individuals with long-standing venous insufficiency also have lymphedema. There is even less evidence and more controversy related to the use of ICP for lymphedema.[211–215] Each client should be carefully examine by an experienced health care professional before pneumatic compression is applied. Blood pressure readings should be taken before each treatment. Increasing total peripheral resistance with pneumatic compression will increase the work of the heart, increasing blood pressure. Individuals with hypertension or a blood pressure reading greater than 140/90 should not receive pneumatic compression treatment. Other contraindications to intermittent compression include acute inflammation or trauma, local infection, presence of thrombus, cardiac or kidney dysfunction, obstructed lymphatic channels, impaired cognitive function.

Positioning

Positioning techniques are used to prevent or support pressure ulcers as well as other types of wounds, edema, lymphedema, and vascular disorders. This important aspect of intervention, as well as PRDs, should not be overlooked or underestimated during treatment planning. Devices and techniques selected should be compatible with the individual's health status as well as the positioning needs of the individual. It is paramount that a personalized positioning and repositioning schedule be developed and prominently displayed for anyone who cannot position or reposition independently. The standard time intervals used for turning schedules (i.e., every 2 hours) are often too long for individuals who are frail, have fragile skin or existing wounds. A turning schedule could be as frequent as every 30 minutes in some cases. Suggestions for patient positioning programs include[216, 217]:

- The patient's heels should be protected and elevated off the surface of the bed.
- The head of bed should not be elevated past 30° unless medically necessary.
- An individualized turning schedule cycling from 30 to 120 minutes should be provided.
- PRDs should be used in conjunction with a turning schedule.
- Positioning with weightbearing directly over the greater trochanter should be avoided.
- Positioning with full weightbearing over an existing wound should be avoided.
- Donut-shaped devices for seating solutions should not be used.
- Pillows and wedges should be used to separate bony prominences from bed and other body parts.

Pressure-Relieving Devices

Pressure has a direct influence on perfusion or vascularity of a wound site. PRDs should be utilized to prevent skin breakdown, during the wound healing phase, and during the self-management phase, for life-long protection and prevention (Fig. 17.49). Along with positioning, patients must be educated about pressure relief and prevention of pressure-related trauma. Advances in pressure reducing support surfaces have made them more sophisticated and effective (Fig. 17.50). Experts in positioning systems are readily available to advise and instruct clinicians working with special populations. Groups such as The Consortium for Spinal Cord Medicine and the U.S. Department of Health and Human Services have made recommendations and algorithms for positioning and pressure relieving devices that can be utilized for intervention planning.[68,93,218,219] See Appendix F for information on Web sites for these agencies.

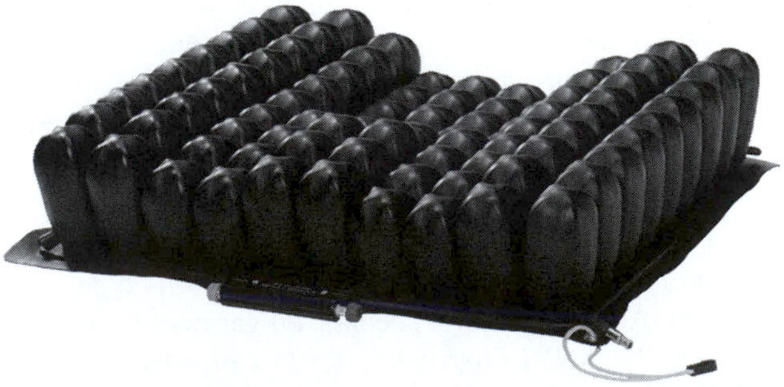

Figure 17.49 CONTOUR SELECT™, a cushion for pressure relief and skin protection. (Courtesy of ROHO, Belleville, IL 62221.)

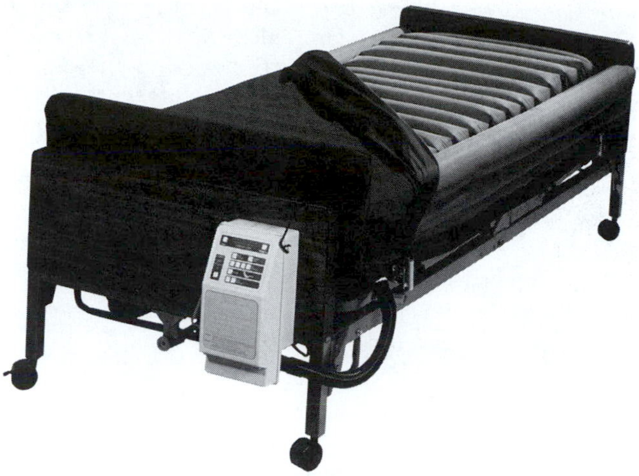

Figure 17.50 *Select*Air® MAX, a low air loss support system for pressure relief. (Courtesy of The ROHO Group, Belleville, IL 62221.)

Exercise

Too often, exercise is neglected in the intervention plan for individuals with vascular, lymphatic, and integumentary disorders, especially those with wounds or edema. The physical therapist should educate patients and promote activities in the POC related to increasing activity levels as appropriate. Exercise may be indicated for a variety of reasons including but not limited to: increase strength and joint ROM, improve quality of movement, increase ADL, improve QoL perceptions, increase blood flow to the extremities, improve calf pump activity, prevent pressure ulcers, and enhance the effects of lymphedema bandaging. Exercise might be contraindicated or planned with caution when medical issues arise such as the need to be nonweightbearing on a foot wound, unstable cardiopulmonary conditions, or related orthopedic problems that would limit activity.

Exercise prescription should be customized to the patient's needs and medical status. A walking program can benefit most individuals who are able to ambulate even short distances. Water-based exercise programs can facilitate the transition from bed or chair to land-based exercise. Individuals with wounds can participate in water-based exercise if it is appropriate to cover the wounds with occlusive dressings. The hydrostatic pressure of water contributes to support of edematous and lymphedematous body regions and creates an ideal setting for exercise for most individuals with swelling.

Orthotics

Splinting

Patients who are immobile may benefit from resting splints to retain, or dynamic splints to regain, functional ROM. Splinting can also prevent skin breakdown by retaining normal positioning of joints during periods of immobility. Extra precautions (i.e., padding) must be taken to protect aging or fragile skin from breakdown when semi-rigid thermoplastic materials are used for splinting. The use of splinting to manage burn scar is covered in Chapter 27. Positioning and splinting pointers found there can also be applied to patients with other types of wounds.

Total Contact Casting

One method for reduction of weightbearing stresses on the foot, is the application of a *total contact cast (TCC)*. This method can be useful for the individual with a neuropathic ulcer on the plantar surface of the foot. After infection and swelling have been controlled, a plaster cast is applied from the toes to below the knee. A specially trained individual uses plaster, padding techniques, and the placement of a rubber insert on the weightbearing part of the cast to complete the application. A total contact cast is usually worn for 7 to 10 days at a time, removed for skin care, and then reapplied. According to Salsich et al, TCC is effective at healing ulcers initially but the rate of reulceration once the cast is removed is high.[220]

Neuropathic Walker

A removable, ankle foot orthosis (AFO) can be custom fabricated or ordered prefabricated to provide weight distribution and cushioning for the individual with an insensate foot, a chronic foot ulcer, or Charcot joint (Fig. 17.51). This option is versatile in fit and allows skin checks, dressing changes, and pressure alterations as needed.

Cast Shoes

Cast shoes or postop shoes can be utilized as an inexpensive, temporary alternative for wound off-loading. These shoes do not provide any means of controlling foot motion and little cushioning protection for the chronic wound. This option should be considered temporary. Patients wearing cast shoes for pressure distribution should be monitored closely for signs of complications.

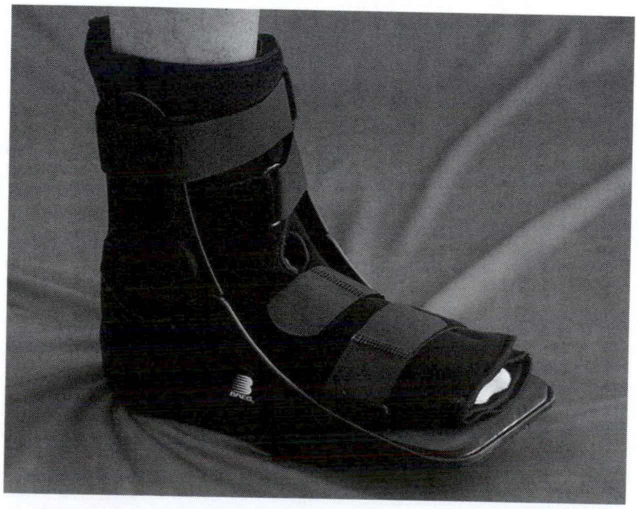

Figure 17.51 An ankle foot orthosis specifically designed to allow distributed weightbearing for individuals with neuropathy.

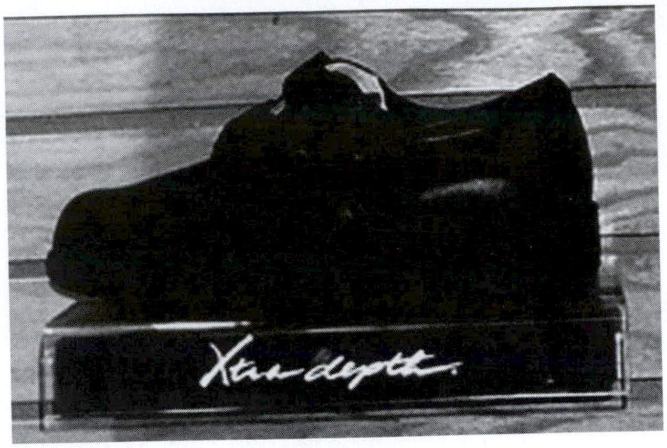

Figure 17.52 Extra-depth shoe.

Extra-Depth Shoes

Extra-depth shoes have features such as a roomy toe box and a deep sole to provide shock absorption and cushion. The shoes should redirect foot pressure away from bony prominences and wounds (Fig. 17.52).[221] Available in many styles, they can be purchased from an Orthotist or at a specialty shoe store. Individuals with insensate feet, with or without wounds, should strongly consider wearing this type of protective shoe to support the health of their feet.

Scar Management

As described earlier in this chapter, scar formation is a component of wound healing. After the wound is filled with collagen, the tissue must be remodeled, and shaped into the finely structured end product. Contraction of scar tissue can lead to disfigurement and loss of function especially if the scar tissue is located over a joint surface. Issues of disfigurement and dysfunction are greatest following thermal injury and are discussed in Chapter 27. Currently, the mechanisms by which scar can be controlled are not completely understood. While some interventions do seem to help, there is room for further investigation into how to have optimal control of scar formation. Most scar tissue is managed by a physical therapist using compression garments, stretching exercises, orthotics, positioning, specific types of massage, and the use of topical adjuncts such as silicone gel sheets (Fig. 17.53) and elastomer putty (Fig. 17.54). Topical creams, oils, and ointments have some positive effects on scar but it is not known if the massaging actions used to apply the agents or the agents themselves provide the therapeutic effects. Early and adequate intervention can prevent most of the complications of scarring. Since the process of scar formation usually continues for 6 to 24 months, follow-up care should be part of the intervention plan. When conservative measures of scar management have not controlled scarring, surgical intervention may be indicated. Following surgery, the individual will have a new wound and subsequent new scar to manage.

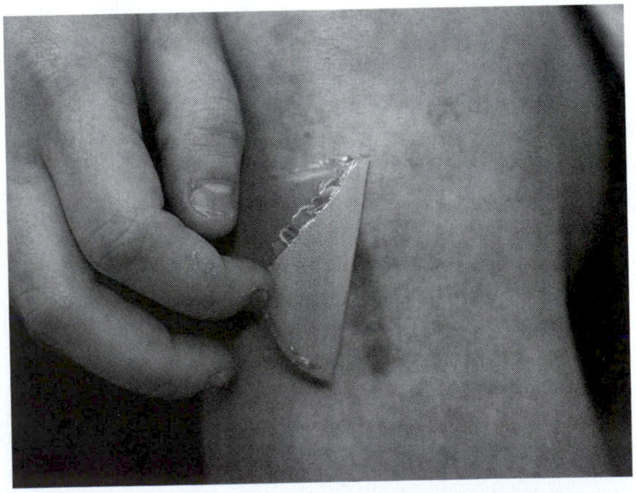

Figure 17.53 Application of a silicon gel sheet to scar tissue during the maturation phase of would healing.

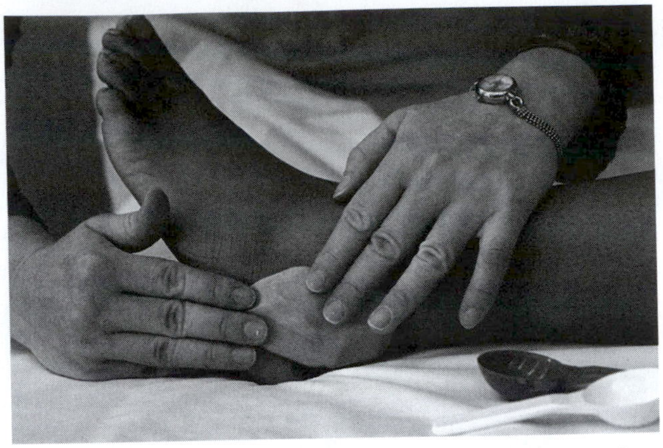

Figure 17.54 Application of elastomer putty to scar tissue during the maturation phase of wound healing.

Summary

These are exciting times for clinicians interested in matters concerning the vascular, lymphatic, and integumentary systems. Skin and wound care practices have changed significantly over the last decade. New information about the microcirculation of blood and lymph has changed treatment strategies. The role of the skin as an organ has gained new respect. It is not surprising that there is an explosion of research, literature, and products to serve the needs of individuals with disorders affecting these systems. Current and future generations are facing healthcare challenges of a magnitude never before seen in our society including an increase in the number of individuals with diabetes, obesity, vascular and lymphatic disease, antibiotic-resistant pathogens, a growing population of older individuals, health care reimbursement challenges, and the growing number of ethical dilemmas in daily practice.

This chapter provides support for clinicians in their efforts to provide excellent patient care. Topics of particular importance include current strategies for wound management, the importance of adequate and appropriate patient education, primary ulcer prevention, ulcer precautions, advanced foot care for individuals with diabetic neuropathy, optimal compression for lymphedema, the essential role of moisture in wound healing, and the importance of exercise as part of the POC.

Ongoing and future research will establish the level of strength of evidence for a variety of topics such as the impact of bio-burden on the wound infection continuum, the preparation of the wound bed, the microbiology of pressure ulcers, the use of exogenous oxygen applications, noncontact US, nonthermal radiofrequency stimulation, cold laser, biosurgery, bioengineered tissue, exogenous growth factors, and topical silver preparations. Wise clinicians must keep abreast of new information and current standards of care, approaching new entries to the field with a strong sense of clinical intuition as well as a firm grasp of the scientific evidence.

Questions for Review

1. Discuss the differences, similarities, and relationships between the arterial, venous, and lymphatic systems. Compare anatomy, method of fluid movement, and function.
2. Outline some of the unique characteristics that can be identified clinically for disorders of the vascular, lymphatic, and integumentary systems.
3. Create a simple diagram to illustrate the normal progression of wound healing using the three phases of wound healing as a guide.
4. List factors that contribute to abnormal wound healing. Divide the list into factors that may be influenced by a physical therapist and factors that may not be influenced by a physical therapist. Discuss why and how the factors in each list may or may not be influenced by a physical therapist.
5. Review the annotated tests and measurements included in this chapter that should be used during a physical therapy examination. Identify tests and measurements routinely performed for patients with vascular, lymphatic, or integumentary disorders.
6. Design a checklist, decision tree, or flow chart for examining a patient with a disorder of the vascular, lymphatic, and/or integumentary systems.
7. Create a general outline of the primary components of a POC for a patient with a wound.
8. Illustrate the interrelatedness of the vascular, lymphatic, and integumentary systems by discussing how one system can impact another.
9. Discuss how a physical therapist should respond to the knowledge that many vascular, lymphatic, and integumentary disorders have a long latency period and require a heightened level of vigilance and proactivity in order to identify symptoms and begin treatment as early as possible.
10. Identify the rationale for each of the following treatments in skin and wound care: moist wound healing, arterial wound hydration, venous wound compression, lymphedema treatment, pressure ulcer prevention, and foot care for the diabetic.

Case Study

REFERRAL

A 78-year-old woman with a primary diagnosis of Alzheimer's disease has been living in a residential facility for 10 months. She is referred to a physical therapist by the physician at the facility.

PAST MEDICAL HISTORY

Unremarkable until onset of symptoms of Alzheimer's 3 years ago.

CURRENT MEDICAL HISTORY

Arteriosclerosis; mild hypertension controlled by medication; treated for pressure ulcer for 4 weeks (30 days) with bid hydrogen peroxide flushes followed by dry gauze 4 × 4s covered with Kerlix and adhesive tape. No changes in wound for 4 weeks. No other intervention in place.

SOCIAL

Husband also resident of same facility, lives in same room. Husband is frail but mobile and contributes to care for wife. No children. Patient enjoys music and trips by wheelchair to activity center in facility.

COGNITIVE

Patient disoriented to place and time. Becomes agitated during wound care. Unable to follow weight shift and turning schedules independently. Follows some instructions when supervised by husband or staff.

HR: 70 BP: 145/90 Resp: 15 Temp: 99°F Weight: 118 lbs

PHYSICAL THERAPY EXAMINATION DATA

Wound

Stage III pressure ulcer over right ischial tuberosity. The wound bed is 50% necrotic yellow tissue and 50% red granulation tissue. The patient has a recent history of positive culture for *Pseudomonas aeruginosa* in the ulcer. The wound is currently contaminated but not infected. Drainage is moderate, yellow-brown and thin. The periwound skin is intact.

Strength and ROM

Patient unable to follow commands consistently but appears to have functional strength and ROM of UEs bilaterally. Gross LE strength is impaired perhaps owing to declining activity levels. Active ROM appears functional in UEs. Bilateral hip flexion contractures of 20° can be reduced to 10° with passive ROM.

Mobility

Patient is either in wheelchair or bed 24 hours/day. Patient is unable to roll independently but can often assist using UEs when instructed. Requires maximum assist of two to pivot transfer. Unable to ambulate at this time.

GUIDING QUESTIONS

1. What are the contributing factors that have most likely led to the chronicity of this wound?
2. What combination of interventions to clean and débride would allow removal of necrotic tissue while protecting granulation tissue?
3. What electromodalities might be appropriate for treatment of this wound?
4. Other than local wound care, what type of intervention will be essential for wound closure?
5. Once progress has been made in wound healing, if the wound were to become dry, what dressing types could be used to create a moist wound environment?
6. If using an occlusive dressing, this patient should be closely monitored for what potential occurrence?
7. Assuming this patient's wounds will close, what are your expectations for the condition of her skin over the wound site?

References

1. Martini, FH: Fundamentals of Anatomy and Physiology, ed 4. Prentice-Hall, Upper Saddle River, NJ, 1998.
2. Kelly, DG: A Primer on Lymphedema. Prentice-Hall, Upper Saddle River, NJ, 2002.
3. McCulloch, JM: Therapeutic modalities stimulate wound management. Biomechanics April: 67, 2004.
4. Eliska, O, and Eliskova, M: Are peripheral lymphatics damaged by high pressure manual massage? Lymphology 28:21, 1995.
5. Casley-Smith, JR: Varying total tissue pressures and the concentration of initial lymphatic lymph. Microvasc Res 25:369, 1983.
6. Mortimer, PS, et al: The measurement of skin lymph flow by isotope clearance-reliability, reproducibility, injection dynamics and the effect of massage. J Invest Dermatol 95 (6):677, 1990.
7. Olszewski, WL, and Engeset, A: Intrinsic contractility of prenodal lymph vessels and lymph flow in human leg. Am J Physiol 239(6):H775, 1980.
8. Smith, A: Lymphatic drainage in patients after replantation of extremities. Plast Reconstr Surg 79:163, 1987.
9. Campton-Johnson, S and Wilson, J: Infected wound management: Advanced technologies, moisture-retentive dressings, and die-hard methods. Crit Care Nurs Q 24(2): 64, 2001.
10. Sen, CK: The general case of redox control of wound repair. Wound Repair Regen 11(6):431, 2003.
11. Knighton, DR, et al: Oxygen as an antibiotic: The effect of inspired oxygen on infection. Arch Surg 119:199, 1984.
12. Gordillo, GM, and Sen, CK: Revisiting the essential role of oxygen in wound healing. The Am J Surg 186:259, 2003.
13. Hopf, H, Hunt, T, and West, J: Wound tissue oxygen tension predicts the risk of wound infection in surgical patients. Arch Surg 132:997, 1997.
14. Grief, R, et al: Supplemental perioperative oxygen to reduce the incidence of surgical wound infection. N Eng J Med 342: 161, 2000.
15. Kurz, A, Sessler, D, and Lenhardt, R: Perioperative normothermia to reduce the incidence of surgical wound infection and shorten hospitalization. N Engl J Med 334: 1209, 1996.
16. Atiyeh, BS, et al: Management of acute and chronic open wounds: The importance of moist environment to optimal wound healing. Curr Pharm Biotechnol 3:179, 2002.
17. Svensjo, T, et al: Accelerated healing of full-thickness skin wounds in a wet environment. Plast Reconstr Surg 106(3): 602, 2000.
18. Eriksson, E, et al: Treatment of chronic, nonhealing abdominal wound in a liquid environment. Ann Plast Surg 36(1): 80, 1996.
19. Dyson, M, et al: Comparison of the effects of moist and dry conditions on dermal repair. J Invest Dermatol 91:434, 1988.
20. Lee, JE, et al: An infection-preventing bilayered collagen membrane containing antibiotic-loaded hyaluronan microparticles: Physical and biological properties. Artif Organs 26(7): 636, 2002.
21. Thomas, DW, et al: Randomized clinical trial of the effect of semi-occlusive dressings on the microflora and clinical outcome of acute facial wounds. Wound Repair Regen 8(4): 258, 2000.
22. Madeo M, et al: A randomized trial comparing Arglaes(a transparent dressing containing silver ions) to Tegaderm (a transparent polyurethane dressing) for dressing peripheral arterial catheters and central vascular catheters. Intens Crit Care Nurs 14(4):187, 1998.
23. Koupil, J, et al: The influence of moisture wound healing on the incidence of bacterial infection and histological changes in healthy human skin after treatment of interactive dressings. Acta Chir Plast 45(3):89, 2003.
24. Hutchinson, JJ, and Lawrence, JC: Wound infection under occlusive dressings. J Hosp Infect 17:83, 1991.
25. Nemeth, AJ, et al: Faster healing and less pain in skin biopsy sites treated with an occlusive dressing. Arch Dermatol 127:1679, 1991.
26. Mechanick, JI: Practical aspects of nutritional support for wound-healing patients. Am J Surg 188 (1), Suppl 1, July: 52, 2004.
27. Shepherd, AA: Nutrition for optimum wound healing. Nurs Stand 18(6):55, 2003.
28. Gray, M: Does oral supplementation with vitamins A or E promote healing of chronic wounds? J Wound Ostom Continen Nurs 30(6):290, 2003.
29. Gray, M: Does vitamin C supplementation promote pressure ulcer healing? J Wound Osteom Continen Nurs 30(5):245, 2003.
30. Collins, N: The right mix: Using nutritional interventions and an anabolic agent to manage a stage IV ulcer. Adv Skin Wound Care 17(1):36, 2004.
31. Collins, N: Diabetes, nutrition and wound healing. Adv Skin Wound Care 16(6):292, 2003.
32. Williams, JZ, and Barbul, A: Nutrition and wound healing. Surg Clin North Am 83:571, 2003.
33. Zulkowski, K, and Albrecht, D: How nutrition and aging affect wound healing. Nursing 33(8):70, 2003.

34. Rodeheaver, G, et al: Wound healing and wound management: Focus on Debridement. Adv Wound Care 7(1):22, 1994.
35. Kirk, SJ, et al: Arginine stimulates wound healing and immune function in elderly human beings. Surgery. 114:155, 1993.
36. Barbul, A, et al: Arginine enhances wound healing and lymphocyte immune responses in humans. Surgery 108:331, 1990.
37. Cartwright, A: Nutritional assessment as part of wound management. Nurs Times 98(44):62, 2002.
38. Bill, TJ, et al: Quantitative swab culture versus tissue biopsy: A comparison in chronic wounds. Ostomy Wound Manage 47(1):34, 2001.
39. Hardy, M: The physiology of scar formation. Phys Ther 69(22):1014, 1989.
40. Kirsner, RS, and Bogensberger, G: The normal process of healing. In Kloth, LC, and McCulloch, JM (eds): Wound Healing: Alternatives in Management, ed 3. FA Davis, Philadelphia, 2002, p 3.
41. Sussman, C, and Bates-Jensen, BM: Wound healing physiology and chronic wound healing. In Sussman, C, and Bates, BM (eds): Wound Care: A Collaborative Practice Manual for Physical Therapists and Nurses, ed 2. Aspen, Gaithersburg, MD, 2001, p 26.
42. Bates-Jensen, BM, and Sussman, C: Tools to measure wound healing. In Sussman, C and Bates, BM (eds): Wound Care: A Collaborative Practice Manual for Physical Therapists and Nurses, ed 2. Aspen, Gaithersburg, MD, 2001, p 142.
43. Weed, T, Ratliff C, and Drake DB: Quantifying bacterial bioburden during negative pressure wound therapy. Ann Plast Surg 52(3):276, 2004.
44. Lindholm, C: Pressure ulcers and infection-Understanding clinical features. Ostomy Wound Manage. 49(5A):4, 2003.
45. Beitz, JM, and Goldberg, E: The lived experience of having a chronic wound: a phenomenologic study. Medsurg Nurs 14(1):51, 2005.
46. Glasper, ER, and Devries, AC: Social structure influences effects of pair-housing on wound healing. Brain Behav Immun 19(1):61, 2005.
47. Detillion, CE, et al: Social facilitation of wound healing. Psychoneuroendocrinology 29(8):1004, 2005.
48. Ebrecht, M, et al: Perceived stress and cortisol levels predict speed of wound healing in healthy male adults. Psychoneuroendocrinology 29(6):798, 2004.
49. Norman, D: The effects of stress on wound healing and leg ulceration. Br J Nurs 10;12(21):1256, 2003.
50. Jones, J: Stress responses, pressure ulcer development and adaptation. Br J Nurs 12(11 Suppl):S17, 2003.
51. Worldwide Wound Management 2002–2012: Products, Technologies & Market Opportunities, Report S200, February 2003, Med-Market Diligence, LLC.
52. Hiatt, WR: Medical treatment of peripheral arterial disease and claudication. N Engl J Med 344(21):1608, 2001.
53. Valencia, IC, et al: Chronic venous insufficiency and venous leg ulceration. J Am Acad Dermatol 44(3): 401, 2001.
54. Kunimoto, B, et al: Best practices for the prevention and treatment of venous leg ulcers. Ostomy Wound Manage 47(2):34, 2001.
55. Seiggreen, MY, and Kline, RA: Vascular ulcers. In Baranoski, S, and Ayello, EA (eds): Wound Care Essentials: Practice Principles. Springhouse, PA: Lippincott Williams & Wilkins, 2004, p 271.
56. Browse, N, and Burnand, K: The cause of venous ulceration. Lancet 2:132, 1982.
57. Kolbach, DN, et al: Severity of venous insufficiency is related to the density of microvascular deposition of PAI-1, uPA and von Willebrand factor. J Vasc Dis 33(1):19, 2004.
58. Berard, A, et al: Risk factors for the first-time development of venous ulcers of the lower limbs: The influence of heredity and physical activity. Angiology 53(6):647, 2002.
59. Sindrup, J, et al: Coexistence of obstructive arterial disease and chronic venous stasis in leg ulcer patients. Clin Exp Dermatol 12:410, 1987.
60. Holloway, GA, Ooi, SK, and Weingarten, MS: Management of Venous Insufficiency and Ulceration: Treatment of Chronic Wounds. Curative Health Services, East Setauket, NY, 1995. Monograph retrieved February 25, 2006 from http://www.curative.com/
61. Kelechi, TJ, et al: Skin temperature and chronic venous insufficiency. J Wound Ostomy Continence Nurs 30(1):17, 2003.
62. Strossenreuther, RHK, et al: Guidelines for the application of MLD/CDT for primary and secondary lymphedema and other selected pathologies. In Foldi, M, Foldi, E, and Kubik, S (eds): Textbook of Lymphology for Physicians and Lymphedema Therapists, ed 5. Elsevier GmbH, Munich, Germany, 2003, p 590.
63. Foldi, E, et al: Lymphostatic diseases. In Foldi, M, Foldi, E, and Kubik, S (eds): Textbook of Lymphology for Physicians and Lymphedema Therapists, ed 5. Elsevier GmbH, Munich, Germany, 2003, p 232.
64. Gaber, Y: Secondary lymphoedema of the lower leg as an unusual side-effect of a liquid silicone injection in the hips and buttocks. Dermatology 208:342, 2004.
65. Sitzia, J, et al: Characteristics of new referrals to twenty-seven lymphoedema treatment units. Eur J Cancer Care 7:255, 1998.
66. Cariati, A, et al: Post-traumatic lymphedema: A survey of two cases. XIX International Congress of Lymphology: Abstract Book. Freiburg, Germany, September 2003.
67. Baumgarten, M, et al: Pressure ulcers and the transition to long-term care. Adv Skin Wound Care 16(6):299, 2003.
68. Pressure Ulcer Prevention and Treatment Following Spinal Cord Injury: A clinical Practice Guideline for Health-Care Professionals. Consortium for Spinal Cord Medicine/Clinical Practice Guidelines. August 2000.
69. Langemo, DK, Anderson, J, and Volden, C: Uncovering pressure ulcer incidence. Nurs Manage 34(10):64, 2003.
70. Scott, EM, et al: Effects of warming therapy on pressure ulcers—a randomized trial. J Perioperative Nurs May, 2001.
71. Reed, RL, et al: Low serum albumin levels, confusion, and fecal incontinence: Are these risk factors for pressure ulcers in mobility-impaired hospitalized adults? Gerontology 49(4):255, 2003.
72. Allman, RM: Pressure ulcers among the elderly. N Engl J Med 320(13):850, 1989.
73. Lyder, C, et al: Quality of care for hospitalized medicare patients at risk for pressure ulcers. Arch Intern Med 161:1549, 2001.
74. Van Rijswijk, L: Full-thickness pressure ulcers: Patient and wound healing characteristics. Decubitus 6(1):16, 1993.
75. Van Rijswijk, L, and Polansky, M: Predictors of time to healing deep pressure ulcers. Ostomy Wound Manage 40(8): 40, 1994.
76. Van Rijswijk, L: The question of outcomes. Ostomy Wound Manage. 49(2):6, 2003.
77. CHA Good Health Report. Fall: 7, 2004. Red Spring(r) Communications, Inc.
78. Cowie, CC, et al: Prevalence of diabetes and impaired fasting glucose in adults—United States, 1999–2000. MMWR Morb Mortal Wkly Rep 52(35):833, 2003.
79. Centers for Disease Control and Prevention: National diabetes fact sheet: general information and national estimates on diabetes in the Unites States, 2003. Atlanta, GA: U.S. Department of Health and Human Services, Centers of Disease Control and Prevention, 2003.
80. American Physical Therapy Association: Guide to Physical Therapist Practice, ed 2. Phys Ther 81(1):S49, 2001.
81. Cornish, BH, et al: Early diagnosis of lymphedema in postsurgery breast cancer patients. Ann NY Acad Sci 904:571, 2000.
82. Mikes, DM, et al: Bioelectrical impedance analysis revisited. Lymphology 32:157, 1999.
83. Cornish, BH, et al: Early diagnosis of lymphedema using multiple frequency bioimpedance. Lymphology 34: 2, 2001.
84. Brennan, MJ, DePompolo, RW, and Garden, FH: Focused review: Postmastectomy lymphedema. Arch Phys Med Rehabil 77:S74, 1996.
85. Lampe, KE: Methods of wound evaluation. In Kloth, LC, and McCulloch, JM (eds): Wound Healing: Alternatives in Management, ed 3. FA Davis, Philadelphia, 2002, p 153.
86. Patterson, GK: Vascular evaluation. In Sussman, C and Bates, BM: Wound Care: A Collaborative Practice Manual for Physical Therapists and Nurses, ed 2. Aspen, Gaithersburg, MD, 2001, p 177.
87. Mehta, T, et al: Disease-specific quality of life assessment in intermittent claudication: Review. Eur J Endovasc Surg 25:202, 2003.
88. Regensteiner, JG, et al: Evaluation of walking impairment by questionnaire in patients with peripheral arterial disease. J Vas Med Biol. 2:142, 1990.
89. Lehert, P: Quality-of-life assessment in comparative therapeutic trials and causal structure considerations in peripheral occlusive arterial disease. Pharmacoeconomics 19(2):121, 2001.
90. Marquis, P, Comte, S, and Lehert, P: International Validation of the CLAUS-S Quality-of-Life Questionnaire for Use in Patients with Intermittent Claudication. Pharmacoeconomics 19(6):667, 2001.

91. Tiedjen, KU, et al: Radiological Diagnostic Procedures in Edema of the Extremities. In Foldi, M, Foldi, E, and Kubik, S (eds): Textbook of Lymphology for Physicians and Lymphedema Therapists, ed 5. Elsevier GmbH, Munich, Germany, 2003, p 434.
92. National Pressure Ulcer Advisory Panel (NPUAP): Pressure ulcers: Prevalence, cost and risk assessment: Consensus development conference statement. Decubitus 2:24, 1989.
93. Bergstrom, N, et al: Pressure Ulcer Treatment, Clinical Practice Guideline, Quick Reference Guide for Clinicians, No. 15. Rockville, MD: U.S. Department of Health and Human Services, Public Health Service Agency, Agency for Health Care Research and Quality. AHRQ Pub. No. 95-0653. Dec. 1994.
94. Thomas, DR, et al: Pressure ulcer scale for healing: Derivation and validation of the PUSH tool. Adv Wound Care 10(5), 1997
95. Wagner, FW: The dysvascular foot: A system for diagnosis and treatment. Foot Ankle. 3:64, 1981.
96. Norton, D, McLaren, R, and Exton-Smith, NA: An Investigation of Geriatric Nursing Problems in Hospitals. Edinburgh, Scotland: Churchill-Livingstone; 1962.
97. Gosnell, DJ: Pressure sore risk assessment: A critique. I: The Gosnell Scale. Decubitis 2(3):40, 1989.
98. Braden, BJ, and Bergstrom, N: A conceptual schema for the study of etiology of pressure sores. Rehabil Nurs 12(1):8, 1987.
99. Braden, BJ, and Bergrstrom, N: Clinical utility of the Braden Scale for predicting pressure sore risk. Decubitis 2:44, 1989.
100. Sussman, C: Wound Care: Patient Education Resource Manual. Aspen, Gaithersburg, MD, 1999.
101. Ehrlich, A, Vinje-Harrewijn, A, and McMahon, E: Living well with lymphedema. Lymph Notes, San Francisco, CA, 2005.
102. Folkedahl, BA, and Frantz, R: Treatment of Pressure Ulcers. Iowa City, IA: University of Iowa Gerontological Nursing Interventions Research Center, Research Dissemination Core; August, 2002.
103. McCulloch, JM, and Boyd, V: The effects of whirlpool and the dependent position on LE volume. J Orthop Sports Phys Ther 16:169, 1992.
104. Sussman, C: Whirlpool. In Sussman, C, and Bates, BM (eds): Wound Care: A Collaborative Practice Manual for Physical Therapists and Nurses, ed 2. Aspen, Gaithersburg, MD, 2001, p 621.
105. Burke, DT, et al: Effects of hydrotherapy on pressure ulcer healing. Am J Phys Med Rehabil 77(5):394, 1998.
106. Luedtke-Hoffmann, KA, and Schafer, DS: Pulsed lavage in wound cleansing. Phys Ther 80:292, 2000.
107. Haynes, LJ, et al: Comparison of Pulsavac and sterile whirlpool regarding the promotion of tissue granulation (abstract). Phys Ther74 (Suppl 5):S4, 1994.
108. Loehne, HB, et al: Aerosolization of microorganisms during pulsatile lavage with suction. Presented at Combined Sections Meeting/American Physical Therapy Association. February 2000; New Orleans, LA.
109. Ovington, LG: Hanging wet-to-dry dressings out to dry. Home Healthc Nurse 19(8):477, 2001.
110. Lawrence, JC: Dressings and wound infection. Am J Surg 167(1A):21S, 1994.
111. Lawrence, JC, Lilly, HA, and Kidson, A: Wound dressings and airborne dispersal of bacteria. Lancet 339:807, 1992.
112. Lim, JK, et al: Normal saline wound dressing-is it really normal? Br J Plast Surg 53:42, 2000.
113. Mosher, BA, et al: Outcomes of 4 methods of debridement using a decision analysis methodology. Adv Wound Care (March); 12(2):81, 1999.
114. Kohr, R: Moist Healing versus wet to dry. Can Nurse 97(1):17, 2001.
115. Colwell, JC, Foreman, MD, and Trotter, JP: A comparison of the efficacy and cost-effectiveness of two methods of managing pressure ulcers. Decubitis 6(4):28, 1993.
116. Capasso, VA, and Munro, BH: The cost and efficacy of two wound treatments. J Perioper Nurs 77(5):984, 2003.
117. Sherman RA, and Pechter, EA: Maggot therapy: A review of the therapeutic applications of fly larvae in human medicine, especially for treating osteomyelitis. Med Vet Entomol 2:225, 1988.
118. Sherman, RA: A new dressing design for use with maggot therapy. Plast Reconstr Surg 100(2):451, 1997.
119. Mumcuoglu, KY: Clinical applications for maggots in wound care. Am J Clin Dermatol 2(4):219, 2001.
120. Prete, PE: Growth effects of Phaenicia sericata larval extracts on fibroblasts: Mechanism for wound healing by maggot therapy. Life Sci 60(8):505, 1997.
121. Wollina, U, et al: Biosurgery in wound healing-the renaissance of maggot therapy. Eur Acad Dermatol Venereol 14:285, 2000.
122. Allen, CS: Merit in maggots. Physical Therapy Products. May/June: 44, 2003.
123. Thomas, S, et al: Using larvae in modern wound management. J Wound Care. 5(2):60, 1996.
124. Thomas, S, and Andrews, A: The effect of hydrogel dressings on maggot development. J Wound Care. 8(2):75, 1999.
125. Burks, RI: Povidone-iodine solution in wound treatment. Phys Ther 78:212, 1998.
126. Rodeheaver, G, et al: Bactericidal activity and toxicity of iodine-containing solutions in wounds. Arch Surg 117:181, 1982.
127. Lineweaver, W: Cellular and bacterial toxicities of topical antimicrobials. Plast Reconstr Surg 75(3):394, 1985.
128. Sussman, C: Appendix A: Guide to topical antiseptics, antifungals, and antibacterials. In Sussman, C, and Bates, BM (eds): Wound Care: A Collaborative Practice Manual for Physical Therapists and Nurses, ed 2. Aspen, Gaithersburg, MD, 2001, p 661.
129. Geronemus, RG, Mertz, PM, and Eaglestein, WH: Wound healing-the effects of topical antimicrobial agents. Arch Dermatol 115:1311, 1979.
130. Popescu, A, and Salcido, R: Wound pain: A challenge for the patient and the wound care specialist. Adv Skin Wound Care 17(1):14, 2004.
131. Nagai, MK, and Embil, JM: Becaplermin: recombinant platelet derived growth factor, a new treatment for healing diabetic foot ulcers. Expert Opin Biol Ther 2(2):211, 2002.
132. Mandracchia, VJ, Sanders, SM, and Frerichs JA: The use of becaplermin (rhPDGF-BB) gel for chronic nonhealing ulcers. A retrospective analysis. Clin Podiatr Med Surg 18(10):189, 2001.
133. Kantor, J, and Margolis, DJ: Treatment options for diabetic neuropathic foot ulcers: A cost-effectiveness analysis. Dermatol Surg 27(4):347, 2001
134. Edmonds, M, et al: New treatments in ulcer healing and wound infection. Diabetes/Metab Res Rev Sept-Oct Suppl 1:S51, 2000.
135. Ladin, D: Becaplermin gel (PDGF-BB) as topical wound therapy. Plastic Surgery Educational Foundation DATA Committee. Plast Reconstr Surg 105(3):1230, 2000.
136. Rees, RS, et al: Becaplermin gel in the treatment of pressure ulcers: A phase II randomized, double-blind, placebo-controlled study. Wound Repair Regen 7(3):141, 1999.
137. Kloth, LC, and McCulloch, JM: Wound Healing: Alternatives in Management, ed 3. FA Davis, Philadelphia, 2002.
138. Sussman, C, and Bates, BM: Wound Care: A Collaborative Practice Manual for Physical Therapists and Nurses, ed 2. Aspen, Gaithersburg, MD, 2001.
139. Kloth, LC: Adjunctive Interventions for Wound Healing. In Kloth, LC, and McCulloch, JM (eds): Wound Healing: Alternatives in Management, ed 3. FA Davis, Philadelphia, 2002, p 316.
140. Sussman, C, and Dyson, M: Therapeutic and Diagnostic Ultrasound. In Sussman, C, and Bates, BM (eds): Wound Care: A Collaborative Practice Manual for Physical Therapists and Nurses, ed 2. Aspen, Gaithersburg, MD, 2001, p 596.
141. McCulloch, J, and Kloth, L: Physical agents in wound repair: What is the evidence?. Course handout. Annual Conference & Exposition of the American Physical Therapy Association, Washington, DC, 2003.
142. McCulloch, J: The integumentary system—repair and management: An overview. Physical Therapy Magazine February: 52, 2004.
143. Doan, N, et al: In vitro effects of therapeutic ultrasound on cell proliferation, protein synthesis, and cytokine production by human fibroblasts, osteoblasts, and monocytes. J Oral Maxillofac Surg 57:409, 1999.
144. Dyson, M: Mechanisms involved in therapeutic ultrasound. Physiotherapy 65:55, 1980.
145. Foulds, IS, and Barker, AT: Human skin battery potentials and their possible role in wound healing. Br J Dermatol 109:515, 1983.
146. Kloth, LC: Electrical stimulation for wound healing: a review of evidence from in vitro studies, animal experiments, and clinical trials. Int J Low Extrem Wounds 4(1):23, 2005.

147. Demir, H, Balay, H, and Kirnap, M: A comparative study of the effects of electrical stimulation and laser treatment on experimental wound healing in rats. J Rehabil Res Dev 41(2):147, 2004.
148. Ojingwa, JC, and Isseroff, RR: Electrical stimulation of wound healing. J Invest Dermatol 121(1):1, 2003.
149. Houghton, PE, et al: Effect of electrical stimulation on chronic leg ulcer size and appearance. Phys Ther 83(1):17, 2003.
150. Edsberg, LE, et al: Topical hyperbaric oxygen and electrical stimulation: Exploring potential synergy. Ostomy Wound Manage 48(1):42, 2003.
151. Kloth, LC: 5 questions—and answers—about electrical stimulation. Adv Skin Wound Care 14(3):156, 158, 2001.
152. Thawer, HA, and Houghton, PE: Effects of electrical stimulation on the histological properties of wounds in diabetic mice. Wound Repair Regen 9(2):107, 2001.
153. Evans, RD, Foltz, D, and Foltz, K:. Electrical stimulation with bone and wound healing. Clinic Podiatr Med Surg 18(1):79, 2001.
154. Kloth, LC: Electrical stimulation for wound healing. In Kloth, LC, and McCulloch, JM (eds): Wound Healing: Alternatives in Management, ed 3. FA Davis, Philadelphia, 2002, p 271.
155. Sussman, C, and Byl, NN: Electrical stimulation for wound healing. In Sussman, C and Bates, BM (eds): Wound Care: A Collaborative Practice Manual for Physical Therapists and Nurses, ed 2. Aspen, Gaithersburg, MD, 2001, p 497.
156. Salzberg, CA, et al: The effect of non-thermal pulsed electromagnetic energy (Diapulse) on wound healing of pressure ulcers in spinal cord injured patients: A randomized, double-blind study. Wounds 7(1):11, 1995.
157. Hill, J, et al: Pulsed short-wave diathermy effects on human fibroblast proliferation. Arch Phys Med Rehabil 83(6):832, 2002.
158. Mayrovitz, H, and Larsen, P: Effects of pulsed electromagnetic fields on skin microvascular blood perfusion. Wounds 4(5):197, 1992.
159. Conner-Kerr, T: Ultraviolet light and wound healing. In Sussman, C and Bates, BM (eds): Wound Care: A Collaborative Practice Manual for Physical Therapists and Nurses, ed 2. Aspen, Gaithersburg, MD, 2001, p 580.
160. Ramsay, C, and Challoner, A. Vascular changes in human skin after ultraviolet irradiation. Br J Dermatol 94:487, 1976.
161. High, AS, and High, JP: Treatment of infected skin wounds using ultraviolet radiation: An in vitro study. Physiotherapy 69(10):359, 1983.
162. Conner-Kerr, T, et al: The effects of ultraviolet radiation on antibiotic-resistant bacteria in vitro. Ostomy Wound Manage 44(10):50, 1998.
163. Conner-Kerr, T, et al: UVC reduces antibiotic-resistant bacterial numbers in living tissue. SAWC Selected Abstracts. Ostomy Wound Manage 45:84, 1999.
164. Thai, T, et al: Ultraviolet light C in the treatment of chronic wounds with MRSA: A case study. Ostomy Wound Manage 48(11):52, 2002.
165. Geronemus, R, et al: The effect of UVC and UVB on epidermal wound healing. Clin Res 50: 586 A, 1982.
166. Nordback, I, et al: Effects of ultraviolet therapy on rat skin wound healing. J Surg Res 48:68, 1990.
167. Boykin, JV: The nitric oxide connection: Hyperbaric oxygen therapy, becaplermin and diabetic ulcer management. Adv Skin Wound Care 13:169, 2000.
168. Quirinia, A, and Viidik, A: The effect of hyperbaric oxygen on different phases of healing of ischemic flap wounds and incisional wounds in skin. Br J Plast Surg 48:583, 1995.
169. Zamboni, WA, et al: Evaluation of hyperbaric oxygen for diabetic wounds: A prospective study. Undersea Hyperb Med J 24:175, 1997.
170. Hammarlund, C, and Sunderberg, T: Hyperbaric oxygen reduced size of chronic leg ulcers: A randomized double-blind study. Plast Reconstr Surg 93:829, 1994.
171. Boykin, JV: Hyperbaric oxygen therapy: A physiological approach to selected problem wound healing. Wounds 8:183, 1996.
172. Kalliainen, L, et al: Topical oxygen as an adjunct to wound healing: A clinical case series. Pathophysiology 9:81, 2003.
173. Edsberg, LE, et al: Topical hyperbaric oxygen and electrical stimulation: Exploring potential synergy. Ostomy Wound Manage 48(11):42, 2002.
174. Landau, Z, and Schattner, A: Topical hyperbaric oxygen and low energy laser therapy for chronic diabetic foot ulcers resistant to conventional treatment. Yale J Biol Med 74:95, 2001.
175. VanOss, CJ, et al: Effect of temperature on the chemotaxis, phagocytic engulfment, digestion and O2 consumption of human polymorphonuclear leukocytes. J Reticuloendothel Soc 27:561, 1980.
176. Doe, PT, et al. A new method of treating venous ulcers with topical radiant warming. J Wound Care 4:87, 1997.
177. Kloth, LC, et al: Effects of a normothermic dressing on pressure ulcer healing. Adv Skin Wound Care 13:69, 2000.
178. Price, P, et al: The effect of a radiant heat dressing on pressure ulcers. J Wound Care 9:203, 2000.
179. Bates-Jensen, BM, et al: Management of the wound environment with advanced therapies. In Sussman, C, and Bates, BM (eds): Wound Care: A Collaborative Practice Manual for Physical Therapists and Nurses, ed 2. Aspen, Gaithersburg, MD, 2001, p 272.
180. Joseph, E, et al: A prospective randomized trial of vacuum-assisted closure versus standard therapy of chronic nonhealing wounds. Wounds 12(3):60, 2000.
181. Gupta, S, Gabriel, A, and Shores, J: The perioperative use of negative pressure wound therapy in skin grafting. Ostomy Wound Manage April;50(4A Suppl):32, 2004.
182. Armstrong, DG, et al: Plantar pressure changes using a novel negative pressure wound therapy technique. J Am Podiatr Med Assoc 94(5): 456, 2004.
183. Mendez-Eastman, S: Determining the appropriateness of negative pressure wound therapy for pressure ulcers. Ostomy Wound Manage April;50(4A Suppl):13, 2004.
184. Wanner, MB, et al: Vacuum-assisted wound closure for cheaper and more comfortable healing of pressure sores: A prospective study. Scan J Plast Reconstr Surg 37(1):28, 2003.
185. Horwitz, LR, Burke, TJ, and Carnegie, D: Augmentation of wound healing using monochromatic infrared energy. Adv Wound Care 12(1):35, 1999.
186. Kochman, AB, Carnegie, DH, and Burke, TJ: Symptomatic reversal of peripheral neuropathy in patients with diabetes. J Am Podiatr Med Assoc 92(3):125, 2002.
187. Leonard, DR, Farooqi, MH, and Myers, S: Restoration of sensation, reduced pain, and improved balance in subjects with diabetic peripheral neuropathy: A double-blind, randomized, placebo-controlled study with monochromatic near-infrared treatment. Diabetes Care 27(1):168, 2004.
188. Powell, MW, Carnegie, DE, and Burke, TJ: Reversal of diabetic peripheral neuropathy and new wound incidence: The role of MIRE. Adv Skin Wound Care 17(6):295, 2004.
189. Noble, JG, Lowe, AS, and Baxter, GD: Monochromatic infrared irradiation (890 nm): effect of a multisource array upon conduction in the human median nerve. J Clin Laser Med Surg 19(6):291, 2001.
190. Burke, TJ: 5 Questions—and answers—about MIRE treatment. Adv Skin Wound Care 16(7):369, 2003.
191. Prendergast, JJ, Miranda, G, and Sanchez, M: Improvement of sensory impairment in patients with peripheral neuropathy. Endocr Pract 10(1):24, 2004.
192. Yusof, NL, et al: Flexible chitin films as potential wound-dressing materials: Wound model studies. J Biomed Mater Res 66A(2):224, 2003.
193. Colletta, V, et al: A trial to assess the efficacy and tolerability of Hyalofill-F in non-healing venous leg ulcers. J Wound Care 12(9):357, 2003.
194. Strossenreuther, RHK, et al: Practical Instructions for Therapists-Manual Lymph Drainage According to Dr. E. Vodder. In Foldi, M, Foldi, E, and Kubik, S (eds): Textbook of Lymphology for Physicians and Lymphedema Therapists, ed 5, Elsevier GmbH, Munich, Germany, 2003, p 496.
195. Franzeck, UK, et al: Combined physical therapy for lymphedema evaluated by fluorescence microlymphography and lymph capillary pressure measurements. J Vascul Res 34:306, 1997.
196. Hwang, JH, et al: Changes in lymphatic function after complex physical therapy for lymphedema. Lymphology 32:15, 1999.
197. Robson, MC: Treating bacterial infections in chronic wounds. Contemp Surg Suppl. Sept:9, 2000.
198. Koksal, C, and Bozkurt, AK: Combination of hydrocolloid dressing and medical compression stockings versus Unna's boot for the treatment of venous leg ulcers. Swiss Med Wkly 133(25-26):364, 2003.
199. Moffat, CJ, et al: Randomized trial comparing two four-layer bandage systems in the management of chronic leg ulceration. Phlebology 14:139, 1999.

200. Leduc, O, Peeters, A, and Borgeois, P: Bandages: Scintigraphic demonstration of its efficacy on colloidal protein reabsorption during muscle activity. Progress in Lymphology-XII. Elsevier, Philadelphia, 1990.
201. Johansson, K, et al: Effects of compression bandaging with or without manual lymph drainage treatment in patients with postoperative arm lymphedema. Lymphology 32:103, 1999.
202. Schmid-Schonbein, GW: Microlymphatics and lymph flow. Physiol Rev 70(4):987, 1990.
203. Simon, DA, Dix, FP, and McCollum, CN: Management of venous leg ulcers. Br Med J 328:1358, 2004.
204. Weiss, J: Treatment of leg edema and wounds in a patient with severe musculoskeletal injuries. Phys Ther 78(10):1104, 1998.
205. Asmussen, PD, and Strossenreuther, RHK: Compression therapy. In Foldi, M, Foldi, E, and Kubik, S (eds): Textbook of Lymphology for Physicians and Lymphedema Therapists, ed 5. Elsevier GmbH, Munich, Germany, 2003, p 528.
206. Yasuhara, H, Shigematsu, H, and Muto, T: A study of the advantages of elastic stocking for leg lymphedema. Int Angiology 15(3):272, 1996.
207. Harris, SR, et al: Clinical practice guidelines for the care and treatment of breast cancer: 11. Lymphedema. Can Med Assoc J 164(2): 191, 2001.
208. Badger, CM, Peacock, JL, and Mortimer, PS: A randomized, controlled, parallel-group clinical trial comparing multiplayer bandaging followed by hosiery versus hosiery alone in the treatment of patients with lymphedema of the limb. Cancer 88(12):2832, 2000.
209. McCulloch, JM, et al: Intermittent pneumatic compression enhances venous ulcer healing. Adv Wound Care 7(4): 22, 1994.
210. Berline,r E, Ozbilgin, B, and Zarin, DA: A systematic review of pneumatic compression for treatment of chronic venous insufficiency and venous ulcers. J Vascul Surg 37(3):539, 2003.
211. Augustine, E: Historical review of external compression for lymphedema management . Summary of presentation at CSM. Rehabil Oncol 16(2):17, 1998.
212. Brennan, MJ, and Miller, LT: Overview of treatment options and review of the current role and use of compression garments, intermittent pumps and exercise in the management of lymphedema. Cancer 83:2821, 1998.
213. Lerner, R: What's new in lymphedema therapy in America? Int Angiology. 7:191, 1998.
214. Ko, D, et al: Effective treatment of lymphedema of the extremities. Arch Surg 133:452, 1998.
215. Petrek, JA, Pressman, PI, and Smith, RA: Lymphedema: Current issues in research and management. CA-A Ca J Clin 50:292, 2000.
216. Brienza, DM, Geyer MJ, and Sprigle, S: Seating, positioning, and support surfaces. In: Baranoski, S, and Ayello, EA (eds): Wound Care Essentials: Practice Principles. Lippincott Williams & Wilkins, Philadelphia, 2004.
217. Panel on the Prediction and Prevention of Pressure Ulcers in Adults. Pressure Ulcers in Adults: Prediction and Prevention. Clinical Practice Guideline, No.3. AHCPR Publication No. 92-0047. Rockville, MD: Agency for Health Care Policy and Research; May 1992.
218. McInnes, E: The use of pressure-relieving devices (beds, mattresses and overlays) for the prevention of pressure ulcers in primary and secondary care. J Tissue Viability. 14(1):4, 2004.
219. Stier, L, et al: Reinforcing organizationwide pressure ulcer reduction on high-risk geriatric inpatient units. Outcomes Manag 8(1):28, 2004.
220. Salsich, GB, et al: Effect of Achilles tendon lengthening on ankle muscle performance in people with diabetes mellitus and a neuropathic plantar ulcer. Phys Ther 85(1):34, 2004.
221. Foto, J, and Birke, J: Evaluation of mulitdensity orthotic materials used in footwear for patients with diabetes. Foot Ankle Int 19:836, 1999.

Supplemental Readings

Baranoski, S, and Ayello, EA: Wound Care Essentials: Practice Principles.Lippincott Williams & Wilkins, Philadelphia, 2004.
National Diabetes Data Group, editors. Diabetes in America, ed 2. Washington, DC: U.S. Department of Health and Human Services, National Institutes of Health, National Institute of Diabetes and Digestive and Kidney Diseases, 1995. NIH Publication No. 95-1468.
Weissleder, H, and Schuchhardt, C: Lymphedema, Diagnosis and Therapy, 2d ed. Kagerer Kommunication, Bonn, Germany, 1997.
Wound Care for the Lymphedema Practitioner. VHS video. Moderator: Fife, Expert Panel. Presented at the 5th Biennial National Lymphedema Network Conference, Chicago, IL August 2002. Can be obtained through the National Lymphedema Network. See contact information in Appendix A.

Appendix A: Web Sites for Selected Specialized Education for Complete Decongestive Therapy including Manual Lymphatic Drainage

Name of Organization	Web Site
National Lymphedema Network	http://www.lymphnet.org
Klose Training	http://www.klosetraining.com
Norton School of Lymphatic Therapy	http://www.nortonschool.com
Dr. Vodder School of North America	http://www.vodderschool.com
Academy of Lymphatic Studies	http://www.acols.com
Casley-Smith Courses in the United States	http://www.lymphoedema.org.au
Lymphology Association of North America	http://www.clt-lana.org

Appendix B: Patient Education: Skin Care and Footwear Instructions

Inspect Your Skin

1. Look at your feet every day. Use a mirror, a magnifying glass, or the help of a family member to help you see all over your feet including between your toes and the bottoms of your feet.
2. Look for these things on your feet: blisters, sores, corns, calluses, red spots, swelling, pain, drainage from a sore, broken toenails, cracked skin, odor. Notify your health care provider if you see any of these things on your feet or if you injure either of your feet.

Take Care of Your Skin

1. Wash your feet gently every day using lukewarm water and mild soap. Test the water temperature with your hand before you wash your feet. If your hand is not sensitive to temperature, use a thermometer. The temperature should be about 85° Fahrenheit.
2. Dry your feet well, especially between your toes.
3. You may want to use a lanolin-based lotion or petroleum jelly to soften dry skin. Do not apply any lotion between your toes. You may use powder or cornstarch between your toes.
4. Never try to treat corns, calluses, or toe nails with sharp instruments, home remedies, or store-bought foot care products. These items can all hurt your skin.
5. Cut toenails straight across; do not cut into corners. Use an emery board for sharp edges. A pumice stone can be used to treat small corns and calluses. Alert your health care provider about your foot care practices.
6. For padding and air circulation, use small bits of lamb's wool between the toes. Change the lamb's wool every day. Be sure to use new pieces after you wash your feet. Do not use cotton or cotton balls because the fibers may irritate your skin.
7. Put on a clean pair of white socks after your skin care routine.
8. Do not walk barefoot.
9. If your feet are cold at bedtime, wear cotton socks; do not use a hot water bottle or heating pad to warm your feet.

Check Your Shoes

1. Check your shoes every day before you put them on. Look inside for small things that could cause a sore on your foot. Alternate shoes each day to allow them to breathe and dry completely.
2. Be sure that your shoes are the right size and width.
3. Do not wear old worn-out shoes or socks.
4. Shop for shoes in the afternoon when your feet are the largest.
5. Break in your new shoes gradually.

See Your Health Care Provider

1. Get help in controlling your diabetes.
2. Have regular appointments with your doctor.
3. Call your health care provider immediately if you find a wound on your foot.

Appendix C: Special Tests for Arterial and Venous Function

Special Tests	Description
Rubor of dependency	A noninvasive test that examined the LE for the presence of ischemia. Following elevation of the limb, lowering of the limb should return the skin of the limb to a pink color. If the color is dark red and takes more than 30 seconds to appear, the test is positive for arterial insufficiency.
Air plethysmography (APG)	A noninvasive test of both the arterial and venous circulation. Changes in leg volume are measured using a pressure cuff that quantifies volume changes during rest, standing, and light walking. Venous obstruction and arterial inflow can be observed with this test.
Transcutaneous oxygen ($TcPo_2$)	A noninvasive examination tool for arterial circulation. A special probe and a heating element measure profusion. Measurement of oxygen at the skin level gives information about what is happening at the cellular level. Also found in the literature as *transcutaneous partial pressure of oxygen* and *transcutaneous oxygen tension measurement*. The results are predictive for healing of ulcers and amputation wounds.
Skin Perfusion Pressure (SPP) measurement	A noninvasive test that measures blood flow in the skin. To take the measurements, a modified laser Doppler probe is secured in the bladder of a specialized blood pressure cuff. Results are predictive for healing of ulcers and amputation wounds.
Venous filling time	The extremity is elevated and then lowered into a dependent position. The time it takes for the veins on top of the foot to refill is recorded. Normal filling time is 15 seconds. Greater than 15 seconds indicates arterial disease while less than 15 indicates venous disease.
Percussion Test	With LE in a dependent position, the greater saphenous vein is palpated distal to the knee with one hand while it is tapped 6 in. proximal to the knee with the other hand. If a wave of fluid is detected under the distal palpation site, this indicates the possibility of valvular incompetency.
Trendelenburg Test	Test measures the time required to refill the veins in the dorsum of the foot. The LE is elevated to allow venous blood to empty. A tourniquet on the thigh prevents backflow. After 1 minute, the individual stands. If veins fully distend within 5 seconds before the tourniquet is released, valvular incompetence in the deep veins is suspected. If distention occurs within 5 seconds after the tourniquet is released, incompetence of superficial veins is suspected.

Appendix D: Pressure Ulcer Scale for Healing (PUSH)

PUSH Tool 3.0

Patient Name ______________________________ Patient ID# ____________

Ulcer Location ______________________________ Date ____________

Directions:

Observe and measure the pressure ulcer. Categorize the ulcer with respect to surface area, exudate, and type of wound tissue. Record a sub-score for each of these ulcer characteristics. Add the sub-scores to obtain the total score. A comparison of total scores measured over time provides an indication of the improvement or deterioration in pressure ulcer healing.

LENGTH × WIDTH (in cm²)	**0** 0	**1** <0.3	**2** 0.3–0.6	**3** 0.7–1.0	**4** 1.1–2.0	**5** 2.1–3.0	**Sub-score**
		6 3.1–4.0	**7** 4.1–8.0	**8** 8.1–12.0	**9** 12.1–24.0	**10** >24.0	
EXUDATE AMOUNT	**0** None	**1** Light	**2** Moderate	**3** Heavy			**Sub-score**
TISSUE TYPE	**0** Closed	**1** Epithelial Tissue	**2** Granulation Tissue	**3** Slough	**4** Necrotic Tissue		**Sub-score**
							TOTAL SCORE

Length × Width: Measure the greatest length (head-to-toe) and the greatest width (side-to-side) using a centimeter ruler. Multiply these two measurements (length x width) to obtain an estimate of surface area in square centimeters (cm^2). Caveat: Do not guess! Always use a centimeter ruler and always use the same method each time the ulcer is measured.

Exudate Amount: Estimate the amount of exudate (drainage) present after removal of the dressing and before applying any topical agent to the ulcer. Estimate the exudate (drainage) as none, light, moderate, or heavy.

Tissue Type: This refers to the types of tissue that are present in the wound (ulcer) bed. Score as a "4" if there is any necrotic tissue present. Score as a "3" if there is any amount of slough present and necrotic tissue is absent. Score as a "2" if the wound is clean and contains granulation tissue. A superficial wound that is reepithelializing is scored as a "1". When the wound is closed, score as a "0".

4 – Necrotic Tissue (Eschar): black, brown, or tan tissue that adheres firmly to the wound bed or ulcer edges and may be either firmer or softer than surrounding skin.
3 – Slough: yellow or white tissue that adheres to the ulcer bed in strings or thick clumps, or is mucinous.
2 – Granulation Tissue: pink or beefy red tissue with a shiny, moist, granular appearance.
1 – Epithelial Tissue: for superficial ulcers, new pink or shiny tissue (skin) that grows in from the edges or as islands on the ulcer surface.
0 – Closed/Resurfaced: the wound is completely covered with epithelium (new skin).

www.npuap.org

PUSH Tool Version 3.0: 9/15/98

Pressure Ulcer Healing Chart

To monitor trends in PUSH Scores over time

(Use a separate page for each pressure ulcer)

Patient Name ______________________________ Patient ID# ____________

Ulcer Location ______________________________ Date ____________

Directions:

Observe and measure pressure ulcers at regular intervals using the PUSH Tool.
Date and record PUSH Sub-scores and Total Scores on the Pressure Ulcer Healing Record below.

	Pressure Ulcer Healing Record													
Date														
Length × Width														
Exudate Amount														
Tissue Type														
PUSH Total Score														

Graph the PUSH Total Scores on the Pressure Ulcer Healing Graph below.

PUSH Total Score	Pressure Ulcer Healing Graph													
17														
16														
15														
14														
13														
12														
11														
10														
9														
8														
7														
6														
5														
4														
3														
2														
1														
Healed = 0														
Date														

www.npuap.org

PUSH Tool Version 3.0: 9/15/98

Appendix E: Sample Wound Examination Form

NAME: ____

B/P ____________ Resp ____________ HR ______________ Temp _______________ Weight ______________________

Date: Orientation to time/place/person? ( ) Yes ( ) No

Arrived: ( ) Ambulatory ( ) Cane ( ) Crutches ( ) Walker ( ) Wheelchair ( ) Stretcher ( ) N/A

( ) Initial Examination Reviewed: Changes in medicine, allergies, or health history since last visit? ( ) Yes ( ) No If yes, indicate changes on flowsheet.

Wound Number				
Wound Location				
Wound Type				
Wound Stage	( ) I ( ) II ( ) III ( ) IV	( ) I ( ) II ( ) III ( ) IV	( ) I ( ) II ( ) III ( ) IV	( ) I ( ) II ( ) III ( ) IV
Length				
Width				
Depth				
Tunnels/ Undermining	( ) Yes ( ) No	( ) Yes ( ) No	( ) Yes ( ) No	( ) Yes ( ) No
Granulation				
Slough				
Eschar	( ) Yes ( ) No	( ) Yes ( ) No	( ) Yes ( ) No	( ) Yes ( ) No
Odor	( ) Yes ( ) No	( ) Yes ( ) No	( ) Yes ( ) No	( ) Yes ( ) No
Drainage Amount	( ) None ( ) Minimal ( ) Moderate ( ) Heavy	( ) None ( ) Minimal ( ) Moderate ( ) Heavy	( ) None ( ) Minimal ( ) Moderate ( ) Heavy	( ) None ( ) Minimal ( ) Moderate ( ) Heavy
Drainage Color	( ) Serous ( ) Sero Sanguineous ( ) Sanguineous ( ) Purulent ( ) Yellow/Green ( ) NA	( ) Serous ( ) Sero Sanguineous ( ) Sanguineous ( ) Purulent ( ) Yellow/Green ( ) NA	( ) Serous ( ) Sero Sanguineous ( ) Sanguineous ( ) Purulent ( ) Yellow/Green ( ) NA	( ) Serous ( ) Sero Sanguineous ( ) Sanguineous ( ) Purulent ( ) Yellow/Green ( ) NA
Wound Margin ( ) Yes ( ) No	( ) Well Defined ( ) Poorly Defined	( ) Well Defined ( ) Poorly Defined	( ) Well Defined ( ) Poorly Defined	( ) Well Defined ( ) Poorly Defined
Exposed Bone	( ) Yes ( ) No	( ) Yes ( ) No	( ) Yes ( ) No	( ) Yes ( ) No
Exposed Muscle/ Tendon/Ligament	( ) Yes ( ) No	( ) Yes ( ) No	( ) Yes ( ) No	( ) Yes ( ) No
Periwound Appearance	( ) Maceration ( ) Intact ( ) Callus ( ) Necrotic ( ) Erythema	( ) Maceration ( ) Intact ( ) Callus ( ) Necrotic ( ) Erythema	( ) Maceration ( ) Intact ( ) Callus ( ) Necrotic ( ) Erythema	( ) Maceration ( ) Intact ( ) Callus ( ) Necrotic ( ) Erythema

(continued)

Pain Management

Pain Scale: None 0 1 2 3 4 5 6 7 8 9 10 Severe

Locations(s):

Described as: ( ) Sharp ( ) Dull ( ) Burning ( ) Throbbing ( ) Radiating ( ) Constant ( ) Intermittent ( ) AM ( ) PM ( ) HS ( ) Only with Dressing Change

Relieved by: ( ) Elevation of Legs/Offloading/Rest ( ) Medication ( ) Standing/Walking ( ) Other_________

Comments: ___________________________________

Pain Management Measures: ( ) LAT ( ) Lidocaine ( ) NA ( ) Refused ( ) Other:

Strength/ROM/ADL/Gait/Transfers/Mobility: ( ) Impaired ( ) Not Impaired Comments:

Other Test Results: ABI: Monofilaments:

Plan of Care

Cleansing:

Dressing:

Modalities:

Débridement:

Exercise:

Education:

Pressure Relief:

Compression:

Other:

Key:
Stage I: skin intact, light skin: nonblanchable red area; dark skin; warm, indurated, hard edema
Stage II: partial thickness skin loss
Stage III: full thickness skin loss
Stage IV: muscle/bone/joint(s) involved

Signature: ___________________________________
Date/Time: ___________________________________

Appendix F: Selected Wound Care Internet Resources

http://www.worldwidewounds.comhttp://medi-smart.com
http://www.woundcare.org
http://www.plasticsurgery.org/medical_professionals
http://www.woundcarenet.comwww.orthopedictechreview.com/issues/junjul99/pg51
http://www.veinsonline.comhttp://medlib.med.utah.edu/kw/derm/pages/woge_12
http://www.smithnephew.com/what/wound.jsp
http://www.christianacare.org/patient_care/patient_care_wound.cfmWoundcareshop.safeshopper.com
http://www.vh.orgwww.woundexpert.com
http://www.harcourtinternational.com/woundcare
http://www.diversifiedtherapy.comwww.internurse.com
http://www.healthproductsforyou.ushttp://ccpe.smsu.edu
http://www.firstmark.com
http://www.healthsystem.virginia.edu/internet/surgicalsc/cwcc.cfm
http://www.allegromedical.com
http://www.bu.edu/woundbiotech/woundcare
http://www.medicaledu.comwww.csmc.edu
http://www.wound.comhttp://gort.ucsd.edu/newjour/a/msg03302
http://www.journalofwoundcare.comhttp://physicaltherapy.about.com
http://www.lww.comwww.aawcone.comwww.uiuc.eduwww.apma.org
http://www.wound.comwww.medline.com
http://www.woundcaresociety.orgwww.eatonhand.com
http://www.internurse.com
http://www.vcp.monashhttp://dir.yahoo.com/Health/Medicine/Wound_Care
http://www.woundcarestrategies.com
http://www.woundcareresources.com
http://www.merck.comwww.emoryhealthcare.org
http://www.wocn.org
http://www.pva.org/res/cpg/contact.htm
http://www.emedicine.com/med
http://www.convatec.com
http://www.vcc.vasculardomain.com
http://www.hhs.gov
http://www.cdc.gov/diabetes/pubs/factsheet.htm

Appendix G: Selected Wound Dressing Manufacturer Web Sites

Augustine Medical	http://www.augustinemedical.com
Bertek Pharmaceuticals	http://www.bertek.com
CarringtonLab	http://www.carringtonlabs.com
Coloplast	http://www.coloplast.com
Convatec	http://www.convatec.com
DeRoyal	http://www.deroyal.com
Healthpoint	http://www.healthpoint.com
Jobst	http://www.jobst-usa.com
Johnson & Johnson	http://www.jnj.com
Kendall	http://www.kendall.com
Smith & Nephew	http://www.smith-nephew.com
Spenco	http://www.spenco.com
3M	www.3m.com/us/healthcare/medicalspecialties

Appendix H: Dressings by Treatment Goal (Purpose) and Wound Type (Indication)

I. Dressing by Treatment Goal

Purpose	Dressing
Space filling (cavities, undermining, tunnels, or sinuses)	Gauze Foams (some) Hydrogels (amorphous/sheets) Alginates Impregnated gauze Absorptive dressings (beads, powders, and pastes) Composite dressings (some)
Mechanical débridement Exudate absorption	Gauze Gauze Foams Absorptive dressings (beads, powders, and pastes) Alginates Hydrocolloids Collagen
Hydration	Hydrogels (amorphous/sheets) Saline-moistened gauze
Autolytic débridement	Transparent films Hydrocolloids Hydrogels (amorphous/sheets) Foams Alginates Impregnated gauze Absorptive dressings (beads, powders, and pastes) Composite
Protection against contamination	Transparent films Hydrocolloids Hydrogel sheets (some) Composite (some) Foams (some)
Hemostasis	Alginates Collagen
Site coverage	Transparent films Hydrocolloids Hydrogel sheets (some) Foams Composite Gauze
Friction reduction	Transparent films Hydrocolloids Hydrogels sheets (some)

Purpose	Dressing
Insulation	Transparent films Hydrocolloids Hydrogels (amorphous/sheet) Foams Composite (some) Gauze
Pain reduction	Transparent films Hydrocolloids Hydrogels (amorphous/sheet) Foams Alginates Composites
Odor reduction	Hydrocolloids Hydrogels (amorphous/sheets) (some) Alginates (some) Foams (charcoal) Absorptive dressings (beads, powders, and pastes) (some)
Cushioning	Hydrocolloids Hydrogel sheets (some) Foams Composite dressings (some) Gauze
Antibacterials	Silver-based dressings Iodine-based dressings Silver sulfadiazine

II. Dressings by Wound Type

Indication	Dressing
Infected wounds	Gauze Alginates Hydrogels Hydrogel sheets Impregnated gauze Foams
Burns	Alginates Hydrocolloids Hydrogels Transparent films Impregnated gauze Foams Biological dressings Collagen
Stage I pressure ulcers	Transparent films Foams
Stage II pressure ulcers	Alginates Hydrocolloids Hydrogels Transparent films Impregnated gauze Foams Collagen

(continued)

Indication	Dressing
Stage III pressure ulcers	Alginates Hydrocolloids Hydrogels Impregnated gauze Foams Collagen
Stage IV pressure ulcers	Alginates Hydrocolloids Hydrogels Impregnated gauze Foams Collagen
Venous ulcers	Alginates Hydrocolloids Hydrogels Foams
Arterial ulcers	Alginates Hydrogels Foams
Diabetic ulcers	Alginates Hydrocolloids Transparent films Foams
Donor sites	Alginates Hydrocolloids Hydrogels Hydrogels sheets Transparent films Impregnated gauze Collagen

CHAPTER

18

LEARNING OBJECTIVES

1. Describe the epidemiology, etiology, pathophysiology, symptomatology, and sequelae of stroke.
2. Identify and describe the examination procedures used to evaluate patients with stroke to establish a diagnosis, prognosis, and plan of care.
3. Describe the role of the physical therapist in assisting the patient in recovery from stroke in terms of interventions, patient/client-related instruction, coordination, communication, and documentation.
4. Identify and describe strategies of intervention during inpatient rehabilitation.
5. Analyze and interpret patient data, formulate realistic goals and outcomes, and develop a plan of care when presented with a clinical case study.

Stroke

Susan B. O'Sullivan, PT, EdD

OUTLINE

Stroke or **brain attack** is the sudden loss of neurological function caused by an interruption of the blood flow to the brain. **Ischemic stroke** is the most common type, affecting about 80 percent of individuals with stroke, and results when a clot blocks or impairs blood flow, depriving the brain of essential oxygen and nutrients. **Hemorrhagic stroke** occurs when blood vessels rupture, causing leakage of blood in or around the brain. The term **cerebrovascular accident (CVA)** is used interchangeably with stroke to refer to the vascular conditions of the brain. Clinically, a variety of focal deficits are possible, including changes in the level of consciousness and impairments of sensory, motor, cognitive, perceptual, and language functions. To be classified as stroke, neurological deficits must persist for at least 24 hours. Motor deficits are characterized by paralysis (**hemiplegia**) or weakness (**hemiparesis**), typically on the side of the body opposite the side of the lesion. The term *hemiplegia* is often used generically to refer to the wide variety of motor problems that result from stroke. The location and extent of brain injury, the amount of collateral blood flow, and early acute care management determine the severity of neurological deficits in an individual patient. Impairments may resolve spontaneously as brain swelling subsides (reversible ischemic neurological deficit), generally within 3 weeks. Residual neurological impairments are those that persist longer than 3 weeks and may lead to permanent disability. Strokes are classified by etiological categories (thrombosis, embolus, or hemorrhage), specific vascular territory (anterior cerebral artery syndrome, middle cerebral artery syndrome, and so forth), and management categories (transient ischemic attack, minor stroke, major stroke, deteriorating stroke, young stroke).

Epidemiology

Stroke is the third leading cause of death and the most common cause of disability among adults in the United States. It affects approximately 700,000 individuals each year; about 500,000 are new strokes and 200,000 are recurrent strokes. There are an estimated 5,400,000 stroke survivors, or 2.6 percent of the population. The incidence of stroke is about 1.25 times greater for males than females. Compared to whites, African-Americans have twice the risk of first-ever stroke; rates are also higher in Mexican-Americans, American Indians, and Alaska Natives.[1] The incidence of stroke increases dramatically with age, doubling in the decade after 65 years of age. For white men 65 to 74 years of age, the incidence is about 14.4 per 1000 population; for ages 75 to 84 it is 24.6 and for 85 and older it is 27.0. Twenty-eight percent of strokes occur in individuals younger than 65 years of age.[2] About 14 percent of persons who survive an initial stroke or TIA will experience another one within 1 year.[1]

About 22 percent of men and 25 percent of women with an initial stroke will die within 1 year, with these rates increasing among people age 65 and older. After 8 years, only about half of patients under the age of 65 are still alive. The type of stroke is significant in determining survival. Of patients with stroke, hemorrhagic stroke account for the largest number of deaths, with mortality rates of 37 to 38 percent at 1 month while ischemic strokes have a mortality rate of only 8 to 12 percent at 1 month.[1] Survival rates are dramatically lessened by increased age, hypertension, heart disease, and diabetes. Loss of consciousness at stroke onset, lesion size, persistent severe hemiplegia, multiple neurological deficits, and history of previous stroke are also important predictors of mortality.[2]

Stroke is the most common cause of chronic disability.[3] Of survivors, an estimated one third will be functionally dependent after 1 year experiencing difficulty with activities of daily living (ADL), ambulation, speech, and so forth.[4] Stroke survivors represent the largest group admitted to inpatient rehabilitation hospitals.[5] Another indicator of disability is the fact that approximately 26 percent of patients with stroke are institutionalized in a nursing home. Direct and indirect costs of stroke in 2005 dollars are estimated at $56.8 billion.[1]

Etiology

Atherosclerosis is a major contributory factor in cerebrovascular disease. It is characterized by plaque formation with an accumulation of lipids, fibrin, complex carbohydrates, and calcium deposits on arterial walls that leads to progressive narrowing of blood vessels. Interruption of blood flow by atherosclerotic plaques occurs at certain sites of predilection. These generally include bifurcations, constrictions, dilation, or angulations of arteries. The most common sites for lesions to occur are at the origin of the common carotid artery or at its transition into the middle cerebral artery, at the main bifurcation of the middle cerebral artery, and at the junction of the vertebral arteries with the basilar artery (Fig. 18.1).

Ischemic strokes are the result of a thrombus, embolism, or conditions that produce low systemic perfusion pressures. The resulting lack of cerebral blood flow (CBF) deprives the brain of needed oxygen and glucose, disrupts cellular metabolism, and leads to injury and death of tissues. A thrombus

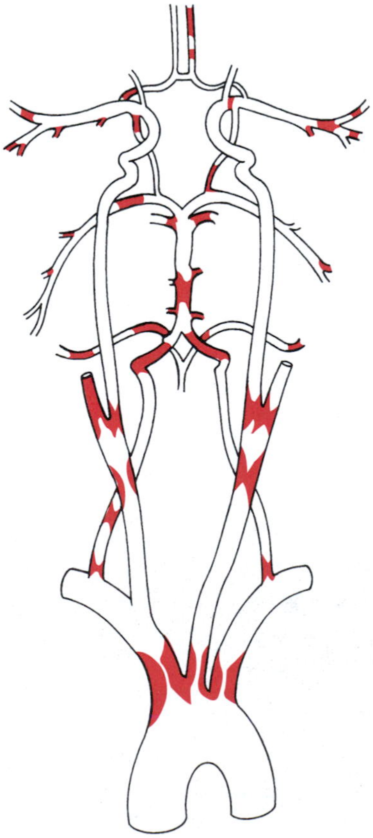

Figure 18.1 Preferred sites for atherosclerotic plaque. (From American Heart Association, Diagnosis and Management of Stroke, 1979, p 4, with permission.)

results from platelet adhesion and aggregation on plaques. **Cerebral thrombosis** refers to the formation or development of a blood clot within the cerebral arteries or their branches. It should be noted that lesions of extracranial vessels (carotid or vertebral arteries) can also produce symptoms of stroke. Thrombi lead to ischemia, or occlusion of an artery with resulting **cerebral infarction** or tissue death (atherothrombotic brain infarction [ABI]). Thrombi can also become dislodged and travel to a more distal site in the form of an intra-artery embolus. **Cerebral embolus (CE)** is composed of bits of matter (blood clot, plaque) formed elsewhere and released into the bloodstream, traveling to the cerebral arteries where they lodge in a vessel, produce occlusion and infarction. The most common source of cerebral embolus is disease of the cardiovascular system. Occasionally systemic disorders may produce septic, fat, or air emboli that affect the cerebral circulation. Ischemic strokes may also result from low systemic perfusion, the result of cardiac failure or significant blood loss with resulting systemic hypotension. The neurological deficits produced with systemic failure are global in nature with bilateral neurological deficits.

Hemorrhagic strokes, with abnormal bleeding into the extravascular areas of the brain are the result of rupture of a cerebral vessel or trauma. Hemorrhage results in increased intracranial pressures with injury to brain tissues and restriction of distal blood flow. **Intracerebral hemorrhage (IH)** is caused by rupture of a cerebral vessel with subsequent bleeding into the brain. Primary **cerebral hemorrhage** (nontraumatic spontaneous hemorrhage) typically occurs in small blood vessels weakened by atherosclerosis producing an **aneurysm. Subarachnoid hemorrhage (SH)** occurs from bleeding into the subarachnoid space typically from a saccular or berry aneurysm affecting primarily large blood vessels. Congenital defects that produce weakness in the blood vessel wall are major contributing factors to the formation of an aneurysm. Hemorrhage is closely linked to chronic hypertension. **Arteriovenous malformation (AVM)** is another congenital defect that can result in stroke. AVM is characterized by a tortuous tangle of arteries and veins with agenesis of an interposing capillary system. The abnormal vessels undergo progressive dilatation with age and eventually bleed in about 50 percent of cases. Sudden and severe cerebral bleeding can result in death within hours, because intracranial pressures rise rapidly and adjacent cortical tissues are compressed or displaced as in brainstem herniation.

Risk Factors and Stroke Prevention

Cardiovascular diseases affecting the brain and heart share a number of common risk factors important to the development of atherosclerosis. Major risk factors for stroke are hypertension, heart disease, and diabetes. In patients with ABI, 70 percent have hypertension, 30 percent coronary heart disease, 15 percent congestive heart disease, 30 percent peripheral arterial disease, and 15 percent diabetes.[2] This coexistence of vascular problems increases significantly with the age of the patient. Stroke risk is increased by four to six times in patients with high blood pressure (elevated above 160/95 mm Hg). Cardiovascular risk is also increased with elevated total blood cholesterol and low-density lipoprotein (LDL) cholesterol and is decreased with higher levels of high-density lipoprotein (HDL) cholesterol.[1] Patients with marked elevations of hematocrits are also at an increased risk of occlusive stroke owing to a generalized reduction of cerebral blood flow. Cardiac disorders such as rheumatic heart valvular disease, endocarditis, or cardiac surgery (e.g., coronary artery bypass graft [CABG]) increase the risk of embolic stroke. Atrial fibrillation is an independent risk factor with five times an increased risk of stroke. Transient ischemic attacks (TIAs) are another important risk factor for stroke. About 10 percent of individuals with TIA will go on to have a major stroke within 90 days; 5 percent will have a major stroke within 2 days.[1,2]

Stroke is largely preventable. Potentially modifiable risk factors include smoking, obesity, lack of exercise, diet, and excess alcohol consumption. Dietary recommendations include control of cholesterol and lipids. Cessation of cigarette smoking significantly decreases risk as does reducing obesity and increasing physical activity. Control of associated diseases, especially diabetes, hypertension, and heart disease, is essential. As with a cardiac risk profile, the more risk factors present or the greater the degree of abnormality of any one factor, the greater the risk of stroke. Stroke risk factors considered nonmodifiable include age (for adults older than 55 the lifetime risk is 1 in 6), gender (the rate for women is slightly higher due to the fact that women live longer), race (African-American), and family history.[1]

Effective stroke prevention also depends on improving public awareness concerning the *early warning signs of stroke*. Only about half of Americans can recognize even one warning sign. Early warning signs identified by The National Stroke Association[6] are listed in Box 18.1.

Box 18.1 Early Warning Signs of Stroke[6]

- Sudden numbness or weakness of the face, arm, or leg, especially on one side of the body
- Sudden confusion, trouble speaking or understanding
- Sudden trouble seeing in one or both eyes
- Sudden trouble walking, dizziness, loss of balance or coordination
- Sudden, severe headaches with no known cause

Other important but less common stroke symptoms include:

- Sudden nausea, fever, and vomiting distinguished from a viral illness by the speed of onset (minutes or hours vs several days)
- Brief loss of consciousness or a period of decreased consciousness (fainting, confusion, convulsions, or coma)

The significance of recognizing early warning signs rests with prompt initiation of emergency care under the rule that "*time is brain*." Patients and families are encouraged to call 911 immediately, even if these symptoms go away quickly or are not painful.[6] Early computed tomography (CT) is used to differentiate between atherothrombotic stroke and hemorrhagic stroke. If the stroke is atherothrombotic, clot-dissolving enzymes (tissue plasminogen activator [t-PA], urokinase, or prourokinase) can be administered. To be effective, thrombolytic therapy such as t-PA must be given within 3 hours of the onset of symptoms and cannot be given with hemorrhagic stroke because the drug may worsen bleeding. Within this window of opportunity, the patient must recognize the situation as a medical emergency, be transported to an appropriate hospital, evaluated by emergency room staff including a CT scan of the brain, and treated. Although this treatment has been available since the mid-1990s and has been shown to be safe and dramatically reduce death and disability,[7,8] current estimates indicate that only 5 percent of individuals experiencing stroke are treated with t-PA.[9] Patients who do receive t-PA are more likely to recover with no disability or minimal disability as compared to those who do not receive the treatment.[10] Major heart and stroke organizations currently promote the use of the term *brain attack* to help individuals recognize the importance of seeking immediate emergency care.

Pathophysiology

Interruption of blood flow for only a few minutes sets in motion a series of pathological events. Complete cerebral circulatory arrest results in irreversible cellular damage with a core area of focal infarction within minutes. The transitional area surrounding the core is termed the *ischemic penumbra* and consists of viable but metabolically lethargic cells. Ischemia triggers a number of damaging and potentially reversible events, termed **ischemic cascade**. The release of excess neurotransmitters (glutamate and aspartate) produces a progressive disturbance of energy metabolism and anoxic depolarization. This results in an inability of brain cells to produce energy, particularly adenosine triphosphate (ATP). This is followed by excess influx of calcium ions and pump failure of the neuronal membrane. Excess calcium reacts with intracellular phospholipids to form free radicals. Calcium influx also stimulates the release of nitric oxide and cytokines. Both mechanisms further damage brain cells. The extension of the infarction into the penumbra area generally takes place over a period of 3 to 4 hours.[11] Research efforts are ongoing toward development of drugs that might restore blood supply and reverse the metabolic changes of the ischemic penumbra area.

Ischemic strokes produce **cerebral edema**, an accumulation of fluids within the brain that begins within minutes of the insult and reaches a maximum by 3 to 4 days. It is the result of tissue necrosis and widespread rupture of cell membranes with movement of water from the blood into brain tissues. The swelling gradually subsides and generally disappears by 2 to 3 weeks. Significant edema can elevate intracranial pressures, leading to intracranial hypertension and neurological deterioration associated with contralateral and caudal shifts of brain structures (**brainstem herniation**). Clinical signs of elevating intracranial pressures (ICP) include decreasing level of consciousness (stupor and coma), widened pulse pressure, increased heart rate, irregular respirations (Cheyne-Stokes respirations), vomiting, unreacting pupils (cranial nerve [CN] III signs), and papilledema. Cerebral edema is the most frequent cause of death in acute stroke and is characteristic of large infarcts involving the middle cerebral artery and the internal carotid artery.[12]

Management Categories

Transient ischemic attack (TIA) refers to the temporary interruption of blood supply to the brain. Symptoms of focal neurological deficit may last for only a few minutes or for several hours, but do not last longer than 24 hours. After the attack is over there is no evidence of residual brain damage or permanent neurological dysfunction. TIAs may result from a number of different etiological factors including occlusive episodes, emboli, reduced cerebral perfusion (arrhythmias, decreased cardiac output, hypotension, overmedication with antihypertensive medications, **subclavian steal syndrome**) or cerebrovascular spasm. The major clinical significance of TIA is as a precursor to susceptibility for both cerebral infarction and myocardial infarction. Patients are classified as having a *major stroke* in the presence of stable, usually severe, impairments. The term *deteriorating stroke* is used to refer to the patient whose neurological status is deteriorating after admission to the hospital. This change in status may be due to cerebral or systemic causes (e.g., cerebral edema, progressing thrombosis). The category of *young stroke* is used to describe a stroke affecting persons younger than the age of 45. Younger individuals may have potential for better recovery.

Vascular Syndromes

Cerebral blood flow (CBF) varies with the patency of the vessels. Progressive narrowing secondary to atherosclerosis decreases blood flow. As in coronary heart disease, symptomatic changes generally result from a restriction of flow greater than 80 percent. The severity and symptoms of stroke are dependent on a number of factors, including (1) the location of the ischemic process, (2) the size of the ischemic area, (3) the nature and functions of the structures involved, and (4) the availability of collateral blood flow.

Presenting symptoms may also depend on the rapidity of the occlusion of a blood vessel because slow occlusions may allow collateral vessels to take over, whereas sudden events do not.

Cerebral Blood Flow

CBF is controlled by a number of *autoregulatory mechanisms* (cerebral) that modulate a constant rate of blood flow through the brain. These mechanisms provide homeostatic balance, counteracting fluctuations in systolic blood pressure while maintaining a normal flow of 50 to 60 ml/100 g of brain tissue per minute. The brain has high energy requirements and very little metabolic reserves. Thus it requires a continuous, rich perfusion of blood to deliver oxygen and glucose to the tissues. Cerebral flow represents approximately 17 percent of available cardiac output. Chemical regulation of CBF occurs in response to changes in blood concentrations of carbon dioxide or oxygen. Vasodilation and increased CBF are produced in response to an increase in $Paco_2$ or a decrease in Pao_2, while vasoconstriction and decreased CBF are produced by the opposite stimuli. Blood flow is also altered by changes in the blood pH. A fall in pH (increased acidity) produces vasodilation, and a rise in pH (increased alkalinity) produces a decrease in blood flow. Neurogenic regulation alters blood flow by vasodilating vessels in direct proportion to local function of brain tissue. Released metabolites probably act directly on the smooth muscle in local vessel walls. Changes in blood viscosity or intracranial pressures may also influence CBF. Changes in blood pressure produce minor alterations of CBF. As pressure rises, the artery is stretched, resulting in contraction of smooth muscle in the vessel wall. Thus, the patency of the vessel is decreased, with a consequent decrease in CBF. As pressure falls, contraction lessens and CBF increases. Following stroke, autoregulatory mechanisms may be impaired.[13]

Knowledge of cerebral vascular anatomy is essential to understand the symptoms, diagnosis, and management of stroke. Extracranial blood supply to the brain is provided by right and left internal carotid arteries and by the right and left vertebral arteries. The internal carotid artery begins at the bifurcation of the common carotid artery and ascends in the deep portions of the neck to the carotid canal. It turns rostromedially and ascends into the cranial cavity. It then pierces the dura mater and gives off the ophthalmic and anterior choroidal arteries before bifurcating into the middle and anterior cerebral arteries. The anterior communicating artery communicates with the anterior cerebral arteries of either side, giving rise to the rostral portion of the **circle of Willis** (Fig. 18.2). The vertebral artery arises as a branch off the subclavian artery. It enters the vertebral foramen of the sixth cervical vertebra and travels through the foramina of the transverse processes of the upper six cervical vertebrae to the

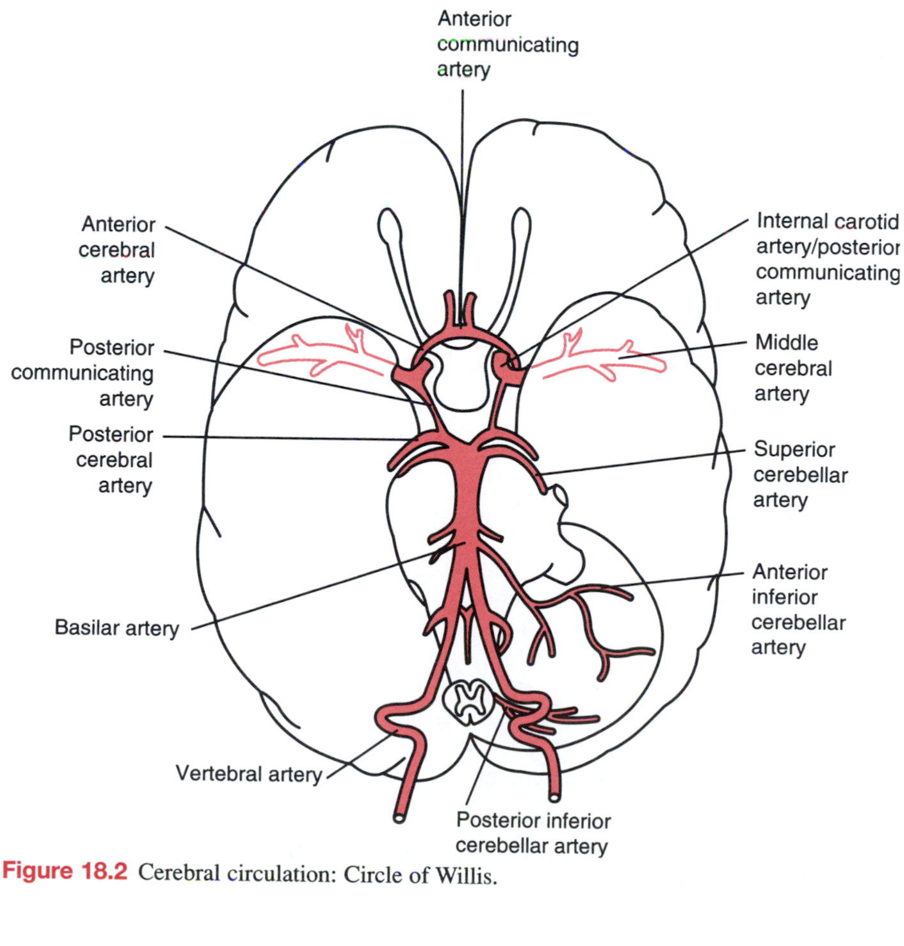

Figure 18.2 Cerebral circulation: Circle of Willis.

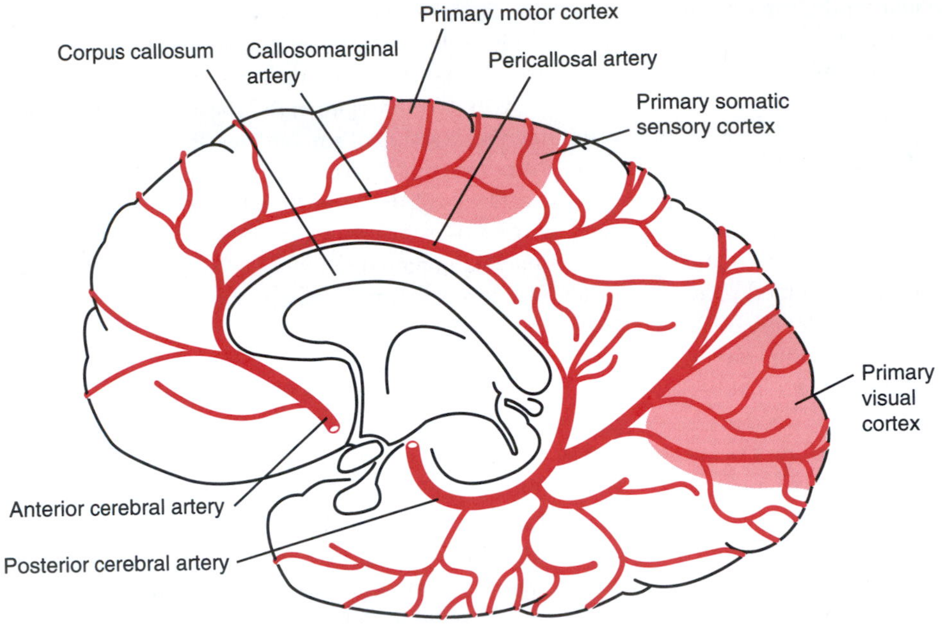

Figure 18.3 Cerebral circulation: A diagram of a midsagittal view of the brain illustrates the distribution of the anterior and posterior cerebral arteries.

foramen magnum and into the brain. There it travels in the posterior cranial fossa ventrally and medially and unites with the vertebral artery from the other side to form the basilar artery at the upper border of the medulla. At the upper border of the pons, the basilar artery bifurcates to form the posterior cerebral arteries and the posterior portion of the circle of Willis. Posterior communicating arteries connect the posterior cerebral arteries with the internal carotid arteries and complete the circle of Willis.

Anterior Cerebral Artery Syndrome

The anterior cerebral artery (ACA) is the first and smaller of two terminal branches of the internal carotid artery. It supplies the medial aspect of the cerebral hemisphere (frontal and parietal lobes) and subcortical structures, including the basal ganglia (anterior internal capsule, inferior caudate nucleus), anterior fornix, and anterior four fifths of the corpus callosum (Fig. 18.3). Because the anterior communicating artery allows perfusion of the proximal anterior cerebral artery from either side, occlusion proximal to this point results in minimal deficit.

More distal lesions produce more significant deficits. Table 18.1 presents the clinical manifestations of *anterior cerebral artery (ACA) syndrome*. The most common characteristic of ACA syndrome is contralateral hemiparesis and sensory loss with greater involvement of the lower extremity because the somatotopic organization of the medial

Table 18.1 Clinical Manifestations of Anterior Cerebral Artery Syndrome

Signs and Symptoms	Structures Involved
Contralateral hemiparesis involving mainly the LE (UE is more spared)	Primary motor area, medial aspect of cortex, internal capsule
Contralateral hemisensory loss involving mainly the LE (UE is more spared)	Primary sensory area, medial aspect of cortex
Urinary incontinence	Posteromedial aspect of superior frontal gyrus
Problems with imitation and bimanual tasks, apraxia	Corpus callosum
Abulia (akinetic mutism), slowness, delay, lack of spontaneity, motor inaction	Uncertain localization
Contralateral grasp reflex, sucking reflex Can be asymptomatic if circle of Willis is competent.	Uncertain localization

LE = lower extremity; UE = upper extremity.

Adapted from Fredericks, C, and Saladin, L: Pathophysiology of the Motor Systems. FA Davis, Philadelphia, 1996, p 504, with permission.

aspect of the cortex includes the functional area for the lower extremity.

Middle Cerebral Artery Syndrome

The middle cerebral artery (MCA) is the second of the two main branches of the internal carotid artery and supplies the entire lateral aspect of the cerebral hemisphere (frontal, temporal, and parietal lobes) and subcortical structures, including the internal capsule (posterior portion), corona radiata, globus pallidus (outer part), most of the caudate nucleus, and the putamen (Fig. 18.4). Occlusion of the proximal MCA produces extensive neurological damage with significant cerebral edema. Increased intracranial pressures typically lead to loss of consciousness, brain herniation, and possibly death. Table 18.2 presents the clinical manifestations of *middle cerebral artery (MCA) syndrome.* The most common characteristics of MCA syndrome are contralateral spastic hemiparesis and sensory loss of the face, upper extremity (UE), and lower extremity (LE), with the face and UE more involved than the LE. Lesions of the parieto-occipital cortex of the dominant hemisphere (usually the left hemisphere) typically produce aphasia. Lesions of the right parietal lobe of the nondominant hemisphere (usually the right hemisphere) typically produce perceptual deficits (e.g., **unilateral neglect**, **anosognosia, apraxia**, and **spatial disorganization**). **Homonymous hemianopsia** (a visual field defect) is also a common finding. The MCA is the most common site of occlusion in stroke.

Internal Carotid Artery Syndrome

Occlusion of the internal carotid artery (ICA) typically produces massive infarction in the region of the brain supplied by the middle cerebral artery. The ICA supplies both the MCA and the ACA. If collateral circulation to the ACA from the circle of Willis is absent, extensive cerebral infarction in the areas of both the ACA and MCA can occur. Significant edema is common with possible uncal herniation, coma, and death (mass effect).

Posterior Cerebral Artery Syndrome

The two posterior cerebral arteries (PCAs) arise as terminal branches of the basilar artery and each supplies the corresponding occipital lobe and medial and inferior temporal lobe (see Fig. 18.3). It also supplies the upper brainstem, midbrain, and posterior diencephalon, including most of the thalamus. Table 18.3 presents the clinical manifestations of *posterior cerebral artery (PCA) syndrome.* Occlusion proximal to the posterior communicating artery typically results in minimal deficits owing to the collateral blood supply from the posterior communicating artery (similar to ACA syndrome). Occlusion of thalamic branches may produce hemianesthesia (contralateral sensory loss) or **central post-stroke (thalamic) pain**. Occipital infarction produces homonymous hemianopsia, **visual agnosia**, **prosopagnosia**, or, if bilateral, cortical blindness. Temporal lobe ischemia results in amnesia (memory loss). Involvement of subthalamic branches may involve

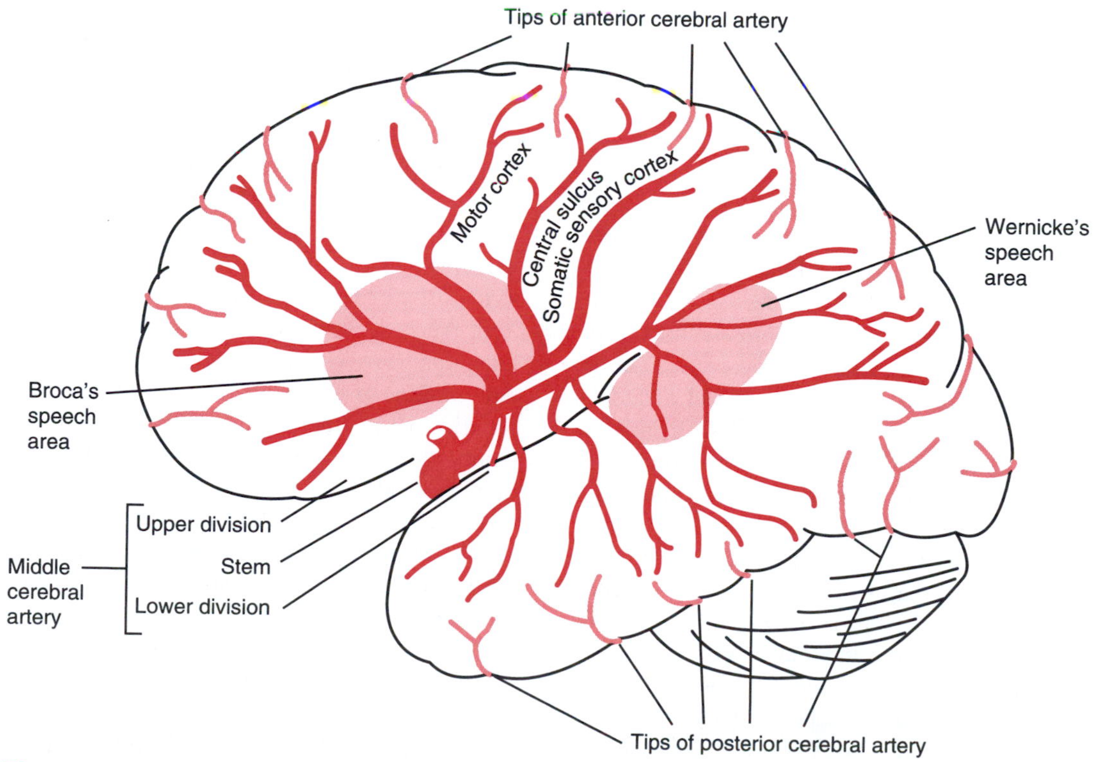

Figure 18.4 Cerebral circulation: Diagram of a lateral view of the brain illustrates the distribution of the middle cerebral artery.

Table 18.2 Clinical Manifestations of Middle Cerebral Artery Syndrome

Signs and Symptoms	Structures Involved
Contralateral hemiparesis involving mainly the UE and face (LE is more spared)	Primary motor cortex and internal capsule
Contralateral hemisensory loss involving mainly the UE and face (LE is more spared)	Primary sensory cortex and internal capsule
Motor speech impairment: Broca's or nonfluent aphasia with limited vocabulary and slow, hesitant speech	Broca's cortical area (third frontal convolution) in the dominant hemisphere, typically the left hemisphere
Receptive speech impairment: Wernicke's or fluent aphasia with impaired auditory comprehension and fluent speech with normal rate and melody	Wernicke's cortical area (posterior portion of the temporal gyrus) in the dominant hemisphere, typically the left
Global aphasia: nonfluent speech with poor comprehension	Both third frontal convolution and posterior portion of the superior temporal gyrus
Perceptual deficits: unilateral neglect, depth perception, spatial relations, agnosia	Parietal sensory association cortex in the nondominant hemisphere, typically the right
Limb-kinetic apraxia	Premotor or parietal cortex
Contralateral homonymous hemianopsia	Optic radiation in internal capsule
Loss of conjugate gaze to the opposite side	Frontal eye fields or their descending tracts
Ataxia of contralateral limb(s) (sensory ataxia)	Parietal lobe
Pure motor hemiplegia (lacunar stroke)	Upper portion of posterior limb of internal capsule

LE = lower extremity; UE = upper extremity.

Adapted from Fredericks, C, and Saladin, L: Pathophysiology of the Motor Systems. FA Davis, Philadelphia, 1996, p 502, with permission.

subthalamic nucleus or its pallidal connections, producing a wide variety of deficits. Contralateral hemiplegia occurs with involvement of the cerebral peduncle.

Lacunar Syndromes

Lacunar syndromes are caused by small vessel disease deep in the cerebral white mater (penetrating artery disease). They are strongly associated with hypertensive hemorrhage and diabetic microvascular disease. Lacunar syndromes are consistent with specific anatomic sites. *Pure motor lacunar stroke* is associated with involvement of the posterior limb of the internal capsule, pons, and pyramids. *Pure sensory lacunar stroke* is associated with involvement of the ventrolateral thalamus or thalamocortical projections. Other lacunar syndromes include *dysarthria/clumsy hand syndrome* (involving the base of the pons, genu of anterior limb or the internal capsule), *ataxic hemiparesis* (involving the pons, genu of internal capsule, corona radiata, or cerebellum), *sensory/motor stroke* (involving the junction of the internal capsule and thalamus), or *dystonia/involuntary movements* (choreoathetosis with lacunar infarction of the putamen or globus pallidus; hemiballismus with involvement of the subthalamic nucleus). Deficits in consciousness, language, or visual fields are not seen in lacunar strokes as the higher cortical areas are preserved. A hypertensive hemorrhage affecting the thalamus can also produce central post-stroke pain.[11–16]

Vertebrobasilar Artery Syndrome

The vertebral arteries arise from the subclavian arteries and travel into the brain along the medulla where they merge at the inferior border of the pons to form the basilar artery. The vertebral arteries supply the cerebellum (via posterior inferior cerebellar arteries) and the medulla (via the medullary arteries). The basilar artery supplies the pons (via pontine arteries), the internal ear (via labyrinthine arteries), and the cerebellum (via the anterior inferior and superior cerebellar arteries). The basilar artery then terminates at the upper border of the pons giving rise to the two posterior arteries (see Fig. 18.2). Occlusions of the vertebrobasilar system can produce a wide variety of symptoms with both ipsilateral and contralateral signs, because some of the tracts in the brainstem will have crossed and others will not. Numerous cerebellar and cranial nerve abnormalities also are present. Table 18.4 presents the clinical manifestations of *vertebrobasilar artery syndromes*.

Locked-in syndrome (LIS) occurs with basilar artery thrombosis and bilateral infarction of the ventral pons. LIS is a catastrophic event with sudden onset. Patients develop

Table 18.3 Clinical Manifestations of Posterior Cerebral Artery Syndrome

Signs and Symptoms	Structures Involved
Peripheral territory	
Contralateral homonymous hemianopsia	Primary visual cortex or optic radiation
Bilateral homonymous hemianopsia with some degree of macular sparing	Calcarine cortex (macular sparing is due to occipital pole receiving collateral blood supply from MCA)
Visual agnosia	Left occipital lobe
Prosopagnosia (difficulty naming people on sight)	Visual association cortex
Dyslexia (difficulty reading) without agraphia (difficulty writing), color naming (anomia), and color discrimination problems	Dominant calcarine lesion and posterior part of corpus callosum
Memory defect	Lesion of inferomedial portions of temporal lobe bilaterally or on the dominant side only
Topographic disorientation	Nondominant primary visual area, usually bilaterally
Central territory	
Central post-stroke (thalamic) pain	
Spontaneous pain and dysesthesias; sensory impairments (all modalities)	Ventral posterolateral nucleus of thalamus
Involuntary movements; choreoathetosis, intention tremor, hemiballismus	Subthalamic nucleus or its pallidal connections
Contralateral hemiplegia	Cerebral peduncle of midbrain
Weber's syndrome	
Oculomotor nerve palsy and contralateral hemiplegia	Third nerve and cerebral peduncle of midbrain
Paresis of vertical eye movements, slight miosis and ptosis, and sluggish pupillary light response	Supranuclear fibers to third cranial nerve

LE = lower extremity; UE = upper extremity.

Adapted from Fredericks, C, and Saladin, L: Pathophysiology of the Motor Systems. FA Davis, Philadelphia, 1996, p 509, with permission.

acute hemiparesis rapidly progressing to tetraplegia and lower bulbar paralysis (CN V through XII are involved). Initially the patient is dysarthric and dysphonic but rapidly progresses to mutism (anarthria). There is preserved consciousness and sensation. Thus the patient cannot move or speak but remains alert and oriented. Horizontal eye movements are impaired but vertical eye movements and blinking remain intact. Communication can be established via these eye movements. Mortality rates are high (59 percent), and those patients that do survive are left with severe impairments associated with brainstem injury.[14,15]

Extracranial injuries to the vertebral arteries as they travel through the cervical spine can also produce vertebrobasilar signs and symptoms. Forceful neck motions (e.g., whiplash or aggressive neck manipulations) are among the more common types of injuries.

Medical Diagnosis of Stroke

History and Examination

An accurate history profiling the timing of neurological events is obtained from the patient or from family members in the case of the unconscious or noncommunicative patient. Of particular importance are the pattern of onset and the course of initial neurological symptoms. An abrupt onset with rapid coma is suggestive of cerebral hemorrhage. Severe headache typically precedes loss of consciousness. An embolus also occurs rapidly, with no warning, and is frequently associated with heart disease and/or heart complications. A more variable and uneven onset is typical with thrombosis. The patient's past history including episodes of TIAs or head trauma, presence of major or

(text continues on page 716)

Table 18.4 Clinical Manifestations of Vertebrobasilar Artery Syndromes

Signs and Symptoms	Structures Involved
Medial medullary syndrome	Occlusion vertebral artery, medullary branch
Ipsilateral to lesion Paralysis with atrophy of half the tongue with deviation to the paralyzed side when tongue is protruded	CN XII, hypoglossal, or nucleus
Contralateral to lesion Paralysis of UE and LE	Corticospinal tract
Impaired tactile and proprioceptive sense	Medial lemniscus
Lateral medullary (Wallenburg's) syndrome	Occlusion of posterior inferior cerebellar artery or vertebral artery
Ipsilateral to lesion Decreased pain and temperature sensation in face	Descending tract and nucleus of CN V, Trigeminal
Cerebellar ataxia: gait and limbs ataxia	Cerebellum or inferior cerebellar peduncle
Vertigo, nausea, vomiting	Vestibular nuclei and connections
Nystagmus	Vestibular nuclei and connections
Horner's syndrome: miosis, ptosis, decreased sweating	Descending sympathetic tract
Dysphagia and dysphonia: paralysis of palatal and laryngeal muscles, diminished gag reflex	CN IX, glossopharyngeal, and CN X, vagus, or nuclei
Sensory impairment of ipsilateral UE, trunk, or LE	Cuneate and gracile nuclei
Contralateral to lesion Impaired pain and thermal sense over 50% of body, sometimes face	Spinal lemniscus—spinothalamic tract
Complete basilar artery syndrome (locked-in syndrome)	Basilar artery, ventral pons
Tetraplegia (Quadriplegia)	Corticospinal tracts bilaterally
Bilateral cranial nerve palsy: upward gaze is spared	Long tracts to cranial nerve nuclei bilaterally
Coma	Reticular activating system
Cognition is spared	
Medial inferior pontine syndrome	Occlusion of paramedian branch of basilar artery
Ipsilateral to lesion Paralysis of conjugate gaze to side of lesion (preservation of convergence)	Pontine center for lateral gaze paramedian pentine reticular formation (PPRF)
Nystagmus	Vestibular nuclei and connections
Ataxia of limbs and gait	Middle cerebellar peduncle
Diplopia on lateral gaze	CN VI, abducens, or nucleus
Contralateral to lesion Paresis of face, UE, and LE	Corticobulbar and corticospinal tract in lower pons
Impaired tactile and proprioceptive sense over 50% of the body	Medial lemniscus

Table 18.4 Clinical Manifestations of Vertebrobasilar Artery Syndromes (continued)

Signs and Symptoms	Structures Involved
Lateral inferior pontine syndrome	Occlusion of anterior inferior cerebellar artery, a branch of the basilar artery
Ipsilateral to lesion	
Horizontal and vertical nystagmus, vertigo, nausea, vomiting	CN VIII, vestibular, or nucleus
Facial paralysis	CN VII, facial, or nucleus
Paralysis of conjugate gaze to side of lesion	Pontine center for lateral gaze (PPRF)
Deafness, tinnitus	CN VIII, cochlear, or nucleus
Ataxia	Middle cerebellar peduncle and cerebellar hemisphere
Impaired sensation over face	Main sensory nucleus and descending tract of fifth nerve
Contralateral to lesion	
Impaired pain and thermal sense over half the body (may include face)	Spinothalamic tract
Medial midpontine syndrome	Occlusion of paramedian branch of the mid-basilar artery
Ipsilateral to lesion	
Ataxia of limbs and gait (more prominent in bilateral involvement)	Middle cerebellar peduncle
Contralateral to lesion	
Paralysis of face, UE, and LE	Corticobulbar and corticospinal tract
Deviation of eyes	PPRF
Lateral midpontine syndrome	Occlusion of short circumferential artery
Ipsilateral to lesion	
Ataxia of limbs	Middle cerebellar peduncle
Paralysis of muscles of mastication	Motor fibers or nucleus of CN V, trigeminal
Impaired sensation over side of face	Sensory fibers or nucleus of CN V, trigeminal
Medial superior pontine syndrome	Occlusion of paramedian branches of upper basilar artery
Cerebellar ataxia	Superior or middle cerebellar peduncle
Internuclear ophthalmoplegia	Medial longitudinal fasciculus
Contralateral to lesion	
Paralysis of face, UE, and LE	Corticobulbar and corticospinal tract

(*continued*)

Table 18.4 Clinical Manifestations of Vertebrobasilar Artery Syndromes (continued)

Signs and Symptoms	Structures Involved
Lateral superior pontine syndrome (occlusion of superior cerebellar artery, a branch of the basilar artery)	
Ipsilateral to lesion	
Cerebellar ataxia of limbs and gait, falling to side of lesion	Middle and superior cerebellar peduncles, superior surface of cerebellum, dentate nucleus
Dizziness, nausea, vomiting	Vestibular nuclei
Horizontal nystagmus	Vestibular nuclei
Paresis of conjugate gaze (ipsilateral)	Uncertain
Loss of optokinetic nystagmus	Uncertain
Horner's syndrome: miosis, ptosis, decreased sweating on opposite side face	Descending sympathetic fibers
Contralateral to lesion	
Impaired pain and thermal sense of face, limbs, and trunk	Spinothalamic tract
Impaired touch, vibration, and position sense, more in LE than UE (tendency to incongruity of pain and touch deficits)	Medial lemniscus (lateral portion)

CN = cranial nerve; LE = lower extremity; UE = upper extremity.

Adapted from Fredericks, C, and Saladin, L: Pathophysiology of the Motor Systems. FA Davis, Philadelphia, 1996, p 505, with permission.

minor risk factors, medications, pertinent family history, and any recent alterations in patient function (either transient or permanent) are thoroughly investigated.

The physical examination of the patient includes a general medical examination as well as a neurological examination. An investigation of vital signs (heart rate, respiratory rate, blood pressure) and signs of cardiac decompensation is essential. The neurological examination stresses function of the cerebral hemispheres, cerebellum, cranial nerves, eyes, and sensorimotor system. The presenting symptoms will help to determine the location of the lesion, and comparison of both sides of the body will reveal the side of the lesion. Bilateral signs are suggestive of brainstem lesions or massive cerebral involvement.

Neurovascular tests are performed. These include:

- *Neck flexion*. Meningeal irritation secondary to subarachnoid hemorrhage will produce resistance or pain with neck flexion.
- *Palpation of arteries*. Both superficial and deep arteries are palpated including temporal, facial, carotid, subclavian, brachial, radial, abdominal aorta, and lower extremity (LE) arteries.
- *Auscultation of heart and blood vessels*. Abnormal heart sounds, murmurs, or bruits may be present and indicate increased flow turbulence and stenosis in a vessel.
- *Ophthalmic pressures*. Abnormal pressures in the ophthalmic artery may indicate problems in the internal carotid artery.

Tests and Measures

A number of routine laboratory and diagnostic tests are performed.[11] These include:

- *Urinalysis*: Detects infection, diabetes, renal failure, or dehydration.
- *Blood analysis*: Provides a complete blood count (CBC), platelet count, prothrombin time, partial thromboplastin time, and erythrocyte sedimentation rate (ESR).
- *Fasting blood glucose level*
- *Blood chemistry profile*: Indicates serum electrolytes and serum cardiac enzyme levels. Electrolyte abnormalities may contribute to extension of infarct to the penumbra area. Elevation of the creatinine phosphokinase isoenzyme (CPK-MB) is indicative of coincidental cardiac infarction.
- *Blood cholesterol and lipid profile*.
- *Thyroid function tests*: Accelerated atherosclerosis can result from hypothyroidism.
- *Full cardiac evaluation*: Includes radiograph of the chest (heart size, lungs); electrocardiograph (ECG) to detect arrhythmias as a source of emboli or coincidental heart

disease. Stroke may also cause ECG abnormalities, typically T-wave inversion, prolonged QT interval, and ST inversion.

- *Echocardiography*: May reveal valvular disease (a source of emboli) or other heart conditions such as congestive heart failure (CHF), recent myocardial infarction (MI).
- *Lumbar puncture*: May be used to diagnosis subarachnoid hemorrhage in the presence of focal neurological deficit and nuchal rigidity.

Imaging

Modern cerebrovascular imaging techniques have vastly improved the accurate diagnosis of stroke. These include:

Computerized Tomography (CT). CT scan is the most commonly used imaging technique. An intravenous iodinated contrast dye may be used to enhance the density of intravascular blood. CT resolution only allows identification of large arteries and veins, and venous sinuses. In the acute phase, the CT scans are used to rule out other brain lesions such as tumor or abscess and to identify hemorrhagic stroke. In the case of suspected stroke, an emergency CT is used to rule out hemorrhage if anticoagulants or clot-busting drugs are to be administered. Many times CT scans during the acute phase are negative with no clear abnormalities. In the subacute phase, CT scans can delineate the development of cerebral edema (within 3 days) and cerebral infarction (within 3 to 5 days) by showing areas of decreased density. It is important to remember that the extent of CT lesion does not necessarily correlate with clinical signs or changes in function (Fig. 18.5).

Magnetic Resonance Imaging (MRI). MRI measures nuclear particles as they interact with a powerful magnetic field. Greater resolution of the brain and its structural detail is obtained with MRI than with a CT scan. Magnetic resonance imaging is more sensitive in the diagnosis of acute strokes, allowing detection of cerebral infarction within 2 to 6 hours after stroke. It is also able to detail the extent of infarction or hemorrhage and can detect smaller lesions than a CT scan. Contrast enhancement (e.g., gadolinium) can be used to document changes in an infarct over the first 2 to 3 weeks.

Positron Emission Tomography (PET). Positron emission from an injected radionuclide is measured. The use of PET allows imaging of regional blood flow and localized cerebral metabolism. PET scanning can be used in the subacute stage to distinguish infracted areas and to identify areas of tissue where ischemia is reversible. The high cost and limited availability of PET scans limit the use in the routine evaluation of stroke.

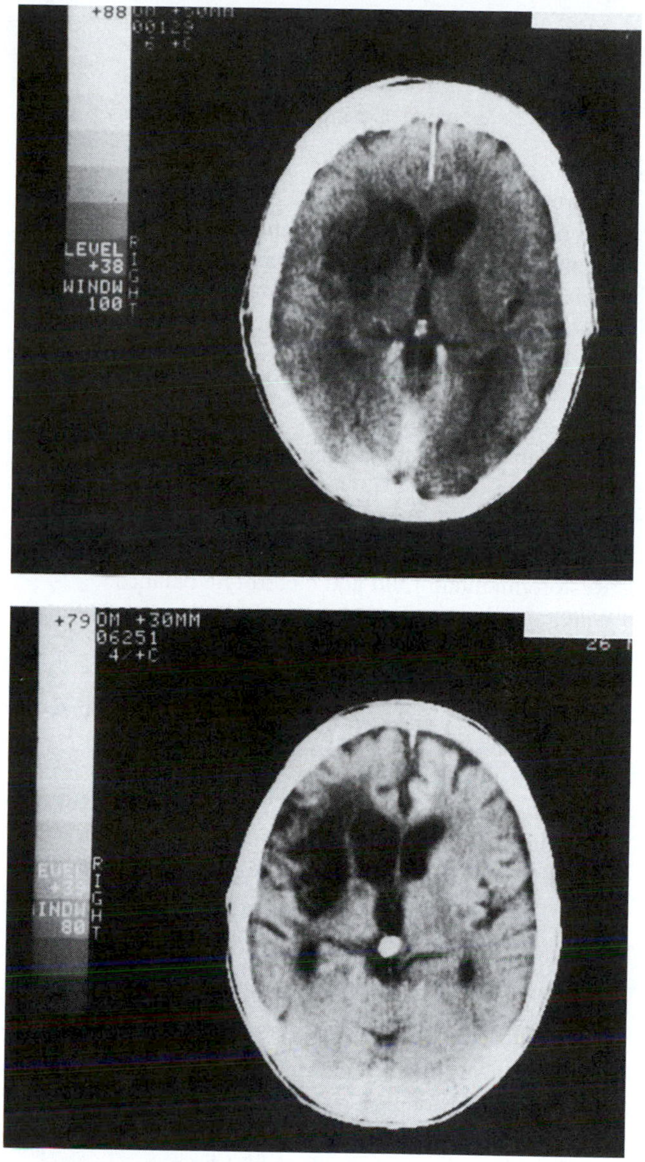

Figure 18.5 Computed tomography scan of a patient with infarction of the middle cerebral artery territory. (From Hackinski, W, and Norris, JW: The Acute Stroke. FA Davis, Philadelphia, 1985, p 194, with permission.)

Transcranial and Carotid Doppler. This technique is used for noninvasive imaging of the neck and chest vessels (carotid, vertebral, and subclavian arteries).

Cerebral Angiography. Cerebral angiography is invasive and involves the injection of radiopaque dye into blood vessels with subsequent radiography. It provides visualization of the vascular system and is often used when surgery is considered (carotid stenosis, arteriovenous malformations). There is associated morbidity and mortality with angiography. CT or MRI scans are more commonly used.

Medical Management

Medical management of completed stroke includes strategies to:

- Improve cerebral perfusion by reestablishing circulation and oxygenation. Oxygen is delivered via mask or nasal cannula. Patients in a coma may require intubation or assisted ventilation and suctioning.
- Maintain adequate blood pressure. Hypotension or extreme hypertension is treated; antihypertension agents have the added risk of inducing hypotension and decreasing cerebral perfusion.
- Maintain sufficient cardiac output. If the causes of stroke are cardiac in origin, medical management focuses on control of arrhythmias and cardiac decompensation.
- Restore/maintain fluid and electrolyte balance.
- Maintain blood glucose levels within the normal range.
- Control seizures and infections.
- Control intracranial pressures and herniation using antiedema agents. Ventriculostomy may be indicated to monitor and drain cerebrospinal fluid.
- Maintain bladder function, which may include urinary catheter. Catheterization is typically short-term but may be long-term with the patient in coma.
- Maintain integrity of skin and joints by instituting protective positioning; a turning schedule every 2 hours; and early physical and occupational therapy.

Pharmacological interventions for completed stroke can include[11]:

- Anticoagulant therapy (heparin, Coumadin): used to improve perfusion and reduce the risk of recurring clots (embolism and thrombosis); clotting times are monitored as there is an increased risk of bleeding.
- Antiplatelet therapy (aspirin): Long-term, low-dose is used to decrease the risk of recurrent stroke; higher doses may be used in place of anticoagulants and may be recommended for patients with atrial fibrillation. Ticlopidine or clopidogrel bisulfate are alternate agents for recurrent stroke prevention.
- Antihypertensive agents.

Neurosurgical intervention may include:

- Endarterectomy which is the surgical removal of the lining and plaque of an artery. Internal carotid artery stenosis affects approximately 25 percent of elderly persons. Endarterectomy is used to prevent strokes but not to treat acute strokes.[11]
- In hemorrhagic stroke, surgery can be used to repair a superficial ruptured aneurysm or AVM, prevent rebleeding, and evacuate a clot (hematoma). Larger, deeper intracranial or brainstem vascular lesions are generally not amendable to surgery.
- Surgery may also be indicated for resection of a superficial unruptured AVM when there is high risk of rupture and stroke.

Primary Impairments

Sensation

Sensation is frequently impaired but rarely absent on the hemiplegic side. Impairments are reported in about 53 percent of patients with stroke and can range from loss of superficial and/or deep sensations to impairments in the combined cortical sensations (see Chapter 5).[2] The type and extent of impairment is related to the location and size of the vascular lesion. Specific localized areas of dysfunction are common with cortical lesions, whereas diffuse involvement throughout one side of the body suggests deeper lesions involving the thalamus and adjacent structures. The most common distribution of loss is a face-UE-LE pattern (reported in 55 percent of cases). Less frequently, impairments may be noted in face-UE (29 percent of cases) or UE-LE (7 percent of cases).[17] Symptoms of crossed anesthesia (ipsilateral facial impairments with contralateral trunk and limb involvement) typify brainstem lesions. Proprioceptive losses are common. In one study, 44 percent of patients with stroke demonstrated significant proprioceptive loss with associated impairments noted in motor control, postural function, and balance.[18] Loss of superficial touch and pain and temperature sensation is also common. Profound hemisensory loss can contribute to unilateral neglect, difficulty with functional tasks, and increased risk of self-injury. The patient may also complain of abnormal sensations such as numbness, dysesthesias, or hyperesthesia.

Pain

Hemorrhagic or ischemic stroke can result in severe headache or neck and face pain. Lesions of the PCA involving the ventral posterolateral thalamus and spinothalamic system can result in central post-stroke (thalamic) pain. This is characterized by constant, severe burning pain with intermittent sharp pains. Patients experience an exaggerated response to stimuli affecting the contralateral half of the body. Paroxysmal spasms of pain may be triggered by simply stroking the skin, pinprick, contact with heat or cold, and pressure (hyperalgesia). Loud noises, bright lights, or other mild irritants may also trigger pain. Thalamic pain is typically delayed in onset and may not appear until a few weeks or months after the onset of stroke. Spontaneous recovery is rare and suffering may be intolerable. Patients may experience little relief from analgesic treatment. The debilitating nature of thalamic pain frequently prevents the patient from actively participating in rehabilitation.[19]

Visual Changes

Homonymous hemianopsia, a visual field defect, occurs with lesions involving the optic radiation in the internal capsule (MCA distribution) or to the primary visual cortex (PCA distribution). It occurs in about 26 percent of patients with stroke. (2) The patient experiences loss of vision in the contralateral half of each visual field; that is, the nasal half of one eye and temporal half of the eye corresponding to the hemiplegic side. Field defects contribute to the patient's overall lack of awareness of the hemiplegic side. Patients who are aware of the problem can compensate with head turning movements. Patients may also experience **visual neglect** (visual inattention) and problems with depth perception, and spatial relationships. See Chapter 29 for a complete discussion of visual and perceptual impairments. Paralysis of conjugate gaze from involvement of frontal lobe eye field area, CN III, or gaze centers in the pontine reticular formation result in **forced gaze deviation**. Unopposed action of eye muscles causes the eyes to deviate in the direction of the intact musculature. Patients with hemispheric lesions may look away from the hemiplegic side, while patients with brainstem lesions may look toward the hemiplegic side. Brainstem strokes affecting the coordination of eye muscles may also produce signs of diplopia, oscillopsia, or visual distortions.

Motor Function

Stages of Motor Recovery

Initially flaccid paralysis is present (stage 1). This is replaced by the development of spasticity, hyperreflexia, and mass patterns of movement, termed **obligatory synergies**. Muscles involved in these synergy patterns are often so strongly linked together that isolated movements outside the obligatory patterns are not possible. During stage 2 (early synergy) facilitatory stimuli will elicit synergies with no or only minimal voluntary movement. As recovery progresses, spasticity is marked with full strong obligatory synergies (stage 3). Synergy influence begins to decline in stage 4 as some movements out-of-synergy emerge, especially if movement takes place in the weaker synergy first. During stage 5, relative independence of synergy, spasticity continues to wane and isolated joint movements become more apparent while during stage 6 patterns of movement are near normal. This general pattern of recovery was initially described by Twitchell[20] and Brunnstrom[21,22] and confirmed by additional investigators[23–26] (Box 18.2). Several important points merit consideration. An overall pattern of motor recovery exists though individual recovery is highly variable. Some patients experience mild involvement with full recovery while other patients demonstrate severe involvement with incomplete recovery. The degree of recovery depends on a number of factors, including lesion location and severity and capacity for adaptation through training. Finally, recovery differs within patients. For example, the UE may be more involved and demonstrate less complete recovery than the LE as is seen in MCA syndrome.

Box 18.2 Sequential Motor Recovery Stages Following Stroke

STAGE 1 Recovery from hemiplegia occurs in a stereotyped sequence of events that begins with a period of *flaccidity* immediately following the acute episode. *No movement of the limbs* can be elicited.

STAGE 2 As recovery begins, the basic limb synergies or some of their components may appear as associated reactions, or *minimal voluntary movement* responses may be present. At this time, spasticity begins to develop.

STAGE 3 Thereafter, the patient gains *voluntary control of the movement synergies,* although full range of all synergy components does not necessarily develop. Spasticity has further increased and may become severe.

STAGE 4 Some *movement combinations that do not follow the paths of either synergy are mastered*, first with difficulty, then with more ease, and *spasticity begins to decline.*

STAGE 5 If progress continues, more *difficult movement combinations are learned* as the basic limb synergies lose their dominance over motor acts.

STAGE 6 With the *disappearance of spasticity, individual joint movements become possible and coordination* approaches normal. From here on, as the last recovery step, normal motor function is restored, but this last stage is not achieved by all, for the recovery process can plateau at any stage.

From Brunnstrom, S: Movement Therapy in Hemiplegia. Harper & Row, New York, 1970, with permission.

Weakness

Weakness (paresis) is found in 80 to 90 percent of all patients after stroke and is a major factor in disability.[17] Patients are unable to generate the force necessary for initiating and controlling movement. The degree of weakness is related to the location and size of the brain injury and varies from a complete inability to achieve any visible contraction to measurable impairments in force production. Deficits on the contralateral, side typically include hemiparesis (opposite UE and LE). Owing to the high incidence of MCA strokes, the UE is frequently more affected than the LE. About 20 percent of individuals with MCA strokes fail to regain any functional use of the affected UE. Typically, distal muscles exhibit greater strength deficits than proximal.[27,28] This can be explained by the greater facilitation of distal muscles than proximal by the corticospinal system.[29] Some researchers have not found this proximal–distal gradient.[30] Mild weakness also occurs on the ipsilateral, "supposedly normal" side.[27,28] This can be explained by the fact that only 75 to 90 percent of the corticospinal fibers cross in the medulla to the contralateral side. The remainder are transmitted to the spinal cord ipsilaterally in the anterior or ventral corticospinal tract. Once in the spinal cord some of these fibers cross while the rest remain uncrossed, thereby explaining bilateral weakness.[29] The amount of weakness experienced by the patient may also vary according to specific functional tasks. Thus, a patient may appear stronger in some tasks than others.

Observed muscle weakness is also associated with a number of changes in both the muscle and the motor unit. Changes occur in muscle composition, including atrophy of muscle fibers. There is a selective loss of type II fast-twitch fibers with an increase in the percentage of type I fibers (a finding also reported in the elderly). This selective loss of type II fibers results in difficulty with initiation and production of rapid, high-force movements. The number of functioning motor units and discharge firing rates also decrease, in one study by as much as 50 percent at 6 months following stroke.[31] This is explained by the presence of transsynaptic degeneration of alpha motoneurons that occurs with loss of corticospinal innervation.[32] Abnormal recruitment of motor units has also been reported.[33–37] Thus patients demonstrate inefficient patterns of muscle activation and difficulty maintaining a constant level of force production. Patients demonstrate increased effort and fatigability with frequent complaints of feelings of weakness. Denervation potentials are common, also the result of denervation changes in the corticospinal tracts.[38] Overall reaction times are increased, a finding also reported in the stronger extremities and for the elderly in general. Movement times are prolonged, a timing abnormality that contributes to impairment of coordinated motor sequences.[39,40] Finally, there is increased coactivation of agonists and antagonists, a timing disorder that limits force production during voluntary movements.[41,42]

Alterations in Tone

Flaccidity (hypotonicity) is present immediately after stroke and is due primarily to the effects of cerebral shock. It is generally short-lived, lasting a few days, or weeks. Flaccidity may persist in a small number of patients with lesions restricted to the primary motor cortex or cerebellum. **Spasticity** (hypertonicity) emerges in about 90 percent of cases and occurs on the side of the body opposite the lesion. Spasticity in UMN syndrome occurs predominately in antigravity muscles (see Chapter 8, Table 8.1). In the patient with stroke, UE, spasticity is frequently strong in scapular retractors; shoulder adductors, depressors, and internal rotators; elbow flexors and forearm pronators; and wrist and finger flexors. In the neck and trunk, spasticity may cause increased lateral flexion to the hemiplegic side. In the LE, spasticity is often strong in the pelvic retractors, hip adductors and internal rotators, hip and knee extensors, plantarflexors and supinators, and toe flexors. Spasticity results in tight (stiff) muscles that restrict volitional movement. Posturing of the limbs (e.g., a tight fisted hand with the elbow bent and held tightly against the chest or a stiff extended knee with a plantarflexed foot) is common with moderate to severe spasticity. Spastic posturing can lead to the development of painful spasms (similar to muscle cramping), degenerative changes, and fixed contractures.[43] The adjustment of postural muscles that occurs normally in preparation for and during a movement task, termed *automatic postural tone,* is also impaired.[44] Thus, patients with stroke may lack the ability to adjust and stabilize proximal limbs and trunk appropriately during movement, with resulting postural abnormalities, balance impairments, and increased risk for falls.

Abnormal Synergy Patterns

Abnormal and highly stereotyped **obligatory synergies** emerge with spasticity. Thus, the patient is unable to perform an isolated movement of a limb segment without producing movements in the remainder of the limb. For example, efforts to bend the elbow also result in shoulder flexion, abduction, and external rotation. The patient is severely limited in the ability to adapt movements to varying task or environmental demands. Obligatory synergies can be elicited either reflexively, as associated reactions, or as minimal voluntary movements. As recovery progresses they become stronger and are linked to spasticity. Two distinct abnormal synergy patterns have been described for each extremity: a flexion synergy and an extension synergy (Table 18.5). An inspection of the synergy components reveals that certain muscles are not usually involved in either synergy. These muscles include the (1) latissimus dorsi, (2) teres major, (3) serratus anterior, (4) finger extensors, and (5) ankle evertors. These muscles, therefore, are generally difficult to activate while the patient is exhibiting these patterns. Obligatory synergies are often incompatible with normal activities of daily living and functional mobility skills (FMS). For example, the patient with a strong LE extensor synergy will have a difficulty walking owing to foot plantarflexion and inversion when the hip and knee are extended. As recovery progresses, spasticity and obligatory synergies begin to disappear and more normal synergies with isolated joint control become possible.[22,45,46]

Abnormal Reflexes

Reflexes are altered and also vary according to the stage of recovery. Initially, stroke results in hypoflexia with flaccidity. When spasticity and synergies emerge, hyperreflexia is seen. Stretch reflexes are hyperactive and patients may demonstrate clonus, clasp-knife response, and a positive Babinski, all consistent findings of UMN syndrome.

Tonic reflexes may appear in a readily identifiable form similar to that seen in other types of neurological insult (e.g., traumatic brain injury, cerebral palsy). Thus, movement of the head or position of the body may elicit an obligatory change in resting tone or movement of the extremities. The most commonly seen is the asymmetric tonic neck reflex (ATNR) in which head rotation causes elbow extension of the UE on the jaw side with elbow flexion of the opposite skull limb.[22,23,47]

Table 18.5 Obligatory Synergy Patterns Following Stroke

	Flexion Synergy Components	Extension Synergy Components
Upper extremity	Scapular retraction/elevation or hyper-extension	Scapular protraction
	Shoulder abduction, external rotation	Shoulder adduction,[a] internal rotation
	Elbow flexion[a]	Elbow extension
	Forearm supination	Forearm pronation[a]
	Wrist and finger	Wrist and finger flexion
	Flexion	
Lower extremity	Hip flexion,[a] abduction, external rotation	Hip extension, adduction,[a] internal rotation
	Knee flexion	Knee extension[a]
	Ankle dorsiflexion, inversion	Ankle plantarflexion,[a] inversion
	Toe dorsiflexion	Toe plantarflexion

[a]Generally the strongest components

Associated reactions are also typically present in patients with stroke who exhibit strong spasticity and obligatory synergies. These consist of unintentional movements of the hemiparetic limb caused by voluntary action of another limb or by the stimulation of yawning, sneezing, or coughing. For example, the patient vigorously contracts the elbow flexors of the stronger UE; the hemiparetic elbow also flexes. Or the patient flexes the hip and lifts the hemiparetic LE in sitting; the hemiparetic UE also flexes. Associated reactions can limit functional performance, especially in the UE.[22,48]

Altered Coordination

Proprioceptive losses can result in sensory ataxia. Strokes affecting the cerebellum typically produce cerebellar ataxia (e.g., lateral medullary syndrome, basilar artery syndrome, pontine syndromes) and motor weakness. The resulting problems with timing and sequencing of muscles can significantly impair function and limit adaptability to changing task and environmental demands. Basal ganglia involvement (posterior cerebral artery syndrome) may lead to slow movements (bradykinesia) or involuntary movements (choreoathetosis, hemiballismus).

Altered Motor Programming

Motor praxis is the ability to plan and execute coordinated movement. Lesions of the premotor frontal cortex of either hemisphere, left inferior parietal lobe, and corpus callosum can produce apraxia. Apraxia is more evident with left hemisphere damage than right and is commonly seen with aphasia. The patient demonstrates difficulty planning and executing purposeful movements that cannot be accounted for by any other reason (i.e., impaired strength, coordination, sensation, tone, cognitive function, communication, or uncooperativeness). There are two main types of apraxia. **Ideational apraxia** refers an inability of the patient to produce movement either on command or automatically and represents a complete breakdown in the conceptualization of the task. The patient has no idea how to do the movement and thus cannot formulate the required motor programs. With **ideomotor apraxia** the patient is unable to produce a movement on command but is able to move automatically. Thus the patient can perform habitual tasks when not commanded to do so and often perseverates, repeating the activity over and over. See Chapter 29 for a more complete discussion of apraxia.

Postural Control and Balance

Balance is disturbed following stroke with impairments in steadiness, symmetry, and dynamic stability common.[49–51] Problems may exist when reacting to a destabilizing external force (reactive postural control) or during self-initiated movements (anticipatory postural control). Thus, the patient may be unable to maintain balance in sitting or standing or to move in a weightbearing posture without loss of balance. Disruptions of central sensorimotor processing lead to an inability to adapt postural movements to changing task and environmental demands and impair motor learning.[52] Patients with stroke typically demonstrate asymmetry with most of the weight in sitting or standing shifted toward the stronger side. They also demonstrate increased postural sway in standing (a finding characteristic of the elderly in general).[53] Delays in the onset of motor activity, abnormal timing and sequencing of muscle activity, and abnormal co-contraction result in disorganization of postural synergies. For example, proximal muscles may be activated in advance of distal muscles or in some patients, very late (a finding also found in many elderly). Compensatory responses typically include excessive hip and knee movements. Corrective responses to perturbations or destabilizing forces are frequently inadequate and result in loss of balance and falls. Patients with hemiplegia typically fall in the direction of weakness.[54,55]

Ipsilateral Pushing

Ipsilateral pushing (also known as **pusher syndrome** [56] **or contraversive pushing** [57]) is an unusual motor behavior characterized by active pushing with the stronger extremities toward the hemiparetic side, leading to a lateral postural imbalance. The end result is a tendency to fall toward the hemiparetic side. Pushing can vary in severity and generally increases with the difficulty of the postural challenge. During sitting, the push results in a strong lateral lean toward the weaker side, often pushing the patient onto the wheelchair arm. In standing, a strong push creates an unstable situation with a high risk of falls because the hemiparetic LE typically cannot support the body weight. The patient shows no fear even when active pushing leads to instability and strongly resists any attempts to passively correct posture to mid-line, symmetrical weightbearing. This pattern is totally opposite the expected postural deficiency seen in most patients after stroke, that is, increased weightbearing to the stronger side to compensate for deficits on the hemiparetic side. Pushing is caused by severe misperception of body orientation in relation to gravity. Karnath et al[57] found patients experienced a misperception of subjective postural vertical position, perceiving their body as vertical when it was actually tilted about 18°. They also found that the visual and vestibular inputs for orientation perception to vertical remained intact as patients were able to align their bodies with the help of visual cues and conscious strategies. Ipsilateral pushing is the result of stroke affecting the posterolateral thalamus[57,58] and a deficit in processing of somesthetic information.[58,59] Pedersen et al[60] identified the behavior in 10 percent of 327 patients with stroke. These researchers also found no significant association between ipsilateral pushing and hemineglect, anosognosia, aphasia, or apraxia. Functional mobility skills are significantly impaired for patients with ipsilateral pushing. Typically the patient demonstrates severe problems in transfers, standing, and gait. The use of a cane during ambulation is problematic because patients use the cane to increase push to the hemiplegic side. Peterson et al[60] demonstrated that patients with ipsilateral pushing have poorer rehabilitation outcomes with longer hospital stays and prolonged recovery times (3.6 weeks longer on average). They also had significantly lower functional scores on admission and discharge with increased levels of dependence at discharge. However with training, the brain can compensate well. The syndrome is rarely still evident at 6 months.[61]

Speech, Language, and Swallowing

Patients with lesions involving the cortex of the dominant hemisphere (typically the left hemisphere) demonstrate speech and language impairments. **Aphasia** is the general term used to describe an acquired communication disorder caused by brain damage and is characterized by an impairment of language comprehension, formulation, and use. Aphasia has been estimated to occur in 30 to 36 percent of all patients with stroke.[2] There are many different types of aphasias; major classification categories are fluent, nonfluent, and global. In **fluent aphasia (Wernicke's/sensory/receptive aphasia)**, speech flows smoothly with a variety of grammatical constructions and preserved melody of speech. Auditory comprehension is impaired. Thus, the patient demonstrates difficulty in comprehending spoken language and in following commands. The lesion is located in the auditory association cortex in the left lateral temporal lobe. In **nonfluent aphasia (Broca's/expressive aphasia)** the flow of speech is slow and hesitant, vocabulary is limited, and syntax is impaired. Speech production is labored or lost completely while comprehension is good. The lesion is located in the premotor area of the left frontal lobe. **Global aphasia** is a severe aphasia characterized by marked impairments of both production and comprehension of language. It is often an indication of extensive brain damage. Severe problems in communication may limit the patient's ability to learn and often impedes successful outcomes in rehabilitation. See Chapter 30 for a complete discussion of these impairments and their management.

Patients with stroke commonly present with **dysarthria** with a reported incidence ranging from 48 to 57 percent.[2] This term refers to a category of motor speech disorders caused by lesions in parts of the central or peripheral nervous system that mediate speech production. Respiration, articulation, phonation, resonance, and/or sensory feedback may be affected. The lesion can be located in the primary motor cortex in the frontal lobe, the primary sensory cortex in the parietal lobe, or the cerebellum. Volitional and automatic actions such as chewing and swallowing and movement of the jaw and tongue are impaired resulting in slurred speech. In patients with stroke, dysarthria can accompany aphasia, complicating the course of rehabilitation (see Chapter 30).

Swallowing difficulty, **dysphagia**, occurs in about 12 percent of patients with lesions affecting the medullary brainstem (CN IX and X), large vessel pontine lesions, as well as in acute hemispheric lesions (especially infarcts in the MCA and PCA).[2] Dysfunction of the lips, mouth, tongue, palate, pharynx, larynx, or proximal esophagus all contribute to dysphagia. The most frequent problem seen with dysphagia is delayed triggering of the swallowing reflex (86 percent of patients) followed by reduced pharyngeal peristalsis (58 percent of patients) and reduced lingual control (50 percent of patients).[62] Altered mental status, altered sensation, poor jaw and lip closure, impaired head control, and poor sitting posture also contribute to the patient's swallowing difficulties. Most patients demonstrate multiple problems that can include drooling, difficulty ingesting food, compromised nutritional status, and dehydration. Dysphagia may be severe enough to require the use of tube feeding, either a nasogastric (NG) tube for short periods of time or an invasive gastrostomy (G) tube for more long-term care. Nutrition can also be provided through an intravenous route (total parenteral nutrition [TPN]). There are numerous risks and complications associated with these feeding methods and difficult clinical decisions are made by the family in conjunction with the medical or dysphagia team.

Perception and Cognition

Stroke can produce visual–perceptual deficits, with a reported incidence ranging from 32 to 41 percent.[2] They are frequently the result of lesions in the right parietal cortex and seen more with left hemiplegia than right. These may include disorders of **body scheme/body image**, **spatial relations**, and **agnosias**. Body scheme refers to a postural model of the body including the relationship of the body parts to each other and the relationship of the body to the environment. Body image is the visual and mental image of one's body that includes feelings about one's body. Both may be distorted following stroke. Specific impairments of body scheme/ body image include **unilateral neglect**, **anosognosia**, **somatoagnosia**, **right–left discrimination**, **finger agnosia**, and **anosognosia**. Spatial relations syndrome refers to a constellation of impairments that have in common a difficulty in perceiving the relationship between the self and two or more objects in the environment. It includes specific impairments in figure–ground discrimination, form discrimination, spatial relations, position in space, and topographical disorientation. Agnosia is the inability to recognize incoming information despite intact sensory capacities. Agnosias can include visual object agnosia, auditory agnosia or tactile agnosia (astereognosis). The reader is referred to Chapter 29 for a more complete discussion of these deficits and their management.

Cognitive deficits are present with lesions involving the cortex and include impairments in alertness, attention, orientation, memory, or executive functions. Premorbid changes associated with pathological aging may also account for some of the dysfunction noted and should be carefully determined from interviews with family, significant others, or caregivers. The patient with acute stroke may be largely unaware of what is going on in the external environment, a problem of impaired alertness that results from lesions in the prefrontal cortex and reticular formation. The patient may also be disoriented and unable to provide information about self, time of day, physical or geographical location, or disability, the result of lesions affecting the prefrontal cortex, limbic system, and limbic cortex. **Attention** is the ability to select and attend to a specific stimulus while simultaneously suppressing extraneous stimuli. Attention disorders include impairments in sustained attention, selective attention, divided attention, or alternating attention. Altered attention results from lesions in the prefrontal cortex and reticular formation. **Memory** is defined as the ability to store experiences and perceptions for later recall. Memory disorders include impairments in immediate recall and short-term or long-term memory. Immediate and short-term memory impairments are common, occurring in about 36 percent of patients with stroke while long-term memory typically remains intact.[2] Thus, the patient cannot remember the instructions for a new task given only minutes or hours ago but can easily remember things done 30 years ago. Short-term memory loss is associated with lesions of the limbic system, limbic association cortex (orbitofrontal areas), or temporal lobes. Long-term memory loss is associated with lesions of the hippocampus of the limbic system. Memory gaps may be filled with inappropriate words or fabricated stories, an impairment termed **confabulation** that also results from lesions in the prefrontal cortex. The patient may be confused, demonstrating disorientation and an inability to understand the specific context of a conversation. Confusion is the result of disruption of the prefrontal cortex and occurs with diffuse, bilateral lesions. **Perseveration** is the continued repetition of words, thoughts, or acts not related to current context. Thus the patient gets "stuck" and repeats words or acts without much success at stopping. Preservation results from lesions in the premotor and/or prefrontal cortex.[63,64]

Executive functions, defined as those capacities that enable a person to engage in purposeful behaviors, include volition, planning, purposeful action, and effective performance. Patients with lesions of the prefrontal cortex typically demonstrate impairments in executive function including some or all of the following: impulsiveness, inflexible thinking, lack of abstract thinking, impaired organization and sequencing, decreased insight, impaired planning ability, and impaired judgment. Patients are unable to realistically appraise their environment and the people and events in it. They also demonstrate difficulty in self-monitoring and self-correcting behaviors, thereby posing enormous safety risks. See Chapter 29 for a complete discussion of these impairments and their management.

Dementia can result from multiple small infarcts of the brain, termed **multi-infarct dementia**. It is characterized by progressive impairments in memory and cognition. These changes are associated with episodes of cerebral ischemia and hypertension. Other contributing factors include arrhythmias, myocardial infarct, TIAs, diabetes, obesity, and smoking. Scattered areas of the brain are involved, evidenced by focal neurological deficits. Onset is frequently abrupt. The patient may fluctuate between periods of impaired function and periods of improved function, demonstrating a stepwise and paroxysmal deterioration of intellectual function. This is in contrast to the gradual onset and more steady, widespread decline seen in Alzheimer's dementia.[65]

Delirium, also known as acute confusional state, can result from a number of factors following acute stroke.

Deprivation of oxygen to the brain, metabolic imbalance, or adverse drug reactions can all induce confusion. Additional contributory factors can include sensory and perceptual losses coupled with an unfamiliar hospital environment and inactivity. Delirium is characterized by a clouding of consciousness or dulling of cognitive processes and impaired alertness. Thus the patient is inattentive, incoherent, and disorganized with fluctuating levels of consciousness. Hallucinations and agitation are also common. Nighttime may be particularly problematic. Patients with significant sensory deficits following stroke may experience sensory deprivation problems evidenced by irritability, confusion, psychosis, delusions, and even hallucinations. These problems are more frequently seen in patients who have been confined to a bed for a long time or whose bed is positioned to limit social interaction (e.g., with the more involved side toward the door). Some patients are equally unable to deal with a sensory overload, produced by too much stimulation. Altered arousal levels are implicated.

Emotional Status

Lesions of the brain affecting the frontal lobe, hypothalamus, and limbic system can produce a number of emotional changes. The patient with stroke may demonstrate **pseudobulbar affect (PBA)**, also known as *emotional lability* or *emotional dysregulation syndrome*. PBA occurs in about 18 percent of cases and is characterized by emotional outbursts of uncontrolled or exaggerated laughing or crying that are inconsistent with mood. The patient quickly changes from laughing to crying with only slight provocation. The patient is typically unable to control these episodes or to inhibit the expression of spontaneous emotions.[66] Frequent crying may also accompany depression. **Apathy** occurs in about 22 percent of cases and is characterized by a shallow affect and blunted emotional responses. In such patients, apathy is frequently misconstrued as depression or poor motivation. Patients can also demonstrate **euphoria** (exaggerated feelings of well-being), increased levels of irritability or frustration, and social inappropriateness. Changes in the ability to sense, move, communicate, think, or act as before are enormously frustrating by themselves and create high stress levels for the patient with stroke. Increased levels of irritability and frustration are the natural outcomes of high stress levels. These behaviors along with a poor social perception of one's self and environment may lead to increasing isolation and social withdrawal.[67,68]

Depression is extremely common, occurring in about one-third of stroke cases.[2] It is characterized by persistent feelings of sadness accompanied by feelings of hopelessness, worthlessness and/or helplessness. Depressed patients may also experience a loss of energy or persistent fatigue, an inability to concentrate, and decreased interest in daily life along with changes in weight and sleep patterns, generalized anxiety, and recurrent thoughts of death or suicide. Depression is seen with lesions in the left frontal lobe (acute stage) and with lesions in the right parietal lobes (subacute stage).[69,70] Most patients remain significantly depressed for many months, with an average time of 7 to 8 months. The period from 6 months to 2 years after a CVA is the most likely time for depression to occur. Depression occurs in both mildly and severely involved patients and thus is not significantly related to the degree of motor impairment. Patients with lesions of the left hemisphere may experience more frequent and more severe depression than patients with right hemisphere or brainstem strokes.[71,72] These findings suggest that post-stroke depression is not simply a result of psychological reaction to disability but rather a direct impairment of the CVA. Prolonged post-stroke depression can interfere with the success of rehabilitation and result in poorer long-term functional outcomes. The reader is referred to Chapter 2 for a more complete discussion of psychosocial impairments and their management.

Hemispheric Behavioral Differences

Individuals with stroke differ widely in their approach to processing information and in their behaviors. Those with *left hemisphere damage* (right hemiplegia) demonstrate difficulties in communication and in processing information in a sequential, linear manner. They are frequently described as cautious, anxious, and disorganized. This makes them more hesitant when trying new tasks and increases the need for feedback and support. They tend, however, to be realistic in their appraisal of their existing problems. Individuals with *right hemisphere damage* (left hemiplegia), on the other hand, demonstrate difficulty in spatial–perceptual tasks and in grasping the whole idea of a task or activity. They are frequently described as quick and impulsive. They tend to overestimate their abilities while acting unaware of their deficits. Safety is therefore a far greater issue with patients with left hemiplegia, where poor judgment is common. These patients also require a great deal of feedback when learning a new task. The feedback should be focused on slowing down the activity, checking sequential steps, and relating it to the whole task. The patient with left hemiplegia frequently cannot attend to visuospatial cues effectively, especially in a cluttered or crowded environment.[73–75] Table 18.6 summarizes the behavioral differences attributed to damage of the left and right hemispheres.

Bladder and Bowel Function

Disturbances of bladder function are common during the acute phase, occurring in about 29 percent of cases.[2] Urinary incontinence can result from bladder hyperreflexia or hyporeflexia, disturbances of sphincter control, and/or sensory loss. A toileting schedule for prompted voiding is often implemented to reduce the incidence of incontinence

Table 18.6 Hemispheric Differences Commonly Seen Following Stroke

Right Brain Injury	Left Brain Injury
Left-side hemiplegia/paresis	Right-side hemiplegia/paresis
Left-side hemisensory loss	Right-side hemisensory loss
Visual–perceptual impairments: Left-side unilateral neglect Agnosia Visuospatial impairments Disturbances of body image and body scheme	Speech and language impairments: (dominant hemisphere/right-handed individuals) Nonfluent (Broca's) aphasia Fluent (Wernicke's) aphasia Global aphasia
Difficulty sustaining a movement	Difficulty planning and sequencing movements Apraxia more common: ideational, ideomotor
Quick, impulsive behavioral style	Slow, cautious behavioral style
Difficulty grasping the overall organization or pattern, problem-solving and synthesizing information	Disorganized problem-solving
Often unaware of impairments Poor judgment Inability to self-correct; increased safety risk	Often very aware of impairments Anxious about poor performance
Rigidity of thought Difficulty with abstract reasoning	Difficulty with processing delays
Difficulty with perception of emotions, expression of negative emotions	Difficulty with expression of positive emotions
Difficulty processing visual cues	Difficulty processing verbal cues, verbal commands
Memory impairments, typically related to spatial-perceptual information	Memory impairments, typically related to language
Dysfunction of either hemisphere depending on lesion location: Visual field defects Emotional abnormalities: lability, apathy, irritability, low frustration levels, depression Cognitive deficits: confusion, short attention span, loss of memory, executive functions	

and to accommodate for factors that cause functional incontinence such as inattention, mental status changes, or immobility. Generally, this problem improves quickly. Persistent incontinence is often due to a treatable medical condition (e.g., urinary tract infection). Absorbent pads and special undergarments or external collection devices may be used if incontinence proves refractory. Urinary retention can be controlled pharmacologically and with intermittent or indwelling catheterization. Early treatment is desirable to prevent further complications such as chronic urinary tract infection and skin breakdown. Patients who are incontinent often suffer embarrassment, isolation, and depression. Persistent incontinence is associated with a poor long-term prognosis for functional recovery.

Disturbances of bowel function can include incontinence and diarrhea or constipation and impaction. Patients who are constipated may require stool softeners and dietary/fluid modifications to resolve this problem. Physical activity is also helpful to improve these problems.

Complications and Indirect Impairments

Musculoskeletal

Loss of voluntary movement and immobility can result in loss of range of movement (ROM) and contractures. Contractures can develop anywhere but are particularly apparent in the paretic limbs. As contractures progress, edema and pain may develop and further restrict mobility. In the UE, limitations in the shoulder motions of flexion, abduction, and external rotation are common. Contractures are likely in the elbow flexors, wrist and finger flexors, and forearm pronators. In the LE, plantarflexion contractures are common. Alterations in alignment coupled with decreased activity of muscles may lead to postural deformity, altered patterns of movement with increased energy expenditure, and excessive effort.

Disuse atrophy and muscle weakness results from inactivity and immobility. Early mobilization stressing out-of-bed upright postures and weightbearing activities along with forced use of the involved extremities are effective strategies in counteracting these effects. Patients recovering from stroke consistently demonstrate the strong negative impact of weakness on functional outcomes. Impairments in gait, balance, falls, UE functional tasks, and manual dexterity have all been linked directly to impairments of strength.[76–79]

Osteoporosis, a bone disease characterized by a loss of bone mass per unit volume, is common in the elderly and results from decreased physical activity, changes in protein nutrition, hormonal deficiency, and calcium deficiency. Patients with stroke who are immobilized and restricted in weightbearing demonstrate increased risk of osteoporosis. Fall risk is also increased with incidence rates ranging between 23 percent and 50 percent for individuals with chronic stroke.[80] Risk of falls in patients with stroke is multifactorial, arising from sensorimotor deficits, impaired balance, confusion, attention deficits, perceptual deficits, visual impairments, behavioral impulsivity, depression, and communication problems.[81–85] Increased risk of fracture, especially vertebral and hip fracture, is the natural outcome of osteoporosis and falls. In patients with stroke, osteoporosis and hip fracture are more likely on the more involved side.[86] Strategies to improve motor function and prevent falls are indicated (for an overview, see Chapter 13).

Neurological

Seizures

Seizures occur in a small percentage of patients with stroke and are slightly more common in occlusive carotid disease (17 percent) than in MCA disease (11 percent). Seizures are common right after stroke during the acute phase (e.g., in about 15 percent of cases with cerebral hemorrhage); late-onset seizures can also occur several months after stroke. They tend to be of the partial motor type.[87] Seizures are potentially life threatening if not controlled. Anticonvulsant medications may be indicated (e.g., phenytoin [Dilantin], carbamazepine [Tegretol], phenobarbital [Solfoton]. Potential adverse side effects include sedation (drowsiness) and ataxia.

Hydrocephalus

Hydrocephalus, an excessive accumulation of cerebral spinal fluid (CSF) within the cranial cavity, is rare but can occur with subarachnoid or intracerebral hemorrhage. The increasing blood volume results in obstruction of CSF circulation. Patients may experience headache, nausea, vomiting, visual impairment, increasing lethargy, and ataxia. Seizures can also occur. Surgical intervention with ventriculostomy and ventricular drainage is necessary in emergency situations. Long-term management is accomplished with the placement of a ventricular peritoneal shunt.[11]

Cardiovascular/Pulmonary

Thrombophlebitis/Deep Vein Thrombosis

Thrombophlebitis and deep venous thrombosis (DVT) are potential complications for all immobilized patients. The incidence of DVT in patients with stroke is as high as 47 percent with an estimated 10 percent of deaths attributed to pulmonary embolism. (2) The dangers are particularly high during the acute phase when venous stasis from bed rest, limb paralysis and decreased activity, hemineglect, and reduced cognitive status significantly elevate the risks. The hallmark clinical signs of DVT include rapid onset of unilateral leg swelling with dependent edema. The patient may report tenderness, a dull ache, or a tight feeling in the calf; pain is usually not severe. About 50 percent of cases do not present with clinically detectable symptoms and can be identified only by radiocontrast venography (the gold standard), impedance plethysmography, or Doppler ultrasonography. Prompt diagnosis and treatment of acute DVT are necessary to reduce the risk of fatal pulmonary embolism. Pharmacological management consists of anticoagulant therapy (blood thinners). Prophylactic use of low-dose heparin (LDH) or low-molecular-weight (LMW) heparin has been shown to reduce the incidence by 45 percent and 79 percent, respectively. Symptomatic treatment of DVT consists of bed rest and elevation of the limb until tenderness subsides (generally 3 to 5 days) to prevent pressure fluctuations within the venous system and emboli. Edema management may include intermittent pneumatic compression and compression stockings.[88] Careful daily monitoring of the lower limbs is essential. Early mobilization and ambulation are important primary prevention measures.

Cardiac Function

The majority of strokes are caused by vascular disease. Patients who suffer a stroke as a result of underlying coronary artery disease (CAD) may demonstrate impaired cardiac output, cardiac decompensation, and serious rhythm disorders. If these problems persist, they can directly alter cerebral perfusion and produce additional focal signs (e.g., mental confusion).[89] Patients with stroke typically exhibit low peak $\dot{V}O_2$ levels during exercise (about half of that achieved by age-matched healthy individuals).[90] These vary according to age, level of disability, number and severity of comorbidities, secondary complications, and medications. Cardiac limitations in exercise tolerance may restrict rehabilitation potential and requires diligent monitoring and careful exercise prescription by the physical therapist.[91]

Most patients with stroke are significantly deconditioned and exhibit low work capacities, the result of acute illness, bedrest, and limited activity levels. Some individuals may have been inactive prior to the stroke. Changes in the cardiovascular system associated with deconditioning include reduced cardiac output, decreased maximal heart rate, increased resting and exercise blood pressures, decreased maximal oxygen uptake, and decreased vital capacity. Changes in the musculoskeletal systems (e.g., decreased muscle mass and strength, decreased bone mass, decreased flexibility) and decreased glucose tolerance also affect exercise tolerance and endurance levels. Decreased activity levels may also be related to depression, a common finding in stroke.[92]

Pulmonary Function

Pulmonary function is often impaired in individuals with stroke. Decreased lung volume, decreased pulmonary perfusion and vital capacity and altered chest wall excursion are all common findings. The decreased respiratory output is accompanied by increased oxygen demands required during altered movement patterns. For example, walking using an orthosis and assistive device dramatically increases the energy demands of the activity. The end result for the patient with stroke is increased fatigue and decreased endurance.

Aspiration, penetration of food, liquid, saliva, or gastric reflux into the airway, occurs in about one third of patients with dysphagia. It is more common during the acute phase of recovery and can occur during any phase of swallowing. Aspiration is an important complication in that it can lead to acute respiratory distress within hours, aspiration pneumonia, and, if left untreated, death. Dysphagia can also lead to dehydration and compromised nutrition. Early examination and treatment of dysphagia is essential to prevent aspiration. Videofluoroscopic examination (a modified barium swallow [MBS]) is the most commonly used technique to examine the preparatory, oral, pharyngeal, and esophageal phases of swallowing. Fiberoptic endoscopic examination of swallowing (FEES) provides information about laryngeal function, hypopharyngeal residue, and airway protection (aspiration).[93]

Integumentary

Ischemic damage and subsequent necrosis of the skin results in skin breakdown and decubitus ulcers. The incidence in patients with stroke is reported to be 14.5 percent.[94] The skin breaks down typically over bony prominences from pressure, friction, shearing, and/or maceration. Intense pressure for a short time or low pressure for a long time results in pressure sores. Friction occurs as the skin rubs or is dragged against the supporting surface, for example, when the patient slides down in bed or is pulled up. Spasticity and contractures can also contribute to increased friction. Shearing occurs from sliding of adjacent structures in opposite directions (skin vs underlying bone), for example, during transfers from bed to stretcher without a pull sheet. Maceration is caused by excess moisture, for example, with urinary incontinence. Additional risk factors include reduced activity (bedfast or chairfast), immobility, decreased sensation, abnormal patterns of movement, poor nutrition, and decreased level of consciousness. The incidence of pressure sores is increased with comorbid medical conditions such as infections, peripheral vascular disease, edema, and diabetes.[2]

Daily systematic inspection of the skin, particularly over high-risk areas is essential in recognizing the early signs of breakdown. The skin needs to be kept clean, dry, and protected from injury. Proper techniques for positioning, turning, and transferring are essential. A positioning schedule is instituted and the time in each position is limited. Assumption of upright postures (sitting and standing) is promoted as soon as possible. Pressure-relieving devices (PRDs) to minimize high concentrations of pressure are used. These may include foam pads, alternating pressure mattress, water mattress, air-fluidized bed, sheepskin, heel and elbow protectors, multipodus boots, and use of a trapeze. Proper positioning (seating) in the wheelchair and use of pressure relieving devices (gel or air cushions) are also critical. Lubricants, protective dressings, and barrier sprays may also be used. Ensuring the patient has adequate nutrition and hydration will also protect against skin breakdown as will early mobilization by the rehabilitation team.

Recovery and Prognosis

Recovery from stroke is generally fastest in the first weeks after onset, with measurable neurological and functional recovery occurring in the first month after stroke. Much of early recovery can be attributed to the resolution of **diachesis**, or transient inhibition of function, that accompanies acute stroke. Thus the reduction of edema, absorption of damaged tissue, and improved local circulation and cellular metabolism allows intact neurons that were previously inhibited to regain function.[95] Patients can continue to make measurable functional gains generally at a reduced rate for months or years after insult. Late recovery of function has been demonstrated for patients with chronic stroke (defined as greater than 1 year post-stroke) who undergo extensive functional training.[96–101] These changes are due largely to function-induced plasticity. A functional training approach that emphasizes use of the more involved extremities and an enriched environment effectively stimulates neural reorganization of the brain. Prolonged recovery with improvements occurring over a period of years is especially apparent in the areas of language and visuospatial function.[2] A more complete discussion of neuroplasticity and function-induced recovery is presented in Chapter 13.

Rates of motor recovery vary across management categories: patients suffering minor stroke recover rapidly with few or no residual deficits whereas severely impaired individuals demonstrate more limited and prolonged recovery. The initial grade of paresis, measured on initial hospital admission, is an important predictor of motor recovery. Motor function often improves after the first few days. In the case of complete paralysis on admission, complete motor recovery occurs in less than 15 percent of patients.[102] Recovery has been demonstrated in a wide variety of patients, including those with extensive central nervous system (CNS) damage and advanced age.[103–112] Patients with small lacunar strokes demonstrate improved motor recovery over patients with large, hemispheric lesions.[113] In an extensive review of the literature, Hendricks et al[102] found no significant difference in potential for motor recovery between type of stroke (hemorrhage vs infarction) and location (brainstem vs hemispheric infarction).

Functional mobility skills are impaired following stroke and vary considerably from individual to individual. During the acute stroke phase, 70 to 80 percent of patients demonstrate mobility problems in ambulation while 6 months to 1 year later the figures are reversed, with only 20 percent of patients needing help to walk independently. Basic ADL skills such as feeding, bathing, dressing, and toileting are also compromised during acute stroke, with 67 to 88 percent of patients demonstrating partial or complete dependence. Independence in ADL also improves with time with only 31 percent of survivors requiring partial or total assistance a year later.[114,115] The ability to perform functional tasks is influenced by a number of factors. Motor and perceptual impairments have the greatest impact on functional performance, but other limiting factors include sensory loss, disorientation, communication disorders, and decreased cardiorespiratory endurance. Enablement factors include high motivation, stable supportive family, financial resources, and intensive training with repetitive practice.

Physical Rehabilitation

Acute Phase

Low-intensity rehabilitation can begin in the acute care facility as soon as the patient is medically stabilized, typically within 72 hours. Patients may be admitted to a stroke unit or a neurological unit that provides comprehensive rehabilitation services. Evidence supports the benefits of such specialized units in significantly improving functional outcomes when compared to patients not receiving specialized care.[116–120] Early mobilization prevents or minimizes the harmful effects of deconditioning and the potential for secondary impairments. Functional reorganization is promoted through early stimulation and use of the hemiparetic side. *Learned nonuse* of the hemiparetic extremities and maladaptive patterns of movement are minimized. Mental deterioration, depression, and apathy can be reduced through the fostering of a positive outlook toward the rehabilitation process. Patients need to be presented early on with an organized plan for rehabilitation that addresses their individual goals and stresses resumption of ADL and independent function. It is equally important that patients and their families receive accurate information about stroke and available support. Current trends are toward shorter acute care hospital stays (average stay is about 7 days). However, early discharge has resulted in an increase in the number of serious medical complications seen during inpatient rehabilitation or at home. The rate of serious medical complications on rehabilitation admission ranges from 22 to 48 percent.[121] These complications in turn may result in delays during active rehabilitation and for some temporary cessation of therapy or transfer back to the acute hospital until medical complications are resolved. Therapists need to be vigilant in monitoring patients for potential risk of medical emergencies (e.g., cardiac arrhythmias, DVT, uncontrolled blood pressure, stroke, and so forth).

Post-Acute Phase

Patients with moderate or severe residual impairments or functional limitations may benefit from intensive inpatient rehabilitation provided in a freestanding rehabilitation facility or in a rehabilitation unit within the acute care hospital. Rehabilitation programs certified by the Commission on Accreditation of Rehabilitation Facilities (CARF) and the Joint Commission on Accreditation of Healthcare Organizations (JCAHO) can be expected to adhere to uniform standards and provide high-quality care.[2] Evidence supports the value of inpatient rehabilitation programs in producing improved functional outcomes for patients with stroke.[122–126] Patients are referred to inpatient rehabilitation if they can tolerate an intensity of services consisting of two or more rehabilitation disciplines, 5 days a week for a minimum of 3 hours of active rehabilitation per day. If the patient requires less intensive services, transfer to a transitional care unit (TCU) within the acute care facility or a skilled nursing facility can be requested. Here rehabilitation services are less intense, ranging from 1 hour of therapy services two to three times per week to daily, short sessions.[2]

The timing of rehabilitation services is an important factor in predicting outcome. In general, a shorter onset-to-admission interval, within the first 20 days, has been shown to significantly improve functional outcomes when compared to longer intervals.[127–130] There is also some evidence to suggest that patients with left hemiplegia who suffer profound cognitive–perceptual deficits may respond less favorably to early rehabilitation. These patients may benefit from additional preadmission time to allow for cognitive and perceptual–motor reorganization so critical for learning.[131] Additional factors that influence the timing of rehabilitation efforts include medical stability, motivation, patient endurance, and recovery. In an era of time-limited payment for comprehensive rehabilitation services, selecting the optimal time for rehabilitation services may prevent unnecessary patient failures and improve long-term functional outcomes.

The preferred practice pattern for patients with stroke from the *Guide to Physical Therapist Practice* is 5 D, *Impaired Motor Function and Sensory Integrity Associated with Nonprogressive Disorders of the Central Nervous System—Acquired in Adolescence or Adulthood.*[132, p 365] In this document the reader will find relevant information on patient/client diagnostic classification; ICD-9-CM codes; examination components; considerations for evaluation, diagnosis, and prognosis; and suggested interventions. Thus the Guide serves as a primary resource to help physical therapists design an appropriate plan of care and document the services provided and outcomes achieved.

A team of rehabilitation specialists including the physician, nurse, physical therapist, occupational therapist, speech–language pathologist, medical social worker, and case manager best provides comprehensive services for the patient with stroke. Additional disciplines may include a neuropsychologist, dietician, ophthalmologist, and recreational or vocational therapist. The patient/client, family, and caregivers are also important members of the team and should be involved in all decision making regarding health, wellness, and fitness needs. Interdisciplinary communication is critical for effective team function and occurs through case conferences, informal interactions, patient care rounds, and patient/client family meetings. Critical tasks for the team include the development of an integrated plan of care with unified goals, interventions, and outcomes that are mutually reinforced by all team members. Effective case management also includes a coordinated education plan, and accurate and effective documentation.

Rehabilitation services during the chronic phase, generally defined to be more than 6 months post-stroke, are typically delivered in an outpatient rehabilitation facility or at home. These services are prescribed for the patient who is discharged from inpatient rehabilitation and in need of continuing rehabilitation. Many of the interventions begun during inpatient rehabilitation are continued and progressed in order to sustain the gains made and improve functional performance. Some patients with mild involvement who did not require intense inpatient rehabilitation may also benefit from outpatient rehabilitation services. A complete record of past medical and rehabilitation services should be made available to these agencies. The intensity of services provided varies but is generally less than that of inpatient rehabilitation (e.g., 60 to 90 minutes per visit, two to three times per week). Outpatient intervention programs that target progressive improvements in flexibility, strength, balance, gait, endurance, and UE function have been shown to be effective in producing meaningful outcomes.[133–138] The patient and family are instructed in a home exercise program (HEP) and educated about the importance of maintaining exercise levels, health promotion, fall prevention, and safety.

The patient can also receive rehabilitation services at home. The challenges of being home can impose additional daily stresses for the patient and family. Difficulties should be addressed promptly as they arise. The therapist needs to emphasize the development of problem-solving skills to ensure successful adaptation to variable home and community environments. Fall risk factors should be eliminated or minimized as appropriate or possible. Examination of the environment and recommendations for modification of the environment are important parts of the preparation for return to home (see Chapter 12).

Finally, the patient should be assisted in the resumption of social and recreational participation. With increasing activity levels, it is important to monitor the patient's endurance levels carefully and provide instruction in energy conservation techniques as needed. A small number of stroke survivors can be evaluated and assisted in return to work. As the patient becomes successful in the home and community environments, services should be gradually phased out. Follow-up visits at periodic intervals are recommended to identify problems as they develop and to ensure long-term maintenance of function.[2]

Examination

The three basic components of a comprehensive physical therapy examination include patient/client history, systems review, and tests and measures. The selection of examination procedures will vary based on a number of factors including patient's age, location and severity of stroke, stage of recovery, data from initial screenings, phase of rehabilitation, home/community/work situation, as well as other factors.

The purposes are to:

- Determine the diagnosis and classification within a specific practice pattern.
- Monitor recovery from stroke.
- Identify patients who are most likely to benefit from rehabilitation services and the most appropriate choice of a setting.
- Develop a specific plan of care, including anticipated goals, expected outcomes, prognosis, and interventions.
- Monitor progress toward projected goals and outcomes through periodic reevaluation.
- Determine if referral to another practitioner is indicated.
- Plan for discharge.

The comprehensive examination provides the main source of information for clinical decision making. Examination findings should be coordinated with those of the rehabilitation team in order to arrive at an integrated plan of care. Box 18.3 presents *Elements of the Examination of*

Box 18.3 Elements of the Examination of the Patient with Stroke[132]

Patient/Client History

- Age, sex, race/ethnicity, primary language, education
- Social history: cultural beliefs and behaviors, family and caregiver resources, social support systems
- Occupation/employment/work
- Living environment: home/ work barriers
- Hand dominance
- General health status: physical, psychological, social, and role function, health habits
- Family history
- Medical/surgical history
- Current conditions/chief complaints
- Medications
- Medical/laboratory test results
- Functional activity level: premorbid

Systems Review

- Neuromuscular
- Musculoskeletal
- Cardiovascular/pulmonary
- Integumentary

Tests and Measures/Impairments

Tests and measures are selected based on their ability to quantify or describe each of the following:

- Level of consciousness, arousal, attention, and cognition: mental status, insight, motivation.
  Primary impairments: impaired alertness and attention, perseveration, confabulation, confusion, disorientation, distractibility, memory deficits, impaired judgment
- Emotional status
  Primary impairments: depression, pseudobulbar affect, apathy, euphoria
- Behavioral style
  Primary impairments: impulsive or cautious behavioral styles; frustration, irritability
- Communication and language: coordinate efforts with the speech–language pathologist
  Primary impairments: fluent, nonfluent or global aphasia, dysarthria.
- Circulation; cardiovascular signs and symptoms.
  Common comorbidities: hypertension, CAD, CHF, diabetes, DVT
- Ventilation and respiration/gas exchange: pulmonary signs and symptoms
  Common comorbidities: chronic pulmonary disease
- Anthropometric characteristics: body mass index, girth, length
  Secondary impairments: edema, common in hand and foot
- Integumentary integrity: skin condition, pressure sensitive areas; effectiveness of protective pressure-relieving devices
  Secondary impairments: altered skin integrity, decubitus ulcers
- Pain: intensity and location
  Primary impairments: central post-stroke pain.
  Secondary impairments: hemiplegic shoulder and/or hand pain
- Cranial and peripheral nerve integrity.
  Primary impairments: dysphagia
- Sensory integrity and integration
  Primary impairments: homonymous hemianopsia, tactile/proprioceptive/kinesthetic losses, astereognosis.
- Perceptual function: coordinate efforts with occupational therapist
  Primary impairments: spatial relations syndrome, body scheme/body image disorders, unilateral neglect, agnosia, topographical disorientation.
- Joint integrity, alignment, and mobility: ROM (active and passive); muscle length and soft tissue extensibility
  Secondary impairments: altered biomechanical alignment; loss of joint ROM, muscle and soft tissue length
- Posture: alignment and position, symmetry (static and dynamic, sitting and standing); ergonomics and body mechanics
  Secondary impairment: altered biomechanical alignment
- Motor function: motor control and motor learning
  Primary impairments:
  Altered reflex integrity: hyperreflexia, tonic reflexes, associated reactions.
  Abnormal tone: flaccidity initially; spasticity: spastic posturing.
  Abnormal (obligatory) synergies: flexion and extension synergy patterns.
  Altered voluntary movement patterns: altered initiation, sequencing, timing of muscle contractions; altered force production.
  Coordination, dexterity, agility: coordination deficits
  Motor planning: ideomotor or ideational apraxia
- Muscle performance: strength, power, and endurance.
  Primary impairments: paralysis or weakness; fatigue
  Secondary impairments: disuse atrophy
- Postural control and balance: sensorimotor integration, balance strategies (static and dynamic); safety
  Primary impairments: altered balance, increased fall risk
- Gait and locomotion: gait pattern and speed, use of assistive devices/orthotic devices, safety
  Primary impairments: altered sequencing, timing, balance, endurance
- Wheelchair management and mobility: safety and endurance
- Aerobic capacity and endurance: functional activity testing, graded exercise testing.
  Secondary impairments: decreased endurance
- Orthotic, protective and supportive devices: fit, alignment, function, use, safety
- Functional status and activity level: performance-based examination of functional skills (FIM level), basic and instrumental ADL; functional mobility skills; home management skills. Assistive or adaptive devices: fit, alignment, function, use; safety
  Primary impairments: loss of independent function
- Work, community, and leisure activities: ability to assume/resume activities, safety

the Patient with Stroke[132] and possible impairments. Many of these examination procedures, tests and measures are discussed in earlier chapters; of special relevance, the reader is referred to Chapter 8. This section discusses relevant tests and measures and *disability-specific instruments* developed for the patient with stroke.

Patient and Client History

Data obtained through interview with the patient/family and review of the medical record should include information on general demographics, medical/surgical history, social and employment history, family history, living environment, general health status, and social and health habits. The patient's current/chief complaints and current functional status, and activity level should be ascertained. Coexisting health problems and medications should also be identified. Data obtained from the history will help focus further in-depth examination and systems review.[79]

Levels of Consciousness

Altered level of consciousness (coma, decreased arousal levels) may occur with extensive brain damage. The Glasgow Coma Scale developed by Teasdale and Jennett[139] is the gold standard used to document level of coma. Three areas of function are examined: eye opening, best motor response, and verbal responses. The therapist should document levels of consciousness using standard descriptive terms: *normal, lethargy, obtundation, stupor*, and *coma*. See Chapter 8. Since the patient's behaviors can be expected to fluctuate widely, frequent repeat observations are necessary.

Communication

The patient's communication abilities should be fully ascertained before proceeding on with other examination procedures. It is not uncommon for family and staff to overestimate the patient's abilities to understand language especially if the patient is cooperative. Close collaboration with the speech–language pathologist is important in making an accurate determination of the patient's communication impairments. Receptive language functions (auditory comprehension, reading comprehension) and expressive language function (word finding, fluency, writing) should be carefully examined. Neuromotor disorders (dysarthria, apraxia) need to be clearly differentiated from aphasia. If communication is severely limited and alternate forms required (gestures, demonstration, communication boards), therapists should be fully knowledgeable of such methods prior to the examination. See Chapter 30.

Cognitive, Emotional, and Behavioral States

It is important to examine cognitive abilities early because it may affect the validity of other tests and measures. An examination of orientation (to person, place, time, and circumstance), attention (selective, sustained, alternating, divided), memory (immediate, short- and long-term), and ability to follow instructions (one-, two-, and three-level commands) can be made from observations of the patient's interactions and responses to specific questions. Higher cortical functions can be examined using tests of simple arithmetic and abstract reasoning (grasp of information, abstract thinking and problem-solving, calculating ability, constructional ability). The *Mini-Mental Status Examination (MMSE)* provides a valid and reliable quick screen of cognitive function.[140] A determination of learning impairments (retention and generalization) usually requires repeat sessions with the patient before a complete picture can be ascertained. Difficulties arise in reaching an accurate determination of cognition when the patient presents with impairments in communication. Close collaboration with the occupational therapist and speech–language pathologist is essential. See Chapters 29 and 30.

Emotional states and behavioral styles can best be examined through observation of the patient in a variety of situations over a number of sessions. It is important to correlate findings with those reported by the family regarding premorbid behaviors and emotional characteristics. Families who report a "personality change" after stroke are likely responding to presenting emotional impairments and disinhibition. Episodes of euphoria and crying should be carefully documented and links to situational or environmental circumstances explored. Duration and frequency of these episodes should also be documented along with strategies that are successful in bringing about an end to the episode. The patient's response to new and stressful situations should also be carefully observed. Depression is common. The *Beck Depression Inventory*[141] is a useful instrument for screening. It consists of 21 statements that are scored on a scale from zero to three (the short version has 13 questions and takes 5 minutes to complete).

Cranial Nerve Integrity

The therapist should examine for facial sensation (CN V), facial movements (CN V, VII), and labyrinthine/auditory function (CN VIII). The presence of swallowing difficulties and drooling necessitates an examination of the motor nuclei of the lower brainstem cranial nerves (CN IX, X, and XII) affecting the muscles of the face, tongue, larynx, and pharynx. This includes determination of motor function of the lips, mouth, tongue, palate, pharynx, and larynx. The gag reflex should be examined because hypoactivity may lead to aspiration into the airway. Adequacy of cough mechanisms should also be carefully examined. A team of specialists, the dysphagia team which typically includes the speech–language pathologist, occupational therapist, and physical therapist, performs detailed examination of swallowing. Therapists need to be able to recognize the presence of swallowing difficulties and initiate prompt referral.

The visual system should be carefully investigated, including tests for visual field defects (CN II, optic radiation, visual cortex), acuity (CN II), pupillary reflexes

(CN II, III), and extraocular movements (CN III, IV, VI). Ocular motility disturbances may be present with brainstem strokes, such as diplopia, oscillopsia, visual distortions, or paralysis of conjugate gaze. Visual field defects (homonymous hemianopsia) need to be differentiated from visual neglect, a perceptual deficit characterized by an inattention to or neglect of visual stimuli presented on the involved side. The patient with pure hemianopsia is typically aware of the deficit and will spontaneously compensate by moving the eyes or head toward the side of deficit; the patient with visual neglect will be unaware (inattentive) of the deficit (see Chapter 29). The use of prescriptive eyeglasses should be determined prior to any testing; the therapist should ensure eyeglasses are worn and clean.

Sensory Integrity

A sensory examination should include testing of superficial sensations (e.g., touch, pressure, sharp or dull discrimination, temperature) and deep sensations (proprioception, kinesthesia, vibration). Combined (cortical) sensations such as stereognosis, tactile localization, two-point discrimination, texture recognition should also be examined (see Chapter 5). Impairments may be evident in one sensory modality and not in others. Differences can also be expected between upper and lower hemiplegic extremities. Comparisons with the intact side can be made, but the therapist should be cognizant that impairments may exist in the supposedly "normal" extremities secondary to effects of comorbid conditions (e.g., neuropathy) or aging. Sensory testing may be difficult or need to be deferred owing to cognitive or communication deficits. Profound sensory impairments will negatively impact on rehabilitation outcomes and goals.

Perception

Significant information on sensory and perceptual deficits will be provided by close collaboration with the occupational therapist. Many tests and formalized test batteries have been developed to examine body scheme, body image, spatial relations, agnosia, and apraxia. These are discussed fully in Chapter 29. Because the patient with left hemiplegia may behave in ways that tend to minimize his or her disabilities, it is easy for staff to overestimate the patient's perceptual abilities. The use of gestures or visual cues may decrease this patient's ability to perform specific perceptual tests, whereas verbal cues may increase chances for success. Carefully structuring the environment to minimize clutter and activity, provide clear boundaries and reference points, as well as provide adequate lighting will also improve performance of the patient who exhibits significant visuospatial impairments.

Problems in unilateral neglect (lack of awareness of part of the body or the external environment) will limit movement and use of the involved extremities (usually the nondominant left side). The patient typically does not react to sensory stimuli (visual, auditory, or somatosensory) presented on the involved side. Careful observation of spontaneous use of affected limbs as well as specific responses to inquiries for movement on or toward the hemiplegic side will provide important information about neglect. Persistent neglect may result in bruising or trauma to the hemiplegic limbs during activity and negatively impacts rehabilitation outcomes.

Joint Integrity and Mobility

An examination of joint integrity and mobility should include both passive and active ROM (AROM), joint hypermobility/hypomobility, and soft-tissue changes (swelling, inflammation, or restriction). The shoulder and wrist should be examined closely because joint malalignment problems are common. Edema of the wrist often produces malaligned carpal bones with resulting impingement during wrist extension. Problems with spasticity may result in inconsistent ROM findings, because fluctuations in tone may occur from one testing session to the next. Thus tonal abnormalities should be noted at the time of examination. AROM tests are invalid for the patient in early or middle recovery when paresis, tonal changes, or obligatory synergies influence performance and preclude the isolated movements required in AROM tests. ROM limitations, developing contracture, and pain should be carefully documented. The therapist needs to carefully identify the nature of the pain and how the pain relates to joint movement and limitation (see Chapter 6).

Tone/Reflexes

For the patient in early and middle recovery, examination of tone and reflexes is essential. Passive motion testing can be used to determine hypotonicity, or spasticity. Patterns of spastic muscles are identified (see Table 8.1). Severity of spasticity can be graded on the basis of resistance to passive stretch using the *modified Ashworth Scale (mAS)*.[142] The position of the affected limbs at rest (resting postures) and during voluntary movements should be observed for tonal influences. An examination of stretch reflexes (hyperreflexia) and pathological reflexes (e.g., Babinski, tonic reflex activity, associated reactions) should also be performed.

Voluntary Movement Patterns

Voluntary movement patterns should be examined for control. Abnormal, obligatory synergies can be expected to dominate performance during early recovery. The therapist must base the examination of synergy dominance on knowledge of the typical components of the synergies (see Table 18.5). It is possible for one limb to vary significantly from the other (e.g., the UE may demonstrate more synergistic dominance than the LE). Synergistic dominance versus isolated joint control may also vary within a limb (e.g., the shoulder may demonstrate more isolated control than the wrist and hand).

During later recovery, movements demonstrate isolated joint control and appear more normal in the absence of spasticity and synergy restrictions. Coordination tests can be used to examine control. The therapist focuses on elements of speed/rate control, steadiness, response orientation, and reaction and movement times. Fine motor control and dexterity should be examined using writing, dressing, and feeding tasks (see Chapter 7). While more significant impairments can be expected on the hemiparetic side, it is important to remember that subtle deficits can occur on the less involved side. Thus, it is important to examine both unilateral and bilateral movements, including symmetrical, asymmetrical, unrelated movements. Performance may vary as the patient moves from supine to sitting to standing positions with the resultant increased postural demands and greater degrees of freedom. Slower than normal movements (bradykinesia), or abnormal involuntary movements (chorea, hemiballismus) may occur with lesions affecting the basal ganglia and should be carefully examined.

Strength

Although an examination of strength is necessary, the traditional manual muscle test may pose problems of validity in the presence of strong spasticity, reflex, and synergy dominance. The patient is often not able to move into the required standard positions or to isolate specific joint actions. In this situation, an estimation of strength can be made from observation of active movements during functional activities (functional strength testing).[143] The patient's self-report can also yield important indicators of weakness and fatigue. The patient in later recovery with improving motor control can be examined using more traditional strength tests and measures (e.g., manual muscle testing [MMT], handheld or isokinetic dynamometry) (see Chapter 6). These can provide accurate information on residual impairments in strength, power, and endurance.

Postural Control and Balance

Postural control and balance should be examined in a variety of postures, especially sitting and standing. The patient's ability to maintain a position (steadiness) as well as postural alignment and position (symmetry) within the base of support are determined. Common asymmetries assumed after stroke include increased weightbearing on the stronger side. Dynamic stability control can be examined by having the patient move within a given posture (weight shift) within his or her limits of stability. The patient should be encouraged to shift weight in all directions, especially to the paretic side where impairments are expected. Functional tasks that utilize moving from one posture to another (e.g., supine-to-sit, sit-to-stand) can also be used to examine dynamic postural control. Both reactive postural control (response to perturbations) and anticipatory postural control (response to voluntary extremity movements) should be examined.[144,145]

Performance-based balance tests and measures can be used to determine balance function following stroke. Stroke specific tests are discussed here while generic tests are discussed in Chapter 8. These include:

- The *Berg Balance Scale (BBS)* was initially developed for use with the acute stroke patient and is now in widespread use. It includes 14 functional tasks that are scored using a 5-point ordinal scale. It examines unsupported sitting and standing, transfers, functional reach, picking objects off the floor, turning, single leg stance and stepping. Descriptive criteria are provided for each scoring level: a score of 4 indicates independent function while a score of 0 indicates unable to perform. A maximum score of 56 points is possible. Both intrarater and interrater reliability are high ($r = 0.95$).[146,147]
- Balance subscale of the *Fugl-Meyer Test (FM-B)*, a subtest of the Fugl-Meyer Assessment of Physical Performance that was developed for use with the acute stroke patient. It includes items of unsupported sitting, standing (with and without support), parachute reactions to both sides, and single limb stance both sides. It is scored using a 3-point ordinal scale (see Appendix A).[148]
- *Postural Assessment Scale for Stroke Patients (PASS)* was developed to examine the postural abilities of the acute stroke patient. It includes 12 items that examine sitting and standing without support, standing on the paretic LE, and changing posture (supine-to-affected side, supine-to-unaffected side, supine-to-sitting, sitting-to-standing, and standing picking a pencil off the floor). It is scored using an ordinal scale with descriptors ranging from cannot perform to perform with little help, to perform without help. It demonstrates good construct validity and high interrater and intrarater reliability (0.88 and 0.72, respectively).[149]

Other performance-based tests and measures (described in Chapter 8) include: *Functional Reach Test (FRT)*[150]; *Performance-Oriented Mobility Assessment—Tinetti (POMA)*[151]; *Timed Up and Go Test*[152]; *Clinical Test of Sensory Interaction and Balance (CTSIB)*[153]; and Dynamic Posturography: *Limits of Stability (LOS) Test®*.[154]

Ambulation and Functional Mobility

Gait is altered following stroke owing to a number of factors. Some of the more common problems in hemiplegic gait and their possible causes are summarized in Box 18.4. An examination of gait typically includes an observational gait analysis (OGA). The therapist examines the movements occurring at the ankle, foot, knee, hip, pelvis, and trunk during walking (kinematic gait analysis). Gait is observed from the different planes of motion and deviations are identified. Videotaping an OGA improves identification of gait deviations, provides a visual record of performance, and offers a useful teaching tool in assisting the patient in remediation of gait problems. Quantitative measures of distance and time, cadence, velocity, and stride times should also be obtained using measured walkways and a stopwatch. Kinetic gait analysis involves the forces

Box 18.4 Gait Deviations Commonly Seen Following Stroke

Stance Phase

Trunk/pelvis

Unawareness of affected side: poor proprioception

Forward trunk:

- Weak hip extension
- Flexion contracture

Hip

Poor hip position (typically adduction or flexion): poor proprioception

Trendelenburg limp: weak abductors

Scissoring: spastic adductors

Knee

Flexion during forward progression:

- Flexion contracture
- Weak hip and knee extensors
- Poor proprioception
- Ankle dorsiflexion range past neutral
- Weakness in extension pattern or in selective motion of hip and knee extensors and plantarflexors

Hyperextension during forward progression:

- Plantarflexion contracture past 90°
- Impaired proprioception: knee wobbles or snaps back into recurvatum
- Severe spasticity in quadriceps
- Weak knee extensors: compensatory locking of knee in hyperextension

Ankle/foot

Equinus gait (heel does not touch the ground): spasticity or contractures of gastrocnemius soleus

Varus foot (patient bears weight on the lateral surface of the foot): hyperactive or spastic anterior tibialis, post tibialis, toe flexors, and soleus

Unequal step lengths: hammer toes caused by spastic toe flexors prevent the patient from stepping forward onto the opposite foot because of pain/weightbearing on flexed toes

Lack of dorsiflexion range on the affected side (approximately 10° is needed)

Swing Phase

Trunk/pelvis

Insufficient forward pelvic rotation (pelvic retraction): weak abdominal muscles

Inclination to sound side for foot clearance: weakness of flexor muscles

Hip

Inadequate flexion:

- Weak hip flexors
- Poor proprioception
- Spastic quadriceps
- Abdominal weakness (hip hikers)
- Hip abductor weakness of opposite site

Abnormal substitutions include circumduction, external rotation/adduction, backward leaning of trunk/dragging toes; momentum/uncontrolled swing

Exaggerated hip flexion: strong flexor synergy

Knee

Inadequate knee flexion:

- Inadequate hip flexion and poor foot clearance
- Spastic quadriceps

Exaggerated but delayed knee flexion: strong flexor synergy

Inadequate knee extension at weight acceptance

- Spastic hamstrings
- Sustained total flexor pattern

Weak knee extensors or poor proprioception

Ankle/foot

Persistent equinus and/or equinovarus

- Plantarflexor contracture or spasticity
- Weak dorsiflexors
- Delayed contraction of dorsiflexors
- Toes drag during midswing

Varus: spastic anterior tibialis, weak peroneals, and toe extensors

Equinovarus: spasticity of post tibialis and/or gastrocnemius soleus

Exaggerated dorsiflexion: strong flexor synergy pattern

Adapted from educational materials used at Rancho Los Amigos Medical Center, Downey, CA, and Spaulding Rehabilitation Hospital, Boston, MA.

involved in gait and requires sophisticated equipment (force plates) to obtain data.[155–157] Stroke specific tests are discussed here while generic tests are discussed in Chapter 10.

Performance-based gait tests can be used to determine gait function following stroke. These include:

- *The 10-Meter Walk Test*: Gait speed is timed using a stopwatch to determine velocity.[158,159]
- The 6-Minute Walk Test: Walking distance is recorded in a specified 6-minute time interval to determine functional gait endurance.[160–163] Shorter distances, e.g., a 2-Minute Walk Test,[163] have been used for patients with acute stroke.
- *Energy expenditure*: Oxygen consumed is measured during a 5-Minute Walk Test.
- *Emory Functional Ambulation Profile (EFAP)*: a walking test that examines walking ability in the patient with stroke[164]; a modified version is also available (mFAP).[165] It includes timed tasks performed over different environmental terrains (hard floor, carpeted floor, obstacle course) as well as items of rising from a chair, timed "up & go", and stair climbing. High interrater and intrarater reliability is reported (ICC = 0.99 and ICC = 0.998, respectively).
- *Walkie-Talkie Test*: determines the ability to divide attention while walking (i.e., holding a conversation while walking).

Box 18.5 **Functional Walking Categories**

Physiological Walker
- Walks for exercise only either at home or in parallel bars during physical therapy.

Household Walker
Limited household walker:
- Relies on walking to some extent for home activities.
- Requires assistance for some walking activities, uses a wheelchair, or is unable to perform others.

Unlimited household walker:
- Able to use walking for all household activities without any reliance on a wheelchair.
- Encounters difficulty with stairs and uneven terrain.
- May not be able to enter or leave the house independently.

Community Walker
Most-limited community walker:
- Can enter and leave the home independently.
- Can ascend and descend a curb independently.
- Can manage stairs to some degree.
- Independent in at least one moderate community activity (i.e., appointments, restaurants) and needs assistance or is unable in no more than one other low-challenge activity (i.e., church, neighborhood, visiting friend).

Least-limited community walker:
- Demonstrates independent stair management.
- Independent in all moderate community activities without assistance or use of wheelchair.
- Independent in either local stores or uncrowded shopping centers.
- Independent in at least two other moderate community activities.

Community walker:
- Independent in all home and community activities.
- Can accept crowds and uneven terrain.
- Demonstrates complete independence in shopping centers.

Note: Patients in each higher category can perform all activities of the previous group as well as the additional level of challenge listed.

From Perry, J, et al[166] p. 985, with permission.

Perry and co-workers[166] constructed a walking ability questionnaire and surveyed a group of 147 patients with chronic stroke about the effects of their limited walking ability. They then developed a classification of walking handicap after stroke (see Box 18.5). The use of functional categories (physiological walker, household walker, and community walker) provides a useful method of identifying customary level of walking at home and in the community. *Walking handicap,* defined as the social disadvantage as a result of limitations in walking ability, can also be identified. Factors that differentiated household from community ambulators included strength, proprioception, isolated knee control (flexion and extension), and velocity. The findings of this study can be used to improve communication among clinicians, treatment planning, and documentation.

Functional Status

Functional measures are used to determine the impact of impairments and the plan of care, monitor progress, ascertain efficacy of stroke rehabilitation efforts, and make recommendations for long-term care or placement. Instruments can include items to examine functional mobility skills (bed mobility, movement transitions, transfers, locomotion, stairs), basic ADL skills (feeding, hygiene, dressing), and instrumental ADL skills (communication, home chores). Information on functional disability following stroke is typically gained through performance-based measures. The *Barthel Index*[167] and its later form the *Functional Independence Measure (FIM)*[168] have been extensively tested and demonstrate excellent reliability, validity, and sensitivity. The FIM is now in widespread use in rehabilitation facilities across the United States. Higher FIM scores have been correlated to successful outcomes, discharge home, and return to the community for patients with stroke.[169] See Chapter 11 for a more detailed discussion of these instruments.

Disability-Specific Instruments

Fugl-Meyer Assessment of Physical Performance (FMA)

The pioneering work of Signe Brunnstrom[21,22] on motor recovery and motor behavior following stroke led to the development of the FMA.[24] This is an impairment-based test with items organized by sequential recovery stages. A three-point ordinal scale is used to measure impairments of volitional movement with grades ranging from 0 (item cannot be performed) to 2 (item can be fully performed). Specific descriptions for performance accompany individual test items. Subtests exist for UE function, LE function, balance, sensation, ROM, and pain. The cumulative test score for all components is 226 with availability of specific subtest scores (e.g., UE maximum score is 66, LE score 34; balance score 14). This instrument has good construct validity and high reliability ($r = 0.99$) for determining motor function and balance.[170] Quantifiable outcome data allow this instrument to be accurately used for research purposes (a gold standard) and document recovery over time. The instrument requires an estimated 30 to 40 minutes to administer (see Appendix A).

National Institutes of Health Stroke Scale (NIHSS)

National Institutes of Health (NIH) developed the NIHSS for initial and serial examination of impairments following acute stroke.[171] The NIH NINDS t-PA Stroke Trial Study Group promotes it use for patients with cerebral infarction. It is an 11-item impairment-based test that uses a variable ordinal scale. Some items are scored 0–2 or 0–3 (level of consciousness, best gaze, visual fields, facial palsy, limb ataxia, sensory, best language, dysarthria, extinction, and inattention) other items items are scored 0–4 (motor arm and motor leg). Specific descriptors are attached to each score.[172] An exam scoring service for the NIHSS is maintained by the National Stroke Association.

Stroke Rehabilitation Assessment of Movement (STREAM)

The STREAM is a clinical measure of voluntary movements and basic mobility following stoke. It consists of 30 items (test movements) distributed equally among three subscales: upper-limb movements, lower-limb movements, and basic mobility items. Voluntary movement items explore out-of-synergy control and are scored using a 3-point ordinal scale (unable to perform, partial performance, complete performance). The basic mobility section includes a variety of items (rolling, bridging, sit-to-stand, standing, stepping, walking, and stairs) and is scored using a 4-point ordinal scale (unable, partial, complete/with aid, complete/no aid). The maximum STREAM score is 70 with each limb subscore worth 20 points and the functional mobility subscore worth 30 points.[173] The instrument has good construct validity and high reliability (r = 0.99).[174] It has been used to document motor recovery over time and predict discharge destination following stroke.[175]

Motor Assessment Scale (MAS)

The MAS was developed by Carr et al[176] to examine functional mobility skills following stroke. It uses a 6-point ordinal scale with descriptors for each item score. It includes eight items of motor function, including movement transitions (supine-to-sidelying, supine-to-sit, sit-to-stand), balanced sitting, walking, upper-arm function, hand movements, and advanced hand function. The ninth item is an impairment item examining muscle tone. This instrument has been shown to be highly reliable (r = 0.89 to .99) with high concurrent validity (0.88 correlated with the Fugl-Meyer Assessment).[177] It can be used to document motor recovery over time.

Goals and Outcomes

Examples of general goals and outcomes for patients with stroke (Preferred Practice Pattern 5D) as adapted from the *Guide to Physical Therapist Practice*[132] are presented in Box 18.6. These general goals will provide the basis for development of specific anticipated goals and expected outcomes for an individual patient.

Box 18.6 Examples of General Goals and Outcomes for Patients with Stroke, Adapted from the *Guide to Physical Therapist Practice*[132]

Impact of pathology/pathophysiology is reduced.
- Patient/client, family, and caregiver knowledge and awareness of the disease, prognosis, and plan of care is enhanced.
- Symptom management is enhanced.
- Changes associated with recovery are monitored.
- Risk of secondary impairments and reoccurrence of condition is reduced.
- Intensity of care is decreased.

Impact of impairments is reduced.
- Cognitive function is improved.
- Communication is improved.
- Sensory awareness and skin integrity are improved.
- Perceptual function is improved.
- Awareness and use of the hemiplegic side is improved.
- Pain is decreased.
- Joint integrity and mobility are improved.
- Motor function (motor control and motor learning) is improved.
- Muscle performance (strength, power, and endurance) is improved.
- Postural control and balance are improved.
- Gait and locomotion are improved.
- Aerobic capacity is increased.

Ability to perform physical actions, tasks, or activities is improved.
- Independence in ADL is increased.
- Tolerance of upright postures and activities is increased.
- Problem-solving and decision making skills are enhanced.
- Safety of patient/client, family, and caregivers is improved.

Disability associated with chronic illness is reduced.
- Ability to assume/resume self-care and home management is improved.
- Ability to assume work (job/school/play), community, and leisure roles is improved.
- Awareness and use of community resources are improved.

Health status and quality of life are improved.
- Sense of well-being is enhanced.
- Stressors are reduced.
- Insight, self-confidence, and self-management skills are improved.
- Health, wellness, and fitness are improved.

Patient/client satisfaction is enhanced.
- Access and availability of services are acceptable to patient/client and family.
- Quality of rehabilitation services is acceptable to patient/client and family.
- Care is coordinated with patient/client, family, caregivers, and other professionals.
- Discharge placement needs are determined.

Physical Therapy Interventions

Framework for Intervention

Neurorehabilitation approaches and therapeutic techniques for the patient with stroke have evolved over the years from a major emphasis on muscle reeducation initially developed for patients with poliomyelitis in the 1940s (e.g., Kenny method) to the neurophysiological/neurodevelopmental approaches first popularized in the 1950s and 1960s. These include *Neurodevelopmental Treatment (NDT)*,[23,56] *Movement Therapy in Hemiplegia—Brunnstrom Approach*,[22] *Proprioceptive Neuromuscular Facilitation (PNF)*,[178,179] and sensory stimulation techniques. Of these, NDT and PNF remain in popular use today. Currently there is increased emphasis on functional/task specific training using intense practice of functional tasks along with behavioral shaping and environmental enrichment (e.g., constraint-induced movement therapy [CIMT] for the paretic UE or locomotor training using *body weight support and treadmill training [BWSTT]*). Compensatory training strategies are also used in some circumstances to promote resumption of function using the less involved extremities. These are indicated for patients who demonstrate severe motor impairment and limited recovery. Motor learning strategies provide a common base for all functional training. These are discussed fully in Chapter 13.

Evidence-Based Practice

There is increasing emphasis on evidence-based practice (EBP) that promotes the use of current best research evidence along with individual clinical expertise in order to reach informed decisions about patient care.[180] EBP allows therapists to identify the best (most effective) techniques and to take responsibility for evaluating their practice on an ongoing basis. Early attempts to validate the success neurodevelopmental/facilitation approaches for the patient with stroke failed to provide convincing evidence. Studies designed to delineate differences between conventional exercise approaches (ROM, functional training) and neurodevelopmental/facilitation approaches failed to demonstrate significant advantages of one approach over another.[181–187] Patients improved regardless of the type of intervention, thus providing evidence about the value of physical therapy as a whole. It should be pointed out that many of these early studies were subject to serious methodological flaws.[188] For example, studies used small sample sizes, failed to include a control group or to control for experimenter bias and co-interventions, and/or utilized poorly defined treatments and/or inappropriate outcome measures. Randomized controlled trials (RCT) that utilize both experimental and control groups and larger sample sizes offer the clinician a higher level of confidence in study findings. Several recent RCTs evaluated the effectiveness of neurodevelopmental/facilitation approaches versus other therapeutic approaches. These are summarized in Box 18.7. Evidence concerning the effectiveness of task-oriented training is presented in Evidence Summary Box 13.1 (Post-Stroke Constraint-Induced Movement Therapy) and Evidence Summary Box 18.8 (Post-Stroke Locomotor Training Using Body Weight Support and Treadmill Training).

Important conclusions to be drawn from these studies are that: (1) collectively they provide consistent evidence for the beneficial effects of physical therapy; (2) studies investigating neurodevelopmental/facilitation approaches have failed to consistently demonstrate superiority over other approaches; and (3) studies on task-oriented training have yielded positive results in terms of improving locomotor function (post-stroke locomotor training studies) and UE function (CIMT training studies). Specificity of training and increased intensity of training are important factors in the positive results of this latter group. It is clear that additional large, multicenter RCT studies (Level I studies) are needed. Finally, it is important to point out that there is no one intervention optimal for all patients with stroke. Because patients with stroke are a diverse group with variable levels of function, interventions must be carefully selected based on individual abilities. Therapists need to select interventions that have the greatest chance of successfully remediating existing impairments and promoting functional recovery. The choice of interventions must also take into consideration a number of other factors, including phase of post-stroke recovery (acute, post-acute, chronic), age of the patient, number of comorbidities, social and financial resources, and potential discharge placement. Early emphasis on improving functional independence provides an important source of motivation for both the patient and family.

Strategies to Improve Sensory Function

Patients who have significant sensory impairments may demonstrate impaired or absent spontaneous movement because of the lack of sensory inputs before and during movement. The more the patient can be encouraged to use the affected side, the greater the chance of increased awareness and function. Conversely, the patient who refuses to use the hemiplegic side contributes to the problems imposed by lack of sensorimotor experience. Without attention during treatment, this learned nonuse phenomenon can contribute to further deterioration.[202] Sensory stimulation is important for recovery. Training focuses on restoring sensitivity of the more affected extremities and requires some residual sensory function. The presentation of repeated sensory stimuli stimulates tactile, mechano- and muscle receptors. For example, stroking, stretch, superficial and deep pressure, and approximation can be used. The selection of sensory inputs should be directly related to a functional task and provided to those body

(text continues on page 740)

Evidence Summary Box 18.7

Post-Stroke Neurodevelopmental/Facilitation Training

Reference	Subjects	Design/Intervention	Duration	Results	Comments
Sunderland, KJ, et al[189] 1992	132 subjects Post-acute stage Mildly affected	Single-blind RCT Compared NDT approach (hands-on PT) with behavioral therapy/motor learning approach Outcome measures: Extended Motricity Index; Motor Club Assessment; PROM; pain; Frenchay Arm Test	4 weeks inpatient therapy and 6 weeks outpatient therapy	At 6 months, behavioral group demonstrated ↑ strength, ROM, and speed of movement No differences in attainment of functional skills	Examinations at 1, 3, and 6 months after stroke Large sample size
Feys, HM, et al[190] 1998	100 subjects post-acute stage, ischemic strokes	Single-blind RCT Exp Gr: received movement training, sensory stimulation, RIP Contr Gr: sham shock wave therapy Outcome measures: FMA Action Research Arm Test BI	5 × week for 6 weeks	No significant difference: improvement noted in both groups Exp Gr better scores on FMA at 6 months No difference on functional tests	Examinations at 1 and 6 weeks, 6 and 12 months Good sample size
Langhammer, B, and Stanghelle, J[191] 2000	61 subjects, acute stage	Double-blind RCT Compared NDT approach with motor learning approach Outcome measures: MAS; BI Nottingham Health Profile Sodring Motor Evaluation Scale	5 × week, 40-minute sessions	Motor learning group had decreased length of stay and improved functional outcome	Examinations at 2 weeks and 3 months Good sample size
Mudie, M, et al[192] 2002	40 subjects	Double-blind RCT Used a reaching task Compared 3 groups: (1) visual feedback group (monitor) (2) NDT group (ROM, tone normalization, balance training); (3) task-training group (functional training) Outcome measures: Weight distribution in sitting and standing; BI	5 × week for 2 weeks	NDT group: improved sitting symmetry Feedback and task training groups: improved sitting symmetry at 12 weeks Task-training group: improved functional gains	Examinations at 2 and 12 weeks Small sample size Outcomes consistent with specificity of training
Basmajian, J, et al[193] 1987	29 subjects post-acute stage	RCT Compared 2 groups receiving behavioral/biofeedback training with NDT training Outcome measures: UE Function Test; Health Belief Survey; Beck's Depression Inventory	3 × week for 5 weeks	Both groups improved; no differences found	Small sample size

BI = Barthel Index; Contr Gr = control group; Exp Gr = experimental group; FMA = Fugl-Meyer Assessment of Physical Performance; MAS = Motor Assessment Scale; PT = physical therapy; RCT = randomized controlled trial; RIP = reflex inhibiting postures; UE = upper extremity.

Evidence Summary Box 18.8

Post-Stroke Locomotor Training Using Body Weight Support and Motorized Treadmill Training

Reference	Subjects	Design/Intervention	Duration	Results	Comments
Visintin, M, et al[101] 1998	100 subjects postacute phase	RCT Treadmill gait training:compared BWS with no-BWS Outcome measures: balance (BBS): motor recovery (STREAM); OG walking speed and endurance	4× week for 6 weeks	BWS group demonstrated significant improvement over no-BWS in functional balance (BBS), motor recovery, OG walking speed and endurance	79% progressed to full weightbearing OG walking; improvements were sustained Good sample size
Hesse, S, et al[194] 1994	9 subjects postacute phase	Nonrandomized cohort design Outcome measures: FAC, Standing Balance Test, Rivermead Motor Assessment, Motricity Index, mAS	15 min/session, 30 min/day, 5×/wk for 5 weeks	Gait capacity improved in all subjects (gait velocity by 3 times, cadence and stride length by 2 times); all but 1 subject progressed to OG walking	No control group; fails to account for recovery and effect of regular ongoing PT Small sample size
Hesse, S, et al[195] 1995	7 subjects, MCA stroke at least 3 mo post-stroke	Case series design: A-B-A Compared TT with BWS with PT based on Bobath approach Outcome measures: FAC, Rivermead Motor Assessment, Motricity Index, mAS	Each session (A-B-A) lasted 3 weeks, 5×/week, 30 min daily	Training using BWS and a treadmill was more effective in improving gait ability and walking velocity	Weekly examinations 5 patients demonstrated unilateral neglect and 3 patients demonstrated pusher syndrome Small sample size
Malouin, F, et al[196] 1992	10 subjects MCA stroke acute stroke (7–14 days post-stroke)	Nonrandomized cohort design Intervention program: early standing (tilt table); weight shifting exercises (limb-load monitor), TT, Kinetron Outcome measures: BI, FMA, treadmill velocity	2× day, 5×/week for 5 weeks	Both treadmill velocity and duration increased	Intensive and graded locomotor training activities were well tolerated Small sample size No control group Double the therapy time of normal
Richards, C, et al[197] 1993	27 subjects	RCT Compared early task-based PT (standing, weightshifting and Kinetron exercises; TT), 1.74 hours/day with conventional PT intervention groups (1.79 hours/day and 0.73 hours/day) Outcome measures: FMA, BI, BBS, gait velocity at 6-month followup	Daily	Significant improvement in gait velocity for task-based therapy group	Small sample size

(continued)

Evidence Summary Box 18.8

Post-Stroke Locomotor Training Using Body Weight Support and Motorized Treadmill Training (continued)

Reference	Subjects	Design/Intervention	Duration	Results	Comments
Sullivan, K, Knowlton, B, and Dobkin, B[198] 2002	24 subjects, chronic stroke	Nonrandomized cohort design Intervention program: walking using BWS and a treadmill, 2 groups of varying speeds (slow speeds 0.22 m/sec; variable speeds 0.22 m/sec to 0.89 m/sec; fast speeds 0.89) Outcome measures: FMA 10-m walk: Self-selected walking speed OG	12 sessions, 20-min duration, over 4–5 weeks	Training at fast speeds was more effective at improving speeds of OG walking than training at slow or variable speeds.	No control group Gains maintained at 3 months Small sample size
Smith, G, et al[199] 1999	14 subjects chronic stroke	Nonrandomized cohort design Intervention program: low-intensity walking using BWS and a treadmill Outcome measures: Dynamometer—reflexive and volitional torque	3× week for 3 months	Training improved volitional torque for both concentric and eccentric contractions	No control group Lacked functional outcome measures Small sample size
Nilsson, L, et al[200] 2001	60 subjects post-acute stage	RCT Compared walking using BWS and a treadmill with OG walking training (motor relearning approach) Outcome measures: FIM FMA FAC 10-m walk test BBS	30 minute/day, 5× week for 2 months	Both groups improved on function (FIM, FAC), balance (BBS), and walking speed	10-month followup Good sample size
Laufer, Y, et al[201] 2001	25 subjects postacute stage	Nonrandomized cohort design Compared walking using BWS and a treadmill wih OG walking Outcome measures: FAC Speed (10-m walk test) stride length (foot switch) EMG activity	3 weeks	Training using BWS and a treadmill improved gait function, stride length and stance on paretic limb	No control group Small sample size

BBS = Berg Balance Scale; BI = Barthel Index; BWS = Body Weight Support using an overhead harness; FAC = Functional Ambulation Category; FIM = Functional Independence Measure; FMA = Fugl-Meyer Assessment of Physical Performance; mAS = Modified Ashworth Scale; MCA = Middle cerebral artery syndrome; OG = overground; PT = physical therapy; RCT = randomized controlled trial; STREAM = Stroke Rehabilitation Assessment of Movement; TT = treadmill training.

surfaces directly used in the task. For example, UE tasks can include stroking the hand with different textured fabrics, pressing objects into the hand (coin, button, key), or drawing shapes/letters/numbers on the skin. During functional training, approximation can be provided to extended UE during weightbearing (e.g., in sitting or standing/modified plantigrade position). Approximation can be added to LE tasks such as standing and stepping. Stimulation should be of sufficient intensity to engage the system but not so strong as to produce adverse effects (e.g., withdrawal). During stimulation, the patient's attention should be focused directly on the stimulation and task. Initial attempts are with eyes closed (EC). If the patient fails to recognize the stimulus, the patient can be allowed to look with eyes open (EO) while the stimulus is made more intense. The therapist needs to provide feedback and encouragement in order to direct the patient's attention and shape the patient's responses.[203,204] Johnstone suggests using inflatable pressure splints to provide additional sensory stimulation (deep pressure, muscle, and joint sensations) during functional training. In more severe cases, she also recommends a program of intermittent pressure therapy to provide alternating stimulation of a limb and overcome the problems of sensory accommodation.[205,206]

A safety education program should be instituted early for patients, family, and caregivers to improve awareness of sensory impairments and ensure protection of anesthetic limbs. This is particularly important for preventing UE trauma during transfer and wheelchair activities.

Patients with hemianopsia or unilateral neglect demonstrate a lack of awareness of the contralesional side. The impairments are more pervasive in patients with neglect and in its most severe form (anosognosia) may extend to a totally unawareness of the disability or the extent of the problems. These patients benefit from training strategies that encourage awareness and use of the environment on the hemiparetic side and use of the hemiparetic extremities. It is important to teach active visual scanning movements through turning of the head and axial trunk rotation to the more involved side. Cueing (e.g., visual, verbal, or motor cues) is used to direct the patient's attention. For example, a red anchor line can be taped on the floor and the patient directed to visually follow the line from one side to the other. Or a red ribbon can be attached to the patient's hemiparetic wrist and the patient directed to keep the red ribbon in sight. Scanning movements can also be stimulated using visual tracking tasks using a computer. Patients are given feedback about the success of their efforts and reinforcement for each successful performance (shaping). Imagery has also been shown to help (e.g., "imagine you are a lighthouse beam; use your beam to sweep and scan the floor from one side to the other"). During therapy, the therapist stimulates and encourages active voluntary movements of the hemiparetic limbs while encouraging the patient to look at his or her limbs while moving. UE exercises that involve crossing the midline toward the hemiparetic side (e.g., reaching activities or PNF chop or lift patterns) are important. Functional activities that encourage bilateral interaction are also valuable (e.g., pouring a drink and drinking from a cup; picking up an object with the more involved hand and placing it in the other; "dusting a tabletop" with a cloth held by both hands). The therapist needs to maximize the patient's attention by providing visual, tactile, or proprioceptive stimuli on the more affected side. These can include stroking, brushing, icing, or vibrating the hemiparetic limbs. The therapist also needs to consistently reorient the patient as inattention develops. Patients with very low levels of arousal are likely to be less responsive to therapy efforts.[207–209]

Strategies to Improve Motor Function

Strategies to Improve Flexibility and Joint Integrity

Soft tissue/joint mobilization and ROM exercises are initiated early to maintain joint integrity and mobility and prevent contractures. AROM and passive ROM (PROM) with terminal stretch should be performed daily in all motions. If a contracture is developing, more frequent ROM (twice daily or more) is necessary and sustained low-load stretching can be considered.

Positioning strategies are also important in maintaining soft tissue length. Effective positioning of the hemiparetic extremities encourages proper joint alignment while positioning the limbs out of the abnormal postures typically assumed. The use of protective devices such as resting splints may be necessary. Coordination with family and caregivers is essential for long-term management (Box 18.9).

In the UE, correct PROM techniques require careful attention to external rotation and distraction of the humerus, especially as ranges approach 90° of flexion or more. The scapula should be mobilized on the thoracic wall with an emphasis on upward rotation and protraction to prevent soft tissue impingement in the subacromial space during overhead movements of the arm (Fig. 18.6) and to prepare for forward reach patterns. The use of overhead pulleys for self-ROM is generally contraindicated because of failure to achieve the above requirements for scapulohumeral movement. Full extension of the elbow is important because the majority of patients with stroke develop tightness in elbow flexors as a result of excess flexor spasticity. Normal length of wrist and finger extensors should also be maintained as tightness is typical in flexion. This can be achieved functionally through sitting, weightbearing on the extended paretic UE with the wrist extended and fingers open and extended. Edema and tonal changes may produce impingement with wrist extension. In this situation, the carpal bones should be mobilized prior to stretching at the wrist. Strategies to teach patients safe self-ROM techniques should be instituted early. Suggested activities include:

- *Arm cradling*: The more affected UE cradles and lifts the less affected UE to 90°; the arm is moved into positions of horizontal abduction and adduction. Active trunk rotation is combined with the arm movements.
- *Table-top polishing*: The affected extremity is positioned in humeral flexion with scapular protraction and elbow extension; both hands are positioned on a towel. The less affected hand moves the paretic hand by pulling on the towel (forward, and side-to-side). Trunk movements and ROM are optimized by placing the chair slightly back from the table.

Box 18.9 Common Malalignments Following Stroke and Positioning Strategies

Common Malalignments

Pelvis/trunk. An asymmetric pelvic position is assumed with more weight borne on the ischial tuberosity on the sound side. This results in lateral flexion of the trunk with the head shifted toward the affected side. A posterior pelvic tilt is common. This results in sacral sitting with a flattened lumbar curve and an exaggerated thoracic curve (kyphosis) and forward head.

Scapula. A position of scapular downward rotation is assumed. Scapular instability (winging) may also be present, especially in weightbearing postures.

Glenohumeral joint. Lateral flexion of the trunk and downward rotation of the scapula result in depression and subluxation.

Upper extremity (UE). The limb is typically held in internal rotation and adduction with elbow flexion, forearm pronation, wrist flexion and ulnar deviation, and finger flexion.

Lower extremity (LE). In standing, a position of pelvic retraction and elevation is assumed, with hip and knee extension and hip adduction/internal rotation (i.e., a scissoring position); in sitting the hip and knee are flexed with hip abduction and external rotation (i.e., a flexor synergy pattern). Ankle plantarflexion is common to both.

Positioning Strategies

Lying in the supine position.
Head/neck: neutral and symmetrical; supported on pillow.
Trunk: aligned in midline.
Affected UE: scapular protracted, shoulder forward; arm supported on a pillow; elbow extended with hand resting on a pillow; wrist neutral, fingers extended, and thumb abducted.
Affected LE: hip forward (pelvis protracted); knee on a small towel roll to prevent hyperextension; nothing against the soles of feet. For persistent plantarflexion, a splint can be used to position the foot and ankle in neutral position.

Sidelying on the nonhemiplegic side.
Head/neck: neutral and symmetrical.
Trunk: aligned in midline; small pillow or towel can be placed under the rib cage to elongate the hemiplegic side.
Affected UE: scapular protracted, shoulder forward; arm on a supporting pillow: elbow extended, wrist neutral, fingers extended, and thumb abducted.
Affected LE: hip and knee flexed, supported on a pillow.

Sidelying on the hemiplegic side.
Head/neck: neutral and symmetrical.
Trunk: aligned in midline.
Affected UE: scapular protracted; shoulder forward; arm placed in slight abduction and external rotation; elbow extended, forearm supinated, wrist neutral, fingers extended, and thumb abducted.
Affected LE: aligned with hip extended and knee flexed. An alternate position is slight hip and knee flexion with pelvic protraction.

Sitting in an armchair or wheelchair.
Head/neck: neutral and symmetrical; head directly above pelvis.
Trunk: spine extension, aligned in midline; equal weightbearing on both buttocks.
Affected UE: shoulder protracted and forward; elbow supported on an arm trough or lapboard; wrist neutral, fingers extended, and thumb abducted.
Both LEs: hips flexed to 90°, positioned in neutral with respect to rotation.

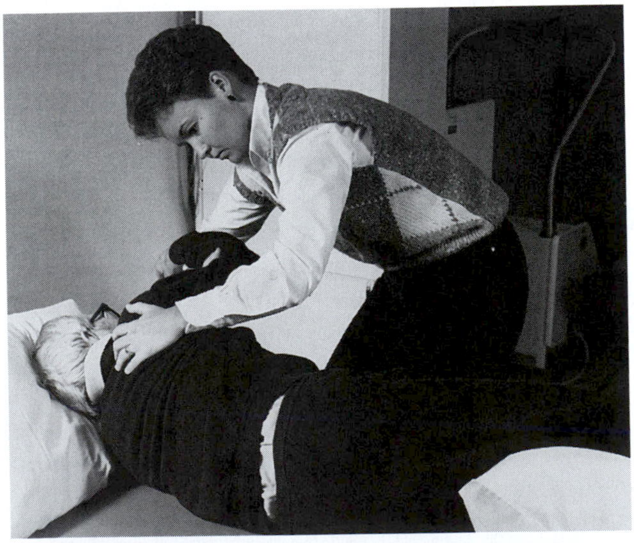

Figure 18.6 Range of motion exercises for the more affected upper extremity. The therapist carefully mobilizes the scapula during arm elevation.

- Sitting, the patient leans forward and reaches both hands down to the floor. This position encourages forward flexion of the humerus with scapular protraction, and extension of the elbow, wrist, and fingers.
- Supine, hands are clasped together and placed behind the head, the elbows fall flat to the mat. This activity should be considered only if scapula upward mobility is present. Hands clasped, self-overhead movements are contraindicated if scapulohumeral rhythm is lacking.

While sitting in a wheelchair, the patient's paretic UE can be positioned on a lap tray or on an arm trough (shallow elbow/forearm support) attached to the armrest. The shoulder is positioned in 5° of abduction and flexion and neutral rotation; elbow in 90° flexion and slightly forward; forearm pronated; and hand in a functional resting position. Splinting the hand can also be considered. A volar resting (pan) splint is commonly used. The forearm, wrist, and fingers are positioned in a functional position (20 to 30° of wrist extension, MP flexion 40 to 45°, IP flexion

10 to 20°, and thumb opposition). A resting splint is more appropriate for nighttime use than daytime when spontaneous function is desired. In the presence of spasticity, tone-reducing devices can be considered (e.g., finger abduction splint, firm cone, spasticity reduction splint, or inflatable pressure splint).

As most patients regain some use of their LEs early in recovery, ROM techniques focus on individual patient needs with attention to several common areas of impairment. For many patients, voluntary movement in the foot and ankle is limited owing to plantarflexor spasticity. Weight-shifting activities in modified plantigrade (forward shift stretches the plantarflexors) or prolonged static positioning using adaptive equipment (i.e., tilt table with toe wedges) can be used to gain range. Facilitation of active contraction of dorsiflexors can also be combined with stretching to provide reciprocal inhibition to plantarflexors. If synergistic influence is strong, the patient can be effectively positioned while supine on a mat with the paretic LE abducted off the side with knee flexed and foot flat on the floor or a stool. This position of hip abduction and extension with knee flexion serves to break-up synergistic dominance and position the limb out of the typical spastic scissoring posture. If the patient spends considerable time sitting in a wheelchair, care should be taken to stretch the hip flexors. If hip flexor contractures are allowed to develop, they can lead to increased difficulty with standing, transfers, and ambulation.

Strategies to Improve Strength

Muscle weakness is a major impairment following stroke. *Active restraint* arising from spastic antagonist muscles has been suggested as a negative influence on movement and a cause of agonist weakness. Bobath,[23] whose theories formed the basis of *Neurodevelopmental Treatment (NDT)*, advocated that strengthening techniques for agonists and excessive effort should be avoided in favor of inhibition techniques designed to reduce spasticity in spastic muscles. This conclusion has been challenged by a number of investigators who have demonstrated that the problems clearly lie with inadequate motor unit recruitment and paresis of agonists.[32,42,43] Patients with stroke can undergo graded strength training without any detrimental increase in spasticity.[210,211] Significant improvements in strength have been demonstrated.[123,210–217] Evidence of carryover effects to improved function is less convincing. Some studies have indicated improvements in function[123,210,215–217] while other studies have failed to demonstrate significant carryover to improved function.[212,214,218,219] Specificity of training may well explain the lack of significant transfer to functional tasks. For excellent comprehensive reviews on this subject the reader is referred to the work of Eng[32] and Morris et al.[79]

Exercise modalities for strengthening include free weights, elastic bands or tubing, and machines (PRE, isokinetics). For patients who are very weak (<3/5), gravity-eliminated exercises using powder boards, sling suspension, or aquatic exercise is indicated. The therapist may need to assist initial movement attempts using active-assisted or facilitated movements (stretch and tracking resistance). Gravity-resisted active movements are indicated for patients who demonstrate 3/5 strength (e.g., arm lifts, leg lifts). Patients who demonstrate adequate strength in gravity-resisted exercise (e.g., 8 to 12 reps) can be progressed to exercise using added resistance (e.g., free weights, bands, or machines). Combining resistance training with functional activities provides additional benefits in terms of improving function (e.g., step-ups or stair climbing while the patient is wearing weighted ankle cuffs). Lifting free weights or using elastic bands places added demands for postural stability and is an important element of training to improve postural control. Many patients with stroke demonstrate poor hand function with no effective grasp. Specially designed gloves may be necessary to ensure maintained contact with exercise equipment (e.g., leather mitts with Velcro®, wrist cuffs). Patients with impaired sensation are at increased risk for injury and should be monitored closely.[91]

In determining a safe exercise prescription, it is important to remember the high incidence of hypertension and cardiac disease in patients with stroke. Exercise is contraindicated in patients with recent stroke and unstable blood pressure (BP). High-intensity strengthening exercises (sustained maximal effort) is generally contraindicated. Isometric exercise accompanied by the Valsalva maneuver and dangerous elevations in BP is also contraindicated. Concentric or eccentric exercises can be used; eccentric exercises will produce less cardiovascular stress than concentric.[220] Dynamic exercises performed in an upright position (sitting) produce less elevations in BP than recumbent/supine exercises. For patients at risk, submaximal protocols using low-intensity exercises (e.g., 30 to 50 percent of maximal voluntary contraction) are appropriate for initial exercise. Varying the exercises (e.g., bench press, leg press, hamstring curl, shoulder press, triceps push-down, biceps curl) is also an effective strategy to reduce risks. The therapist needs to ensure that warm-ups and cool-downs are adequate and the overall exercise progression is gradual.

Careful monitoring of exercise is essential. For patients at risk, BP, heart rate (HR), and ratings of perceived exertion (RPE) should be taken after each exercise set initially. As exercise progresses, less frequent monitoring can be implemented. The therapist also needs to monitor breathing rate and form, ensuring breath holding and Valsalva do not occur. Patients should be instructed in how to measure their own HR and RPE. They should also be taught the warning signs for when to stop exercising. These include:[91]

- Lightheadedness or dizziness.
- Chest heaviness, pain, or tightness; angina.
- Palpitations or irregular heart beat.

- Sudden shortness of breath not due to increased activity.
- Discomfort or stiffness in muscles persisting for several days after exercise.

Patients who are on medications that limit cardiac output (e.g. beta-blockers) will demonstrate reduced heart rate responses and lower peak heart rates. Patients taking diuretics to reduce fluid volume may demonstrate altered electrolyte balance with resulting dysrhythmias. Patients taking vasodilators may require a longer cool-down period after exercise to prevent post-exercise hypotension.[90]

Patients with stroke and older adults who have been immobilized for long periods of time demonstrate increased risk of muscle injury with exercise. Heavy-resistance strength training is therefore contraindicated. The risk of muscle injury is greatest with eccentric exercise.[221] In order to reduce this risk, the therapist needs to begin training with low-intensity exercises and gradually increase intensity to patient tolerance. It is important to ensure adequate rest periods using distributed practice to start, and provide a variety of exercises. Careful monitoring of fatigue and muscle soreness is necessary.[32] Episodes of prolonged or unusual fatigue and delayed-onset muscle soreness (DOMS, 24 to 48 hours after exercise) should be avoided. Progression to higher training levels should proceed only in the absence of DOMS and fatigue.

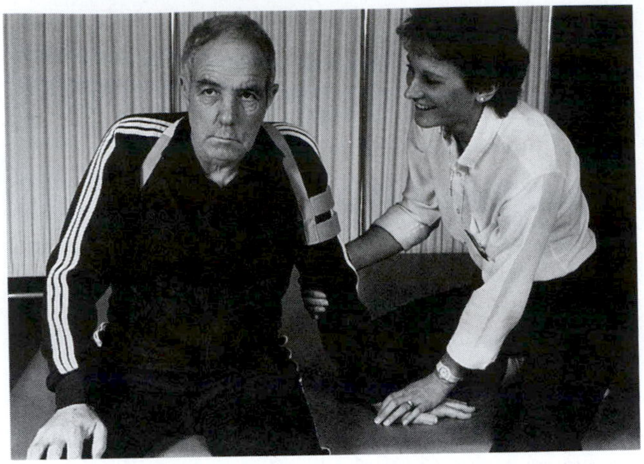

Figure 18.7 Sitting, with extended arm support. The patient is wearing a humeral cuff sling to prevent subluxation of the shoulder. The therapist assists in stabilizing the elbow and fingers in extension.

Strategies to Manage Spasticity

Patients who demonstrate spasticity benefit from interventions designed to modify or reduce tone. These include early mobilization combined with elongation of spastic muscles and sustained stretch through positioning. The technique of rhythmic rotation (a passive manual technique) can be effective in gaining initial range. The therapist slowly moves the limb into the lengthened range while gently rotating it back and forth. Once full range is achieved, the limb is positioned in the lengthened position. For example, the shoulder is extended, abducted, and externally rotated with the elbow, wrist, and fingers extended and positioned in weightbearing (see Fig. 18.7). The patient then needs to maintain the position for an extended time (e.g., 5 to 10 minutes of sustained stretching). Additional inhibitory effects are attained from prolonged pressure on the long flexor tendons of the hand. Slow rocking movements (rocking the body over the elongated limb) also increase the inhibitory effects through adding influences of slow vestibular stimulation. Spasticity in the quadriceps can be similarly inhibited through prolonged pressure and weightbearing in kneeling or quadruped positions (Fig. 18.8). A reduction in truncal tone can be promoted using techniques of rhythmic rotation or rhythmic initiation combined with axial trunk rotation (e.g., in sidelying, sitting or hooklying, segmental trunk rotation). PNF upper trunk patterns (chopping or lifting) that emphasize rotational movements of the trunk can also be effective in maintaining reduced trunk tone.[179] Sidesitting on the hemiparetic side provides sustained stretch to the spastic side flexors. The patient and family member or caregiver should be taught specific stretching techniques that focus on spastic muscles.

Training strategies should include activation of the antagonist muscles using slow and controlled movements. Local facilitation techniques can be added to activate very weak antagonist muscles and are effective in reducing agonist tone through the effects of reciprocal inhibition. Thus in the UE efforts are directed toward active contractions of the elbow extensors in the presence of flexor spasticity while in the LE efforts are directed toward active contractions of the knee flexors with extensor spasticity. Reciprocal relationships are not always within a normal range, however, particularly in the presence of strong spasticity and spastic co-contraction.[23] Additional modalities and/or splinting can be effective in reducing tone. Cold in the

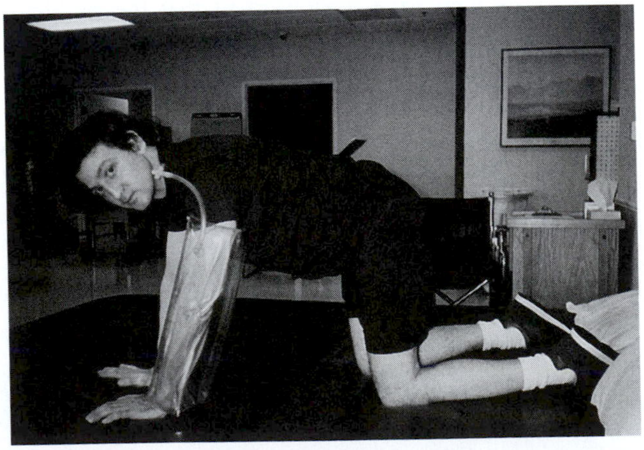

Figure 18.8 Use of a pressure splint applied to support the elbow in extension during weightbearing in the quadruped position. Weightbearing is on the hands and knees.

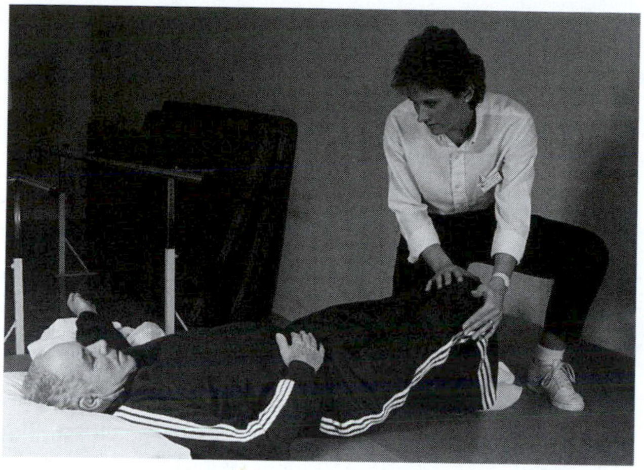

Figure 18.9 Inhibition of truncal tone through lower trunk rotation. The therapist uses the technique of rhythmic initiation to increase mobility.

form of ice wraps or ice packs can be used to temporarily dampen neural firing rates and therefore spasticity. Electrical stimulation to the antagonist muscles or vibration have also been used with some success. Soothing verbal commands and cognitive relaxation techniques (mental imagery) provide an overall calming influence and generally relax tone. Pain syndromes have the opposite effect.

As mentioned earlier, Johnstone[206] advocates the use of inflatable pressure splints (air splints) to stabilize and maintain an extremity in an elongated position and provide tone inhibition. Splints also help to control unwanted synergistic movements and associated reactions, and assist in early weightbearing. Figure 18.8 demonstrates the use of an air splint to stabilize elbow extension in the quadruped position while Figure 18.10 demonstrates its use in the modified plantigrade position. Patients with a flaccid, hypotonic limb may also benefit from the use of pressure splints to provide sensory input and initial stabilization. Long or full limb pressure splints also assist in controlling edema, a common problem of paralyzed limbs. Positioning the splinted limb in elevation can assist in reducing edema.

Strategies to Improve Initial Movement Control

Activities that promote normal postural alignment and control and functional use of the extremities are the primary focus of initial movement training. Patients with stroke typically present with loss of dissociated or fractionated movements with obligatory synergy patterns and associated reactions.[222] For example, coordinated grasp and manipulation are lost as the fingers respond with strong flexion when lifting the arm results in elbow flexion with flexion, abduction, and external rotation of the shoulder. Inter- and intralimb control is also abnormal with movements of one limb strongly linked to movements of the other. During initial training, the therapist needs to focus on *dissociation* of different body segments (the ability to move the different parts of the body or limb separately) and *selective* (out-of-synergy) movement patterns. For example, the more affected UE is stabilized in an extended weightbearing position while the patient practices stepping movements in modified plantigrade position.

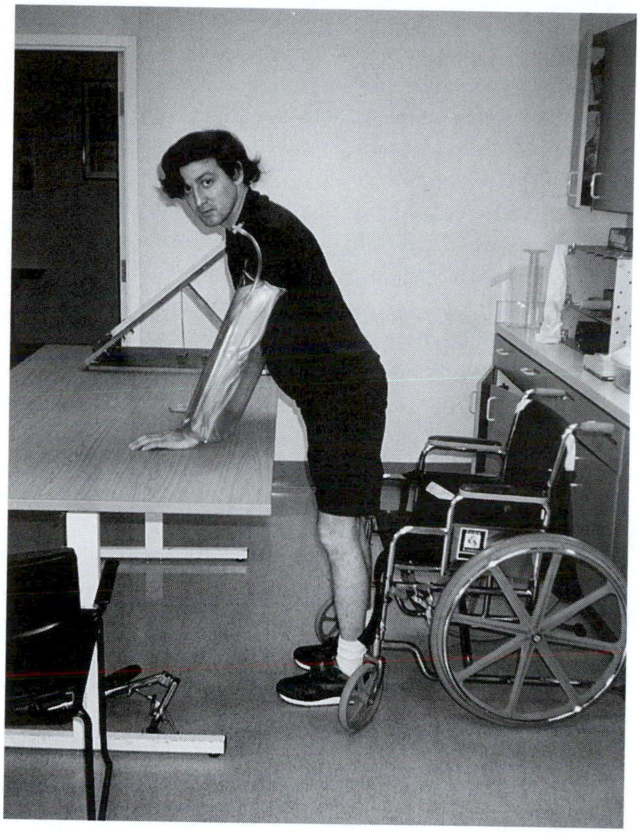

Figure 18.10 Use of a pressure splint applied to support the elbow in extension during weightbearing in the modified plantigrade position. Weightbearing is on the hands and feet.

The linking together of the proper components of movement and the refinement of isolated control requires a great deal of mental concentration and volitional control. Movements that are performed too quickly or with too much force will be ineffective in producing the control needed. Thus the therapist needs to instruct the patient to avoid excessive effort and unnecessary force during movement. The therapist should aim for as much normalcy in movement as possible and select postures that assist the desired movements through optimal biomechanical stabilization and/or use of the optimal point in the range. As control develops, postures can be changed to more difficult ones that challenge developing control. For example, initial elbow extension can be first attempted in sidelying with the shoulder flexed to 90°. The posture can then be changed to sitting, and finally standing. Movements may start out assisted (guided) but should shift to active control as soon as possible. Often the resistance of gravity acting on the body, or slight manual (tracking) resistance, is enough to initiate or facilitate correct movement responses through proprioceptive loading. If the patient's motor responses are very weak and or unable to activate, direct facilitation using a variety of different stimuli may be necessary to assist the patient in initiation of movement. For example, the patient who lacks adequate control of elbow extension can be positioned in sitting with the affected UE weightbearing. Tapping can be applied over the triceps to facilitate holding in extension. The work of Davies provides an excellent resource for early training activities.[56,223]

Functional tasks are the main focus of training (e.g., reaching and manipulation, walking, stair climbing). Normal function implies variability of movements. Muscles need to be activated in varied activities using varied types of contractions. All three types—eccentric, isometric, and concentric—are important to include in an exercise program. For the patient with stroke who demonstrates very weak movements, eccentric contractions should be practiced before concentric contractions as they utilize elastic elements and muscle spindle support more efficiently. For the same amount of tension, fewer motor units are required. Practice of functional tasks that utilize variations of contractions should also be implemented. For example, the patient who practices sit-to-stand, stabilizing in stance, and then stand-to-sit is utilizing sequences of concentric-isometric-eccentric contractions. Weak muscles (typically antagonistic to strong spastic muscles) should be activated first in unidirectional movements. As control develops, exercises can shift to include slow active reciprocal contractions of agonist and antagonist muscles first in limited ranges, then in full range. This emphasis on balanced interaction of both agonists and antagonists is crucial for normal coordination and function. Proprioceptive neuromuscular facilitation (PNF) patterns using reversal of antagonists and proprioceptive loading through light, tracking resistance are ideal for this.[179] See Chapter 13 for an expanded discussion.

Strategies to Improve Motor Learning

Motor skill learning is based on the brain's capacity for recovery through mechanisms of reorganization, and adaptation. An effective rehabilitation plan capitalizes on this potential and encourages active participation—*the patient must be fully engaged*. Activities are selected that are meaningful and important to the patient. Optimal motor learning can be promoted through attention to a number of factors, most importantly, strategy development, feedback, and practice. Carr and Shepherd[224] describe many of these strategies in their book entitled *Motor Relearning Programme for Stroke*.

Strategy Development

The therapist first assists the patient in learning the desired task (cognitive stage). More specifically, critical task elements and successful goals and outcomes are identified. The desired task is demonstrated at the ideal performance speeds. The patient then begins to practice. If the task has a number of interrelated steps, practice of component parts may precede practice of the whole task. It is important, however, not to delay practice of the integrated task because this may interfere with effective transfer of learning. The therapist should give clear, simple verbal instructions and not overload the patient with excessive or wordy commands. Correct performance should be reinforced and intervention provided when movement errors become consistent. Active participation is essential for learning; *there is no learning with passive movements*. Practicing the movements on the less affected side first can yield important transfer effects. Simultaneous practice of similar movements on both sides (bimanual task practice) have also been shown to improve learning and promote integration of the two sides of the body. Visualization of the movement components (mental practice) can help some patients in initially organizing the movement if cognition is intact.

As initial practice progresses, the patient is asked to self-examine performance and identify problems, specifically, what difficulties exist, what can be done to correct the difficulties, and what movements can be eliminated or refined. If a complex task is practiced, the patient is asked to identify if the correct components were performed, how the individual components fit together, and if they were appropriately sequenced. If the patient is unable to provide an accurate assessment of problems, the therapist can prompt the patient in decision making using guiding questions and utilize demonstration to help identify problems. For example, if the patient consistently falls to the right while standing, questions can be directed toward this problem (e.g., "In what direction did you fall?" "What do you need to do to prevent yourself from falling?"). The patient is thus actively involved in developing problem-solving skills (self-monitoring and self-correction of movements). These skills are essential in ensuring independence and generalizability of learning to other environments and variations.

Feedback

Feedback can be intrinsic (naturally occurring as part of the movement response) or extrinsic (provided by the therapist). During early motor learning the therapist provides extrinsic feedback (e.g., verbal cueing, manual cueing) to shape performance. It is important to monitor performance carefully and provide accurate feedback. The patient's attention should be directed to naturally occurring intrinsic feedback. During early intervention visual inputs are critical for motor learning. This can be facilitated by having the patient look at the movement (a central concept of PNF). Use of a mirror can be an effective adjunct for some patients to improve visual feedback, especially during postural and positioning activities. It is, however, contraindicated in patients with marked visuospatial perceptual impairments. During later learning (associative phase), proprioception becomes important for movement refinement. This can be encouraged by early and carefully reinforced weightbearing (approximation) on the more affected side during upright activities. Additional proprioceptive inputs (manual contacts, tapping, stretch, tracking resistance, antigravity postures, or vibration) can be used to improve feedback and stimulate learning. The patient should be encouraged to "feel the movement" while learning to distinguish correct movement responses from incorrect ones. Surface electromyography (EMG) can also be used to provide augmented feedback. Exteroceptive inputs (light rubbing, stroking) may be used to provide additional sources of sensory inputs, particularly where distortions of proprioception exist. As treatment progresses, the emphasis again shifts from extrinsic to intrinsic feedback and to self-monitoring and correcting movement responses. Great care must be taken to avoid sensory bombardment or feedback dependence (i.e., movements that occur only if stimulated). This requires careful consideration during each treatment session. Therapists should also limit use of immediate feedback to allow the patient adequate time for introspection. Pain and fatigue (either mental or physical) should be avoided, as each can result in decreased performance and learning.

Practice

Practice, practice, and more practice is essential for motor skill learning and recovery. The therapist needs to organize the patient's therapy session to ensure optimal practice. Constant repetition of the desired task (blocked practice) will improve initial performance and motivation. Most hospitalized patients initially require a distributed practice schedule with adequate rest periods owing to limited endurance. The patient should be encouraged to self-monitor practice sessions and recognize when fatigue may be setting in and rest is required. The therapist needs to progress the patient to variable practice (practice of similar or related tasks using serial or random practice orders) as soon as possible. Variable practice also improves performance and more importantly results in better retention of learned skills, adaptability (modification of tasks), and generalizability to different contexts (environments). Patient, staff, and family efforts should be coordinated to ensure continued and consistent practice during off-therapy times.

Careful attention to the learning environment will also yield important therapeutic gains. Distractions should be reduced and a consistent and comfortable environment provided in which the patient can learn. For many patients with stroke, this will initially be a closed environment with limited distractions. Later the environment can be varied, providing an appropriate level of *contextual interference*. Thus the patient is progressed toward performing the same skill in more open, variable and real-life environments. The addition of *Easy Street Environments* to many rehabilitation centers provides an important tool to simulate community environments.

Motivation is key to successful learning. The patient should be fully involved in collaborative goal-setting from the beginning and continually reminded of the goal, the task, where they are, and what they are striving for (expected outcomes). Treatment sessions should include positive experiences, ensuring the patient experiences success in therapy and instilling self-confidence. Beginning and ending the therapy session on a positive note is a helpful strategy. Self-efficacy ratings can be used to monitor progress (e.g., "What successes did you achieve in therapy today?"). Supportive strategies should be discussed with family and caregivers. Finally, the therapist should continually communicate support and encouragement to the patient. Recovery from stroke is an extremely stressful experience and will challenge the coping abilities of both patient and family.

Strategies to Improve Postural Control and Functional Mobility

The loss of sensory and motor function on one side will present a tremendous challenge for the patient struggling to relearn postural control and functional mobility. Initial treatment strategies should focus on trunk symmetry and use of both sides of the body. Progression is from guided movements to active movements as soon as the patient is able to assume independent control.

Suggested functional training activities include:

Rolling

Rolling to both sides should be practiced; rolling onto the less affected side will prove more difficult. Extremity movement patterns (e.g., PNF D1 flexion of the LE) can be used to enhance the movement. Care must be take to ensure the patient does not leave the more affected UE behind but rather brings it forward. This can be accomplished by having the patient clasp the hands together in a prayer position first. The more affected LE can also be used to assist in rolling by pushing off from a flexed and adducted, hooklying position (Fig. 18.11). Rolling onto the

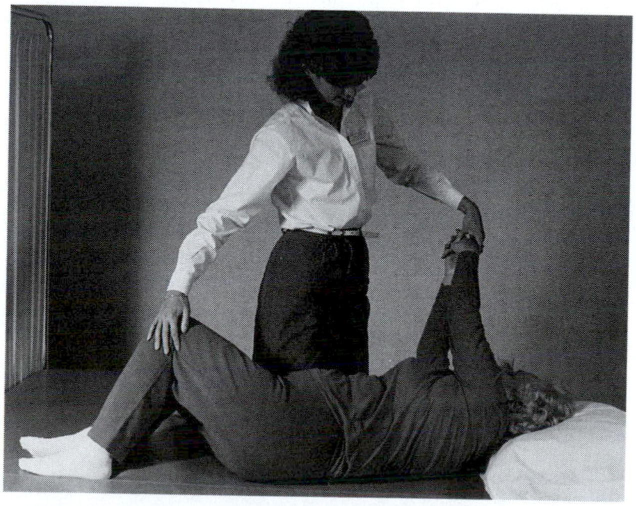

Figure 18.11 Early mobility activities: rolling onto the unaffected side. The therapist guides the movement and assists the upper extremity pattern of prayer position.

more affected side and into a sidelying-on-elbow position is important to promote early weightbearing. This position also has the added benefit of elongating the lateral trunk flexors, which may be spastic.

Supine-to-Sit and Sit-to-Supine

The patient should practice moving from supine-to-sitting from both sides, with an emphasis on rising from the more involved side. The therapist can provide assistance from sidelying on the more affected side by shifting the LEs over the edge of the bed or mat while the patient pushes up into sitting using both UEs for support. Controlled lowering should also be practiced.

Sitting

Early training in sitting should focus on achieving a symmetrical posture with proper spine and pelvic alignment. The pelvis should be neutral, spine straight. Feet should be flat on the support surface. Typically, patients with stroke will sit asymmetrically with weight borne more on the less affected side, pelvis in a posterior tilt, and upper trunk flexed (kyphotic). Lateral flexion to the affected side is also common. The therapist can manually guide the patient into the correct sitting position and provide verbal and tactile cues. Early sitting can be assisted by having the patient use the UEs for bilateral support (at sides or in front: on table top, a large ball, or the therapist's shoulders with the therapist sitting directly in front of the patient). Sitting on a therapy ball can also be used to promote pelvic alignment and mobility (pelvic rotations) and trunk upright alignment (gentle bouncing). Sitting control should be progressed from first holding steady in the posture (stability) to moving in the posture (dynamic stability), and finally to dynamic challenges (reaching). A common problem with hemiplegia is the inability of the upper trunk to move independently of the lower trunk (dissociate). Upper trunk mobility with reciprocal flexion/extension, lateral flexion, and rotation movements should therefore be practiced. Lateral weight shifts to the more affected side typically are the most difficult. Manual contacts in the direction of the movement combined with gentle resistance can provide important early learning cues. PNF patterns of chop/reverse chop or lift/reverse lift are excellent examples of patterns that promote trunk rotation, bilateral UE activity, and crossing the midline (important for unilateral neglect). The patient should also practice scooting in sitting ("butt walking") to ensure mobility for dressing (putting pants on) and sit-to-stand transitions (coming to the edge of the seat to place the feet back and under the body).

Bridging

Bridging activities help develop trunk and hip extensor control important for use of a bedpan, pressure relief on the buttocks, initial bed mobility (scooting), and sit-to-stand transfers. It also develops advanced LE out-of-synergy control (hip extension with knee flexion), and stimulates early weightbearing through the foot (Fig. 18.12). Bridging activities include independent assumption of the posture, holding in the posture, and moving in the posture (lateral weight shifts, bridge-and-placing hips to one side). If the more affected LE is unable to hold in a hooklying position, the therapist will need to assist by stabilizing the foot. Lifting the less affected foot off the surface (placing it on a small ball) while maintaining the pelvis level significantly increases the difficulty and can be used to increase demands on the more affected side. Difficulty can also be increased by varying the position of the UEs, from extended and abducted at the sides, to arms folded across the chest or hands clasped together overhead in a prayer position.

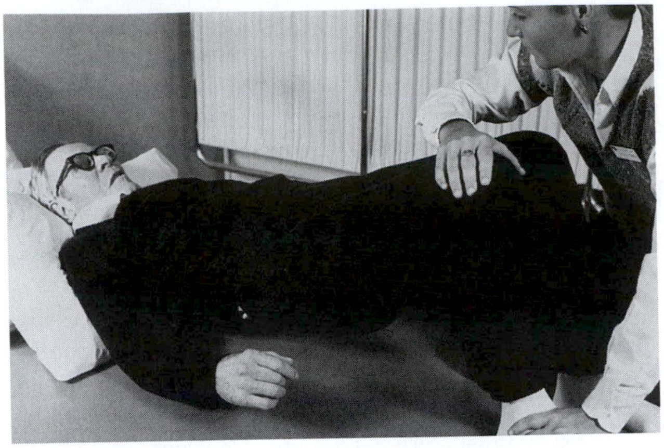

Figure 18.12 Early mobility activities: bridging. The patient combines hip extension with knee flexion. The therapist assists in stabilizing the affected knee in flexion with foot flat.

Sit-to-Stand (STS) and Sit-Down Transfers

STS transfers should be practiced with a focus on symmetrical weightbearing, coordinated muscular responses, and adequate timing (Fig. 18.13). Initially the patient must actively flex the trunk and use momentum to shift the body mass forward (*flexion-momentum phase*). The feet should be placed well back to allow ankle dorsiflexors to assist with forward rotation. The patient with stroke typically demonstrates decreased forward movement and momentum. The therapist should focus the patient's eyes on a visual target directly in front at eye level and use verbal cues to facilitate the desired movements ("move your shoulders forward and stand up"). The patient can be assisted in this phase by swinging both hands forward or reaching forward with both UEs, hands clasped together in a prayer position. If the patient is apprehensive of falls, both hands can be positioned on a large therapy ball while the therapist stabilizes and moves the ball forward in time with the forward weight shift. Pushing off with both hands on the support surface is not effective in producing the forward weight shift and should be discouraged. The patient's movements must then be directed into the *extension phase* which requires hip and knee extensors to produce vertical movement into the upright position. Weakness and incoordination of these muscles typically result in incomplete

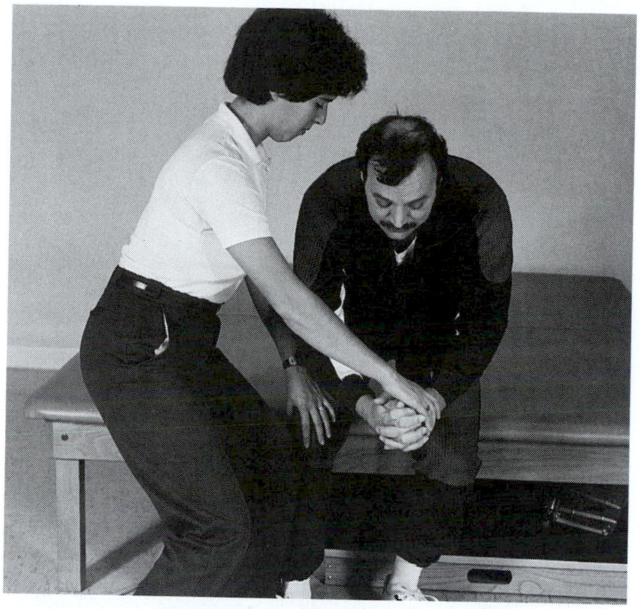

Figure 18.13 Sit-to-stand movement transitions. The therapist assists the patient in straightening his affected knee while he brings his center of mass forward. Hands are held together in a prayer position.

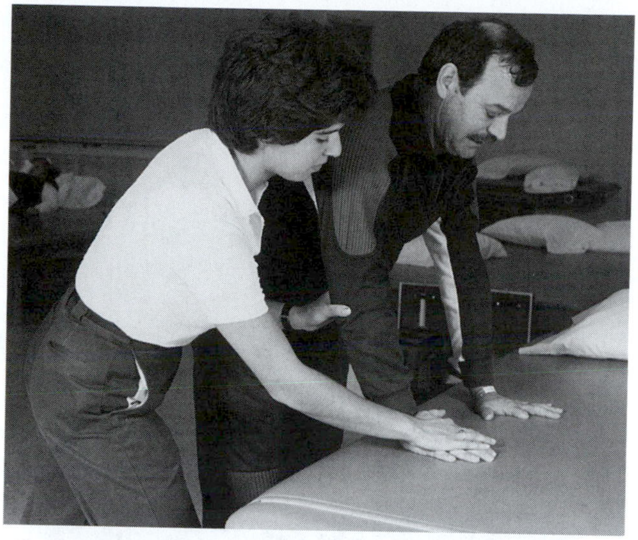

Figure 18.14 Early weightbearing in modified plantigrade with extended UEs. The therapist assists elbow and finger extension of the affected right UE.

extension and inability to stand up independently. The height of the seat can be elevated at first to decrease the extensor force required. Progression is then to lower seat heights. Increased weightbearing on the stronger LE can be achieved by varying the initial foot position, placing the stronger foot slightly behind the weaker foot. As the patient improves, the position of the feet can be reversed to focus attention on increased use of the weaker side. The patient with stroke typically accomplishes standing up very slowly. With repetitive practice, the patient should be encouraged to focus on increasing the speed of the movement and to not pause between the two phases. Using a prayer position (hands clasped together and held straight ahead with elbows extended) reduces UE push-off. The patient with stroke also demonstrates decreased control in sitting down owing to lack of eccentric control and will sit down abruptly after moving partially through the range. Eccentric movements (small range movements) can be practiced with the patient positioned back against a wall doing partial wall squats. Lower trunk rotation can be promoted by having the patient practice STS using a platform mat. From standing, the patient shifts the pelvis laterally to the more affected side, and then sits down. By using this activity, the patient can move all the way around the mat alternating standing and controlled sitting, focusing on moving toward the weaker side.

Standing, Modified Plantigrade

Modified plantigrade is an ideal early standing posture to develop postural and extremity control. The more affected UE is extended and weightbearing (an out-of- synergy posture), while the more affected LE is holding in extension (also an out-of-synergy pattern of hip flexion with knee extension). The forward trunk position creates an extension moment at the knee, thus assisting weak knee extensors. In addition, the posture has a wide (four-limb) base of support and is very stable (Fig. 18.14). Progression should again be from holding in the posture to moving in the posture (weight shifts) to reaching tasks.

Standing

Initial upright standing can be enhanced using fingertip light touch down support on a high table or wall. As soon as possible, the patient should be encouraged to practice standing with unilateral UE support (more affected side) and then free standing (no UE support). As in other postures, an appropriate progression includes first holding in the posture, to moving in the posture (weight shifts), and finally withstanding challenges to dynamic balance (e.g., reaching in all directions, stepping). The patient is instructed in proper symmetry and alignment. Gentle resistance can be applied to assist in holding, using the PNF technique of rhythmic stabilization. Weight shifts should incorporate moving forward-backward, side-to-side, and diagonally (incorporating upper trunk rotation). Lateral weight shifts to the more affected side are the most difficult. Manual contacts in the direction of the movement combined with gentle resistance can provide important early learning cues. Early weightbearing on the more affected limb can be achieved using a half-sitting position (Fig. 18.15).

Transfers

During early transfers, the patient may require maximal assistance. Adjusting the hospital bed to the height of the chair or wheelchair will help to decrease the difficulty of the transfer. Staff often emphasize the sound

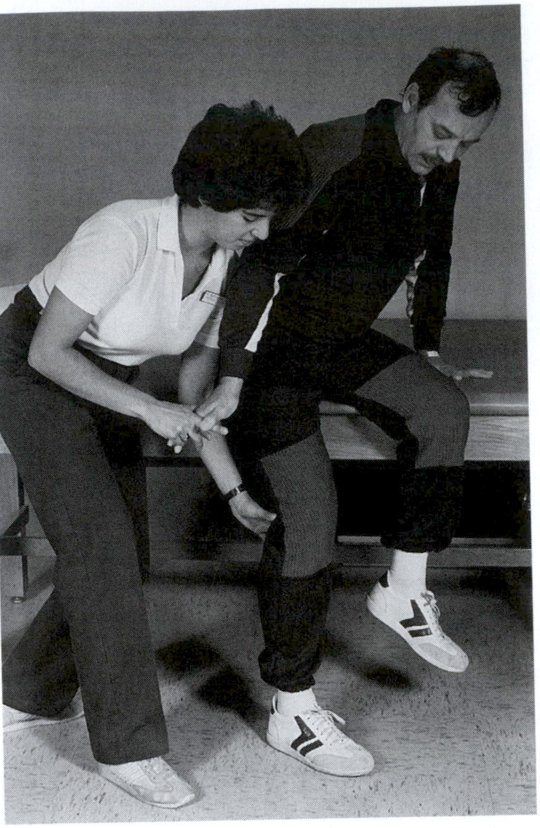

Figure 18.15 Early weightbearing on the affected LE. The therapist assists controlled, small-range flexion and extension movements of the knee. The affected UE is maintained in an inhibitory position.

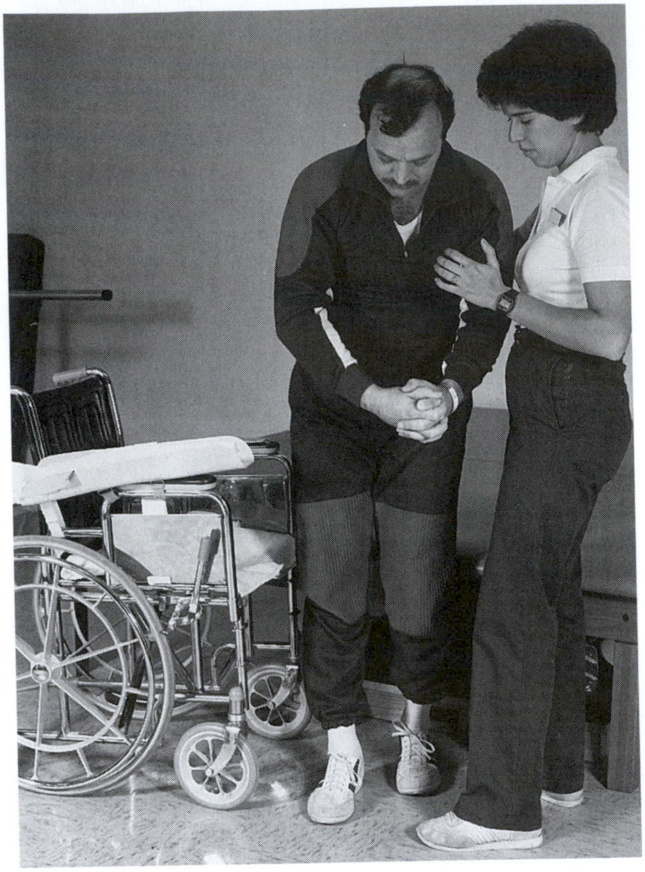

Figure 18.16 Transferring to the affected side. The patient learns to control standing up and pivoting with the affected LE leading. The therapist assists in balance.

side by placing the chair to that side and having the patient stand and pivot a quarter turn on the stronger LE before sitting down. Although this compensatory strategy promotes early transfers, it neglects the weaker side and may make subsequent training more difficult. The patient should be taught to transfer to both sides, with emphasis on moving toward the more affected side. Practice to both sides has functional significance, as most bathrooms are not large enough to allow positioning of the wheelchair on both sides of a tub or toilet. Also, the patient is not likely to be able to reposition the wheelchair once he or she transfers into bed so that a transfer toward the same side can be achieved when getting out of bed. When transferring, the patient's affected arm can be stabilized in extension and external rotation against the therapist's body. Alternately, the patient's UEs (hands in prayer position) can be placed in front or to one side on the therapist's shoulders. (Fig. 18.16). The therapist can then assist in STS by using manual contacts, either at the upper trunk or pelvis. The more affected LE may be stabilized by the therapist's knee exerting a counterforce on the patient's knee as needed. Transfer training should include practice in transferring to various different surfaces and heights (e.g., wheelchair, toilet, tub seat, car).

Functional mobility training is begun early and continued throughout the course of rehabilitation. Training activities and postures are varied according to individual needs. Additional postures such as modified prone-on-elbows (table top weightbearing), quadruped, side-sitting, kneeling, and half-kneeling may be appropriate and can be used to increase the level of difficulty and focus on specific body segments and deficiencies in control. Some postures may not be appropriate (e.g., prone-on-elbows for the patient with cardiorespiratory compromise or a flaccid, subluxed UE, or kneeling for the patient with osteoarthritis). Advanced functional training should include practice in getting down to and up from the floor in the event of a fall. See Davies[56,223] and O'Sullivan and Schmitz[225] for additional functional training activities.

The Patient with Ipsilateral Pushing (Pusher Syndrome)

The patient with ipsilateral pushing presents with an entirely different set of postural control problems. The patient sits or stands asymmetrically, but with most of the weight shifted toward the weaker side. The patient uses the stronger UE or LE to push over to the weaker side, often resulting in instability and falls. Efforts by the therapist to passively correct the patient's tilted posture often result in the patient pushing stronger. Training needs to emphasize vertical positions with *active* movement shifts to the stronger side. Use of visual stimuli is effective as patients retain the ability to correct posture with such stimuli but may not be able to do so spontaneously. Patients should be asked to look at their posture and see if they are upright. Environmental prompts can be used to assist orientation. These can include use of a mirror if visuospatial deficits are not present or vertical structures in the environment. For example, the therapist can sit on the patients less involved side and instruct the patient to "lean over to me." Or the patient can be positioned with the stronger side next to a wall and instructed to "lean toward the wall."[61] Therapists can provide verbal and tactile cues for postural orientation. To improve sitting posture, training activities can include sitting on a therapy ball to promote symmetry and sitting, crossing the weaker LE over the stronger LE. In early standing the weaker LE is often flexed and has difficulty supporting the body on that side. Extension can be assisted by the use of an air-splint or a posterior leg splint or by direct tapping over the quadriceps muscle.[56] The modified plantigrade position is effective for early supported standing; however, the therapist should focus on unilateral support using the weaker UE. Again, an airsplint can be used to assist extension of the weaker arm. If a cane is used, it can be shortened to encourage weight shift to the stronger side. An environmental boundary can be used to achieve symmetrical standing (e.g., standing in a doorway or corner standing). It is important to limit pushing with the sound extremities. For example, in sitting or standing, the therapist should block the stronger limb from drifting laterally into abduction and extension and pushing. Motor learning strategies are very effective in reducing the effects of this disorder and enhancing recovery. In particular, the therapist should demonstrate correct orientation to vertical, provide consistent feedback about body orientation, and practice correct orientation and weight shifts. The patient should be fully involved in problem-solving. For example, the therapist should ask questions such as "what direction are you tilted? "and "what direction do you have to move in order to achieve vertical?". Karnath and Broetz[61] indicate that the potential for minimizing the impact of ipsilateral pushing is good with effective training.

Strategies to Improve Upper Extremity Function

Patients with severe sensory, motor, and functional impairments (recovery stage 3 or less) are generally less responsive to remedial interventions than patients demonstrating more advanced recovery. These patients will benefit from early mobilization, ROM, and positioning strategies, previously discussed in this chapter. Compensatory training strategies and environmental adaptations should be considered to maximize function. For patients with more advanced recovery (stage 4 or higher), training strategies that focus on repetitive and intense use of tasks can be expected to produce meaningful improvements in function. Activities to retrain UE postural support, reaching, and manipulation are essential elements of training. Enhanced training programs along with behavioral training methods (e.g., constraint-induced movement therapy) have demonstrated promising gains in recovery of function. The greatest treatment effects are seen in those patients with some initial active movement control while those with more severe involvement demonstrate poorer final outcomes.[226,227] Training to improve UE function should be closely coordinated with the occupational therapist.

UE as a Postural Support

Extended arm weightbearing with stabilized hand on a support surface is an important early activity to promote proximal stabilization and counteract the effects of excess flexor hypertonus and a dominant flexion synergy. Approximation can be used to increase stimulation of shoulder/scapular stabilizers and elbow extensors. Weightbearing activities are performed in sitting (see Fig. 18.7), modified plantigrade (see Fig. 18.14), and standing positions. The quadruped posture provides the greatest challenge for UE stabilization control but may be too difficult for some patients. Control should progress from holding to dynamic stabilization activities. For example, the patient stabilizes with the more affected UE while performing weight shifts and functional tasks with the stronger UE (e.g., reaching).[228] As previously mentioned, the more affected UE should also be recruited for postural assistance during functional training activities (e.g., pushing up from sidelying into sitting).

Reaching

Patients with stroke have difficulty regaining control of scapular upward rotation and protraction, elbow extension, and wrist and finger extension. Reaching and manipulation also requires accurate processing and use of visual–perceptual information. Patients with minimal voluntary control can practice initial reaching forward in a sideling position, where the patient's UE is supported by the therapist in shoulder flexion with elbow extension. The UE is mobilized forward and the patient is asked to hold this position. If holding is successful, then eccentric and reciprocal movements are attempted. Supported reaching can be also practiced in sitting with the hand resting on a tabletop. The patient is encouraged to slide the hand forward over tabletop, recruiting shoulder flexors, scapular protractors, and elbow extensors. A cloth can be used to decrease friction effects as the patient practices wiping or polishing a table. The patient can also practice reaching forward and downward touching the floor. Advanced reaching activities include independent lifting and reaching forward (e.g., UE placed into a shirt sleeve), overhead, or sidewards. A PNF D1 thrust pattern can be practiced (reverse thrust is contraindicated as the limb is moving into a flexion synergy pattern). Combining reaching with increased balance challenges in standing should also be incorporated (e.g., standing and reaching to pick an object up off a shelf, a low stool or the floor; modified push-ups in standing). Varying the height and distance reached, increasing the weight of objects held in the hand or increasing the speed and accuracy requirements can increase difficulty. Strategies used for substitution when the patient is unable to reach include trunk or head lateral movements and should not be allowed. Excessive shoulder elevation should also be discouraged.[228,229]

Manipulation and Dexterity

Meaningful task-oriented practice involving grasp and manipulation is important for stimulating recovery. Initial hand movements typically include gross grasp and release while advanced hand patterns (fine motor control) may not be present unless there is more advanced recovery. Voluntary release is generally much more difficult to achieve than voluntary grasp, and stretching/positioning and inhibitory techniques may be necessary to facilitate extension movements. Initial hand tasks can include using the more affected hand to stabilize (e.g., hand stabilizes paper while the stronger hand writes, hand stabilizes food while the stronger hand cuts) or holding a book with both hands for reading. The patient should be encouraged to use the weaker hand to assist in ADL (e.g., washing the upper body with a washcloth, bringing food to mouth). Forks, toothbrushes, and pens may need to have built-up handles for grasp. Task training should combine reach patterns with hand activity (e.g., picking sock off floor, reaching for an object off a shelf). Advanced hand activities include practice of wrist and finger extension, opposition, and manipulation of objects (e.g., using utensils to eat, drinking from a cup, writing, picking up and reorienting coins, paperclips or other objects). Pronation often predominates while active supination without elbow and shoulder flexion is difficult to achieve. The therapist must observe movements carefully and assist in eliminating those aspects of movement patterns that interfere with effective and efficient control. Graded physical assist and use of mental practice/imagery techniques can be helpful to improve learning and performance.[228]

Enhanced Training Activities

Constraint-induced movement therapy (CIMT) is discussed in Chapter 13 (see Evidence Summary Box 13.1). Gains in motor function following CIMT have been demonstrated in patients with stroke and are associated with changes in brain organization as evidenced by functional magnetic resonance imaging (fMRI). These include an apparent shift in motor cortical activation toward other ipsilateral areas and the contralesional hemisphere.[230] Figure 18.17 illustrates a training session using CIMT.

Bilateral arm training with rhythmic auditory cueing (BATRAC) has been shown to improve motor function in patients with chronic stroke.[231] This repetitive training program utilizes a customized bilateral arm trainer in which the patient holds onto T-bar handles and moves them in a nearly friction-free environment forward in the transverse plane (simulating forward reaching and its reverse motion). The bilateral movements are timed to an auditory metronome set at the patient's preferred speed. Significant improvements were noted in functional motor performance of the weaker UE that were sustained 2 months after training.

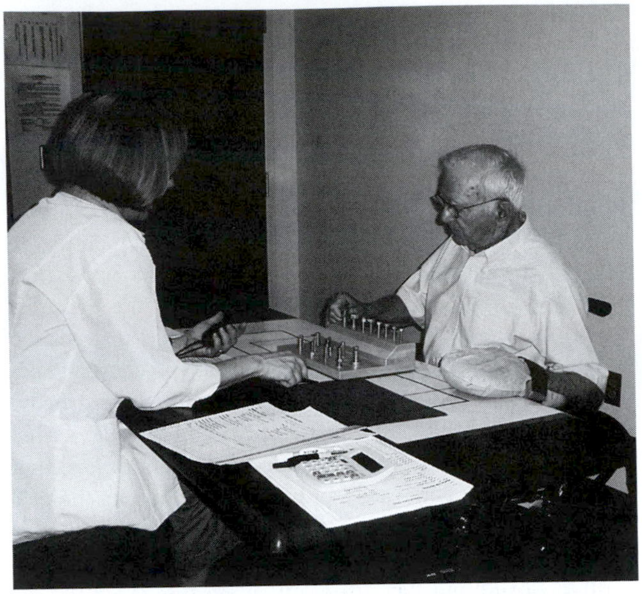

Figure 18.17 Constraint-induced-movement therapy (CIMT). The patient practices a pegboard task using the affected UE while the sound hand is constrained with a mitt. The therapist times the activity while encouraging the patient.

Electromyographic biofeedback (EMG-BFB) has been used to improve motor function in patients following stroke. This technique allows patients to alter motor unit activity based on augmented audio and visual feedback information. Training can focus on voluntary inhibition of spastic muscles (e.g., reducing firing frequency of spastic finger flexors), or on increasing kinesthetic awareness and recruitment of motor units in weak, hypoactive muscles (e.g., wrist/forearm extensor muscles). Patients in the chronic stage (1 year post-stroke) or patients in late recovery for whom spontaneous recovery is more or less complete (6 months post-stroke) have demonstrated positive results that have been attributed to biofeedback therapy.[232–236] Reported benefits include improvements in ROM, voluntary control, and function. Most researchers indicate that effectiveness of biofeedback neuromuscular reeducation is greatest when used as an adjunct to task-specific training.

Neuromuscular electrical stimulation (NMES) has been used with patients recovering from stroke to reduce spasticity, improve sensory awareness, and volitional limb movements.[237] NMES has been shown to increase the ability of muscle to exert force by preferentially activating the fast-contracting motor units.[238] Effective treatment results have been reported for improving function in wrist extensors,[239] and the deltoid and supraspinatus muscles. In the latter example, glenohumeral alignment was improved and subluxation reduced.[240,241] As with the biofeedback research, optimal results have been obtained when combined with task-specific training.

Management of Shoulder Pain

Hemiplegic shoulder pain (HSP) is a common complication after stroke, with incidence rates ranging from 38 to 84 percent of cases.[242,243] Pain is described as sharp and stabbing and is more common on movement than rest. Early on, pain can be intermittent and limited to just the shoulder. During later stages pain is constant and can progress to severe pain in more than just the shoulder. Several causes of HSP have been identified, that can be broadly divided into flaccid and spastic presentations. In the flaccid stage, proprioceptive impairment, lack of tone, and muscle paralysis reduce the support and normal seating action of the rotator cuff muscles, particularly the supraspinatus. The ligaments and capsule thus become the shoulder's sole support. The normal orientation of the glenoid fossa is upward, outward, and forward, so that it keeps the superior capsule taut and stabilizes the humerus mechanically. In the absence of supporting musculature, any abduction or forward flexion of the humerus, or scapular depression and downward rotation, reduces this stabilization and causes the humerus to sublux. Initially the *subluxation* is not painful, but mechanical stresses resulting from traction and gravitational forces produce persistent malalignment and pain. Glenohumeral friction–compression stresses also occur between the humeral head and superior soft tissues during flexion or abduction movements in the absence of normal scapulohumeral rhythm (*shoulder impingement syndrome*). During the spastic stage, abnormal muscle tone may contribute to poor scapular position (depression, retraction, and downward rotation) and contributes to subluxation and restricted movement. Secondary tightness in ligaments, tendons, and joint capsule can develop quickly. *Adhesive capsulitis* (intracapsular inflammation: "frozen shoulder") is a common finding. Poor handling and positioning of the more affected UE have been implicated in producing joint microtrauma and pain. Activities that traumatize the shoulder include PROM without adequate mobilization of the scapula (promoting normal scapulohumeral rhythm), pulling on the UE during a transfer, or using reciprocal pulleys.[244,245] An incorrectly aligned joint can significantly impair the patient's ability to move.

Prolonged soft tissue injury can result in *chronic regional pain syndrome (CRPS-type I),* also known as reflex sympathetic dystrophy (RSD). This pain typically has a diffuse onset and is characterized as aching throughout the limb. CRPS-1 is associated with a range of other symptoms. The wrist tends to assume a flexed position with intense pain likely during wrist extension movements. The elbow is not involved. Early *stage 1* vasomotor changes include discoloration (pale pink or cool) and alterations in temperature. The skin may be hypersensitive to touch, pressure, or temperature variations. The patient typically guards against movement attempts. *Stage 2* is characterized by subsiding pain and early dystrophic changes: muscle and skin atrophy, vasospasm, hyperhidrosis (increased sweating), and course hair and nails. There is radiographic evidence of early osteoporosis. In *stage 3,* the atrophic phase, pain and vasomotor changes are rare. There is progressive atrophy of the skin, muscles, and bones (severe osteoporosis is evident). Pericapsular fibrosis and articular changes become pronounced. The hand typically becomes contracted in a clawed position with metacarpophalangeal (MP) extension and interphalangeal (IP) flexion (similar to the intrinsic minus hand). There is marked atrophy of thenar and hypothenar muscles with flattening of the hand. Chances of reversal of signs and symptoms are high for stage 1 and variable for stage 2, while stage 3 changes are largely irreversible.[246]

Early diagnosis and identification of factors that cause HSP is essential. Interventions are selected based examination findings. Because of close daily contact with the patient, the therapist is frequently one of the first to recognize and report early signs and symptoms. In the flaccid stage, the arm should be supported at all times. Proper positioning and handling is essential. In supine and sitting the scapula/shoulder should be protracted with the arm forward in slight abduction and neutral rotation. Interventions aimed at reducing subluxation include NMES therapy, and use of supportive devices (see section below). Interventions aimed at normalizing tone and reducing pain include appropriate mobilization techniques (gentle grade 1 to 2 mobilizations, gentle stretching), cryotherapy, EMG biofeedback, and relaxation training. Interventions for adhesive capsulitis include mobilization and PROM techniques, and ultrasound. The therapist needs to ensure that everyone involved in assisting the patient (e.g., family member, caregiver, nurses, and aides) has been instructed in proper handling/mobilization of the UE, and recognizes the importance of avoiding trauma and traction injuries during PROM, transfers, and wheelchair activities. Active assisted range of motion (AAROM) and active movements of the UE and trunk are facilitated in order to optimize functional recovery. Interventions to manage edema may also be a consideration. Persistent pain may be managed with oral analgesics or local injection techniques (e.g., triamcinolone acetonide). Repeat steroid injections are not recommended due to likely weakening of the rotator cuff. With intractable pain, surgical nerve blocks may also be considered.[244,245]

Supportive Devices

A patient with hypotonia is at increased risk of *traction injury*. Care must be taken not to pull on a flaccid UE during position changes or let it hang unsupported. Slings can prevent soft tissue stretching (e.g., capsular stretching) and relieve pressure on the neurovascular bundle. However, slings do little to reduce subluxation or improve shoulder function, especially if scapular and trunk malalignment are not adequately addressed. Most slings have the additional negative feature of positioning the arm close to the body in adduction, internal rotation, and elbow flexion. With prolonged use, contractures and increased flexor tone may develop. Slings also impair trunk mobility, balance, sensory input, and body image and may increase body neglect. Slings block spontaneous use of the UE and can contribute to learned nonuse. There are considerable differences in the effectiveness of the various types of supports.[247] A pouch sling or single strap hemisling with two cuffs that support the elbow and wrist provides minimal mechanical support of the humerus. An alternate approach to the traditional sling is a humeral cuff sling. This device has an arm cuff on the distal humerus supported by a figure-eight harness. It provides humeral support with slight external rotation while allowing elbow extension, and may also provide some reduction of subluxation (see Fig. 18.7). This style of sling can be worn for longer periods because it does not restrict the elbow in a flexed position or limit distal function.[248,249]

Gillen[228] suggests the following guidelines are appropriate to consider when prescribing a sling:

- Slings are appropriate for initial transfer and gait training, but overall use should be minimized during rehabilitation.
- Slings that position the UE in flexion are less desirable and should be used only for select upright activities and only for short time periods.
- No one sling is appropriate for all patients; selection and use should be carefully evaluated.
- Effective alternatives to use of a sling should be considered: taping (strapping) to facilitate or inhibit musculature surrounding the scapula; NMES. The hand can also be positioned in a garment pocket.

The patient, family members, and caregivers should be instructed in and allowed to practice proper use of the support. As recovery progresses and spasticity and voluntary movement emerge, spontaneous reduction of shoulder subluxation typically occurs. Slings have no value at this point in recovery.

For patients using a wheelchair, an arm board or lap tray can provide support for the flaccid arm. A lateral elbow guard and/or straps may be necessary if the patient's arm slips off the side. Patients with decreased sensation are at risk for hand injury if the hand becomes stuck in the spokes of the wheelchair; elbow trauma can occur if the elbow slips off the side (e.g., the elbow hits as the patient is going through a doorway).

Strategies to Improve Lower Extremity Function

LE training activities essentially prepare the patient for the appropriate gait. This requires breaking up the obligatory synergy patterns. For example, during midstance hip and knee extensors need to be activated with hip abductors and dorsiflexors. Suggested activities include PNF LE D1 extension pattern; holding against elastic band resistance around the upper thighs in supine or standing positions; and standing, lateral side-steps. Hip adduction should be stressed during flexion movements of the hip and knee. Suggested activities include supine, PNF LE D1flexion pattern; sitting, crossing and uncrossing the more affected LE over the less affected; and standing, step-ups. Hip extension with knee flexion is needed to allow for toe-off at the end of stance. Activities that can be used to promote knee flexion with hip extension include bridging, supine hip extension with knee flexion over the side of the mat pushing down through the heel, or standing, posterior foot rises. Pelvic control is important and can be promoted through lower trunk rotation activities that emphasize forward pelvic rotation (protraction); post-stroke, the patient typically demonstrates a retracted and elevated pelvis. Rotation can be practiced in sidelying; supine, modified hooklying; kneeling; or standing. Sitting on a therapy ball, pelvic shifting is another useful activity to promote pelvic control. Control of knee motions is often problematic; post-stroke, the patient with knee weakness typically exhibits hyperextension when standing. Reciprocal action (smooth reversals of flexion and extension movements) should be stressed early, beginning first in supine (e.g., foot slides in hooklying), sitting (e.g., foot slides under the chair), partial sitting (see Fig. 18.15), or partial wall squats in standing.

An effective progression increases the challenge to the patient gradually by modifying postures while reducing synergy influence (e.g., hip abduction can be performed first in hooklying, then supine, sidelying, modified plantigrade, and finally standing). Dorsiflexors can be activated in sitting by first having the patient hold and slowly let the forefoot move down, then pull the forefoot up. This simulates the functional expectations of the normal gait cycle as the foot goes from swing phase through stance. The sequence can then be repeated in standing, a much more difficult position in which to control dorsiflexors. Voluntary control of eversion is often the most difficult motion to achieve because these muscles do not function in either synergy. The application of stretch and resistance to these muscles during an activity that recruits dorsiflexors and evertors may be effective in initiating a response (e.g., in bridging, knee rocks side-to-side).

Strategies to Improve Balance

Balance Training

Stroke results in significant changes in balance. Patients typically exhibit delayed, varied, or absent balance responses with impairments in latency, amplitude, and timing of muscle activity. It is therefore important to proceed slowly in training and to select challenges appropriate for the patient's level of control. Once postural alignment and static stability is achieved in upright postures, the patient is ready for center-of-mass (COM) control training. In sitting and standing, the patient is instructed to explore his or her limits of stability (LOS) through low-frequency weight shifting. The patient learns how far in any one direction he or she can safely move and how to align the COM within the base of support (BOS) to maintain upright stability. The therapist needs to stress symmetrical weightbearing, as well as activities that promote shifting toward the more affected side. Weightbearing on the more affected hip (sitting) and foot (standing) is encouraged while unnecessary activity of the less affected limbs (grabbing for support) is discouraged. The therapist can increase the difficulty of the activity by manipulating:

- Base of support: sitting, LEs uncrossed to crossed; standing, wide to narrow to tandem position; standing on one LE
- Support surface: sitting on a mat to sitting on a therapy ball; standing on the floor to standing on dense foam
- Sensory inputs: EO to EC; feet on firm surface or foam
- UE position/support: light touch down support; UEs extended out to the side to UEs across the chest
- UE movements: single UE raises to bilateral UE raises (symmetrical, asymmetrical); reaching; picking objects off table, stool, floor
- LE movements: single LE raises, stepping (forward–backward, side; step-ups); marching in place; foot on ball, moving ball
- Trunk movements: head and trunk rotations; looking up at ceiling or down to floor
- Destabilizing functional activities: sit-to-stand, sit-down, turning, floor-to-standing
- Dual task training: standing while catching or kicking a ball; standing while talking; standing while holding a tray with a glass of water
- Environmental conditions: closed to open environments

The goals of training are to increase the consistency, range, and speed of self-initiated movements while encouraging symmetry and maximum use of the more affected side. Supportive devices such as a posterior leg splint, gait belt, or body-weight support harness can be used to assist in early standing to instill confidence and prevent falls.

Postural strategy training is an important component of intervention. Ankle strategies can be promoted through small range anterior–posterior shifts or by applying a small perturbation at the hips (forward–backward). Standing on a half-foam roller or wobble board also promotes ankle strategies, but may be too advanced for some patients during early rehab. Hip strategies can be promoted through larger anterior–posterior shifts or stronger perturbations. Medial–lateral hip strategies are promoted by tandem stance (on floor or foam roller). Stepping strategies are promoted by increased displacements of the COM (e.g., forward, backward, or sideward leans that move the COM

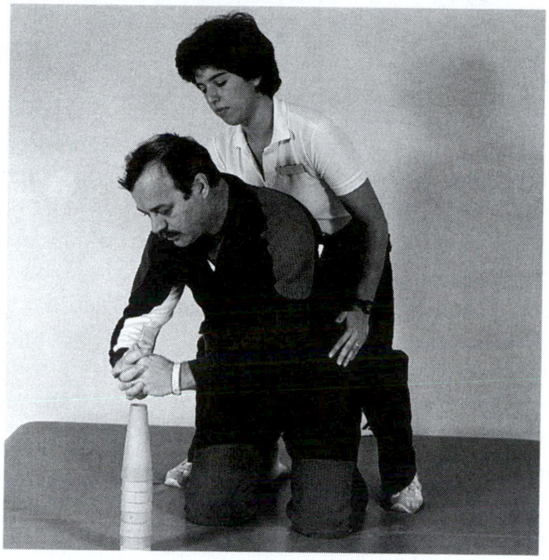

Figure 18.18 Balance training in kneeling. The therapist assists in maintenance of the kneeling posture while encouraging the patient in the weight shift and cone-stacking task.

outside of the BOS). The therapist can apply an elastic band around the hips, offering resistance to the forward lean. Resistance that is quickly released once the patient achieves the desired lean will necessitate a step to control balance. Step-ups (small step to large; foam surface) should also be practiced.[250]

The patient's full attention and concentration is required and should be directed toward completion of the task at hand (task-specific training vs a focus on balance in general) (Fig. 18.18). The therapist provides well-timed feedback to help the patient correct alignment and adjust postural control while minimizing hands-on support (only as needed). Balance training should encourage active problem-solving. The patient is presented with challenges, is able to identify potential problems, and recruits safe strategies to maintain balance. Thus adaptability of skills needed for successful community reentry is promoted. Safety education about fall prevention is a critical factor in ensuring maintenance of the patient's hard-won functional independence (see Chapter 13).

Enhanced Training Activities. Force platform biofeedback (center-of-pressure biofeedback) provided to the patient while standing on a computerized force-plate system can be used to improve balance. The patient practices voluntary movement shifts in response to computer generated visual feedback. Patients can also practice responding to unexpected platform tilts (perturbations) in order to improve reactive balance control. A safety harness may be required during early training; holding on with one or both hands is discouraged. Improvements with biofeedback/forceplate training have been found in steadiness (reduced sway),[251,252] postural symmetry,[251,252] and dynamic stability.[252-254] Nichols[255] points out that the evidence is stronger and more consistent for the latter two parameters than for changes in steadiness. There is limited evidence of carryover of improved balance during functional skills, specifically transfer skills and endurance,[254] functional reach,[256] and measures of ADL and mobility.[252] Carryover to improved locomotor performance has not been demonstrated.[251,254,256] Failure to find significant correlations to gait is most likely related to specificity of training, specifically a dissimilarity between training mode and outcome measure. Studies comparing conventional balance training with biofeedback/forceplate training based on improvements on functional balance measures (Berg Balance Scale, Timed Up-and-Go) have failed to show any differences between the training modes; both interventions were effective in improving balance.[257,258]

Strategies to Improve Locomotion

Locomotor Training

While locomotor control is distributed across discrete regions of the CNS, walking is primarily a brainstem and spinal cord function. For example, locomotor central pattern generators (CPG) have been identified as existing in the ventral spinal cord while integrating command centers have been identified in the medial medullary reticular formation. Thus patients with cortical stroke may be able to regain the ability to walk. The CNS is responsive to training-induced plastic changes in locomotor function and recovery. Thus, patients with limited recovery who lack voluntary isolated control can still be trained to walk. While sensation is normally used for walking, patients can also learn to walk with limited sensation.

Locomotor training using body weight support from an overhead harness and a motorized treadmill allows the clinician to stimulate automatic walking using intensive task-oriented training (Fig. 18.19). Normal kinematics and phase relationships of the full gait cycle are promoted, including limb loading in midstance and unweighting and stepping during swing. Initially manual assistance is provided by trainers to normalize gait in the presence of muscle weakness and impaired balance. For example, one therapist provides manual assistance to foot placement during stepping movements of the weaker LE while a second therapist stands behind the patient and provides manual assistance to pelvic rotation movements. An overhead harness is used to support a portion of the patient's weight (e.g., 30 percent progressing down to 20 percent, and 10 percent). The harness controls the upright position of the patient in the absence of good postural stability and reduces fear of falling. The use of a harness also eliminates the need for adaptive UE support to compensate for LE weakness (e.g., as seen with the use of a walker). As improvements in walking occur, the harness is removed and full weight-bearing is allowed. At this point, the patient is practicing supervised walking on a treadmill. Initially the treadmill speeds are slow (e.g., 0.52 mph [0.23 m/sec]) and are gradually increased as the patient's walking ability is improved (e.g., 0.95 mph [0.42 m/sec)[101] Sullivan et al[198] trained three groups at different speeds and found that training at fast speeds (0.98 m/sec) was more effective at improving speeds of overground walking than training at slow (0.22 m/sec) or variable speeds (0.22 m/sec to 0.89 m/sec). It is important to keep in mind that the functional speeds required for community ambulation (normal healthy population) average 2.8 mph (1.3 m/sec).[166] Stepping movements are triggered by LE muscle and joint receptors (e.g., stretch on hip flexors and plantarflexors at the end of the support phase triggers stepping) while load receptors in the stance limb trigger extensors.[259] Patients train on average 30 minutes/day, 5 days per week for durations of 6 to 12 weeks. This form of locomotor training has been shown to be a safe and effective task-oriented training activity that allows the patient to regain walking ability. Specificity and intensity of training is directly related to reported outcomes. These include improvements in walking speed,[101,194–198,200] distance,[101,196] endurance,[101] functional balance (Berg Balance Scale)[101,200] and motor recovery (STREAM).[101] Walking also results in improvements in muscular and cardiovascular endurance.[260] See Evidence Summary Box 18.8. Progression is to overground walking.

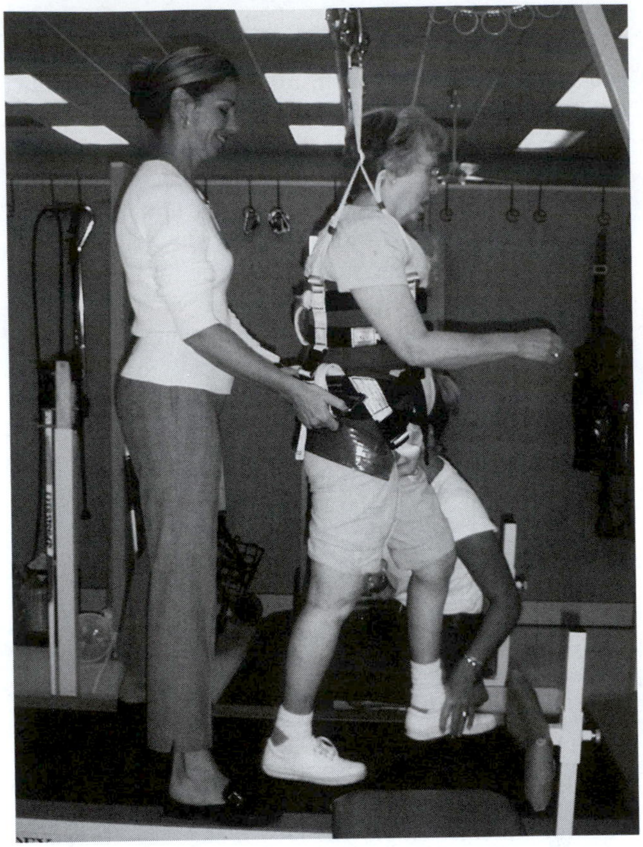

Figure 18.19 Locomotor training using body weight support and a treadmill. One therapist manually assists pelvic motions while a second therapist assists stepping of the affected left LE.

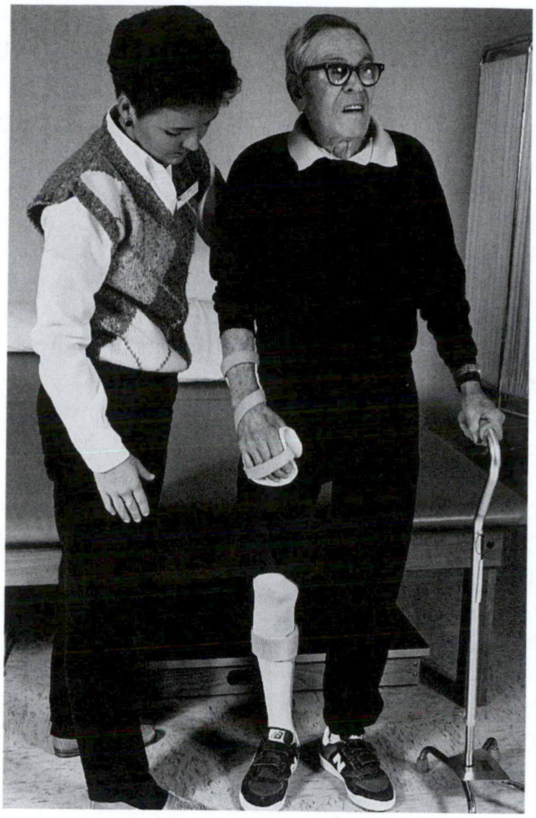

Figure 18.20 Assisted ambulation using a plastic ankle-foot orthosis and a quad cane. A resting pan splint supports the patient's affected hand.

Gait Training

Conventional gait training focuses on improving the mechanics and quality of walking. Parallel bars and ambulation aids (e.g., walkers, hemiwalkers, quad canes) can assist in early gait stability and safety (see Fig. 18.20). However, prolonged use of these devices can be problematic for a patient who has the potential to walk without the device. There is increased loading on UE and the stronger LE. With prolonged use, the patient also fails to develop appropriate balance mechanisms while asymmetry is promoted. There is an excessive weight shift toward the less affected side with the use of a hemiwalker or quad cane. Prolonged use of a walker encourages a forward trunk position with maximum loading on the UEs. Gait is typically slower with assistive devices and overall locomotor rhythm is impaired. It is important to progress patients as quickly as possible to the least restrictive device and to no device whenever possible. Gait practice with an overhead harness and partial body weight support provides the least interference with balance and walking. Consideration should be given to maintaining the natural rhythm of walking and speed. The patient should be encouraged to take even steps. This can be facilitated by the use of rhythmic auditory cues (e.g., verbal cues, metronome) and foot markers placed on the floor. Progression is to longer steps and increased overall distances with faster speeds. The patient should also practice walking in varying environments that encourage adaptation to natural environments.

An accurate analysis of gait abnormalities is critical (see Box 18.5 Gait Deviations Commonly Seen Following Stroke). These abnormalities arise as a result of impairments in flexibility, strength, coordination, and balance. Gait activities should focus on improving specific gait impairments and modifying key elements. Critical areas of stance phase control that will need to be addressed include initial weight acceptance, midstance control, and forward weight advancement during stance on the more involved limb. During swing, control of knee and foot for toe clearance and foot placement are key requirements. Finally, persistent posturing of the UE in flexion and adduction during gait should be addressed. This latter problem can be effectively controlled through positioning the hemiplegic UE in extension and abduction with the hand open (Fig. 18.21).

The patient should practice functional, task-specific locomotor skills: walking forward, backward, sideward, and in crossed stepping (e.g., sidestepping, braiding). Elevation activities (e.g., step-up/step-down activities; lateral step-ups; stair climbing, step-over-step) and

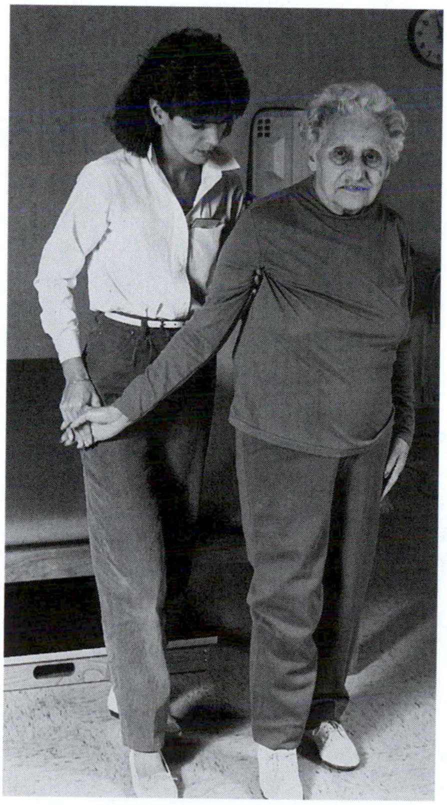

Figure 18.21 Assisted ambulation. The therapist provides support and assists in the lateral weight transfer onto the affected side. The UE is maintained in an inhibitory position (extension abduction and external rotation).

community activities (e.g., walking on ramps, curbs, uneven terrain, over and around obstacles) and those with coincident timing requirements (e.g., crossing the street; stepping on and off elevators or escalators; walking through automatic doors) should be practiced. Initially gait will be slow and deliberate. As control develops, the patient should be encouraged to improve gait speed while maintaining safety. Dual-task activities (e.g., holding a ball, bouncing a ball, carrying a tray, carrying on a conversation) and balance activities (e.g., tandem walking on a line, walking on foam) can be incorporated into the training program as control improves. Timing and reciprocity of LE movements can be improved with the use of progressive treadmill, cycle ergometer, and Kinetron® isokinetic training.

An important goal of training is to have the patient be able to monitor his or her performance and recognize and initiate corrective actions. The patient should be able to vary walking speed and direction, navigate changes in the support surface and the environment while walking. Functional practice in real-life environments will assist the patient in developing the confidence needed for meeting the demands of community reentry.

Enhanced Training Activities. *Limb load monitors* provide biofeedback about the amount of loading or weightbearing on the hemiparetic limb and have been effective in improving stance and gait. Patients receiving this training demonstrate more symmetrical weightbearing and increased stance times on their more affected limb with increased swing times on their less affected limb.[261]

NMES has been used to improve dorsiflexor function and prevent drop foot.[262-264] Multichannel FES (MFES) uses a program developed from individual profiles of EMG and anthropometric measurements to stimulate antagonistic groups of muscles. Significant improvements of gait in patients with stroke have been reported.[265–268] Because the patients had limbs that had been paralyzed for more than 6 months, the results suggest a significant training effect as a result of the intervention.

Orthotics

An orthosis may be required when persistent problems prevent safe ambulation (e.g., inadequate ankle dorsiflexion during swing, mediolateral ankle instability, and insufficient push-off during late stance). Prescription will depend on the unique problems each patient presents. The pattern of instability and weakness at the ankle and knee, and the extent and severity of spasticity and sensory deficits of the limb are major considerations when prescribing an orthosis. Temporary devices (e.g., dorsiflexor assists) may be used during the early stages while recovery is proceeding to allow the patient to practice standing and walking. Use of a temporary orthosis also provides insight into the type of components that will most effectively address the patient's needs. Permanent devices are prescribed once the patient's status stabilizes. Consultation with a certified orthotist and clinic team is initiated if a permanent orthosis is needed.

Foot–Ankle Controls. An ankle–foot orthosis (AFO) is commonly prescribed to control impaired ankle/foot function. These may include a custom molded polypropylene AFO (posterior leaf spring, modified AFO, or solid ankle AFO), or conventional double upright/ dual channel AFO. The least restrictive AFO is the posterior leaf spring (PLS) used to control drop foot. A modified AFO has a slightly wider lateral brim and can provide additional control of calcaneal and forefoot inversion and eversion. A solid ankle molded AFO provides maximum stabilization through its lateral trim lines that project more anteriorly. Movement in all planes (dorsiflexion, plantarflexion, inversion, and eversion) is limited. The conventional double upright metal AFO may be indicated for patients who cannot tolerate plastic AFOs owing to sensory impairments, girth fluctuations, or diabetic neuropathy, or who require additional controls. A posterior stop can be added to limit plantarflexion while a spring assist can be added to assist dorsiflexion (Klenzak joint). Advantages of a conventional AFO include better stabilization of the ankle, allowing improved heelstrike and push-off.[269] Disadvantages include heavier weight, less cosmetic appearance, and increased difficulty donning and doffing. An air-stirrup brace can be used to provide medial–lateral stability at the subtalar joint while allowing dorsiflexion and plantarflexion.[270]

Knee Controls. Knee instability following stroke can be controlled with an AFO by adjusting the position of the ankle. An ankle set in 5° dorsiflexion limits knee hyperextension, while an ankle set in 5° plantarflexion decreases the flexor moment and stabilizes the knee during midstance.[271] A patient with knee hyperextension without foot and/or ankle instability may benefit from the application of a Swedish Knee Cage to protect the knee. Extensive bracing using a knee–ankle–foot orthosis (KAFO) is rarely indicated or successful. The added weight and restrictions in normal knee joint motion significantly increase energy costs and limit independent function.

The therapist must frequently reexamine the patient's motor function and recovery. The need for an orthosis or a particular type of orthosis may change with continuing recovery. The therapist may need to recommend a change in prescription or discontinuing the use of a device. With limited reimbursements, ordering a new orthosis may prove problematic and speaks to the need to anticipate changes when ordering the initial device. For example, a good option for the patient who needs a custom molded solid AFO is to order a hinged AFO with a plantarflexion stop. As the patient regains sufficient knee and dorsiflexor control, the device can be adjusted to remove the stop and allow the hinges to work. Orthotic training should be initiated and includes donning and doffing, skin inspections, and education in safe use of the device during gait. See Chapter 31 for a more complete description of orthotic devices.

Wheelchairs

Most patients require the use of a wheelchair for mobility at some point during their recovery. Patients with stroke exhibit typical postural asymmetries, which need to be carefully evaluated. These include:

- Trunk laterally flexed to the weaker side; head may also be flexed to the weaker side.
- Pelvic posterior tilt with some obliquity (lower on the unaffected side).
- LE rolled out into abduction and external rotation; if spasticity is present, increased hip extension, adduction, and internal rotation with knee extension may occur; foot is typically plantarflexed and inverted.
- UE held flexed and adducted to the trunk with increased elbow, wrist, and finger flexion. With flaccidity, the shoulder is subluxed with the hand dangling in a dependent position.

Positioning in a wheelchair needs to correct for these postural asymmetries and ensure correct sitting posture. The reader is referred to Chapter 33 for a more complete discussion of general seating principles and wheelchair adaptations.

A patient with stroke can learn to propel a wheelchair using the stronger UE and LE. The seat-to-floor height is critical in ensuring successful use of the foot for steering and propulsion. A *hemi-height wheelchair* with a lower seat to floor height (17.5 in.) may be required. A standard wheelchair has a seat to floor height of 19.5 in. One-arm drive chairs in which both handrims are placed on one wheel were designed for individuals with only one functional UE. The patient with stroke is rarely successful in using this type of chair as it takes a great deal of strength and coordination to propel the wheelchair in a forward direction. It is contraindicated in patients with significant perceptual and coordination impairments. A power wheelchair may be required for some individuals who cannot successfully use a manual wheelchair and will depend upon a wheelchair as their primary means of locomotion. The therapist needs to consider individual needs and reimbursement policies when ordering a wheelchair. It is important to balance both present and future needs as providers restrict frequent reordering of a new wheelchair. It is also important to remember that prolonged used of a wheelchair contributes to learned non-use and may limit recovery, especially if walking is a primary goal of therapy.

Wheelchair training activities include patient and caregiver instruction in the use, maintenance, and safety of all parts of the wheelchair (e.g., brakes, legrests, removable armrests). The patient needs to be instructed in methods of propulsion and given the opportunity to practice on level and varied surfaces (e.g., ramps, outdoor terrain). Transfers (to and from bed, toilet, tub, car) should also be practiced once the patient receives the prescriptive wheelchair.

Strategies to Improve Aerobic Function

Patients with stroke demonstrate decreased levels of physical conditioning following periods of prolonged immobility and reduced activity. The energy costs to complete many functional tasks are higher than normal owing to the abnormal ways in which the activities are performed.[272–275] Many patients also demonstrate concomitant cardiovascular disease and may be recovering from acute cardiac events at the same time.[276] These patients require careful determination of cardiopulmonary responses during exercise and appropriate monitoring. Vital signs, heart rate, and ratings of perceived exertion (RPE) are all important measures of cardiopulmonary adaptation to exercise. Signs and symptoms of exertional intolerance (i.e., excessive fatigue, dyspnea, dizziness, diaphoresis, nausea, vomiting, chest pain) should be monitored closely and can signal an inappropriate level of exercise intensity and cardiac decompensation.[277] Some patients may also require electrocardiographic monitoring to ensure safety during training.

Individuals recovering from stroke can benefit from endurance (aerobic) training to improve cardiovascular function. During the early stages of inpatient rehabilitation, functional activities are appropriate for training (e.g., overground walking). During the postacute stage, patients/clients may be able to engage in more traditional exercise training modes such as treadmill walking or stationary cycling. Patients with balance impairments will benefit from treadmill training or overground walking with a safety harness, or a recumbent cycle ergometer. To ensure safety, patients should receive a thorough examination and supervised exercise test before starting a training program (e.g., symptom-limited graded exercise test). Prescriptive elements include mode (type of exercise), frequency, intensity, and duration (see Chapter 16: Heart Disease). Choice of training mode depends upon the individual's abilities and interests. Intensities are typically in the range of 40 percent to 70 percent of maximal oxygen uptake. Suggested frequency is three times per week for 20 to 60 minutes per session. Frequency may be increased to daily if lower intensities are used. Because of the level of deconditioning, patients with stroke should begin with intermittent training protocols but can be progressed to 30 minutes of continuous exercise.[90,91] The use of a training log or exercise diary is an excellent way to keep track of prescriptive elements, objective measurements (heart rate, blood pressure), and subjective reactions (RPE, perceived enjoyment). Adequate supervision, monitoring, and safety education about warning signs for impending stroke and heart attack are critical components.

Endurance training programs for patients with stroke have been shown to yield significant improvements in physical fitness, functional status, psychological outlook, and self-esteem.[278–280] Regular exercise may also have the additional benefit of reducing risk of recurrent stroke or heart attack. Finally, patients who participate in a regular conditioning program may be more successful in adopting continuing, life-long exercise habits and in moving beyond the disability associated with stroke.

Strategies to Improve Feeding and Swallowing

A multidisciplinary team, including the speech-language pathologist, occupational therapist, physical therapist, nutritionist, and physician manages dysphagia. The goals/outcomes of dysphagia management are to (1) improve strength, coordination, and range of oral musculature; (2) promote normal feeding through graduated resumption of activities; (3) promote volitional control through effective verbal coaching; and (4) provide effective education and support.

A critical component of dysphagia management is positioning. Posture should be normally aligned with the head held in a chin-down (tucked) position rather than extended or tipped back. This reduces the chances of aspiration or choking and promotes normal swallowing through appropriate alignment of the necessary structures. If the patient lacks adequate head control, the head should be supported either manually or with supports.

Oral exercises including movements of the lips, tongue, cheeks, and jaw should be practiced. The patient is instructed to purse lips and hold a tongue depressor between the lips. Tongue movements in all directions are practiced and can be resisted manually (using a sterile gauze or glove to cover finger or with a moist tongue depressor). Firm pressure applied to the anterior third of the tongue with a tongue depressor can be used to stimulate posterior elevation of the tongue. Cheek exercises include practice in puffing, blowing bubbles, and drinking thick liquids through a straw. Vibrating or pressing above the upper lip for closure and under the lower lip for opening can stimulate jaw movements.[281]

Food presentation is an important part of dysphagia management. Food should be positioned at an appropriate height and distance from the patient and within the patient's visual field. Adapted utensils, plate guards, and nonslip mats can be used to assist in the transfer of food to the mouth. Some guiding may be required to self-feed with more involved UE. Food should be at first semimoist (e.g., pureed food, pasta, boiled chicken), progressing to regular textures and foods rich in taste, smell, and texture, qualities that assist in facilitating the swallowing reflex. Favorite foods should be employed whenever possible. Verbal cues should be given, encouraging the patient to swallow each mouthful and to eat slowly. Stroking the neck can be used to stimulate swallowing. Massaging the check may be helpful in clearing the cheek of a food bolus. Resisted sucking can be promoted using a straw and very thick liquids (slushes, shakes), or by holding the open end of the straw against the finger. As sucking ability improves, the patient can be presented with thinner liquids. Modification of the eating environment is also an important consideration. Every effort should be made to ensure that the environment is pleasant, free from distraction, devoid of unpleasant sights and smells, and provides adequate lighting. The patient's full attention should be directed to the task by using appropriate and consistent verbal cues. The importance of mealtime for social interaction should not be overlooked.[93,281]

Patient/Client-Related Instruction

Stroke represents a major health crisis for patients and their families. Ignorance about the cause of the illness or the recovery process and misconceptions concerning the rehabilitation program and potential outcomes can negatively influence coping responses and progress in rehabilitation. Frequently the problems seem unmanageable and overwhelming for the family, especially when faced with alterations in the patient's behavior, cognition, and emotion. Patients may feel depressed, isolated, irritable, or demanding. Families often demonstrate reactions that include initial relief and hope for full recovery, followed by feelings of entrapment, depression, anger, or guilt when complete recovery does not occur. These changes and feelings can strain even the best of relationships. Therapists can often have a dramatic influence on this situation because of the high frequency of contact and the often close relationships that develop with patients and their families. There are a number of important guidelines to follow when planning educational interventions[2]:

- Give accurate, factual information; counsel family members about the patient's capabilities and limitations; *avoid* predictions that categorically define expected function or future recovery.
- Structure interventions carefully, giving only as much information as the patient or family need or can assimilate; provide reinforcement and repetition.
- Adapt interventions to ensure they are appropriate to the educational and cultural background of the patient and family.
- Offer a variety of educational interventions: didactic sessions, books, brochures, and videotapes, and family participation in therapy. (See Appendix B.)
- Provide a forum for open discussion and communication.

- Be supportive, sensitive, and maintain a positive, hopeful manner.
- Assist patients and families in confronting alternatives and developing problem-solving abilities.
- Motivate and provide positive reinforcement in therapy; enhance patient satisfaction and self-esteem.
- Refer patients and families to support and self-help groups such as the following national associations:

  American Stroke Association—A Division of the American Heart Association
  7272 Greenville Avenue
  Dallas, TX 75231
  1–800–AHA–USA1 (1–800–242–8721)

  National Stroke Association
  9707 East Easter Lane
  Englewood, CO 80112
  1–800–STROKES (1–800–787–6537)

Psychotherapy and counseling (e.g., sexual, leisure, vocational) can assist in improving overall quality of life and should be recommended as needed.

Discharge Planning

Planning for discharge begins early in rehabilitation and involves the patient and family. Potential placement (safe place of residence), level of family and community support, and need for continued medical and rehabilitation services should all be explored. Family members should regularly participate in therapy sessions to learn exercises and activities designed to support the patient's independence. Discharge should be considered when reasonable treatment goals/outcomes are attained. Indication of the attainment of a functional ceiling can be considered when there is lack of evidence of progress at two successive evaluations over a period of 2 weeks. Home visits should be made prior to discharge to determine the home's physical structure and accessibility. Potential problems can be identified and corrective measures initiated. Home adaptations, assistive devices, and supportive services should be in place before the patient is discharged to home. Several trial home stays may be helpful in smoothing the transition from rehabilitation center to home. Patients with residual impairments or functional limitations who will be receiving outpatient or home therapy should be given all the necessary information concerning these services. Community services should be identified and information provided to the patient and family. Long-term follow-up at regularly scheduled intervals should be initiated in order to maintain patients at their highest possible functional level.

Stroke Rehabilitation Outcomes

Most patients with stroke regain their independent living status following discharge. The Copenhagen Stroke Study, based on 1197 patients, revealed that 64 percent of patients were discharged to home, 15 percent were discharged to a nursing home, and 21 percent of patients died during their hospital stay. After rehabilitation, 11 percent of survivors still exhibited severe or very severe deficits, 11 percent had moderate deficits, and 78 percent had mild or no deficits.[282] Functional recovery was completed within 12.5 weeks of stroke onset in 95 percent of patients.[110] Recovery of walking function occurred in 61 percent of survivors (50 percent were independent while 11 percent required assistance).[111] Only 30 to 60 percent of stroke survivors regain independence in ADL. Major problems in stroke outcome studies include the heterogeneity of patients admitted for rehabilitation, lack of consistency in outcome measures, and differences in duration, type, and onset of rehabilitation programs. Patients who demonstrate less successful rehabilitation outcomes tended to include those with (1) advanced age; (2) severe motor impairments (prolonged paralysis, apraxia); (3) persistent medical problems (incontinence); (4) impaired cognitive function (decreased alertness, poor attention span, judgment, memory), severe language disturbances, and an inability to learn new tasks or follow simple commands; (5) severe visuospatial hemineglect; and (6) other less well-defined social and economic problems.[283–285]

Summary

Stroke can result from a number of different vascular events that interrupt cerebral circulation and impair brain function, including cerebral thrombosis, emboli, or hemorrhage. The location and size of the ischemic process, the nature and functions of the structures involved, the availability of collateral blood flow, and effectiveness of early emergency medical management all influence the symptomatology that evolves. For many patients, stroke represents a major cause of disability, with diffuse problems affecting widespread areas of function. From a practical standpoint, patients with stroke present a tremendous challenge for clinicians. Effective rehabilitation should take advantage of the brain's capacity for repair and recovery. Rehabilitation interventions seek to promote recovery and independence through neurofacilitation, functional, and compensatory training strategies. Interventions also focus on the prevention of secondary impairments. The utilization of effective motor learning strategies with task-oriented training for real-life environments is critical for the successful attainment of functional outcomes.

Questions for Review

1. Differentiate between each of the following vascular syndromes: anterior cerebral artery, middle cerebral artery, internal carotid artery, posterior cerebral artery, lacunar, and vertebrobasilar artery. What are the differences that can be expected between hemispheric lesions?
2. What are the major causes of stroke? Define and explain each.
3. What diagnostic measures are used to confirm stroke? Describe the role of the CT scan in the implementation of emergency medical measures.
4. Describe the normal recovery process in stroke including expected stages of motor recovery. Give an example of how this knowledge may influence selection of interventions.
5. What are the major communication, cognitive, and emotional impairments that can result from stroke? Where are the likely lesions?
6. Differentiate between the following stroke-specific instruments: the Fugl-Meyer Assessment of Physical Performance (FMA) and the Stroke Rehabilitation Assessment of Movement (STREAM).
7. Identify three motor learning strategies important for treating the patient with stroke.
8. What are the major goals for reestablishing postural control? Identify three training activities that could be used during the post-acute stage to reestablish postural control and functional mobility.
9. What are the essential elements of an intervention program designed to improve UE function? Identify three training activities.
10. What are the essential elements of an intervention program designed to improve LE function? Identify three training activities.
12. Describe the benefits of locomotor training using body weight support and a treadmill. How should training be progressed?
13. Identify and describe common LE orthotic devices used for the patient with stroke. What are the major indications and contraindications for each?
14. Differentiate between the focus of rehabilitation efforts during the acute and postacute phases of stroke rehabilitation.
15. What are the essential elements included in an educational program for the patient with stroke and family members?

Case Study

HISTORY

The patient/client is a 41-year-old man admitted to an acute care hospital with a diagnosis of CVA with R hemiparesis (L MCA). Admitted to a rehabilitation facility 10 days later.

PAST MEDICAL HISTORY

- Seizure disorder since childhood. Dilantin was discontinued 5 years ago.
- History of mild hypertension well controlled with medication.
- Smokes 1 pack/day; 20-year history.

MEDICATIONS

Persantine 50 mg po tid
Tenormin 25 mg po qd
Aspirin 10 grains po bid

TESTS

- Carotid angiography: complete occlusion of left internal carotid artery.
- Cardiac ultrasound: intermittent mitral valve prolapse.
- EKG: nonspecific ST wave changes.
- CT scan: initial scan unremarkable; repeat CT scan consistent with a large left middle cerebral artery ischemic infarction.

SOCIAL HISTORY

Patient lives with his wife and three teenage children and was independent and active prior to CVA. He has a college education and has worked for 20 years as a computer programmer. There is a two-step access to a rented, single-family house.

COGNITION

- Disoriented to time.
- Good attention span for 30- to 45-minute treatment session.
- Difficult to examine further owing to language impairment; cognitive deficits likely.
- Patient has difficulty following directions for motor responses; two- or three-step commands.

LANGUAGE/COMMUNICATION

- Auditory comprehension: moderate to severe decrease in understanding words and simple concrete sentences; unreliable yes/no responses.
- Verbal expression: severely decreased to nonfunctional; limited to only occasional automatic words.
- Reading comprehension: severely decreased to nonfunctional at a word level. Unable to match word to object.

- Written expression: to be determined.
- Gestures: spontaneous use of gestures not evident.

PHYSICAL THERAPY EXAMINATION

PROM

- BUEs WNL; R shoulder pain at end ranges
- BLEs WNL except R dorsiflexion 0 to 5°

Tone

- RUE increased tone (moderate to severe) in elbow flexors; shoulder adductors and internal rotators.
- RLE increased tone (moderate) in hip and knee extensors, plantar flexors.

Motor Control

- RUE: partial motion (1/2 range) in extensor synergy pattern (shoulder and elbow extension); no voluntary motion of hand; cannot perform flexor synergy pattern.
- Demonstrates RUE neglect and often lets UE drop off the wheelchair.
- RLE: full motion in both extensor and flexor synergy patterns with extensor pattern dominating; extensor synergy achieved with associated reaction of RUE (extensor synergy).
- LUE and LLE: full isolated movement with G+ to N strength.

Sensory

- RUE: impaired, severity difficult to determine owing to communication deficits.
- No apparent sensation to sharp/dull stimuli; moderate decrease in light touch sensitivity.
- RLE: few consistent responses to sharp/dull stimuli proximally; moderate to severe decrease distally; no sensation noted on dorsum of foot.
- Patient reports pain in both RUE and RLE.
- Proprioception: inappropriate responses; difficult to determine owing to patient's difficulty with understanding of questions being asked.

Coordination

- LUE and LLE intact.
- RUE and RLE unable to test.

Postural Control/Balance

- Head control: good
- Sitting static control: good, able to maintain balance without support; maintains centered alignment (COM) for 5 minutes.
- Sitting dynamic control: fair, able to maintain balance; weight shifting with reduced limits of stability (LOS); shifts to R are reduced 50%; shifts to L are normal.
- Standing static control: fair, able to maintain independent standing in parallel bars for up to 1 minute with LUE handhold.
- Standing dynamic control: poor; unable to weight shift to R without loss of balance; weight shifts to L are reduced 50%.

Motor Planning

Appears to have mild motor apraxia; difficult to determine owing to communication impairments.

Endurance

Tolerates 3/4-hour treatment session with occasional rests.

Functional Status

- Rolls to R: Independent with bed rail
- Rolls to L: Min assist
- Scoots up in bed: Supervision
- Supine-to-sit: Min assist
- Sit-to-supine: Min assist
- Transfers bed-to-chair: Stand pivot transfer, Mod assist (FIM 3)
- W/C mobility: propels 150 ft with supervision (FIM 5); uses LUE and L foot for propulsion
- Locomotion: ambulates 10 ft in parallel bars with max assist of one (FIM 1).
  Requires assist in initiation of movement of RLE.
  Requires assist with R knee control for extension.
  R foot is plantarflexed and supinated during stance, foot drop during swing.
  AFO ordered (solid ankle AFO)
- Stairs: to be determined at a later date.
- Eating: Supervision (FIM 5)
- Bathing: Mod assist RUE and RLE (FIM 3)
- Dressing: Mod assist RUE and RLE (FIM 3)

(FIM = Functional Independence Measure)

PSYCHOSOCIAL

Patient is motivated and cooperative. He appears anxious about his future and exhibited a brief episode of crying during the initial therapy session. Family is supportive and anxious to have him home again.

GUIDING QUESTIONS

1. Identify/categorize this patient's problems in terms of:
   a. Direct impairments.
   b. Indirect impairments.
   c. Functional limitations/disabilities
2. Identify anticipated goals (remediation of impairments) and expected outcomes (remediation of functional limitations/disability) for this patient.
3. Formulate five treatment interventions with one progression that could be used during the first 3 weeks of therapy. Provide a brief rationale that justifies your choice.
4. Identify relevant motor learning strategies appropriate for the initial physical therapy sessions with this patient.

References

1. American Heart Association: Heart and Stroke Statistical—2005 Update. American HeartAssociation, Dallas, 2005.
2. Post-Stroke Rehabilitation Guideline Panel: Post-Stroke Rehabilitation Clinical Practice Guideline. Aspen, Gaithersburg, MD, 1996 (formerly published as AHCPR Publication No. 95-0662, May 1995).
3. Wolfe, C: The impact of stroke. Br Med Bul 56:275, 2000.
4. Murray, C, and Lopez, A: The Global Burden of Disease: A Comprehensive Assessment of Mortality and Disability from Diseases, Injuries, and Risk Factors in 1990 and Projected to 2020. Harvard University Press, Boston, 1996.
5. Granger, C, and Hamilton, B: The Uniform Data System for Medical Rehabilitation report of first admissions for 1992. Am J Phys Med Rehabil 73:51, 1994.
6. American Stroke Association: Stroke Warning Signs. American Heart Association, Dallas Texas, 2000.
7. The National Institute of Neurological Disorders and Stroke rt-PA Study Group: Tissue plasminogen activator for acute ischemic stroke. N Engl J Med 333:1581, 1995.
8. Hack, W, et al, for the European Cooperative Acute Stroke Study (ECASS) Group: Intravenous thrombolysis with recombinant tissue plasminogen activator for acute hemispheric stroke. JAMA 274:1017, 1995.
9. Wehrmacher, W, Iqbal A, and Messmore, H: Brain attack: Who will write the orders for thrombolytics? Arch Int Med 160:119, 2000.
10. Kwiatkowski, T, et al: Effects of tissue plasminogen activator or acute ischemic stroke at one year. N Engl J Med 340:1781, 1999.
11. Gilroy, J: Basic Neurology, ed 3. McGraw-Hill, New York, 2000.
12. Hachinski, V and Norris, J: The Acute Stroke. FA Davis, Philadelphia, 1985.
13. Curtis, S, and Porth, C: Disorders of brain function. In Porth, C (ed): Pathophysiology, ed. 5. Lippincott, Philadelphia, 1998, p 879.
14. Haig, A, et al: Locked-in syndrome: A review. Curr Concepts Rehabil Med 2:12, 1986.
15. Haig, A, et al: Mortality and complications of the locked-in syndrome. Arch Phys Med Rehabil 68:24, 1987.
16. Kaplan, P, Cailliet, R, and Kaplan, C: Rehabilitation of Stroke. Butterworth-Heinemann, Woburn, MA, 2003.
17. Bogousslavsky, J, et al: The Lausanne stroke registry: Analysis of 1,000 consecutive stroke patients. Stroke 19: 1083, 1988.
18. Smith, D, et al: Proprioception and spatial neglect after stroke. Age Ageing 12:63, 1983.
19. Fields, H: Pain. McGraw-Hill, New York, 1987.
20. Twitchell, T: The restoration of motor function following hemiplegia in man. Brain 47:443, 1951.
21. Brunnstrom, S: Motor testing procedures in hemiplegia based on recovery stages. J Am Phys Ther Assoc 46:357, 1966.
22. Brunnstrom, S: Movement Therapy in Hemiplegia. Harper & Row, New York, 1970.
23. Bobath, B: Adult Hemiplegia: Evaluation and Treatment, ed 2. Heinemann, London, 1978.
24. Fugl-Meyer, A, et al: The post stroke hemiplegic patient, 1. A method for evaluation of physical performance. Scand J Rehabil Med 7:13, 1976.
25. Gray, C, et al: Motor recovery following acute stroke. Age Ageing 19:179, 1990.
26. Wade, D, et al: Recovery after stroke: The first 3 months. J Neurol Neurosurg Psychiatry 48:7, 1985.
27. Colebatch, J, and Gandevia, S: The distribution of muscular weakness in upper motor neuron lesions affecting the arm. Brain 112:749, 1989.
28. Adams, R, Gandevia, S, and Skuse, N: The distribution of muscle weakness in upper motoneuron lesions affecting the lower limb. Brain 113: 1459, 1990.
29. Davidoff, R: The pyramidal tract. Neurology 40:332, 1990.
30. Andrews A, and Bohannon, R: Distribution of muscle strength impairments following stroke. Clinical Rehab 14:79, 2000.
31. McComas, A, et al: Functional changes in motoneurons of hemiparetic patients. J Neurol Neurosurg Psychiatry 36: 183, 1973.
32. Eng, J: Strength training in individuals with stroke. Physiother Can, 56:189, 2004.
33. Weightman, M: Motor unit behavior following cerebrovascular accident. Neurology Report (now JNPT) 18:26, 1994.
34. Dattola, R, et al: Muscle rearrangement in patients with hemiparesis after stroke: An electrophysiological and morphological study. Eur Neurol 33:109, 1993.
35. Tang, A, and Rymer, W: Abnormal force: EMG relations in paretic limbs of hemiparetic human subjects. J Neurol Neurosurg Psychiatry 44:690, 1981.
36. Rosenfalck, A, and Andreassen, S: Impaired regulation of force and firing pattern of single motor units in patients with spasticity. J Neurol Neurosurg Psychiatry 43:907, 1980.
37. Canning, C, Ada, L, and O'Dwyer, N: Slowness to develop force contributes to weakness after stroke. Arch Phys Med Rehabil 80:66, 1999.
38. Spaans, F, and Wilts, G: Denervation due to lesions of the central nervous system: An EMG study in cases of cerebral contusion and cerebrovascular accidents. J Neurol Sci 57:291, 1982.
39. Dickstein, R, et al: Reaction and movement times in patients with hemiparesis for unilateral and bilateral elbow flexion. Phys Ther 73:37, 1993.
40. Buonocore, M, et al: Psychomotor skills in hemiplegic patients: Reaction time differences related to hemispheric lesion side. Neurophysiol Clin 20:203, 1990.
41. Gowland, C, et al: Agonist and antagonist activity during voluntary upper-limb movement in patients with stroke. Phys Ther 72:624, 1992.
42. Knutsson, E, and Martensson, C: Dynamic motor capacity in spastic paresis and its relationship to prime mover dysfunction, spastic reflexes and antagonistic co-ordination. Scand J Rehabil Med 12:93, 1980.
43. Hufschmidt, A, and Mauritz, K: Chronic transformation of muscle in spasticity: A peripheral contribution to increased tone. J Neurol Neurosurg Psychiatry 48:676, 1985.
44. Schenkman, M, and Butler, R: Automatic postural tone in posture, movement, and function. Forum on physical therapy issues related to cerebrovascular accident. American Physical Therapy Association, Alexandria, VA, 1992.
45. Michels, E: Synergies in hemiplegia. Clin Manage 1:9, 1981.
46. Sahrmann, S, and Norton, B: The relationship of voluntary movement to spasticity in the upper motor neuron syndrome. Ann Neurol 2:460, 1977.
47. Bobath, B: Abnormal Postural Reflex Activity Caused by Brain Lesions, ed 3. Heinemann, London, 1985.
48. Mulley, G: Associated reactions in the hemiplegic arm. Scand J Rehabil Med 14:17, 1982.
49. Horak, F, et al: The effects of movement velocity, mass displaced and task certainty on associated postural adjustments made by normal and hemiplegic individuals. J Neurol Neurosurg Psychiatry 47:1020, 1984.
50. Dickstein, R, et al: Foot-ground pressure pattern of standing hemiplegic patients: Major characteristics and patterns of movement. Phys Ther 64:19, 1984.
51. Mizrahi, J, et al: Postural stability in stroke patients: Vectorial expression of asymmetry, sway activity, and relative sequence of reactive forces. Med Bio Eng Comput 27:181, 1989.
52. DiFabio, R, and Badke, M: Relationship of sensory organization to balance function in patients with hemiplegia. Phys Ther 70:543, 1990.
53. Shumway-Cook, A, Anson, D, and Haller, S: Postural sway biofeedback: Its effect on reestablishing stance stability in hemiplegic patients. Arch Phys Med Rehabil 69:395, 1988.
54. Badke, M, and DiFabio, R: Balance deficits in patients with hemiplegia: Considerations for assessment and treatment. In Duncan, P (ed): Balance: Proceedings of the APTA Forum. American Physical Therapy Association, Alexandria, VA, 1990, p 73.
55. Duncan, P, and Badke, M: Determinants of abnormal motor control. In: Duncan, P, and Badke, M (eds): Stroke Rehabilitation: The Recovery of Motor Control. Year Book Medical, Chicago, 1987, p 135.

56. Davies, P: Steps to Follow: The Comprehensive Treatment of Patients with Hemiplegia, ed 2. Springer-Verlag, New York, 2000.
57. Karnath, H, Ferber, S, and Dichgans, J: The origin of contraversive pushing: Evidence for a second graviceptive system in humans. Neurology 55:1298, 2000.
58. Karnath, H, Ferber, S, and Dichgans, J: The neural representation of postural control in humans. PNAS 97:13931, 2000.
59. Perennou, D, et al: Understanding the pusher behavior of some stroke patients with spatial deficits: A pilot study. Arch Phys Med Rehabil 83:570, 2002.
60. Pedersen, P, et al: Ipsilateral pushing in stroke: Incidence, relation to neuropsychological symptoms, and impact on rehabilitation. The Copenhagen stroke study. Arch Phys Med 77:25, 1996.
61. Karnath, H, and Broetz, D: Understanding and treating "pusher syndrome." Phys Ther 83:1119, 2003.
62. Veis, S, and Logemann, J: Swallowing disorders in persons with cerebrovascular accident. Arch Phys Med Rehabil 66:372, 1985.
63. Arnadottir, G: Impact of neurobehavioral deficits on activities of daily living. In Gillen, G, and Burkhardt, A (eds): Stroke Rehabilitation: A Function-Based Approach, ed 2. CV Mosby, St. Louis, 2005, p 285.
64. Starkstein, S, and Robinson, R: Neuropsychiatric aspects of stroke. In Coffey, C, and Cummings, J (eds): Textbook of Geriatric Neuropsychiatry. American Psychiatric Press, Washington, DC, 1994, p 457.
65. Hibbard, MR, and Gordon, WA: The comprehensive psychological assessment of individuals with stroke. J Neurol Rehabil 2:9, 1992.
66. Robinson, R, et al: Pathological laughing and crying following stroke: Validation of a measurement scale and a double-blind study. Am J Psychiatry 150:286, 1993.
67. Binder, L: Emotional problems after stroke. Stroke 15:174, 1984.
68. Robinson, R, et al: A two-year longitudinal study of post-stroke mood disorders: Diagnosis and outcome at one and two years. Stroke 18:837, 1987.
69. Remer-Osborn, J: Psychological, behavioral, and environmental influences on post-stroke recovery. Top Stroke Rehabil 5(2) 45, 1998.
70. Robinson, R: An 82-year-old woman with mood changes following a stroke. JAMA 283(12):1607, 2000.
71. Robinson, R, and Price, T: Post-stroke depressive disorders: A follow-up study of 103 patients. Stroke 13:635, 1982.
72. Robinson, R, and Benson, D: Depression in aphasic patients: Frequency, severity, and clinical-pathological correlations. Brain Lang 14:282, 1981.
73. Diller, L: Perceptual and intellectual problems in hemiplegia: Implications for rehabilitation. Med Clin North Am 53:575, 1969.
74. American Heart Association: How Stroke Affects Behavior. American Heart Association, Dallas, 1994.
75. Geschwind, N: Specialization of the human brain. Sci Am 241:80, 1979.
76. Bohannon, R: Selected determinants of ambulation capacity in patients with hemiplegia. Clin Rehab 3:47, 1989.
77. Bohannon, R: Correlation of lower limb strengths and other variables in standing performance in stroke patients. Physiother Can 41:198, 1989.
78. Hamrin, E, et al: Muscle strength and balance in post stroke patients. Ups J Med Sci 87:11, 1982.
79. Morris, S, Dodd, K, and Morris, M: Outcomes of progressive resistance strength training following stroke: A systematic review. Clin Rehab 18:27, 2004.
80. Harris, J, et al: Relationship of balance and mobility to fall incidence in people with chronic stroke. Phys Ther 85:150, 2005.
81. Byers, V, Arrington, M, and Finstuen, K: Predictive risk factors associated with stroke patient falls in acute care settings. J Neurosci Nurs 22: 147, 1990.
82. Nyberg, L, and Gustafson, Y: Patient falls in stroke rehabilitation: A challenge to rehabilitation strategies. Stroke 26:838, 1995.
83. Teasall, R, et al: The incidence and consequences of falls in stroke patients during inpatient rehabilitation: Factors associated with high risk. Arch Phys Med Rehabil 83:329, 2002.
84. Tutuarima, J, et al: Risk factors for falls of hospitalized stroke patients. Stroke 28:297, 1997.
85. Forster, A, and Young, J: Incidence and consequences of falls due to stroke: A systematic inquiry. Br Med J 311:83, 1995.
86. Ramnemark, A, et al.: Fractures after stroke. Osteoporos Int 8:92, 1998.
87. Cocito, L, et al: Epileptic seizures in cerebral arterial occlusive disease. Stroke 13:189, 1982.
88. Clagett, GP, et al: Prevention of venous thromboembolism. Chest 102(Suppl):391, 1992.
89. Buck, L: The coincidence of heart disease and stroke: Pathogenesis and considerations for therapy. Neurology Report (now JNPT) 18:29, 1994.
90. Palmer-McLean, K, and Wilberger, J: Stroke and head injury. In American College of Sports Medicine: ACSM's Exercise Management for Persons with Chronic Diseases and Disabilities. Human Kinetics, Champaign IL, 1997, p 169.
91. Rimmer, J, and Nicola, T: Stroke. In American College of Sports Medicine: ACSM's Resources for Clinical Exercise Physiology: Musculoskeletal, Neuromuscular, Neoplastic, Immunologic, and Hematologic Conditions. Lippincott, Williams & Wilkins, Philidelphia, 2002, p 3.
92. Mol, V, and Baker, C: Activity intolerance in the geriatric stroke patient. Rehabil Nurs 16:337, 1991.
93. Avery-Smith, W: Dysphagia management. In Gillen, G, and Burkhardt, A (eds): Stroke Rehabilitation: A Function-Based Approach, ed 2. CV Mosby, St. Louis, 2004, p 514.
94. Roth, EJ: Medical complications encountered in stroke rehabilitation. Phys Med Rehabil Clin North Am 2:563, 1991.
95. Stein, D, Brailowsky, S, and Will, B: Brain Repair. Oxford University Press, New York, 1995.
96. Wolf, S, et al: Forced use of hemiplegic upper extremities to reverse the effect of learned nonuse among chronic stroke and head-injured patients. Exp Neurol 104:125, 1989.
97. Liepert, J, et al: Motor cortex plasticity during constraint-induced movement therapy in stroke patients. Neurosci Lett 250:5, 1998.
98. Miltner, W, et al: Effects of constraint-induced movement therapy on patients with chronic motor deficits after stroke: A replication. Stroke 30: 586, 1999.
99. Kunkel, A, et al: Constraint-induced movement therapy for motor recovery in chronic stroke patients. Arch Phys Med Rehabil 80:624, 1999.
100. Taub, E, et al: Technique to improve chronic motor deficit after stroke. Arch Phys Med Rehabil 74:347, 1993.
101. Visintin, M, et al.: A new approach to retrain gait in stroke patients through body weight support and treadmill stimulation. Stroke 29:1122, 1998.
102. Hendricks, H, et al.: Motor recovery after stroke: A systematic review of the literature. Arch Phys Med Rehabil 83:1629, 2002.
103. Dombovy, M, and Bach-y-Rita, P: Clinical observations on recovery from stroke. Adv Neurol 47:265, 1988.
104. Kelly-Hayes, M, et al: Time course of functional recovery after stroke: The Framingham Study. J Neurol Rehabil 3:65, 1989.
105. Duncan, P, et al: Measurement of motor recovery after stroke. Outcome assessment and sample size requirements. Stroke 23:1084, 1992.
106. Kwakkel, G, et al: Predicting disability in stroke—A critical review of the literature. Age Ageing 25:479, 1996.
107. Andrews, K, et al: The rate of recovery from stroke—and its measurement. Int Rehabil Med 3:155, 1981.
108. Binkofski, F: Recovery of motor functions following hemiparetic stroke—a clinical and magnetic resonance morphometric study. Cerebrovasc Dis 11:273, 2001.
109. Bonita, R, and Beaglehole, R: Recovery of motor function after stroke. Stroke:19:1497, 1988.
110. Jorgenson, H, et al: Outcome and time course of recovery. Part II: Time course of recovery. The Copenhagen Stroke Study. Arch Phys Med Rehabil 76:406, 1995.
111. Jorgensen, H, et al: Recovery of walking function in stroke patients: The Copenhagen Stroke Study. Arch Phys Med Rehabil 76:27, 1995.
112. Nakayama, H, et al: Compensation in recovery of upper extremity function after stroke: The Copenhagen Stroke Study. Arch Phys Med Rehabil 75:852, 1994.
113. Samuelsson, M, Soderfeldt, B, and Olsson, G: Functional outcome in patients with lacunar infarction. Stroke 27:842, 1996.
114. Ferrucci, L, et al: Recovery of functional status after stroke: A postrehabilitation follow-up study. Stroke 24:200, 1993.

115. National Stroke Association: The Complete Guide to Stroke. National Stroke Association, Englewook, CO, 2003.
116. Langhorne, P, et al: Do stroke units save lives? Lancet 342:395, 1993.
117. Hayes, S, and Carroll, S: Early intervention care in the acute stroke patient. Arch Phys Med Rehabil 67:319, 1986.
118. Strand, T, et al: A non-intensive stroke unit reduces functional disability and the need for long-term hospitalization. Stroke 16:29, 1985.
119. Hamrin, E: Early activation in stroke: Does it make a difference? Scand J Rehabil Med 14:101, 1982.
120. Stroke Unit Trialists' Collaboration: Organised inpatient (stroke unit) care after stroke (Cochrane Review). The Cochrane Library, Issue 3. John Wiley & Sons, Ltd, Chichester, UK, retrieved August 20, 2005 from: http://www.cochrane.org/reviews/en/ab000197.html.
121. Kalra, L, et al: Medical complications during stroke rehabilitation. Stroke 26:990, 1995.
122. Dombovy, M, Sandok, B, and Basford, J: Rehabilitation for stroke: A review. Stroke 17:363, 1986.
123. Inaba, M, et al: Effectiveness of functional training, active exercise, and resistive exercise for patients with hemiplegia. Phys Ther 53:28, 1973.
124. Ernst, E. A review of stroke rehabilitation and physiotherapy. Stroke, 21:1081, 1990.
125. Kwakkel, G, et al: Intensity of leg and arm training after primary middle-cerebral-artery stroke: A randomized trial. Lancet 354:191, 1999.
126. Miller, K, Garland, S, and Koshland, G: Techniques and efficacy of physiotherapy poststroke. Phys Med Rehabil 12:473, 1998.
127. Paolucci, S, et al: Early versus delayed inpatient stroke rehabilitation: A matched comparison conducted in Italy. Arch Phys Med Rehabil 81:695, 2000.
128. Feigenson, J, et al: Factors influencing outcome and length of stay in a stroke rehabilitation unit. Part 1: Analysis of 248 unscreened patients. Medical and functional prognostic indicators. Stroke 8:651, 1977.
129. Shay, S, Vanclay, F, and Cooper, B: Predicting discharge status at commencement of stroke rehabilitation. Stroke 20:766, 1989.
130. Novack, T, Satterfield, W, and Connor, M: Stroke onset and rehabilitation: Time lag as a factor in treatment outcome. Arch Phys Med Rehabil 65:316, 1984.
131. Johnston, M, and Keister, M: Early rehabilitation for stroke patients: A new look. Arch Phys Med Rehabil 65:437, 1984.
132. American Physical Therapy Association: Guide to Physical Therapist Practice, ed 2. Phys Ther 81:1, 2001.
133. Duncan, P, et al: Randomized clinical trial of therapeutic exercise in subacute stroke. Stroke 34:2173, 2003.
134. Werner, R, and Kessle, S: Effectiveness of an intensive outpatient rehabilitation program for post acute stroke patients. Am J Phys Med Rehabil 75:114, 1996.
135. Rodriquez, A, et al: Gait training efficacy using a home-based practice model in chronic hemiplegia. Arch Phys Med Rehabil 77:801, 1996.
136. von Koch, L, et al: A randomized controlled trial of rehabilitation at home after stroke in southwest Stockholm: Outcome at six months. Scand J Rehab Med 32:80, 2000.
137. Geddes, J, and Chamberlain, A: Home-based rehabilitation for people with stroke: A comparative study of six community services providing co-ordinated, multidisciplinary treatment. Clin Rehabil 15:589, 2001.
138. Eng, J, et al: A community-based group exercise program for persons with chronic stroke. Med Sci Sports Exerc 35:1271, 2003.
139. Teasdale, G, and Jennett, B: Assessment of coma and impaired consciousness: A practical scale. Lancet 13:2, 1974.
140. Folstein, MF, et al: Mini mental state: A practical method for grading the cognitive state of patients for the clinician. J Psychiatr Res 12:189, 1975.
141. Beck, A, and Beck, R: Screening depressed patients in family practice: A rapid technique. Postgrad Med 52:81, 1972.
142. Bohannon, R, and Smith, M: Interrater reliability of a modified Ashworth scale of muscle spasticity. Phys Ther 67:206, 1987.
143. Bohannon, R: Measurement and treatment of paresis in the geriatric patient. Top Geriatr Rehabil 7:15, 1991.
144. Badke, M, and DiFabio, R: Balance deficits in patients with hemiplegia: Considerations for assessment and treatment. In Duncan, P (ed): Balance: Proceedings of the APTA Forum. American Physical Therapy Association, Alexandria, VA, 1990, p 23.
145. Badke, M, and Duncan, P: Patterns of rapid motor responses during postural adjustments when standing in healthy subjects and hemiplegic patients. Phys Ther 63:13, 1983.
146. Berg, KO, et al: Measuring balance in the elderly: Preliminary development of an instrument. Physiother Can 41:304, 1989.
147. Berg, KO, et al: Measuring balance in the elderly: Validation of an instrument. Can J Public Health 83 (Suppl):7, 1992.
148. Fugl-Meyer, A: Post-stroke hemiplegia assessment of physical properties. Scand J Rehabil Med 7:85, 1980.
149. Benaim, C, et al: Validation of a standardized assessment of postural control in stroke patients: The Postural Assessment Scale for Stroke Patients (PASS). Stroke 30 (9): 1862, 1999.
150. Duncan, P, et al: Functional reach: A new clinical measure of balance. J Gerontol 45:192, 1990.
151. Tinetti, ME: Performance-oriented assessment of mobility problems in elderly patients. J Am Geriatr Soc 34:119, 1986.
152. Podsiadlo, D, and Richardson, S: The timed "Up and Go": A test of basic functional mobility for frail elderly persons. J Am Geriatr Soc 39:142, 1991.
153. Shumway-Cook, A, and Horak, F: Assessing the influence of sensory interaction on balance: Suggestion from the field. Phys Ther 66:1548, 1986.
154. Nashner, LM: Sensory, neuromuscular, and biomechanical contributions to human balance. In Duncan, P (ed): Balance: Proceedings of the APTA Forum. American Physical Therapy Association, Alexandria VA, 1990, p 4.
155. Richards, C, Malouin, F, and Dean, C: Gait in stroke: Assessment and rehabilitation. Clin Geriatr Med 15:833, 1999.
156. Turnbull, G, and Wall, J: The development of a system for the clinical assessment of gait following a stroke. Physiotherapy 71:294, 1985.
157. Holden, M, et al: Clinical gait assessment in the neurologically impaired: Reliability and meaningfulness. Phys Ther 64:35, 1984.
158. Salbach, N, et al: Responsiveness and predictability of gait speed and other disability measures in acute stroke. Arch Phys Med Rehabil 82:1204, 2001.
159. Dean, C, Richards, C, and Malouin, F: Walking speed over 10 meters overestimates locomotor capacity after stroke. Clin Rehabil 15:415, 2001.
160. Sadaria, K, and Bohannon, R: The 6-Minute Walk Test: A brief review of literature. Clin Exerc Physiol 3:127, 2001.
161. Harada, N, Chiu, V, and Stewart, A: Mobility-related function in older adults: Assessment with a 6-Minute Walk Test. Arch Phys Med Rehabil 80:837, 1999.
162. Kervio, G, Carre, F, and Ville, N: Reliability and intensity of the Six-Minute Walk Test in healthy elderly subjects. Med Sci Sports Exer 35:169, 2003
163. Miller, P, Moreland, J, and Stevenson, T: Measurement properties of a standardized version of the Two-Minute Walk Test for Individuals with Neurological Dysfunction. Physiother Can 54(4):241, 2002.
164. Wolf, S, et al: Establishing the reliability and validity of measurements of walking time using the Emory Functional Ambulation Profile. Phys Ther 79:1122, 1999.
165. Baer, H, and Wolf, S: Modified Emory Functional Ambulation Profile. Stroke 32:973, 2001.
166. Perry, J, et al: Classification of walking handicap in the stroke population. Stroke 26:982. 1995.
167. Mahoney, F, and Barthel, D: Functional evaluation: Barthel Index. Md State Med J 14:61, 1965.
168. Keith, RA, et al: The Functional Independence Measure. Adv Clin Rehabil 1:6, 1987.
169. Uniform Data Service, Data Management Service: UDS Update. State University of New York at Buffalo, 1993.
170. Duncan, P, et al: Reliability of the Fugl-Meyer Assessment of Sensorimotor Recovery following cerebrovascular accident. Phys Ther 63:1606, 1983.
171. Wityk, RJ, Pessin, MS, and Kaplan, RF: Serial assessment of acute stroke using the NIH stroke scale. Stroke 25(2):362, 1994.

172. Goldstein, LB, and Samsa, GP: Reliability of the national institutes of health stroke scale. Stroke 28: 307, 1997.
173. Daley, K, et al.: The Stroke Rehabilitation Assessment of Movement (STREAM): Refining and validating the content. Physiother Can 49:269, 1997.
174. Daley, K, Mayo, N, and Wood-Dauphinee, S: Reliability of scores on the Stroke Rehabilitation Assessment of Movement (STREAM) measure. Phys Ther 79:8, 1999.
175. Ahmed, S, et al: The Stroke Rehabilitation Assessment of Movement (STREAM): A comparison with other measures used to evaluate effects of stroke and rehabilitation. Phys Ther 83: 617, 2003.
176. Carr, J, et al: Investigation of a new motor assessment scale for stroke patients. Phys Ther 65:175, 1985.
177. Pool, J, and Whitney, S: Motor Assessment Scale for stroke patients: Concurrent validity and interrater reliability. Arch Phys Med Rehabil 69:195, 1988.
178. Voss, D, et al: Proprioceptive Neuromuscular Facilitation, ed 3. Harper & Row, Philadelphia, 1985.
179. Adler, S, et al: PNF in Practice, ed 2. Springer-Verlag, Berlin, 2003.
180. Sackett, D, et al: Evidence-based Medicine, ed 2. Churchill Livingstone, New York, 2000.
181. Ernst, E: A review of stroke rehabilitation and physiotherapy. Stroke 21:1082, 1990.
182. Logigian, M, et al: Clinical exercise trial for stroke patients. Arch Phys Med Rehabil 64:364, 1983.
183. Stern, P, et al: Effects of facilitation exercise techniques in stroke rehabilitation. Arch Phys Med Rehabil 51:526, 1970.
184. Lord, J, and Hall, K: Neuromuscular reeducation versus traditional programs for stroke rehabilitation. Arch Phys Med Rehabil 67:88, 1986.
185. Dickstein, R, et al: Stroke rehabilitation: Three exercise therapy approaches. Phys Ther 66:1233, 1986.
186. Jongbloed, L, et al: Stroke rehabilitation: Sensorimotor integrative treatment versus functional treatment. Am J Occup Ther 43:391, 1989.
187. Wagenaar, R, et al: The functional recovery of stroke: A comparison between neuro-developmental treatment and the Brunnstrom method. Scand J Rehabil Med 22:1, 1990.
188. Ashburn, A, et al: Physiotherapy in the rehabilitation of stroke: A review. Clin Rehabil 7:337, 1993.
189. Sunderland, KJ, et al: Enhanced physical therapy improves recovery of arm function after stroke: A randomized controlled trial. J Neurol Neurosurg 55(7):530, 1992.
190. Feys, HM, et al: Effect of a therapeutic intervention for the hemiplegic upper limb in the acute phase after stroke. Stroke 29 (4): 785, 1998.
191. Langhammer, B, and Stanghelle, J: Bobath or motor relearning programme? A comparison of two different approaches of physiotherapy in stroke rehabilitation: A randomized controlled study. Clin Rehabil 14 (4):361, 2000.
192. Mudie, M, et al: Training symmetry of weight distribution after stroke: A randomized controlled pilot study comparing task-related reach, Bobath and feedback training approaches. Clin Rehabil 16(4):361, 2002.
193. Basmajian, J, et al: Stroke treatment: Comparison of integrated behavioral physical therapy vs traditional physical therapy programs. Arch Phys Med Rehabil 68:267, 1987.
194. Hesse, S, et al: Restoration of gait in nonambulatory hemiparetic patients by treadmill training with partial body-weight support. Arch Phys Med Rehabil 75:1087, 1994.
195. Hesse, S, et al: Treadmill training with partial body weight support compared with physiotherapy in nonambulatory hemiparetic patients. Stroke 26:976, 1995.
196. Malouin, F, et al: Use of an intensive task-oriented gait training program in a series of patients with acute cerebrovascular accidents. Phys Ther 72:781, 1992.
197. Richards, C, et al: Task-specific physical therapy for optimization of gait recovery in acute stroke patients. Arch Phys Med Rehabil 74 (6) 612, 1993.
198. Sullivan, K, Knowlton, B, and Dobkin, B: Step training with body weight support: Effect of treadmill speed and practice paradigms on poststroke locomotor recovery. Arch Phys Med Rehabil 83(5):683, 2002.
199. Smith, G, et al: Task-oriented exercise improves hamstring strength and spastic reflexes in chronic stroke patients. Stroke 30(10):2112, 1999.
200. Nilsson, L, et al: Walking training of patients with hemiparesis at an early stage after stroke: A comparison of walking training on a treadmill with body weight support and walking training on the ground. Clin Rehabil 15(5):515, 2001.
201. Laufer Y, et al: The effect of treadmill training on the ambulation of stroke survivors in the early stages of rehabilitation: A randomized study. J Rehabil Res Dev 38 (1):69, 2001.
202. Taub, E: Somatosensory deafferentation research with monkeys. In Ince, L (ed): Behavioral Psychology in Rehabilitation Medicine: Clinical Applications. Williams & Wilkins, Baltimore, 1980, p 371.
203. Dannenbaum, R, and Dykes, R: Sensory loss in the hand after sensory stroke: Therapeutic rationale. Arch Phys Med Rehabil 69:833, 1988.
204. Weinberg, J, et al: Training sensory awareness and spatial organization in people with right brain damage. Arch Phys Med Rehabil 60:491, 1979.
205. Johnstone, M: Therapy for Stroke. Churchill Livingstone, New York, 1991.
206. Johnstone, M: Restoration of Normal Movement After Stroke. Churchill Livingstone, New York, 1995.
207. Bailey, M, Riddoch, M, and Crome, P: Treatment of visual neglect in elderly patients with stroke: A single-subject series using either a scanning and cueing strategy or a left-limb activation strategy. Phys Ther 82(8):782, 2002.
208. Bailey, M, and Riddoch, M: Hemineglect in stroke patients. Part 2. Rehabilitation techniques and strategies: A summary of recent studies. Phys Ther Rev 4:77, 1999.
209. Wiart, L, et al: Unilateral neglect syndrome rehabilitation by trunk rotation and scanning training. Arch Phys Med Rehabil 78:424, 1997
210. Sharp, SA, and Brouwer, BJ: Isokinetic strength training of the hemiparetic knee: Effects on function and spasticity. Arch Phys Med Rehabil 78:1231, 1997
211. Badics, E, et al: Systematic muscle building exercises in the rehabilitation of stroke patients. Neuro Rehab 17:211, 2002.
212. Kim, CM, et al: Effects of isokinetic strength training on walking in persons with stroke: A double-blind controlled pilot study. J Stroke Cerebrovasc Dis 10:265, 2001.
213. Carr, M, and Jones, J: Physiologic effects of exercise on stroke survivors. Top Stroke Rehabil 9:57, 2003.
214. Bourbonnais, D, et al: Effect of force-feedback treatments in patients with chronic motor deficits after a stroke. Am J Phys Med Rehabil 81:890, 2002.
215. Engardt, M, et al: Dynamic muscle strength training in stroke patients: Effects on knee extension torque, electromyographic activity, and motor function. Arch Phys Med Rehabil 76:419, 1995.
216. Weiss, A, et al: High intensity strength training improves strength and functional performance after stroke. Am J Phys Med Rehabil 79:369, 2000.
217. Butefisch, C, et al: Repetitive training of isolated movements improves the outcome of motor rehabilitation of the centrally paretic hand. J Neurol Sci 103:59, 1995.
218. Moreland, JD, et al: Progressive resistance strengthening exercises after stroke: A single-blind randomized controlled trial. Arch Phys Med Rehabil 84:1433, 2003.
219. Glasser, L: Effects of isokinetic training on the rate of movement during ambulation in hemiparetic patients. Phys Ther 66:672, 1986.
220. Overend, TJ, et al: Cardiovascular stress associated with concentric and eccentric isokinetic exercise in young and older adults. J Gerontol A Biol Sci Med Sci 55:177, 2000.
221. McCully, KK: Exercise-induced injury to skeletal muscle. Fed Proc 45:2933, 1986.
222. Howle, J: Neuro-Developmental Treatment Approach—Theoretical Foundations and Principles of Clinical Practice. NDTA Assoc, Laguna Beach, CA, 2002.
223. Davies, P: Right in the Middle—Selective Trunk Activity in the Treatment of Adult Hemiplegia. Springer-Verlag, New York, 1990.

224. Carr, J, and Shepherd, R: A Motor Relearning Programme for Stroke, ed 2. Aspen, Gaithersville, MD, 1987.
225. O'Sullivan, S, and Schmitz, T: Physical Rehabilitation Laboratory Manual: Focus on Functional Training. FA Davis, Philadelphia, 1999.
226. Sunderland, A et al: Enhanced physical therapy improves recovery of arm function after stroke: A randomized controlled trial. J Neurol Neurosurg Psychiatry 55:530, 1992.
227. Woldag, H, and Hummelsheim, H: Evidence-based physiotherapeutic concepts for improving arm and hand function in stroke patients: A review. J Neurol 249(5):518, 2003.
228. Gillen, G: Upper extremity function and management. In Gillen, G, and Burkhardt, A (eds): Stroke Rehabilitation: A Function-Based Approach, ed 2. CV Mosby, St. Louis, 2004, p 172.
229. Carr, J, and Shepherd, R: Stroke Rehabilitation—Guidelines for Exercise and Training to Optimize Motor Skill. Butterworth Heinemann, Elsevier, Philadelphia, 2003.
230. Schaechter, JD, et al: Motor recovery and cortical reorganization after constraint-induced movement therapy in stroke patients: A preliminary study. Neurorehabil Neural Repair 16(4):326, 2002.
231. Whitall, J, et al: Repetitive bilateral arm training with rhythmic auditory cueing improves motor function in chronic hemiparetic stroke. Stroke 31:2390, 2000.
232. Wolf, S, and Binder-Macleod, S: Electromyographic biofeedback applications to the hemiplegic patient—changes in lower extremity neuromuscular and functional status. Phys Ther 63:1404, 1983.
233. Prevo, A, et al: Effect of EMG feedback on paretic muscles and abnormal co-contraction in the hemiplegic arm, compared with conventional physical therapy. Scand J Rehabil Med 14:121, 1982.
234. Tries, J: EMG feedback for the treatment of upper extremity dysfunction: Can it be effective? Biofeedback Self Regul 14(1):21, 1989.
235. Schleenbaker, RE, and Mainous, AG: Electromyographic biofeedback for neuromuscular education in the hemiplegic stroke patient: A meta-analysis. Arch Phys Med Rehabil 74(12):1301,1993.
236. Glantz, M, et al: Biofeedback therapy in post-stroke rehabilitation: A meta-analysis of the randomized controlled trials. Arch Phys Med Rehabil 76:508, 1995.
237. Smith, L: Restoration of volitional limb movement in hemiplegia following patterned functional electrical stimulation. Percept Mot Skills 71:851, 1990.
238. Trimble, M, and Enoka, R: Mechanisms underlying the training effects associated with neuromuscular electrical stimulation. Phys Ther 71:273, 1991.
239. Bowman, B, et al: Positional feedback and electrical stimulation: An automated treatment for the hemiplegic wrist. Arch Phys Med Rehabil 60:497, 1979.
240. Baker, L, and Parker, K: Neuromuscular electrical stimulation of the muscles surrounding the shoulder. Phys Ther 66:1930, 1986.
241. Price, C, and Pandyan, A: Electrical stimulation for preventing and treating post-stroke shoulder pain (Cochrane review). The Cochrane Library, Issue 3. John Wiley & Sons, Chichester, UK, retrieved July 20, 2005 from: http://www.cochrane.org/reviews/en/ab000197.html.
242. Roy, C: Shoulder pains in hemiplegia: A literature review. Clin Rehabil 2:35, 1988.
243. Jespersen, HF, et al: Shoulder pain after a stroke. Int J Rehabil Res 18A:273, 1995.
244. Turner-Stokes, L, and Jackson, D: Shoulder pain after stroke: A review of the evidence base to inform the development of an integrated care pathway. Clin Rehabil 16:276, 2002.
245. Snels, I, et al: Treating patients with hemiplegic shoulder pain. Am J Phys Med Rehabil 81(2):150, 2002.
246. Tepperman, P, et al: Reflex sympathetic dystrophy in hemiplegia. Arch Phys Med Rehabil 65:442, 1984.
247. Zorowitz, R, et al: Shoulder subluxation after stroke: A comparison of four supports. Arch Phys Med Rehabil 76:763, 1995.
248. Brooke, M, et al: Shoulder subluxation in hemiplegia: Effects of three different supports. Arch Phys Med Rehabil 72:582, 1991.
249. Bernath, V: Shoulder supports in patients with hypotonicity following stroke. Centre for Clinical Effectiveness, Clayton Australia, Jan 2001. Retrieved August 20, 2005 from http://www.med.monash.edu.au/healthservices/cce/evidence/pdf/c/470.pdf.
250. Rose, D: Fall Proof: A Comprehensive Balance and Mobility Training Program. Human Kinetics, Champaign, IL, 2003.
251. Winstein, C, et al: Standing balance training: Effect on balance and locomotion in hemiparetic adults. Arch Phys Med Rehabil 70:755, 1989.
252. Sackley, C, and Lincoln, N: Single blind randomized controlled trial of visual feedback after stroke: Effects on stance symmetry and function. Disabil Rehabil 19:536, 1997.
253. Hamman, R, et al: Training effects during repeated therapy sessions of balance training using visual feedback. Arch Phys Med Rehabil 73:738, 1992.
254. McRae, J, et al: Rehabilitation of hemiplegia: Functional outcomes and treatment of postural control. Phys Ther 74(Suppl):S119, 1994.
255. Nichols, D: Balance retraining after stroke using force platform biofeedback. Phys Ther 77:553, 1997.
256. Fishman, M, et al: Comparison of functional upper extremity tasks and dynamic standing. Phys Ther 76(Suppl):79, 1996.
257. Walker, C, Brouwer, B, and Culham, E: Use of visual feedback in retraining balance following acute stroke. Phys Ther 80:886, 2000.
258. Geiger, R, et al: Balance and mobility following stroke: Effects of physical therapy interventions with and without biofeedback/force-plate training. Phys Ther 81:995, 2001.
259. Shepherd, R, and Carr, J: Treadmill walking in neurorehabilitation. Neurorehabil Neural Repair 13:171, 1999.
260. Macko, RF, et al: Treadmill aerobic exercise training reduces the energy expenditure and cardiovascular demands of hemiparetic gait in chronic stroke patients; A preliminary report. Stroke 28(2):326, 1997.
261. Binder, S, et al: Evaluation of electromyographic biofeedback as an adjunct to therapeutic exercise in treating the lower extremities of hemiplegic patients. Phys Ther 61:886, 1981.
262. Cranstam, B, et al: Improvement of gait following functional electrical stimulation. Scand J Rehabil Med 9:7, 1977.
263. Merlitte, R, et al: Clinical experience of electronic peroneal stimulators in 50 hemiparetic patients. Scand J Rehabil Med 11:111, 1979.
264. Cozean, C, et al: Biofeedback and functional electric stimulation in stroke rehabilitation. Arch Phys Med Rehabil 69:401, 1988.
265. Bogataj, U, et al: The rehabilitation of gait in patients with hemiplegia: A comparison between conventional therapy and multichannel functional electrical stimulation therapy. Phys Ther 75:490, 1995.
266. Jacobs-Daly, J, et al: Electrically induced gait changes post stroke, using an FNS system with intramuscular electrodes and multiple channels. J Neurol Rehab 7:17, 1993.
267. Bogataj, U, et al: Restoration of gait during two to three weeks of therapy with multichannel electrical stimulation. Phys Ther 69:319, 1989.
268. Stanic, U, et al: Multichannel electrical stimulation for the correction of hemiplegic gait. Scan J Rehabil Med 10:75, 1978.
269. Gok, H, et al: Effects of ankle-foot orthoses on hemiparetic gait. Clin Rehabil 17:137, 2003.
270. Burdett, R, et al: Gait comparison of subjects with hemiplegia walking unbraced, with ankle-foot orthosis, and with air-stirrup brace. Phys Ther 68:1197, 1988.
271. Lehmann, J, et al: Knee movements: Origin in normal ambulation and their modification by double-stopped ankle-foot orthoses. Arch Phys Med Rehabil 63:345, 1982.
272. Corcoran, P, et al: Effects of plastic and metal braces on speed and energy cost of hemiparetic ambulation. Arch Phys Med Rehabil 5:69, 1970.
273. Hirschberg, G, and Ralston, H: Energy cost of stairclimbing in normal and hemiplegic subjects. Am J Phys Med 44:165, 1965.
274. Fisher, S: Energy cost of ambulation in health and disability: A literature review. Arch Phys Med Rehabil 59:124, 1978.
275. Roth, E, et al: Cardiovascular response to physical therapy in stroke rehabilitation. NeuroRehab 2:7, 1992.
276. Buck, L: The coincidence of heart disease and stroke: Pathogenesis and considerations for therapy. Neurology Report (now JNPT) 18:29, 1994.
277. Monga, T, et al: Cardiovascular response to acute exercise in patients with cerebrovascular accidents. Arch Phys Med Rehabil 69:937, 1988.

278. Macko, RF, et al: Treadmill aerobic exercise training reduces the energy expenditure and cardiovascular demands of hemiparetic gait in chronic stroke patients. Stroke 28(2):326, 1997.
279. Potempa, K, et al: Physiological outcomes of aerobic exercise training in hemiparetic stroke patients. Stroke 26:101, 1995.
280. Brinkman, J, and Hoskins, T: Physical conditioning and altered self-concept in rehabilitated hemiplegic patients. Phys Ther 59:859, 1979.
281. Carr, E: Assessment and treatment of feeding difficulties after stroke. Top Geriatr Rehabil 7:35, 1991.
282. Jorgensen, H, et al: Outcome and time course of recovery in stroke. Part I: Outcome. The Copenhagen Stroke Study. Arch Phys Med Rehabil 76:406, 1995.
283. Meijer, R, et al: Prognostic factors for ambulation and activities of daily living in the subacute phase after stroke. A systematic review of the literature. Clin Rehabil 17(2): 119, 2003.
284. Galski T, et al: Predicting length of stay, functional outcome, and aftercare in the rehabilitation of stroke patients. Stroke 24:1794, 1993.
285. Granger, C, and Hamilton, B: Measurement of stroke rehabilitation outcome in the 1980s. Stroke 21(Suppl II):1146, 1990.

Supplemental Readings

Carr, J, and Shepherd, R: Stroke Rehabilitation. Butterworth Heinemann, New York, 2003.
Davies, P: Steps to Follow: The Comprehensive Treatment of Patients with Hemiplegia, ed 2. Springer-Verlag, New York, 2000.
Davies, P: Right in the Middle—Selective Trunk Activity in the Treatment of Adult Hemiplegia. Springer-Verlag, New York, 1990.
Gillen, G, and Burkhardt, A (eds): Stroke Rehabilitation: A Function-Based Approach, ed 2. CV Mosby, St. Louis, 2004.
Johnston, M: Restoration of Normal Movement After Stroke. Churchill Livingstone, New York, 1995.
Reyerson, S, and Levit, K: Functional Movement Reeducation. Churchill Livingstone, New York, 1997.
Refshauge, K, Ada, L, and Ellis, E (eds): Science-Based Rehabilitation—Theories into Practice. Butterworth-Heinemann, New York, 2005.

Appendix A: Fugl-Meyer Assessment of Physical Performance

SUMMARY OF SCORES

MOTOR

Upper arm	______		Maximum Score	36
Wrist & hand	______	______	Maximum Score	30
TOTAL UPPER EXTREMITY SCORE		______	MAXIMUM SCORE	66
TOTAL LOWER EXTREMITY SCORE		______	MAXIMUM SCORE	34

TOTAL MOTOR SCORE	______	TOTAL MAXIMUM SCORE	100	PERCENTAGE OF RECOVERY ______
BALANCE				
TOTAL SCORE	______	MAXIMUM SCORE	14	
SENSATION				
TOTAL SCORE	______	MAXIMUM SCORE	24	
JOINT RANGE OF MOTION				
TOTAL SCORE	______	MAXIMUM SCORE	44	
PAIN				
TOTAL SCORE	______	MAXIMUM SCORE	44	

TOTAL FUGL-MEYER SCORE	______	TOTAL MAXIMUM SCORE	226	PERCENTAGE OF RECOVERY ______

Appendix A: Fugl-Meyer Assessment of Physical Performance (continued)

Area	Test	Scoring Criteria	Maximum Possible Score	Attained Score
	Motor			
UPPER EXTREMITY (sitting)	I. Reflexes a. biceps _____ b. triceps _____	0—No reflex activity can be elicited. 2—Reflex activity can be elicited.	4	
	II. Flexor Synergy elevation _____ shoulder retraction _____ abduction (at least 90°) _____ external rotation _____ elbow flexion _____ forearm supination _____	0—Cannot be performed at all. 1—Performed partly. 2—Performed faultlessly.	12	
	III. Extensor Synergy shoulder adduction/internal rotation _____ elbow extension _____ forearm pronation _____	0—Cannot be performed at all. 1—Performed partly. 2—Performed faultlessly.	6	
	IV. Movement Combining Synergies a. Hand to lumbar spine _____ b. Shoulder flexion to 90° elbow at 0° _____ c. Pronation/supination of forearm with elbow at 90° and shoulder at 0° _____	a. 0—No specific action performed. 1—Hand must pass anterior superior iliac spine. 2—Action is performed faultlessly. b. 0—Arm is immediately abducted or elbow flexes at start of motion. 1—Abduction or elbow flexion occurs in later phase of motion. 2—Faultless motion. c. 0—Correct position of shoulder and elbow cannot be attained, and/or pronation or supination cannot be performed at all. 1—Active pronation or supination can be performed even within a limited range of motion, and at the same time the shoulder and elbow are correctly positioned. 2—Complete pronation and supination with correct positions at elbow and shoulder.	6	
	V. Movement Out of Synergy a. Shoulder abduction to 90° elbow at 0° and forearm pronated _____ b. Shoulder flexion, 90–180° elbow at 0° and forearm in mid position _____ c. Pronation/supination of forearm elbow at 0° and shoulder between 30–90° of flexion _____	a. 0—*Initial* elbow flexion occurs or any deviation from pronated forearm occurs. 1—Motion can be performed partly, or if during motion, elbow is flexed or forearm cannot be kept in pronation. 2—Faultless motion. b. 0—Initial flexion of elbow or shoulder abduction occurs. 1—Elbow flexion or shoulder abduction, occurs during shoulder flexion. 2—Faultless motion. c. 0—Supination and pronation cannot be performed at all or elbow and shoulder position cannot be attained. 1—Elbow and shoulder properly positioned and pronation and supination performed in a limited range. 2—Faultless motion.	6	

(*continued*)

Appendix A: Fugl-Meyer Assessment of Physical Performance (continued)

Area	Test	Scoring Criteria	Maximum Possible Score	Attained Score
UPPER EXTREMITY	*Motor* VI. Normal Reflex Activity biceps and/or finger flexors and triceps _____	(This stage, which can render the score of two, is included only if the patient has a score of 6 in stage V.) 0—At least 2 of the 3 phasic reflexes are markedly hyperactive. 1—One reflex markedly hyperactive or at least 2 reflexes are lively. 2—No more than one reflex is lively and none are hyperactive.	2	
WRIST	VII. a. Stability, elbow at 90°, shoulder at 0° b. Flexion/extension, elbow at 90°, shoulder at 0° _____ c. Stability, elbow at 0°, shoulder at 30° _____ d. Flexion/extension, elbow at 0°, shoulder at 30° _____ e. Circumduction _____	a. 0—Patient cannot dorsiflex wrist to required 15°. 1—Dorsiflexion is accomplished, but no resistance is taken. 2—Position can be maintained with some (slight) resistance. b. 0—Volitional movement does not occur. 1—Patient cannot actively move the wrist joint throughout the total ROM. 2—Faultless, smooth movement. c. Scoring is the same as for item a. d. Scoring is the same as for item b. e. 0—Cannot be performed. 1—Jerky motion or incomplete circumduction. 2—Complete motion with smoothness.	10	
HAND	VIII. a. Finger Mass Flexion _____ b. Finger Mass Extension _____ c. Grasp #1—MP joints extended and PIPS & DIPS are flexed. Grasp is tested against resistance. d. Grasp #2—Patient is instructed to adduct thumb, 1st carpometacarpophalangeal and interphalangeal joint at 0° e. Grasp #3—Patient opposes the thumb pad against the pad of index finger. A pencil is interposed _____ f. Grasp #4—The patient should grasp a cylinder shaped object (small can), the volar surface of the 1st and 2nd finger against each other _____ g. Grasp #5—A spherical grasp.	a. 0—No flexion occurs. 1—Some flexion, but not full motion. 2—Complete active flexion (compared with unaffected hand). b. 0—No extension occurs. 1—Patient can release an active mass flexion grasp. 2—Full active extension. c. 0—Required position cannot be acquired. 1—Grasp is weak. 2—Grasp can be maintained against relatively great resistance. d. 0—Function cannot be performed. 1—Scrap of paper interposed between the thumb and index finger can be kept in place, but not against a slight tug. 2—Paper is held firmly against a tug. e. Scoring procedures are the same as for Grasp #2. f. Scoring procedures are the same as for Grasp #2 and #3. g. Scoring procedures are the same as for Grasp #2, 3, and 4.	14	
HAND	IX. Coordination/Speed—Finger-to-nose (five repetitions in rapid succession). a. Tremor _____ b. Dysmetria _____ c. Speed _____	a. 0—Marked tremor. 1—Slight tremor. 2—No tremor. b. 0—Pronounced or unsystematic dysmetria. 1—Slight or systematic dysmetria. 2—No dysmetria. c. 0—Activity is more than 6 seconds longer than unaffected hand. 1—2 to 5 seconds longer than unaffected hand. 2—Less than 2 seconds difference.	6	
		TOTAL MAXIMUM UPPER EXTREMITY SCORE	66	

LOWER EXTREMITY (supine)	I. Reflex activity—tested in suprine position. Achilles _____ Patellar _____	0—No reflex activity 2—Reflex activity	4	
Supine	II. a. Flexor Synergy Hip flexion _____ Knee flexion _____ Ankle dorsiflexion _____ b. Extensor synergy—(motion is resisted) Hip extension _____ Adduction _____ Knee extension _____ Ankle plantarflexion _____	a. 0—Cannot be performed 1—Partial motion 2—Full motion b. 0—No motion 1—Weak motion 2—Almost full strength compared to normal	6 8	
SITTING (knees free of chair)	III. Movement Combining Synergies a. Knee flexion beyond 90° _____ b. Ankle dorsiflexion _____	a. 0—No active motion 1—From slightly extended position knee can be flexed but not beyond 90° b. 0—No active flexion 1—Incomplete active flexion 2—Normal dorsiflexion	4	
STANDING	IV. Movement Out of Synergy Hip at 0° a. Knee flexion _____ b. Ankle dorsiflexion _____	a. 0—Knee cannot flex without hip flexion 1—Knee begins flexion without hip flexion, but doesn't get to 90°, or hip flexes during motion 2—Full motion as described b. 0—No active motion 1—Partial motion 2—Full motion	4	
SITTING	V. Normal Reflexes Knee flexors _____ Patellar _____ Achilles _____	0—2 of the 3 are markedly hyperactive 1—One reflex is hyperactive or 2 reflexes are lively 2—No more than 1 reflex lively	2	
(SUPINE)	VI. Coordination/Speed Heel to opposite knee (5 repetitions in rapid succession) a. Tremor _____ b. Dysmetria _____ c. Speed _____	a. 0—Marked tremor 1—Slight tremor 2—No tremor b. 0—Pronounced or unsystematic 1—Slight or systematic 2—No dysmetria c. 0—Six seconds slower than unaffected side 1—Two to 5 seconds slower 2—Less than 2 seconds difference	6	
		TOTAL MAXIMUM LOWER EXTREMITY SCORE	34	

(*continued*)

Appendix A: Fugl-Meyer Assessment of Physical Performance (continued)

Area	Test	Scoring Criteria	Maximum Possible Score	Attained Score
BALANCE	a. Sit without support _____ b. Parachute reaction, non-affected side _____ c. Parachute reaction, affected side _____ d. Supported standing e. Stand without support f. Stand on unaffected side _____ g. Stand on affected side _____	a. 0—Cannot maintain sitting without support 1—Can sit unsupported less than 5 minutes 2—Can sit longer than 5 minutes b. 0—Does not abduct shoulder or extend elbow 1—Impaired reaction 2—Normal reaction c. Scoring is the same as #2 d. 0—Cannot stand 1—Stands with maximum support of others 2—Stands with minimum support of one for 1 minute e. 0—Cannot stand 1—Stands less than 1 minute or sways 2—Stands with good balance more than 1 min. f. 0—Cannot be maintained longer than 1–2 sec. 1—Stands balanced 4–9 seconds 2—Stands balanced more than 10 sec. g. 0—Scoring is the same as #6		
		MAXIMUM BALANCE SCORE	14	
UPPER AND LOWER EXTREMITIES	*Sensation* I. Light Touch a. Upper arm _____ b. Palm of hand _____ c. Thigh _____ d. Sole of foot _____ II. Proprioception a. Shoulder _____ b. Elbow _____ c. Wrist _____ d. Thumb _____ e. Hip _____ f. Knee _____ g. Ankle _____ h. Toe _____	Light Touch Scoring 0—Anesthesia 1—Hyperaesthesia/dyesthesia 2—Normal Proprioception Scoring 0—No sensation 1—Three quarter of answers are correct, but considerable difference in sensation compared with unaffected side. 2—All answers are correct, little or no difference	8 16	

		Motion/Pain Motion	Pain			
SHOULDER	Flexion	____	____	**Motion Scoring**	Motion	
	Abduction to 90°	____	____	0—Only a few degrees of motion	44	
	External rotation	____	____	1—Decreased passive range of motion		
	Internal rotation	____	____	2—Normal passive range of motion		
ELBOW	Flexion	____	____			
	Extension	____	____	**Pain Scoring**		
WRIST	Flexion	____	____	0—Marked pain at end of range or pain through range	44	
	Extension	____	____	1—Some pain		
FINGERS	Flexion	____	____	2—No pain		
	Extension	____	____			
FOREARM	Pronation	____	____			
	Supination	____	____			
HIP	Flexion	____	____			
	Abduction	____	____			
	External rotation	____	____			
	Internal rotation	____	____			
KNEE	Flexion	____	____			
	Extension	____	____			
ANKLE	Dorsiflexion	____	____			
	Plantarflexion	____	____			
FOOT	Pronation	____	____			
	Supination	____	____			

Appendix B: Web-Based Resources for Clinicians, Families, and Patients with Stroke

American Heart Association	http://www.americanheart.org/
American Stroke Association-a division of the American Heart Association	http://www.strokeassociation.org/
National Stroke Association	http://www.stroke.org/
American Stroke Foundation	http://www.americanstroke.org/
International Stroke Society	http://www.internationalstroke.org
Stroke Association—UK	http://www.stroke.org.uk/
Heart and Stroke Foundation of Canada	http://www.heartandstroke.ca/
Veterans Affairs—stroke	http://www.va.gov/
Americans with Disabilities Act: ADA home page	http://www.usdoj.gov/crt/ada
Medicare information	http://www.cms.hhs.gov
Social Security Online	http://www.ssa.gov
National Institute of Neurological Disorders and Stroke	http://www.ninds.nih.gov
National Library of Medicine	http://www.nlm.nih.gov
American Association of Physical Medicine and Rehabilitation	http://www.aapmr.org/condtreat/rehab/stroke.htm
American Academy of Neurology (ANA)	http://www.aan.com/professionals http://www.aan.com/public (public education) http://www.neurology.org (Journal of Neurology)
National Rehabilitation Information Center (NARIC)	http://www.naric.com
Stroke rehab forum at Med Help	http://www.medhelp.org/forums/stroke Rehab/
Rehabilitation Research & Training Center on Stroke Rehabilitation	http://www.rrtc-stroke.org
Internet Handbook of Neurology	http://www.neuropat.dote.hu/stroke1.htm
Stroke and depression	http://www.nimh.nih.gov/publicat/depstroke.cfm
National Aphasia Association	http://www.aphasia.org
National Easter Seal Society	http://www.easter-seals.org
Disease prevention	http://www.everydaychoices.org
The Neurology Channel—stroke	http://www.neurologychannel.com/stroke/
Agency for Healthcare Research & Quality	http://www.ahrq.gov/consumer/strokecon.htm
Brain attack- stroke prevention & treatment—USFDA	http://www.fda.gov/fdac/features/2005/205_stroke.html
Stroke Information Directory	http://www.stroke-info.com
Clinical trials—National Institutes of Health (NIH)—stroke	http://www.clinicaltrials.gov/search/term=stroke
Stroke survivors	http://www.stroke-survivors.com
Resource center for clinicians and families	http://www.strokehelp.com/
The Stroke Network, Inc	http://www.strokenetwork.org
National Family Caregivers Association (NFCA)	http://www.nfcacares.org
Well Spouse Foundation	http://www.wellspouse.org
Ability Hub—assistive technology solutions	http://www.abilityhub.com
ABLEDATA—assistive technology information	http://www.abledata.com
Disabled Online	http://www.disabledonline.com

CHAPTER

19

Multiple Sclerosis

Susan B. O'Sullivan, PT, EdD

LEARNING OBJECTIVES

1. Describe the etiology, epidemiology, pathophysiology, signs and symptoms, diagnosis, and course of multiple sclerosis (MS).
2. Describe elements of the medical management of patients with MS.
3. Identify and describe the examination procedures used to evaluate patients with MS to establish the physical therapy diagnosis, prognosis, and plan of care.
4. Describe the role of the physical therapist in the management of patients with MS in terms of direct interventions and patient/client-related instruction to maximize function and quality of life.
5. Describe appropriate elements of the exercise prescription for patients with MS.
6. Review current research findings concerning the rehabilitation of patients with MS.
7. Identify the psychosocial impact of MS and describe appropriate interventions.
8. Analyze and interpret patient data, formulate realistic goals and outcomes, and develop a plan of care when presented with a clinical case study.

OUTLINE

Multiple sclerosis (MS) is a chronic inflammatory, demyelinating disease of the central nervous system (CNS). It affects largely young adults between the ages of 20 and 40, and is often referred to as the "great crippler of young adults." It was described as early as 1822 in the diaries of an English nobleman and further depicted in an anatomy book in 1858 by a British medical illustrator. Dr. Jean Cruveilhier, a French physician, first used the term "islands of sclerosis" to describe areas of hardened tissue discovered on autopsy. However, it was Dr. Jean Charcot in 1868 who defined the disease by its clinical and pathological characteristics: paralysis and the cardinal symptoms of intention tremor, scanning speech, and nystagmus, later termed **Charcot's triad**. Using autopsy studies he identified areas of hardened plaques and termed the disease *sclerosis in plaques*.[1]

Epidemiology

The onset of MS typically occurs between the ages of 15 and 50 years, with the peak at age 30. The disease is rare in children, as is the onset of symptoms in adults older than the age of 50 years. It affects approximately 400,000 individuals in the United States. The disease is more common in woman than in men by a ratio of 2:1, a difference especially evident at the younger ages. There are well reported ethnic differences. MS affects predominately white populations; African Americans demonstrate approximately half the risk of acquiring the disease. Low rates are also reported in Asians and Native Americans.

Epidemiological studies have revealed a geographical pattern of distribution of MS with areas of high, medium, and low frequency. High-frequency areas include the temperate zones of the northern United States, Scandinavian countries, northern Europe, southern Canada, New Zealand, and southern Australia, with the incidence reported at rates of 30 to 80 per 100,000 population. Areas of medium frequency closer to the equator include the southern United States and Europe, and the rest of Australia with a reported incidence of 10 to 25 per 100,000. Low-frequency tropical areas (Asia, Africa, and South America) have reported rates of less than 5 per 100,000.[2,3] Migration studies indicate the geographical risk associated with an individual's birthplace is retained if emigration occurs after the age of 15 years. Individuals migrating before this age assume the risk of their new location.[4] There have been reported epidemics of MS in the literature, one in the Faroe Islands off the coast of Scotland and one in Iceland following occupation by soldiers during World War II. These epidemiological studies lend support to a theory that exposure to an unidentified infectious agent transmitted person-to-person, such as a slow-acting virus, predisposed individuals to the development of MS later on.[5,6]

Etiology

The precise etiology of MS is unknown. The most widely accepted theory is that it is an autoimmune disease induced by a viral or other infectious agent. In particular, herpes viruses (I, II, and VI) and chlamydial pneumonia are agents of greatest interest in an infectious hypothesis.[7,8] The presence of increased immunoglobulin (IgG) and oligoclonal bands in the cerebrospinal fluid (CSF) of 65 to 95 percent of MS patients provides convincing evidence of a precipitating infection eliciting an autoimmune response with resulting pathological changes.[9] Viral infection has been shown to precipitate about 33 percent of relapses in MS. Genetics also plays a role in the acquisition of MS. Approximately 15 percent of patients have a positive family history (first-degree relative, such as a parent or sibling with MS). The risk is 3 to 5 percent for a fraternal co-twin but rises to 26 percent for an identical co-twin.[10] Genetic studies have revealed multiple markers in multiplex families, defined as families in which several members have MS. In particular, major histocompatibility complex (MHC) proteins, encoded on chromosome 6, have been linked to antibody production (class I antigens) and MS. It appears that although individuals do not inherit the disease, they may inherit a genetic susceptibility to immune system dysfunction.[11]

Pathophysiology

In patients with MS, the immune response triggers the production of T-lymphocytes, macrophages, and immunoglobulins (antibodies). In turn, a command or trigger protein, the antigen, is activated, producing autoimmune cytotoxic effects within the CNS (this process can be viewed as a form of "friendly fire"). The blood–brain barrier fails and myelin-sensitized T-lymphocyte cells enter and attack the myelin sheath that surrounds the nerve. **Myelin** serves as an insulator, speeding up the conduction along nerve fibers from one node of Ranvier to another (termed *saltatory conduction*). It also serves to conserve energy for the nerve because depolarization occurs only at the nodes. Disruption of the myelin sheath produces active **demyelination**, slowing neural transmission and causing nerves to fatigue rapidly. With severe disruption, conduction block occurs with resulting disruption of function. Local inflammation, edema, and infiltrates surround the acute lesion and can cause a *mass effect* (abnormally high pressures), further interfering with the conductivity of the nerve fiber. Conceivably, this inflammation (which gradually subsides) may, in part, account for the pattern of fluctuations in function that characterize this disease. During the early stages of MS, *oligodendrocytes* (myelin-producing cells) survive the initial insult and can produce remyelination. This process is often incomplete and as the disease becomes more chronic, stalls altogether. Eventually the oligodendrocytes become involved and myelin repair cannot occur. One form of MS, primary-progressive MS, appears to be associated exclusively with disease of the oligodendrocytes.[7] Demyelinated areas eventually become filled with fibrous astrocytes and undergo a process called gliosis. **Gliosis** refers to the proliferation of neuroglial tissue within the CNS and results in glial scars *(plaques)*. At this stage, the axon itself becomes interrupted and undergoes retrograde degeneration (dying axonopathy). Axonal loss varies from 10 to 20 percent in milder forms of the disease to as much as 80 percent in severe MS.[12] In advanced cases, there are both acute and chronic lesions of varying size scattered throughout the CNS (brain, brainstem, cerebellum, and spinal cord). They primarily affect white matter early, with lesions of gray matter evident in more advanced disease. There are certain areas of predilection, such as the optic nerves, periventricular white matter, spinal cord (corticospinal tracts, posterior white columns), and cerebellar peduncles.[7]

Clinical Course

MS is highly variable and unpredictable from person-to-person and within a given individual over time. At one end of the continuum, there is *benign MS,* defined as disease in which the patient remains fully functional in all neurological systems 15 years after onset. Benign MS affects fewer than 20 percent of cases. At the other end of the continuum, there is *malignant MS (Marburg disease),* a relatively rare disease course characterized by rapid onset and almost continual progression leading to significant disability or death within a relatively short time after onset. *Relapsing-remitting MS (RRMS)* is the most common course, affecting approximately 70 percent of patients with MS. It is characterized by clearly defined disease *relapses,* periods of acute worsening of neurological function, followed by *remissions,* defined as periods without disease progression and partial or complete abatement of signs and symptoms. About 80 percent of RRMS cases go on to develop *secondary progressive MS (SPMS)*. SPMS begins with a relapsing-remitting course followed by progression with or without occasional relapses, minor remissions, and plateaus. *Progressive-relapsing MS (PRMS)* begins with a progressive disease course from the onset, with clear, acute relapses that may or may not resolve with full recovery. The intervals between relapses are marked by continuing disease progression. *Primary progressive MS (PPMS)* is a rare form occurring in about 10 percent of cases. It is characterized by a nearly continuous worsening of the disease from the onset without distinct relapses. Some individuals do have occasional plateaus or temporary minor improvements. PPMS typically has a later onset, usually after age 40. Permanent neurological disability results from relapses with incomplete remissions, progression of the disease, or both. Because the course of the disease may alter, clinicians need to be alert to changes in signs or symptoms in terms of severity and frequency.[13,14] Box 19.1 summarizes the categories of multiple sclerosis.

Box 19.1 Definitions and Terminology Used to Describe Categories of Multiple Sclerosis

- **Relapsing-remitting MS (RRMS):** Characterized by relapses with either full recovery or some remaining neurological signs/symptoms and residual deficit upon recovery; the periods between relapses are characterized by lack of disease progression.
- **Primary-progressive MS (PPMS):** Characterized by disease progression from onset, without plateaus or remissions or with occasional plateaus and temporary minor improvements.
- **Secondary-progressive MS (SPMS):** Characterized by initial relapsing-remitting course, followed by progression at a variable rate that may also include occasional relapses and minor remissions.
- **Progressive-relapsing MS (PRMS):** Characterized by progressive disease from onset but without clear acute relapses that may or may not have some recovery or remission; commonly seen in people who develop the disease after 40 years of age.
- **Benign MS:** Characterized by mild disease in which patients remain fully functional in all neurological systems 15 years after disease onset.
- **Malignant MS (Marburg's variant):** Characterized by rapid progression leading to significant disability or death within a relatively short time after onset.

Exacerbating Factors

MS relapses (exacerbations) are defined by new and recurrent MS symptoms that last at least 24 hours and are unrelated to another etiology. Several factors have been identified. Avoiding these aggravating factors is important in ensuring the patient's optimal function. An individual whose overall health deteriorates is more likely to have a relapse than one who remains healthy. Viral or bacterial infections (e.g., cold, flu, urinary tract infection, sinus infection) and diseases of major organ systems (e.g., hepatitis, pancreatitis, asthma attacks) are associated with relapses of disease. There is also a modest link between stress and acute attacks. Both major life stress events (divorce, death, losing a job, trauma) and minor stresses (exhaustion, dehydration, malnutrition, and sleep deprivation) can affect the immune system and an already compromised nervous system.[15]

Pseudoexacerbation refers to the temporary worsening of MS symptoms. The episode typically comes and goes quickly, usually within 24 hours. The overwhelming majority of individuals with MS demonstrate an adverse reaction to heat, known as **Uthoff's symptom**. Anything that raises the body temperature can bring on a pseudo-attack. External heat stressors include sun exposure, hot muggy environmental temperatures, or a hot bath. Internal elevations in temperature can be produced by fever or prolonged exercise. The effects are usually immediate and dramatic in terms of reduced function and increased fatigue. Most pseudo-attacks resolve within 24 hours of cooling off and/or the end of a fever.

Clinical Manifestations

Signs and symptoms of MS vary considerably, depending on the location of specific lesions. Early symptoms typically include minor visual disturbances (e.g., episodes of double vision) and paresthesias progressing to numbness, weakness, and fatigability. In more advanced stages, patients demonstrate multiple symptoms with varying involvement. Common symptoms in MS are presented in Box 19.2.[15,16] The onset of symptoms can develop rapidly over a course of minutes or hours; less frequently, onset is insidious, occurring over a period of weeks or months. An early remission may lead the individual to postpone initial neurological workup for months or longer.

Sensory Changes

Complete loss of any single sensation (anesthesia) is rare. Focal deficits can produce limited areas of diminished sensation. Altered sensations are far more common and can include *paresthesias* (pins and needles sensation) or numbness of the face, body, or extremities. Disturbances

Box 19.2 Common Symptoms in Multiple Sclerosis[15,16]

Sensory Symptoms
Hypoesthesia, numbness
Paresthesias

Pain
Dysesthesias
Optic or trigeminal neuritis
Lhermitte's sign
Chronic pain

Visual Symptoms
Blurred or double vision
Diminished acuity/loss of vision
Scotoma
Nystagmus

Cognitive Symptoms
Memory or recall problems
Decreased attention, concentration
Diminished abstract reasoning
Diminished problem solving, judgment
Diminished speed of information processing
Diminished visual–spatial abilities

Emotional Symptoms
Depression
Pseudobulbar affect
Anxiety

Motor Symptoms
Weakness or paralysis
Fatigue
Spasticity
Incoordination
Intention tremor
Impaired balance
Gait disturbances

Bladder Symptoms
Urinary urgency, frequency
Nocturia
Incontinence
Urinary hesitancy, dribbling

Sexual Symptoms
Impotence
Decreased libido
Decreased vaginal lubrication
Impaired ability to achieve orgasm

Bowel Symptoms
Constipation
Diarrhea
Incontinence

Speech and Swallowing
Dysarthria
Diminished verbal fluency
Dysphonia
Dysphagia

Cardiovascular dysautonomia

Pattern of Symptoms
Vary greatly from person-to-person
Vary over time in each individual affected
First symptoms usually transient
Early symptoms are typically sensory and visual
Involves more than one functional component of the CNS

in position sense are also common, as are lower extremity (LE) impairments of vibratory sense.

Pain

Approximately 80 percent of patients with MS experience pain, with clinically significant pain occurring in about 55 percent. Almost half experience chronic pain.[17] Patients often experience acute, paroxysmal pain characterized by sudden and spontaneous onset. The pains are described as intense, sharp, shooting, electric shock-like, and burning. The most common types are trigeminal neuralgia, paroxysmal limb pain, and headache. *Trigeminal neuralgia* (tic douloureux) results from demyelination of the sensory division of the trigeminal nerve innervating the face, cheek, and jaw. Eating, shaving, or simply touching the face may trigger painful episodes. A common sign of posterior column damage in the spinal cord is **Lhermitte's sign** in which flexion of the neck produces an electric shock-like sensation running down the spine and into the LEs. Paroxysmal limb pain presents as abnormal burning, aching pain (dysesthesias) that can affect any part of the body but is more common in the LEs. It is the most common type of pain in MS and is worse at night and after exercise. It can be aggravated by temperature elevations. *Hyperpathia*, a hypersensitivity to minor sensory stimuli, can occur. For example, a light touch or light pressure stimulus elicits a severe pain reaction. Headache is more frequent in MS than in the general population and can be migraine or tension type. Chronic *neuropathic pain* can result from demyelinating lesions in spinothalamic tracts or in the sensory roots. It is more common in patients with minimum disability and is described as a burning pain similar to pain described by individuals with disk herniation. Musculoskeletal pain associated with muscle and ligament strain can develop from mechanical stress, abnormal postures, and immobility, often the result of weak muscles, powerful spasticity, and tonic spasms. Anxiety and fear can worsen pain symptoms.[18]

Visual Changes

Visual symptoms are common with MS and are found in approximately 80 percent of patients. Involvement of the optic nerve produces altered visual acuity; blindness is rare. *Optic neuritis,* inflammation of the optic nerve, is a common problem, and produces an ice-pick like pain behind the eye with blurring or graying of vision, or blindness in one eye. A *scotoma* or dark spot may occur in the center of the visual field. Neuritis rarely affects both eyes, and is usually self-limiting. Vision generally improves within 4 to 12 weeks. Damage to the optic nerve will also affect light reflexes. **Marcus Gunn pupil** often develops with MS in individuals who have had an episode of optic neuritis. Shining a bright light into the healthy eye will produce reflex contraction in both eyes (consensual light reflex). If the light is then shone in the affected eye, a paradoxical widening (dilation) of both pupils occurs.

Eye movements can be disturbed in a variety of ways. *Nystagmus* is common in patients with MS and results from lesions affecting the cerebellum or central vestibular pathways. This involves involuntary cyclical movements of the eyeball (horizontal or vertical) that develop when the patient looks to the sides or vertically (gaze-induced nystagmus) or when the patient moves the head. *Internuclear ophthalmoplegia* (INO) produces incomplete eye adduction (lateral gaze palsy) on the affected side and nystagmus of the opposite abducting eye with gaze to one side. It is caused by demyelination of the pontine medial longitudinal fasciculus (MLF). Additional impairments in conjugate gaze and control of eye movements may also be present with brainstem lesions affecting cranial nerves III, IV, and VI or the MLF. *Diplopia,* double vision, occurs when the muscles that control the eyes are not well coordinated. Visual disturbances frequently remit and are seldom the primary cause of disability. The effects of impaired vision on balance and movement should be carefully examined.

Motor Dysfunction

Weakness

Patients with corticospinal lesions demonstrate signs and symptoms of upper motor neuron (UMN) involvement. Paresis, spasticity, brisk tendon reflexes, involuntary flexor and extensor spasms, clonus, Babinski's sign, exaggerated cutaneous reflexes, and loss of precise autonomic control all characterize UMN involvement[19] (see Chapter 8). Movements are slow, stiff, and weak, the result of loss of orderly recruitment and reduced firing rate modulation of motoneurons. Reduced muscle strength, power, and endurance, along with impaired synergistic relationships are evident. Patients with cerebellar lesions demonstrate asthenia or generalized muscle weakness along with ataxia. Patients can also experience muscle weakness secondary to inactivity. Muscle weakness can vary from a mild paresis, often transient at first, to total paralysis of the involved extremities.

Fatigue

Fatigue has been defined by the Panel on Fatigue of the MS Council for Clinical Practice Guidelines as "a subjective lack of physical and/or mental energy that is perceived by the individual or caregiver to interfere with usual and desired activities."[20, p 1] Fatigue is a daily event, experienced by 75 percent to 95 percent of individuals with the disease. Approximately 50 percent to 60 percent of patients report that fatigue is one of their most troubling symptoms. Patients consistently report that fatigue interferes with physical functioning (79 percent of patients), overall role performance (67 percent of patients), and perceived health status.[21–23] Fatigue comes on abruptly, without warning, and resembles an overwhelming flu-like exhaustion. Severity of disease does not seem to be related to fatigue severity; that is, individuals mildly affected by disease (ambulatory patients) report disabling fatigue as often as more severely disabled patients.[24] Fatigue is the result of central activation failure (*central fatigue*) and failure in excitation–contraction coupling. Precipitating factors contributing to fatigue include physical exertion, exposure to heat and humidity (reported by 92 percent of patients), depression and sleep disorders, low self-esteem and mood disorders, medical conditions and secondary complications of MS (e.g., respiratory impairment, infection). Side effects of medications also impact fatigue, including analgesics, anticonvulsants, antidepressants, antihistamines, antihypertensive agents, and anti-inflammatory agents.[20] Environmental mastery (sense of control) is a strong psychosocial predictor of fatigue. Individuals with a low sense of environmental mastery reported significantly more fatigue and fatigue-related distress.[25]

Spasticity

Spasticity is an extremely common problem in patients with MS, occurring in 80 percent of all cases. Spasticity can range from mild to severe, depending on the progression of the disease, and occurs most frequently in the muscles of the upper and lower extremities. Clinical indications of spasticity include impaired voluntary control of movement (abnormal co-contraction); increased deep tendon reflexes (DTRs), clonus, flexion or extension synergy patterns, and decreased range of motion (ROM). Spasticity also results in increased fatigue, impaired functional mobility, and impaired activities of daily living (ADL). Spasticity can cause pain, disabling contractures, abnormal posturing, and problems in maintaining skin integrity. Spasticity fluctuates on a daily basis and can be exacerbated by certain factors, such as fatigue, stress, extremes of temperature and humidity, infections, or noxious stimuli (e.g., tight clothing).[26] Certain antidepressant agents (serotonin-reuptake inhibitors such as fluoxetine, sertraline, and paroxetine) can exacerbate spasticity and should be used cautiously.[27] Spasticity does not typically abate during spontaneous remissions. In patients with advanced disease, spasticity can be quite disabling and difficult to manage.

Balance and Coordination

Demyelinating lesions in the cerebellum and cerebellar tracts are common in MS, producing cerebellar symptoms. Clinical manifestations include ataxia, postural and intention tremors, hypotonia, and truncal weakness. Ataxia is a general term used to describe uncoordinated movements characterized by **dysmetria**, **dyssynergia**, and **dysdiadochokinesia**. Progressive ataxia of the trunk and LEs is often apparent. During sitting or standing, when a limb or the body must be supported against gravity, the patient typically presents with *postural tremor* (shaking, back-and-forth oscillatory movements). *Intention (action) tremors* are involuntary, rhythmic, shaking movements that occur when purposeful movement is attempted and results from the inability of the cerebellum to dampen motor movements. Tremors vary in severity from slight, barely perceptible quivering (fine tremor) to wide oscillations (gross tremors). Severe tremors impose significant limitations in performance of functional activities, particularly in such areas as eating, speaking clearly, writing, personal hygiene, and walking. Tremor can be exacerbated by stress, excitement, and anxiety, all adrenalin-releasing conditions producing a temporary aroused condition.[28] Severe numbness of the feet can contribute to difficulty with standing balance or walking (sensory ataxia).[15]

Dizziness is a common symptom of MS and results from lesions affecting the cerebellum (archicerebellum) or central vestibular pathways. Patients typically experience difficulties with balance (dysequilibrium), vertigo, nausea, and so forth. Symptoms are precipitated or made worse by movements of the head or eyes. Patients can also experience a paroxysmal attack or sudden onset of symptoms. This can be brought on by a period of hyperventilation.[29]

Ambulation and Mobility

Individuals with MS experience difficulty walking as a result of weakness, fatigue, spasticity, impaired sensation, visual problems, and ataxia. Approximately half of patients with RRMS will require some form of assistance during walking within 15 years of their diagnosis.[30] Staggering, uneven steps, poor foot placement and uncoordinated limb movements, and frequent loss of balance characterize gait. It is often mistaken for drunkenness, a finding that frequently results in the patient revealing the disease for the first time ("outing").

Speech and Swallowing Dysfunction

Speech problems are the result of muscle weakness, spasticity, tremor, or ataxia and affect as many as 40 percent of individuals with MS. **Dysarthria** is characterized by slurred or poorly articulated speech with low volume, unnatural emphasis, and slow rate. **Dysphonia** is characterized by changes in vocal quality including harshness, hoarseness, breathiness, or hypernasal sounds. Poor coordination of the tongue and oral muscles can also result in **dysphagia** or difficulty in swallowing. Signs of swallowing dysfunction include difficulty chewing and maintaining a lip seal, inability to swallow (ingest food), and spitting or coughing during or after meals. Aspiration pneumonia is a serious complication that can develop if foods or liquids are inhaled into the trachea. Signs of this include a wet voice quality with gurgling or sounds of congestion, and fever. The patient is also at risk for poor nutritional intake and dehydration and may experience weight loss. Poor coordination of breath control and posture contributes to speech and feeding difficulties.[31]

Cognitive and Affective Changes

Cognitive Impairments

Cognitive impairments in MS are common, seen in approximately 50 percent of patients. The impairments typically range from mild to moderate impairment, with only 10 percent of patients experiencing problems severe enough to interfere with daily activities. Cognitive impairments are related to the specific distribution of the lesions rather than to the overall severity of the disease, its course, or the patient's disability status. Changes in cognitive function include impaired attention and concentration (especially alternating and divided attention), slowed information processing, impaired recent memory, and impaired executive functions (concept formation, abstract reasoning, problem solving, and planning and sequencing).[32] Focal frontal lobe lesions can produce cognitive inflexibility. Significant mental deterioration (global dementia) is relatively rare and may be seen in rapidly progressing disease (malignant MS) or in patients with significant cerebral lesions. Level of cognitive dysfunction is a major factor in determining quality of life, social functioning, employment status, and function in ADL.[33,34]

Depression

Depression is common in patients with MS, with at least 50 percent of individuals experiencing a major depressive episode.[35] Depressive symptoms can include feelings of hopelessness or despair, diminished interest or pleasure in activities, changes in appetite and significant weight loss or gain, insomnia or hypersomnia, feelings of lethargy or worthlessness, fatigue or loss of energy, decreased concentration, and recurrent thoughts of death and suicide.[35] It can occur as a direct result of MS lesions, as a side effect of some drugs (e.g., steroids, adrenocorticotrophic hormone [ACTH], interferon medications), or as a psychological reaction to the stresses of this far-reaching and unpredictable disease.[36] Anxiety, denial, anger, aggression, or dependency can also occur. Patients with MS face enormous issues related to the ambiguity of their health status, the unpredictable course of disease activity, unpredictable future status, and the loss of effective functioning during the prime of their lives. Feelings of learned helplessness and low self-efficacy are common and have been linked to depression.[37] Moreover, many of the symptoms of MS (tremor, scanning speech, incontinence) are socially embarrassing, causing additional emotional distress.

Affective Changes

Affective disorders occur in approximately 10 percent of cases and can include changes in mood, feelings, emotional expression, and control.[38] **Pseudobulbar affect** (*emotional lability, emotional dysregulation syndrome*) is characterized by sudden loss of emotional control (laughing or crying or both) on multiple occasions that is typically unrelated to external circumstances, depression, or underlying mood. It tends to be associated with more progressive disability and greater intellectual impairment.[39] **Euphoria** consists of an exaggerated feeling of well-being, a sense of optimism incongruent with the patient's incapacitating disability. It also is found primarily in patients with advanced disease.[36] Bipolar affective disorders (alternating periods of depression and mania) can occur. Affective symptoms have been linked to diffuse, bilateral cerebral involvement (especially prefrontal cortex and corticobulbar tracts involved in the control of emotional expression).[40]

Autonomic Changes

Cardiovascular Dysautonomia

Cardiovascular dysautonomia is caused by involvement of the autonomic nervous system and results in problems with cardioacceleration and reduction in blood pressure response during exercise. Some individuals with MS can also have either attenuated or absent sweating responses.

Bladder Dysfunction

Urinary bladder dysfunction occurs in about 80 percent of patients.[41] Loss in volitional and synergistic control of the micturition reflex is produced by demyelinating lesions affecting the lateral and posterior spinal tracts unmasking the sacral reflex arc. Types of bladder dysfunction in MS can include a small, spastic bladder (a failure to store problem), a flaccid or big bladder (a failure to empty problem), or a dyssynergic bladder. The dyssynergic or conflicting bladder represents a problem with coordination between the bladder contraction and sphincter relaxation.[15] Common symptoms include urinary urgency, urinary frequency, hesitancy in starting urination, nocturia (frequency at night), dribbling, and incontinence. The severity of bladder symptoms is associated with severity of other neurological symptoms, particularly pyramidal tract involvement. Progressive loss of functional mobility (e.g., hand skills, sitting balance and transfer skills, ambulation) contributes to personal hygiene problems, emotional distress, and functional incontinence (inability to toilet or manage dysfunction). Emptying dysfunction with large residual urine volume increases the risk of recurrent urinary tract infections (UTI) and kidney damage from frequent UTIs.[42]

Bowel Dysfunction

Constipation is the most common bowel complaint in MS and results from lesions affecting control of the gastrocolic reflex. It is associated with the presence of spasticity of the pelvic floor muscles and is also a frequent consequence of inactivity, lack of fluid intake, poor diet and bowel habits, depression, and medication side effects. Bowel impaction is a serious complication that requires immediate attention. Diarrhea and incontinence is less of a problem but can also occur as a result of loss of rectal control, sphincter abnormalities, or as the result of secondary problems (gastroenteritis, inflammatory bowel disease).[43]

Sexual Dysfunction

Sexual dysfunction is common, affecting as many as 91 percent of men and 72 percent of women. In women, symptoms can include changes in sensation, vaginal dryness, trouble reaching orgasms, and loss of libido. In men, symptoms can include impotence, decreased sensation, difficulty or inability to ejaculate, and loss of libido. Sexual activity is also affected by the appearance of other symptoms such as spasticity, uncontrollable spasms, pain, weakness and fatigue, bladder or bowel incontinence, losses in functional mobility, and changes in self-image. Psychological factors have a large impact on function. Sexual dysfunction has tremendous functional and psychosocial implications for both patient and partner.[15]

Diagnosis

The diagnosis of MS is made by a neurologist based on history, clinical findings, and supportive clinical tests, including magnetic resonance imaging (MRI); CSF; and evoked potentials (EP). Diagnostic criteria for MS are outlined in Table 19.1.[44]

Imaging

MRI is a sensitive tool for confirming disease when used along with other clinical and CSF data. MRI detects both acute and chronic lesions, small and large, with high resolution. Gadolinium is a chemical compound given during MRIs (Gd-MRI). These scans are used to help distinguish new lesions with active inflammation that occur during the preceding 6 weeks or so. Lesions are seen as areas of increased signal intensity, "bright spots." T2 scans are used to detect more long-term disease activity (i.e., loss of myelin and axons, gliosis). These lesions are seen as "black holes" on the MRI; the darker the lesion, the more extensive the tissue damage. Approximately 95 percent of patients with clinically defined MS have well defined MRI changes. Excessive MRI activity includes three or more enhancements on repeat scans separated by at least quarterly intervals (*scattered in time and place*). Lesions revealed on MRI do not always correlate with clinical disability. "Silent attacks" documented by MRI changes outnumber the attacks that cause active symptoms such as paralysis or vision loss by 10:1. Misdiagnosis can occur as 5 percent of individuals with confirmed MS do not exhibit MRI changes. In addition, other diseases can cause similar lesions evident on MRI (e.g., disseminated encephalomyelitis) and some healthy individuals can exhibit bright spots on MRI. Current neurology guidelines call for MRIs to be performed at predefined intervals to document disease progression and response to disease-altering medications.[44]

Cerebrospinal Fluid

Patients with MS show elevated total immunoglobulin in spinal fluid and the presence of oligoclonal IgG bands (seen in 85 to 90 percent of patients). Patients with PPMS have higher levels of immunoglobulins in spinal fluid than patients with RRMS.

Evoked Potentials

Up to 90 percent of individuals with MS demonstrate abnormal evoked potentials. The presence of demyelinating

Table 19.1 Tip Sheet: McDonald Diagnostic Criteria for Multiple Sclerosis (MS)

What Is an Attack?

- Neurological disturbance of the kind seen in MS
- Subjective report or objective observation
- 24 hours duration, minimum
- Excludes pseudoattacks, single paroxysmal episodes

Determining Time Between Attacks

- 30 days between onset of event 1 and onset of event 2

How is "Abnormality" in Paraclinical Tests Determined?	
Magnetic resonance imaging (MRI)	Three out of four: • 1 Gd-enhancing **or** 9 T2 hypertense lesions if no Gd-enhancing lesion • 1 or more Infratentorial lesions • 1 or more juxtacortical lesions • 3 or more periventricular lesions (1 spinal cord lesion = 1 brain lesion)
Cerebrospinal fluid	• Oligoclonal IGG bands in CSF (and not serum) • or elevated IgG index
Evoked potentials	• Delayed but well-preserved wave form

What Provides MRI Evidence of Dissemination in Time?

A Gd-enhancing lesion demonstrated in a scan done at least 3 months following onset of clinical attack at a site different from attack,

or

In absence of Gd-enhancing lesions at 3-month scan, follow-up scan after an additional 3 months showing Gd-lesion or new T2 lesion.

Steps in Making a Diagnosis of MS[a]	
• 2 or more attacks • 2 or more objective clinical lesions	None; clinical evidence will suffice (additional evidence desirable but must be consistent with MS)
• 2 or more attacks • 1 objective clinical lesion	Dissemination in *space,* demonstrated by • MRI[c,d] • Positive CSF and 2 or more MRI lesions consistent with MS • **or** Further clinical attack, different site
• 1 attack • 2 or more objective clinical lesions	Dissemination in *time*, demonstrated by • MRI • **or** second clinical attack
• 1 attack • 1 objective clinical lesion (monosymptomatic presentation)	Dissemination in *space*, demonstrated by • MRI[c,d] • **or** positive CSF and 2 or more MRI lesions consistent with MS **and** Dissemination in *time* demonstrated by • MRI • Second clinical attack

(continued)

Table 19.1 Tip Sheet: McDonald Diagnostic Criteria for Multiple Sclerosis (MS) (continued)

Insidious neurological progression suggestive of MS (primary progressive MS)[b]	Positive CSF **and** Dissemination in *space* demonstrated by • MRI evidence of 9 or more T2 brain lesions • **or** 2 or more spinal cord lesions • **or** positive VEP with 4–8 MRI lesions • **or** positive VEP with <4 brain lesions plus 1 spinal cord lesion **and** Dissemination in *time* demonstrated by • MRI • **or** continued progression for 1 year

From National Multiple Sclerosis Society, with permission.

[a]McDonald et al: Recommended diagnostic criteria for multiple sclerosis: Guidelines from the International Panel on the Dianosis of Multiple Sclerosis. Ann Neurol 50(1):121, 2001.

[b]Thompson et al: Diagnostic criteria for primary progressive MA: A position paper. Ann Neurol 47:832, 2000.

[c]Barkhof et al: Comparison of MR imaging criteria at first presentation to predict conversion to clinically define MS. Brain 120:2059, 1997.

[d]Tintore et al: Isolated demyelinating syndromes: comparison of different imaging criteria to predict conversion to clinically define MS. Am J Radiology 21:702, 2000.

lesions on visual, auditory, somatosensory, or motor pathways produce slowed or abnormal conduction.

It is important to remember that these remain general guidelines and cannot be used to describe outcomes for individual patients.

Prognosis

Only a small percentage of patients actually die as a consequence of the disease. For most individuals, life expectancy is not reduced, with 74 percent of patients surviving 25 years after onset of symptoms. However, only a minority of individuals with MS are still in the workforce 10 years after onset. At 15 years, 50 percent of patients will require the use of an assistive device to walk, and at 20 years, 50 percent will require a wheelchair.[16]

Despite its variable course, certain prognostic factors have been identified in MS.

- *Symptoms*: Onset with only one symptom is one of the strongest indicators of a favorable prognosis.
- *Course of disease*: Benign and RRMS are associated with a more favorable prognosis whereas PPMS is generally considered more ominous.
- *Age*: Young age at onset is more favorable than onset after age 40, which is associated with a PPMS course and increased disability.
- *Neurological findings at 5 years* are one of the most important prognostic factors; significant pyramidal and cerebellar signs with involvement at multiple sites at 5 years is associated with a poorer prognosis and more severe disability.
- *MRI findings*: Favorable prognostic factors include low total lesion burden, low active lesion formation, and negligible myelin or axon loss.

Medical Management

Disease-Modifying Agents

Advances in pharmacotherapy have produced synthetic interferon drugs (interferon beta-1b [Betaseron], interferon beta 1-a [Avonex and Rebif]) that have substantial immunomodulating properties. These are close copies of a naturally occurring human chemical, interferon beta. Interferons slow down the immune system response by reducing inflammation, swelling, and rapid proliferation of T and B cells. They also block activated T cells from crossing the blood–brain barrier and damaging myelin. Other disease-modifying drugs include Glatiramer acetate (Copaxone) and Novantrone. Copaxone is also an immunomodulator that acts as a decoy, clogging T cell receptors. Novantrone is an immunosuppressant and has a limited lifetime dose to prevent heart damage.[45] Table 19.2 presents an overview of the disease-modifying drugs.

For most patients receiving disease-modifying drugs, treatment is only partially effective in controlling their disease. Some patients have shown reduced relapses (by about 30 percent when compared to placebo treatment), reduced severity of attack as evidenced by acquired neurological deficits, fewer and smaller damaged areas on MRI, and a slower rate of disease progression.[46] Continued, frequent relapses or excessive MRI activity may indicate the need to switch drug therapy to higher doses and more

Table 19. 2 Disease-Modifying Drugs[49]

Brand Name Generic Name FDA Approval	Delivery System Frequency Dose
Betaseron Interferon beta—1b Approved 1993,[a]	SC injection Every other day 250 mcg
Avonex Interferon beta-1a Approved 1996,[a and b]	IM injection Once/week 30 mcg
Copaxone Glatiramer acetate Approved 1996,[a]	SC injection Every day 20 mg (20,000 mcg)
Novantrone mitoxantrone Approved 2000,[a and c]	IV infusion in a medical facility Lifetime limit: 8–12 doses 12 mg/m2 every 3 months
Rebif Interferon beta-1a Approved 2002,[a]	SC injection 3 times/week 44 mcg

Approved by the FDA for treatment of
[a] = relapsing-remitting MS
[b] = single clinical episode if MRI features consistent with MS
[c] = progressive-relapsing or secondary-progressive MS
IM = intramuscular injection; IV = intravenous; SC = subcutaneous injection (just under the skin).

frequently administered beta-interferons or combination therapies. However, these agents cannot reverse existing deficits.[47] Clinical trials have primarily included ambulatory patients with RRMS as these drugs are not indicated for PPMS.

Common adverse effects of the interferon drugs include injection-site skin reactions (soreness, redness, pain, bruising, or swelling) and flu-like symptoms following injection that lessen over time (fever, chills, sweating, muscle aches, and fatigue). Injection sites are varied to reduce adverse effects. Rarer and more severe adverse reactions include depression, allergic reactions, and liver reactions. Copaxone can produce similar injection site reactions and an initial flushing reaction immediately after injection (anxiety, chest pain, palpitations, shortness of breath). It has the advantage of not causing flu-like symptoms or depression. Patients receive Novantrone by IV infusion in a medical facility and must be closely monitored for serious heart and liver damage. An additional disadvantage is the significant annual cost of these drugs (in the thousands of dollars) that is not covered by many private insurance plans.[48]

Problems with adherence using immunomodulating agents are well documented. Approximately 38 percent of patients with RRMS are not on immunomodulatory therapy. Health professionals can have a significant impact on promoting acceptance and maintenance of immunomodulating therapy. In discussions with the patient the therapist needs to support the patient's hope for a positive outcome including a benign disease course and a positive effect from drug therapy. Benefits of early treatment and the importance of consistency in management should be emphasized.[49]

Management of Relapses and Symptoms

Prompt management of flare-ups and symptomatic and supportive treatment are essential elements of care. The clinician should have a thorough understanding of the medications the patient is taking, the expected benefit, and potential adverse reactions.

Corticosteroid therapy (e.g., prednisone, methylprednisolone) is used to treat acute disease relapses, shortening the duration of the episode. These drugs exert powerful anti-inflammatory and immunosuppressive effects, diminishing swelling within the CNS and temporarily repairing the blood–brain barrier. They may also prevent circulating toxins or immunoactive cells from entering the CNS. These drugs do not modify the disease course or degree of recovery. Typically corticosteroids are given in high doses (1000 mg/day), administered intravenously for a brief course (e.g., 3 to 5 days), followed by tapered dosage of oral medication over a period of 10 days to 5 to 6 weeks. They are associated with adverse side effects, which can include agitation, nervousness, and insomnia; increased sweating, appetite, and susceptibility to infection; and GI distress including heartburn and diarrhea or constipation. ACTH (adrenocorticotropic hormone) can also be used to provide long-term suppression of the immune system, either alone or in combination with steroids (e.g., cyclophosphamide and ACTH). Potentially serious adverse effects can occur with these powerful im-munosuppressant drugs, including suppression of blood production by bone marrow, bleeding disorders, and increased risk of infection.[15]

Spasticity

Management of spasticity and spasms includes the use of muscle relaxants. Oral baclofen (Lioresal) is typically the first drug of intervention. Dosage is progressed gradually to obtain optimal effects. Other oral agents used include tizanidine (Zanaflex), dantrolene (Dantrium), and diazepam (Valium). The reduction in spasticity must be balanced with the possibility of adverse effects with overdosing, including sedation (drowsiness), weakness, and fatigue. The therapist must be alert to these changes and communicate with the physician to achieve optimal dosing for rehabilitation. The therapist must also recognize that at times spasticity can be used to enhance function, substituting for lack of strength. For example, extensor spasticity can be used to assist standing during a stand-pivot transfer. Significant reduction of spasticity with medications might only serve to produce loss of function. Carbamazepine (Tegretol) can be effective in reducing paroxysmal (sudden, sharp onset) spasms. Patients who do not adequately respond to conservative drug treatment (e.g., those with intractable spasticity or spasms) may benefit from intrathecal administration of baclofen directly into the CSF of the lumbar spine via a catheter. A programmable implanted pump controls the dosage. Significant reduction in spasticity and spasms has been reported in the LEs and trunk with less improvement reported in the UEs. Adverse effects include pump failure, infection, and lead displacement.[50,51]

Surgical interventions are indicated for more severe spasticity. The typical surgical candidate has had spastic paralysis for many years resulting in a nonfunctional limb and serious complications (e.g., contractures and skin breakdown). The techniques include severing tendons (*tendonotomy*), nerves (*neurectomy*), or nerve roots (*rhizotomy*). Phenol nerve blocks are also used to decrease severe spasticity and can be effective for up to 6 months. Botulism toxin (Botox) is a paralytic agent that can cause a temporary blockage of a nerve and muscle that has a similar limited time frame for effectiveness. Repeat injections are then given.[15]

Pain

Pain is managed according to the pathogenesis. Paroxysmal pain responds best to carbamazepine (Tegretol), amitriptyline (Elavil), phenytoin (Dilantin), diazepam (Valium), or gabapentin (Neurontin). Dysesthesias are managed with low doses of amitriptyline (Elavil), imipramine (Tofranil) or desipramine (Norpramin). A wide variety of drugs are used to manage chronic pain. The discomfort and pain associated with spasticity and spasms may be managed with over-the-counter or prescription anti-inflammatory drugs. Pain and numbness can sometimes be successfully managed with a brief course of corticosteroids. Sometimes antidepressants such as amitriptyline (Elavil) are used, or pain is managed with mild painkillers (acetaminophen or ibuprofen. Narcotic analgesics are problematic and not typically prescribed.[18]

Fatigue

Symptomatic treatment of fatigue can also include the use of drugs. Amantadine hydrochloride (Symmetrel) is the recommended first-line therapy in the Clinical Practice Guidelines of the MS Council.[20] This is an antiviral and dopamine agonist shown to have a significant impact on lessening fatigue. Modafinil (Provigil) has also shown efficacy. Although sometimes prescribed, pemoline (Cylert) is a CNS stimulant that has undesirable side effects (e.g., anorexia, irritability, insomnia).

Tremor

Agents to improve tremor have been used with varying degrees of success. Some patients respond well to a single drug, some to combinations of drugs, and some find no benefit. Medications used to decrease tremor include hydroxyzine (Atarax, Vistaril), clonazepam (Klonopin]), propranolol (Inderal), buspirone (Buspar), ondansetron (Zofran), and primidone (Mysoline). Dizziness and vertigo can be managed with antinauseant drugs (Meclizine [Antivert]) or with scopolamine patches). Severe cases may require the administration of a short course of corticosteroids. Severe tremor can also be treated with neurosurgery (thalamotomy) or deep brain stimulation (DBS) that involves implanting electrodes into the thalamus. DBS was developed for patients with Parkinson's disease and remains experimental for patients with MS.[28]

Cognitive and Emotional Problems

Agents approved by the FDA for the treatment of Alzheimer's disease (donepezil [Aricept]) have been used to slow cognitive decline in patients with MS. Modest benefits in memory deficits have been observed.[32] Depression can be managed with any of a number of antidepressant medications (e.g., fluoxetine [Prozac], Paxil, sertraline [Zoloft]). Some antidepressants can also decrease fatigue. Stimulant medications (e.g., methylphenidate [Ritalin], pemoline [Cylert], dextroamphetamine [Dexedrine]) can also be used but may be habit forming. Patients with pseudobulbar affect can be effectively treated with the antidepressant medication amitriptyline (Elavil). Professional counseling and participation in support groups often help the patient cope with the stresses of this unpredictable disease. An active life-style also helps reduce depression and anxiety.[35]

Bladder and Bowel Problems

Urinary problems require a complete urodynamic work-up to identify the specific cause of the problem and to arrive at the appropriate course of treatment. Treatment for an overactive, spastic bladder (storage dysfunction) typically involves pharmacological management with anticholinergic medications (propantheline [Pro-Banthine], oxybutynin [Ditropan], imipramine [Tofranil]) to regulate bladder emptying. Adverse effects can include dry mouth, tachycardia, and accommodation disturbances. Dietary recommendations include drinking 8 glasses of fluid per day (water) while limiting intake of caffeine or alcohol. A flaccid bladder (emptying dysfunction) is managed with alternate techniques for emptying, including instruction in the *Crede maneuver* (the application of manual downward pressure over the lower abdomen) or intermittent self-catheterization (ISC). Dietary recommendations include limiting intake of citrus juices while drinking cranberry juice daily or taking cranberry tablets. A dyssynergic bladder (combined dysfunction) is managed with alpha-adrenergic blocking agents (e.g., terazosin [Hytrin], prazosin [Minipress], tamsulosin [Flow Max]) and antispasticity agents (e.g., baclofen [Lioresal], tizanidine hydrochloride [Zanaflex]). On rare occasions when bladder symptoms cannot be controlled with medication and/or ISC, continuous catheterization (indwelling or Foley catheter; condom, or Texas catheter) or surgical urinary diversion (suprapubic catheter) may be necessary. For example, the patient with advanced disease and significant ataxia of the upper extremities may be unable to manually perform self-catheterization. Urinary tract infections result from retention of urine in the bladder and from catheterization procedures. Antibiotic therapy is the mainstay of treatment.[42]

Constipation is a common problem and is typically managed with dietary changes. These include increased fluid intake and fiber in the diet, and can also include bulk-forming supplements (Metamucil, FiberCon, Citrucel), or stool softeners (dioctyl sodium sulfosuccinate [Colace]). Regular or continuous use of stimulant laxatives and enemas is not recommended. Incontinence management includes dietary changes such as avoidance of irritants (caffeine, alcohol), adjustment of medications used to reduce spasticity which can contribute to the problem, or addition of medications to control bowel spasms (tolterodine [Detrol], propantheline [Pro-Banthine]).[43]

Framework for Rehabilitation

The chronicity of this disease, along with its variable and unpredictable course, may lead some to view individuals with MS as poor rehabilitation candidates. While the disease cannot be altered by rehabilitation, there is a growing body of evidence that indicates significant gains in reducing impairments and promoting functional mobility and independence can be achieved. In addition, known complications of MS can be reduced or prevented while quality of life is enhanced.[52–71]

According to the National MS Society's Medical Advisory Board, rehabilitation referral should be initiated whenever there is an "abrupt or gradual worsening of function or an increase in impairment that has a significant impact on the individual's mobility, safety, independence, and/or quality of life.[72, p1]

Individuals with neurodegenerative diseases such as MS benefit from **restorative intervention,** aimed at remediating or improving impairments, functional limitations, and disabilities.[73] Direct CNS impairments may be less responsive to intervention, especially in the late stages of the disease. However, during the early and middle stages of the disease, a focus on remediating impairments can result in meaningful improvements in function (e.g., strength training results in improved balance and gait). Indirect impairments caused by evolving multisystem dysfunction from inactivity and disuse (Fig. 19.1) or comorbidities are also an important focus of restorative care. This is especially true in the later stages of the disease when these impairments may evolve quickly and require prompt treatment. Goals and outcome statements reflective of restorative intervention focus on remediating impairments and regaining functional independence while promoting self-management skills. As the disease progresses, important goals and outcomes also include assisting the patient in effective coping skills by promoting acceptance and adjustment to limitations and disabilities and enhancing quality of life. The enhancement of quality of life may in

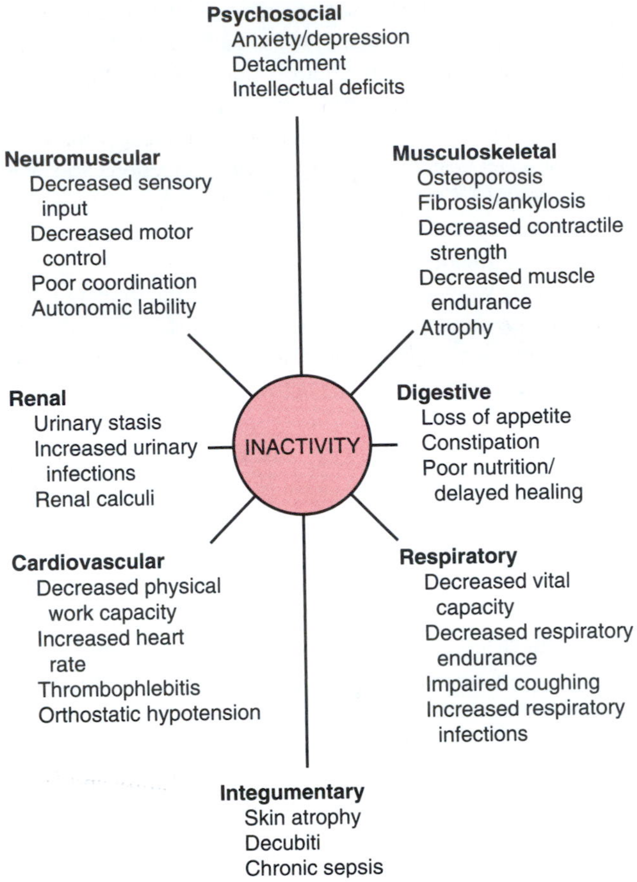

Figure 19.1 Clinical manifestations of inactivity.

fact be the most meaningful outcome for patients in the face of chronic neurodegenerative disease.

Preventative intervention is aimed at minimizing potential complications, impairments, functional limitations, or disabilities as the disease progresses. This includes prevention of a disease in a susceptible or potentially susceptible population, termed *primary prevention.* Preventive efforts for the patient with MS are geared toward decreasing the duration and severity of symptoms or delaying the emergence of disease sequelae through early detection and intervention, termed *secondary prevention.* Prevention is also aimed at minimizing the degree of disability, termed *tertiary prevention.* Goal and outcome statements reflective of preventative intervention focus on promotion of health, wellness, fitness, and preservation of optimal function.[73]

Compensatory intervention is aimed at modifying the task, activity, or environment in order to allow the patient to remain fully functional within the scope of existing impairments and limitations. Goal and outcome statements reflective of compensatory intervention focus on regaining/maintaining function.

Maintenance therapy is defined as a series of occasional clinical, educational, and administrative services designed to maintain the patient's current level of function.[111] Individuals with MS who benefit from maintenance therapy typically are in the late stages of the disease (EDSS stages

7.0 to 9.5). Maintenance programs are typically not well funded by private insurance. Medicare, which covers services for the elderly and the disabled, will cover maintenance therapy if the skills of a therapist (specialized knowledge and judgment) are needed to manage a patient because of identified dangers. For example, risk of secondary impairment and loss of functional capabilities is reduced or safety of caregivers is enhanced. The therapist examines and evaluates the patient, designs an intervention program appropriate to the capacity and tolerance of the patient and the objectives of medical management, implements the plan of care, and periodically reevaluates the plan as required by the patient's condition. A variety of interventions are used to achieve goals and outcomes, including limited direct interventions, patient/client-related instruction, and supportive counseling. The primary focus is to teach patients, family, and caregivers the management skills necessary to carry out the maintenance program.[74,75]

A coordinated interdisciplinary team is necessary to oversee the comprehensive examination and management needed to address the patient's complex and multifaceted problems. The team typically includes the physician, nurse, physical therapist, occupational therapist, speech–language pathologist, nutritionist, and social worker. As with any team, the patient is the central figure, with family and caregivers being key members. The ideal rehabilitation program considers the patient's disease history, course and symptoms, including impairments, functional limitations, and disability. Of equal importance are the patient's abilities (assets), priorities, and resources (e.g., family, home, community). The focus is on long-range planning with anticipated episodes of care, including hospital-based, outpatient, and home/community-based care. Dal Bello-Haas[76] discusses a continuum of care based on disease stage (early, middle, and late) for individuals with neurodegenerative diseases.

Physical Therapy Examination

Because many different areas of the CNS may be affected, it is imperative that a careful examination is performed to determine the extent of neurological and functional involvement. Subsequent reexamination at specified intervals are used to distinguish change in status as well as effects of treatment. It may not always be possible to differentiate change in status associated with remission of symptoms from treatment outcomes. Considering the variability of symptoms of any individual patient, it is often beneficial to perform the initial examination over a period of a few days to obtain a representative sample of baseline functioning. Fatigue and exacerbating factors should be taken into account when scheduling the examination.

Physical therapy examination data can be obtained through the patient's history and systems review, and relevant tests and measures. The selection of examination procedures and level of inquiry are determined by the patient's unique status. The severity of problems, stage of disease (acute, subacute, chronic), age, phase and setting of rehabilitation, and other factors must all be taken into account in structuring the examination.

Patient/Client History

Data obtained through interview with the patient/family and review of the medical record should include information on general demographics, medical/surgical history, social and employment history, family history, living environment, general health status, and social and health habits. The patient's current/chief complaints and current functional status, and activity level should be ascertained. Coexisting health problems and medications should also be identified. Data obtained from the history will help focus further in-depth examination and systems review (Box 19.3).

Tests and Measures

The following are specific areas and relevant tests and measures that can be used to examine function in patients with MS (for more detailed descriptions, see earlier chapters in this text focusing on examination).

Cognition

Memory function, attention, concentration, conceptual reasoning, problem solving, speed of information processing should be examined as well as the effects of fatigue on cognitive performance. An expert panel convened by the Consortium of MS Centers in 2001 developed the *Minimal Examination of Cognitive Function in MS (MACFIMS)*. This comprehensive battery includes seven neuropsychological tests examining processing speed/working memory, learning and memory, executive function, visual—spatial processing, and word retrieval. The MACFIMS takes approximately 90 minutes to administer.[77] A brief screen of cognitive function can be achieved using the *Mini Mental Status Exam (MMSE)*.[78]

Affective and Psychosocial Function

Emotional stability should be examined. The presence of emotional lability, euphoria, emotional dysregulation; depression (symptoms, severity, length, effect on functional performance); level of stress and anxiety, coping strategies; and presence of sleep disorders should be documented. A useful instrument is the *Beck Depression Inventory*.[79]

Sensation

Superficial and deep sensations (touch, pressure, temperature, pain, proprioceptive) and combined or cortical sensations (stereognosis, tactile localization, two-point discrimination) should be examined. The presence of acute, paroxysmal pain (Lhermitte's sign, dysesthesias) and chronic pain including pain behaviors and reactions during specific

Box 19.3 **Elements of the Examination of the Patient with Multiple Sclerosis[73]**

Patient/Client History
- Age, sex, race/ethnicity, primary language, education
- Social history: cultural beliefs and behaviors, family and caregiver resources, social support systems
- Occupation/employment/work
- Living environment: home/work barriers
- Hand dominance
- General health status: physical, psychological, social, and role function, health habits
- Family history
- Medical/surgical history
- Current conditions/chief complaints
- Medications
- Medical/laboratory test results
- Functional status and activity level: premorbid and current

Systems Review
- Neuromuscular
- Musculoskeletal
- Cardiovascular/pulmonary
- Integumentary

Tests and Measures/Impairments
- Cognition: mental status, memory
- Communication
- Anthropometric characteristics: body mass index, girth, length
- Circulation: response to position change/degree of orthostatic hypotension
- Aerobic capacity and endurance: during functional activities and standardized exercise protocols. Cardiovascular signs and symptoms in response to exercise and activity. Pulmonary signs and symptoms in response to exercise and activity.
- Ventilation and gas exchange
- Integumentary integrity: skin condition, pressure sensitive areas; activities, positioning, and postures to relieve pressure
- Sensory integrity and integration
- Pain: intensity and location
- Perceptual function: visuospatial skills
- Joint integrity, alignment, and mobility: range of motion (active and passive); muscle length, and soft tissue extensibility
- Posture: alignment and position, symmetry (static and dynamic, sitting and standing); ergonomics, and body mechanics
- Muscle performance: strength, power, and endurance
- Motor function: motor control and motor learning.
- Postural control and balance: degree of postural instability, balance strategies; safety
- Gait and locomotion: gait pattern and speed, safety
- Functional status and activity level: performance-based examination of functional skills (FIM level), basic and instrumental ADL; functional mobility skills; home management skills
- Psychosocial function: motivation
- Assistive or adaptive devices: fit, alignment, function, use; safety
- Environment, home, and work barriers
- Work, community, and leisure activities: ability to participate in activities, safety

movements and provoking stimuli should be documented. The *McGill Pain Questionnaire*[80] or the *Dallas Pain Questionnaire*, developed to examine the effects of chronic spinal pain on daily activities, anxiety–depression, and social interest, can be used.[81]

Visual Acuity

Acuity, tracking, and accommodation should be examined; the presence of visual deficits (blurred vision, field defects [scotoma], diplopia) should be documented.

Cranial Nerve Integrity

Motor and sensory cranial nerve function should be examined; the presence of deficits (optic pain [optic neuritis], oculomotor dyscontrol, dysphagia, impaired gag reflex, trigeminal neuralgia) should be documented.

Range of Motion (ROM)

Passive (PROM) and active (AROM) range of motion should be examined; the presence of specific ROM deficits should be documented.

Muscle Performance

Functional strength using manual muscle testing (MMT) and dynamometers (isokinetic, grasp and pinch dynamometers) should be examined; strong spasticity may be a contraindication to standard MMT positions.

Fatigue

The frequency, duration, and severity of fatigue should be examined; precipitating factors; activity levels and efficacy of rest attempts should be documented. The *Modified Fatigue Impact Scale (MFIS)* was developed by Fisk et al[82,83] and is included in the National Multiple Sclerosis Society Clinical Practice Guidelines on Fatigue.[84] It is a structured, self-report 21-item questionnaire addressing the effects of fatigue on cognitive, physical, and psychosocial function using a 5-point ordinal scale with 0 equal to never and 4 equal to almost always. Each area (subscale) can be scored separately; the total MFIS score range is from 0 to 84 (see Appendix A). The MFIS can be downloaded in PDF format from http://www.nationalmssociety.org/MUCS_fatigue.asp. An abbreviated version of the MFIS has five items (the *MFIS-5*).

Temperature Sensitivity

The degree of temperature sensitivity and its effect on fatigue and weakness should be examined. A tympanic membrane thermometer (ear thermometer) can be used before, during, and after moderate-intensity exercise. A determination of the correlation between temperature changes and worsening of neurological symptoms can be made.

Motor Function

The therapist should examine for the presence of corticospinal signs (paresis, spasticity, hyperactive DTRs, positive Babinski's sign, and involuntary spasms [flexor or extensor]). The *Amended Motor Club Examination (AMCA)* was developed to examine the nature and degree of motor and functional deficits in patients with MS.[85]

Spasticity can be examined using a subjective rating scale. The *Ashworth Spasticity Scale*[86] led to the more widely used the *Modified Ashworth Scale*.[87] These are ordinal scales designed to measure tone intensity; the modified Ashworth has an additional grade at the lower end allowing for more discrete rating. A determination should be made of the differences between lower limbs versus upper limbs, right and left sides; and factors that influence tone.

The therapist should examine for the presence of cerebellar signs (ataxia, intention tremor, nystagmus, dysarthria). The effects of position change (e.g., sitting-to-standing) may produce an increase in ataxic movements with increased demands for postural stability and should be documented.

The therapist should examine for the presence of vestibular dysfunction (dizziness, vertigo, nystagmus, blurred vision with head and body movements, and postural imbalance).

Posture

Static and dynamic postural control in various different positions (e.g. sitting, standing) should be examined. The presence of postural abnormalities and postural tremor should be documented. Instruments can include posture grids, plumb lines, still photography with light-emitting diodes.

Balance, Gait, and Locomotion

The therapist should examine static and dynamic balance, reactive and anticipatory control, sensory interaction, and synergistic strategies. Useful instruments include the *Clinical Test for Sensory Interaction in Balance,*[88] dynamic posturography,[89,90] the *Berg Balance Scale,*[91,92] and the *Tinetti Performance Oriented Mobility Examination (POMA)*.[93]

Gait parameters and characteristics should be examined including gait speed, kinematics, stability, safety, and endurance. Examination of patients with significant ataxia can be enhanced through the use of videotaped performance. Useful tests include timed walk tests (10-meter Walk Test or 6-Minute Walk Test); the *Dynamic Gait Index*[94]; and the *Ambulation Index (AI)*.[95] The *Rivermead Visual Gait Examination (RVGA)*[96] was developed to examine gait in patients with MS.

Alignment and fit, safety, practicality and ease of use of orthotic and assistive devices should be examined along with energy conservation and expenditure. Wheelchair skills including functional mobility, management, safety, transfer skills, and energy conservation and expenditure should be examined.

Aerobic Capacity and Endurance

Vital signs (heart rate, blood pressure, respiratory rate) and breathing patterns should be examined at rest and during exercise. Exertional symptoms (dyspnea, elevated blood pressure, heart rate, respiratory rate) and perceived exertion during and after activity should be documented. Useful scales include the *Rating of Perceived Exertion Scale (the Borg RPE scale)*[97] and the *Dyspnea Scale*.[98]

Skin Integrity and Condition

Skin integrity and condition should be examined. The presence of areas of insensitivity, bruising, moisture build-up, and skin breakdown should be documented along with level of urinary continence; bed and wheelchair positioning, effectiveness of pressure relieving compensatory strategies and pressure-relieving devices (PRDs); and cognitive status and safety awareness.

Functional Status

An examination of functional mobility skills (FMS), basic activities of daily living (BADL) and instrumental activities of daily living (IADL) is indicated along with social functioning; community and work adaptive skills. A commonly used instrument for patients undergoing active rehabilitation is the *Functional Independence Measure (FIM)*.[99,100]

Environment (Home, Community, and Work)

Physical space for barriers, access, safety should be examined; a specific task-analysis (patient performance-based examination) in relevant environments (home, work) may be included (see Chapter 12).

General Health

General health measures are used to examine outcomes across a broad spectrum of global or long-term health outcomes. Instruments involve self-report of the patient's perceptions of physical limitations and quality of life (e.g., physical and social function, general health and vitality, emotional well-being, bodily pain, and so forth). The *Health Status Questionnaire (SF-36)*[101] is widely acknowledged as the gold standard of generic measures of health status. The properties of this instrument have been investigated in patients with MS. Freeman et al[102] found limitations in evaluating change in moderate to severely disabled patients participating in inpatient rehabilitation with significant floor and ceiling effects in four of eight SF-36 dimensions. The *Sickness Impact Profile,*[103] and the *Examination of Motor and Process Skills (AMPS)*[104] are also general health measures.

Disease-Specific Measures

Disease-specific measures are designed to examine attributes common in a specific disease entity. Items are included to provide information about the disease process and outcomes, and ideally document clinically meaningful change over time. Thus the instruments have greater responsiveness or sensitivity to change than general health measures.

Expanded Disability Status Scale (EDSS) for Patients with Multiple Sclerosis

In 1955, Kurtzk developed a 10-point scale for rating overall disability in MS (the Disability Status Scale or DSS).[105] This scale was expanded in 1983 to increase its clinical sensitivity by including half-point increments, becoming the EDSS (Appendix B).[106] This scale has been widely adopted by clinicians and has been used to standardize MS research. Based on a standard neurological examination, patients are first graded on presenting symptoms in seven specific functional systems including pyramidal, cerebellar, brainstem, sensory, bowel and bladder, visual, mental, plus other functions. Functional system scores (FSS) are obtained using an ordinal clinical rating scale ranging from 0 to 5 or 6. The EDSS is based on the grades obtained from the FSS and uses a 0 to 10 ordinal scale graded in half-point increments, with 0 equal to normal neurological function and 10.0 equal to death owing to MS. For example, patients classified in EDSS step 2.5 demonstrate minimal disability in two FSS (two FSS grade 2, others 0 or 1). The EDSS focuses on ambulation as the primary indicator of disability (see scores 3.0 through 6.5 for levels of ambulation; patients with scores 7.0 or greater are unable to walk). Criticisms of the EDSS include its lack of sensitivity to changes that do not include functional mobility (ambulation) and problems in interrater reliability with patients whose performance is less impaired (scores in the lower ranges, ambulation less impaired).[107] Copies of the EDSS can be obtained from the National Multiple Sclerosis Society at http://www.nationalmssociety.org/MUCS_FSS.asp.

The Minimum Record of Disability (MRD)

The MRD was developed by the International Federation of Multiple Sclerosis Societies in 1985.[108] This instrument has three subscales: the EDSS with FSS, the *Incapacity Status Scale (ISS),* and the *Environmental Status Scale (ESS).* It is widely used and includes classification of dysfunction according to World Health Organization terminology. Thus, the instrument addresses impairments (the FS and EDSS), disability (ISS), and handicap (ESS). The ISS includes 16 items that address functional disability in ADL. The ESS measures social performance including work status, financial and economic status, place of residence, personal assistance, transportation, community assistance, and social activity. Solari et al[109] examined the validity of the self-administered version of the MRD and found that determination of ambulatory ability, ADL skills, and social activities was both accurate and cost-effective.

MS Functional Composite (MSFC)

The MSFC is a 21-item test that includes 3 different functional subtests including the Timed 25-Foot Walk (T23-FW), 9-Hole Peg Test (9HPT), and the Paced Auditory Serial Addition Test (PASAT). The MSFC Administration and Scoring Manual can be obtained from the National Multiple Sclerosis Society at http://www.nationalmssociety.org/MUCS_MSFC.asp.

Multiple Sclerosis Quality of Life—54 (MSQOL)

The test is a modification of the generic *Health Status Questionnaire (SF-36)* with the addition of items relevant to people with MS. It omits one item in the SF-36 (graphic representation of quality of life) and instead uses a semantic differential scale. There are 11 subscales: physical health, role limitations due to physical problems (RLPP), role limitations due to emotional problems (RLEP), pain, emotional well-being, energy, health perceptions, social function, cognitive function, health distress, and sexual function.[110]

MS Quality of Life Inventory (MSQLI)

The MSQLI was developed as a comprehensive outcomes examination package by the Consortium of Multiple Sclerosis Centers, Health Science Research Subcommittee.[111] In includes a battery of 10 self-report scales (138 items) that provide information about health-related quality of life in MS, including the Health Status Questionnaire (SF-36), the Modified Fatigue Impact Scale (MFIS), the MOS Pain Effects Scale (PES), Sexual Satisfaction Scale (SSS), Bladder Control Scale (BLCS), Bowel Control Scale (BWCS), Impact of Visual Impairment Scale (IVIS), Perceived Deficits Questionnaire (PDQ), Mental Health Inventory (MHI) and the MOS Modified Social Support Survey (MSSS). The battery can be administered in approximately 45 minutes in most cases. Abbreviated versions of some of the scales can reduce the set to 81 items requiring approximately 30 minutes to administer. A User's Manual can be obtained from http://www.nationalmssociety.org/MUCS_MSQLI.asp.

Functional Examination of Multiple Sclerosis (FAMS)

The FAMS is a 59-item index of health-related quality of life measure developed by Cella et al.[112] There are six subscales (mobility, symptoms, emotional well-being [depression], general contentment, thinking/fatigue, and family/social well-being). The mobility subscale strongly correlates with the Kurtzke EDSS.

Multiple Sclerosis Impact Scale (MSIS-29)

The MSIS-29 measures the physical and psychological impact of MS.[113] The scale was primarily developed for

Box 19.4 Examples of General Goals and Outcomes for Patients with Progressive Disorders of the Central Nervous System

Impact of pathology/pathophysiology is reduced.
- Patient/client, family, and caregiver knowledge and awareness of the disease, prognosis, and plan of care is enhanced.
- Symptom management is enhanced.
- Risk of secondary impairment is reduced.
- Intensity of care is decreased.

Impact of impairments is reduced.
- Cognitive function is improved.
- Joint integrity and mobility are improved.
- Sensory awareness and skin integrity are improved.
- Pain is decreased.
- Motor function is improved.
- Muscle performance (strength, power, and endurance) is improved.
- Postural control and balance are improved.
- Gait and locomotion are improved.
- Management of fatigue is enhanced.
- Aerobic capacity is increased.

Ability to perform physical actions, tasks, or activities is improved.
- Independence in activities of daily living is increased.
- Tolerance of positions and activities is increased.
- Activity pacing and energy conservation are enhanced.
- Problem-solving and decision making skills are enhanced.
- Safety of patient/client, family, and caregivers is improved.

Disability associated with chronic illness is reduced.
- Ability to assume/resume self-care and home management is improved.
- Ability to assume work (job/school/play), community, and leisure roles is improved.
- Patient/client and family knowledge and awareness of personal and environmental factors associated with worsening of the condition is enhanced.
- Awareness and use of community resources are improved.

Health status and quality of life are improved.
- Sense of well-being is enhanced.
- Stressors are reduced.
- Insight, self-confidence, and self-management skills are improved.
- Health, wellness, and fitness are improved.

Patient/client satisfaction is enhanced.
- Access and availability of services are acceptable to patient/client and family.
- Quality of rehabilitation services is acceptable to patient/client and family.
- Care is coordinated with patient/client, family, caregivers, and other professionals.

Adapted from the *Guide to Physical Therapist Practice.*[73]

community-based populations though testing with hospital-based populations (patients admitted for inpatient rehabilitation, IV corticosteroid treatment for MS relapses, and patients with PPMS) revealed consistency of psychometric properties.[114]

Goals and Outcomes

The general goals and outcomes for patients with progressive disorders of the central nervous system, adapted from the *Guide to Physical Therapist Practice,*[73] are presented in Box 19.4. These general goals will provide the basis for the development of specific anticipated goals and expected outcomes for an individual patient.

The preferred practice pattern for patients with multiple sclerosis from the *Guide for Physical Therapist Practice* is 5 E, *Impaired Motor Function and Sensory Integrity Associated with Progressive Disorders of the Central Nervous System.* In this document the reader will find relevant information on patient/client diagnostic classification; ICD-9-CM codes; examination components; considerations for evaluation, diagnosis, and prognosis; and suggested interventions. Thus the Guide serves as a primary resource to help physical therapists design an appropriate plan of care and document the services provided and outcomes achieved. Additional resources for effective documentation of functional outcomes include the works of Quinn and Gordon[115] and Dittmar and Gresham.[116]

Physical Therapy Interventions

Management of Sensory Deficits and Skin Care

Strategies should be instituted to increase awareness of sensory deficits, compensate for sensory loss, and promote safety. It is important to remember that sensory deficits may remit, so ongoing examination is necessary. The success of compensatory training strategies depends on the availability of other intact sensory systems. For example, visual compensation techniques can be instituted when deficits in proprioception produce imbalance and place the patient at risk for falls. If multiple sensory systems are involved (e.g., vision is also impaired), sensory compensatory strategies are not likely to be successful.

Patients with proprioceptive losses demonstrate impairments in movement control and motor learning. They require increased use of other sensory systems, especially vision. Tapping, verbal cueing, and/or biofeedback can all be effective forms of augmented feedback. Proprioceptive loading through exercise, light tracking resistance, resistance bands or weights, and the use of a pool may heighten residual proprioceptive function and improve movement awareness.

Visual loss will interfere with movement and postural control. Blurred vision, especially at night or in low light situations, can occur after episodes of optic neuritis. It is therefore important to instruct the patient in maintaining adequate lighting at all times (e.g., use of a bright light at night) and reducing clutter to improve safety. Adding contrast between items in the environment (e.g., stair markings) can also improve safety. Double vision is the frequent result of impaired coordination and weak eye muscles. It can be controlled by placing a patch over one eye and is an important strategy for improving reading, driving, or watching television. However, eye patching should not be used all the time as it will prevent possible adaptation of the CNS. Eye patching also interferes with depth perception. The symptoms of visual blurring and double vision also fluctuate and can be heightened with fatigue, an increase in temperature, stress, and infection. Management of these symptoms can be an important strategy to improve vision.[15] If low vision persists, the patient should be referred to a low-vision specialist or one of the national service organizations that provide help to individuals with vision impairments (National Association for Visually Handicapped, National Federation of the Blind, American Foundation for the Blind).

Patients with deficits in superficial sensations risk damage to insensitive areas of skin. The development of decubitus ulcers becomes a major concern in individuals with chronic, progressive disease. Changes in skin turgor, static posturing, and prolonged pressure over bony prominences increase the likelihood of skin breakdown. Patients may not feel the discomfort of prolonged positioning or may be unable to shift position because of weakness or spasticity. In addition, spasticity and/or spasms may cause friction effects between the skin and supporting surfaces. Awareness, protection, and care of desensitized parts should be taught early in the rehabilitation process and consistently reinforced by all members of the team. The patient/family/caregiver should be educated in the following principles of skin care:

- The skin should be kept clean and dry. Soiled skin should be cleansed and dried promptly.
- The skin should be inspected regularly (at least once a day) and carefully, with particular attention to persistent areas of redness and over bony prominences.
- Clothing should be breathable and comfortable (soft, not too loose or wrinkled, or too tight). Seams, buttons, and pockets should not press on the skin, particularly in weightbearing areas.
- Regular pressure relief is essential. Patients should be instructed to change their position or be changed frequently, typically every 2 hours in bed and every 15 minutes when sitting in a wheelchair. Wheelchair push-ups or repositioning maneuvers should be taught to relieve pressure.

Pressure-relieving devices (PRDs) may be necessary to protect insensitive areas and should be implemented as appropriate. These can include mattresses (water, gel, air, or alternating pressure) to distribute body weight and reduce shear and friction in bed. Sheepskins, air or foam cushions, cuffs, and/or boots may be necessary to protect body areas prone to breakdown (shoulder blades, elbows, ischial tuberosities, sacrum, trochanters, knees, malleoli, or heels). Cushions (foam; fluid or air pressure-relieving cushions) are necessary for patients who spend prolonged periods of time sitting in their wheelchair.

Prevention is the best strategy. Important measures for maintaining skin integrity and function include maintaining good nutrition and drinking plenty of fluids. The patient must be cautioned against activities that might traumatize the skin. Dragging, bumping, or scraping body parts during a transfer or bed mobility activities can injure the skin. Thermal injury can result from contact with hot water or hot objects. If skin redness develops (lasting longer than 30 minutes) patients should be instructed to stay off the area until the redness disappears. Blisters, blue areas, or open sores indicate more serious injury and require immediate attention. This may include systemic antibiotic therapy for infection and wound management techniques (cleansing and débridement, topical antibiotic agents, and protective dressings).[15]

Management of Pain

The management of pain depends on an accurate determination of its causes. Musculoskeletal strain or joint malalignment from chronically weakened muscles are important considerations and are responsive to physical therapy intervention. Patients may experience relief of pain with regular stretching or exercise, massage, and ultrasound. Postural retraining and correction of faulty movement patterns along with orthotic and/or adaptive seating devices can reduce malalignment and pain. Stabbing pain from Lhermitte's sign may be relieved with a soft collar to limit neck flexion. Hydrotherapy or pool therapy using *lukewarm* water may have a beneficial effect on painful dysesthesias. Pressure stockings or gloves can also be used to relieve pain, converting the sensation of pain to one of pressure. Neutral warmth may be a factor in the pain relief experienced with stockings or gloves. Patients with chronic pain will benefit from referral to a total management approach for chronic pain, for example, the *multidisciplinary pain clinic* (see Chapter 28). Stress management techniques, relaxation training, biofeedback, meditation, and so forth are often helpful in reducing both anxiety and pain. The use of transcutaneous electrical nerve stimulation (TENS) to modulate pain in patients with MS has had conflicting results, with some patients experiencing improvement and some a worsening of symptoms.[15]

Exercise Training

Muscle weakness and decreased endurance are common findings in patients with MS. In addition, patients with MS often adopt a sedentary lifestyle and limit their physical activity, sometimes on the mistaken advice of health care professionals who seek to minimize relapses and symptoms of fatigue.[72] The benefits of exercise have been firmly established in terms of producing meaningful physiological and psychological changes, improving function while lessening disability, and enhancing quality of life.[117–125] Individuals with minimal to moderate impairments (i.e., EDSS scores between 1 and 6) and stable disease demonstrate the best exercise tolerance. This speaks to the need to institute exercises early in the course of the disease. Exercise responses of the patient with MS are influenced by a host of factors that require careful attention during exercise, including fatigue, spasticity, incoordination, impaired balance, sensory loss and numbness, tremor, and heat intolerance. Depression may affect adherence. Therapists therefore need to provide constant reinforcement and a positive environment. Box 19.5 presents a summary of research on *Exercise and Multiple Sclerosis*.

Strength and Conditioning

Maximal muscle force during sustained isometric or isokinetic exercise is lower for persons with MS secondary to reduced ability to activate muscles (reduced force/unit muscle mass), reduced muscle metabolic responses, and muscle weakness secondary to muscle fiber atrophy, spasticity, and disuse.[126] Determining an appropriate exercise prescription to improve strength and endurance is challenging and needs to be carefully individualized for each patient. Prescription is based on four interrelated elements: frequency of exercise, intensity of exercise, type of exercise, and time or duration (the *FITT equation*). The following guidelines can be used[127,128]:

- Exercise sessions should be scheduled on alternate (nonendurance) days and during optimal times, such as in the morning, when body core temperatures tend to be lowest and before fatigue sets in.[128] Patients with greater neurological involvement may require more frequent exercise (e.g., daily exercise time).
- Submaximal exercise intensities (moderate intensities 50 to 70 percent MVC) are tolerated, whereas maximal exercise is generally not well tolerated.[117]
- Resistance training modes can include weight machines, free or pulley weights, elastic resistance bands, or isokinetic machines.[117,118]
- Circuit training, in which improved work capacity is developed through the use of various different stations that alternate work between upper and lower extremities, distributes the load among muscles and may prove best for reducing the likelihood of fatigue.[118]
- Sessions should involve discontinuous work, carefully balancing exercise with adequate rest periods.
- Progression is generally slower than with healthy individuals.[127]
- Precautions should be taken to prevent the deleterious effects of overwork. Exercising to the point of fatigue is contraindicated and can result in worsening of symptoms, most notably increased weakness. This may have additional adverse effects on the continuing motivation of the patient.[127]
- Precautions should be taken to monitor the effects of fatigue. *Time-to-fatigue* varies greatly among individuals with MS and is *not* correlated with the level of physical impairment or disability.[126]
- Precautions should be taken to manage core body temperature and prevent overheating. Environmental temperatures should be carefully controlled. Air conditioning is a medical necessity in many climates. Additional cooling can be achieved through the use of fans,[122] wet neck wraps, and spray bottles for misting the skin with cool water, and immersion in cool water with aquatic exercises.[118,120,121,128,129] Surface cooling devices have emerged as effective tools in managing body temperatures, controlling fatigue, and improving function. These include cooling suits[130–132] or vests.[133]
- Precautions should be taken with certain impairments. Tactile and proprioceptive losses or incoordination and tremors may make the use of some equipment (e.g., free weights) unsafe. Visual feedback, when intact, should be used to monitor exercise performance. An alternate suggestion would be to use synchronized arm/leg ergometers to control limb movements.[126]
- Precautions should be taken with cognitive and memory impairments. Individuals may require written or posted exercise instructions/diagrams including reminders of the number of repetitions, proper form, and correct use of equipment.[126]
- Functional training activities (e.g., closed chain exercises) can be used to promote strength and functional endurance. Individuals with balance problems require the use of more stable postures (e.g., plantigrade, quadruped, or supported sitting).[134]
- Group exercise classes can provide valuable motivation and social support. The therapist's primary role is one of educator and group leader. Successful management of group classes requires careful, individualized examination of group members to determine specific goals and exercises. Significant improvements have been demonstrated in patients with MS not in active exacerbations.[135]
- Outcome measures include MMT, isokinetic dynamometry, body composition, fatigue (MFIS), functional tests, and quality of life measures (HRQL).

Cardiovascular Conditioning

Individuals with MS demonstrate expected physiological responses to submaximal aerobic exercise, that is, heart rate (HR), blood pressure (BP), and oxygen uptake (Vo_2)

(text continues on page 798)

Evidence Summary Box 19.5

Exercise and Multiple Sclerosis

Reference	Subjects	Design/ Intervention	Duration	Results	Comments
White, LJ, et al[117] 2004	8 subjects with MS, mild-mod disability; EDSS scores between 1 and 5; baseline BMI = 27% (overweight category)	Nonrandomized, cohort design Resistance training (RT) progressing from 50% to 70% MVIC; Outcome measures: MVIC on isokinetic dynamometer, MRI thigh muscles, body composition, 25-ft Walk Test, MFIS, EDSS	8 weeks, 2×/week	Significant ⇑ in strength of knee ext (7%), plantarflexion (52%) Stepping performance ⇑ (8.7%); fatigue ⇓ on MFIS (24%); self-report disability (EDSS) ⇓ from 3.7 > 3.2; no change BME; no MS exacerbations reported	Lacked control group; RT resulted in ⇑ strength and ambulatory function; RT is a safe, well tolerated intervention; small sample size
Surakka J, et al[118] 2004	95 with MS, mild-mod disability; EDSS scores between 1 and 5.5; exercise group = 46; Non-exercise group = 48	Randomized control trial 5 supervised resistance and 5 aerobic exercise sessions; aerobic exercises in pool (temp 28˚C), 65–70% age-predicted HR_{max}; resistance training (RT) = circuit training UE and LE Ms, 50–60% 1 RM; home exercise program (HEP): RT used elastic bands; aerobic training, walking; subjects kept daily diary; Outcome measures: Ms torque (dynamometer); Fatigue (FI, FSS, AFI)	Supervised exercise = 3 weeks; HEP = 23 weeks	Significant ⇓ in motor fatigue in women (*n* = 30) but not men (*n* = 17) after 6 months of aerobic and strength exercise; exercise activity of women was 25% more than men.	Long training period (6 months) may have masked disease progression, especially in men. Men more likely to have PPMS then RRMS.
Mostert, S, and Kesselring, J[119] 2002	37 subjects with MS, mild-mod disability, inpatient rehabilitation; EDSS scores between 2.5–6.5; MS-Exercise group =13; MS–no intervention group = 13; Healthy control group = 26	Randomized control trial Aerobic exercise training: leg cycle ergometry; Outcome measures: Max GXT; tests of lung function (FVC); spasticity LEs (mAS); EDSS Baecke Activity Questionnaire; SF-36 Health Survey; FSS	4 weeks, 5×/week, 30 min sessions	MS training group ⇑ aerobic threshold, improved health perception (vitality ⇑ 46%, social interaction ⇑ 36%); ⇑ activity of level (17%); tendency for less fatigue; $M\dot{V}o_2$ and lung function did not change	Aerobic training is safe and improves aerobic capacity; symptom exacerbation lower than expected (6%); compliance of MS training group was low (65%); stresses need for motivational setting; MS patients less fit than healthy controls; more disabled MS patients improved more than less impaired patients; small sample size.

Evidence Summary Box 19.5

Exercise and Multiple Sclerosis (continued)

Reference	Subjects	Design/ Intervention	Duration	Results	Comments
Roehrs, T, and Karst, G[120] 2004	31 subjects with primary or secondary progressive MS	Nonrandomized, cohort design Aquatics exercise program (water temp. 83–85°F) including aerobic, strength, balance, and flexibility exercises Outcome measures: SF-36, MSQLI	12 weeks, 2×/week, 1-hour sessions	Significant improvement noted in domains of social functioning (SF-36, MSSS) and fatigue (MFIS)	Aquatic exercise appears safe in PPMS and SPMS; lacked control group; small sample size; 19 subjects completed intervention; 12 individuals withdrew from study; 6 before any participation and 6 during participation due to multiple reasons; barriers to exercise need to be anticipated
Sutherland, G, Andersen, M, and Stoove, M[121] 2001	22 subjects, with MS, mild-mod disability; EDSS of 5.0 or less; no-special-activity group = 11; exercise group = 11	Randomized control trial Exercise intervention: land-based weight training; water aerobics, water jogging Outcome measures: Submax GXT; HRQOL	10 weeks, 3×/week 45 min sessions	Exercise group ⇑ in physical fitness (not significant); Reported ⇑ energy and vigor, mood, better social and sexual functioning; less bodily pain and fatigue.	Exercise improved psychological health and quality of life; use of water-based aerobics can be effective in patients with MS who have spasticity and coordination deficits; small sample size.
Petajan, J, et al[122] 1996	46 subjects with MS, mild-mod disability; EDSS scores between 1 and 4; exercise group = 21; nonexercise group = 25	Randomized control trial Aerobic training, combined leg and arm ergometry Outcome measures: GXT: $\dot{V}o_2$ max; isometric strength; body composition, blood lipids, daily activities, POMS, SIP, FSS	15 weeks, 3×/week, 40 min sessions	Significant ⇑ in $\dot{V}o_2$ max (22%); workload (10%); UE and LE strength; significant ⇓ in skinfolds, triglycerides, VLDL; significant ⇓ in POMS depression and anger scores, and fatigue; significant ⇑ in social interaction, emotional behavior, total SIP scores; EDSS scores unchanged except for improved bowel and bladder scores	Exercise training improved fitness and had a large, positive impact on quality of life factors; small sample size; 7 patients experienced an exacerbation during training (4 exercise; 4 non-exercise); cooling provided with large fans.
Ponichterra-Mulcare, et al[123] 1997	23 subjects with MS, mild-mod disability; 11 = AMB group (ambulatory), EDSS scores of 1–4.5; 8 = SEMI group (semi-ambulatory), EDSS scores of 5.0–6.5; 4 = controls	Nonrandomized, cohort design Recumbent or upright cycle ergometry, combined UE/LE; training HR = 65–70% HR_{max} Outcome measures: GXT, Vo_2 max	6 months, 3×/week, 30 min sessions	Significant ⇑ in $\dot{V}o_2$ max (20% AMB; 5% SEMI); control group declined 12%.	Exercise improves cardiovas. fitness; may not apply to more severely involved; small sample size; exacerbation of symptoms in 2 subjects in SEMI group; cooling provided with large fans.

(continued)

Evidence Summary Box 19.5

Exercise and Multiple Sclerosis (continued)

Reference	Subjects	Design/ Intervention	Duration	Results	Comments
Ponichtera-Mulcare, J, et al[124] 1991	10 subjects with MS (6 females, 4 males), mild-mod disability; EDSS scores of 1–4.5; matched to 10 non-MS subjects (age, gender, height, weight, exercise level, lifestyle)	Nonrandomized, cohort design Exercise testing with arm ergometry (ARM), leg ergometry (LEG) or combined LEG/ARM), discontinuous protocol Outcome measures: GXT, $\dot{V}o_2$ peak HR_{max}	3 tests using the different modes, 72 hours apart	$\dot{V}o_2$ peak significantly higher for non-MS group for ARM and LEG/ARM tests but not for LEG tests; HR_{max} during ARM, LEG, LEG/ARM was 89%, 86%, and 91% of predicted HR_{max} for MS group; 96% for all, non-MS group.	Combined LEG/ARM design may be a more effective testing and training for patients with MS; used recumbent cycle ergometer with back support; toe and heel straps for legs; separate flywheel for arms; distributes exercise load better.

AFI = Ambulatory Fatigue Index (500-m walk test); BMI = body mass index; EDSS = Kurtzke Expanded Disability Status Scale; FI = Fatigue Index; FSS = Fatigue Severity Scale; GXT = Graded Exercise Test; HRQOL = Health-related Quality of Life; LE = lower extremity; mAS = Modified Ashworth Scale; MHR = maximal heart rate; MFIS = Modified Fatigue Impact Scale; Ms = muscle; MVIC = maximal voluntary isometric contraction; POMS = Profile of Mood States; PPMS = primary progressive multiple sclerosis; RRMS = Relapsing remitting multiple sclerosis; SIP = Sickness Impact Profile; 1–RM = 1-repetition maximum contraction; UE = upper extremity; VLDL = very-low-density lipoprotein; $\dot{V}o_2$ max = maximal oxygen uptake.

all increase in a linear fashion in response to increasing workloads. Respiratory responses (respiratory rate [RR] and minute ventilation) also increase.[126] However, HR and BP responses may be blunted secondary to cardiovascular dysautonomia.[136,137] Reported incidence of these changes has been as high as 50 percent of patients with MS. A direct relationship exists between the duration and extent of disease and the likelihood of autonomic cardiovascular dysfunction. Patients with mild disease typically do not exhibit these responses, whereas patients with significant long-standing disease are much more likely to demonstrate autonomic dysfunction.[138] Patients with MS can also demonstrate respiratory muscle dysfunction (weakness, dyssynergia), contributing to reduced exercise tolerance.[139]

Exercise tolerance and maximal aerobic power ($\dot{V}O_{2max}$) are reduced in individuals with reduced cardiorespiratory fitness secondary to physical inactivity. Decreased physical work capacity, decreased vital capacity, increased heart rate at rest and in response to exercise, decreased muscular strength, increased fatigue, increased anxiety, and depression are common findings.

Determining an appropriate exercise prescription to improve cardiovascular conditioning is challenging and needs to be carefully individualized for each patient. The following guidelines for *clinical exercise testing* can be used.[128]

- The preferred mode is either an upright or recumbent leg cycle ergometer. A recumbent device is indicated if sitting balance is impaired. Combination leg and arm ergometry or UE ergometry may be necessary with increased LE involvement. Toe clips and heel straps are recommended to control foot placement especially in patients with spasticity, tremor, or weakness.
- Performance measures include: HR, ratings of perceived exertion (RPE), BP, and expired gas analysis ($\dot{V}O_2$). Using the RPE scale, peripheral exertion is consistently rated as more stressful (higher) than central exertion.
- A continuous or discontinuous protocol (3- to 5-minute stages) can be used; the discontinuous protocol is indicated with symptomatic disease, especially fatigue.
- A submaximal test should be used. Most individuals with MS can achieve 70 to 85 percent of their age-predicted maximal heart rate (HR_{max}).
- Recommendations for increasing workloads for each stage are: 12 to 25 watts for LE work and 8 to 12 watts for combined UE and LE work.[128]
- Termination criteria include achievement of peak HR, fatigue, significant BP changes (SBP > 200 mm Hg or DPB > 115 mm Hg or a hypotensive response), or a decrease in oxygen uptake with increasing work rate.
- Precautions should be taken to monitor for attenuated HR or BP responses during exercise.
- Precautions should be taken to manage core body temperature and prevent overheating.
- Precautions should be taken to monitor the effects of fatigue.
- Precautions should be taken to prevent the deleterious effects of overwork.
- Precautions should be taken with certain medications that can affect results: Amantadine HCl may temporarily reduce fatigue; baclofen and amitriptyline HCl may cause muscle weakness; prednisone can also cause

muscle weakness along with reduced sweating and hypertension.
- Morning is the optimal time for testing.

Individuals with stable MS appear to be good candidates for *exercise training* (see Evidence Summary Box 19.5). Prescription is again based on the four interrelated elements of the FITT equation. Recommendations for exercise programming to improve cardiovascular conditioning include[127,128]:

- Recommended training frequency is three sessions/week, on alternate days. Daily exercise at lower levels of intensity is recommended for individuals with more limited exercise capacities (e.g., 3 to 5 metabolic equivalent [METs]).
- Training intensity should be limited to 60 to 75 percent peak HR or 50 to 65 percent peak $\dot{V}O_2$.[126]
- Type of exercise can include cycling, walking, swimming, or water aerobics.[118,119–124,140,141]
- Circuit training may prove best for optimizing training.
- Individuals with balance problems or sensory loss will require non-weightbearing activities.
- Recommended duration is 30 min/session or for more involved individuals, three 10-min sessions/day.
- Exercise precautions: discussed in previous section.
- Depression may affect adherence requiring constant support and planned reinforcement for the patient.
- Outcome measures include graded exercise testing (GXT), HR (which may be difficult to monitor with dysautonomia; sensory loss in the fingers may make self-monitoring difficult), tests of lung function (FVC), body composition, RPE, fatigue (FI, MFIS), functional status, and quality of life measures (HRQL).

Patient education is particularly important as the overall success of a fitness program is influenced by the individual's level of understanding of the basic principles of training, independence in self-monitoring, and skill in decision-making relative to level of impairment and exercise modifications required, lifestyle, and general health and safety considerations.[141]

Flexibility Exercises

Flexibility (stretching) and ROM exercises are necessary to ensure adequate joint ROM and to counteract the effects of spasticity. Sedentary or inactive persons who are dependent on wheelchairs often develop tightness in hip flexors, adductors, hamstrings, and heel cords. Limited overhead ROM is seen with tightness in the pectoralis major/minor, and latissimus dorsi and is associated with a slumped, forward posture. Patients confined to bed typically present with tightness in hip/knee extensors and plantarflexors. Both PROM and AROM exercises should be performed daily for short periods. Supported positions (seated or lying down) should be used to decrease the impact of balance problems. More active patients may benefit from Tai Chi that provides additional important benefits of relaxation and balance training.[126] Goniometry is an appropriate outcome measure.

Management of Fatigue

Fatigue is one of the most debilitating symptoms of MS and is characterized by overwhelming sleepiness, excessive tiredness, and sense of weakness that comes on suddenly and severely. Aversion to activity for fear of bringing on fatigue is also common.[23] The resultant lowered activity levels have important implications for diminished health status and deconditioning. Therapists are faced with a balancing act, on one hand prescribing exercise, while on the other hand avoiding overwork and the development of fatigue.[142] Aerobic exercise training (previously discussed) and *energy effectiveness strategies (ESS)* are central to any intervention plan to lessen fatigue.[143]

Patients are often instructed to keep an *activity diary* in which they record how they slept the night before, daily activities by hour, and how costly those activities were. For each activity, they can be asked to rate their level of fatigue (F), the value or importance of the activity (V), and satisfaction perceived with performance of the activity (S) by assigning a number between 1 and 10 with 1 being very low and 10 being very high. For example, the activity might be fixing lunch. Scores reported for this activity might be $F = 7$, $V = 3$, and $S = 2$. Aggravating factors associated with increasing fatigue (e.g., heat stress) and MS symptoms that appear or worsen during the day are also recorded. An *MS Daily Activity Diary* is presented in Appendix C.[143]

Based on this information, therapists can initiate training sessions, teaching energy effectiveness strategies. **Energy conservation** refers to the adoption of strategies that reduce overall energy requirements of the task and overall level of fatigue. These can include modifying the task or modifying the environment to ensure successful completion of daily activities. For example, a motorized scooter or powered wheelchair can be considered for community or home mobility to help conserve energy and maintain independence. Other mobility equipment such as walkers, and crutches, or orthotics can also be considered. Activities that are difficult or have high energy needs can be broken down into component parts, requiring accurate activity analysis. **Activity pacing** refers to the balancing of activity with rest periods interspersed throughout the day. For the patient with chronic fatigue, *rest–activity ratios* are developed, with periodic rest periods planned in advance. Time-outs with complete rest should be instituted if an activity becomes exhaustive. Overall levels of energy can be improved if patients learn to set priorities and limit their activities, saving their energy for those activities that are truly important to them (e.g., activities that are enjoyable and meaningful in terms of the individual's lifestyle). The occupational therapist addresses EES and can provide valuable suggestions in terms of planning, work simplification, and developing energy-efficient activities for self-care and home management. The vocational rehabilitation counselor can provide useful strategies for behavioral modification and vocational rehabilitation. Team efforts with the physical therapist and others are important for consistency and reinforcement. Weekly review of activities and recommended modifications is used to evaluate progress. The MFIS should be administered on a regular basis to monitor ongoing fatigue status (Appendix A).

The OT/PT team should complete a direct environmental examination of the home and/or job site (see Chapter 12). A number of adaptations may be considered to improve efficiency and safety, including air-conditioning, home or work modifications, or ergonomic equipment. The patient/family/caregivers should be educated as to the importance of these recommendations for improved function. Periodic review of equipment and environmental modifications is also recommended.

During an acute exacerbation, the patient will fare better if he or she is allowed to rest for a few days. Allowing the patient to continue the same level of exercise or ambulation is not helpful. Therapy can be reinstituted when the deterioration has stabilized and no new symptoms are appearing. The focus and pace of therapy must be readjusted according to the patient's specific abilities and needs at that time. Finally, stress management techniques are important components of symptom management.

Management of Spasticity

Spasticity is functionally limiting and contributes to the development of a number of secondary impairments such as contractures, postural deformity, and decubitus ulcers. A variety of physical therapy interventions can be utilized, including cryotherapy, hydrotherapy, therapeutic exercise, positioning, or any combination thereof. The responses to these interventions must be monitored closely and carefully balanced with pharmacological interventions. The therapist must closely monitor the effects of the antispasticity medications prescribed and optimize physical therapy interventions with the dosing cycle. For example, patients on baclofen will respond better to stretching techniques if they are applied in the middle of the dosing cycle rather than at the end or beginning. Physical therapists must also recognize contributing factors that impact tone and respond appropriately. For example, infection or fever that increases tone may require a referral to the physician. It is important to reduce or eliminate all factors that can aggravate spasticity (e.g., heat, humidity, stress).

Topical cold (ice packs or wraps) or hydrotherapy (cool bath) can temporarily reduce spasticity by decreasing tendon reflex excitability and clonus, and by slowing conduction of impulses in nerves and muscles. The effects of cryotherapy are relatively short-lived, although some patients may experience enhanced ability to move that lasts for minutes or hours. It is important to remember that some patients, particularly those with intact sensation, may react to the unpleasant sensation of cold with *fight or flight* (autonomic nervous system) responses, such as increased heart rate, respiratory rate, or nausea. Cryotherapy may be contraindicated in these patients.

ROM exercises begun early in the course of the disease and continued daily can help patients maintain joint integrity and mobility. In the face of unremitting spasticity, stretching techniques are indicated to increase extensibility of the muscle tendon unit and connective tissue. Intermittent static stretching held a minimum of 30 to 60 seconds should be applied, ideally for 5 to 10 repetitions. Combining stretching movements with rhythmic rotation (gentle rotation of the limb) or PNF facilitated stretching techniques (hold–relax active contraction [HRAC], contract–relax active contraction [CRAC]) are also effective strategies to assist in gaining range. See Chapter 13 for a discussion of these techniques. Maintained stretch, held for 30 minutes to 3 hours, also can be used and has been shown to decrease stretch reflex activity.[144] Maintained stretch can be achieved with prolonged positioning (e.g., tilt table standing with toe wedges), low-load weights applied using skin traction, or serial casts. Air splints also provide an effective mechanism to maintain limbs in lengthened, out of spasticity positions. Patients/family members/clients should be taught stretching exercises as part of a home exercise program (HEP). Caution must be used to prevent fast, ballistic stretching movements, because spasticity is velocity sensitive. Stretching movements need to proceed slowly to gradually achieve the desired range. Typically the LEs demonstrate stronger spasticity than the UEs, especially in the extensor antigravity muscles. Although spasticity varies greatly from person-to-person, muscles that require particular emphasis during stretching include the quadriceps, adductors, and plantarflexors. For patients who spend prolonged times sitting in a wheelchair, stretching should also address the hamstrings and hip flexors.

Active exercises at slow or self-selected speeds should focus on expanding the available ROM. Emphasis on contracting the antagonist muscles can assist through mechanisms of reciprocal inhibition. Electrical stimulation of muscles antagonist to the spastic muscles can also be used to decrease spasticity. Movements that encourage or utilize abnormal postures should be discouraged. In patients with minimal to moderate spasticity, exercise combined with low doses of baclofen resulted in significant improvements in overall levels of tone.[145] Patients with problems with abnormal co-contraction may benefit from exercises focused on improving motor control (timing exercises) or biofeedback. Tai Chi, yoga, and aquatic exercises combined with cool water temperatures (less than 85°F) can also be helpful in producing desired relaxation.[146]

Functional activities aimed at reducing tone should concentrate on trunk and proximal segments, as many patterns of hypertonus seem to be fixed from the action of the stronger proximal muscles. Extensor tone seems to predominate, so activities that stress LE flexion with trunk rotation are generally the most effective. For example, lower trunk rotation (LTR) in sidelying or hooklying can be effective in reducing extensor tone. One very effective strategy is to position the patient in hooklying with a therapy ball under the flexed legs and gently rock the ball back and forth. Moving from quadruped position to side-sitting can also be effective in reducing extensor tone in some patients as the activity combines LTR with prolonged inhibitory pressure on the quadriceps.[134] A more generalized decrease in tone may be achieved through techniques aimed at decreasing overall CNS central activity while promoting relaxation (e.g., slow rocking, relaxation training).

For the patient with limited functional mobility (EDSS levels of 7.0 or above) positioning out of abnormal, spastic postures is an important component of the management program. In general, prolonged or static positioning in any fixed posture can be deleterious to the patient with strong spasticity and should be avoided. For example, the patient who remains in bed all day with the LEs positioned in extension, adduction, and plantarflexion may be unable to flex enough at the hips and knees to sit in a wheelchair. Similarly, the feet will remain fixed in plantarflexion and cannot be positioned on the footpedals. A positioning schedule using varied positions (in bed, chair or wheelchair) will help keep the patient from getting stuck in any one posture. Mechanical positioning devices (e.g., resting splints, toe spreader, finger spreader, ankle splint) are helpful in maintaining position and preserving joint structures.

Management of Coordination and Balance Deficits

Cerebellar deficits are common in MS and can be difficult to manage. Interventions directed at promoting static postural control should first focus on static control (holding) in weightbearing, antigravity postures (e.g., sitting, quadruped, kneeling, plantigrade, and standing). Progression through a series of postures is used to gradually increase postural demands by varying the base of support (BOS), raising the center of mass (COM), and increasing the number of body segments (degrees of freedom) that must be controlled. Specific exercise techniques that can be used to promote stability include joint approximation applied through proximal joints (shoulders or hips) or head and spine, and rhythmic stabilization (PNF). Patients with significant ataxia will not be able to hold steady and may benefit from the application of the technique of PNF dynamic reversals (slow reversals), progressing through decrements of range.[147] Dynamic postural control can be challenged by incorporating activities such as weight shifting or reaching (UE) or stepping (LE). For example, in sitting a resisted PNF chop pattern that combines UE movements with trunk movements (flexion with rotation or extension with rotation) can be used. The patient should also practice important functional movements, such as bridging, sit-to-stand, scooting, and wall squats.[134]

The pool is an important therapeutic medium to practice static and dynamic postural control in both sitting and standing. Water provides graded resistance that slows down the patient's ataxic movements, while the buoyancy aids in upright balance. Water aerobics have been shown effective in improving strength, decreasing muscular fatigability, and increasing endurance in patients with MS.[118,121] In addition, the use of moderate or cool water temperatures (no greater than 85°F [29°C]) can help moderate spasticity.

An important goal of therapy is to promote safe and functional balance. Effective training should involve a variety of tasks that challenge balance. As training progresses, tasks are modified (e.g., wide base to narrow base to tandem stance, stable surface to moveable surface) to promote adaptation of skills. Sensory conditions are also varied to promote adaptive control in various different perceptual contexts (e.g., eyes open to eyes closed, firm surface to thick foam surface). The intervention program can also utilize force platform training (e.g., SMART Balance Master® [NeuroCom International, Inc., Clackamas, OR 97015]). Limits of stability training is also important. The patient with ataxia needs to learn how to reduce excess postural sway (frequency and amplitude) and to control center of alignment position. The added biofeedback from visual and/or auditory feedback displays on these machines is especially useful for patients with somatosensory deficits. Prolonged latencies (onset of responses) should be expected. Functional balance control should also be challenged using real-life tasks within simulated real-life environments. For example, self-initiated movements using reaching, turning, or bending can be practiced in both sitting and standing. Movement transitions (e.g., sit-to-stand transfers) can also be practiced. A moveable surface can be used to challenge balance. For example, sitting activities on a therapy ball are an excellent way to promote dynamic balance control.[134] Some patients with MS may benefit from vestibular training exercises to reduce the effects of central vestibular dysfunction. While evidence is limited on the effect of such balance training programs for patients with MS, a positive trend toward balance improvement is a consistent finding.[148,149]

Control of ataxic limb movements (tremor and dysmetria) can be achieved through proprioceptive loading and light resistance. For example, the therapist can use PNF extremity patterns using the technique of dynamic reversals with light tracking resistance to modulate force output and reciprocal actions of muscles.[147] Ataxic movements have sometimes been helped by the application of elastic resistance bands or light weights to stabilize movements. Velcro® weight cuffs (wrist or ankle), weighted boots, or a weighted jacket or belt can reduce tremors of the limbs or trunk. The extra weights will also increase energy expenditure, and must therefore be carefully balanced against the increased fatigue they might cause. Weighted canes or walkers can be used to reduce ataxic UE movements that interfere with the use of an assistive device during ambulation. Weighted spoons or forks can be used to enhance eating. For patients with significant tremor, these devices may mean the difference between dependent and independent function. External devices (braces or splints) can be used to stabilize ataxic limbs but also have the undesirable effect of adding weight to limb movements. Air splints can also stabilize limb movements and should be considered as they are less energy costly. A soft neck collar can be used to stabilize head and neck tremors. All these strategies, however, should be viewed as temporary and compensatory. Once the devices are removed, ataxic movements will return or in some cases may actually temporarily worsen.

Frenkel's exercises were originally developed in 1889 to treat patients with tabes dorsalis and problems of sensory ataxia owing to a loss of proprioception. These exercises have been applied in the treatment of individuals with MS. The exercises are performed in supine, sitting, and standing. Each activity is performed slowly with the patient using vision to carefully guide correct movement. The exercises require a high degree of mental concentration and effort and are, therefore, not appropriate for all patients with MS. For those patients with the prerequisite abilities, they may be helpful in regaining control of movement through cognitive compensation strategies. Patients with partial sensation can progress to practicing exercises with eyes closed. Frenkel's exercises are presented in Box 19.6.

Unwanted movements are worse under conditions of stress, anxiety, and excitement. The increased arousal, the result of adrenalin pumping through the system, increases existing tremors while decreasing function. Stress management techniques are therefore an important component of the plan of care. In general, patients do better in a low-stimulus environment that allows full concentration on control of movements. They benefit from augmented feedback (verbal cueing of knowledge of results and knowledge of performance; biofeedback) and repetition to improve motor learning. The patient with MS is often restricted in practice by neuromuscular fatigue and neurological deficits that impair sensory feedback, attention, memory, and concentration. The successful therapist will need to carefully identify the patient's resources and abilities and capitalize on them to maximize learning.

Locomotor Training

Walking ability is frequently impaired. However, at least 65 percent of patients with MS are still walking after 20 years.[15] Early gait problems often include poor balance and heaviness of one or more limbs. Patients frequently report difficulty lifting their legs (hip flexor weakness). Weak dorsiflexors are also common, resulting in foot drop. Problems with foot clearance may result in a circumducted gait pattern. Later problems evolve owing to clonus, spasticity, sensory loss, and/or ataxia. Weakness generally extends to

Box 19.6 Frenkel's Exercises

General instructions: Exercises can be performed with the part supported or unsupported, unilaterally or bilaterally. They should be practiced as smooth, timed movements, performed to a slow, even tempo by counting out loud. Consistency of performance is stressed and a specified target can be used to determine range. Four basic positions are used: lying, sitting, standing, and walking. The exercises progress from postures of greatest stability (lying, sitting) to postures of greatest challenge (standing, walking). As voluntary control improves, the exercises progress to stopping and starting on command, increasing the range and performing the same exercises with eyes closed. Concentration and repetition are the keys to success. A similar progression of exercises can be developed for the upper extremities.

Examples:

1. Half-lying: hip and knee flexion and extension of each limb, foot flat on mat
2. Half-lying: hip abduction and adduction of each limb with the foot flat, knee flexed; then with knee extended
3. Half-lying: hip and knee flexion and extension of each limb, heel lifted off mat
4. Half-lying: heel of one limb to opposite leg (toes, ankle, shin, patella)
5. Half-lying: heel of one limb to opposite knee, sliding down crest of tibia to ankle
6. Half-lying: hip and knee flexion and extension of both limbs, legs together
7. Half-lying: reciprocal movements of both limbs—flexion of one leg during extension of the other
8. Sitting: knee extension and flexion of each limb; progress to marking time
9. Sitting: hip abduction and adduction
10. Sitting: alternate foot placing to a specified target (using floor markings or a grid)
11. Standing up and sitting down: to a specified count
12. Standing: foot placing to a specified target (floor markings or grid)
13. Standing: weight shifting
14. Walking: sideways or forward to a specified count. (parallel lines, or floor markings may be used as targets to control foot placement, stride length, and step width)
15. Walking: turning around to a specified count. (Floor markings can be helpful in maintaining a stable base of support.)

include the quadriceps and hip abductors. Quadriceps weakness typically results in hyperextension of the knee and forward flexion of the trunk with increased lumbar lordosis. Hip abductor weakness results in a Trendelenburg gait pattern with a strong lateral lean to the weak side.

A well-designed exercise program of tone reduction, stretching, and strengthening exercises can improve gait. Standing and walking activities should stress safety and maintaining a stable base of support; maximum weight-bearing through the LEs; and adequate weight transfer and forward progression with trunk, limb, and pelvic kinematics consistent with normal walking. Verbal and manual cueing can assist the patient in the correct mechanics of gait. The pool is an important medium that can also be used to assist training while reducing tone and fatigue and controlling for ataxia.

Locomotor training using an overhead harness to support body weight and a motorized treadmill has been the focus of increasing attention in the literature and used extensively to improve gait in patients with spinal cord injury and stroke[150–153] (see discussion in Chapter 13). Application to other chronic neurological conditions is limited but emerging.[154] This task-oriented intervention was used as part of a comprehensive 12-week program by Fulk to improve gait speed, endurance, and balance in a patient with MS (EDSS score of 2.5).[155] The amount of body weight support was reduced (20 percent to 0 percent) while gait speed increased by 21 percent (10 meter walk test) and 24.6 percent (6 minute walk test). Scores on the Berg Balance Scale (BBS), and Activities-Specific Balance Confidence (ABC) scale, and the Modified Fatigue Impact Scale—5-item test (MFIS-5) also improved. Perhaps most important of all, the patient reported feeling safer and better able to engage in daily social activities. Thus this form of locomotor training appears to be a feasible and safe intervention producing significant positive effects and deserving of additional research.

Patients with MS typically require orthotic devices as ambulation skills decline. Ankle–foot stability can be achieved by the addition of an ankle–foot orthosis (AFO). Improvements in energy efficiency and safety are also important outcomes. AFOs are prescribed for foot drop, poor knee control (especially hyperextension), minimal to moderate spasticity, and poor somatosensation. The most common type used is the standard polypropylene AFO which is lightweight and has the added benefit of cosmesis. An AFO with an articulated joint can be prescribed to provide more rigid control for the ankle with the addition of a plantarflexion stop. Relative contraindications to the prescription of these devices include severe spasticity, foot edema, and weakness (nonfunctional grades of LE muscles, especially hip flexors). Although knee–ankle–foot orthoses (KAFOs) can provide additional stabilization control of the knee, they are rarely used because of the increased energy expenditure required. Rocker shoes (modified Danish clogs) have been successful with selected patients with MS in compensating for lost ankle mobility. Gait patterns appeared more normal, with a significant savings in energy cost (150 percent over ambulation without rocker shoes).[156]

Canes, forearm crutches, or a walker may be necessary to compensate for deficits in fatigue, strength, sensory loss (numbness), or balance. For many patients acceptance of an assistive device involves full recognition of their disability. They need to be convinced that use of these devices is far safer than “wall-walking” or “furniture walking.” Devices also provide recognition to the community at large that patients are not staggering or losing their balance because they are “drunk,” a frequent occurrence with many patients. The devices may be the difference between community participation or remaining homebound because of fear of falling. Patients should be encouraged to try different devices out to determine which works best for them. For example, the patient with significant fatigue levels may benefit from a large-wheeled walker with locking hand brakes and a seat that allows for frequent rests. Cosmesis is an important factor in promoting acceptance. There are many innovations in assistive technology that make the choices easier. For example, designer canes now come in many different colors and styles, including clear Lucite. ABLEDATA (http://www.abledata.com) is a federally funded project that offers product information, resources, and links to manufacturers.[157]

As the disease progresses, many patients benefit from a wheeled mobility device (powered scooter or wheelchair). The course and progression of the disease and presenting symptoms should be taken into consideration when deciding on a device. For patients with adequate trunk stability, UE function, and appropriate visual, perceptual, and cognitive skills, a scooter provides needed mobility while conserving energy. Scooters also do not carry the same negative stigma as that of a wheelchair. Both three- and four-wheel scooters are available. Four-wheel scooters have superior outdoor and uneven terrain performance, but are not as easily transported. Features that should be recommended include a seat that rotates for easy mounting and dismounting, easy dismantling for loading into the car, and steering mechanisms that minimize the work of the UEs. One disadvantage of scooters is that seating cannot always be customized. They are often not designed for prolonged sitting or for patients with moderate to severe postural instability. Some new three-wheeled scooters are designed to turn in very small areas while others have a wide turning radius and may not be suitable for in-home use.

A wheelchair should be considered when postural demands necessitate increased support. A standard wheelchair is often not much help to patients with MS because of the energy expenditure and coordination required for propulsion. A power wheelchair should be considered when impairments prevent or limit manual propulsion. Power wheelchairs are more costly, more difficult to repair, and require specialized transportation by a wheelchair-accessible van or bus. Most patients will navigate using a joystick. For patients with impaired hand strength and sensation, the joystick can be adjusted to increase sensitivity. Wheelchair seating should ensure proper alignment of the pelvis, trunk and head, and limbs while enhancing function. Common malalignments include posterior tilting of the pelvis (sacral sitting) with kyphosis, typically the result of spasticity in the hamstring muscles. This can be improved with the addition of a cushion with a solid base of support (solid seat or wood insert) to prevent hammocking of the wheelchair upholstery. Postural alignment can also be assisted by the addition of contoured seating (custom built) or a contoured wheelchair cushion (e.g., contoured cushion with gel). A solid back support and adjustable lateral trunk supports may be needed to enhance postural alignment and upright sitting. Footrests should be positioned to ensure that the thighs are parallel to the floor. If extensor spasms are strong, they can actually propel the patient out of the chair. A strong lap belt that secures firmly around the pelvis is necessary for safety. For patients who present with strong adductor spasticity, a medial knee block (pommel) may be necessary. Heel loops and straps may be required to maintain foot position on the footrests. Patients who no longer demonstrate adequate trunk and head stability require an alternate seating design. For some patients, the tilt-in-space wheelchair with head/neck support is a better option than a reclining wheelchair with high back and elevating leg rests. The former maintains the normal hip sitting angle; the latter produces extension of the hips and may feed into strong extensor spasticity. Elevating leg rests tend to stretch hamstring muscles and may cause posterior pelvic tilting when spasticity is present. The reclining wheelchair with elevating leg rests also creates greater environmental access problems. Motorized control of the seat back (available in either tilt-in-space or reclining wheelchairs) will allow the patient to make easy adjustments in position, thus preventing skin breakdown.

Patients should be instructed in transfer and wheelchair mobility/management skills. A transfer board or hydraulic lift may be necessary as UE function deteriorates. Attention to good sitting posture and pressure relief techniques is essential to maintain alignment and prevent skin breakdown. Patients should be encouraged to balance time in the wheelchair with other activities, such as walking or exercising, and should be extra diligent in stretching muscles that tend to contract as a result of prolonged sitting (e.g., hip and knee flexors).

One of the constraints the therapist will have to deal with is financial reimbursement for the changing mobility needs of the patient with chronic MS. Private or public insurance organizations require a statement of medical necessity for payment. As symptoms are not static in MS but rather typically exacerbate or remit, the therapist needs to provide clear and convincing documentation of need, stressing improved function and safety. Many third-party payers will not reimburse for new wheelchairs prescribed within specified time intervals or may be hesitant to finance expensive specialty wheelchairs such as the tilt-in-space chair or a second lightweight chair for traveling. The therapist will need to provide careful documentation of potential adverse outcomes in order to justify the cost of the new chair. For example, a likely deleterious outcome for a patient who is denied reimbursement for a tilt-in-space chair may be skin breakdown. The costs of nursing and surgical care for decubitus ulcers can then be compared to the cost of the new wheelchair, which can be justified as a preventive measure. It is equally important to anticipate future needs as they relate to rate of disease progression when ordering equipment.

Functional Training

Functional training should focus on problem solving and the development of appropriate decision making skills required to meet the challenges of being disabled. Skills should be adapted and practiced to ensure safe performance in both the home and community environments. Training in functional mobility skills (e.g., bed mobility, transfers, locomotion) is typically directed by the physical therapist while ADL training (e.g., dressing, personal hygiene, bathing, toileting, and feeding) is directed by the occupational therapist and training in communication skills by the speech–language pathologist. Close communication and coordination among team members is necessary to ensure that training methods are consistently applied and successful. Full participation of the patient in all phases of planning and training will increase personal involvement, while decreasing dependency and passivity.

The majority of patients with MS will use multiple adaptive devices. This requires careful attention to appropriate prescription of devices and environmental modifications to assist the patient in conserving energy and maintaining function. Adaptive equipment can include bed or bathroom grab bars, overhead trapeze, raised seats, transfer board, or hydraulic lift. Wrist rests to facilitate writing or typing, and plates and cups with lips to minimize spills are often helpful in assisting with hand function. Long-handled shoe horns, reachers, button hooks, sock aids, or Velcro® closures can assist in dressing. Effective communication may require built-up writing utensils or a universal cuff for written communication or more sophisticated computerized devices. Patients with severe speech problems may require voice amplification devices, electronic aids, or computer-assisted alternative communication systems. The team must recognize when a device is indicated, and assist the patient in acceptance and in learning how to use the device *before* significant deterioration of function occurs.

Management of Speech and Swallowing

Shallow respiratory patterns contribute to speech difficulties and recurrent respiratory infections. Thus, respiratory muscle training is an important component of the plan of care for patients with chronic MS, and should be combined with activities to improve trunk stability, head control, and sitting balance. Respiratory patterns can be facilitated through the use manual contacts, resistance, and incentive spirometry. The therapist should focus on diaphragmatic and segmental chest expansion, expiratory training, and effective coughing. A significant increase in expiratory muscle strength was demonstrated following a 3-month training program in patients with MS.[158]

When dysphagia or difficulty in swallowing is present, physical therapy efforts should be closely coordinated with those of the speech–language pathologist and occupational therapist. A detailed examination is necessary, including video-fluoroscopy for dysphagia. The physical therapist can assist in the management plan by improving sitting position, head control, and oral-motor coordination. An upright posture with a slightly forward head position and chin parallel to table or slightly tucked is necessary to achieve good swallowing and avoid aspiration. Oral–motor exercises can improve mouth function and include specific exercises for lip closure, tongue movements, and jaw control. Stretch and resistance can be used to strengthen weak muscle actions.

Swallowing reflexes can be stimulated by using icy beverages such as a shake, sherbet, or fruit slush. Patients are instructed to begin meals with something cold and to take single small sips, never trying consecutive swallowing. Resistive sucking through a straw can also be helpful. Thicker liquids, which provide some resistance and therefore some facilitation of muscle action, are generally easier to swallow than thin liquids such as water. Moist foods (with sauces, broth, water, or milk) are easier to manage than dry ones. Semisolid and pureed foods are easier than regular solids. Foods that irritate the throat (e.g., vinegar) and crumbly or stringy foods (e.g., cake, cookies, potato chips, celery, cheeses) should be avoided. Patients are instructed to focus their efforts on chewing food thoroughly and not attempt to talk during eating. Maintaining a quiet and peaceful environment during meals is important. Fatigue can affect food intake. When the patient starts slowing down during a meal, he or she is instructed to switch back to something icy. Late in the day, patients should consume thick liquids while saving thin liquids for early in the day. Patients may benefit from reducing the size of meals and eating multiple small meals throughout the day. The speech–language pathologist also teaches swallowing techniques, including the power swallow. This involves having the person first inhale and then hold his or her breath, thereby closing the airway. The person then swallows, exhales, and swallows again. Feeding tubes may become necessary with severe dysphagia. For overall safety, it is important that family members and caregivers are taught the Heimlich maneuver.[15,159]

Cognitive Training

Cognitive impairments can present major difficulties for the patient and for the rehabilitation team in general. Referral to a neuropsychologist may be indicated to determine the patient's strengths and weaknesses and to assist in the adaptive process. Compensatory strategies for memory deficits can be helpful. These include the use of memory aids, timing devices, and environmental strategies. Memory can be assisted by making lists of things to do, using a memory notebook to log daily events and reminders, and listening to audiotapes. A pill dispenser can assist the patient in maintaining a correct medication schedule. Cueing devices such as an alarm clock, bell timer, or watch alarm can help patients remember when to do certain tasks (e.g., taking medications, performing pressure relief). Structuring and labeling the environment is also an effective strategy to assist memory (e.g., labeled drawers, cabinets). Directions for functional tasks (e.g., transfers, self-stretching techniques) should be carefully written down for both patients and caregivers. Complex tasks can be broken down with clear written directions provided for each step. Directions can be posted in different areas of the home (e.g., steps for toilet or tub transfer posted in the bathroom). Additional cognitive strategies that may be helpful include mental rehearsal, requesting assistance, maximizing alertness, avoidance of difficult situations, and mental exercises. Poor follow-through should be expected among patients with severe cognitive deficits, as often there is very little insight. In this situation, the efforts of family and caregivers must be fully maximized.[36]

Psychosocial Issues

Individuals with MS and their families experience a variety of loses such as loss of social functioning, interpersonal relationships, employment status, independence, and functional skills. Disabilities emerge as the disease progresses over time. Various different psychosocial adaptations can be seen including anger, denial, depression, and so forth. The unique feature of a relapsing-remitting disease course is that it requires continual readjustment every time a new set of symptoms appear. Patients who appear well adjusted at one stage may regress as the disease worsens. The uncertainty of MS produces significant cognitive and emotional stress. Patients often feel out of control and unsure of themselves. Matson and Brooks point out that living with MS requires not only initial acceptance, but also a tremendous flexibility to deal with this lack of closure.[160] Patients also experience the cumulative effects of smaller, everyday stresses that are associated with inability to perform ADL, dependency on others, architectural barriers, and so forth.[161,162] Many factors play a role in determining how an individual reacts to MS. These include the overall effect of the disease on daily life functioning, previous coping skills, perceived self-efficacy, extent of social support, and spiritual well-being. They may experience attitudes of "wait and see" or "nothing can be done." This may explain why an estimated 42 percent of individuals with MS still do not take medications to help control their MS despite medical guidelines recommending disease-modifying drugs. The longer they are influenced by these attitudes, the less likely they are to seek help.[163] Learned helplessness, low self-efficacy, and lack of environmental mastery have been identified as major factors contributing to depression and fatigue.[25] **Self-efficacy** is the belief that an individual will be able to deal with particular situations that may contain novel, unpredictable, and stressful elements.[164] Strategies that promote self-efficacy and self-management empower the patient with MS. The use of stress reduction techniques (e.g., progressive relaxation techniques, cognitive imagery, meditation) can also be helpful in promoting effective coping.

Depression is extremely common and in some individuals may also be part of the disease process. Depression does not necessarily correlate to the severity of the disease. For example, a person with mild disease can be severely depressed, whereas the person with severe disability is not. The therapist must be alert to the signs of depression and intervene as appropriate. Chapter 2 presents a complete discussion of this topic.

Patient and Family/Caregiver Education

The primary roles of the clinician can be categorized as caring professional, teacher expert, and competent professional.[165] A positive, affirming attitude can effectively influence patients' attitudes and assist them to view rehabilitation from a more positive perspective. The development of a strong collaborative relationship with the patient and family/caregivers in which there is respect, compassion, and effective communication is key to successful rehabilitation outcomes.[166] The overall focus should be on the maintenance of *hope* and *encouragement* tempered with *realism*.

As an educator, the therapist has an important role in assisting the patient and family/caregivers in providing information on:

- The disease process, clinical manifestations, and their significance in terms of management.
- Prevention of secondary complications, indirect impairments, and functional limitations.
- The rehabilitation process, the plan of care (POC), and its specific interventions.
- The home exercise program (HEP) including interventions that can be carried out independently.
- Monitoring the effects and possible adverse reactions of medications.
- Use of assistive devices and adaptive equipment.
- General health and stress management techniques.
- Community resources.

Prompt referral to community resources including a support group can provide a necessary stabilizing base for patients and their families/caregivers. Within this environment individuals can gain accurate and useful information about the disease, discuss common problems and methods of coping, and share anxieties and resources. Thus, it provides a valuable forum to assist in the continual adjustment process. The National Multiple Sclerosis Society (http://www.nationalmssociety.org) provides education, emotional support, and a variety of programs and services to individuals with MS and their families through their local chapters.[167] Other organizations and Web-based resources are provided in Appendix D.

A significant number of patients with MS (one out of every two patients) will require the assistance of another person at some point in the course of their disease.[168] This places an extra burden on family members and on the financial resources of the patient if outside caregivers must be utilized. The majority of caregivers experience moderate levels of stress associated with their caregiving duties. As the level and duration of physical care increases, caregivers can experience a variety of signs and symptoms, including physical (e.g., fatigue, headache, sleep disturbances, appetite changes), psychological (e.g., anxiety, depression, frustration), social (e.g., family conflicts, decreasing social experiences or "lack of life"), and spiritual changes (e.g., hopeless and meaningless life and work).[166] The therapist will need to be sensitive to these changes and to conflicts, problems, and tensions as they develop. Considerable time and energy will be devoted to counseling and educating caregivers and coordinating home management.

Summary

Timely referral to neurorehabilitation services is the key to successful management of functional limitations, disability, and quality of life issues in patients with MS. Too often services are not begun until the individual becomes severely disabled. A comprehensive plan of care that addresses the needs of the whole patient and emphasizes meaningful functional activities, patient education, and self-management is ideal for such a complex neurodegenerative disorder. Activities that prove attainable and safe ensure patient success and build self-efficacy. Many patients with MS report that they lack the knowledge and skills needed to exercise safely.[169] Promoting mastery can be achieved through supervised programs that focus on regular exercise, activity pacing, energy conservation, and overall healthy behaviors. Comprehensive efforts of the interdisciplinary team are needed to provide the coordinated and continuing care required with anticipated inpatient, outpatient, and home/community episodes of care.

Questions for Review

1. What are the pathophysiological processes involved in MS? Primary areas of CNS involvement? Common signs and symptoms?
2. Differentiate among the various clinical courses MS can take. How will they influence the rehabilitation plan of care?
3. How is the diagnosis of MS established? What tests and measures are used to confirm the diagnosis?
4. Identify the disease-modifying drugs used in the medical management of MS. What are their indications and potential adverse effects?
5. What components should be included in a physical therapy examination? Describe three disability-specific measures developed for use with the patient with MS.
6. Discuss the components of an effective exercise prescription for the patient with MS to improve both strength and aerobic performance.
7. Discuss the problem of fatigue in MS. How will it influence the design of an exercise program?
8. What are the clinical effects of prolonged inactivity for the patient with chronic, progressive MS? Identify three strategies that can be used to counteract these effects.
9. Differentiate between restorative, preventative, and compensatory interventions. Give an example of each.
10. What are the general considerations in ordering a wheelchair for a person with chronic progressive MS?
11. How can psychosocial adjustment and self-efficacy be facilitated in the patient with relapsing-remitting MS?

Case Study

HISTORY

The patient is a 27-year-old graduate student who was admitted to an acute care facility with a chief complaint of double vision for 2 weeks. She reported that both lower extremities (LEs) seemed weaker recently. Four months earlier, she had noticed persistent tingling of her fingers on the left hand and some numbness on the left side of her face.

Neurological examination showed a scotoma in the upper field of the left eye, weakness of the left medial rectus muscle, horizontal nystagmus on left lateral gaze, and mild weakness of the left central facial muscles. All other muscles had normal strength. The deep tendon reflexes were normal on the right and brisk on the left, and there was a left extensor plantar response. The sensory system was unremarkable. A diagnosis of suspected MS was made. The patient was discharged a few days later, seemingly improved after corticosteroid treatment.

The patient was readmitted to a neurological service 10 months later because she noticed increased difficulty in walking and her speech had become thickened.

NEUROLOGIST REPORT

Patient presents with wide-based ataxic gait, minor slurring of speech, bilateral tremor in the finger-to-nose test, and dysdiadochokinesia. CT scan is within normal limits. MRI scan reveals numerous white areas indicative of lesions. Lumbar puncture shows 56 mg of protein with increased level of gamma-globulin. All other CSF findings are normal. Treatment with high doses of intravenous corticosteroids seemed to improve the neurological symptoms. Patient was discharged home with a referral for outpatient rehabilitation.

Two months later, the patient's symptoms worsened and she is now admitted for intensive rehabilitation.

MEDICATIONS

Prednisone 20 mg po qid
Maalox 30 cc po qid
Valium 10 mg qid

SOCIAL HISTORY

Patient has been living on her own for several years until her recent illness. She has taken a medical leave from graduate school and had returned home to live with her parents. They are both supportive and would like some advice as to how to modify their two-story home. There are five entry stairs with a handrail on both sides. There is a first floor bathroom, and they plan to convert the first floor study into a bedroom. Her parents are both in their early 60s, in good health, and very anxious about their daughter's rapidly deteriorating condition.

PHYSICAL THERAPY EXAMINATION FINDINGS

Mental Status

Alert, oriented
Memory: min. impairment
At times lacks insight, seems unaware of the seriousness of her condition

Euphoric at times; other times she is depressed and cries easily

Communication

Speech is dysarthric, difficult to understand at times

Vision

Transient double vision
Gaze-evoked nystagmus to both left and right
Ocular dysmetria
Upper field defect of left eye

Endurance/Fatigue

Moderate impairment
Tolerance to activity is approximately 10 minutes before rest is required

Skin

WNL except for small bruise on right lateral malleolus

ROM

WNL except for 0° right dorsiflexion; 0 to 5° left dorsiflexion

Tone

Moderate extensor spasticity (2 on the modified Ashworth Scale) in both lower extremities (BLEs), left greater than right
Occasional extensor spasms, which are a major safety risk when they occur during transfers

Sensation

Paresthesias in BLEs with moderate proprioceptive losses, ankle joints greater than proximal joints
Both upper extremities (BUEs): mild decrease in light touch, left greater than right

Strength

Moderate weakness in BLEs; generally functional muscle grades (able to move against gravity), with the greatest weakness noted at the hips
Standard MMT positions not used owing to spasticity
BUEs 3+/5 (fair+) to 4/5 (good) strength

Coordination

BUEs: Intention tremors with mild limb ataxia; voluntary movements are hypermetric
RAM are moderately impaired
BLEs: Movements restricted by spasticity and spasms; unable to test

Balance

Sitting Balance

Static: With eyes open (EO), able to maintain position independently up to 5 minutes with minimal postural tremor; with eyes closed (EC), truncal ataxia is pronounced
Dynamic: With EO, able to weight shift to left and right to about 40 percent of limits of stability (LOS); with EC, experiences loss of balance (LOB) with minimal weight shifts

Standing Balance

Static: Able to maintain standing position in parallel bars with min assist × 1 for up to 3 minutes; during standing, patient is unable to maintain centered alignment; demonstrates moderate postural tremor; with EC, sway is increased dramatically and patient quickly loses her balance
Tends to keep her hips and knees stiff in extension/hyperextension
Dynamic: Unable to weight shift or step without bilateral handhold.

Functional

Functional Independence Measure (FIM)

Eating: FIM 6; requires adaptive equipment.
Grooming: FIM 6; requires adaptive equipment.
Bathing: FIM 5; requires set-up and adaptive equipment.
Dressing—upper and lower: FIM 4; min assist
Toileting: FIM 4; min assist for balance
Sphincter control—Bladder FIM 6; Bowel FIM 6
Transfers—bed, chair, wheelchair: FIM 4, min contact assist for stand pivot transfers
Transfers—toilet and tub: FIM 4; min contact assist
Locomotion—walk: FIM 4; min contact assist, uses walker
Locomotion—stairs: FIM 2; less than 4 to 6 stairs, max assist
Locomotion—wheelchair: FIM 5; supervision, uses manual wheelchair for distances up to 150 ft; posture in wheelchair: sacral sitting
Requires a lap belt due to extensor spasms, which can cause her to fling out of the chair
Communication—expression: FIM 6; requires extra time, mild dysarthria
Communication—comprehension: FIM 6; complete understanding, requires extra time for processing
Social interaction: FIM 7
Problem solving: FIM 6; requires extra time, slight difficulty initiating decisions
Memory: FIM 6; slight difficulty remembering daily routines and executing requests without need for repetition

Expanded Disability Status Scale (EDSS) score: 6.5

PATIENT'S GOALS

She would like to regain ambulation skills and independent living status. She recognizes the need to live with her parents for the time being but sees this as only temporary.

GUIDING QUESTIONS

1. Develop a problem list: identify/categorize this patient's problems in terms of:
   - Direct impairments
   - Indirect impairments

- Functional limitations
- Disability

2. Identify two outcomes (the remediation of functional limitations and disability) and two goals (remediation of impairments) for this patient.
3. Formulate four treatment interventions that could be used at the start of therapy to achieve the stated outcomes and goals. Provide a brief rationale for each.
4. What strategies can be used to develop self-management skills and promote self-efficacy and quality of life?

References

1. Dean, G: The multiple sclerosis problem. Sci Am 223:40, 1970.
2. Anderson, D, et al: Revised estimate of the prevalence of multiple sclerosis in the United States. Ann Neurol 31:333, 1992.
3. Kurland, LT: The evolution of multiple sclerosis epidemiology. Ann Neurol 36(Suppl 1): S2, 1994.
4. Alter, M, et al: Migration and risk of multiple sclerosis. Neurology 28:1089, 1978.
5. Kurtzke, J, and Hyllested, K: Multiple sclerosis in the Faroe Islands: I. Clinical and epidemiological features. Ann Neurol 5:6, 1979.
6. Weinshenker, B: Epidemiology of multiple sclerosis. Neurol Clin 14:291, 1996.
7. Herndon, R: The pathology of multiple sclerosis and its variants. In Herdon, R (ed): Multiple Sclerosis: Immunology, Pathology and Pathophysiology. Demos Medical Publishers, New York, 2003, p 184.
8. Johnson, R: The virology of demyelinating disease. Ann Neurol 36(Suppl):S54, 1994.
9. Chelmicka-Schoor, E, and Arnason, B: Nervous system-immune system interactions and their role in multiple sclerosis. Ann Neurol 36(Suppl 1):S29, 1994.
10. Sadovnick, A, and Ebers, G: Genetics of multiple sclerosis. Neurol Clin 13:99, 1995.
11. Kahana, E, et al: Multiple sclerosis: Genetic versus environmental aetiology: Epidemiology in Israel updated. J Neurol 241:341, 1994.
12. Matthews, WB, et al: McAlpine's Multiple Sclerosis. Churchill Livingstone, Edinburgh, 1991.
13. Lassmann, H, Suchanek, G, and Ozawa, K: Histopathology and the blood—cerebrospinal fluid barrier in multiple sclerosis. Ann Neurol 36 (Suppl 1): S42, 1994.
14. Lublin, F, and Reingold, S: Defining the clinical course of multiple sclerosis: Results of an international survey. Neurology 46:907, 1996.
15. Shapiro, R: Managing the Symptoms of Multiple Sclerosis, ed 4. Demos Medical Publishers, New York, 2003.
16. Lechtenberg, R: Multiple Sclerosis Fact Book, ed 2. FA Davis, Philadelphia, 1995.
17. Shapiro, R: Symptom management in multiple sclerosis. Ann Neurol 36:S1230, 1994.
18. Maloni, H: Pain in Multiple Sclerosis, Clinical Bulletin. National Multiple Sclerosis Society, New York, 1999.
19. Katz, R, and Rymer, Z: Spastic hypertonia: Mechanisms and measurement. Arch Phys Med Rehabil 70:144, 1989.
20. Schapiro, R, and Schneider, D: Management of fatigue in multiple sclerosis (Clinical Bulletin). National Multiple Sclerosis Society, New York, 2004.
21. Krupp, L, et al: Fatigue in multiple sclerosis. Arch Neurol 45:435, 1988.
22. Freal, J, et al: Symptomatic fatigue in multiple sclerosis. Arch Phys Med Rehabil 65:135, 1984.
23. Packer, T, et al: Fatigue secondary to chronic illness: Postpolio syndrome, chronic fatigue syndrome, and multiple sclerosis. Arch Phys Med Rehabil 75:1122, 1994.
24. Fisk, J, et al: The impact of fatigue on patients with multiple sclerosis. J Can Sci Neurol 21:9, 1994.
25. Schwartz, C, et al: Psychosocial correlates of fatigue in multiple sclerosis. Arch Phys Med Rehabil 77:165, 1996.
26. Kushner, S, and Brandfass, K: Spasticity (Clinical Bulletin). National Multiple Sclerosis Society, New York, 2004.
27. Stolp-Smith, K, et al: Management of impairment, disability, and handicap due to multiple sclerosis. Mayo Clin Proc 72:1184, 1997.
28. Smedman, L: Tremor, Multiple Sclerosis Basic Facts Series. National Multiple Sclerosis Society, New York, 2004.
29. Herrera, W: Vestibular and other balance disorders in multiple sclerosis. Neurol Clin 5:407, 1990.
30. Clinical Education Committee: Gait and Walking Problems. National Multiple Sclerosis Society, New York, 2004.
31. Clinical Education Committee: Speech and Swallowing. National Multiple Sclerosis Society, New York, 2004.
32. Schiffer, R: Cognitive Loss in Multiple Sclerosis, A Clinical Bulletin for Health Professionals. National Multiple Sclerosis Society, New York, 2004.
33. Petersen, R, and Kokmen, E: Cognitive and psychiatric abnormalities in multiple sclerosis. Mayo Clin Proc 64:657, 1989.
34. Franklin, G, et al: Cognitive loss in multiple sclerosis. Arch Neurol 46:162, 1989.
35. Samuel, L, and Cavallo, P: Emotional Issues of the Person with MS, A Clinical Bulletin for Health Professionals. National Multiple Sclerosis Society, New York, 2004.
36. Brassington, J, and Marsh, N: Neuropsychological aspects of multiple sclerosis. Neuropsychol Rev 8:43, 1998.
37. Shnek, Z, et al: Helplessness, self-efficacy, cognitive distortions and depression in multiple sclerosis and spinal cord injury. Ann Behav Med 19:287, 1997.
38. Minden, S: Pseudobulbar Affect, A Clinical Bulletin for Health Professionals. National Multiple Sclerosis Society, New York, 2004.
39. Feinstein, A, et al: Prevalence and neurobehavioral correlates of pathological laughing and crying in multiple sclerosis. Arch Neurol 54:1116, 1997.
40. Minden, S, and Schiffer, R: Affective disorders in multiple sclerosis. Arch Neurol 47:98, 1990.
41. Andrews, K, and Husmann, D: Bladder dysfunction and management in multiple sclerosis. Mayo Clin Proc 72:1176, 1997.
42. Kalb, R: Urinary Dysfunction and MS: A Guide for People with Multiple Sclerosis. National Multiple Sclerosis Society, New York, 2002.
43. Clinical Education Committee: Bowel Problems. National Multiple Sclerosis Society, New York, 2004.
44. McDonald, W, et al: Recommended diagnostic criteria for multiple sclerosis: Guidelines from the International Panel on the Diagnosis of Multiple Sclerosis. Ann Neurol 50(1): 121, 2001.
45. King, M: Immunology for the rest of us. Inside MS. Spring: 50–59, 2002.
46. Goodin, D, et al: Disease modifying therapies in multiple sclerosis: Subcommittee of the American Academy of Neurology and the MS Council for Clinical Practice Guidelines. Neurology 58:169, 2002.
47. Cook, S: Changing Therapy in Relapsing Multiple Sclerosis: Considerations and Recommendations of a Task Force of the National Multiple Sclerosis Society. Consensus Statement. National Multiple Sclerosis Society, New York, 2004.
48. Clinical Monograph: Comparing The Disease-Modifying Drugs. National MS Society, New York, 2005. Retrieved June 25, 2005, from http://www.nationalmssociety.org/Brochures-Comparing (revised 2/28/05).
49. Holland, N: Improving Adherence to Therapy with Immunomodulating Agents. National Multiple Sclerosis Society, New York, 2004.
50. Abel, N, and Smith, R: Intrathecal Baclofen for treatment of intractable spinal spasticity. Arch Phys Med Rehabil 75:54, 1994.
51. Orsnes, G, et al: The effect of Baclofen on the transmission in spinal pathways in spastic multiple sclerosis patients. Clin Neurophysiol 111:1372, 2000.

52. Thompson, A: The effectiveness of neurological rehabilitation in multiple sclerosis. J Rehabil Res Dev 37(4): 455, 2000.
53. Baker, N, and Tickle-Degnen, L: The effectiveness of physical, psychological, and functional interventions in treating clients with multiple sclerosis: A meta-analysis. Am J Occup Ther 55(3):324, 2001.
54. Craig, J, et al: A randomized controlled trial comparing rehabilitation against standard therapy in multiple sclerosis patients receiving steroid treatment. J Neurol Neurosurg Psychiatry 74:1225, 2003.
55. Di Fabio, R, et al: Health-related quality of life for persons with progressive multiple sclerosis: Influence of rehabilitation. Phys Ther 77(12):1704, 1997.
56. DiFabio, R, et al: Extended outpatient rehabilitation: Its influence on symptom frequency, fatigue, and functional status for persons with progressive multiple sclerosis. Arch Phys Med Rehabil 79:141, 1998.
57. Feigenson, JS, et al: The cost-effectiveness of multiple sclerosis rehabilitation: A model. Neurology 31:1316, 1981.
58. Freeman, J, et al: The impact of inpatient rehabilitation on progressive multiple sclerosis. Ann Neurol 42(2):236, 1997.
59. Freeman, J, et al: Inpatient rehabilitation in multiple sclerosis: Do the benefits carry over into the community? Neurology 52(1): 50, 1999.
60. Fuller, K, Dawson, K, and Wiles, C: Physiotherapy in chronic multiple sclerosis: A controlled trial. Clin Rehabil 10:195, 1996.
61. Greenspun, B, et al: Multiple sclerosis and rehabilitation outcome. Arch Phys Med Rehabil 68:434, 1987.
62. Kidd, D, et al: The benefit of inpatient neurorehabilitation in multiple sclerosis. Clin Rehabil 9:198, 1995.
63. KoKo, C: Effectiveness of rehabilitation for multiple sclerosis. Clin Rehabil 13(1):33, 1999.
64. Kraft, G: Rehabilitation still the only way to improve function in multiple sclerosis. Lancet 354:2016, 1999.
65. Langdon, D, and Thompson, A: Multiple sclerosis: A preliminary study of selected variables affecting rehabilitation outcome. Mult Scler 5:94, 1999.
66. Liu, C, Playford, E, and Thompson, A: Does neurorehabilitation have a role in relapsing remitting multiple sclerosis? J Neurol 250(10): 1214. 2003.
67. Patti, F, et al: Effects of a short outpatient rehabilitation treatment on disability of multiple sclerosis patients—A randomized controlled trial. J Neurol 250(7):861, 2003.
68. Slade, A, Tennant, A, and Chamberlain, M: A randomized controlled trial to determine the effect of intensity of therapy upon length of stay in a neurological rehabilitation setting. J Rehabil Med 34 (6): 260, 2002.
69. Solari, A, et al: Physical rehabilitation has a positive effect on disability in multiple sclerosis patients. Neurology 52:57, 1999.
70. Wiles C, et al: Controlled randomized crossover trial of the effects of physiotherapy on mobility in chronic multiple sclerosis. J Neurol Neurosurg Psychiatry 70:174, 2001.
71. Sutherland, G, and Andersen, M: Exercise and multiple sclerosis: Physiological, psychological, and quality of life issues. J Sports Med Phys Fitness 41:421, 2001.
72. Kraft, G, and Schapiro, R (Co-Chairs) National MS Society's Medical Advisory Board: Rehabilitation: Recommendations for Persons with Multiple Sclerosis. National Multiple Sclerosis Society, New York, 2004.
73. American Physical Therapy Association: Guide to physical therapist practice. Phys Ther 81:1, 2001.
74. Moffa-Trotter, M, and Anemaet, W: Addressing functional maintenance programs in home care. Advance, August 24, 1998.
75. Mertin, J: Rehabilitation in multiple sclerosis. Ann Neurol 36:S130, 1994.
76. Dal Bello-Haas, V: A framework for rehabilitation of neurodegenerative diseases: Planning care and maximizing quality of life. Neurology Report (now JNPT) 26(2):115, 2002.
77. Benedict, R, et al: Minimal neuropsychological examination of MS patients: A consensus approach. Clin Neuropsychol 16 (3):381, 2002.
78. Folstein, M: Mini-mental state: A practice of method for grading the cognitive state of patients for the clinician. J Psychiatr Res 12:189, 1975.
79. Beck, A, and Beck, R: Screening depressed patients in family practice: A rapid technique. Postgrad Med 52:81, 1972.
80. Melzack, R: The McGill Pain Questionnaire: Major properties and scoring methods. Pain 1:227, 1975.
81. Lawlis, G, et al: The development of the Dallas pain questionnaire. Spine 14(5):511, 1989.
82. Fisk, JD, et al: The impact of fatigue on patients with multiple sclerosis. Can J Neurol Sci 21(1): 9, 1994.
83. Fisk, JD, et al: Measuring the functional impact of fatigue: Initial validation of the fatigue impact scale. Clin Infect Dis Suppl 1:S79. 1994.
84. National Multiple Sclerosis Society: Clinical Practice Guidelines: Fatigue and Multiple Sclerosis, National Multiple Sclerosis Society, New York, 2004.
85. De Souza, L, and Ashburn, A: Examination of motor function in people with multiple sclerosis. Physiother Res Int 1:98, 1996.
86. Lee, K, et al: The Ashworth Scale: A reliable and reproducible method of measuring spasticity. J Neuro Rehab 3:205, 1989.
87. Bohannon, R, and Smith, M: Interrater reliability of a modified Ashworth scale of muscle spasticity. Phys Ther 67:206, 1987.
88. Shumway-Cook, A, and Horak, F: Assessing the influence of sensory interaction on balance. Phys Ther 66:1548, 1986.
89. Nelson, S, et al: Vestibular and sensory interaction deficits assessed by dynamic platform posturography in patients with multiple sclerosis. Ann Otol Rhinol Laryngol 104:62, 1995.
90. Jackson, R, et al: Abnormalities in posturography and estimations of visual vertical and horizontal in multiple sclerosis. Am J Otol 16:88, 1995.
91. Berg, K, et al: Measuring balance in the elderly: Preliminary development of an instrument. Physiother Can 41:304, 1989.
92. Berg, K, et al: Measuring balance in the elderly: Validation of an instrument. Can J Public Health Suppl 2(Jul–Aug):S7-11, 1992.
93. Tinetti, M: Performance-oriented examination of mobility problems in elderly patients. J Am Geriatr Soc 34:119, 1986.
94. Shumway-Cook, A, and Woollacott, M: Motor Control Theory and Practical Applications, ed 2. Lippincott Williams & Wilkins, Philadelphia, 2001.
95. Schwid, S, et al: The measurement of ambulatory impairment in multiple sclerosis. Neurology 49:1419, 1997.
96. Lord, SE, et al: Visual gait analysis: The development of a clinical examination and scale. Clin Rehabil 12:107, 1998.
97. Borg, G: Psychophysical bases of perceived exertion. Med Sci Sports Exerc 14:377, 1982.
98. American College of Sports Medicine: ACSM's Guidelines for Exercise Testing and Prescription, ed 6. Lippincott Williams & Wilkins, Philadelphia, 2000.
99. Guide for the Uniform Data Set for Medical Rehabilitation including the FIM instrument, Version 5.0. State University of New York at Buffalo, Buffalo, 1996.
100. Granger, C, et al: Functional examination scales: A study of persons with multiple sclerosis. Arch Phys Med Rehabil 71:870, 1990.
101. Stewart, A, Hays, R, and Ware, J: The MOS short-form general health survey. Reliability and validity in a patient population. Med Care 26(7):724, 1988.
102. Freeman, JA, et al: Clinical appropriateness: A key factor in outcome measure selection: The 36 item short form health survey in multiple sclerosis. J Neurol 68(2):150, 2000.
103. Gilson, B, et al: The Sickness Impact Profile: Development of an outcome measure of health care. Am J Public Health 65:1304, 1975.
104. Doble, S, et al: Functional competence of community-dwelling persons with multiple sclerosis using the Examination of Motor and Process Skills. Arch Phys Med Rehabil 75:843, 1994.
105. Kurtzke, J: On the evaluation of disability in multiple sclerosis. Neurology 11:686, 1961.
106. Kurtzke, J: Rating neurological impairment in multiple sclerosis: An expanded disability status scale (EDSS). Neurology 33:1444, 1983.
107. Noseworthy, J, et al and Canadian Cooperative MS Study Group: Interrater variability with the Expanded Disability Status Scale (EDSS) and Functional Systems (FS) in a multiple sclerosis clinical trial. Neurology 40:971, 1990.
108. Haber, A, and LaRocca, N (eds): M.R.D. Minimal Record of Disability for Multiple Sclerosis. National Multiple Sclerosis Society, New York, 1985.

109. Solari, A, et al: Accuracy of self-examination of the minimal record of disability in patients with multiple sclerosis. Acta Neurol Scand 87:43, 1993.
110. Vickrey, BG, et al: A health-related quality of life measure for multiple sclerosis. Qual Life Res 4:187, 1995.
111. Consortium of Multiple Sclerosis Centers, Health Science Research Subcommittee: Multiple Sclerosis Quality of Life Inventory: A User's Manual. National Multiple Sclerosis Society, New York, 1997.
112. Cella, DF, et al: Validation of the Functional Examination of Multiple Sclerosis quality of life instrument. Neurology 47(1):129, 1996.
113. Hobart, JC, et al: The Multiple Sclerosis Impact Scale (MSIS-29): A new patient-based outcome measure. Brain 124:962, 2001.
114. Riazi, A, et al: Multiple Sclerosis Impact Scale (MSIS-29): Reliability and validity in hospital based samples. J Neurol Neurosurg Psychiatry 73(6):701, 2002.
115. Quinn, L, and Gordon, J: Functional Outcomes Documentation for Rehabilitation. WB Saunders, Philadelphia, 2003.
116. Dittmar, S, and Gresham, G: Functional Examination and Outcome Measures for the Rehabilitation Health Professional. Aspen, Gaithersburg, MD, 1997.
117. White, LJ, et al: Resistance training improves strength and functional capacity in persons with multiple sclerosis. Mult Scler 10:668, 2004.
118. Surakka, J, et al: Effects of aerobic and strength exercise on motor fatigue in men and women with multiple sclerosis: A randomized control trial. Clin Rehabil 18:737, 2004.
119. Mostert, S, and Kesselring, J: Effects of a short-term exercise training program on aerobic fitness, fatigue, health perception, and activity level of subjects with multiple sclerosis. Mult Scler 8:161, 2002.
120. Roehrs, T, and Karst, G: Effects of an aquatics exercise program on quality of life measures for individuals with progressive multiple sclerosis. JNPT 28(2):63, 2004.
121. Sutherland, G, Andersen, M, and Stoove, M: Can aerobic exercise training affect health-related quality of life for people with multiple sclerosis? J Sport Exerc Psychol 23:122, 2001.
122. Petajan, J, et al: Impact of aerobic training on fitness and quality of life in multiple sclerosis. Ann Neurol 39:432, 1996.
123. Ponichtera-Mulcare, J, et al: Change in aerobic fitness of patients with multiple sclerosis during a 6-month training program. Sports Med Train Rehab 7:265, 1997.
124. Ponichtera-Mulcare, J, et al: Maximal aerobic exercise of individuals with multiple sclerosis using three modes of ergometry. Clin Kinesiol 46:12, 1992.
125. Gehlsen, G, et al: Effects of an aquatic fitness program on the muscular strength and endurance of patients with multiple sclerosis. Phys Ther 64:653, 1984.
126. Mulcare, J, and Petajan, J: Multiple Sclerosis. In American College of Sports Medicine: ACSM's Resources for Clinical Exercise Physiology: Musculoskeletal, Neuromuscular, Neoplastic, Immunologic, and Hematologic Conditions. Lippincott, Williams & Wilkins, Philadelphia, 2002, p 29.
127. Costello, E, et al: Exercise prescription for individuals with multiple sclerosis. Neurology Report 20:24, 1996.
128. Mulcare, J: Multiple Sclerosis. In American College of Sports Medicine: ACSM's Exercise Management for Persons with Chronic Diseases and Disabilities. Human Kinetics, Champaign IL, 1997, p 189.
129. White, AT, et al: Effect of precooling on physical performance in multiple sclerosis. Mult Scler 6:176, 2000.
130. Erland, C, et al: Effects of the Mark VII personal cooling system on selected symptoms of multiple sclerosis. Neurology Report 19:23, 1995.
131. Kinnman, J, et al: Cooling suit for multiple sclerosis: functional improvement in daily living? Scan J Rehabil Med 32:20, 2000.
132. Flensner, G, and Lindencrona, C: The cooling-suit: Case studies on its influence on fatigue among eight individuals with multiple sclerosis. J Adv Nur 37(6): 541, 2002.
133. Ku, YE, et al: Physiologic and functional responses of MS patients to body cooling. Am J Phys Med Rehabil 79:427, 2000.
134. O'Sullivan, S, and Schmitz, T: Physical Rehabilitation Laboratory Manual: Focus on Functional Training. FA Davis, Philadelphia, 1999.
135. DeSouza, L: A different approach to physiotherapy for multiple sclerosis patients. Physiotherapy 70:428, 1984.
136. Anema, J, et al: Cardiovascular autonomic function in multiple sclerosis. J Neurol Sci 104:129, 1992.
137. Sterman, A, et al: Disseminated abnormalities of cardiovascular autonomic functions in multiple sclerosis. Neurology 35:1665, 1985.
138. Pentland, B, and Ewing, D: Cardiovascular reflexes in multiple sclerosis. Eur Neurol 26:46, 1987.
139. Foglio, K, et al: Respiratory muscle function and exercise capacity in multiple sclerosis. Eur Respir J 7:23, 1994.
140. Gappmaier, E, et al: Aerobic exercise in multiple sclerosis. Neurology Report 19:41, 1995.
141. Kirsch, N, and Myslinski, MJ: The effect of a personally designed fitness program on the aerobic capacity and function for two individuals with multiple sclerosis. Phys Ther Case Rep 2:19, 1999.
142. McComas, A, et al: Fatigue brought on by malfunction of the central and peripheral nervous systems. In Simon, C, et al (eds): Fatigue. Plenum Press, New York, 1995, p 495.
143. Multiple Sclerosis Council for Clinical Practice Guidelines: Fatigue and Multiple Sclerosis: Evidence-Based Management Strategies for Fatigue in Multiple Sclerosis. Paralyzed Veterans of America, New York, 1998.
144. Meythaler, JM (ed): Spastic hypertonia. Phys Med Rehabil Clin N Am. 12 (4): November, 2001.
145. Brar, S, et al: Evaluation of treatment protocols on minimal to moderate spasticity in multiple sclerosis. Arch Phys Med Rehabil 72:186, 1991.
146. Kushner, S, and Brandfass, K: Spasticity—A clinical bulletin for health professionals. National Multiple Sclerosis Society, New York, 2004.
147. Adler, S, Beckers, D, and Buck, M: PNF in Practice, ed 2. Springer, New York, 2003.
148. Kasser, S, Rose, D, and Clark, S: Balance training for adults with multiple sclerosis: Multiple case studies. Neurology Report (now JNPT) 23(1): 5, 1999.
149. Hammon, RG, et al: Training effects during repeated therapy sessions of balance training using visual feedback. Arch Phys Med Rehabil 73:738, 1992.
150. Behrman, AL, and Harkema, SJ: Locomotor training after human spinal cord injury: A series of case studies. Phys Ther 80:688, 2000.
151. Nymark, J, et al: Body weight support treadmill gait training in the subacute recovery phase of incomplete spinal cord injury. J Neuro Rehab 12:119, 1998.
152. Visintin, M, et al: A new approach to retain gait in stroke patients through body weight support and treadmill stimulation. Stroke 29:1122, 1998.
153. Sullivan, KJ, Knowlton, GJ, and Dobkin, BH: Step training with body weight support: Effect of treadmill speed and practice paradigms on poststroke locomotor recovery. Arch Phys Med Rehabil 83:683, 2002.
154. Miyai, I, et al: Treadmill training with body weight support: Its effect on Parkinson's disease. Arch Phys Med Rehabil 81:849, 2000.
155. Fulk, G: Locomotor training and virtual reality-based balance training for an individual with multiple sclerosis: A case report. JNPT 29(1):34, 2005
156. Perry, J, et al: Rocker shoe as walking aid in multiple sclerosis I. Arch Phys Med Rehabil 62:59, 1981.
157. National Multiple Sclerosis Society (Basic Facts Series): Gait or Walking Problems. National Multiple Sclerosis Society, New York, 2003.
158. Smeltzer, S, Lavietes, M, and Cook, S: Expiratory training in multiple sclerosis. Arch Phys Med Rehabil 77:909, 1996.
159. National Multiple Sclerosis Society (Basic Facts Series): Speech and Swallowing. National Multiple Sclerosis Society, New York, 2004.
160. Matson, R, and Brooks, N: Adjusting to multiple sclerosis: An exploratory study. Soc Sci Med 11:245, 1977.
161. Pulton, T: Multiple sclerosis social psychological perspective. Phys Ther 57:170, 1977.

162. Cervera-Deval, J, et al: Social handicaps of multiple sclerosis and their relation to neurological alterations. Arch Phys Med Rehabil 75:1223, 1994.
163. Kraft, G, et al: Disability, disease duration, and rehabilitation services needs in multiple sclerosis: Patient perspective. Arch Phys Med Rehabil 67:164, 1986.
164. Shnek, Z, et al: Helplessness, self-efficacy, cognitive distortions, and depression in multiple sclerosis and spinal cord injury. Ann Behav Med 19:287, 1997.
165. Leino-Kilpi, H, et al: Elements of empowerment and MS patients. J Neurosci Nurs 30:116, 1998.
166. Bello-Hass, V, Bene, M, and Mitsumoto, H: End of life: Challenges and strategies for the rehabilitation professional. Neurology Report (now J Neurol Phys Ther) 26(4):174, 2002.
167. Hertz, D, and Holland, N: Community Resources for Your Patients with MS (Resource Bulletin, Information for Health Professionals). National Multiple Sclerosis Society, New York, 2004.
168. Price, G: The challenge to the family. Am J Nurs 80:283, 1980.
169. Stuifbergen, A, and Roberts, G: Health promotion practices of women with multiple sclerosis. Arch Phys Med Rehabil 78(Suppl 5):S-3, 1997.

Supplemental Readings

Blackston, M: First Year—Multiple Sclerosis: An Essential Guide for the Newly Diagnosed. Marlow and Co, New York, 2002.

Burks, JS, and Johnson, KP (eds): Multiple Sclerosis: Diagnosis, Medical Management, and Rehabilitation. Demos Medical Publishers, New York, 2000.

Cohen, JA, and Rudick, RA (eds): Multiple Sclerosis Therapeutics, ed. 2 Martin Dunitz, London, 2003.

Coyle, PK, and Halper, J: Meeting the Challenge of Progressive Multiple Sclerosis. Demos Medical Publishers, New York, 2001.

Holland, NJ, Murray, TJ, and Reingold, SC: Multiple Sclerosis: A Guide for the Newly Diagnosed, ed 2. Demos Medical Publishing, New York, 2002.

Kalb, R (ed): Multiple Sclerosis: A Guide for Families. Demos Medical Publishing, New York, 1998.

Draft, GH, and Catanzaro, M: Living with Multiple Sclerosis: A Wellness Approach, ed. 2. Demos Medical Publishing, New York, 2000.

Kraft, GH: Rehabilitation principles for patients with multiple sclerosis. J Spinal Cord Med 21(2):117, 1998.

McDonald, WI, et al: Recommended diagnostic criteria for multiple sclerosis: Guidelines from the International Panel on the Diagnosis of Multiple Sclerosis. Ann Neurol 50:121, 2001.

Miller, A, Lublin, F, and Coyle, PK: Multiple Sclerosis in Clinical Practice. Martin Dunitz, London, 2003.

Northrop, DE, and Cooper, S: Health Insurance Resource Manual: Options for People with Chronic Disease and Disability. Demos Medical Publishing, New York, 2003.

Paty, DW, and Ebers, GC (eds): Multiple Sclerosis. FA Davis, Philadelphia, 1998.

Shapiro, R: Managing the Symptoms of Multiple Sclerosis, ed 4. Demos Medical Publishing, New York. 2003.

Appendix A: Modified Fatigue Impact Scale (MFIS)

Fatigue is a feeling of physical tiredness and lack of energy that many people experience from time to time. But people who have medical conditions like MS experience stronger feelings of fatigue more often and with greater impact than others.

Following is a list of statements that describe the effects of fatigue. Please read each statement carefully, then *circle the one number* that best indicates how often fatigue has affected you in this way during the *past 4 weeks.* (If you need help in marking your responses, *tell the interviewer the number* of the best response.) *Please answer every question.* If you are not sure which answer to select, choose the one answer that comes closest to describing you. Ask the interviewer to explain any words or phrases that you do not understand.

Name: ______________________________ Date: _____/_____/_____

ID#: ______________________________ Test: 1 2 3 4

Because of my fatigue during the past 4 weeks. . .

	Never	Rarely	Sometimes	Often	Almost always
1. I have been less alert.	0	1	2	3	4
2. I have had difficulty paying attention for long periods of time.	0	1	2	3	4
3. I have been unable to think clearly.	0	1	2	3	4
4. I have been clumsy and uncoordinated.	0	1	2	3	4
5. I have been forgetful.	0	1	2	3	4
6. I have had to pace myself in my physical activities.	0	1	2	3	4
7. I have been less motivated to do anything that requires physical effort.	0	1	2	3	4
8. I have been less motivated to participate in social activities.	0	1	2	3	4
9. I have been limited in my ability to do things away from home.	0	1	2	3	4
10. I have trouble maintaining physical effort for long periods.	0	1	2	3	4
11. I have had difficulty making decisions.	0	1	2	3	4
12. I have been less motivated to do anything that requires thinking.	0	1	2	3	4
13. My muscles have felt weak.	0	1	2	3	4
14. I have been physically uncomfortable.	0	1	2	3	4
15. I have had trouble finishing tasks that require thinking.	0	1	2	3	4
16. I have had difficulty organizing my thoughts when doing things at home or at work.	0	1	2	3	4
17. I have been less able to complete tasks that require physical effort.	0	1	2	3	4
18. My thinking has been slowed down.	0	1	2	3	4
19. I have had trouble concentrating.	0	1	2	3	4
20. I have limited my physical activities.	0	1	2	3	4
21. I have needed to rest more often or for longer periods.	0	1	2	3	4

Instructions for Scoring the MFIS

Items on the MFIS can be aggregated into three subscales (physical, cognitive, and psychosocial), as well as into a total MFIS score. All items are scaled so that higher scores indicate a greater impact of fatigue on a person's activities.

Physical Subscale

This scale can range from 0 to 36. It is computed by adding raw scores on the following items: 4 + 6 + 7 + 10 + 13 + 14 + 17 + 20 + 21.

Cognitive Subscale

This scale can range from 0 to 40. It is computed by adding raw scores on the following items: 1 + 2 + 3 + 5 + 11 + 12 + 15 + 16 + 18 + 19.

Psychosocial Subscale

This scale can range from 0 to 8. It is computed by adding raw scores on the following items: 8 + 9.

Total MFIS Score

The total MFIS score can range from 0 to 84. It is computed by adding scores on the physical, cognitive, and psychosocial subscales.

From: Multiple Sclerosis Council for Clinical Practice Guidelines,[143] with permission.

Appendix B: An Expanded Disability Status Scale (EDSS) for Patients with Multiple Sclerosis

Functional Systems

Pyramidal Functions

0. Normal.
1. Abnormal signs without disability.
2. Minimal disability.
3. Mild or moderate paraparesis or hemiparesis; severe monoparesis.
4. Marked paraparesis or hemiparesis; moderate quadriparesis; or monoplegia.
5. Paraplegia, hemiplegia, or marked quadriparesis.
6. Quadriplegia.

V. Unknown.

Cerebellar Functions

0. Normal.
1. Abnormal signs without disability.
2. Mild ataxia.
3. Moderate truncal or limb ataxia.
4. Severe ataxia, all limbs.
5. Unable to perform coordinated movements due to ataxia.

V. Unknown.

X. Is used throughout after each number when weakness (grade 3 or more on pyramidal) interferes with testing.

Brainstem Functions

0. Normal.
1. Signs only.
2. Moderate nystagmus or other mild disability.
3. Severe nystagmus, marked extraocular weakness, or moderate disability of other cranial nerves.
4. Marked dysarthria or other marked disability.
5. Inability to swallow or speak.

V. Unknown.

Sensory Functions (revised 1982)

0. Normal.
1. Vibration or figure-writing decrease only, in one or two limbs.
2. Mild decrease in touch or pain or position sense, and/or moderate decrease in vibration in one or two limbs; or vibratory decrease alone in three or four limbs.
3. Moderate decrease in touch or pain or position sense, and/or essentially lost vibration in one or two limbs; or mild decrease in touch or pain and/or moderate decrease in all proprioceptive tests in three or four limbs.
4. Marked decrease in touch or pain or loss of proprioception, alone or combined, in one or two limbs; or moderate decrease in touch or pain and/or severe proprioceptive decrease in more than two limbs.
5. Loss (essentially) of sensation in one or two limbs; or moderate decrease in touch or pain and/or loss of proprioception for most of the body below the head.
6. Sensation essentially lost below the head.

V. Unknown.

Bowel and BladderFunctions (revised 1982)

0. Normal.
1. Mild urinary hesitancy, urgency, or retention.
2. Moderate hesitancy, urgency, retention of bowel or bladder, or rare urinary incontinence.
3. Frequent urinary incontinence.
4. In need of almost constant catheterization.
5. Loss of bladder function.
6. Loss of bowel and bladder function.

V. Unknown.

Visual (or Optic) Functions

0. Normal.
1. Scotoma with visual acuity (corrected) better than 20/30.
2. Worse eye with scotoma with maximal visual acuity (corrected) of 20/30 to 20/59.
3. Worse eye with large scotoma, or moderate decrease in fields, but with maximal visual acuity (corrected) of 20/60 to 20/99.
4. Worse eye with marked decrease of fields and maximal visual acuity (corrected) of 20/100 to 20/200; grade 3 plus maximal acuity of better eye of 20/60 or less.
5. Worse eye with maximal visual acuity (corrected) less than 20/200; grade 4 plus maximal acuity of better eye of 20/60 or less.
6. Grade 5 plus maximal visual acuity of better eye of 20/60 or less.

V. Unknown.

X. Is added to grades 0 to 6 for presence of temporal pallor.

Cerebral (or Mental) Functions

0. Normal.
1. Mood alteration only (does not affect DSS score).
2. Mild decrease in mentation.
3. Moderate decrease in mentation.
4. Marked decrease in mentation; chronic brain syndrome: moderate.
5. Dementia or chronic brain syndrome: severe or incompetent.

V. Unknown.

Other Functions

0. None.
1. Any other neurologic findings attributed to MS (specify).

V. Unknown.

Expanded Disability Status Scale (EDSS)

0 = Normal neurologic exam (all grade 0 in functional systems [FS]; cerebral grade 1 acceptable).

1.0 = No disability, minimal signs in one FS (i.e., grade 1 excluding cerebral grade 1).

1.5 = No disability, minimal signs in more than one FS (more than one grade 1 excluding cerebral grade 1).

2.0 = Minimal disability in one FS (one FS grade 2, others 0 or 1).

2.5 = Minimal disability in two FS (two FS grade 2, others 0 or 1).

3.0 = Moderate disability in one FS (one FS grade 3, others 0 or 1), or mild disability in three or four FS (three/four FS grade 2, others 0 or 1) though fully ambulatory.

3.5 = Fully ambulatory but with moderate disability in one FS (one grade 3) and one or two FS grade 2; or two FS grade 3; or five FS grade 2 (others 0 or 1).

4.0 = Fully ambulatory without aid, self-sufficient, up and about some 12 hours a day despite relatively severe disability consisting of one FS grade 4 (others 0 or 1), or combinations of lesser grades exceeding limits of previous steps. Able to walk without aid or rest some 500 meters.

4.5 = Fully ambulatory without aid, up and about much of the day, able to work a full day, may otherwise have some limitation of full activity or require minimal assistance; characterized by relatively severe disability, usually consisting of one FS grade 4 (others 0 or 1) or combinations of lesser grades exceeding limits of previous steps. Able to walk without aid or rest for some 300 meters.

5.0 = Ambulatory without aid or rest for about 200 meters; disability severe enough to impair full daily activities (e.g., to work full day without special provisions). (Usual FS equivalents are one grade 5 alone, others 0 or 1; or combinations of lesser grades usually exceeding specifications for step 4.0.)

5.5 = Ambulatory without aid or rest for about 100 meters; disability severe enough to preclude full daily activities. (Usual FS equivalents are one grade 5 alone, others 0 or 1; or combinations of lesser grades usually exceeding those for step 4.0.)

6.0 = Intermittent or unilateral constant assistance (cane, crutch, or brace) required to walk about 100 meters with or without resting. (Usual FS equivalents are combinations with more than two FS grade 3+.)

6.5 = Constant bilateral assistance (canes, crutches, or braces) required to walk about 20 meters without resting. (Usual FS equivalents are combinations with more than two FS grade 3+.)

7.0 = Unable to walk beyond about 5 meters even with aid, essentially restricted to wheelchair; wheels self in standard-wheelchair and transfers alone; up and about in wheelchair some 12 hours a day. (Usual FS equivalents are combinations with more than one FS grade 4+; very rarely, pyramidal grade 5 alone.)

7.5 = Unable to take more than a few steps; restricted to wheelchair; may need aid in transfer, wheels self but cannot carry on in standard wheelchair a full day; may require motorized wheelchair. (Usual FS equivalents are combinations with more than one FS grade 4+.)

8.0 = Essentially restricted to bed or chair or ambulated in wheelchair, but may be out of bed itself much of the day; retains many self-care functions; generally has effective uses of arms. (Usual FS equivalents are combinations, generally grade 4+ in several systems.)

8.5 = Essentially restricted to bed much of the day; has some effective use of arm(s); retains some self-care functions. (Usual FS equivalents are combinations, generally 4+ in several systems.)

9.0 = Helpless bed patient; can communicate and eat. (Usual FS equivalents are combinations, mostly grade 4+.)

9.5 = Totally helpless bed patient; unable to communicate effectively or eat/swallow. (Usual FS equivalents are combinations, almost all grade 4+.)

10.0 = Death due to MS.

From Kurtzke,[105] with permission.

Appendix C: MS Daily Activity Diary

Instructions

1. At the top of the day's diary, describe how you slept the night before.
2. Assign a number value from **1 to 10** (1 being very low and 10 being very high) for:
   - Your level of fatigue **(F)**
   - The value or importance of the activity you are doing **(V)**
   - The satisfaction you feel with your performance of the activity **(S)**

   You can compute the "value" of an activity by comparing it to other activities you would like to do during the course of the day.
   For example:
   1 pm: F = 7 V = 3 S = 2 Activity: Fixing lunch standing 15 minutes (hot);
   Comment: Blurred vision
3. Always describe the physical work done in the **Activity** section (e.g., stood to shower 10 minutes, went up 20 stairs, walked 200 feet).
4. Note the **external temperature** of the environment under Activity.
5. List under **Comments** all MS symptoms as they appear or worsen during the day, including cognitive problems, visual problems, weakness, dizziness, dragging foot, pain, numbness, burning, and so forth.
6. Make notes **every hour.**

Name: ______________________________ Date: ______________________________

Describe sleep last night: ______________________________

Time	F	V	S	Activity	Comment
6:00 AM					
7:00					
8:00					
9:00					
10:00					
11:00					
12:00 PM					
1:00					
2:00					
3:00					
4:00					
5:00					
6:00					
7:00					
8:00					
9:00					
10:00					
11:00					

Appendix D: Web-Based Resources for Clinicians and Patients/Families Living with Multiple Sclerosis

National Multiple Sclerosis Society	http:/www.nationalmssociety.org
Americans with Disabilities Act: ADA home page	http://www.usdoj.gov/crt/ada
Medicare information	http://cms.hhs.gov
Social Security Online	http://www.ssa.gov
National Institute of Neurological Disorders and Stroke	http://www.ninds.nih.gov
National Library of Medicine	http://www.nim.nih.gov
Archives of Neurology	http://archneur.ama-assn.org
Neurology	http://www.neurology.org
CenterWatch Clinical Trials Listing Service	http://www.centerwatch.com
Veterans Affairs MS Centers of Excellence	http://www.va.gov/ms
CLAMS: Computer Literate Advocates for Multiple Sclerosis	http://www.clams.org
Consortium of Multiple Sclerosis Centers	http://www.mscare.org
The Heuga Center—MS Can Do program	http://www.heuga.org
Multiple Sclerosis International Federation	http://www.msif.org
Amgen—drug manufacturer of Novantrone	http://www.amgen.com http://www.novantrone.com http://www.msactivesource.com
Biogen—drug manufacturer of Avonex	http://www.biogen.com www.avonex.com
Berlex—drug manufacturer of Betaseron	http://www.berlex.com www.betaseron.com
Teva Neurosciences—drug manufacturer of Copaxone	http://www.tevaneuroscience.com http://www.mswatch.com
Serono Group—drug manufacturer of Rebif	http://www.serono.com http://www.rebif.com
MSWorld	http://www.msworld.org/communications.htm
The Myelin Project—MS research	http://www.myelin.org
Rocky Mountain MS Center	http://www.mscenter.org
National Family Caregivers Association (NFCA)	http://www.nfcacares.org
Well Spouse Foundation	http://www.wellspouse.org
American Academy of Neurology (ANA)	http://www.aan.com (ANA members, professionals) http://www.aan.com/public (public education)
National Rehabilitation Information Center (NARIC)	http://www.naric.com
Paralyzed Veterans of America (PVA)	http://www.pva.org
Ability Hub-assistive technology	http://www.abilityhub.com
ABLEDATA-assistive technology	http://www.abledata.com
Disabled Online	http://www.disabledonline.com
Apple Computer Accessibility	http://www.apple.com/accessibility
IBM Accessibility	http://www.306.ibm.com/able
Microsoft Accessibility Technology for Everyone	http://www.microsoft.com/enable

CHAPTER

20

LEARNING OBJECTIVES

1. Describe the epidemiology, etiology, pathogenesis, diagnosis, and general prognosis of amyotrophic lateral sclerosis (ALS).
2. Compare and contrast the El Escorial diagnostic criteria for ALS.
3. Differentiate among impairments related to lower motor neuron pathology, upper motor neuron pathology, and bulbar impairments.
4. Discuss the medical and health care management of individuals with ALS.
5. Outline a framework for rehabilitation for individuals with ALS.
6. Describe the components of the physical therapy examination for individuals with ALS.
7. Describe the role of the physical therapist in the management of an individual with ALS and the factors that influence intervention options.
8. Compare and contrast overwork damage and disuse atrophy as it relates to ALS.
9. Summarize the literature related to exercise and ALS.
10. Describe considerations that must be taken into account when designing an exercise program for the individual with ALS
11. Discuss problems commonly seen in individuals with ALS and the physical therapy interventions for these common problems.
12. Determine the anticipated goals and expected outcomes for an individual with ALS based on physical therapist examination findings.
13. Design an intervention program for the individual with ALS based on the physical therapist examination findings.

Amyotrophic Lateral Sclerosis

Vanina Dal Bello-Haas, BScPT, PhD

OUTLINE

Motor neuron diseases (MND) include a heterogeneous spectrum of inherited and sporadic (no family history) clinical disorders of the upper motor neurons (UMNs), lower motor neurons (LMNs), or a combination of both[1] (Table 20.1). **Amyotrophic lateral sclerosis** (ALS),[a] commonly known as Lou Gehrig's disease, is the most common and devastatingly fatal motor neuron disease among adults. ALS is characterized by the degeneration and loss of motor neurons in the spinal cord, brain stem, and brain, resulting in a variety of UMN and LMN clinical signs and symptoms.[2]

[a]The term MND is used to describe the disease in the United Kingdom, whereas the term ALS is used in North America and Europe. In Europe, ALS is also called Charcot's disease.

Table 20.1 Motor Neuron Disorders

Subtype	Nervous System Pathology
Amyotrophic lateral sclerosis	Degeneration of the corticospinal tracts, neurons in the motor cortex and brainstem, and anterior horn cells in the spinal cord
Primary lateral sclerosis	Degeneration of upper motor neurons
Progressive bulbar palsy	Degeneration of motor neurons of cranial nerves IX to XII
Progressive muscular atrophy	Loss or chromatolysis of motor neurons of the spinal cord and brainstem

Adapted in part from: Rowland, LP.[1]

Epidemiology

It is estimated that 30,000 individuals in the United States have ALS at any one time and 15 cases of the disease are diagnosed per day. Except in a very few areas, such as Guam and the Kii Peninsula of Japan, more recent studies report the overall incidence of ALS to be in the range of 0.4 to 2.4 cases per 100,000, with the incidence increasing with each decade of life, until at least the seventh decade. The prevalence of ALS has been reported to be higher than the incidence, 4 to 10 cases per 100,000.[3–7]

Although ALS can occur at any age, the average age at onset is the mid-to-late 50s.[4,5,7,8] Most studies have found that the disease affects men slightly more than women, with an approximate ratio of 1.7:1[3,5,6]; however, after the age of 65, this gender-related incidence is less pronounced.[3] In 5 percent to 10 percent of individuals with ALS, the disease is inherited as an autosomal dominant trait *(familial ALS [FALS])*,[3,9,10] although rare cases of juvenile onset ALS are inherited in an autosomal recessive pattern.[11] Of the hereditary ALS cases, approximately 20 percent are a result of more than 90 mutations in *SOD1*,[12,13] a gene that encodes the copper-zinc superoxide dismutase enzyme (CuZnSOD). The very large majority of adult individuals with ALS have no family history of the disease *(sporadic ALS)*, and a very small percentage of individuals with sporadic ALS also have a mutation in *SOD1*.[14,15]

Approximately 70 to 80 percent of individuals develop *limb-onset ALS*, with initial involvement in the extremities; while 20 to 30 percent develop *bulbar-onset ALS*, with initial involvement in the bulbar muscles.[6,16,17] Bulbar-onset ALS is more common in middle-aged women, and initial symptoms may include difficulty speaking, chewing, or swallowing.[2,6]

Etiology

Other than a small percentage of cases, etiology for the most part is unknown. It is hypothesized that no one single mechanism, but rather multiple mechanisms, may be responsible for neuron degeneration in ALS.[13] Possible pathological mechanisms include:

1. *Superoxide dismutases (SODs)* are a group of enzymes that eliminate oxygen free radicals, that, although products of normal cell metabolism, have been implicated in neurodegeneration. There are three isoforms of SOD in humans: *cytosolic copper-zinc superoxide dismutase (CuZnSOD), mitochondrial manganese superoxide dismutase (MnSOD)*, and *extracellular superoxide dismutase (ECSOD). SOD1*, a gene on chromosome 21, encodes CuZnSOD. Genetic studies of individuals with adult-onset FALS have determined that about 20 percent of these individuals have mutations in *SOD1*; however, the primary gene defect is unknown. When the SOD enzyme activity is decreased, as has been observed in individuals with FALS with *SOD1* mutations, free radicals may accumulate causing damage.[13,18,19] Most mutations identified in FALS show modest loss in enzyme activity,[20] suggesting the mutant SOD-1 protein may have toxic properties that cause motor neurons to die, the mechanism of which has yet to be determined.[13]
2. *Glutamate*, an excitatory neurotransmitter, has also been implicated in neurodegeneration. Excess glutamate triggers a cascade of events leading to cell death.[13] Increased levels of glutamate in the cerebrospinal fluid (CSF), plasma, and in postmortem tissue of individuals with ALS has been reported.[21,22] In 1995, a deficiency in EAAT2, a specific glutamate transporter protein, in the motor cortex and spinal cord of postmortem ALS tissue was reported and lends support to the theory of excitotoxicity causing neurodegeneration.[23,24]
3. Clumping of neurofilament proteins into spheroids in the cell body and proximal axon is one of the histopathological characteristics of ALS.[13,25,26] Whether or not abnormal accumulation is secondary to the pathology or if it contributes to motor neuron degeneration has yet to be determined.[13]
4. Several studies have implicated an autoimmune reaction in the etiology of ALS.[7,27–29] For example, serum factors toxic to anterior horn motor neurons in individuals with ALS have been reported,[27] and antibodies to calcium channels have been identified in individuals with ALS.[29]
5. It has been hypothesized that a lack of neurotrophic factors could contribute to the development of ALS and other neurodegenerative disorders.[30] In vivo experiments and experiments with isolated motor neurons in cell culture have shown neurotrophic factors are important in motor neuron survival.[31,32] However, factor deficits in

ALS have not been conclusive. For example, a postmortem study found decreased amounts of ciliary neurotrophic factor (CNTF) in the ventral horn of the spinal cord, but not in the motor cortex; nerve growth factors were decreased in the motor cortex, but increased in the lateral column of the spinal cord.[33]

6. Other potential theories that have been thought to contribute to neurodegeneration in ALS, which have limited or indirect evidence, include exogenous or environmental factors,[34] *apoptosis,* programmed cell death,[35] and viral infections.[36]

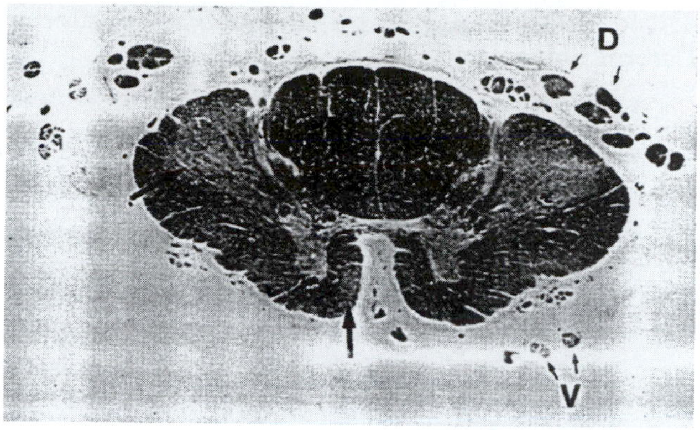

Figure 20.1 Luxol Fast B stained cross section of spinal cord at the high cervical level from a patient with classical ALS. Marked pallor, secondary to degeneration of the lateral and anterior corticospinal tracts, can be seen (large arrows). The ventral roots (V, small arrows) are atrophied, especially compared to the dorsal roots (D, small arrows). [From King, PH, and Mitsumoto H: Neuropathology of amyotrophic lateral sclerosis. In Belsh, JM, and Schiffman, PL (eds): Amyotrophic Lateral Sclerosis: Diagnosis and Management for the Clinician. Blackwell Publishing, Oxford, UK, 1996, p 205, with permission.]

Pathophysiology

Amyotrophic lateral sclerosis is characterized by a progressive degeneration and loss of motor neurons in the spinal cord, brainstem, and motor cortex (Fig. 20.1). UMNs in the cortex are affected, as are the corticospinal tracts. Brainstem nuclei for cranial nerves V (trigeminal), VII (facial), IX (glossopharyngeal), X (vagus), and XII (hypoglossal) and anterior horn cells in the spinal cord are also involved.[2] Brainstem nuclei for cranial nerves controlling external ocular muscles (III: occulomotor, IV: trochlear, and VI: abducens) are usually spared, and if degeneration occurs, it does so late in the course of the disease.[37] Motor neurons of the *Onufrowicz nucleus (Onuf's nucleus),* located in the ventral margin of the anterior horn in the second sacral spinal level, are also generally spared; if they are affected, it is to a very limited extent.[38,39] These neurons control striated muscles in the pelvic floor, including anal and external urethral sphincters.[40]

The sensory system and spinocerebellar tracts are also generally spared in ALS. Some studies suggest that sensory neurons may be involved in ALS, but to a much lesser extent than the motor neurons. Morphological studies have found peripheral sensory nerves exhibit axonal atrophy, demyelination, and degeneration[41,42]; dorsal root ganglia cells at autopsy reveal loss of large ganglion cells.[43] Degeneration of Clarke's neurons and of the spinocerebellar tracts has also been reported.[44–46] Degeneration of the spinocerebellar tracts is a well-recognized pathological feature of FALS and has been described in sporadic ALS, although it is rare.[44] Posterior column degeneration is more common in FALS, but rare in sporadic ALS.[47] As motor neurons degenerate, they can no longer control the muscle fibers they innervate. Healthy, intact surrounding axons can sprout and reinnvervate the partially denervated muscle[48] (Fig. 20.2), in essence assuming the role of the degenerated motor neuron and preserving strength and function early in the disease; however, the surviving motor units undergo enlargement.[49,50] Reinnervation can compensate for the progressive degeneration until motor unit loss is about 50 percent[49,50] and electromyography (EMG) studies have found evidence of motor unit reinnervation in individuals with ALS.[51,52] As the disease progresses, reinnervation cannot compensate for the rate of degeneration,[51] and a variety of impairments develop (Table 20.2).

The progression of ALS is thought to spread in a *contiguous* manner, within spinal cord segments (e.g., cervical segments to cervical segments), before developing rostral or caudal symptoms.[17,53] Thus, signs and symptoms spread

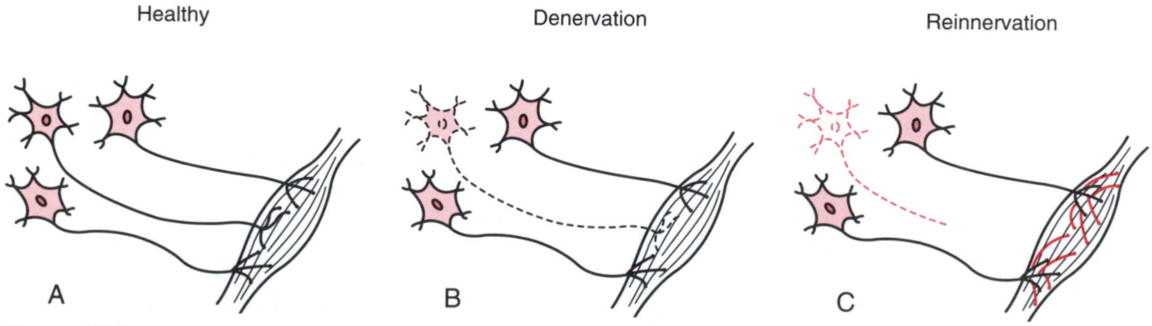

Figure 20.2 Sprouting: (*A*) Normal motor neurons; (*B*) Denervation; (*C*) Reinnervation.

Table 20.2 Common Impairments Associated with Amyotrophic Lateral Sclerosis

Type of Impairment/Location	Clinical Manifestation of Pathology
Impairments related to LMN pathology	Muscle weakness, hyporeflexia, hypotonicity, atrophy, muscle cramps, fasciculations
Impairments related to UMN pathology	Spasticity, pathological reflexes, hyperreflexia, muscle weakness
Impairments related to bulbar pathology	Dysphagia, dysarthria, sialorrhea, pseudobulbar affect
Respiratory impairments	Exertional dyspnea, nocturnal respiratory difficulty, orthopnea, hypoventilation
Other impairments	Dementia, cognitive impairments
Rare impairments	Sensory impairments, bowel and bladder dysfunction, ocular palsy
Indirect and composite impairments	Fatigue, weight loss, cachexia, decreased range of motion, tendon shortening, joint contracture, joint subluxation, adhesive capsulitis, pain, balance and postural control impairments, gait disturbances, deconditioning, depression, anxiety

Adapted in part from Swash, M.[2]
LMN = Lower motor neuron; UMN = upper motor neuron.

locally within a region (e.g., bulbar, cervical, thoracic, lumbosacral) before moving to other regions. Caudal-to-rostral spread within the spinal cord and spread from the cervical to bulbar region appears to occur faster than rostral-to-caudal spread within the spinal cord.[17,53]

Clinical Manifestations

Clinical manifestations of ALS vary depending on the localization and extent of motor neuron loss, the degree and combination of LMN and UMN loss, pattern of onset and progression, body region(s) affected and stage of the disease. At onset, signs or symptoms are usually asymmetrical and focal[2] and progression of the disease leads to increasing numbers and severity of impairments.

Impairments Related to LMN Pathology

The most frequent presenting impairment is focal, asymmetrical weakness beginning in the lower extremity (LE) or upper extremity (UE), or weakness in the bulbar muscles, occurring in a majority of patients.[3,7] Muscle weakness is considered the cardinal sign of ALS and may be caused by LMN or UMN loss. The weakness associated with LMN loss causes more significant dysfunction than the UMN loss weakness.[54] Initial muscle weakness usually occurs in isolated muscles, most often distally, and is followed by progressive weakness and functional limitations.[2,54] For example, at onset an individual may notice difficulty with fine motor movements, such as buttoning, pinching, or writing, or may notice foot "slapping" or increased frequency of tripping while walking. Individuals with bulbar onset may notice changes in their voice, difficulty moving the tongue, decreased ability to move the lips, or open or close the mouth.

In ALS, cervical extensor weakness is typical.[2,54] Individuals may initially notice neck stiffness, feel "heavy-headed" after reading or writing, or may have difficulties stabilizing the head with unanticipated movements, such as in an accelerating car. As weakness progresses, the head may begin to fall forward, and in more advanced stages the neck becomes completely flexed with the head dropped forward, causing cervical pain and impairments in ambulation and feeding (Fig. 20.3).

Muscle weakness typically leads to decreased range of motion (ROM), predisposing the patient to joint subluxation (e.g., shoulder), tendon shortening (e.g., Achilles), joint contractures (commonly claw-hand deformity) and adhesive capsulitis. Weakness also results in ambulation difficulties, deconditioning, and impaired postural control and balance. Foot drop, secondary to distal weakness, and instability, secondary to proximal weakness, are common. The pattern and progression of LE weakness is characterized by greater losses of muscle force in distal muscles compared to proximal muscles.[55,56] A retrospective study found that decreases in walking ability from independent walking, to walking in the community with assistance, to walking only at home, to being unable to walk were precipitated by relatively small changes in muscle force.[56] Falls are also common, reported to occur in 46 percent of individuals with ALS.[57]

Several factor impact fatigue levels in patients with ALS. As motor neurons die, the remaining neurons or sprouted neurons are overburdened. Weak muscles must work at a higher percentage of their maximal strength to perform the same activity. This hastens muscle fatigue.[58]

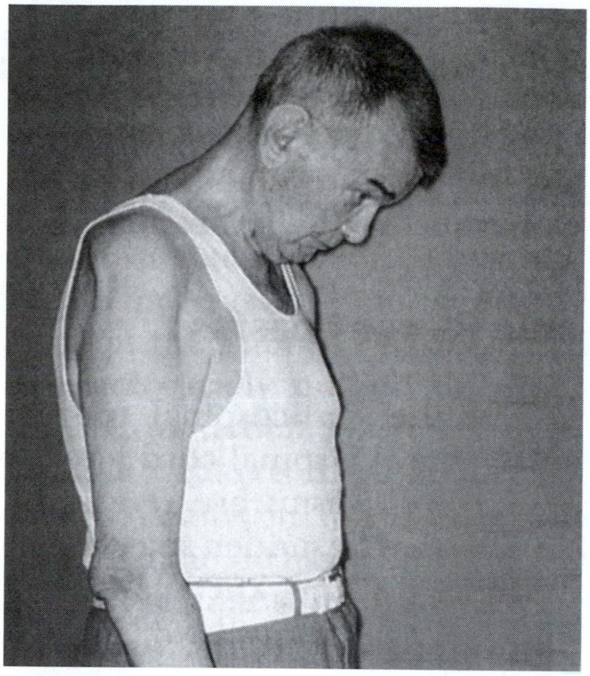

Figure 20.3 Marked head droop in a 65-year-old man with ALS who first developed progressive weakness in both upper extremities. (From Mitsumoto, H, Chad, DA, and Pioro, EK,[54] p 52, with permission.)

Fatigue may also be related to sleep disturbances, respiratory impairments, hypoxia, and depression. Sanjak et al. demonstrated that individuals with ALS have abnormal physiological and metabolic responses to single bouts of exercise.[59] Sharma and colleagues found that in individuals with ALS, tetanic and maximal voluntary force during sustained contraction were decreased compared to controls. No impairment was found in the muscular membrane or neuromuscular transmission, suggesting that muscle fatigue in ALS, in part, is due to impaired contraction activation.[60]

As muscle fibers progressively denervate, their volume decreases resulting in atrophy. Fasciculations are common in individuals with ALS, although they are rarely an initial symptom. The etiology of fasciculations remains unclear and is thought to be related to hyperexcitability of motor axons.[54]

Other LMN signs include hyporeflexia, decreased or absent reflexes, decreased muscle tone or flaccidity, and muscle cramping.[2,54] The etiology of muscle cramping is not well understood and is also thought to be related to hyperexcitability of motor axons. In individuals with ALS, muscle cramps can occur in uncommon sites such as the tongue, jaw, neck, abdomen, as well as in the UEs, hands, and calf or thigh.[2]

Sensory pathways are spared for the most part in ALS; however, some patients may complain of ill-defined paresthesia or pain in the limbs. Pain can occur, especially when muscle weakness and spasticity lead to immobility, adhesive capsulitis, or contractures. Cramps and spasticity are other sources of pain, as is increased pressure on the skin, bones, and joints owing to immobility.[2,54]

Impairments Related to UMN Pathology

UMN loss may also cause muscle weakness, but is characterized by spasticity, hyperflexia, clonus, and pathological reflexes, such as a Babinski or Hoffmann sign. As the disease progresses, UMN signs may decrease.[2,54]

Spasticity can eventually lead to contractures and deformities, as well as cause dyssynergic movement patterns, abnormal timing, loss of dexterity, and fatigue, all of which impact motor control and function.[61,62] For example, difficulties with the swing phase of gait secondary to distal spasticity and decreased balance secondary to generalized spasticity are often seen in individuals with ALS.

Impairments Related to Bulbar Pathology

As UMNs and LMNs of the bulbar muscles degenerate, *spastic bulbar palsy* or *flaccid bulbar palsy* (respectively) develops. In individuals with ALS a mixed palsy, that includes both flaccid and spastic components is common.[54]

Dysarthria, impaired speech, can occur with either spastic or flaccid palsy, owing to weakness of the tongue and muscles of the lip, jaw, larynx, and pharynx. Initial symptoms include the inability to project the voice (e.g., shouting, singing) and problems with enunciation. In spastic dysarthria, the voice sounds forced, as more effort is needed to move air through the upper airway; whereas in flaccid dysarthria, the voice sounds hoarse or breathy. With pharyngeal weakness, air in the mouth leaks into the nose during enunciation, resulting in a nasal tone. As the disease progresses, speech becomes more difficult and unintelligible, and eventually the individual becomes **anarthric**.[2,54]

Dysphagia, impaired chewing or swallowing, can also occur with either spastic or flaccid palsy. Manipulating food inside the mouth or moving food into the esophagus is difficult, and swallowing is impaired. With flaccid bulbar palsy, liquids may regurgitate into the nose because of pharyngeal weakness, and the cough reflex may be weak or absent greatly increasing the risk of aspiration. Individuals with spastic bulbar palsy will have uncoordinated closure of the epiglottis, that may allow liquids or solids to pass to the larynx.[2,54] Choking and slowed eating pattern are associated with dysphagia placing the patient at risk for less than optimal fluid and caloric intake that results in weight loss and potentially cachexia.[54]

Individuals with ALS frequently experience **sialorrhea**, excessive saliva and drooling, because of an absence of automatic, spontaneous swallowing to clear excessive saliva, or because the lower facial muscles are too weak to close the lips tightly to prevent leakage.[54] Individuals with bulbar-onset will experience this symptom relatively early.

Initially, the individual may begin to notice drooling at night (e.g., the pillow is wet in the morning); this eventually requires repeated use of a tissue to wipe away the saliva.

Pseudobulbar affect, a term used to describe poor or pathological emotional control,[63] is commonly seen in individuals with spastic bulbar palsy.[2,54] Spontaneous crying or laughter occurs in the absence of emotional triggers or emotional responses are exaggerated,[63] and can occur in as many as 50 percent of individuals.[64]

Respiratory Impairments

Respiratory impairments in ALS are related to loss of respiratory muscle strength and a decrease in vital capacity (VC). A VC reduced to 50 percent of predicted is often associated with respiratory symptoms.[65] Early signs and symptoms of respiratory muscle weakness may include fatigue, dyspnea on exertion, difficulty sleeping in supine, and frequent awakening at night, recurrent sighing, excessive daytime sleepiness, and morning headaches due to hypoxia.[66,67] Patients experiencing a gradual increase in respiratory muscle weakness will not complain of respiratory symptoms because they tend to decrease their overall level of physical activity owing to muscle weakness in the extremities.[68] Although the decline of respiratory muscle strength differs among individuals, for the most part it tends to progress at a linear rate.[69] As weakness progresses, truncated speech, orthopnea, dyspnea at rest, paradoxical breathing, accessory muscle use, and a weak cough are typically evident. A VC of less than 25 percent to 30 percent of predicted indicates significant risk of impending respiratory failure or death.[65] If an individual does not receive ventilatory support, eventual CO_2 retention will lead to acidosis, coma, and respiratory failure.[68]

Cognitive Impairments

Although once considered rare outside the western Pacific region, cognitive impairments ranging from mild deficits[70] to severe *frontotemporal dementia (FTD)*,[71] have been reported. A recent large prospective study found that 35.6 percent of patients with ALS showed clinically significant cognitive impairment,[72] and it has been suggested that FTD now be considered a component of the pathological spectrum of ALS.[73] ALS-associated FTD has been characterized by cognitive decline, executive functioning impairments, difficulties with planning, organization and concept abstraction, and personality and behavior changes.[71,74–76] Individuals with ALS, without FTD, have been reported to have a variety of cognitive impairments including difficulties with verbal fluency, language comprehension, memory, abstract reasoning, and generalized impairments in intellectual function.[72,76–78] Studies have found that patients with bulbar-onset ALS are more likely to have cognitive impairments than patients with limb-onset disease.[76,78]

Rare Impairments

Sensory pathways are spared, for the most part, in ALS. Some individuals may complain of vague, ill-defined sensory symptoms of paresthesia or focal pain in the limbs.[54] External ocular muscles are usually spared in ALS; and if degeneration occurs, it does so late in the course of the disease.[37] Patients who have been maintained on ventilators for long periods of time may develop the inability to voluntarily close the eyes or *ophthalmoplegia,* complete ocular paralysis.[37]

Motor neurons controlling the anal and vesicourethral sphincter muscles and muscles of the pelvic floor are generally spared. Urinary symptoms, such as urgency, obstructive micturition, or both have been reported, suggesting that supranuclear control over sympathetic, parasympathetic, and somatic neurons may be abnormal in ALS.[54]

Diagnosis

With the exception of one genetic test, no definitive diagnostic test or diagnostic biological marker exists for ALS. For individuals with a clinical presentation of ALS laboratory studies, EMG, nerve conduction velocity (NCV) studies, muscle and nerve biopsies, and neuroimaging studies are used to support the diagnosis of ALS and to exclude other diagnoses.

The diagnosis of ALS requires the *presence* of (1) LMN signs by clinical, electrophysiological, or neuropathological examination; (2) UMN signs by clinical examination; and (3) progression of the disease within a region or to other regions by clinical examination or via the medical history; and the *absence* of (1) electrophysiological and pathological evidence of other diseases that may explain the UMN and LMN signs; and (2) neuroimaging evidence of other disease processes that may explain the observed clinical and electrophysiological signs.[79]

Because of the variability in clinical findings in the early stages of ALS and the lack of absolute biological diagnostic markers, the World Federation of Neurology Research Group on Motor Neuron Diseases established the *El Escorial criteria* in 1994, and revised them in 1998.[79] These widely accepted criteria are considered standard for the diagnosis of ALS for clinical practice, therapeutic trials, and other research purposes. In the absence of pathological evidence, the diagnosis of ALS is classified into *clinically definite, clinically probable, clinically probable with laboratory support,* and *possible* categories (Fig. 20.4).[79] A diagnosis of *clinically definite ALS* is defined as both UMN and LMN findings in at least three of four regions (bulbar, cervical, thoracic, or lumbosacral) or UMN and LMN signs in the bulbar region and at least two spinal regions. Clinically probable ALS

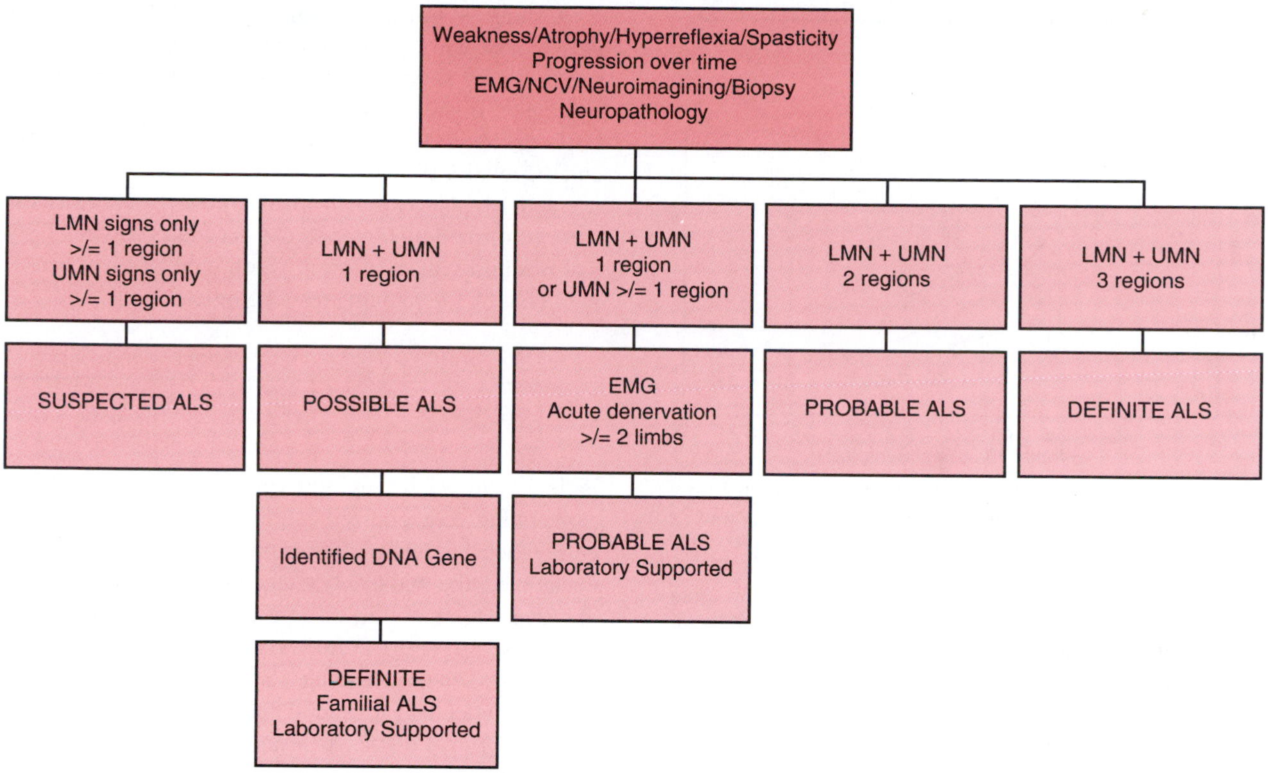

Figure 20.4 El Escorial Criteria for the Diagnosis of ALS. (From The World Federation of Neurology, London, UK. Retrieved March 23, 2003 from http://www.wfneurology.org, with permission. *Note*: The Suspected ALS category was removed when the El Escorial criteria were revised.)

is defined as UMN and LMN signs in two regions, with at least one UMN finding rostral to the LMN findings. Clinically probable, laboratory-supported ALS is defined as UMN and LMN clinical signs in one region only, or UMN signs alone present in one region and LMN signs defined by EMG criteria present in at least two regions. The EMG criteria include signs of active denervation, such as fibrillation potentials and positive sharp waves; and, signs of chronic denervation such as large motor unit potentials (increased duration, increased proportion of polyphasic potentials, increased amplitude) and unstable motor unit potentials. Clinically possible ALS is defined as UMN and LMN signs found together in only one region, or UMN signs found alone in two or more regions, or LMN signs found rostral to UMN signs and the inability to establish a diagnosis of clinically probable, laboratory-supported ALS.[79]

Disease Course

ALS has a progressive and deteriorating disease trajectory, and the progression from pathology to impairments to functional limitations to disabilities is inevitable. Although the disease course varies among individuals, with time from onset to death ranging from several months to 20 years, studies have found the average duration of ALS to be between 27 and 43 months, and the median duration to be between 23 and 52 months.[3,5,7,80,81] Five-year and ten-year survival rates range from 9 to 40 percent and 8 to 16 percent, respectively.[7,80,82,83] A 50 percent survival probability after the first symptom of ALS appears is slightly greater than 3 years, unless mechanical ventilation is used to sustain breathing.[6] In most patients, death occurs within 3 to 5 years after diagnosis and usually results from respiratory failure[5] (Fig. 20.5).

Prognosis

Age at time of onset has the strongest relationship to prognosis. Studies have found that patients less than 35 to 40 years of age at onset had better 5-year survival rates than older individuals.[5,6,81,84,85] Individuals with limb-onset ALS have a better prognosis than those with bulbar-onset; 5-year survival rates were reported to be 37 percent and 44 percent, compared to survival rates of 9 percent and 16 percent for patients with bulbar-onset ALS.[84,85] Less severe involvement at the time of diagnosis, a longer interval between onset and diagnosis, and no symptoms of dyspnea at onset are other factors associated with a better prognosis.[5,6,86]

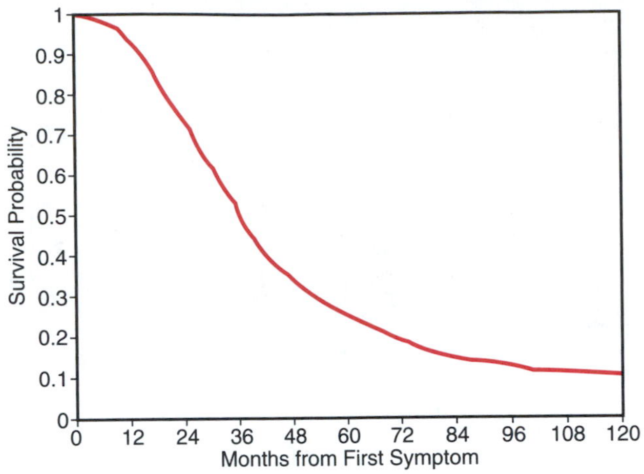

Figure 20.5 Kaplan-Meier curve describing survival in ALS. The number of patients known alive at date of first symptom and at yearly intervals thereafter: 831, 738, 504, 302, 170, 103, 69, 42, 31, 17, 13. (Figure 30-1 from "Amyotrophic Lateral Sclerosis" by Appel, Smith, Lai, Mosier and Haveerkamp, from Prognosis of Neurological Disorders, ed 2, edited by Randolph W. Evans, et al, copyright 1992, 2000 by Oxford University Press, Inc. Used by permission of Oxford University Press, Inc.)

A study of 144 individuals with ALS found that those individuals with psychological well-being had significantly longer survival times compared to those with psychological distress. Mortality rates were found to be 6.8 times greater in those experiencing psychological distress, and the relationship was independent of age, disease severity, and length of time from diagnosis.[87] These findings were confirmed in a later study that found degree of physical disability, disease progression, and survival could be predicted by the patient's psychological status.[88]

Management

Patients with ALS may receive care in a variety of health care settings. Specialized centers or clinics that provide a comprehensive and multidisciplinary approach to care are considered the most advantageous considering the progressive nature of the disease and continually, changing patient status (Fig. 20.6). A recent study comparing a cohort of patients attending a multidisciplinary clinic versus those attending a general neurology practice found the median survival of the ALS clinic cohort was 7.5 months longer than for patients in the general neurology cohort.

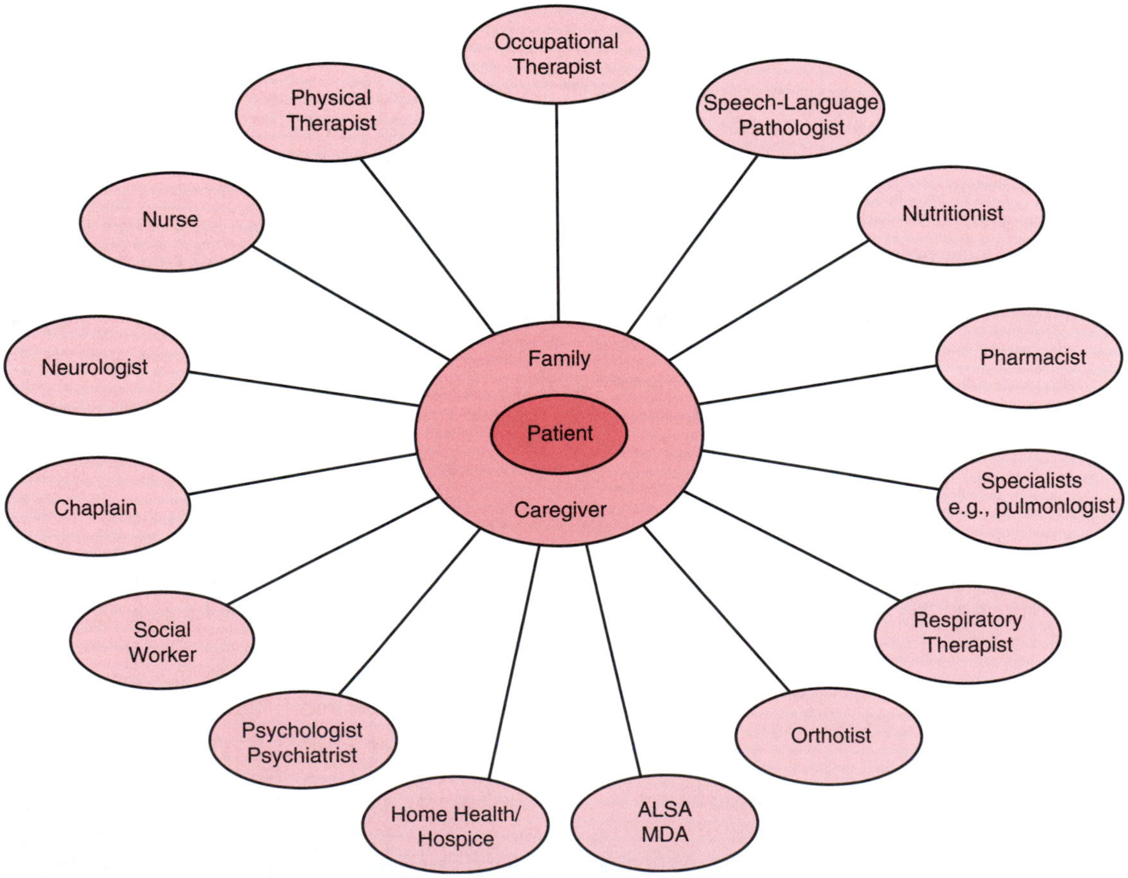

Figure 20.6 Multidisciplinary approach to the care of the individual with ALS. ALSA = Amyotrophic Lateral Sclerosis Foundation; MDA = Muscular Dystrophy Association.

The findings indicated that attendance at the ALS clinic was an independent covariate of survival, suggesting active and aggressive management enhances survival.[89]

The Amyotrophic Lateral Sclerosis Association (ALSA) and the Muscular Dystrophy Association (MDA), non-profit voluntary health agencies, have developed standards for ALS clinics and centers. Clinics and centers that meet ALSA's standards and pass a rigorous application and site visit are certified as ALSA Centers. MDA centers that conduct ALS research and have staff with expertise in dealing with ALS earn special designations as MDA ALS Research and Clinical Centers.

Disease-Modifying Agents

Currently, there is no cure for ALS, although a number of clinical drug trials are being conducted. In 1995, the Food and Drug Administration approved *Riluzole (Rilutec),* a glutamate inhibitor, for the treatment of ALS. The standard dose of Riluzole is one 50 mg tablet two times a day, and side effects include liver toxicity (which requires discontinuation), asthenia, nausea, vomiting, and dizziness. Evidence suggests the effects of Riluzole to be modest, extending survival for 2 to 3 months.[90,91]

Symptomatic Management

Disease-modifying agents currently available are not curative and may extend survival for a very short time. Because the pathological process cannot be reversed and is progressive in nature, the context of medical management for individuals with ALS may be considered palliative. As defined by the World Health Organization, palliative care is "... the active total care of patients *whose disease is not responsive to curative treatment*. Control of pain, of other symptoms, and of psychological, social, and spiritual problems is paramount. The goal of palliative care is achievement of the best possible quality of life for patients and their families."[92, p 11]

Although there is no cure for ALS, it is still considered a "treatable disease" and rehabilitation plays an integral role in the overall comprehensive care of the patient. Medical management is symptomatic and individualized and involves supportive care to address impairments as they arise. Medical management may include the prescription of anticramping and antispasticity agents, drying agents for sialorrhea, and antidepressants; recommendations and referrals for *percutaneous endoscopic gastrostomy (PEG)* tubes and ventilatory support (noninvasive ventilation, tracheostomy); and discussion of advanced care directives.[2,54]

In 1999 a multidisciplinary task force was established to develop recommendations for management of ALS.[93] The task force examined the research and clinical evidence of five areas related to the care of individuals with ALS: (1) informing the patient and family about the diagnosis and prognosis; (2) symptom management of *sialorrhea* and *pseudobulbar affect;* (3) nutrition management and PEG decisions; (4) management of respiratory insufficiency and ventilation decisions; and (5) advance directives and palliative care. Medical decision-making algorithms (practice patterns) developed by the task force for the management of sialorrhea, nutrition, and respiratory symptoms are presented in Figures 20.7 to 20.9.

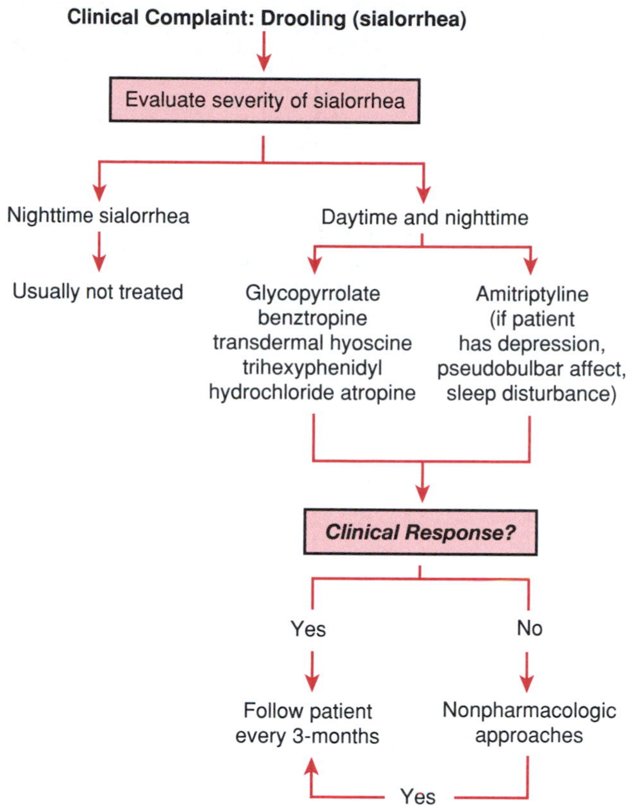

Figure 20.7 Algorithm for sialorrhea management. (From Miller, RG, et al,[93] p 1315, with permission.)

Management of Sialorrhea and Pseudobulbar Affect

Management of *sialorrhea* is directed at anticholinergic medications that decrease saliva production, such as glycopyrrolate (Robinul), benztropine (Cogentin), transdermal hyoscine (scopolamine), atropine, and trihexyphenidyl hydrochloride (Artane). For patients with associated thick mucus production, beta-blockers such as propranolol (Inderal) or metoprolol (Toprol) are used. For patients with pseudobulbar affect, the tricyclic antidepressant, amitriptyline (Elavil) or selective serotonin reuptake inhibitors (SSRIs), such as fluvoxamine (Luvox) are prescribed, secondary to their dual action.[93]

Nonpharmacological treatment for sialorrhea includes manually assisted coughing techniques and use of a suction or *mechanical insufflation–exsufflation (MI-E) device*[93] (Fig. 20.10). The MI-E device is designed to inflate the

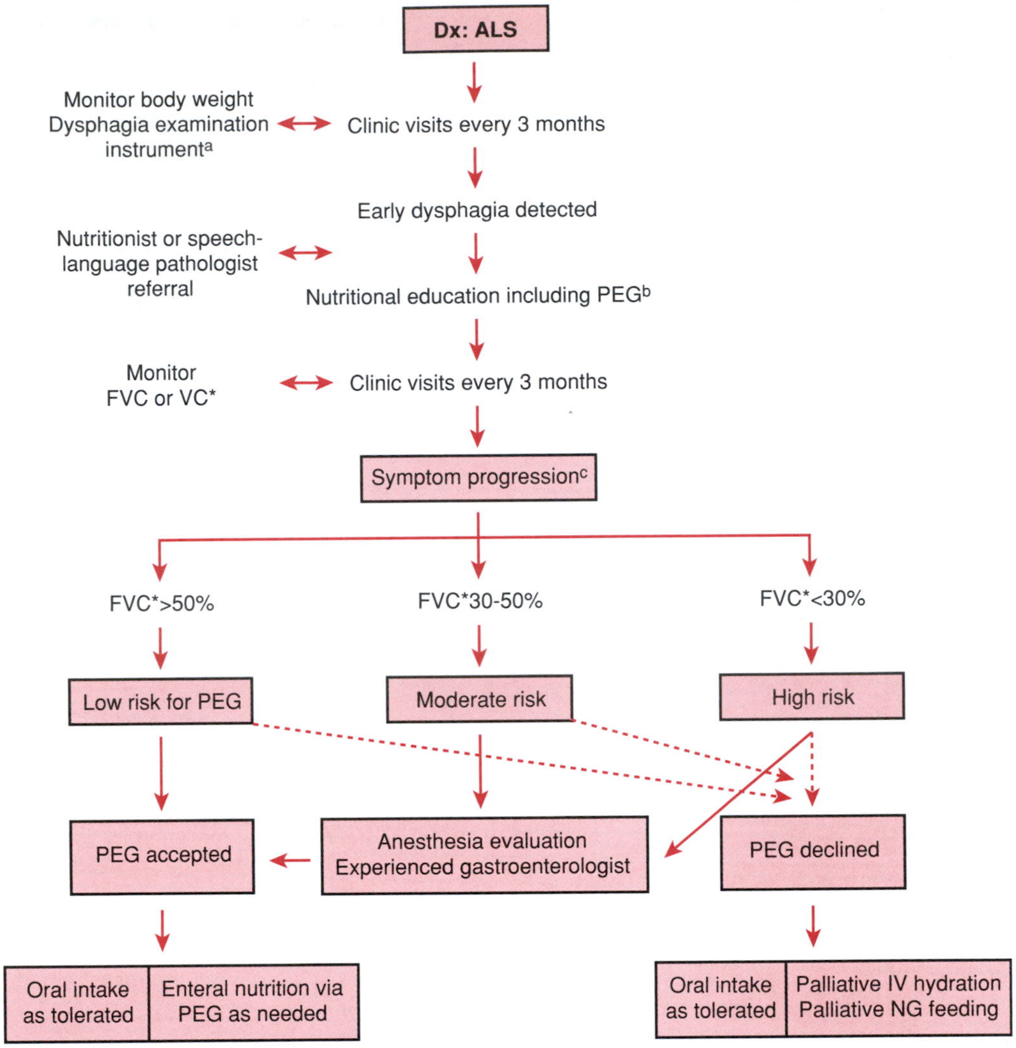

Figure 20.8 Algorithm for nutrition management. [a]For example, Colorado Dysphagia Disability Inventory, bulbar questions in the ALS Functional Rating Scale, or other instrument. [b]Rule out contraindications. [c]Prolonged mealtime, ending meal prematurely because of fatigue, accelerated weight loss due to poor caloric intake, family concern about feeding difficulties. *Forced vital capacity (FVC) or vital capacity (VC) can be used. VC may be more accurate in patients with bulbar dysfunction. Dx = diagnosis; PEG = percutaneous endoscopic gastrostomy. (From Miller, RG, et al,[93] p 1316, with permission.)

lung with positive pressure and assist cough with negative pressure through the flip of a switch. A positive-pressure breath of 30 to 50 cm H_2O over a 1- to 3-second period via an oral–nasal mask or tracheal airway is provided. The airway pressure is then reversed abruptly to –30 to –50 cm H_2O and maintained for 2 to 3 seconds. A peak expiratory "cough" flow within normal range is achieved, thereby assisting with the clearance of secretions.[94]

Management of Dysphagia

Early, mild **dysphagia** is addressed by a nutritionist or registered dietician together with a speech-language pathologist (SLP). SLPs conduct swallowing examinations such as video fluoroscopy to determine the degree and nature of the swallowing impairment and to assist in formulating a plan of care. Nutritionists provide counseling and diet management throughout the course of the disease.

Nutrition status has been identified as a prognostic factor for survival and disease complications.[95] A study of 1600 hospitalized patients with ALS found the most common concurrent diagnosis was dehydration and malnutrition, present in 36 percent of patients.[96] This finding emphasizes the need for careful attention to nutritional and hydration status.

Initial treatment of dysphagia is directed toward (1) dietary modifications, such as adapting foods and fluid consistencies for easier and safer swallowing; (2) patient education regarding dietary strategies for maximizing calories and nutrients and maintaining adequate hydration; and (3) adaptations to promote swallowing such as tucking the chin down during swallowing or performing a clearing cough after each swallow.[97]

As dysphagia progresses, the time required to consume a meal gradually increases owing to fatigue, increased difficulty chewing, and frequent choking. It is not uncommon

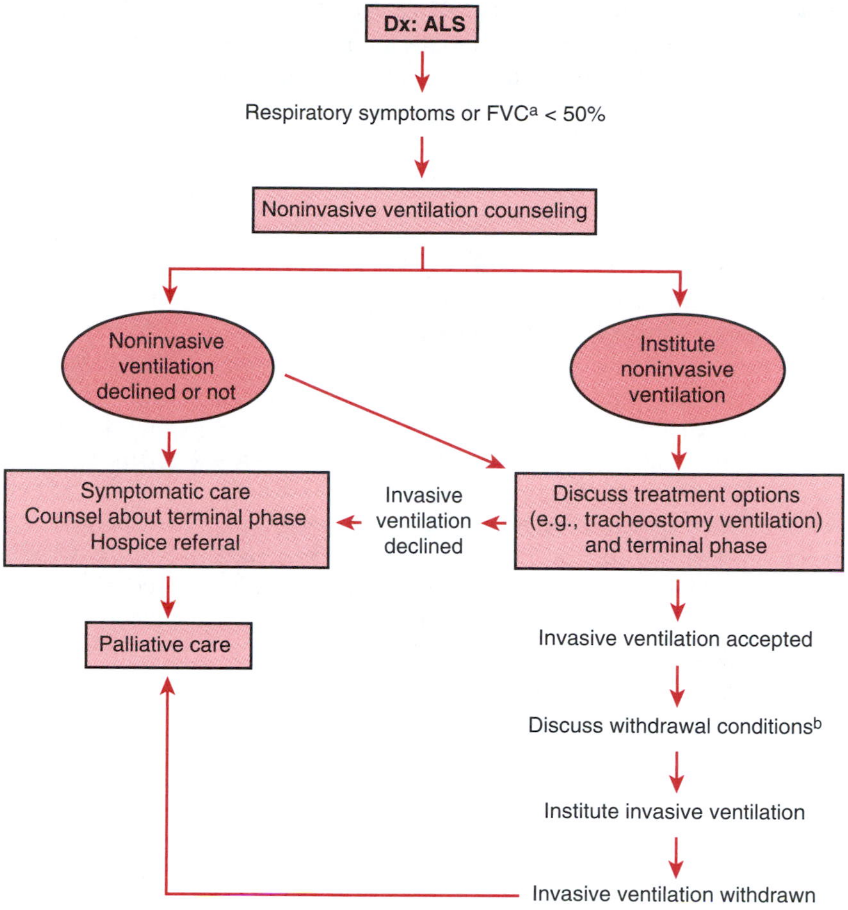

Figure 20.9 Algorithm for respiratory management. [a]Forced vital capacity (FVC) or vital capacity (VC) can be used. VC may be more accurate in patients with bulbar dysfunction. [b]Agreement needed for conditions of withdrawal prior to or concurrent with instituting invasive ventilation (e.g., locked in state, coma, etc.). Dx = diagnosis. (From Miller, RG, et al,[93] p 1317, with permission.)

for these eating difficulties to cause an accelerated weight loss. In these circumstances a percutaneous endoscopic gastrostomy (PEG) may be recommended. A PEG is a type of gastrostomy tube inserted via endoscopic surgery that creates a permanent opening into the stomach for the introduction of food. For optimal safety and efficacy the PEG procedure should be offered to the patient and completed before the individual's vital capacity (VC) falls below 50 percent of predicted.[93] Studies have found PEG insertion may prolong survival. Patients with PEG were found to live 1 to 4 months longer than those individuals who refused PEG or were deemed ineligible for the procedure. Survival was greatest for patients with a VC greater than 50 percent predicted at the time of the procedure.[98,99] It is important to note that a PEG does not prevent the risk of aspiration.[100,101]

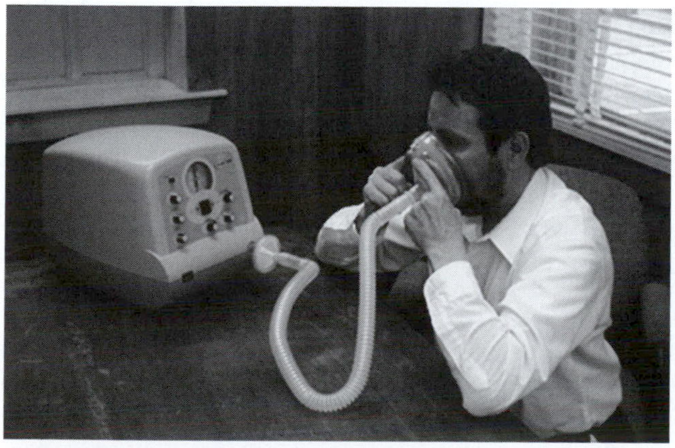

Figure 20.10 Mechanical insufflation-exsufflation (MI-E) device. (Courtesy of JH Emerson Co., Cambridge, MA 02140.)

Management of Respiratory Impairments

Respiratory impairments place the patient at risk for respiratory tract infections. Important management considerations include: (1) pneumococcal and yearly influenza vaccinations[68]; (2) prevention of aspiration; and (3) effective oral and pulmonary secretion management. Supplemental oxygen must be used with caution because it can suppress respiratory drive, exacerbate hypoventilation, and ultimately lead to hypercarbia and respiratory arrest. Typically, supplemental oxygen is recommended only for individuals with concomitant pulmonary disease or as a comfort measure for patients who decline ventilatory support.[68]

When VC decreases to 50 percent of predicted, positive-pressure noninvasive ventilation (NIV) is recommended.[68,93] NIV has been shown to decrease symptoms of hypoventilation and increase survival time by several months.[102–105] When NIV can no longer be tolerated or it is no longer effective, a decision must be made between invasion ventilation (IV) with tracheostomy via surgical intervention or hospice care to address late-stage respiratory symptoms.

Owing to the emotional, social, and financial burden of IV, patients and families must be carefully informed of the multiple costs and benefits of the intervention. Conditions for withdrawal of ventilation are discussed prior to, or at the time of, instituting IV because the patient may become unable to communicate his or her wishes as the disease progresses.[68,93]

Management of Dysarthria

Dysarthria impairments are managed primarily by a speech–language pathologist. Initial speech changes are usually managed with intelligibility strategies, such as having the individual exaggerate articulation or decrease the rate of speech; and, environmental modifications, such as decreasing background noise. As the severity of dysarthria progresses, management will focus on decreasing the patient's dependence on speech as the primary method of communication. Interventions first include "low-tech" devices, such as using a writing board or pad and pen for patients with adequate hand function or using an alphabet board. A progression is then made to more "high-tech" devices, such as computers with voice synthesizers or single-switch, scanning computerized communication systems.[106,107]

A *palatal lift prosthesis* may be prescribed for individuals with good articulation but who have a breathy voice quality or decreased loudness because of excessive air loss through the nose. The device, a dental appliance designed to attach to the existing teeth and to elevate the soft palate, is custom-made by a prosthodontist. It allows the soft palate to close around the surrounding structures such as the pharynx, making verbal communication more understandable by reducing or eliminating hypernasal speech. The device also lowers the hard palate which reduces tongue movement allowing speech to be less fatiguing.[107] Findings from a retrospective study of 25 patients with ALS treated with a palatal lift indicated 21 patients showed improvement in their dysarthria, specifically in reduction of hypernasality, with 19 patients benefitting at least moderately for 6 months.[108]

Management of Muscle Cramps, Spasticity, Fasciculations, and Pain

Anticonvulsant medication such as phenytoin (Dilantin) and carbamazepine (Atretol, Tegretol) may be prescribed for muscle cramps, if they are not relieved with a program of muscle stretching and adequate hydration and nutrition. Both of these medications can cause gastrointestinal upset and rash, and carbamazepine can cause sedation. Benzodiazepines, such as diazepam (Valium), clonazepam (Klonopin), or lorazepam (Ativan), can also be prescribed for muscle cramps, and side effects may include sedation, dizziness, respiratory depression, and increased weakness. Benzodiazepines, especially diazepam, may also be prescribed for spasticity, although baclofen (Lioresal) and tizanidine (Zanaflex) are more commonly used. Side effects include weakness, fatigue, sedation, and hypotension.[54,108]

Patients with brisk, widespread fasciculations are generally instructed to avoid or minimize caffeine and nicotine. Lorazepam (Ativan) may be prescribed to decrease the intensity of the fasciculations.[54] Depending on the etiology of pain, a variety of management strategies may be utilized. Mild pain or pain associated with joint discomfort is usually addressed with analgesics, such as acetaminophen or nonsteroidal anti-inflammatory drugs. For more severe refractory pain, narcotics such as codeine, hydrocodone, or methadone may be prescribed. In the terminal stages of ALS, morphine may be administered to provide analgesia, sedation, and relief from respiratory distress.[54,108]

Management of Anxiety and Depression

Anxiety and depression can greatly impact a patient's and his or her family's quality of life, as well as the ability to cope with and adapt to the progressive changes and losses of the disease. Thus, pharmacotherapy and psychological counseling are important management strategies for addressing the anxiety and depression that can develop. Individuals with depression may be prescribed an SSRI, such as fluoxetine (Prozac) or sertraline (Zoloft). It is important to note that antidepressant effects may not occur for several weeks after initiation of the medications, and side effects may include agitation and insomnia. If the patient presents with depression and insomnia or agitation, a tricyclic antidepressant, such as amitriptyline (Elavil) or imipramine (Tofranil) is preferred.[54]

Benzodiazepines, such as chlordiazepoxide (Librium), clorazepate, diazepam, and flurazepam (Dalmane) may be prescribed for anxiety or for patients with depression and insomnia. For patients whose respiratory status is affected, a nonbenzodiazepine anxiolytic, such as buspirone (BuSpar), is preferred.[54,108]

Framework for Rehabilitation

The course of ALS cannot be altered and eventually the individual will become dependent in essentially all aspects of mobility and self-care. However, appropriate rehabilitation programs should be designed and implemented to allow the individual to maintain his or her independence and function for as long as possible, within the context of his or her goals and resources, throughout the disease and across health care settings. Because of the progressive nature of ALS, it is imperative that the physical therapist not only address an individual's current problems, but also plan ahead for future problems.[109,110]

A large body of evidence to help guide physical therapy decision-making is currently unavailable. As identified earlier, ALS has a progressive and deteriorating disease trajectory, with inevitable progression to disability. However, there is great variability among individuals. Staging ALS into *early, middle* (early-middle and late-middle), and *late*

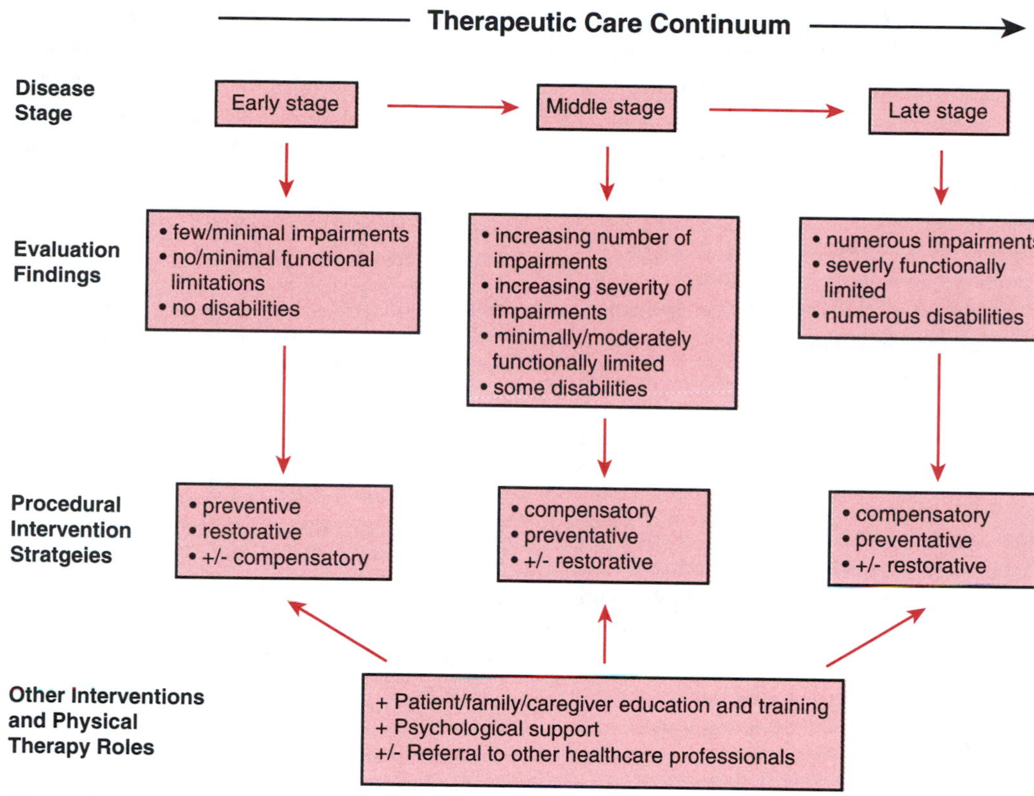

Figure 20.11 Framework for Rehabilitation for Individuals with ALS. (From Dal Bello-Haas, V,[110] p 116, with permission.)

stages based on limitations, functional impairments, and disabilities may assist the therapist in designing appropriate and realistic interventions throughout the disease process as well as anticipate the evolving needs of individual patients[110] (Fig. 20.11).

In the *early* stage of the disease, ALS will manifest as a variety of signs and symptoms recognized by the patient as abnormal. The resultant impairments may or may not cause minor functional limitations and no disabilities will be present. In the *middle* stage of ALS, the patient experiences increasing signs and symptoms and develops an increase in number of impairments or severity of impairments. Minimal to moderate functional limitations will be noted and as a result disabilities will develop. In the *late* stage of ALS, disease progression leads to numerous and increasingly more severe impairments. The patient becomes increasingly more functionally limited owing to lack of voluntary motor control and numerous disabilities ensue. The patient becomes dependent in essentially all aspects of mobility and self-care, and may require mechanical ventilation to address respiratory compromise, if not already ventilated.[110]

Within this framework, impairments, functional limitations and disabilities are managed through restorative, compensatory, or preventative physical therapy interventions. These interventions should be tailored to the stage of the disease and grounded in evidence-based research whenever possible. The patient's goals must be considered as well as the psychosocial factors that may impact the patient's decision making such as acceptance of the diagnosis and social and financial resources.[110]

Physical Therapy Examination

At any one time, a variety of body regions can be affected by ALS and in various combinations. Impairments may occur as a direct result of the pathology (*direct impairment*), as sequelae to the pathology (*indirect impairment*), or may be the result of multiple underlying origins *(composite impairments)*. Therefore, a careful and comprehensive examination is required to determine the extent of involvement, and the impact of involvement on functional limitations and disabilities. Reexamination at regular intervals is necessary to determine the extent and rate of progression of the disease. However, at times it may be difficult to differentiate between the progressive course of the disease and the lack of impact of the interventions. In considering the tests and measures to include in a reexamination, the physical therapist needs to weigh the benefits against the psychological impact of repeating tests and measures when the patient is progressively deteriorating. This is especially true in the late-middle and late stage of the disease. It is important for the physical therapist to reexamine, monitor, and evaluate changes, as some medical decision-making may be based on the physical therapist's findings, for example, the patient's percent predicted VC and the timing of PEG placement.

The patient's goals and individual psychosocial factors, rate of disease progression, extent and area of involvement, stage of the disease, respiratory and bulbar involvement that may impact on the patient's ability to participate all need to be taken into account when structuring the initial examination. The types of data generated from the patient history and interview are presented in Chapter 1. When collecting these data, determining what is important, relevant, and valued by the individual patient is key. By understanding what is most meaningful to a patient, the physical therapist can narrow the gap between a patient's expectations and hopes and actual experiences through realistic and appropriate interventions. For example, a young mother with ALS may inform the physical therapist her priority is caring for her children rather than maintaining employment. Thus, the initial examination would be structured around abilities and activities related to home, rather than work.

Many of the tests and measures described in this text are generally appropriate components of a comprehensive examination for an individual with ALS. However, selection is always based on specific patient need. The tests and measures frequently applicable to patients with ALS include examination of: sensory function, muscle performance, coordination, motor function, gait, functional status and activity level, the environment, and cognitive function (see Chapters 5, 6, 7, 8, 10, 11, 12, and 29). The following section presents areas that typically warrant emphasis during the examination.

Cognition

No ALS-specific cognitive test or measure exists. If dementia or cognitive impairments are suspected, executive functioning, language comprehension, memory, and abstract reasoning should be examined. The Mini-Mental State[111] examination has been used in clinical studies. Referral for a neuropsychological evaluation may be indicated.

Psychosocial Function

As depression and anxiety are common in individuals with ALS, screening is important and referral to a psychologist or psychiatrist for further evaluation may be indicated. The *Beck's Depression Inventory*,[112] the *Center of Epidemiologic Study-Depression Scale*,[113] the *Hospital Anxiety and Depression Scale (HADS)*,[114] and the *State-Trait Anxiety Inventory*[115] have been used in clinical studies.

Pain

Pain is common in individuals with ALS and should be examined subjectively and objectively, using a *Visual Analogue Scale* for example. Pain is not necessarily a direct impairment of ALS, but rather an indirect (decreased ROM, adhesive capsulitis) or a composite impairment (joint malalignment secondary to spasticity). Further examination of underlying causes of pain is often required.

Joint Integrity, Range of Motion, and Muscle Length

Functional range of motion (ROM), active, active-assisted, and passive range ROM, muscle length, and soft tissue flexibility and extensibility should be examined using standard methods.

Muscle Performance

Specific deficits of muscle strength, power and endurance, and muscle performance during functional activities should be determined. Specific deficits can be measured with manual muscle testing (MMT), isokinetic muscle strength testing, or hand-held dynamometry. In clinical trials, muscle strength is often examined as Maximum Voluntary Isometric Contraction (MVIC) using a strain gauge tensiometer system.[116] This method eliminates muscle length and velocity as factors in testing and produces reliable, valid, interval data.[116–119] MVIC is considered the most direct technique for investigating motor unit loss, and has been used extensively for examining muscle strength in individuals with ALS for the past 10 years. Its range and sensitivity have been validated by several natural history studies.[5,17,120] However, MVIC testing requires specialized equipment and training in its use.

A recent study compared test reliability of MMT and MVIC scores among uniformly trained physical therapists at several institutions. Reproducibility between MMT and MVIC was found to be equivalent. Sensitivity to detect progressive muscle strength changes in individuals with ALS favored MMT. However, 6 muscles were tested with MVIC and 34 muscles were tested with MMT; thus, the difference in detecting change was largely accounted for by the number of muscles sampled by MMT versus MVIC.[121]

Motor Function

Impairments in dexterity, coordination of large movement patterns as well as gross and fine motor control may be evident owing to spasticity and muscle weakness. Hand function and initiation, modification and control of movement patterns should be examined.

Tone and Reflexes

Muscle tone may be examined using the *Modified Ashworth Scale*.[122] Deep tendon and pathological reflexes should be tested to distinguish between UMN and LMN involvement.

Cranial Nerve Integrity

The cranial nerves commonly affected by ALS include: V, VII, IX, X, and XII. Cranial nerves should be tested to determine the extent of bulbar involvement. Screening for oral motor function, phonation, and speech production can be accomplished through the interview and observation. Referral to a speech–language pathologist is recommended.

Sensation

If the patient complains of sensory symptoms or if sensory involvement is suspected, sensory testing should be completed.

Postural Alignment, Control, and Balance

Static and dynamic postural alignment and body mechanics during self-care, functional mobility skills, functional activities, and work conditions and activities should be examined. Postural stability, reactive control, anticipatory control, and adaptive postural control should also be determined. No ALS-specific balance test or measure exists. A variety of balance status measures are available originally designed for use with other patient populations, including the *Tinetti Performance Oriented Mobility Assessment (POMA)*,[123] the *Berg Balance Scale*,[124] the *Timed Up and Go Test*,[125] and the *Functional Reach Test*.[126] Low total *Tinetti Balance Test* scores, indicating impaired balance, were found to be moderately to strongly related to LE muscle weakness and functional disabilities in individuals with ALS,[127] Kloos et al suggest that the Tinetti Balance Test is a reliable measure for individuals in the early or early-middle stages of ALS.[128]

Gait

No ALS-specific gait test or measure exists. Gait stability, safety and endurance should be examined. Energy expenditure, alignment, fit, practicality, safety and ease of use of orthotic and assistive devices should also be examined at regular intervals.

Respiratory Function

Determination of respiratory status and function includes examination of respiratory symptoms and muscle function, breathing pattern, chest expansion, respiratory sounds, cough effectiveness, and vital capacity or forced vital capacity using a hand-held spirometer. Aerobic capacity and cardiovascular–pulmonary endurance may be tested in the early stages of ALS using standardized protocols to evaluate and monitor responses to aerobic conditioning.

Integument

In general, even in the late stage of ALS skin integrity is rarely a problem. Skin inspection should be used to examine contact points between the body and assistive, adaptive, orthotic, protective, and supportive devices, mobility devices, as well as the sleeping surface. Such inspection is especially important when the patient's mobility becomes increasingly more dependent. If present, swelling should also be examined and monitored. Swelling of the distal limb may develop owing to lack of muscle pumping action in a weakened extremity.

Functional Status

Functional mobility skills, safety, and energy expenditure are important considerations. Basic and instrumental activities of daily living and the need for adaptive equipment should be examined. The *Functional Independence Measure (FIM™)*[129] has been used to document functional status in clinical trials.

The *Schwab and England Activities of Daily Living Scale*[130] is an 11-point global measure of functioning that asks the rater to report activities of daily living (ADL) function from 100 percent (normal) to 0 percent (vegetative functions only), and has been used to examine function in individuals with ALS (Appendix A). The ALS CNTF Treatment Study Group found the scale to have excellent test–retest reliability, to correlate well with qualitative and quantitative changes in function, and to be sensitive to changes over time.[131]

Environmental Barriers

The patient's home and work environments should be examined for current and potential barriers, access, and safety.

Fatigue

Fatigue is very common in individuals with ALS. No ALS-specific measures exist; the *Fatigue Severity Scale*[132] has been used in clinical trials.

Disease-Specific and Quality of Life Measures

Disease-Specific Measures

The *ALS Functional Rating Scale (ALSFRS)*[131] and the revised version, ALSFRS-R[133] (Appendix B) examine the functional status of patients with ALS. The patient is asked to rate his or her function using a scale from 4 (normal function) to 0 (unable to attempt the task). The original scale, the ALSFRS, correlated positively with objective measures of upper and lower extremity muscle strength and was found to be valid and reliable for measuring the decline in function that results from loss of muscular strength.[131] The ALSFRS-R was expanded to include additional respiratory items, and was found to have internal consistency, construct validity, and to have retained the properties of the original scale.[133] Other disease specific scales include the *Appel ALS Scale (AALS),*[134] the *ALS Severity Scale (ALSSS),*[135] and the *Norris Scale.*[136]

Quality of Life Measures

Quality of life in individuals with ALS has been examined with generic measures, such as the *SF-36,*[137] the *Schedule for Evaluation of Individual Quality of Life-Direct Weighting (SEIQoL-DW),*[138] and the *Sickness Impact Profile (SIP).*[139]

The *ALSAQ-40,*[140] an ALS-specific quality of life measure, contains 40 items that represent five distinct areas of health: mobility (10 items), activities of daily living (10 items), eating and drinking (3 items), communication (7 items), and emotional functioning (10 items). The questions refer to the patient's condition during the past 2 weeks and responses are given on a five-point Likert scale. The *ALSAQ-40* measures health status in each domain using a summary score from 0 (best health status) to 100 (worst health status). The validity and reliability of this instrument have been examined and reported.[140,141] The *ALSAQ-40* has been shortened to 11 items and also appears valid and reliable.[142]

Physical Therapy Interventions

The role of the physical therapist in management of individuals with ALS and the extent of interventions provided vary depending on whether or not the therapist is working as a member of a neuromuscular team specialized in ALS care or as an independent or clinic-based therapist. Additional variables include the availability of other health care professionals in the practice setting and the reason the individual is seeking physical therapy (e.g., specific ALS-related problem vs a comorbidity problem such as arthritis).

Restorative intervention is directed toward remediating or improving impairments and functional limitations. In the early and middle stages of ALS, restorative interventions are temporary at best because disease progression is expected and permanent loss of function and disability is likely. Restorative interventions in the late stage of ALS are for the most part directed solely toward remediation of impairments that result from other systems pathology (e.g., pressure sores, edema, pneumonia, atelectasis, adhesive capsulitis).

Compensatory intervention is directed toward modifying activities, tasks or the environment to minimize functional limitations and disabilities. In the early and middle stages of ALS, tasks, or activities may be adapted to achieve function. As the disease progresses, increasing environmental adaptations will be necessary to maintain and promote function.[110]

In the early and early–middle stages of ALS, **preventative intervention** is directed toward minimizing potential impairments such as loss of ROM, aerobic capacity, or strength, preventing pneumonia or atelectasis, and functional limitations. Beginning an early prevention program may alter impairments and maintain physical function temporarily, and may also improve well-being and decrease fatigue as well as the secondary effects of immobility. In the late-middle and late stages, the pathology is more advanced and mobility becomes progressively restricted. In these stages, it may be extremely difficulty or impossible to prevent impairments and functional limitations that are directly related to the nervous system pathology. Thus, the role of prevention is *tertiary,* in order to mitigate the effects of the pathology that lead to impairments in other systems. For example, educating caregivers about a passive ROM exercise program to prevent adhesive capsulitis in the shoulder.[110] In general, the role of the physical therapist includes:

- Promoting independence and maximizing function throughout the stages of the disease, through restorative and compensatory interventions that address impairments, functional limitations, and disabilities;
- Promoting health and wellness in the early and early-middle stages of the disease through restorative interventions;
- Providing alternative means of carrying out functional activities with adaptive equipment and alternate methods for performing tasks and activities as the disease progresses;
- Minimizing or preventing complications through preventative interventions throughout the course of the disease; and
- Providing education, psychological support, and recommendations for equipment and community resources to assist in adaptations to the disease progression.[110]

Owing to the individual variability of the disease, patients with ALS will present with unique and different sets of problems; thus, interventions will vary. As mentioned earlier, interventions are directed mainly toward addressing functional limitations and disabilities because often times the impairments causing the limitations and disabilities cannot be altered. However, in the early and early–middle stages of ALS, it may be possible to direct treatment toward the underlying CNS impairments, and perhaps postpone the onset of functional limitations. For example, a preliminary study of patients in the early stages of ALS who performed muscle strengthening exercises demonstrated increases in MVIC for several muscle groups. In addition, over the study period, they had less absolute decreases and percentage decreases per month in ALSFRS scores, Schwab and

England function scores, SF-36 Physical Function scores and forced vital capacity (FVC) compared to a matched control group who performed stretching exercises only.[143] Patients and therapists must understand that any beneficial effects of an early prevention program will be short term and will not have an impact on the overall course of the disease. Much more research into the effectiveness of interventions for individuals with ALS is needed.

In developing a plan of care (POC), in addition to the patient's goals, the therapist must also consider the rate of disease progression, the extent and area of involvement, stage of the disease, respiratory and bulbar factors that may impact participation, timing of the intervention, patient acceptance and motivation, life support choices, availability of psychosocial support, and resources.

Some patients may view the need to use adaptive equipment, an ambulatory assistive device or wheelchair as a definitive marker for disease progression and impending death. This may cause the patient to be hesitant to accept the recommended aid or device as a means of maintaining some aspect of control over the disease. The physical therapist will be required to maintain a balance between being realistic about what can be achieved and providing a sense of hope, not helplessness, when discussing intervention options. An overview of ALS disease stages and general intervention strategies is presented in Table 20.3. Common impairments and functional limitations associated with ALS and their respective interventions are described below.

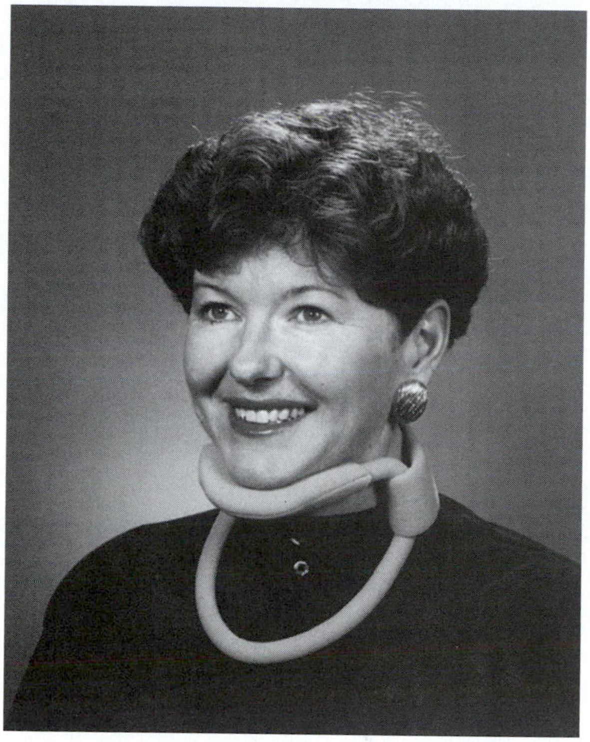

Figure 20.12 The Headmaster Collar. (Courtesy of Symmetric Designs, Salt Spring Island, BC, Canada, V8K 1C9.)

Cervical Muscle Weakness

Progressive cervical extensor weakness will cause the head to fall forward, resulting in overstretching of the posterior musculature and soft tissues. This may cause bouts of acute pain or develop into chronic cervical syndromes, and anterior muscle tightness. Some patients will compensate for the forward head position by increasing lordosis, as they attempt to maintain their posture during ambulation.

For mild to moderate cervical weakness, a soft foam collar may be worn during specific activities. Soft collars are comfortable and usually well tolerated. However, wear-induced compressibility requires they be replaced frequently. For moderate to severe weakness, a semirigid or rigid collar is prescribed. These are usually made of padded rigid plastic or leather and provide very firm support. Patients may find the collars very warm; may experience discomfort at points of body contact, such as the chin, mandible, sternum, or over clavicles; may feel pressure on the trachea; and, may feel confined. Several types of collars are presented in Figures 20.12 and 20.13, and the pros and cons of individual collar types are summarized in Table 20.4.

Some patients with combined cervical and upper thoracic weakness may benefit from a cervical-thoracic orthosis, or a

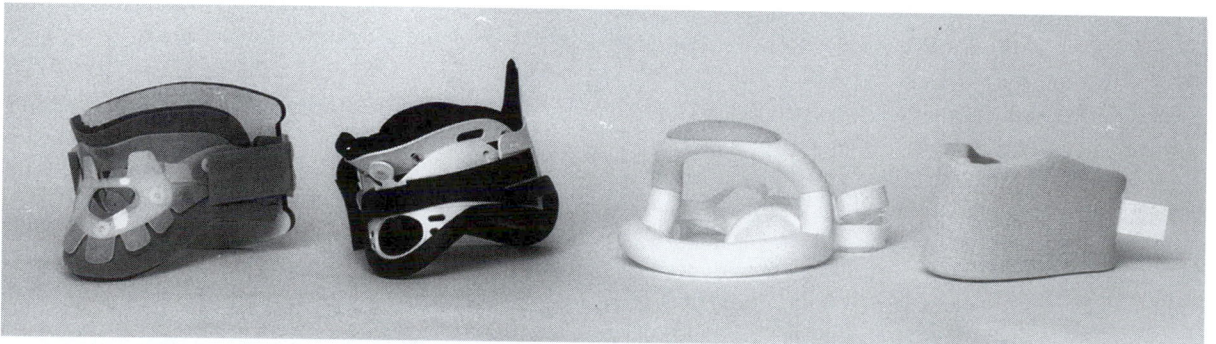

Figure 20.13 Types of Collars. From left to right: Aspen Collar, Miami-J Collar, Executive Collar, and Soft Collar.

Table 20.3 Amyotrophic Lateral Sclerosis Disease Stages and Common Intervention Strategies: Framework for Rehabilitation for Individuals with ALS

Stage	Common Impairments and Functional Limitations	Interventions
Early	Mild to moderate weakness in specific muscle groups Difficulty with ADLs and mobility toward the end of this stage	**Restorative/Preventative** • Strengthening exercises[a142,169,170] • Endurance exercises[171] • Active ROM,[172] Active-assisted ROM, stretching exercises **Compensatory** • Determine potential need for adaptive or assistive devices • Determine potential need for ergonomic modifications of home/workplace • Energy conservation • Educate the patient about the disease process, energy conservation, and support groups
Middle	Progressive decrease in mobility throughout stage Wheelchair needed for long distances; increased wheelchair use toward end of stage Severe muscle weakness in some groups; mild to moderate weakness in other groups Progressive decrease in ADL skills throughout stage Pain	**Compensatory** • Support weak muscles (assistive and supportive devices, adaptive equipment, slings, orthoses) • Modifications to workplace/home (e.g., install ramp, move bedroom to first floor) • Wheelchair prescription • Education of caregivers regarding functional training **Preventative** • Active[172] active-assistive, and passive ROM, stretching exercises • Strengthening exercises[142,169,170] (early middle) • Endurance exercises[171] (early middle) • Determine need for pressure-relieving devices (e.g., pressure distributing mattress)
Late	Wheelchair dependent or restricted to bed Complete dependence with ADLs Severe weakness of UE, LE, neck and trunk muscles Dysarthria, dysphagia Respiratory compromise Pain	**Preventative** • Passive ROM • Pulmonary care[a] • Hospital bed and pressure-relieving devices • Skin care, hygiene[a] **Compensatory** • Caregiver education regarding transfers, positioning, turning, skin care • Mechanical lift

[a]May be restorative.

From Dal Bello-Haas, V,[110] p 123, with permission.

ADL = activities of daily living; LE = lower extremity; ROM = range of motion; UE = upper extremity.

Sterno-occipital Mandibular Immobilizer (SOMI). These devices provide greater support, but are more expensive and heavy and may be difficult to don and doff. For severe or intractable neck weakness, referral to an orthotist for a custom-made device may be necessary.

In addition to wearing collars, individuals with cervical weakness may also benefit from taking frequent rest periods, supportive seating such as high back chairs or recliners; tilt-in-space or reclining wheelchairs; elevating reading material; and education about good arm support for prolonged sitting, proper use of head rest when riding in a car, and ergonomic changes for work centers. It is important to note that when trunk weakness accompanies neck weakness positioning for head support becomes more challenging.

Dysarthria and Dysphagia

In collaboration with the speech–language pathologist, the physical therapist can play a role in managing dysarthria

Table 20.4 Types of Semirigid and Rigid Cervical Collars

Type	Examples	Advantages	Disadvantages
Collars without anterior neck access	Philadelphia® Collar[a]	Offers good support	Patient may feel confined May cause pressure on trachea Patient may experience difficulty breathing or swallowing Can be uncomfortably warm
Collars with anterior neck access (for tracheostomy)	Miami-J® Collar[b] Aspen Collar[c] Malibu Collar[d]	Padding absorbs and wicks moisture away from skin Suitable for individuals with cervical weakness in all 3 planes	Patient may feel confined May be uncomfortably warm More expensive
	Canadian Collar[e] Headmaster Collar[e]	Open design allows for circulation of air Lightweight No pressure on trachea Some patients consider collar more cosmetically appealing	May put pressure on chin and sternum Some models more expensive Some models require custom cutting Not adequate if rotation and lateral flexion weakness is also present

[a]Philadelphia® Cervical Collar Co, Thorofare, NJ 08086.
[b]Jerome Medical, Moorestown, NJ 08057-3239.
[c]Aspen Medical Products Inc, CA, 92618-5202.
[d]Seattle Systems, Poulsbo, WA 98370.
[e]Symmetric Designs Ltd, Salt Spring Island, BC, Canada.

and dysphagia by addressing the patient's head and trunk control and position in sitting. In addition, the physical therapist can reinforce the use of strategies for eating and swallowing and the use of prescribed communication devices with the patient. Because patients are at risk for aspiration, education of the patient, family, and caregiver is imperative (see Respiratory Muscle Weakness below).

UE Muscle Weakness

Weakness of the UEs greatly impacts the patient's ability to carry out activities of daily living. There is a large variety of adaptive equipment available that may assist the patient prolong function for as long as possible (see Activities of Daily Living below).

Patients with a painful shoulder subluxation may benefit from a sling, similar to those used with patients following stroke with decreased tone, although subluxation cannot be corrected completely. Splinting of the wrist or hand may be indicated to prevent contractures or to improve the patient's function, such as the ability to grasp.

Shoulder Pain

Individuals with ALS may develop shoulder pain and present with capsular patterns of restriction. Pain may be caused by several factors: abnormal scapulohumeral rhythm secondary to spasticity or weakness causing imbalance that may lead to impingement; overuse of strong muscles; muscle strain; poor resting position; glenohumeral subluxation secondary to weakness; or a fall. Depending on the cause of the shoulder pain, interventions may include modalities, ROM exercises, passive stretching, joint mobilizations, and education about proper joint support and protection.

A recent report described a 20 percent incidence of adhesive capsulitis in individuals with ALS. Recommendations for managing the pain and decreased ROM included a protocol of an intra-articular analgesic and anti-inflammatory cocktail injection, followed by a course of aggressive ROM exercises. Some patients reported an acute resolution of pain, while others reported improvements over 2 to 3 weeks.[144]

Respiratory Muscle Weakness

Education is extremely important. Patients and caregivers must be taught how to balance activity and rest and educated about energy conservation techniques. Patients and caregivers should also be educated about signs and symptoms of aspiration; positioning to avoid aspiration, such as upper cervical spine flexion during eating; causes and signs of respiratory infection; and strategies for managing oral secretions or choking episodes, such as the Heimlich maneuver. Breathing exercises and positioning to optimize ventilation/perfusion matching may also be incorporated, although their effectiveness in ALS has not been determined. Airway clearance techniques may be necessary when conditions that cause secretion retention, such as pneumonia or atelectasis, arise.

To compensate for a weakened cough, the patient and caregiver may be instructed in the use of manually assisted coughing techniques or mechanical insufflation–exsufflation. Again, the effectiveness of these techniques or device has not been demonstrated in ALS, but case reports have described the benefits from regular use of a mechanical insufflation device.[145,146] A recent study examining cough flows and pressures during cough augmentation found manual assistance increased flow 11 percent in bulbar and 13 percent in nonbulbar ALS patients, and MI-E increased flow 26 percent in bulbar and 28 percent in nonbulbar ALS patients. The greatest improvements were in patients with the weakest coughs.[147]

LE Muscle Weakness and Gait Impairments

Orthoses may be recommended to improve function by offering support to weakened muscles and the joints they surround, decrease the stress on remaining functioning or compensatory muscles, conserve energy, or minimize local or general muscle fatigue. Controlling knee impairments can often be achieved through an ankle orthosis, and thus addressing the ankle should be considered first. It is also important to consider the weight of the orthosis as individuals with ALS will have energy expenditure issues, and it may be more fatiguing for the patient to ambulate with a heavy orthosis than to ambulate without the impairment being corrected. For this reason, a knee–ankle–foot orthosis (KAFO) is usually not recommended.

Deciding between a premanufactured versus custom orthosis is certainly dependent on the patient's resources, but the rate of disease progression should also be considered. For an individual with rapidly progressive ALS and who is likely to use the orthosis for limited time, a premanufactured orthosis may suffice. Solid ankle–foot orthoses (AFOs) are a good choice for patients who have mediolateral instability of the ankle with quadriceps weakness. The fixed ankle position, combined with the quadriceps weakness may make it difficult for sit-to-stand transfers, climbing stairs, and negotiating inclines. Hinged AFOs allow dorsiflexion and may be appropriate for the patient with adequate knee extensor strength with mild ankle strength loss.

The type of ambulatory assistive device prescribed is dependent on the degree of proximal muscle strength or instability, function of the UEs, the pattern, extent, and rate of disease progression, acceptance by the patient, and financial constraints. Again, weight of the device is an important factor to consider in decision making, while also taking into account which device will ensure optimal function and safety. Wheeled walkers, which do not require the patient to lift the device, are usually recommended. In general, crutches are rarely used by individuals with ALS. If used, Loftstrand (Canadian) crutches are preferred.

Activities of Daily Living

A large variety of adaptive equipment is available to assist individuals with muscle weakness perform everyday tasks. However, the benefits and effectiveness of adaptive equipment for ALS have not been evaluated systematically. No one type of device is suitable for every patient or for every stage of the disease. Reimbursement for the equipment is variable and although a piece of adaptive equipment can help the patient maintain independence, limited financial resources may prevent recommending or purchasing the item. For example, in the

Table 20.5 Common Types of Adaptive Equipment

Feeding and Eating	Foam tubing to increase the size of utensil handles; utensils and cups with modified handles or holders; long-levered jar opener; plate guard; serrated or rocker knife; wrist splint/adapted cuff (for holding tools and instruments); mobile arm support; Dycem®
Self-Care and Bathing	Bathing benches; bath tub seats; shower commode; handheld shower head; grab bars; raised toilet seat; long handled sponge; electric toothbrush or shaver; strap-fitted hairbrushes
Dressing	Zipper pulls or hooks; button hooks; long-handled shoe horn; Velcro® clothing closures; elastic shoe laces
Writing and Reading	Foam tubing to increase the size of the pen or pencil; triangular pencil grip; pen holders; book holders; automatic page turner; adjustable angle table
Other	Key holders; doorknob adapters; lamp extension switch; personal alarm system; switch-operated environmental controls; speaker phone with automatic dialing; telephone holder; use of telecommunication devices for the deaf (TDD)

early stages of ALS a Universal cuff with a pocket for writing or feeding utensils may be beneficial. As the disease progresses and proximal shoulder weakness increases, a mobile arm support may be incorporated to allow the patient to maintain independence in eating. In the late stage of ALS when the patient is dependent on the caregiver for eating, a long straw and straw holder may be recommended to assist the caregiver with the activity. Examples of adaptive equipment that may be beneficial for performing activities of daily living are presented in Table 20.5.

Decreased Mobility

Patients with LE weakness may have difficulty with sit-to-stand or car transfers. Simple interventions include placing a firm cushion 2 to 3 inches thick under the buttocks in the chair or elevating the chair by placing the legs in prefabricated blocks (Fig. 20.14). Self-powered lifting cushions are relatively inexpensive and portable, but the individual needs adequate trunk control and balance in order to use the device safely (Fig. 20.15). Powered seat lift recliner chairs may also be recommended, but are more expensive. All these interventions increase the biomechanical advantage and make it easier for the patient to rise from a sitting position.

Caregivers will need to be educated regarding assisting the patient with transitional movements. Transfer boards may be used for transfers once the individual is unable to stand, either alone if the person has adequate arm strength and good sitting balance, or the caregiver can be instructed in how to assist the patient. Other useful devices to assist the patient's mobility are transfer belts and swivel cushions or seats. Transfer belts ease the burden of the transfer for the caregiver and prevent potential pulling on the patient's UEs. Swivel cushions are lightweight, cushioned seats that swivel in both directions and make getting in and out of a car easier (Fig. 20.16).

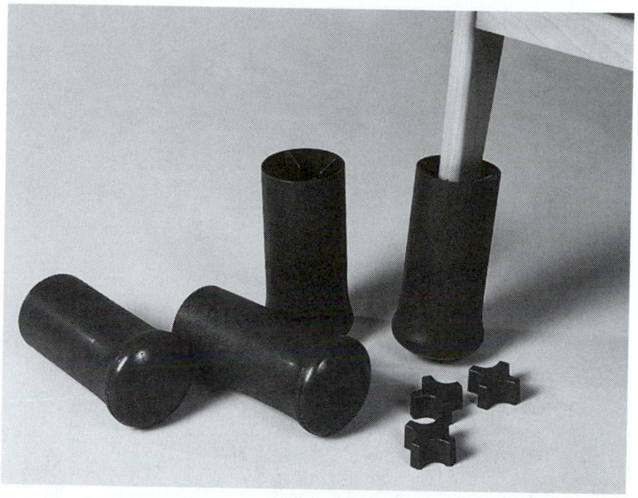

Figure 20.14 Pre-fabricated blocks. (Courtesy of Homecraft AbilityOne, Kirkby-in-Ashfield, Nottinghamshire, England NG17 7ET.)

Once an individual cannot perform transfers, even with the assistance of a caregiver, a hydraulic or mechanical lift is required. Commonly recommended lifts devices include the Easy Pivot™ (Rand-Scot Inc, Fort Collins, CO 80524), and the Hoyer Lift® (Sunrise Medical, Longmont, CO 80503). Use of an electric hospital bed may facilitate bed mobility and transfers both for the patient and caregiver and, depending on resources, home modifications and automobile adaptations may also be considered.

Chair glides or stairway lifts can be suggested for those individuals who live in multi-level homes, but who cannot or should not climb stairs (see Chapter 12). These lifts are measured and custom-made for individual staircases and are very expensive. Insurance companies usually do not reimburse for stairway lifts, but some medical supply companies offer "rent-to-own" options. In addition, local ALS Association (ALSA) chapters or Muscular Dystrophy

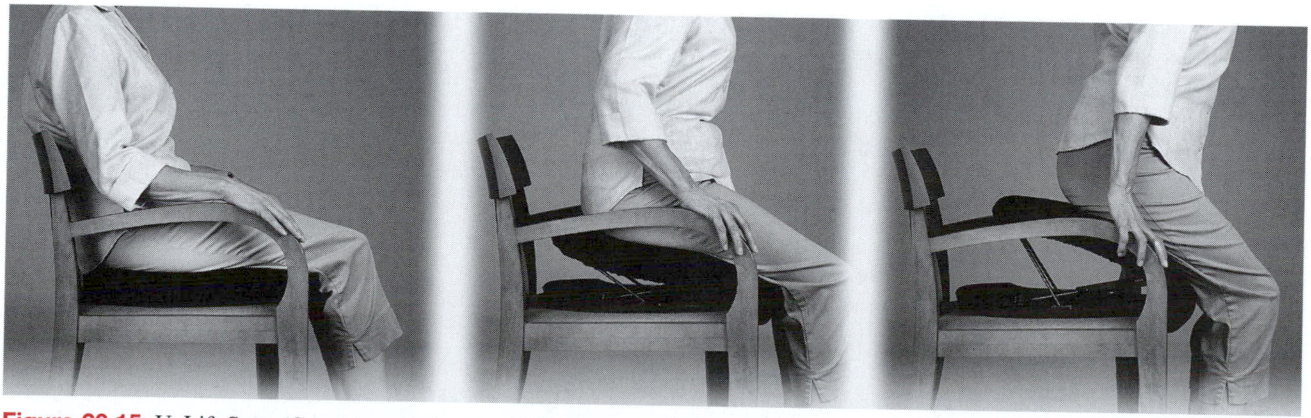

Figure 20.15 UpLift Seat. (Courtesy of Uplift Technologies Inc., Dartmouth, NS, Canada, B3B 1M2.)

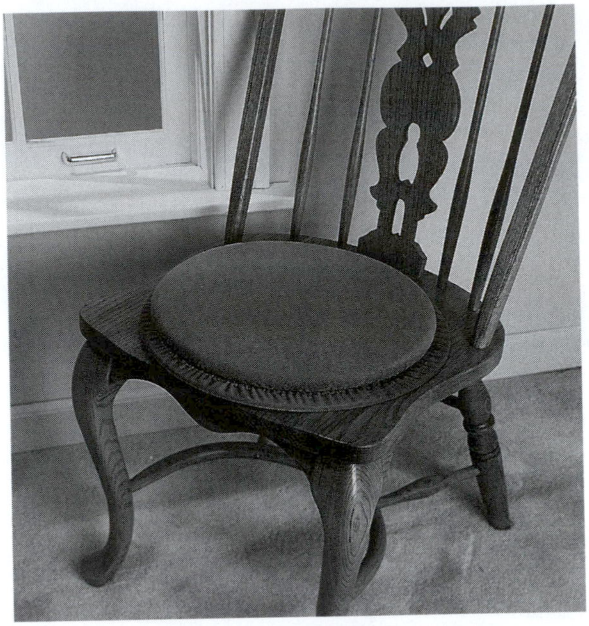

Figure 20.16 Swivel cushion. (Courtesy of Sammons Preston Rolyan Canada, Mississauga, Ontario, Canada, L4Y 4C5.)

Association (MDA) chapters may have lifts that have been recycled.

At some time point as the disease progresses, the extent of muscle weakness or the energy requirements for ambulation will necessitate wheelchair use for mobility. In the early or early-middle stage of ALS, a manual wheelchair, preferably lightweight, may be used for traveling long distances as an energy conservation technique. This wheelchair should be rented on a short-term basis or loaned from a local ALSA or MDA chapter or other source, as most insurance companies will reimburse for only one wheelchair purchase. As the disease progresses, a power wheelchair system tailored to the patient's current needs and potential future needs will be necessary. Numerous customized wheelchair features and options are available that can assist the individual in maintaining a maximum level of independence and comfort. A referral to a wheelchair and seating clinic may be the best option owing to the numerous, specialized, and evolving needs of the individual with ALS.

Trail and colleagues surveyed 42 patients with ALS and moderate disability, as documented on the AALS, about the wheelchair features they found most beneficial. Sixty-one percent of patients reported that their wheelchairs allowed them to maintain their previous activity levels. In order of priority, manual wheelchair users cited a lightweight frame, small turning radius, high reclining back and supports for the head, trunk, and extremities as most desirable; undesirable features included low, sling, nonreclining back; nonmotorized; static, nonadjustable leg rests; heaviness or large size; and, nonremovable armrests. Desirable features for patients who used powered wheelchairs included independent mobility, maneuverability, overall comfort and tilt-in-space/recline features; undesirable features included low, nonreclining back, heaviness or large size, uncomfortable seat, nonadjustable leg rests, and general discomfort.[148]

Although power scooters may be suitable for a patient with adequate UE and trunk strength in the earlier stages of ALS, the vehicle becomes limiting as the disease progresses and should not be prescribed. If the patient has already been reimbursed for a scooter, most insurance companies will not pay for a power wheelchair, because the scooter is considered a power mobility device. If a scooter is to be recommended at all, the patient should rent or borrow the device for short-term use.

Muscle Cramps and Spasticity

Muscle cramps may be alleviated with massage and a stretching program. Cold can temporarily decrease spasticity. Physical therapists can perform and instruct caregivers in slow prolonged stretches and passive ROM exercises to address spasticity. In addition, postural and positioning techniques can be incorporated to decrease spasticity and splinting may be necessary to prevent contractures. A recently published Cochrane review describes one study that found patients with ALS who engaged in moderate intensity exercise had decreased spasticity, as measured by the *Modified Ashworth Scale*.[149]

Psychosocial Issues

A diagnosis of ALS is devastating for both the patient and family-caregiver unit. Because of the progressive nature of the disease, impairments readily lead to functional limitations and disabilities, which may impact quality of life. The emotional responses of the person experiencing the disease, family members, and individuals caring for the patient are multifaceted and may fluctuate throughout the stages of the disease. Much is lost when living with a terminal, progressive disease: physical health and abilities, body image, work and family roles, identity, family and social networks, lifestyle, independence, control, hope, meaning, and the anticipated future.[150,151] The physical therapist must be able to recognize the patient's ability to cope and adapt, and his or her psychological reactions, level of acceptance, and willingness and ability to integrate therapeutic recommendations. It is also imperative that the physical therapist be able to differentiate between normal reactionary grief to losses or a change in physical function and the presence of clinical anxiety and depression, and refer the patient to the appropriate health care team member, when necessary.[152]

When pervasive, anxiety and depressive symptoms need to be treated aggressively with pyschopharmacological medications, because left untreated these psychosocial impairments can adversely affect an individual's ability to adapt, cope, and participate in the plan of care (POC). Depression may also lead to suicide. In addition, anxiety and depression may also be prevalent among family members or caregivers.[152]

Exercise and ALS

Despite the high incidence of muscle weakness in individuals with ALS, the effects of exercise programs have not been extensively studied, and thus, are not well understood. Often physical therapy programs involve ROM and stretching exercises only. Despite the lack of research evidence, some discourage exercise programs because of fear of overuse weakness and believe that no exercise other than everyday activities is indicated.

Studies of individuals with other neuromuscular diseases (NMD) such as poliomyelitis, Duchenne's muscular dystrophy, myotonic dystrophy, hereditary motor and sensory neuropathy, spinal muscular atrophy, and limb-girdle, Becker, and fascioscapulohumeral dystrophy have found that exercise programs are beneficial and do not produce overuse weakness.[153–160] The research evidence in these patient populations suggests:

- Overuse weakness does not occur in muscles with a Manual Muscle Test (MMT) grade of 3 (fair) or greater out of 5 (normal).
- Moderate resistance exercises can increase strength in muscles with a MMT grade of 3 or greater out of 5.
- Strength gains are proportional to initial muscle strength.
- Heavy eccentric exercise should be avoided.
- Exercise may produce functional benefits.
- Psychological benefits have yet to be determined.[153–160]

When prescribed appropriately, exercise may be beneficial, especially in the early stages of the disease. Exercise may not improve the strength of muscles already weakened by ALS, certainly not those below grade 3. However, general active ROM and stretching of affected joints, resistive strengthening exercises of unaffected muscles with low to moderate weights, and aerobic activities, such as swimming, walking, and bicycling, at submaximal levels, may be prescribed.

When designing a strengthening exercise program for a patient with ALS, the physical therapist must take into consideration the balance between overuse fatigue and disuse atrophy. Evidence from patients with other neuromuscular diseases suggests that highly repetitive or heavy resistance exercise can cause prolonged loss of muscle strength in weakened, denervated muscle.[161,162] Some animal studies have found that neuromuscular activity has inhibitory effects on sprouting in partially denervated muscle,[163–165] whereas other studies have reported no effect[166,167] or that activity can promote sprouting or reinnervation.[168,169]

On the other hand, a marked reduction in activity level secondary to ALS can lead to cardiovascular deconditioning and disuse weakness beyond the amount caused by the disease itself. Therefore, the type and intensity of the exercise program should be carefully monitored and adjusted by the physical therapist in order to prevent excessive fatigue, while at the same time promoting optimal use of intact muscle groups. Patients should be advised not to carry out any activities to the point of extreme fatigue, and should keep track of *symptoms of overuse*, such as, the inability to perform daily activities following exercise due to exhaustion or pain, increased fasciculations or increased muscle cramping. They may also be advised to exercise for several brief periods throughout the day, with sufficient rest in between.

Disuse Atrophy

Reduced physical activity, particularly if prolonged, reduces function of the neuromuscular system, in addition to the skeletal and other organ systems. With insufficient activity, disuse atrophy develops when muscle contractions are less than 20 percent of the total tension a muscle is capable of producing. As contractile proteins are lost, the muscle weakness progresses at a rate of 3 percent per day.[170] Strength loss through inactivity and disuse can significantly debilitate individuals with ALS, making them highly susceptible to deconditioning, and muscle and joint tightness leading to contractures and pain.

Overuse Fatigue

The potential for inducing overwork damage in individuals with ALS through excessive exercise is a common concern. Sanjak et al. demonstrated that individuals with ALS demonstrate abnormal physiological and metabolic responses to single bouts of exercise. Oxygen consumption during submaximal exercise was increased in individuals with ALS compared to controls, and $\dot{V}O_{2max}$ and work capacity were decreased. In addition, it was found that several metabolic substrates of plasma and muscle compartments did not increase to the same level as untrained control subjects, indicating that the availability of substrate for energy production is affected.[59]

In individuals with ALS, the safe range for therapeutic exercise narrows, and the degree to which the range narrows is dependent on the extent of disease involvement and the rate of disease progression. A weak or denervated muscle is more susceptible to overwork damage because it is already functioning close to its maximal limits. Activities of daily living alone may cause impaired muscles to act as though in training and exercise that would improve normal muscles may actually cause overwork damage in impaired muscles. The remaining motor units will respond to training, and these motor units must work harder to handle a given amount of exercise stress.[170] Thus, special attention must be paid to developing an exercise program for patients with ALS, and physical therapists should prescribe exercise training at moderate to low intensities.

The literature related to exercise in individuals with ALS is limited. Two early case studies demonstrated positive effects of specific strengthening and endurance exercises.[171,172] More recently, the effects of exercise in individuals with ALS have been evaluated with larger samples. Both of these studies found significantly less decline in function scores and other outcome measures[173,174] in the exercise group. Two recent animal studies found that endurance exercise training at moderate intensities slowed disease progression[175,176]; whereas, a third study found that high endurance exercise training had detrimental effects on male mice only.[177] The evidence related to exercise and ALS is presented in Evidence Summary Box 20.1 (human studies) and Evidence Summary Box 20.2 (animal studies).

Patient/Client-Related Instruction

A diagnosis of ALS is devastating for individuals and their families. They are faced with continual, multiple changes and losses, and eventual death. Assisting the individual and his or her family and caregivers to come to terms with the impact of the disease is an important role for the physical therapist, and providing psychological support and opportunities for expression of feelings, frustrations and concerns is imperative. Collaborating with and educating the patient, family, and caregiver in an open and encouraging environment may empower patients in their efforts to cope with their disease, foster a sense of purpose and self-efficacy, and enhance the overall effectiveness of the intervention by increasing compliance.[110]

Evidence Summary Box 20.1

Exercise and ALS: The Evidence from Human Studies

Reference	Subject(s)	Methods	Duration	Results
Bohanon, RW[171] 1983	56-year-old nonambulatory woman	Case study UE resistive exercises using PNF patterns	75 days	14 muscle groups increased in strength from 7% to 96% 4 muscle groups lost strength by 10–21%
Sanjak, M, Reddan, W, and Brooks, BR[172] 1987	46-year-old man	Case study Air-Dyne bicycle ergometer	6 weeks	Isokinetic strength and cardiopulmonary responses to exercise improved in the UEs, but not in the LEs
Pinto, AC, Alves, M, and Nogueira, A[173] 1999	20 Ss, E = 8 Mean age E: 62 ± 14 years C: 64 ± 16 years	Prospective, controlled single blind; C: no endurance protocol E: Bruce or Naughton treadmill protocol, while using BiPap; exercise to anaerobic threshold until stop parameters reached	12 months	E: significantly greater FIM scores ($p < 0.03$); slower Spinal Norris Score decline ($p < 0.02$); significant difference in the slope of FVC decline ($p < 0.008$)
Drory, VE, et al[174] 2001	25 male Ss, E = 14 Mean age E: 58.0 ± 13.2 years C: 60.7 ± 16.4 years	Randomly assigned to 2 groups: C: usual daily activities E: limb and trunk exercises against modest loads	2 times/day for 15 minutes 12 months	At 3 months, E: significantly less decline in ALSFRS ($p <$ 0.001) and Ashworth Spasticity Scale scores ($p =$ 0.005); no significant differences in MMT, FSS, pain, SF-36 scores; at 6 months, no significant differences between groups

ALSFRS = Amyotrophic Lateral Sclerosis Functional Rating Scale; BiPap = Bidirectional positive airway pressure ventilation; C = control; E = experimental; FIM = Functional Independence Measure; FSS = Fatigue Severity Scale; FVC = forced vital capacity; LE = lower extremity; Ss = subjects; UE = upper extremity.

Evidence Summary Box 20.2

Exercise and ALS: The Evidence from Animal Studies

Reference	Animals	Methods	Duration	Results
Kirkinezos, IG, et al[175] 2003	7-week old G93A-SOD1 transgenic mice	E: running on a treadmill (30 min at 13 m/min initially; speed and duration decreased stepwise) C: sedentary	5 days/week until unable to keep up with a speed of 7 m/min	E: overall, significant increase in lifespan of G93A-SOD1 mice ($p = 0.007$); significant increase in male mice lifespan ($p = 0.02$); trend toward increase in female mice lifespan, but not significant ($p = 0.1$)
Veldink, JH, et al[176] 2003	8-week old transgenic low-copy hSOD1 mice and wild-type littermates	E: running on a treadmill (45 min at 16 m/min) C: sedentary	Until too ill to run	E: exercise delayed onset of disease in female, but not male hSOD1 mice; exercise prolonged survival in female mice
Mahoney, DJ, et al[177] 2004	40-day-old G93A and wild-type littermate control mice	E: running on a treadmill (20 min/day at 9 m/min for week 1; 25 min/day for week 2; 30 min/day for week 3; progressive increase in intensity week 2 and 3; 45 min/day at 22 m/min) C: sedentary	3 days/week for first 3 weeks; 5 days/week for remainder	E: onset of disease not affected in female and male mice; exercise hastened death in male, but not female mice ($p < 0.0001$)

C = control; E = experimental; min = minutes.

Patient and family/caregiver education is integral throughout the stages of the disease. The scope of education can include, but is not limited to:

- Providing accurate, factual information about the disease process and clinical manifestations, and their significance in terms of management. Give only as much information as the patient, family, and caregivers need; information should be provided in manner appropriate to their understanding.
- Instructing patients, family members, and caregivers regarding interventions that can be carried out independently such as monitoring the effects and side effects of medications, use of assistive devices and adaptive equipment, and preventing secondary complications.
- Advising the patient about methods to promote general health. Instruction regarding energy conservation, balancing rest and activity, and relaxation techniques may be beneficial in assisting the patient to cope with the daily constraints of the disease.
- Counseling regarding care and life decisions, if the patients asks about these issues.
- Referring patients to support groups or psychological counseling.
- Providing information on health and available social and support services.[110]

The ALS Association and the Muscular Dystrophy Association are the two national voluntary organizations that provide many functions and programs for individuals with ALS and their families and caregivers, including the provision of written and video educational materials, local education programs, patient and caregiver support groups, equipment loan programs, respite programs, transportation programs, advocacy programs, and ALS Awareness Programs. Patients can explore these resources through the following contact information:

Amyotrophic Lateral Sclerosis Association
27001 Agoura Road, Suite 150
Calabasas Hills, CA 91301-5104
(818) 880-9007; (800) 782-474
http://www.alsa.org

The Muscular Dystrophy Association
3300 East Sunrise Drive
Tucson, AZ 85718-3208
(520) 529-2000; (800) 572-1717
http://www.mdausa.org

Summary

Amyotrophic lateral sclerosis, the most common and devastatingly fatal motor neuron disease among adults, causes a progressive increase in the number and severity of impairments, functional limitations, and disabilities. Other than a small percentage of cases, etiology for the most part is unknown, and it is hypothesized that multiple mechanisms may be responsible for the disease. Although there is no cure for ALS and its course cannot be altered, it should be considered a "treatable disease." Medical management is primarily symptomatic, and a team approach to care is considered optimal. Rehabilitation management is focused on maximizing function and promoting independence to the highest level possible, and ensuring optimal quality of life throughout the course of the disease and across health care settings.

The physical therapist plays an integral role in designing and implementing therapeutic interventions for individuals with ALS that will allow them to maintain independence and function for as long as possible. The selection of interventions, grounded in evidence-based research whenever possible, is based on the stage and progression of the disease and may be restorative, compensatory, or preventative. These interventions should take into consideration the individual's goals; psychosocial factors that may impact decision making such as the individual's acceptance of the diagnosis and the individual's social and financial resources. Because of the progressive nature of the ALS, the physical therapist must not only address the patient's current problems, but also plan for the patient's future needs.

Acknowledgments

Special thanks to Liz Scott and Erica Poole for their extraordinary typing, administrative and editorial skills, and to Peggy Ingels-Allred for her thoughtful and critical review.

Questions for Review

1. Describe the clinical manifestations of ALS. Differentiate among impairments associated with upper and lower motor neuron pathology and bulbar pathology.
2. What examination procedures are used to help support the diagnosis of ALS?
3. Identify and define the major classifications of ALS included in the El Escorial criteria developed by the World Federation of Neurology Research Group on Motor Neuron Diseases.
4. Describe the disease course of ALS. What factors have shown a relationship to prognosis?
5. Considering the variety of impairments associated with ALS, what physical therapy tests and measures should be included in a comprehensive examination?
6. Differentiate among *restorative, compensatory,* and *preventive* interventions.
7. When designing an exercise program for a patient with ALS, what factors need to taken into consideration?
8. What information should be considered and included when developing a plan for patient and family education following the diagnosis of ALS?

Case Study

The patient is a right-handed 36-year-old white man recently diagnosed with ALS.

HISTORY

Seven months ago, the patient experienced cramping in his left calf and a few months later noted that his left foot slapped and that he "caught his toes" and tripped while playing basketball or walking on the golf course. He also noticed painless twitching of the muscles in his right hand, forearm, and upper arm and reported difficulty fastening the snaps on his youngest son's pajamas.

PAST MEDICAL HISTORY

No significant past medical history.

SOCIAL HISTORY

The patient has been married for 10 years. He has a 3-year-old and a 9-month-old son, and his wife is pregnant with their third child. He lives in a two-story house with 4 steps up to the front door (no railing), 12 stairs between levels (bilateral railing), and 10 stairs to the basement with a railing on the right.

He stopped playing basketball and baseball because he is embarrassed about the frequent tripping, but continues to play golf on the weekend. He uses a golf cart because he is "unable to keep up with his friends on the golf course." He would like to be more active.

OCCUPATION

He is a manager at a computer graphics business and reports his voice becomes hoarse on occasion after long presentations. He reports significant fatigue if he works on the computer for long periods of time or if he has to stand for long periods for presentations. He attributes this to "getting older."

DIAGNOSTIC TESTS

Electromyographic studies showed: (1) low compound motor action potentials in all extremities; (2) normal sensory nerve conduction; (3) fibrillations and fasciculations in all extremities; and (4) widespread neurogenic changes in motor unit action potentials, abnormal recruitment patterns in the distal leg musculature and mild to moderate changes in the upper extremities.

PHYSICAL EXAMINATION FINDINGS

Observation: Marked wasting of the interossei regions bilaterally.

Speech: No abnormalities noted.

ROM: WNL for all joints, except the thumbs and the L ankle. Patient was only able to oppose thumbs to the third digits. He lacks 5° of L dorsiflexion.

Strength: Bilateral LE strength graded as 5/5, except for the hip flexor group (R = 4/5; L = 4+/5) and the L ankle dorsiflexors (3–/5). Shoulder muscle strength graded as 4+/5 (R) and 4/5 (L); elbow muscle strength graded as 4/4 (R) and 4+/5 (L).

Hand strength: R = 12 lbs; L = 24 lbs (hand-held dynamometer).

Pinch strength: R-tripod = 2 lbs; lateral = 3 lbs; L-tripod = 5 lbs; lateral = 3 lbs (see below for normative data on grip and pinch strength).

Coordination: Purdue Pegboard Testing, R—6 peg holes in 30 seconds; L—3 peg holes in 30 seconds.

Tone: 1 for both UEs and 1+ for both LEs (Modified Ashworth spasticity scores).

Reflexes: A clonic jaw reflex; hyperreflexia in both UEs; hyporeflexia in both LEs; positive Babinski reflex bilaterally.

Gait: independent of assistive devices; positive for L foot drop and hip hiking; 15-ft walk test = 3.6 seconds

Balance (standing): unilateral stance/eyes open, R = 25 seconds; L = 6 seconds.

Respiratory: Forced vital capacity and maximum inspiratory pressure (MIP) are within normal limits.

Functional status: The patient rated himself at 90 percent on the Schwab and England Rating Scale (see Appendix A). ALSFRS-R scores (see Appendix B):

ALSFRS-R Scores

Item	Score
Speech	4
Salivation	3
Swallowing	3
Handwriting (pre-ALS dominant hand)	3
Cutting food and handling utensils (patients without gastrostomy)	3
Dressing and hygiene	3
Turning in bed; adjusting bed clothes	4
Walking	3
Climbing stairs	3
Dyspnea	3
Orthopnea	4
Respiratory insufficiency	4

Grip and Pinch Strength Values (Pounds) for Men 35 to 39 (n = 25)

	Hand	Mean	SD	SE	Low	High
Grip	R	119.7	24.0	4.8	76	176
	L	112.9	21.7	4.4	73	157
Tip	R	18.0	3.6	.73	12	27
	L	17.7	3.8	.76	10	24
Palmar	R	26.1	3.2	.65	21	32
	L	25.6	3.9	.77	18	32
Lateral (Key)	R	26.2	4.1	.83	19	36
	L	25.9	5.4	1.17	14	40

From: Mathiowetz, V, et al: Grip and pinch strength: Normative data for adults. Arch Phys Med Rehabil 66:69, 1984.

GUIDING QUESTIONS

1. What El Escorial diagnostic criteria would you anticipate documented in the patient's medical record?
2. Identify the patient's problems in terms of direct, indirect, and composite impairments.
3. What impact do the impairments have on the patient's ability to function (i.e., functional limitations)?
4. What additional tests and measurements should be conducted; what consultations should be recommended?
5. At present, what are the key areas of patient education that should be addressed initially?
6. Identify the general elements of a physical therapy plan of care for the patient.

References

1. Rowland, LP: Diverse forms of motor neuron disease. Adv Neurol 36:1, 1982.
2. Swash, M: Clinical features and diagnosis of amyotrophic lateral sclerosis. In Brown, R Jr, Meininger, V, and Swash, M (eds): Amyotrophic Lateral Sclerosis. Martin Dunitz Ltd, London, 2000, p 3.
3. Norris, F, et al: Onset, natural history and outcome in idiopathic adult motor neuron disease. J Neurol Sci 118(1):48, 1993.
4. Pradas, J, et al: The natural history of amyotrophic lateral sclerosis and the use of natural history controls in therapeutic trials. Neurology 43(4):751, 1993.
5. Ringel, SP, et al: The natural history of amyotrophic lateral sclerosis. Neurology 43(7):1316, 1993.
6. Haverkamp, LJ, Appel, V, and Appel, SH: Natural history of amyotrophic lateral sclerosis in database population: Validation of a scoring system and a model for survival prediction. Brain 118:707, 1995.
7. Gubbay, SS, et al: Amyotrophic lateral sclerosis: A study of its presentation and prognosis. J Neurol 232:295, 1985.
8. Appel, SH, et al: Amyotrophic lateral sclerosis: Associated clinical disorders and immunological evaluations. Arch Neurol 43:234, 1986.
9. Mulder, DW, et al: Familial adult motor neuron disease: Amyotrophic lateral sclerosis. Neurology 36:511, 1987.
10. Strong, MJ, Hudson, AJ, and Alvord, WG: Familial amyotrophic lateral sclerosis, 1850-1989: A statistical analysis of the world literature. Can J Neurol Sci 18:45, 1991.
11. Hamida, MB, and Hentati, F: Juvenile amyotrophic lateral sclerosis. In Brown, R Jr, Meininger, V, and Swash, M (eds): Amyotrophic Lateral Sclerosis. Martin Dunitz Ltd, London, 2000, p 59.
12. Rosen, DR, et al: Mutations in Cu/Zn superoxide dismutase gene are associated with familial amyotrophic lateral sclerosis. Nature 362:59, 1993.
13. Jackson, M, and Rothstein, JD: Amyotrophic lateral sclerosis. In Marcoux, FW, and Choi, DW (eds). Central Nervous System Neuroprotection. Springer, New York, 2002, p 423.
14. Jackson, M, et al: Analysis of chromosome 5q13 genes in amyotrophic lateral sclerosis: Homozygous NAIP deletion in a sporadic case. Ann Neurol 39:796, 1996.
15. Robberecht, W, et al: D90 A heterozygosity in the SOD1 gene is associated with familial and apparently sporadic amyotrophic lateral sclerosis. Neurology 47:1336, 1996.
16. Caroscio, JT, Calhoun, WF, and Yahr, MD: Prognostic factors in motor neuron disease: A prospective study of longevity. In Rose, FC (ed): Research Progress in Motor Neuron Disease. Pitman, London, 1984, p 34.
17. Brooks, BR, et al: The natural history of amyotrophic lateral sclerosis. In Williams, AC (ed): Motor Neurone Disease. Chapman and Hall, London, 1994, p 121.
18. Hosler, BA, and Brown, RH: Copper/zinc superoxide dismutase mutations and free radical damage in amyotrophic lateral sclerosis. Adv Neurol 680:41, 1995.
19. Rothstein, JD, et al: Chronic inhibition of superoxide dismutase produces apoptotic death of spinal neurons. Proc Natl Acad Sci USA 91:4155, 1994.
20. Borchelt, DR, et al: Superoxide dismutase 1 with mutations linked to familial amyotrophic lateral sclerosis possesses significant activity. Proc Natl Acad Sci USA 91:8292, 1994.
21. Plaitakis, A, and Carosio, JT: Abnormal glutamate metabolism in amyotrophic lateral sclerosis. Ann Neurol 22(5):575, 1987.
22. Rothstein, JD, Tsai, G, and Kuncl, RW: Abnormal excitatory amino acid metabolism in amyotrophic lateral sclerosis. Ann Neurol 28:18, 1990.
23. Rothstein, JD, Martin, LJ, and Kuncl, RW: Decreased glutamate transport by the brain and spinal cord in amyotrophic lateral sclerosis. N Engl J Med 236:1464, 1992.
24. Rothstein, JD, et al: Selective loss of glial glutamate transporter GLT-l in amyotrophic lateral sclerosis. Ann Neurol 38:73, 1995.
25. Carpenter, S: Proximal axonal enlargement in motor neuron disease. Neurology 18:841, 1968.
26. Hirano, A, et al: Fine structural observations of neurofilamentous changes in amyotrophic lateral sclerosis. J Neuropathol Exp Neurol 43:461, 1984.
27. Wolfgang, F, and Myers, L: Amyotrophic lateral sclerosis: Effect of serum on anterior horn cells in tissue culture. Science 179:579, 1973.
28. Troost, D, Van Den Oord, JJ, and Vianney DeJong, JMB: Immunohistochemical characterization of the inflammatory infiltrate in amyotrophic lateral sclerosis. Neuropathol Applied Neurobiol 16:401, 1990.
29. Smith, RB, et al: Serum antibodies to L-type calcium channels in patients with amyotrophic lateral sclerosis. N Engl J Med 327:1721, 1992.
30. Appel, SH: A unifying hypothesis for the cause of amyotrophic lateral sclerosis, parkinsonism, and Alzheimer disease. Ann Neurol 10:499, 1981.
31. Lindsay, RM: Brain-dervied neurotrophic factor: An NGF-related neurotrophin. In Loughlin, SE, and Fallon, JH (eds): Neurotrophic Factors. Academic Press, San Diego, 1993, p 257.
32. Thoenen, H, Hughes, RA, and Sendtner, M: Trophic support of motoneurons: Physiological, pathophysiological, and therapeutic implications. Exp Neurol 124:47, 1993.
33. Anand, P, et al: Regional changes in ciliary neurotrophic factor and nerve growth factor levels in postmortem spinal cord and cerebral cortex from patients with motor neuron disease. Nat Med 1:168, 1995.
34. Strong, MJ: Exogenous neurotoxins. In Brown, R Jr, Meininger, V, and Swash, M (eds): Amyotrophic Lateral Sclerosis. Martin Dunitz Ltd, London, 2000, p 279.
35. Brown, R, Jr: Apoptosis in amyotrophic lateral sclerosis: A review. In Brown, R Jr, Meininger, V, and Swash, M (eds): Amyotrophic Lateral Sclerosis. Martin Dunitz Ltd, London, 2000, p 363.
36. Mitsumoto, H, Chad, DA, and Pioro, EK: Hypotheses for viral and other transmissable agents in amyotrophic Lateral Sclerosis. In Mitsumoto, H, Chad, DA, and Pioro, EK (eds): Amyotrophic Lateral Sclerosis. F.A. Davis, Philadelphia, 1998, p 239.
37. Mizutani, T, et al: Amyotrophic lateral sclerosis with ophthalmoplegia and multisystem degeneration in patients on long-term use of respirators. Acta Neuropathol 84:372, 1992.
38. Iwata, M, and Hirano, A: Sparing of the Onufrowicz nucleus in sacral anterior horn lesions. Ann Neurol 4:245, 1978.
39. Mannen, T, et al: Preservation of a certain motoneurone group of the sacral cord in amyotrophic lateral sclerosis: Its clinical significance. J Neuropathol Exp Neurol 47:642, 1988.
40. Barr, ML, and Kiernan, JA: The Human Nervous System: An Anatomical Viewpoint, ed 6. J.B. Lippincott Co., Philadelphia, 1993.

41. Bradley, WG, et al: Morphometric and biochemical studies of peripheral nerves in amyotrophic lateral sclerosis. Ann Neurol 14:267, 1983.
42. Heads, T, et al: Sensory nerve pathology in amyotrophic lateral sclerosis. Acta Neuropathol 82:316, 1991.
43. Kawamura, Y, et al: Morphometric comparison in the vulnerability of peripheral motor and sensory neurons in amyotrophic lateral sclerosis. J Neuropathol Exp Neurol 40:667, 1988.
44. Swash, M, et al: Selective and asymmetric vulnerability of corticospinal and spinocerebellar tract in motor neuron disease. J Neuro Neurosurg Psychiatry 51:785, 1988.
45. Averback, P, and Crocker, P: Regular involvement of Clarke's nucleus in sporadic amyotrophic lateral sclerosis. Arch Neurol 39:155, 1982.
46. Takahaski, H, et al: Clarke's column in sporadic amyotrophic lateral sclerosis. Acta Neuropathol 84:465, 1992.
47. Hudson, AJ: Amyotrophic lateral sclerosis and its association with dementia, parkinsonism and other neurological disorders: A review. Brain 104:217, 1981.
48. Wohlfart, G: Collateral regeneration in partially denervated muscles. Neurology 8:175, 1958.
49. Hansen, S, and Ballantyne, JP: A quantitative electrophysiological study of motor neuron disease. J Neurol Neurosurg Psychiatry 41:773, 1978.
50. McComas, AJ, et al: Functional compensation in partially denervated muscles. J Neurol Neurosurg Psychiatry 34:453, 1971.
51. Swash, M, and Schwartz, MS: A longitudinal study of changes in motor units in motor neuron disease. J Neurol Sci 56:185, 1982.
52. Swash, M, and Schwartz, MS: Staging motor neurone disease: Single fibre EMG studies of asymmetry, progression and compensatory reinnervation. In Rose, FC (ed): Research Progress in Motor Neuron Disease. Pitman, London, 1984, p 123.
53. Brooks, BR, et al: Natural history of amyotrophic lateral sclerosis: Quantification of symptoms, signs, strength and function. In Serratrice, G, and Munsat, TL (eds): Advances in Neurology: Pathogenesis and Therapy of Amyotrophic Lateral Sclerosis. Lippincott-Raven, Philadelphia, 1995, p 163.
54. Mitsumoto, H, Chad, DA, and Pioro, EK: Clinical features: Signs and symptoms. In Mitsumoto, H, Chad, DA, and Pioro, EK (eds): Amyotrophic Lateral Sclerosis. F.A. Davis, Philadelphia, 1998, p 47.
55. Brooks, BR: Natural history of ALS: Symptoms, strength, pulmonary function, and disability. Neurology 47(suppl):S71, 1996.
56. Jette, DU, et al: The relationship of lower-limb muscle force to walking ability in patients with amyotrophic lateral sclerosis. Phys Ther 79(7):672, 1999.
57. Dal Bello-Haas, V, et al: Development, analysis, refinement and utility of an interdisciplinary amyotrophic lateral sclerosis database. Amyotroph Lateral Scler Other Motor Neuron Disord 2(1):39, 2001.
58. Kilmer, DD: The role of exercise in neuromuscular disease. Physical Medicine and Rehabilitation Clinics of North America 9(1):115, 1998.
59. Sanjak, M, et al: Physiologic and metabolic response to progressive and prolonged exercise in amyotrophic lateral sclerosis. Neurology 37:1217, 1987.
60. Sharma, KR, et al: Physiology of fatigue in amyotrophic lateral sclerosis. Neurology 45:733, 1995.
61. Sahrmann, SA, and Norton, BJ: The relationship of voluntary movement to spasticity in the upper moor neuron syndrome. Ann Neurol 2:460, 1977.
62. Mayer, NH: Clinicophysiologic concepts of spasticity and motor dysfunction in adults with an upper motoneuron lesion. Muscle Nerve 6:S1, 1997.
63. Schiffer, RB, Cash, J, and Herndon, RM: Treatment of emotional lability with low-dosage tricyclic antidepressants. Psychosomatics 24:1094, 1983.
64. Gallagher, JP: Pathologic laughter and crying in ALS: A search for their origin. Acta Neurol Scand 80:114, 1989.
65. Fallat, RJ, et al: Spirometry in amyotrophic lateral sclerosis. Arch Neurol 36:74, 1979.
66. Rochester, DF, and Esau, SA: Assessment of ventilatory function in patients with neuromuscular disease. Clin Chest Med 14:751, 1994.
67. Vitacca, M, et al: Breathing pattern and respiratory mechanics in patients with amyotrophic lateral sclerosis. Eur Respir J 10:1614, 1997.
68. Krivickas, L: Pulmonary function and respiratory failure. In Mitsumoto, H, Chad, DA, and Pioro, EK (eds): Amyotrophic Lateral Sclerosis. F.A. Davis, Philadelphia, 1998, p 382.
69. Schiffman, PL, and Belsh, JM: Pulmonary function at diagnosis of amyotrophic lateral sclerosis: Rate of deterioration. Chest 103:508, 1993.
70. Abe, K, et al: Cognitive function in amyotrophic lateral sclerosis. J Neurol Sci 14:95, 1997.
71. Kew, JJM, et al: The relationship between abnormalities of cognitive function and cerebral activation in amyotrophic lateral sclerosis: A neuropsychological and positron emission tomography study. Brain 116:1399, 1993.
72. Massman, PJ, et al: Prevalence and correlates of neuropsychological deficits in amyotrophic lateral sclerosis. J Neurol Neurosurg Psychiatry 61:450, 1996.
73. Wilson, CM, et al: Cognitive impairment in sporadic ALS: A pathological continuum underlying a multisystem disorder. Neurology 57:651, 2001.
74. Lomen-Hoerth, C, et al: Are amyotrophic lateral sclerosis patients cognitively normal? Neurology 60(7):1094, 2003.
75. Neary, D, et al: Frontal lobe dementia and motor neuron disease. J Neurol Neurosurg Psychiatry 53:23, 1990.
76. Strong, MJ, et al: A prospective study of cognitive impairment in ALS. Neurology 53:1665, 1999.
77. Abrahams, S, et al: Verbal fluency and executive dysfunction in amyotrophic lateral sclerosis. Neuropsychologia 38(6):734, 2000.
78. Abrahams, S, et al: Relationship between cognitive dysfunction and pseudobulbar palsy in amyotrophic lateral sclerosis. J Neurol Neurosurg Psychiatry 62:464, 1997.
79. Brooks, BR, et al: El Escorial revisited: Revised criteria for the diagnosis of amyotrophic lateral sclerosis. Amyotroph Lateral Scler Other Motor Neuron Disord 1(5):293, 2000.
80. Juergens, SM, et al: ALS in Rochester, Minnesota. Neurology 30:463, 1980.
81. Caroscio, JT, Mulvihil, MN, and Sterling, R: Amyotrophic lateral sclerosis: Its natural history. Neurol Clin 5:108, 1987.
82. Kristensen, O, and Melgaard, B: Motor neuron disease: Prognosis and epidemiology. Acta Neurol 56:299, 1977.
83. Granieri, E, et al: Motor neuron disease in the province of Ferrara, Italy, in 1964-1982. Neurology 38:1604, 1988.
84. Tysnes, OB, Vollset, SE, and Aarli, JA: Epidemiology of amyotrophic lateral sclerosis in Hordaland County, western Norway. Acta Neurol Scan 83:280, 1991.
85. Rosen, AD: Amyotrophic lateral sclerosis: Clinical features and prognosis. Arch Neurol 35:638, 1978.
86. Tysnes, OB, et al: Prognostic factors and survival in amyotrophic lateral sclerosis. Neuroepidemiology 13:225, 1994.
87. McDonald, ER, et al: Survival in amyotrophic lateral sclerosis: The role of psychological factors. Arch Neurol 51:17, 1994.
88. Johnston, M, et al: Mood as a predictor of disability and survival in patients diagnosed with ALS/MND. Br J of Health Psych 4:122, 1999.
89. Traynor, BJ, et al: Effect of a multidisciplinary amyotrophic lateral sclerosis (ALS) clinic on ALS survival: A population based study, 1996–2000. Neurol Neurosurg Psychiatry 74:1258, 2003.
90. Bensimon, G, Lacomblez, L, and Meininger, V: A controlled trial of riluzole in amyotrophic lateral sclerosis: ALS/Riluzole Study Group. N Engl J Med 330:585, 1994.
91. Lacomblez, L, et al: The Amyotrophic Lateral Sclerosis/Riluzole Study Group II. Dose-ranging study of riluzole in amyotrophic lateral sclerosis. Lancet 347:1425, 1996.
92. The World Health Organization (WHO) Expert Committee: Cancer pain relief and palliative care. WHO, Geneva, Switzerland, 1990.
93. Miller, RG, et al (ALS Practice Parameters Task Force): The care of the patient with amyotrophic lateral sclerosis (an evidence-based review). Report of the quality Standards Subcommittee of the American Academy of Neurology. Neurology 52(7):1311, 1999.
94. Bach, JR: Respiratory muscle aids for the prevention of pulmonary morbidity and mortality. Semin Neurol 15:72, 1995.
95. Desport, JC, et al: Nutritional status is a prognostic factor for survival in ALS patients. Neurology 53(5):1059, 1999.

96. Lechtzin, N, et al: Hospitalization in amyotrophic lateral sclerosis: Causes, costs, and outcomes. Neurology 56(6):753, 2001.
97. Hillel, AD, and Miller, R: Bulbar amyotrophic lateral sclerosis: Patterns of progression and clinical management. Head Neck 11:51, 1989.
98. Mathus-Vliegen, LMH, et al: Percutaneous endoscopic gastrostomy in patients with amyotrophic lateral sclerosis and impaired pulmonary function. Gastrointest Endosc 40:463, 1994.
99. Mazzini, L, et al: Percutaneous endoscopic gastrostomy and enteral nutrition in amyotrophic lateral sclerosis. Neurology 242:695, 1995.
100. Jarnagin, WR, et al: The efficacy and limitations of percutaneous endoscopic gastrostomy. Arch Surg 127:261, 1992.
101. Kadakia, SC, Sullivan, HO, and Starnes, E: Percutaneous endoscopic gastrostomy or jejunostomy and the incidence of aspiration in 79 patients. Am J Surg 164:114, 1992.
102. Piper, AJ, and Sullivan, CE: Effects of long-term nocturnal nasal ventilation on spontaneous breathing during sleep in neuromuscular and chest wall disorders. Eur Respir J 9:1515, 1996.
103. Cazzolli, PA, and Oppenheimer, EA: Home mechanical ventilation for amyotrophic lateral sclerosis: Nasal compared to tracheostomy-intermittent positive pressure ventilation. J Neurol Sci 139(suppl):123, 1996.
104. Pinto, AC, et al: Respiratory assistance with a non-invasive ventilator (Bipap) in MND/ALS patients: Survival rates in controlled trials. J Neurol Sci 129(suppl):19, 1995.
105. Aboussouan, LS, et al: Effect of noninvasive positive-pressure ventilation on survival in amyotrophic lateral sclerosis. Ann Intern Med 127:450, 1997.
106. Yorkston, KM, et al: Speech deterioration in amyotrophic lateral sclerosis: Implications for the timing of intervention. J Med Speech-Language Pathol 1:35, 1993.
107. Adams, L, and Kazandjian, M: Managing communication and swallowing difficulties. In Mitsumoto, M, and Munsat, T (eds): Amyotrophic Lateral Sclerosis: A Guide for Patients and Families, ed 2. Demos Medical Publishing, Inc., New York, 2001, p 133.
108. Esposito, SJ, Mitsumoto, H, and Shanks, M: Use of palatal lift and palatal augmentation prostheses to improve dysarthria in patients with amyotrophic lateral sclerosis: A case series. J Prosthet Dent 83(1):90, 2000.
109. Gelinas, DF, and Miller, RG: A treatable disease: A guide to the management of amyotrophic lateral sclerosis. In Brown, R Jr, Meininger, V, and Swash, M (eds): Amyotrophic Lateral Sclerosis. Martin Dunitz Ltd, London, 2000, p 405.
110. Dal Bello-Haas, V: A framework for rehabilitation in degenerative diseases: Planning care and maximizing quality of life. Neurology Report (now JNPT) 26(3):115, 2002.
111. Folstein, MF, Folstein, SE, and McHugh, PR: Mini-mental State: A practical method for grading the cognitive state of patients for the clinician. J Psychiatr Res 12(3):189, 1975.
112. Beck, AT, Ward, CH, and Mendelson, M: An inventory for measuring depression. Arch Gen Psych 4:561, 1961.
113. Radloff, LS: CES-D scale: A self-report depression scale for research in the general population. Appl Psychol Meas 1:385, 1977.
114. Zigmond, AS, and Snaith, RP: The Hospital Anxiety and Depression Scale. Acta Psychiatra Scandinavica 67:361, 1983.
115. Spielberger, CS, Gorsuch, RL, and Lushene, RE: Manual for the State Trait Anxiety Inventory. Consulting Psychologists Press, Palo Alto, CA, 1970.
116. Andres, PL, et al: Quantitative motor assessment in amyotrophic lateral sclerosis. Neurology 36:937, 1986.
117. deBoer, A, Boukes, RJ, and Sterk, JC: Reliability of dynamometry in patients with neuromuscular disorders. N Engl J Med 11:169, 1982.
118. Scott, DM, et al: Quantification of muscle function in children: A prospective study in Duchenne muscular dystrophy. Muscle Nerve 5:291, 1982.
119. Munsat, TL, Andres, P, and Skerry, L: Therapeutic trials in amyotrophic lateral sclerosis: Measurement of clinical deficit. In Rose, C (ed): Amyotrophic Lateral Sclerosis. Demos Publications, New York, 1990, p 65.
120. Brooks, BR, Sufit, PL, and DePaul, R: Design of clinical therapeutic trials in amyotrophic lateral sclerosis. Adv Neurol 56:521, 1991.
121. Great Lakes ALS Study Group: A comparison of muscle strength testing techniques in amyotrophic lateral sclerosis. Neurology 61(11):1503, 2003.
122. Bohannon, RW, and Smith, MB: Interrater reliability of a modified Ashworth scale of muscle spasticity. Phys Ther 67: 206, 1987.
123. Tinetti, ME: Performance-oriented assessment of mobility problems in elderly patients. J Am Geriatr Soc 34:119, 1986.
124. Berg, KO, et al: Measuring balance in the elderly: Validation of an instrument. Can J Public Health 83(2 Suppl):S7, 1992.
125. Podsiadlo, D, and Richardson, S: The timed "Up & Go": A test of basic functional mobility for frail elderly persons. JAGS 9:142, 1991.
126. Duncan, PW, et al: Functional reach: A new clinical measure of balance. J Gerontol 45:M192, 1990.
127. Kloos, A, et al: Validity of the Tinetti Balance Assessment in individuals with amyotrophic lateral sclerosis. Proceedings of the 9th International Symposium on ALS/MND. Munich, Germany, November 1998, p 149.
128. Kloos, AD, et al: Interrater and Intrarater reliability of the Tinetti Balance Test for Individuals with Amyotrophic Lateral Sclerosis. JNPT 28(1):12, 2004.
129. Guide for the Uniform Data System for Medical Rehabilitation (Adult FIM™), version 4.0. State University of New York at Buffalo, Buffalo, NY, 1993.
130. Schwab, R, and England, A: Projection technique for evaluating surgery in Parkinson's disease. In Gillingham, J, and Donaldson, I: Third Symposium on Parkinson's Disease. Livingstone, Edinburgh, Scotland, 1969.
131. The ALS CNTF Treatment Study (ACTS) Phase I-II Study Group: The amyotrophic lateral sclerosis functional rating scale: Assessment of activities of daily living in patients with amyotrophic lateral sclerosis. Arch Neurology 53: 141, 1996.
132. Krupp, LB, et al: The fatigue severity scale: Application to patients with multiple sclerosis and systemic lupus erythematosus. Arch Neurology 46: 1121, 1989.
133. Cedarbaum, JM, et al: The ALSFRS-R: A revised ALS functional rating scale that incorporates assessments of respiratory function. J Neurol Sci 169:13, 1999.
134. Appel, V, et al: A rating scale for amyotrophic lateral sclerosis. Ann Neurol 22:328, 1987.
135. Hillel, AD, et al: Amyotrophic Lateral Sclerosis Severity Scale. Neuroepidemiology 8:142, 1989.
136. Norris, F, et al: The administration of guanidine in amyotrophic lateral sclerosis. Neurology 24:721, 1974.
137. Ware, JE, et al: SF-36 Health Survey: Manual and Interpretation Guide. Health Institute, New England Medical Center, Boston, 1993.
138. Hickey, AM, et al: A new short form individual quality of life measure (SEIQoL-DW): Application in a cohort of individuals with HIV/AIDS. Br Med Journal 313:29, 1996.
139. Bergner, M, et al: The Sickness Impact Profile: Development and final revision of a health status measure. Med Care 19:787, 1981.
140. Jenkinson, C, et al: Development and validation of a short measure of health status for individuals with amyotrophic lateral sclerosis/motor neuron disease: The ALSAQ-40. J. Neurol 246:16, 1999.
141. Jenkinson, C, et al: Evidence for the validity and reliability of the ALS assessment questionnaire: The ALSAQ-40. Amyotroph Lateral Scler Other Motor Neuron Disord 1:33, 1999.
142. Jenkinson, C, and Fitzpatrick, R: Reduced item set for the amyotrophic lateral sclerosis assessment questionnaire: Development and validation of the ALSAQ-5. J Neurol Neurosurg Psychiatry 70(1):70, 2001.
143. Dal Bello-Haas, VP, et al: A preliminary study: The effects of a strengthening program on maximum voluntary isometric contraction, functional abilities, fatigue and quality of life in patients with amyotrophic lateral sclerosis. Amyotroph Lateral Scler Other Motor Neuron Disord 2(S2):93, 2001.
144. Ingels, PL, et al: Adhesive capsulitis: A common occurrence in patients with ALS. Amyotroph Lateral Scler Other Motor Neuron Disord 2(S2):60, 2001.
145. Lahrmann, H, et al: Expiratory muscle weakness and assisted cough in ALS. Amyotroph Lateral Scler Other Motor Neuron Disord 4(1):49, 2003.

146. Hanayama, K, Yuka, I, and Bach, JR: Amyotrophic lateral sclerosis: Successful treatment of mucous plugging by mechanical insufflation-exsufflation. Am J Phys Med Rehabil 76:338, 1997.
147. Mustfa, N, et al: Cough augmentation in amyotrophic lateral sclerosis. Neurology 61(9):1285, 2003.
148. Trail, M, et al: Wheelchair use by patients with amyotrophic lateral sclerosis: A survey of user characteristics and selection preferences. Arch Phys Med Rehabil 82(1):98, 2001.
149. Ashworth, NL, Satkunam, LE, and Deforge, D: Treatment for spasticity in amyotrophic lateral sclerosis/motor neuron disease (Cochrane Review). In: The Cochrane Library, (Issue 4). John Wiley & Sons, Ltd., Chichester, UK, 2004.
150. Kemp, C: Psychosocial needs, problems, and interventions: The individual. In Terminal Illness: A Guide to Nursing Care, ed 2. Lippincott, Philadelphia, 1999, p 17.
151. Doka, KJ: Mourning psychosocial loss: Anticipatory mourning in Alzheimer's, ALS, and irreversible coma. In Rando, TA (ed): Clinical Dimensions of Anticipatory Mourning: Theory and Practice in Working With the Dying, Their Loved Ones, and Their Caregivers. Research Press, Champaign, IL, 2000, p 477.
152. Dal Bello-Haas, V, DelBene, M, and Mitsumoto, H: End of life: Challenges and strategies for the rehabilitation professional. Neurology Report (now JNPT) 26(4): 174, 2002.
153. Kilmar, DD, et al: The effect of a high resistance exercise program in slowly progressive neuromuscular disease. Arch Phys Med Rehabil 75:560, 1994.
154. Lindeman, E, et al: Strength training in patients with myotonic dystrophy and hereditary motor and sensory neuropathy: A randomized clinical trial. Arch Phys Med Rehabil 76:612, 1995.
155. Aitkens, SG, et al: Moderate resistance exercise program: Its effect in slowly progressive neuromuscular disease. Arch Phys Med Rehabil 74:711, 1993.
156. Milner-Brown, HS, and Miller, RG: Muscle strengthening through high resistance weight training in patients with neuromuscular disorders. Arch Phys Med Rehabil 69:14, 1988.
157. Florence, JM, and Hagberg, JM: Effects of training on the exercise response of neuromuscular disease patients. Med Sci Sports Ex 16(5):460, 1984.
158. Vignos, PJ, Jr: Physical models of rehabilitation in neuromuscular disease. Muscle Nerve 6(5):323, 1983.
159. Einarsson, G: Muscle conditioning in late poliomyelitis. Arch Phys Med Rehabil 72:11, 1991.
160. McCartney, N, et al: The effects of strength training in patients with selected neuromuscular disorders. Med Sci Sports Exerc 20(4):362, 1988.
161. Bennett, RL, and Knowlton, GC: Overwork weakness in partially denervated skeletal muscle. Clin Orthop 12:711, 1958.
162. Johnson, EW, and Braddom, R: Overwork weakness in fasioscapulohumeral muscular dystrophy. Arch Phys Med Rehabil 52:333, 1971.
163. Tam, SL, et al: Increased neuromuscular activity reduces sprouting in partially denervated muscles. J Neurosci 21(2):654, 2001.
164. Gardiner, PF, Michel, RN, and Iadeluca, G: Previous exercise training influences functional sprouting of rat hindlimb motoneurons in response to partial denervation. Neurosci Lett 45:123, 1984.
165. Rafuse, VF, Gordon, T, and Orozco, R: Proportional enlargement of motor units after partial denervation of cat triceps surae muscles. J Neurophysiol 68:1261, 1992.
166. Michel, RN, and Gardiner, PF: Influence of overload on recovery of rat plantaris from partial denervation. J Appl Physiol 66:732, 1989.
167. Seburn, KL, and Gardiner, PF: Properties of sprouted rat motor units: Effects of period of enlargement and activity level. Muscle Nerve 19:1100, 1996.
168. Ribchester, RR: Activity-dependent and independent synaptic interactions during reinnervation of partially denervated rat muscle. J Physiol (Lond) 401:53, 1988.
169. Einsiedel, LJ, and Luff, AR: Activity and motor unit size in partially denervated rat medial gastrocnemius. J Appl Physiol 76:2663, 1994.
170. Coble, NO, and Maloney, FP: Effects of exercise in neuromuscular disease. In Maloney, FP, Burks, JS, and Ringel, SP (eds): Interdisciplinary Rehabilitation of Multiple Sclerosis and Neuromuscular Disorders. JB Lippincott, New York, 1985, p 228.
171. Bohanon, RW: Results of resistance exercise on a patient with amyotrophic lateral sclerosis. Phys Ther 63(6):965, 1983.
172. Sanjak, M, Reddan, W, and Brooks, BR: Role of muscular exercise in amyotrophic lateral sclerosis. Neurol Clinics 5(2):251, 1987.
173. Pinto, AC, Alves, M, and Nogueira, A: Can amyotrophic lateral sclerosis patients with respiratory insufficiency exercise? J Neurol Sci 169:69, 1999.
174. Drory, VE, et al: The value of muscle exercise in patients with amyotrophic lateral sclerosis. J Neurol Sci 191:133, 2001.
175. Kirkinezos, IG, et al: Regular exercise is beneficial to a mouse model of amyotrophic lateral sclerosis. Ann Neurol 53:804, 2003.
176. Veldink, JH, et al: Sexual differences in onset of disease and response to exercise in a transgenic model of ALS. Neuromuscular Disease 13: 737, 2003.
177. Mahoney, DJ, et al: Effects of high-intensity endurance exercise training in the G93A mouse model of amyotrophic lateral sclerosis. Muscle Nerve 29: 656, 2004.

Supplemental Readings and Resources

Albom, M: Tuesdays with Morrie—An Old Man, A Young Man, And Life's Greatest Lesson. Bantam Doubleday Dell, New York, 1997.
Amyotrophic Lateral Sclerosis Association: Living With ALS© Manuals and Videos, http://www.alsa.org
Amyotrophic Lateral Sclerosis Society of Canada: A Manual for People Living with ALS, http://www.als.ca
Dal Bello-Haas, V, Kloos, A, and Mitsumoto, H: Physical therapy for the stages of amyotrophic lateral sclerosis: A case report. Phys Ther 78(12):1312, 1998.
Feigenbaum, D (ed): Journeys with ALS: Personal Tales of Courage and Coping With Lou Gehrig's Disease. DLRC Press, Virginia Beach, 1998.
Kazandjian, M (ed): Communication and Swallowing Solutions for the ALS/MND Community. Singular Publishing Group, San Diego, 1997.
Mitsumoto, M, and Munsat, T (eds): Amyotrophic Lateral Sclerosis: A Guide for Patients and Families, ed 2. Demos Medical Publishing, New York, 2001.
Muscular Dystrophy Association: ALS: A Guide to Related Materials on MDA's Web Site, http://www.mdausa.org/publications/alsmats.html
National Institute of Neurological Disorders and Stroke, National Institutes of Health (NIH), U.S. Department of Health and Human Services Web site, http://www.ninds.nih.gov
World Federation of Neurology Amyotrophic Lateral Sclerosis Web site, http://www.wfnals.org
Yorkston KM, et al: Management of Speech and Swallowing in Degenerative Diseases, ed 2. Pro Ed, Austin, 2004.

Appendix A: Schwab and England Activities of Daily Living Scale

100% =	Completely independent; able to do all chores without slowness, difficulty, or impairment; essentially normal; unaware of any difficulty
90% =	Completely independent; able to do all chores with some degree of slowness, difficulty, and impairment; may take twice as long as usual; beginning to be aware of difficulty
80% =	Completely independent in most chores; takes twice as long as normal; conscious of difficulty and slowness
70% =	Not completely independent; more difficulty with some chores; takes three to four times as long as normal in some; must spend a large part of the day with some chores
60% =	Some dependency; can do most chores, but exceedingly slowly and with considerable effort and errors; some chores impossible
50% =	More dependent; needs help with half the chores, slower, etc.; difficulty with everything
40% =	Very dependent; can assist with all chores but does few alone
30% =	With effort, now and then does a few chores alone or begins alone; much help needed
20% =	Does nothing alone; can be a slight help with some chores; severe invalid
10% =	Totally dependent and helpless; complete invalid
0% =	Vegetative functions such as swallowing, bladder and bowels are not functioning; bedridden

From Schwab R, and England, A,[130] with permission.

Appendix B: Amyotrophic Lateral Sclerosis Functional Rating Scale-Revised[a]

1. SPEECH

4 Normal speech processes.
3 Detectable speech disturbance.
2 Intelligible with repeating.
1 Speech combined with nonvocal communication.
0 Loss of useful speech.

2. SALIVATION

4 Normal.
3 Slight but definite excess of saliva in mouth; may have nighttime drooling.
2 Moderately excessive saliva; may have minimal drooling.
1 Marked excess of saliva with some drooling.
0 Marked drooling; requires constant tissue or handkerchief.

3. SWALLOWING

4 Normal eating habits.
3 Early eating problems—occasional choking.
2 Dietary consistency changes.
1 Needs supplemental tube feeding.
0 NPO (exclusively parenteral or enteral feeding).

4. HANDWRITING

4 Normal.
3 Slow or sloppy; all words are legible.
2 Not all words are legible.
1 Able to grip pen but unable to write.
0 Unable to grip pen.

5a. CUTTING FOOD AND HANDLING UTENSILS ***(patients without gastrostomy)***

4 Normal.
3 Somewhat slow and clumsy, but no help needed.
2 Can cut most foods, although clumsy and slow; some help needed.
1 Food must be cut by someone, but can still feed slowly.
0 Needs to be fed.

OR

5b. CUTTING FOOD AND HANDLING UTENSILS ***(alternate scale for patients with gastrostomy)***

4 Normal.
3 Clumsy but able to perform all manipulations independently.
2 Some help needed with closures and fasteners.
1 Provides minimal assistance to caregiver.
0 Unable to perform any aspect of task.

6. DRESSING & HYGIENE

4 Normal function.
3 Independent and complete self-care with effort or decreased efficiency.
2 Intermittent assistance or substitute methods.
1 Needs attendant for self.
0 Total dependence.

7. TURNING IN BED AND ADJUSTING BED CLOTHES

4 Normal.
3 Somewhat slow and clumsy, but no help needed.
2 Can turn alone or adjust sheets, but with great difficulty.
1 Can initiate, but not turn or adjust sheets alone.
0 Helpless.

8. WALKING

4 Normal.
3 Early ambulation difficulties.
2 Walks with assistance.
1 Nonambulatory functional movement only.
0 No purposeful leg movement.

9. CLIMBING STAIRS

4 Normal.
3 Slow.
2 Mild unsteadiness or fatigue.
1 Needs assistance.
0 Cannot do.

10. DYSPNEA

4 None.
3 Occurs when walking.
2 Occurs with one or more of the following: eating, bathing, dressing (ADL)
1 Occurs at rest, difficulty breathing when either sitting or lying.
0 Significant difficulty, considering using mechanical respiratory support.

11. ORTHOPNEA

4 None.
3 Some difficulty sleeping at night due to shortness of breath, does not routinely use more than two pillows.
2 Needs extra pillows in order to sleep (more than two).
1 Can only sleep sitting up.
0 Unable to sleep.

12. RESPIRATORY INSUFFICIENCY

4 None.
3 Intermittent use of BiPAP.
2 Continuous use of BiPAP during the night.
1 Continuous use of BiPAP during the night and day.
0 Invasive mechanical ventilation by intubation or tracheostomy.

From Cedarbaum, JM, et al,[133] with permission.

[a]Original ALSFRS consists of items 1 through 9 and the original item 10 below:

10. BREATHING

4 Normal.
3 Shortness of breath with minimal exertion (e.g., walking, talking).
2 Shortness of breath at rest.
1 Intermittent (e.g. nocturnal) ventilatory assistance.
0 Ventilator dependent.

BiPAP = bidirectional positive airway pressure; NPO = *non per os*, nothing by mouth.

CHAPTER

21

LEARNING OBJECTIVES

1. Describe the etiology, pathophysiology, clinical manifestations, and sequelae of Parkinson's disease.
2. Identify and describe the examination procedures used to evaluate patients with Parkinson's disease to establish a diagnosis, prognosis, and plan of care.
3. Describe the role of the physical therapist in assisting a patient with Parkinson's disease in terms of direct interventions and patient and family/caregiver-related instruction to maximize function.
4. Describe appropriate elements of the exercise prescription for patients with Parkinson's disease.
5. Identify the neuropsychological effects and social impact of Parkinson's disease and describe appropriate interventions to maximize quality of life.
6. Analyze and interpret patient data, formulate realistic goals and outcomes, and develop a plan of care when presented with a clinical case study.

Parkinson's Disease

Susan B. O'Sullivan, PT, EdD

OUTLINE

Parkinson's disease (PD) is a chronic, progressive disease of the nervous system characterized by the cardinal features of **rigidity**, **bradykinesia**, **tremor**, and postural instability. In addition, the disease may cause a variety of other symptoms including movement and gait disturbances; sensory changes; speech, voice, and swallowing disorders; cognitive and behavioral changes; autonomic nervous system dysfunction; gastrointestinal changes, and cardiopulmonary changes. Onset is insidious with a slow rate of progression. Disruption in daily functions, roles and activities, and depression is common in individuals with PD.

Epidemiology

PD is a very common neurodegenerative disease that affects more than 2 percent of the population older than 65 years of age. Average age of PD onset is approximately 50 to 60 years. The incidence increases dramatically with increasing age. There are less than 10 new cases per 100,000 under age 50 while there are at least 300 new cases per 100,000 ages 80 to 99 years annually. A small percentage (4 to 10 percent) develop *young-onset PD*, which is defined by the appearance of initial symptoms before the age of 40. Men and women are affected almost equally.[1]

Etiology

The term **parkinsonism** is used to refer to a group of disorders that produce abnormalities of basal ganglia (BG) function. PD, or idiopathic parkinsonism, is the most common form, affecting approximately 78 percent of patients. *Secondary parkinsonism* results from a number of different identifiable causes, including virus, toxins, drugs, tumors, and so forth (see Box 21.1). The term *parkinsonism-plus syndromes* refers to those conditions that mimic PD in some respects, but the symptoms are caused by other neurodegenerative disorders.

Box 21.1 Classification of Parkinsonism

Idiopathic Parkinson's Disease
Late-onset (>40 years; generally sporadic)
Early-onset (<40 years; often familial)
  Young-onset (>21 years)
  Juvenile (<21 years)

Parkinsonism Due to Identifiable Causes
Virus (e.g., encephalitis lethargica)
Toxins (e.g., carbon monoxide, manganese, methylphenyltetrahydropyridine [MPTP])
Drugs (e.g., phenothiazines, reserpine, butyrophenones, metoclopramide)
Vascular disease (multi-infarct)
Tumors of basal ganglia
Normal pressure hydrocephalus
Hemiparkinsonism, hemiatrophy
Metabolic
  Wilson's disease
  Hepatocerebral degeneration
  Hallervorden-Spatz disease
  Hypoparathyroidism

Parkinsonism in Other Neurodegenerative Disorders
Progressive supranuclear palsy
Cortical–basal ganglionic degeneration
Disorders with cerebellar/autonomic/pyramidal manifestation:
  Multiple system atrophy
  Striatonigral degeneration
  Shy-Drager syndrome
  Olivopontocerebellar atrophy
  Machado-Joseph disease
Disorders with prominent and often early dementia:
  Diffuse cortical Lewy body disease
  Alzheimer's disease with parkinsonism
Parkinsonism–dementia–ALS complex of Guam
  Pallidopontonigral degeneration/disinhibition–dementia-parkinsonism–amyotrophy complex

From Pal, P, et al: Cardinal features of early Parkinson's disease. In Factor, S, and Weiner, W (eds): Parkinson's Disease—Diagnosis and Clinical Management. New York, Demos Medical Publishing, 2002, p 42, with permission.

Parkinson's Disease

True PD or paralysis agitans was first described as "the shaking palsy" by James Parkinson in 1817.[2] Etiology is idiopathic or unknown. Two distinct clinical subgroups have been identified. One group includes individuals whose dominant symptoms include postural instability and gait disturbances (*postural instability gait disturbed [PIGD]*). Another group includes individuals with tremor as the main feature (*tremor predominant*). Patients who are tremor predominant typically demonstrate few problems with bradykinesia or postural instability.[3]

Secondary Parkinsonism

Postinfectious Parkinsonism

The influenza epidemics of encephalitis lethargica that occurred from 1917 to 1926 affected large numbers of individuals. The onset of parkinsonian symptoms typically occurred after many years, giving rise to the theory that a slow virus was infecting the brain. There has been no recent recurrence of this influenza and the incidence of this type of parkinsonism is slowly decreasing in frequency.[4] Moving case histories of these individuals are portrayed in the book *Awakenings* by Oliver Sacks.[5] The development of parkinsonism with other encephalitic conditions is rare.

Toxic Parkinsonism

Parkinsonian symptoms occur in individuals exposed to certain industrial poisons and chemicals (manganese, carbon disulfide, carbon monoxide, cyanide, methanol). The most common of these toxins is manganese, which represents a serious occupational hazard to many miners. Severe and lasting classic parkinsonian has been inadvertently produced in individuals who injected a synthetic heroin containing the chemical MPTP.[6]

Drug-Induced Parkinsonism (DIP)

A variety of drugs can produce extrapyramidal dysfunction that mimics the signs of PD. These drugs are thought to interfere with dopaminergic mechanisms either presynaptically or postsynaptically. They include (1) *neuroleptic drugs* such as chlorpromazine (Thorazine), haloperidol (Haldol), thioridazine (Mellaril), and thiothixene (Navane); (2) *antidepressant drugs* such as amitriptyline (Triavil), amoxapine (Asendin), and trazodone (Desyrel); and (3) *antihypertensive drugs* such as methyldopa (Aldomet) and reserpine. High doses of these medications are particularly problematic in the elderly. Withdrawal of these agents usually reverses the symptoms within a few weeks, although in some cases the effects can persist and may be related to subclinical PD.[7]

Metabolic Causes

Parkinsonism can be caused in rare cases by metabolic conditions, including disorders of calcium metabolism that result in BG calcification. These include hypothyroidism, hyperparathyroidism, hypoparathyroidism, and Wilson's disease.

Parkinson-Plus Syndromes

A group of neurodegenerative diseases can affect the substantia nigra and produce parkinsonian symptoms along with other neurological signs. These diseases include striatonigral degeneration (SND), Shy-Drager syndrome, progressive supranuclear palsy (PSPO), olivopontocerebellar atrophy (OPCA), and cortical–basal ganglionic degeneration (CBGD). In addition, parkinsonian symptoms can be exhibited in patients with multi-infarct vascular disease, Alzheimer's disease, diffuse Lewy body disease (DLBD), normal pressure hydrocephalus (NPH), Creutzfeldt-Jakob disease (CJD), Wilson's disease (WD), and juvenile Huntington's disease. Many of these conditions are rare and affect relatively small numbers of individuals. Early in their course, these diseases may present with rigidity and bradykinesia indistinguishable from PD. However, other diagnostic symptoms eventually appear (e.g., cognitive impairment in Alzheimer's disease). Another diagnostic feature is that Parkinson-plus syndromes typically do not show measurable improvement from the administration of anti-Parkinson medications such as levodopa (L-dopa) therapy (termed the *apomorphine test*).[7,8]

Pathophysiology

The basal ganglia (BG) are a collection of interconnected gray matter nuclear masses deep within the brain. It is composed of the caudate and putamen (collectively termed the striatum) plus the globus pallidus, subthalamic nucleus, and the substantia nigra (Fig. 21.1). The main input structure of the BG is the striatum. Input is received from all parts of the cerebral cortex via corticostriate projection. The striatum also receives input from the substantia nigra (substantia nigra pars compacta, SNc). Output is channeled primarily through the globus pallidus (globus pallidus internum, GPi) and the substantia nigra (substantia nigra pars reticulata, SNr) to the thalamus and back to the cortex, completing the loop. There are both direct and indirect pathways. The direct pathway facilitates BG output to the thalamus and motor areas of the cortex while the indirect pathway provides disinhibition to the subthalamic nucleus (STN), and in turn suppression of some movements. Parts of the globus pallidus project to the brainstem and in turn to the motor neurons in the brainstem and spinal cord (Fig. 21.2). Neurons in the BG discharge before movement begins.[9,10]

The BG plays an important role in the planning and programming of movement by selecting and inhibiting specific motor synergies. Motor programs are consolidated into efficient goal-directed motor plans, translating thought into willed movements and regulating levels of kinetic activity, muscle tone, and muscle force.[9] The BG also play a role in some cognitive processes, primarily the caudate nucleus, including awareness of body orientation in space, ability to adapt behavior as task requirements change, and motivation.[11]

PD is associated with degeneration of dopaminergic neurons that produce *dopamine*. They have their cell bodies in the SNpc and send their axons to the striatum. Clinical signs begin to emerge with 30 to 60 percent degeneration of neurons. Nigral cell loss is estimated at 10 percent per year and is more prevalent in the ventral cell group. Loss of the melanin-containing neurons produces characteristic changes in depigmentation (Fig. 21.3). There are other deficiencies in neurotransmitters as well (e.g., serotonin, norepinephrine). The effects of these depletions are less well understood. As

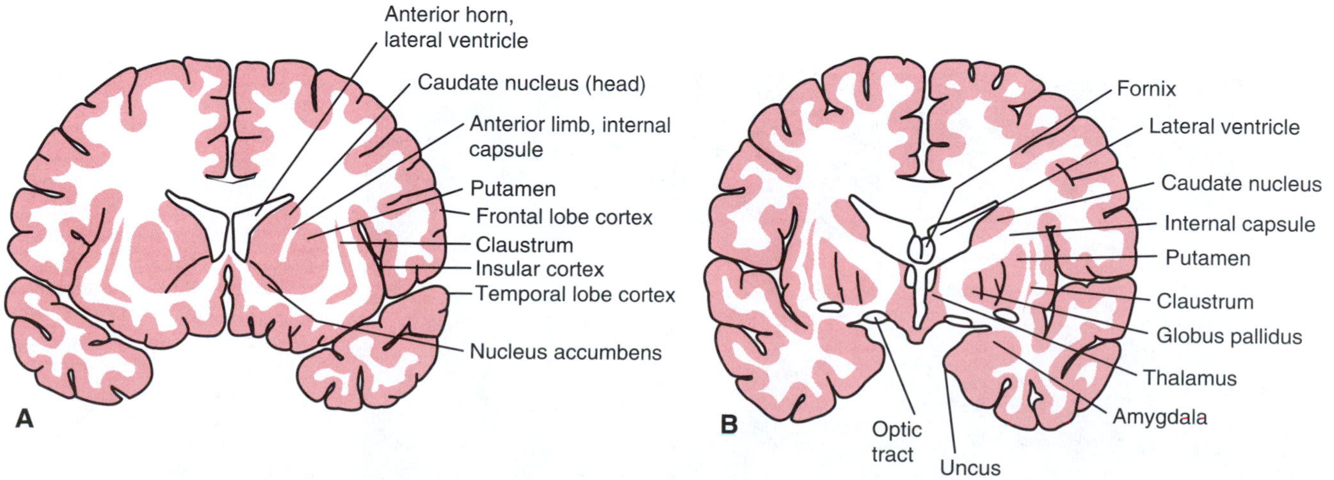

Figure 21.1 The major structures of the basal ganglia.

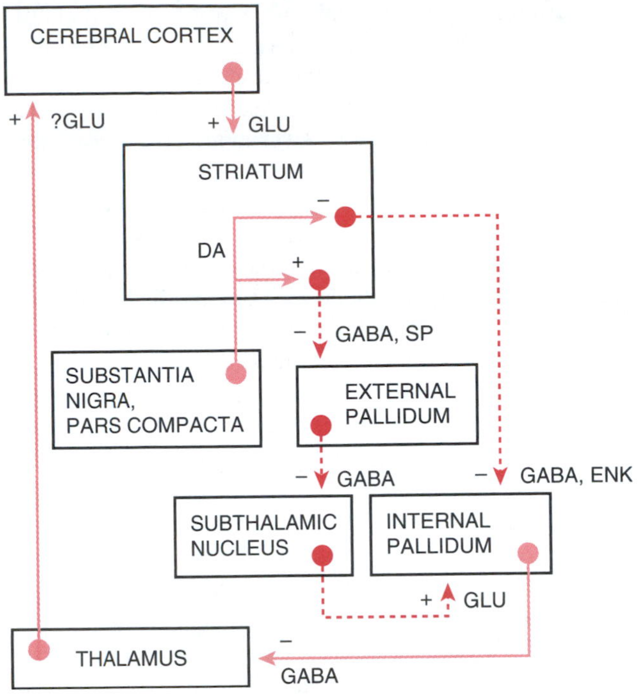

Figure 21.2 Schematic diagram of some connections of the basal ganglia, showing excitatory (+) and inhibitory (–) synapses and neurotransmitters. The direct striopallidal projection is bold shaded and the indirect projection is dashed. Corticonigral and corticosubthalamic projections, which are excitatory, are not shown in the diagram. (From Kiernan, JA: Barr's The Human Nervous System: An Anatomical Viewpoint, ed 7. Lippincott-Raven, Philadelphia, 1998, p 255, with permission.)

the disease progresses and neurons degenerate, they develop characteristic cytoplasmic inclusion bodies, called Lewy bodies. Other sites of predilection include the dorsal motor nucleus of the vagus, the hypothalamus, the locus ceruleus, the cerebral cortex, and the autonomic ganglia.[11] Loss of dopamine results in an overactive indirect pathway that is though to underlie akinesia and rigidity. An underactive direct pathway is thought to be responsible for bradykinesia. Other BG disorders produce hyperkinesias, characterized by excessive or abnormal movements (e.g., hemiballismus, chorea). These are thought to result from underactive indirect pathways while dyskinesias, dystonia, or athetosis are thought to result from an overactive direct pathway.[9] Tremor is viewed as a release phenomena, representative of loss of inhibitory influences within the BG. Significant changes in striatal dopamine receptors also occurs, resulting in decreased binding sites for dopamine in the BG. This may explain the loss of clinical effectiveness of L-dopa (a dopamine [DA] substitution treatment) during later stages of the disease.[12,13]

Clinical Presentation

Cardinal Features

Rigidity

Rigidity is one of the clinical hallmarks of PD. Patients frequently complain of "heaviness" and "stiffness" of their limbs. Rigidity is defined as increased resistance to passive motion. It is felt uniformly in both agonist and antagonist muscles and in movements in both directions. Spinal stretch reflexes are normal. Rigidity is fairly constant regardless of the task, amplitude, or speed of movement. Two types are identified: cogwheel or leadpipe. **Cogwheel rigidity** is a jerky, ratchetlike resistance to passive movement as muscles alternately tense and relax. **Leadpipe rigidity** is more sustained resistance to passive movement, with no fluctuations. Rigidity is often asymmetrical, especially in the early stages of PD. It typically affects proximal muscles first, especially the shoulders and neck, and it progresses to involve muscles of the face and extremities. Rigidity may initially affect the left or right side, eventually spreading to involve the whole body. As the disease progresses, rigidity becomes more severe. Rigidity decreases the ability to move easily. For example, loss of bed mobility or loss of reciprocal arm

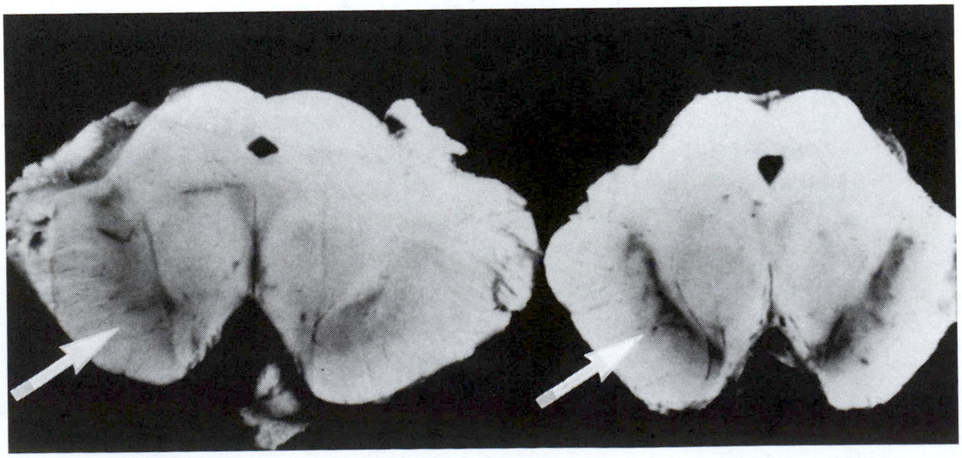

Figure 21.3 The substantia nigra in PD. The upper layer (zona compacta) of the substantia nigra normally has many melanin-containing neurons. In the transverse section through the midbrain (*left*), the substantia nigra of a patient with PD shows a marked depletion of melanin-containing nerve cells. This produces a characteristic pallor (depigmentation) compared with a normal control (*right*). (From Rowland, LP [ed]: Merritt's Textbook of Neurology, ed 8. Copyright Lea & Febiger, Philadelphia, 1989, p 659, with permission.)

swing during gait are often related to the degree of truncal rigidity. Active movement, mental concentration, or emotional stress may all increase rigidity. Prolonged rigidity results in decreased range of motion (ROM) and serious secondary complications of contracture and postural deformity. Rigidity also has a direct impact on increasing resting energy expenditure and fatigue levels.

Bradykinesia

Patients with PD demonstrate problems with voluntary movement. Akinesia refers to absence of movement. Moments of **freezing** may occur and are characterized by a sudden break or block in movement. Akinesia represents a deficit in the preparatory phase of movement control and can be directly influenced by the degree of rigidity as well as stage of disease and fluctuations in drug action. Disturbances in attention and depression can also compound problems with akinesia. **Hypokinesia** refers to reduced amplitude of movement. Bradykinesia refers to slowness and difficulty maintaining movement. Movements are typically reduced in speed, range, and amplitude. Rigidity and depression can also influence bradykinesia. Often it is the most disabling symptom of PD, with the slowness and prolonged movement times leading to increased dependence in daily tasks.

Tremor

Tremor is the initial symptom of PD in about 70 percent of patients.[7] It is an involuntary oscillation of a body part occurring at a slow frequency of 4 to 6 Hz. Parkinsonian tremor is described as a resting tremor, because it is typically present at rest and disappears with voluntary movement. This is usually manifest as a pill-rolling tremor of the hand, although resting tremors may also be seen in the forearm (pronation–supination), jaw, or tongue. Tremor in the lower limbs is most apparent while the patient is supine. Tremor of the head and trunk, **postural tremor**, can be seen when muscles are used to maintain an upright position against gravity. Tremor tends to be less severe when the patient is relaxed and unoccupied; it is diminished by voluntary effort, and disappears completely during sleep. It is aggravated by emotional stress or fatigue. In the early stages, tremor is usually unilateral, quite mild and occurs for only short periods, whereas in later stages tremor can become severe, interfering with daily function. Fluctuations in frequency and intensity are common.[14]

Postural Instability

Patients with PD demonstrate abnormalities of posture and balance. These changes are rare in the early years of PD (i.e., the first 5 years after diagnosis). As the disease progresses, abnormal and inflexible postural responses along with increased body sway are seen. Narrowing of the base of support (tandem stance or single-limb stance) or competing attentional demands (divided attention situations) increases postural instability. Patients also experience increasing difficulty during dynamic destabilizing activities such as self-initiated movements (e.g., functional reach, walking, turning) and perform poorly under conditions of perturbed balance.[15] The response to instability is an abnormal pattern of coactivation, resulting in a rigid body and an inability to utilize normal postural synergies to recover balance.[16,17] Patients also demonstrate difficulty in regulating feed-forward, anticipatory adjustments of postural muscles during voluntary movements.[18,19] Contributing factors include rigidity, decreased muscle torque production, loss of available ROM particularly of trunk motions, and weakness. Extensor muscles of the trunk demonstrate greater weakness than flexor muscles, contributing to the adoption of a flexed, stooped posture with increased flexion of the neck, trunk, hips, and knees.[20] This results in a significant change in the center-of-alignment position, positioning the individual at the forward limits of stability (Fig. 21.4). Patients with PD also demonstrate an inability to adapt movement strategies to changing sensory conditions, a problem in sensorimotor adaptation.[16] Visuospatial impairment has been identified in patients with PD and correlated with lower scores in mobility.[21] Some patients are unable to perceive the upright or vertical position, which may indicate an abnormality in processing of vestibular, visual, and proprioceptive information contributing to balance.

Frequent falls and fall injury are the result of progressive loss of balance, with about two thirds of patients with

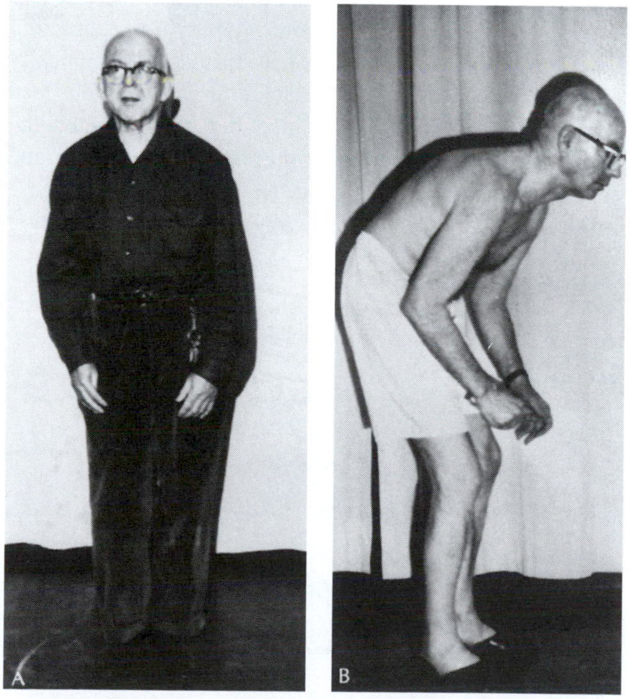

Figure 21.4 Posture and PD. The body posture of a patient with PD. (*A*) Front view. (*B*) Side view. (From Rowland, LP [ed]: Merritt's Textbook of Neurology, ed 8. Copyright Lea & Febiger, Philadelphia, 1989, p 529, with permission.)

PD experiencing falls and 13 percent falling more than once a week.[22,23] The rate of fall injury is about 40 percent, although most injury is not serious. Disease severity including freezing, poor gait, and balance impairments are clearly linked to increased risk for falls. Other risk factors include dementia, depression, postural hypotension, and involuntary movements associated with long-term use of antiparkinsonian medication.[24] Falls can lead to "fear of falling" with increasing levels of immobility and dependency with a deteriorating quality of life.

Torque production is decreased at all speeds resulting in functional limitations and muscle weakness.[25–27] It is thought to be caused by insufficient neural activation of agonist muscles. Electromyography (EMG) studies reveal that motor unit recruitment is delayed and that once initiated is characterized by asynchronization; that is, pauses and an inability to smoothly increase firing rate as contraction continues.[28,29] These difficulties are compounded during the production of complex movements. As the disease progresses, disuse weakness evolves, increasing movement difficulties.[30,31] Patients who are in an *"off" state,* characterized by reduced levels of L-dopa medication and diminished effectiveness, typically experience increased muscle weakness, especially in extensor muscles.[25]

In patients with PD, *fatigue* is among the most common symptoms reported. The patient has difficulty in sustaining activity and experiences increasing weakness and lethargy as the day progresses. Repetitive motor acts may start out strong but decrease in strength and amplitude as the activity progresses. Movements then become arrhythmic with frequent hesitations and arrests. For example, the first few words spoken may be loud and strong but diminish rapidly as speech progresses. Performance decreases dramatically with great physical effort or mental stress. Rest or sleep may restore mobility. When L-dopa therapy is initiated, the patient may notice a dramatic improvement initially and feel significantly less fatigued. In long-standing disease and drug therapy, fatigue typically reappears. A common perception among patients is an increased sense of effort associated with movement that is manifested by difficulty activating and sustaining responses.

Most patients with PD are elderly and show the effects of generalized musculoskeletal deconditioning, especially as the disease progresses. *Contractures* commonly develop in hip and knee flexors, hip rotators and adductors, plantarflexors, dorsal spine and neck flexors, shoulder adductors and internal rotators, and elbow flexors. Function becomes progressively more limited by these musculoskeletal constraints. *Kyphosis* is the most common postural deformity (see Fig. 21.4). Some patients may develop *scoliosis,* the result of unequal distribution of rigidity in the trunk. Older individuals with reduced activity levels and poor diet are likely to develop *osteoporosis*.

Motor Planning

Motor planning deficits are present with this disease. Movement preparation (i.e., the when, where, and how to initiate movement) is significantly prolonged (a finding also seen with advanced age). This **start hesitation** is especially evident as the disease progresses. Movement times are also prolonged but not to the same degree.[32] Patients experience difficulty performing complex, sequential or simultaneous movements. These are linked to deficits in response programming. For example, the patient is slow and hesitant or unable to initiate movement during a transfer sequence. Overall control is also impaired in routine actions representative of ingrained motor programs. For example, patients with PD typically demonstrate **micrographia**, an abnormally small handwriting that is difficult to read (Fig. 21.5).

Freezing episodes (motor blocks) occur and can be triggered by confrontation of competing stimuli. For example, the patient slows or stops walking when exposed to a narrowed space or an obstacle. These episodes are linked to bradykinesia and decreased circulating levels of

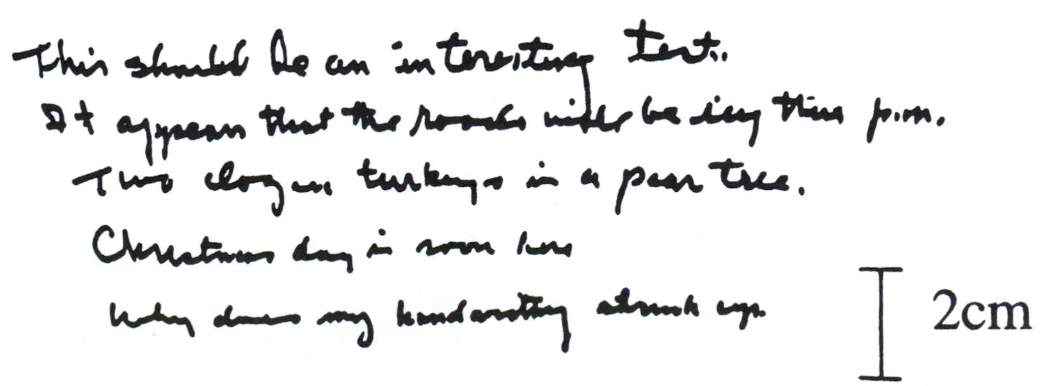

Figure 21.5 Micrographia in PD. Patients with PD may have problems maintaining the scale of their movements. (From Phillips, JG, et al: What can indices of handwriting quality tell us about parkinsonian handwriting? Hum Move Sci 10:301, 1991, with permission.)

neurotransmitters (specifically norepinephrine and serotonin). Freezing episodes are typically short-lived and usually can be overcome by attentional strategies or "behavioral tricks" using external cues (e.g., dropping a tissue initiates a stepping response). Stress can exacerbate freezing episodes. In advanced PD, freezing episodes can severely limit function.[33]

Patients with PD demonstrate **poverty of movement**, described as an overall decrease in the total number and amplitude of movements. For example, patients with moderate or severe PD present with **hypomimia**, a reduction in the expressiveness of the face. The patient demonstrates a *masked face* with infrequent blinking and dimished animation and expression. Smiling may be possible only on command or with volitional effort. As task complexity increases, movement difficulty increases. This provides evidence of a central deficit in motor planning.[34] Rotation movements are reduced, resulting in movements that are basically uniplanar (in one plane of motion). Constantly combating the effects of bradykinesia, rigidity, and movement impoverishment can lead to mental fatigue and loss of motivation.

Motor Learning

Procedural learning deficits are common in patients with PD while declarative learning is usually intact. However procedural deficits are not universal. Deficits in motor skill learning have been demonstrated for complex and sequential tasks but not for relatively simple movement tasks.[35,36] Thus the processing requirements of the procedural task are critical in determining the degree of expected learning deficits. Learning is also impaired with random presentations of stimulus conditions (random practice order) while blocked practice order reduces learning difficulty. Thus context interference degrades learning in patients with PD.[37] Deficits can be expected to be severe if multiple motor programs are required either simultaneously or sequentially (i.e., switching among different motor programs). For example, the patient freezes up when asked to carry out another motor task while walking (dual tasking). Compounding variables that degrade learning include the severity of disease, dementia, and visual perceptual deficits. Differences in learning can also be expected based on medication levels. Motor learning is degraded when patients are "off" state medication.[38]

Gait

Approximately 13 to 33 percent of patients present with postural instability and gait disturbances as their initial motor symptom and comprise a postural instability gait disturbed (PIGD) group. Gait disturbances are also a common feature of late-onset or advanced PD.[33] The patient with PD demonstrates a number of significant gait changes resulting from impoverished movement (Box 21.2). An abnormal stooped posture contributes to development of a *festinating gait,* characterized by a progressive increase in speed with a shortening of stride. Thus, the patient takes multiple short steps to catch up with his or her center of mass (COM) to avoid falling, and may eventually break into a run or trot. Gait can be *anteropulsive* (a forward festinating gait) or less commonly *retropulsive* (a backward festinating gait). Some patients are able to stop only when they come in contact with an object or a wall. Patients who are toe-walkers owing to plantarflexion contractures exhibit an additional postural instability from narrowing of their base of support. Turning or changing direction is particularly difficult and typically accomplished by taking multiple small steps. Problems with controlling posture and balance limit independence, community ambulation, and safety.[39–41] Patients who are in the "off" state experience a deterioration in gait performance while gait patterns are reproducible when peak medication prevails.[42] Most patients with gait deficits can compensate at least partially using external cues and attentional strategies.[40]

Sensation

Patients with PD do not suffer from primary sensory loss. However, as many as 50 percent experience paresthesias and pain, including sensations of numbness, tingling, coldness, aching pain, and burning. These symptoms are typically intermittent, and vary in intensity and location. The BG is thought to participate in sensorimotor integration, with primarily inhibitory output directed toward the thalamus and neurons that project to cortical areas involved in somatosensory function. Some patients report their pain is linked to the motor fluctuations experienced during L-dopa therapy (e.g., pain is more intense in an "off" state). Pain may also be increased in patients experiencing depression.[43] In is also important to remember that some of the discomfort and pain can result from *postural stress syndrome* secondary to lack of movement, muscle rigidity, faulty posture, or ligamentous strain. For example, back pain may occur as a result of a stooped, kyphotic posture.

Some patients experience **akathisia**, a sense of an inner restlessness and need to move. This motor restlessness and agitation affects as many as 25 percent of patients and is relieved with movement (e.g., walking or moving the limbs while seated). It can interfere with relaxation and sleep. Akathisia is associated with advanced PD and is more commonly seen in the "off" state medication.[44]

Proprioceptive regulation of voluntary movement may also be impaired. Patients with PD perform significantly worse than control subjects on tests of kinesthesia. Without visual guidance, patients demonstrate increased difficulty in accurately perceiving the extent of movement, consistently underscaling their movements.[45–47]

Box 21.2 Cardinal Features and Clinical Manifestations of Parkinson's Disease

Cardinal Features
Rigidity
Bradykinesia
Tremor
Postural instability

Clinical Manifestations

Motor Performance
Decreased torque production
Fatigue
Contractures and deformity common

Motor Planning
Start hesitation
Freezing episodes
Poverty of movement
Masked face
Micrographia

Motor Learning
Procedural learning deficits for complex and sequential tasks

Gait
Reduced stride length; increased step-to-step variability
Reduced speed of walking
Cadence (steps per minute) typically intact; may be reduced in advanced PD
Increased time: double limb support
Insufficient hip, knee, and ankle flexion: shuffling steps
Insufficient heel strike with increased forefoot loading
Reduced trunk rotation: decreased or absent arm swing
Festinating gait: anteropulsion common
Freezing of gait (FOG)
Difficulty turning: increased steps per turn
Difficulty with dual tasking: simultaneous motor and/or cognitive tasks
Difficulty with attentional demands of complex environments

Posture
Kyphosis with forward head
Leaning to one side with tonal asymmetries
Increased fall risk

Sensation
Paresthesias
Pain
Akathisia

Speech, Voice, and Swallowing Disorders
Hypokinetic dysarthria
Dysphagia

Cognition Function and Behavior
Dementia
Bradyphrenia
Visuospatial deficits
Depression
Dysphoric mood

Autonomic Nervous System
Excessive sweating
Abnormal sensations of heat and cold
Seborrhea
Sialorrhea
Constipation
Urinary bladder dysfunction

Cardiopulmonary Function
Low resting blood pressure (BP)
Compromised cardiovascular response to exercise
Impaired respiratory function

Conventional drugs (e.g., anticholinergic drugs) used in PD can cause visual disturbances (e.g., blurred vision and photophobia). These drugs can also worsen the normal visual changes associated with aging (presbyopia). Conjugate gaze and saccadic eye movements may also be impaired. Eye pursuit movements may have a jerky, cogwheeling quality. Decreased blinking can produce bloodshot, irritated eyes that burn and itch.[43]

Speech, Voice, and Swallowing

Dysphagia, impaired swallowing, is present in as many as 95 percent of patients and is the result of rigidity, reduced mobility, and restricted range of movement.[47] It is often an early symptom of the disease though it is present in all stages. Individuals with PD experience problems in all four phases of swallowing: oral preparatory, oral, pharyngeal, and esophageal. Thus the patient demonstrates abnormal tongue control, and problems with chewing, bolus formation, delayed swallow response, and peristalsis. Dysphagia can lead to choking or aspiration pneumonia and impaired nutrition with significant weight loss. Nutritional inadequacy can contribute to the fatigue and exhaustion typically experienced by patients with PD. Patients also typically experience excessive drooling *(sialorrhea)* as a result of increased salivary production and decreased spontaneous swallowing. Drooling is particularly problematic while sleeping or initiating speech and in advanced cases increases the risk of aspiration. Excessive drooling has important negative social implications.[47,48]

Speech is impaired in 75 to 89 percent of patients and is the result of primary symptoms of PD (rigidity, bradykinesia, hypokinesia, and tremor).[47] Patients with PD experience *hypokinetic dysarthria,* which is characterized by decreased voice volume, monotone/monopitch speech, imprecise or distorted articulation, and uncontrolled speech rate. Vocal quality is degraded with speech described as hoarse, breathy, and harsh. In addition, patients experience timing difficulty of vocal onsets and offsets. Reduced mobility, restricted range of movement, and uncontrolled rate of movement of muscles controlling respiration, phonation, resonation, and articulation is present. Reduced vital capacity results in reduced air expended during phonation. In advanced cases, the patient may speak in whispers or not at all, demonstrating **mutism**. Sensory problems may also contribute to speech difficulties. Patients who are instructed to upscale their speech sounds to produce loud speech consistently describe their speech as "too loud." Speech difficulties contribute to social isolation and impaired activity participation.[47]

Cognitive Function and Behavior

Impairments in cognitive function can be mild (e.g., mildly impaired memory) or severe. PD dementia occurs in approximately 20 to 40 percent of the patients. Older patients appear to be at greatest risk for dementia, with reported rates 4.4 times higher for individuals 80 years of age or older.[49] Dementia is associated with increased mortality rates. Coexisting Alzheimer's disease or multi-infarct dementia secondary to atherosclerotic disease are also common in the elderly and may be contributory factors in some patients. Dementia associated with PD is characterized by loss of executive functions (planning, reasoning, abstract thinking, judgment, and so forth) and changes in visuospatial skills, memory, and verbal fluency. **Bradyphrenia**, a disorder of intellectual function, can be seen in patients with PD dementia. It is characterized by a slowing of thought and information processing. Patients typically demonstrate problems with selective attention and in shifting attention. Cognitive performance is degraded in the "off" state.[49,50] Hallucinations and delusions are common complications owing to L-dopa toxicity.

Deficits in visuospatial skills are also present in this disease. Patients demonstrate significantly more errors than normal on visual perception tasks involving spatial organization. The BG, in association with the frontal lobe, appear to play an important role in the integration of sensory information. Deficits have been reported in vertical perception, topographic orientation, body scheme, and spatial relations. Motor tasks involving gestural movements, delayed double tasks, tracking, and constructional ability may be impaired.[21]

Depression is common in patients with PD. Major depression is reported to occur in approximately 40 percent of patients.[50] A significant number of patients develop depression prior to or just after onset of motor symptoms, suggesting an endogenous cause that may be related to underlying deficiencies of dopamine, serotonin, and norepinephrine. Patients demonstrate a variety of symptoms, including feelings of guilt, hopelessness, and worthlessness; loss of energy; poor concentration; deficits in short term memory; loss of ambition or enthusiasm; and disturbances in appetite and sleep. Suicidal thoughts may also be present. Hypomimia, a reduction in facial expressiveness, can give the appearance of depression.[50,51] Patients can also demonstrate a *dysthymic disorder* characterized by variability in dysphoric mood, or a wide range of anxiety disorders, including panic disorder and phobias that occur at higher than expected rates for an elderly population. Social withdrawal (social phobia) can result from the embarrassment patients experience from PD symptoms. Finally, greater anxiety is experienced with patients who are in the "off" medication state.[52]

Autonomic Nervous System

Autonomic nervous system dysfunction **(dysautonomia)** occurs with PD. Thermoregulatory dysfunction includes excessive sweating and abnormal or uncomfortable sensations of warmth and coldness. Patients in the "off" state experience impaired peripheral vasodilation with difficulty dissipating body heat. Seborrhea (increased oil secretion of the sebaceous glands of the skin) and seborrheic dermatitis (oily, chafing, and reddened skin) are common. Patients with PD exhibit abnormally slow pupillary responses to light and pain and reduced overall response to changes in light. Gastrointestinal dysfunction includes poor motility, changes in appetite, sialorrhea, and weight loss. Constipation is a common problem for most patients with PD. Urinary bladder dysfunction occurs with common symptoms of urinary frequency, urgency, urge incontinence, and nocturia. Many of these problems occur in the aging population in general and in men with benign prostatic hypertrophy. Sexual dysfunction is often present, including impotence and reduced rates of sexual activity.[53]

Cardiopulmonary Function

Orthostatic hypotension is common. Patients complain of light-headedness and blurred vision with position changes (e.g., supine-to-sit or sit-to-stand) or following exercise. Oral L-dopa medication can exaggerate symptoms of orthostatic hypotension. Patients with advanced PD also exhibit low resting blood pressure (BP).[53] Cardiovascular reflexes can be compromised, causing abnormal cardiac responses to exercise. For example, tachycardia in response to exercise may be suppressed.[54,55] Cardiac arrhythmias can occur and are associated with most antiparkinsonian medication.

Patients with PD demonstrate respiratory impairments, reported in as many as 84 percent of patients. Airway obstruction (e.g., air trapping, lung insufflation) is the most frequently reported pulmonary problem and has been linked to episodes of pulmonary failure. The etiology remains unknown but may be linked to bradykinetic disorganization of respiratory movements. Restrictive lung dysfunction is common and is linked to the decreased chest expansion that occurs as a result of rigidity of the trunk muscles, loss of musculoskeletal flexibility, and kyphotic posture. Patients with PD demonstrate lower forced vital capacity (FVC), lower forced expiratory volume (FEV_1), and higher residual volume (RV) and airway resistance (RAW) values when compared to age-matched controls. Daily function and activity participation are reduced in patients with pulmonary dysfunction.[56,57]

A sedentary lifestyle with decreased activity levels contributes to cardiopulmonary deconditioning. Limited research suggests that patients with mild to moderate PD do not appear to demonstrate significantly different exercise capacity (maximal heart rate, maximal oxygen consumption) when compared to age-matched controls.[58,59] However, these patients did demonstrate decreased peak power, and higher submaximal heart rates and oxygen consumption rates than controls.[59,60]

In long-standing disease, the lower extremities may exhibit circulatory changes owing to venous pooling as a result of decreased mobility and prolonged sitting. Thus, patients can present with mild to moderate edema of the feet and ankles, which usually subsides during sleep.

Table 21.1 Hoehn and Yahr Classification of Disability

Stage	Character of Disability
I	Minimal or absent; unilateral if present.
II	Minimal bilateral or midline involvement. Balance not impaired.
III	Impaired righting reflexes. Unsteadiness when turning or rising from chair. Some activities are restricted, but patient can live independently and continue some forms of employment.
IV	All symptoms present and severe. Standing and walking possible only with assistance.
V	Confined to bed or wheelchair.

From Hoehn and Yahr,[62] p 433, with permission.

Medical Diagnosis

Early diagnosis at onset of PD is difficult with accurate diagnosis possible only with continued observation of evolving clinical signs and symptoms. There is no single definitive test or group of tests used to diagnose the disease. The diagnosis is made on the basis of history and clinical examination. Handwriting samples, speech analysis, interview questions that focus on developing symptoms, and physical examination are used in the preclinical stage to detect early manifestations of the disease. A diagnosis of PD can be made if at least two of the four cardinal features are present. Exclusion of Parkinson-plus syndromes is necessary. The presence of extrapyramidal signs that are bilateral symmetrical and do not respond to L-dopa and dopamine agonists (apomorphine test) is suggestive of these syndromes, not PD.[8] Imaging can be used to rule out other pathologies. In vivo functional imaging (magnetic resonance imaging, MRI) using chemical markers to identify dopaminergic deficits in PD and related disorders identifies dopamine deficiency but does not discriminate between PD and other causes of parkinsonism. Positron emission tomography (PET) and single-photon emission computerized tomography (SPECT) scans are emerging technologies that have been used in human studies but not in routine diagnosis.

Clinical Course

The disease is slowly progressive, with a long subclinical period (without apparent clinical manifestations), estimated to be at least 5 years.[61] Before L-dopa therapy, 28 percent of patients became severely disabled (functionally dependent) or died within 5 years of diagnosis, 61 percent within 10 years, and 83 percent within 15 years. Following L-dopa therapy, only 9 percent had become disabled or had died at 5 years, 21 percent at 10 years, and 37.5 percent at 15 years. Overall the mean survival has increased by about 5 years since the introduction of L-dopa.[62] There is variability of the rate of progression. Patients who have a young age at onset or who are tremor predominant typically demonstrate a more benign progression and a relatively good prognosis. Patients with PD who present with postural instability and gait disturbances (the PIGD group) tend to have more pronounced deterioration with a more rapid disease progression. Neurobehavioral disturbances and dementia are also more common in this group. Mortality is usually due to cardiovascular disease or pneumonia.[3,61] An estimate of the stage and severity of the disease can be made using a staging scale. The most widely used is the *Hoehn-Yahr Classification of Disability Scale* (Table 21.1).[62] It provides a useful measure for charting the progression of the disease. Stage I is used to indicate minimal disease involvement, whereas stage V is indicative of severe deterioration in which the patient is confined to bed or a wheelchair.

Medical Management

There is no cure for PD. Medical management is directed at slowing of disease progression, and symptomatic treatment of motor features, motor complications, and non-motor features. Most anti-parkinsonian medications became available in the 1960s and have become the mainstay of management. Nutritional management is also an important consideration. Some patients benefit from surgical intervention. With effective management, the effects of the disease and complications can be minimized.

Pharmacological Management

Drug management can be divided into early neuroprotective therapy and symptomatic therapy (see Table 21.2).

Neuroprotective Therapy

Monoamine Oxidase Inhibitors (MAOs)

Patients in the early stages of PD may be given MAOs to improve metabolism of intracerebral dopamine (e.g., selegiline [SD-Deprenyl]). Clinically, selegiline has been shown to delay the primary endpoint at which patients need to start taking levodopa by about 9 months and may slow the overall progression of the disease. Selegiline also appears to have a mild symptomatic benefit in early PD, improving performance on measures of disability and motor impairment. Once levodopa therapy is started, selegiline in combination permits a lower dose to be used. There are few adverse effects; an increase in dyskinesias and orthostatic hypotension may be seen when selegiline is combined with levodopa therapy.[63–65]

Symptomatic Therapy

Levodopa

Levodopa (L-dopa) is the mainstay of symptomatic treatment for PD. It was first introduced in 1961 as an experimental drug and came into widespread clinical use by 1967. It is a metabolic precursor of dopamine that is able to cross the blood–brain barrier and raise the level of striatal dopamine in the basal ganglia; thus, administration of the drug represents an attempt to correct the essential neurochemical imbalance. Most of L-dopa (almost 99 percent) is metabolized before reaching the brain, requiring administration of high doses that can produce numerous side effects. Today, L-dopa is commonly administered with carbidopa, a decarboxylase inhibitor that allows a higher percentage of L-dopa to enter the CNS. Thus, lower doses of L-dopa can be used with fewer adverse side effects. Sinemet is the most common carbidopa/L-dopa medication. Its primary benefit is in alleviating bradykinesia and rigidity with less effect on tremor. It does not appear to have a direct impact on postural instability. The initial functional improvement is often dramatic. This is sometimes referred to as the *honeymoon period,* in which there is clear-cut drug effectiveness. Sinemet is available in immediate-release (IR) and controlled-release (CR) formulations. The IR form has a short half-life requiring multiple oral dosing throughout the day. The CR form is a long-acting, sustained release preparation. Both are equally effective.[65]

There are numerous adverse effects of L-dopa therapy. Adjusting the dosage and administering the medication in combination with other drugs can manage most symptoms. The most common disturbances are (1) gastrointestinal (anorexia, nausea, vomiting, constipation), (2) cognitive (confusion and hallucinations), (3) cardiovascular (hypotension and arrhythmias), (4) genitourinary (dysuria), (5) neuromuscular (motor fluctuations and dyskinesias), and (6) sleep disturbances (insomnia, sleep fragmentation).[63] During the initial dosing, patients may feel so much better that they may engage in sudden overactivity, seriously overtaxing their musculoskeletal and/or cardiovascular systems. The therapist needs to watch for this and to pace the patient accordingly.

A deterioration of the overall therapeutic effectiveness of L-dopa can be expected over time with a reported increase motor complications of 10 percent per year.[64] For many patients the therapeutic window is 5 to 7 years before optimal benefit wears off. This is thought to result from a progressive nigrostriatal degeneration. Thus, there is an ongoing debate of whether levodopa therapy should be initiated early or reserved for individuals who are in the later stages of the disease. Wearing-"off" state or **end-of-dose deterioration** is a worsening of symptoms during the expected time-frame of medication effectiveness. Freezing episodes, or sudden episodes of immobility, may appear. Random fluctuations in motor performance, termed **"on–off" phenomenon**, occur in about 50 percent of patients treated for more than 2 years and can be very disabling. Involuntary movements, **dyskinesias**, often emerge in tandem with end-of-dose deterioration. Initially these may appear as facial grimacing with twitching of the lips and tongue protrusion. With time the involuntary movements become more prevalent, vigorous, and more extensive, involving the limbs, trunk, and neck. Patients may also experience disabling psychiatric toxicity (visual hallucinations, delusions, and paranoia), depression, anxiety, abnormal sleep patterns, early morning akinesia, and pain. These changes are dose related and indicate the need for drug modification. Deprenyl can be administered with L-dopa to control mild wearing "off" phenomena. Unsupervised reduction or sudden discontinuation of L-dopa is contraindicated and may produce dangerous, life-threatening adverse effects.[63,65]

Dopamine Agonists

Dopamine agonists (DA) are a class of drugs designed to act directly on the postsynaptic dopamine receptors. They are administered along with L-dopa, allowing lower doses to be administered with prolonged effectiveness (i.e., L-dopa-sparing therapy). Patients with moderate to advanced PD who demonstrate declining responses to L-dopa therapy may benefit from DA drugs such as bromocriptine (Parlodel), ropinirole (Requip), and pramipexole (Mirapex). The greatest benefit of these drugs is on reducing rigidity and bradykinesia; they can also be used to reduce motor fluctuations. Adverse effects are similar to those of L-dopa with orthostatic lightheadedness and nausea being the most common.[66,67]

Anticholinergic Agents

Anticholinergic agents are used in early, untreated PD or as an adjunct for patients on levodopa. They block cholinergic function and have the most benefit moderating tremor and rigidity; they have little or no effect on bradykinesia, and postural instability. They may be given in conjunction with L-dopa to smooth motor fluctuations. Trihexyphenidyl (Artane), benztropine (Cogentin), ethopropazine (Parsidol), and procyclidine (Kemadrin) are commonly prescribed drugs in this group. Anticholinergic adverse effects include blurred vision, dry mouth, dizziness, constipation, and urinary retention. Central toxicity is indicated by impaired memory, confusion, hallucinations, and delusions.[63]

Amantadine (Symmetrel) is an antiviral agent that has anti-Parkinson effects. It potentiates the action of dopamine in the CNS. Patients taking amantadine demonstrate modest improvement in tremor, rigidity, and bradykinesia.

Implications for the Physical Therapist

The therapist needs to be fully aware of each of the medications the patient is taking and potential adverse effects. It is important to remember that patients on levodopa therapy may demonstrate fluctuations related to medication cycle. Optimal performance can be expected at peak dosage whereas worsening performance is associated with end-of-dose cycle and medication depletion. Therapists are involved in monitoring drug effectiveness on motor performance, function, and activity participation. As the disease progresses, patients may develop a tolerance for a particular medication, necessitating a change in prescription. Often, it is the therapist who first notices a change in functional status as the patient's system adapts to either the amount or type of drug prescribed. Accurate observation, examination, and reporting of these changes greatly assists the physician in modifying a drug prescription. Therapists may also be involved with clinical drug trials as new medications or combinations are developed. Table 21.2 presents an overview of the pharmacology of PD.

Nutritional Management

A high-protein diet can block the effectiveness of L-dopa. The dietary amino acids in protein compete with L-dopa absorption. This is particularly problematic in patients with chronic disease who exhibit fluctuations in motor performance. Thus patients are generally advised to follow a high-calorie, low-protein diet. Generally no more than 15 percent of calories should come from protein. Dietary recommendations may also include shifting the intake of daily protein to the evening meal when patients are less

Table 21.2 Pharmacology of Parkinson's Disease

Drug Class	Example	Average Dosage[a]	Side Effects
Anticholinergics	Trihexyphenidyl Bentropin	2 mg tid 1 mg bid	Dry mouth, dizziness, blurred vision Tachycardia, dry mouth, nausea, vomiting, confusion
Dopamine replacement	Levodopa/carbidopa Sinemet Sinemet CR	10/100 tid/qid 25/100 tid/qid 25/250 tid 25/100 tid 25/200 bid	Dystonia Abnormal, involuntary movements Nausea, vomiting Confusion Dreams, hallucinations
Dopamine agonists	Pergolide Bromocriptine	1 mg tid 5 mg bid	Nervousness, dyskinesias, insomnia, hallucinations, nausea, confusion, erythromelalgia Nausea, headache, dizziness, fatigue, cramps/constipation, confusion, pulmonary/peritoneal fibrosis
Amantadine		100 mg bid	Lightheadedness, livedo reticularis, edema
MAOI-B[b]	Seligiline	5 mg bid	Nausea, dreams, hallucinations, confusion, dyskinesias

[a]bid = twice a day, tid = three times a day; qid = four times a day.
[b]MAOI-B, monoamine oxidase inhibitor, type B.
From Cutson, T, et al,[67] p 367, with permission.

active. These modifications minimize motor fluctuations and maximize responsiveness to L-dopa therapy. The patient is encouraged to eat a variety of foods and may be advised to take dietary supplements to ensure adequate intake of vitamins and minerals. Patients are also advised to increase their daily intake of water and dietary fiber to alleviate problems of constipation.[68]

Rigidity and bradykinesia can limit upright posture and upper extremity (UE) feeding movements. Learned motor plans, for example, using a cup or eating utensils, may also be difficult. Occupational therapy intervention to improve feeding and recommended adaptive eating devices is of considerable importance in helping to maintain nutrition and general health status. The speech–language pathologist also has an important role in the evaluation of dysphagia and the recommendation of strategies to assist with swallowing dysfunction. Patient, family and caregiver education should focus on the importance of maintaining good nutritional intake.

Surgical Management

Surgery is an accepted treatment for patients with advanced PD who respond poorly to medication or who experience complications related to pharmacotherapy. There are three main surgical approaches: ablative surgery, deep brain stimulation (DBS), and neural transplantation.

Ablative Surgery

Stereotactic surgery, the surgical lesioning of the brain, was pioneered in the 1950s, and is in current renewed use owing to the increased accuracy of imaging and surgical equipment.[69] **Pallidotomy** involves producing a destructive lesion in the sensorimotor portion of the globus pallidus internus (GPi). The lesion reduces excessive GPi inhibitory activity that results in tonic thalamic hypoactivity. It is indicated for L-dopa-induced dyskinesias, severe "on–off" state fluctuations, rigidity, and tremor while balance, gait disturbances, freezing, and hypophonia are less responsive. Effects are contralateral and benefits appear to be long lasting.[70] **Thalamotomy** involves producing a destructive lesion within the ventral intermediate nucleus (VIM) of the thalamus. It has been shown to effectively reduce longstanding tremor that is unresponsive to drug treatment and may offer some improvement of rigidity. It is not effective on symptoms of bradykinesia or gait disturbances.[69] Bilateral surgical lesions are usually not recommended because of a high rate of motor complications, especially speech and swallowing difficulties. Reported adverse effects of surgery include hemorrhage, infarction, infection, seizures, confusion, depression, dysarthria, or death.[65]

Deep Brain Stimulation

Deep brain stimulation (DBS) involves the implantation of electrodes into the brain where they block nerve signals that cause symptoms. Stimulation of the VIM of the thalamus is commonly done with severe and uncontrolled UE tremors that are unresponsive to medication. A pacemaker is implanted in the chest, with a thin wire that goes under the skin to the brain electrodes. High-frequency stimulation is provided. The patient can control the pacemaker's "on-off" switch while the physician determines the amount of stimulation it delivers, tailoring it to the individual's needs. Total suppression of tremor is observed in one-third to one-half of patients.[71] Thalamic stimulation is not indicated for other PD symptoms. Its major advantage is its potential to alter tremor without producing an irreversible brain lesion. DBS has also been shown to significantly improve patient performance on instrumental activities of daily living (IADL), with the greatest improvement noted when control is for tremor in the dominant hand.[72] More recently DBS of the globus pallidus (GPi) and the subthalamic nucleus (STN) has been used to successfully control other PD symptoms of motor overactivity (i.e., on-state dyskinesias, akinesia, rigidity) along with tremor.[73,74] STN simulation has been shown to reduce the medication requirements in PD.[75]

Neural Transplantation

Transplantation of cells capable of surviving and delivering dopamine into the striatum of patients with advanced PD is an experimental treatment and currently under investigation. Studies involve the grafting of embryonic stem cells from umbilical cord blood or fetal cells. Ethical considerations are posed with the use of human embryonic tissue. Sustained clinical improvements have been observed in some patients and not in others. Variability in terms of efficacy and outcome may be due to cell therapy techniques. Younger patients in the early stages of the disease appear to show some improvement in motor function. Adverse side effects such as serious dyskinesias in more than 50 percent of patients have been reported.[76] Patients usually undergo immunosuppression following surgery to reduce the risks of graft rejection. Currently under investigation are techniques to expand cell production and use genetically engineered cells.[77] Availability of transplantation procedures is very limited.

Framework for Rehabilitation

Rehabilitation has an important role in reducing functional limitations while promoting activity participation and independence. In addition, known complications of PD can be reduced or prevented while quality of life is promoted. Optimal management involves a coordinated interdisciplinary team to oversee a comprehensive plan of care can address the patient's individual clinical problems, concerns, and needs. The team typically includes the physician, nurse, physical therapist, occupational therapist, speech-language pathologist, and social worker. Referral to other specialists may also be necessary, for example, psychologist, nutritionist, gastroenterologist, urologist, pulmonologist, and so forth. As with any team, the patient is the central figure with family and caregivers being key members.

The ideal rehabilitation program considers the patient's disease history, course and symptoms, together with impairments, functional limitations, and disability. Of equal importance are the patient's abilities (assets), priorities, and resources including family, home, and community resources. Deterioration of condition and medication-induced fluctuations in performance should be expected. The overall focus is on long-range planning, with anticipated episodes of care including hospital-based, outpatient, and home/community-based care. A continuum of care based on disease stage (early, middle, late) is an effective way to organize care and is presented in Table 21.3. Interventions are restorative (aimed at improving impairments, functional limitations, and disabilities), preventative (aimed at minimizing potential complications and indirect impairments), and compensatory (aimed at modifying the task, activity, or environment to improve function). See discussion in Chapter 1. It is critical for the whole team to provide a supportive environment to assist patients and their family members in the difficult adjustment to living with a chronic and progressive disease.

Physical Therapy Examination and Evaluation

A comprehensive examination is required to determine the level of impairments and degree of function. Subsequent reexamination at specified intervals is used to distinguish change in status as well as effects of treatment. Data are obtained from the patient's history, systems review, and relevant tests and measures (Box 21.3). The selection of examination procedures and level of inquiry is determined by the patient's unique status. The severity of problems, stage of disease, age, phase and setting of rehabilitation, and other factors must all be taken into account in structuring the examination and evaluating data. During the early and middle stages of PD, measures of impairment and physical performance are relatively stable.[78] During late stages of the disease and under conditions of fluctuating symptoms with pharmacological instability, measures can be expected to be less stable.

This section presents strategies for examination as well as relevant tests and measures. A complete description of many of the tests and measures identified are provided in earlier chapters focusing on examination.

Table 21.3 Overview of Parkinson's Disease Management

		Treatment Considerations		
Stage	**Characteristics**	**Pharmacological Agents**	**Physical**	**Psychosocial**
Early	Fully functional May have unilateral tremor, rigidity	Anticholinergics (tremor) Seligiline (possible neuro-protection)	Preventative exercise program	Education Information
Early middle	Symptoms bilateral, bradykinesia, rigidity Mild speech impairment Axial rigidity, stooped posture, stiffness Gait impairments begin	Levodopa/carbidopa Seligiline	Corrective exercise program	Counseling Support group Monitor for depression
Late middle	All symptoms worse but independent in ADL[a] May need minor assistance Balance problems	Levodopa/carbidopa Dopamine agonists Seligiline Antidepressants	Compensatory and corrective exercise Speech-language therapy Occupational therapy	Caregiver issues (medications, mobility) Monitor for dementia
Late	Severely disabled, impaired Dependent with ADL	Levodopa/carbidopa Dopamine agonists Antidepressants	Compensatory exercise Dietary concerns Skin care Hygiene Pulmonary function	Dementia Depression

[a]ADL = activities of daily living

From Cutson, T, et al,[67] p 370, with permission.

Box 21.3 Elements of the Examination for a Patient with Parkinson's Disease[79]

Patient/Client History
- Age, sex, race/ethnicity, primary language, education
- Social history: cultural beliefs and behaviors, family and caregiver resources, social support systems
- Occupation/employment/work
- Living environment: home/ work barriers
- Hand dominance
- General health status: physical, psychological, social, and role function, health habits
- Family history
- Medical/surgical history
- Current conditions/chief complaints
- Medications
- Medical/laboratory test results
- Functional status and activity level: premorbid and current

Systems Review
- Neuromuscular
- Musculoskeletal
- Cardiovascular/pulmonary
- Integumentary

Tests and Measures/Impairments
- Cognition: mental status, memory: hesitation, slowness of thought processes
- Oromotor function: communication (fluctuations, reduced volume), swallowing
- Psychosocial function: motivation, anxiety, depression
- Anthropometric characteristics: body mass index, girth, length; edema
- Circulation: response to position change, orthostatic hypotension
- Aerobic capacity and endurance: during functional activities and standardized exercise protocols including cardiovascular and pulmonary signs and symptoms
- Ventilation and gas exchange
- Integumentary integrity: skin condition, pressure sensitive areas; activities, positioning, and postures to relieve pressure
- Autonomic nervous system integrity: thermal responses, sweating
- Sensory integrity and integration
- Pain: intensity and location
- Perceptual function: visuospatial skills
- Joint integrity, alignment, and mobility: range of motion (active and passive); muscle length, and soft tissue extensibility
- Posture: alignment and position, symmetry (static and dynamic); ergonomics, and body mechanics
- Muscle performance: strength, power, and endurance
- Motor function: motor control and motor learning: tone, voluntary movement patterns; involuntary movements; hesitation, slowness, arrests of movements; poverty of movements
- Procedural learning for complex and sequential tasks
- Postural control and balance: degree of postural instability, balance strategies; safety
- Gait and locomotion: gait pattern and speed, safety
- Functional status and activity level: performance-based examinement of functional skills (FIM level), basic and instrumental ADL; functional mobility skills; home management skills
- Assistive or adaptive devices: fit, alignment, function, use; safety
- Environment, home, and work barriers
- Work, community, and leisure activities: ability to participate in activities, safety

Cognitive Function

Memory, orientation, conceptual reasoning, problem solving, and judgment should be examined. Speed of information processing, attention, and concentration are particularly important to determine if bradyphrenia is suspected. A brief screen of cognitive function can be obtained using the *Mini-Mental Status Exam (MMSE)*.[80]

Psychosocial Function

The therapist should determine overall levels of stress and anxiety, and available coping strategies. It is important to ask the patient about the presence of depressive symptoms such as sadness, apathy, passivity, insomnia, anorexia, weight loss, inactivity and dependency, inability to concentrate and impaired memory, or suicidal ideation. Useful instruments include the *Geriatric Depression Scale*[81] or the *Beck Depression Inventory*.[82] The patient's premorbid interests, abilities, and daily activities should be investigated in order to translate them into a treatment program that will engage the patient's full cooperation.

Sensation

A screening examination of sensation is indicated (superficial and deep sensations, combined cortical sensations). Sensory changes can be expected with aging (blunting of touch sensations and proprioception with greater losses in lower extremities than upper, and distal more than proximal). The patient should be asked about the presence of paresthesias (sensations of numbness or tingling). Specific areas of sensory loss may be indicative of comorbid pathology, for example, stroke, diabetic neuropathy, and so forth.

An examination of vision should include a determination of acuity, peripheral vision, tracking, accommodation, light and dark adaptation, and depth perception. Visual changes can be expected with aging such as loss of visual acuity, inability to focus on printed word (presbyopia), decreased adaptation to light, sensitivity to light and glare, and loss of color discrimination. Patients with PD may experience blurring of vision and difficulty reading that is not improved by corrective lenses as well as problems with eye pursuit (cogwheeling). Specific deficits may be indicative of comorbid pathologies that are common in the elderly, such as cataracts (clouding of central vision first, then peripheral), glaucoma (early loss of peripheral vision), senile macular degeneration or diabetic retinopathy (early loss of central vision), and cerebrovascular accident (homonymous hemianopsia). Medications may also produce impaired or fuzzy vision, for example, antidepressants and anticholinergics.

An examination of the presence of pain is indicated. Mild aching and cramplike sensations are common in patients with PD and are often poorly localized. It is important to examine for postural stress syndrome (pain linked to lack of movement, faulty movements or posture, and ligamentous strain). Frequent pain or excruciating pain are not common but may also occur. Useful instruments include *The McGill Pain Questionnaire*[83] and the *visual analogue scale* (VAS).

Musculoskeletal Function

Flexibility

An examination of musculoskeletal ROM and flexibility is important. The therapist can document specific ROM impairments (AROM, passive ROM [PROM]) using goniometric measurement. Patients with PD are likely to present with losses in hip and knee extension, dorsiflexion, shoulder flexion, elbow extension, dorsal spine and neck extension, and axial rotation. To a lesser extent, many of these changes are also experienced by the elderly in general. It is particularly important to examine spinal ROM (ability to rotate, flex, and extend the spine) because patients with PD have been shown to exhibit impairments in this area.[84] All segments of the spine should be examined, including cervical, thoracic, and lumbar segments. The mobility of the spine should be examined during a series of functional movements, such as axial rotation (looking behind) and walking. Hamstring length can be determined using a straight leg test.

Posture

An examination of resting posture and changes in posture that occur with movement is indicated. The therapist can use posture grids/plumb lines, still photography, or videotape to document changes. Patients with PD typically assume a flexed, stooped posture (kyphosis with forward head) with the center of mass placed forward within the limits of stability.

Muscle Performance

An examination of strength and endurance is indicated. The therapist can measure strength using manual muscle testing (MMT). Hand-held and isokinetic dynamometry can be used to quantify peak force (torque output). Patients with PD have been shown to exhibit impairments in the rate of force development and in maximum torque production capability. Isokinetic dynamometry can also be used to document muscle endurance and has been suggested for documenting tremor, using slow speeds of movement (25 mm/s) and low torques.[85]

Motor Function

Rigidity

Rigidity is usually equal in both agonist and antagonist muscle groups. It can be sustained (lead pipe) or intermittent (cogwheel). Distribution of rigidity is often asymmetric especially in the early stages of the disease and can vary during the course of the day and with stress. It is therefore important to determine which body segments are affected and the severity of involvement. Tone changes in the neck and shoulders are suggestive of early disease, whereas tone changes in the trunk and extremities are typically present with more extensive disease. Deficits in functional mobility and postural reactions should be suspected in the presence of significant trunk rigidity. The patient should be examined for facial immobility (hypomimia or masked face); the ability to smile or use the muscles of facial expression should also be examined. A determination of severity of rigidity can be made based on criteria of resistance to passive movement and availability of ROM. For example, a determination of severe rigidity is made if ROM can only be achieved with difficulty (see Appendix A). An inspection of voluntary repetitive movements should be performed to determine active limitations imposed by rigidity.

Bradykinesia

Initially movements are slowed, then movements decrease in amplitude (hypokinesia), and in later stages, movements become arrhythmic with frequent hesitations and arrests (akinesia). A stopwatch can be used to quantify detectable slowing of movement (*movement time*) and movement hesitancy or *reaction time* (elapsed time between the patient's desire to move and the actual movement response). The therapist should examine overall amplitude of movement and changes in amplitude. For example, amplitude of arm swing during walking can be examined. As the disease progresses, marked slowness, poverty, and small amplitude of movement should be expected. Timed tests for rapid alternating movements (RAM) can be used to determine the effects of bradykinesia. These include repeated opposition of the forefinger and thumb, alternating pronation–supination, opening and closing of hands, and tapping (finger or foot tapping). Dexterity in complex motor tasks (e.g., writing, dressing, skilled object manipulation) can be expected to be impaired and should be examined (e.g., *Purdue Peg Board Test*). This is also true for motor tasks involving simultaneous use of both sides (e.g., rapid alternating pronation–supination of both arms).[7]

More sophisticated methods have been used to study movement in patients with PD, largely in the research setting. EMG has been used to quantify the effects of rigidity and bradykinesia on motor performance. Long-latency EMG responses (50 to 120 msec) have been observed when muscles are subjected to sudden stretch. Abnormal patterns of motor unit recruitment have also been observed.[85]

Tremor

The location, persistence, and severity (amplitude) of tremor should be recorded. The therapist should determine if tremor is present at rest (the typical pattern) or present with action and interferes with function. This latter pattern may occur in severe, long-standing disease. UE functional skills such as writing, feeding, and dressing should be closely examined for effects of tremor. Tremor in the lower extremities is generally only seen when the patient is supine and usually disappears with walking. As stress increases tremor, simultaneous cognitive tasks such as serial seven subtractions (i.e., counting backward from 100 by 7) can be used to test for tremor in apparently uninvolved limbs.[86]

Postural Instability

A thorough examination of balance is indicated including an examination of orientation to vertical. The patient's perception of vertical should be ascertained as some patients will says they are fully upright when actually is leaning forward. A plumb line and grid with still photographs can be used to document position.

Balance control can be expected to degrade under conditions of narrowing base of support, or in response to perturbations. The patient should be asked to maintain steady standing while varying the base of support (e.g., feet apart, feet together, tandem stance, step stance, and single-limb stance). Perturbation tasks that can be used to challenge balance include self-initiated movements (e.g., arm raise, bend-reach, *Functional Reach Test (FR)*[87] or the *Multidirectional Reach Test (MDRT)*[88] and step tests). In addition, the *retropulsion test,* sudden sternum push or shoulder pull, can be used. Patients with PD especially in the early stages of the disease may not demonstrate balance impairments in response to steady standing/normal BOS or self-initiated movements as along as their attention is fully directed to the task at hand. However, if competing attentional demands are instituted (i.e., dual tasking such as talking while balancing), instability can be expected. Self-initiated tasks with a timing component (number of steps per minute) will also likely reveal balance impairments as will responding to unexpected perturbations. With continued deterioration, greater impairments in balance control will be noted. Smithson et al[89] demonstrated strong temporal stability of performance (repeatability of measurements) on balance tests in a group of 20 patients with idiopathic PD during the "on" phase of the medication cycle. When comparing fallers with non-fallers, some of the tests proved more discriminating in identifying fallers (e.g., tandem stance, single-limb stance, functional reach, and the retropulsion test).

Dynamic posturography uses a standardized and reproducible postural perturbation from a moving platform that can reveal deficits in placement of the center of mass (COM), increased postural sway, and unstable responses to platform perturbation.[90] Variability of responses in patients with PD has been demonstrated, especially during the "on" phase of medication.[91] Available postural strategies and reactions to challenges should be carefully documented (e.g., ankle, hip, and stepping strategies). The patient with PD typically exhibits coactivation patterns (rigid body) with an inability to recover a stable posture.[16] Responses to perturbation typically include delayed responses for recovery (start hesitation) or absence of postural responses (patient would fall if not caught by examiner or body support harness).

The patient with PD can be expected to exhibit problems with sensory organization related to difficulty changing sensory conditions. This can be examined using the *Clinical Test for Sensory Integration in Balance (CTSIB).* Six different sensory conditions are examined, including (1) eyes open, stationary surface (EOSS); (2) eyes closed, stationary surface (ECSS); (3) visual conflict (moving surround), stationary surface (VCSS); (4) eyes open, moving surface (EOMS); (5) eyes closed, moving support surface (ECMS), and (6) visual conflict, moving surface (VCMS).[92,93] In the absence of posturography equipment, the patient can stand on dense foam instead of a moving platform and a visual dome can substituted for the moving visual screen.[94] A *Modified Test for Sensory Integration in Balance (m-CTSIB)* uses four different sensory conditions: EOSS, ECSS, EOFS (foam surface), and ECFS and proves a useful quick clinical screening measure.[95]

There are a number of clinical balance tests that examine functional limitations related to balance. Many of these instruments have been developed for use with the elderly and correlate well with frequency of falls.

The *Timed Up and Go Test*[96] is a particularly valuable instrument for patients with PD because it includes tasks that are typically problematic. The individual rises from a chair, walks 10 ft, turns, and then returns to the chair. It uses time as an outcome measure. Scores within 10 seconds are normal for most adults; scores of 11 to 20 seconds are within normal limits for frail elderly or disabled patients; scores greater than 20 seconds are considered abnormal and indicate need for further examination and intervention.

Tinetti's *Performance-Oriented Mobility Assessment (POMA)*[97] includes both static and dynamic balance items, organized into two subtests of balance (nine items) and gait (six items). It has a total possible score of 28; patients who score less than 19 are considered at high risk for falls while those who score between 19 and 24 are at moderate risk for falls. The gait subtest was found to be a useful screening instrument in identifying gait dysfunction in patients with PD from healthy elderly, but was not sensitive enough to distinguish performance across conditions of varying instructional sets (i.e., "swing your arms," "walk fast," "take large steps").[98]

Gait

An examination of gait is indicated. Parameters and characteristics of gait that should be examined during straight line walking include speed of walking, stride length, cadence, stability, variability, and safety. A *10-Meter Walk Test* can be used to determine speed, average stride, and cadence or more sophisticated kinetic analysis can be obtained from embedded force plates, body markers, and computerized equipment (motion analysis systems typically seen in the laboratory setting). Patients with PD typically demonstrate difficulty attaining and sustaining walking speed and may have difficulty with foot clearance onto force plates with shuffling gait patterns seen in advanced disease.[41] Gait should be examined for kinematic or qualitative changes, including reductions in hip, knee, and ankle motions that result in a short-stepped, shuffling gait pattern with reduced trunk rotation and arm swing. Postural abnormalities that contribute to the development of a festinating gait pattern should be documented (i.e., flexed, stooped posture). Gait should be examined in all movement directions: forward, backward, and sideward. A complex gait pattern like cross-stepping or braiding can be used to examine deficits in motor planning. Patients with PD experience difficulty with adaptability and cannot easily vary walking in complex or open environments. Walking should therefore be examined using varied surfaces (e.g., community environment) or negotiating an obstacle course. Increased difficulty in walking is also experienced in response to varying attentional demands and sets. Changes observed during dual task walking (e.g., *Walkie-Talkie Test,* walking while carrying objects on a tray), turns on command, or walking in response to varying attentional sets (i.e., "swing your arms," "walk fast," "take large steps") should be documented.[99] Freezing episodes should be investigated in terms of frequency, duration, and triggering stimuli (auditory or visual cues) that release the patient and allow initiation of movement.

A determination of fall history and fall injuries is an important component of the examination of balance and gait function. There is a strong association between duration and severity of PD with increased risk of falls. Of particular significance are balance and walking impairments, freezing, and the presence of involuntary movements (dyskinesias). Other linked factors include postural hypotension, dementia, depression, and prior history of falls.[21,100] A *fall risk diary* can be used to assist the patient and family/caregivers in accurately recording a fall event and the context of daily life in which the fall occurred. For example, activity at the time of the fall, timing and effectiveness of medication, timing of food intake, type of footwear, degree of fatigue and injury, and other risk factors all should be documented.[100] The need for assisted gait and frequency of contact guarding from family members or caregivers during walking should also be documented.

Swallowing and Speech

An examination of swallowing function, feeding, and speech is important. Referral to a speech–language pathologist is indicated if the patient demonstrates functional limitations in any of these areas.

Autonomic Function

The therapist should examine for problems with autonomic dysfunction. Excessive drooling (salivation) or sweating, greasy skin, and abnormalities in thermoregulation should be noted. Excessive sweating and flushing during the "On" state is linked to the presence of dyskinesias. Episodes of orthostatic hypotension should also be carefully documented, with blood pressures taken at rest and after position change. A change in BP of greater than 15 mm Hg is significant. In patients with advanced PD, blood pressures are significantly lower in the "on" state than in the "off" state, leading to frequent hypotension and complaints of dizziness.[101]

Cardiopulmonary Function

Endurance may be reduced as a result of impaired cardiorespiratory function and long-standing inactivity, both common problems in chronic PD. An examination of respiratory function should include inspection of rib cage compliance, chest wall mobility, and thoracic expansion. Visual inspection of breathing patterns and an examination of the influence of posture on breathing should be performed. Ventilation parameters (respiratory rate, minute ventilation, inspiratory time) should be determined. Changes in breathing pattern with activity should also be noted. Objective measurements can include circumferential measurements of the chest and abdomen. Relevant pulmonary function tests include spirometry: flow-volume, lung volumes, and airway resistance (e.g., forced vital capacity [FVC], forced expiratory volume [FEV], maximal expiratory flow [MEF], maximal inspiratory flow [MIF], total lung capacity [TLC], residual volume [RV], and airway resistance [RAW]).[57]

The therapist should examine vital signs (heart rate, blood pressure, and respiratory rate) at rest and following exercise or activity. Patients with mild to moderate PD may be able to be tested using standard exercise performance tests (*12-Minute Walk Test* or *6-Minute Walk Test,* treadmill test, cycle ergometer test).[58] These tests may prove too exhausting for the patient with advanced PD. Light and co-workers[102] used a *2-Minute Walk Test* to evaluate walking endurance in patients with advanced PD (Hoehn and Yahr Stages III and IV) and found it to be a sensitive and feasible test.

Reduced maximal heart rate and maximal oxygen consumption along with higher submaximal heart rates should be expected with deconditioning and moderate to severe PD.[59,60] However, these changes have not been found with milder disease manifestations.[58] Exertional symptoms (dyspnea, dizziness or confusion, excessive fatigue, pallor, and so forth) should be carefully documented. Perceived exertion can be recorded using *Borg's Rating of Perceived Exertion Scale (RPE scale)*.[103] The patient should be questioned regarding level of fatigue or exhaustion experienced during daily activity (the fall risk diary can be used to document these findings). Knowledge and use of energy conservation and activity pacing strategies should also be determined.

Integumentary Integrity

The therapist should examine the patient closely for areas of bruising and skin breakdown. Patients who are severely disabled may be restricted to bed, wheelchair, or both. Incontinence may occur during late stage disease. The effect of these problems on skin integrity should be carefully documented. Use and effectiveness of pressure-relieving strategies and devices should also be documented.

Functional Status

An examination of functional status is indicated, including performance of functional mobility skills, basic activities of daily living (BADL), and instrumental activities of daily living (IADL). For patients undergoing inpatient rehabilitation, the *Functional Independence Measure (FIM)* is commonly administered.[104] Need for and appropriate use of protective and supportive devices is an important component of the functional status examination. Close collaboration with the occupational therapist is essential.

During functional performance tests, each skill should be analyzed to determine the impact of direct and indirect impairments on performance. For example, sit-to-stand transfers typically present a significant challenge for patients with moderate to severe PD as evidenced by increased time and increased falls. These changes have been attributed to hypokinesia, decreased rates of force production, and changes in distal muscle timing.[105,106] The approach used in treatment to improve sit-to-stand function will be very different depending on correct identification of the source of problem. Patients with PD typically demonstrate greatest difficulty in those activities having a rotational component, such as rolling or turning in bed or sitting up. The time it takes to initiate and to complete an activity should be recorded. Because these patients experience increased fatigue with resultant fluctuations in performance, examination sessions should be kept brief. Repeat sessions should be undertaken at the same time of day and at the same time in the medication cycle. An accompanying videotape can provide an objective record of functional performance. An examination of functional performance in the home (or work) environment is also indicated. The patient's physical environment is examined for barriers, access, and safety.

Global Health and Disease-Specific Measures

Global health measures can be used to determine individual outcomes across a broad spectrum. Instruments typically include items that examine ability to perform routine daily activities and quality of life (e.g., physical and social function, general health and vitality, emotional well-being, bodily pain, and so forth). General health measures have been used to study large populations and are most useful in determining long-term health outcomes. They lack the sensitivity needed to document short-term outcomes of treatment.[107] Commonly used measures of general health status include: *Rand 36-Item Health Survey SF-36*[108] and the *Sickness Impact Profile*.[109]

Disease-specific measures are designed to determine attributes unique to a specific disease entity. Items are included that provide information about the disease process and outcomes, and ideally document clinically meaningful change over time. Thus these instruments have greater responsiveness or sensitivity to change than general health measures. Examples of instruments developed specifically for the examination of patients with PD include the Unified Parkinson's Disease Rating Scale and Parkinson's Disease Questionnaire (PDQ-39).

The *Unified Parkinson's Disease Rating Scale (UPDRS)*[110] was originally devised to document the overall effects of the disease (Appendix A). It is a composite scale, consisting of six sections. Part I includes four items examining mental status, behavior, and mood. Part II includes 13 items that examine activities of daily living as well as ratings of difficulty walking, tremor, and sensory symptoms. A determination of "on/off" performance is indicated. Part III, motor examination, includes 14 items that examine speech, facial expression, finger and hand movements, posture, gait, and the effects of tremor, rigidity, and bradykinesia. Part IV investigates the complications of therapy including dyskinesias, dystonia, clinical fluctuations ("on/off" performance), nausea or vomiting, sleep disturbances, and orthostatic hypotension. Unless otherwise stated, items are graded on a scale of 0 to 4, with 0 being normal and 4 being severely affected. Part V is a modified *Hoehn and Yahr Staging*. Disease severity is divided over 5 stages into unilateral or bilateral signs; higher numbered stages represent progressively more difficulty with mobility and balance. Part VI is the *Schwab and England Activities of Daily Living Scale*. Estimates are made in terms of percent impairment (0 percent = vegetative functions (bedridden) to 100 percent = completely independent). The UPDRS is the most commonly used scale to examine PD disease severity and progression as well as the patient's response to drug therapy. Overall, the scale has

Box 21.4 Examples of General Goals and Outcomes for Patients with Progressive Disorders of the Central Nervous System,[a] adapted from the *Guide to Physical Therapist Practice*[79]

Impact of pathology/pathophysiology is reduced.
- Patient/client, family, and caregiver knowledge and awareness of the disease, prognosis, and plan of care is enhanced.
- Symptom management is enhanced.
- Risk of secondary impairment is reduced.
- Intensity of care is decreased.

Impact of impairments is reduced.
- Cognitive function is improved.
- Joint integrity and mobility are improved.
- Sensory awareness and skin integrity are improved.
- Pain is decreased.
- Motor function is improved.
- Muscle performance (strength, power, and endurance) is improved.
- Postural control and balance are improved.
- Gait and locomotion are improved.
- Management of fatigue is enhanced.
- Aerobic capacity is increased.

Ability to perform physical actions, tasks, or activities is improved.
- Independence in activities of daily living is increased.
- Tolerance of positions and activities is increased.
- Activity pacing and energy conservation skills are enhanced.
- Problem-solving and decision-making skills are enhanced.
- Safety of patient/client, family, and caregivers is improved.

Disability associated with chronic illness is reduced.
- Ability to assume/resume self-care and home management is improved.
- Ability to assume work (job/school/play), community, and leisure roles is improved.
- Patient/client and family knowledge and awareness of personal and environmental factors associated with worsening of the condition are enhanced.
- Awareness and use of community resources are improved.

Health status and quality of life are improved.
- Sense of well-being is enhanced.
- Stressors are reduced.
- Insight, self-confidence, and self-management skills are improved.
- Health, wellness, and fitness are improved.

Patient/client satisfaction is enhanced.
- Access and availability of services are acceptable to patient/client and family.
- Quality of rehabilitation services is acceptable to patient/client and family.
- Care is coordinated with patient/client, family, caregivers, and other professionals.

[a]Anticipated goals and expected outcomes are specific to the individual patient.

good interrater reliability (r = 0.98) with some individual items demonstrating less reliability (i.e., facial expression, estimating severity of sensory symptoms and bradykinesia).[111]

The *Parkinson's Disease Questionnaire (PDQ-39)* is a 39-item questionnaire developed from in-depth interviews with patients with PD.[112] It focuses on the subjective report of the impact of PD on daily life and addresses eight health-related quality of life dimensions (mobility, ADL, emotional well-being, stigma, social support, cognition, communication, and bodily discomfort). The PDQ-39 produces a profile of scores on the eight individual dimensions. A summary score (the Parkinson's Disease Summary Index [PDSI]) can also be determined, with scores that range from 0 (perfect health) to 100 (worst health). It provides a useful indication of the global impact of PD on health status. Internal and test–retest reliability were found to be moderate to high with reported ranges from 0.68 to 0.96. Construct validity was examined by comparing the PDSI with other measures of health. Significant and high correlations were found between the PDQ-39 and the SF-36 and the Hoehn and Yahr staging score.[113,114]

A determination of goals and outcomes is based on careful examination and evaluation of the patient's individual abilities, impairments, functional limitations, and disability (Box 21.4).

Physical Therapy Intervention

A combined approach of physical therapy and pharmacological intervention plays a key role in the management of the patient with PD. For most patients, physical therapy is not prescribed until the disease has progressed to the point when function has declined. A variety of interventions are used to achieve goals and outcomes, including direct interventions, supervision of assistive personnel, patient/family/caregiver instruction, environmental modification, and supportive counseling. Early intervention is critical in preventing the devastating musculoskeletal impairments these patients are so prone to develop. Interventions also focus on improvement of motor function, exercise capacity, functional performance, and activity participation. Education of patients, family members, and caregivers is critical to attaining optimal outcomes.

Motor Learning Strategies

Patients with PD typically demonstrate motor learning deficits, including impairments in learning long and complex movement sequences, simultaneous motor/cognitive tasks, and movements dependent on internally generated cues versus external cues.[115–117] In the early stages of the disease, practice can be expected to improve learning and performance while in the more advanced stages and in the presence of pronounced cognitive deficits, training will likely be less successful.[37,38,118–120] The therapist needs to structure treatment sessions to optimize motor learning.

Critical elements of practice include a large number of repetitions to develop procedural skills. Long and complex movement sequences should be avoided or broken down into component parts. Random practice order (i.e., practice in which the patient switches back and forth between tasks) should be avoided in favor of a blocked practice order, thereby reducing the effects of contextual interference. Tasks should be modified to minimize competing cognitive demands. Thus the patient is instructed to avoid dual tasking in order to improve movement performance. The environment should also be modified to reduce clutter and competing attentional demands that may trigger freezing episodes. The therapist should instruct the patient to deliberately focus his or her full attention on the desired movement. Use of *structured instructional sets* has been shown to improve movement speed and consistency.[99,121] For example, walking patterns can be improved with focused instructions of "swing your arms," "walk fast," or "take large steps." For the patient with advanced disease and cognitive deficits, repetitive drill-like practice should be used along with an increased focus on caregiver training to ensure safety.[99]

External cues have been shown effective in triggering sequential movements and improving movement characteristics in individuals with mild to moderate PD (see Evidence Summary Box 21.5). *Visual cues* include stationary floor markings (e.g., brightly colored lines on the floor placed perpendicular to the gait path and spaced about one step length apart) and dynamic transportable cues (e.g., a straight cane inverted and held so the patient steps over the handle).[129–132] A subject-mounted light device (a laser device attached to the chest that projects two laser lines to the floor in front of the patient) has also been used successfully to trigger stepping.[133] Visual targets have been shown to improve stride length and velocity while cadence was relatively unchanged. Freezing episodes are also reduced with the use of visual cues.[126,130–133] UE movements were improved by reaching toward a moving target (e.g., a rolling ball descending down a track).[123] *Rhythmic auditory stimulation (RAS)* includes use of a metronome beat or a steady beat from a musical listening device. Auditory cues have also been shown to improve gait.[127,128,134–137] These stimuli appear to have a greater influence on the temporal components of movement (e.g., gait cadence, stride synchronization) rather than on spatial components. *Pulsed cues* to the earlobe or the hand, a form of tactile cueing, have also been shown to improve gait.[125] *Multisensory cueing* (use of both visual and auditory cueing) has been used for patients with PD. When sensory enhanced therapy using multisensory cueing was compared with conventional therapy, significant improvements were found in the sensory training group.[138,139] When simultaneous use of auditory and visual cues was compared to use of both cues individually, they were not found to offer significant benefit in improving gait over use of each cue alone.[140]

External cues appear to facilitate movement by utilizing different brain areas.[137] For example, the premotor cortex is active in the generation of movement in response to visual or auditory stimuli. Normally the supplementary motor area (SMA) with inputs from the BG is involved in the initiation of self-generated movements and the performance of well-learned, repetitive movement sequences.[125] External cues heighten patient attention through a common mode of action, that is, to bypass the diminished internal cueing of the basal ganglia. Thus focus is shifted to less automatic movement using alternative, more conscious motor control pathways. This is supported by the finding that when patients were requested to carry out a secondary task while walking (dual-tasking), the beneficial effects of visual and attentional cues was reduced.[126] Selection of the type of cue and successful use will depend on the individual patient. Dietz et al[131] found that the predicted long-term benefit of a particular type of cue was dependent on its initial success.

External cues are clearly not effective for all patients with PD. For patients with advanced disease and severe reductions in stride length, cueing is not effective.[133] When cueing is withheld, performance can be expected to deteriorate. Focused attention with cueing requires constant vigilance and is cognitively demanding. Thus cueing is not suitable for patients with dementia. Cueing may also not be effective when medication instability and disease fluctuations are present.[136] However, for many patients, use of external cues is a valid treatment strategy and one in which improved performance can be anticipated.[141]

Exercise Training

Relaxation Exercises

Gentle rocking can be used to produce generalized relaxation of excessive muscle tension due to rigidity. Professor Charcot, who noted dramatic improvement in patients with PD following rides in bumpy, horse-drawn carriages, first described this effect almost 100 years ago in Paris. Following this observation he constructed a vibrating chair to use with his patients.[142] Although the exact mechanism underlying rigidity has not been identified, the beneficial effects of slow rocking on excess tone have been demonstrated.[143,144] Following Charcot's lead, a rocking chair can be used to temporarily reduce rigidity and enhance sit-to-stand transfers. During therapy, slow, rhythmic, rotational movements of the extremities and trunk can be considered and should precede interventions such as ROM, stretching, and functional training.[145] For example, hooklying, lower trunk rotation, or sidelying rolling, or upper and lower trunk segmental rotations can be used to promote relaxation. The

(text continues on page 876)

Evidence Summary Box 21.5

External Cues and Motor Performance in Patients with Parkinson's Disease

Reference	Subjects	Design/Intervention	Duration	Results
Lehman, D, et al[121] 2005	Part 1: 5 subjects, no controls Part 2: 11 subjects with early stage PD (Hoehn & Yahr Stage 2–2.5; UPDRS scores 1–2); normal mentation (MMSE) Patients stable, within 1–2 hours on PD meds Training group = 6 Control group = 5	Nonexperimental, cohort study Protocol: Exp. group: walked 30 ft using verbal cuing "take long steps" 10 times/session; Control group: walking with no verbal cueing Outcome measures: step length, velocity, and cadence, preferred walking (Gait Rite® electronic walkway).	3 training sets/day for 10 days	Significantly increased gait velocity and step length and reduced cadence; significant effects noted in both groups but more pronounced in exp. group
Mak, M, and Hue-Chan, C,[122] 2004	15 subjects with PD (Hoehn & Yahr Stage severity score of 2.5) Patients stable, within 1 hour on PD medication 15 healthy controls matched for age, gender, weight, height (no PD)	Nonexperimental, cohort study Protocol: 2 conditions of sit-to-stand (STS) (1) self-initiated; (2) using auditory cues (verbal commands) and visual cues (circular light at eye level) Outcome measures: force through feet (force plate); kinematic analysis of movements (reflective markers, high speed video camera)	2 test trials: STS, self-initiated STS, cue-initiated	PD group: STS-self-initiated had signif. dec. in hip flexion and ankle dorsiflexion torques; dec. horizontal and vertical velocities; prolonged movement time to complete STS STS—cued signif. inc. all torque values; time to peak torque reduced by 23–27%; no improvement in peak velocity; signif. dec movement time. Control group: STS— cued had small but signif. inc. knee ext torque
Majsak, M, et al[123] 1998	6 subjects with PD (Hoehn & Yahr Stage 3) 6 healthy controls (no PD disease)	Nonexperimental, cohort study Protocol: 2 conditions of reaching task (1) self-regulated reach and grasp stationary ball as fast as possible; (2) reach and grasp a rolling ball (visually cued) Outcome measures: 2-dimensional kinematic analysis of reaching movements (video camera, reflective markers)	6 practice trials; 6 test trials	PD group: in response to visually cued target, inc. speed and acceleration of reaching (comparable to control group); decreased movement time; movement accuracy maintained Healthy controls had comparable reaching times under both conditions
McIntosh, G, Flanagan, J, and Gentile, A[124] 1995	31 subjects with PD (Hoehn & Yahr Stages II, III, and IV): 21 on meds within 1 – 1 1/2 hours of dosing; 10 "off" meds (24 hours after last dose) 10 healthy controls	Nonexperimental, cohort study Protocol: 4 conditions of walking: (1) self-selected speed; (2) with rhythmic auditory stimulation (RAS) matched to baseline cadence; (3) RAS 10% faster than baseline; (4) without RAS RAS = instrumental music, 50 msec square wave Outcome measures: gait velocity, cadence, stride length (computerized foot switch system)	Warm-up 2-min walk, 20 m 4 gait trials, each 30-m walk	Faster RAS produced significant improvement in mean gait velocity, cadence, and stride length of all groups. No RAS: all PD patients showed abnormal gait patterns: "off" group > than "on" group Inc. in gait velocity, cadence, and stride length persisted during last uncued walking trial with only a small decay rate (1–5%)

Evidence Summary Box 21.5

External Cues and Motor Performance in Patients with Parkinson's Disease (continued)

Reference	Subjects	Design/Intervention	Duration	Results
Burleigh-Jacobs, A, et al[125] 1997	6 subjects with PD (Hoehn & Yahr Stages III–IV when off) Tested both "off" meds (overnight) and "on" meds (within 1 hour of dosing) 2 healthy matched controlled	Nonexperimental, cohort study Protocol: 3 test conditions (1) self-generated step; (2) step to cue (pulsed cue to earlobe or hand); (3) step to perturbation (horizontal backward surface translation) Outcome measures: ground reaction forces (force plate); body kinematics—COM position, step length (motion analysis system)	5 practice trials; 1 test trial	When "off," all PD patients had marked difficulty walking with freezing episodes compared to "on" and healthy controls. Both PD and normal subjects inc. force and velocity of movement in response to cutaneous cueing. Step to perturbation: both PD and normal subjects improve speed of postural adjustments; PD subjects did not inc. force of push-off.
Morris, M, et al[126] 1996	54 subjects with PD	Nonexperimental cohort study 3 trials: walking with use of (1) visual floor markers (2) attentional strategies (3) secondary tasks of inc. levels of complexity Outcome measures: computerized stride analysis: spatial (distance) and temporal (timing) parameters	20 min training using repeat 10 m walks, set at control stride length Gait patterns monitored every 15 min for 2 hours	Both visual cues and attentional strategies were effective in producing a normal stride length. Secondary tasks reduced stride length.
Thaut, M, et al[127] 1996	Exp. group: 15 subjects with PD 2 control groups: 11 subjects	Nonexperimental, cohort study Exp. group: training with rhythmic auditory stimulation (RAS) Control groups: self-paced training, and no training RAS = instrumental music Outcome measures: EMG patterns, gait velocity, cadence, stride length (computerized foot switch system)	3-week home-based gait training program	Patients who trained with RAS signif. improved gait velocity (25%), stride length (12%), and step cadence (10%) more than self-paced subjects. No-training group dec. velocity by 7%. In RAS group, signif. changes in EMG patterns.
Freeman, J, et al[128] 1993	9 subjects with PD, on routine medication; mild to moderate impairment 12 healthy controls	Nonexperimental, cohort study Protocol: 2 conditions (1) auditory cues of target tapping frequencies over 30-s period; (2) auditory cues of target tapping frequencies first 10 sec only (30-s period) Outcome measures: Finger tapping test (computer analysis of frequency); tremor recordings	4 trials: 2 each hand	Healthy controls were able to duplicate target frequencies and sustain frequencies during withdrawal of stimulation. PD patients less accurate in duplicating target frequencies, especially at lower and higher end of frequencies; withdrawal of auditory stimulation resulted in marked impairment of rhythm.

COM = center of mass; COP = center of pressure; dec. = decrease; inc. = increase; meds = medications; MMSE = Mini-Mental State Exam; PD = Parkinson's disease; RAS = rhythmic auditory stimulation; signif. = significant; UPDRS = Unified Parkinson Disease Rating Scale.

PNF technique of *rhythmic initiation (RI)*, in which movement progresses from passive to active-assistive to lightly resisted or active movement was specifically designed to help overcome the effects of rigidity in PD.[146]

Additional strategies to promote relaxation include an emphasis on diaphragmatic breathing during exercise. For example, bilateral symmetrical PNF D2 flexion patterns are important patterns that can be used to expand the restricted chest and promote shoulder ROM. The patient's attention can be focused on deep inspiration during D2F ("breathe in deeply") while during D2E patterns attention is focused on expiration ("breathe out deeply").[146] Patients may also benefit from cognitive imaging or meditation techniques (e.g., the relaxation response of Benson[147]) or conscious recognition and release of muscle tension (e.g., progressive relaxation techniques[148]). Relaxation audiotapes can be used at home as part of the home exercise program (HEP). Gentle yoga and Tai Chi can be effective for patients with PD because of the emphasis on combining slow, steady stretching with maintenance of postures and movement forms.

Stress management techniques are an important adjunct to relaxation training. A daily schedule needs to be planned to accommodate the restrictions of the disease and the functional needs of the patient. Lifestyle modifications and time management techniques reduce anxiety associated with movement difficulties and prolonged times required to complete basic functional tasks.

Flexibility Exercises

Both active and passive ROM exercises are used to improve flexibility. Ideally ROM exercises emphasize active motions that are performed two to three times a day. Exercises should focus on strengthening the weak, elongated extensor muscles, while lengthening the shortened, tight flexor muscles. Passive ROM exercises work within the patient's available ROM to maintain range. Because these patients have a minimum of energy to expend and multiple clinical problems, they may benefit from ROM exercises in physiological patterns of motion. For example, PNF patterns combine several motions at once while emphasizing rotation, a movement component typically lost early in PD. In the upper extremities, bilateral symmetrical D2 flexion patterns are ideal in promoting upper trunk extension and in counteracting kyphosis. In the lower extremities, hip and knee extension should be emphasized, ideally in a D1 extension pattern (hip extension, abduction, internal rotation) to counteract the typical flexed, adducted position of the lower extremities. Specific muscle contractures may respond to active muscle inhibition techniques such as the PNF hold–relax (HR) or contract–relax (CR) techniques.[146] Of the two, CR is the preferred technique because it combines autogenic inhibition from isometric contraction of the tight agonist muscle with active rotations of the limb. ROM exercises should also emphasize restoring range in the neck and trunk and can be performed in combination with rotational exercises to promote relaxation.

Traditional stretching techniques can also be used to elongate muscles. Special consideration should be given to the gentle stretching of elbow flexors, hip and knee flexors, and ankle plantarflexors. Stretching can be combined with joint mobilization techniques to reduce tightness of the joint capsule or of ligaments around a joint. By using selected grades of accessory movement, both improved ROM and decreased pain can be achieved.[149] Stretching techniques are an important component of the HEP. The patient and caregiver should be instructed in the appropriate stretching exercises and the importance of maintaining the stretch force for at least 20 to 30 seconds. Ideally the stretches are repeated at least three to five times. Ballistic stretches (high-intensity bouncing stretches) should be avoided because they are linked to increased injury. Muscle tears or ruptures of weakened tissues are especially prevalent in elderly, sedentary individuals. Vigorous stretching can stimulate pain receptors and cause rebound muscle contraction. Patients with PD who are elderly and have long-standing disease must be considered at risk for osteoporosis and therefore must be stretched accordingly. The therapist should also use caution when stretching edematous tissue, a common lower extremity (LE) problem associated with immobility as risk of injury is also increased in this situation.[150]

Passive positioning, a long duration technique to improve flexibility, can also be used to stretch tight muscles and soft tissues. Patients in late-stage PD are likely to demonstrate severe flexion contractures of the trunk and limbs. The "phantom pillow" posture may develop in supine; that is, the head and shoulders are flexed as if there were a pillow present. Early on, the patient may benefit from daily positioning in pronelying. As the disease progresses and significant postural deformity and cardiorespiratory impairments develop, the patient may not tolerate this position. The patient with a developing lateral curvature can be positioned in sidelying with a small pillow under the lateral trunk. Mechanical low load stretching can also be used. For example, the patient who is bedridden may benefit from weights applied to reduce hip and knee flexion contractures. This approach utilizes a weighted pulley and traction setup with low load weights (e.g., 5 to 15 lbs or 5 to 10 percent of body weight). The stretch is prolonged, with times ranging from 20 to 30 minutes to several hours. Additional mechanical stretching can be achieved through the use of a tilt table, for example, the patient is positioned with fixed leg straps to reduce hip and knee flexion contractures and toe wedges to reduce plantarflexion contractions.[150]

Strength Training

Strengthening exercises are indicated for patients with primary muscle weakness and insufficient central activation of the motor unit as well as for disuse weakness associated with prolonged inactivity. Specific effects of weakness include postural changes (e.g., a flexed, stooped posture) and functional deficits (e.g., inability to get out of a chair). Weakness also contributes to postural instability, falls, and fall injury as well as increased sense of effort.[151] The benefits of strength training in the frail elderly have been well documented by the Frailty and Injuries: Cooperative Studies of Intervention Techniques (FICSIT) trials.[152–155] Collectively these studies have shown that the frail elderly improve on measures of strength, functional mobility, balance, gait, fall risk, and quality of life following interventions that include strength training. Strength training has also been shown to improve strength and motor function in patients with mild to moderate PD.[156–158] Hirsch et al[157] compared two different exercise training programs for patients with PD. They found significantly greater improvements in balance and strength using a combined program of balance training and high-intensity resistance training for knee extensors and flexors, and ankle plantarflexors as compared to balance training alone.

While patients with mild to moderate PD can benefit from exercise training to improve strength and power as well as subjective well-being, specific guidelines for exercise prescription are lacking. Corcos et al[25] found a significant interaction between medication and strength. Withdrawal of L-dopa during an "off" state period caused a decrease in strength and rate of force development. Exercise training should therefore optimally be timed for "on" periods when the patient is at his or her best (i.e., 45 minutes to 1 hour after medication has been taken). Exercising during an "off" period may not be possible or pose great difficulty for the patient. The patient should consistently exercise at the same time after a medication dose on alternate days. Greater changes have also been noted in force production during isokinetic contractions rather than isometric contractions. As patients with PD already demonstrate too much coactivation, isometric training may be contraindicated. Exercise machines may be safer than free weights as the movements are more controlled, especially for the patient who demonstrates dyskinesias at peak dose or cognitive changes.[159] Functional training activities (see next section) and pool exercises are also effective interventions to improve strength.

Functional Training

An exercise program should be based on focused practice of functional skills. The overall emphasis is on improving mobility function with specific emphasis on improving mobility of axial structures, the head, trunk, hips, and shoulders. Progression to more difficult motor activities should be gradual. The more severely involved patient may benefit initially from assisted movements progressing to active movements (e.g., the PNF technique of RI) to improve initial motor performance.[160]

Moving in bed (i.e., rolling, supine-to-sit transitions) are essential skills that are often very difficult owing to truncal rigidity and bradykinesia. Sidelying rolling activities that emphasize segmental rotation patterns (i.e., isolated upper and lower trunk rotations) should be practiced rather than a log-rolling pattern. Patients with very stiff trunks may benefit from compensatory rolling strategies using the UE or LE to reach over and initiate the movement (e.g., D1F patterns of the UE or LE). Rolling should be practiced on different surfaces progressing from firm to soft and finally simulating the patient's bed surface at home. Transitions to sitting that utilize the sidelying-on-elbow position as an interim posture improve the level of trunk rotation and lateral flexion and should be practiced.

Sitting posture can be facilitated through exercises designed to improve pelvic mobility as the patient with PD typically sits with a stiff and posteriorly tilted pelvis (i.e., sacral sitting position) along with a flexed upper trunk. Anterior and posterior tilts, side-to-side tilts, pelvic clock exercises can be practiced while sitting on a therapy ball. These activities can then be progressed to sitting on a stationary surface such as a mat table using an inflatable disc to finally no apparatus. Sitting activities should include weight shifting emphasizing upper trunk rotations and reaching. PNF extremity patterns in sitting can be used to enhance trunk mobility. For example, bilateral symmetrical UE D2F and D2E patterns are ideal to promote upper trunk extension. Or a lift/reverse lift pattern can be used to promote upper trunk extension with rotation.

Sit-to-stand transitions are also very difficult for many patients with PD. Initial rocking forward and backward can be used to promote relaxation and enhance the patient's ability to move weight forward. The patient should be instructed to scoot forward to the edge of the seat and tuck the feet underneath. Cueing strategies such as counting can be used to assist forward rocking movements. Practice from a firm raised seat can help promote ease of rise. Progression is then to lower, standard height seats. Strengthening of the hip and knee extensors can be achieved using modified wall squats and can be an important preparatory lead-up activity to sit-to-stand training. Standing up to a modified plantigrade position with the UEs extended forward on a wall (shoulders flexed to 90° and hands weightbearing) can be used to improve initial stability in standing for the patient who is unable to stop forward progression.

Standing training activities can model the progression used in sitting. The patient needs to first gain the fully upright position with symmetrical weightbearing over the base of support (BOS). Tactile cueing or light resistance to hip extensors on the anterior pelvis can be used to promote full extension in standing. Once standing, weight shifts and rotational movements of the trunk should be practiced (e.g., reciprocal arm swings or reaching movements). Weight shifting and stepping movements that incorporate pelvic rotation should also be practiced. Lateral side steps or step-ups using a low platform step can be used to improve abductor function. Standing with UEs extended and hands weightbearing on a wall can be used to promote upper trunk extension (e.g., standing wall push-ups or corner push-ups).

Patients with PD typically experience a high number of falls and should be taught how to get up after a fall. To that end, skills in quadruped creeping should be practiced so the patient is able to move to a nearby stable chair or couch at home. The patient should also practice transitions moving from quadruped to kneeling to half-kneeling and finally to standing using UE support.

Mobilizing facial muscles is another important component of the exercise program because the patient will have limited social interaction and poor feeding skills in the presence of marked facial rigidity and bradykinesia. These factors can greatly influence the patient's overall psychological state, motivation, and social participation. Use of massage, stretch, manual contacts, and verbal cueing can be used to enhance facial movements. The patient can be instructed to practice lip pursing, movements of the tongue, swallowing, and facial movements such as smiling, frowning, and so forth. A mirror can be used to provide visual feedback. In cases where eating is impaired by immobility, the movements of opening and closing the mouth and chewing should be combined with neck stabilization in a neutral position. Verbal skills should be practiced in association with breath control.

Adaptive and Supportive Devices

Attention should be directed toward needs for adaptive and supportive devices that can improve function. To promote bed mobility, the patient can be helped to assume a sitting position by elevating the head of the bed with commercially available blocks of approximately 4 in. (10 cm), or by using an electronic hospital bed. A simpler solution might include attaching a knotted rope to the end of the bed to pull on. The bed should be stable and the mattress firm to facilitate mobility. Satin sheets and pajamas have sometimes been helpful to enhance bed mobility. Patients should be instructed to select firm chairs with armrests and avoid soft, low seats such as a low sofa. The chair can be raised (i.e., 4 in. [10 cm] and secured with blocks, or tilted forward by elevating only the back legs about 2 in. [5 cm]). Some patients benefit from the use of a rocking chair to facilitate independent sit-to-stand transfers. Chairs that have spring-loaded seats that push the patient into standing are heavily marketed to the geriatric population but should be used with caution. The patient is propelled into standing but may have difficulty stopping the movement and/or getting his or her balance within an appropriate time frame when first reaching the standing position. A raised toilet seat and toilet rails are also essential devices to facilitate ease of sit-to-stand transitions in the bathroom.

Loose-fitting clothing and sneakers with Velcro® closures can be used to facilitate dressing. If the patient demonstrates a shuffling gait, shoes should have leather or hard composition soles, because shoes with crepe or rubber soles will not slide easily and can result in falls. A festinating gait can sometimes be alleviated by the addition of modified heel or shoe wedges. A flat heel or toe wedge may slow down a propulsive gait, whereas a raised heel or heel wedge may diminish a retropulsive gait pattern. The use of assistive devices can be problematic owing to movement difficulties. A cane or walker can be helpful for patients with mild to moderate disease to assist in balance or cue stepping (inverted walking stick). It is important that the height of the device not promote increased flexion of the trunk. Vertical poles can also be helpful during walking (i.e., pole striding) to improve upright posture during walking. Patients with more pronounced movement difficulties and poor balance are not likely to benefit from assistive devices. Walkers with wheels are particularly hazardous, and are likely to increase a festinating gait; hand brakes are an essential requirement.

Most patients use adaptive devices to assist in ADL. Reachers can be used to provide assistance in dressing as well as for other activities. Eating can be facilitated in a number of ways. The patient should be seated properly, close to the table, with good posture. Specially adapted utensils, plate guards, and enlarged handles can aid the patient's efforts. Because eating time will be prolonged, heated plates or pads may help keep food warm and palatable. Drooling and/or spills should be anticipated and clothing protected. Extra time should be planned, and the patient should not feel rushed.

Balance Training

It is important to recall that learning is task and context specific. Thus, a balance training program should include a variety of activities that alter task demands and expose the patient to varying environmental conditions. Whenever possible the therapist should try to duplicate the conditions the patient will encounter in everyday life. The level of challenge is important. A therapist should know the limitations of the patient and the specific demands of the task and environment in order to select and progress tasks accordingly and ensure patient safety. The reader is referred to Chapter 13 for a more complete discussion of balance and gait training.

An important focus of balance training for the patient with PD is center-of-mass (COM) and limits of stability (LOS) control training. Patients should be instructed in how COM influences balance and how to improve posture in sitting, standing, and during dynamic movement tasks.[95] Patients should also explore their LOS and practice working toward expanding them in both sitting and standing. In standing, patients with PD typically demonstrate restricted LOS with forward displacement of center of foot pressure. Patients should be instructed in how to improve postural alignment and in ways to avoid postural disturbances and falls. The therapist can assist with postural and safety awareness by using appropriate verbal, tactile or proprioceptive cues to facilitate the desired responses. For example, the patient is instructed to "sit tall" or "stand tall" and a mirror is used to provide feedback concerning upright posture. A standing platform training device (i.e., posturography system) can be valuable in providing COM position and LOS biofeedback.

Balance training should emphasize practice of dynamic stability tasks (e.g., weight shifts, reaching, axial rotation of the head and trunk, axial rotation combined with reaching, and so forth). Seated activities can include sitting on a compliant surface (inflatable disc) or a therapy ball. Challenges to balance can be introduced by varying arm position (i.e., arms out to side, arms folded across chest), varying foot/leg position (i.e., feet apart, feet together) or adding voluntary movements (e.g., arm clapping, arms overhead, single leg raises, head and trunk rotations). In addition, balance can be challenged by the addition of stepping or marching in place, and functional reach. Movement transitions such as sit-to-stand or half-kneeling-to-standing can also be used to challenge the postural control system. Training should focus on achieving faster initiation and execution movement times supported by the use of appropriate cueing strategies.[118] Externally induced perturbations in the form of gentle manual displacements of the patient's COM are generally contraindicated for many patients with PD as they can produce an increase in postural stiffness and fixation. Strategies for varying environmental demands include altering the support surface (e.g., standing on foam), visual inputs (e.g., reduced lighting, eyes closed), or challenging the patient with a variable open environment (e.g., busy clinic setting).

Adequate strength and ROM are important components needed to withstand the challenges of balance. The patient can be instructed in standing exercises to enhance balance, including heel-rises and toe-offs, partial wall squats and chair rises, single-limb stance with side-kicks or back-kicks, and marching in place. Collectively these exercises are sometimes referred to as the *"kitchen sink exercises"* and are important components of the HEP for patients with balance deficiencies. The patient is instructed to maintain light touch-down support of the hands in order to stabilize and progresses from bilateral support to unilateral.

Locomotor Training

Locomotor training focuses on primary gait impairments which typically include slowed speed, shuffling gait pattern, diminished arm swing and trunk movements, and an overall attitude of flexion while walking. Training programs are designed to lengthen stride, broaden base of support, improve stepping, improve heel–toe gait pattern, increase contralateral trunk movement and arm swing, increase speed, and provide a program of regular walking.

Strategies for improving upright alignment include having the patient walk with vertical poles (pole walking) and verbal cues to "walk tall." Gait training using an overhead harness also assists upright posture. The harness eliminates the need for UE weightbearing inherent with the use of assistive devices, a practice that promotes the forward flexed posture. The harness also protects patients from falls and allows faster speeds than normally achieved. In studies of patients with PD that combined use of an overhead harness with walking on a motorized treadmill, both walking speed and stride length were improved.[161,162] Miyai et al[162] provided support for up to 20 percent of body weight while Pohl et al[161] used the harness for safety and did not support patient weight. In a follow-up study, Miyai et al[163] found that gains in walking speed and number of steps following this type of training were maintained at 4 months. The researchers state that attentional strategies were not used and speculate that the enhancement of gait might be due to activation of central pattern generators as is thought the case in stroke and SCI studies.

Gait training strategies to normalize step length, velocity, and arm swing excursion include the use of verbal instructional sets (e.g., "walk fast," "take large steps," "walk while swinging both arms"). Behrman et al[164] found that commands for large step and arm swing were more effective instructional strategies than the command to walk fast. As previously discussed, visual and auditory cues are also effective in improving gait speed and step length. Strategies to improve foot placement can include use of floor grids or footprints on the floor. Strategies to improve step height include practice of marching in place progressing to walking using an exaggerated high stepping pattern. Brisk marching music can be used to enhance pace. Sidestepping and crossed-step walking should be practiced. The PNF activity of braiding, which combines sidestepping with alternate crossed-stepping, is an ideal training activity for the patient with PD because it emphasizes lower trunk rotation with stepping and side-stepping movements. It can be practiced with the patient holding on lightly to a dowel held jointly with therapist or as a free walking pattern. Two dowels (held by the patient and therapist, one in each hand) can be used to facilitate reciprocal arm swing during gait. The therapist uses his or her arm swing to assist the patient's. Task specific training should also include practice in changing directions, turns, and negotiating obstacles.

Strategies for varying environmental demands include altering the support surface (e.g., walking on a tile floor to walking on carpet, to walking outdoors on a grassy terrain), and stepping on and off varied surfaces (e.g., foam). Visual inputs should be varied (e.g., reduced lighting, eyes closed). The patient should be challenged with walking in a variable open environment (e.g., community walking). The patient can also practice stair climbing, up and down curbs, and ramp walking.

Patients in the advanced stage of the disease will be limited in terms of the task and environmental variations that can be utilized. The overall goal is to promote regular walking while maintaining safety and preventing falls. Compensatory training strategies are indicated. Freezing episodes are common and are often resistant to drug therapy. The therapist and patient should identify and practice strategies for unfreezing gait. For example, rotational stimulation or "trick" movements such as dropping a tissue that the patient must step over can be successful in reducing freezing.[165]

Cardiopulmonary Training

Respiratory dysfunction is linked to morbidity and mortality in patients with PD. Both obstructive and restrictive ventilatory deficits are present as the disease becomes more advanced.[58,166] For these patients, a comprehensive pulmonary rehabilitation program should be instituted. Components include diaphragmatic breathing exercises, air-shifting techniques, and exercises that recruit neck, shoulder, and trunk muscles. The patient should be instructed in deep breathing exercises to improve chest wall mobility and vital capacity. Air shifts are promoted to lesser-ventilated areas of the lung. For example, basal expansion can be promoted using manual stretch and resistance to those segments. Upper body resistance training exercises are indicated. These can include raising and lowering a dowel with light weights added to increase resistance (e.g., 1 lb [453.5 g]). Weights are increased as function improves. As previously mentioned, chest wall mobility can be improved by using PNF UE bilateral symmetrical D2 flexion and extension patterns. Light weights (wrist cuffs) can also be added to these exercises. Patients are encouraged to coordinate breathing with UE movement. Exercises are performed in unsupported sitting to promote trunk stabilization. A focus on improving trunk extension is especially important in improving breathing patterns in patients with postural kyphosis. Pulmonary training programs have been shown to be safe and effective for patients with PD in improving pulmonary function (i.e., oxygen consumption [VO_2], minute ventilation [V_E], respiratory rate, inspiratory muscle strength)[167,168] and perception of dyspnea.[169]

Individuals with mild to moderate PD demonstrate a maximal exercise capacity that is similar to healthy adults.[58,59] They also demonstrate a peak aerobic capacity that occurs at a lower work level than healthy adults.[60] Standardized graded exercise testing can be used to safely determine the patient's level of fitness prior to commencing an aerobic exercise program.[59] An individualized exercise prescription is developed based on the ACSM guidelines for frequency, intensity, duration, and progression.[170] Intensities will be less than normal training intensities or submaximal (i.e., 55 to 65 percent of maximum heart rate or 40 to 50 percent oxygen uptake reserve) for the patient with a low-fitness level, sedentary lifestyle, and moderate disease. When lower intensities are used, longer-duration or more frequent exercise sessions are necessary to improve fitness. Careful monitoring is indicated, as autonomic dysfunction is common. L-Dopa can produce arrhythmias and orthostatic hypotension along with dyskinesias. The therapist should monitor ECG changes, heart rate, blood pressure, RPE, fatigue levels, and symptoms of exertional intolerance (e.g., significant dyspnea, hypotensive response, serious dysrhythmias, and so forth). Training modes typically include LE ergometry, UE ergometry, and walking. Selection will depend on the specific abilities of the patient; for example, postural instability and increased risk of falls may rule out use of a treadmill without an overhead harness. Recumbent or seated LE ergometry is a suitable alternative. For most patients a program of regular walking is recommended. The duration, speed, and terrain covered can be modified, based on individual ability. Accessibility to a supervised walking program using an indoor walking track is important for some to ensure safety. For outdoor walkers, a shopping mall can provide an acceptable environment in case of inclement weather. A supervised aerobic pool program can also provide an acceptable mode for some patients. The warmth of the water may be relaxing and the buoyancy may enhance movement. The minimum recommended exercise frequency is 3 to 5 days per week. Daily walking with short bouts throughout the day is recommended for individuals with lower functional capacity. Intermittent exercise with repetitive exercise-rest periods is indicated for those patients who are elderly and deconditioned, and who present with pulmonary dysfunction. Aerobic training programs have been shown to be safe and effective for patients with PD in improving aerobic capacity.[58,155,169]

Group and Home Exercises

Group exercise classes can be valuable for patients with PD. Patients benefit from the positive support, camaraderie, and communication the group situation offers. Careful evaluation of each patient prior to admission into a group is essential. Patients should be able to perform the therapeutic core of the class. Selecting patients with similar levels of disability is often advisable because the sense of competition can frequently be a key factor in motivating groups. The ratio of staff to patients should be kept small (ideally 1:8 or 1:10), and extra staff should be added if patients are unable to work on their own. A variety of activities can be used to stimulate and motivate patients. The patients can begin in the seated position and progress to standing, using light, touch-down support of the back of the chair. Stretching exercises or calisthenics involving large joints can be used as initial warm-up activities. Progression is to combination movements (upper and lower extremities with axial trunk rotation). Well-structured, low-impact aerobics are an appropriate focus for a group class. For example, patients can march in place, first in sitting, then in standing. The group can then practice walking with an emphasis on taking large, high steps. Music is used to provide necessary stimulation to movement and movement pacing. Exercise stations (e.g., stationary bicycle, mats, pulleys, and so forth) can also be used. Exercises done by the whole group together should focus on important exercise goals (e.g., improving ROM, mobility, and so forth). Recreational activities can follow the aerobic portion, such as line dancing, ball activities, beanbag toss, and so forth. The activities selected should be interesting and varied. Finally, a relaxation training segment should be incorporated into each class.[171]

The HEP includes many of the interventions already discussed, with exercises designed to improve relaxation, flexibility, strength, and cardiopulmonary function. A key element is stressing the importance of regular daily exercise and avoidance of prolonged periods of inactivity. The HEP should be realistic and of moderate duration and intensity. The patient should be cautioned against overdoing activity, which could result in excessive fatigue. Early morning warm-up calisthenics are often helpful in reducing the increased stiffness patients may experience upon arising. Stretching and strengthening exercises are performed in supine, sitting, and standing positions. Home ROM exercises can often be assisted by use of adaptive equipment. For example, to reduce the effects of forward head and kyphotic posture, the patient can be instructed to hang by the hands using an overhead bar. Standing, corner wall stretches can also be used to provide a maintained stretch on the upper trunk flexors. Use of a wand or cane can be effective in promoting overhead motions. In standing, a countertop or back of a sturdy chair can be used to assist in stabilization during standing calisthenics and balance activities.[172] Lun et al[173] compared the effectiveness of a self-supervised home exercise program with a physical therapist-supervised exercise program and found both were equally effective in improving motor symptoms in PD.

Psychosocial Issues

The progressive nature of PD necessitates frequent personal and social adjustments, and affects all aspects of life for both the patient and family. Disruption in daily functions, roles, and activities are experienced. Some of the changes associated with PD are socially isolating (masked face, progressive immobility, and unintelligible speech) whereas other changes (increased salivation, perspiration, decreased sexual function) are distressing and can be socially embarrassing. The patient may feel increasingly isolated and family relationships may suffer. Depression is extremely common.[174] A comprehensive evaluation is needed to determine each individual's unique situation and emotional resources.

The principal goal for team members is to assist the patient and family in their understanding of the disease and in developing insights and adjustments that lead to more effective self-management. Some individuals are able to successfully deal with the changes associated with the disease; others are not. Coping skills can be facilitated. First and foremost education is the key to assisting patients and family members assume responsibility. Feelings of hopelessness and dependency are reduced as the patient develops a sense of control over his or her own life. Self-management skills that should be promoted include advanced planning of activities, effective time management strategies, and stress management techniques. It is equally important to ensure that patients do not become isolated and that appropriate services are available. Team members must be vigilant regarding their assumptions and expectations. A condescending or pessimistic and limiting attitude can become a self-fulfilling prophecy. Patients and family members need reassurances and encouragement. An overall emphasis on what patients *can do* rather than what they cannot do helps to empower patients. Therapists need to provide a message of *hope tempered with realism.*

Patient, Family and Caregiver Education

The interdisciplinary team provides information about a variety of topics related to living with PD. These are presented in Box 21.6. Interventions can take the form of direct one-on-one instruction, group sessions, printed materials, and video or computer presentations. The therapist's overall approach needs to be positive and supportive.

Box 21.6 Elements of a Patient, Family and Caregiver Education Program

- Parkinson's disease: clinical presentation, strategies to manage symptoms
- Medications: purpose, dosage, possible adverse side effects, signs of either over- or undermedication
- Preventative measures to minimize the secondary complications and impairments
- Impact of PD on movement and effective strategies to manage movement problems
- Barriers to exercise and effective solutions to regular exercise participation
- Impact of PD on function and effective strategies to maintain independent function in home, community, or work environments.
- Strategies for energy conservation and activity pacing
- Strategies for ensuring activity participation in valued leisure and family activities
- Community resources for patients: support groups, in-home interventions, community training programs, day programs
- Community resources for caregivers: counseling, support groups, exercise programs, respite care

Community support groups are available for patients and their families. They disseminate information and offer a chance to discuss common issues, problems, and management tips. They also can provide a stabilizing influence, assisting patients and families to focus on healthy behaviors, coping skills, and effective self-management. For some patients in the early stages of the disease, participation in a support group may increase levels of anxiety as they observe more disabled patients. Groups particularly targeted to patients with early stage disease and similar ages may be more helpful.

Educational pamphlets, newsletters, and location of support groups can be obtained through national PD associations.

National Parkinson Foundation (NPF)
1501 Northwest 9th Street (Bob Hope Road)
Miami, FL 33136-1407
Web site: http://www.parkinson.org
Ph: (800) 327-4545
E-mail: mailbox@parkinson.org

Parkinson's Disease Foundation (PDF)
1359 Broadway, Suite 1509
New York, NY 10018
Web site: www.pdf.org
Ph: (800) 457-6676
E-mail: info@pdf.org

The American Parkinson Disease Association (APDA)
1250 Hylan Boulevard Suite 4-B
Staten Island, New York 10305
Web site: http://www.apdaparkinson.org
Ph: (800) 223-2732
E-mail: apda@apdaparkinson.org

Web-based resources for clinicians and patients/families living with PD are presented in Appendix B. A listing of sample educational and video materials can be found in Supplemental Readings and Materials.

Management Considerations by Stage of Disease

In the early stages of the disease, patients are functional and independent. They are typically seen on an outpatient basis. Medical therapies may include the administration of Selegiline to stay the need for L-dopa and other drugs designed to provide symptomatic relief. A referral for physical therapy is often delayed at this stage, although benefits could clearly be obtained. During the early stages, interventions are indicated that focus on prevention or reversal of musculoskeletal and cardiorespiratory impairments and improvement of general health status. Early education for patient and family can provide meaningful assistance in understanding the disease and its ramifications. Early referral to support groups is also helpful.[67]

During the middle stages of the disease, symptoms are more readily apparent and functional limitations emerge. The patient may still be independent in gait and many ADL, although performance is slowed and less efficient. Some assistance may be required. Treatment with L-dopa is typically delayed until the early middle stages, although individual differences exist. Once placed on L-dopa patients may exhibit a dramatic improvement in symptoms, most notably in rigidity and bradykinesia. The alleviation of these symptoms does not always produce a similar level of improvement in function, however; poor habits and faulty posture may have developed. Exercise training programs have been shown to be effective for patients with mild to moderate PD in improving motor performance.[157,158,175–178] Perceived quality of life and subjective well-being is also improved.[158,179] Family and caregiver instruction is intensified to assist the patient in remaining functionally mobile.

Patients with late-stage disease typically demonstrate a number of complications including pharmacological intolerance, increased primary symptoms, fixed musculoskeletal impairments, a decline in cognitive functioning, sleep disturbances, incontinence, malnutrition, significant cardiopulmonary compromise, and severe immobility. Patients are dependent in many or most of their daily functional mobility skills and ADL. They may be wheelchair bound or bedridden. Family and community resources are vital in maintaining the patient in the home. Some patients may require placement in a chronic care facility. At this stage of disease, patients generally do not respond as well to medical management and experience decreasing effectiveness of pharmacological interventions, fluctuations in performance, and adverse side effects of long-term L-dopa medication. These changes can be a source of great frustration to the patient and family. Goals and expectations need to be restructured. During late-stage disease, the therapist needs to focus on skin care to avoid breakdown and pressure wounds, pulmonary hygiene to avoid pneumonia, and assistance in positioning and feeding to avoid malnutrition, aspiration, and pneumonia. Caregiver training becomes increasingly important. Safety for both the caregiver and the patient becomes a primary concern as patients are assisted in position changes in bed or during transfers. Patients should be encouraged and assisted to maximize out-of-bed time and to move as much as possible and not allow everything to be done for them. Often, environmental adaptations may mean the difference between total dependence and partial independence. The rehabilitation team should be supportive of the patient's efforts no matter how small they may be. Patients in late-stage PD demonstrate extremely limited skills to interact with their environment, with increasing social isolation and withdrawal. Families also suffer from the increasing demands of care, burnout, and social isolation. Therapists need to maximize psychosocial support and be readily available for consultation.

Summary

PD is a chronic, progressive disorder of the basal ganglia characterized by the cardinal features of rigidity, bradykinesia, tremor, and postural instability. Additional impairments include the development of abnormal fixed postures, poverty of movement, fatigue, masked face, contractures, a festinating gait pattern, swallowing and communication difficulties, visual and sensorimotor disturbances, cognitive and behavioral dysfunction, autonomic dysfunction, and cardiopulmonary changes. Pharmacological interventions have become the mainstay of treatment and provide protective and symptomatic treatment. Effective rehabilitation focuses on the patient's stage of disease and symptoms, functional limitations, and residual abilities and assets. Interventions are restorative; that is, rehabilitation is focused on the improvement of strength, ROM, functional skills, endurance, and so forth. Individuals with PD also benefit from functional maintenance programs designed to manage the effects of progressive disease. Strategies are developed to prevent or reduce indirect impairments, and promote regular exercise, good health, and self-management skills. A comprehensive team approach including active involvement of patient and family provides optimal benefits. Team members need to be active during all stages of the disease, assisting the patient and family in maintenance of function and providing psychosocial support as needed.

Questions for Review

1. What are the major CNS structures involved in PD? How is the function of these structures altered?
2. What are the cardinal features of PD? Additional impairments and complications?
3. What components should be included in a physical therapy examination? Identify four standardized measures that would be appropriate to use with the patient with PD.
4. Describe the drug therapy used in PD. How might a physical therapy program be influenced by L-dopa drug management?
5. What are the major goals and outcomes of physical therapy intervention? How might they vary by stage of disease?
6. What are the effects of prolonged inactivity for the patient with PD? Identify three interventions that can be used to counteract these effects.
7. Identify three interventions that can be used to relax the patient and improve flexibility.
8. What interventions strategies can be used to improve cardiorespiratory fitness?
9. Describe the gait impairments common in patients with PD. What interventions can be used to improve locomotor function?
10. What types of interventions are appropriate for the patient with advanced disease who is relatively unresponsive to drug management?
11. Differentiate between a rehabilitation program with a restorative focus versus one with a functional maintenance focus. Consider goals, outcomes, and overall training approach.
12. What are the major considerations in providing psychosocial support ? Patient, family and caregiver education?

Case Study

The patient is a 60-year-old woman with a 7-year history of PD. Lately she has experienced increasing severity of symptoms and is referred for outpatient physical therapy and a home exercise program (HEP).

HISTORY

The patient first presented with tremor of her left hand that progressed to include stiffness and awkwardness of her left UE and LE. Her family physician referred her to a neurologist who found moderate tremor and rigidity on the left side. He prescribed Artane, which was helpful for a while. Eventually the tremor became worse, especially under conditions of stress when she was unable to use her left UE at all. She was then started on Sinemet and referred for an initial episode of physical therapy as an outpatient. Once Sinemet began to work and her symptoms dramatically lessened, she stopped doing her HEP. Over the next few years as her symptoms increased, her dose of Sinemet was increased.

CURRENT STATUS

The patient is currently taking Sinemet and Bromocriptine. She reports bouts of dyskinesia about 45 minutes into taking her Sinemet that involve involuntary writhing movements of her shoulders and neck. Her chief complaints are:

1. Difficulty walking, especially when she has to go through a narrow doorway, or walk in a crowded place.
2. Episodes of gait blocks; if she tries to do something while walking like take a tissue out of her pocket, she stops abruptly in her tracks. The harder she tries to move, the worse it gets. Episodes of freezing have lasted up to 20 minutes.
3. Postural instability: over the past few years she has experienced increasing bouts of uncontrolled or unsteady balance. This is particularly disturbing to her because if it occurs while she is walking, it causes her to fall. She has fallen seven times in the past month, with no residual fall injury. Because of her increased fear of falling, she has stopped going out by herself.
4. She is experiencing increased difficulty rolling over in bed, getting out of bed, and standing up from a chair independently. Her husband now has to provide assistance 90 percent of the time to accomplish these activities.
5. She reports having trouble sleeping at night. She has stopped drinking coffee but this has not helped. She wakes four to five times a night, and requires assistance from her husband to go to the bathroom at night. She also has hallucinated at night, claiming to see bugs on the wall. During these periods she becomes extremely frightened.
6. She complains her medication seems to be helping less and less. If she plans to go out, she takes an extra Sinemet. She revisited her neurologist in hopes that he would increase her dosage. Instead he told her the symptoms were most likely the result of excess medication. He instructed her not to take the extra Sinemet and has adjusted her dosage.

EXAMINATION FINDINGS

Cognition

Alert, oriented × 3; she is displaying mild impairments in short-term memory.

Psychosocial

She is showing signs of depression; she is less interested in going out and socializing; she reports "it is just too much effort."

Speech

Mild dysarthria, hypophonia.

Sensation

Slightly decreased proprioception bilaterally in both ankles; otherwise intact.

Tone

Rigidity (cogwheel type) moderate in all extremities L > R.
Marked rigidity throughout neck and trunk.
Masklike face.

ROM

Decreased due to moderate rigidity; limitations noted in:
- Bilateral elbow extension (10 to 140°)
- Bilateral hip extension (0 to 10°)
- Bilateral knee extension (10 to 120°)
- Bilateral ankle dorsiflexion (0 to 15° RLE; 0 to 10° LLE).

Strength

Generally fair (3/5) to good minus (4−/5).
Poor (2/5) dorsiflexor muscle grades noted in both ankles.

Motor Function

Moderate to severe resting tremors, L hand > R hand.
Bradykinesia: marked slowness, poverty of movement.
Hesitation on initiation of movement; frequent arrests of ongoing movement.

Posture

Forward head position; flexed; kyphotic spine.
Stands with flexion of hips and knees.

Gait

Ambulates independently with a shuffling gait pattern with decreased step length and arm, trunk, hip and knee motions; tendency for propulsive gait.
Frequent freezing of gait.

Balance

Decreased limits of stability.
Patient's forward alignment increases her tendency to fall forward.
Sitting static control: good (able to maintain balance without handhold).
Sitting dynamic control: fair (accepts minimal challenge; able to lift both arms).
Standing static control: good (able to maintain balance without handhold).
Standing dynamic control: poor (unable to accept minimal challenge without handhold).
She has slowed reactions to loss of balance with decreased rotational movements of head/trunk and ineffective use of stepping strategies.
Timed Up & Go score is 36 seconds.
Patient is fearful of falling.

Functional Mobility

Generally decreased.
Requires moderate assist: rolling in bed, supine-to-sit transfers, sit-to-stand transfers.
Unable to bridge secondary to hip flexion contractures.
Patient has good safety awareness.

Self-Care

Requires minimal assistance to supervision for feeding.
Requires minimal to moderate assist for dressing/bathing.

Cardiopulmonary Function/Endurance

Shallow (upper respiratory) breathing pattern.
Generally decreased functional capacity (estimated functional work capacity [FWC] is 6 metabolic equivalents [METs]).
Patient fatigues easily and requires frequent rest periods.
Mild edema both ankles.

Skin

Intact, no areas of breakdown.
Experiences bouts of increased perspiration.

GUIDING QUESTIONS

1. Identify/categorize this patient's problems in terms of:
   a. Direct impairments
   b. Indirect impairments
   c. Functional limitations
   d. Activity restrictions/disability
2. Identify two outcomes (the remediation of functional limitations and disability) and two goals (remediation of impairments) for this patient.
3. Determine four treatment interventions that could be used at the start of therapy to achieve the outcomes and goals provided for question 2. Provide a brief rationale for each.
4. What motor learning strategies would you use to assist in improving her motor function?
5. What strategies would you use to assist in the development of self-management skills and to promote quality of life?

References

1. Rajput, M, and Rajput, A: Epidemiology of Parkinsonism. In Factor, S, and Weiner, W (eds): Parkinson's Disease—Diagnosis and Clinical Management. Demos Medical Publishung, New York, 2002, p 31.
2. Parkinson, J: An Essay on the Shaking Palsy. Sherwood Neely & Jones, London, 1817.
3. Zetusky, W, et al: The heterogeneity of Parkinson's disease: Clinical and prognostic implications. Neurology 35:522, 1985.
4. Koller, W: Classification of Parkinsonism. In Koller, W (ed): Handbook of Parkinson's Disease. Marcel Dekker, New York, 1987, p 51.
5. Sacks, O: Awakenings. HarperCollins, New York, 1990.
6. Langston, JW, and Ballard, P: Chronic parkinsonism in humans due to a product of meperidine-analog synthesis. Science 219:976, 1983.
7. Pal P, Samii, A, and Calne, D: Cardinal features of early Parkinson's disease. In Factor, S, and Weiner, W (eds): Parkinson's Disease—Diagnosis and Clinical Management. Demos Medical Publishing, New York 2002, p 41.
8. Bakheit, AMO: Early diagnosis of Parkinson's disease. Postgrad Med J 71:151, 1995.
9. Hallett, M: Physiology of basal ganglia disorders: An overview. Can J Neurol Sci 20:177, 1993.
10. Bear, M, Connors, B, and Paradiso, M: Neuroscience—Exploring the Brain, ed 2. Lippincott Williams & Wilkins, Baltimore, 2001.
11. Alexander, G, Brutcher, M, and DeLong, M: Basal ganglia—thalamocortical circuits: Parallel substrates for motor oculomotor, "prefrontal" and "limbic" functions. Prog Brain Res 85:119, 1990.
12. Forno, L: Neuropathology of Parkinson's disease. J Neuropathol Exp Neurol 55:259, 1996.
13. Ma, TP: The basal ganglia. In Haines, D (ed): Fundamental Neuroscience. Churchill Livingstone, New York, 1997, p 364.
14. Cohen, A: Tremors and the Parkinson patient. Parkinson Report. National Parkinson Foundation Inc, Miami, FL, 1991.
15. Smithson, F, et al: Performance on clinical tests of balance in Parkinson's disease. Phys Ther 78:577, 1998.
16. Horak, F, et al: Postural instability in Parkinson's disease: Motor coordination and sensory organization. Neurology Report (now JNPT) 12:54, 1988.
17. Bloem, B, et al: Postural reflexes in Parkinson's disease during 'resist' and 'yield' tasks. J Neurol Sci 129:109, 1995.
18. Traub, M, et al: Anticipatory postural reflexes in Parkinson disease and other akinetic-rigid syndromes and in cerebellar ataxia. Brain 103:393, 1980.
19. Rogers, M: Disorders of posture, balance, and gait in Parkinson's disease. In Studenski, S (ed): Clinics in Geriatric Medicine. Gait Balance Disord 12:825, 1996.
20. Bridgewater, K, and Sharpe, M: Trunk muscle performance in early Parkinson's disease. Phys Ther 78:566, 1998.
21. Maeshima, S, et al: Visuospatial impairment and activities of daily living in patients with Parkinson's disease. Am J Phys Med Rehabil 76:383, 1997.
22. Wood, B, et al: Incidence and prediction of falls in Parkinson's disease: A prospective multidisciplinary study. J Neurol Neurosurg Psychiatry 72:721, 2002.
23. Koller, W, et al: Falls and Parkinson's disease. Clin Neuropharmacol 12:98, 1989.
24. Gray, P, and Hildebrand, K: Fall risk factors in Parkinson's disease. J Neurosci Nursing 32:222, 2000.
25. Corcos, D, et al: Strength in Parkinson's disease: Relationship to rate of force generation and clinical status. Ann Neurol 39:79, 1996.
26. Pedersen, S, and Oberg, B: Dynamic strength in Parkinson's disease: Quantitative measurements following withdrawal of medication. Eur Neurol 33:97, 1993.
27. Stelmach, G, et al: Force production characteristics in Parkinson's disease. Exp Brain Res 76:165, 1989.
28. Milner-Brown, H, et al: Electrical properties of motor units in parkinsonism and a possible relationship with bradykinesia. J Neurol Neurosurg Psychiatry 42:35, 1979.
29. Dengler R, et al: Behavior of motor units in parkinsonism. Adv Neurol 53:167, 1990.
30. Bennett, K, et al: A kinematic study of the reach to group movement in a study with hemi-Parkinson's disease. Neuropsychologia 31:713, 1993.
31. Yanagawa, S, et al: Muscular weakness in Parkinson's disease. Adv Neurol 53:259, 1990.
32. Marsden, C: What do the basal ganglia tell premotor cortical areas? Ciba Found Symp 132:282, 1997.
33. Giladi, N: Gait disturbances. In Factor, S and Weiner, W (eds): Parkinson's Disease —Diagnosis and Clinical Management. Demos Medical Publishing, New York 2002, p 57.
34. Rogers, M, and Chan, C: Motor planning is impaired in Parkinson's disease. Brain Res 438:271, 1988.
35. Agostino, R, Sanes, J, and Hallett, M: Motor skill learning in Parkinson's disease. J Neurol Sci 139:218, 1996.
36. Fattapposta, F, et al: Preprogramming and control activity of bimanual self-paced motor task in Parkinson's disease. Clin Neurophys 111:873, 2000.
37. Haaland, K, et al: Cognitive–motor learning in Parkinson's disease. Neuropsychology 11:180, 1997.
38. Soliveri, P, et al: Learning manual pursuit tracking skills in patients with Parkinson's disease. Brain 120:1325, 1997.

39. Pederson, S, et al: Gait analysis, isokinetic muscle strength measurement in patients with Parkinson's disease. Scand J Rehabil Med 29:67, 1997.
40. Morris, M, et al: The biomechanics and motor control of gait in Parkinson disease. Clin Biomech 16:459, 2001.
41. Melnick, M, Radtka, S, and Piper, M: Gait analysis and Parkinson's disease. Rehab Manage Aug/Sept:48, 2002.
42. Morris, M, et al: Temporal stability of gait in Parkinson's disease. Phys Ther 76:763, 1996.
43. Zewig, R: Sensory symptoms. In Factor, S and Weiner, W (eds): Parkinson's Disease —Diagnosis and Clinical Management. Demos Medical Publishing, New York 2002, p 67.
44. Koller, W: Sensory Symptoms in Parkinson's Disease. Parkinson Report. National Parkinson Foundation, Miami, 1985.
45. Jobst, E, et al: Sensory perception in Parkinson disease. Arch Neurol 54:450, 1997.
46. Demirci, M, et al: A mismatch between kinesthetic and visual perception in Parkinson's disease. Ann Neurol 41:781, 1997.
47. Ramig, L, et al: Speech, voice, and swallowing disorders. In Factor, S, and Weiner, W (eds): Parkinson's Disease—Diagnosis and Clinical Management. Demos Medical Publishing, New York 2002, p 75.
48. Robbins, J, et al: Swallowing and speech production in Parkinson's disease. Ann Neurol 19:282, 1986.
49. Marder, K, and Jacobs, D: Dementia. In Factor, S, and Weiner, W (eds): Parkinson's Disease—Diagnosis and Clinical Management. Demos Medical Publishing, New York 2002, p 125.
50. Mayeux, R: Behavioral and cognitive dysfunction. In Cohen, A, and Weiner, W (eds): The Comprehensive Management of Parkinson's Disease. Demos Medical Publishing, New York, 1994, p 119.
51. Chow, T, Masterman, D, and Cummings, J: Depression. In Factor, S, and Weiner, W (eds): Parkinson's Disease—Diagnosis and Clinical Management. Demos Medical Publishing, New York 2002, p 145.
52. Richard, I, and Kurlan, R: Anxiety and panic. In Factor, S and Weiner, W (eds): Parkinson's Disease—Diagnosis and Clinical Management. Demos Medical Publishing, New York 2002, p 161.
53. Hubble, J, and Weeks, C: Autonomic nervous system dysfunction. In Factor, S, and Weiner, W (eds): Parkinson's Disease—Diagnosis and Clinical Management. Demos Medical Publishing, New York 2002, p 95.
54. Ludin, S, Steiger, M, and Ludin, H: Autonomic disturbances and cardiovascular reflexes in idiopathic Parkinson's disease. J Neurol 235:10, 1987.
55. Piha, S, et al: Autonomic dysfunction in recent onset and advanced Parkinson's disease. Clin Neurol Neurosurg 90:221, 1988.
56. Hovestadt, A, et al: Pulmonary function in Parkinson's disease. J Neurol Neurosurg Psychiatry 52:329, 1989.
57. Sabate, M, et al: Obstructive and restrictive pulmonary dysfunction increases disability in Parkinson disease. Arch Phys Med Rehabil 77:29, 1996.
58. Canning, C, et al: Parkinson's disease: An investigation of exercise capacity, respiratory function, and gait. Arch Phys Med Rehabil 78:199, 1997.
59. Protas, E, et al: Cardiovascular and metabolic responses to upper- and lower-extremity exercise in men with idiopathic Parkinson's disease. Phys Ther 76:34, 1996.
60. Stanley, R, Protas, E, and Jankovic, J: Exercise performance in those having Parkinson's disease and healthy normals. Med Sci Sports Exerc 31(6):761, 1999.
61. Feigin, A, and Eidelberg, D: Natural history. In Factor, S, and Weiner, W (eds): Parkinson's Disease—Diagnosis and Clinical Management. Demos Medical Publishing, New York, 2002, p 109.
62. Hoehn, M, and Yahr, M: Parkinsonism: Onset, progression and mortality. Neurology 17:427, 1967.
63. Golbe, L, and Sage, J: Medical treatment of Parkinson's disease. In Kurlan, R (ed): Treatment of Movement Disorders. JB Lippincott, Philadelphia, 1995, p 1.
64. Ward, C: Does selegiline delay progression of Parkinson's disease? A critical re-evaluation of the DATATOP study. J Neurol Neurosurg Psychiatry 57:217, 1994.
65. Rascol, O, et al: Treatment interventions for Parkinson's disease: An evidence based assessment. Lancet 359:1589, 2002.
66. Kuntzer, T: Treatment of Parkinson's disease. Eur Neurol 36:396, 1996.
67. Cutson, T, et al: Pharmacological and nonpharmacological interventions in the treatment of Parkinson's disease. Phys Ther 75:363, 1995.
68. Mantero-Atienza, E, et al: Nutritional Considerations of Parkinson's Disease. National Parkinson Foundation, Miami, 1990.
69. Park, J, Lozano, A, and Lang, A: Stereotaxic pallidotomy and thalamotomy. In Factor, S, and Weiner, W (eds): Parkinson's Disease—Diagnosis and Clinical Management. Demos Medical Publishing, New York, 2002, p 531.
70. Bronstein, J, et al: Stereotactic pallidotomy in the treatment of Parkinson disease: An expert opinion. Arch Neurol 56:1964, 1999.
71. Koller, W, et al: High-frequency unilateral thalamic stimulation in the treatment of essential and Parkinsonian tremor. Ann Neurol 42:292, 1997.
72. Hariz, G, et al: Examinement of ability/disability in patients treated with chronic thalamic stimulation for tremor. Mov Disord 13:78, 1998.
73. Byrd, D, Marks, W, and Starr, P: Deep brain stimulation for advanced Parkinson's disease. AORN J 72:385, 2000.
74. Houeto, J, et al: Subthalamic stimulation in Parkinson disease: A multidisciplinary approach Arch Neurol 57:461, 2000.
75. Molinuevo, J, et al: Levodopa withdrawal after bilateral subthalamic nucleus stimulation in advanced Parkinson disease. Arch Neurol 57:983, 2000.
76. Sanchez-Ramos, J: Embryonic stem cells, fetal cells, and Parkinson disease. Parkinson Report Fall:12, 2003.
77. Arenas, E: Stem cells in the treatment of Parkinson's disease. Brain Res Bull 57:795, 2002.
78. Schenkman, M, et al: Reliability of impairment and physical performance measures for persons with Parkinson's disease. Phys Ther 77:19, 1997.
79. American Physical Therapy Association: Guide to Physical Therapist Practice, ed 2. Phys Ther 81:383, 2001.
80. Folstein, M, et al: Mini-Mental Status: A practical method for grading the cognitive state of patients for the clinician. J Psychiatr Res 12:189, 1975.
81. Yesavage, J, and Brink, T: Development and validation of a geriatric depression screening scale: A preliminary report. J Psychiatr Res 17:41, 1983.
82. Gallagher, D: The Beck Depression Inventory and older adults review of its development and utility. In Brink, T (ed): Clinical Gerontology: A Guide to Examinement and Intervention. Haworth Press, New York, 1986, p 149.
83. Melzack, R: The McGill Pain Questionnaire: Major properties and scoring methods. Pain 1:277, 1975.
84. Bridgewater, K, and Sharpe, M: Trunk muscle performance in early Parkinson's disease. Phys Ther 78:566, 1998.
85. Dengler, R, et al: Behavior of motor units in parkinsonism. Adv Neurol 53:167, 1990.
86. Bohannon, R: Documentation of tremor in patients with central nervous system lesions. Phys Ther 66:229, 1986.
87. Duncan, P, et al: Functional reach: A new clinical measure of balance. J Gerontol 45:M192, 1990.
88. Newton, R: Validity of the Multi-Directional Reach Test. J Gerontol A Biol Sci Med Sci 56(4):M248, 2001.
89. Smithson, F, Morris, M, and Iansek, R: Performance on clinical tests of balance in Parkinson's disease. Phys Ther 78:577, 1998.
90. Goldie, et al: Force platform measures for evaluating postural control: Reliability and validity. Arch Phys Med Rehabil 70:510, 1989.
91. Bloem, B: Clinimetrics of postural instability in Parkinson's disease. J Neurol 245:669, 1998.
92. Nashner, L, Woollacott, M, and Tuma, G: Organizataion of rapid responses to postural and locomotor-like perturbations of standing man. Exp Brain Res 36:463, 1979.
93. Peterka, R, and Black, F: Age-related changes in human posture control: Sensory organization tests. J Vestib Res 1:73, 1990.
94. Shumway-Cook, A, and Horak, F: Examining the influence of sensory interaction on balance. Phys Ther 66:1548, 1986.
95. Rose, D: Fall Proof—A Comprehensive Balance and Mobility Training Program. Human Kinetics, Champaign, IL, 2003.
96. Podsiadlo, D, and Richardson, S: The timed "up and go": A test of basic functional mobility for frail elderly patients. J Am Geriatr Soc 39:142, 1991.

97. Tinetti, M: Performance-oriented assessment of mobility problems in elderly patients. J Am Geriatr Soc 34:119, 1986.
98. Behrman, A, Light, K, and Miller, G: Sensitivity of the Tinetti Gait Assessment for detecting change in individuals with Parkinson's disease. Clin Rehabil 16:399, 2002.
99. Morris, M, and Iansek, R: Gait disorders in Parkinson's disease: A framework for physical therapy practice. Neurology Report (now JNPT) 21:125, 1997.
100. Hildebrand, K: Fall risk factors in Parkinson's disease. J Neurosci Nursing 32:222, 2000.
101. Sage, J: Fluctuations of nonmotor symptoms. In Factor, S, and Weiner, W (eds): Parkinson's Disease—Diagnosis and Clinical Management. Demos Medical Publishing, New York 2002, p 455.
102. Light, K, et al: The 2-Minute Walk Test: A tool for evaluating walking endurance in clients with Parkinson's disease. Neurology Report (now JNPT) 21:136, 1997.
103. Borg, G: Psychophysical bases of perceived exertion. Med Sci Sports Exerc 14:377, 1982.
104. Guide for the Uniform Data Set for Medical Rehabilitation including the FIM instrument, Version 5.0. State University of New York at Buffalo, Buffalo, 1996.
105. Bishop, M, et al: Changes in distal muscle timing may contribute to slowness during sit to stand in Parkinson's disease. Clin Biomech 20:112, 2005.
106. Ramsey, V, Miszko, T, and Horvat, M: Muscle activation and force production in Parkinson's patients during sit to stand transfers. Clin Biomech 19:377, 2004.
107. Dittmar, S, and Gresham, G: Functional Assessment and Outcome Measures for the Rehabilitation Professional. Aspen, Gaithersburg, MD, 1997.
108. McHorney, C, et al: The MOS 36-Item Short-Form Health Survey (SF-36) II. Psychometric and chemical and clinical tests of validity in measuring physical and mental health constructs. Med Care 31:247, 1993.
109. Gilson, B, et al: The Sickness Impact Profile: Development of an outcome measure of health care. Am J Publ Health 65:1304, 1975.
110. Fahn, S, and Elton, R: Unified Parkinson's disease rating scale. In: Fahn, S, et al (eds): Recent Developments in Parkinson's Disease, Vol 2. Macmillan Health Care Information, Florham Park, NJ, 1987.
111. Martinez-Martin, P, et al: The cooperative multicentric group: Unified Parkinson's Disease Rating Scale Characteristics and Structure. Mov Disord 9:76, 1994.
112. Petro, V, et al: The development and validation of a short measure of functioning and well being for individuals with Parkinson's disease. Qual Life Res 4:241, 1995.
113. Jenkinson, C, et al: Self-reported functioning and well-being in patients with Parkinson's disease: Comparison of the Short-form Health Survey (SF-36) and the Parkinson's Disease Questionnaire (PDQ-39). Age Ageing 24:505, 1995.
114. Fitzpatrick, R, et al: Health-related quality of life in Parkinson's disease: A study of outpatient clinic attenders. Mov Disord 12:916, 1997.
115. Harrington, D, et al: Procedural memory in Parkinson's disease: Impaired motor but not visuoperceptual learning. J Clin Exp Neuropsychol 12:323, 1990.
116. Jackson, G, et al: Serial reaction time learning and Parkinson's disease: Evidence for a procedural learning deficit. Neuropsychologia 33:577, 1995.
117. Brown, R, and Marsden, C: Dual task performance and processing resources in normal subjects and patients with Parkinson's disease. Brain 114:215, 1991.
118. Behrman, A, Cauraugh, J, and Light, K: Practice as an intervention to improve speeded motor performance and motor learning in Parkinson's disease. J Neurol Sci 174:127, 2000.
119. Platz, T, et al: Training improves the speed of aimed movements in Parkinson's disease. Brain 121:505, 1998.
120. Swinnen, S, et al: Motor learning and Parkinson's disease: Refinement of within-limb and between-limb coordination as a result of practice. Behav Brain Res 111:45, 2000.
121. Lehman, D, et al. Training with verbal instructional cues results in near–term improvement of gait in people with Parkinson disease. JNPT 29:2, 2005.
122. Mak, M, and Hue-Chan, C: Audiovisual cues can enhance sit-to-stand in patients with Parkinson's disease. Mov Disord 19:1012, 2004.
123. Majsak, M, et al: The reaching movements of patients with Parkinson's disease under self-determined maximal speed and visually cued conditions. Brain 121:755, 1998.
124. McIntosh, G, Flanagan, J, and Gentile, A: Modulation of ballistic reaching movements in Parkinson's disease: The effects of a moving versus a stationary target. Neurology Report (now JNPT) 19:47, 1995.
125. Burleigh-Jacobs, A, et al: Step initiation in Parkinson's disease: Influence of levodopa and external sensory triggers. Mov Disord 12:206, 1997.
126. Morris, M, et al: Stride length regulation in Parkinson's disease. Normalization strategies and underlying mechanisms. Brain 119:551, 1996.
127. Taut, M, et al: Rhythmic auditory stimulation in gait training for Parkinson's disease patients. Move Disord 11:193, 1996.
128. Freeman, J, et al: The influence of external timing cues upon the rhythm of voluntary movements in Parkinson's disease. J Neurol Neurosurg Psychiatry 56: 1078, 1993.
129. Dibble, L, and Nicholson, D: Sensory cueing improves motor performance and rehabilitation in persons with Parkinson's disease. Neurology Report (now JNPT) 21:117, 1997.
130. Bagely, S, et al: The effect of visual cues on the gait of independently mobile Parkinson's patients. Physiotherapy 77:415, 1991.
131. Dietz, M, et al: Evaluation of a modified inverted walking stick as a treatment for Parkinsonian freezing episodes. Mov Disord 5:243, 1990.
132. Dunne J, Hankey, G, and Edis, R: Parkinsonism: Upturned walking stick as an aid to locomotion. Arch Phys Med Rehabil 68:380, 1987.
133. Lewis, G, Byblow, W, and Walt, S: Stride length regulation in Parkinson's disease: The use of extrinsic visual cues. Brain 123:2077, 2000.
134. Eni, G: Gait improvements in parkinsonism: The use of rhythmic music. Int J Res 11:272, 1988.
135. Enzensberger, W, and Fischer, P: Metronome in Parkinson's disease. Lancet 347:1337, 1996.
136. Freedland, R, et al: The effects of pulsed auditory stimulation on various gait measurements in persons with Parkinson's disease. Neuro Rehabil 17:81, 2002.
137. Jahanshahi, M, et al: Self-initiated versus externally triggered movements. 1. An investigation using measurement of regional cerebral blood flow with PET and movement-related potentials in normal and Parkinson's disease subjects. Brain 118:913, 1995.
138. Dam, M, et al: Effects of conventional and sensory enhanced physiotherapy on disability of Parkinson's disease patients. Adv Neurol 69:551, 1996.
139. Muller, V, et al: Short-term effects of behavioral treatment on movement initiation and postural control in Parkinson's disease: A controlled clinical trial. Mov Disord 12:306, 1997.
140. Suteerawattananon, M, et al: Effects of visual and auditory cues on gait in individuals with Parkinson's disease. J Neurol Sci 219:63, 2004.
141. Nieuwboer, A, et al: Is using a cue the clue to the treatment of freezing in Parkinson's disease. Physiother Res Int 2:125, 1997.
142. Tyler, W: History of Parkinson's disease. In Koller, W (ed): Handbook of Parkinson's Disease. Marcel Dekker, New York, 1987.
143. Pederson, D: The soothing effects of rocking as determined by the direction and frequency of movement. Can J Behav Sci 7:237, 1975.
144. Peterson, B, et al: Changes in response of medial pontomedullary reticular neurons during repetitive cutaneous, vestibular, cortical and fectal stimulation. J Neurophysiol 39:564, 1976.
145. Schenkman, M, et al: Management of individuals with Parkinson's disease: Rationale and case studies. Phys Ther 69:944, 1989.
146. Voss, D, et al: Proprioceptive Neuromuscular Facilitation, ed 3. Harper & Row, New York, 1985.
147. Benson, H: The Relaxation Response. Avon, New York, 1975.
148. Jacobson, E: Progressive Relaxation. University of Chicago Press, Chicago, 1938.
149. Kaltenborn, F: Mobilization of the Extremity Joints: Examination and Basic Treatment Techniques. Olaf Norlis Bokhandel, Oslo, Norway, 1989.
150. Kisner, C, and Colby, L: Therapeutic Exercise Foundations and Techniques, ed 4. FA Davis, Philadelphia, 2002.

151. Glendinning, D: A rationale for strength training in patients with Parkinson's disease. Neurology Report (now JNPT) 21:132, 1997.
152. Fiatarone, M, et al: High-intensity strength training in nonagenarians. Effects on skeletal muscle. JAMA 263:3029, 1990.
153. Judge, J, et al: Effects of resistive and balance exercises on isokinetic strength in older persons. J Am Geriatr Soc 42:937, 1994.
154. Tinnetti, M, et al: A multifactorial intervention to reduce the risk of falling among elderly people living in the community. N Engl J Med 331:821, 1994.
155. Wolfson, L, et al: Balance and strength training in older adults: Intervention gains and Tai Chi maintenance. J Am Geriatr Soc 44:498, 1996.
156. Scandalis, T, et al: Resistance training and gait function in patients with Parkinson's disease. Am J Phys Med Rehabil 80:38, 2001.
157. Hirsch, M, et al: The effects of balance training and high-intensity resistance training on persons with idiopathic Parkinson's disease. Arch Phys Med Rehabil 84:1109, 2003.
158. Reuter, I, et al: Therapeutic value of exercise training in Parkinson's disease. Med Sci Sports Exerc 31:1544, 1999.
159. Stanley, R, and Protas, E: Parkinson's Disease. In American College of Sports Medicine: ACSM's Resources for Clinical Exercise Physiology. Lippincott Williams & Wilkins, Philadelphia, 2002, p 38.
160. O'Sullivan, S, and Schmitz, T: Physical Rehabilitation Laboratory Manual. FA Davis, Philadelphia, 1999.
161. Pohl, M et al: Immediate effects of speed-dependent treadmill training on gait parameters in early Parkinson's disease. Arch Phys Med Rehabil 84:1760, 2000.
162. Miyai, I, et al: Treadmill training with body weight support: Its effect on Parkinson's disease. Arch Phys Med Rehabil 81: 849, 2000.
163. Miyai, I, et al: Long-term effect of body weight-supported treadmill training in Parkinson's disease: A randomized controlled trial. Arch Phys Med Rehabil 83:1370, 2002.
164. Behrman, A, Teitelbaum, P, and Cauraugh, J: Verbal instructional sets to normalize the temporal and spatial gait variables in Parkinson's disease. J Neurol Neurosurg Psychiatry 65:580, 1998.
165. Van Vaerenbergh, J, Vranken, R, and Baro, F: The influence of rotational exercises on freezing in Parkinson's disease. Funct Neurol 18:11, 2003
166. Tzelepis, G, et al: Respiratory muscle dysfunction in Parkinson's disease. Am Rev Respir Dis 138:266, 1988.
167. Koseoglu, F, et al: The effects of a pulmonary rehabilitation program on pulmonary function tests and exercise tolerance in patients with Parkinson's disease. Funct Neurol 12:319, 1997.
168. Inzelberg, R, et al. Inspiratory muscle training and the perception of dyspnea in Parkinson's disease. Can J Neurol Sci 32:213, 2005.
169. Bergen, J, et al: Aerobic exercise intervention improves aerobic capacity and movement initiation in Parkinson's disease patients. NeuroRehabilitation 17:161, 2002.
170. American College of Sports Medicine: ACSM's Guidelines for Exercise Testing and Prescription, ed 6. Lippincott Williams & Wilkins, Baltimore, 2000.
171. Pedersen, S, et al: Group training in parkinsonism: Quantitative measurements of treatment. Scand J Rehabil Med 22:207, 1990.
172. Hurwitz, A: The benefit of a home exercise regimen for ambulatory Parkinson's disease patients. J Neurosci Nurs 21:180, 1989.
173. Lun, V, et al: Comparison of the effects of a self-supervised home exercise program with a physiotherapist-supervised exercise program on the motor symptoms of Parkinson's disease. Mov Disord 20:971, 2005.
174. Abuli, S, et al: Parkinson's disease symptoms: Patient's perceptions. J Adv Nurs 25:54, 1997.
175. Comella, C, et al: Physical therapy and Parkinson's disease: A controlled clinical trial. Neurology 44:376, 1994.
176. Viliani, T, et al: Effects of physical training on straightening-up processes in patients with Parkinson's disease. Disabil Rehabil 21:68, 1999.
177. De Goede, C, et al: The effects of physical therapy in Parkinson's disease: A research synthesis. Arch Phys Med Rehabil 82:509, 2001.
178. Schenkman, M, et al: Exercise to improve spinal flexibility and function for people with Parkinson's disease: A randomized, controlled trial. J Am Geriatr Soc 46:1207, 1998.
179. Baatile, J, et al: Effect of exercise on perceived quality of life of individuals with Parkinson's disease. J Rehabil Res Dev 37:529, 2000.

Supplemental Readings and Materials

Clinical Monograph: Fitness Counts, ed 2. National Parkinson Foundation, Inc, Miami, FL, 2004. Retrieved June 25, 2005 from http://www.parkinson.org.

StEP (Stalevo Educational Programs) initiative: Managing Parkinson's Disease (http://www.stepkit.net). Novartis, developed in consultation with the National Parkinson Foundation, the American Parkinson Disease Association and the Parkinson Alliance.

Motivating Moves for People with Parkinson's (video divided into three sections: "How to Do Motivating Moves" [45 min], "The Exercise Class" [36 min], and "Practical Tips for Daily Living" [4 min]). Available from the Parkinson Disease Foundation, New York, NY, http://www.pdf.org.

The PDF Exercise Program. Available from the Parkinson Disease Foundation, New York, NY, http://www.pdf.org.

Levine, C. Always on Call: When Illness Turns Families into Caregivers, ed 2. Vanderbilt University Press, Nashville, TN, 2004.

Appendix A: Unified Parkinson's Disease Rating Scale (UPDRS), Version 3.0: February 1987[a]

I. Mentation, Behavior and Mood

1. *Intellectual impairments:*
   - 0 = None.
   - 1 = Mild. Consistent forgetfulness with partial recollection of events and no other difficulties.
   - 2 = Moderate memory loss, with disorientation and moderate difficulty handling complex problems. Mild but definite impairment of function at home with need of occasional prompting.
   - 3 = Severe memory loss with disorientation for time and often to place. Severe impairment in handling problems.
   - 4 = Severe memory loss with orientation preserved to person only. Unable to make judgments or solve problems. Requires much help with personal care. Cannot be left alone at all.
2. *Thought disorder* (due to dementia or drug intoxication):
   - 0 = None.
   - 1 = Vivid dreaming.
   - 2 = "Benign" hallucinations with insight retained.
   - 3 = Occasional to frequent hallucinations or delusions; without insight; could interfere with daily activities.
   - 4 = Persistent hallucinations, delusions, or florid psychosis. Not able to care for self.
3. *Depression:*
   - 0 = Not present.
   - 1 = Periods of sadness or guilt greater than normal, never sustained for days or weeks.
   - 2 = Sustained depression (1 week or more).
   - 3 = Sustained depression with vegetative symptoms (insomnia, anorexia, weight loss, loss of interest).
   - 4 = Sustained depression with vegetative symptoms and suicidal thoughts or intent.
4. *Motivation/initiative:*
   - 0 = Normal.
   - 1 = Less assertive than usual; more passive.
   - 2 = Loss in initiative or disinterest in elective (non-routine) activities.
   - 3 = Loss of initiative or disinterest in day-to-day (routine) activities.
   - 4 = Withdrawn, complete loss of motivation.

II. Activities of Daily Living (determine for "on/off")

5. *Speech:*
   - 0 = Normal.
   - 1 = Mildly affected. No difficulty being understood.
   - 2 = Moderately affected. Sometimes asked to repeat statements.
   - 3 = Severely affected. Sometimes asked to repeat statements.
   - 4 = Unintelligible most of the time.
6. *Salivation:*
   - 0 = Normal.
   - 1 = Slight but definite excess of saliva in mouth; may have nighttime drooling.
   - 2 = Moderately excessive saliva; may have minimal drooling.
   - 3 = Marked excess of saliva with some drooling.
   - 4 = Marked drooling, requires constant tissue or handkerchief.
7. *Swallowing:*
   - 0 = Normal.
   - 1 = Rare choking.
   - 2 = Occasional choking.
   - 3 = Requires soft food.
   - 4 = Requires nasogastric tube or gastrotomy feeding.
8. *Handwriting:*
   - 0 = Normal.
   - 1 = Slightly slow or small.
   - 2 = Moderately slow or small; all words are legible.
   - 3 = Severely affected; not all words are legible.
   - 4 = The majority of words are not legible.
9. *Cutting food and handling utensils:*
   - 0 = Normal.
   - 1 = Somewhat slow and clumsy, but no help needed.
   - 2 = Can cut most foods, although clumsy and slow; some help needed.
   - 3 = Food must be cut by someone, but can still feed slowly.
   - 4 = Needs to be fed.
10. *Dressing:*
    - 0 = Normal.
    - 1 = Somewhat slow, but no help needed.
    - 2 = Occasional assistance with buttoning, or with getting arms in sleeves.
    - 3 = Considerable help required, but can do some things alone.
    - 4 = Helpless.
11. *Hygiene:*
    - 0 = Normal.
    - 1 = Somewhat slow, but no help needed.
    - 2 = Needs help to shower or bathe; or very slow in hygienic care.

3 = Requires assistance for washing, brushing teeth, combing hair, going to bathroom.
4 = Foley catheter or other mechanical aids.

12. *Turning in bed and adjusting bed clothes:*
0 = Normal.
1 = Somewhat slow and clumsy, but no help needed.
2 = Can turn alone or adjust sheets, but with great difficulty.
3 = Can initiate, but not turn or adjust sheets alone.
4 = Helpless.

13. *Falling (unrelated to freezing):*
0 = None.
1 = Rare falling.
2 = Occasionally falls, less than once per day.
3 = Falls on average of once daily.
4 = Falls more than once daily.

14. *Freezing when walking:*
0 = None.
1 = Rare freezing when walking; may have start-hesitation.
2 = Occasional freezing when walking.
3 = Frequent freezing. Occasionally falls from freezing.
4 = Frequent falls from freezing.

15. *Walking:*
0 = Normal.
1 = Mild difficulty; may not swing arms or may tend to drag leg.
2 = Moderate difficulty, but requires little or no assistance.
3 = Severe disturbance of walking, requiring assistance.
4 = Cannot walk at all, even with assistance.

16. *Tremor:*
0 = Absent.
1 = Slight and infrequently present.
2 = Moderate; bothersome to patient.
3 = Severe; interferes with many activities.
4 = Marked; interferes with most activities.

17. *Sensory complaints related to parkinsonism:*
0 = None.
1 = Occasionally has numbness, tingling, or mild aching.
2 = Frequently has numbness, tingling, or aching; not distressing.
3 = Frequent painful sensations.
4 = Excruciating pain.

III. Motor Examination

18. *Speech:*
0 = Normal.
1 = Slight loss of expression, diction, and/or volume.
2 = Monotone, slurred but understandable; moderately impaired.
3 = Marked impairment, difficult to understand.
4 = Unintelligible.

19. *Facial expression:*
0 = Normal.
1 = Minimal hypomimia, could be normal "poker face."
2 = Slight but definitely abnormal diminution of facial expression.
3 = Moderate hypomimia; lips parted some of the time.
4 = Masked or fixed facies with severe or complete loss of facial expression; lips parted ¼ in or more.

20. *Tremor at rest:*
0 = Absent.
1 = Slight and infrequently present.
2 = Mild in amplitude and persistent; or moderate in amplitude, but only intermittently present.
3 = Moderate in amplitude and present most of the time.
4 = Marked in amplitude and present most of the time.

21. *Action or postural tremor of hands:*
0 = Absent.
1 = Slight; present with action.
2 = Moderate in amplitude, present with action.
3 = Moderate in amplitude with posture holding as well as action.
4 = Marked in amplitude; interferes with feeding.

22. *Rigidity* (judged on passive movement of major joints with patient relaxed in sitting position; cogwheeling to be ignored):
0 = Absent.
1 = Slight or detectable only when activated by mirror or other movements.
2 = Mild to moderate.
3 = Marked; but full range of motion easily achieved.
4 = Severe; range of motion achieved with difficulty.

23. *Finger taps* (patient taps thumb with index finger in rapid succession with widest amplitude possible, each hand separately):
0 = Normal.
1 = Mild slowing and/or reduction in amplitude.
2 = Moderately impaired; definite and early fatiguing; may have occasional arrests in movement.
3 = Severely impaired; frequent hesitation in initiating movements or arrests in ongoing movement.
4 = Can barely perform the task.

24. *Hand movement* (patient opens and closes hands in rapid succession with widest amplitude possible, each hand separately):
0 = Normal.
1 = Mild slowing and/or reduction in amplitude.
2 = Moderately impaired; definite and early fatiguing; may have occasional arrests in movement.
3 = Severely impaired; frequent hesitation in initiating movements or arrests in ongoing movement.
4 = Can barely perform the task.

25. *Rapid alternating movements of hands* (pronation-supination movements of hands, vertically or horizontally, with as large an amplitude as possible, both hands simultaneously):
  0 = Normal.
  1 = Mild slowing and/or reduction in amplitude.
  2 = Moderately impaired; definite and early fatiguing; may have occasional arrests in movement.
  3 = Severely impaired; frequent hesitation in initiating movements or arrests in ongoing movement.
  4 = Can barely perform the task.
26. *Foot agility* (patient taps heel on ground in rapid succession, picking up entire leg; amplitude should be about 3 inches):
  0 = Normal.
  1 = Mild slowing and/or reduction in amplitude.
  2 = Moderately impaired; definite and early fatiguing; may have occasional arrests in movement.
  3 = Severely impaired; frequent hesitation in initiating movements or arrests in ongoing movement.
  4 = Can barely perform the task.
27. *Arising from chair* (patient attempts to arise from a straight-backed wood or metal chair with arms folded across chest).
  0 = Normal.
  1 = Slow; or may need more than one attempt.
  2 = Pushes self up from arms of seat.
  3 = Tends to fall back and may have to try more than one time, but can get up without help.
  4 = Unable to arise without help.
28. *Posture:*
  0 = Normal erect.
  1 = Not quite erect, slightly stooped posture; could be normal for older person.
  2 = Moderately stopped posture, definitely abnormal; can be slightly leaning to one side.
  3 = Severely stooped posture with kyphosis; can be moderately leaning to one side.
  4 = Marked flexion with extreme abnormality of posture.
29. *Gait:*
  0 = Normal.
  1 = Walks slowly, may shuffle with short steps, but no festination or propulsion.
  2 = Walks with difficulty, but requires little or no assistance; may have some festination, short steps, or propulsion.
  3 = Severe disturbance of gait, requiring assistance.
  4 = Cannot walk at all, even with assistance.
30. *Postural stability* (response to sudden posterior displacement produced by pull on shoulders while patient is erect with eyes open and feet slightly apart; patient is prepared):
  0 = Normal.
  1 = Retropulsion, but recovers unaided.
  2 = Absence of postural response; would fall if not caught by examiner.
  3 = Very unstable, tends to lose balance spontaneously.
  4 = Unable to stand without assistance.
31. *Body bradykinesia and hypokinesia* (combining slowness, hesitancy, decreased armswing, small amplitude, and poverty of movement in general):
  0 = None.
  1 = Minimal slowness, giving movement a deliberate character; could be normal for some persons. Possibly reduced amplitude.
  2 = Mild degree of slowness and poverty of movement that is definitely abnormal. Alternatively, some reduced amplitude.
  3 = Moderate slowness, poverty, or small amplitude of movement.
  4 = Marked slowness, poverty, or small amplitude of movement.

IV. Complications of Therapy (in the past week)

A. Dyskinesias

32. *Duration: What proportion of the waking day are dyskinesias present?* (historical information)
  0 = None.
  1 = 1–25% of day.
  2 = 26–50% of day.
  3 = 51–75% of day.
  4 = 76–100% of day.
33. *Disability: How disabling are the dyskinesias?* (historical information; may be modified by office examination)
  0 = Not disabling.
  1 = Mildly disabling.
  2 = Moderately disabling.
  3 = Severely disabling.
  4 = Completely disabled.
34. *Painful dyskinesia: how painful are the dyskinesias?*
  0 = No painful dyskinesias.
  1 = Slight.
  2 = Moderate.
  3 = Severe.
  4 = Marked.
35. *Presence of early morning dystonia* (historical information):
  0 = No
  1 = Yes

B. Clinical fluctuations

36. *Are any "off" periods predictable as to timing after a dose of medication?*
  0 = No
  1 = Yes
37. *Are any "off" periods unpredictable as to timing after a dose of medications?*
  0 = No
  1 = Yes

38. *Do any of the "off" periods come on suddenly, for example, over a few seconds?*
    0 = No
    1 = Yes
39. *What proportion of the waking day is the patient "off" on average?*
    0 = None.
    1 = 1–25% of day.
    2 = 26–50% of day.
    3 = 51–75% of day.
    4 = 76–100% of day.

C. Other complications.

40. *Does the patient have anorexia, nausea, or vomiting?*
    0 = No
    1 = Yes
41. *Does the patient have any sleep disturbances, for example, insomnia or hypersomnolence?*
    0 = No
    1 = Yes
42. *Does the patient have symptomatic orthostasis?*
    0 = No
    1 = Yes

Record the patient's blood pressure, pulse, and weight on the scoring form

V. Modified Hoehn and Yahr Staging

Stage 0 = No signs of disease.
Stage 1 = Unilateral disease.
Stage 1.5 = Unilateral plus axial involvement.
Stage 2 = Bilateral disease, without impairment of balance.
Stage 2.5 = Mild bilateral disease, with recovery on pull test.
Stage 3 = Mild to moderate bilateral disease; some postural instability; physically independent.
Stage 4 = Severe disability; still able to walk or stand unassisted.
Stage 5 = Wheelchair bound or bedridden unless aided.

VI. Schwab and England Activities of Daily Living Scale

100%—Completely independent. Able to do all chores without slowness, difficulty, or impairment. Essentially normal. Unaware of any difficulty.
90%—Completely independent. Able to do all chores with some degree of slowness, difficulty, and impairment. Might take twice as long. Beginning to be aware of difficulty.
80%—Completely independent in most chores. Takes twice as long. Conscious of difficulty and slowness.
70%—Not completely independent. More difficulty with some chores. Three to four times as long in some. Must spend a large part of the day with chores.
60%—Some dependency. Can do most chores, but exceedingly slowly and with much effort. Errors; some impossible.
50%—More dependent. Help with half, slower, and so forth. Difficulty with everything.
40%—Very dependent. Can assist with some chores, but does few alone.
30%—With effort, now and then does a few chores alone, or begins alone. Much help needed.
20%—Nothing done alone. Can be a slight help with some chores. Severe invalid.
10%—Totally dependent, helpless. Complete invalid.
0%—Vegetative functions, such as swallowing, bladder and bowel functions, not functioning. Bedridden.

From Fahn, S, et al:[110] pp 36–41 with permission.
[a]Definition of 0–4 scale.

Appendix B: Web-Based Resources for Clinicians and Patients/Families Living with Parkinson's Disease

National Parkinson Foundation (NPF)	http://www.parkinson.org
Parkinson's Disease Foundation (PDF)	http://www.pdf.org
American Parkinson Disease Association (APDA)	http://www.apdaparkinson.com
World Parkinson Disease Association (WPDA)	http://www.wpda.org
Parkinson Society Canada	http://www.parkinson.ca
Young Onset Parkinson's Association	http://www.yopa.org
Young Parkinson's Information and and Referral Center	http://www.youngparkinsons.org
Michael J. Fox Foundation for Parkinson's Research	http://www.michaeljfox.org
The Parkinson Alliance	http://www.parkinsonalliance.net
Parkinson's Action Network	http://www.ParkActNet@AOLcom
The Parkinson's Institute	http://www.parkinsoninstitute.org
People Living with Parkinson's	http://www.plwp.org
Understanding Parkinson's	http://www.understandingparkinson's.com
Americans with Disabilities Act: ADA home page	http://www.usdoj.gov/crt/ada
Medicare information	http://cms.hhs.gov
Social Security Online	http://www.ssa.gov
National Institutes of Health	http://www.ninds.nih.gov/medlineplus/parkinsonsdisease.Html
National Library of Medicine	http://www.nim.nih.gov
Archives of Neurology	http://archneur.ama-assn.org
Neurology	http://www.neurology.org
Veterans Affairs	http://www.va.gov
National Family Caregivers Association (NFCA)	http://www.nfcacares.org
Parkinson's disease Caregiver Information	http://www.myparkinsons.org
Well Spouse Foundation	http://www.wellspouse.org
American Academy of Neurology (ANA)	http://www.aan.com (ANA members, professionals)
	http://www.aan.com/public (public education)
National Rehabilitation Information Center (NARIC)	http://www.naric.com
Ability Hub- assistive technology	http://www.abilityhub.com
ABLEDATA—assistive technology	http://www.abledata.com
Disabled Online	http://www.disabledonline.com

CHAPTER

22

LEARNING OBJECTIVES

1. Describe the pathophysiology of traumatic brain injury.
2. Describe the interdisciplinary team concept used in the rehabilitation of individuals with traumatic brain injury.
3. Identify the different team members involved in the management of the patient with traumatic brain injury and differentiate their respective roles.
4. Describe two clinical rating scales and their usefulness.
5. Describe commonly seen deficits that result from traumatic brain injury.
6. Describe the role of the physical therapist in the different episodes of care of the patient with traumatic brain injury.
7. Explain cognitive considerations required during physical therapy examination and intervention.
8. Identify the components of a physical therapy examination for the patient with traumatic brain injury.
9. Describe treatment interventions available to the physical therapist in working with the patient with traumatic brain injury at the various stages of rehabilitation.
10. Analyze and interpret patient data, formulate realistic goals and outcomes, and develop a plan of care when presented with a clinical case study.

Traumatic Brain Injury

George D. Fulk, PT, PhD

OUTLINE

The traumatic brain injury (TBI) population is one of the most challenging that a physical therapist may encounter. Because of the multiple body systems affected by a brain injury and the strong likelihood of secondary impairments, a physical therapist must be proficient in a wide variety of examination procedures and intervention techniques. Owing to behavioral difficulties encountered during recovery, a physical therapist working with this population must also possess strong interpersonal skills, be able to react quickly and effectively to suddenly changing situations, and have keen observation skills. These factors and others can make working with this population both challenging and exhausting, both emotionally and physically. However, the rewards of assisting a patient with a severe brain injury to return home or to school vastly outweigh the challenges of rehabilitation.

The patient with a brain injury is treated across a wide continuum of care, which includes acute hospitalization, rehabilitation centers, community reentry programs, outpatient therapy, schools, vocational rehabilitation, and assisted living centers.[1] Because of the wide variety of impairments and complications arising from a brain injury, it is vital that a strong team concept be employed when treating this population. A physical therapist is an important member of this team in any setting. It is crucial that there be open communication between all team members to ensure safe, timely, and consistent treatment. Regardless of the setting, it is important to remember that the patient is the key member of the team.

Epidemiology

TBI is a common and devastating occurrence in American society. It is a leading cause of death and disability in young adults in the United States. An estimated 1.5 to 2 million people will incur a TBI each year.[2] Approximately 50,000 individuals will die each year as a result of a TBI, while over 230,000 are hospitalized and survive.[3] Of those individuals, 80,000 to 90,000 people will develop intellectual, behavioral, and/or physical disabilities that will prevent return to a normal, independent lifestyle.[4] This has resulted in between 2.5 and 6.5 million Americans living with the consequences of a TBI.[2]

Motor vehicle accidents cause approximately one half of all traumatic brain injuries, with falls accounting for 25 percent, assaults and violence for 15 percent, and sports and recreation for 10 percent.[4] Men are injured more often than women. The typical patient is between the ages of 15 and 24 years at the time of injury.

The economic impact of TBI is substantial, for both the individual and society. The annual cost of acute care and rehabilitation for new brain injuries in the United States is about $9 to $10 billion. Estimates for average lifetime cost of care for a patient with severe TBI range from $600,000 to $1,872,000.[2] Vangel et al found motor disability and improvement during inpatient rehabilitation were significant predictors of costs after traumatic brain injury.[5] Because there is no "cure" for a brain injury, it is important that health care professionals become involved in preventative measures. This may involve community outreach and educating high-risk groups, particularly teenagers. One example is *Think First* (http://www.thinkfirst.org/home.html), an association whose mission is to prevent brain injury, spinal cord injury, and other traumatic injuries through education. The group targets teens and children and educates them on the devastating effects of a brain injury or spinal cord injury. The program teaches students the basics about how the brain and spinal cord work. Students are also instructed on preventative measures such as wearing bike helmets and seat belts, the dangers of driving while intoxicated, and the importance of using proper protective equipment during athletics. Perhaps the most effective tool used by the *Think First* program is having brain injury survivors participate in the presentations. They are able to tell the students firsthand about the debilitating effects of a brain injury. Seeing and hearing their stories have a much more profound effect on the students than listening to a lecture on the dangers of drinking and driving.

Pathophysiology

A variety of pathophysiological mechanisms result from a TBI, each a result of external forces acting on brain tissue. Acceleration, deceleration, and rotational forces of the brain relative to the bony skull cause compression, strain, shearing, and displacement of brain tissue. For example, damage to the prefrontal area of the brain may occur as a result of a motor vehicle accident. The moving body and head suddenly stop but the brain continues to move inside the skull and strikes the inner surface of the cranium. Damage from a penetrating object, such as a bullet, can cause tissue lacerations and contusions. Injuries can be both focal and diffuse.

Focal Injury

Focal brain injury is localized to the area of the brain under the site of impact on the skull. The damage may be in the form of a hematoma, edema, contusion, or laceration, or a combination of the four. A severe blow to the head may result in brain damage not only directly under the site of impact, but also directly opposite the site of impact. This results from the brain "bouncing" and making contact with the skull at a site opposite from the site of initial impact. Such an injury is referred to as **coup-contrecoup injury**. Common sites of focal brain injury are the anterior–inferior temporal lobes and prefrontal lobes.

Diffuse Axonal Injury

Acceleration, deceleration, and rotational forces cause **diffuse axonal injury (DAI)**, which is characterized by widespread shearing and retraction of damaged axons. Axonal changes eventually lead to their separation from the soma. Diffuse axonal injury may be severe enough to cause coma and correlates with less clinical recovery. In addition to cortical white matter, it often involves the corpus callosum, basal ganglia, brainstem, and cerebellum.

Hypoxic–Ischemic Injury

Hypoxic–ischemic injury (HII) results from a lack of oxygenated blood flow to the brain tissue. It can be caused by systemic hypotension, anoxia, or damage to specific vascular territories of the brain. Hypoxic ischemic injury can lead to global damage and is associated with poorer cognitive function and lower expected outcomes.

Increased Intracranial Pressure

Because the rigid skull surrounds the brain, swelling or abnormality of brain fluid dynamics often results in increased **intracranial pressure (ICP)**. Elevated ICP may also result from hematomas. Hematomas are usually classified according to their site (**epidural**, **subdural**, or **intracerebral**). Normal ICP is 4 to 15 mm Hg. Even mildly increased ICP is associated with increased morbidity in survivors. Severely increased ICP may result in herniation of the brain. Table 22.1 presents common types of brain herniation syndromes and their effects. Increased ICP is also correlated with poorer expected outcomes and higher mortality rates.

Secondary cell death can also occur as a result of a variety of cellular events that follow tissue damage. These include glutamate neurotoxicity, influx of calcium and other

Table 22.1 Herniations of the Brain

Type	Location	Cause	Anatomic Structures Involved	Clinical Effects
Uncal	Tentorial notch, midbrain	Mass lesion in temporal lobe or middle fossa	Hippocampal gyrus and uncus Oculomotor nerve Cerebral peduncle Midbrain ascending reticular activating system Posterior cerebral artery	 Paresis of nerve III Hemiparesis Coma Homonymous hemianopia
Central (transtentorial)	Tentorial notch, midbrain	Mass lesion in frontal, parietal, or occipital lobe Progression of uncal herniation	Midbrain and pons Ascending reticular activating system	Decerebrate rigidity Coma
Tonsillar (foramen magnum)	Foramen magnum, medulla	Mass lesion in posterior fossa Progression of uncal or transtentorial herniation	Cerebellar tonsils Indirect activation pathways Ascending reticular activating system Vasomotor centers	Neck pain and stiffness Flaccidity Coma Alteration of pulse, respiration, blood pressure

From Daube, JR, et al: Medical Neurosciences, ed 2. Little, Brown, & Co., Boston, 1986, p 368, with permission.

ions, free radical release, and cytokines that can lead to cell death.

Diagnosis

A variety of neuroimaging techniques are available to aid in the diagnosis and identification of neuroanatomical structures and systems damaged as a result of the injury. The most commonly available technologies are the computerized tomography (CT) scan and the magnetic resonance imaging (MRI) scan. More technologically advanced, but less readily available techniques include positron emission tomography (PET), single-photon emission computerized tomography (SPECT), and functional magnetic resonance imaging (fMRI).

CT scans are useful in identifying hematomas, ventricular enlargement, and atrophy. However, comparisons of CT and MRI confirm that CT is relatively insensitive to many of the lesions present after trauma. MRI provides superior soft tissue discrimination compared to CT. CT and MRI findings correlate moderately with pathology and outcomes.[1] Professionals and family members should be aware that a lack of significant abnormalities on CT does not rule out the presence of extensive brain damage. In particular, DAI may be undetectable on CT or MRI.

PET, SPECT, and fMRI are functional neuroimaging techniques able to detect regional cerebral blood flow, metabolism, cerebral perfusion, or increases in neuronal activity.[1] These imaging techniques are becoming more widely used in research centers to investigate the effects of rehabilitation interventions on cerebral function.

Neuropsychological testing is often done as well to provide further insight into cognitive and behavioral deficits. These tests can also aid in establishing the prognosis and expected outcomes after TBI.

Sequelae of TBI

TBI is associated with a wide variety of neuromuscular, cognitive, and behavioral impairments that lead to functional limitations and disability. Table 22.2 identifies some of the prevalent impairments associated with TBI. Although physical therapists are primarily concerned with improving neuromuscular function, the cognitive and behavioral changes associated with TBI are usually the most disabling in the long run.

Neuromuscular Impairments

The patient with TBI often presents with abnormal tone. Primitive postures may include those associated with

Table 22.2 Impairments Associated with Traumatic Brain Injury

Neuromuscular • Abnormal tone • Sensory impairments • Motor function (motor control and motor learning) impairments • Impaired balance • Paresis/paralysis **Cognitive** • Altered level of consciousness/alertness • Memory loss • Altered orientation • Attentional deficits • Impaired insight and safety awareness • Problem solving/reasoning impairments • Perseveration • Impaired executive functioning **Visual** **Perceptual**	**Behavioral** • Disinhibition • Impulsiveness • Physical and verbal aggressiveness • Apathy • Lack of concern • Sexual inappropriateness • Irritability • Egocentricity **Communication** • Receptive aphasia • Expressive aphasia • Dysarthria • Auditory deficits • Impaired reading comprehension • Impaired written expression • Impaired pragmatics (use of language) **Dysphagia**

decorticate or **decerebrate rigidity**. In decorticate rigidity, the upper extremities are in a flexed posture and the lower extremities are extended. This is indicative of a lesion at or above the upper brainstem (above the superior colliculus). With decerebrate rigidity, both the upper and lower extremities are positioned in extension. The lesion is located in the brainstem between the vestibular nucleus and the superior colliculus.[6] Abnormal tone may take the form of spastic hypertonus. This may range from spasticity that severely affects the entire body and greatly inhibits normal, functional movement, to lesser levels of tone that affect individual muscle groups and function.

Alterations in sensation are common following TBI and may include impairments in light touch, pain, deep pressure, and temperature. Proprioception and kinesthesia may also be impaired and are of particular concern to the physical therapist. Ambulation and other mobility skills can be secondarily impaired if the individual does not know where his or her body is in space. Impaired proprioception, along with visual or vestibular impairments, will affect balance.

Motor control impairments can take many forms. They include monoparesis, hemiparesis, tetraparesis (quadriparesis), and/or abnormal reflexes. Individuals with TBI may also exhibit impairments in coordination, timing, and sequencing of movement. This is particularly true with damage to the cerebellum. Motor control deficits and abnormal tone are highly variable, both between patients and with day-to-day fluctuations in individual patients. Chapter 8 provides an in-depth discussion of motor control impairments and examination procedures.

Many patients who experience a TBI will exhibit balance impairments, as cerebellar injury is common. These deficits may be subtle in patients with minor brain injuries. Owing to the cognitive impairments described below, neuromuscular impairments may become magnified in an open and distracting environment.

Cognitive Impairments

Altered level of consciousness occurs consistently with acceleration–deceleration type injuries (DAI) and may occur with some focal injuries. Consistent use of terminology in dealing with altered consciousness is important. According to Jennett and Teasdale, *coma* is defined as not obeying commands, not uttering words, and not opening the eyes.[7] The Glasgow Coma Scale (GCS) score can be used to identify coma, with a score of 8 or less defining coma. Patients in coma have no spontaneous eye opening and do not respond to vigorous sensory stimulation. It is important to note that coma usually lasts only a few weeks at most. Patients with a decreased level of awareness with intact eye opening and sleep–awake cycles but no ability to follow commands or speak are described as being in a *vegetative state*. Patients in a *persistent vegetative state* have no meaningful motor or cognitive function and a complete absence of awareness of self or the environment.[8] This is typically defined as greater than 1 year for TBI and greater than 3 months for anoxic brain injury.

It is important to distinguish patients who are in a vegetative state from those who are in a **minimally conscious state (MCS)**. The MCS is defined as severely altered consciousness with minimal but definite evidence of self or environmental awareness.[8] Cognitive-mediated behavior occurs inconsistently, but is reproducible or sustained to distinguish it from reflexive behavior that is present with the vegetative state. For example, a patient in a vegetative state may exhibit nonpurposeful movement and withdraw from noxious stimuli. A patient in a MCS will localize to noxious stimuli and reach for objects.

Commonly used terms to describe other altered levels of consciousness states are *stupor* and *obtunded*. Stupor is described as an unresponsive state from which the patient can be aroused only briefly with vigorous, repeated sensory stimulation. The obtunded patient sleeps often and when aroused exhibits decreased alertness and interest in the environment and delayed reactions.

Orientation and memory deficits are common cognitive impairments. The patient is often disoriented to person, place, and time. Memory deficits can include both *retrograde* and/or *anterograde amnesia*. *Posttraumatic amnesia (PTA)* describes the time between the injury and the time when the patient is again able to remember ongoing events, such as what was eaten for breakfast or what happened the previous day. While the patient has PTA, it is as though each moment exists in isolation. There is no carryover of information from hour-to-hour or day-to-day. The implications for functional training are obvious and can be frustrating for the patient and rehabilitation team members. It is difficult to relearn functional skills without memory.

There is a difference between **declarative** and **procedural memory**. Declarative memory is the ability to recall facts and previous events and is used in explicit learning. Procedural memory is related to the knowledge of how to do motor tasks and is used in implicit learning. This refers to learning tasks that can be performed without attention or conscious thought, such as a habit.[9] Repeated practice of a motor task may lead to procedural memory. Patients with declarative memory deficits may learn (or relearn) motor skills using procedural memory. A patient with PTA is unable to describe memories (declarative memory) or verbalize the steps necessary to complete a task. However, he or she may, at times, show carryover of skills that do not require verbal explanation (procedural memory). For example, with repeated practice a patient may improve the ability to transfer from sit-to-stand but could not describe the steps necessary to complete the task.

Impaired attention also plays a role in the rehabilitation process. Patients may exhibit hyperactivity, impulsiveness, and a decreased attention span. Patients may be easily distractible. The distraction can be externally mediated, or in some cases, internally. This can also contribute to difficulty in reacquiring functional skills. Patients may not be able to focus on a task for a long enough period of time to facilitate learning. Individuals with TBI may also lack insight into their impairments and demonstrate diminished safety awareness. This can be especially problematic with patients that have fair to good physical skills but still require some physical assistance. The patient may not realize that he or she cannot transfer out of bed or ambulate across a street safely without supervision or physical assistance.

Executive function cognitive skills refer to four overlapping capabilities: volition, planning, purposive action, and effective performance.[10] Executive function skills allow the individual to successfully develop and carry out purposeful goal oriented behavior. An in-depth discussion of cognitive impairments associated with neurological injuries is provided in Chapter 29.

Behavioral Impairments

Research and clinical experience have established that behavioral disorders are the most enduring and socially disabling of any of the impairments commonly seen after TBI.[11] Long-term changes in behavior such as sexual disinhibition, emotional disinhibition, apathy, aggressive disinhibition, low frustration tolerance, and depression often affect social skills and make re-integration back into society difficult. Factors to be considered in the evaluation and management of behavioral impairments are (1) the person's premorbid personality; (2) the physical, cognitive, and emotional effects of the injury; and (3) the nature of the social environment. Typically, neuropsychologists skilled in the evaluation and treatment of behavioral disorders play a leading role in determining behavioral programs. However, to achieve a successful outcome, behavior programs need to be generalized across all treatment settings.

Communication Impairments

Numerous types of communication deficits are noted with patients following brain injury, and these can have a significant impact on rehabilitation. Expressive or receptive aphasia, reading comprehension and written expression, language skill deficits, and dysarthria may be present to varying degrees. See Chapter 30 for a discussion of these impairments.

Visual–Perceptual Impairments

Damage to cranial nerves or the occipital lobes can cause visual impairments. This can include hemianopsia or on rare occasions cortical blindness. Perceptual impairments can include spatial neglect, apraxia, spatial relations syndrome, somatagnosia, and right–left discrimination deficits. See Chapter 29 for a discussion of perceptual deficits.

Swallowing Impairments

Following TBI, many individuals commonly experience **dysphagia**. Swallowing deficits can be caused by damage to cranial nerves, motor control impairments, apraxia, and poor postural control. A speech–language pathologist is the primary team member in treating this impairment (see Chapter 30).

Indirect Impairments

Owing to the complex nature of TBI and prolonged immobility, patients are likely to suffer from a variety of indirect

Box 22.1 Indirect Impairments Associated with Traumatic Brain Injury

- Soft tissue contractures
- Skin breakdown, decubitus ulcer
- Deep vein thrombosis
- Heterotropic ossification
- Decreased bone density
- Muscle atrophy
- Decreased endurance
- Infection
- Pneumonia

impairments as well. Box 22.1 presents the more common indirect impairments associated with TBI.

Clinical Rating Scales

Outcome measures are extremely important for the rehabilitation professional. Valid and reliable outcome measures can be used by physical therapists to assist in predicting outcomes or in making a diagnosis. They are used to evaluate change in the patient over time, which also provides a means for determining the effectiveness of the interventions provided. When data for large groups of patients are presented in aggregate form, the findings can provide information regarding the cost effectiveness of physical therapy and other rehabilitation interventions. Some of the most commonly used clinical rating scales designed for individuals with a TBI are briefly described below.

Glasgow Coma Scale

The *Glasgow Coma Scale (GCS)*, developed by Teasdale and Jennett, is the most widely used clinical scale that measures level of consciousness and helps define and classify the severity of injury.[12] The GCS is comprised of three response scores: motor response, verbal response, and eye opening (Table 22.3). The scores from the separate responses are summed to provide a score between 3 and 15. Coma is commonly defined as scores ≤8. Scores ≤8 are classified as a severe brain injury, scores between 9 and 12 are defined as moderate and 13 to 15 are classified as mild brain injury. The GCS has high inter-rater reliability[13] and can be used as a prognostic measure.[14]

Galveston Orientation and Amnesia Test

The *Galveston Orientation and Amnesia Test (GOAT)* is a measure of posttraumatic amnesia (PTA).[15] Duration of PTA has been shown to be a valid predictor of long-term outcome after TBI.[16,17] The GOAT is administered by asking a series of standardized questions related to orientation

Table 22.3 Glasgow Coma Scale

Activity	Score
Eye Opening	
Spontaneous	4
To speech	3
To pain	2
No response	1
Best Motor Response	
Follows motor commands	6
Localizes	5
Withdraws	4
Abnormal flexion	3
Extensor response	2
No response	1
Verbal Response	
Oriented	5
Confused conversation	4
Inappropriate words	3
Incomprehensible sounds	2
No response	1

From Jennett and Teasdale,[7] p 78, with permission.

and the ability to recall events prior to and after the injury. Scores between 100 and 76 are considered normal and patients with scores below are considered to have PTA. The GOAT has high interrater reliability.[15]

Rancho Los Amigos Level of Cognitive Functioning

The *Rancho Los Amigos Level of Cognitive Functioning (LOCF)* scale is a descriptive scale used to examine cognitive and behavioral recovery in individuals with TBI (Box 22.2) as they emerge from coma.[18] This scale does not address specific cognitive deficits, but is useful for communicating general cognitive and/or behavioral status and for treatment planning. The eight categories describe typical cognitive and behavioral progress after a brain injury. Clients may plateau at any level. The LOCF has been shown to be a reliable and valid measure of cognitive and behavioral function for individuals with brain injury.[19,20] This scale, together with the GCS, is among the most widely used in clinical facilities.

Glasgow Outcome Scale

The *Glasgow Outcome Scale (GOS)* is used as a general outcomes measure after a TBI.[21] It is often used in prognostic studies at discharge and 6 months to a year after injury. The GOS consists of five categories: dead, vegetative, severely disabled, moderately disabled, and good recovery. The extended GOS expands the severely disabled, moderately disabled, and good recovery categories (Table 22.4). This scale has good reliability.[22,23]

Box 22.2 Rancho Los Amigos Levels of Cognitive Functioning (LOCF)[a]

I. No Response
Patient appears to be in a deep sleep and is completely unresponsive to any stimuli.

II. Generalized Response
Patient reacts inconsistently and nonpurposefully to stimuli in a nonspecific manner. Responses are limited and often the same regardless of stimulus presented. Responses may be physiological changes, gross body movements, and/or vocalization.

III. Localized Response
Patient reacts specifically but inconsistently to stimuli. Responses are directly related to the type of stimulus presented. May follow simple commands such as closing eyes or squeezing hand in an inconsistent, delayed manner.

IV. Confused–Agitated
Patient is in a heightened state of activity. Behavior is bizarre and nonpurposeful relative to immediate environment. Does not discriminate among persons or objects; is unable to cooperate directly with treatment efforts. Verbalizations frequently are incoherent and/or inappropriate to the environment; confabulation may be present. Gross attention to environment is very brief; selective attention is often nonexistent. Patient lacks short- and long-term recall.

V. Confused–Inappropriate
Patient is able to respond to simple commands fairly consistently. However, with increased complexity of commands or lack of any external structure, responses are nonpurposeful, random, or fragmented. Demonstrates gross attention to the environment but is highly distractible and lacks ability to focus attention on a specific task. With structure, may be able to converse on a social automatic level for short periods of time. Verbalization is often inappropriate and confabulatory. Memory is severely impaired; often shows inappropriate use of objects; may perform previously learned tasks with structure but is unable to learn new information.

VI. Confused–Appropriate
Patient shows goal-directed behavior but is dependent on external input or direction. Follows simple directions consistently and shows carryover for relearned tasks such as self-care. Responses may be incorrect due to memory problems, but they are appropriate to the situation. Past memories show more depth and detail than recent memory.

VII. Automatic–Appropriate
Patient appears appropriate and oriented within the hospital and home settings; goes through daily routine automatically, but frequently robotlike. Patient shows minimal to no confusion and has shallow recall of activities. Shows carryover for new learning but at a decreased rate. With structure is able to initiate social or recreational activities; judgement remains impaired.

VIII. Purposeful-Appropriate
Patient is able to recall and integrate past and recent events and is aware of and responsive to environment. Shows carryover for new learning and needs no supervision once activities are learned. May continue to show a decreased ability relative to premorbid abilities, abstract reasoning, tolerance for stress, and judgement in emergencies or unusual circumstances.

[a]Condensed form. From Professional Staff Association, Rancho Los Amigos Hospital,[18] pp 87–88, with permission.

Table 22.4 Glasgow Outcome Scale

Extended Scale		Original Scale	
Dead		Dead	Dead
Vegetative		Vegetative	Dependent
Degree of disability:	5	Severely disabled	
	4		
	3		Independent
	2	Moderately disabled	
	1		
	0	Good recovery	
Total Categories 8		5	3

From Jennett and Teasdale,[7] p 306, with permission.

Table 22.5 Disability Rating Scale

Category	Item
Arousability, awareness and responsivity	Eye opening[1] Verbalization[2] Motor response[3]
Cognitive ability for self-care	Feeding[4] Toileting[4] Grooming[4]
Dependence on others	Level of functioning[5]
Psychosocial adaptability	"Employability"[6]

[1]Eye Opening		[2]Best Verbal Response		[3]Best Motor Response		[4]Cognitive ability for self-care (Does patient know how and when? Ignore motor disability.)	
Spontaneous	0	Oriented	0	Obeying	0	Complex	0
To speech	1	Confused	1	Localizing	1	Partial	1
To pain	2	Inappropriate	2	Withdrawing	2	Minimal	2
None	3	Incomprehensive	3	Flexing	3	None	3
		None	4	Extending	4		
				None	5		

[5]Level of Functioning		[6]"Employability"	
Completely independent	0	Not restricted	0
Independent in special environment	1	Selected jobs	1
Mildly dependent[a]	2	Sheltered workshop	2
Moderately dependent[b]	3	Not employable	3
Markedly dependent[c]	4		
Totally dependent[d]	5		

Disability Categories	
Total DR Score	**Level of Disability**
0	None
1	Mild
2–3	Partial
4–6	Moderate
7–11	Moderately severe
12–16	Severe
17–21	Extremely severe
22–24	Vegetative state
25–29	Extreme vegetative state
30	Death

Condensed form. From Rappaport,[24] p 119, with permission.
[a]Needs limited assistance (nonresident helper).
[b]Needs moderate assistance (person in home).
[c]Needs assistance with all major activities at all times.
[d]24-hour nursing care required.

Disability Rating Scale

Rappaport's Disability Rating Scale (DRS) covers a wide range of functional areas and is used to classify levels of disability ranging from death to no disability (Table 22.5).[24] It can be used to track individual progress from coma through community integration. The maximum score is a 29, indicating extreme vegetative state, while the lowest possible score is a 0, indicating no disability. The DRS has good reliability as well.[19,24]

Functional Independence Measure and Functional Assessment Measure

The *Functional Independence Measure (FIM™)*[25–27] is a commonly used measure of functional mobility and ADL function. The FIM™ was designed to measure level of disability in individuals undergoing in-patient rehabilitation, and is useful for monitoring patient progress and evaluating outcomes. The *Functional Assessment Measure (FAM)* was developed as an adjunct to the FIM™. It includes functional areas not addressed in the FIM™ that are important for individuals with TBI and stroke. The other items include community access, reading, writing, safety, employability, and adjustment to limitations.[28,29] The FIM™ in combination with the FAM are valid and reliable measures of disability after TBI.[30,31]

Prognosis and Goal Setting

Owing to the wide range of cognitive, motor, and neurobehavioral impairments that accompany brain injury, it can be difficult to establish and predict long-term outcomes and set goals for these patients, even for an experienced clinician. When setting goals, the patient, family, caregivers, and entire interdisciplinary team should be consulted. The patient's potential for cognitive and behavioral improvement will greatly affect future motor ability and social participation.

Outcomes research has identified some factors that help predict outcome after a TBI. Initial severity of injury as measured on the GCS,[32,33] duration of coma,[16,17] and length of PTA[16,17] have all been shown to be predictors of disability. In one study by Katz,[17] all of the subjects whose duration of coma was greater than 2 weeks were left with moderate or severe disability, as measured on the GOS, at 1 year post-injury. The majority of subjects who experienced a coma of less than 1 week duration had either moderate disability or a good recovery. Similar results were associated with duration of PTA. If PTA lasted greater than 12 weeks, then all of the subjects demonstrated moderate to severe disability. The majority of subjects with PTA lasting 4 weeks or less had a good recovery or moderate disability after one year. The above described factors that assist with predicting outcome after a TBI should be used as general guidelines with individual patients. Because of the widespread neurological damage and range of resulting impairments and functional limitations, it is difficult to use these predictors with precision for individual patients.

Medical Management

Medical treatment for a patient with a TBI starts at the scene of the accident. Early resuscitation with the goal of stabilizing the cardiovascular and respiratory systems is important in order to maintain sufficient blood flow and oxygen to the brain.[34] Patients who are unresponsive should be intubated and ventilated.

Once the patient arrives at the medical center, the primary goals are to stabilize vital signs, perform a complete examination of the injury, and establish a comprehensive monitoring system.[34] The GCS is used to determine the severity of the brain injury. A complete neurological examination is also done. Additional information about the extent of the injury is obtained through X-ray films and neuroimaging studies such as CT and MRI of the head, spine, thorax, and abdomen. Large intracranial hematomas or other mass lesions are surgically evacuated.

Intracranial pressure (ICP) is monitored. This can be done via a catheter placed in the lateral ventricle, a screw in the skull inserted into the subarachnoid space, or a transducer placed directly in the epidural space. Normal values for ICP are between 4 and 15 mm Hg. Medical intervention aims to maintain an ICP below 20 mm Hg.[34] Elevated ICP is treated with the use of sedating medications, moderate head up positioning (head elevated to 30°), ventricular drainage, osmotherapy, hypothermia, surgical decompression, and barbiturates.[34]

Medical scientists are researching the effectiveness of various medications to prevent the pathophysiological mechanisms that cause secondary brain damage. No drug has achieved this goal so far. However, glutamate receptor antagonists, free radical scavengers, calcium antagonists, and cyclosporin have shown promise.[34]

Owing to the severity of the injury and the potential for concomitant injuries, such as long bone fractures, patients with TBI often present with a variety of medical complications that can interfere with rehabilitation and the recovery process. One study found that 56 percent of patients with severe brain injury exhibited neurological problems, 50 percent developed gastrointestinal difficulties, 45 percent developed genitourinary problems, 34 percent had respiratory problems, 32 percent had cardiovascular problems, and 21 percent had dermatological complications.[35] Examples of specific conditions include ventricular dilatation, **posttraumatic seizures**, impaired liver function tests, urinary tract infections, hypertension, and decubitus ulcers.

Medications may be used to treat these and other complications that may arise. The physical therapist typically spends more time with the patient as compared to the medical doctor, allowing the therapist an advantageous position of alerting the physician regarding a host of varied medical problems that can be treated with medications. This serves to enhance the patient's medical status, which in turn maximizes the patient's ability to participate in therapy sessions. Areas that the therapist might logically provide recommendations include pain management, spasticity, motor restoration, and cognitive issues including level of consciousness, awareness, attention quality, speech, memory, and disinhibited emotional, physical, and sexual behaviors. The physician has a similar responsibility to inform the rehabilitation team when doses are increased or when new medications are started. Because patients with brain injury are often on several medications at one time, all team members typically take an active role in monitoring side effects and determining the impact of the medications. Refer to Appendix A for some commonly prescribed medications with comments and side effects for each medication.

Rehabilitation Perspective

Interdisciplinary Team

The rehabilitation of patients with TBI occurs across a continuum of care in a variety of settings (Fig. 22.1). Patients who are in a minimally conscious state or in coma may receive on-going therapy in a nursing home or other

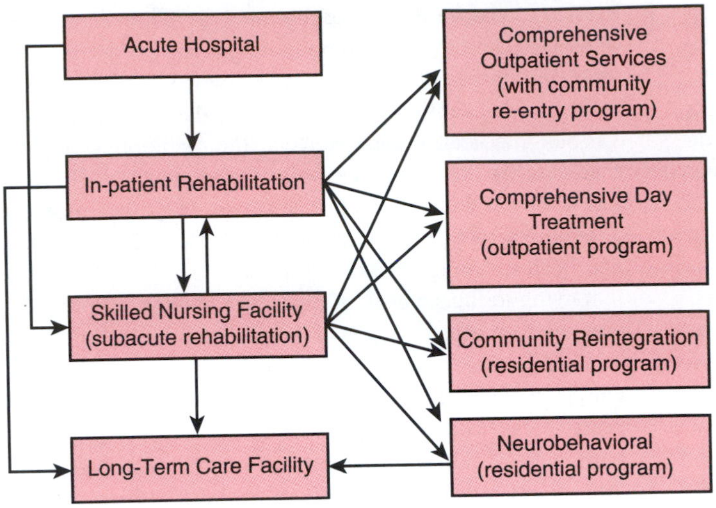

Figure 22.1 Rehabilitation settings for individuals with TBI across the continuum of care.

long-term care facility once they are medically stable. Patients who are beginning to recover from coma with moderate to severe cognitive, behavioral, and physical impairments often continue rehabilitation in either an acute or subacute in-patient rehabilitation facility. As patients progress in recovery, they will be discharged to other community-based settings depending on the needs of the individual patient.

As mentioned earlier, the foundation for successful rehabilitation of the patient with a brain injury is an *interdisciplinary team*. No one person could possibly have the knowledge and skills necessary to treat all aspects of a brain injury. An interdisciplinary team approach is essential to providing the most comprehensive care that will lead to maximizing the patient's functional recovery. Although most research conducted in this area is not controlled, an interdisciplinary approach to rehabilitation for this population has been shown to be effective for improving function and participation in society.[36–39]

Within the context of the team, individual members collaborate, contributing their expertise in a specific area, thereby enhancing the team's overall effectiveness. Communication and open mindedness are key to any team. The different members must share their skills and findings with the whole team and be willing to learn from other team members to promote optimal return of function. The physical therapist must be willing to share a unique knowledge of motor control, but be open to learning from other team members such as the speech–language pathologist about cognitive deficits. All team members should take what they have learned from other team members and incorporate it into their treatment. This will lead to a consistent and complete approach to care.

Some members may play more prominent roles depending on the setting. For example, a recreational therapist will not likely be involved with a patient in the acute hospital, but would play a vital role in a community reentry setting. The following section identifies some of the team members involved in the care of brain injury survivors and their roles in an acute rehabilitation hospital.

Patient and Family

It cannot be stressed enough that the most important members of the team are the patient and his or her family. Both the patient's and the family's lives are likely to be dramatically changed as a result of the injury. Familial roles may change. The patient who previously took care of the children may now be on the receiving end of care. The team must garner information regarding the patient's work, school, financial status, and social history. Family members should be questioned to obtain information on the patient's lifestyle, favorite hobbies, and other likes and dislikes. Information about the family dynamics should be ascertained. Who is the head of the household? Who is the breadwinner in the family? Is the patient responsible for taking care of the children? What grade is the patient in? Is the patient in college or working full time? All of these and many other similar questions should be answered to develop a comprehensive plan of care.

Education is another essential aspect of care that should begin as soon as possible with the family and patient, when appropriate. The great majority of lay people are unaware of the implications of a brain injury. They may think their loved one will wake up from a coma and return to his or her previous lifestyle with little difficulty, like in a television movie. Unfortunately, this is rarely the case. It is the job of the entire interdisciplinary team to begin educating the family and patient about the affects of a brain injury and the long, arduous road to recovery. The family should be introduced to the Ranchos Los Amigos LOCF Scale and what to expect at the different stages. It is often beneficial to provide educational material for the patient and family. The physical therapist should begin education on basic components of care such as how to perform passive range of motion (PROM), to more complex issues, such as why spasticity develops and how the brain controls movement.

Family members often ask if the patient will return to a "normal" life, or how much function he or she will regain. During the initial stages of recovery in the acute hospital and acute rehabilitation hospital, this question is difficult to answer. Every patient recovers differently and at different rates. An effective way to help answer family questions and concerns is through education.

Physician

In the acute rehabilitation hospital, the physician overseeing the care of the patient with a brain injury is usually a physiatrist or neurologist. The physiatrist has expertise and training in physical medicine, rehabilitation, and function. A neurologist's skills lie in the realm of the brain and nervous system. A neurologist will have particular knowledge related to how the brain may recover, and what impairments are likely to be seen given the location and the extent of the injury. Both a physiatrist and neurologist have vast knowledge in neuropharmacology, an extremely important part of management with this patient population. Certain medications may have harmful side effects that may not be readily apparent. For example, a physiatrist or neurologist may be able to prescribe a less sedating drug than would normally be used in a different patient population to treat a certain clinical problem.

Speech–Language Pathologist

Because of to the nature of a brain injury, the speech–language pathologist (SLP) plays an important and diverse role in the rehabilitation of the patient. The SLP examines, evaluates, and treats communication, swallowing, and cognitive impairments in the patient. As can be seen from the presentation of impairments in Table 22.2, this can be a challenging task. It is important for the physical therapist to be in close communication with the SLP to provide consistency of care in relation to cognitive, swallowing, and communication impairments. With the guidance of the SLP, the team will be able to devise the most effective and consistent way to communicate with the patient. He or she will also be able to instruct the team in how the patient's cognitive impairments may impede new learning, which in turn will affect everyone's interactions with the patient and the treatment plan.

Occupational Therapist

The occupational therapist (OT) examines, evaluates, and treats the patient's diminished ability to perform activities of daily living (ADL), visual/perceptual impairments, upper extremity (UE) functional loss, and sensory integration problems, and will often work with the SLP in treating cognitive impairments. Basic ADL (BADL) includes dressing, self-feeding, bathing, and grooming. Instrumental ADL (IADL) includes home management, housekeeping, grocery shopping, driving, and telephone use. In the rehabilitation hospital, the occupational and physical therapists often work very closely together. A useful treatment approach is co-treatments with the OT. Having two trained professionals working at the same time with the patient can be very productive. Many times two sets of experienced and trained hands are needed to effectively treat the patient. This is especially true with patients that have severe motor control and cognitive deficits. The OT will also work closely with the nursing staff to educate them on the best ways to assist the patient with ADL.

Rehabilitation Nurse

In a rehabilitation hospital, the nurse is responsible for dispensing medications and closely monitoring their effects. The nurse will initiate a bowel and bladder retraining program to assist the patient in learning to become continent again. Bowel and bladder control is extremely important for self-esteem and is related to discharge placement. The nurse performs daily monitoring of vital signs to make sure the patient remains medically stable. The nurse will inspect the patient's skin daily to ensure there are no signs of skin breakdown. The nurse also has the difficult task of consistently following through with the team's treatment plan throughout the day. For example, the third nursing shift needs to continue to follow splinting schedules established by the physical and occupational therapists. The nurse often has the most interaction on a regular basis with the patient's family.

Case Manager/Team Coordinator

The case manager acts as the coordinator for the team. The case manager is often a nurse, medical social worker, or other health professional. The case manager will direct team meetings, schedule family conferences, and act as a liaison with third-party payers. He or she must promote good communication among all team members to ensure that the rehabilitation care being provided is truly team oriented. The case manager will also be in constant communication with the patient and family to ensure their needs are being met and that questions and concerns are adequately addressed. The case manager will coordinate payment and insurance benefit issues with the case manager from the patient's insurance company. In addition, the case manager is responsible for setting up follow-up and discharge services for the patient and family.

Medical Social Worker

The medical social worker (MSW) provides much needed support to both the family and patient. During the first few days after the initial injury, the family is in a state of crisis. They are thrown into a world that they, most likely, never knew existed. The MSW can support the family with education and counseling. As the patient progresses with recovery, the MSW will also provide counseling for the patient. This is particularly important as the patient begins to develop greater awareness and insight into his or her deficits. If the patient has behavioral impairments, the MSW can be pivotal in assisting both the patient and family. By providing counseling to both the patient and family, the MSW assists in the development of coping strategies for what may be a lifelong disability.

Neuropsychologist

The neuropsychologist plays an important role on the team. He or she will often perform neuropsychological testing when appropriate to determine the patient's baseline cognitive functioning. He or she will also assist the team in developing a behavioral management program. When the patient with a brain injury has severe behavioral impairments, the neuropsychologist assumes the role of the team leader.

Other Team Members

Many patients with severe brain injury may require ventilatory support. The *respiratory care practitioner* is a vital participant in the evaluation and treatment of respiratory impairments. In the rehabilitation hospital, the respiratory therapist contributes to monitoring the patient's pulmonary status and providing appropriate treatment.

A *recreational therapist* assists the patient's return to activities enjoyed prior to the accident, or in helping identify new activities that the patient will find rewarding. This is an extremely important part of rehabilitation. Being able to participate in some type of leisure or recreational activities is a significant step in returning to a fulfilling lifestyle. Unfortunately, many insurance companies no longer reimburse for the services of a recreational therapist.

Physical Therapy Examination and Treatment

A patient with a moderate to severe TBI is likely to require extensive rehabilitation services across a variety of settings along a continuum of care (Fig. 22.1). A physical therapist is likely to be involved in the rehabilitation management in all of these settings. However, the role of the physical therapist will vary depending on the setting and the needs of the individual patient.

The complex and diverse nature of the impairments, functional limitations, and cognitive and behavioral problems associated with TBI calls for an organized approach to exploring physical therapy examination techniques and interventions. The following section adopts the Ranchos Los Amigos LOCF scale as a framework to address specific elements of physical therapy examination and treatment. The reader should bear in mind that physical recovery does not always mirror cognitive and behavioral recovery. For example, just because a patient is moving from level IV to level V on the LOCF scale it does not mean that he or she will begin to show a similar gain in physical function. Two patients with brain injury may be in stage V of recovery, but one may have severe physical impairments and need to use a wheelchair, while the other may be able to ambulate independently and have minimal physical impairments.

Ranchos Los Amigos Levels I, II, and III: Decreased or Low-Level Response Levels of Recovery

Examination

At these early stages of recovery, the patient is likely to be in an acute hospital. However, the patient might also be seen in an in-patient rehabilitation setting. A patient with a chronic injury who has not progressed beyond these stages may be seen in a long-term care facility. In Level I, the patient is unresponsive to stimuli. In Level II, the patient reacts inconsistently to stimuli. The response may be total body movements, vocalizations, or physiological changes. The response is often the same regardless of the stimuli. Level III is characterized by a localized response that is directly related to the type of stimuli presented (see Box 22.2).

The first step in beginning an examination at these stages of recovery is to conduct a complete chart review. Because the patient may not be medically stable, as well as the prevalence of various precautions and complications seen in this patient population, it is important to obtain all of the critical information from the chart before actually seeing the patient. The patient may be on a ventilator, monitoring of ICP may be ongoing, he or she may have weight-bearing precautions and range of motion (ROM) restrictions owing to orthopedic injuries, open wounds, or an external fixator may be present. By doing a complete chart review, the therapist can begin to form a comprehensive picture of the patient, and have a complete understanding of the precautions and contraindications that must be observed during the examination and subsequent treatment. Because the patient's medical status may be dynamic at these stages it is important to check with the patient's primary nurse before beginning any session.[40] The therapist should ascertain what the patient's vital signs are, if the patient is running a temperature, how alert the patient is, and if there are any contraindications or precautions in effect. Owing to the possibility of various infections, team members should always observe universal precautions and may need to wear gowns, gloves, and/or masks when treating the patient.

After reviewing the chart and receiving an update on the patient's status from the nursing staff, the physical therapist is ready to begin the examination. The initial portion of the examination should focus on observing the patient and documenting how he or she responds to stimuli in the environment. Key questions to address include:

- What posture is the patient in? Is there evidence of primitive postures or reflexes?
- Are the patient's eyes open or closed?
- Is the patient able to track to auditory or visual stimulation?

- Is the patient able to vocalize?
- Does the patient exhibit any active movement? Is the movement purposeful or nonpurposeful?
- Does the patient react to tactile/painful stimulation?
- Do the patient's vital signs change when external stimulation is presented?

Primitive postures may include those associated with **decorticate** or **decerebrate** rigidity, described earlier. Chapter 8 presents a detailed description of other primitive reflex patterns and postures associated with neurological insult.

Examination of PROM and muscle tone should be completed. Patients with TBI are at a high risk of developing contractures[41] owing to prolonged periods of immobilization and abnormal reflexive posturing. Because of these risk factors it is particularly important to document tone and PROM measurements. One common clinical tool used to examine muscle tone is the *modified Ashworth Scale*[42–45] (Table 22.6). Using the modified Ashworth Scale involves moving the patient's limb through the available ROM and determining the amount of resistance to passive movement at the joint.

If it is not medically contraindicated, the examination should include an attempt to sit the patient up on the side of the bed with assistance. The therapist should monitor vital signs and document any changes in tone or head and trunk control. When it is appropriate, the patient should be transferred into a wheelchair. The patient may require the assistance of two to three people to transfer at this stage. In most cases, a reclining or tilt-in-space wheelchair is the best option for positioning, with a specialized pressure-reducing cushion. Often it may require several treatment sessions to complete the entire examination. Whenever the therapist is working with the patient, signs of progress or regression should be carefully monitored.

Table 22.6 Modified Ashworth Scale for Grading Spasticity

Grade	Description
0	No increase in muscle tone.
1	Slight increase in muscle tone, manifested by a catch and release or by minimal resistance at the end of the ROM when the affected part(s) is moved in flexion or extension.
1+	Slight increase in muscle tone, manifested by a catch, followed by minimal resistance throughout the remainder (less than half) of the ROM.
2	More marked increase in muscle tone through most of the ROM, but affected part(s) easily moved.
3	Considerable increase in muscle tone, passive movement difficult.
4	Affected part(s) rigid in flexion or extension.

From Bohannon and Smith,[43] p 207, with permission.

Evaluation, Prognosis, and Plan of Care

The data gathered during the initial examination is used to evaluate the patient's status and develop a prognosis and plan of care (POC). Schenkman et al[46] provide a clinically useful model to assist the clinical reasoning and management process for patients with neurological impairments. This clinical decision-making tool follows Nagi's model of disablement from pathology to impairment to functional limitation to disability. Based on the findings from the initial examination, primary and secondary impairments contribute to the patient's functional limitations, which lead to disability. Goals and specific interventions are then established based on the impairments and functional limitations of the patient. See Chapter 1 for a more thorough discussion of this topic.

When working with patients who are slow to recover and minimally conscious, it is important to consider that not all of these individuals will emerge from their coma or minimally conscious state. As discussed earlier in the chapter, the longer the duration of coma the less likelihood of functional recovery. Patients who remain in this stage of recovery are often placed in long-term residential nursing home facilities where they receive custodial care. It may be difficult to find an appropriate long-term setting for these patients.

The following is a list of general goals and outcomes anticipated for patients in Levels I, II, and III (LOCF) adapted from the American Physical Therapy Association's *Guide to Physical Therapist Practice*.[47] They can be used to guide the development of specific anticipated goals and expected outcomes for an individual patient.

- Physical function and level of alertness are increased.
- The risk of secondary impairments is reduced.
- Motor control is improved.
- The effects of tone are managed.
- Postural control is improved.
- Tolerance of activities and positions is increased.
- Joint integrity and mobility are improved or remain functional.
- Family and caregivers are educated on patient's diagnosis, physical therapy interventions, goals, and outcomes.
- Care is coordinated among all team members.

Intervention

Whenever possible, interventions should be selected that address several goals at once. For example, when PROM is performed joint mobility and integrity are improved, risk of secondary impairments is reduced, and sensory stimulation is provided.

Preventing Indirect Impairments

Because of the patient's inability to move at these levels, he or she is susceptible to indirect impairments such as contractures, decubiti, pneumonia, and deep vein thrombosis.[35] If this is not addressed early in rehabilitation, these impairments are likely to impede future progress, and can even be life threatening. Proper positioning both in bed and in a wheelchair is essential. Good positioning will assist in preventing skin breakdown, contractures, improve pulmonary hygiene and circulation, and may modify muscle tone.[48] When the patient is in bed, the head should be kept in neutral. This will help prevent neck contractures and may lessen the effects of tonic neck reflexes (Fig. 22.2). The hips and knees should be slightly flexed, but ROM should be monitored to ensure that contractures do not develop. The nurses and family members should be instructed in how to properly position and turn the patient. Turning may help prevent skin breakdown and pneumonia. Patients should be turned every 2 hours when in bed. Specialized air mattresses are another effective way to assist with the prevention of pressure sores.[49] Table 22.7 presents strategies for positioning and handling.

Proper wheelchair positioning is important.[50] Because of reduced postural control at these levels, a reclining wheelchair or a tilt-in-space wheelchair is typically required. Proper pelvic and head positioning are the key elements in promoting good posture in a wheelchair (Fig. 22.3). Refer to Chapter 33 for further discussion of this topic. Splints may also be used to assist in positioning. Multipodus boots can be used to position the foot to prevent foot drop and skin breakdown on the heel (Fig. 22.4).

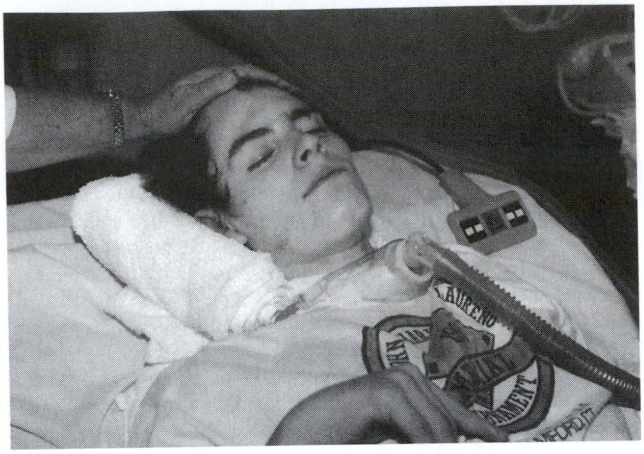

Figure 22.2 Head and neck positioned in neutral using towels. (From Chapman, PE,[40] p 286, with permission.)

Table 22.7 Techniques to Decrease Abnormal Posturing and Primitive Reflexes

Area	Positioning	Handling
Head	• Neutral position • Roll placed behind neck to support head and neck curvature • Roll parallel to head to prevent lateral flexion and rotation	• Gentle range of motion when ICP and cerebral perfusion stable • Hands at base of skull or on sides of head
Trunk	• Rolls behind shoulders • Roll behind hip if rotation is occurring • Normal alignment needs to be maintained	• Hand on scapula, arm supported, rhythmical protraction/retraction, elevation/depression • Hand on posterior pelvis, leg supported, rhythmical elevation and depression (rotation) • When patient stable: rolling segmentally
Upper extremity	• Roll behind shoulder • Cone in hand if fingers in flexion • Wedges between fingers if adducted • When stable: turn onto side for weight-bearing into arm	• Relaxation of scapula (1 above) • Hand placed in patient's hand from ulnar side to help decrease flexor tone of elbow, wrist, and hand • Range of motion of fifth finger or thumb to help break up flexor tone • Hand placed over biceps when increased extensor tone and over the triceps when increased flexor tone
Lower extremity	• Hips and knees supported in a slightly flexed position • No pressure on ball of foot medially • Roll between legs if strong adduction or internal rotation	• Hand on lateral side sole of foot for range of motion of foot, knee, and hip • Hands placed above and below knee, medially for external rotation, hip and knee flexion • Hand behind knee for flexion and external rotation of hip, flexion of knee

ICP = intracranial pressure.
From Chapman, PE,[40] with permission.

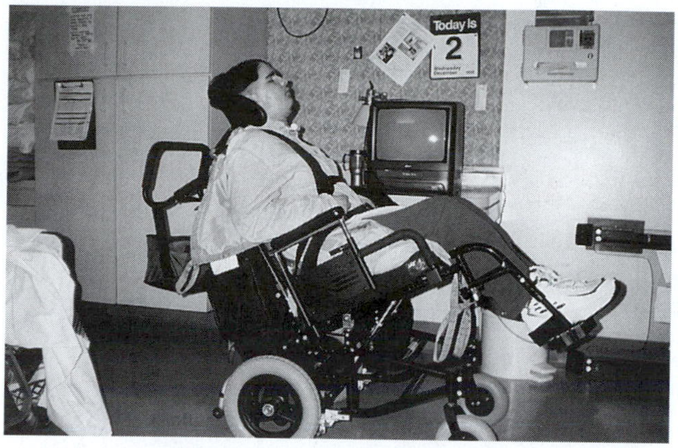

Figure 22.3 Wheelchair positioning using a tilt-in-space wheelchair. The wheelchair is tilted to assist in maintaining the patient's posture. The headrest maintains the head in an upright and neutral position. The chest straps keep the patient sitting upright when the seat is tilted forward. The tilt-in-space aspect allows for pressure relief when the angle of tilt is changed. The pad underneath the patient is used with a lift for transfers. Also, in the background against the wall in the lower right-hand corner, is a lap tray that can be used to better position the upper extremities. Photographs of the patient's family and friends are taped to the tray.

Respiratory care practitioners, physical therapists, and nurses often use postural drainage, percussion, vibration, and positioning to prevent pulmonary complications and improve pulmonary function.[51] The presence of increased ICP should be viewed as a contraindication for the use of these techniques.[52]

PROM helps prevent contractures, decreases hypertonicity,[53–55] and provides sensory stimulation. When moving the UEs during PROM, care should be taken to mobilize the scapula, and to maintain proper joint mechanics at the glenohumeral joint. If this is not done, the humerus is likely to impinge in the glenoid fossa, causing pain and destabilization of the joint capsule. With the lower extremities, it is essential to maintain the ROM at all joints. However, the ankle and hips are especially important as decreased ROM at these joints can greatly impact functional activities such as transfers, sitting, wheelchair positioning, ambulation, and stair climbing. When performing ROM, forceful or aggressive motions should be avoided. There is some indication that forceful PROM,[56] increased muscular tone, paresis,[57] and trauma[58] may be risk factors for **heterotopic ossification**. Heterotopic ossification is the abnormal formation of bone in muscle and other soft tissue. It usually occurs at the more proximal joints (shoulders, hips, and knees), has an incidence in individuals with TBI between 11 and 77 percent[59,60] and is associated with poor outcomes.[61]

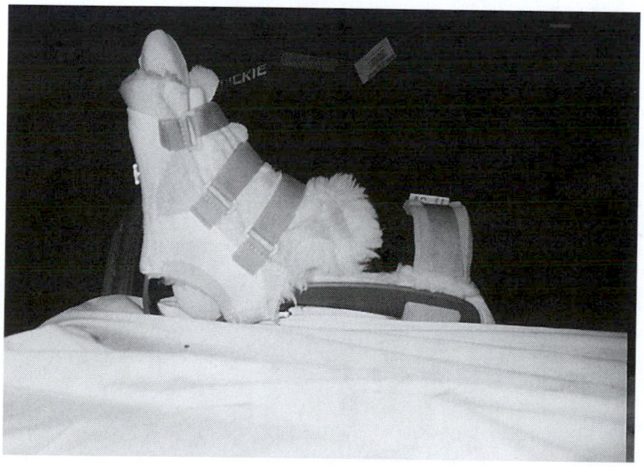

Figure 22.4 Multipodus boot used for foot and ankle positioning and to prevent skin breakdown on the heel. This type of positioning device may not be beneficial for the patient with moderate to severe tone at the ankle; it is not strong enough to prevent the ankle from plantarflexing and may even increase tone.

Improving Arousal Through Sensory Stimulation

Sensory stimulation is an intervention used in an attempt to increase the level of arousal and elicit movement in individuals in a coma or persistent vegetative state. The theory is that by providing stimulation in a controlled, multisensory manner, with a balance of stimulation and rest, the reticular activating system may be stimulated causing a general increase in arousal. The value of sensory stimulation for patients who are slow to recover remains unproven. Theoretical support for such programs comes from research in four areas: (1) effects of sensory deprivation on neurological recovery; (2) effects of "enriched" environments on behavior and nervous system structure and function; (3) nervous system plasticity; and (4) effects of environmental input during sensitive periods of neurodevelopment.[62]

In general, multisensory stimulation involves the presentation of sensory stimulation in a highly structured and consistent manner. The following sensory systems are systematically stimulated: auditory, olfactory, gustatory, visual, tactile, kinesthetic, and vestibular.[63–66] During this type of intervention, the patient must be closely monitored for subtle responses such as changes in heart rate, blood pressure, rate of respiration, or diaphoresis. Various motor responses, such as eye movements, facial grimacing, changes in posture, head turning, or vocalization, should be documented. Evidence Summary Box 22.3 presents recent studies examining the effectiveness of sensory stimulation in individuals at these early levels of recovery.[63–68] As seen from review of the available evidence, the effectiveness of this type of intervention is still in question. A recent systematic review published by the Cochrane library suggests there is no reliable evidence to support or rule out the effectiveness of sensory stimulation programs for this patient population.[69]

Patient and Family Education

Family members and caregivers of patients who have experienced a TBI play a critical role in the recovery

(text continues on page 912)

Evidence Summary Box 22.3

Selected Studies Examining the Effectiveness of Coma Stimulation

Reference	Subjects	Methods	Duration	Results	Comments
Lippert-Gruner, M, et al[68] 2003	Ss = 24 Mean age: 38 years Mean initial GCS: 4.6; Mean length of coma: 32.4 days	Pretest, posttest design; Multimodal early onset stimulation (MEOS) started 15.8 days after injury; this included consistent and structured sensory stimulation provided by the rehabilitation team; Outcome measures taken at 12 months after injury	MEOS provided 4–5 hours/day for a mean of 46.6 days	At 1 year follow- up: 6 Ss died; 3 Ss in vegetative state; 6 Ss with severe disability (GOS: 3); 6 Ss with moderate disability (GOS: 4); 3 Ss with minimal disability (GOS: 5); of the 18 Ss who lived: 15 unable to work, 2 returned to previous profession, 1 to a less challenging job	No control or comparison group; no results provided after MEOS intervention period
Grüner, ML, and Terhaag, D[63] 2000	Ss = 16 Mean age: 43.6 years; Mean GCS at start of study: 6.5	Pretest, posttest design (A–B–A design); Multimodal early onset stimulation (MEOS) after injury; this included consistent and structured sensory stimulation provided by the rehabilitation team; HR, RR, skin temperature measured in an A–B–A format while MEOS interventions provided; A phases consisted of 10 min of no stimulation; B phase consisted of individual stimulation of the different sensations; GOS and return to work measured at 2 years after injury	Two 1-hour sessions/day of MEOS until preset maximum score on GCS reached; mean of 9.8 days	Increases in HR during tactile and acoustic stimulation; 12 Ss followed up at 2 years: 1 Ss in vegetative state, 2 Ss with severe disability (GOS: 3), 6 with moderate disability (GOS: 4), 3 with minimal disability (GOS: 5)	No control or comparison group; authors made conclusions that HR significantly increased during sensory stimulation, but only A-B-A data from one Ss presented; no results provided after MEOS intervention period
Johnson, DA, et al[66] 1993	Ss = 14 males Mean age: 29.6 years; Mean GCS of 4.8	Randomized clinical trial to examine efficacy of multisensory stimulation program; E: 7 Ss, 1 hour of treatment/day; each treatment session consisted of 20 min pretreatment, 20 min of sensory stimulation and 20 min posttreatment; order of stimulus was randomized; C: 7 Ss, no stimulation during treatment time	Unclear; 6 days for both groups or 8.1 days for E and 3.7 days for C	No significant differences in outcome measures at post treatment between groups except for lower levels of 3-methoxy, 4-hydroxyphenylglycol in the E group; when Ss divided into groups of survivors and deceased, there were significantly lower levels of 3-methoxy, 4-hydroxyphenylglycol and acetylcholinesterase in the survivors	Small sample size; sensory stimulation provided for a relatively short period of time

Evidence Summary Box 22.3

Selected Studies Examining the Effectiveness of Coma Stimulation (continued)

Reference	Subjects	Methods	Duration	Results	Comments
		Dependent outcome measures were: catecholamine levels, serotonin levels, acetylcholinesterase levels, 3-methoxy, 4-hydroxyphenylglycol levels, HR and skin conductance; these were taken prior to pretreatment and after treatment			
Mitchell, S, et al[65] 1990	E: Ss = 12 Mean age of 22.3 years; GCS range 4-6; C: Ss = 12 Mean age of 22.75 years; GCS range 4–6	Pretest, posttest nonequivalent control group design; Ss in control group matched to experimental group for age, gender, type and location of brain injury, surgical intervention, and GCS on admission E: Received coma arousal procedure (CAP) a mean of 7.08 days after injury; CAP consisted of sensory stimulation C: No CAP at any time Outcome measures included GCS and duration of coma	1–2 hours/day for 4 weeks; Ss family encouraged to provide CAP as well	Duration of coma significantly shorter in E group compared to C group; 22 days vs. 26.9 days; No significant difference in GCS at 4 weeks between the groups	No randomization
Kater, KM[64] 1989	Ss = 30 Mean age 28 years	Pretest, posttest nonequivalent control group design; control group matched to experimental group for age, sex, location of brain injury, and GCS on admission E: 15 Ss, duration of coma ranged from 4 days to 6 months; received structured sensory stimulation (SSS) C: 15 Ss, duration of coma ranged from 1 week to 6 months; received normal nursing care; outcome measures used were GCS and RLA LOCF scale at 2 weeks and 3 months post injury	Two 45 min sessions of SSS/day for 1–3 months; Ss family encouraged to provide SSS as well	Ss who received SSS had significantly higher RLA LOCF score (mean 6.33 vs. 4.40) at 3 months	No randomization; Parametric tests used for data analysis; as the RLA LOCF score is ordinal data, nonparametric tests would have been more appropriate; GCS outcomes between groups not reported

(continued)

Evidence Summary Box 22.3

Selected Studies Examining the Effectiveness of Coma Stimulation (continued)

Reference	Subjects	Methods	Duration	Results	Comments
Pierce, JP, et al[67] 1990	Ss = 31 Mean age 24 years	Pretest, posttest non-equivalent control group design; E: 31 Ss in a coma or vegetative state for at least 2 weeks after initial injury; received vigorous, multisensory stimulation (MSS); Outcome measures were length of coma, defined as ability to follow "simple command" on two consecutive occasions at least 24 hours apart, and GOS at 10–12 months post-injury; outcomes compared to a historical reference group consisting of 135 patients in prolonged coma	Up to 8 hours of MSS/day for 2-32 weeks; MSS provided by Ss family	No significant differences in length of coma or GOS at follow up between groups	No randomization; interventions for historical reference group not reported; data on actual amount and duration of MSS not reported

C = control group; E = experimental group; GCS = Glasgow Coma Scale; GOS = Glasgow Outcome Scale; HR = heart rate; RLA LOCF = Ranchos Los Amigos Levels of Cognitive Function RR = respiratory rate; Ss = subjects.

process. Family members commonly experience a high level of stress related to worries about the future, less free time, and increased conflict.[70,71] Family education is an important component of the POC.[72,73] The goal of patient and family education is to teach the family about the stages of recovery and what can be expected in the future. By becoming informed, the family may not feel so helpless. The family can also become involved in performing ROM exercises, positioning, and sensory stimulation.[65] Although it is difficult to predict long-term outcome at these early levels of recovery, families should be informed of possible outcomes. The therapist should be realistic but provide hope for the family. It is often beneficial to have a medical social worker consult with the family to provide support and guidance.

Managing the Effects of Abnormal Tone and Spasticity

Abnormal tone is a common problem throughout the continuum of care for many patients with TBI. A wide variety of methods are available to the therapist and rehabilitation team to treat the adverse affects of abnormal tone. Interventions used to manage tone are discussed in a later section.

Early Transition to Sitting Postures

Upright sitting is extremely important because it addresses elements of treatment goals for the early levels of recovery. As soon as medically stable, the patient should be transferred to a sitting position and out of bed to a wheelchair or chair. All precautions should be observed. The head should be properly supported, as the patient is not likely to have adequate neck and head control to maintain an upright posture without support. Often, it is beneficial to perform co-treatments with an occupational therapist when first sitting and transferring the patient. This approach allows two skilled professionals to assist the patient, as maximal assistance is often required. Use of a tilt table is also advantageous because it allows early weightbearing through the lower extremities. The upright position, both on a tilt table and in a wheelchair, may improve overall level of alertness.

When attempting early functional tasks, such as sitting and grooming activities, *therapeutic guiding techniques*, such as those described by Davies,[74] may be effective. The therapist assists the patient in interacting with the environment. The goal is to promote movement and learning by guiding the patient's body in the performance of a functional task. Guided movements provide tactile, proprioceptive, and kinesthetic stimulation when performing a task. It also allows continuous monitoring of the patient's abilities, as the therapist's hands can directly feel the quality of movement.[74]

Documentation

Documentation of progress can be very challenging. The patient may progress at a slower rate than other patient populations and the changes are often more difficult to quantify. To ensure ongoing reimbursement from available sources, it is important to effectively document changes to indicate progress toward achievement of goals and to justify treatment. Examples of documentation at these levels of recovery include:

1. Patient's neck is rotated to left with left UE abducted, elbow extended in possible asymmetric tonic neck reflex posture (ATNR).
2. Patient inconsistently tracks to right to auditory stimulation.
3. Patient exhibits active, nonpurposeful movement in right upper and lower extremities.
4. Patient withdraws to painful stimuli on right side of body.
5. No reaction to painful stimuli on left side of body.

Ranchos Los Amigos Level IV: The Confused–Agitated Level of Recovery

As the patient begins to emerge from coma, he or she often experiences a period of acute posttraumatic agitation.[75,76] The confusion, amnesia, and disorientation during Level IV often results in agitation, aggression, noncompliance, and combative behavior.[77] As described earlier, damage to certain neuroanatomical areas also contributes to these behaviors during the acute and chronic stages.

Examination

It is extremely challenging to examine the patient who is in the confused–agitated level of recovery. The patient may be markedly agitated and prone to emotional outbursts. These may range from verbally acting out to physically attempting to hurt themselves or others, to sexually inappropriate behaviors. The patient is often confused. He or she will have poor memory, usually both short- and long-term. The patient will have a decreased attention span and be easily distracted. Refer to Box 22.2 for further description of this level. Again, it is often helpful to have another therapist assist with the examination. This could be another physical therapist, an occupational therapist, or a speech–language pathologist.

It may be difficult to gather data from examination procedures, such as PROM or strength, because the patient will often be unable to cooperate; the therapist must utilize observation skills and the ability to estimate. The therapist should examine functional mobility, balance both in sitting and standing if appropriate, ROM, strength, motor control, tone, sensation, and reflexes. The physical therapist should also begin to determine the patient's cognitive abilities in this level of recovery. This will include orientation, attention span, memory, insight, safety awareness, and alertness. Key questions to address include:

- Is the patient able to follow commands: one-step, two-step, or multistep commands?
- Is the patient oriented to person, place, or time?
- Does the patient recognize family members?
- It is beneficial to consult with other team members, especially the speech–language pathologist, to obtain additional information about the patient's cognitive status.

Evaluation, Prognosis, and Plan of Care

The following is a list of general goals and outcomes anticipated for patients in Level IV adapted from the American Physical Therapy Association's *Guide to Physical Therapist Practice*[47]: They can be used to guide the development of specific anticipated goals and expected outcomes for an individual patient.

- Patient's endurance is improved.
- Joint mobility and integrity are maintained.
- Risk of secondary impairments is reduced.
- Tolerance of activities is increased.
- The patient's family is educated regarding patient's diagnosis, prognosis, physical therapy interventions, and outcomes.
- Care is coordinated among all team members.

The overall goals of physical therapy at this level of recovery are to maintain the patient's functional capabilities. The most important goal the whole team strives to achieve in this level of recovery is to prevent agitated outbursts and to assist the patient to control his or her behavior.

Intervention

The therapist should incorporate creativity and flexibility when designing and providing interventions during this level of recovery. Generally, the therapist should work near the patient's physical level of function and attempt to improve endurance, rather than progress to more challenging skills that would require new learning, as the patient does not have the capacity for new learning at this level of recovery. The neuropsychologist can assist the team by providing insight into different ways to manage the patient's agitated behavior and may set up a behavioral modification program. Behavioral modification techniques such as positive reinforcement using a point or reward system, redirection, and compliance training are useful in managing these inappropriate behaviors and improving participation in therapy.[77] Different medications may be effective in helping the patient manage behavior as well.[78] The following special considerations are offered for management of patients at this level of recovery.

Consistency
Consistency is important. All team members, including family members, should interact and address inappropriate behaviors in a consistent manner. Remember that the patient is confused. To help decrease confusion, the patient should be seen by the same person at the same time and in the same location every day. Establishing a daily routine is very important. It is calming and reassuring to have a sense of familiarity. Additionally, orientation (i.e., person, place, and time) should be provided frequently and in a nonthreatening manner. At this level, it is often better to provide orientation information than to challenge the patient to provide it, particularly if the patient is not expected to succeed.

Expect No Carryover
Teaching new skills at this level is unrealistic. The patient may begin to perform a functional task, such as brushing teeth or ambulating. However, this does not indicate a general learning ability, as brushing one's teeth and especially walking are automatic skills with an ingrained neural network. The use of charts or graphs may be useful to help the patient progress each day. Without the use of such aids, the patient is likely to have no recall of the previous day's performance.

Model Calm Behavior
The patient is likely to perceive, and may reflect, the demeanor of the caregiver. Therefore, it is important for the therapist to assume a calm and focused affect. The patient may not be able to control his or her behavior and may not feel safe. To help the patient feel safe, it is important for the therapist to be perceived as in control of his or her emotions and behavior.

Expect Egocentricity
At this level of recovery, the patient cannot be expected to see another's point of view. He or she will tend to think only of him- or herself and, at this point, it is unwise to stress the patient with attempts to do otherwise.

Flexibility/Options
The patient will have a limited attention span and may not be able to concentrate on any given activity for a very long time. It is important to be prepared with numerous activities. If the patient cannot be redirected to the selected task, it is appropriate to attempt to engage him or her in another. Treat the patient at an appropriate age level. Give control to the patient when it is safe and appropriate. Control can be given while maintaining focus on therapeutic goals by phrasing questions as, "Would you rather play ball or go for a walk?" This prevents situations where the patient chooses an undesirable or unrealistic activity if asked, "What would you like to do?" or the case where the patient simply answers "No" when asked, "Would you like to . . . ?" Provide safe choices for the patient. This allows the patient to feel that he or she has some control over the situation. This is important, as the patient typically feels considerable loss of control during prolonged hospitalization.

Safety
Owing to the patient's often unpredictable and inappropriate behaviors, it is important to keep the patient and those interacting with him or her safe. In addition to utilizing some of the above-mentioned behavioral strategies, patients in this level of recovery may be kept on a locked unit of the hospital. Patients may require one-to-one staff supervision and assistance throughout the day.

Patient and Family Education
As described previously, it is difficult to provide education for the patient at this level; the patient has very little, if any, ability for new learning. However, it is extremely important to provide education for the patient's family. Above all, the family should understand that the patient does not have control of his or her behavior. The patient is not striking out or swearing because of intent to hurt others, but because of agitation and confusion. Many times families do not understand why a patient is performing these behaviors. They must be told that these behaviors are a symptom of the brain injury just as the patient's inability to walk or eat is. It is important to educate the family that entering this level of recovery is a good sign because it indicates the patient is moving toward the next level of recovery. Aggressive behaviors are usually short lived, typically lasting only a few weeks at most. Family members should also be taught to use the above strategies when interacting with their loved one. Consistency is important for everyone, including family members. If a behavioral plan is being implemented, the family should be a part of devising it and carrying it out.

Documentation
Documentation may read as follows:

1. Passive ROM appears to be within functional limits bilaterally in lower extremities except for right ankle dorsiflexion, which appears to lack 10° from neutral.
2. Patient exhibits full active ROM at all joints, except for right ankle dorsiflexion.
3. Active movement in all four extremities is nonpurposeful and uncoordinated.
4. Patient exhibits impaired safety awareness and is disoriented to place and time.
5. Unable to examine formally owing to patient's decreased ability to follow commands and behavioral outbursts.
6. Patient unable to participate in physical therapy today due to aggressive behavioral outbursts.

Ranchos Los Amigos Levels V and VI: Confused–Inappropriate and Confused–Appropriate Levels of Recovery

Examination
At Levels V and VI, the patient is confused, but with structure is able to follow simple commands, which makes a

more formal and accurate physical therapy examination possible. Refer to Box 22.2 for a description of patient behavior at these levels of recovery. The examination methods may need to be modified because the patient may still have difficulty when asked to perform complex tasks in an open environment. It is important to obtain concise and objective data at this point since accuracy may have been compromised during earlier attempts at data collection. As in earlier levels of recovery, the examination process may take more than one session and should be ongoing.

The examination should include the following: attention and cognition, cranial nerve integrity, balance (in both sitting and standing), gait, skin integrity, joint mobility, motor control, muscle strength, sensorimotor integration, pain, ROM, reflexes, ADL skills (including functional mobility), and sensory integrity. Other areas may need to be examined, depending on the status of the individual patient. Determination of the patient's functional abilities should be done in a variety of environments, as some patients may perform well in the closed environment of a private room, but performance may deteriorate in an open environment with multiple distractions. The earlier section of this chapter on clinical rating scales provides information on standardized outcome measures useful for examining attention and cognition. Chapters 4 to 8 and 10 to 12 provide a detailed description of procedures and tools for examining the above-mentioned areas. A brief description of some of the more clinically useful outcome measures for individuals with TBI follows.

The Balance Scale developed by Berg and colleagues[79] (provided in Chapter 8, Appendix A) has been shown to be a valid and clinically useful measure of balance in individuals with TBI.[80,81] Two studies demonstrated that the Balance Scale, along with functional status measured using the Functional Independence Measure (FIM™), was a useful method of predicting in-patient rehabilitation length of stay, falls during rehabilitation stay, and functional gains during rehabilitation.[80,81]

There are many different methods of examining gait and walking ability. Physical therapists use observational gait analysis (OGA) as a preferred method in the clinic.[82] One instrument used clinically is the Ranchos Los Amigos OGA system.[83] Refer to Chapter 10 for a further discussion of this instrument. This OGA instrument gathers data on the cyclical movements of walking that occur from one stride cycle to the next. The gait cycle is divided into the stance and swing phases. Clinicians visually analyze a patient's walking pattern, looking for asymmetries and deviations from normal. Based on these observations, physical therapists determine which impairments may be the cause of the deviations. Specific interventions are then designed to address the possible causes of the gait deviations. Gait speed,[84–86] measured over a 10-m walk, and gait endurance,[87,88] measured over a 6-minute walk, are two other clinically useful measures of walking ability.

Examination of motor control should include tone, coordination, and movement patterns. Most standardized measures of motor control validated for individuals with neurological deficits were designed for use following stroke. Although individuals with TBI may present with hemiparesis, physical therapists should exercise caution when using these tests with this population. Some of these measures include the Fugl-Meyer Assessment of Motor Recovery[89,90] and the Chedoke-McMaster Stroke Assessment.[91] Chapter 18 contains more information on these and other similar tests. Owing to impairments in motor control that these patients exhibit, care should be taken when testing strength using standard manual muscle testing procedures. Abnormal tone and motor control deficits may mask strength impairments.

Functional status, including the ability to perform ADL, transfers, bed mobility, stairs and locomotion, is commonly measured using the FIM™ and FAM as described earlier. In addition to measuring the amount of physical assistance required to perform a functional task, the therapist should also analyze how the patient performs the task. Key questions to ask include:

- How well does the patient maintain his or her balance throughout the task?
- How long does it take the patient to initiate and complete the task?
- Is the patient able to perform the task consistently?
- Does the patient perform the task efficiently, with a minimal amount of energy expenditure?
- Can the patient shift his or her weight forward enough and maintain normal body alignment while transferring from sitting to standing?

Another important consideration is the level of family support and projected place of discharge. Individuals with moderate to severe brain injury often require continued care and rehabilitation after discharge from the hospital. The amount of care needed ranges from supervision because of cognitive deficits to physical assistance in performing basic ADL skills such as transfers, bathing, and dressing. Many times family members must provide this care, so it is essential to ascertain the level of family support early in the rehabilitation process.

Evaluation, Prognosis, and Plan of Care

The following is a list of general goals and outcomes anticipated for patients in Levels V and VI adapted from the American Physical Therapy Association's *Guide to Physical Therapist Practice*.[47] They can be used to guide the development of specific anticipated goals and expected outcomes for an individual patient.

- Performance of functional mobility and ADL skills is increased.
- Gait, mobility, and balance are improved.
- Motor control and postural control are increased.

- Risk of secondary impairments is reduced.
- Strength and endurance are increased.
- Safety with functional mobility tasks and ADL skills is improved.
- Patient and family are educated on diagnosis, prognosis, physical therapy interventions, and goals.
- Tolerance of activities is improved.
- Care is coordinated among all team members.

The overall goals during this stage of the rehabilitation process are to maximize functional recovery of the individual and prepare him or her and the family for discharge home and to the community.

Interventions

Some of the same strategies regarding the patient's behavior discussed in Level IV should be considered when working with individuals in Levels V and VI. Individuals at these levels will still present with behavioral and cognitive deficits that will impede the reacquisition of motor skills. Treatment sessions should be thoughtfully planned to maximize the patient's motor learning capabilities. Practice should be distributed. Owing to cognitive impairments, these patients may experience mental as well as physical fatigue during treatment sessions. Signs of mental fatigue may include increased irritability, decreased attention and concentration, deterioration in performance of physical skills, and delayed initiation. Treatment sessions should include sufficient rest periods to minimize both physical and mental fatigue and maximize motor relearning. Feedback is also very important. Owing to cognitive, sensory, and perceptual impairments, explicit feedback may be more beneficial in the early stages of motor learning as opposed to intrinsic feedback.[92] However, care should be taken not to overwhelm the patient with feedback. Refer to Chapter 13 for an in-depth discussion of motor learning principles.

As discussed earlier, an early, interdisciplinary approach to rehabilitation after TBI has been shown to be beneficial.[38,39,93] There are many intervention approaches available to the physical therapist that can promote functional recovery following brain injury. Two basic treatment strategies are a *compensatory* and a *restorative* approach. The compensatory approach seeks to improve functional skills by compensating for the lost ability. A simple example of this would be teaching one-handed dressing techniques if a patient presented with a hemiparetic UE. The restorative approach seeks to restore the "normal" use of the affected UE.

No studies to date have identified what types of interventions are most beneficial. Current research has demonstrated that task specific interventions with large amounts of practice can induce beneficial neuroplastic changes in the central nervous system and restore function. Studies involving monkey and rat models of brain injury have demonstrated the importance of intensive, task-oriented training on neuroplastic changes in the motor cortex and functional recovery.[94,95] Current theories of motor control and motor learning advocate for a task-oriented approach to interventions for individuals with neurological deficits.[9,96] Locomotor training, utilizing body weight support (BWS) and a treadmill,[97–99] and constraint induced (CI) movement therapy for improving UE function[100,101] are two interventions that have shown potential. See Chapter 13.

Locomotor training with BWS and a treadmill involves suspending the client in a parachute like overhead harness that allows for a percentage of body weight to be relieved. Therapists assist the patient by providing trunk/pelvic stabilization, assistance with weight shifting, and advancing the lower extremities. Locomotor training with BWS is commonly combined with treadmill ambulation (Fig. 22.5), but can be done overground as well. Locomotor training with BWS and a treadmill allows for repetitive training throughout a complete gait cycle. Progressively decreasing the amount of BWS and increasing the treadmill speed allows the physical therapist to gradually increase the difficulty of the task as walking ability improves. In two separate case reports, researchers have documented improvement in walking ability in individuals with brain injury using this approach.[97,99] Locomotor training with BWS

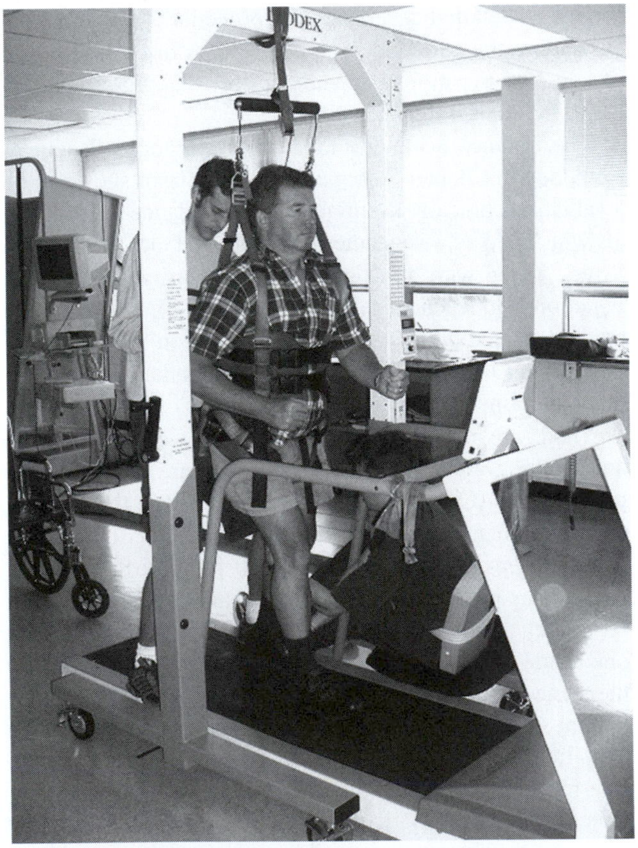

Figure 22.5 Locomotor training utilizing a body weight support system and treadmill. One trainer is assisting with trunk and pelvic stability and weight shifting, while another trainer is facilitating stepping at the left LE.

and a treadmill has a solid theoretical basis and has been more extensively studied in individuals with stroke and incomplete spinal cord injury.

Constraint induced (CI) movement therapy involves promoting the use of the most affected UE for up to 90 percent of waking hours and reducing the use of the least affected UE. Intensive, task oriented training is provided for the affected UE for up to 6 hours per day over a 2- to 3-week period.[102] Two small studies have examined the effectiveness of CI movement therapy in individuals with chronic TBI. Shaw and colleagues reported improvement in the amount of use and caregivers' evaluation of use of the more affected UE in seven individuals with chronic TBI, after CI movement therapy.[101] Page and Levine implemented a modified CI movement therapy program with three individuals with chronic brain injury. The subjects demonstrated an improvement in the amount and quality of UE use and functional use of the UE.[100]

Some treatment approaches utilize the developmental sequence and muscle facilitation techniques. Developmental postures can be used to facilitate and help restore movement and functional mobility. Table 22.8 identifies different postures in the developmental sequence and the benefits derived from working in each posture. Figures 22.6 and 22.7 depict sample treatment activities with a patient using modifications of the developmental postures. Because of indirect impairments and accessory injuries such as long bone fractures, it may be necessary to adapt activities.

Because individuals with TBI present with many different physical, cognitive, and emotional impairments, therapists should be well versed in a variety of treatment options, not just one approach. No matter which intervention technique is chosen, an emphasis should be placed on shaping the task to the patient's abilities (cognitive as well as physical) to optimize success while progressively increasing the complexity and demands of the task and relating the intervention to a meaningful functional goal.

Patient and Family Education

It is important to emphasize safety awareness education with the patient. The individual is beginning to exhibit improved mobility skills at these levels, but may lack the insight to recognize that he or she may not yet be safe to ambulate or transfer alone. Family members should learn how to assist the patient with functional mobility. This typically includes training in bed mobility, transfers, ambulation, and wheelchair mobility skills. They should be instructed in proper body mechanics when assisting with functional mobility, so as to avoid risking injury to the patient or themselves. Family members should also be educated about how to assist the patient with strengthening exercises and PROM. Family members and caregivers should also be aware of methods to enhance decision-making skills and safety awareness. All of these skills are important for family members to learn, as they may become the primary caregiver for the patient upon discharge to home.

Table 22.8 Developmental Sequence Postures and Treatment Benefits

Posture	Treatment Benefits
Prone-on-elbows	• Improve upper trunk, UE and neck/head control • Increase ROM at hip extensors • Improve shoulder stabilizers strength • Wide BOS, low COG
Quadruped	• Improve upper trunk, lower trunk, LE, UE, and neck/head control • Weightbearing through hips • Increase hip stabilizers strength • Decrease extensor tone at knees by weight-bearing • Increase shoulder stabilizers strength • Weight-bearing through shoulders, elbows, and wrists • Increase extensor ROM at wrists and fingers • Wide BOS, low COG
Bridging	• Improve lower trunk and LE control • Increase hip stabilizers strength • Weightbearing through feet and ankles • Lead up activity for bed mobility • Wide BOS, low COG
Sitting	• Improve upper trunk, lower trunk, LE, and head/neck control • Weightbearing through UE • Functional posture • Improve balance reactions • Medium BOS, Medium COG
Kneeling and half-kneeling	• Improve head/neck, upper trunk, lower trunk, and LE control • Weightbearing through hips • Inhibit extensor tone at knees • Increase hip stabilizers strength • Improve balance reactions • Weightbearing through ankle in half-kneeling • Narrow BOS, high COG (kneeling) • Wide BOS, high COG (half-kneeling)
Modified plantigrade	• Improve head/neck, upper trunk, lower trunk, UE, and LE control • Weightbearing through UE and LE • Improve balance reactions • Functional posture • Increase extensor ROM at wrists and fingers • Wide BOS, high COG
Standing	• Improve head/neck, upper trunk, lower trunk, and LE control • Weightbearing through LE • Improve balance reactions • Functional posture • Narrow BOS, high COG

BOS = base of support; COG = center of gravity; LE = lower extremity; ROM = range of motion; UE = upper extremity.

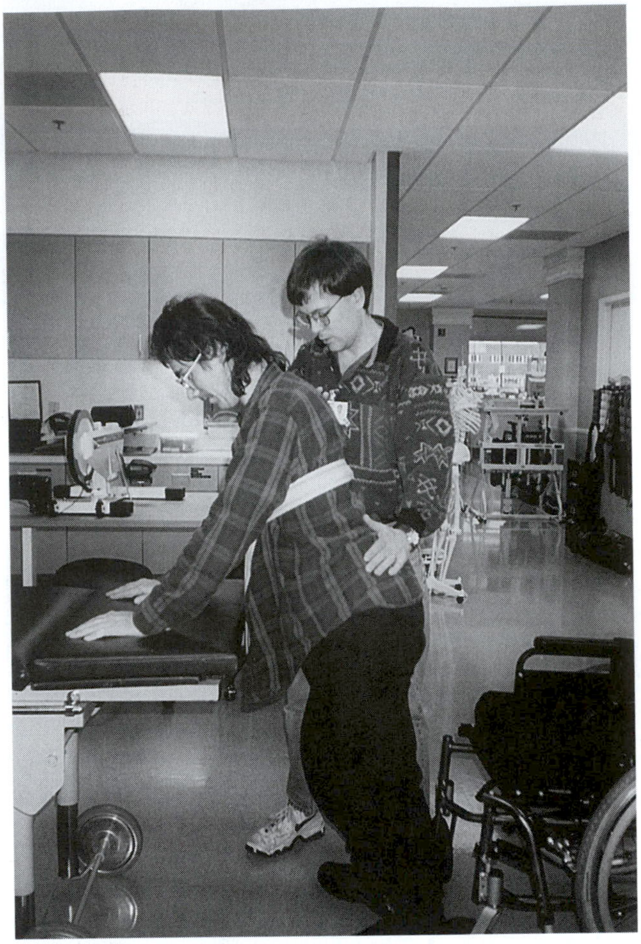

Figure 22.6 Modified plantigrade. Owing to long bone fractures and increased tone, the patient is not able to maintain this posture in good alignment. However, it is still a beneficial posture because it allows for weightbearing on all four extremities and will improve trunk and extremity control.

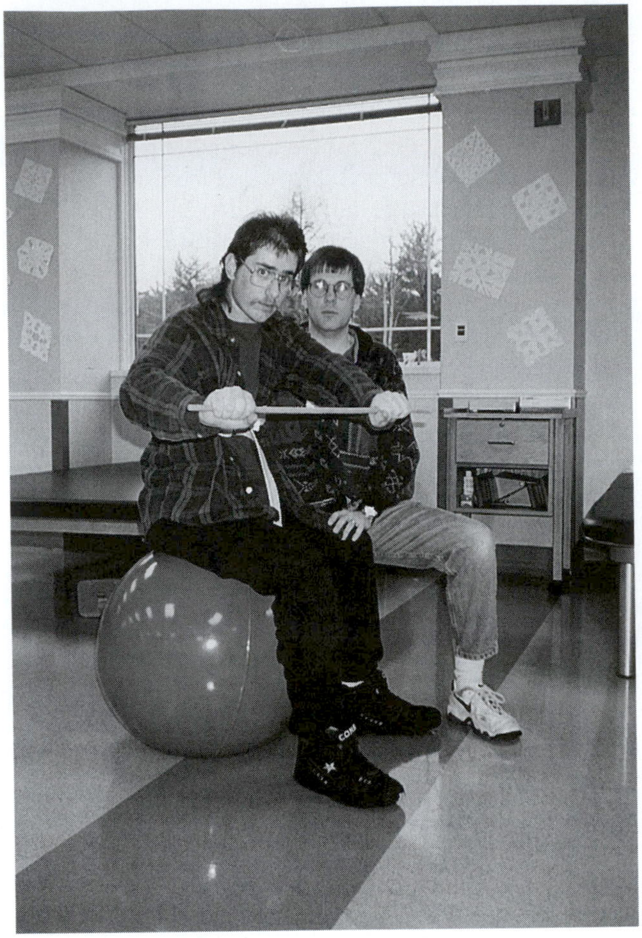

Figure 22.7 Sitting on therapy ball and rotating to either side will improve the patient's balance, upper trunk rotation, trunk control, and posture. The dowel is used to isolate upper trunk rotation.

Documentation

Examples of documentation include:

1. Patient able to ambulate 75 ft with minimal assistance in a closed environment, without device. However, in an open environment, such as the physical therapy gym, patient requires moderate assistance and multiple verbal cues to ambulate 75 ft.
2. Patient able to transfer from wheelchair to bed with minimal assistance with two to three verbal cues for brake management and safety precautions. However, in an open environment, patient requires moderate assistance to transfer from wheelchair to bed and multiple verbal cues for safety precautions.
3. Patient exhibits increased extensor tone in right lower extremity (LE), 3 on modified Ashworth scale.
4. Patient presents with decreased safety awareness and is highly distractible. These traits are increased in an open environment.

Ranchos Los Amigos Levels VII and VIII: Appropriate Response Levels of Recovery

It is usually in the late confused-appropriate and early automatic-appropriate levels that the patient is discharged from in-patient rehabilitation. Box 22.2 provides a description of the patient's behavior at these stages. Prior to discharge, it is crucial to begin to wean the patient from the external structure provided by the hospital setting that was so important in the early stages of recovery. As the patient becomes better able to control him or herself, external control provided by the environment should be lessened.

Therapy is often delivered in a comprehensive day treatment setting, with an interdisciplinary emphasis on community re-entry, return to work or school, and cognitive, behavioral, and psychosocial issues.[37,103,104] In this setting, the patient goes to therapy throughout the day for 4 to 5 days a week and returns home in the late afternoon. Individuals with more severe physical impairments may continue their rehabilitation in a residential based community reentry program, while those with continued, severe behavioral issues may require a residential neurobehavioral program (see Fig. 22.1).

Examination, Evaluation, Prognosis, and Plan of Care and Interventions

At these levels of recovery, the restoration of physical function is not significantly different from the preceding level. The same examination procedures discussed in Levels V and VI should be used. The following is a list of general goals and outcomes for patients in Levels VII and VIII (LOCF) adapted from the American Physical Therapy Association's *Guide to Physical Therapist Practice*[47]: They can be used to guide the development of specific anticipated goals and expected outcomes for an individual patient.

- Patient and family are educated about diagnosis, prognosis, physical therapy intervention, and goals.
- Safety of patient and family is improved.
- Ability to perform physical tasks related to ADL skills, community and work reintegration, and leisure activities is increased.
- Functional mobility is improved.
- Motor control, balance, and postural control are improved.
- Self-management of symptoms is increased.
- Strength and endurance are increased.
- Level of supervision and assistance for task performance is decreased.

The major goal of treatment at Levels VII and VIII is to assist the patient in integrating the cognitive, physical, and emotional skills necessary to function in the community. Skills in judgment, problem solving, planning, self-awareness, health and wellness, and social interaction are emphasized.

For the demands of treatment to approximate the demands of the real world, treatment focuses on advanced activities such as community skills, social skills, and daily living skills. Examples of these skills are presented in Table 22.9. The interdisciplinary team emphasizes patient assumption of self-responsibility. Because the patient now has some insight into his or her own strengths and weaknesses, it is important to involve the individual in decision-making. The patient is now working to reintegrate him or herself back into home and community. Therefore, the focus of treatment is to maintain and improve performance while decreasing external structure and supervision. Independent as well as cooperative work with others is encouraged. Group treatment sessions are often the basis of interventions. Honest feedback from the therapist and support group is crucial for the patient to learn how to function in society with his or her present abilities and limitations. Trial periods of independent living and supported work are important. Adaptations are often required by the family, work, and school to accommodate to the needs of the individual.

Table 22.9 Components of Community Skills, Social Skills, and Daily Living Skills Programs

Daily Living	Social Skills	Community Skills
Food preparation Housekeeping Money management Meal planning Telephone use Time management	Introductions Nonverbal communication Assertiveness Listening skills Giving/receiving feedback	Shopping Public transport Map reading Leisure planning Community resources

Patient and Family Education

At these levels of recovery, the patient should be educated in how to best compensate for residual impairments or disabilities. The patient and family should contact local support groups. Talking to another survivor of brain injury who has gone through some of the same difficulties can be of great benefit. If necessary, the patient and family members should continue with regular counseling provided by a medical social worker or neuropsychologist. There are many community resources available to assist the patient and family in making the transition to home and the community, and many resources can be found on the Internet. The Brain Injury Association of America is a national organization that provides community service information and resources, participates in legislative advocacy, facilitates prevention awareness, sponsors educational programs, and encourages research. The association can be contacted at:

Brain Injury Association of America, Inc.
8201 Greensboro Dr.
McLean, VA 22102
(800) 444-6443
http://www.biausa.org

Most states have local chapters that can provide information and support as well.

Another important aspect of patient education is wellness and prevention. Individuals with TBI should be encouraged to participate in a regularly scheduled fitness/exercise program. Research has shown that an aerobic exercise program is beneficial for improving exercise capacity as well as psychosocial and general health status.[105–108]

Documentation

Examples of documentation for Levels VII and VIII include:

1. Patient requires three to four verbal cues to safely ambulate across a street at a cross walk with an ankle foot orthosis (AFO) on right LE.

2. Patient requires minimal assistance and two to three verbal cues to locate two objects in grocery store aisle; patient exhibits nystagmus in eyes bilaterally when turning head upward and to right to look for objects.
3. Patient requires three verbal cues to safely find way from hospital entrance to physical therapy gym.

Special Considerations

Abnormal Tone

Individuals with TBI often present with abnormalities in muscle tone. One study reported that among individuals with TBI who are undergoing in-patient rehabilitation, up to 84 percent developed contractures due to spastic hypertonia.[41] The clinical characteristics of spasticity are brisk deep tendon reflexes, involuntary flexor and extensor spasms, Babinski sign, and velocity dependent increase in stretch reflexes. Increased tone may have beneficial as well as detrimental effects. Increased tone may make personal hygiene difficult, lead to contractures and pressure sores, and be painful to the individual. Full body spasms may interfere with transfers. In other instances, increased tone may help improve function. An increase in LE extensor tone may allow an individual to bear enough weight through the LEs to facilitate an independent bed transfer, or make the transfer easier for the caregiver. Clinicians should weigh the potential risks and benefits to the individual patient before proceeding with treatment.

The foundations of spasticity management are therapeutic stretching and strengthening exercises with adjunctive modalities and functional retraining. PROM and selective strengthening of the antagonist muscles can help to decrease spasticity.[53,54] Positioning is an important adjunct in the management of tone abnormalities.[48] Maintaining the head and neck in a neutral position is important for minimizing the effects that primitive postures may have in increasing tone. Keeping the whole body in proper alignment is also important. Refer to Table 22.7 for positioning strategies.

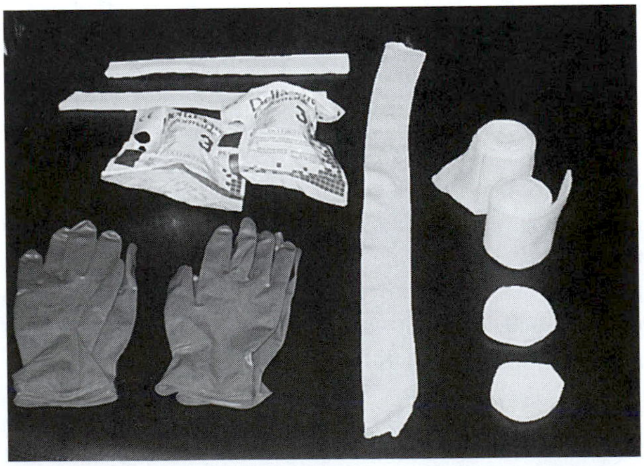

Figure 22.8 Materials used for serial casting: fiberglass casting material, rubber gloves, stockinette, a layer of padding to wrap around the lower leg, and padding for the malleoli and proximal and distal ends of the cast.

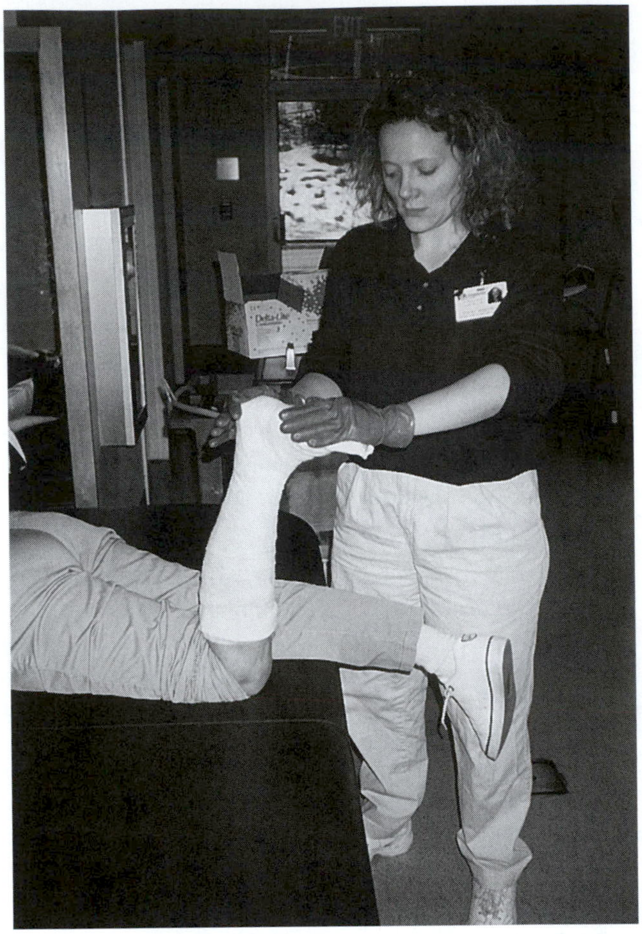

Figure 22.9 Serial casting: first a layer of padding is wrapped around the lower leg and foot.

Serial casting is another intervention that may help decrease hypertonia.[109–112] Serial casting is often used for plantarflexor or biceps contractures resulting from either increased tone or prolonged shortening of the muscle. With a plantarflexion contracture, the ankle is stretched into as much dorsiflexion as possible and then a short leg cast is applied. In approximately 1 week the cast is removed. The muscle is stretched again and another cast is applied (Figs. 22.8, 22.9, and 22.10). This procedure is repeated until satisfactory gains in ROM have been achieved, or no further progress is made. Precise ROM measurements should be taken between each casting. Because the individual with brain injury is likely to have impaired sensation and communication and behavioral deficits, there is a risk of skin breakdown or the patient hurting him or herself or others with the cast. The decision to use casts should be made carefully. The benefits and possible side effects should be thoroughly discussed with input from appropriate team members. Hands-on experience under the supervision of

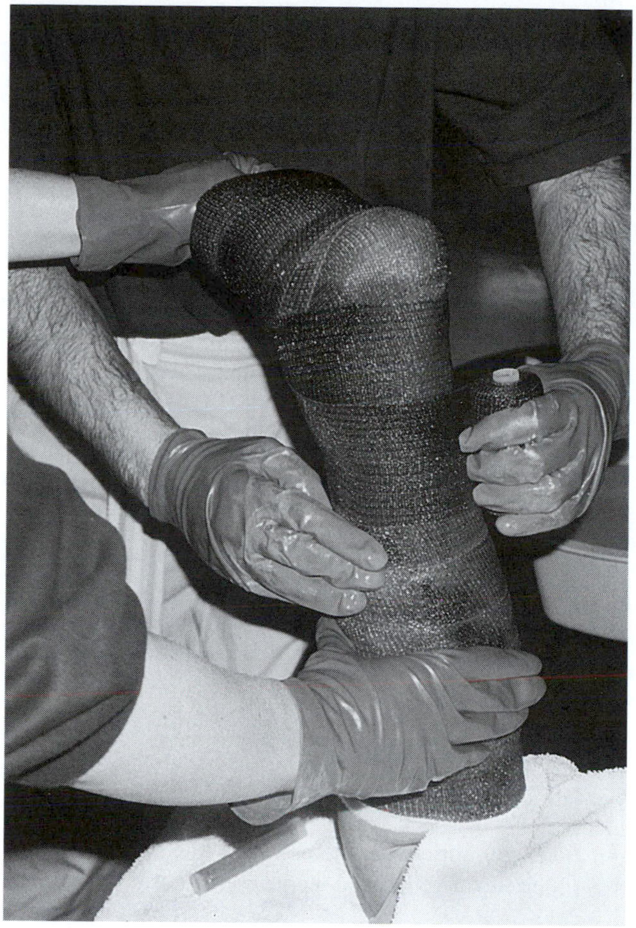

Figure 22.10 Serial casting: then the fiberglass casting material is wrapped around the lower leg and foot. One clinician does the wrapping, while another holds the leg and foot in the proper position.

a skilled clinician is recommended before attempting cast applications.

The consistent, prolonged stretch and the warmth and total pressure supplied by the cast provide theoretical support for the use of serial casting.[113,114] A systematic review on the effectiveness of serial casting for individuals with TBI concluded that there is strong evidence to support the use of serial casts to improve PROM. However, there is limited evidence for its effectiveness to decrease tone and improve function.[115] Other modalities that may help reduce hypertonia include cryotherapy[116] and air splints.[117,118] However, the effect of both of these modalities is temporary.

Various medications may also help reduce spasms and increased muscle tone. Oral medications used to modify the effects of increased tone include baclofen, diazepam, dantrolene, gabapentin, and tizanidine.[1,119,120] However, these medications may produce a variety of side effects that can be especially detrimental for individuals with TBI. Potential side effects include fatigue, weakness, sedation, and drowsiness. Intramuscular injections of phenol and botulinum toxin have local effects, which are shorter lived, on reducing spasticity[1,121,122] (Appendix A).

Rehabilitation Technology

Owing to the wide variety of impairments, functional limitations, and disability associated with brain injury, the patient may benefit from the use of adaptive equipment to increase social participation and independence. Today's advanced adaptive equipment can range from computer based augmented communications systems to environmental control units (ECU)[123] that will allow the individual to open doors, answer the telephone, turn on the television, as well as perform other tasks from a wheelchair. Pocket computers are being used to assist with community reintegration[124] and as memory aids.[125–127] A wheelchair is a form of adaptive equipment that the physical therapist is likely to prescribe to enhance functional mobility.[50] Wheelchairs can range from manual to power. A power wheelchair can be controlled in a variety of ways. These include a joystick, sip and puff mechanism, head control, tongue control, or even a single switch. Seating systems can be adapted so the patient can perform independent pressure relief using a power system (Fig. 22.11). It must be kept in mind, however, that using a power wheelchair, especially one controlled with just one switch, requires a great deal of cognitive skill. Refer to Chapter 33 for further discussion on this topic.

In addition to helping compensate for lost function, rehabilitation technologies are being used as interventions to restore function for individuals with TBI. Preliminary

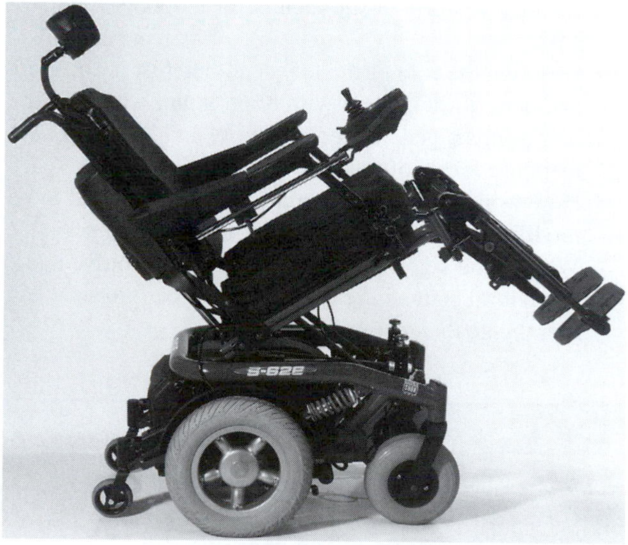

Figure 22.11 Power wheelchair with a power tilt-in-space seating system that allows the patient to independently perform pressure relief. Using the wheelchair joystick, the patient can tilt the seat back to change positions and redistribute pressure. (Courtesy of Sunrise Medical, Carlsbad, CA 92008.)

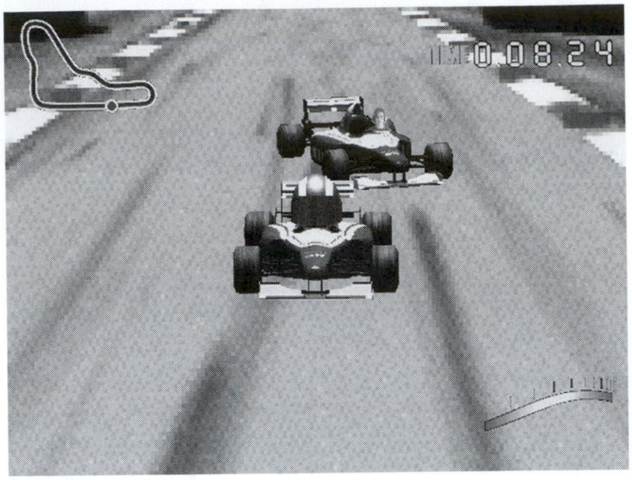

Figure 22.12 Visual image presented to a patient while performing balance training in a virtual environment with the IREX system. Using a camera-based tracking system, the patient is able to see him or herself on a screen. The patient's image is superimposed into the virtual racecar and he or she "steers" the virtual car by weight shifting to avoid objects in the car's path. (Courtesy of JesterTek, Inc, Port Jefferson, NY 11731.)

research indicates that virtual reality[128] technologies are beneficial for improving cognition,[129] ADL function,[130] driving skills,[131] UE function,[132] and balance[133] (Fig. 22.12).

Summary

A TBI is a devastating and life-changing event for the individual and his or her family. The resulting impairments make working with the patient with brain injury extremely rewarding and challenging. There are a multitude of issues to consider. The physical therapist must adapt traditional physical therapy examination procedures and interventions to the unique motor control, cognitive, and behavioral challenges presented. The interdisciplinary team offers a unique opportunity for the physical therapist to learn. By working together with a team, the physical therapist is able to provide appropriate care that will help the individual with a brain injury reach maximum functional potential.

Questions for Review

1. Describe three different pathophysiological mechanisms that may be involved with a TBI.
2. Describe how each of the following rating scales is utilized: Glasgow Coma Scale, Rancho Los Amigos Levels of Cognitive Functioning Scale, FIM in combination with the FAM, and Glasgow Outcome Scale.
3. Identify three neuroimaging techniques used in the diagnosis of patients with TBI.
4. Identify key prognostic factors for individuals with TBI.
5. Describe the role of the physical therapist in the management of the patient with brain injury who is in the no response, generalized response, and localized response levels of recovery (LOCF).
6. How would a physical therapy plan of care need to be modified for a patient with post-traumatic amnesia?
7. What is the significance of a patient's cognitive and behavioral status in relation to his or her physical therapy goals and outcomes?
8. List and describe key elements in planning interventions appropriate for the patient in the confused–inappropriate and confused–appropriate levels of recovery (LOCF V, VII).
9. How does knowledge of a patient's ability or inability to learn new information affect a physical therapist's plan of care?
10. Describe the importance of the team approach in treating the patient with brain injury. Describe the roles of key members of the team in the acute rehabilitation setting.
11. List the important aspects of patient and family education in the low, middle, and high levels of recovery.
12. Why is it important to monitor the effects of different medications in this patient population?
13. List and describe key elements in planning interventions appropriate for the patient in the confused-agitated stage of recovery (LOCF IV).

Case Study

Note: The case study is divided into the following sections: Part A (guiding questions 1–3), Part B (guiding questions 4–6), and Part C (guiding questions 7 and 8).

PART A

The patient is a 34-year-old female who was involved in a motor vehicle accident (MVA). She was struck by another car as she exited her car. The patient suffered a severe closed brain injury. She was taken to a local hospital. CT scan revealed a right temporal parietal hemorrhage, a left parietal hemorrhage, diffuse edema, and multiple contusions. At the acute hospital, the patient underwent a ventriculostomy, gastrostomy tube placement, and tracheostomy. Her ICP was slightly elevated. The ventriculostomy was removed approximately

2 weeks after the initial injury. Approximately 6 weeks after her injury, the patient was transferred to an acute rehabilitation hospital.

PAST MEDICAL HISTORY

Healthy, 34-year-old woman with no significant past medical history.

SOCIAL HISTORY

Patient worked as an administrative assistant at a college. She was very active in the community. She enjoyed outdoor activities and was president of the local Sierra Club chapter. She has a very supportive husband (who was at the scene of the accident) and mother. Patient is right handed.

PHYSICAL THERAPY EXAMINATION FINDINGS

Arousal/Consciousness

Patient's eyes are open with random eye movements, but not able to track to auditory or visual stimuli. Patient does blink eyes when startled.
Patient does not respond to verbal commands.
Patient not able to vocalize, or make any attempt at communication.

Vital Signs

Heart rate: 72
Blood pressure: 124/72
Respiratory rate: 12

Motor Control

Patient presents with decorticate posturing
Nonpurposeful movement in UEs and LEs bilaterally, more movement on right side than left
No active dorsiflexion (DF) exhibited on either side
Increased extensor tone bilaterally in LEs, 3 on left and 2 on right (modified Ashworth scale)
Increased flexor tone bilaterally in UEs, 3 on left and 2 on right (modified Ashworth scale)
Multibeat continuous clonus left plantarflexors, and 2 to 3 beat clonus right plantarflexors

Joint Integrity and Passive Range of Motion

LEs bilaterally within normal limits (WNL) except right DF: lacks 15° from neutral and left DF: lacks 25° from neutral
Right UE WNL
Left UE WNL except shoulder abduction: 0–85°, flexion: 0–95°, external rotation: 0–45°, elbow extension: lacks 20°. One finger subluxation left shoulder

Postural Control and Balance

Patient requires maximal assistance of one to sit on edge of bed.
Requires minimal to moderate assistance to maintain head control in sitting.
Patient inconsistently exhibits delayed equilibrium and protective reactions in sitting.
Patient tolerated sitting for approximately 5 minutes, then exhibited increase in tone and respiratory rate.

Functional Mobility

Patient is dependent for all mobility. This includes rolling, moving to and from supine and sitting, transfers, and wheelchair mobility.
Patient is not able to stand.
FIM scores: bed/chair transfers: 1, walk: 1, wheelchair: 1, stairs: 1.

MEDICATIONS

Vancomyacin: 250 mg via IV q 12 hours for 5 days, for the infection.
Heparin: 5000 U, subcutaneous q 12 hours, to prevent DVT.
Ativan: 1 mg via G-tube, PRN, q 6 hours, in case of increased agitation.

OTHER FINDINGS

Patient has tracheostomy intact.
The patient exhibits dysphagia and is NPO (nothing by mouth) except for trial feedings with the speech–language pathologist.
Patient has stage three decubiti on both heels.
She also has an infection, *methicillin-resistant staphylococcus aureus* (MRSA), in lungs; as a result, patient is on contact precautions; gown, gloves, and mask should be worn when working with the patient.

GUIDING QUESTIONS

1. Categorize the patient's level of consciousness upon admission to the acute rehabilitation hospital based on the Glasgow Coma Scale and level of cognitive functioning based on the Ranchos Los Amigos Levels of Cognitive Functioning (LOCF).
2. Create a problem list and differentiate direct impairments, indirect impairments, and functional limitations.
3. Describe three physical therapy interventions that would be appropriate for this patient at this time. Include at least one related to family education.

PART B

The patient described above has continued to progress. She is still in the acute rehabilitation hospital and it is now 7 weeks later, 13 weeks post-injury.

PHYSICAL THERAPY EXAMINATION FINDINGS

Motor Control

Increased extensor tone left LE, 2 on modified Ashworth scale. Left UE flexor tone, 2 on modified Ashworth scale. Right UE and LE tone, WNL

Patient exhibits full active range of motion (AROM) for all muscle groups in right UE and LE.

Strength is in G/G– (4/4–) range at all muscle groups on right except DF is F– (3–) and hip abduction is F+(3+).

Patient exhibits partial (1/2 to 3/4) AROM against gravity in left upper and LE for all muscle groups except DF, which is trace.

Patient exhibits impaired coordination in all four extremities, greater on left than right.

Delayed initiation, dysdiadochokinesia, and slower speed of movement on left; accuracy decreases with increased speed of movement with all four extremities; minimally ataxic gait pattern.

Passive Range of Motion

WNL all four extremities except right DF: 0°, left DF: lacks 10° from neutral (patient has a full weightbearing short leg serial cast on left), left elbow flexion: 5°–150° (lacks the last 5° of full extension)

Sensation

Intact throughout for light touch, pinprick, deep pressure, hot/cold, and proprioception.

Postural Control/Balance

Sitting: static, patient able to maintain sitting balance with moderate challenges; dynamic, patient able to reach slightly outside LOS and maintain balance.

Standing: static, patient able to stand for 3 to 5 minutes with minimal assistance; dynamic, patient requires moderate assistance to ambulate 35 ft; decreased weightbearing on left LE; Berg Balance Scale score: 8/56.

Patient exhibits protective reactions in sitting, delayed on both left and right, slower on left than right; patient also exhibits righting reactions both sitting and standing; both are moderately delayed, greater delay in standing than sitting.

Functional Mobility

Bed mobility: Rolling to left, independent; rolling to right, minimal assistance; supine-to-sit, minimal to moderate assistance; sit-to-supine, supervision; patient requires two to three verbal cues to ensure correct technique with all the above, except for rolling to left.

Transfers: Bed to and from W/C, moderate assistance using stand pivot to left or right; patient requires two to three verbal cues to correctly position W/C and to lock brakes.

Wheelchair mobility: Patient able to propel W/C 150 ft with supervision and verbal cues; patient uses both LEs to propel W/C.

Ambulation: Patient able to ambulate 35 ft with moderate assistance, forearm crutch in right UE, and hinged ankle foot orthosis (AFO) with plantarflexion stop set at 0° on right LE.

Stairs: Unable to perform at this time.

FIM scores: Bed/chair transfers: 3, walk: 1, W/C: 5, stairs: 1

Cognition

Patient exhibits short-term memory impairments. She is inconsistently disoriented to place and time and oriented to person 100% of the time. Patient able to follow two- to three-step commands when in a closed environment. When in an open environment, the patient is only able to follow one-step commands. Patient exhibits decreased insight into impairments and diminished safety awareness. Patient is easily distracted, able to attend to a task for only 5 minutes at best.

Communication

Patient exhibits expressive aphasia. She is able to make basic needs known using verbal language and gestures. She exhibits severe word retrieval deficits. Her receptive language skills are WNL.

Vision and Perception: WNL

OTHER INFORMATION

Patient's infection is cleared. The only medication the patient is taking is bromocriptine. She has a custom-fit hinged AFO with a plantarflexion stop for her right foot, and her left foot and ankle are casted in a full weightbearing short leg serial cast. She wears a bivalve elbow extension brace on her left elbow at night. She had previously undergone serial casting at her left elbow. Her skin on both heels is now intact.

GUIDING QUESTIONS

4. Describe how this patient's memory impairments will affect physical therapy interventions and how the physical therapist should adapt interventions to maximize the patient's motor learning abilities.
5. List five possible goals for this patient.
6. Describe two interventions appropriate for this patient based on stated goals.

PART C

It is now approximately 5 months after the initial accident. The same patient is now discharged home with her husband. She returns to the rehabilitation hospital to participate in the day treatment program from 8:30 to 3:30 Monday through Friday. The patient requires 24-hour supervision owing to continuing cognitive, communication, and mobility impairments.

PHYSICAL THERAPY EXAMINATION FINDINGS

Motor Control

Tone: WNL all four extremities

Coordination: Impaired in both UEs and LEs; slowed movement, accuracy decreases with increased speed, greater on left than right; minimally ataxic gait pattern

Strength: Right UE WNL; right LE WNL except DF: F+; left UE G for all muscle groups; left LE G for all muscle groups except DF: F– and hip abduction: F–.

Passive Range of Motion

WNL all four extremities except right DF, 0–10°; left DF, 0°.

Postural Control

Sitting: static, WNL; dynamic, WNL; balance reactions WNL.

Standing: static, able to maintain balance with minimal challenges; dynamic balance reactions minimally delayed; Berg Balance Scale score: 40/56.

Functional Mobility

Bed mobility: Rolling to left and right, independent. Moving to and from sitting and supine, independent.

Transfers: W/C to and from bed requires supervision with one to two verbal cues for safety and locking brakes; floor-to-stand, moderate assistance.

Wheelchair mobility: Independent in the home.

Ambulation: Supervised 300 ft (91 m) in a closed environment (home or in the hospital) with bilateral hinged AFOs. Patient uses a forearm crutch in the right UE; in an open environment, the patient requires contact guard to minimal assistance to ambulate; gait speed: 0.65 m/s (2 ft/s) gait endurance over a 6-minute walk: 574 ft (175 m).

Stairs: Contact guard up and down one flight with bilateral AFOs and one railing.

FIM + FAM scores: Bed/chair transfers: 5, walk: 5, wheelchair: 5, stairs: 4, car transfer: 5, community access: 3.

Cognition

Patient oriented to person, place, and time 100% of the time. While patient has shown improvement in short-term memory and new learning, she is still impaired in this area. She is able to follow four- to five-step commands in a closed environment. Patient performs best in a highly structured environment. In an open environment, patient becomes easily distracted, needing verbal cues to complete a task. Patient's insight and safety awareness have improved, but are still impaired. For example, she requires verbal reminders not to transfer or ambulate independently.

Communication

Patient exhibits moderate word finding deficits and anomia (inability to remember names of objects).

GUIDING QUESTIONS

7. List and prioritize the patient's direct impairments, indirect impairments, and functional limitations.
8. Describe two interventions appropriate for this patient. At least one intervention should focus on community reentry.

References

1. Dobkin, B: The Clinical Science of Neurologic Rehabilitation, ed 2. Oxford University Press, Oxford, 2003.
2. Consensus Conference: Rehabilitation of persons with traumatic brain injury. NIH Consensus Development Panel on Rehabilitation of Persons with Traumatic Brain Injury. JAMA 282:974, 1999.
3. Thurman, D, and Guerrero, J: Trends in hospitalization associated with traumatic brain injury. JAMA 282:954, 1999.
4. Thurman, DJ, et al: Traumatic brain injury in the United States: A public health perspective. J Head Trauma Rehabil 14:602, 1999.
5. Vangel, SJ, et al: Long-term medical care utilization and costs among traumatic brain injury survivors. Am J Phys Med Rehabil 84(3):153, 2005.
6. Mayer, N, et al: Hypertonicity and movement disorders. In Rosenthal, M, et al (eds): Rehabilitation of the Adult and Child with Traumatic Brain Injury, ed 2. FA Davis, Philadelphia, 1999, p 503.
7. Jennett, B, and Teasdale, G: Management of Head Injuries. FA Davis, Philadelphia, 1981.
8. Giacino, JT, et al: The minimally conscious state: Definition and diagnostic criteria. Neurology 58:349, 2002.
9. Shumway-Cook, A, and Woollacott, MH: Motor Control: Theory and Practical Applications, ed 2. Lippincott Williams & Wilkins, Philadelphia, 2001.
10. Lezak, MD: Neuropsychological assessment, ed 3. Oxford University Press, New York 1995.
11. Rappaport, M, et al: Head injury outcome up to ten years later. Arch Phys Med Rehabil 70:885, 1989.
12. Teasdale, G, and Jennett, B: Assessment of coma and impaired consciousness. A practical scale. Lancet 2:81, 1974.
13. Teasdale, G, et al: Observer variability in assessing impaired consciousness and coma. J Neurol Neurosurg Psychiatry 41:603, 1978.
14. Thornhill, S, et al: Disability in young people and adults one year after head injury: Prospective cohort study. Br Med J 320:1631, 2000.
15. Levin, HS, et al: The Galveston Orientation and Amnesia Test: A practical scale to assess cognition after head injury. J Nerv Ment Dis 167:675, 1979.
16. Katz, DI, and Alexander, MP: Traumatic brain injury: Predicting course of recovery and outcome for patients admitted to rehabilitation. Arch Neurol 51:661, 1994.
17. Katz, DI: Neuropathology and neurobehavioral recovery from closed head injury. J Head Trauma Rehabil 7:1, 1992.
18. Ranchos Los Amigos Hospital. Rehabilitation of the Head Injured Adult. Downey, CA: Professional Staff Association, 1979.
19. Gouvier, WD, et al: Reliability and validity of the Disability Rating Scale and the Levels of Cognitive Functioning Scale in monitoring recovery from severe head injury. Arch Phys Med Rehabil 68:94, 1987.
20. Cifu, DX, et al: Acute predictors of successful return to work 1 year after traumatic brain injury: A multicenter analysis. Arch Phys Med Rehabil 78:125, 1997.
21. Jennett, B, and Bond, M: Assessment of outcome after severe brain damage. Lancet 1:480, 1975.
22. Anderson, SI, et al: Glasgow Outcome Scale: An inter-rater reliability study. Brain Inj 7:309, 1993.
23. Jennett, B, et al: Disability after severe head injury: Observations on the use of the Glasgow Outcome Scale. J Neurol Neurosurg Psychiatry 44:285, 1981.
24. Rappaport, M, et al: Disability rating scale for severe head trauma: Coma to community. Arch Phys Med Rehabil 6:118, 1982.
25. Guide for the Uniform Data Set for Medical Rehabilitation: UB Foundation Activities, Inc, Buffalo, NY, 2002.

26. Dodds, TA, et al: A validation of the functional independence measurement and its performance among rehabilitation inpatients. Arch Phys Med Rehabil 74:531, 1993.
27. Stineman, MG, et al: The Functional Independence Measure: Tests of scaling assumptions, structure, and reliability across 20 diverse impairment categories. Arch Phys Med Rehabil 77:1101, 1996.
28. Hall, KM, et al: Characteristics and comparisons of functional assessment indices: Disability Rating Scale, Functional Independence Measure, and Functional Assessment Measure. J Head Trauma Rehabil 8:60, 1993.
29. Gurka, JA, et al: Utility of the functional assessment measure after discharge from inpatient rehabilitation. J Head Trauma Rehabil 14:247, 1999.
30. Hobart, JC, et al: Evidence-based measurement: Which disability scale for neurologic rehabilitation? Neurology 57:639, 2001.
31. Donaghy, S, and Wass, PJ: Interrater reliability of the Functional Assessment Measure in a brain injury rehabilitation program. Arch Phys Med Rehabil 79:1231, 1998.
32. Levin, HS, et al: Neurobehavioral outcome 1 year after severe head injury. Experience of the Traumatic Coma Data Bank. J Neurosurg 73:699, 1990.
33. Ono, J, et al: Outcome prediction in severe head injury: Analyses of clinical prognostic factors. J Clin Neurosci 8:120, 2001.
34. Clausen, T, and Bullock, R: Medical treatment and neuroprotection in traumatic brain injury. Curr Pharm Des 7:1517, 2001.
35. Kalisky, Z, et al: Medical problems encountered during rehabilitation of patients with head injury. Arch Phys Med Rehabil 66:25, 1985.
36. Malec, JF, and Basford, JS: Postacute brain injury rehabilitation. Arch Phys Med Rehabil 77:198, 1996.
37. Malec, JF: Impact of comprehensive day treatment on societal participation for persons with acquired brain injury. Arch Phys Med Rehabil 82:885, 2001.
38. Semlyen, JK, et al: Traumatic brain injury: Efficacy of multidisciplinary rehabilitation. Arch Phys Med Rehabil 79:678, 1998.
39. Braverman, SE, et al: A multidisciplinary TBI inpatient rehabilitation programme for active duty service members as part of a randomized clinical trial. Brain Inj 13:405, 1999.
40. Chapman, P: Physical therapy in the intensive care unit. In MacKay, L (ed): Maximizing Brain Injury Recovery Integrating Critical Care and Early Rehabilitation. Aspen, Gaithersburg, MD, 1997, p 271.
41. Yarkony, GM, and Sahgal, V: Contractures: A major complication of craniocerebral trauma. Clin Orthop 219:93, 1987.
42. Shaw, J, et al: Clinical and physiological measures of tone in chronic stroke. Neurology Report (now JNPT) 23:19, 1999.
43. Bohannon, RW, and Smith, MB: Interrater reliability of a modified Ashworth scale of muscle spasticity. Phys Ther 67:206, 1987.
44. Gregson, JM, et al: Reliability of measurements of muscle tone and muscle power in stroke patients. Age Ageing 29:223, 2000.
45. Gregson, JM, et al: Reliability of the Tone Assessment Scale and the modified Ashworth scale as clinical tools for assessing post-stroke spasticity. Arch Phys Med Rehabil 80:1013, 1999.
46. Schenkman, M, et al: Multisystem model for management of neurologically impaired adults: An update and illustrative case. Neurology Report (now JNPT) 23:145, 1999.
47. American Physical Therapy Association: Guide to Physical Therapist Practice, ed 2. APTA, Alexandria, VA, 2001.
48. Chatterton, HJ, et al: Positioning for stroke patients: A survey of physiotherapists' aims and practices. Disabil Rehabil 23:413, 2001.
49. Still, JM, et al: A retrospective study to determine the incidence of pressure ulcers in burn patients using an alternating pressure mattress. Burns 29:505, 2003.
50. Kanyer, B: Meeting the seating and mobility needs of the client with traumatic brain injury. J Head Trauma Rehabil 7:81, 1992.
51. Ciesla, ND: Chest physical therapy for patients in the intensive care unit. Phys Ther 76:609, 1996.
52. American Association for Respiratory Care Clinical Practice Guideline: Postural drainage therapy. Respir Care 36:1418, 1991.
53. Schmit, BD, et al: Stretch reflex adaptation in elbow flexors during repeated passive movements in unilateral brain-injured patients. Arch Phys Med Rehabil 81:269, 2000.
54. Al Zamil, ZM, et al: Reduction of elbow flexor and extensor spasticity following muscle stretch. J Neurol Rehabil 9:161, 1995.
55. Hale, LA, et al: Prolonged static muscle stretch reduces spasticity. S Afr J Physiother 51: 3, 1995.
56. Michelsson, JE, et al: Myositis ossificans following forcible manipulation of the leg: A rabbit model for the study of heterotopic bone formation. J Bone Joint Surg Am 62:811, 1980.
57. Tsur, A, et al: Relationship between muscular tone, movement and periarticular new bone formation in postcoma-unaware (PC-U) patients. Brain Inj 10:259, 1996.
58. Garland, DE: Clinical observations on fractures and heterotopic ossification in the spinal cord and traumatic brain injured populations. Clin Orthop 233:86, 1988.
59. Sazbon, L, et al: Widespread periarticular new-bone formation in long-term comatose patients. J Bone Joint Surg Br 63:120, 1981.
60. Garland, DE, et al: Periarticular heterotopic ossification in head-injured adults: Incidence and location. J Bone Joint Surg Am 62:1143, 1980.
61. Johns, JS, et al: Impact of clinically significant heterotopic ossification on functional outcome after traumatic brain injury. J Head Trauma Rehabil 14:269, 1999.
62. Ansell, BJ: Slow-to-recover brain-injured patients: Rationale for treatment. J Speech Hear Res 34:1017, 1991.
63. Grüner, ML, and Terhaag, D: Multimodal early onset stimulation (MEOS) in rehabilitation after brain injury. Brain Inj 14:585, 2000.
64. Kater, KM: Response of head-injured patients to sensory stimulation. West J Nurs Res 11:20, 1989.
65. Mitchell, S, et al: Coma arousal procedure: A therapeutic intervention in the treatment of head injury. Brain Inj 4:273, 1990.
66. Johnson, DA, et al: Biochemical and physiological parameters of recovery in acute severe head injury: Responses to multisensory stimulation. Brain Inj 7:491, 1993.
67. Pierce, JP, et al: The effectiveness of coma arousal intervention. Brain Inj 4:191, 1990.
68. Lippert-Gruner, M, et al: Outcome of prolonged coma following severe traumatic brain injury. Brain Inj 17:49, 2003.
69. Lombardi, F, et al: Sensory stimulation for brain injured individuals in coma or vegetative state. Cochrane Database Syst Rev, 2002.
70. Florian, V, et al: Impact of traumatic brain damage on family dynamics and functioning: A review. Brain Inj 3:219, 1989.
71. Kreutzer, JS, et al: Traumatic brain injury: Family response and outcome. Arch Phys Med Rehabil 73:771, 1992.
72. Tyerman, A, and Booth, J: Family interventions after traumatic brain injury: A service example. Neurorehabilitation 16:59, 2001.
73. Smith, MS, and Testani-Dufour, L: Who's teaching whom? A study of family education in brain injury. Rehabil Nurs 27:209, 2002.
74. Davies, PM: Starting again: Early rehabilitation after traumatic brain injury. Springer-Verlag, Berlin, 1994.
75. Sandel, ME, and Mysiw, WJ: The agitated brain injured patient. Part 1: Definitions, differential diagnosis, and assessment. Arch Phys Med Rehabil 77:617, 1996.
76. Brooke, MM, et al: Agitation and restlessness after closed head injury: A prospective study of 100 consecutive admissions. Arch Phys Med Rehabil 73:320, 1992.
77. Slifer, KJ, et al: Antecedent management and compliance training improve adolescents' participation in early brain injury rehabilitation. Brain Inj 11:877, 1997.
78. Kim, E: Agitation, aggression, and disinhibition syndromes after traumatic brain injury. Neurorehabil 17:297, 2002.
79. Berg, K, et al: Measuring balance in the elderly: Preliminary development of an instrument. Physiother Can 41:304, 1989.
80. Feld, JA, et al: Berg balance scale and outcome measures in acquired brain injury. Neurorehabil Neural Repair 15:239, 2001.
81. Juneja, G, et al: Admission balance and outcomes of patients admitted for acute inpatient rehabilitation. Am J Phys Med Rehabil 77:388, 1998.
82. Krebs, DE, and Edelstein, JE: Reliability of observational kinematic gait analysis. Phys Ther 65:1027, 1985.

83. The Pathokinesiology Service and the Physical Therapy Department Ranchos Los Amigos Medical Center: Observational Gait Analysis. Los Amigos Research and Education Institute, Inc, Downey, CA, 1996.
84. Richards, CL, et al: Gait in stroke: Assessment and rehabilitation. Clin Geriatr Med 15:833, 1999.
85. Holden, MK, et al: Clinical gait assessment in the neurologically impaired: Reliability and meaningfulness. Phys Ther 64:35, 1984.
86. Holden, MK, et al: Gait assessment for neurologically impaired patients: Standards for outcome assessment. Phys Ther 66:1530, 1986.
87. Mossberg, KA: Reliability of a timed walk test in persons with acquired brain injury. Am J Phys Med Rehabil 82:385, 2003.
88. Sadaria, KS, and Bohannon, RW: The 6-Minute Walk Test: A brief review of literature. Clin Exerc Physiol 3:127, 2001.
89. Gladstone, DJ, et al: The Fugl-Meyer assessment of motor recovery after stroke: A critical review of its measurement properties. Neurorehabil and Neural Repair 16:232, 2002.
90. Fugl-Meyer, AR, et al: The post-stroke hemiplegic patient: A method for evaluation of physical performance. Scand J Rehab Med 7:13, 1975.
91. Gowland, C, et al: Measuring physical impairment and disability with the Chedoke-McMaster Stroke Assessment. Stroke 24:58, 1993.
92. Haring, LD, et al: Motor learning patterns of patients with traumatic brain injury and impaired memory function: Learning a sequential motor task under a high versus low frequency of feedback. Neurol Rep 25:143, 2001.
93. Mackay, LE, et al: Early intervention in severe head injury: Long-term benefits of a formalized program. Arch Phys Med Rehabil 73:635, 1992.
94. Kolb, B: Overview of cortical plasticity and recovery from brain injury. Phys Med Rehabil Clin North Am 14:S7, 2003.
95. Nudo, RJ: Functional and structural plasticity in motor cortex: Implications for stroke recovery. Phys Med Rehabil Clin North Am 14:S57, 2003.
96. Carr, J, and Shepherd, R: Movement Science: Foundations for Physical Therapy In Rehabilitation, ed 2. Aspen, Gaithersburg, MD, 2000.
97. Wilson, DJ, and Swaboda, JL: Partial weight-bearing gait retraining for persons following traumatic brain injury: Preliminary report and proposed assessment scale. Brain Inj 16:259, 2002.
98. Hunter, DL, et al: The effects of harness support on lower extremity muscle activity of able-bodied and traumatic brain injured subjects during gait. Phys Ther 77:S84, 1997.
99. Seif-Naraghi, AH, and Herman, RM: A novel method for locomotion training. J Head Trauma Rehabil 14:146, 1999.
100. Page, S, and Levine, P: Forced use after TBI: Promoting plasticity and function through practice. Brain Inj 17:675, 2003.
101. Shaw, SE, et al: Constrain-induced movement therapy to improve upper extremity function in subjects following traumatic brain injury. Neurology Report (now JNPT) 24:172, 2000.
102. Taub, E, et al: Improved motor recovery after stroke and massive cortical reorganization following Constraint-Induced Movement therapy. Phys Med Rehabil Clin North Am 14:S77, 2003.
103. Klonoff, PS, et al: Outcomes from milieu-based neurorehabilitation at up to 11 years post-discharge. Brain Inj 15:413, 2001.
104. Ekstam, MH: Step by step: The road to independence following a traumatic brain injury: An outpatient/day treatment approach. Inside Case Manag 10:3, 2003.
105. Jankowski, LW, and Sullivan, SJ: Aerobic and neuromuscular training: Effect on the capacity, efficiency, and fatigability of patients with traumatic brain injuries. Arch Phys Med Rehabil 71:500, 1990.
106. Wolman, RL, et al: Aerobic training in brain-injured patients. Clin Rehabil 8:253, 1994.
107. Gordon, WA, et al: The benefits of exercise in individuals with traumatic brain injury: A retrospective study. J Head Trauma Rehabil 13:58, 1998.
108. Bateman, A, et al: The effect of aerobic training on rehabilitation outcomes after recent severe brain injury: A randomized controlled evaluation. Arch Phys Med Rehabil 82:174, 2001.
109. Moseley, AM, et al: The effect of casting combined with stretching on passive ankle dorsiflexion in adults with traumatic head injuries. Phys Ther 77:240, 1997.
110. Pohl, M, et al: Effectiveness of serial casting in patients with severe cerebral spasticity: A comparison study. Arch Phys Med Rehabil 83:784, 2002.
111. Childers, MK, et al: Inhibitory casting decreases a vibratory inhibition index of the H-reflex in the spastic upper limb. Arch Phys Med Rehabil 80:714, 1999.
112. Lehmkuhl, LD, et al: Multimodality treatment of joint contractures in patients with severe brain injury: Cost, effectiveness, and integration of therapies in the application of serial/inhibitive casts. J Head Trauma Rehabil 5:23, 1990.
113. Stoeckmann, T: Casting for the person with spasticity. Top Stroke Rehabil 8:27, 2001.
114. Watkins, CA: Mechanical and neurophysiological changes in spastic muscles: Serial casting in spastic equinovarus following traumatic brain injury. Physiother 85:603, 1999.
115. Mortenson, PA, and Eng, JJ: The use of casts in the management of joint mobility and hypertonia following brain injury in adults: A systematic review. Phys Ther 83:648, 2003.
116. Price, R, et al: Influence of cryotherapy on spasticity at the human ankle. Arch Phys Med Rehabil 74:300, 1993.
117. Robichaud, JA, and Agostinucci, J: Air-splint pressure effect on soleus muscle alpha motoneuron reflex excitability in subjects with spinal cord injury. Arch Phys Med Rehabil 77:778, 1996.
118. Robichaud, JA, et al: Effect of air-splint application on soleus muscle motoneuron reflex excitability in nondisabled subjects and subjects with cerebrovascular accidents. Phys Ther 72:176, 1992.
119. Francisco, GE, et al: GABA agonists and gabapentin for spastic hypertonia. Phys Med Rehabil Clin North Am 12:875, 2001.
120. Nance, PW: Alpha adrenergic and serotonergic agents in the treatment of spastic hypertonia. Phys Med Rehabil Clin North Am 12:889, 2001.
121. Yablon, SA: Botulinum neurotoxin intramuscular chemodenervation: Role in the management of spastic hypertonia and related motor disorders. Phys Med Rehabil Clin North Am 12:833, 2001.
122. Zafonte, RD, and Munin, MC: Phenol and alcohol blocks for the treatment of spasticity. Phys Med Rehabil Clin North Am 12:817, 2001.
123. Graf, M, et al: Environmental control unit considerations for the person with high-level tetraplegia. Top Spinal Cord Inj Rehabil 2:30, 1997.
124. Ried, S, et al: Computers, assistive devices, and augmentative communication aids: Technology for social inclusion. J Head Trauma Rehabil 10:80, 1995.
125. Hart, T, et al: Clinician expectations for portable electronic devices as cognitive-behavioural orthoses in traumatic brain injury rehabilitation. Brain Inj 17:401, 2003.
126. Hart, T, et al: Use of a portable voice organizer to remember therapy goals in traumatic brain injury rehabilitation: A within-subjects trial. J Head Trauma Rehabil 17:556, 2002.
127. Wright, P, et al: Comparison of pocket-computer memory aids for people with brain injury. Brain Inj 15:787, 2001.
128. Johnson, DA, et al: Virtual reality: A new prosthesis for brain injury rehabilitation. Scott Med J 43:81, 1998.
129. Christiansen, C, et al: Task performance in virtual environments used for cognitive rehabilitation after traumatic brain injury. Arch Phys Med Rehabil 79:888, 1998.
130. Zhang, L, et al: A virtual reality environment for evaluation of a daily living skill in brain injury rehabilitation: Reliability and validity. Arch Phys Med Rehabil 84:1118, 2003.
131. Lengenfelder, J, et al: Divided attention and driving: A pilot study using virtual reality technology. J Head Trauma Rehabil 17:26, 2002.
132. Holden, MK, et al: Retraining movement in patients with acquired brain injury using a virtual environment. Stud Health Tech Informatics 81:192, 2001.
133. Sveistrup, H, et al: Experimental studies of virtual reality-delivered compared to conventional exercise programs for rehabilitation. Cyberpsychology Behav 6:245, 2003.

Supplemental Readings

Carr, J, and Shepherd, R: Neurological Rehabilitation: Optimizing Motor Performance. Butterworth Heinemann, Oxford, 1998.

Carr, J, and Shepherd, R: Movement Science: Foundations for Physical Therapy in Rehabilitation, ed 2. Aspen, Gaithersburg, MD, 2000.

Cicerone, KD, et al: Evidence-based cognitive rehabilitation: Recommendations for clinical practice. Arch Phys Med Rehabil 81:1596, 2000.

Consensus Conference: Rehabilitation of persons with TBI. NIH Consensus Development Panel on Rehabilitation of Persons with TBI. JAMA 282:974, 1999.

Dobkin, B: The Clinical Science of Neurologic Rehabilitation, ed 2. Oxford University Press, Oxford, 2003.

Gennarelli, TA, and Graham, DI: Neuropathology of the Head Injuries. Semin Clin Neuropsychiatry 3:160, 1998.

Koller, WC, et al: Posttraumatic movement disorders: A review. Mov Disord 4:20, 1989.

The Multi-Society Task Force on PVS: Medical aspects of the persistent vegetative state. N Engl J Med 330:1572, 1994.

Rosenthal, M, et al: Rehabilitation of the Adult and Child with TBI, ed 3. FA Davis, Philadelphia, 1999.

Shumway-Cook, A, and Woollacott MH: Motor Control: Theory and Practical Applications, ed 2. Lippincott, Williams & Wilkins, Philadelphia, 2001.

Appendix A: Commonly Prescribed Medications

Analgesics

NSAIDs (Nonsteroidal Anti-inflammatory Drugs)

Examples	Mechanism of Action	Clinical Use	Comments
Aspirin, naproxen, ibuprofen, indomethacin	Inhibits prostaglandin synthesis; thus NSAID exhibit anti-inflammatory, analgesic, and antipyretic properties.	Used to produce: (1) analgesia, (2) anti-inflammatory effect, (3) antipyresis, and (4) inhibition of platelet aggregation (e.g., in prophylaxis of unstable angina).	The most important adverse effect is gastric bleeding or gastritis. Most commonly used NSAID, aspirin, is toxic when overdosed. It may cause tinnitus, central hyperventilation, metabolic acidosis, fever, dehydration, hypoprothrombinemia, coma, vascular collapse, and renal and respiratory failure. Aspirin binds very avidly with plasma albumins, displacing other drugs from their protein binding sites. Therefore, co-administration of aspirin with other drugs (such as tolbutamide, chlorpropamide, methotrexate, or phenytoin) may cause sudden elevation of plasma concentration. Aspirin is contraindicated in children who suffer from varicella or influenza infection, as it is believed that aspirin use is related to Reye's syndrome (brain and liver damage).

Acetaminophen

Examples	Mechanism of Action	Clinical Use	Comments
Acetaminophen (generic name)	It is postulated that acetaminophen inhibits a third, not yet characterized, cyclooxygenase (COX-3) that is expressed in the CNS. This action is assumed to be responsible for antipyretic and analgesic properties.[a]	Induces analgesia and antipyresis. Contrary to NSAIDs, acetaminophen does not possess anti-inflammatory properties, and does not affect platelet aggregation.	Acetaminophen may cause fatal hepatic and renal necroses when overdosed. Successful detoxification can be achieved by prompt administration of *N*-acetylcysteine.

Opioids

Examples	Mechanism of Action	Clinical Use	Comments
(1) Strong agonists: morphine, methadone, fentanyl, oxymorphone, meperidine; (2) Moderate agonists: codeine, oxycodone, propoxyphene, diphenoxylate; (3) Mixed agonists-antagonists: buprenorphine, pentazocine; (4) Antagonists: naloxone.	Act through μ, κ, and λ receptors. Effects of opioids include: (1) analgesic effect; changes perception and response to pain; pain may be still perceived, but emotional response to it is abolished; (2) euphoria; (3) sedation; (4) respiratory depression by inhibition of the respiratory center; cough suppression; (5) miosis; (6) truncal rigidity; (7) nausea and vomiting; (8) constipation; (9) constriction of smooth muscles in the biliary tract; (10) depression of renal function due to decrease in renal plasma flow; (11) may prolong labor [mechanism unknown].	(1) analgesia, (2) acute pulmonary edema, (3) cough, (4) diarrhea, (5) anesthesia [especially when minimizing cardiovascular effects of anesthesia is important], and (6) opioids are also used in epidural and subarachnoid spinal anesthesia.	Opioids induce development of tolerance and dependence. Tolerance develops to all effects of opioids except: miosis, constipation, and seizure induction potential. Opioids are contraindicated for patients (1) with head injury [induced respiratory depression leads to carbon dioxide retention and cerebral vasodilatation that in turn causes an increase in intracranial pressure]; (2) with impaired pulmonary function; (3) pregnant women [opioids may induce dependence in the fetus; administration during delivery may cause respiratory depression in a newborn]; (4) with renal and biliary colic [pain may increase due to contraction of smooth muscles]; Note: Administration of naloxone, an opioid antagonist, quickly reverses all the toxic symptoms of opioids; administration of naloxone to an individual dependent on opioids induces withdrawal reaction.

Insomnia

Sedatives–Hypnotics

Examples	Mechanism of Action	Clinical Use	Comments
(1) Benzodiazepines [diazepam, lorazepam, clonazepam, nitrazepam, alprazolam, flunitrazepam]; (2) barbiturates [phenobarbital, pentobarbital, secobarbital].	These drugs act through the GABA receptor, facilitating action of this neurotransmitter. Benzodiazepine antagonist, flumazenil, antagonizes sedative–hypnotics action at the receptor site, and may be used in drug overdosing.	(1) sedation, (2) decreases time to fall asleep, (3) anesthesia, (4) anticonvulsant effect, (5) muscle relaxation, and (6) anxiolysis	Prolonged administration of these drugs (several weeks) induces tolerance and dependence (psychological and physical). Withdrawal syndrome may be life threatening; symptoms include: restlessness, anxiety, weakness, orthostatic hypotension, hyperactive reflexes, and seizures.

Zolpidem, Zaleplon

Examples	Mechanism of Action	Clinical Use	Comments
Zolpidem, Zaleplon	Both drugs are structurally unrelated to benzodiazepines or barbiturates. They both bind to the benzodiazepine receptor, facilitating inhibitory action of GABA.	Hypnosis	Flumazenil antagonizes action of zolpidem. Both drugs exhibit hypnotic action. Zolpidem has minimal sedative and muscle relaxing properties, and has much smaller potential to induce dependence and tolerance than benzodiazepines. With the use of zaleplon, no development of tolerance and withdrawal syndrome have been reported.

Depression

Examples	Mechanism of Action	Clinical Use	Comments
(1) Selective serotonin reuptake inhibitors (SSRI) (fluoxetine, sertraline, paroxetine, fluvoxamine); (2) tricyclic antidepressants (TCA) (imipramine, desimipramine, nortriptyline, clomipramine); (3) Monoamine oxidase inhibitors (MAOI) (tranylcypromine, phenelzine).	It is believed that antidepressive agents exert their effects through increasing monoamine neurotransmission (dopamine, serotonin, norepinephrine).	Depression, panic disorder, obsessive–compulsive disorder, enuresis, chronic pain, bulimia, social phobia, attention deficit disorder.	*SSRI:* Are the most well tolerated antidepressants. Compared with TCA and MAOI, SSRI have lowest sedative, anticholinergic, and orthostatic hypotensive action. However, they may cause nausea, headache, neuromuscular restlessness similar to akathisia, insomnia or sedation, delayed ejaculation or anorgasmia. Combination of SSRI with MAOI may cause fatal serotonin syndrome, due to markedly elevated serum serotonin concentration. *TCA:* The most common adverse effects include: (1) cardiovascular effects—orthostatic hypotension, conduction defects, arrhythmias; (2) antimuscarinic effects—blurred vision, constipation, confusion, urinary hesitancy; (3) sexual dysfunction—in men impotence, in women decreased arousal; (4) neurologic effects—seizures. *MAOI:* Improper diet (food containing tyramine—cured meat or fish, beer, red wine, cheese, overripe fruit) may lead to severe hypertensive crisis with potential myocardial infarction or stroke. Many over the counter cold and pain remedies that increase monoaminergic transmission have to be avoided. MAOI may cause orthostatic hypotension. Phenelzine may cause somnolence, and tranylcypromine insomnia and agitation.

Antiseizure

Examples	Mechanism of Action	Clinical Use	Comments
Carbamazepine, valproic acid, phenytoin, ethosuximide, lamotrigine	Antiseizure agents act on neurons depressing their activity by: (1) increasing GABAergic transmission (direct action on the GABA channel: benzodiazepines, barbiturates; decreasing reuptake or metabolism of GABA: gabapentin, tiagabine, vigabatrin), (2) refractory period prolongation of the voltage-gated Na channel (phenytoin, carbamazepine, topiramate), (3) reducing T-channel C-current in thalamic neurons (ethosuximide).	The goal of the medical therapy is to prevent seizures without inducing any side effects, preferably using a single agent. Antiseizure drugs have different effectiveness against different type of seizures. Therefore, the choice of an antiseizure medication depends on the diagnosed seizure type. The first line agents for tonic–clonic seizure are: valproic acid and lamotrigine; for partial seizures: carbamazepine, phenytoin, valproic acid, lamotrigine; for absence seizure: ethosuximide, and valproic acid. There are many other alternative agents.	Adverse effects. Carbamazepine: ataxia, dizziness, diplopia, vertigo, aplastic anemia, leucopenia, GI irritation, hepatotoxicity, hyponatremia. Valproic acid: ataxia, sedation, tremor, hepatotoxicity, thrombocytopenia, GI irritation, weight gain, transient alopecia, hyperammonemia; when administered to a pregnant woman, induces neural tube defects in 2% of fetuses. Phenytoin: dizziness, diplopia, ataxia, incoordination, confusion, gingival hyperplasia, lymphadenopathy, hirsutism, osteomalacia, facial coarsening, skin rash. Ethosuximide: ataxia, lethargy, headache, GI irritation, skin rash, bone marrow suppression. Lamotrigine: dizziness, diplopia, sedation, ataxia, headache, skin rash, Steven-Johnson syndrome.

Antipsychotic

Examples	Mechanism of Action	Clinical Use	Comments
Chlorpromazine, haloperidol, clozapine.	Depression of the dopaminergic neuron in the brain.	(1) Schizophrenia, (2) mania in bipolar disorder, (3) Tourette's syndrome; (4) disturbed behavior in Alzheimer's disease, (5) psychotic features in depression, (6) antiemetic [chlorpromazine], (7) antipruritic; and (8) preoperative sedation.	In healthy subjects, antipsychotic drugs cause unpleasant combined sensation of sleepiness, restlessness, and autonomic effects. Healthy subjects show impaired psychomotor performance. However, psychotic patients show better performance as the psychosis subsides. Adverse effects include (1) pseudo-depression due to drug induced akinesia [usually responds to antiparkinsonism treatment]; (2) Parkinsonism; (3) akathisia; (4) dystonia; (5) tardive dyskinesia; (6) seizures [clozapine]; (7) anticholinergic reactions [urinary retention, dry mouth, blurred vision]; (8) orthostatic hypotension; (9) agranulocytosis [clozapine]; (10) may deposit in the cornea [chlorpromazine] or retina [thioridazine]; and (11) neuroleptic malignant syndrome [life threatening].

Antiemetic Drugs

Antihistamines

Examples	Mechanism of Action	Clinical Use	Comments
Diphenhydramine, hydroxyzine	Antihistaminic activity at H1 receptor.	These drugs have strong antiemetic activity, and are particularly effective for the nausea and vomiting related to motion sickness. This predilection may be due to depression of the vestibulo-cerebellar pathway.	Their use may be limited by pronounced adverse effects: sedation, dizziness, confusion, dry mouth, urinary retention, cycloplegia. Diphenhydramine is most commonly used in conjunction with other drugs in treatment of emesis due to chemotherapy.
Scopolamine	Muscarinic receptor antagonist.	Excellent agent for prevention of motion sickness.	When administered orally or parenterally, exhibits strong anticholinergic effects. Therefore, it is better tolerated in the form of transdermal patches.

Phenothiazines

Examples	Mechanism of Action	Clinical Use	Comments
Prochlorperazine, promethasine	Block histaminic, dopamine, and muscarinic receptors. Sedative properties are due to antihistaminic activity. Antiemetic properties are mediated by blockade of dopamine and muscarinic receptors in the proemetic chemoreceptor trigger zone located in the floor of the fourth ventricle (area postrema).	These drugs are mainly used as antipsychotic agents, but due to their strong antiemetic properties are also used to prevent nausea and vomiting in selected clinical situations (sedation for endoscopic procedures, postoperative nausea and vomiting).	The most common adverse effect is dystonia. It can be decreased by concomitant administration of diphenhydramine.

Metoclopramide

Examples	Mechanism of Action	Clinical Use	Comments
Metoclopramide	Releases acetylcholine from myenteric plexus neurons through stimulation of 5-HT_4 receptors. Metoclopramide is a potent dopamine (D_2) antagonist in the chemoreceptor trigger zone of the medulla.	Gastrointestinal reflux disease, postsurgical delayed gastric emptying, diabetic gastroparesis, prevention and treatment of nausea and vomiting.	The drug stimulates esophageal clearance, raises lower esophageal sphincter pressure, stimulates gastric emptying and shortens small intestine transit time. The most common adverse effects include: somnolence, nervousness, and dystonia. It may also induce parkinsonism and tardive dyskinesia, especially in the elderly. Increased release of prolactin from the pituitary with resulting galactorrhea and amenorrhea have been reported as well.

5-HT_3 Inhibitors

Examples	Mechanism of Action	Clinical Use	Comments
Ondansetron, granisetron, dolasetron	Antiemetic action is mainly mediated through blockade of peripheral 5-HT_3 receptor on gastrointestinal vagal afferents, although central 5-HT_3 receptor blockade may play an important role as well.	These drugs are important in cancer chemotherapy, owing to their ability to prevent nausea and emesis associated with the administration of chemotherapeutics. These drugs are also effective in controlling post-radiation and post-operative nausea and vomiting.	Emesis induced by vagal stimulation is controlled well. Emesis produced by other stimuli (e.g., motion sickness) is poorly controlled. These drugs are well tolerated and are remarkably safe.

Spasmolytics

Examples	Mechanism of Action	Clinical Use	Comments
Gabapentin	An antiseizure drug that facilitates GABA action	It is an antiseizure drug that exhibits antispasmodic properties in patients with multiple sclerosis.	Adverse effects may include drowsiness, dizziness, headache, fatigue, and ataxia.
Diazepam	See sedative–hypnotic	Exhibits antispasmodic action	See sedative–hypnotic
Baclofen	Baclofen is an agonist of GABA-B receptor. It has been suggested that it has a presynaptic inhibitory function.	It is as effective as diazepam in reducing spasticity, but produces less sedation. Appears to be more effective in spasticity caused by spinal cord damage than cerebral damage.	In patients with epilepsy, baclofen may increase seizure activity. Its adverse effects include drowsiness, confusion, headache, muscle weakness, and lethargy.
Dantrolene	Dantrolene blocks the ryanodine receptor. Ryanodine receptor is a calcium channel that releases calcium from the sarcoplasmic reticular cysterns. Blockage of this channel prevents muscle contraction.	Reduce spasticity; special indication includes malignant hyperthermia	In addition to antispasmotic action, it may cause muscle weakness, sedation, and, rarely, hepatitis.

Botulinum toxin	This toxin is produced by bacteria *Clostridium botulinum*. The toxin inhibits acetylcholine release from the axon terminals of motor neurons. The toxin uptake by peripheral and cranial nerves is mediated by a receptor localized to the axon terminals.	This agent is used in treatment of spasticity cerebral palsy, stroke and blepharospasm. A single toxin injection relieves muscle spasm for several months.	Adverse effects may include pain at injection site, muscle weakness in injected muscle, hematoma, muscle necrosis, and phlebitis.
Cyclobenzaprine	Cyclobenzaprine is a prototype drug for the large group of compounds used for treatment of acute spasm. The exact mechanism of action is unknown, but the drug exerts its action at the level of the brainstem and spinal cord.	Used to treat an acute muscle spasm.	Cyclobenzaprine is not effective in cerebral palsy and spinal cord injury. The drug has strong antimuscarinic properties responsible for severe sedation, confusion, and hallucinations.
Tizanidine	An $alpha_2$-receptor agonist. Increases pre- and postsynaptic inhibition.	Beneficial in patients with traumatic brain injury, stroke, spinal cord injury, multiple sclerosis, and cerebral palsy.	Similar to clonidine, but produces less cardiovascular effects. Adverse effects include drowsiness, hypotension, dry mouth, asthenia. Equal in effectiveness as baclofen and diazepam, but more favorably tolerated.

[a]From Botting RM: Mechanism of action of acetaminophen: Is there a cyclooxygenase-3? Clin Infect Dis 31:S202, 2000. Table prepared by Maciej Markowski, MD, PhD.

CHAPTER

23

LEARNING OBJECTIVES

1. Identify the major etiological factors associated with traumatic spinal cord injury.
2. Describe the clinical presentation following damage to the spinal cord.
3. Describe the indirect impairments and complications associated with spinal cord injury.
4. Identify the expected functional outcomes for patients with spinal cord injury at various lesion levels.
5. Identify and explain the relevant systems review and tests and measures included in the examination process.
6. Describe appropriate treatment interventions for the acute, active rehabilitation, and chronic phases of management.
7. Analyze and interpret patient data, formulate anticipated goals and expected outcomes, and develop a plan of care when presented with a clinical case study.

Traumatic Spinal Cord Injury

George D. Fulk, PT, PhD
Thomas J. Schmitz, PT, PhD
Andrea L. Behrman, PT, PhD

OUTLINE

Spinal cord injury (SCI) is a low-incidence, high-cost disability requiring tremendous changes in an individual's lifestyle. It is estimated that approximately 11,000 new cases of SCI occur in the United States annually. A gross estimate indicates that there are between 225,000 and 288,000 individuals with SCI currently living in the United States.[1]

Demographics

Statistics from the National Spinal Cord Injury Database (NSCID) provide important demographic information about traumatic spinal cord injury. The NSCID was established in 1973 and contains information on more than 22,000 individuals who sustained traumatic SCIs. Twenty-five federally funded Model SCI Care Systems have provided data to the NSCID. Information from the NSCID provide many of the statistical references reported in the following sections.[1,2]

Etiology

Spinal cord injuries can be grossly divided into two broad etiological categories: *traumatic* injuries and *nontraumatic* damage. Traumas are by far the most frequent cause of injury in adult rehabilitation populations. They result from damage caused by a traumatic event such as a motor vehicle accident, fall, or gunshot wound. Because of their higher incidence, management of traumatic injuries will be described in this chapter; however, the treatment principles discussed will have direct application to nontraumatic lesions as well.

Statistics from the NSCID indicate that accidents involving motor vehicles are the most frequent cause of traumatic SCI (45.6 percent), followed by falls (19.6 percent), acts of violence (17.8 percent), recreational sports injuries (10.7 percent), and other etiologies (6.3 percent).[3]

Nontraumatic damage in adult populations generally results from disease or pathological influence. Several examples of nontraumatic conditions that may damage the spinal cord are vascular malfunctions (arteriovenous malformation [AVM], thrombosis, embolus, or hemorrhage); vertebral **subluxations** secondary to rheumatoid arthritis or degenerative joint disease, infections such as syphilis or transverse myelitis, spinal neoplasms, syringomyelia, abscesses of the spinal cord, and neurological diseases such as multiple sclerosis and amyotrophic lateral sclerosis. Statistics that detail the incidence of nontraumatic cord damage are not currently available. However, it is estimated that nontraumatic etiologies account for 30 percent of all spinal cord injuries.

Distribution by the National Spinal Cord Injury Database (NSCID) Variables

The NSCID has collected data on multiple patient variables. The most salient statistics are presented here. Of the patients for whom data were collected, 81.0 percent were men, representing a slightly higher than 4:1 ratio of men to women. More than half of the population (51.6 percent) was between the ages of 16 and 30 years, with a mean age at time of injury of 33.3 years. Ethnic distributions indicate that whites represented 66.6 percent of the database, followed by African-Americans (21.0 percent), Hispanics (9.7 percent), and others (3.5 percent).[3]

Fifty-one percent of patients experienced cervical lesions, 34.6 percent had thoracic lesions, and 10.8 percent had lumbosacral lesions. At discharge from the rehabilitation hospital, 18.6 percent had neurologically incomplete paraplegia, 29.4 percent of patients had neurologically incomplete tetraplegia, 26.3 percent had neurologically complete paraplegia, and 20.7 percent had neurologically complete tetraplegia. The proportion of patients with neurologically incomplete injuries has increased since 1973 from 45.9 percent to 55.3 percent in 2004. This trend can be partially attributed to the improvement in emergency medical services delivered at the scene of the injury.[2]

Data were also collected on employment status, residence, marital status, length of hospital stay, and life expectancy. At the time of injury, 63.0 percent of the patients were employed. Postinjury employment status is slightly higher among individuals with paraplegia as compared to those with *tetraplegia* (preferred over the term *quadriplegia*). Follow-up information indicates that at 10 years postinjury, 31.7 percent of individuals with paraplegia were employed as compared to 26.4 percent of those with tetraplegia. At time of discharge, the majority of patients (88.3 percent) returned to a private residence (most to their homes) and 5.1 percent were discharged to nursing homes. Because the majority of individuals with SCIs are young adults, more than half (53.0 percent) were single at the time of injury. The average length of hospital stay in an acute care unit was 15 days and the average stay in a rehabilitation unit was 40 days. This is a decrease compared to 1974 when acute care hospitalization lasted an average of 25 days and rehabilitation stays lasted an average of 115 days.[1]

Life expectancy has increased over the years but is still less than for individuals without a SCI. Factors that influence life expectancy are age at injury and level and extent of neurological injury. For example, an individual who was injured at 30 years of age with a high cervical injury (C1–C4) would have a life expectancy of 58.4 years, whereas a 30-year-old with paraplegia would have a life expectancy of 66.8 years.[2]

The financial impact of SCI is extremely high. The disability is characterized by lengthy hospitalization, medical complications, extensive follow-up care, and recurrent hospitalizations. The costs of medical care during the first year postinjury were $682,957 for high tetraplegia (C1–C4), $441,025 for low tetraplegia (C5–C8), and $249,549 for paraplegia. Average lifetime costs for an individual injured at 25 years of age were $2,693,887 for high tetraplegia (C1–C4), $1,523,204 for low tetraplegia (C5–C8), and $900,085 for paraplegia. These numbers do not take into account lost wages, fringe benefits, and productivity.[1]

This brief presentation of demographic information provides some important general perspectives on characteristics of SCI. It is a relatively low-incidence disability affecting a predominantly young population and is associated with lengthy and costly care.

Classification of Spinal Cord Injuries

Spinal cord injuries typically are divided into two broad functional categories: tetraplegia and paraplegia. **Tetraplegia** refers to complete paralysis of all four extremities and trunk, including the respiratory muscles, and results from lesions of the cervical cord. **Paraplegia** refers to complete paralysis of all or part of the trunk and both lower extremities (LEs), resulting from lesions of the thoracic or lumbar spinal cord or cauda equina.

Before considering designation of spinal cord lesions, it is useful to review briefly the anatomical relationship of the spinal cord and nerve roots to the vertebral bodies (Fig. 23.1).[4] There are 31 pairs of spinal nerves: 8 cervical, 12 thoracic, 5 lumbar, 5 sacral, and 1 coccygeal. The upper cervical nerves are relatively horizontal as they exit the intervertebral foramina. However, the remaining nerves exit in a downward direction and do not emerge at the corresponding vertebral level. During fetal development the cord fills the entire length of the vertebral canal, and the spinal nerves run in a horizontal direction. As the vertebral column elongates with growth, the spinal cord, which does not elongate at the same rate or as much, is drawn upward. The roots assume an

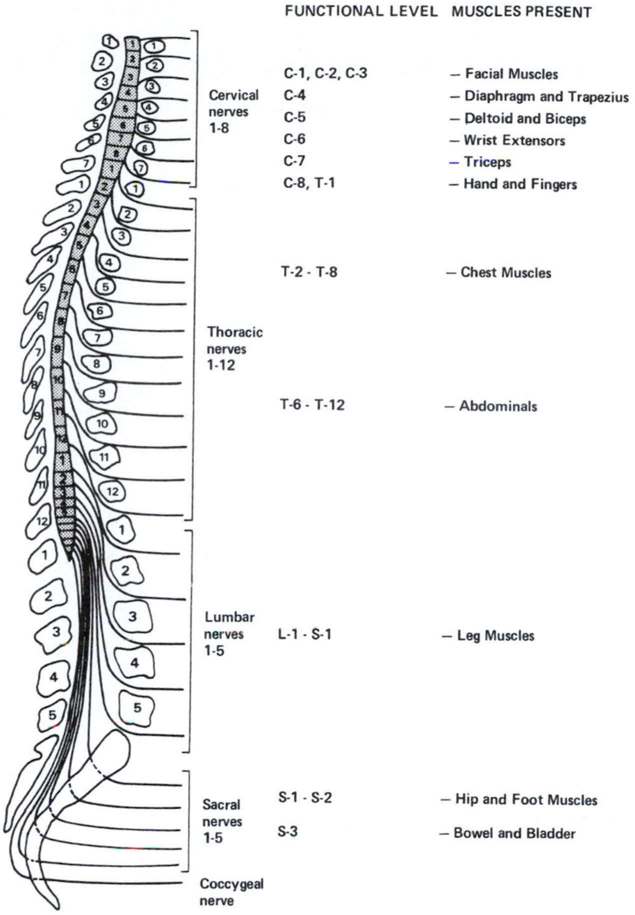

Figure 23.1 Relationship between the spinal cord and nerve roots to vertebral bodies and innervation of major muscle groups. (From Coogler, CE,[4, p 150], with permission.)

increasingly oblique and downward direction, running in an almost vertical direction in the lumbar area, giving the appearance of a "horse's tail" (cauda equina).

Designation of Lesion Level

It is extremely important for clinicians and researchers to be able to accurately determine the extent of neurological impairment in terms of motor and sensory loss when working with individuals with SCI. The extent of motor and sensory function after injury has a large impact on the medical and rehabilitation needs of the individual. The American Spinal Injury Association (ASIA) created the International Standards of Neurological Classification of Spinal Cord Injury (ISNCSCI)[5] (Fig. 23.2) in an effort to standardize the way in which severity of injury is determined and documented.[5] The ISNCSCI provides a standardized examination method to determine the extent of motor and sensory function loss after a SCI. It allows for better communication between and among professionals, provides guidance for establishing the prognosis, and is an important tool for clinical research trials.

The **neurological level** is defined as the most caudal level of the spinal cord with normal motor and sensory function on both the left and right sides of the body. **Motor level** is referred to as the most caudal segment of the spinal cord with normal motor function bilaterally. **Sensory level** is defined in the same way except in terms of sensory function. Sensory level is typically determined by testing the patient's sensitivity to light touch and pin prick on the left and right side of the body at key dermatomes (see Fig. 23.2). Scoring of sensation is based on a 3-point ordinal scale where 0 = absent, 1 = impaired, and 2 = normal. Motor level is determined by testing the strength of a key muscle on the right and left side of the body at myotomes adjacent to the suspected level of impairment (see Fig. 23.2 for key muscles). Key muscle strength is scored using the 6-point ordinal scale commonly used for manual muscle testing.[5,6]

Assigning a single muscle to represent one myotome is a generalization. Most muscles are innervated by more than one segmental nerve root; usually two nerve roots innervate each muscle. For example, the extensor carpi radialis longus receives innervation from the C6 and C7 spinal nerve roots. For the purpose of determining motor and neurological level, the key muscle is defined as having intact innervation if it has a manual muscle test score of at least 3/5 (fair) and the next most rostral key muscle exhibits 5/5 (normal) strength on the manual muscle test. If the rostral key muscle does not demonstrate 5/5 strength, but the therapist feels that the muscle would test normally except for factors that would impede normal testing (e.g., pain with testing or difficulty with positioning), then this information should be carefully documented. For myotomes that are not clinically testable (i.e., C1–C4, T2–L1, and S2–S5) the motor level is defined as the same as the sensory level.[5]

In determining neurological level there may be differences in terms of level of sensory and motor function and between the left and right sides of the body. For example, a patient's sensory level may be at C5 on the left, C8 on the right and the motor level may be C5 on the left and T1 on the right. In these cases, it is not appropriate to assign a single neurological level, as this can be misleading. Each of the sensory and motor levels on the right and left sides of the body should be documented separately.[5]

Complete Injuries, Incomplete Injuries, and Zone of Partial Preservation

A complete anatomical transection of the spinal cord is rare. However, even if the injury is not anatomically complete, it may present clinically as complete. The ISNCSCI defines a **complete injury** as having no sensory or motor function in the lowest sacral segments (S4 and S5). Sensory and motor function at S4 and S5 are determined by anal sensation and voluntary external anal sphincter contraction. An **incomplete injury** is classified as having motor and/or sensory function below the neurological level

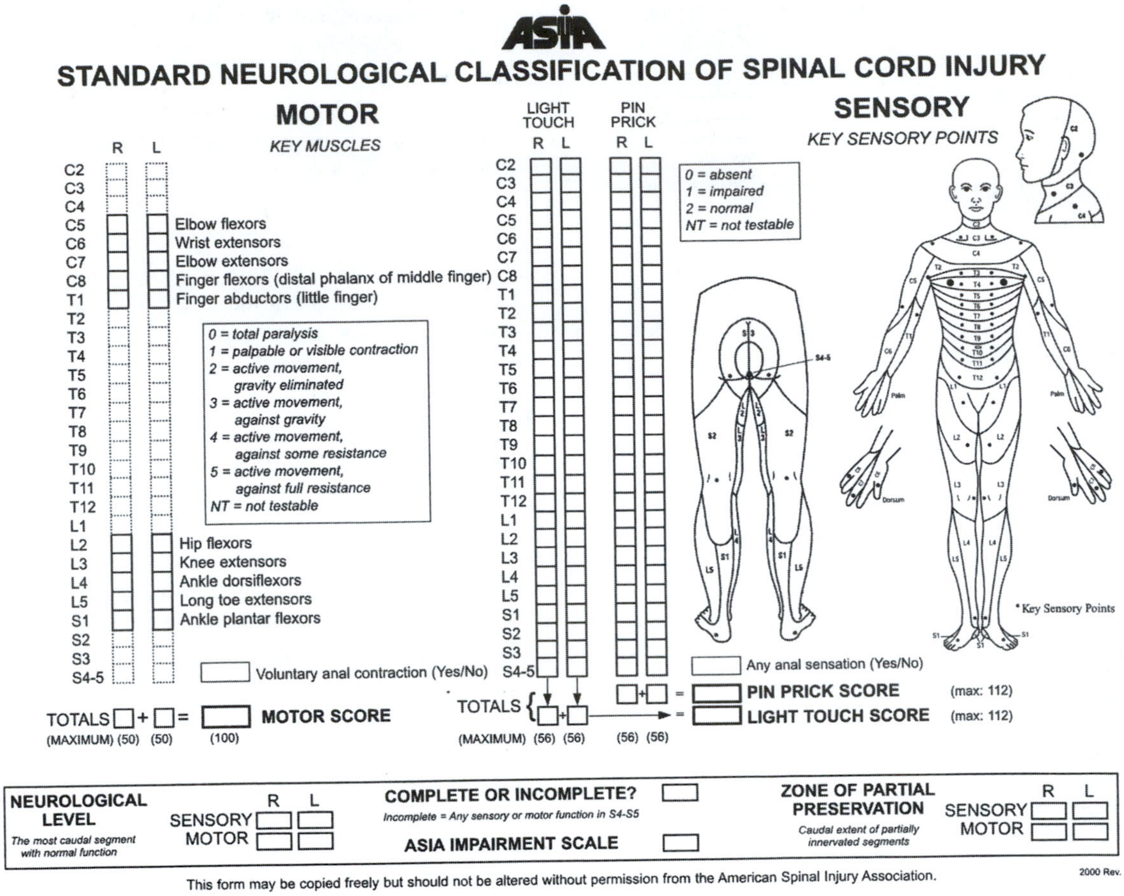

Figure 23.2 Motor and sensory examination form recommended by ASIA. (From American Spinal Injury Association,[5, p 27] with permission.)

including sensory and/or motor function at S4 and S5. If an individual has motor and/or sensory function below the neurological level, but does not have function at S4 and S5 then the areas of intact motor and/or sensory function below the neurological level are termed **zones of partial preservation**.[5]

ASIA Impairment Scale

Individuals with incomplete injuries may have variable clinical presentations in terms of motor and/or sensory function below the neurological level. For example, one patient may have close to normal sensory and motor function below the level of the lesion while another with the same lesion level may have impaired sensation and no motor function below the neurological level. The ASIA impairment scale (Table 23.1)[5] was created so that clinicians and researchers could better communicate the degree of impairment of individuals with spinal cord injuries.

Clinical Syndromes

Despite the uncertainty associated with recovery of incomplete lesions, several syndromes have emerged with

Table 23.1 Impairment Scale

- ☐ A = **Complete:** No motor or sensory function is preserved in the sacral segments S4 to S5.
- ☐ B = **Incomplete:** Sensory but not motor function is preserved below the neurological level and includes the sacral segments S4 to S5.
- ☐ C = **Incomplete:** Motor function is preserved below the neurological level, and more than half of key muscles below the neurological level have a muscle grade less than 3.
- ☐ D = **Incomplete:** Motor function is preserved below the neurological level, and at least half of key muscles below the neurological level have a muscle grade of 3 or more.
- ☐ E = **Normal:** Motor and sensory function is normal.

Clinical Syndromes

- ☐ Central cord
- ☐ Brown-Sequard
- ☐ Anterior cord
- ☐ Conus medullaris
- ☐ Cauda equina

From American Spinal Cord Injury Association,[5] p 28, with permission.

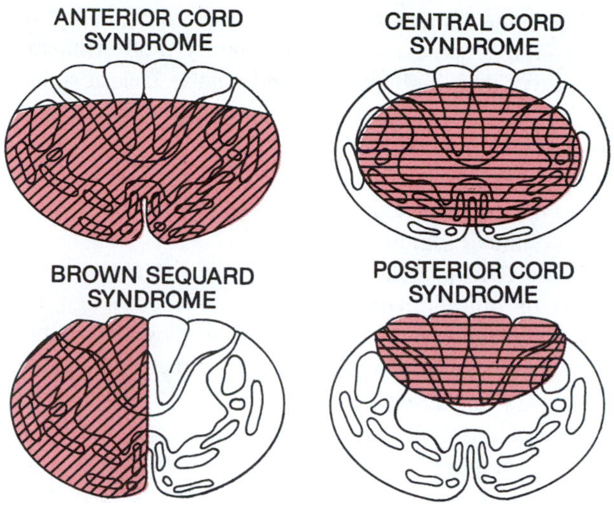

Figure 23.3 Areas of spinal cord damage in incomplete cord syndromes. (From Rieser, TV, et al[7, p 14] with permission.)

consistent clinical features. Information related to the anticipated sensory and motor functions of these syndromes is useful in establishing goals, outcomes, and plan of care (POC). The area of cord damage of each syndrome is presented in Figure 23.3.[7]

Brown-Sequard Syndrome

Brown-Sequard syndrome occurs from hemisection of the spinal cord (damage to one side) and is typically caused by penetration wounds, i.e., gunshot or stab. Partial lesions occur more frequently; true hemisections are rare. The clinical features of this syndrome are asymmetrical. On the *ipsilateral* (same) side as the lesion, there is loss of sensation in the dermatome segment corresponding to the level of the lesion. Owing to lateral column damage, there are decreased reflexes, lack of superficial reflexes, clonus, and a positive Babinski sign. As a result of dorsal column damage, there is loss of proprioception, kinesthesia, and vibratory sense. On the side *contralateral* (opposite) to the lesion, damage to the spinothalamic tracts results in loss of sense of pain and temperature. This loss begins several dermatome segments below the level of injury. This discrepancy in levels occurs because the lateral spinothalamic tracts ascend two to four segments on the same side before crossing.[7–9]

Anterior Cord Syndrome

Anterior cord syndrome is frequently related to flexion injuries of the cervical region with resultant damage to the anterior portion of the cord and/or its vascular supply from the anterior spinal artery. There is typically compression of the anterior cord from fracture, dislocation, or cervical disk protrusion. This syndrome is characterized by loss of motor function (corticospinal tract damage) and loss of the sense of pain and temperature (spinothalamic tract damage) below the level of the lesion. Proprioception, kinesthesia, and vibratory sense are generally preserved, because they are mediated by the posterior columns with a separate vascular supply from the posterior spinal arteries.[7–10]

Central Cord Syndrome

Central cord syndrome most commonly occurs from hyperextension injuries to the cervical region. It also has been associated with congenital or degenerative narrowing of the spinal canal.[7] The resultant compressive forces give rise to hemorrhage and edema, producing damage to the most central aspects of the cord. There is characteristically more severe neurological involvement of the upper extremities (UEs)(cervical tracts are more centrally located) than of the LEs (lumbar and sacral tracts are located more peripherally).[11,12] Varying degrees of sensory impairment occur[13] but tend to be less severe than motor deficits. With complete preservation of sacral tracts, normal sexual, bowel, and bladder function will be retained. Patients with central cord syndrome typically recover the ability to ambulate with some remaining distal UE weakness. Surgical intervention to relieve the source of compression has produced significant improvement in some patients.

Posterior Cord Syndrome

Posterior cord syndrome is an extremely rare syndrome resulting in deficits of function served by the posterior columns.[14] The clinical picture includes preservation of motor function, sense of pain, and light touch.[7] There is loss of proprioception and epicritic sensations (e.g., two-point discrimination, graphesthesia, stereognosis) below the level of lesion. A wide-based steppage gait pattern is typical. In the past, this syndrome was seen with tabes dorsalis, a condition found with late-stage syphilis.

Sacral Sparing

Sacral sparing refers to an incomplete lesion in which the most centrally located sacral tracts are spared. Varying levels of innervation from sacral segments remain intact. Clinical signs include perianal sensation and external anal sphincter contraction. These are important neurological findings and often the first signs that a cervical lesion is incomplete.[7,10]

Cauda Equina Injuries

The spinal cord tapers distally to form the conus medullaris at the lower border of the first lumbar vertebra. Although some anatomical variations exist, this is the typical termination point of the spinal cord. Below this level is the collection of long nerve roots known as the *cauda equina*. Complete transections in this area may occur. However, **cauda equina lesions** are frequently incomplete owing to the great number of nerve roots involved and the comparatively large surface area they encompass (i.e., it would be unlikely that an injury to this region would involve the entire surface area and all the nerve roots).

Cauda equina lesions are peripheral nerve **(lower motor neuron [LMN])** injuries. As such, they have the same potential to regenerate as peripheral nerves elsewhere in the body. However, full return of innervation is not common because (1) there is a large distance between the lesion and the point of innervation; (2) axonal regeneration may not occur along the original distribution of the nerve; (3) axonal regeneration may be blocked by glial-collagen scarring; (4) the end organ may no longer be functioning once reinnervation occurs; and (5) the rate of regeneration slows and finally stops after about 1 year.

Mechanisms of Injury

Various mechanisms, often in combination, produce injuries to the spinal cord. Spinal cord injury most frequently occurs from indirect forces produced by movement of the head and trunk and less often from direct injury to a vertebra.[15] Common mechanisms operating in SCI include flexion, compression, hyperextension, and flexion–rotation. These forces result in either a fracture and/or **dislocation**. The intensity and combination of forces imposed have direct influence on the type and location of fracture(s), the amount of dislocation, and the extent of soft tissue damage.[16]

The spine demonstrates various degrees of susceptibility to injury. Some areas are inherently more vulnerable because of their high mobility and relative lack of stability as compared with other segments of the spine (e.g., the rigid thoracic region).[17] The areas of the spine that demonstrate the highest frequency of injury are between C5 and C7 in the cervical region and between T12 and L2 in the thoracolumbar region.

Table 23.2 presents a summary of the major mechanisms of injury involved in SCI.[15,17–19] Although these forces typically occur in combination, they are presented individually inasmuch as each has characteristic patterns of primary and associated injuries.

Two additional contributing mechanisms involved in SCI are shearing and distraction. *Shearing* occurs when a horizontal force is applied to the spine relative to the adjacent segment.[10] Shearing frequently disrupts ligaments and is associated with fracture dislocations of the thoracolumbar region.[15] *Distraction* involves a traction force and is the least common mechanism. It occurs when significant momentum of the head is created, as in whiplash injuries. This momentum creates a tensile force in the cervical spine as the head is pulled away from the body.[10,15]

Table 23.2 Mechanisms of Injury[15,17,18,19]

Force	Etiology	Associated Fractures	Potential Associated Injuries
Flexion	• Head-on collision in which head strikes steering wheel or windshield. • Blow to back of head or trunk. • Most common mechanism of SCI.	• Wedge fracture of anterior vertebral body (vertebral body compressed). • High percentage of injuries occur from C4 to C7 and from T12 to L2.	• Tearing of posterior ligaments. • Fractures of posterior elements: spinous processes, laminae, or pedicles. • Disruption of disk. • Anterior dislocation of vertebral body.
Compression	• Vertical or axial blow to head (diving, surfing, or falling objects). • Closely associated with flexion injuries.	• Concave fracture of endplate. • Explosion or burst fracture (comminuted). • Teardrop fracture.	• Bone fragments may lodge in cord. • Rupture of disk.
Hyperextension	• Strong posterior force such as a rear-end collision. • Falls with chin hitting a stationary object (more commonly seen in elderly populations).	• Fractures of posterior elements: spinous processes, laminae, and facets. • Avulsion fracture of anterior aspect of vertebrae.	• Rupture of anterior longitudinal ligament. • Rupture of disk. • Associated with cervical lesions; only of minor influence in thoracolumbar injuries.
Flexion-rotation	Posterior to anterior force directed at rotated vertebral column (e.g., rear-end collision with passenger rotated toward driver).	Fracture of posterior pedicles, articular facets, and laminae (fracture is very unstable if posterior ligaments rupture).	• Rupture of posterior and interspinous ligaments. • Subluxation or dislocation of facet joints. • In thoracic and lumbar regions, facets may "lock."

Clinical Manifestations

Spinal Shock

Immediately following SCI there is a period of areflexia called **spinal shock**. This period of transient reflex depression is not clearly understood. It is believed to result from the very abrupt withdrawal of connections between higher centers and the spinal cord.[7,8,20] It is characterized by absence of all reflex activity, flaccidity, and loss of sensation and motor function below the level of the lesion. It may last for several days to several weeks.[21] In addition to the loss of deep tendon reflexes there is a loss of the bulbocavernosus reflex, the cremasteric reflex, and a delayed plantar response. These reflexes evolve over several days to weeks after SCI.[22] One of the first indicators that spinal shock is resolving is the presence of a positive bulbocavernosus reflex. This test is part of the neurologist's examination. During a digital rectal examination, this reflex is elicited by pressure applied to the glans penis or glans clitoris or by intermittently "tugging" on an indwelling catheter. If positive, a reflex contraction of the anal sphincter around the examining digit will be evident.[23] A bulbocavernosus reflex, cremasteric reflex, or a normal plantar response may be present several weeks before deep tendon reflexes are apparent in the LEs.

Motor and Sensory Impairments

Following SCI there will be either complete or partial loss of muscle function below the level of the lesion. Disruption of the ascending sensory fibers following SCI results in impaired or absent sensation below the level of the lesion.

The clinical presentation of motor and sensory impairments depends on the specific features of the lesion. These include the neurological level, the completeness of the lesion, and the symmetry of the lesion (transverse or oblique).

Autonomic Dysreflexia

Autonomic dysreflexia (hyperreflexia) is a pathological autonomic reflex that typically occurs in lesions above T6 (above sympathetic splanchnic outflow). However, it has been reported in patients with injuries at T7 and T8.[24,25] Incidence of this problem varies. One study[26] found a 48 percent occurrence in a group of 213 patients. Rosen[27] estimates that as many as 85 percent of those with tetraplegia and high-level paraplegia experience this problem during the course of rehabilitation. Episodes of autonomic dysreflexia gradually subside over time and are relatively uncommon, but not rare, 3 years following injury.[27] It is seen in patients with both complete and incomplete lesions.[28]

This clinical syndrome produces an acute onset of autonomic activity from noxious stimuli below the level of the lesion. Afferent input from these stimuli reach the lower spinal cord (lower thoracic and sacral areas) and initiate a mass reflex response resulting in elevation of blood pressure. Normally, the impulses stimulate the receptors in the carotid sinus and aorta, which signal the vasomotor center to readjust peripheral resistance. Following SCI, however, impulses from the vasomotor center cannot pass the site of the lesion to counteract the hypertension by vasodilation.[27,29,30] This is a critical, emergency situation. Owing to the lack of inhibition from higher centers, hypertension will persist if not treated promptly. Death may result.

Initiating Stimuli

The most common cause of this pathological reflex is bladder distention (urinary retention). Other precipitating stimuli include rectal distention, pressure sores, urinary stones, bladder infections, noxious cutaneous stimuli, kidney malfunction, urethral or bladder irritation, and environmental temperature changes.[26] Episodes of autonomic dysreflexia also have been reported following passive stretching at the hip.[31]

Symptoms

The symptoms of autonomic dysreflexia include hypertension, bradycardia, headache (often severe and pounding), profuse sweating, increased spasticity, restlessness, vasoconstriction below the level of lesion, vasodilation (flushing) above the level of the lesion, constricted pupils, nasal congestion, piloerection (goose bumps), and blurred vision.[26,32]

Intervention

The onset of symptoms should be treated as a medical emergency. If lying flat, the patient should be brought to a sitting position, inasmuch as blood pressure will be lowered in this position. Because bladder distention is a primary cause of autonomic dysreflexia, the drainage system should be examined immediately. If the patient is wearing a clamped catheter, it should be released. The drainage tubes also should be checked for internal or external blockage or twisting. The patient's body should be checked for irritating stimuli such as tight clothing, restricting catheter straps, or abdominal binders.

If symptoms do not subside, or if the source of irritation cannot be located, medical and/or nursing assistance should be sought immediately. Additional measures may include bladder irrigation (a higher-level block may exist), removal and replacement with a new catheter, and examination for bowel impaction. Drug therapy (antihypertensives) may be indicated to control these episodes if more conservative approaches are unsuccessful.

The attending physician, nursing staff, and other team members should always be notified of occurrences of autonomic dysreflexia. This will allow careful monitoring of the patient for several days following the episode and will alert others to the risk of future occurrences. The individual patient's symptoms, precipitating stimuli, and methods of relief should be documented.

Postural Hypotension

Postural hypotension (orthostatic hypotension) is a decrease in blood pressure that occurs when assuming an erect or vertical position (e.g., lying-to-sitting or sitting-to-standing). It is caused by a loss of sympathetic vasoconstriction control. The problem is enhanced by lack of muscle tone, causing peripheral venous and splanchnic bed pooling. Reduced cerebral blood flow and decreased venous return to the heart typically occurs, producing symptoms of lightheadedness, dizziness, or fainting.[33]

Inasmuch as many patients may be immobilized for several weeks, episodes of postural hypotension are a fairly common occurrence during early progression to a vertical position. They tend to occur more frequently with lesions of the cervical and upper thoracic regions. Patients will often describe the onset as feelings of "dizziness," "faintness," or impending "blackout." Although the exact mechanism is not clearly understood, the cardiovascular system, over time, gradually reestablishes sufficient vasomotor tone to allow assumption of the vertical position.[34]

A related problem is edema of the legs, ankles, and feet, which is usually symmetric and pitting in nature. It occurs secondary to the above problems and is complicated by decreased lymphatic return.[33]

To minimize these effects, the cardiovascular system should be allowed to adapt gradually by a slow progression to the vertical position. This frequently begins with elevation of the head of the bed and progresses to a reclining wheelchair with elevating leg rests and use of a tilt table. Vital signs should be monitored carefully, and the patient should always be moved very slowly. Use of compressive stockings and an abdominal binder will further minimize these effects. Pharmacological therapy may be indicated (e.g., ephedrine to increase blood pressure or low-dose diuretics to relieve persistent edema of legs, ankles, or feet).[33] As vasomotor stability returns, tolerance to the vertical position will gradually improve.

Impaired Temperature Control

After damage to the spinal cord the hypothalamus can no longer control cutaneous blood flow or level of sweating. This autonomic (sympathetic) dysfunction results in loss of internal thermoregulatory responses. The ability to shiver is lost; vasodilation does not occur in response to heat nor does vasoconstriction occur in response to cold. There is absence of thermoregulatory sweating, which eliminates the normal evaporative cooling effects of perspiration in warm environments. This lack of sweating is often associated with excessive compensatory *diaphoresis* above the level of lesion. Patients with incomplete lesions may also demonstrate "spotty" areas of localized sweating below the lesion level.[35]

Changes in thermal regulation result in body temperature being significantly influenced by the external environment. This is a more frequent problem with cervical lesions than with thoracic or lumbar involvement. Patients must rely heavily on sensory input from the head and neck regions to assist in determining appropriate environmental temperatures. Although some improvement in thermoregulatory responses occurs over time, patients with tetraplegia typically experience long-term impairment of body temperature regulation, especially in response to extreme environmental changes.[10]

Respiratory Impairment

Respiratory function varies considerably, depending on the level of lesion. With high spinal cord lesions between C1 and C3, phrenic nerve innervation and spontaneous respiration are significantly impaired or lost. An artificial ventilator or phrenic nerve stimulator is required to sustain life. In contrast, lumbar lesions present with full innervation of both primary (diaphragm) and secondary (neck, intercostal, and abdominal) respiratory muscles.

All patients with tetraplegia and those with high-level paraplegia demonstrate some compromise in respiratory function. The level of respiratory impairment is directly related to the lesion level, residual respiratory muscle function, and additional trauma sustained at time of injury, as well as premorbid respiratory status. Respiratory involvement represents a particularly serious and life-threatening feature of SCI. Pulmonary complications (especially bronchopneumonia and pulmonary embolism) are responsible for a high mortality during the early stages of tetraplegia.[36,37]

There is a progressively greater loss of respiratory function with increasingly higher lesion levels. Multiple respiratory changes occur that are related to both the inspiratory and expiratory phases of ventilation. The primary muscles of inspiration are the diaphragm and external intercostals. As the diaphragm contracts and descends, the intercostals normally elevate the ribs and increase the lateral anterior–posterior diameter of the thorax.[38] Paralysis of the intercostals results in decreased chest expansion and a lowered inspiratory volume. With progressively higher-level lesions, increased involvement of the accessory muscles of respiration will be noted. These muscles assist with elevation of the ribs and include the sternocleidomastoid, trapezii, scaleni, pectoralis minor, and serratus anterior.

The primary muscles of expiration are the abdominals and internal intercostals. Normally, relaxed expiration is essentially a passive process that occurs through elastic recoil of the lungs and thorax. However, the abdominals and internal intercostals contribute several important functions related to movement of air out of the lungs. Loss of these muscles significantly decreases expiratory efficiency.

When fully innervated, the abdominal muscles play an important role in maintaining intrathoracic pressure for effective respiration. They support the abdominal viscera[39,40] and assist in maintaining the position of the diaphragm. They also function to push the diaphragm upward during forced expiration. With paralysis of the abdominals this support is lost, causing the diaphragm to assume an unusually low position in the chest.[41] This lowered position and lack of abdominal pressure to move the diaphragm upward during forced expiration results in a decreased expiratory reserve volume. This subsequently decreases cough effectiveness and the ability to expel secretions.

Paralysis of the external obliques also influences expiration. Their normal function is to depress the ribs and compress the chest wall to assist with forceful expulsion of air.[39,40] With higher-level lesions this function becomes less efficient, with a further reduction in the patient's ability to cough and to expel secretions. These factors combine to make the patient with SCI particularly susceptible to retention of secretions, atelectasis, and pulmonary infections.[36]

Paralysis also results in the development of an altered breathing pattern.[38,42,43] This pattern (Fig. 23.4)[38] is characterized by some flattening of the upper chest wall, decreased chest wall expansion, and a dominant epigastric rise during inspiration. With relaxation of the diaphragm, a negative intrathoracic pressure gradient moves air into the lungs.[38,43] Over time, this breathing pattern will lead to permanent postural changes.

Two additional factors may further impair the respiratory status of the patient: additional trauma sustained at the time of injury, and premorbid respiratory problems.

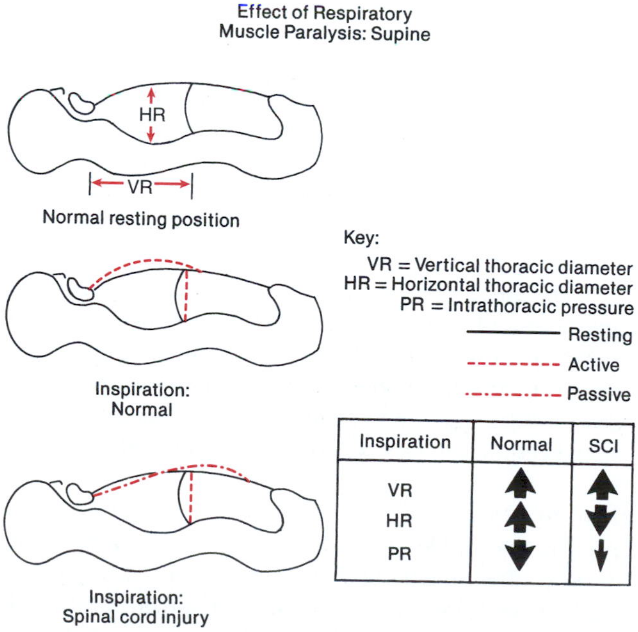

Figure 23.4 Effect of paralysis on thoracic volume and breathing pattern. (From Alvarez, SE, Peterson, M, and Lunsford, BR,[38, p 1738] with permission.)

Fractures (e.g., ribs, sternum, or extremities), lung contusions, or soft tissue damage will also compound respiratory problems. These secondary injuries are particularly problematic if long periods of immobility are required for healing or if pain inhibits full lung expansion. Premorbid respiratory problems, such as existing pulmonary disease, allergies, asthma, or a history of smoking, will further compromise respiratory function.

Spasticity

Spasticity results from release of intact reflex arcs from central nervous system control and is characterized by hypertonicity, hyperactive stretch reflexes, and clonus. It typically occurs below the level of lesion after spinal shock subsides. There is a gradual increase in spasticity during the first 6 months and a plateau is usually reached 1 year after injury. Spasticity is increased by multiple internal and external stimuli, including positional changes, cutaneous stimuli, environmental temperatures, tight clothing, bladder or kidney stones, fecal impactions, catheter blockage, urinary tract infections, decubitus ulcers, and emotional stress.[10,44]

Spasticity varies in the degree of severity. Patients with minimal to moderate involvement may learn to trigger the spasticity at appropriate times to assist in functional activities. However, strong spasticity interferes with many aspects of rehabilitation and can be a deterrent to independent function. In these situations, spasticity is often managed first through drug therapy. Drugs typically used include muscle relaxants and spasmolytic agents such as diazepam (Valium),[14] baclofen (Lioresal),[45] and dantrolene sodium (Dantrium).[33] Pharmacological management is usually not completely successful in alleviating spasticity, and its benefits must be weighed against potentially adverse side effects. In addition, patients often develop a tolerance to prolonged use of individual drugs.

Injected chemical agents also have been used to decrease spasticity. Generally, these are considered only if results obtained from pharmacological management are deemed inadequate. The two approaches used are *peripheral nerve blocks* and *intrathecal injections*. In nerve blocks, the chemical injection is used peripherally to selectively block transmission of the motor nerve to a spastic muscle and therefore to interrupt the intact reflex arc peripherally. With intrathecal injections, a central (within the spinal canal) chemical injection is used. These procedures provide a temporary reduction in spasticity and include (1) phenol peripheral nerve blocks and (2) phenol motor point blocks.[33]

Surgical approaches also have been used to combat spasticity in more severe cases. They range from relatively simple orthopedic procedures to complex neurosurgery. Orthopedic surgical procedures used include **myotomy**, a sectioning or release of a muscle; **neurectomy**, a partial or complete severance of a nerve; or *tenotomy,* a sectioning of a tendon that allows subsequent lengthening (e.g., heel cords). Each of these procedures decreases spasticity by altering the contraction potential of the muscle.[33,46]

A number of more radical neurosurgical interventions are used to eliminate extremely severe spasticity. These destructive approaches (neural tissue is damaged) result in permanent and profound alterations in spasticity. These procedures are useful when spasticity is at an intolerable level and prohibits or significantly limits functional activities. Examples of these interventions include severance of nerve roots (**rhizotomy**) or of spinal cord nerve fibers (**myelotomy**).

Bladder and Bowel Dysfunction

Bladder Dysfunction

The effects of bladder dysfunction following SCI pose a serious medical complication requiring consistent and long-term management. Urinary tract infections (UTIs) are among the most frequent medical complication during the initial medical-rehabilitation period. During the stage of spinal shock, the urinary bladder is flaccid. All muscle tone and bladder reflexes are absent.[47] Medical considerations during this period are focused on establishing an effective system of drainage and prevention of urinary retention and infection.

The spinal integration center for **micturition** is the conus medullaris. Primary reflex control originates from the sacral segments of S2, S3, and S4 within the conus medullaris. Following spinal shock, one of two types of bladder conditions will develop, depending on location of the lesion. Patients with lesions that occur within the spinal cord above the conus medullaris typically develop a *spastic* or reflex (automatic) bladder. Following a lesion of the conus medullaris or cauda equina, a *flaccid* or nonreflex (autonomous) bladder develops.[48]

A spastic or reflex (upper motor neuron [UMN]) bladder contracts and reflexively empties in response to a certain level of filling pressure. An UMN bladder occurs with SCI above the micturition reflex center (S2–S4), generally involving T11–T12 vertebral injury or above. The reflex arc is intact with this type of injury. Reflex emptying may be triggered by manual stimulation techniques such as stroking, kneading, or tapping the suprapubic region[46] or thigh, and lower abdominal stroking, pinching, or hair pulling.[49]

A flaccid or nonreflex (LMN lesion) bladder is essentially flaccid because there is no reflex action of the detrusor muscle. A LMN bladder occurs with SCI at the micturition reflex center (S2–S4), generally involving T12 vertebral injury or below. This type of bladder can be emptied by increasing intra-abdominal pressure using a Valsalva maneuver or by manually compressing the lower abdomen using the **Crede maneuver**. Characteristics of spastic and flaccid urinary dysfunction are presented in Table 23.3.[48]

Bladder Training Programs

The primary goal of bladder training programs is to allow the patient to be free of a catheter and to control bladder function. Because urinary incontinence has very strong psychosocial implications for the patient, a coordinated approach to this problem is particularly important. Knowledge of and participation in the bladder-training program is an important consideration for the physical therapist.

The bladder-training program most frequently used with a reflex bladder is *intermittent catheterization.* The purpose of this program is to establish reflex bladder emptying at regular and predictable intervals in response to a certain level of filling. Briefly stated, the program involves establishing a fluid intake pattern restricted to approximately 2000 ml/d. Fluid intake is monitored at 150 to 180 ml/h from morning until early evening. Intake is stopped late in the day to reduce the need for catheterization during the night. Initially, the patient is catheterized every 4 hours. Prior to catheterization, the patient attempts to void in combination with one or more of the manual stimulation techniques. The catheter is then inserted and residual volume drained. A record is maintained of voided and residual urine. As bladder emptying becomes more effective, residual volumes will decrease and time intervals between catheterizations can be expanded.[50]

A *timed voiding program* is another method of bladder training and is indicated for the autonomous or nonreflex bladder. This program involves first establishing the patient's pattern of incontinence. The residual urine volume is then checked to ensure that it is within safe limits. Once the pattern of incontinence has been established, it is compared with the patterns of intake. This information provides the basis for establishing a new intake and voiding schedule. The bladder gradually becomes accustomed or "trained" to empty at regular, predictable intervals. As incontinence decreases, the schedule is readjusted to expand the intervals between voiding. Fluid intake is avoided late in the day to decrease the risk of **nocturia.** Stimulation techniques are also incorporated into this type of training program.

It should be noted that not all bladder-training programs are successful. Some patients will require long-term use of either an external (condom) or indwelling catheter. For male patients, the condom catheter is preferred because it provides decreased risk of infection. For female patients, an indwelling catheter is currently the only option.

Bowel Dysfunction

As with the bladder, the neurogenic bowel conditions that develop after spinal shock subsides are of two types. In cord lesions above the conus medullaris there is a spastic or reflex bowel (UMN lesion), and in conus medullaris or cauda equina lesions a flaccid or nonreflex bowel (LMN lesion) develops.[49] Table 23.4[48] presents the characteristics

Table 23.3 Characteristics of Spastic and Flaccid Urinary Dysfunction

	Spastic (Automatic) Urinary Dysfunction (Upper Motor Neuron)	Flaccid (Autonomous) Urinary Dysfunction (Lower Motor Neuron)
Level of cord injury	Occurs above micturition reflex center (S2–S4) located within the conus medullaris.	Involves micturition reflex center (S2–S4) in the conus medullaris and/or sacral nerve roots in the cauda equina.
Level of innervation:		
1. Local	Stretch receptors in bladder wall and afferent neuron intact.	Same as UMN.
2. Spinal micturition reflex (S2–S4)	Micturition reflex intact. Parasympathetic innervation to detrusor muscle and bladder neck sphincter (internal) intact.	Micturition reflex center in conus medullaris and/or sacral nerve roots destroyed.
3. Sympathetic innervation cord segments T1 to T2	Reflexes may be intact depending on level of cord injury.	Same as for UMN.
4. Brain/higher centers • Motor	• Nerve pathways between brain and spinal micturition reflex center (S2-S4) interrupted; loss of inhibiting influences on spinal reflexes from higher centers.	• Loss of final common pathway for transmission of impulses between CNS and detrusor muscle and bladder sphincters (internal and external).
• Sensory	• Ascending sensory pathways interrupted; loss of sensation of bladder distention and urge to urinate.	• Same as for UMN.
Results of pathology	• Loss of UMN innervation. • Intact micturition reflexes. • Spastic bladder dysfunction.	• Loss of LMN innervation. • Loss of micturition reflexes. • Flaccid bladder dysfunction.
Prognosis for bladder control[a]	Bladder training is aimed at using micturition reflexes and "trigger" stimulus to establish planned reflex voiding.	Unable to establish reflex voiding, intermittent bladder catheterization may be best method for bladder management.

From Dolan,[48] p 629, with permission.

[a]Bladder training depends on many factors, such as level of injury, prior bladder habits, patient/family/caregiver motivation, and teamwork.

CNS = central nervous system; LMN = lower motor neuron; UMN = upper motor neuron.

of each type of bowel dysfunction together with treatment implications.

Bowel Programs

Typically, reflex bowel management requires use of suppositories and digital stimulation techniques to initiate defecation. Digital stimulation involves manual stretch of the anal sphincter, either with a lubricated gloved finger or an orthotic digital stimulator. This stretch stimulates peristalsis of the colon and evacuation of the rectum (mediated by S2, S3, and S4).[33] Nonreflex bowel management relies heavily on straining with available musculature and manual evacuation techniques.

The major goal of a bowel program for the patient with a SCI is establishment of a regular pattern of evacuation. This is achieved through multiple interventions, including diet, fluid intake, stool softeners, suppositories, digital stimulation, and manual evacuation.

As with bladder programs, bowel management is an emotionally laden issue and an extremely high priority for most patients. Lack of bowel control may negate other rehabilitation efforts because it will seriously limit the patient's involvement.

Sexual Dysfunction

"Sexual information is as vital and as normal a part of the rehabilitation process as is providing other information to enable the patient to better understand and adapt to his medical condition."[51] For many years, physical disability was assumed to depress or to eliminate sex drives. This erroneous attitude fostered considerable neglect of sexual function as a component of the rehabilitation process.[52] Today, sexual disturbances are recognized as a complex rehabilitation issue. Characterized by physiological dysfunction, and sensory and motor impairment, these disturbances are often accompanied by social and psychological distress.[53,54] Greater numbers of SCI care centers now include a sexual counselor as a component team member. This individual may be a physician or a psychologist with a specialty in this area or a nonphysician specialist trained in the treatment of sexual dysfunction.[53] Many rehabilitation

Table 23.4 Characteristics of Spastic and Flaccid Bowel Dysfunction

	Spastic Bowel Dysfunction (Upper Motor Neuron)	Flaccid Bowel Dysfunction (Lower Motor Neuron)
Level of cord injury	Occurs above defecation reflex center (S2–S4) located within the conus medullaris.	Involves defecation reflex center (S2–S4) in the conus medullaris and/or sacral nerve roots in the equina.
Level of vertebral injury	Involves T11 to T12 vertebra or above.	Involves T12 vertebra or below.
Levels of innervation:		
1. Local	Intrinsic (myenteric plexus) intact; responsible for weak peristaltic activity, which is not of sufficient strength by itself to produce a large bowel movement.	Same as for UMN.
2. Spinal defecation reflex center S2 to S4	Defecation reflex intact; parasympathetic tone to descending and sigmoid colon, rectum, and internal anal sphincter intact.	Defecation reflex center in the conus medullaris and/or sacral nerve roots destroyed.
3. Brain/higher centers • Motor	• Nerve pathways between brain and spinal defecation reflex center (S2–S4) interrupted: loss of inhibitory influences on spinal reflexes from higher centers.	• Loss of final common pathway for transmission of impulses between CNS and descending and sigmoid colon, rectum, and anal sphincters.
• Sensory	• Ascending sensory pathways interrupted: loss of sensation of fullness in bowel and urge to defecate.	• Same as for UMN.
Results of pathology	• Loss of UMN innervation. • Intact spinal defecation reflexes. • Spastic bowel dysfunction with spastic contraction of bowel and anal sphincters.	• Loss of LMN innervation. • Loss of spinal defecation reflexes. • Flaccid bowel dysfunction.
Prognosis for bowel control[a]	With intact defecation reflexes, bowel training is aimed at using these reflexes to evacuate the bowel. Bowel and anal sphincters respond to rectal/anal stimulation, enabling a planned bowel regimen, which empties the rectum and prevents incontinence. Prognosis is excellent for good bowel control.	With loss of spinal defecation reflex activity and LMN innervation, the bowel and anal sphincters are flaccid. They do not respond to planned rectal or anal stimulation. Arrival of feces in the rectum results in incontinence. Bowel training is deployed to evacuate stool from rectum. Presence of stool in rectum precipitates incontinence. Prognosis is favorable for bowel control providing a routine of regular bowel evacuation removes the stimulus for bowel emptying.
Bowel incontinence	Rarely occurs with good bowel management. Incontinence is due to spastic contraction. Diet is a significant factor in effective bowel management.	Occasionally occurs even with good bowel management, due to flaccid sphincters. As with spastic bowel dysfunction, diet is a significant factor in effective bowel management.
Bowel training program	Regularly scheduled evacuation, usually every other day.	Evacuation necessary on a daily basis to keep rectum clear of feces and prevent incontinence.
Use of medications including suppositories and laxatives	Responsive to a combination of laxatives (milk of magnesia), stool softener (dioctyl sodium sulfosuccinate [docusate, Colace]), and suppositories (Dulcolax).	Response to medications less effective than with spastic bowel dysfunction.
Digital stimulation	Used to initiate a planned reflex bowel evacuation.	Nonresponsive to digital stimulation, manual removal of stool from rectum may be required.

From Dolan,[48] p 627, with permission.

[a]Successful bowel training depends on many factors, such as level of injury, prior bowel habits, patient/family/caregiver motivation, teamwork.

CNS = central nervous system; LMN = lower motor neuron; UMN = upper motor neuron.

centers also offer structured programs to assist patients with sexual adjustment.[51,55] Although the format of these programs varies, common shared goals include (1) direct patient care including examination, prognosis, treatment, and counseling; (2) education of the patient and his or her partner; and (3) preparation of staff members to deal with sexual concerns.

Male Response

A gradually expanding body of literature is available on the male sexual response following SCI.[56–64] Sexual response is directly related to level and completeness of injury. As with bowel and bladder function, sexual capabilities are broadly divided between UMN (damage to the cord above the conus medullaris) and LMN lesions (damage to the conus medullaris or cauda equina).

Statistics related to sexual capacity provide important general information regarding anticipated function following a given type of injury. However, these statistics must be considered cautiously. Owing to the inherent methodological difficulties in collecting these types of data and the close relationship between sexual activity and self-image, some discrepancy may exist between reported and actual sexual function.[65]

Erectile Capacity

In a review of the literature on sexual response after SCI, Higgins[65] presented two consistent findings: (1) erectile capacity is greater in UMN lesions than in LMN lesions, and (2) erectile capacity is greater in incomplete lesions than in complete lesions.

There are two types of erections: reflexogenic and psychogenic. Reflexogenic erections occur in response to external physical stimulation of the genitals or perineum. An intact reflex arc is required (mediated through S2, S3, and S4). Psychogenic erections occur through cognitive activity such as erotic fantasy. They are mediated from the cerebral cortex either through the thoracolumbar or sacral cord centers.[66]

An early study by Comarr[67] examined erectile capability in 525 patients with UMN lesions. His findings indicated that 93 percent of the patients with complete lesions and 98 percent of those with incomplete lesions had reflexogenic erections. Data were also collected on 154 patients with LMN lesions. In the group with complete LMN lesions, 74 percent had no erections and 26 percent had erections only by psychogenic stimuli. With incomplete LMN lesions, 83 percent had erections, but all by psychogenic means. Drug intervention may also be used to improve erectile function in some patients.

Ejaculation

There is a higher incidence of ejaculation with (1) LMN lesions than with UMN lesions, (2) lower-level versus higher-level cord lesions, and (3) incomplete as compared with complete lesions.[65,67] Historically, relatively few patients with SCI were able to sire children. This low level of fertility was associated with impaired spermatogenesis and an inability to ejaculate.[66] However, vibratory stimulation may improve ejaculatory response and promote higher semen quality.[56–58] The semen samples produced are used for intrauterine inseminations.

Orgasm

Orgasm and ejaculation are two separate events. Orgasm is a cognitive, psychogenic event, whereas ejaculation is a physical occurrence. Relatively little information is available related to the effects of SCI on orgasm. This again relates to inherent difficulties in collecting such data. Higgins[65] also suggests that the few studies that have been done have demonstrated serious methodological flaws. He identifies the major problems in these studies as a lack of criteria for defining orgasm, considering ejaculation and orgasm as identical events, and a lack of reported data on how subjects achieved orgasm. Accurate data on the effects of SCI on male orgasm are not available.

Female Response

Relatively little literature exists addressing the impact of SCI on sexual function in women. This may be a function of women remaining capable of sexual intercourse following SCI. It also may be related to the fact that fertility is unaffected, or, perhaps, because of the proportionately lower number of female patients.[68] Trieschmann[52] also believes that this relates to the traditionally passive sexual roles ascribed to women. Historically, sexual functions of women following SCI have been considered relatively unimpaired and given comparatively little attention. However, there is a growing interest in female sexual response following SCI.[69–74]

Female sexual responses also follow a pattern related to location of lesion. In patients with UMN lesions, the reflex arc will remain intact. Therefore, components of sexual arousal (vaginal lubrication, engorgement of the labia, and clitoral erection) will occur through reflexogenic stimulation, but psychogenic response will be lost. Conversely, with LMN lesions, psychogenic responses will be preserved and reflex responses lost.

Menstruation

The menstrual cycle typically is interrupted for a period of 1 to 3 months following injury. After this time, normal menses return.

Fertility and Pregnancy

The potential for conception remains unimpaired. Pregnancy is possible under close medical supervision inasmuch as the patient is placed at high risk for impaired respiratory function. In addition, owing to impaired sensation the initiation of labor may not be perceived. Labor also may precipitate the onset of autonomic dysreflexia. Consequently, patients are frequently hospitalized for a period of time prior to the expected delivery date to monitor cervical dilation.[68] Although uterine contractions are hormonally controlled and not affected by paralysis, patients with an inability to bear down during the final stages of delivery[68] or who experience prolonged or difficult labor may be candidates for cesarean section.[23]

A major consideration for the physical therapist regarding sexual dysfunction is that a patient will often direct questions to the individuals with whom he or she feels most comfortable. It is not uncommon for such a discussion to arise during a physical therapy session. These questions or issues should be addressed openly and honestly. In addition, the therapist must anticipate and be prepared for these situations by (1) obtaining accurate information about the patient's physiological state and anticipated sexual function, and (2) having knowledge of referral options and support services available to the patient for appropriate examination and counseling.

Indirect Impairments and Complications

Individuals with SCI are at great risk for secondary complications during acute hospitalization and rehabilitation because of prolonged immobilization and the wide-ranging effects of the SCI on multiple body systems. The National Spinal Cord Injury Statistical Center reported that only 18.3 percent of patients did not experience a secondary medical complication. The three most common secondary complications were pneumonia (34.3 percent of patients) followed by **pressure ulcers** (33.5 percent) and **deep vein thrombosis** (15.0 percent).[2]

Respiratory Complications

Respiratory system diseases are the most common cause of death for individuals with SCI, with 71.2 percent of these cases being pneumonia.[2] Weak and/or paralyzed muscles of inspiration leads to reduced ventilation of the lungs. Inadequate or absent strength of coughing muscles makes it difficult to clear secretions. This inability to clear secretions leads to a build up of fluid in the lungs, which can result in atelectasis and pneumonia.

Pressure Sores

Pressure sores (decubitus ulcers) are ulcerations of soft tissue (skin or subcutaneous tissue) caused by unrelieved pressure and shearing forces. They are subject to infection, which can migrate to bone. Pressure sores are a serious medical complication, a major cause of delayed rehabilitation, and may even lead to death. Pressures sores are among the more frequent medical complications following SCI[75] and are an important factor in increasing duration and subsequently cost of hospital stay.

Impaired sensory function and the inability to make appropriate positional changes are the two most influential factors in the development of pressure sores. Other important factors are (1) loss of vasomotor control, which results in a lowering of tissue resistance to pressure; (2) spasticity, with resultant shearing forces between surfaces; (3) skin **maceration** from exposure to moisture (e.g., urine); (4) trauma, such as adhesive tape or sheet burns; (5) nutritional deficiencies (low serum protein and anemia will reduce tissue resistance to pressure); (6) poor general skin condition; and (7) secondary infections.[76,77] Another primary factor in the development of pressure sores is the intensity and duration of the pressure. The higher the intensity of pressure, the shorter the time required for anoxia of the skin and soft tissues to occur.

Pressure sores will develop over any bony prominence subjected to excessive pressure.[78,79] Among the more common sites of involvement are the sacrum, heels, trochanters, and ischium. Other areas susceptible to skin breakdown are the scapula, elbows, anterior iliac spines, knees, and malleoli.

By far the most important intervention for eliminating the potential development of pressure sores is prevention. This involves a coordinated approach, and it is a responsibility shared by each member of the rehabilitation team. Initially, the patient will be turned every 2 hours by the nursing staff on a 24-hour schedule. Skin condition should be monitored on a continual basis. If a reddened area occurs, the patient's position must be altered immediately to alleviate the pressure. As the rehabilitation program progresses, the patient gradually assumes responsibility for skin care. Preparation for assumption of this responsibility will include patient education about the potential risks of pressure sores, and instruction in skin inspection techniques and the use of pressure relief equipment and procedures.

Deep Vein Thrombosis

Deep venous thrombosis (DVT) results from development of a thrombus (abnormal blood clot) within a vessel. The occurrence of such a clot is a dangerous medical complication. It has the potential to break free of its attachment and float freely within the venous bloodstream. Such mobile clots are known as *emboli*. They are particularly likely to block pulmonary vessels (pulmonary emboli), which can result in death.[35]

The most important factor contributing to the development of DVT following SCI is loss of the normal "pumping" mechanism provided by active contraction of LE musculature. This slows the flow of blood, allowing higher concentrations of procoagulants (e.g., thrombin) to develop in localized areas. This in turn results in a predisposition to thrombus formation. Normally, these procoagulants are rapidly mixed with large quantities of blood and removed in the liver.[80] The risks of DVT are heightened with age and prolonged pressure (e.g., extended contact against the bed or supporting surface). Prolonged pressure can damage the vessel wall and precipitate initiation of the clotting process. In addition, loss of vasomotor tone and immobility further enhance the potential development of DVT. Other contributing factors include immobility leading to venous stasis, sepsis, hypercoagulability, and trauma.[47,81,82] DVT most frequently occurs within the first 2 months following injury.

The formation of a thrombus results in inflammation (thrombophlebitis) with characteristic clinical features of local swelling, erythema, and heat. These signs are similar to those of early ectopic bone formation and long bone fractures.[83] Differential diagnosis is made on the basis of venous flow studies and venography.[83,84]

The clinical manifestations of DVT have been estimated to occur in approximately 15 percent of patients with SCI.[84] However, one study reported an incidence as high as 40 percent.[85] Studies using iodine-125 fibrinogen scanning have yielded a much higher incidence. Fibrinogen scanning is sensitive to fibrin deposits and can detect the presence of an active thrombotic process in the absence of clinical manifestations.[86] Using this technique, incidence of DVT in patients with acute SCI has been reported at 90 percent in one group of 10 patients[87] and 100 percent in a group of 14 patients.[86]

Management of this secondary complication focuses on prevention. Prophylactic anticoagulant drug therapy is typically initiated following the acute onset of injury and routinely continued for 2 to 3 months[85,88,89] or for up to 6 months for patients at high risk.[90] Other preventative measures include (1) a turning program designed to avoid pressure over large vessels, (2) passive range of motion (PROM) exercises, (3) elastic support stockings,[47] and (4) positioning of the LEs to facilitate venous return.

Contractures

Contractures develop secondary to prolonged shortening of structures across and around a joint, resulting in limitation in motion. Contractures initially produce alterations in muscle tissue but rapidly progress to involve capsular and pericapsular changes. Once the tissue changes have occurred, the process is irreversible. A combination of factors places the patient with SCI at particularly high risk for developing joint contractures. Lack of active muscle function eliminates the normal reciprocal stretching of a muscle group and surrounding structures as the opposing muscle contracts.[83] Spasticity often results in prolonged unopposed muscle shortening in a static position. Flaccidity may result in gravitational forces maintaining a relatively consistent joint position. In addition, faulty positioning, heterotopic ossification, edema, and imbalances in muscle pull (either active or spastic) contribute to the specific direction and location of contracture development.

Contractures are strongly influenced by the existing pattern of spasticity and the positioning methods used. The hip joint is particularly prone to flexion deformities and typically includes components of internal rotation and adduction. The shoulder may develop tightness in flexion or extension (depending on early positioning). Both patterns at the shoulder are associated with internal rotation and adduction. All joints of the body are at risk for contractures, including the elbows, wrist and fingers, knees, ankles, and toes.

The most important management consideration related to the potential development of contractures is prevention. A consistent and concurrent program of ROM exercises, positioning, and, if appropriate, splinting effectively maintains joint motion.

Heterotopic (Ectopic) Ossification

Heterotopic ossification is osteogenesis in soft tissues below the level of the lesion.[83,91,92] The etiology of this abnormal bone growth is unknown. However, multiple theories have been proposed, including tissue hypoxia secondary to circulatory stasis,[93] abnormal calcium metabolism, local pressure, and microtrauma related to overly aggressive range of motion (ROM) exercises.[94]

Heterotopic ossification is always extra-articular and extracapsular.[95] It may develop in tendons, connective tissue between muscle, aponeurotic tissue, or the peripheral aspects of muscle.[83,94,95] It must be differentiated from myositis ossificans, which results from injury to a muscle and is characterized by bony deposits within muscle tissue. No relationships have been found between the development of heterotopic bone formation and level of injury, amount of exercise, or degree of spasticity or flaccidity.[93,96]

Heterotopic ossification typically occurs adjacent to large joints, with the hips and knees most commonly involved.[91] Other joints that have demonstrated involvement include the elbows,[83] shoulders, and spine.[91] Early symptoms of heterotopic ossification resemble those of thrombophlebitis, including swelling, decreased ROM, erythema, and local warmth near a joint.[97] Early onset is also characterized by elevated serum alkaline phosphatase levels and negative radiographic findings.[98] During later clinical stages, soft tissue swelling subsides and radiographic findings are positive.[98]

For many patients the development of heterotopic ossification will pose no significant functional limitations. However, a serious complication affecting 20 percent of patients is joint ankylosis, with the hip most commonly affected.[83]

Management of ectopic bone formation utilizes several approaches, including pharmacological therapy, physical therapy, and, with severe functional limitations, surgery. Pharmacological therapy (diphosphates) has been used to inhibit the formation of calcium phosphate and to prevent ectopic bone formation.[83] These agents, however, have no effect on mature ectopic bone. Physical therapy is important in maintaining ROM and preventing deformity. Early research discouraged the use of ROM, indicating that the exercise increased ectopic bone formation.[95] However, other studies have shown no increase in the formation of bone deposition with ROM exercises.[91,93,96] A logical approach to maintaining functional ROM appears to be a combination of pharmacological therapy with regular exercises during the early formation stages of ectopic development. Finally, surgery is used when extreme limitations in function impede rehabilitation. This generally involves resection of the ectopic bone.[83]

Pain

Pain is a common occurrence following SCI.[99,100] Several classification systems have been developed to describe this pain. These classifications are related to the source and type of pain as well as to the length of time since onset (acute vs chronic pain).

Traumatic Pain

Initially, pain experienced following acute traumatic injury is related to the extent and type of trauma sustained as well as to the structures involved. Pain may arise from fractures, ligamentous or soft tissue damage, muscle spasm, or early surgical interventions. This acute pain generally subsides with healing in 1 to 3 months. Typical management includes immobilization and use of analgesics.[33] Transcutaneous electrical nerve stimulation (TENS) also has been found effective in reducing this type of acute, postinjury pain.[101]

Nerve Root Pain

Pain or irritation may arise from damage to nerve roots at or near the site of cord damage. Pain can be caused by acute compression or tearing of the nerve roots,[102] or it may arise secondary to spinal instability, periradicular scar tissue and adhesion formation, or improper reduction.[33] Nerve root pain is often described as sharp, stabbing, burning, or shooting and typically follows a dermatomal pattern. It is most common in cauda equina injuries, in which a high distribution of nerve roots is present.[99]

Management of nerve root pain is a challenging clinical problem. Multiple approaches have been suggested, with varying degrees of success. Conservative management involves pharmacological therapy[102] and TENS. Surgical interventions for more severe, debilitating pain include nerve root sections (neurectomy) and posterior rhizotomies.[33]

Spinal Cord Dysesthesias

It is not uncommon for patients to experience many peculiar, often painful sensations *(dysesthesias SCI)* below the level of the lesion. The sensations tend to be diffuse and usually do not follow a dermatome distribution.[33] They occur in body parts that otherwise lack sensation and are often described by the patient as burning, numbness, pins and needles, or tingling feelings. Occasionally, they involve abnormal proprioceptive sensations, causing the individual to perceive a limb in other than its actual position. Dysesthesias have been described as "phantom" pains or sensations similar to those experienced following amputation.[103] The exact etiology of this pain is not well understood. However, it is theorized to be related to scarring at the distal end of the severed spinal cord.[33] These sensations are present following the acute onset of injury and typically subside over time. However, they tend to be more persistent and long-standing in cauda equina lesions.

Dysesthesia pain is particularly resistant to treatment. It is important that the complaints be acknowledged as real and that the patient be educated as to the legitimacy of the pain. Gentle handling of the patient's limbs and careful positioning frequently make the pain more tolerable. Pharmacological management using carbamazepine (Tegretol) and phenytoin (Dilantin) has been found effective in reducing dysesthesia pain.[102] Narcotic analgesics are usually discouraged because of the danger of addiction.

Musculoskeletal Pain

Pain also may occur above the level of lesion and frequently involves the shoulder joint.[104,105] Pathological changes at the shoulder often are related to faulty positioning and/or inadequate ROM, resulting in tightening of the joint capsule and surrounding soft tissue structures. In addition, the shoulder muscles are excessively challenged in their role as tonic stabilizers to substitute for lack of trunk innervation. This situation may be complicated by muscle imbalances around the joint, inflammation, or upper extremity (UE) fractures sustained at the time of injury.

Prevention of secondary shoulder involvement is critical, considering the importance of this joint in self-care and functional activities. Shoulder pain and limitation of ROM will significantly delay the rehabilitation process. The most important preventative measures include a regular program of ROM exercise and a positioning program designed to facilitate full motion at the shoulder.

Osteoporosis and Renal Calculi

Changes in calcium metabolism following SCI lead to *osteoporosis* below the level of the lesion and development of renal calculi.[106] Normally, there is a dynamic balance between the bone resorption activity of osteoclasts and the role of osteoblasts in laying down new bone. Following SCI, there is a net loss of bone mass because the rate of resorption is greater than the rate of new bone formation.[83] Consequently, there is a greater susceptibility to fracture. As a result of this resorption there are large concentrations of calcium present in the urinary system (hypercalciuria), creating a predisposition to stone formation.

The highest incidence of bone mass changes and hypercalciuria occurs during the first 6 months following SCI.[107,108] After this period, changes gradually diminish and assume a constant low-normal level after approximately 1 year.[108,109]

The exact mechanism causing bone mass changes following paralysis is not clearly understood. However, immobility and lack of stress placed on the skeletal system through dynamic weightbearing activities are well accepted as major contributing factors.

Treatment consists primarily of dietary management and early and continuing weightbearing activities (e.g., tilt-table). Dietary considerations include calcium-restricted foods and vigorous hydration (especially increased amounts of water). Excessive intake of foods such as milk, ice cream, and other dairy products high in calcium is generally discouraged. High-protein foods such as meats, whole-grain products, eggs, and vitamin-rich foods such as cranberries or dried fruit (e.g., prunes or plums) are encouraged. In addition, the risk of calculi formation will be reduced by prevention of urinary tract infections and careful maintenance of bladder drainage to prevent urinary stasis.[110]

Prognosis

One of the most common questions that patients and families have after a SCI is how much recovery of motor function will occur. The potential for recovery from SCI is directly related to the extent of damage to the spinal cord and/or nerve roots. Donovan and Bedbrook[110] have identified three primary influences on potential for recovery: (1) the degree of pathological changes imposed by the trauma, (2) the precautions taken to prevent further damage during rescue, and (3) prevention of additional compromise of neural tissue from hypoxia and hypotension during acute management.

Formulation of a prognosis is initiated after spinal shock has subsided and is guided by whether or not the lesion is complete. Following spinal shock, a lesion is generally considered complete in the absence of any sensory or motor function below the level of cord damage, with no anal sensation or motor function present. Early appearance of reflex activity in these instances is considered a poor prognostic indicator.[111] With complete lesions, no motor improvement is expected other than that which may occur from nerve root return.

An incomplete lesion indicated by motor function below the neurological level of the lesion with sensation and/or motor anal function intact are good prognostic indicators of a likelihood of significant recovery of motor function.[112–114] It is important to note that with most incomplete lesions improvement begins almost immediately following cessation of spinal shock. Many patients will have some progressive improvement of muscle return. It may be minimal or, less frequently, dramatic and usually becomes apparent during the first several months following injury. With a consistent progression of returning function (daily, weekly, or even monthly) further recovery can be expected at the same rate, or a slightly slower rate. Meticulous and frequent examination of sensory and motor functions during this period will provide important information about the progression of recovery.

In time, the rate of recovery will decrease, and a plateau will be reached. When the plateau is reached and no new muscle activity is observed for several weeks or months, no additional recovery can be expected.

The remainder of this chapter is divided into the acute medical management and active rehabilitation stages. The section on acute management addresses treatment interventions from the onset of injury until the fracture site is stable and upright activities can be initiated. The rehabilitation phase includes suggested treatment activities following initial orientation to the vertical position through preparation for discharge from the rehabilitation facility.

Acute Medical Management Phase

Emergency Care

Ideally, management of SCI begins at the location of the accident. Techniques used in moving and managing the patient immediately following the trauma can influence prognosis significantly. Rescue personnel must be adept at questioning and examining for signs of SCI before moving the individual. When a SCI is suspected, efforts should be made to avoid both active and passive movements of the spine.[110] Movement of the spine can be averted by strapping the patient to a spinal backboard or a full-body adjustable backboard, use of a supporting cervical collar, and assistance from multiple personnel in moving the patient to safety. These measures will assist in maintaining the spine in a neutral, anatomical position and will prevent further neurological damage.[110] Administration of high doses of methylprednisolone within 3 to 8 hours of injury for 24 to 48 hours can modestly improve motor[115,116] and functional recovery.[117]

On arrival at the emergency room, initial attention is focused on stabilizing the patient medically. A complete neurological examination is performed. Radiographic and imaging[118] studies, assist in determining the extent of damage and plans for management. Attention is directed toward preventing progression of neurological impairment by restoration of vertebral alignment and early immobilization of the fracture site. Cardiac, hemodynamic, and respiratory status are closely monitored.[119] A urinary catheter typically is inserted, and secondary injuries are addressed. Unstable spinal fractures require early reduction and fixation. Symptoms of instability may include pain and tenderness at the fracture site, radiating pain, increasing neurological signs, and decreasing motor function.

Fracture Stabilization

Reduction and immobilization of spinal injuries can be achieved via conservative or operative methods. There is no clear evidence supporting the use of closed reduction over open reduction or vice versa.[1–3] Animal studies have demonstrated improved neurological recovery after early decompression; however, exact time frames for surgical intervention in humans has not been determined.[1,4] Closed reduction can be achieved with the use of traction devices. Traction can be applied by the use of tongs attached to the outer skull (Fig. 23.5) or by a halo device (Figs. 23.6 and 23.7).

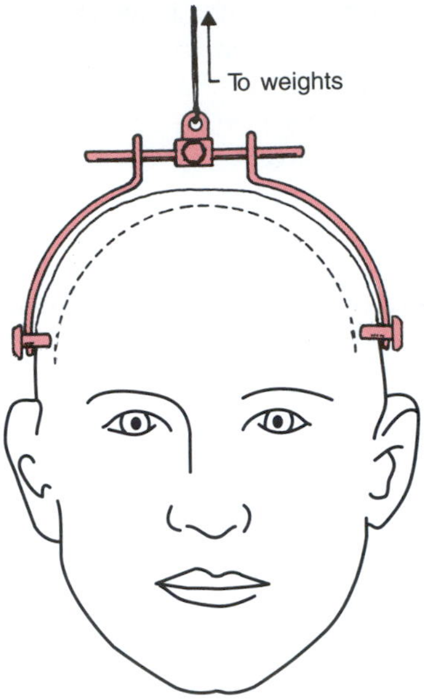

Figure 23.5 Cervical tongs. (Adapted from Judd, E [ed]: Nursing Care of the Adult. FA Davis, Philadelphia, 1983, p 482, with permission.)

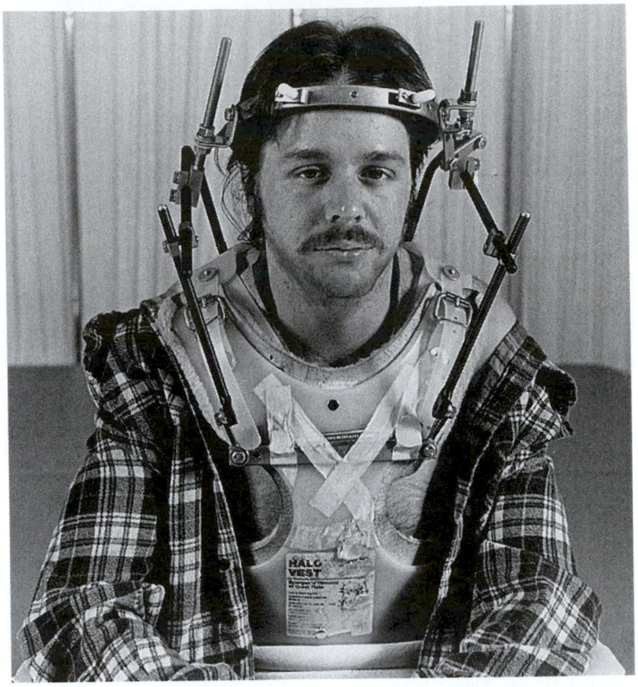

Figure 23.6 Halo device on an individual with a cervical cord lesion.

Surgical decompression and stabilization may be indicated in patients with deteriorating neurological status, instability following closed reduction, unstable fracture site, and bilateral facet dislocation.[4,5,120,121] Operative treatment usually consists of an anterior or posterior arthrodesis with plate or rod fixation. Surgical intervention may occur as early as within the first 24 hours postinjury. Prolonged bed rest in traction is only recommended when other treatment options are not available.[2]

Immobilization

Following reduction of the fracture site, through either conservative or surgical means, the spine is immobilized for a period of time through the use of tongs, halo devices, turning frames, beds, and orthoses to allow for healing.

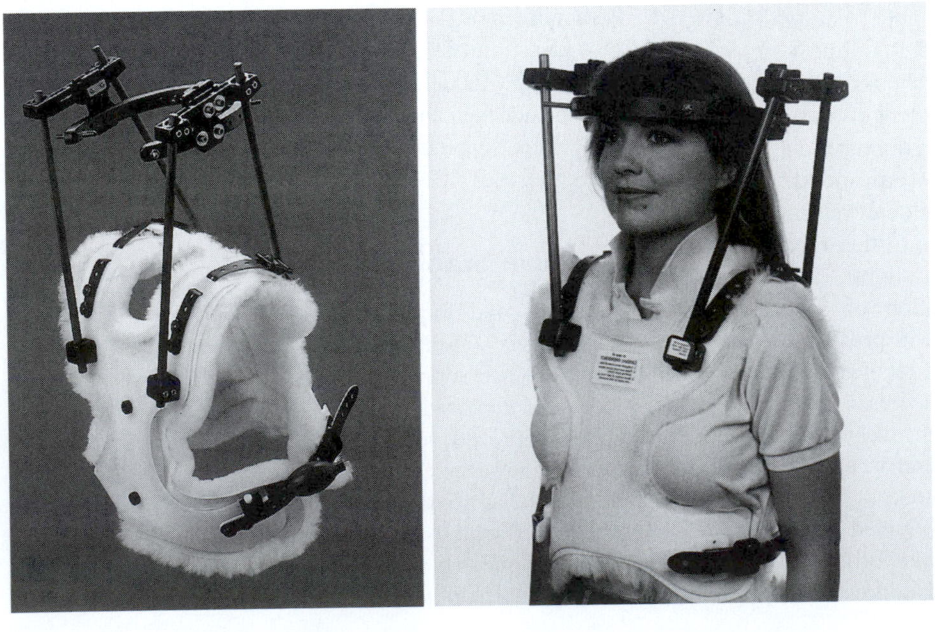

Figure 23.7 The Progress Mankind Technology (PMT) graphite halo system that is MRI compatible. (Courtesy PMT Corp, Chanhassen, MN 55317.)

Tongs

Several types of tongs are available (e.g., Crutchfield, Barton, Vinke, Gardner-Wells), each with a slightly different design. The tongs or calipers are inserted laterally on the outer table of the skull (see Fig. 23.5). Traction is accomplished by attachment of a traction rope to the skull fixation. With the patient in a supine position, this rope is threaded through a pulley or traction collar with weights attached distally. The weights hang freely without touching the floor. Tongs are used primarily as a temporary mode of skeletal traction with replacement using a halo device.

Halo Devices

Halo devices are used commonly to immobilize cervical fractures. These traction devices (see Figs. 23.6 and 23.7) consist of a halo ring with four steel screws that attach directly to the outer skull. The halo is attached to a body jacket or vest by four vertical steel posts. Owing to their structural configuration, these devices are contraindicated with severe respiratory involvement.

Halo devices have several important advantages. They assist in reducing the secondary complications of prolonged bed rest, permit earlier progression to upright activities, allow earlier involvement in a rehabilitation program, and reduce the length and cost of hospital stay.[122] In addition, for patients without neurological involvement, discharge from the hospital may occur days after application if the halo device. These patients are then followed on an outpatient basis.[123]

Skeletal traction devices are left in place until radiographic findings indicate stability has been achieved (approximately 12 weeks). Following removal, a cervical orthosis is applied during a transitional period (approximately 4 to 6 weeks) until unrestricted movement is allowed. The sterno–occipital–mandibular immobilizer (SOMI) cervical orthosis, hard collar (Fig. 23.8), or custom-made plastic collars are frequently used during the transition period, with progression to a soft foam collar prior to resuming unsupported movement.

Turning Frames and Beds

Several types of frames and beds are used for immobilization during the acute phase of care. Each has different design characteristics and functions. Among the most commonly used turning frame is the Stryker frame. It consists of an anterior and posterior frame attached to a turning base (Fig. 23.9). In turning from a supine position, the anterior frame is placed on top of the patient. A circular ring clamps in place to secure the two frames during turning. Safety straps provide additional security. Rotation to the prone position is accomplished by manually turning the two frames as a unit. The uppermost frame is then removed. Return to the supine position is accomplished in the same manner. The primary benefit of these devices is that they allow positional changes while maintaining anatomical alignment of the spine. Turning can be accomplished without interruption of the cervical traction. A disadvantage of turning frames is that positioning is limited to prone and supine. This is particularly problematic for patients with a low tolerance for the prone position (e.g., cardiac or respiratory involvement). In addition, these frames cannot accommodate obese

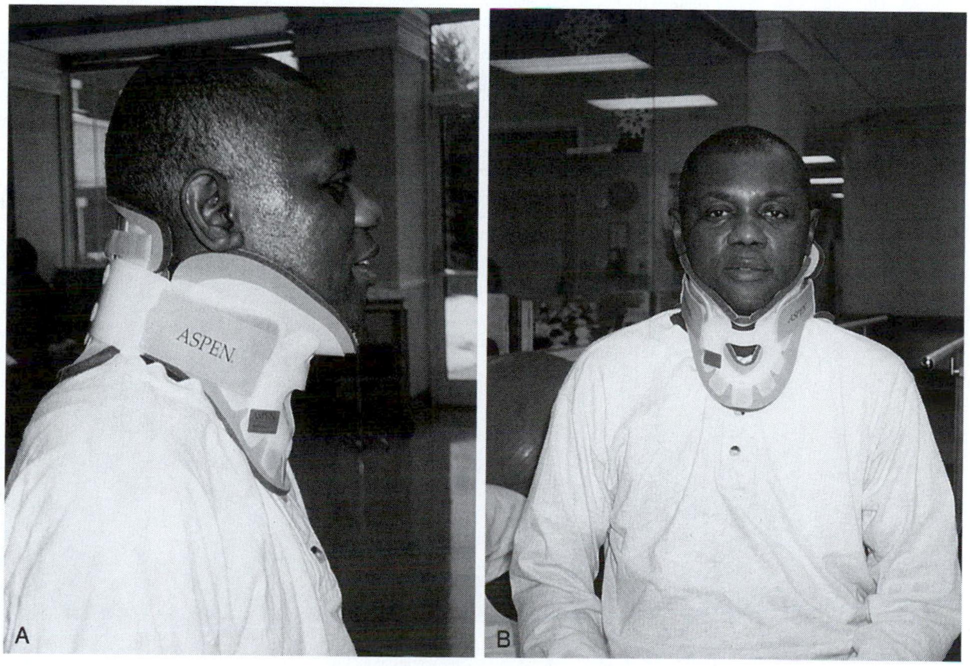

Figure 23.8 Lateral (*A*) and anterior (*B*) views of the hard collar.

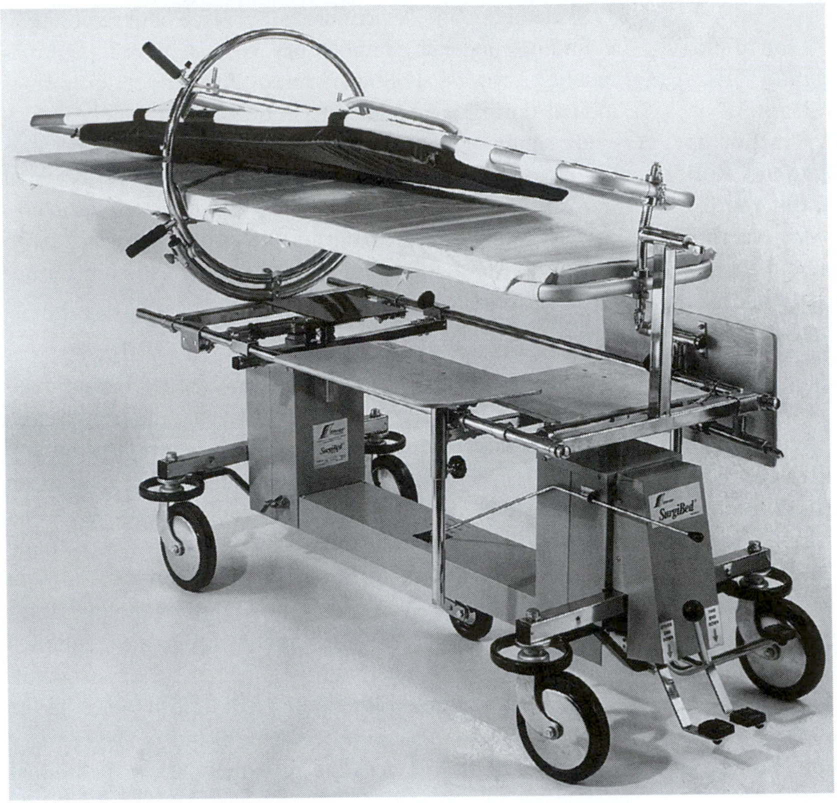

Figure 23.9 Stryker turning frame (Courtesy of Stryker Corp, Kalamazoo, MI 49048.)

patients and are unsuitable for unconscious patients. Although once the norm for managing spinal fractures, frames are now used primarily as a temporary method of immobilization.[124]

Finally, in some facilities standard hospital beds are used. Any of a variety of special pressure-relieving mattresses (gel, sand, water, air, or foam) are used for pressure relief. Positional changes are accomplished by log rolling.

Thoracolumbosacral Orthoses

A thoracolumbosacral orthosis (TLSO) is commonly used to immobilize the spine in patients with thoracic or lumbar injuries. The plastic body jacket (Fig. 23.10) functions to immobilize the spine and allow earlier involvement in a rehabilitation program. Body jackets are typically bivalved to allow for removal during bathing and skin inspection.

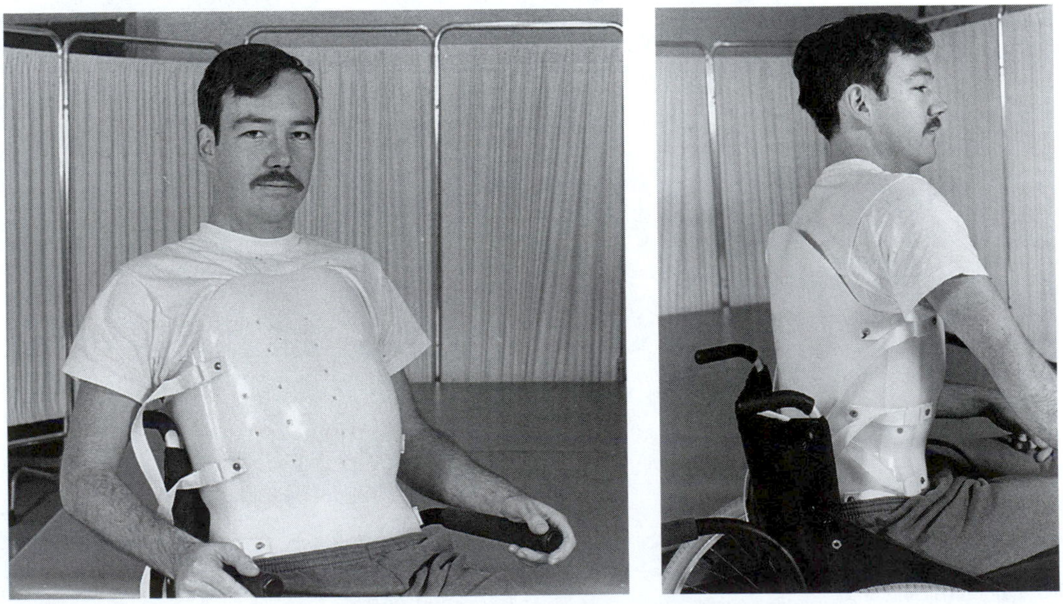

A B

Figure 23.10 Anterior and lateral view of bivalved, plastic body jacket.

Physical Therapy Examination

During the acute medical management phase a general physical therapy examination of the patient is indicated, including respiratory function, skin condition, sensation, tone, muscle strength, and functional mobility. Results will assist the therapist in determining the lesion level, identifying general functional expectations, and formulating appropriate treatment goals. As noted earlier, the lesion level is considered to be the lowest segmental level in which normal muscle strength and sensation are present bilaterally. During the acute stage, spinal instability often precludes a thorough physical therapy examination. However, gross screening will provide important initial data until the patient is medically stable and cleared for further activity.

Useful tools for documenting results of the examination are the ISNCSCI (Fig. 23.2) and the ASIA Impairment Scale (Table 23.1) developed by ASIA. These tools improve standardization of the examination process for patients with SCI and were described earlier.

Respiratory Examination

Details of respiratory status and function are essential. The areas listed below should be addressed.

Function of Respiratory Muscles

Muscle strength and tone of the diaphragm, abdominals, and intercostals should be examined; respiratory rate should be noted.

Chest Expansion

Circumferential measurements should be taken at the level of the axilla and xiphoid process using a cloth tape measure. Chest expansion is recorded as the difference in measurement between maximum exhalation and maximum inhalation. Normally, chest expansion is approximately 2.5 to 3 in. (6.4 to 7.6 cm) at the xiphoid process.[41]

Breathing Pattern

A determination should be made of muscles that are functioning and their contributions to respiration. This may be accomplished by manual palpation over the chest and abdominal region and by observation. Particular attention should be directed toward use of accessory neck muscles and alteration in breathing pattern when the patient is talking or moving.[38]

Cough

Coughing allows the patient to remove secretions. Ineffective cough function will necessitate suctioning to avoid pulmonary complications. Alvarez et al[38] have defined three cough classifications: (1) *functional,* strong enough to clear secretions; (2) *weak functional,* adequate force to clear upper respiratory tract secretions in small quantities; assistance is required to clear mucus secondary to infection; and (3) *nonfunctional,* unable to produce any cough force.

Vital Capacity

Initial measures may be taken with a hand-held spirometer.[38] Vital capacity measures also can be used as a baseline for defining respiratory muscle weakness.

Integument

During the acute phase, meticulous and regular skin inspection is a shared responsibility of the patient and the entire medical/rehabilitative team. As management progresses into the active rehabilitation phase, the patient will gradually assume greater responsibility for this activity. Patient education related to skin care is crucial and should be initiated early. Frequent position changes and skin inspection may be viewed by the patient as bothersome or distracting from sleep if there is not adequate awareness of the importance and purpose of these activities. Skin inspection combines both visual observation and palpation.[76] The patient's entire body should be observed regularly with particular attention to areas most susceptible to pressure (Table 23.5). Palpation is useful for identifying skin temperature changes that may be indicative of a hyperemic reaction. This is particularly important in examining individuals with dark skin, because early skin responses to pressure

Table 23.5 Areas Most Susceptible to Pressure in Recumbent Positions

Supine	Prone	Sidelying
• Occiput • Scapulae • Vertebrae • Elbows • Sacrum • Coccyx • Heels	• Ears (head rotated) • Shoulders (anterior aspect) • Illiac crest • Male genital region Patella • Dorsum of feet	• Ears • Shoulders (lateral aspect) • Greater trochanter • Head of fibula • Knees (medial aspect from contact between knees) • Lateral malleolus Medial malleolus (contact between malleoli)

may not be readily apparent. Skin reactions to excess pressure include redness, local warmth, local edema, and small open or cracked skin areas. Careful attention should be directed toward accidental skin abrasions or bruises, which increase the potential for skin breakdown.[76] If the patient is wearing a halo, vest, or other orthotic device, contact points between the body and the appliance must also be inspected.

Sensation

A detailed examination of superficial and deep sensations should be completed (see Chapter 5). Particular emphasis should be placed on pin prick and light touch responses (typically used to identify sensory level of lesion) as well as proprioceptive responses. As noted previously, the sensory level of injury may not correspond to the motor level of injury.

Tone and Deep Tendon Reflexes

Muscle tone should be examined (see Chapter 8) with reference to quality, muscle groups involved, and factors that appear to increase or to decrease tone. An examination of deep tendon reflexes is indicated. Level of the lesion will influence the specific tendons selected for testing. The deep tendon reflexes most commonly examined and their levels of innervation are the biceps (C5), extensor carpi radialus longus (C6), triceps (C7), quadriceps (L3), and gastrocnemius (S1).[68]

Manual Muscle Test and Range of Motion

In addition to testing the key muscles identified in the ISNCSCI (see Fig. 23.2), other muscle groups should be tested throughout the myotomes that have intact innervation. For example, if the C5 myotome is intact as indicated by a normal strength in the biceps then the strength of other muscles such as the deltoids and supraspinatus that are innervated by the C5 nerve root should also be determined. Standard techniques should be used for the manual muscle test (MMT)[6] and ROM.[125] Because of limited mobility and surgical precautions during the acute phase, deviations from standard positioning may be necessary and should be carefully documented. In cases of spinal instability, extreme caution should be used when performing gross muscle and ROM tests, because movements of this sort may place undue stress on the fracture site. Discretion should be used in applying resistance around the shoulders in tetraplegia and around the lower trunk and hips in paraplegia.

Functional Status

A detailed, accurate, and specific determination of functional skills is usually delayed until the active rehabilitation stage when the patient is medically stable and cleared for activity. An initial screening of functional ability may be done during the early acute stage, but the therapist must be aware of any contraindications or precautions to movement necessitated by healing and potentially unstable fracture sites.

Physical Therapy Intervention

During the acute phase, emphasis is placed on respiratory management, prevention of indirect impairments and complications, maintaining ROM, and facilitating active movement in available musculature. Pending orthopedic clearance, limited strengthening activities also may be initiated during this early phase.

Respiratory Management

Respiratory care will vary according to the level of injury and individual respiratory status. Primary goals of management include improved ventilation, increased effectiveness of cough, and prevention of chest tightness and ineffective substitute breathing patterns.[38] Depending on the individual patient the following treatment activities may be appropriate:

Deep-Breathing Exercises

Diaphragmatic breathing should be encouraged. To facilitate diaphragmatic movement and increase vital capacity, the therapist can apply light pressure during both inspiration and expiration. Manual contacts can be made just below the sternum. This will assist the patient to concentrate on deep breathing patterns even in the absence of thoracic and abdominal sensation. To facilitate expiration, manual contacts are made over the thorax with the hands spread wide. This creates a compressive force on the thorax, resulting in a more forceful expiration followed by a more efficient inspiration.[46] Patients immobilized in traction devices or limited to recumbent positions may benefit from use of a mirror to provide visual feedback during these activities. Inflation hold and incentive spirometry are also useful adjuncts to deep breathing exercises.[126]

Glossopharyngeal Breathing

This activity is often appropriate for patients with high-level cervical lesions. The technique utilizes accessory muscles of respiration to improve vital capacity. The patient is instructed to inspire small amounts of air repeatedly, using a "sipping" or "gulping" pattern, thus utilizing available facial and neck muscles. By using this technique, enough air is gradually inspired to improve chest expansion despite paralysis of the primary muscles of respiration.

Airshift Maneuver

This technique provides the patient with an independent method of chest expansion. Closing the glottis after a maximum inhalation, relaxing the diaphragm, and allowing air to shift from the lower to upper thorax. Airshifts can increase chest expansion by 0.5 to 2 in. (1.3 to 5.1 cm).

Strengthening Exercises

Progressive resistive exercises can be used to strengthen the diaphragm. This can be accomplished by manual contacts over the epigastric area below the xiphoid process or by use of weights. Strengthening exercises for innervated abdominal and accessory musculature are also indicated.

Assisted Coughing

To assist with coughing and movement of secretions, manual contacts are placed over the epigastric area. The therapist pushes quickly in an inward and upward direction as the patient attempts to cough.[127]

Abdominal Support

An abdominal corset or binder is indicated for patients whose abdomen protrudes, allowing the diaphragm to "sag" into a poor position for function. The corset will support the abdominal contents and improve the resting position of the diaphragm. In addition, abdominal supports provide the secondary benefits of maintaining intrathoracic pressure and decreasing postural hypotension.

Stretching

Mobility and compliance of the thoracic wall can be facilitated by manual stretching of pectoral and other chest wall muscles.

In addition to these respiratory approaches, intermittent positive pressure breathing may be utilized to assist in maintenance of lung compliance. Modified postural drainage and percussion techniques also may be indicated to assist with mobilizing and eliminating secretions.

Range of Motion and Positioning

While the patient is immobilized in bed or on a turning frame, full ROM exercises should be completed daily except in those areas that are contraindicated or require selective stretching. With paraplegia, motion of the trunk and some motions of the hip are contraindicated. Generally, straight leg raising more than 60° and hip flexion beyond 90° (during combined hip and knee flexion) should be avoided. This will avert strain on the lower thoracic and lumbar spine. If possible, ROM exercises should be completed in both the prone and supine positions (prone positioning may be contraindicated for some patients owing to fracture and/or respiratory compromise in this position). In the prone position, attention should be directed toward shoulder and hip extension and knee flexion. With tetraplegia, motion of the head and neck is contraindicated pending orthopedic clearance. Stretching of the shoulders should be avoided during the acute period; however, the patient should be positioned out of the usual position of comfort, in which there is internal rotation, adduction and extension of the shoulders, elbow flexion, forearm pronation, and wrist flexion. Full ROM exercises are generally included for both LEs.

Patients with SCIs do not require full ROM in all joints. Some joints benefit from allowing tightness to develop in certain muscles to enhance function. For example, with tetraplegia, tightness of the lower trunk musculature will improve sitting posture by increasing trunk stability; tightness in the long finger flexors will provide an improved tenodesis grasp. Conversely, some muscles require a fully lengthened range. After the acute phase, the hamstrings will require stretching to achieve a straight leg raise of approximately 100°. This ROM is required for many functional activities such as sitting, transfers, and LE dressing. Care should be taken not to overstretch the hamstring muscles as some tightness in this muscle group provides passive pelvic stabilization in sitting. This process of understretching some muscles and full stretching of others to improve function is referred to as *selective stretching*.

Positioning splints for the wrist, hands, and fingers are an important early consideration. Alignment of the fingers, thumb, and wrist must be maintained for functional activities or future dynamic splinting. For high-level lesions the wrist is positioned in neutral, the web space is maintained, and the fingers are flexed.[128] If the wrist extensors are functional (fair muscle grade), a C-bar or short-opponens splint is usually sufficient.

Ankle boots or splints are indicated to maintain alignment and to prevent heel cord tightness and pressure sores. Ankle boots designed to suspend the heel in space and distribute pressure evenly along the lower leg are available commercially (Fig. 23.11). Sandbags or towel rolls also may be required to maintain a position of neutral hip rotation.

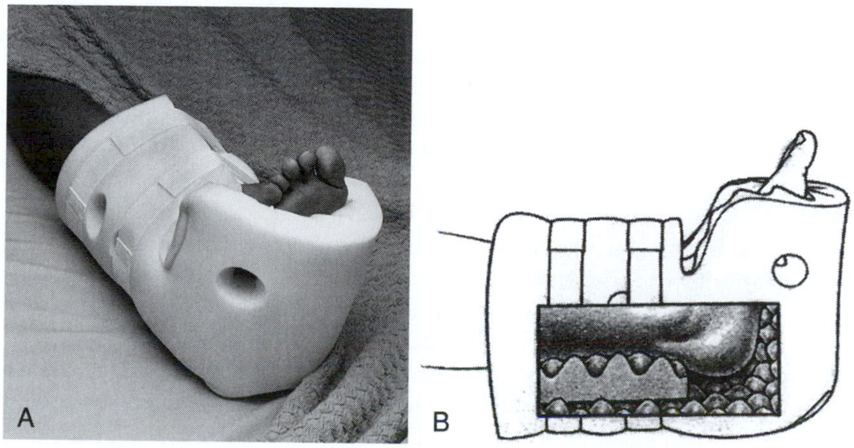

Figure 23.11 Ankle boot designed to distribute pressure along lower leg (*A*) and suspend the heel in space (*B*). (Courtesy of DM Systems, Inc, Evanston, IL 60201.)

Following orthopedic clearance, the patient typically is placed on a schedule to increase tolerance to the prone position. For patients wearing a halo device, one or two pillows under the chest will allow assumption of the prone position. The ankles should be positioned at a 90° angle. Tolerance to the prone position should be increased gradually until the patient is able to sleep all, or at least part, of the night in this position. This routine will assist with prevention of pressure sores on posterior aspects of the body and development of flexor tightness at the hips and knees.

Selective Strengthening

During the course of rehabilitation, all remaining musculature will be strengthened maximally. However, during the acute phase certain muscles must be strengthened very cautiously to avoid stress at the fracture site. During the first few weeks following injury, application of resistance may be contraindicated to (1) musculature of the scapula and shoulders in tetraplegia and (2) musculature of the pelvis and trunk in paraplegia.

An important consideration in planning exercise programs during the acute phase is to emphasize bilateral UE activities because these will avoid asymmetric, rotational stresses on the spine. Several forms of strengthening exercises are appropriate during this early phase: bilateral manually resisted motions in straight planes, bilateral UE proprioceptive neuromuscular facilitation (PNF) patterns, and progressive resistive exercises using cuff weights or dumbbells. Biofeedback training also may be a useful adjunct during early exercise programs. With tetraplegia, emphasis should be placed on strengthening the anterior deltoid, shoulder extensors, biceps, and lower trapezius. If present, the radial wrist extensors, triceps, and pectorals should also be emphasized because they will be of key importance in improving functional capacity. With paraplegia, all UE musculature should be strengthened, with emphasis on shoulder depressors, triceps, and latissimus dorsi, which are required for transfers and ambulation.

Early involvement in functional activities should be stressed. In addition to their intrinsic value, many activities afford the important benefit of progressive strengthening. For example, self-feeding and involvement in limited personal care activities will assist with strengthening the shoulder and elbow flexors. Another example of a functional activity (although not appropriate during the acute phase) with important strengthening benefits is wheelchair propulsion (deltoids, biceps, and shoulder rotators).

Orientation to the Vertical Position

Once radiographic findings have established stability of the fracture site, or early fracture stabilization methods are complete, the patient is cleared for upright activities. As discussed, the patient typically will experience symptoms of postural hypotension if approach to management has required some period of immobility. A very gradual acclimation to upright postures is most effective. The use of an abdominal binder and elastic stockings will retard venous pooling. During early upright positioning, elastic wraps are often used in combination with (placed over) the elastic stockings.

Initially, upright activities can be initiated by slowly elevating the head of the bed and progressing to a reclining or tilt-in-space wheelchair with elevating leg rests. Use of the tilt-table provides another option for orienting the patient to a vertical position. Vital signs should be monitored carefully and documented during this acclimation period. Patients who have been immobilized in halo devices or undergone surgical spine stabilization will not be confined to recumbent positions for prolonged periods. For these patients, the same progression is used, although a more rapid advance to the vertical position can be anticipated.

Active Rehabilitation Phase

Specific functional goals must be established as part of overall rehabilitation planning. Reasonable functional expectations, at various lesion levels, for a young, healthy patient with a complete lesion and unimpaired by secondary complications are shown in Table 23.6. This information may provide a useful guide in establishing realistic goals. However, it is important not to adhere too closely to established "norms" and, hence, to limit the patient by your own expectations. Goals should be established individually for each patient on the basis of examination findings in accordance with the level and extent of injury.

The term *key muscles* is a common expression in the management of patients with SCI and is used in Table 23.6. Key muscles are those that add significantly to a patient's functional capability at each successive level of lesion. It is also important to note that the neurological level of innervation may vary slightly from source to source. These key muscles are not to be confused with the key muscles identified in the ISNCSCI.

Physical Therapy Examination

All the examination procedures completed during the acute phase will be continued at regular intervals during the active rehabilitation phase. Inasmuch as greater patient mobility is now allowed, more complete testing of muscle strength, ROM, and functional skills can be performed. During MMT the therapist must be alert to the distinction between true voluntary contraction and movement associated with spasticity or substitution.

A variety of standardized outcome measures are available to the physical therapist. Some of the more frequently used tools are discussed here. The *Functional Independence Measure (FIM™)* is used to measure

(text continues on page 965)

Table 23.6 Functional Expectations for Patients with Spinal Cord Injury[a]

Most Distal Nerve Root Segments Innervated and Key Muscles	Available Movements	Functional Capabilities	Equipment and Assistance Required
C1, C2, C3 Face and neck muscles (cranial innervation)	Talking Mastication Sipping Blowing	Bed skills ADL • Total dependence in ADL	Dependent Mechanical ventilator: may use phrenic nerve stimulator during the day *Full-time attendant required*
		• Activation of light switches, page turners, call buttons, electrical appliances, and speaker phones	Environmental control units
		Wheelchair skills	Independent with power wheelchair (typical components include an electronically controlled seating system, a seatbelt and trunk support); a portable ventilator is typically attached; microswitch or sip-and-puff controls may be used
		Transfers	Dependent
C4 Diaphragm Trapezius	Respiration Scapular elevation	Bed skills ADL • Limited self-feeding	Dependent Mobile arm supports (possibly with powered elbow orthotic), powered flexor hinge hand splint Adapted eating equipment (long straws, built-up handles on utensils, plate guards, and so forth) Plexiglas lapboard
		• Typing	Computer keyboard using head or mouth stick or sip-and-puff controls; another option is a rubber-tipped stick held in hand by a splint (in combination with mobile arm supports and powered splints)
		• Page turning	Head or mouth stick Environmental control unit for powered page turner
		• Activation of light switches, call buttons, electrical appliances, and speaker phones	Environmental control units
		Wheelchair skills	Independent with power wheelchair with head, mouth, chin, breadth, or sip-and-puff controls
		• Pressure relief	Power tilt-in-space wheelchair
		• Transfers	Dependent
		Skin inspection	Dependent
		Cough with glossopharyngeal breathing	Dependent
		Recreation	Head or mouth stick
		• Table games such as cards or checkers	Built-up playing pieces
		• Painting and drawing	*Full-time attendant required*

(*continued*)

Table 23.6 Functional Expectations for Patients with Spinal Cord Injury[a] (continued)

Most Distal Nerve Root Segments Innervated and Key Muscles	Available Movements	Functional Capabilities	Equipment and Assistance Required
C5 Biceps Brachialis Brachioradialis Deltoid Infraspinatus Rhomboid (major and minor) Supinator	Elbow flexion and supination Shoulder external rotation Shoulder abduction to 90° Limited shoulder flexion	Bed skills	Some assistance required
		ADL • Able to accomplish all activities of a C4 tetraplegic with less adaptive equipment and more skill	Assistance is required in setting up patient with necessary equipment; patient can then accomplish activity independently
		• Self-feeding	Mobile arm supports, deltoid aid Adapted utensils and splinting
		• Typing	Computer keyboard Hand splints Adapted typing sticks Some patients may require mobile arm supports or slings
		• Page turning	Same as above
		• Limited UE dressing	Assistance required
		• Limited self-care (i.e., washing, brushing teeth, and grooming)	Hand splints Adapted equipment (wash mitt, adapted toothbrush, and so forth)
		Wheelchair skills	Independent with manual wheelchair with plastic- coated handrim projections Power wheelchair with joystick or adapted UE controls
		Transfer activities	Dependent Overhead swivel bar Sliding board
		Skin inspection	Dependent
		Pressure relief	Independent with power tilt-in-space wheelchair
		Cough with manual pressure to diaphragm	Assistance required
		Driving	Van with hand controls *Part-time attendant required*
C6 Extensor carpi radialis Infraspinatus Latissimus dorsi Pectoralis major (clavicular portion) Pronator teres Serratus anterior Teres minor	Shoulder flexion, extension, internal rotation, and adduction Scapular abduction and upward rotation Forearm pronation Wrist extension (tenodesis grasp)	Bed skills	Some assistance to independent with use of side rails on bed or overhead triangle
		ADL • Self feeding	Universal cuff Intertwine utensils in fingers Adapted utensils
		• Dressing	Utilizes momentum, button hooks, zipper pulls, or other clothing adaptations; dependent on momentum to extend limbs Cannot tie shoes
		• Self care	Flexor hinge splint Universal cuff Adaptive equipment
		Wheelchair skills	Independent with manual wheelchair with projection or friction surface hand rims; power wheelchair may be required for long distances and community mobility
		Transfers	Independent with sliding board on level surfaces
		Skin inspection and pressure relief	Independent

Table 23.6 Functional Expectations for Patients with Spinal Cord Injury[a] (continued)

Most Distal Nerve Root Segments Innervated and Key Muscles	Available Movements	Functional Capabilities	Equipment and Assistance Required
		Bowel and bladder care	Can be independent with equipment depending on bowel and bladder routine
		Cough with application of pressure to abdomen	Independent
		Driving	Automobile with hand controls and U-shaped cuff attached to steering wheel Usually requires assistance in getting wheelchair into car
		Wheelchair sports	Limited participation (i.e., bowling, fishing)
		Meal preparation	Can be independent with occasional light meals with adaptive equipment
C7 Extensor pollicus longus and brevis Extrinsic finger extensors Flexor carpi radialis Triceps	Elbow extension Wrist flexion Finger extension	Bed skills	
		ADL	Independent
		• Self-feeding	Independent
		• Dressing	Independent Button hook may be required
		• Self-care	Shower chair Hand-held shower nozzle Adapted handles on bathroom items may be required
		Wheelchair skills	Independent with manual wheelchair with friction surface hand rims
		Transfers	Independent (with or without sliding board)
		Bowel and bladder care	Independent with appropriate equipment (digital stimulator, suppositories, raised toilet seat, urinary drainage device, and so forth)
		Manual cough	Independent
		Housekeeping	Light kitchen activities Requires wheelchair accessible kitchen and living environment Adapted kitchen tools
		Driving	Automobile with hand controls Able to get wheelchair in and out of car
C8 to T1 Extrinsic finger flexors Flexor carpi ulnaris Flexor pollicis longus and brevis Intrinsic finger flexor	Full innervation of UE muscles including fine coordination and strong grasp	Bed skills	
		ADL	Independent Independent in all self-care and personal hygiene Some adaptive equipment may be required (e.g., tub seat, grab bars, and so forth)
		Wheelchair skills	Independent with manual wheelchair with standard hand rims
		Housekeeping	Independent in light housekeeping and meal preparation Some adaptive equipment may be required (e.g., reachers) Requires a wheelchair-accessible living environment
		Transfers	Independent
		Driving	Automobile with hand controls
		Employment	Able to work in a building free of architectural barriers

(continued)

Table 23.6 Functional Expectations for Patients with Spinal Cord Injury[a] (continued)

Most Distal Nerve Root Segments Innervated and Key Muscles	Available Movements	Functional Capabilities	Equipment and Assistance Required
T4 to T6 Top half of intercostals Long muscles of back (sacrospinalis and semispinalis)	Improved trunk control Increased respiratory reserve Pectoral girdle stabilized for lifting objects	Bed skills ADL Wheelchair skills • Curb climbing in wheelchair • Wheelchair sports Transfers Physiological standing (not practical for functional ambulation) Housekeeping	Independent Independent in all areas Independent with manual wheelchair Able to negotiate curbs using a "wheelie" technique Full participation Independent Standing table or frame Bilateral knee–ankle-foot orthoses (KAFOs) with spinal attachment Some patients may be able to ambulate for short distances with assistance Independent with routine activities Requires a wheelchair accessible living environment
T9 to T12 Lower abdominals All intercostals	Improved trunk control Increased endurance	Household ambulation Wheelchair skills	Bilateral AFOs and crutches or walker (high energy consumption for ambulation) Wheelchair used for energy conservation
L2, L3, L4 Gracilis Iliopsoas Quadratus lumborum Rectus femoris Sartorius	Hip flexion Hip adduction Knee extension	Functional ambulation Wheelchair skills	Bilateral KAFOs and crutches Wheelchair used for convenience and energy conservation
L4, L5 Extensor digitorum Low back muscles Medial hamstrings (weak) Posterior tibialis Quadriceps Tibialis anterior	Strong hip flexion Strong knee extension Weak knee flexion Improved trunk control	Functional ambulation Wheelchair skills	Bilateral AFOs and crutches or canes Wheelchair used for convenience and energy conservation

[a] This table presents general functional expectations at various lesion levels. Each progressively lower segment includes the muscles from the previous levels. Although the key muscles listed frequently receive innervation from several nerve root segments, they are listed here at the neurological levels where they add to functional outcomes.

functional ability in a variety of activities of daily living (ADL) such as dressing and grooming, transfers, locomotion, and toileting. The FIM™ has been shown to be a reliable and valid measure of functional ability for individuals with SCI.[129–132] Chapter 11 provides more detail regarding the FIM™.

Most individuals with SCI will rely on a wheelchair as their primary means of locomotion in their home and community. As such, it is important to examine the patient's ability to perform wheelchair skills. This includes setting and releasing the wheel locks, removing footrests and armrests, propelling the wheelchair on level surfaces, performing wheelies, ascending and descending curbs, and various other wheelchair skills necessary for independent mobility in the community. The *Wheelchair Skills Test* (Fig. 23.12) developed by Kirby and colleagues is an outcome measure designed to examine a manual wheelchair user's skills in performing 57 representative wheelchair skills.[133–135] Different skills are categorized according to three levels: *indoor*, *community*, and *advanced*; that reflect difficulty and the setting in which the skills are most often used. The *Wheelchair Skills Test* can be used as a diagnostic measure to determine which wheelchair skills need to be addressed in therapy and to document improvement during rehabilitation.

In addition to examining wheelchair mobility, the physical therapist should perform a thorough seating and wheelchair examination to determine the most appropriate seating system and wheelchair for the patient. More detail on this process is provided below; Chapter 33 provides a comprehensive review of this topic.

Regaining the ability to walk is a common goal for most individuals with SCI (see later section on gait training). Two commonly used outcome measures designed to examine walking ability after SCI are the *Walking Index for Spinal Cord Injury (WISCI)*[136] and the *Spinal Cord Injury Functional Ambulation Inventory (SCI-FAI)*[137] (Fig. 23.13).

Physical Therapy Intervention

During the active rehabilitation phase, the emphasis of treatment is on maximizing functional independence. Initially this includes basic skills such as bed mobility, transfers, and wheelchair mobility skills. As the patient progresses, these interventions are expanded to include skills necessary for work, home, and community reentry. Individuals who are not able to accomplish a specific functional task independently owing to the lesion level should be educated on how to instruct another person to perform the task for them. Individuals who are not able to perform basic ADL such as dressing, bed mobility tasks, and transfers independently require a personal care attendant. For example, an individual with a high cervical lesion who is not able to turn in bed or feed him- or herself independently must to be able to instruct a personal care attendant on how to perform the task.

Continuing Activities

During the active rehabilitation phase, many of the treatment activities initiated during the acute period will be continued. Interventions designed to address respiratory management, ROM, and positioning will continue. The patient also will be involved in a continuing and expanded program of resistive exercises for all muscles that remain innervated (e.g., PNF, progressive resistance exercise [PRE] using manual resistance, weights, wall pulleys, sling suspension, and group exercise classes). Development of motor control and muscle reeducation techniques directed at appropriate muscles (based on lesion level) are indicated. Emphasis is also placed on regaining postural control and balance by substituting upper body control and vision (for lost proprioception). This phase of treatment will also focus on improved cardiovascular response to exercise. This can effectively be accomplished by use of interval training using an UE aerobic activity (e.g., UE ergometer).[128]

Skin Inspection

During this phase of management, the patient will be instructed gradually to assume responsibility for skin inspection. This will involve practice in use of long-handled (Fig. 23.14) or adapted mirrors to allow inspection of areas not easily visible. Wall mirrors adjacent to the bed may assist in achieving independence with this activity. Patients with high-level lesions may be incapable of skin inspection. It is important that these patients be instructed in how to direct others to complete this examination. Continued emphasis by the therapist should be placed on the importance of skin inspection and the rationale for pressure relief. Skin inspection and care must become a regular and lifelong component of the patient's daily routine.

Mat Programs

Mat activities constitute a major component of treatment during the rehabilitation phase. The sequence of activities typically progresses from achievement of stability within a posture and advances through controlled mobility to skill in functional use.[138] Early activities are bilateral and symmetrical. A progression is then made to weight shifting and movement within the posture. A gradual emphasis is placed on improved timing and speed.

Mat activities are often individual components of more complex functional skills. They should be sequenced from easiest to most difficult so that the patient is performing activities within, or almost within, the sphere of mastery. As mastery of the various components of more complex and difficult activities is achieved, the patient should be asked to perform these tasks in the current living environment (i.e., hospital room, or eventually, home on weekends).

The therapist must determine the appropriate mat activities for each patient based on level of injury and medical status. It is important to note that complete mastery of an activity is not always necessary before moving on to the

(text continues on page 968)

Wheelchair Skills Test (Manual) 3.2 Report

NAME: DATE:

TEST INFORMATION: WST: [X] WST-Q: [ ]	SUBJECT: Wheelchair User: [X] Caregiver: [ ]

Wheelchair used:

	Group	#	Skill	L	Score	R	Comments:
ADVANCED	Wheelies on level terrain	56,57	Moving turns backward	□		□	
		54,55	Moving turns forward	□		□	
		52,53	Turns in place	□		□	
		51	Rolling backward		□		
		50	Rolling forward		□		
		49	Stationary		□		unable to hold wheelie for full 10s.
		48	No-hands rest		□		
	Level changes	47	15cm wheelie fwd descent		□		
		46	15cm descent		■		
		45	15cm ascent		■		
	Inclines	42	7.5° wheelie fwd descent		□		
COMMUNITY	Level changes	44	5cm descent		■		
		43	5cm ascent		■		
	Inclines	41	5° descent		■		
		40	5° ascent		■		
	Pot-Holes	39	30cm across		■		used left foot to help bridge gap.
		38	15cm across		■		
	↑ Rolling Resistance	37	Gravel		■		
	Cross-Slope	34,35		■		■	
	Obstacles	33	13cm high		■		
	Fold/Unfold	29	Unfold		□		seat rails not fully opened into seat saddles.
	Wheelchair	28	Fold		■		
	Rolling	14	Street crossing		■		Speed: 0.77 m/s pass≥0.33m/s
INDOOR	↑ Rolling resistance	36	Carpet		■		
	Obstacles	32	2cm high		■		
	Doors	31	Open toward		■		
		30	Open away		■		
	Transfers	27	Into wheelchair		■		
		26	Out of wheelchair		■		
	Reaching	25	High object		■		
		24	Ground		■		
	Sideways Manuevering	22,23		■		■	
	Moving	20,21	Backwards	■		■	
	Turns	18,19	Forwards	■		■	
	Turns in Place	16,17		■		■	
	Rolling	15	Backward		■		
		13	Forward		■		
	Footrests	11,12	Restore	N/P		N/P	reports never uses
		9,10	Move Away	N/P		N/P	
	Armrests	7,8	Restore	N/P		N/P	
		5,6	Move Away	N/P		N/P	
	Brakes	3,4	Release		■		
		1,2	Apply		■		

See Wheelchair Skills Program for explanations. Available at www.wheelchairskillsprogram.ca.

Scores:	TOTAL	INDOOR	COMMUNITY	ADVANCED	Codes
Percentage	73.5	100.0	92.3	14.3	■ Pass (1)
# passed / (total possible-NPs) X 100%					□ Not able to complete (0)
TESTER:					N/P No part

Figure 23.12 Wheelchair Skills Test,[133–135] with permission.

SCI Functional Ambulation Inventory (SCI-FAI)

Name: Session: Date:

PARAMETER	CRITERION	L	R
A. Weight shift	Shifts weight to stance limb.	1	1
	Weight shift absent or only onto assistive device.	0	0
B. Step width	Swing foot clears stance foot on limb advancement.	1	1
	Stance foot obstructs swing foot on limb advancement.	0	0
	Final foot placement does not obstruct swing limb.	1	1
	Final foot placement obstructs swing limb.	0	0
C. Step rhythm (relative time needed to advance swing limb)	At heel strike of stance limb, the swing limb:		
	begins to advance in <1 second *or*	2	2
	requires 1–3 seconds to begin advancing *or*	1	1
	requires >3 seconds to begin advancing	0	0
D. Step height	Toe clears floor throughout swing phase *or*	2	2
	Toe drags at initiation of swing phase only *or*	1	1
	Toe drags throughout swing phase	0	0
E. Foot contact	Heel contacts floor before forefoot *or*	1	1
	Forefoot or foot flat first contact with floor.	0	0
F. Step length	Swing heel placed forward of stance toe *or*	2	2
	Swing toe placed forward of stance toe *or*	1	1
	Swing toe placed rearward of stance toe.	0	0
	Parameter total		Sum /20

ASSISTIVE DEVICES		L	R
Upper extremity balance/weightbearing devices	None	4	4
	Cane(s)	3	3
	Quad cane(s), Crutch(es) (forearm/axillary)	2	2
	Walker	2 (L and R combined)	
	Parallel bars	0 (L and R combined)	
Lower extremity assistive devices	None	3	3
	AFO	2	2
	KAFO	1	1
	RGO	0	0
	Assistive device total		Sum /14

TEMPORAL/DISTANCE MEASURES			
Walking mobility (typical walking practice as opposed to W/C use)	Walks...		
	regularly in community (rarely/never use W/C)	5	
	regularly in home/occasionally in community	4	
	occasionally in home/rarely in community	3	
	rarely in home/never in community	2	
	for exercise only	1	
	does not walk	0	
	Walking mobility score		Sum/5
Two-minute walk test (distance walked in 2 minutes)	Distance walked in 2 minutes = ...	feet/ minute	meters/ minute

AFO: ankle-foot orthosis; KAFO: knee-ankle-foot orthosis; RGO: reciprocal gait orthosis; W/C: wheelchair.

Figure 23.13 Spinal Cord Injury Functional Ambulation Inventory (SCI-FAI),[137] with permission.

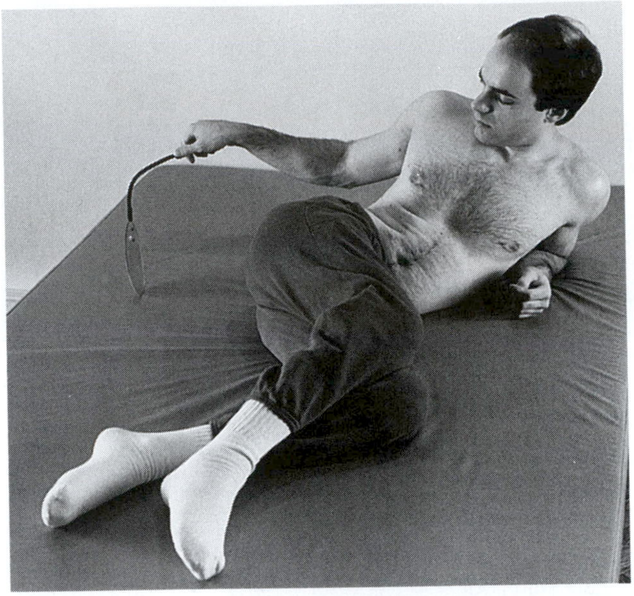

Figure 23.14 Skin inspection with use of long-handled mirror.

next. At some points in treatment, several components of the mat progression will be worked on concurrently.

Mat activities should be initiated as soon as the patient is cleared for activity. Progression through the sequence of mat activities develops improved strength and functional ROM, improves awareness of the new center of gravity, promotes postural stability, facilitates dynamic balance, and assists with determining the most efficient and functional methods for accomplishing specific tasks. It also provides the opportunity to develop functional patterns of movement (e.g., use of innervated musculature or momentum to move body parts that lack active movement).

The following section represents a sample progression of selected mat activities. The degree to which they can be performed independently and the time needed to learn them vary considerably with the level of lesion and the individual. Each component of the mat progression is presented with its functional implications and several suggested treatment activities to facilitate accomplishment of the activity. It is important to note that the exact method of performing a functional activity may vary for individual patients depending on many factors other than neurological lesion level such as psychological adjustment, body weight, body type (i.e., short arms) fear, and cardiovascular conditioning. The therapist and patient often must experiment with different methods of performing the task or intervention to come up with a specific method that works well for the patient. Chapter 13, *Physical Rehabilitation Laboratory Manual: Focus on Functional Training*,[138] and *Spinal Cord Injury: Functional Rehabilitation*[21] provide additional and more in-depth treatment suggestions.

Rolling

Rolling is of functional significance for improved bed mobility, preparation for independent positional changes in bed (for pressure relief) and LE dressing. Rolling is a frequent starting point of mat programs for patients with SCI and provides an early lesson in developing functional patterns of movement. It requires the patient to learn to use the head, neck, and UEs, as well as momentum, to move the trunk and/or LEs. It is usually easiest to begin rolling activities from the supine position, working toward the prone position. If asymmetric involvement exists, rolling should be initiated with movement toward the weaker side.

The activity is initially taught on a mat. However, rolling must also be mastered on the surface of a bed similar to the one that the patient will use at home. To develop maximum independence, bed rails, ropes, canvas "ladders," or overhead devices such as trapezes should be avoided, if possible. However, if these adaptive devices allow the patient to perform the task independently when they could not otherwise do the task then they should be incorporated into the overall plan of care (POC). In addition, the patient should achieve independent rolling when covered by sheets and blankets. To begin training and facilitate rolling, several approaches can be used.

- Flexion of the head and neck with rotation may be used to assist movement from supine to prone positions.
- Extension of the head and neck with rotation may be used to assist movement from prone to supine positions.
- Bilateral, symmetrical UE rocking with outstretched arms produces a pendular motion when moving from supine to prone positions. The patient rhythmically rocks the outstretched arms and head from side-to-side and then forcefully "tosses" them to the side to which the patient is rolling. The trunk and hips will follow (Fig. 23.15). Use of wrist cuff weights (2 to 3 lbs) may be used initially to increase kinesthetic awareness and momentum.
- Crossing the ankles will also facilitate rolling (see Fig. 23.15). The therapist crosses the patient's ankles so that the upper limb is toward the direction of the roll (e.g., the right ankle would be crossed over the left when rolling toward the left). Rolling can be promoted further by flexing the hip and knee of the top LE and placing it over the opposite limb (e.g., the hip and knee of the right LE would be flexed and placed over the left when rolling toward the left).
- In moving from the supine position to the prone position, pillows may be placed under one side of the pelvis (or scapula, if needed) to create initial rotation in the direction of the roll. The activity can be started with two pillows, progress to one, and then to rolling without the use of pillows. If difficulty is encountered in initiating the roll, the activity can be started from a sidelying position. To facilitate movement from prone to supine positions, pillows may be placed under one side of the chest and/or pelvis. Again, the number and height of pillows should be reduced gradually and eventually eliminated.
- Several PNF patterns are useful during early rolling activities. The UE patterns of D1 flexion, D2 extension,

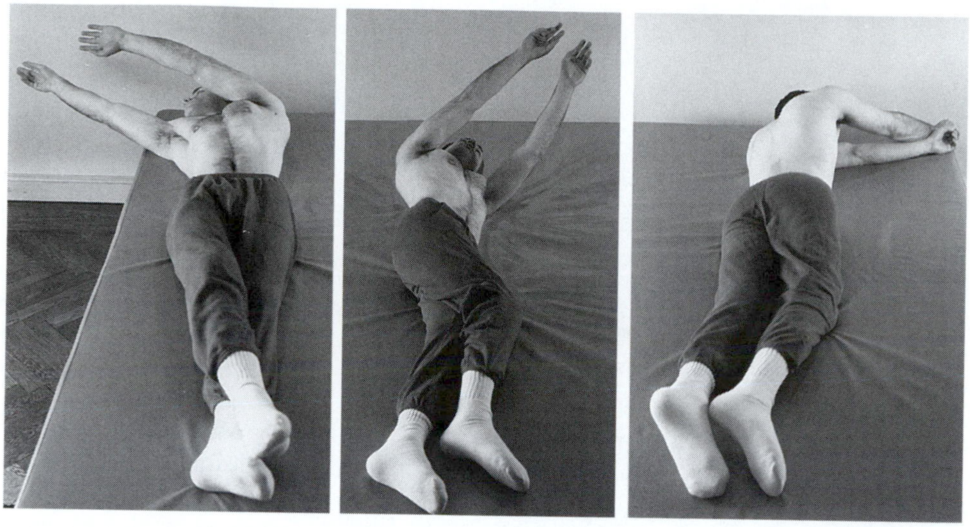

Figure 23.15 Rolling from supine position to prone position facilitated by UE momentum and crossing of the ankles.

and reverse chop will facilitate rolling toward the prone position. The UE lift pattern will facilitate rolling toward the supine position from sidelying.

Prone-on-Elbows Position

The functional implications of this activity are improved bed mobility and preparation for assuming the quadruped and sitting positions. This component of the mat progression facilitates head and neck control as well as proximal stability of the glenohumeral and scapular musculature via co-contraction. Scapular strengthening exercises also can be accomplished in this position. At first, the patient may require the therapist's assistance in assuming the prone-on-elbows position. To assume this position independently (from prone), the patient places the elbows close to the trunk and the hands near the shoulders and pushes the elbows down into the mat while lifting the head and upper trunk. From this position, one of two maneuvers can be used: (1) weight shifting from elbow-to-elbow will allow progressive movement of the elbows forward until they are under the shoulders; (2) or body weight can be shifted posteriorly until the elbows are under the shoulders.

The prone-on-elbows position must be used with caution, particularly following thoracic and lumbar injuries. Some patients may find it difficult to tolerate the increased lordotic curve imposed by this position.

- Weightbearing in the prone-on-elbows position will improve stability at the shoulders through joint approximation. Weight shifting assists with the development of controlled mobility and is usually easiest in a lateral direction with a progression to anterior or posterior movements.
- Rhythmic stabilization may be used to increase stability of the head, neck, and scapula.
- Manually applied approximation can be used to facilitate stabilization of proximal musculature.
- Unilateral weightbearing on one elbow (static dynamic activity) can be achieved in the prone-on-elbows position by having the patient lift one arm. This further facilitates co-contraction in the weightbearing limb.
- Movement within this posture can be achieved by an on-elbows forward, backward, and side-to-side progression.
- Strengthening of the serratus anterior and other scapular muscles can be achieved with prone-on-elbows push-ups. This is accomplished by having the patient push the elbows down into the mat and tuck in the chin while lifting and rounding out the shoulders and upper thorax (Fig. 23.16). This is similar to the "cat/camel" maneuver used in the quadruped position. The patient lowers the chin and upper chest to the mat again by allowing the scapula to adduct.

Prone-on-Hands Position (with Paraplegia)

The functional carryover of this position (Fig. 23.17) includes development of the initial hyperextension of the hips and low back for patients who will require this postural alignment during ambulation, and standing from a wheelchair or rising from the floor with crutches and bilateral knee–ankle–foot orthoses (KAFOs).

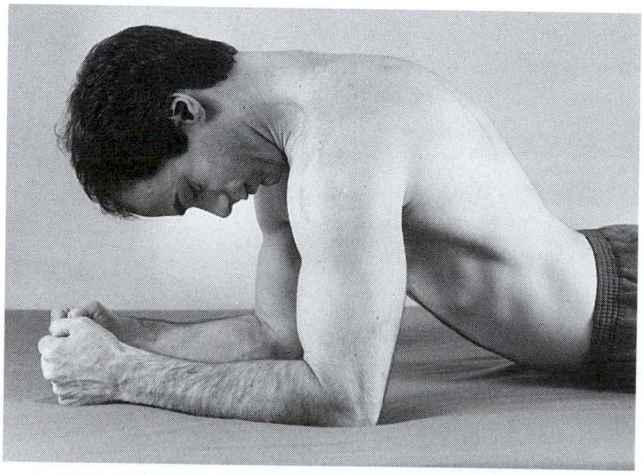

Figure 23.16 The prone-on-elbows position can be used for strengthening the serratus anterior and other scapular muscles.

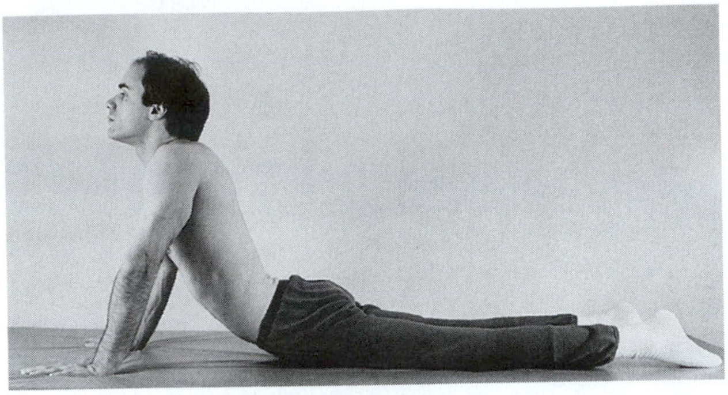

Figure 23.17 Prone-on-hands position.

Some patients may have difficulty assuming this position initially, and a gradual acclimation may be indicated (strong pectoralis major and deltoid muscles are required to accomplish this activity). A gradual progression can be made by supporting the patient's upper trunk with a wide, firm bolster, wedge, or a sling suspension system. As the patient gradually becomes accustomed to the new position, the height of the support can be increased (if gradual acclimation is needed) and eventually removed.

Hand placement for the prone-on-hands position is similar to a standard push-up position except that the hands are slightly more lateral and the arms are externally rotated.

It should be noted that this position would not be appropriate for every patient with paraplegia owing to the excessive lordosis required to assume and to maintain the position.

- Lateral weight shifting with weight transfer between hands will increase joint approximation.
- Additional approximation force can be applied through manual contacts to facilitate tonic holding of proximal musculature further.
- Scapular depression and prone push-ups may be utilized as strengthening exercises.

Supine-on-Elbows Position

The purpose of this activity is to assist with bed mobility and to prepare the patient to assume a long sitting position (Fig. 23.18). There are several approaches to assuming the supine-on-elbows position. If control of abdominal muscles is present, the patient may have sufficient strength to achieve the position by pushing the elbows into the mat and lifting into the position.

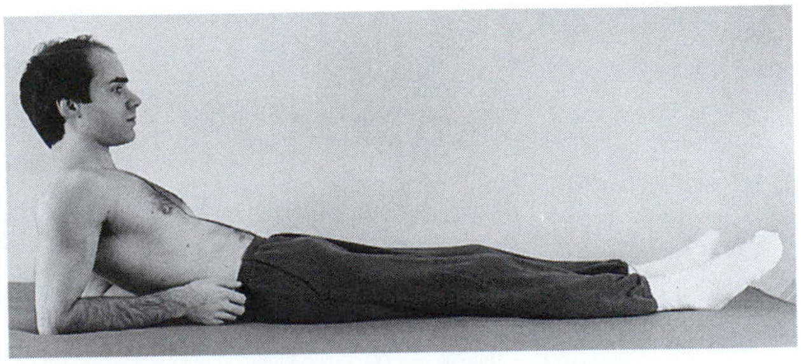

Figure 23.18 Supine-on-elbows position.

A more common technique is for the patient to "wedge" the hands under the hips or to hook the thumbs into pants pockets or belt loops. By contracting the biceps and/or wrist extensors, the patient can pull up partially into the posture. By shifting weight from side-to-side, the elbows can then be positioned under the shoulders.

Finally, some patients may find it easiest to assume this position from sidelying. The lower elbow is first positioned and pushed into the mat. The patient then rolls toward the supine position and quickly extends the upper arm, landing on the elbow as close to the shoulder as possible. By weight shifting, placement of the elbows can then be adjusted.

Much of the inherent benefit of this activity is achieved in learning to assume the posture and then move into long sitting. In addition to its direct functional significance, this activity is also an important strengthening exercise for shoulder extensors and scapular adductors.

- Lateral weight shifting can be practiced in this position.
- Side-to-side movement in this posture will enhance the patient's ability to align the trunk with the LEs when in bed or in preparation for positional changes.
- Precautions should be taken with this posture as it may cause increased shoulder pain due to the pressure exerted on the anterior shoulder joint capsule.

Pull-Ups (with Tetraplegia)

The purpose of pull-ups is to strengthen the biceps and shoulder flexors in preparation for wheelchair propulsion. The patient is positioned in the supine position. The therapist assumes the high-kneeling position with one LE on each side of the patient's hips. The therapist grasps the patient's supinated forearms just above the wrists. The patient pulls to sitting and then lowers back to the mat. Alternately, an overhead trapeze bar can be used for training.

Sitting

Both long (Fig. 23.19) and short (Fig. 23.20) sitting positions are essential for many activities of daily living, such

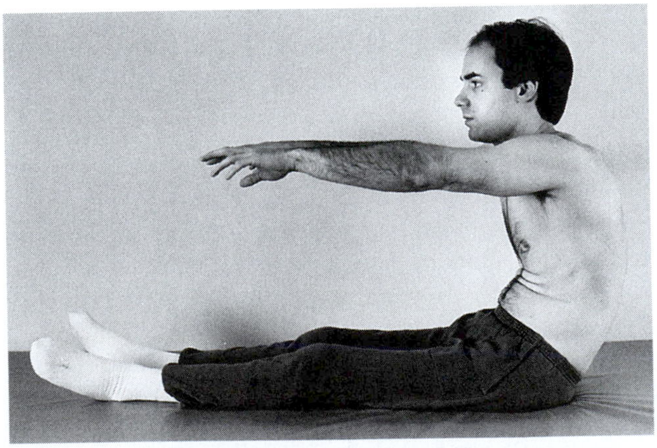

Figure 23.19 Individual with a T4 complete paraplegia in long-sitting position without UE support.

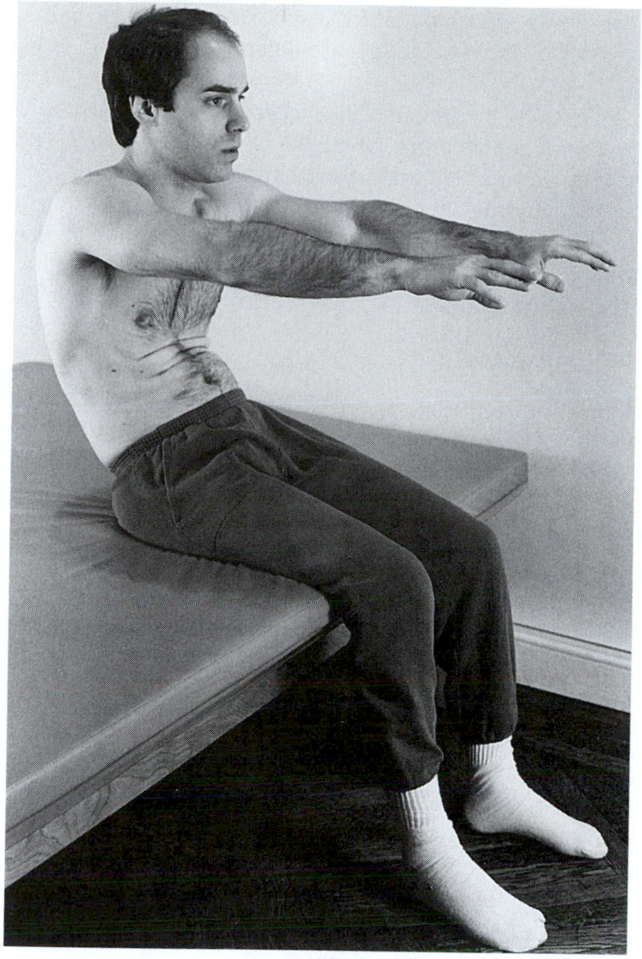

Figure 23.20 Individual with a T4 complete paraplegia in short-sitting position without UE support.

as dressing, self-ROM, transfers, and wheelchair mobility. Good sitting balance and the ability to move within this posture are also critical prerequisite skills to standing.

Patients with tetraplegia require approximately 100° of straight-leg ROM to assume a long-sitting position. Without this available motion, hamstring tension will cause a posterior tilting of the pelvis. This will result in the patient's sitting on the sacrum (*sacral sitting*), with resultant stretching of the lower back musculature.

It is important to note that sitting posture will vary considerably with lesion level. Patients with low thoracic lesions can be expected to sit with a relatively erect trunk. Individuals with low cervical and high thoracic lesions will maintain sitting balance by forward head displacement and trunk flexion. Patients with high cervical lesions will demonstrate poor sitting posture.

For patients with triceps and abdominal musculature (paraplegia), the sitting position can generally be assumed without difficulty. Patients with tetraplegia initially are taught to assume a stable sitting position by placing the shoulders in hyperextension and external rotation, and the elbows and wrists in extension with the fingers flexed (flexion of the fingers is particularly important to avoid overstretching, which will interfere with a functional tenodesis grasp). Weight is then borne on the base of the hand. Patients without triceps function can be taught to lock the elbows mechanically, using shoulder girdle musculature. The patient first tosses the shoulder into hyperextension with the forearm supinated. Once the base of the hand makes contact with the mat, the humerus is flexed to cause the elbow to extend since the arm is in a closed kinetic chain. This is followed by rapid shoulder depression to maintain elbow extension. This technique will stabilize the arm in hyperextension and external rotation.

There are two basic approaches to instructing the patient to assume the sitting position. Starting in the supine-on-elbows position, the patient is instructed to shift weight from side-to-side. Once sufficient momentum is achieved, the patient tosses one arm behind and shifts the weight onto that extended arm. The opposite arm is then tossed behind into an extended position. From this point, the patient "walks" the arms forward until a stable sitting position is achieved.

From a prone-on-elbows position, the patient creeps sideward, using the elbows and forearms. This will position the trunk in flexion and allow the patient to reach the LEs. The patient then hooks the uppermost forearm under the knee, pulls forward with this arm using the biceps, and then quickly tosses the opposite extremity behind. The UE originally placed under the knee is then also thrown into an extended position. The patient then "walks" forward until a stable sitting position is achieved.

Numerous patients have developed their own variations on these basic techniques. Often patient-devised approaches may be the most appropriate for the individual and should be examined in terms of safety, function, and energy expenditure. In addition, during the early stages of rehabilitation, adaptive equipment such as an overhead trapeze, rope ladders, or graduated loops hanging from over-bed frames may be used judiciously to facilitate movement into sitting.

Several suggestions that can be utilized in a sitting position are listed below.

- Initial activities will focus on practice in maintaining the position. During early sitting, a mirror may provide important visual feedback.
- Manual approximation force may be used at the shoulders to promote co-contraction.
- A variety of PNF techniques may be used. Specifically, alternating isometrics and rhythmic stabilization are important in promoting early stability in this posture.
- Balancing activities may be practiced in sitting. The base of support provided by the UEs can be gradually decreased, progress to single limb support, or, with some patients, be eliminated (see Figs. 23.19 and 23.20). The patient's limits of stability can be challenged progressively in each position. Activities such as ball throwing or tapping a balloon between the patient and therapist

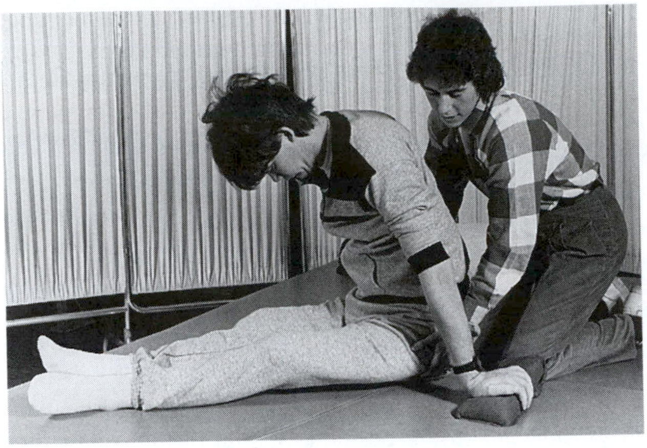

Figure 23.21 Individual with a C5 incomplete quadriplegia in long-sitting position. Push-ups are initially facilitated by manual assistance from the therapist with use of sandbags for weightbearing. Note that hand placement maintains finger flexion during wrist extension to avoid stretching of the long finger flexors.

(with or without cuff weights) also may be incorporated into a progression of sitting activities.

- Sitting push-ups are an important preliminary activity for transfers and ambulation. For tetraplegia, the patient is positioned with the shoulders in extension, the elbows locked, and the hands posterior to the hips. The patient leans forward and depresses the shoulders to clear the buttocks. Initially this activity may be facilitated by manual assistance from the therapist and/or by use of sandbags or small, hard bolsters to provide a firmer weightbearing surface for the UEs (Fig. 23.21). For paraplegia, a progression can be achieved by initiating the activity with weightbearing on the base of the hands placed directly on the mat and then using push-up blocks (Fig. 23.22) with graded increments in height.
- Movement within this posture can be accomplished by using a sitting push-up in combination with momentum created by movement of the head and upper body. This momentum is created by throwing the head and shoulders forcefully in the direction opposite to the desired direction of motion (head-hips relationship). For example, while performing a sitting push-up on the mat from a long sitting position, simultaneous rapid and forceful extension of the head and shoulders will move the LEs forward; movement in a posterior direction can be achieved by use of a sitting push-up with simultaneous rapid and forceful flexion of the head and trunk. This same progression of movement is used with the swing-to and swing-through gait patterns. Early mobility activities in both long and short sitting should emphasize adequate clearance of the buttocks for skin protection.

Quadruped Position

The functional implication of this all-fours position is its importance as a lead-up activity to ambulation. It is the first position in the mat sequence that allows weightbearing through the hips and is useful for facilitating initial control of the available musculature of the lower trunk and hips.

Generally the patient is instructed to assume a quadruped position from the prone-on-elbows position. From this position the patient can "walk" backward on elbows, progressing to weightbearing on hands, one at a time. Forceful flexion of the head, neck, and upper trunk while pushing into the mat with the elbows or hands will assist with elevating the pelvis. The patient continues to "walk" backward until the hips are positioned over the knees.

A second technique is to assume the quadruped posture from long sitting. In this approach the patient rotates the trunk to allow weightbearing on the hands with the elbows extended. From this sidesitting position the patient then moves into the quadruped position by a combination of UE and available trunk strength and momentum from the head and shoulders (moving opposite the direction of the hips).

Several suggested activities that can be utilized in the quadruped position are listed below.

- Initial activities will involve practice in maintaining the position; rhythmic stabilization can be used to facilitate co-contraction.
- Manual application of approximation force also can be used to facilitate co-contraction.
- Weight shifting can be practiced in a forward, backward, and side-to-side direction.
- Rocking through increments of range (forward, backward, side-to-side, and diagonally) will promote development of balance responses.

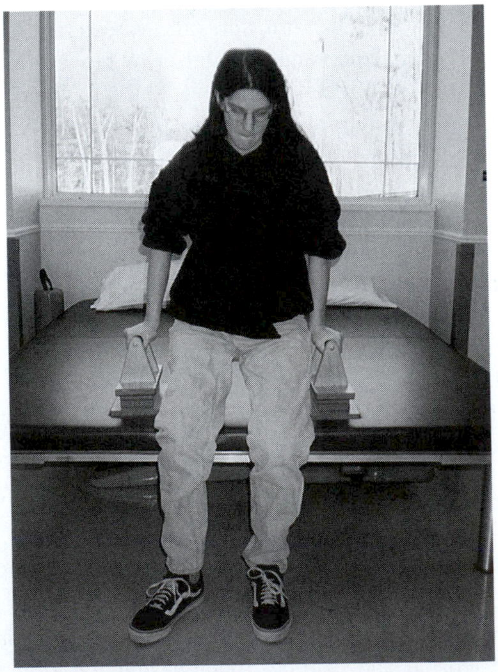

Figure 23.22 Individual with a complete lesion at T12 using push-up blocks in preparation for transfers and ambulation.

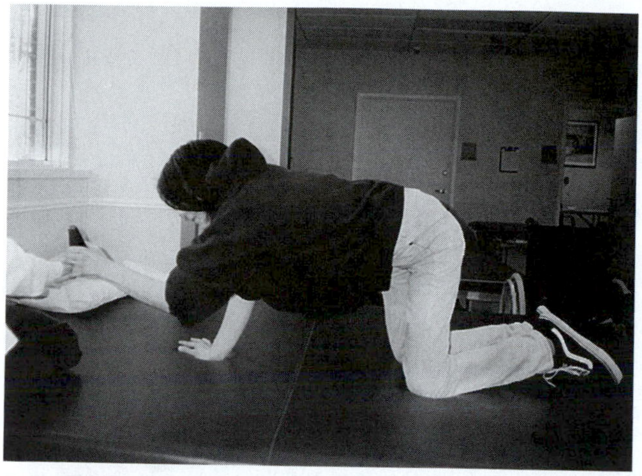

Figure 23.23 Static–dynamic activity. Freeing one UE from a weightbearing position will promote dynamic stability owing to reduction in the overall base of support and the shift of center of gravity over the support limbs.

- Alternately freeing one UE from a weightbearing position may be used in the quadruped position (Fig. 23.23). This static-dynamic control activity provides greater joint approximation forces on the supporting extremity and increased tonic holding of the available postural muscles (e.g., moving the dynamic limb in a diagonal pattern).
- Movement within the quadruped position (creeping) has important implications for ambulation. Creeping can be used to improve strength (resisted forward progression), to facilitate dynamic balance reactions, and to improve coordination and timing.

Kneeling Position

This position is particularly important for establishing functional patterns of trunk and pelvic control and for further promoting upright balance control. It is an important lead-up activity to ambulation using crutches and bilateral knee-ankle-foot orthoses.

It is usually easiest to assist the patient into the kneeling position from the quadruped position. From the quadruped position, the patient moves or "walks" the hands backward until the knees further flex and the pelvis drops toward the heels. The patient will be "sitting" on the heels. From this position the patient may be assisted to kneeling by using the UEs to climb stall bars (wall ladder) while the therapist guides the pelvis. Another method is for the therapist to assume a heel-sitting position directly in front of the patient. The patient's UEs are supported on the therapist's shoulders while the therapist manually guides the pelvis. In time, the patient can be taught to assume a kneeling position using mat crutches (Fig. 23.24) or other support device.

Several suggested activities that can be utilized during kneeling are listed below.

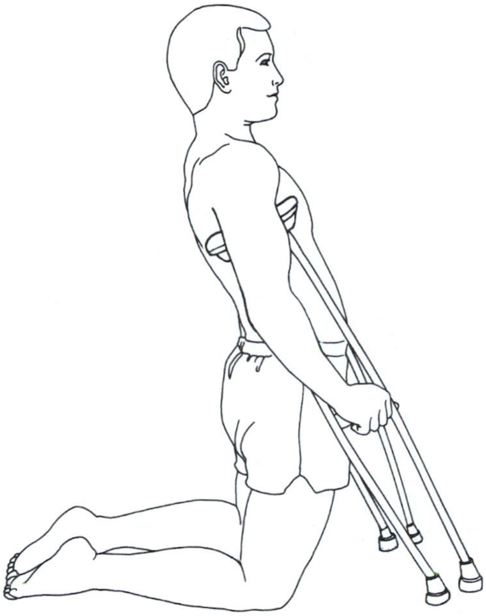

Figure 23.24 Kneeling position with use of mat crutches.

- Initial activities will concentrate on maintaining the position using available musculature and postural alignment (hips fully extended with the pelvis slightly anterior to the knees).
- The patient's balance may be challenged in this position. Balancing activities may progress from support with both UEs to support from only one.
- A variety of mat crutch activities can be used in the kneeling position; examples include weight shifting anteriorly, posteriorly, and laterally, with emphasis on lower trunk and pelvic control; placing the crutches forward, backward, and to the side with weight shifts in each direction, alternately raising one crutch at a time and returning it to the mat; hip hiking; instruction in gait pattern; and forward progression using crutches.

Transfers

Transfer training is generally initiated once the patient has achieved adequate sitting balance. It is a necessary prerequisite skill to many other functional activities, such as tub transfers, ambulation, and driving. Training is usually initiated on a firm mat surface and progresses to alternate surfaces such as a bed, toilet, bathtub, car, chair-to-floor (and reverse), and so forth. Patients with SCI most frequently use some variation of a lateral scoot transfer (with or without the use of a transfer board) (Fig. 23.25). Some experimentation and problem solving between the patient and therapist are generally required to determine the most efficient and safest method for an individual patient. Patients using wheelchairs with tubular footrests attached directly to the frame (nonremovable, fixed front end) typically transfer with the feet remaining on the tubular foot support (Fig. 23.26).

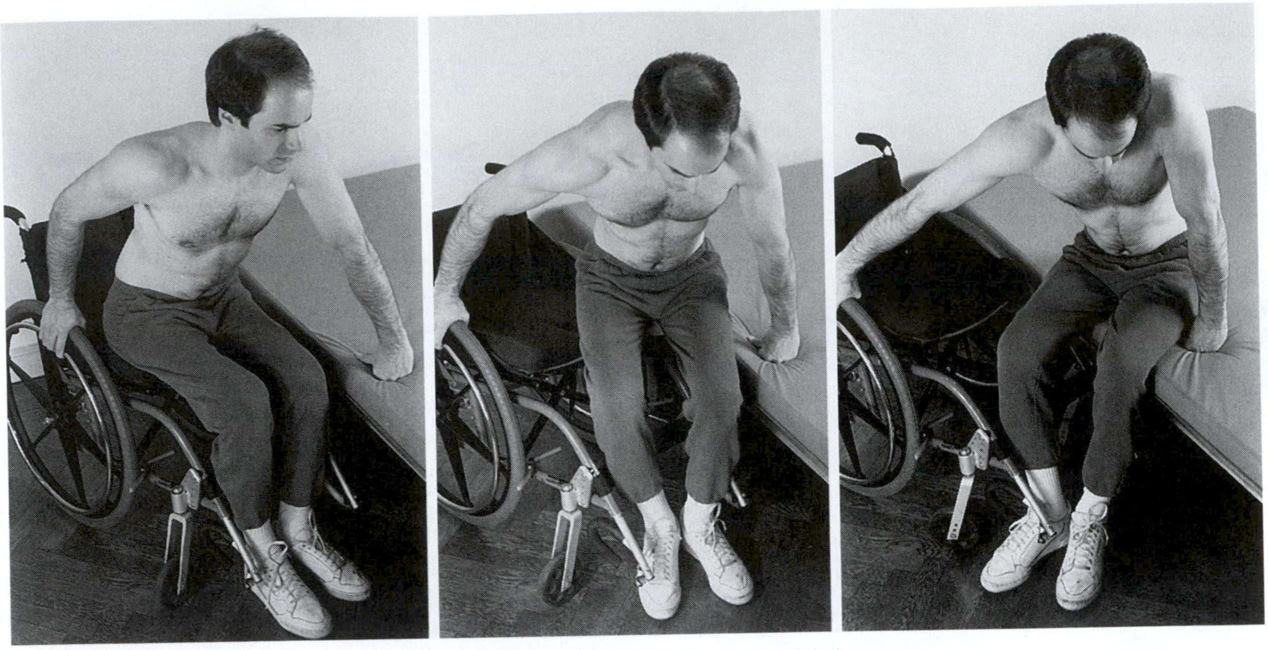

Figure 23.25 Individual with a T4 complete paraplegia transferring from wheelchair to mat with feet placed on floor.

In addition to neurological lesion level, three important components of transfer skills are momentum, muscle substitution, and head–hips relationship. Momentum can be used to facilitate movement at a joint(s) when the surrounding musculature is weak. Muscle substitution can also be used in this way. For example, an individual with a neurological level of C6 without triceps innervation can lock the elbows to assist with a transfer. This is done by placing the hand on the mat (or other surface) and using deltoid and pectoralis musculature to flex and adducted the humerus. This closed chain action at the UE causes the forearm to move medially and anteriorly, effectively locking the elbow. The *head–hips relationship* can be viewed as a first class lever. When the patient moves the head in one direction the buttocks will move in the opposite direction as he or she pivots at the shoulders. For example when attempting to transfer, a patient must lift body weight off the buttocks. To assist with this, the patient can place the hands on the transfer surface and rock the head forward and down. This movement will cause the buttocks to lift up.[21]

It is important to note there is more to a transfer than just the physical aspect of moving the body from one surface to another. As with all functional skills, the patient must be instructed in the component parts of the activity (e.g., positioning the wheelchair, locking the brakes,

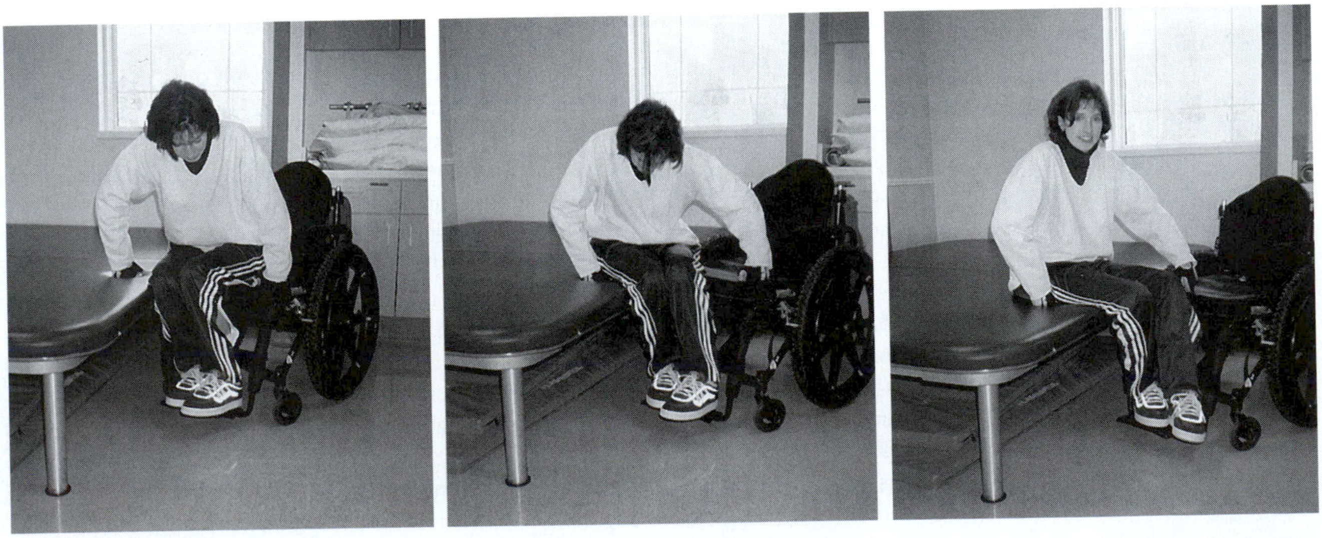

Figure 23.26 Transfer with feet remaining on permanently attached tubular foot supports.

removing the armrests, placing the sliding board) before the entire sequence is attempted.

Prescriptive Wheelchair

Most patients with SCI will use a wheelchair as the primary means of mobility. Even the patient with paraplegia who has mastered ambulation with crutches and orthoses will choose to use a wheelchair as a primary means of locomotion because it provides a lower energy expenditure and greater speed and safety. Because most patients will be using a wheelchair extensively, it should be custom-ordered (prescribed) for each individual. When prescribing a wheelchair consideration should be given to the patient's goals and characteristics as well as the activities and environment in which it will be used.

The first choice is between a power and manual wheelchair. Generally, individuals with intact triceps function are able to independently propel a manual wheelchair. Individuals with a C6 or C5 level injury may also be able to independently propel a manual wheelchair, but they may not have the endurance or strength for community wheelchair mobility. Individuals with higher cervical injuries generally rely on a power wheelchair for their mobility needs (see Table 23.6).

There are two basic frames for manual wheelchairs, a *folding* or a *rigid* frame. Lightweight folding chairs are an important consideration for patients who plan to transfer into a car as they can be folded compactly for storage without having to remove parts. Folding frames typically incorporate a below-seat crossbar and generally provide a smoother ride on uneven surfaces. Potential drawbacks include: more moveable parts causing it to be less energy efficient and slightly less lateral stability.

A rigid frame is more energy efficient, usually lighter weight and often has an adjustable seat-to-back angle. This type of frame may be more difficult to store in a car as both wheels must be removed (on some models the entire seating system also lifts off) for storage. This design allows placement of the wheelchair into and out of a car as components rather than as one large unit. Although rigid frames are generally less smooth riding on uneven surfaces, some models incorporate shock absorbing springs to minimize this effect (Fig. 23.27).

Advances in rehabilitation technologies have created a new class of wheelchairs that fall between manual and power wheelchairs, *push rim activated power assist wheelchairs* (PAPAW). A PAPAW is a manual wheelchair to which power assist wheels have been added. When the user applies force to the pushrims the motor is activated, which provides assist to the wheels. Propelling a PAPAW requires less energy, lower stroke frequency, and less shoulder ROM than a manual wheelchair.[139,140] A PAPAW may be beneficial for individuals with mid to lower level cervical injuries (C5–C6) who may not have the endurance or strength to use a manual wheelchair all the time.[141]

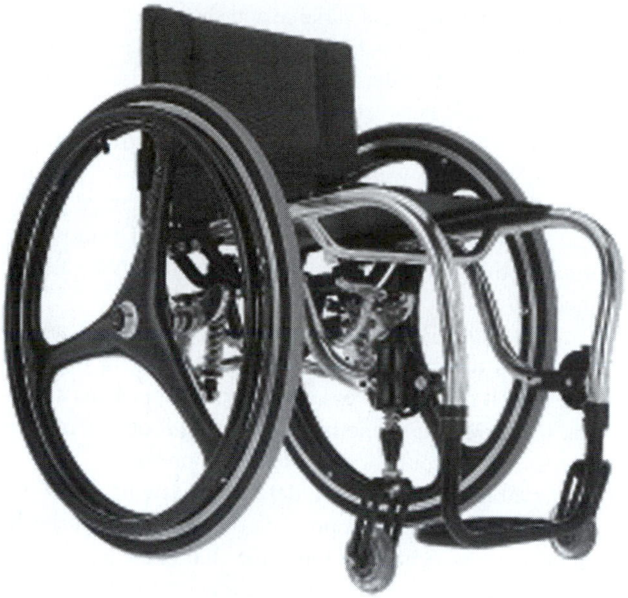

Figure 23.27 Rigid frame with four wheel independent suspension providing shock absorption on uneven terrain. (Courtesy of Colors in Motion, Anaheim, CA 92806.)

Power wheelchairs are indicated for all patients with C4 lesions and above. Patients with C5 level lesions may also elect to use power wheelchairs, particularly for community mobility. A tilt-in-space or reclining seating system provides improved postural control and it allows the user to independently perform pressure relief. There are various types of controls. They range from a hand-operated joystick to a sip-and-puff control.

A wheelchair prescription will vary according to the level and extent of injury. More specific information is presented in Chapter 33; however, some general considerations follow:

1. Seat depth should be approximately 1 to 2 in. (2.5 to 5.1 cm) back from the popliteal space to allow an even weight distribution on the thighs and to prevent excessive pressure on the ischial tuberosities.
2. Floor-to-seat height is important. If a chair has a sling-type seat, a seat cushion will be required (some contoured, custom-designed seats eliminate the need for a seat cushion). The type and dimensions of the cushion or custom-seat must be known so that seat height can be measured accurately, allowing adequate (2 in. [5.1 cm]) clearance from the floor to the foot pedals, and can provide slightly greater than a 90° angle at the hips.
3. Back height is also a consideration. If the patient will not be pushing the wheelchair, a high back may be desired for added comfort and stability. A patient with tetraplegia who will be pushing the wheelchair requires a back height that is below the inferior angle of the scapula so that the axilla is free of the handles during functional activities. Most patients with paraplegia prefer a lower back height, especially if they have intact abdominal muscles.

4. Seat width and depth is variable and should be fitted to the anthropometric characteristics of the patient. The patient should be fitted in the narrowest chair possible, but have adequate space between the lateral edges of the thighs and wheelchair armrests or wheels to avoid skin irritation. The patient's previous weight should be considered, especially if there has been a significant loss since the initial injury, and potential exists to regain the weight. If orthoses or thick clothing in cold climates are worn, they must also be included in the consideration of width.
5. Patients with LE spasticity may require heel loops and/or toe loops on the footrests to keep the feet in place. A pelvic belt may be necessary for extensor spasms affecting the lower trunk and hips. Elevating footrests may be necessary if circulatory problems are present.
6. Removable armrests and detachable swing-away leg rests are important components of wheelchairs used by many patients with SCI. On some chairs, the leg rests do not detach and the armrests are of a "flip-up" design. The suitability of these features must be considered with respect to the transfer capabilities and techniques used by the individual patient.

Additional wheelchair accessories may be required to meet specific patient needs. Several features that warrant consideration include enlarged release mechanisms on the leg rests, a friction surface on the hand rims, brake extensions, anti-tipping devices, and grade aids (which decrease backward movement of the chair while ascending inclined surfaces).

Some patients may require more than one wheelchair. Many standard lightweight "everyday" chairs are suitable for sport and recreational activities. However, depending on the interests of the patient, a second chair specifically designed for a particular sport such as tennis (Fig. 23.28) or racing (Fig. 23.29 A and B) may be required. Other examples of sport and recreational chairs are presented in Chapter 33.

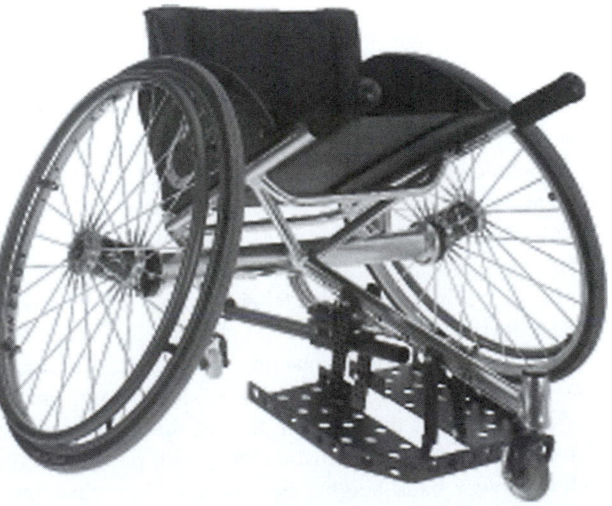

Figure 23.28 Wheelchair designed specifically for sports such as tennis. (Courtesy of Colors in Motion, Anaheim, CA 92806.)

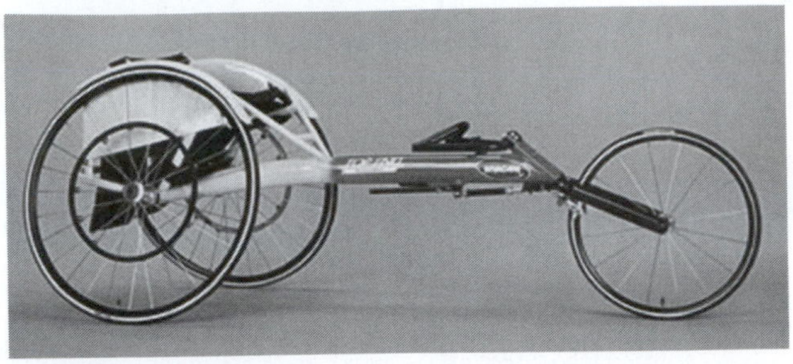

A

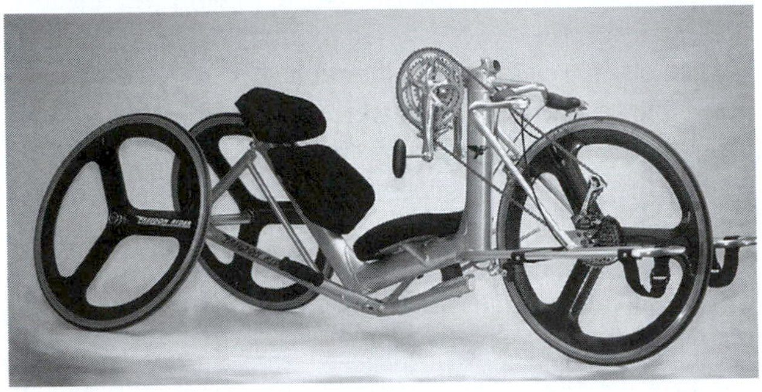

B

Figure 23.29 Wheelchairs designed specifically for racing (*A* Courtesy of Invacare, Elyria, OH 44035; *B* Courtesy of Brike International, Ltd, Tualatin, OR 97062.)

Because patients with SCI are at high risk for skin breakdown, a customized seating system including a wheelchair cushion will be required. A large variety of cushion styles are commercially available. The cushion should be comfortable, and provide a stable seating surface for functional use of the UEs. Figure 23.30 presents several styles of available seat cushions.

Wheelchair Skills

The patient should be taught how to operate all the specific parts of the wheelchair. Management of the brakes, arms, and pedals is crucial for all transfer activities. Many patients with limited hand function are able to propel the wheelchair by using the base of the hand against the hand rim. Some patients require assistive devices to aid in propulsion. Vertical or horizontal hand rim projections (Fig. 23.31) are useful for patients with poor hand function. The use of cycling gloves will protect the skin and also will improve the patient's grip on the hand rims.

Wheelchair mobility activities should begin on level surfaces (including doorways and elevators) and progress to outdoor, uneven surfaces. Patients with sufficient UE strength and upper trunk control also should be instructed in "wheelies," which involve balancing on the back wheels of the chair with the casters off the floor. Wheelies are required for independent curb climbing. Many facilities utilize canvas straps secured to the ceiling to assist with teaching this technique. The distal end of each strap has a C-clamp, which attaches to the push handle of the wheelchair. This allows safe practice by eliminating the danger of a posterior fall.

In addition to developing the *Wheelchair Skills Test* described earlier, Kirby and colleagues also developed the

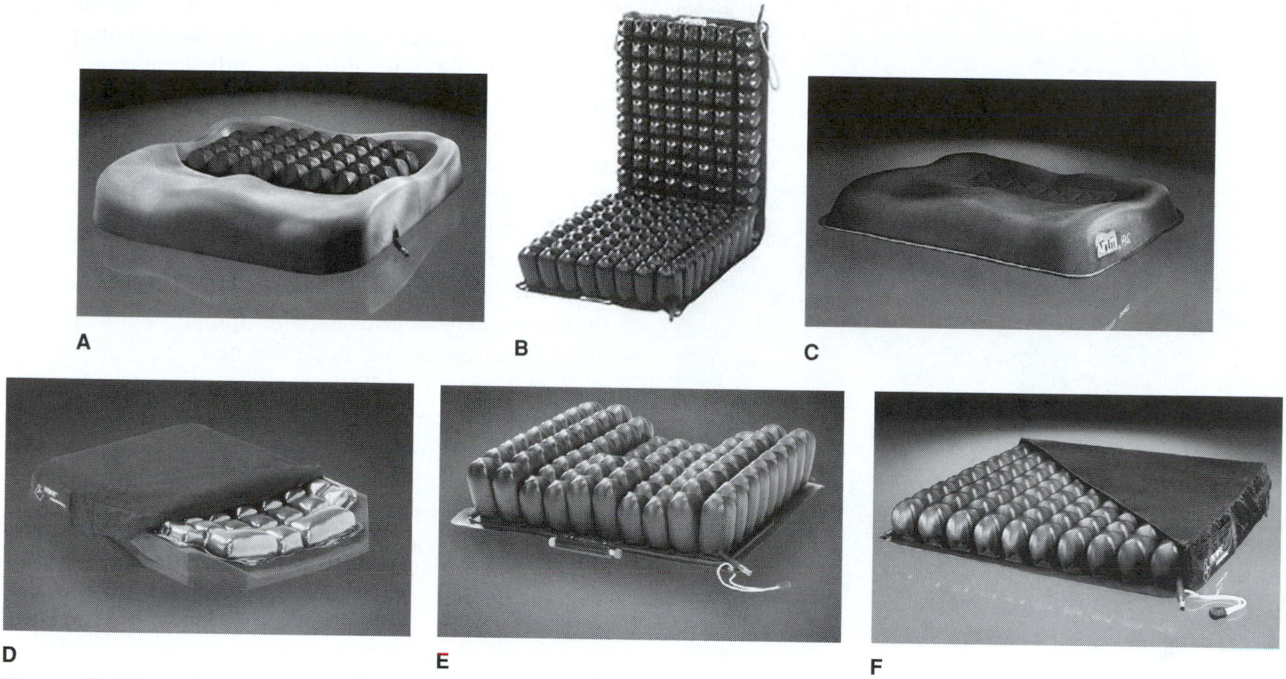

Figure 23.30 A large variety of wheelchair cushion styles are available. Shown here are (*A*) a contoured foam base cushion with a dry floatation® support pad, (*B*) dry floatation® recliner cushion, (*C*) contoured foam base cushion with a sealed air support pad, (*D*) dry floatation® cushion with a pre-contoured foam base, (*E*) a contoured air chamber cushion, and (*F*) a low profile air chamber cushion. (Courtesy of ROHO, Inc, Belleville, IL 62221.)

Wheelchair Skills Training Program. Based on the skills of the *Wheelchair Skills Test* and principles of motor learning, the Wheelchair Skills Training Program was designed to improve manual wheelchair user performance and safety. Research studies have shown it to be a safe and effective training method for new wheelchair users,[142] community-based wheelchair users,[143] occupational therapy students[144] and caregivers.[145] Detailed information on both the *Wheelchair Skills Test* and Wheelchair Skills Training Program can be obtained on the Inernet at: http://www.wheelchairskillsprogram.ca/.

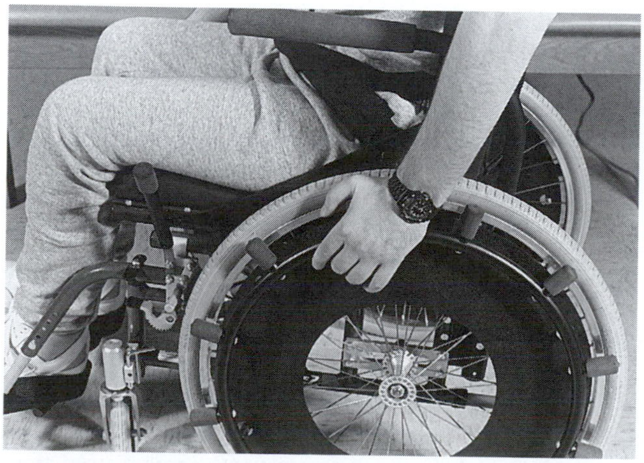

Figure 23.31 Hand rim projections assist with forward propulsion of wheelchair for patients with limited hand function.

The patient should be instructed in pressure relief techniques from a sitting position. Ten to 15 seconds of pressure relief (or tissue redistribution) for every 10 minutes of sitting should become part of the patient's daily routine. Although many patients will develop their own techniques, several common approaches to these activities include (1) wheelchair push-ups (Fig. 23.32), (2) hooking an elbow or

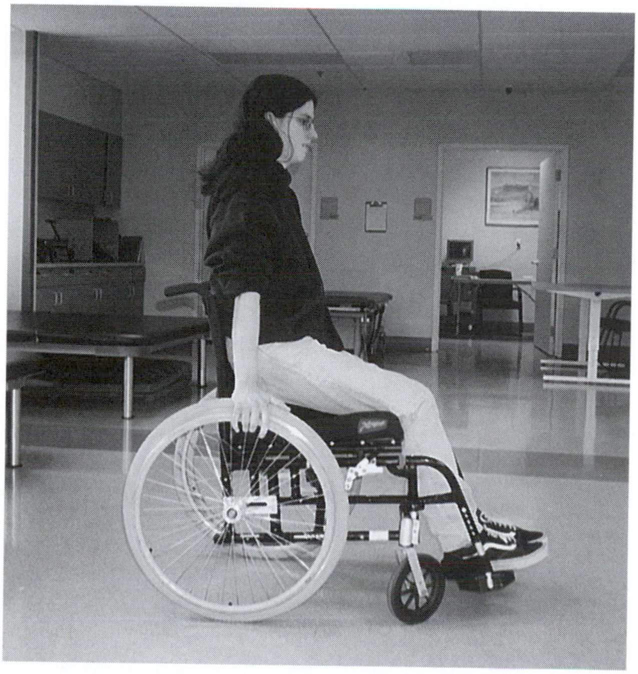

Figure 23.32 Wheelchair push-ups for pressure relief.

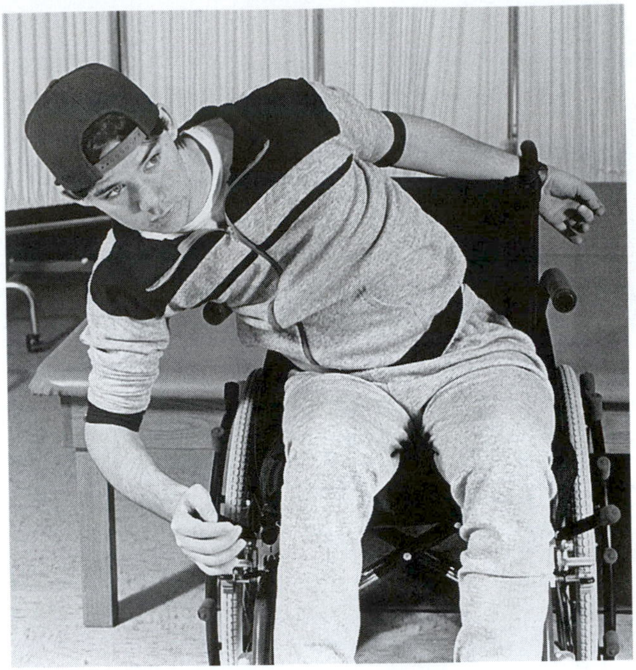

Figure 23.33 Lateral weight shift for pressure relief.

wrist around the push handle and leaning toward the opposite wheel (Fig. 23.33), and (3) hooking one elbow or wrist around the push handle and leaning forward (if triceps are available, hooking the elbow or wrist will be unnecessary).

Those patients who will be driving a car must learn how to fold and/or disassemble the wheelchair and slide it in and out of the car as well as learn to drive with hand controls. Transfer techniques should be considered with respect to the type of car the patient will drive. Vans with self-contained ramps (Fig. 23.34) or lifting platforms are a great asset for patients with tetraplegia and can increase their functional independence significantly.

Ambulation After Spinal Cord Injury

Regaining the ability to walk is a common goal for most individuals following a SCI. A number of factors will influence the success or failure in attaining this goal. Patients must possess adequate muscle strength, postural alignment, ROM, and sufficient cardiovascular endurance to initiate gait training. Becoming a functional ambulator following SCI is very difficult. Walking with orthoses and assistive devices is slower and requires more energy than normal ambulation. Many individuals with SCI who learn to walk with these devices may not continue walking once they stop rehabilitation.

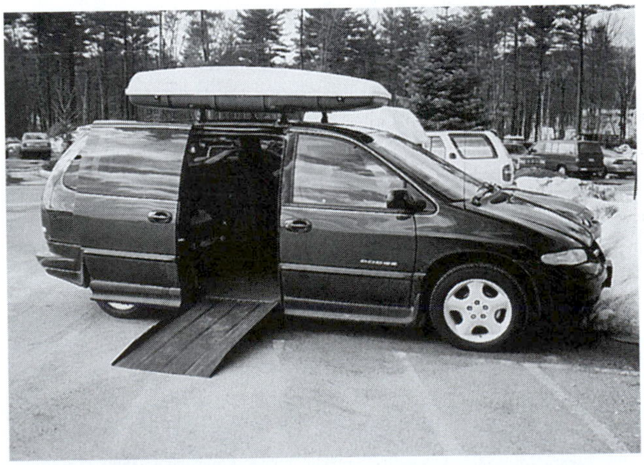

Figure 23.34 Ramp allows entry to van while individual remains seated in a wheelchair.

When initiating a gait training program therapists should be realistic with patients and provide a clear picture of the costs and potential benefits. Patients who wish to learn to ambulate following a SCI should be given this option even if their potential for functional ambulation is small. Although some patients may not become functional ambulators standing alone may provide other important benefits such as improved circulation, skin integrity, bowel and bladder function, sleep and well-being.[146]

Individuals with complete SCI must rely on orthotic devices, assistive devices, adequate ROM, and strengthening neurologically intact musculature for standing and walking. Inasmuch as spinal bracing is too restrictive, heavy, and impractical for functional ambulation, adequate ROM and postural alignment are crucial in achieving stability of the trunk. Full ROM in hip extension is essential in attaining balance in the upright position. The patient learns to lean into the anterior ligaments of the hip to stabilize the trunk or pelvis. The absence of knee flexion and plantarflexion contractures is also important in attaining upright standing balance.

Adequate cardiovascular endurance also is a criterion for functional ambulation.[147] Because the energy cost of ambulation for a patient with paraplegia is two to four times greater than normal walking, endurance becomes an important factor in determining success or failure as a functional ambulator. Although some training effects can be attained with a program of endurance training for the UEs, the patient's age, body weight, and history of cardiovascular disease or respiratory problems can restrict the amount that can be achieved.

Other factors that may restrict ambulation include severe spasticity, loss of proprioception (particularly at the hips and knees), pain, and the presence of secondary complications such as decubitus ulcers, heterotopic bone formation at the hips, or deformity. In addition, the patient's motivation plays a key role in determining success or failure in ambulation. A highly motivated patient can learn to ambulate with limited residual function. However, these patients may eventually find that the energy cost of ambulation is too great.

Follow-up studies of long-term continuation of ambulation have not been extensive. Mikelberg and Reid[148] surveyed 60 individuals with SCI for whom orthotics had been prescribed. From this group, 60 percent used their wheelchairs as the primary means of mobility. Thirty-one

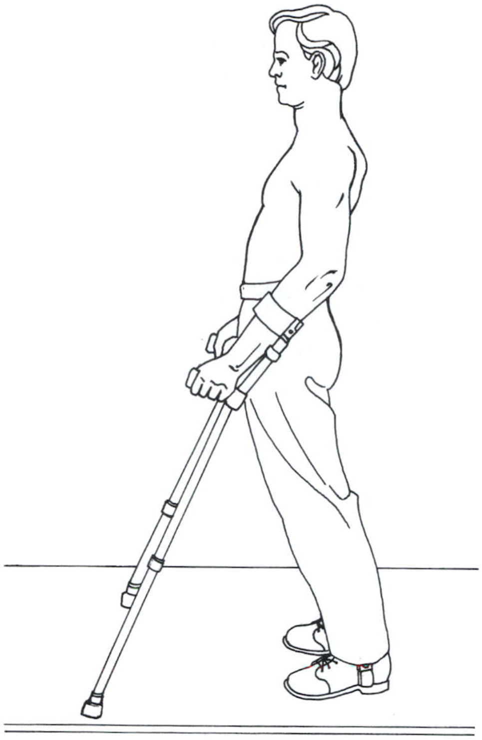

Figure 23.35 Standing alignment using bilateral knee-ankle-foot orthoses. Note that the upright position is maintained by leaning into the anterior Y ligaments, creating hyperextension at the hips.

percent completely discarded their orthoses. Those who did use their orthoses reserved them primarily for standing and exercise activities. Considering the high cost of orthoses and ambulatory training, the authors suggest careful individual consideration of each patient before orthoses are prescribed. They also suggest delaying decisions about ambulation; training might reasonably occur during later, follow-up care.

Degree of incomplete SCI is an important prognostic factor for determining ambulation potential. In a group of 105 patients classified as ASIA C or D tetraplegia (see Table 23.1) within 72 hours of injury, Burns and colleagues[149] found that 100 percent of patients with ASIA D injury, 91 percent of patients younger than 50 years old with ASIA C injury, and 42 percent of ASIA C injury 50 years or older were ambulatory by discharge. In a study with 246 patients with complete paraplegia and incomplete paraplegia and tetraplegia, only 5 percent of individuals with complete paraplegia were community ambulators 1 year after injury, while 76 percent of individuals with incomplete paraplegia where community ambulators.[150] Alander and colleagues[151] found that in patients 50 years of age or older with tetraplegia no patients with ASIA A classification could walk, 20 percent with ASIA B classification could walk, 85 percent with ASIA C classification could walk, and 90 percent ASIA D classification could walk at follow-up.

Gait Training for Individuals with Complete Spinal Cord Injury

For patients with complete SCI training emphasis is on strengthening available musculature, using assistive devices and orthoses to support weak or denervated muscles, and learning new, compensatory methods of walking.

Orthotic Prescription. The orthotic prescription varies according to the lesion level. Usually only ankle and/or knee control bracing is necessary. Patients with complete thoracic lesions will require KAFOs. Conventional KAFOs include bilateral metal uprights, posterior thigh and calf bands, an anterior knee flexion pad, drop-ring or bail locks, adjustable locked ankle joints, a heavy-duty stirrup, and a cushion heel. The ankle joints are usually locked in 5 to 10° of dorsiflexion to assist hip extension at heel strike. Orthotic hip control is not necessary, because the braces allow the patient to balance weight over the feet with the hips hyperextended (Fig. 23.35). The center of gravity is kept posterior to the hip joints but anterior to the ankles.

The Scott–Craig orthosis[152] is another type of KAFO that is frequently prescribed for patients with paraplegia (see Chapter 31). These orthoses consist of standard double uprights, an offset knee joint providing improved biomechanical alignment, bail locks, a posterior thigh band, an anterior tibial band, adjustable ankle joint, and a sole plate that extends beyond the metatarsal heads. A modification of this orthosis (Fig. 23.36) includes a plastic solid

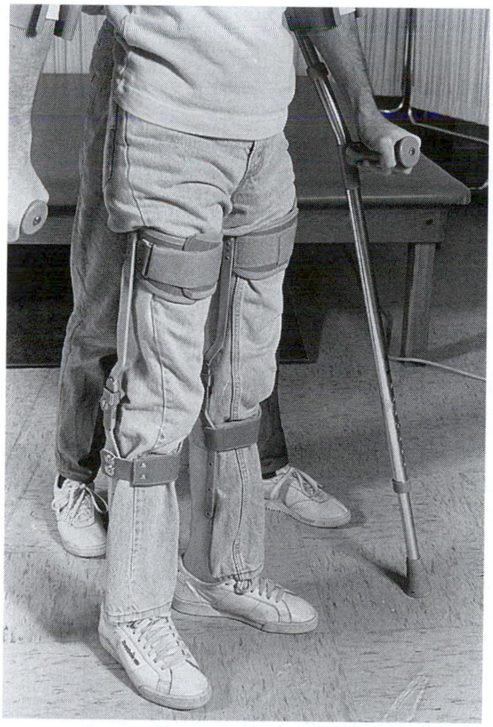

Figure 23.36 New England Regional Spinal Cord Injury Center (NERSCIC) orthosis (modification of the Craig-Scott orthosis). Note that patient is wearing orthoses over clothing for purposes of demonstration.

ankle section in place of the metal ankle joint and sole plate. This change decreases overall weight of the orthosis, improves cosmesis, and eliminates the need for custom-made shoes.[153]

Another type of orthotic device available to patients with SCI is the reciprocating gait orthosis (RGO) (see Chapter 31). The RGO is composed of two plastic KAFOs that are joined by a molded pelvic band with thoracic extensions. The RGO has a dual-cable system that runs posteriorly and attaches at the hip joints. These cable attachments transmit forces between LEs and provide reciprocal movement. Movement at the hip in one direction facilitates movement in the opposite direction on the contralateral hip. For example, as weight is shifted onto the left LE the right is moved forward. The dual-cable system allows control of both flexion and extension. These cables function to "coordinate" action between the two extremities during ambulation. As the advancing leg is unloaded, it is assisted into flexion while the stance leg is simultaneously pushed into extension. Thus, the orthosis allows for unilateral leg advancement and a reciprocating gait pattern. With this orthosis, a two- or four-point gait pattern can be used in combination with crutches or a reciprocating walker. Movement to a seated position is accomplished by unlocking the drop lock at the knee joint.[154–156]

Pelvic bands and spinal attachments are rarely prescribed for use with conventional KAFOs. These attachments severely restrict dressing activities, movement from sitting-to-standing, and ambulation, by reducing trunk and pelvis flexibility and by adding extra weight (often as much as 4 lbs). Furthermore, the use of these components makes gait slow, laborious, and usually nonfunctional. Patients who would require these attachments are usually not candidates for orthotic prescription. Instead, these patients can achieve physiological standing with the use a standing frame (Fig. 23.37).

Ankle–foot orthoses (AFOs) are often appropriate for patients with lower-level lesions (e.g., L3 and below). Either a conventional metal-upright or plastic AFO may be indicated.

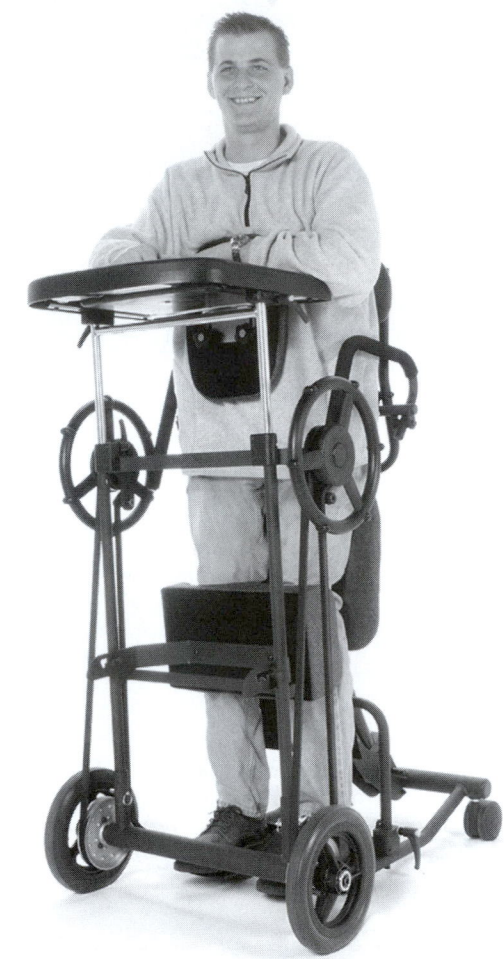

Figure 23.37 A standing frame provides mobility within environment. This unit is a supportive sit-to-stand stander; the posterior seat moves slowly between a seat configuration and an upright posterior support to facilitate transfers and promote upright standing. (Courtesy of Altimate Medical, Morton, MN 56270.)

Gait Training Strategies. A swing-through type of gait pattern (Fig. 23.38) should be the ultimate goal for functional ambulators with KAFOs. In teaching this pattern, it is important to stress a smooth, even cadence. Crutches should be placed equidistant from both toes at toe-off and be equidistant from both heels at heel strike. It is important to establish an overall rhythm, as improved timing will result in improved energy efficiency and cosmesis. Relevant training activities include those described below.

- *Putting on and removing orthoses.* The patient is first taught the correct way to don and doff the orthoses. The entire procedure is usually done in the supine or sitting position. The patient must be cautioned to continuously monitor for pressure areas, particularly after brace removal.
- *Sit-to-stand activities.* These activities should be practiced in the parallel bars using a wheelchair. The patient must learn to slide to the edge of the chair and lock and unlock the orthoses. Initially the patient is taught to pull to standing, using the parallel bars (a progression is made to using the wheelchair armrests to push to standing). Once in an upright position, the patient pushes down on the hands and tilts the pelvis forward in front of the shoulders. Return to sitting is a reversal of this procedure.
- *Trunk balancing.* The patient learns to balance the trunk in the hips-extended position, keeping the weight balanced over the feet, and learns to remove first one hand then both from the support. Placing hands forward and backward behind the hips while maintaining a stable position should also be practiced. Chapter 14 should be consulted for a more detailed description of suggestions for early parallel bar activities.
- *Push-ups.* This includes lifting the body off the floor using shoulder depression, ducking the head to gain added height, and controlled lowering of the body.

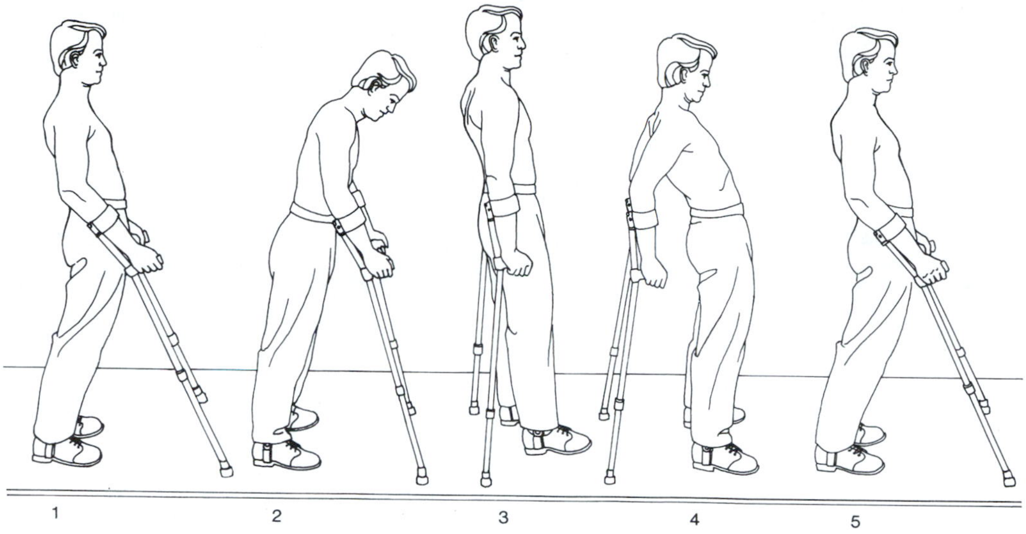

Figure 23.38 Swing-through gait pattern.

- *Turning around.* This involves lifting and lowering the body in 90° turns and changing hands from one bar to another.
- *Jack-knifing.* This entails controlling the pelvic position using UE support and positioning the head and shoulders forward ahead of the pelvis. This is an unstable position, and the patient must be taught recovery to overcome and/or to prevent this from happening during ambulation.
- *Ambulation activities in the parallel bars.* Four- and two-point gaits require hip flexion or hip hiking. Patients with high lesions may learn this movement using the secondary hip hikers (internal and external obliques and latissimus dorsi). Those with low lesions will have the quadratus lumborum intact. Trunk rotation on the swing side or lateral flexion toward the stance side will facilitate forward progression. *Note:* Swing-to and swing-through gaits require varying degrees of body elevation and push off. These gait patterns involve some jack-knifing and recovery. At push off, the head ducks to gain increased height, and at foot contact the head and back arch to help regain stability.
- *Assistive device.* Forearm crutches are most often selected for patients with paraplegia. These crutches provide several advantages. They are lightweight; they allow use of the hand without the crutch becoming disengaged; they fit more easily into an automobile; and, most importantly, they improve function in ambulation and stair climbing by allowing full hip extension and unrestricted movement at the shoulders.
- *Standing from the wheelchair with crutches.* To begin this activity the patient first places the crutches behind the chair, leaning against the push handle(s). To assume a standing position with crutches, the patient moves forward in the chair, locks both knee joints, crosses one leg over the other (Fig. 23.39), and then rotates the trunk and pelvis. Hand placements on the armrest are reversed and the patient pushes to standing by pivoting around to face the chair. The reverse of this technique is used to return to the chair.
- *Crutch balancing.* Initially, the patient must learn to become secure in the tripod stance. This is best achieved by first balancing in the parallel bars or against a wall. Weight shifting, alternating lifting one crutch off the floor, and jack-knifing should be practiced.
- *Ambulation activities.* Four-point, two-point, swing-to, and swing-through gaits should be practiced. They demonstrate a progression from a slow, steady gait pattern to a faster, unstable one. A gradual emphasis should be placed on improved timing and speed.
- *Travel activities.* The patient should become proficient in walking sideward and backward, turning, and walking through doorways. Changes in floor surface (e.g., carpeting, tile) and terrain (sidewalks and grass) may present problems for the patient if they are not introduced during training. All patients will require proficiency in ambulation on level surfaces to master these more difficult activities successfully.
- *Elevation activities.* The easiest pattern of ascent or descent of stairs is usually upstairs backward (Fig. 23.40) and downstairs forward (Fig. 23.41). Most patients will use a handrail; only the very exceptional patient can manage stairs without one. Once some degree of proficiency is attained, going upstairs forward and downstairs backward can be practiced as well. The use of graduated steps will help make the initial task of learning easier. The therapist needs to guard and to support the patient adequately. The use of a properly fitting guarding belt is essential. Curbs should be attempted last, because this is usually the most difficult elevation activity. Using graduated platforms or curbs will assist the patient in mastery of this task. A four-point gait pattern, going up backward and down forward is the slower, more

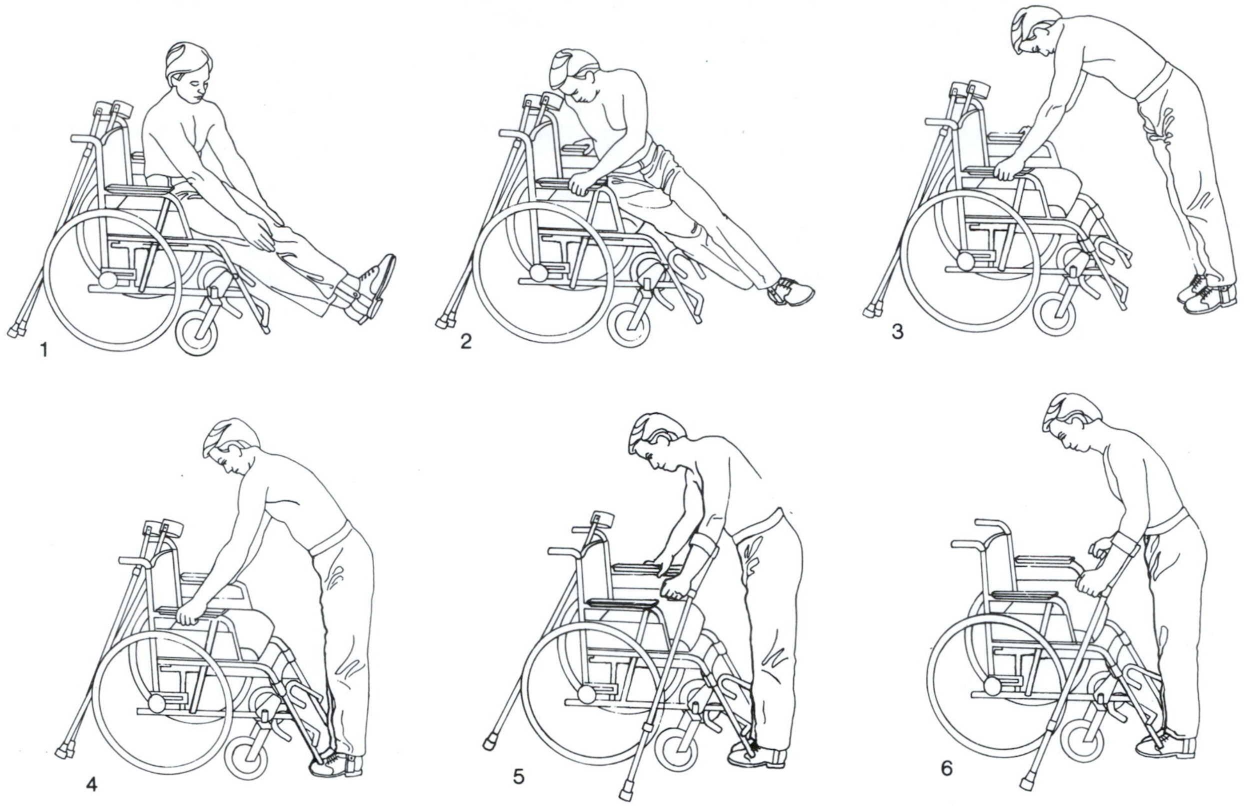

Figure 23.39 Standing from wheelchair using crutches and bilateral knee-ankle-foot orthoses. The reverse sequence is used to return to the chair.

stable method. Swinging both legs up together takes considerable balance and is for the more advanced ambulator.

- *Falling.* Controlled falling and getting up from the floor are important considerations for patients expected to become functional ambulators.

Locomotor Training for Individuals with Incomplete Spinal Cord Injury

Locomotor training using partial body weight support (BWS), a treadmill (TM), and manual assistance by trainers is a relatively new therapeutic intervention to retrain walking after SCI. Terms to describe this training include *body weight supported treadmill training*, *partial body weight supported treadmill training*, or *weight supported treadmill training*. These terms emphasize the exercise or training equipment that is currently advocated for retraining walking by medical equipment manufacturers and by some clinicians and researchers, however, the terms fail to describe the critical elements of the

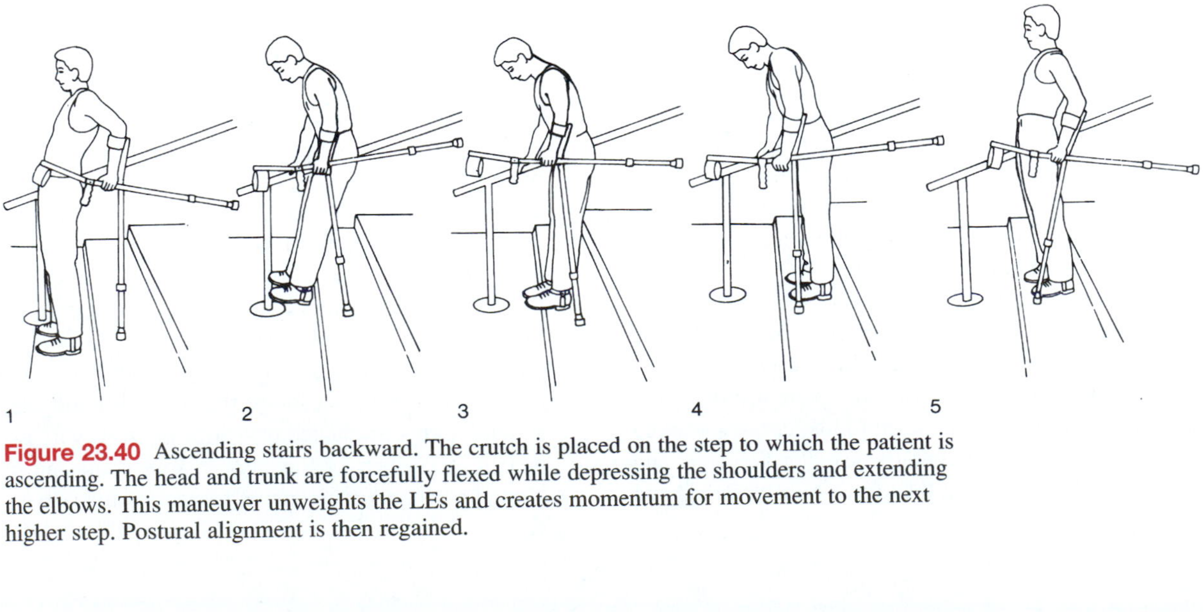

Figure 23.40 Ascending stairs backward. The crutch is placed on the step to which the patient is ascending. The head and trunk are forcefully flexed while depressing the shoulders and extending the elbows. This maneuver unweights the LEs and creates momentum for movement to the next higher step. Postural alignment is then regained.

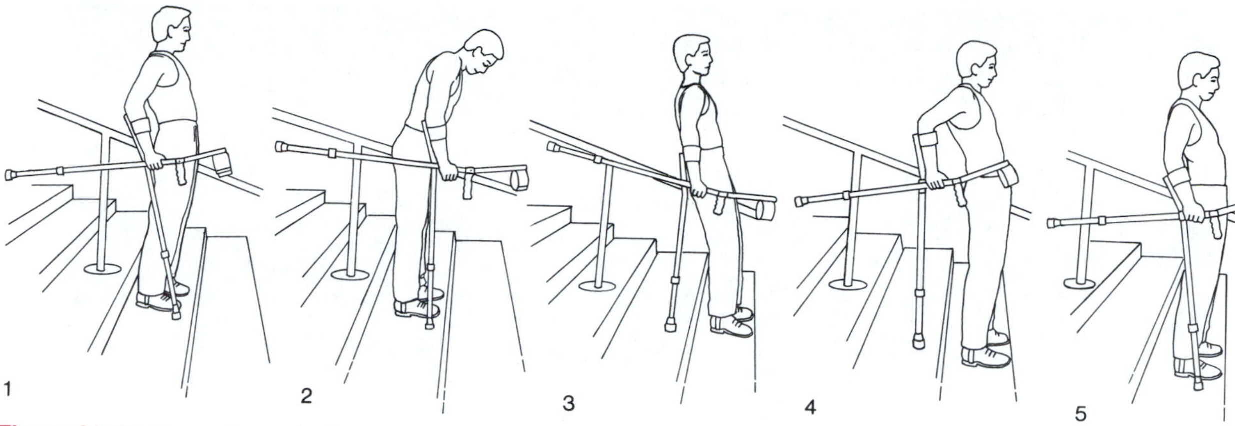

Figure 23.41 Descending stairs forward. To begin, the crutch remains on the step that the patient is leaving. Initial flexion of the head and trunk is immediately followed by forceful extension while depressing the shoulders and extending the elbow. This procedure unweights the LEs and creates momentum for the movement to the next lower step. The crutch is then lowered and postural alignment regained.

training. What does a therapist actually do with a patient to retrain walking using this equipment? As this intervention is relatively new, its use is in transition from an experimental intervention to that of an evidence-based intervention. This section describes: (1) locomotor training and how it differs from conventional gait training approaches for persons with SCI; (2) the clinical guidelines for selection and use of locomotor training strategies; and (3) evidence supporting use of locomotor training following SCI.

Locomotor training is a product of *translational research* or *bridge research*. Knowledge gained by basic science researchers concerning the neurobiological control of walking laid the foundation for developing a therapeutic intervention with application to human, clinical populations. Basic scientists seeking to understand the role and contribution of the spinal cord to the control of walking used an animal model of complete SCI for their inquiries. They discovered that when mid-thoracic spinalized cats were placed on a treadmill, suspended by a sling, and repetitively trained for hind-limb stepping with assistance of trainers for loading and limb placement that the animals learned to hind-limb step (on the treadmill) independent of supraspinal input.[157,158] Furthermore, this intense training was task-specific in that the spinalized cats could be trained to stand, or to step, but that training to perform one task did not transfer to performance of the other task.[159] Seminal research in this arena stimulated a neuroscientist and physical therapist, Hugues Barbeau, to attempt the same strategy for retraining walking in humans after traumatic SCI: translational research.

Barbeau and co-workers published the first studies in which humans were partially suspended with a body weight support apparatus over a treadmill to examine its impact on gait[160,161] and then provided training similar to that experienced by the cats for persons with SCI.[162] Though a suspension system and treadmill appear to be strong common denominators of the training, the equipment is likely not the dominant, critical component. The equipment provides an effective and controlled environment for consistent and intense practice of walking that can closely approximate the sensory experience of walking. The successes of the spinalized cats and improvements in walking by humans after incomplete SCI were attributed to activity-dependent plasticity of the neural axis.[163] Activity-dependent plasticity or the responsiveness of the spinal cord to task-specific practice and its capacity to learn were new concepts and revolutionary for the rehabilitation of persons after SCI.[164] The spinal cord and neural axis were responsive to the ensemble of sensory information specific to walking and generated a motor response for stepping. Many researchers and clinicians, including Barbeau, continue to translate knowledge from basic science into developing a rehabilitation intervention to retrain walking after neurologic injury or disease.[165–169] In parallel, other researchers focus on testing this intervention's efficacy and effectiveness for the recovery of walking after SCI.[170–175]

Historically, rehabilitation for ambulation after SCI has been built on the premise that the spinal cord is neither "plastic" (adaptable), nor can it can learn. After SCI, clinicians thus set goals to maximize use and strength of the musculature remaining under voluntary control and to substitute for weak or paralyzed muscles with braces and/or assistive devices. Thus, therapists taught alternative strategies for ambulation that incorporated braces and assistive devices and compensatory gait patterns. In contrast, locomotor training is a means of intensely practicing the distinct and specific task of walking (providing the sensory experience of walking) with the aim of tapping into the intrinsic neural pathways responsible for generating steps. This strategy may be viewed as a relative "bottom-up" approach, emphasizing the sensory experience of walking to drive the motor response of walking. In contrast, teaching new strategies to walk, such as "brace-walking" is a relative "top-down" approach requiring the development of a new skill with which to be upright and to ambulate

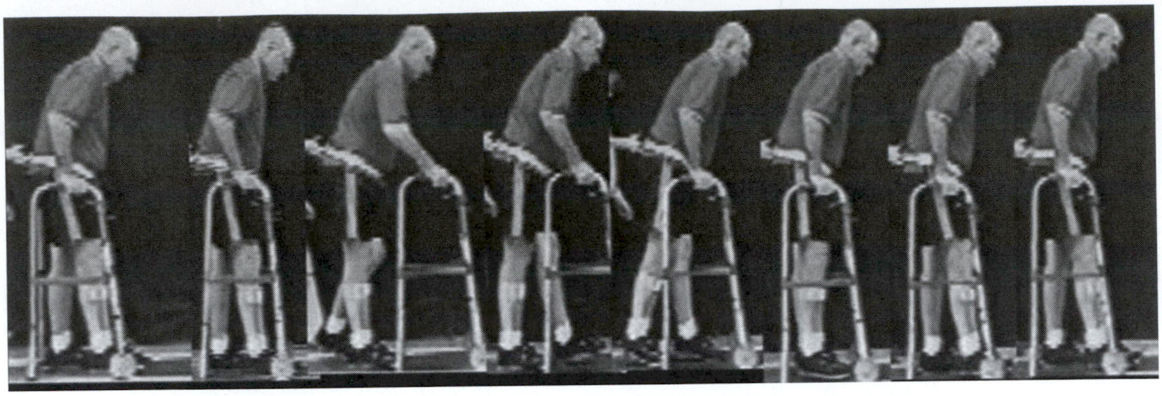

Figure 23.42 Gait pattern of a person with an incomplete spinal cord injury using a rolling walker and right ankle foot orthosis.

(see previous section). Certainly, sensory and cognitive processing is required for both strategies, however the relative emphasis may differ.

Locomotor training is to *train like you walk*. It requires defining the task of walking, its kinematics, kinetics, spatial–temporal pattern, posture, balance, and adaptability. It also requires an environment to experience the specific task of walking and intense practice, with progression toward independence in the task of walking.

Figure 23.42 contains a series of photos of a person walking with a rolling walker and a right AFO at a walking speed of 0.13 m/s using a traditional approach to gait retraining after SCI. Is this individual effectively practicing the task of walking? What elements are consistent with the task of walking and what elements are inconsistent with the task of walking? For instance, moving from point A to point B while upright is consistent with the task of walking. However, a forward flexed trunk and head aimed at the ground, weightbearing through the arms, hip extension to neutral, uneven step lengths, hiking the right hip, vaulting on the left toe, no knee flexion on the right, and the slow walking speed are not consistent with the task of walking.

Train like you walk translates into the following practical training guidelines: (1) the LEs are maximally loaded for weightbearing, minimizing or eliminating loading of the arms; (2) the posture, trunk, pelvis, and limb kinematics are coordinated and specific to the task of walking, and (3) compensatory strategies for movement (i.e., hip hiking) are minimized or eliminated.[174] As with learning any skill, practice and repetition are important and carryover beyond the clinic is critical. Persons with incomplete SCI may exhibit compromised balance; weakness in the trunk, upper limbs, and lower limbs; increased or decreased muscle activity in flexors or extensors; symmetrical or asymmetrical impairments; and in some, an inability to stand without lower or upper limb support. To practice the specific task of walking for this population, a training environment must afford safety, support, task-specific repetition of walking, and a means to challenge and progress abilities.

An appropriate BWS system and TM provide this opportunity. The patient wearing a trunk/pelvis harness is supported by an overhead and adjustable suspension system over a TM. Trainers require access to the trunk/pelvis and lower limbs to facilitate upright posture, weight shift, and limb movements. This environment affords control of the amount of lower limb loading, assists in upright posture and balance, and allows control of the speed of walking (Fig. 23.43).[176] With 35 percent BWS, manual assistance at the trunk and pelvis to promote upright posture and minimize hip hiking, and lower limb trainers promoting step symmetry, hip extension, and hip/knee flexion on the right, the individual is able to walk at a speed of 0.8 to 1.0 m/sec. The therapist must determine what elements of practice are consistent with the task of walking and what elements are inconsistent with the task of walking. If the aim is task-specific training then this is perhaps a good starting point for training. Each of these parameters then becomes a means of progression[176] by adjusting load, treadmill speed, and amount of manual assistance (independence). As with any training protocol, intensity is required, thus achieving 20 to 30 minutes of total stepping time is recommended, with increasing duration of each training bout. Goals must also be set to address adaptability for negotiating the environment and for meeting the behavioral demands of the individual for walking.[177]

The same training principles should be applied outside of the BWS system and TM environment. Adaptations can be made for training overground to *train like you walk*. In the example from figure 23.42, the rolling walker can afford speed, however, this individual's posture and inability to flex his right knee preclude any faster speed. The lack of upright posture also limits hip extension range and loading, likely necessary precursors to initiating swing. Several suggestions are to have this individual practice upright standing with his back to a wall and his walker to load his legs as opposed to his arms (Fig. 23.44), to have him stand weightbearing solely on the left and with his right leg flexed on a stool or chair (Fig. 23.45A and B), and to elevate the height of his walker to encourage upright posture.[176] Certainly, use of

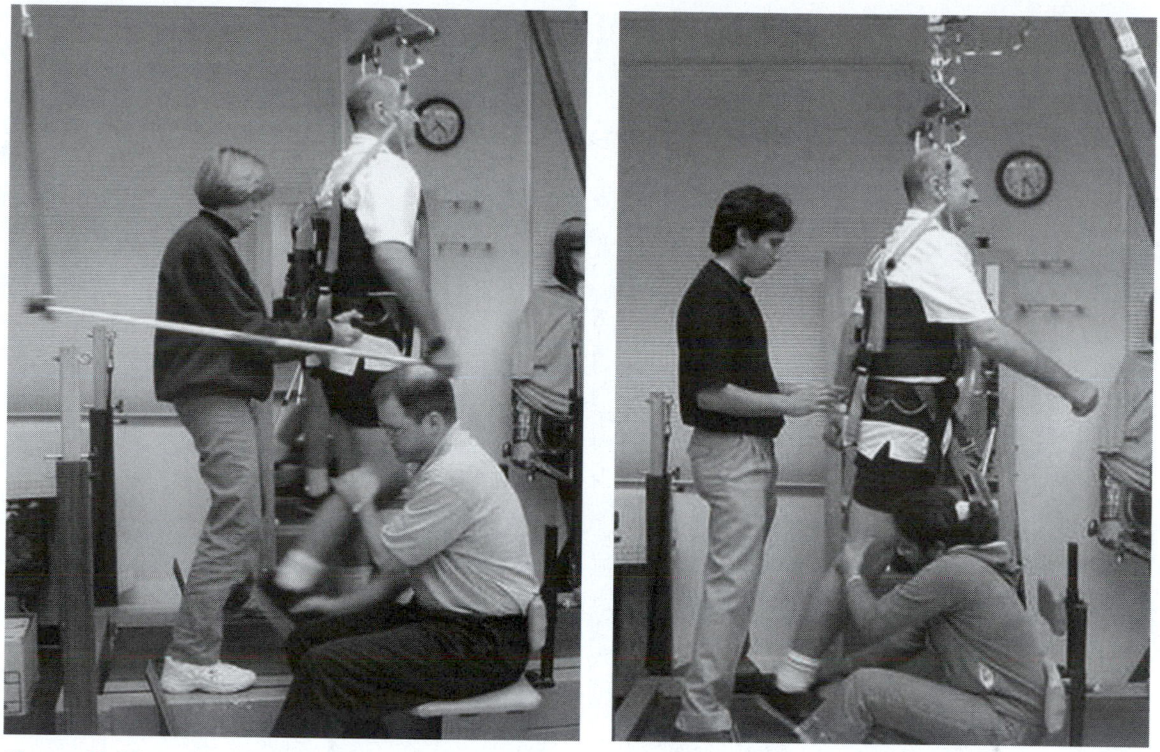

Figure 23.43 Locomotor training for a person with an incomplete SCI using the body weight support, treadmill, and manual assistance by trainers.

the BWS system and TM has advantages and may be the optimal environment for consistent practice, but the transition and application to community ambulation is also critical (Fig. 23.46).

Locomotor training principles can thus be applied while on the TM with a BWS system and overground for community ambulation and encompasses both of these environments. Transferring skills acquired in one environment to another is an important element for learning and can be reinforced by a daily examination of the walking abilities overground and on the treadmill with BWS.[176] Modifying the parameters of training in both environments will challenge the use of new skills, reinforce new patterns and independence, and afford information for goal-setting across environments.

Clinical guidelines for locomotor training and for safe and effective use of the BWS system and TM as therapeutic equipment are essential to the practice of evidence-based physical therapy for rehabilitation following SCI. Such guidelines have not yet been developed; research is in the early stages of examining efficacy and effectiveness. As research findings are published, clinicians should seek information to guide their decision-making and practice. Clinicians should seek information from the literature that will identify: (1) who will benefit from locomotor training with the aim of improving the ability to walk, i.e., persons classified according to ASIA A, B, C, or D impairments (see Table 23.1); persons who already walk, but not well; persons who have a particular clinical motor or sensory presentation; or persons at a particular neurological

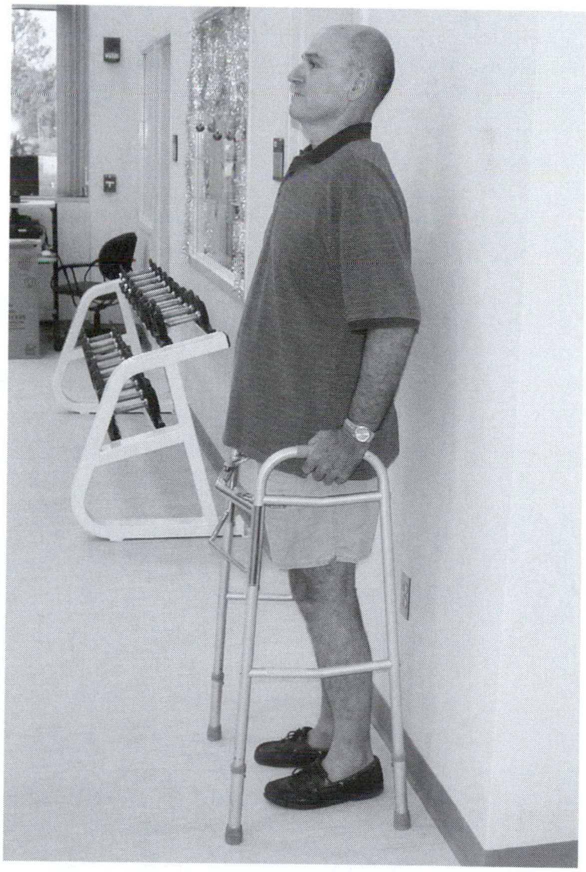

Figure 23.44 Locomotor training principles applied to the task of standing with upright posture for a person with incomplete SCI.

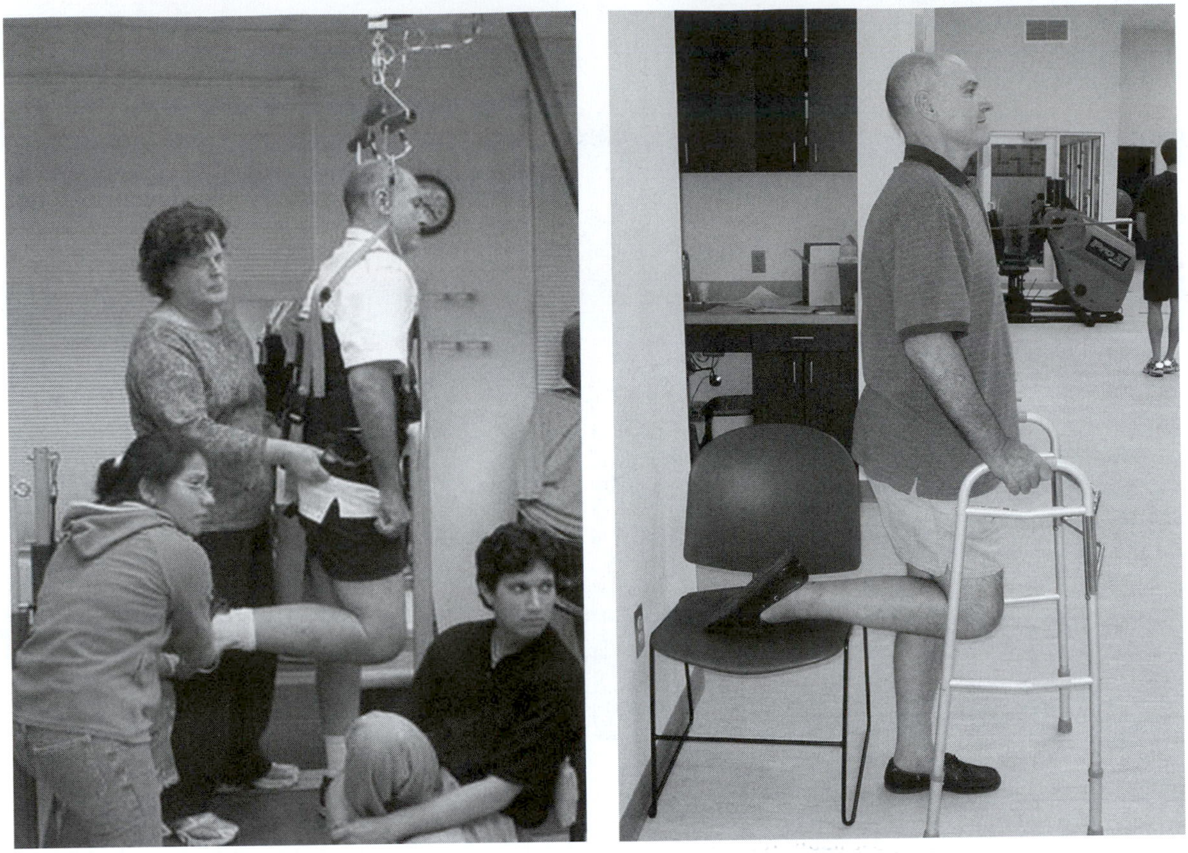

A B

Figure 23.45 Locomotor training principles applied to standing upright while practicing loading and extension on the left lower limb while the right lower limb is unloaded and flexed on the treadmill with body weight support (*A*) and overground with a walker (*B*).

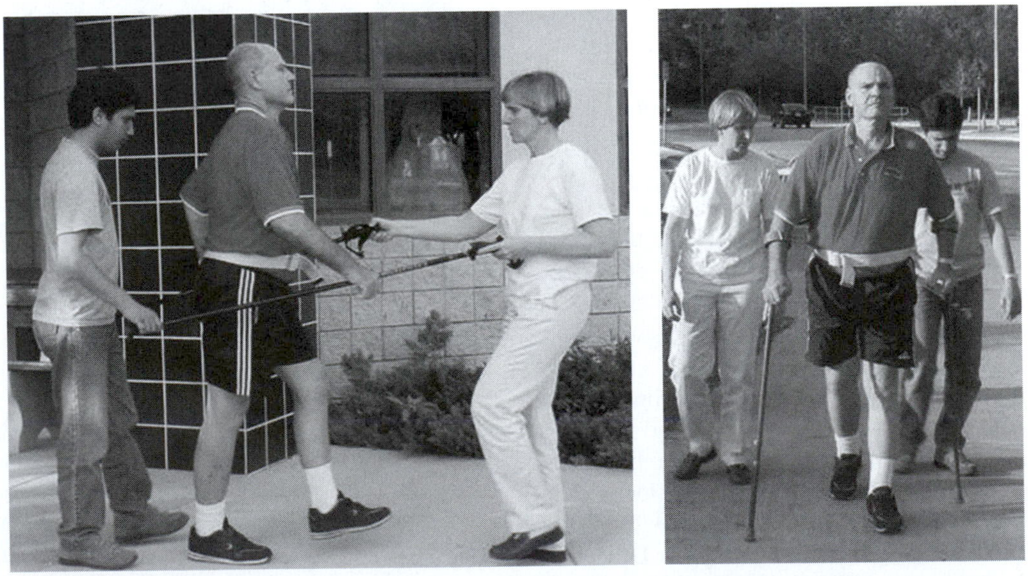

Figure 23.46 Translation of skills acquired on the treadmill to walking overground and community ambulation

level of injury, thus the severity of injury[178]; (2) when is the best time post-injury to provide an intervention for optimal recovery of walking, i.e., in the acute stage of rehabilitation, after discharge from rehabilitation, or how long after SCI and thus, the appropriate time after injury[178]; (3) what is the optimal dose of therapy, i.e. intensity, frequency, and duration of the training; (4) how to train and progress a patient, how to use the BWS system and TM equipment, how to examine new training equipment as it reaches the market (i.e., suspension systems, robotic devices), how to monitor the trainers' body ergonomics during training; (5) any medical precautions and safety issues for persons with SCI and their effect on locomotor training, i.e., autonomic dysreflexia, skin, bowel and bladder, falling, osteoporosis, spasticity, cardiovascular health; (6) what therapies may augment locomotor training or what combined therapies enhance the recovery of walking, i.e., strengthening, functional electrical stimulation[179–183]; and the (7) cost–benefit; i.e., cost to provide this intervention in the clinic including equipment and personnel; reimbursement policies; and outcomes and value to the patient and community.

Currently, the literature (case studies, small n, efficacy studies) indicates that following locomotor training (LT) or gait therapy that incorporated use of a BWS system and TM in subacute[173] and post-acute rehabilitation that persons with incomplete SCI (ASIA Impairment Scale classification C and D [see Table 23.1]) improved in balance, gait speed, endurance, stair-climbing, and independence[170–172,174,175] (see Evidence Summary Box 23.1). Safety and feasibility for providing LT to persons with incomplete SCI during acute rehabilitation has also been established.[184] For instance, clinical adaptations were required to safely train persons having a halo, a catheter and drainage bag or bladder/bowel impairments, sensory impairment, and susceptibility to orthostatic hypotension or autonomic dysreflexia. The question of whether providing LT has benefit during the active rehabilitation phase warrants further investigation.

Another important area for research is the benefits of LT to a person's health after SCI. Does LT decrease the risk of pressure sores or bladder infections; reduce bone loss or muscle atrophy? Do benefits for health warrant increased access to LT? Can robotic devices provide an avenue to cost-effectively provide this service?

The advent of locomotor training represents a new era in spinal cord rehabilitation. This era, brought forth by partnership among basic scientists, rehabilitation scientists, physicians, and clinicians, encompasses knowledge of the neurobiological control of walking and the physiological promise of activity-dependent plasticity as bases for developing new interventions and advancing the potential for recovery after SCI.

Functional Electrical Stimulation

Functional electrical stimulation (FES) is the application of low-level electrical current to improve function in paralyzed and/or weak muscles. FES can be used for a variety of purposes to improve function and quality of life for individuals with SCI; these include: cardiovascular training,[185–187] breathing,[188–190] UE function,[191–194] ambulation,[195–199] transfers and standing,[200] and bowel and bladder function.[201] FES can be applied using surface electrodes, percutaneous electrodes or surgically implanted electrodes. The electrical stimulation is interfaced with a computer, which controls the timing and onset of stimulation. Research regarding the use and design of these systems is ongoing.

Prevention, Health Promotion, Fitness, and Wellness

Improvements in medical care, rehabilitation techniques and technology have increased the life span of individuals with SCI. Because of the variety of secondary complications that these individuals are at risk for developing throughout their life span, it is important to develop effective prevention and fitness strategies that can be carried out after patients have finished their rehabilitation.

Shoulder Pain

Shoulder pain is relatively common after SCI.[202,203] The cause of shoulder pain is associated with a variety of factors. These factors include: duration of injury, weightbearing, wheelchair use, poor seated posture, age, body mass index, level of injury, muscle imbalance at the shoulder joint complex, and decreased ROM.[202–205] Generally speaking the pain is biomechanical in nature. The method in which an individual with a SCI must perform ADLs and mobility (i.e., transfer with weightbearing on the UEs, reach overhead from a seated position in a wheelchair in an internally rotated shoulder posture to reach objects on a counter, and propel a wheelchair for locomotion) cause the shoulder complex to be under greater mechanical stress than in persons without SCI. Functions that are normally performed by the trunk and LEs must now be performed by the UEs. Prevention of shoulder pain is vital. Proper postural alignment is a key factor as well as strengthening and stretching shoulder musculature.[202,206]

Exercise

Just as with individuals without disability, exercise is important for individuals with SCI. A well designed endurance training and resistance training program has been shown to improve function, strength, endurance, respiratory function, perceived health, and quality of life.[206–209] The American College of Sports Medicine recommends exercising three to five times a week at 50 to 80 percent of peak HR. Common endurance exercise modalities include: UE ergometer, wheelchair propulsion, swimming, and circuit resistance training.[206] Strength training recommendations include 8 to 12 repetitions per exercise for two sessions per

Evidence Summary Box 23.1

Selected Studies Examining the Use of Locomotor Training

Reference	Subjects	Methods/Procedure	Results	Comments
Wernig, A, et al[170] 1995	E Ss=45 acute injury, within "weeks" of injury E Ss=44 chronic injury, median time since injury: 12 months C Ss=40 acute injury C Ss=24 chronic injury, median time since injury: 24 months	Quasi-experimental with historical controls, E outcomes in E group compared to historical group (C group) that received conventional PT previously. Acute E group received BWSTT for 30 min/day, 5 days/week for 4 months. Chronic E group received BWSTT for 30 min/day, 5 days/week for 2.5 months. Acute C group received "conventional PT" for 4 months Chronic C group received "conventional PT" for 2.5 months	Acute E group: 92% improved in walking ability to a 3–5 on FAC. Chronic E group: 78% improved in walking ability to a 3–5 on FAC. Acute C group: 50% improved in walking ability to a 3–5 on FAC. Chronic C group: 7% improved in walking ability to a 3–5 on FAC.	Authors did not describe well how the actual BWSTT was carried out in terms of manual assistance and TM speed. There was not a concomitant increase in LE strength with improvement in walking ability in the E groups.
Nymark, J, et al[173] 1998	Ss=5, ASIA B–D, mean 36 days s/p injury, undergoing active rehabilitation in rehab hospital. Initially none of the subjects could ambulate.	Case series. Ss received BWSTT 3 days/week for 12 weeks. Initial BWS 26%–83%, 3 Ss progressed to 0% BWS by end. Initial TM training speed: 0.15–0.30 m/s, final TM training speed: 0.2–0.6 m/s. Mean duration of each training walk initially: 3–7 min, final: 6–9 min.	All subjects demonstrated improvement in walking ability on the COVS ambulation subscore. 4 of 5 subjects demonstrated increase in strength.	Specifics in terms of how manual assistance provided during BWSTT not provided.
Gardner, MB, et al[171] 1998	Ss=1, 28 years old, 7 months post- injury. Incomplete C5–C6 injury. Able to ambulate independently without AD or orthosis.	Single subject design: A1 phase: 6 weeks of no intervention, B phase: 6 weeks of 3 ×/week of BWSTT of 20 min of training using a modified Bruce protocol, A2 phase: 3 weeks of no intervention.	Ss demonstrated improvement in comfortable walking and fast walking gait speed during B phase and maintained during A2 phase.	No manual assistance provided during training. ASIA score of subject not provided. High functioning Ss prior to treatment.
Behrman, AL, and Harkema, SJ[174] 2000	Ss=4. Ss 1: 20 years old T5 SCI, ASIA A, 1 year post-injury, nonambulatory. Ss 2: 20 years old T5 SCI, ASIA C, 1 months post-injury, nonambulatory. Ss 3: 43 years old C6 SCI, ASIA C, 8 months post-injury. Ss 4: 45 years old T9 SCI, ASIA D, 3 months post-injury.	Case series. LT × 3 week. Ss1: 85 sessions of LT with BWS and TM Ss2: 64 sessions of LT with BWS and TM, 44 sessions of LT overground. Ss3: 27 sessions of LT with BWS and TM, 15 sessions of LT overground. Ss 4: 5 sessions of LT on TM, subject did not require BWS. Initial BWS ranged from 45% to 0%, final BWS ranged from 25% to 0%. TM speed of 0.75–1.25 m/s. Goal of three 10-minute walks/session.	Ss1: able to take 3–10 consecutives steps on TM with 10% BWS with manual assistance only for foot placement. Ss2: FIM walking score improved from 1 to a 6, gait speed improved to 0.53 m/s, and 2-min walk distance improved to 67 m. Ss3: FIM walking score stayed constant (6 at both pre- and posttest), but pre-treatment used W/C as primary means of mobility and	LT protocol well described. Ss also demonstrated improvement in measures of handicap after training.

Evidence Summary Box 23.1

Selected Studies Examining the Use of Locomotor Training (continued)

Reference	Subjects	Methods/Procedure	Results	Comments
			posttreatment walking was primary means of mobility, gait speed improved from 0.09 m/s to 0.33 m/s, and 2-min walk distance improved from 12 m to 68 m. Ss 4: walking speed improved from 0.6 m/s to 1.6 m/s.	
Protas, EJ, et al[175] 2000	Ss=3, T8–T12 SCI, ASIA C-D, 2–13 years post-injury	Case Series. STAT 1 hour/day, 5 days/week for 12 weeks. Targeted a total of 20 min of walking/session. Overground walking attempted after 3 weeks of training.	Improvement in walking speed, pretest mean=0.12 m/s, posttest mean=0.32 m/s; and distance in 5-min walk: pretest mean=20.3 m, posttest mean=63.5 m.	Ss also demonstrated improvement in $\dot{V}O_2$ consumption, balance and self-reported handicap.
Field-Fote, EC[180] 2001	Ss=19, ASIA C 56 months post-injury (median)	Before and after comparison. 36 sessions (3 days/week for 12 weeks) of combined BWS with FES. FES to the peroneal nerve to elicit a flexor withdrawal at terminal stance with up to 30% BWS.	Improvement in walking speed, pretest mean=0.12 m/s, posttest mean=0.21 m/s.	Ss did not receive manual assistance when training. FES used to facilitate stepping.

AD = Assistive device; ASIA = American Spinal Injury Association; BWS = body weight support; BWSTT = body weight support treadmill training; C = control group; COVS = clinical outcome variables; E = experimental group; FAC = functional ambulation category; FES = functional electrical stimulation; FIM = functional independence neasure; LT = locomotor training; m = meters; m/s = meters/second; SCI = spinal cord injury; Ss = subjects; STAT = supported treadmill ambulation training; TM = treadmill; W/C = wheelchair.

week using one of the following exercise modalities: free weights, weight machines or elastic tubing.[206]

Education

An important aspect of long-range rehabilitation planning involves educating the patient in lifelong management of the disability. This will focus on community reintegration and methods of maintaining the optimal state of health and function achieved during rehabilitation. Consideration must be given to multiple issues, including housing, nutrition, transportation, finances, maintaining functional skills and level of physical fitness, employment or further education, and methods for involvement in desired social or recreational activities. Each of these issues must be addressed early in the course of rehabilitation in consultation with the patient, family, and appropriate team members. Educating the patient will allow him or her to make informed decisions regarding medical care and life style choices throughout the lifespan. There are a plethora of resources available on the Internet. Patients should be encouraged to contact and to explore the available resources. Appendix B lists some of the many resources available both for patients and clinicians.

Finally, a coordinated plan should be developed for long-term periodic medical and rehabilitation follow-up.

Summary

This chapter has presented the principal clinical manifestations, indirect impairments, and secondary complications of traumatic SCI. Emphasis has been placed on physical therapy intervention during both the acute medical management and active rehabilitation stages of recovery. Anticipated goals, expected outcomes, and treatment interventions have been addressed. Each must be tailored to meet the needs of an individual patient. This will be achieved through a process of careful examination with specific attention to length of time since onset, lesion level, method(s) of fracture stabilization, premorbid interests, psychosocial factors, and presence of secondary complications.

Management of the patient with SCI is a complex and challenging task in which continuity of care is critical to achieving the overall goals of rehabilitation. Frequent and open communication among team members, patient, family, and caregivers is vital to maintaining an organized and highly individualized approach to both rehabilitation and reintegration of the patient into the community.

Questions for Review

1. Identify the clinical features of Brown-Sequard, anterior, central, and posterior cord syndromes.
2. Define spinal shock.
3. Describe the impairments associated with spinal cord injury. Your description should address alterations that occur in each of the following areas:
    - Motor function
    - Sensory function
    - Temperature control
    - Respiratory function
    - Muscle tone
    - Bladder and bowel function
4. What is autonomic dysreflexia? Describe the initiating stimuli and symptoms of this syndrome. What action would you take if a patient experienced an onset of symptoms during a physical therapy treatment?
5. What is heterotopic ossification? Describe the early symptoms. Where does it most commonly develop following SCI?
6. Describe the clinical features of deep venous thrombosis. Why are patients with SCI at risk for development of this secondary complication?
7. Suggest a positioning program to prevent limitations in ROM at the shoulders for a patient with tetraplegia during the acute phase of management.
8. Identify three primary factors affecting prognosis following spinal cord injury.
9. Describe the major advantages of halo devices as compared with tongs for immobilizing cervical fractures.
10. What is included in a physical therapy examination during the acute medical management phase of recovery? How might some of the standard examination techniques need to be modified?
11. What is meant by the term *selective stretching*?
12. Identify the primary goals of respiratory care during the acute phase of management. Suggest potential treatment activities to meet these goals.
13. What forms of strengthening exercises are appropriate during the acute phase? Why are bilateral UE activities emphasized?
14. Outline sample mat progressions for two patients, one with a C6 tetraplegia and one with a T12 paraplegia. Assume that both patients have complete lesions. Describe the specific mat sequence and activities you would include. Identify the functional significance of each. What type of progressive strengthening activities would you suggest for each patient as an adjunct to the mat program?
15. Describe how you would modify training parameters when performing locomotor training utilizing a BWS and TM system for an individual with an incomplete SCI.

Case Study

HISTORY

The patient is a 21-year-old white man who was transferred to a rehabilitation hospital yesterday. He suffered a traumatic cervical spinal cord injury 8 days ago. He was given methylprednisolone in the ER. He had surgery to stabilize fracture site, internal fixation and decompression using a R iliac bone graft. He was discharged to your facility yesterday and is currently wearing a Philadelphia collar. He is able to extend his elbows but cannot flex his fingers in either hand. He is a senior at college, computer science major. Lives in on-campus apartment, not w/c accessible. His parents live in the next state.

MEDICATIONS

Lovenox, midodrine, amitriptyline, OxyContin, and Dulcolax.

PHYSICAL THERAPY EXAMINATION

Cardiopulmonary

HR: 75
BP: supine: 110/72; sitting: 100/66
Forced vital capacity: 2.2 liters
Weak, nonproductive cough

Communication/Cognition

Alert, oriented × 3, able to follow multistep commands

Muscle Performance

Bilateral: biceps: 5/5, wrist extensors: 5/5, triceps: 4/5, no active contraction below C7

Sensory Integrity

Intact pin prick and light touch C2–T4, absent below T4.
Intact anal sensation.
Proprioception intact in bilateral UEs, absent below.

Functional Mobility

Bed mobility: moderate assistance to roll to the left and right
Supine ↔ short sit: maximal assistance
Supine ↔ long sit: maximal assistance
Transfer wheelchair ↔ bed: FIM score 2 (requires maximal assistance with transfer board)
Transfer wheelchair ↔ toilet: FIM score 2 (requires maximal assistance with transfer board)

Locomotion

Unable to ambulate.
Able to propel wheelchair 150 ft on level surface with minimal assistance

Wheelchair Skills

Requires assistance with locking wheel locks, removing footrests and armrests, and to perform pressure relief. Wheelchair Skills Test score: 4%.
Currently using a loaner folding wheelchair with contoured high back and gel filled cushion.
Tolerates sitting in wheelchair for 20 to 30 minutes

Balance

Long sitting: able to maintain balance on mat for 1 minute with UEs in weightbearing position with supervision
Short sitting: able to maintain balance on edge of mat for 1 minute with UEs in weightbearing position with minimal assistance

Motor Function

Increased spasticity in bilateral hip flexors, 2 on modified Ashworth Scale

PROM

WNL except bilateral ankle dorsiflexion is 10° from neutral.

Skin Integrity

Stage 1 wound on right heel.

Self-Care

Dressing upper body: FIM score 2 (requires maximal assistance)
Dressing lower body: FIM score 1 (dependent)
Bathing: FIM score 1 (dependent using shower chair)
Feeding: FIM score 3 (moderate assistance with adapted utensils)
Grooming: FIM score 3 (moderate assistance with adapted utensils)
Toileting: FIM score 2 (maximal assistance)

Bowel and Bladder

Bladder: FIM score 1 (just began intermittent catheterization program and requires total assist to manage)
Bowel: FIM score 1 (just began bowel training program with nursing, has been incontinent of bowel during the past day)

GUIDING QUESTIONS

1. What is the patient's neurological level of injury, motor level of injury, and sensory level of injury? What is the patient's ASIA impairment classification?
2. Identify/categorize this patient's problems in terms of
   - Direct impairments
   - Indirect impairments
   - Composite impairments (combined effects of both direct and indirect impairments)
   - Functional limitations/disabilities
3. Identify three anticipated goals and three expected outcomes (remediation of functional limitations/disability) for this patient.
4. Formulate three treatment interventions with one progression that could be used during the first 3 weeks of therapy. Provide a brief rationale that justifies your choice.
5. Identify relevant motor learning strategies appropriate for the initial physical therapy sessions with this patient.

References

1. National Spinal Cord Injury Statistical Center: Spinal Cord Injury: Facts and Figures at a Glance, August 2004. National Spinal Cord Injury Statistical Center. University of Alabama, Birmingham, AL 35249-7330. Retrieved March 12, 2006 from http://www.spinalcord.uab.edu/show.asp?durki=21446.
2. National Spinal Cord Injury Statistical Center: The 2004 Annual Statistical Report for the Model Spinal Cord Injury Care Systems. National Spinal Cord Injury Statistical Center, University of Alabama, Birmingham, AL 35249-7330. Retrieved March 12, 2006 from http://images.main.uab.edu/spinalcord/pdffiles/2004StatReport.pdf.
3. Jackson, AB, et al: A demographic profile of new traumatic spinal cord injuries: Change and stability over 30 years. Arch Phys Med Rehabil 85:1740, 2004.
4. Coogler, CE: Clinical decision making among neurologic patients: Spinal cord injury. In Wolf, SL (ed): Clinical Decision Making in Physical Therapy. FA Davis, Philadelphia, 1985, p 149.

5. American Spinal Injury Association: International Standards for Neurological Classification of Spinal Cord Injury. American Spinal Injury Association, Chicago Illinois, 2002.
6. Hislop, HJ, and Montgomery, J: Daniels and Worthingham's Muscle Testing: Techniques of Manual Examination, ed 7. WB Saunders, Philadelphia, 2002.
7. Rieser, TV, et al: Orthopedic evaluation of spinal cord injury and management of vetebral fractures. In Adkins, HV (ed): Spinal Cord Injury. Churchill Livingstone, New York, 1985, p 1.
8. Gilman, S, and Newman, SW: Maner and Gatz's Essentials of Clinical Neuroanatomy and Neurophysiology, ed 10. FA Davis, Philadelphia, 2003.
9. Lundy-Ekman, L: Neuroscience: Fundamentals for Rehabilitation, ed 2. WB Saunders, Philadelphia, 2002.
10. Atrice, MB, et al: Traumatic spinal cord injury. In Umphred, DA (ed): Neurological Rehabilitation, ed 4. CV Mosby, St. Louis, 2001, p 477.
11. Levi, AD, Tator, CH, and Bunge, RP: Clinical syndromes associated with disproportionate weakness of the upper versus the lower extremities after cervical spinal cord injury. Neurosurgery 38:179, 1996.
12. Alexeeva, N, et al: Central cord syndrome of cervical spinal cord injury: Widespread changes in muscle recruitment studied by voluntary contractions and transcranial magnetic stimulation. Exp Neurol 148:399, 1997.
13. Brodkey, JS, Miller, CF, Jr, and Harmody, RM: The syndrome of acute central cervical spinal cord injury revisited. Surg Neurol 14:251, 1980.
14. Esses, SI: Textbook of Spinal Disorders. JB Lippincott, Philadelphia, 1995.
15. Rogers, LF: Fractures and dislocations of the spine. In Calenoff, L (ed): Radiology of Spinal Cord Injury. CV Mosby, St. Louis, 1981.
16. McKinnis, LN: Fundamentals of Orthopedic Radiology. FA Davis, Philadelphia, 1997.
17. Buchanan, LE: An overview. In Buchanan, LE, and Nawoczenski, DA (eds): Spinal Cord Injury: Concepts and Management Approaches. Williams & Wilkins, Baltimore, 1987, p 1.
18. Buchanan, LE: Emergency care. In Buchanan, LE, and Nawoczenski, DA (eds):, Spinal Cord Injury: Concepts and Management Approaches. Williams & Wilkins, Baltimore, 1987, p 21.
19. English, E: Mechanisms of cervical spine injuries. In Tator, CH (ed): Early Management of Acute Spinal Cord Injury. Raven Press, New York, 1982, p 25.
20. Young, PA, and Young, PH: Basic Clinical Neuroanatomy. Williams & Wilkins, Baltimore, 1997.
21. Somers, MF: Spinal Cord Injury: Functional Rehabilitation, ed 2. Prentice-Hall, Upper Saddle River, NJ, 2001.
22. Ko, HY, et al: The pattern of reflex recovery during spinal shock. Spinal Cord 37:402, 1999.
23. Edibam, RC: Medical management. In Bedbrook, G (ed): The Care and Management of Spinal Cord Injuries. Springer-Verlag, New York, 1981, p 109.
24. Comarr, AE: Autonomic dysreflexia (hyperreflexia). J Am Paraplegia Soc 7:53, 1984.
25. Moeller, BA, and Scheinberg, D: Autonomic dysreflexia in injuries below the sixth thoracic segment. JAMA 224:1295, 1973.
26. Lindan, R, et al: Incidence and clinical features of autonomic dysreflexia in patients with spinal cord injury. Paraplegia 18:285, 1980.
27. Rosen, JS: Autonomic dysreflexia. In Calenoff, L (ed): Radiology of Spinal Cord Injury. CV Mosby, St. Louis, 1981, p 554.
28. Comarr, AE, and Eltorai, I: Symposium on autonomic dysreflexia. J Spinal Cord Med 20:345, 1996.
29. Comarr, AE: Autonomic dysreflexia. In Pierce, D, and Nickel, VH (ed): The Total Care of Spinal Cord Injuries. Little, Brown, Boston, 1977, p 181.
30. Yeo, JD: Recent research in spinal cord injuries. In Bedbrook, G (ed): The Care and Management of Spinal Cord Injuries. Springer-Verlag, New York, 1981, p 285.
31. McGarry, J, Woolsey, RM and Thompson, CW: Autonomic hyperreflexia following passive stretching to the hip joint. Phys Ther 62:30, 1982.
32. Erickson, RP: Autonomic hyperreflexia: Pathophysiology and medical management. Arch Phys Med Rehabil 61:431, 1980.
33. Rosen, JC: Rehabilitation process. In Calenoff, L (ed): Radiology of Spinal Cord Injury. CV Mosby, St. Louis, 1981, p 309.
34. Belson, P: Autonomic nervous system dysfunction in recent spinal cord injured patients: A physical therapist's perspective. In Eisenberg, MG, and Falconer, JA (eds): Treatment of the Spinal Cord Injured. Charles C Thomas, Springfield, IL, 1978, p 34.
35. Guyton, AC, and Hall, JE: Human Physiology and Mechanisms of Disease, ed 6. WB Saunders, Philadelphia, 1997.
36. Lemons, VR, and Wagner, FC: Respiratory complications after cervical spinal cord injury. Spine 19:2315, 1994.
37. Jackson, AB, and Groomes, TE: Incidence of respiratory complications following spinal cord injury. Arch Phys Med Rehabil 75:270, 1994.
38. Alvarez, SE, Peterson, M, and Lunsford, BR: Respiratory treatment of the adult patient with spinal cord injury. Phys Ther 61:1737, 1981.
39. Moore, KL: Clinically Oriented Anatomy, ed 3. Williams & Wilkins, Baltimore, 1992.
40. Smith, LK, et al: Brunnstrom's Clinical Kinesiology, ed 5. FA Davis, Philadelphia, 1996.
41. Nixon, V: Spinal Cord Injury: A Guide to Functional Outcomes in Physical Therapy Management. Aspen, Rockville, MD, 1985.
42. Bach, JR, and Wang, TG: Pulmonary function and sleep disordered breathing in patients with traumatic tetraplegia: A longitudinal study. Arch Phys Med Rehabil 75:279, 1994.
43. Wetzel, J: Respiratory evaluation and treatment. In Adkins, HV (ed): Spinal Cord Injury. Churchill Livingston, New York, 1985, p 75.
44. Seidel, AC: Spinal cord injury. In Logigian, MK (ed): Adult Rehabilitation: A Team Approach for Therapists. Little, Brown, Boston, 1982, p 325.
45. Campbell, SK, et al: The effects of intrathecally administered baclofen on function in patients with spasticity. Phys Ther 75:352, 1995.
46. Bromley, I: Tetraplegia and Paraplegia, ed 3. Churchill Livingston, New York, 1985.
47. Ditunno, JF, and Buchanan, LE: Acute care: Medical/surgical management. In Buchanan, LE, and Nawoczenski, DA (eds): Spinal Cord Injury: Concepts and Management Approaches. Williams &Wilkins, Baltimore, 1987, p 35.
48. Dolan, JT: Clinical management of the patient with a spinal disorder. In Ruppert, SD, et al (eds): Dolan's Critical Care Nursing: Clinical Management Through the Nursing Process. F.A. Davis, Philadelphia: 1991, p 613.
49. Cardenas, DD, Kelly, E, and Mayo, ME: Manual stimulation of reflex voiding after spinal cord injury. Arch Phys Med Rehabil 66:459, 1985.
50. Zejdlik, CP: Maintaining urinary function. In Zejdlik, CP (ed): Management of Spinal Cord Injury. Jones and Bartlett, Boston, 1992, p 353.
51. Comarr, AE, and Vigue, M: Sexual counseling among male and female patients with spinal cord and/or cauda equina injury. Am J Phys Med 57:107, 1978.
52. Trieschmann, RB: Spinal Injuries: Psychological, Social and Vocational Adjustment, ed 2. Demos Medical Publishing, New York, 1988.
53. Miller, S, Szasz, G, and Anderson, L: Sexual health care clinician in an acute spinal cord injury unit. Arch Phys Med Rehabil 62:315, 1981.
54. Weitzenkamp, DA, et al: Spouses of spinal cord injury survivors: The added impact of caregiving. Arch Phys Med Rehabil 78:822, 1997.
55. Dunn, KL: Sexuality education and the team approach. In Sipski, ML, and Alexander, CJ (eds): Sexual Function in People with Disabilities and Chronic Illness. Aspen, Gaithersburg, MD, 1997, p 381.
56. Brackett, NL, et al: An analysis of 653 trials of penile vibratory stimulation in men with spinal cord injury. J Urol 159:1931, 1998.
57. Pryor, JL, et al: Vibratory stimulation for treatment of anejaculation in quadriplegic men. Arch Phys Med Rehabil 76:59, 1995.
58. Brackett, NL, Padron, OF, and Lynne, CM: Semen quality of spinal cord injured men is better when obtained by vibratory stimulation versus electroejaculation. J Urol 157:151, 1997.
59. Brackett, NL, et al: Sperm from spinal cord injured men lose motility faster than sperm from normal men: The effect is exacerbated at body compared to room temperature. J Urol 157:2150, 1997.

60. Brackett, NL, Santa-Cruz, C, and Lynne, CM: Male fertility following spinal cord injury: Facts and fiction. Phys Ther 76:1221, 1996.
61. Brackett, NL, Bloch, WE, and Lynne, CM: Predictors of necrospermia in men with spinal cord injury. J Urol 159:844, 1998.
62. Kreuter, M, Sullivan M, and Siosteen, A: Sexual adjustment and quality of relationship in spinal paraplegia: A controlled study. Arch Phys Med Rehabil 77:541, 1996.
63. Chao, R, and Clowers, DE: Experience with intracavernosal tri-mixture for the management of neurogenic erectile dysfunction. Arch Phys Med Rehabil 75:276, 1994.
64. Brackett, NL, et al: Treatment by assisted conception of severe male factor infertility due to spinal cord injury or other neurologic impairment. J Assist Reprod Genet 12:210, 1995.
65. Higgins, GE: Sexual response in spinal cord injured adults: A review of the literature. Arch Sex Behav 8:173, 1979.
66. Gott, LJ: Anatomy and physiology of male sexual response and fertility as related to spinal cord injury. In Sha'ked, A (ed): Human Sexuality and Rehabilitation Medicine: Sexual Functioning Following Spinal Cord Injury. Williams & Wilkins, Baltimore, 1981, p 67.
67. Comarr, AE: Sexual function in patients with spinal cord injury. In Pierce, D, and Nickel, VH (eds): The Total Care of Spinal Cord Injuries. Little, Brown, Boston, 1977, p 67.
68. Hanak, M, and Scott, A: Spinal Cord Injury: An Illustrated Guide for Health Care Professionals. Springer-Verlag, New York, 1983.
69. Baker, ER, and Cardenas, DD: Pregnancy in spinal cord injured women. Arch Phys Med Rehabil 77:501, 1996.
70. Cross, LL, et al: Pregnancy, labor and delivery post spinal cord injury. Paraplegia 30:890, 1992.
71. Baker, ER, Cardenas, DD, and Benedetti, TJ: Risks associated with pregnancy in spinal cord-injured women. Obstet Gynecol 80:425, 1992.
72. Sipski, ML, and Alexander, CJ: Sexual activities, response and satisfaction in women pre- and post-spinal cord injury. Arch Phys Med Rehabil 74:1025, 1993.
73. Westgren, N, et al: Pregnancy and delivery in women with a traumatic spinal cord injury in Sweden, 1980–1991. Obstet Gynecol 81:926, 1993.
74. Sipski, ML, Alexander, CJ, and Rosen, RC: Orgasm in women with spinal cord injuries: A laboratory-based assessment. Arch Phys Med Rehabil 76:1097, 1995.
75. Levi, R, et al: The Stockholm spinal cord injury study: 1. Medical problems in a regional SCI population. Paraplegia 33:308, 1995.
76. Zejdlik, CP: Maintaining protective functions of the skin. In Zejdlik, CP (ed): Management of Spinal Cord Injury. Jones and Bartlett, Boston, 1992, p 451.
77. Nettina, SM: The Lippincott Manual of Nursing Practice, ed 6. Lippincott, Philadelphia, 1996.
78. Patterson, RP, et al: The impaired response of spinal cord injured individuals to repeated surface pressure loads. Arch Phys Med Rehabil 74:947, 1993.
79. Kernozek, TW, and Lewin, JE: Seat interface pressures of individuals with paraplegia: Influence of dynamic wheelchair locomotion compared with static seated measurements. Arch Phys Med Rehabil, 79:313, 1998.
80. Guyton, AC, and Hall, JE: Human Physiology and Mechanisms of Disease, ed 6. WB Saunders, Philadelphia, 1997.
81. McCagg, C: Postoperative management and acute rehabilitation of patients with spinal cord injuries. Orthop Clin North Am 17:171, 1986.
82. Turpie, A: Thrombosis prevention and treatment in spinal cord injured patients. In Bloch, R, and Basbaum, M (eds): Management of Spinal Cord Injuries. Williams & Wilkins, Baltimore, 1986, p 212.
83. Hendrix, RW: Soft tissue changes after spinal cord injury. In Calenoff, L (ed): Radiology of Spinal Cord Injury. CV Mosby, St. Louis, 1981, p 438.
84. Neiman, HL: Venography in acute spinal cord injury. In Calenoff, L (ed): Radiology of Spinal Cord Injury. CV Mosby, St. Louis, 1981, p 298.
85. van Hove, E: Prevention of thrombophlebitis in spinal injury patients. Paraplegia 16:332, 1978.
86. Todd, JW, et al: Deep venous thrombosis in acute spinal cord injury: A comparison of 125I fibrinogen leg scanning, impedance plethysmography and venography. Paraplegia 14:50, 1976.
87. Brach, BB, et al: Venous thrombosis in acute spinal cord paralysis. J Trauma 17:289, 1977.
88. Green, D, et al: Prevention of thromboembolism in spinal cord injury: Role of low molecular weight heparin. Arch Phys Med Rehabil 75:290, 1994.
89. Merli, GJ, et al: Etiology, incidence, and prevention of deep vein thrombosis in acute spinal cord injury. Arch Phys Med Rehabil 74:1199, 1993.
90. El Masri, WS, and Silver, JR: Prophylactic anticoagulant therapy in patients with spinal cord injury. Paraplegia 19:334, 1981.
91. Wharton, GW: Heterotopic ossification. Clin Orthop 112:142, 1975.
92. Lal, S, et al: Risk factors for heterotopic ossification in spinal cord injury. Arch Phys Med Rehabil 70:387, 1989.
93. Stover, SL, Hataway, CJ, and Zeiger, HE: Heterotopic ossification in spinal cord-injured patients. Arch Phys Med Rehabil 56:199, 1975.
94. Rossier, AB, et al: Current facts of para-osteo-arthropathy (POA). Paraplegia 11:38, 1973.
95. Damanski, M: Heterotopic ossification in paraplegia: A clinical study. J Bone Joint Surg Br 43:286, 1961.
96. Wharton, GW, and Morgan, TH: Ankylosis in the paralyzed patient. J Bone Joint Surg Am 52:105, 1970.
97. Cioschi, H, and Staas, WE: Follow-up care. In Buchanan, LE, and Nawoczenski, DA (eds): Spinal Cord Injury: Concepts and Management Approaches. Williams & Wilkins, Baltimore, 1987, p 219.
98. Nicholas, JJ: Ectopic bone formation in patients with spinal cord injury. Arch Phys Med Rehabil 54:354, 1973.
99. Nepomuceno, C, et al: Pain in patients with spinal cord injury. Arch Phys Med Rehabil 60:605, 1979.
100. Yezierski, RP: Pain following spinal cord injury: The clinical problem and experimental studies. Pain 68:185, 1996.
101. Richardson, RR, Meyer, PR, Jr, and Cerullo, LJ: Transcutaneous electrical neurostimulation in musculoskeletal pain of acute spinal cord injuries. Spine 5:42, 1980.
102. Davis, R: Pain and suffering following spinal cord injury. Clin Orthop 112:76, 1975.
103. Bors, E: Phantom limbs of patients with spinal cord injury. AMA Arch Neurol Psychiatry 66:610, 1951.
104. Ohry, A, et al: Shoulder complications as a cause of delay in rehabilitation of spinal cord injured patients: Case reports and review of the literature. Paraplegia 16:310, 1978.
105. Scott, JA, and Donovan, WH: The prevention of shoulder pain and contracture in the acute tetraplegic patient. Paraplegia 19:313, 1981.
106. Cole, J: The pathophysiology of the autonomic system in spinal cord injury. In Illis, L (ed): Spinal Cord Dysfunction: Assessment. Oxford University Press, New York, 1988, p 201.
107. Burr, RG: Urinary calculi composition in patients with spinal cord lesions. Arch Phys Med Rehabil 59:84, 1978.
108. Claus-Walker, J: Calcium excretion in quadriplegia. Arch Phys Med Rehabil 53:14, 1972.
109. Hancock, DA, Reed, GW, and Atkinson, PJ: Bone and soft tissue changes in paraplegic patients. Paraplegia 17:267, 1979.
110. Donovan, WH, and Bedbrook, G: Comprehensive management of spinal cord injury. Clin Symp 34:2, 1982.
111. Holdsworth, F: Fractures, dislocations, and fracture-dislocations of the spine. J Bone Joint Surg Am 52:1534, 1970.
112. Poynton, AR, et al: Sparing of sensation of pin prick predicts recovery of motor segment after injury to the spinal cord. J Bone Joint Surg 79:952, 1977.
113. Waters, RL, et al: Motor and sensory recovery following incomplete paraplegia. Arch Phys Med Rehabil 75(1):67, 1994.
114. Waters, RL, et al: Motor and sensory recovery following incomplete paraplegia. Arch Phys Med Rehabil 75(3):306, 1994.
115. Bracken, MB: Methylprednisolone and acute spinal cord injury: An update of the randomized evidence. Spine 26:S47, 2001.
116. Bracken, MB: Pharmacological interventions for acute spinal cord injury. The Cochrane Database of Systematic Reviews, 2000.
117. Bracken, MB, and Holford, TR: Neurological and functional status 1 year after acute spinal cord injury: Estimates of functional recovery in National Acute Spinal Cord Injury Study II from results modeled in National Acute Spinal Cord Injury Study III. J Neurosurg Spine 96:259, 2002.

118. Marciello, MA, et al: Magnetic resonance imaging related to neurologic outcome in cervical spinal cord injury. Arch Phys Med Rehabil 74:940, 1993.
119. Management of acute central cervical spinal cord injuries. Neurosurgery 50(3 Suppl):S166, 2002.
120. Cerullo, LJ: Surgical stabilization of spinal cord injuries: Section A: Cervical spine. In Calenoff, L (ed): Radiology of Spinal Cord Injury. CV Mosby, St. Louis, 1982, p 202.
121. Meyer, PR: Surgical stabilization of spinal cord injury: Section B: Thoracic and lumbar spine. In Calenoff, L (ed): Radiology of Spinal Cord Injury. CV Mosby, St. Louis, 1981, p 202.
122. Tator, CH: Halo devices for the treatment of acute spinal cord injury. In Tator, CH (ed): Early Management of Acute Spinal Cord Injury. Raven Press, New York, 1982, p 231.
123. Edmonds, VE, and Tator, CH: Coordination of a halo program for an acute spinal cord unit. In Tator, CH (ed): Early Management of Acute Spinal Cord Injury. Raven Press, New York, 1982, p 263.
124. Bohlman, HH: Complications and pitfalls in the treatment of acute cervical spinal cord injuries. In Tator, CH (ed): Early Management of Acute Spinal Cord Injury. Raven Press, New York, 1982, p 373.
125. Norkin, CC, and White, DJ: Measurment of Joint Motion: A Guide to Goniometry, ed 3. FA Davis, Philadelphia, 2003.
126. Clough, P, et al: Guidelines for routine respiratory care of patients with spinal cord injury: A clinical report. Phys Ther 66:1395, 1986.
127. Jaeger, RJ, et al: Cough in spinal cord injured patients: Comparison of three methods to produce cough. Arch Phys Med Rehabil 74:1358, 1993.
128. Lamont, LS, et al: A comparison of two arm exercises in patients with paraplegia. Cardiopulmonary Phys Ther 7:3, 1996.
129. Dodds, TA, et al: A validation of the functional independence measurement and its performance among rehabilitation inpatients. Arch Phys Med Rehabil 74:531, 1993.
130. Hamilton, BB, et al: Relation of disability costs to function: Spinal cord injury. Arch Phys Med Rehabil 80:385, 1999.
131. Heinemann, AW, et al: Relationships between disability measures and nursing effort during medical rehabilitation for patients with traumatic brain and spinal cord injury. Arch Phys Med Rehabil 78:143, 1997.
132. Granger, CV, et al: Performance profiles of the functional independence measure. Am J Phys Med Rehabil 72:84, 1993.
133. Kirby, RL: Wheelchair Skills Program (WSP): Version 3.1 Manual, Dalhousie University. Retrieved December 12, 2004 from http://www.wheelchairskillsprogram.ca/downloads/WSP_Manual_3_1_4.pdf.
134. Kirby, RL, et al: The Wheelchair Skills Test: A pilot study of a new outcome measure. Arch Phys Med Rehabil 83:10, 2002.
135. Kirby, RL, et al: The wheelchair skills test (version 2.4): Measurement properties. Arch Phys Med Rehabil 85:794, 2004.
136. Ditunno, JF, et al: Walking index for spinal cord injury (WISCI): An international multicenter validity and reliability study. Spinal Cord 38:234, 2000.
137. Field-Fote, EC, et al: The Spinal Cord Injury Functional Ambulation Inventory (SCI-FAI). J Rehabil Med, 33:177, 2001.
138. O'Sullivan, SB, and Schmitz, TJ: Physical Rehabilitation Laboratory Manual: Focus on Functional Training. FA Davis, Philadelphia, 1999.
139. Cooper, RA, et al: Evaluation of a pushrim-activated, power-assisted wheelchair. Arch Phys Med Rehabil 82:702, 2001.
140. Algood, SD, et al: Impact of a pushrim-activated power-assisted wheelchair on the metabolic demands, stroke frequency, and range of motion among subjects with tetraplegia. Arch Phys Med Rehabil 85:1865, 2004.
141. Somers, MF, and Wlodarczyk, S: Use of a pushrim-activated, power-assisted wheelchair enhanced mobility for an individual with cervical 5/6 tetraplegia. Neurol Rep 27:22, 2001.
142. MacPhee, AH, et al: Wheelchair skills training program: A randomized clinical trial of wheelchair users undergoing initial rehabilitation. Arch Phys Med Rehabil 85:41, 2004.
143. Best, KL: Efficacy of the Wheelchair Skills Training Program for community-based manual wheelchair users. Dalhousie University, 2004.
144. Coolen, AL, et al: Wheelchair skills training program for clinicians: A randomized controlled trial with occupational therapy students. Arch Phys Med Rehabil 85:1160, 2004.
145. Kirby, RL, et al: The manual wheelchair-handling skills of caregivers and the effect of training. Arch Phys Med Rehabil 85:2011, 2004.
146. Eng, JJ, et al: Use of prolonged standing for individuals with spinal cord injuries. Phys Ther 81:1392, 2001.
147. Hirokawa, S, et al: Energy expenditure and fatiguability in paraplegic ambulation using reciprocating gait orthosis and electric stimulation. Disabil Rehabil 18:115, 1996.
148. Mikelberg, R, and Reid, S: Spinal cord lesions and lower extremity bracing: An overview and follow-up study. Paraplegia 19:379, 1981.
149. Burns, SP, et al: Recovery of ambulation in motor-incomplete tetraplegia. Arch Phys Med Rehabil 78:1169, 1997.
150. Waters, RL: Functional prognosis of spinal cord injuries. J Spinal Cord Med 19:89, 1996.
151. Alander, DH, et al: Intermediate-term outcome of cervical spinal cord-injured patients older than 50 years of age. Spine 22:1189, 1997.
152. Scott, BA, Parker, J, and Stauffer, ES: Engineering principles and fabrication techniques for the Scott-Craig long leg brace for paraplegics. Orthop Pros 25:14, 1971.
153. Lobley, S, et al: Orthotic design from the New England Regional Spinal Cord Injury Center: Suggestion from the field. Phys Ther 65:492, 1985.
154. Franceschini, M, et al: Reciprocating gait orthoses: A multicenter study of their use by spinal cord injured patients. Arch Phys Med Rehabil 78:582, 1997.
155. Sykes, L, et al: The reciprocating gait orthosis: Long-term usage patterns. Arch Phys Med Rehabil 76:779, 1995.
156. Bernardi, M, et al: The efficiency of walking of paraplegic patients using a reciprocating gait orthosis. Paraplegia 33:409, 1995.
157. Lovely, RG, et al: Effects of training on the recovery of full-weight-bearing stepping in the adult spinal cat. Exp Neurol 92:421, 1986.
158. Barbeau, H, and Rossignol, S: Recovery of locomotion after chronic spinalization in the adult cat. Brain Res 412:84, 1987.
159. Edgerton, VR, et al: Use-dependent plasticity in spinal stepping and standing. Adv Neurol 72:233, 1997.
160. Barbeau, H, Wainberg, M, and Finch, L: Description and application of a system for locomotor rehabilitation. Med Biol Eng Comput 25:341, 1987.
161. Finch, L, Barbeau, H, and Arsenault, B: Influence of body weight support on normal human gait: Development of a gait retraining strategy. Phys Ther 71:842, 1991.
162. Barbeau, H, et al: The effects of locomotor training in spinal cord injured subjects: A preliminary study. Restor Neurol Neurosci 5:81, 1993.
163. Hodgson, JA, et al: Can the mammalian lumbar spinal cord learn a motor task? Med Sci Sports Exerc 26:1491, 1994.
164. Edgerton, VR, et al: A physiological basis for the development of rehabilitative strategies for spinally injured patients. J Am Paraplegia Soc 14:150, 1991.
165. Visintin, M, and Barbeau, H: The effects of body weight support on the locomotor pattern of spastic paretic patients. Can J Neurol Sci 16:315, 1989.
166. Visintin, M, and Barbeau, H: The effects of parallel bars, body weight support, and speed on the modulation of the locomotor pattern of spastic paretic gait: A preliminary communication. Paraplegia 32:540, 1994.
167. Harkema, SJ, et al: Human lumbosacral spinal cord interprets loading during stepping. J Neurophysiol 77:797, 1997.
168. Beres-Jones, JA, and Harkema, SJ: The human spinal cord interprets velocity-dependent afferent input during stepping. Brain 127:2232, 2004.
169. Ferris, DP, et al: Muscle activation during unilateral stepping occurs in the nonstepping limb of humans with clinically complete spinal cord injury. Spinal Cord 42:14, 2004.
170. Wernig, A, et al: Short communication: Laufband therapy based on 'rules of spinal locomotion' is effective in spinal cord injured persons. Eur J Neurosci 7:823, 1995.
171. Gardner, MB, et al: Partial body weight support with treadmill locomotion to improve gait after incomplete spinal cord injury: A single-subject experimental design. Phys Ther 78:361, 1998.
172. Wernig, A, Nanassy, A, and Muller, S: Laufband (treadmill) therapy in incomplete paraplegia and tetraplegia. J Neurotrauma 16:719, 1999.

173. Nymark, J, et al: Body weight support treadmill gait training in the subacute recovery phase of incomplete spinal cord injury. J Neuro Rehab 12:119, 1998.
174. Behrman, AL, and Harkema, SJ: Locomotor training after human spinal cord injury: A series of case studies. Phys Ther 80:688, 2000.
175. Protas, EJ, et al: Supported treadmill ambulation training after spinal cord injury: A pilot study. Arch Phys Med Rehabil 82:825, 2001.
176. Behrman, AL, et al: Locomotor training progression and outcomes after incomplete spinal cord injury. Phys Ther 85(12):1356, 2005.
177. Barbeau, H, et al: Walking after spinal cord injury: Evaluation, treatment, and functional recovery. Arch Phys Med Rehabil 80:225, 1999.
178. Barbeau, H: Locomotor training in neurorehabilitation: Emerging rehabilitation concepts. Neurorehabil Neural Repair 17:3, 2003.
179. Ladouceur, M, and Barbeau, H: Functional electrical stimulation-assisted walking for persons with incomplete spinal injuries: Longitudinal changes in maximal overground walking speed. Scand J Rehabil Med 32:28, 2000.
180. Field-Fote, EC: Combined use of body weight support, functional electric stimulation, and treadmill training to improve walking ability in individuals with chronic incomplete spinal cord injury. Arch Phys Med Rehabil 82:818, 2001.
181. Field-Fote, EC, and Tepavac, D: Improved intralimb coordination in people with incomplete spinal cord injury following training with body weight support and electrical stimulation. Phys Ther 82:707, 2002.
182. Barbeau, H, et al: The effect of locomotor training combined with functional electrical stimulation in chronic spinal cord injured subjects: Walking and reflex studies. Brain Res Rev 40:274, 2002.
183. Edgerton, VR, et al: Plasticity of the spinal neural circuitry after injury. Annu Rev Neurosci 27:145, 2004.
184. Dobkin, BH, et al: Methods for a randomized trial of weight-supported treadmill training versus conventional training for walking during inpatient rehabilitation after incomplete traumatic spinal cord injury. Neurorehabil Neural Repair 17:153, 2003.
185. Raymond, J, et al: Oxygen uptake and heart rate responses during arm vs combined arm/electrically stimulated leg exercise in people with paraplegia. Spinal Cord 35:680, 1997.
186. Hooker, SP, et al: Peak and submaximal physiologic responses following electrical stimulation leg cycle ergometer training. J Rehabil Res Dev 32:361, 1995.
187. Bremner, LA, et al: A clinical exercise system for paraplegics using functional electrical stimulation. Paraplegia 30:647, 1992.
188. Mitsuyama, T, et al: Diaphragm pacing with the spinal cord stimulator. Acta Neurochir Suppl 87:89, 2003.
189. DiMarco, AF: Neural prostheses in the respiratory system. J Rehabil Res Dev 38:601, 2001.
190. Baer, GA, et al: Phrenic nerve stimulation in tetraplegia: A new regimen to condition the diaphragm for full-time respiration. Scand J Rehabil Med 22:107, 1990.
191. Peckham, PH, et al: An advanced neuroprosthesis for restoration of hand and upper arm control using an implantable controller. J Hand Surg Am 27:265, 2002.
192. Peckham, PH, et al: Efficacy of an implanted neuroprosthesis for restoring hand grasp in tetraplegia: A multicenter study. Arch Phys Med Rehabil 82:1380, 2001.
193. Grill, JH, and Peckham, PH: Functional neuromuscular stimulation for combined control of elbow extension and hand grasp in C5 and C6 quadriplegics. IEEE Trans Rehabil Eng 6:190, 1998.
194. Bryden, AM, et al: Perceived outcomes and utilization of upper extremity surgical reconstruction in individuals with tetraplegia at model spinal cord injury systems. Spinal Cord 42:169, 2004.
195. Brissot, R, et al: Clinical experience with functional electrical stimulation-assisted gait with Parastep in spinal cord-injured patients. Spine 25:501, 2000.
196. Johnston, TE, et al: Functional electrical stimulation for augmented walking in adolescents with incomplete spinal cord injury. J Spinal Cord Med 26:390, 2003.
197. Johnston, TE, et al: Implanted functional electrical stimulation: An alternative for standing and walking in pediatric spinal cord injury. Spinal Cord 41:144, 2003.
198. Wieler, M, et al: Multicenter evaluation of electrical stimulation systems for walking. Arch Phys Med Rehabil 80:495, 1999.
199. Gallien, P, et al: Restoration of gait by functional electrical stimulation for spinal cord injured patients. Paraplegia 33:660, 1995.
200. Agarwal, S, et al: Long-term user perceptions of an implanted neuroprosthesis for exercise, standing, and transfers after spinal cord injury. J Rehabil Res Dev 40:241, 2003.
201. Jezernik, S, et al: Electrical stimulation for the treatment of bladder dysfunction: Current status and future possibilities. Neurol Res 24:413, 2002.
202. Hastings, J, and Goldstein, B: Paraplegia and the shoulder. Phys Med Rehabil Clin N Am 15:vii, 2004.
203. Dyson-Hudson, TA, and Kirshblum, SC: Shoulder pain in chronic spinal cord injury, part I: Epidemiology, etiology, and pathomechanics. J Spinal Cord Med 27:4, 2004.
204. Ballinger, DA, Rintala, DH, and Hart, KA: The relation of shoulder pain and range-of-motion problems to functional limitations, disability, and perceived health of men with spinal cord injury: A multifaceted longitudinal study. Arch Phys Med Rehabil 81:1575, 2000.
205. Nawoczenski, DA, et al: Three-dimensional shoulder kinematics during a pressure relief technique and wheelchair transfer. Arch Phys Med Rehabil 84:1293, 2003.
206. Jacobs, PL, and Nash, MS: Exercise recommendations for individuals with spinal cord injury. Sports Med 34:727, 2004.
207. Jacobs, PL, Nash, MS, and Rusinowski, JW: Circuit training provides cardiorespiratory and strength benefits in persons with paraplegia. Med Sci Sports Ex 33:711, 2001.
208. Finley, MA, et al: Impact of physical exercise on controlling secondary conditions associated with spinal cord injury. Neurology Report (now JNPT) 26:21, 2002.
209. Hicks, AL, et al: Long-term exercise training in persons with spinal cord injury: Effects on strength, arm ergometry performance, and psychological well-being. Spinal Cord 41:34, 2003.

Supplemental Readings

Amador, MJ, and Guest, JD: An appraisal of ongoing experimental procedures in human spinal cord injury. J Neurol Phys Ther 29(2):70, 2005.

Beekhuizen, KS: New perspectives on improving upper extremity function after spinal cord injury. J Neurol Phys Ther 29(3):157, 2005.

Britton, D, et al: Baclofen pump intervention for spasticity affecting pulmonary function. J Spinal Cord Med 28(4):343, 2005.

Chan, SK, and Man, DW: Barriers to returning to work for people with spinal cord injuries: A focus group study. Work 25(4):325, 2005.

Chiodo, A: Pain management with interventional spine therapy in patients with spinal cord injury: A case series. J Spinal Cord Med 28(4):338, 2005.

Cohen, LJ, et al: Development of the seating and mobility script concordance test for spinal cord injury: Obtaining content validity evidence. Assist Technol 17(2):122, 2005.

Como, JJ, et al: Characterizing the need for mechanical ventilation following cervical spinal cord injury with neurologic deficit. J Trauma 59(4):912, 2005.

Dobkin, B: The Clinical Science of Neurologic Rehabilitation, ed 2. Oxford University Press, New York, 2003.

Durfee, WK, and Rivard, A: Design and simulation of a pneumatic, stored-energy, hybrid orthosis for gait restoration. J Biomech Eng 127(6):1014, 2005.

Giuliano, F, et al: Efficacy and safety of vardenafil in men with erectile dysfunction caused by spinal cord injury. Neurology 66(2):210, 2006.

Haran, MJ, et al: Health status rated with the Medical Outcomes Study 36-Item Short-Form Health Survey after spinal cord injury. Arch Phys Med Rehabil 86(12):2290, 2005.

Haubert, LL, et al: A comparison of shoulder joint forces during ambulation with crutches versus a walker in persons with incomplete spinal cord injury. Arch Phys Med Rehabil 87(1):63, 2006.

Henderson, CE: Application of ventilatory strategies to enhance functional activities for an individual with spinal cord injury. J Neurol Phys Ther 29(2):107, 2005.

Lechner, HE, Frotzler, A, and Eser, P: Relationship between self- and clinically rated spasticity in spinal cord injury. Arch Phys Med Rehabil 87(1):15, 2006.

Livneh, H, and Martz, E: Psychosocial adaptation to spinal cord injury: A dimensional perspective. Psychol Rep 97(2):577, 2005.

Myslinski, MJ: Evidence-based exercise prescription for individuals with spinal cord injury. J Neurol Phys Ther 29(2):104, 2005.

Nash, MS: Exercise as a health-promoting activity following spinal cord injury. J Neurol Phys Ther 29(2):87, 2005.

National Spinal Cord Injury Statistical Center: Spinal cord injury: Facts and figures at a glance. J Spinal Cord Med 28(4):379, 2005.

Noreau, L, et al: Participation after spinal cord injury: The evolution of conceptualization and measurement. J Neurol Phys Ther 29(3):147, 2005.

Paker N, et al: Reasons for rehospitalization in patients with spinal cord injury: 5 years' experience. Int J Rehabil Res 29(1):71, 2006.

Post, M, and Noreau, L: Quality of life after spinal cord injury. J Neurol Phys Ther 29(3):139, 2005.

Rigby, P, et al: Impact of electronic aids to daily living on the lives of persons with cervical spinal cord injuries. Assist Technol 17(2):89, 2005.

Smith, PM, and Jeffery, ND: Spinal shock—comparative aspects and clinical relevance. J Vet Intern Med 19(6):788, 2005.

Somers, MF: Spinal Cord Injury: Functional Rehabilitation, ed 2. Prentice-Hall, Upper Saddle River, NJ, 2001.

Tasiemski, T, et al: The association of sports and physical recreation with life satisfaction in a community sample of people with spinal cord injuries. NeuroRehabilitation 20(4):253, 2005.

van der Salm A, et al: Comparison of electric stimulation methods for reduction of triceps surae spasticity in spinal cord injury. Arch Phys Med Rehabil 87(2):222, 2006.

Appendix A: Sample of Available Internet Resources for Patients and Clinicians

Foundations/Associations Information Resources

Spinal Cord Injury Information Network	http://www.spinalcord.uab.edu/
Christopher Reeve Paralysis Foundation	http://www.christopherreeve.org/index.cfm
Model Spinal Cord Injury System Dissemination Center	http://www.mscisdisseminationcenter.org/
Wheelchair Net	http://www.wheelchairnet.org/index2.html
Wheelchair Skills Program	http://www.wheelchairskillsprogram.ca/
Disability Resources	http://www.disabilityresources.org/
National Council on Independent Living	http://www.ncil.org/
American Paraplegia Society	http://www.apssci.org/
American Spinal Injury Association	http://www.asia-spinalinjury.org/home/index.html
National Spinal Cord Injury Association	http://www.spinalcord.org/
Paralyzed Veterans of American	http://www.pva.org/
Dangerwood (site to survive spinal cord injury and paralysis)	http://www.survivingparalysis.com/
Think First	http://www.thinkfirst.org/
Northeast Passage	http://www.nepassage.org/
Woodrow Wilson Rehabilitation Center	http://www.wwrc.net/Default.htm
Sports'n Spokes	http://www.pvamagazines.com/sns/
New Mobility	http://www.newmobility.com/
Good Shepherd	http://www.goodshepherdrehab.org/
Shake-A-Leg	http://www.shakealeg.org/
The Cleveland Center	http://fescenter.case.edu/
Society to Increase Mobility	http://www.thestim.org/index.html
The Miami Project to Cure Paralysis	http://www.miamiproject.miami.edu/
disAbility Information and Resources	http://www.makoa.org/

Model Spinal Cord Injury Systems

UAB Model Spinal Cord Injury Care System	http://main.uab.edu/show.asp?durki=10712
California Model Spinal Cord Injury System	http://www.tbi-sci.org/sci.html
Regional Spinal Cord Injury Care System of Southern California	http://www.rancho.org/
Rocky Mountain Regional Spinal Injury System	http://www.craighospital.org/Research/SCIModelsystems.asp
Southern Florida Regional Spinal Cord Injury Model System	http://www.SCI.med.miami.edu
Georgia Regional Spinal Cord Injury Care System	http://www.shepherd.org/
New England Regional Spinal Cord Injury Center	http://www.bmc.org/rehab/spinalcord.html
University of Michigan Model Spinal Cord Injury Care System	http://www.med.umich.edu/pmr/model_sci/
Missouri Model Spinal Cord Injury System	http://www.hsc.missouri.edu/~momscis
Northern New Jersey Spinal Cord Injury System	http://www.kmrrec.org/KM/nnjscis/index.php3
Mount Sinai Spinal Cord Injury Model System	http://www.mssm.edu/rehab/spinal/
Regional Spinal Cord Injury Center of the Delaware Valley	http://www.spinalcordcenter.org
University of Pittsburgh Model Center on Spinal Cord Injury	http://www.upmc-sci.org
Texas Model Spinal Cord Injury System	http://www.bcm.edu/pm&r/sci/research/modelsystem/
VCU Model Spinal Cord Injury System	http://www.sci.pmr.vcu.edu
Northwest Regional Spinal Cord Injury System	http://depts.washington.edu/rehab/sci/

CHAPTER

24

LEARNING OBJECTIVES

1. Identify and differentiate vestibular symptom pathology from other manifestations of vertigo, dizziness, and dysequilibrium.
2. Identify and describe the examination procedures used to evaluate patients with vestibular dysfunction to establish a diagnosis, prognosis, and plan of care.
3. Analyze and interpret examination data and determine appropriate interventions for the clinical problems presented.
4. Describe appropriate elements of the rehabilitation program for patients with vestibular dysfunction.

Vestibular Disorders

Michael C. Schubert, PT, PhD

OUTLINE

Physical therapists are likely to encounter patients with vestibular disorders in a variety of clinical settings. It is estimated that the incidence of dizziness in the United States is 5.5 percent, or greater than 15 million people per year who develop the symptom.[1] The reported prevalence of dizziness as a medical complaint in community-dwelling adults varies based on subjects' age, gender, and definition of the complaint (1 to 35 percent).[2–6] Dizziness is one of the most common complaints adults report to their physicians and prevalence increases with age.[7,8]. For patients older than 75 years of age, dizziness is the most common reason to see a physician.[9] Patients who experience dizziness report a significant disability that reduces their quality of life.[10–12] Furthermore, it has been reported that greater than 70 percent of patients with initial complaints of dizziness will not have a resolution of symptoms at a 2-week follow-up. Of patients with persistent dizziness, 63 percent reported recurrent symptoms continuing beyond 3 months.[13]

Cawthorne[14] and Cooksey[15] were the first clinicians to advocate exercises for persons suffering from dizziness and vertigo. It has only been within the last two decades, however, that our knowledge of vestibular function and related disorders has profoundly changed the approaches toward rehabilitation. Once an accurate diagnosis involving the vestibular pathways has been made, functional limitations are minimized and progression toward disability can be prevented.

The peripheral vestibular system serves as the primary focus of this chapter because it is the most common origin for patient signs and symptoms. The physical therapist, however, must recognize patterns of signs and symptoms from a central pathology as well. To appreciate the complexity of the vestibular system and its vital role in human function, a brief synopsis of anatomy and physiology is provided. Once the normally functioning vestibular system is understood, the reader will be able to discern anomalies of the system and begin to formulate effective rehabilitation strategies.

Anatomy

Peripheral Vestibular System

The three primary functions of the peripheral vestibular system include: (1) stabilization of visual images on the fovea of the retina during head movement to allow clear vision; (2) maintaining postural stability, especially during movement of the head; and (3) providing information used for spatial orientation.

Semicircular Canals

Within the petrous portion of each temporal bone lies the membranous vestibular labyrinth. Each labyrinth contains five neural structures that detect head acceleration: three *semicircular canals* and two otolith organs (Fig. 24.1). The three semicircular canals (SCC) (horizontal, posterior, and anterior) respond to angular acceleration and are orthogonal with respect to one another. Alignment of the SCC in the temporal bone is such that each canal has a contralateral coplanar mate. The horizontal canals form a coplanar pair while the posterior and contralateral anterior SCC form coplanar pairs. The anterior aspect of the horizontal SCC is inclined 30° upward from a plane connecting the external auditory canal to the lateral canthus. The posterior and anterior SCCs are inclined about 92° and 90° from the plane of the horizontal SCC.[16] Angular head rotation stimulates each canal to varying degrees.[17]

The SCCs are filled with *endolymph* that has a density slightly greater than water.[18] Endolymph moves freely within each canal in response to the direction of the angular head rotation. The SCCs enlarge at one end to form the ampulla. Within the ampulla lies the cupula, a gelatinous barrier that contains the sensory hair cells (Fig. 24.2). The kinocilia and stereocilia of the hair cells are seated in the crista ampullaris. Deflection of the stereocilia caused by motion of the endolymph results in an opening (or closing) of the transduction channels of hair cells, which results in changes in the membrane potential of the hair cells. Deflection of the stereocilia toward the kinocilia in each hair cell leads to excitation (*depolarization*) and deflection of the stereocilia away from the kinocilia leads to inhibition (*hyperpolarization*).

Each of the SCCs responds best to motion in its own plane with coplanar pairs exhibiting a push–pull dynamic. For example, as the head is turned to the right, the hair cells in the right horizontal SCC are excited, while hair cells in the left horizontal SCC are inhibited. The brain detects the direction of head movement by comparing input from the coplanar labyrinthine mates.

Otolith Organs

The saccule and utricle make up the *otolith organs* of the membranous labyrinth and respond to linear acceleration and static head tilt. Sensory hair cells project into a gelatinous material that has calcium carbonate crystals (otoconia) embedded in it, which provide the otolith organs with an inertial mass (Fig. 24.3). Similar to the SCC, motion toward the kinocilia causes excitation, while motion away leads to inhibition. Utricular excitation occurs during horizontal linear acceleration and/or static head tilt and saccular excitation occurs during vertical linear acceleration.

Central Vestibular System

Many vestibular reflexes are controlled by processes that exist primarily within the brainstem. Tracing techniques

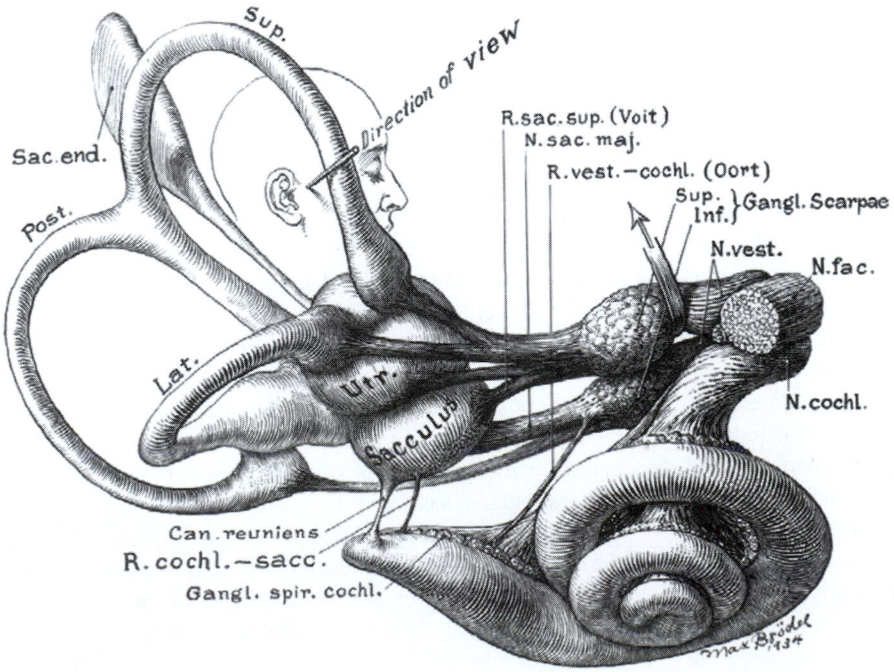

Figure 24.1 Anatomy of the vestibular labyrinth. Structures include the utricle (Utr.), sacculus, anterior (or superior) semicircular canal (Sup.), posterior semicircular canal (Post.), and the lateral semicircular canal (Lat.). The three semicircular canals (SCCs) are orthogonal with each other. Note the superior vestibular nerve innervating the anterior and lateral semicircular canals as well as the utricle. The inferior vestibular nerve innervates the posterior semicircular canal and the saccule. The cell bodies of the vestibular nerves are located in Scarpa's ganglion (Gangl. Scarpae). Also note that the semicircular canals enlarge at one end to form the ampulla. (Drawing from the Max Brödel Archives [No. 933]. Reproduced with permission of the Department of Art as Applied to Medicine, Johns Hopkins University, Baltimore, MD.)

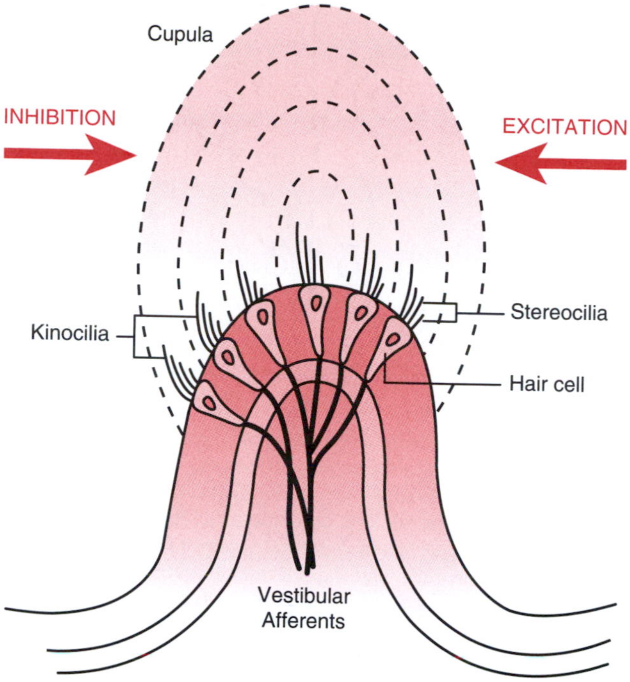

Figure 24.2 The cupula of the ampulla is a flexible, gelatinous barrier that partitions the canal. The crista ampullaris contains the kinocilia and stereocilia sensory hair cells. The hair cells generate action potentials in response to cupular deflection. Deflection of the stereocilia toward the kinocilia causes excitation; deflection in the opposite direction causes inhibition.

however, have identified extensive connections between the vestibular nuclei and the reticular formation, thalamus, and cerebellum[19–21] (Fig. 24.4). In addition, vestibular pathways appear to terminate in a unique cortical area. Primate studies have identified the junction of the parietal and insular lobes as the location for a vestibular cortex.[22–24] Recent evidence in human studies using functional magnetic

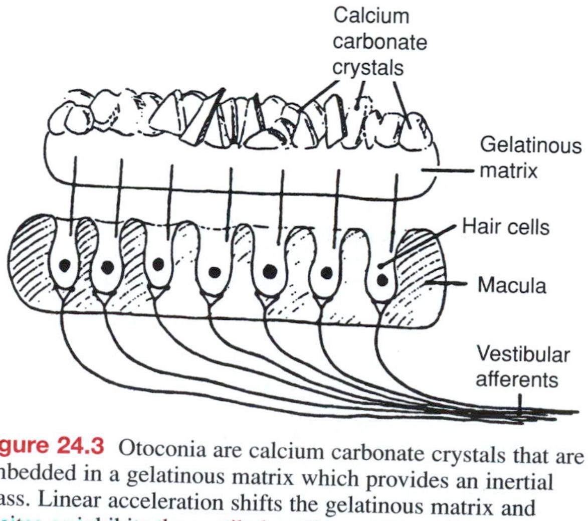

Figure 24.3 Otoconia are calcium carbonate crystals that are embedded in a gelatinous matrix which provides an inertial mass. Linear acceleration shifts the gelatinous matrix and excites or inhibits the vestibular afferents depending on the direction in which the stereocilia are deflected. (Adapted from Baloh, RW, and Hornrubia, V,[30] p 4, by permission of Oxford University Press, Inc.)

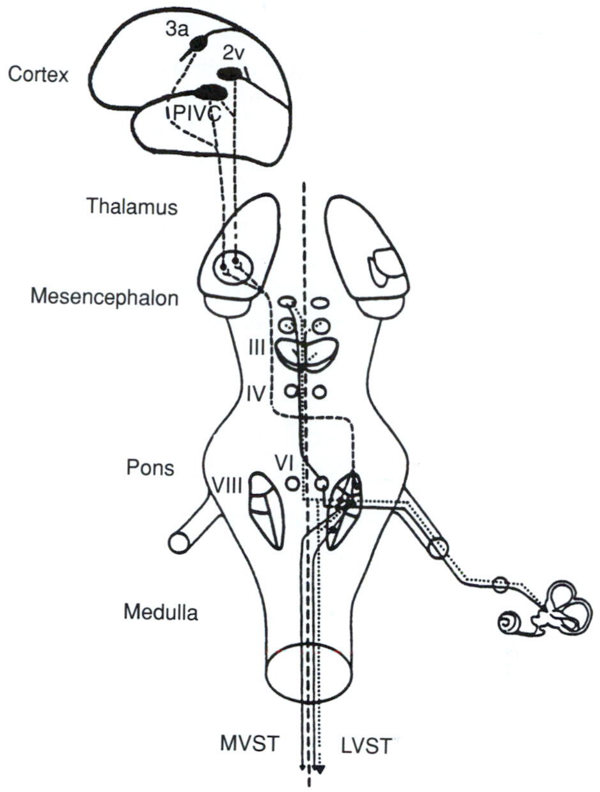

Figure 24.4 The semicircular canal (angular) and otolith (linear) input is sent to the vestibular nuclei. From the vestibular nuclei, the input travels to the ocular motor nuclei (III, IV, VI) for mediation of the vestibulo-ocular reflex. For arousal and conscious awareness of the head and body in space, information proceeds further to the thalamus and cortex. For maintenance of postural control, the peripheral vestibular input is sent distally as the medial and lateral vestibulo-spinal tracts (MVST, LVST). PIVC = Parieto-insular vestibular cortex. (Adapted from Brandt, T, and Dieterich, M,[27] p 343, with permission.)

resonance imaging (fMRI) appears to confirm the parietal and insular regions as the cortical location for processing vestibular information.[25] Connections with the vestibular cortex, thalamus, and reticular formation enable the vestibular system to contribute to the integration of arousal and conscious awareness of the body, as well as to discriminate between movement of self and the environment.[26,27] The cerebellar connections help maintain calibration of the vestibulo-ocular reflex (VOR), contribute to posture during static and dynamic activities, and influence the coordination of limb movements.

Physiology and Motor Control

Knowledge of basic vestibular neurophysiology is important for understanding the signs and symptoms of vestibular dysfunction. Important principles of the vestibular system include the tonic firing rate, VOR, push–pull mechanism, inhibitory cutoff, and the velocity storage system (VSS).

Tonic Firing Rate

In primates, primary vestibular afferents of the healthy vestibular system have a resting firing rate that is typically 70 to 100 spikes/s.[28,29] The presence of the high tonic firing rate means each vestibular system can detect head motion through excitation or inhibition. During angular head rotations, ipsilateral vestibular afferents and ipsilateral central vestibular neurons are excited.[28] Such head movements also result in inhibition of peripheral afferents and of many central vestibular neurons receiving innervation from the contralateral labyrinth.

Vestibulo-Ocular Reflex and Vestibulo-Ocular Reflex Gain and Phase

The **vestibulo-ocular reflex (VOR)** is responsible for maintaining stability of an image on the fovea of the retina during rapid head movements. To do this, the VOR must generate rapid compensatory eye movements in the direction opposite the head rotation. The VOR achieves this with relatively simple patterns of connectivity in the central vestibular pathways. In its most basic form, the pathways controlling the VOR can be described as a three-neuron arc. In the case of the anterior SCC, primary vestibular afferents from the anterior SCC synapse in the ipsilateral vestibular nuclei. Secondary vestibular neurons receiving innervation from the ipsilateral labyrinth decussate and synapse in the contralateral oculomotor nucleus. Motoneurons from the oculomotor nucleus then synapse at the neuromuscular junction of the ipsilateral superior rectus and the contralateral inferior oblique muscles respectively (Fig. 24.5). Similar patterns of connectivity exist for the vertical SCC and the eye muscles that receive innervations from them (Table 24.1). See Figure 24.6 for insertions of the ocular muscles.

Normally, as the head moves in one direction, the eyes move in the opposite direction with equal velocity. This relationship of eye velocity to head velocity is expressed as the gain (*VOR gain*) of the vestibular system (eye velocity/head velocity = −1). For example, when the head is moved down the anterior SCCs are stimulated. Excitation of the anterior SCC afferents rotates both eyes in the direction opposite the angular head movement, or up (Fig. 24.5). *VOR Phase* is a second useful measure of the vestibular system and represents the timing relationship for eye and head position. Ideally, eye position should arrive at a point in time that is equal with the oppositely directed head position. By convention, this is described as zero phase shift.

In individuals with healthy oculomotor function, for head velocities below 60° per second *gaze stability* can be maintained fairly well using *smooth pursuit*.[30] In situations where head velocity is greater than 60°/s the vestibular system is primarily responsible for generating eye movement

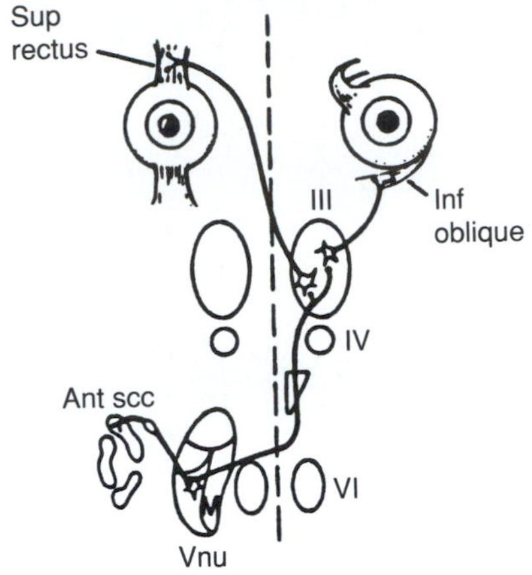

Figure 24.5 From the anterior semicircular canal (Ant SCC), afferent input travels to the vestibular nuclei (VNu). The signal continues to the contralateral oculomotor nuclei (III). From there, motoneurons synapse with the superior rectus muscle that moves the eye upward, and the inferior oblique muscle that moves the eye upward and torsionally. Also shown are the oculomotor nuclei IV, and VI. (Adapted from Baloh, RW, and Honrubia, V,[30] p 52, by permission of Oxford University Press, Inc.)

Table 24.1 Innervation Pattern of Excitatory Input from the Semicircular Canals

Primary Afferent	Secondary Neuron[a]	Extraocular Motoneuron	Muscle
Lateral (right)	Medial vestibular nucleus	Right oculomotor nucleus[b] →	Right medial rectus
		Left abducens nucleus →	Left lateral rectus
Anterior (or superior) (right)	Lateral vestibular nucleus	Left oculomotor nucleus →	Left inferior oblique
		↘	Right superior rectus
Posterior (or inferior) (right)	Medial vestibular nucleus	Left trochlear nucleus →	Right superior oblique
		Left oculomotor nucleus →	Left inferior rectus

[a]Ascending secondary neurons travel in the medial longitudinal fasciculus.

[b]For the lateral semicircular canal, secondary neurons also travel in the ascending tract of Dieters.

From Schubert, MC, and Minor, LB: Vestibulo-ocular physiology underlying vestibular hypofunction. Phys Ther 84:373, 2004, p 378, with permission.

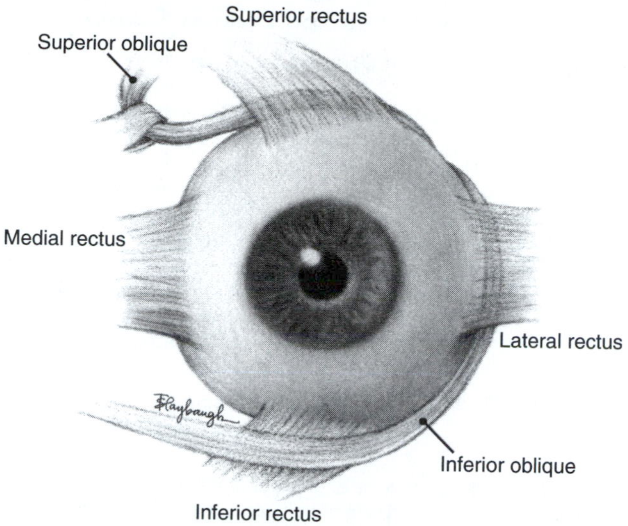

Figure 24.6 Muscle insertions of the left eye. Six extraocular muscles insert into the sclera and can be considered as complementary pairs. The medial and lateral rectus muscles rotate the eyes horizontally, the superior and inferior rectus muscles rotate the eyes vertically, and the superior and inferior oblique muscles rotate the eyes torsionally with some vertical component. By convention, the torsional rotation is noted as it relates to the superior poles of the eyes. The superior oblique muscle rotates the eye downward and toward the nose, whereas the inferior oblique muscle rotates the eye upward and away from the nose. The superior oblique muscle travels through the fibrous trochlea, which attaches to the anteromedial superior wall of the orbit. (From Schubert, MC, and Minor, LB: Vestibulo-ocular physiology underlying vestibular hypofunction. Phys Ther 84:373, 2004, p 378, with permission.)

(in the direction opposite the head movement) to maintain *gaze* on the target.[31] The VOR operates at head velocities as great as 350 to 400°/s.[32]

Push-Pull Mechanism

The brain detects head movement and direction through comparison of inputs between the two vestibular systems. The SCCs each work in coplanar fashion as mentioned earlier; as the head is turned to the right, the right horizontal SCC will have an increased firing rate while the left horizontal SCC has a decreased firing rate. This is called the *push–pull mechanism* (Fig. 24.7). The brain is then responsible for recognizing the difference and interpreting movement. A faulty interpretation will lead to difficulties with gaze stabilization, postural stability, and motion perception.

Inhibitory Cutoff

Recall that during angular head rotations ipsilateral vestibular afferents can be excited up to 400 spikes/s.[32] A concomitant hyperpolarization of the opposite labyrinth also occurs. However, the hyperpolarization of the hair cells in the opposite labyrinth can only decrease the firing rate to zero, at which point the inhibition is cut off (*inhibitory cutoff*). The response to head movements that hyperpolarize the hair cells is limited to a velocity range up to 70 to 100°/s. For example, if the tonic firing rates of the vestibular afferents are 80 spikes/s, with a rotation to the right of 120°/s the vestibular afferents increase their firing rate from 80 to 200 spikes/s (tonic firing rate + rotational velocity). In contrast, the left ear will decrease from 80 to zero, not to negative 40 (−40).* Because the resting discharge rate of these afferents and central vestibular neurons averages 70 to 100 spikes/s, inhibitory cutoff is more likely to occur than is excitation saturation.

Velocity Storage System

The signal generated by movement of the cupula is brief, lasting only as long as the cupula is deflected.[33] The response is sustained, however, by a circuit of neurons in the medial vestibular nucleus and lasts longer than 10 seconds in people with normal vestibular function. The purpose of sustaining the vestibular input is thought to assist the brain in detecting low frequency head rotation.

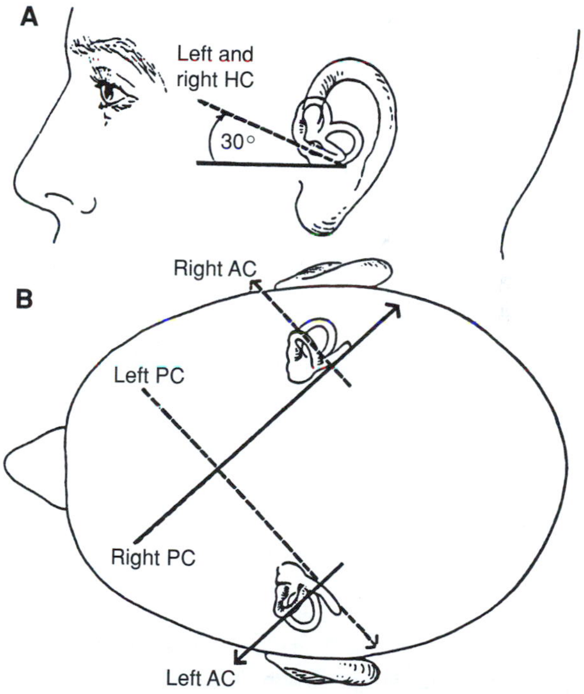

Figure 24.7 (*A*) Orientation of the horizontal semicircular canals (HC) in situ, with the head neutrally aligned. (*B*) The semicircular canals (ipsilateral anterior and contralateral posterior, and each horizontal) work in pairs. The arrows indicate the angular pitch direction of individual SCC stimulation. The dashed and continuous lines illustrate each SCC has an equally opposing SCC, sensitive to the opposite angular pitch direction of the head, for example, the right anterior canal (right AC) is paired with the left posterior canal (left PC). (Adapted from Baloh, RW, and Hornrubia, V,[30] p 27, by permission of Oxford University Press, Inc.)

*It is generally recognized that a 1:1 ratio exists between head velocity and spikes per second neuronal firing rate.

Examination

History

Physical therapists examining people who report dizziness and imbalance have the difficult task of sorting through potential causes. Capturing a thorough history is a critical component of the process. Key elements of taking the history are identification of symptoms as well as their duration and the circumstances under which the symptoms occur.

Identification of Symbols

Many patients and clinicians use the imprecise term "dizziness" to describe a vague sensation of light-headedness or a feeling that they have a tendency to fall. The imprecision of the term can entangle clinical management decisions. It is essential to determine what the patient is experiencing when the term **dizziness** is used. Most complaints of being "dizzy" can be categorized as vertigo, light-headedness, dysequilibrium, or oscillopsia. Generally, dizziness is vaguely defined as the sensation of whirling or feeling a tendency to fall. Ideally, patients should be directed away from using the word.

Vertigo is defined as an illusion of movement. Many patients use the term "vertigo" incorrectly and thus the clinician must be certain to inform patients of the true definition as well as identify their unique experience. Patients may describe that they sense their environment is moving or that they see the environment moving (spinning). Vertigo tends to be episodic and to indicate pathology at one or more places along the vestibular pathways. It is most common during the acute stage of a unilateral vestibular hypofunction (UVH), but may also manifest itself via displaced otoconia (benign paroxysmal positional vertigo), or an acute unilateral brainstem lesion affecting the root entry zone of the peripheral vestibular neurons or the vestibular nuclei.

Lightheadedness is often defined as a feeling that fainting is about to occur and can be caused by nonvestibular factors such as hypotension, hypoglycemia, or anxiety.[34] Lightheadedness is vague and less localizing than vertigo.

Dysequilibrium is defined as the sensation of being off balance. Typically, acute and chronic vestibular lesions will produce dysequilibrium. Often, however, this symptom is associated with nonvestibular problems such as decreased somatosensation or weakness in the lower extremities (Table 24.2).

Oscillopsia is the subjective experience of motion of objects in the visual environment that are known to be stationary. Oscillopsia can occur with head movements in patients with vestibular hypofunction since the vestibular system is not generating an adequate compensatory eye velocity during the head motion. Such a deficit in the VOR results in motion of images on the fovea and in a decline in visual acuity. The severity of gaze instability however, varies across individuals with vestibular hypofunction.[35–38]

Table 24.2 Symptom and Possible Causes

Symptom	Possible Cause
Vertigo	BPPV, UVH, unilateral central lesion affecting the vestibular nuclei
Lightheadedness	Orthostatic hypotension, hypoglycemia, anxiety, panic disorder
Dysequilibrium	BVH, chronic unilateral vestibular hypofunction, lower extremity somatosensation loss, upper brainstem/vestibular cortex lesion, cerebellar and motor pathway lesions

BPPV = Benign paroxysmal positional vertigo; BVH = bilateral vestibular hypofunction; UVH = unilateral vestibular hypofunction.

Duration and Circumstances of Symptoms

The clinician must determine how recently the patient has had an acute attack of vertigo, lightheadedness, dysequilibruim, or oscillopsia and whether the symptom is constant or episodic. If the symptom is episodic, the clinician must attempt to determine the average duration of the episodes in seconds, minutes, or hours. For example, vertigo lasting seconds to minutes commonly suggests benign paroxysmal positional vertigo. In contrast, vertigo lasting minutes to hours suggest Ménière's disease, while vertigo lasting for days implies vestibular neuronitis or migraine associated dizziness.

The physical therapist must also determine under what circumstances the patient experiences symptoms. It is important to discern whether the patient experiences symptoms with particular movements, positions, or at rest. For example, is the patient sensitive to motion as the passenger in a moving car? Or, does the patient experience a vigorous vertigo when the head is moved into certain positions?

Tests and Measures

Visual Analogue Scale

Use of a *visual analogue scale (VAS)* is an effective technique to obtain subjective intensity ratings of vertigo, lightheadedness, dysequilibrium, and oscillopsia.[39,40] The patient is asked to answer a question and mark on a 10-cm line where the symptoms exist at that moment. The clinician then measures the line and obtains a quantified value.

Dizziness Handicap Inventory

The *Dizziness Handicap Inventory (DHI)* is a popular tool used to measure a patient's self-perceived handicap as a result of vestibular disorders (Table 24.3).[41] The DHI has excellent test-retest reliability ($r = 0.97$) and good internal consistency reliability ($r = 0.89$). Patients respond to 25 questions,

Table 24.3 Final Alpha Version of Dizziness Handicap Inventory with Corrected Item-Total Correlation Coefficients

Dizziness Handicap Inventory[a]

Instructions: The purpose of this scale is to identify difficulties that you may be experiencing because of your dizziness or unsteadiness. Please answer "yes," "no," or "sometimes" to each question. *Answer each question as it pertains to your dizziness or unsteadiness problem only.*

Item	Item Total
P1. Does looking up increase your problem?	.54
E2. Because of your problem, do you feel frustrated?	.34
F3. Because of your problem, do you restrict your travel for business or recreation?	.76[b]
P4. Does walking down the aisle of a supermarket increase your problem?	.39
F5. Because of your problem, do you have difficulty getting into or out of bed?	.50
F6. Does your problem significantly restrict your participation in social activities such as going out to dinner, going to movies, dancing, or to parties?	.69
F7. Because of your problem, do you have difficulty reading?	.44
P8. Does performing more ambitious activities like sports, dancing, or household chores such as sweeping or putting dishes away increase your problem?	.54
E9. Because of your problem, are you afraid to leave your home without having someone accompany you?	.43
E10. Because of your problem, have you been embarrassed in front of others?	.46
P11. Do quick movements of your head increase your problem?	.51
F12. Because of your problem, do you avoid heights?	.49
P13. Does turning over in bed increase your problem?	.43
F14. Because of your problem, is it difficult for you to do strenuous housework or yardwork?	.58
E15. Because of your problem, are you afraid people may think you are intoxicated?	.30
F16. Because of your problem, is it difficult for you to go for a walk by yourself?	.62
P17. Does walking down a sidewalk increase your problem?	.58†
E18. Because of your problem, is it difficult for you to concentrate?	.49†
F19. Because of your problem, is it difficult for you to walk around your house in the dark?	.48
E20. Because of your problem, are you afraid to stay home alone?	.27
E21. Because of your problem, do you feel handicapped?	.41
E22. Has your problem placed stress on your relationships with members of your family or friends?	.46
E23. Because of your problem, are you depressed?	.41
F24. Does your problem interfere with your job or household responsibilities?	.56
P25. Does bending over increase your problem?	.57

[a]A "yes" response is scored 4 points. A "sometimes" response is scored 2 points. A "no" response is scored 0 points.

[b]Questions with the highest corrected item-total correlation for each subscale. F indicates functional subscale; E, emotional subscale; P, physical subscale.

From Jacobsen, GP, and Newman, CW,[41] p 424, with permission.

subgrouped into functional, emotional, and physical components. The DHI provides quantification of the patient's perception of dysequilibrium and its impact on daily activities. It is useful to establish subjective improvement. Measures of subjective impairment and physiological improvement have not been correlated[42,43]; therefore, it is likely that factors other than organic recovery of vestibular function are responsible for subjective impairment.

Functional Disability Scale

The *Functional Disability Scale* was developed to determine a patient's response to physical therapy (Table 24.4).[44] The scale is administered before and after rehabilitation. The authors reported that patients who believed their vestibular disorders were more disabling did not improve as much as those patients who perceived themselves to be less disabled.

Motion Sensitivity Quotient

The *Motion Sensitivity Quotient (MSQ)* was developed to provide a subjective score of an individual's dizziness.[45] The test involves placing patients into positions

Table 24.4 Functional Disability Scale

0	No disability-negligible symptoms
1	No disability-bothersome symptoms
2	Mild disability-performs usual duties
3	Moderate disability-disrupts usual duties
4	Recent severe disability-medical leave
5	Established severe disability

Note: The physical therapist assigns the patient a score before and after treatment, based on interview history (from Telian et al,[44] p 90, with permission).

incorporating head or entire body motion to determine whether the movement reproduces dizziness (Fig. 24.8). If the patient reports an increased symptom intensity moving into a provoking position, the intensity is assigned a point, graded by the patient between 1 (mild) and 5 (severe). The duration of symptoms are also assigned points from 0 to 3 (0 to 4 seconds = 0; 5 to 10 seconds = 1; 11 to 30 seconds = 2; >30 seconds = 3). The symptom intensity and duration values are then added together for a score. The MSQ is calculated by multiplying the number of positions that provoked symptoms by the score. This number is then divided by 2048. An MSQ score of zero indicates no symptoms while a score of 100 means severe dizziness in all positions.

Eye Movements

Owing to the direct relationship between vestibular receptors in the inner ear and eye movements produced by the VOR, the examination of eye movements can be of primary importance in defining and localizing vestibular pathology. The key tests include observation for nystagmus, examination of the VOR at high acceleration (head thrust test), head-shaking induced nystagmus (HSN), positional testing, and the dynamic visual acuity (DVA) test.

Nystagmus is the primary diagnostic indicator used in identifying most peripheral and *central vestibular lesions*. An involuntary eye movement, nystagmus due to a *peripheral vestibular lesion* is composed of both slow and fast component eye movements. The direction of the nystagmus

Name: ______________________ Age: ________ Gender: ________ Date: ________

Baseline Symptoms	INTENSITY	DURATION	SCORE
1. Sitting-to-supine			
2. Supine-to-left side			
3. Supine-to-right side			
4. Supine-to-sit			
5. Left Hallpike-Dix test			
6. Return from Hallpike-Dix test			
7. Right Hallpike-Dix test			
8. Return from Hallpike-Dix test			
9. Sitting: nose toward left knee			
10. Return to sitting			
11. Sitting: nose toward right knee			
12. Return to sitting			
13. Sitting: head rotation 5×			
14. Sitting: head flexion and extension 5×			
15. Standing: turn right (180°)			
16. Standing: turn left (180°)			

Intensity: rated from 0 to 5 (0 = no symptoms; 5 = severe symptoms)

Duration: rated from 0 to 3 (5-10 sec = 1 point, 11-30 sec = 2 points, ≥30 sec = 3 points)

Motion sensitivity quotient: $\frac{\text{\#Provoking positions} \times \text{score} \times 100}{2048} =$ ________ Total

Note: An MSQ score of zero means no symptoms and 100 means severe dizzines in all positions.

Figure 24.8 Motion sensitivity quotient. (Adapted from Smith-Whcclock, M, et al,[45] p 221, with permission.)

is named by the direction of the fast component. For individuals with a unilateral vestibular lesion, the slow component is due to relative excitation of one side of the vestibular system. The fast component is generated from the parapontine reticular formation in the brainstem and repositions the eye to the center of the orbit. For example, in left-beating nystagmus, the eyes move slowly to the right (VOR), and the resetting eye movement is to the left (fast component). Therefore, the direction opposite the quick component of the nystagmus localizes the side of the vestibular lesion.

Nystagmus due to a vestibular lesion is most commonly seen after an acute unilateral insult, spontaneous (at rest) nystagmus. This type of nystagmus occurs in the absence of motion because of the asymmetry between the functioning and nonfunctioning vestibular systems. The brain perceives the asymmetry as active stimulation from the healthy side. Resolution of *spontaneous nystagmus* in the light typically occurs within 3 to 7 days but may vary, and it can last as long as 2 months.[46,47] Spontaneous nystagmus may always be present in the dark after a unilateral loss of vestibular function. Regardless, resolution of spontaneous nystagmus in the light or dark occurs when symmetry between the resting firing rates of both vestibular systems is reestablished.[48]

Observation for Nystagmus

Vestibular nystagmus can be suppressed in light and when a person visually fixates on a target.[49] As a result, the observation of nystagmus should be performed under conditions in which the person cannot see the surrounding environment. This can be achieved with Frenzel lenses or an infrared camera system. Frenzel lenses are goggles that have magnifying lenses enabling the clinician to observe for nystagmus yet preventing the patient from fixating on a target. An infrared camera uses infrared light to illuminate the eye though the patient is unable to see.

Head Thrust Test

The head thrust test is a widely accepted clinical tool that is used to examine semicircular canal function.[50–54] Cervical range of motion (ROM) should be determined prior to performing the head thrust test and the clinician should explain why the head must be moved quickly. The head thrust test is performed by having the patient first fixate on a near target (e.g., the clinician's nose). When testing the horizontal SCC, the head is flexed 30°. Patients are asked to keep their eyes focused on a target while their head is manually rotated in an unpredictable direction using a small-amplitude (5° to 15°), high-acceleration (3000 to 4000°/s^2) angular thrust (Fig. 24.9). When the VOR is functioning normally, the eyes move in the direction opposite to the head movement and gaze will remain on the target. In a patient with a loss of vestibular function, the VOR will not move the eyes as quickly as the head rotation and the eyes move off the target. The patient will make a corrective **saccade** to reposition the eyes (fovea) on the target. A corrective saccade is a rapid eye movement used to reposition the eyes to the target of interest. The appearance of corrective saccades indicates vestibular hypofunction as determined by the head thrust test and occurs because inhibition of vestibular afferents and central vestibular neurons on the intact side (persons with unilateral vestibular hypofunction) are less effective in encoding the amplitude of a head movement than excitation (inhibitory cutoff). A patient who has a unilateral peripheral lesion or pathology of the central vestibular neurons will not be able to maintain gaze when the head is rotated quickly toward the side of the lesion. A patient with a bilateral loss of vestibular function will make corrective saccades after a head thrust to either side. The head thrust test provides a sensitive indication of vestibular hypofunction in patients with complete loss of function in the affected labyrinth that occurs following ablative surgical procedures, such as labyrinthectomy.[50,53–55] The test is less sensitive in detecting hypofunction in patients with incomplete loss of function.[56–59]

Head-Shaking Induced Nystagmus

The **head-shaking induced nystagmus (HSN)** test is a useful aid in the diagnosis of a unilateral peripheral vestibular defect. During this test vision is occluded. The patient is instructed to close his or her eyes. The clinician flexes the head 30° and oscillates the head horizontally for 20 cycles at a frequency of 2 repetitions per second (2 Hz). Upon stopping the oscillation, the patient opens the eyes and the clinician checks for nystagmus. In subjects with normal vestibular function, nystagmus will not be present. An asymmetry between the peripheral vestibular inputs to central vestibular nuclei, however, may result in HSN. Typically, a person with a UVH will manifest a horizontal HSN, with the quick phases of the nystagmus directed toward the healthy ear and the slow phases directed toward the lesioned ear.[60] Not all patients with a UVH will have HSN. Patients with a complete loss of vestibular function bilaterally will not have HSN because neither system is functioning. As a result, there is no asymmetry between the tonic firing rates. The presence of vertical nystagmus after either horizontal or vertical head shaking suggests a central lesion.

Positional Testing

Positional testing is commonly used to identify whether otoconia have been displaced into the SCC, causing a condition referred to as **benign paroxysmal positional vertigo (BPPV)**. The addition of the otoconia into the endolymph makes the semicircular canals sensitive to changes in head position. The **Hallpike-Dix test** is the most common positional test used to examine for BPPV.[61] The patient is moved from sitting with the head rotated 45° to one side, to a supine position with the head extended 30° beyond horizontal, head still rotated 45° (Fig. 24.10). The maneuver places each of the SCC in a gravity dependent position and the clinician should observe the eyes for nystagmus. The direction of the nystagmus is unique to the involved SCC. The direction and duration of the resultant nystagmus can help determine whether the patient has

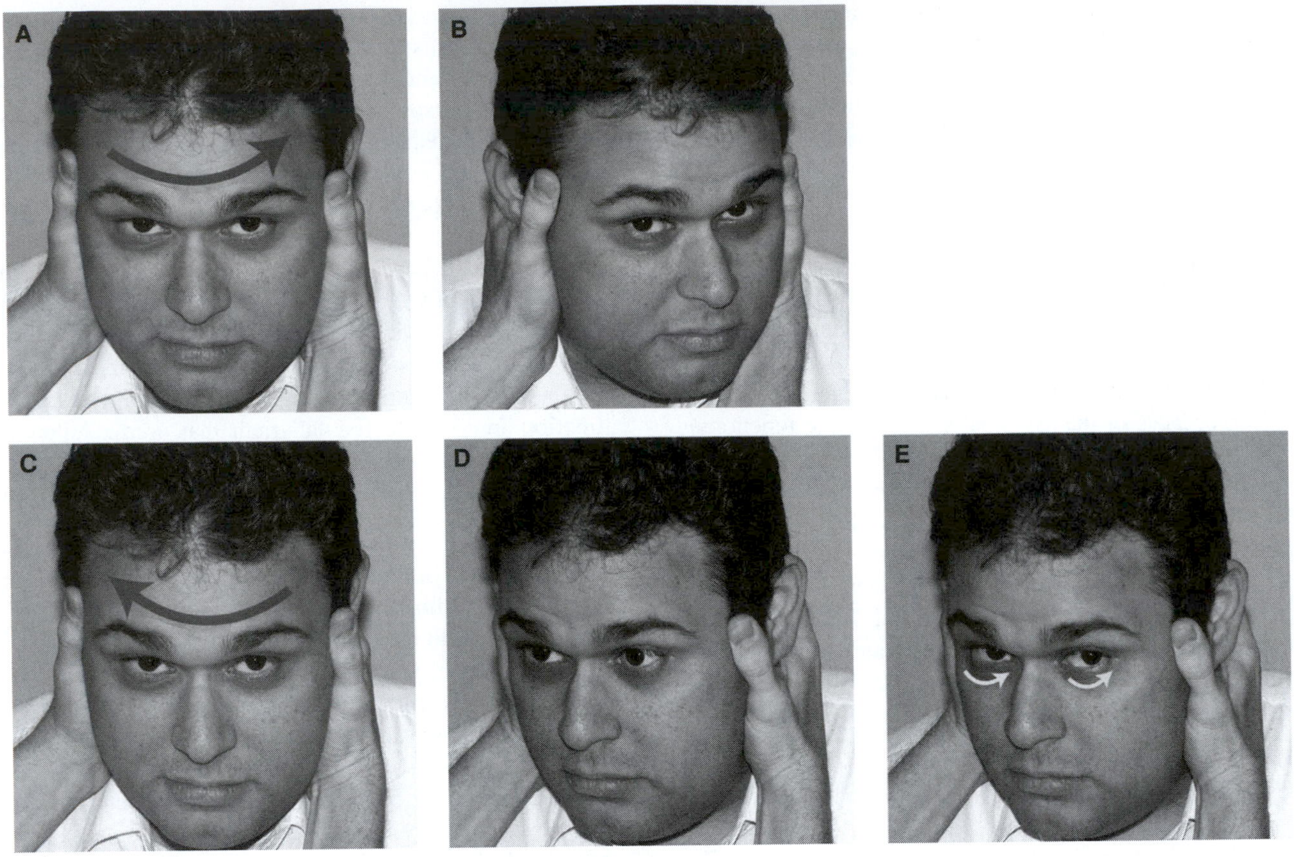

Figure 24.9 Normal head thrust test to the left (*A, B*), abnormal to the right (*C-E*). Large arrow denotes direction the head will be thrust. (*A*) Initial starting position places subject's head into cervical flexion; eyes are focused on the target. (*B*) Upon stopping the head thrust, the eyes are still on target and no corrective saccade is observed. In photographs *A* and *B*, the subject's eyes stay fixed on the examiner's nose throughout the test. (*C*) Initial starting position places subject's head into cervical flexion; eyes are focused on the target. (*D*) As the head is thrust rapidly to the right, the eyes fall off the target and move with the head. (*E*) The subject must make a corrective saccade (small arrows) to bring the eyes back to the target of interest. (From Schubert, MC, et al,[59] p 153, with permission.)

BPPV or a central lesion. An alternative form of the Hallpike-Dix test asks the patient to move into a sidelying position (Fig. 24.11). In both versions illustrated, the ear toward the ground is the labyrinth being tested. If horizontal SCC BPPV is suspected, the roll test can be used instead (Fig. 24.12). In this test, the patient is positioned supine with the head flexed 20°. Rapid rotations to the sides are done separately and the clinician observes for nystagmus.

Dynamic Visual Acuity Test

Dynamic visual acuity (DVA) is the measurement of visual acuity during horizontal motion of the head. A "bedside" and computerized form of the test can be used to identify the functional significance of the vestibular hypofunction.[62,63] Head velocities need to be greater than 100°/s at the time DVA is measured to ensure that the vestibular afferents from the contralateral side are driven into inhibition and the letters are not identified with a **smooth pursuit** eye movement. To perform the test, static visual acuity is determined first. The patient is asked to "Read the lowest line you can see" on a wall-mounted acuity chart. Lighthouse EDTRS™ (Early Treatment Diabetic Retinopathy Study) wall charts are recommended as they provide uniform light luminance for each of the letters. The patient then attempts to read the chart while the clinician horizontally oscillates the patient's head at a frequency of 2 Hz. A metronome can be useful to ensure correct frequency of the oscillation. For patients with loss of vestibular function, the eyes will not be stable in space during head movements. This causes a decrement in DVA compared with visual acuity when the head is still. A three or more line decrement in visual acuity during head movement is suggestive of vestibular hypofunction.[63] For people with normal vestibular function, head movement results in little or no change of visual acuity compared with the head still (<1 line difference). Computerized DVA has been found to correctly identify the side of lesion in patients with unilateral hypofunction for self-generated and unpredictable head motion.[63,64]

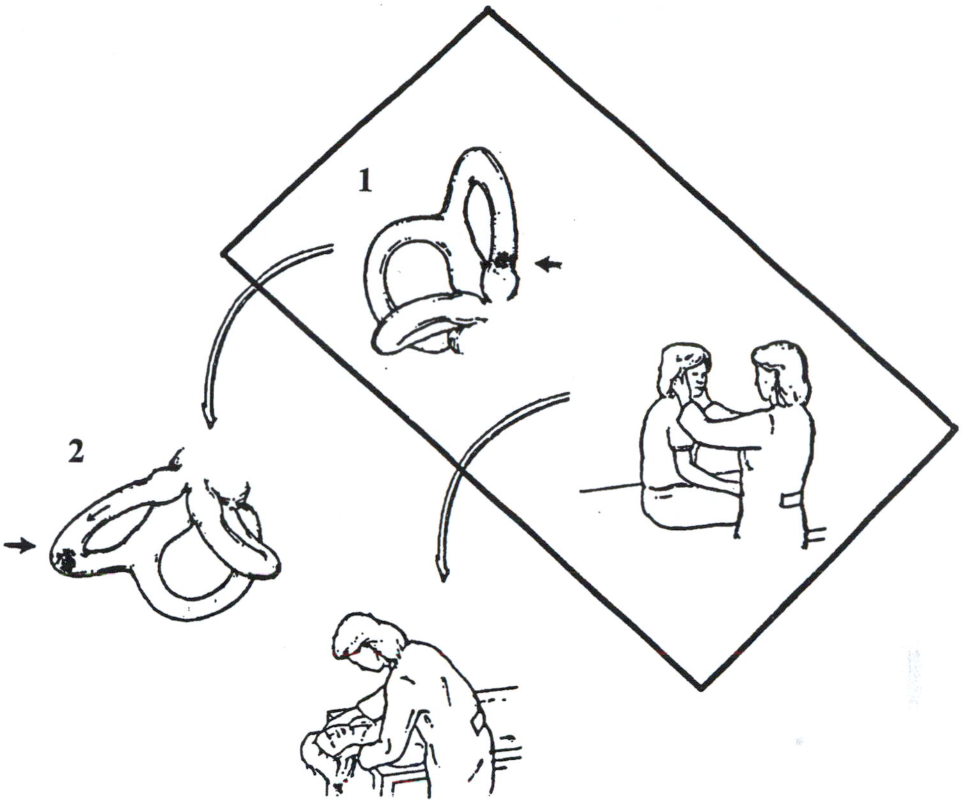

Figure 24.10 The Hallpike-Dix test. (*1*) The patient sits on the examination table and the clinician turns the head horizontally 45°. (*2*) As the examiner maintains the 45° rotation, the patient is quickly brought to a supine position with the neck extended 30° beyond the horizontal. The examiner must look for nystagmus and ask the patient if vertigo is being experienced. The patient is then slowly brought back to the starting position, and the other side is tested. The side that reproduces nystagmus and vertigo is the side that has the benign paroxysmal positional vertigo (BPPV). Shown here for testing right posterior or right anterior semicircular canal BPPV. (Adapted from Tusa, RJ: Canalith Repositioning for Benign Positional Vertigo. Education Program Syllabus. American Academy of Neurology, St. Paul, MN, 1998, p 6, with permission.)

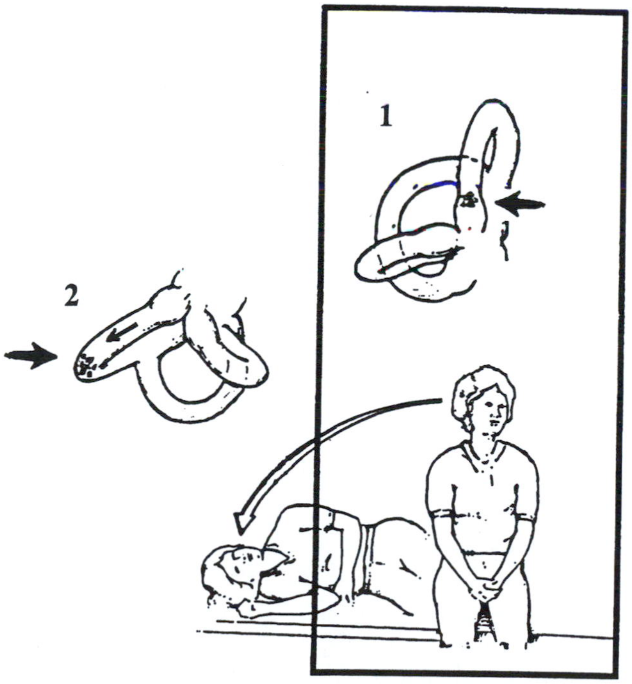

Figure 24.11 The Hallpike-Dix test (sidelying). (*1*) The patient sits on the edge of the examination table. The clinician turns the head horizontally 45°. (*2*) As the examiner maintains the 45° rotation, the patient is quickly brought down to the side opposite the head rotation (pictured here as the right side). The examiner checks for nystagmus and vertigo, and then slowly brings the patient to the starting position. The other side is then tested. (Adapted from Tusa, RJ: Canalith Repositioning for Benign Positional Vertigo. Education Program Syllabus. American Academy of Neurology, St. Paul, MN, 1998, p 6, with permission.)

Gait and Balance Testing

Examination of gait and balance problems is important for determination of a patient's functional status. Testing should address both static and dynamic balance (e.g., weight shifting, automatic postural responses, and ambulation). Gait and balance tests cannot uniquely identify pathology within the vestibular system. Table 24.5 includes common balance tests and expected results.

Vestibular Function Tests

Semicircular Canal Tests

The more common vestibular function tests include caloric testing and rotary chair tests. *Caloric testing* involves infusing the external auditory canal with air or water. This stimulus introduces a temperature gradient. In the presence of gravity, this temperature gradient results in the convective flow of endolymph that deflects the cupula and generates nystagmus within the horizontal SCC. This test is particularly useful for determining the side of the deficit, because each labyrinth is stimulated separately. A variation with ice water is useful to determine whether minimal function exists in the vestibular system for patients with severe loss. However, the caloric test provides limited information because only the horizontal SCCs are stimulated and that stimulation corresponds to a frequency (0.025 Hz) that is much lower than the natural frequencies of head movement (1 to 20 Hz).[65,66]

The rotary chair test stimulates each vestibular system by rotating subjects in the dark. In subjects with normal

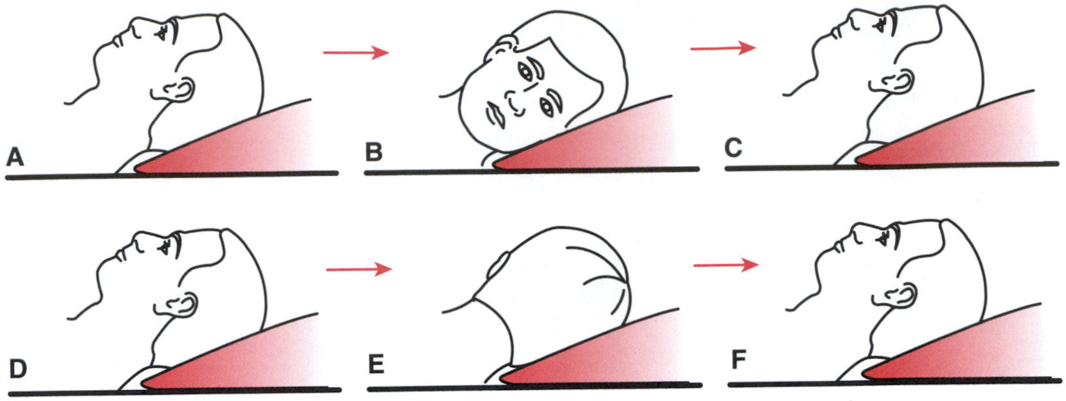

Figure 24.12 Roll Test for Horizontal Semicircular Canal BPPV. Initially, the patient's head should be placed in 20° cervical flexion. (*A*) The patient is positioned in supine. (*B*) The head is quickly turned 90° to the left side. The clinician then checks for nystagmus and vertigo. (*C*) The head is then gently returned to the neutral starting position. (*D–F*) The test is repeated to the other side, (head is quickly turned 90° to the right side). The therapist again must check for nystagmus and vertigo.

vestibular function, nystagmus should be generated by the rotations. In the presence of a vestibular disorder, the extent of pathology can be determined by comparing VOR gain and phase from rotations toward one ear with rotations toward the opposite ear. In addition, VOR gain and phase of people with normal vestibular function can be compared with that of people with suspected vestibular hypofunction. Rotary chair testing is limited because only the horizontal SCCs are routinely tested to determine extent of pathology.

Otolith Tests

Recent advances in vestibular diagnostic testing have extended the region of identifiable pathology to include the otolith organs.[67–69] The *vestibular-evoked myogenic potentials (VEMP)* test has gained broad clinical use in recent years.[67] The VEMP test exposes patients to a series of loud (95-dB) clicks. During the sound application, the ipsilateral sternocleidomastoid (SCM) muscle is tested for myogenic potentials. In people with healthy vestibular function, an initial inhibitory potential (occurring at a latency of 13 msec after the click) is followed by an excitatory potential (occurring at a latency of 21 msec after the click). For patients with vestibular hypofunction, the VEMPs are absent on the side of the lesion. The saccule has been implicated as the site of afferent stimulation during VEMP testing because saccular afferents provide ipsilateral inhibitory disynaptic input to the SCM muscle,[70] are responsive to click noise,[71–73] and are positioned close to the footplate of the stapes and therefore are subject to mechanical stimulation.[68,71]

The *subjective visual vertical (SVV)* and *subjective visual horizontal (SVH)* tests are used to examine otolith function, though they cannot be used to uniquely detect saccular or

Table 24.5 Common Balance Tests and Expected Results Related to Specific Diagnosis

Test	BPPV	UVL	BVL	Central Lesion
Romberg	Negative	Acute: positive Chronic: negative	Acute: positive Chronic: negative	Often negative
Tandem Romberg	Negative	Positive, eyes closed	Positive	Positive
Single-legged stance	Negative	May be positive	Acute: positive Chronic: negative	May be unable to perform
Gait	Normal	Acute: wide-based, slow, decreased arm swing and trunk rotation Compensated: normal	Acute: wide-based, slow, decreased arm swing and trunk rotation Compensated: mild gait deviation	May have pronounced ataxia
Turn head while walking	May produce slight unsteadiness	Acute: may not keep balance Compensated: normal	May not keep balance or slows cadence to perform	May not keep balance, increased ataxia

BPPV = Benign paroxysmal postural vertigo; BVL = bilateral vestibular lesion; UVL = unilateral vestibular lesion.

utricular pathology. During the SVV test, patients are asked to align a dimly lit luminous bar (in an otherwise darkened room) with what they perceive as being vertical. The SVH test asks patients to align a bar with what they perceive as being horizontal. Subjects without vestibular problems typically align the bar within 1.5° of true vertical or horizontal, whereas patients with UVH generally align the bar more than 2° from true vertical or horizontal with the bar tilted toward the lesioned side.[69,74,75]

Vestibular System Dysfunction

Peripheral Pathology

Mechanical

The most common cause of vertigo, BPPV, is a biomechanical disorder. Symptoms of BPPV include vertigo with change in head position, nausea with or without vomiting, and dysequilibrium. In the most common form, a latency of onset of the vertigo and nystagmus occurs within 15 seconds once the head is in the provoking position. The duration is usually less than 60 seconds. The vertigo and nystagmus are direct impairments caused by the misplaced otoconia. Many individuals also experience nausea, vomiting, and imbalance. BPPV is believed to occur via one of two mechanisms: *cupulolithiasis* and *canalithiasis*. Both of the theories involve the otoliths becoming dislodged from the utricle and falling into the SCCs. Schuknecht first theorized that fragments of otoconia break away and adhere to the cupula of one of the SCCs (cupulolithiasis).[76] When the head is moved into certain positions, the weighted cupula is deflected by the pull of gravity. This abnormal signal results in vertigo and nystagmus, which persists as long as the patient is in the provoking position. Cupulolithiasis, therefore, does not explain the brief duration of the vertigo common in BPPV.[77] A second theory was proposed in 1979, canalithiasis, in which the otoconia are floating freely in one of the SCCs.[78] When a patient changes head position, the pull of gravity causes the freely floating otoconia to move inside the SCC resulting in endolymph movement and deflection of the cupula. Figure 24.13 illustrates BPPV occurring from cupulolithiasis or canalithiasis.

Decreased Receptor Input

The most common causes of UVH leading to decreased or eliminated receptor input are viral insults, trauma, and

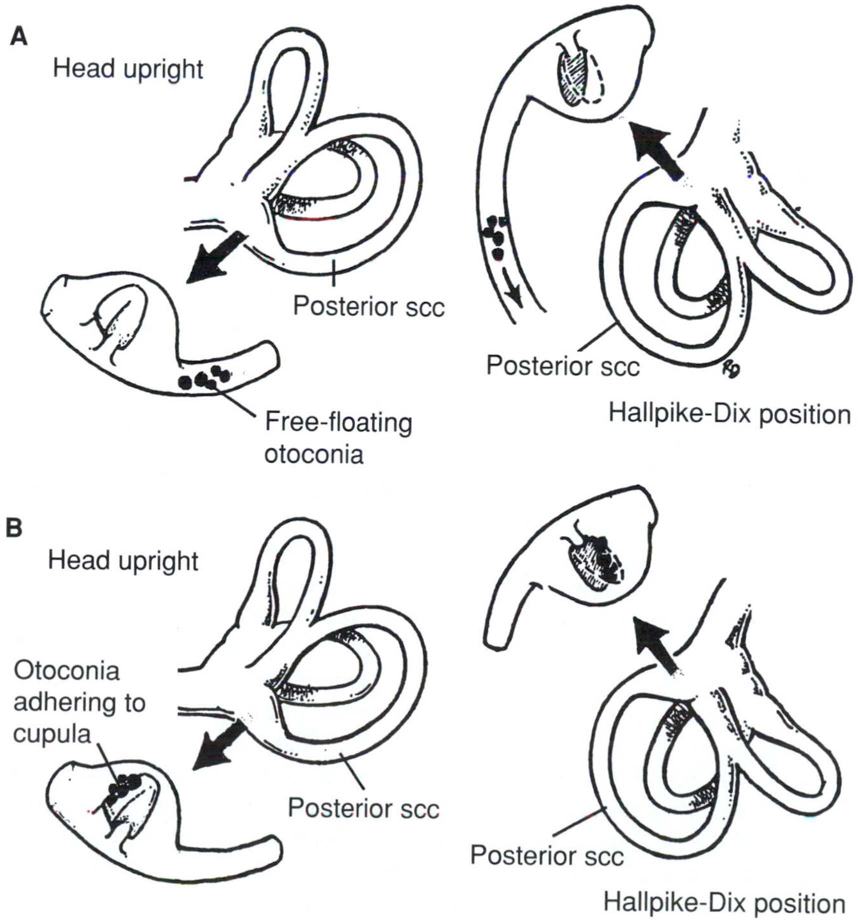

Figure 24.13 Illustrated is benign paroxysmal positional vertigo of the posterior SCC, note the cupular deflection. (*A*) Canalithiasis indicates free-floating otoconia within the SCC. When the head is moved into a position that places the SCC parallel to the pull of gravity, the free-floating otoconia move to the dependent position within the canal. The movement of the free-floating otoconia results in deflection of the cupula. (*B*) Cupulolithiasis indicates otoconia adhering to the cupula. When the head is moved to a position placing one of the SCC parallel to the pull of gravity, the cupula is continually displaced. Illustrated is BPPV of the posterior SCC, also note the cupular deflection. Note that the cupula is drawn with the superior aspect detached from the ampulla.

vascular events.[79,80] Patients who sustain a UVH will experience direct impairments of vertigo, spontaneous nystagmus, oscillopsia with head movements, postural instability, and dysequilibrium. Initially, the patient will experience the vertigo and nystagmus impairments due to the asymmetry created when one vestibular system is no longer functioning. This resolves within 3 to 7 days assuming the patient is exposed to common daylight conditions.[81] Spontaneous nystagmus beyond this time period should alert the clinician to a possible central lesion or an unstable peripheral vestibular lesion. The direct impairments of visual blurring, postural instability, and dysequilibrium respond to physical therapy intervention. Because vertigo owing to asymmetry typically resolves within 7 days, persistent symptoms of vertigo beyond 2 weeks should be considered chronic, also necessitating vestibular rehabilitation.

The most common cause of a bilateral vestibular hypofunction (BVH) is **ototoxicity**. Certain classes of antibiotics such as aminoglycosides (gentamicin, streptomycin) are readily taken up by the hair cells of the vestibular apparatus and continue to build in the system even after the person has stopped using the antibiotic. Less common causes of BVH include meningitis, autoimmune disorders, head trauma, tumors on each eighth cranial nerve (including bilateral vestibular schwannoma), transient ischemic episodes of vessels supplying the vestibular system, and sequential unilateral vestibular neuronitis.[82–84] The primary complaint is dysequilibrium though oscillopsia and gait ataxia are common clinical signs with a BVH diagnosis, all direct impairments. Unless the BVH is asymmetric, the patient will not experience nausea or vertigo, because there is no asymmetry in the tonic firing rate of the vestibular neurons. Halmagyi et al reported that patients with gentamicin ototoxicity have posture and gait abnormalities, decreased visual acuity with head movement, and reduced VOR gains resulting in a positive head thrust test.[85] These impairments are likely permanent though patients with BVH can return to high levels of activity.

Central Nervous System Pathology

Various central nervous system (CNS) injuries can affect the vestibular system.[86] Cerebrovascular insults involving the *anterior-inferior cerebellar artery (AICA), posterior-inferior cerebellar artery (PICA),* and *vertebral artery* may cause vertigo, though other signs associated with these infarcts are present and help clarify the site of pathology. Signs and symptoms between an AICA and PICA infarct can be difficult to distinguish though hearing loss is usually more common with AICA infarcts. Lesions of the vertebral artery may affect the cerebellum only and can mimic a peripheral vestibular hypofunction in its clinical presentation. Most patients with cerebellar lesions however, will have associated signs such as dysdiadochokinesia or past pointing.[87] Individuals with transient ischemic attacks may present with sudden vertigo that lasts minutes and also include complaint of hearing loss. For more thorough reading discerning types of central vestibular pathology, see Brandt and Dieterich[86] and Delaney.[87]

Patients who have sustained a traumatic brain injury (TBI) due to labyrinthine or skull fractures may complain of vertigo.[88] As much as 78 percent of patients sustaining a mild head injury had acute complaints of vertigo, and 20–37 percent still experienced the vertigo 6 months to 5 years later.[89,90] Abnormal central processing as well as reduced receptor input may cause the perseveration of the vertigo reported in patients with TBI.

Signs and symptoms associated with *vertebrobasilar insufficiency (VBI)* typically don't involve the classic signs and symptoms of vestibular pathology. Rather, symptoms such as *drop attacks* (sudden loss of muscle tone resulting in a fall), transient blindness, or dysarthria are associated with VBI. One study identified visual dysfunction, drop attacks, and unsteadiness/incoordination as the three most common symptoms associated with VBI.[91]

Demyelinating diseases such as multiple sclerosis (MS) can affect cranial nerve VIII where it enters the brainstem. In such a case, signs and symptoms may be identical to a UVH. A magnetic resonance image scan will need to be performed to ensure an accurate diagnosis of MS.

Discerning Peripheral Vestibular Pathology from Central Vestibular Pathology

Observation of nystagmus is a useful tool for assisting in determining a diagnosis of CNS pathology. Nystagmus from a cerebellar lesion may be in a pure vertical direction.[92] The nystagmus may not have a slow component and the eyes therefore oscillate at equal speeds, called *pendular nystagmus.* Pendular nystagmus is often indicative of congenital disorders, such as the absence of central vision (cortical visual processing). Another clue to discern a central versus a peripheral vestibular pathology is the recovery time. Unlike nystagmus following a peripheral vestibular lesion, nystagmus from a central vestibular lesion may never resolve.

Vertigo can be a symptom with central pathology but is rare and if present, is often much less intense than with a peripheral vestibular lesion.[93] Patients with lesions of the vestibular nuclei can present with vertigo, nystagmus, and dysequilibrium similar to the patient with a peripheral vestibular lesion. However, central lesions above the level of the vestibular nuclei will manifest lateropulsion, head tilt, and visual perceptual difficulties as well as oculomotor signs. *Lateropulsion* refers to the person's tendency to fall to one side.

Brandt et al classify central vestibular syndromes from a clinical consensus of establishing perceptual, ocular motor, and postural signs.[94] They report that the most sensitive signs of unilateral brainstem infarct are tilt of the patient's SVV and ocular torsion. *Ocular torsion* refers to both eyes rotating downward toward the direction of tilt.

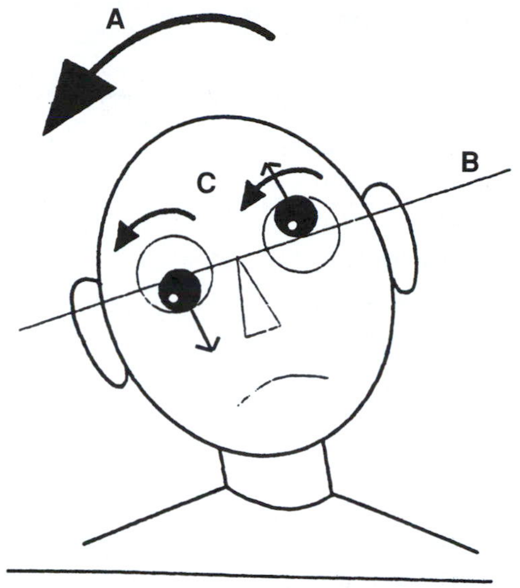

Figure 24.14 The ocular tilt reaction (OTR) consists of a triad of signs: (*A*) Head tilting to the right, indicated with the large arrow. (*B*) Skew deviation of the eyes (right eye is down, left eye is up), indicated with the bisecting line and straight arrows. (*C*) Torsion of the eyes to the right, indicated with the two smaller rounded arrows. (Adapted from Brandt, T, and Dieterich, M,[27] p 339, with permission.)

Ocular torsion combined with *head tilting* and skew deviation encompass a triad of signs termed a complete *ocular tilt reaction (OTR)*.[95] *Skew deviation* of the eyes appears as one eye being superiorly displaced in comparison with the other eye. In a study of patients with Wallenberg's (PICA infarct) syndrome, one-third of these patients demonstrated a complete OTR (Fig. 24.14).[96]

"Red flags" that should alert the clinician to a central vestibular etiology include horizontal or vertical **diplopia** lasting longer than 2 weeks after the onset of signs or symptoms thought to be due to UVH, persistent pure vertical *positional nystagmus* (anterior canal cupulolithiasis should be ruled out), and a spontaneous up beating nystagmus (rare). The therapist should refer a patient with these manifestations to a neurologist.

It is not within the scope of this chapter to expand on the differential diagnosis within the CNS, identifying the site of lesion. However, the physical therapist must recognize the difference between central and peripheral vestibular dysfunction because this guides the treatment strategy. Table 24.6 can be used as a guide to discern central vestibular pathology from peripheral vestibular pathology.

Interventions

Benign Paroxysmal Positional Vertigo

The development of specific anticipated goals and expected outcomes for the individual patient with BPPV is based on the following general goals:

- The otoconia will be returned into the vestibule.
- The patient will demonstrate reduced vertigo associated with head motion.
- The patient will demonstrate improved balance.

Table 24.6 Common Symptoms Associated with Central versus Peripheral Vestibular Pathology

Central Vestibular Pathology	Peripheral Vestibular Pathology
Ataxia often severe.	Ataxia mild.
Abnormal smooth pursuit and abnormal saccadic eye movement tests.	Smooth pursuit and saccades usually normal; positional testing may reproduce nystagmus.
SX usually do not include hearing loss; if so, it is often sudden and permanent. SX might include diplopia, altered conscious, lateropulsion.	SX may include hearing loss (insidious-may recover), fullness in ears, tinnitus.
SX of acute vertigo not usually suppressed by visual fixation.	SX of acute vertigo usually suppressed by visual fixation. SX of acute vertigo usually intense (more than central vestibular pathology).
Pendular nystagmus (eyes oscillate at equal speeds).	Nystagmus will incorporate slow and fast phases (jerk nystagmus).
Pure persistent vertical nystagmus persists regardless of positional testing (persistent downbeat nystagmus in Hallpike-Dix may indicate anterior canal BPPV).	Spontaneous horizontal nystagmus usually resolves within 7 days in a patient with UVH.

BPPV = Benign paroxysmal postural vertigo; SX = symptoms; UVH = unilateral vestibular hypofunction.

Table 24.7 Type of Nystagmus Based on SCC Location and Mechanism of BPPV

SCC[a]	Mechanism	Nystagmus[b]	Incidence (%)[c]
Right posterior	Cupulolithiasis Canalithiasis	Persistent UBN and right torsion[d] Transient UBN and right torsion	63
Left posterior	Cupulolithiasis Canalithiasis	Persistent UBN and left torsion Transient UBN and left torsion	
Right anterior	Cupulolithiasis Canalithiasis	Persistent DBN and right torsion Persistent DBN and right torsion	12
Left anterior	Cupulolithiasis Canalithiasis	Persistent DBN and left torsion Persistent DBN and left torsion	
Horizontal[e]	Cupulolithiasis Canalithiasis	Persistent ageotropic Transient geotropic	1

[a]Testing for BPPV in the SCC assumes the patient is in the appropriate positional test.

[b]Nystagmus is labeled by the direction of the fast component (UBN means the fast component of the nystagmus is beating upwards, DBN = down beat nystagmus).

[c]Twenty-four percent of cases were indistinguishable between posterior and anterior SCC BPPV.[98]

[d]The torsional rotation is noted as it relates to the superior poles of the eyes, from the perspective of the examiner.

[e]When BPPV occurs in the horizontal SCC, nystagmus will be present when the head is positioned to either side.

Ageotropic nystagmus = fast component beats away from the ground; geotropic nystagmus = fast component beats toward the ground.

- The patient will demonstrate enhanced decision-making skills regarding self-treatment strategies as a form of prophylaxis.
- The patient will demonstrate independence in daily activity (BADL; IADL) involving head motion.

Because BPPV is the most common peripheral vestibular pathology, physical therapists should be familiar with treatment of this disorder. Nystagmus, generated as result of placing the SCC in gravity dependent positions, dictates which SCC is involved (Table 24.7) and directs the clinician to choose an appropriate treatment approach. Three different treatment approaches have been developed, each based on pathophysiologic theories of this disorder. The techniques include the canalith repositioning maneuver, the Liberatory (Semont) maneuver, and Brandt–Daroff exercises.

The *canalith repositioning maneuver (CRM)* is based on the canalithiasis theory of free-floating debris in the SCC.[97] The patient's head is moved into different positions in a sequence that will move the debris out of the involved SCC and into the vestibule (general term for the location of the utricle and saccule; see Fig. 24.1). Once the debris is in the vestibule, the signs and symptoms should resolve. The positions used in the treatment of posterior and anterior SCC canalithiasis are the same. Figure 24.15 illustrates the CRT as applied to either the left posterior or left anterior SCC. After the treatment, the patient may be fit with a soft collar as a reminder to avoid vertical head movements that may again dislodge the otoconia. It is important to instruct the patient that horizontal movement of the head should be performed to prevent stiff neck muscles. CRM has also been adapted for application to the horizontal SCC (Fig. 24.16), although BPPV is much less common in either the horizontal or anterior SCC.[98] The original post-CRM instructions asked patients to remain upright for one to two nights (sleep in a recliner chair) and then to avoid sleeping on the involved side for five additional nights. Evidence shows that sleeping upright for greater than 1 night has no effect on remission of symptoms.[99] Recurrence of BPPV is very low.[100,101]

The *Liberatory (Semont) maneuver* was first offered as a treatment for posterior SCC BPPV based on the cupulolithiasis theory.[102] It involves rapidly moving the patient through positions designed to dislodge the debris from the cupula (Fig. 24.17). Recent evidence shows it is effective as an alternative treatment for canalithiasis, though it is more difficult for the patient to tolerate.[103,104]

Brandt–Daroff exercises were originally designed to habituate the CNS to the provoking position.[105] They may also act to dislodge debris from the cupula or by causing debris to move out of the canal. Figure 24.18 illustrates the exercises. The exercise should be performed for 5 to 10 repetitions, three times a day until the patient has no vertigo for 2 consecutive days. If the patient has severe vertigo or complaints of nausea, decreasing the number of repetitions to three, performed three times a day, may render the exercises more tolerable. It is important to explain to the patient that the movements must be performed rapidly and that this will

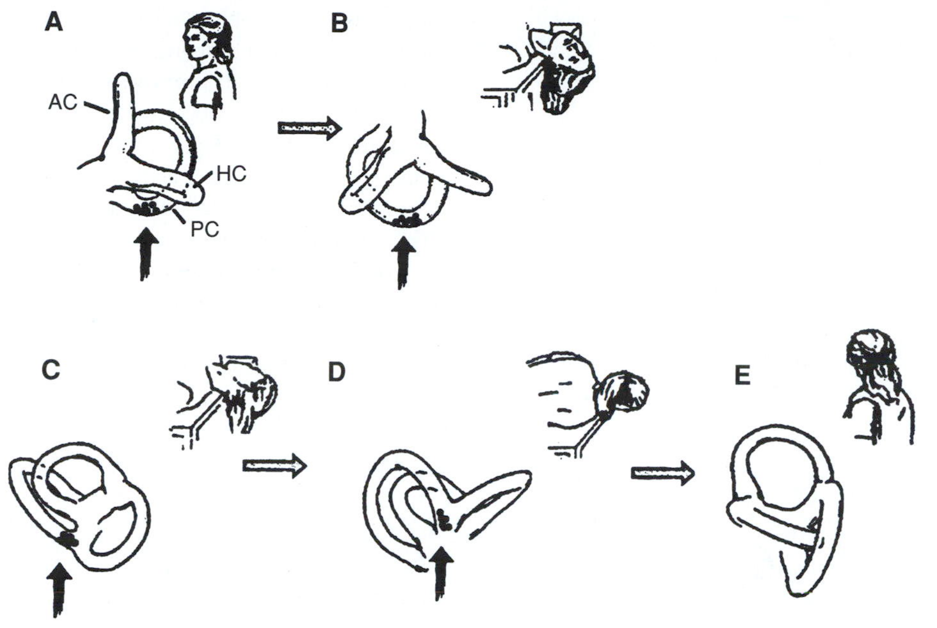

Figure 24.15 Canalith repositioning treatment (CRT) for posterior or anterior semicircular canal BPPV. (*A*) The patient's head is first rotated 45° toward the involved side, pictured here as the left. (*B*) The patient is then moved into the Hallpike-Dix position with the affected left ear toward the ground. (*C*) Next, the head is rotated 90° to the right. It is important to maintain the 30° neck extension during this step. The head should now be positioned 45° to the right. (*D*) The patient is rolled onto the right shoulder and (*E*) slowly brought up to sitting position, head still rotated 45° to the right. The patient may then be fitted with a soft collar. Note the orientation of the labyrinth for each stage. The arrow points to the free-floating debris and shows its movement through the canal into the common crus (*D*). AC = Anterior SCC; PC = posterior SCC; HC = horizontal SCC. Between each step, the clinician should wait 1 to 2 minutes or until the vertigo and nystagmus has stopped to ensure otoconia flow through the canal. (From Tusa, RJ: Canalith Repositioning for Benign Positional Vertigo. Education Program Syllabus. American Academy of Neurology, St. Paul, MN, 1998, p 13, with permission.)

probably provoke the patient's vertigo. Patient education should also include informing the patient that it is normal to have some residual symptoms of dysequilibrium and nausea on completing the exercise. The residual symptoms are usually temporary and patients need to continue the exercises.

The physical therapy goal of performing CRT and liberatory procedures are to replace the otoconia into the vestibule, where the calcium crystals can be reabsorbed. The Brandt–Daroff exercises, although originally designed to habituate the peripheral vestibular response, have also led to a complete remission of symptoms, sometimes after the first exercise session.[105] Physical therapy outcomes should also include teaching the patient how to use the appropriate techniques at home, in the case of recurrence. See Table 24.8 for suggested guidelines for use of the CRT, the Liberatory (Semont) maneuver, or Brandt–Daroff exercises.

Unilateral Vestibular Hypofunction

The development of specific anticipated goals and expected outcomes for the individual patient with UVH is based on the following general goals:

- The patient will demonstrate improved stability of gaze during head movement.
- The patient will demonstrate diminished sensitivity to motion.
- The patient will demonstrate improved static and dynamic postural stability.

Table 24.8 Benign Paroxysmal Positional Vertigo Treatment Techniques

Treatment Procedure	Diagnosis/Symptoms
CRT	BPPV due to canalithiasis Posterior SCC canalithiasis is the most common
Liberatory maneuver	BPPV due to cupulolithiasis Posterior SCC cupulolithiasis is the most common
Brandt-Daroff exercises	Persistent/residual or mild vertigo (even after CRT) For the patient who may not tolerate CRT

BPPV = Benign paroxysmal positional vertigo; CRT = canalith repositioning treatment; SCC = semicircular canal.

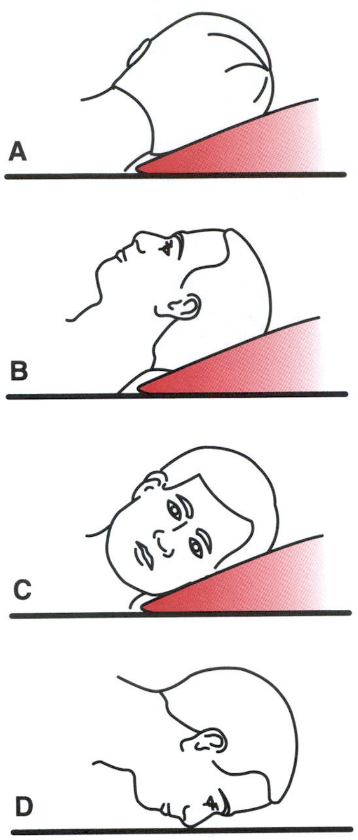

Figure 24.16 Canalith repositioning treatment (CRT) for right horizontal semicircular canal BPPV. Initially, the patient's head should be placed in 20° cervical flexion. (*A*) For treating a right-sided horizontal canal BPPV, the patient's head is initially placed 90° to the right. (*B*) Next, the head is rotated 90° to the left. The therapist should wait in this position for 15 seconds or until the vertigo and nystagmus stops. (*C*) The head should then be rotated another 90° to the left, again the therapist must wait for 15 seconds or until the vertigo and nystagmus stops. (*D*) The patient must then roll into prone position and await the signs or symptoms to stop. The therapist must attempt to keep the head in 20° flexion during the transition from C to D. If the CRT has been successful, nystagmus and vertigo should resolve once the patient is in the prone position. The patient may need assistance to sit up from the prone position.

- The patient will be independent in proper performance of a home exercise program (HEP) that includes walking.

Patients with UVH should be informed that recovery time upon initiating vestibular rehabilitation averages 6 to 8 weeks. To ensure compliance with the vestibular rehabilitation exercises, patients should be encouraged frequently and the mutually agreed upon goals and outcomes regularly reinforced.

Gaze Stability

The purpose of these exercises is to improve the VOR and other systems that are used to assist gaze stability with head motion. Vestibular adaptation exercises are designed to expose patients to **retinal slip**. Retinal slip occurs when the image of an object moves off the fovea of the retina, resulting in visual blurring. Retinal slip is necessary as this is the signal used to improve the response of the residual vestibular system. Because the brain can tolerate small amounts of retinal slip yet see a target clearly, the patient must try to keep the target in focus. Otherwise, head motion that is too rapid will result in excessive retinal slip. The two primary paradigms of vestibular adaptation are ×1 (times 1) and ×2 (times 2) exercises.[106] In the ×1 exercise the patient is asked to move the head horizontally (and vertically if appropriate) as quickly as possible while maintaining focus on a stable target. The patient must learn to slow the head movement if the target becomes blurred. A good target to use is a business card, asking the patient to focus on a word or a letter within a word. The starting

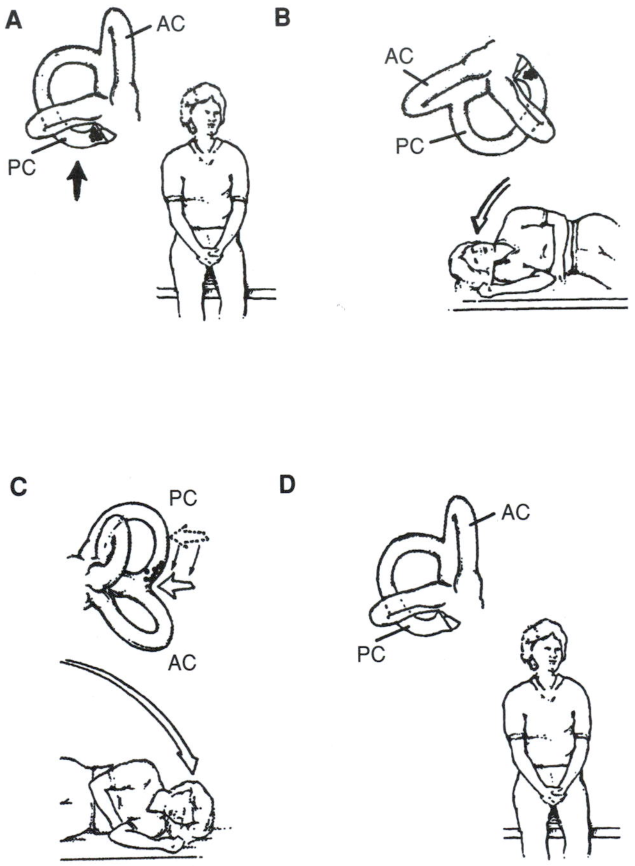

Figure 24.17 Liberatory (Semont) maneuver for right posterior SCC BPPV. The physical therapist should assist the patient through this positioning procedure. Note the otoconia adherent to the cupula in A and B. (*A*) The head is rotated 45° to the left side. (*B*) With assistance, the patient is then moved from sitting to right sidelying and stays in this position for 1 minute. (*C*) The patient is then rapidly moved 180°, from right sidelying to left sidelying. The head should be in the original starting position, left rotated (nose down in final position) in this example. Note the otoconia have been dislodged from the cupula. After 1 minute in this position, (*D*) the patient returns to sitting and may be fitted with a soft collar. AC = Anterior SCC; PC = posterior SCC. (Adapted from Johnson, R, and Griffin, J,[106] p 10, with permission.)

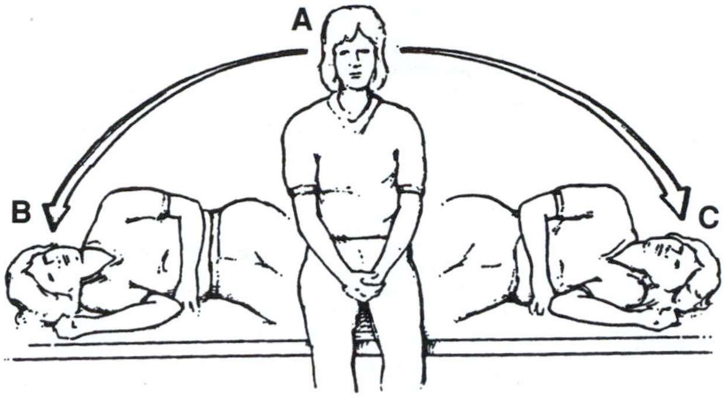

Figure 24.18 Brandt-Daroff treatment for posterior SCC BPPV. (*A*) The patient starts in a sitting position and turns the head 45° to one side (*left*) then quickly lies down on the opposite shoulder (*right*). (*B*) The patient should be instructed to remain in this position for 30 seconds or until the vertigo stops. The patient then slowly returns to the starting position (*A*), maintaining the head rotation (*left*) until sitting upright. Next, the patient turns the head to the opposite direction (*right*) and lies down on the other shoulder (*left*) (*C*), observing the similar 30-second time guidelines. The exercise should be done 10 to 20 times, three times per day until the patient is without vertigo for two consecutive days. (Adapted from Johnson, R, and Griffin, J,[106] p 10, with permission.)

target distance should be an arm's length away. The ×2 paradigm requires the patient to move the head and target in opposite directions (Fig. 24.19). Both paradigms should be made increasingly more difficult as the patient improves. Examples of increasing difficulty include the use of a distracting background while the patient attempts to read the letter or word (checkerboard, venetian blinds), varying the distance from which the patient performs the exercises, moving the head more rapidly, and performing the exercise while standing. The *computerized DVA* test is a useful measure of improved gaze stability for individuals with UVH and TBI.[63,107]

Postural Stability

The purpose of postural stability exercises is to improve balance by encouraging the development of balance strategies within the limitations of the patient, be they somatosensory, visual, or vestibular. The exercises should challenge the patient and be safe enough to perform independently (Table 24.9). Exercises must be updated and progressed to incorporate more challenges (Fig. 24.20). In addition, it is important to incorporate head movement into the exercises because many patients with vestibular loss tend to decrease their head movement.

Motion Sensitivity

Habituation training is warranted when a patient with a UVH has continual complaints of dizziness. *Habituation* is defined as the reduction in response to a repeatedly performed movement. These exercises were the first successful methods used to treat persons with vestibular disorders. Various investigators[45,108] have developed versions of positional tests based on the original work of Cawthorne,[14] Cooksey,[15] Norre and DeWeerdt,[109] and Dix.[110,111] As our knowledge of the vestibular system improves, however, we are able to provide more specific exercises than what habituation offers. Clinicians should not treat all vestibular patients with habituation exercises.

To determine which habituation exercises to prescribe, the physical therapist must determine the provoking positions first (Fig. 24.8). When a position elicits a mild to moderate dizziness, the patient remains in the provoking position for 30 seconds or until the symptoms abate, whichever comes first.[108] The patient is provided with a home exercise program (HEP) based on the results of the positional test.[45,108] The provoking exercises are performed from three to five times each, two to three times a day. Figure 24.21 provides an example of a HEP using vestibular habituation training. The exercises are designed to

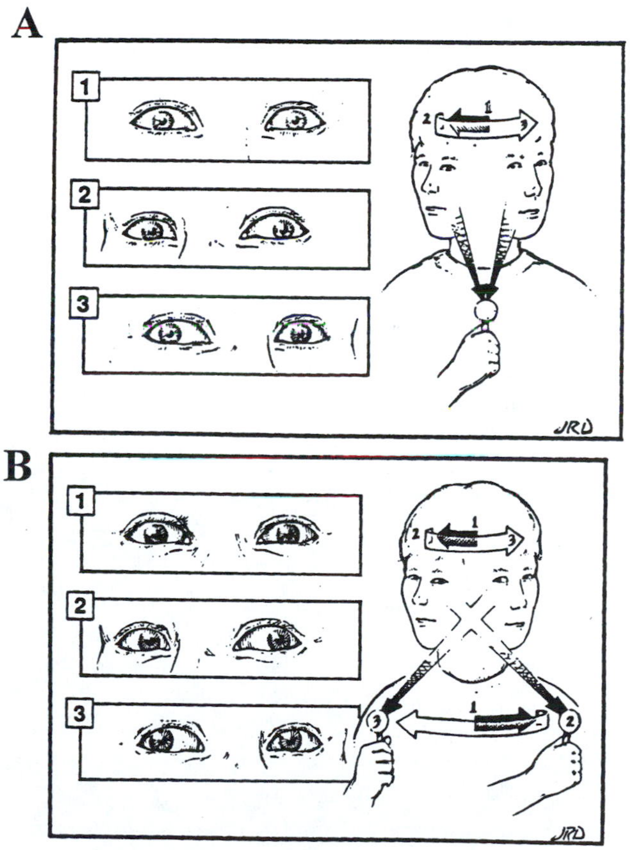

Figure 24.19 Gaze stability exercises. (*A*) ×1 paradigm: The patient is instructed to focus the eyes on a near target. While maintaining focus on the target, the patient horizontally rotates the head keeping the target still. (*B*) ×2 paradigm: The patient is instructed to focus the eyes on a near target. While the focus is maintained, the patient horizontally rotates the head and the target in *opposite* directions. Both ×1 and ×2 paradigms require vigilance of the patient to ensure clear vision during the motions. Both exercises are typically performed for 1 to 2 minutes, five times a day. It can be repeated using vertical head movements. (From Johnson, R, and Griffin, J,[106] p 12, with permission.)

Table 24.9 Balance Exercises and Progressions

Begin With	Progress To	Purpose
1. Stand with feet shoulder-width apart, arms across the chest.	Bring feet closer together. Close eyes. Stand on a sofa cushion or foam.	Enhance the use of vestibular cues for balance by decreasing base of support. Eyes closed increases reliance on vestibular cues for balance.
2. Practice ankle sways: medial–lateral and anterior-posterior.	Doing circle sways. Close eyes.	Teaches the patient to use a correct ankle strategy.
3. Attempt to walk with heel touching toe on firm surface.	Do the same exercise on carpet.	Enhance the use of vestibular cues for balance by decreasing base of support. Doing the exercise on carpet alters proprioceptive input, increasing difficulty.
4. Practice walking five steps and turning 180^0 (left and right).	Making smaller turns. Close eyes.	Turning provides a greater challenge to the vestibular system.
5. Walk and move the head side-to-side, up and down.	Counting backwards from 100 by threes.	Use distracting cognitive or motor demands to challenge balance.

Note: This table presents a limited number of exercises that are effective at improving functional balance. Each of the balance exercises should be performed three times a day for 1–2 minutes each repetition.

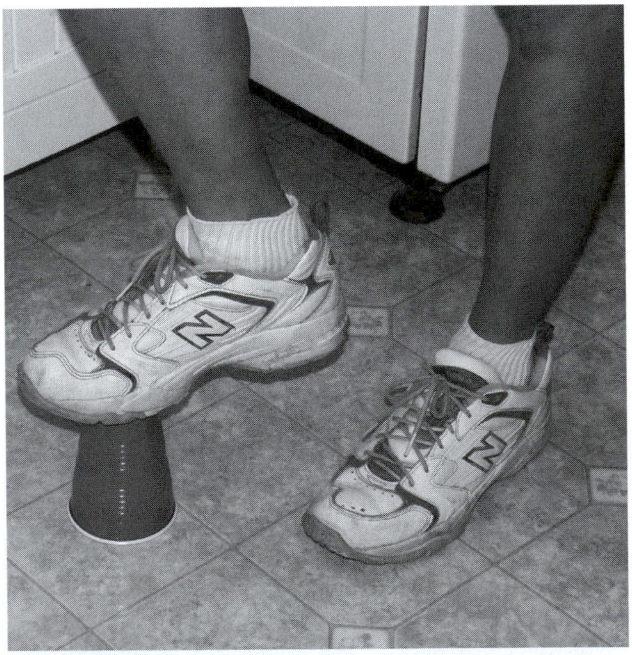

Figure 24.20 Example of a more difficult balance exercise. Instruct the patient to gently place foot on a plastic cup and maintain their balance without crushing the cup. Initially, the patient should be advised to use a handhold. The exercise can be progressed to eyes closed, no hand hold, or stepping while alternating foot placement on the cup.

reproduce the dizziness and the patient should be encouraged that the symptoms normally decrease within 2 weeks. If after 2 weeks the symptoms are no better, the habituation exercises should first be changed. If this is not helpful, the patient should be referred to either a physical therapist with special training in vestibular rehabilitation and/or a physician for further evaluation.

Bilateral Vestibular Hypofunction

The development of specific anticipated goals and expected outcomes for the individual patient with BVH is based on the following general goals:

- The patient will demonstrate reduced subjective complaints of gaze instability.
- The patient will demonstrate improved static and dynamic balance.
- The patient will be independent in proper performance of a HEP that includes walking.
- The patient will demonstrate enhanced decision making skills regarding performance of daily activity (BADL; IADL) made more challenging owing to the disorder.

Treatment of patients with a BVH is designed to address the primary complaints of gaze instability during head motion, dysequilibrium, and gait ataxia. Gaze stability exercises can be similar to the ×1 paradigm described in treatment for UVH. Use of the ×2 paradigm is not recommended for a patient with a BVH because this exercise may cause excessive retinal slip in patients with BVH.

Instructions for the Patient:
Once in the provoking position, wait for 10 seconds to determine if the dizziness will occur. If you experience symptoms of dizziness, remain in the position for an additional 20 seconds (30 seconds total) or until the dizziness abates, whichever comes first. If you do not experience any symptoms you may return to your starting position. Now that you have returned to your starting position, remain here for 10 seconds to monitor your dizziness. If you are dizzy, remain in the return position for an additional 20 seconds (30 seconds total) or until the symptoms abate, whichever comes first. Repeat five times.

Example of Exercises:
1.) Quickly move from sitting upright to bending at the trunk as if to touch your nose to your knee.
2.) Quickly move from sitting at the edge of the bed to lying flat.
3.) In supine, roll onto your left then right side.

Guidelines for the Therapist:
Often, the patient may complain of a certain movement that provokes the symptoms which the examination does not incorporate. This movement can be adapted to be a part of the patient's home exercise program.

	Mon	Tues	Wed	Thur	Fri	Sat	Sun
Duration (0–30 seconds)							
Intensity (0–5)							

Figure 24.21 Example of a home exercise program using habituation therapy.

Instead, exercises that incorporate sequenced eye and head movements and the use of imaginary targets may improve gaze stability by enhancing central preprogramming of eye movements, Table 24.10.

Patients with BVH depend on somatosensation and/or vision to maintain postural stability. Balance exercises should enhance the use of these cues. Care must be taken that the exercises are performed safely because people with BVH are more likely to fall.[112] It is imperative to begin the patient on a walking program, daily if tolerated. This can be progressed to ambulating on different surfaces (grass, gravel, sand) and in different environments (grocery store, mall). Recovery from a lesion involving both vestibular systems takes much longer than a unilateral lesion. Patients should be informed that as long as 2 years may be necessary to ensure as complete a recovery as possible. For this reason, patient education emphasizing daily activity is a high priority. Daily activity must continue beyond the course of vestibular rehabilitation. Other recommended activities include exercises in a pool and Tai Chi. The pool provides an environment of reduced gravity, allowing the patient to move safely without the risk of falling quickly to the ground. Tai Chi incorporates slow, controlled motions used to improve balance, flexibility, and increase strength. In most cases, a person with a BVH will incur a functional disability. Certain activities may always be limited, such as walking in the dark, night driving, or sports involving quick movements of the head.[113] Older patients may have to use an assistive device such as a cane for safe ambulation at night or on uneven surfaces. Habituation exercises do not work for the patient with a bilateral vestibular loss.[44]

Table 24.10 Bilateral Vestibular Lesion Exercises to Improve Central Preprogramming of Eye Movements

Begin With	Progress To
1. Hold two targets at arm's length from your head. Look with your eyes first, then turn your head toward the target. Attempt to do this for 60 seconds.	Progress to increasing the distance used to see the target. Use a busy background (checkerboard, venetian blinds).
2. Perform exercise 1 in the vertical direction.	Same as above.
3. Hold one target at arm's length from your head. Close your eyes and turn your head away from the target, attempting to keep your eyes focused on the target. Open your eyes only after having turned your head.	Progress to doing this standing. Progress to decreasing base of support.

Vestibular adaptation exercises are an excellent starting point for rehabilitation of patients with vestibular hypofunction (UVH and BVH). Research supports the beneficial effects of vestibular adaptation exercises on gait, posture, and DVA (Evidence Summary Box 24.1).

Central Vestibular Hypofunction

The development of specific anticipated goals and expected outcomes for the individual patient with a central vestibular lesion is based on the following general goals:

- The patient will demonstrate enhanced decision making skill regarding fall prevention strategies and necessary

(text continues on page 1023)

Evidence Summary Box 24.1

Outcome Studies Using Vestibular Adaptation Exercises to Improve Gait, Balance, and Dynamic Visual Acuity in Subjects with Vestibular Hypofunction

Reference	Subjects	Design/ Intervention	Duration	Results	Comments
Horak, FB, et al[114] 1992	25 subjects; randomly assigned to 1 of 3 groups (1 E and 2 C groups) E (N = 13) C-1 (N = 4) C-2 (N = 8)	RCT; treatment outcome study; 2 control groups E: vestibular rehabilitation (VR) C-1: general conditioning exercises and pain prevention (GC/PP) C-2: medication only (MO)	E = VR: 2×/week for 1 hour using adaptation and habituation exercises, general conditioning, balance retraining, and pain control interventions; C-1 = GC/PP C-2 = MO	VR group showed reduced sway for conditions 5 and 6 of CDP and increased time SOLEO and SOLEC compared with medication-only group	GC/PP group size too small to use for comparisons (authors' observation); specific exercises not listed; first study to report outcomes using vestibular adaptation exercises; habituation exercises also used; thus, cannot differentiate effect of either exercise type
Krebs, DE, et al[115] 1993	8 subjects E (N = 4) BVH Mean age 67.3 ± 15.9 C (N = 4) BVH Mean age 61.1 ± 12.2	RCT; treatment outcome study; control group E: Vestibular adaptation and substitution exercises C: Isometric exercises and general conditioning	Each group: outpatient PT once per week and HEP 1 or 2×/day	E: quicker preferred gait velocity, reduced time in double support; tolerated COM to deviate from the COP for increased distance; no change in rotary chair test, caloric test, VVOR test, or DHI scores for either E or C groups	First controlled study investigating efficacy of vestibular rehabilitation in patients with BVH
Szturm, T, et al[116] 1994	23 subjects E: (N = 11); 8 UVH, 2 BVH, 1 Normal C: (N = 12); 8 UVH, 1 BVH, 3 Normal	RCT; control group pretest/posttest E: Vestibular adaptation, OKS, and balance exercises C: Smooth pursuit and head exercises (Cawthorne-Cooksey exercises); no specific vestibular adaptation	E = 45 minutes outpatient PT 3×/week for 12 weeks; custom HEP similar to exercises supervised in clinic C = Exercises done at home (HEP) 3–4×/day for 15–20 minutes	E: Significant fall reduction over training time; improvement in condition 3 and 4 of CDP; improved VOR gain symmetry during 60°/s rotary chair test; no difference in OKN, peak slow eye velocities, or time constant during rotary chair tests for either E or C groups	Inclusion of subject with normal vestibular function in the E group possibly affected outcome; recovery of 60°/s VOR gains possibly due to peripheral vestibular recovery; questionable interaction effect due to C group not having clinic visits

Evidence Summary Box 24.1

Outcome Studies Using Vestibular Adaptation Exercises to Improve Gait, Balance, and Dynamic Visual Acuity in Subjects with Vestibular Hypofunction (continued)

Reference	Subjects	Design/ Intervention	Duration	Results	Comments
Herdman, SJ, et al[117] 1995	E: ($N = 11$); UVH due to AN resection; mean age 59.3 ± 10.9 years; C: ($N = 8$); mean age 47.9 ± 10.4 years; EC: patients with noncerebellar and/or brainstem tumor encroachment or musculoskeletal deficits	RCT; pretest/posttest treatment study with control group; E: Vestibular adaptation exercises, ambulation exercises C: Smooth pursuit exercises (placebo) and ambulation exercises	Exercises started on POD 3 Each group performed exercises (adaptation or smooth pursuit) for 1 minute, 5×/day for a total of 20 minutes per day	CDP main outcome measure E: less disequilibrium; at POD 3: 64% E subjects could do RomEC vs. 25% controls; at POD 3: E had less A-P sway for conditions 4–6 of CDP; at POD 6, 80% E subjects could do RomEC vs. 57% controls	First study advocating VR as an early post-operation intervention for AN; each subject (E and C) was age-matched due to significant difference in age
Strupp, M, et al[118] 1998	39 patients with stable UVH due to neuritis E: ($N = 19$); mean age 51.7 ± 11.1 C: ($N = 20$); mean age 52.4 ± 9.9 EC: reduced visual acuity, diseases impairing mobilization, central vestibular disorders, prior history of vestibulopathy	RCT; pretest/posttest with control group; intervention: both groups received general walking program; E group also performed saccades, VOR, smooth pursuit, balance exercises, and cervico-ocular reflex enhancement	E: performed unique exercises 3×/day for 30 minutes each for 5–7 days; to be continued independently for 3 weeks via video instruction C: received walking program; encouragement	No difference in ocular torsion, subjective visual vertical, or mean slow eye velocity due to caloric irrigation; E group showed greater reduction in total sway path during stance on platform posturography	Outcome measures examined central vestibular function
Cohen, HS, and Kimball, KT[119] 2003	53 subjects with chronic vestibulopathy; assigned to 1 of 3 groups EC: Ménière's disease, BPPV, acute vestibular neuritis or labyrinthitis, orthopaedic limitations, head trauma, neurological disease, otologic disease, use of vestibular suppressant medication	RCT; pretest/posttest non-controlled; Each group performed exercises at home only (HEP); Group 1: slow head rotation while seated without visual fixation Group 2: quick head rotation with visual fixation, seated and standing Group 3: same as Group 2 with phone call follow-up for encouragement	All 3 groups: 5–10 minutes of exercise 5×/day at home (HEP); posttest after 4 weeks of HEP	No difference between 3 groups in reduction of vertigo intensity, vertigo frequency, or symptoms generated during ADL skills	HEP beneficial for patients with vestibular hypofunction; outcome measures all subjective making functional significance uncertain; difficult to discern that results are not due to natural recovery without a true control group (i.e., no treatment or no head rotation)

(*continued*)

Evidence Summary Box 24.1

Outcome Studies Using Vestibular Adaptation Exercises to Improve Gait, Balance, and Dynamic Visual Acuity in Subjects with Vestibular Hypofunction (continued)

Reference	Subjects	Design/ Intervention	Duration	Results	Comments
Krebs, DE, et al[120] 2003	84 subjects UVH: (N = 33); mean age 59.42 ± 20.37 BVH: (N = 51); mean age 59.56 ± 18.97 EC: BPPV, Ménière's disease, unstable vestibulopathy	RCT; double blind with control; gait stability measures at baseline, 6 weeks, 12 weeks, 1 year E: Vestibular adaptation and substitution exercises; balance retraining exercises; VR HEP C: Isometric exercises and general conditioning; outpatient VR	E: outpatient PT 1×/week for 6 weeks; then 6 weeks of VR HEP C: outpatient PT 1×/week for 6 weeks; then 6 weeks of VR (1×/week)	At 6 weeks measure, only E group had significantly increased preferred gait velocity, reduced BOS, reduced double support time, reduced M-L sway, reduced lateral velocity, increased distance subjects tolerated their COM to deviate from the COP; 61% of E group demonstrated these improvements; at 1 year, significant treatment effects noted for preferred gait velocity, reduced BOS, reduced M-L sway, and reduced lateral velocity	First long-term study to document VR benefits; BVH subjects recovered by similar amounts as the UVH subjects
Patten et al, C[121] 2003	20 subjects E: (N = 10) patients with BVH; mean age 69 ± 13.2. C: (N = 10) healthy controls; mean age 68.9 ± 13.03; height and body mass were matched EC: CNS dysfunction, neuromusculoskeletal impairment, CVA, peripheral nerve deficit, visual impairment	RCT; pretest/posttest with control group E: cites exercises similar to Krebs 1993 study C: no exercise	Study cites exercise duration similar to Krebs 1993	Significant improvement in head pitch coordination; comparable to healthy controls	Authors recommend VR goals include exercises to enhance head stability during gait

Evidence Summary Box 24.1

Outcome Studies Using Vestibular Adaptation Exercises to Improve Gait, Balance, and Dynamic Visual Acuity in Subjects with Vestibular Hypofunction (continued)

Reference	Subjects	Design/ Intervention	Duration	Results	Comments
Herdman, SJ, et al[39] 2003	21 patients with UVH E: $N = 13$; Mean age 65.1 ± 16.5 C: $N = 8$; Mean age 64.9 ± 16.2	RCT; double blind; repeated measures with control; E: VOR adaptation exercises and balance retraining C: smooth pursuit and balance exercises; DVA measured weekly for 4 weeks	E and C groups exercised 4–5×/day for 20 to 30 minutes in addition to 20 minutes of balance exercises	12 of 13 individuals in the E group demonstrated DVA that returned to age matched normal values; no change in DVA for control group; only the type of exercise contributed to change in DVA	Important first study showing the beneficial effect of VOR adaptation exercises to improve gaze stability in persons with UVH as measured by the DVA

AN = Acoustic neuroma; BOS = base of support; BPPV = benign paroxysmal positional vertigo; BVH = bilateral vestibular hypofunction; C = control group; CDP = computerized dynamic posturography; CNS = central nervous system; COM = center of mass; COP = center of pressure; CVA = cerebral vascular accident; DHI = dizziness handicap inventory; DVA = dynamic visual acuity; E = experimental group; EC = exclusion criteria; HEP = home exercise program; M-L = medial–lateral; OKN = optokinetic nystagmus; OKS = optokinetic stimulation; POD = post-operation day; PT = physical therapy; RomEC = Romberg eyes closed; SOLEC = stand on one leg eyes closed; SOLEO = stand on one leg eyes open; UVH = unilateral vestibular hypofunction; VVOR = visual vestibular interaction (visual vestibulo-ocular reflex).

safety precautions to allow safe functioning within the home and community.

- The patient will demonstrate enhanced decision making skills regarding use of compensatory strategies to assist in gaze stability.
- The patient will be independent in performance of a HEP that includes walking.

Once an accurate diagnosis of central vestibular pathology is made, the physical therapist must be careful in choosing rehabilitation strategies. Expectations for recovery should be described initially to the patient. Generally, the time to recover will be 6 months or more, and may be incomplete.[122] Many of the adaptive mechanisms thought responsible for recovery of the vestibular system are central processes that may have been damaged in the initial central lesion. Physical therapists treating patients with TBI must be careful not to be too aggressive thereby greatly exacerbating the patients symptoms. Though vestibular rehabilitation offers promise for treating persons with TBI,[123] it may not always be the treatment of choice owing to its irritating nature.

The physical therapy intervention for a *central vestibular lesion* at the level of the brainstem (vestibular nuclei) likely will be similar to a UVH, with the same expectations for recovery. Vestibular cortical lesions may also recover, similar to the process a cerebral vascular accident might.

As many patients with central vestibular lesions complain of dizziness, a good treatment to start with is habituation exercises. However, the exercises should not be too aggressive, thereby aggravating the patient's condition. In addition, gait and balance exercises designed to incorporate somatosensory, visual, and vestibular contributions are also effective means with this patient population.

Patient Education

The vestibular system requires movement to recover from most lesions. This basic tenet should be thoroughly discussed when educating patients about returning to daily activity, exercising independently at home, and as a general guideline for their recovery. The vestibular system will not improve maximally without head motion. The challenge for both the outpatient and inpatient physical therapist is determining the amount of exertion the patient can tolerate, creating an effective vestibular rehabilitation strategy without causing deleterious effects.

Diagnoses Involving the Vestibular System

Ménière's Disease

Ménière's disease is diagnosed by a documented low-frequency hearing loss and episodic vertigo. The patient may also complain of a sense of fullness in the ear and tinnitus. The symptoms gradually increase in severity and then last 1 to 2 hours per episode. Chronic Ménière's disease, however, can result in a UVH, for which rehabilitation is appropriate. The pathophysiology of Ménière's disease probably involves an increase in endolymphatic fluid causing distension of the membranous tissues.[124] Medical treatment is therefore directed toward reducing or preventing fluid buildup. Many patients can manage the symptoms well with a controlled diet. Patients with Ménière's disease are often placed on a 2 g/d or less sodium diet. This is the most important dietary restriction to follow. Other substances to be avoided are caffeine and alcohol. Sometimes medical management includes use of a diuretic to control the amount of water in the body. Surgery to either prevent the fluid buildup in the inner ear (endolymphatic shunt placement) or to stop the abnormal vestibular signal (vestibular nerve section, or transtympanic gentamicin injection) may be indicated if the episodes are frequent enough to disturb daily function. Physical therapy is most beneficial in treating the effects of a UVH owing to chronic Ménière's disease, although the therapy will not stop the episodes of vertigo. Gaze and postural stability exercises may be appropriate. Physical therapy is also useful in the treatment of dysequilibrium occurring after a vestibular neurectomy.

Perilymphatic Fistula

Perilymphatic fistula (PLF) is most commonly caused by a rupture of the oval or round windows, membranes that separate the middle and inner ear. A rupture of these membranes results in leakage of the perilymph into the middle ear. The result is vertigo and hearing loss. Normally, perilymph bathes the SCCs and serves as a protective barrier between the bony and membranous labyrinth. PLF usually is caused from a traumatic event, such as excessive pressure changes as in deep-water diving, blunt head trauma without skull fracture, or extremely loud noise.[125] This diagnosis is much debated and the treatment for PLF is similarly ambiguous. Patients often are treated first with bed rest in hopes of allowing the membrane to heal. Surgical patches of the fistula are also performed. Physical therapy is contraindicated for most patients with PLF; however, it can be beneficial in those patients who have continual dysequilibrium or develop a vestibular hypofunction postoperatively. Medical management will likely include strict limitations on activities, warranting good communication between physical therapist and physician.

Acoustic Neuroma

Acoustic neuroma, also called vestibular schwannomma, is a benign tumor located on cranial nerve VIII. Complaints include progressive hearing loss, **tinnitus**, and dysequilibrium. Treatment usually involves surgical excision of the tumor. Preoperatively, vertigo is often not present because the tumor is slow growing and the central vestibular system compensates to the gradual reduction in function. Postoperatively, many patients experience vertigo because the procedure often requires sacrificing all or part of the vestibular nerve. Optimally, physical therapy is initiated during the early postoperative period to help the patient resolve symptoms of dysequilibrium and oscillopsia.[117] Outpatient treatment should be considered similar to the treatment for a unilateral vestibular loss.

Motion Sickness

Motion sickness is a normal sensation, that in some people becomes debilitating. The predominate explanation for motion sickness is the *sensory conflict theory.*[126] The three sensory inputs of proprioception, vestibular, and visual information do not match stored neural patterns the brain expects to recognize. As a result, persons experience pallor, nausea, emesis, diaphoresis, and motion sensitivity. Physical therapy has been successfully used to reduce motion sensitivity.[127] Other methods reported to combat motion sickness include the use of cognitive–behavioral management, medications, biofeedback, and habituation training using ground and flight situations.[128–131]

Migraine-Related Dizziness

Migraine-related dizziness can be deceptively similar to a peripheral vestibular lesion. The reason being the vascular event occurs in a vestibular structure such as the vestibular nuclei. Migraine related symptoms include vertigo, dizziness, and motion sickness. The prevalence of migraine is significant, affecting 6 percent of men and 15 to 18 percent of women between the ages of 25 and 55.[132] The clinical examination will provide the differential diagnosis between vestibular pathology and migraine. If the therapist suspects migraine the patient should be referred to a neurologist, preferably one with a special interest in headache. Migraine is often well controlled with medication and diet.

Multiple Sclerosis

Multiple sclerosis (MS) can affect cranial nerve VIII where it enters the brainstem and causes identical symptoms to a unilateral vestibular pathology. A magnetic resonance image (MRI) scan will ensure an accurate diagnosis of MS.

Multiple System Atrophy

Multiple system atrophy (MSA) is a progressive degenerative disease of the nervous system involving four clinical domains: cerebellar ataxia, autonomic dysfunction, Parkinson's disease like symptoms, and corticospinal dysfunction. MSA has been found to be a cause of dizziness and imbalance.[133] The effect of physical therapy for persons with MSA has not been investigated.

Cervical Vertigo

Cervical vertigo is a diagnosis commonly used in Europe yet controversial in the United States. A large percentage of persons suffering from motor vehicle accidents, however, do report symptoms of dizziness warranting further investigation into the source. The mechanisms of involvement are believed to be from at least two sources. First, the upper cervical spine sends proprioceptive input to the contralateral vestibular nucleus.[134] Soft tissue injury and joint dysfunction might alter the afferent input contributing to spatial orientation. Vestibular rehabilitation may be warranted for these individuals.[135] Second, a patient might have vertebrobasilar insufficiency (VBI). If VBI is suspected, vascular compromise must first be ruled out as a cause of the patient's symptoms. The VBI test can be performed while the subject is seated. The patient leans forward and extends the neck. The neck is then rotated 45° to the suspicious side. Symptoms of VBI include diplopia, dysarthria, syncope, headache, and visual field deficits as well as vertigo and nystagmus. Persons suspected of having VBI should be referred to a neurologist immediately. Repeated episodes of vertigo without the associated VBI symptoms usually suggests a peripheral vestibular diagnosis.

Contraindications to Vestibular Rehabilitation

Physical therapy is not appropriate for unstable vestibular disorders such as Ménière's disease (with the exception mentioned above) and PLF. Other contraindications the clinician should be alert to include sudden loss of hearing, increased feeling of pressure or fullness to the point of discomfort in one or both ears, and severe ringing in one or both ears. When treating patients who have had a surgical procedure, the clinician must be observant for discharge of fluid from the ears or nose, which may indicate cerebrospinal fluid leak. Patients with acute neck injuries may not be able to tolerate some components of the physical exam, the CRM, or some of the gaze stability exercises.

Summary

Physical therapists must recognize signs and symptoms associated with vestibular disorders because of high incidence and prevalence rates. It is essential to differentiate a peripheral pathology from a central one. Peripheral and central lesions have separate manifestations and may require different intervention strategies. In addition, all vestibular disorders should not be treated similarly. The most common form of vertigo, BPPV, is a biomechanical problem readily treated with a single maneuver. This is in stark contrast to a patient with a BVH, which requires a greater rehabilitation effort. Evidence supports the use of vestibular adaptation exercises for patients with vestibular hypofunction.

The *Vestibular Disorders Association (VEDA)* has a list of physical therapists in each state, interested in treating patients with vestibular disorders. VEDA can be contacted via phone number (800) 837-8428 (24-hour voice mail) (503) 229-7705 (answering machine) or e-mail http://www.vestibular.org.

The supplemental reading list contains other excellent literature for the reader interested in pursuing a greater depth of knowledge in vestibular rehabilitation.

Questions for Review

1. Differentiate the two movement sensors of the vestibular system.
2. Describe the physiologic manifestation causing a corrective saccade after the head thrust test.
3. Why does the patient with an acute unilateral vestibular lesion experience spontaneous nystagmus?
4. What is the pathology of BPPV due to cupulolithiasis?
5. What are the key elements in taking a history?
6. Explain inhibitory cut off.
7. Differentiate the ×1 exercise paradigm from the ×2 exercise paradigm.
8. In a patient with vestibular nystagmus, which part of the eye movement (slow or fast) is from the vestibular system? Why?
9. Describe how the Hallpike-Dix test would elicit nystagmus for posterior SCC BPPV.
10. Differentiate between adaptation and habituation training for patients with vestibular dysfunction.
11. Differentiate between the canalith repositioning maneuver and Brandt-Daroff exercises for patients with BPPV.

Case Studies

CASE STUDY 1

You are performing an initial examination of a patient with complaints of imbalance and dizziness. In a sitting position, at rest, the patient is observed to have a purely vertical and pendular nystagmus with head tilting to the left. The nystagmus is not altered with any change in head position, and the head-shaking–induced nystagmus test (HSN) is negative.

GUIDING QUESTIONS

1. Do you suspect a central or peripheral pathology as a cause of the imbalance and dizziness?
2. Is physical therapy appropriate at this time?

CASE STUDY 2

On your patient's return to sitting up after you have performed the canalith-repositioning maneuver (CRM) for a left posterior canalithiasis, you notice down-beating and left torsional nystagmus. The patient is complaining of vertigo.

GUIDING QUESTIONS

1. Where is the otoconia now located?
2. How will you treat for benign paroxysmal positional vertigo (BPPV) the second time?
3. Following the second treatment for BPPV, the patient complains of dizziness and neck pain. The vertigo and nystagmus are gone. Can you prescribe any other forms of exercise for the remaining dizziness? What about the neck pain?

CASE STUDY 3

A patient with a unilateral vestibular hypofunction (UVH) complains of feeling worse after 7 days of starting a vestibular rehabilitation program. The patient has had no falls. The complaints consist of increased dizziness with head motion, nausea, and fatigue.

GUIDING QUESTIONS

1. Is your rehabilitation program making the patient worse?
2. How can you modify the program?
3. What information will you tell your patient with a UVH regarding time to recover? What will you tell patients with BPPV, BVH, or central nervous system pathology regarding times to recover?

CASE STUDY 4

Three weeks after initiating vestibular rehabilitation for a patient with a BVH, the patient falls at home but is not injured.

GUIDING QUESTIONS

1. Will you modify the physical therapy intervention?
2. Was your home exercise program too rigorous?

References

1. Kroenke, K, and Mangelsdorff, AD: Common symptoms in ambulatory care: Incidence, evaluation, therapy, and outcome. Am J Med 86(3):262, 1989.
2. Yardley, L, et al: Prevalence and presentation of dizziness in a general practice community sample of working age people. Br J Gen Pract 48(429):1131, 1998.
3. Sloane, PD: Dizziness in primary care. Results from the National Ambulatory Medical Care Survey. J Fam Pract 29(1):33, 1989.
4. Tinetti, ME, et al: Dizziness among older adults: A possible geriatric syndrome. Ann Intern Med 132(5):337, 2000.
5. Colledge, NR, et al: The prevalence and characteristics of dizziness in an elderly community. Age Ageing 23(2):117, 1994.
6. Sloane, PD, et al: Dizziness in a community elderly population. J Am Geriatr Soc 37:101, 1989.
7. Sloane, PD, et al: Dizziness: State of the science. Ann Intern Med 134:823, 2001.
8. Kroenke, K, et al: How common are various causes of dizziness? A critical review. South Med J 93:160, 2000.
9. Koch, H, and Smith, MC: Office-based ambulatory care for patients 75 years old and over: National Ambulatory Medical Care Survey, 1980 and 1981. NCHS Advance Data No 110, US Department of Health and Human Services, Public Health Service, National Center for Health Statistics, Washington, DC, 1985, p. 6.
10. Grimby, A, and Rosenhall, U: Health related quality of life and dizziness in old age. Gerontology 41:286, 1995.
11. National Institute on Deafness and other Communication Disorders (NIDCD): A Report of the Task Force on the National Strategic Research Plan, NIDCD, National Institutes of Health, Bethesda, Maryland, 1989, p 74.
12. Clark, MR, et al: Psychiatric and medical factors associated with disability in patients with dizziness. Psychosomatics 34(5):409, 1993.
13. Kroenke, K, et al: Causes of persistent dizziness: A prospective study of 100 patients in ambulatory care. Ann Intern Med 117(11):898, 1992.
14. Cawthorne, T: The physiological basis for head exercises. J Charter Soc Physiother 30:106, 1944.
15. Cooksey, FS: Rehabilitation in vestibular injuries. Proc R Soc Med 39:273, 1946.
16. Della Santina, CC, et al: Orientations of human vestibular labyrinth semicircular canals. In Proceedings of the 2004 Midwinter Meeting of the Association for Research in Otolaryngology; Daytona Beach, FL(February 22–26, 2004). Association for Research in Otolaryngology, Mt Royal, NJ, 2004.
17. Cremer, PD, et al: Semicircular canal plane head impulses detect absent function of individual semicircular canals. Brain 121:699, 1998.
18. Smith, CA, et al: The electrolytes of the labyrinthine fluids. Laryngoscope 64:141, 1954.
19. Troiani, D, et al: Relations of single semicircular canals to the pontine reticular formation. Arch Ital Biol Nov 114(4):337, 1976.
20. Buttner, U, and Henn, V: Thalamic unit activity in the alert monkey during natural vestibular stimulation. Brain Res Feb 13; 103(1):127, 1976.
21. Brodal, A, and Brodal, P: Observations on the secondary vestibulocerebellar projections in the macaque monkey. Exp Brain Res 58:62, 1985.

22. Buttner, U, and Buettner, UW: Parietal cortex (2v) neuronal activity in the alert monkey during natural vestibular and optokinetic stimulation. Brain Res 153:392, 1978.
23. Grusser, OJ, et al: Localization and responses of neurones in the parieto-insular vestibular cortex of awake monkeys (Macaca fascicularis). J Physiol 430:537, 1990.
24. Their, P, and Erickson, RG: Vestibular input to visual-tracking neurons in area MST of awake rhesus monkeys. Ann NY Acad Sci 656:960, 1992.
25. Brandt, T, et al: Visual-vestibular and visuovisual cortical interaction: new insights from fMRI and PET. Ann NY Acad Sci 956:230, 2002.
26. Dieterich, M, et al: fMRI signal increases and decreases in cortical areas during small-field optokinetic stimulation and central fixation. Exp Brain Res 148:117, 2003.
27. Brandt, T, and Dieterich, M: Vestibular syndromes in the roll plane: Topographic diagnosis from brainstem to cortex. Ann Neurol 36:337, 1994.
28. Goldberg, JM, and Fernandez C: Physiology of peripheral neurons innervating semicircular canals of the squirrel monkey, I: Resting discharge and response to constant angular accelerations. J Neurophysiol 34:635, 1971.
29. Lysakowski, AM, et al: Physiological identification of morphologically distinct afferent classes innervating the cristae ampullares of the squirrel monkey. J Neurophysiol 73:1270, 1995.
30. Baloh, RW, and Honrubia, V: Clinical neurophysiology of the vestibular system. FA Davis, Philadelphia, 1990.
31. Meyer, CH, et al: The upper limit of human smooth pursuit velocity. Vision Res 25:561, 1985.
32. Fernandez, C, and Goldberg, JM: Physiology of peripheral neurons innervating semicircular canals of the squirrel monkey, II: Response to sinusoidal stimulation and dynamics of peripheral vestibular system. J Neurophysiol 34:661, 1971.
33. Dai, M, et al: Model-based study of the human cupular time constant. J Vestib Res 9(4):293, 1999.
34. Baloh, RW: Dizziness: Neurological emergencies. Neurol Clin 16:305, 1998.
35. Gillespie, MB, and Minor LB: Prognosis in bilateral vestibular hypofunction. Laryngoscope 109:35, 1999.
36. Telian, SA, et al: Bilateral vestibular paresis: Diagnosis and treatment. Otolaryngol Head Neck Surg 104:67, 1991.
37. Belal, A Jr: Dandy's syndrome. Am J Otol 1:151, 1980.
38. Bhansali, SA, et al: Oscillopsia in patients with loss of vestibular function. Otolaryngol Head Neck Surg 109:120, 1993.
39. Herdman, SJ, et al: Recovery of dynamic visual acuity in unilateral vestibular hypofunction. Arch Otolaryngol Head Neck Surg 129(8):819, 2003.
40. Dixon, JS, and Bird, HA: Reproducibility along a 10 cm vertical visual analog scale. Ann Rheum Dis 40:87, 1981.
41. Jacobsen, GP, and Newman, CW: The development of the dizziness handicap inventory. Arch Otolaryngol Head Neck Surg 116:424, 1990.
42. Robertson, D, and Ireland, D: Dizziness handicap inventory correlates of computerized dynamic posturography. J Otolaryngol 24:118, 1995.
43. Jacobson, GP, and McCaslin, DL: Agreement between functional and electrophysiologic measures in patients with unilateral peripheral vestibular system impairment. J Am Acad Audiol 14(5):231, 2003.
44. Telian, SA, et al: Habituation therapy for chronic vestibular dysfunction: Preliminary results. Otolaryngol Head Neck Surg 103(1):89, 1990.
45. Smith-Wheelock, M, et al: Physical therapy program for vestibular rehabilitation. Am J Otol May 12(3):218, 1991.
46. Fetter, M, and Dichgans, J. Adaptive mechanisms of VOR compensation after unilateral peripheral vestibular lesions in humans. J Vestib Res 1:9, 1990.
47. Cass, SP, et al: Patterns of vestibular function following vestibular nerve section. Laryngoscope 102:388, 1992.
48. Maioli, C, et al: Short- and long-term modifications of vestibulo-ocular response dynamics following unilateral vestibular nerve lesions in the cat. Exp Brain Res 50:259, 1983.
49. Watabe, H, Hashiba, M, and Baba, S: Voluntary suppression of caloric nystagmus under fixation of imaginary or after-image target. Acta Otolaryngol Suppl 525:155, 1996.
50. Halmagyi, GM, and Curthoys, IS: A clinical sign of canal paresis. Arch Neurol 45:737, 1998.
51. Halmagyi, GM, et al: The human horizontal vestibulo-ocular reflex in response to high-acceleration stimulation before and after unilateral vestibular neurectomy. Exp Brain Res 81:479, 1990.
52. Minor, LB, et al: Symptoms and signs in superior canal dehiscence syndrome. Ann N Y Acad Sci 942:259, 2001.
53. Aw, ST, et al: Unilateral vestibular deafferentation causes permanent impairment of the human vertical vestibulo-ocular reflex in the pitch plane. Exp Brain Res 102:121, 1994.
54. Cremer, PD, et al: Semicircular canal plane head impulses detect absent function of individual semicircular canals. Brain 121:699, 1998.
55. Foster, CA, et al: Functional loss of the horizontal doll's eye reflex following unilateral vestibular lesions. Laryngoscope 104:473, 1994.
56. Harvey, SA, and Wood, DJ: The oculocephalic response in the evaluation of the dizzy patient. Laryngoscope 106:6, 1996.
57. Harvey, SA, et al: Relationship of the head impulse test and head-shake nystagmus in reference to caloric testing. Am J Otol 18:207, 1997.
58. Beynon, GJ, et al: A clinical evaluation of head impulse testing. Clin Otolaryngol 23:117, 1998.
59. Schubert, MC, et al: Optimizing the sensitivity of the head thrust test for identifying vestibular hypofunction. Phys Ther 84:151, 2004.
60. Hain, TC, et al: Head-shaking nystagmus in patients with unilateral peripheral vestibular lesions. Am J Otolaryngol 8:36, 1987.
61. Dix, R, and Hallpike, CS: The pathology, symptomatology and diagnosis of certain common disorders of the vestibular system. Ann Otol Rhinol Laryngol 6:987, 1952.
62. Longridge, NS, and Mallinson, AI: The dynamic illegible E (DIE) test: A simple technique for assessing the ability of the vestibulo-ocular reflex to overcome vestibular pathology. J Otolaryngol 16:97, 1987.
63. Herdman, SJ, et al: Computerized dynamic visual acuity test in the assessment of vestibular deficits. Am J Otol 19:790, 1998.
64. Tian, JR, et al: Dynamic visual acuity during passive and self-generated transient head rotation in normal and unilaterally vestibulopathic humans. Exp Brain Res 142(4):486, 2002.
65. Grossman, GE, et al: Frequency and velocity of rotational head perturbations during locomotion. Exp Brain Res 70:470, 1988.
66. Das, VE, et al: Head perturbations during walking while viewing a head-fixed target. Aviat Space Environ Med 66:728, 1995.
67. Colebatch, JG, and Halmagyi GM: Vestibular evoked potentials in human neck muscles before and after unilateral vestibular deafferentation. Neurology 42:1635, 1992.
68. Halmagyi, GM, et al: Tapping the head activates the vestibular system: A new use for the clinical reflex hammer. Neurology 45:1927, 1995.
69. Curthoys, IS, et al: Human ocular torsional position before and after unilateral vestibular neurectomy. Exp Brain Res 85:218, 1991.
70. Kushiro, K, et al: Saccular and utricular inputs to sternocleidomastoid motoneurons of decerebrate cats. Exp Brain Res 126:410, 1999.
71. Young, ED, et al: Responses of squirrel monkey vestibular neurons to audio-frequency sound and head vibration. Acta Otolaryngol 84:352, 1977.
72. Murofushi, T, et al: Responses of guinea pig primary vestibular neurons to clicks. Exp Brain Res 103:174, 1995.
73. Murofushi, T, et al: Response of guinea pig vestibular nucleus neurons to clicks. Exp Brain Res 111:149, 1996.
74. Bohmer, A, et al: Can a unilateral loss of otolithic function be clinically detected by assessment of the subjective visual vertical? Brain Res Bull 41:423, 1996.
75. Tabak, S, et al: Deviation of the subjective vertical in long-standing unilateral vestibular loss. Acta Otolaryngol 117:1, 1997.
76. Schuknecht, HF: Cupulolithiasis. Arch Otolaryngol 90:765, 1969.
77. Furuya, M, et al: Experimental study of speed-dependent positional nystagmus in benign poaroxysmal positional vertigo. Acta Otolaryngol 123(6):709, 2003.
78. Hall, SF, et al: The mechanics of benign paroxysmal vertigo. J Otolaryngol 8(2):151, 1979.

79. Cooper, CW: Vestibular neuronitis: A review of a common cause of vertigo in general practice. Br J Gen Pract 43:164, 1993.
80. Jayarajan, V, and Rajenderkumar, D. A survey of dizziness management in general practice. J Laryngol Otol 117(8):599, 2003.
81. Fetter, M, and Dichgans, J: Adaptive mechanisms of VOR compensation after unilateral peripheral vestibular lesions in humans. J Vestib Res 1:9, 1990.
82. Baloh, RW: Vertebrobasilar insufficiency and stroke. Otolaryngol Head Neck Surg 112:114, 1995.
83. Schuknecht, HF, and Witt, RL: Acute bilateral sequential vestibular neuritis. Am J Otolaryngol 6:255, 1985.
84. Barber, HO, and Dionne, J: Vestibular findings in vertebro-basilar ischemia. Ann Otol Rhinol Laryngol 80:805, 1971.
85. Halmagyi GM, et al: Gentamicin vestibulotoxicity. Otolaryngol Head Neck Surg 111:571, 1994.
86. Brandt, T, and Dieterich, M: Vestibular syndromes in the roll plane: Topographic diagnosis from brainstem to cortex. Ann Neurol 36:337, 1994.
87. Delaney KA: Bedside diagnosis of vertigo: Value of the history and neurological examination. Acad Emerg Med 10(12):1388, 2003.
88. Berman, J, and Frederickson, J: Vertigo after head injury: A five year follow-up. J Otolaryngol 7:237, 1978.
89. Tuohimma, P: Vestibular disturbances after acute mild head injury. Acta Otolaryngol Suppl (Stockh) 359:7, 1978.
90. Masson, F, et al: Prevalence of impairments 5 years after a head injury, and their relationship with disabilities and outcome. Brain Inj 10(7):487, 1996.
91. Grad, A, and Baloh, RW: Vertigo of vascular origin. Clinical and electronystagmographic features in 84 cases. Arch Neurol 46(3):281, 1989.
92. Leigh, RJ, and Zee, DS: Diagnosis of central disorders of ocular motility. In Leigh, RJ and Zee, DS (eds): The Neurology of Eye Movements, ed 3. Oxford University Press, New York, 1999, p 415.
93. Kluge, M, et al: Epileptic vertigo: Evidence for vestibular representation in human frontal cortex. Neurology 55(12):1906, 2000.
94. Brandt, T, et al: Vestibular cortex lesions affect the perception of verticality. Ann Neurol 35:403, 1994.
95. Brandt, T, et al: Plasticity of the vestibular system: Central compensation and sensory substitution for vestibular deficits. Brain Plast Adv Neurol 73:297, 1997.
96. Dieterich, M, and Brandt, T: Wallenberg's syndrome: Lateropulsion, cyclorotation, and subjective visual vertical in thirty-six patients. Ann Neurol 31:399, 1992.
97. Epley, JM: The canalith repositioning procedure: For treatment of benign paroxysmal positional vertigo. Otolaryngol Head Neck Surg 107:399, 1992.
98. Herdman, SJ, et al: Eye movement signs in vertical canal benign paroxysmal positional vertigo. In Fuchs, AF, et al (eds): Contemporary Ocular Motor and Vestibular Research: A Tribute to David A. Robinson. George Thieme Verlag, Stuttgart, 1994, p 385.
99. Tusa, RJ, and Schubert, MC: Canalith repositioning for benign paroxysmal positional vertigo. Publication 7BS.002. American Academy of Neurology, St. Paul, MN, 2002.
100. Simhadri, S, Freyss, G, and Vitte, E: Efficacy of particle repositioning maneuver in BPPV: A prospective study. Am J Otolaryngol 24(6):355, 2003.
101. Sakaida, M, Freyss, G, and Vitte, E: Long-term outcome of benign paroxysmal positional vertigo. Neurology 60(9):1532, 2003.
102. Semont, A, Freyss, G, and Vitte, E: Curing the BPPV with a liberatory maneuver. Adv Otorhinolaryngol 42:290, 1988.
103. Campanini, A, and Vicini, C: Semont maneuver vs. particle repositioning maneuver: Comparative study. Acta Otorhinolaryngol Ital 21(6):331, 2001.
104. Campanini, A, et al: Efficacy of the Semont maneuver in benign paroxysmal positional vertigo. Arch Otolaryngol Head Neck Surg 129(6):629, 2003.
105. Brandt, T, and Daroff, RB: Physical therapy for benign paroxysmal positional vertigo. Arch Otolaryngol 106:484, 1980.
106. Johnson, R, and Griffin, J: Current Therapy in Neurologic Disease. Mosby Year-Book, St. Louis, 1993.
107. Gottshall, K, et al: Objective vestibular tests as outcome measures in head injury patients. Laryngoscope 113(10):1746, 2003.
108. Shumway-Cook, A, and Horak, FB: Vestibular rehabilitation: An exercise approach to managing symptoms of vestibular dysfunction. Semin Hearing 10:196, 1989.
109. Norre, ME, and DeWeerdt, W: Treatment of vertigo based on habituation. J Laryngol Otol 94:971, 1980.
110. Dix, MR: The rationale and technique of head exercises in the treatment of vertigo. Acta Otorhinolaryngol Belg 33:370, 1979.
111. Dix, MR: The physiological basis and practical value of head exercises in the treatment of vertigo. The Practitioner 217:919, 1976.
112. Herdman, SJ, et al: Falls in patients with vestibular deficits. Am J Otol 21:847, 2000.
113. Cohen, HS, et al: Driving disability and dizziness. J Safety Res 34(4):361, 2003.
114. Horak, FB, et al: Effects of vestibular rehabilitation on dizziness and imbalance. Otolaryngol Head Neck Surg 106(2):175, 1992.
115. Krebs, DE, et al: Double-blind, placebo-controlled trial of rehabilitation for bilateral vestibular hypofunction: Preliminary report. Otolaryngol Head Neck Surg 109(4):735, 1993.
116. Szturm, T, et al: Comparison of different exercise programs in the rehabilitation of patients with chronic peripheral vestibular dysfunction. J Vestib Res 4(6):461, 1994.
117. Herdman, SJ, et al: Vestibular adaptation exercises and recovery: Acute stage after acoustic neuroma resection. Otolaryngol Head Neck Surg 113:77, 1995.
118. Strupp, M, et al: Vestibular exercises improve central vestibulospinal compensation after vestibular neuritis. Neurology 51(3): 838, 1998.
119. Cohen, HS, and Kimball, KT: Increased independence and decreased vertigo after vestibular rehabilitation. Otolaryngol Head Neck Surg 128(1):60, 2003.
120. Krebs, DE, et al: Vestibular rehabilitation: Useful but not universally so. Otolaryngol Head Neck Surg 128(2):240, 2003.
121. Patten, C, et al: Head and body center of gravity control strategies: Adaptations following vestibular rehabilitation. Acta Otolaryngol 123(1):32, 2003.
122. Shepard, NT, et al: Vestibular and balance rehabilitation therapy. Ann Otol Rhinol Laryngol 102:198, 1993.
123. Gurr, B, and Moffat, N: Psychological consequences of vertigo and the effectiveness of vestibular rehabilitation for brain injury patients. Brain Inj 15(5):387, 2001.
124. Arenberg, IK: Ménières disease: Diagnosis and management of vertigo and endolymphatic hydrops. In Arenberg, IK (ed): Dizziness and Balance Disorders. Kugler Publications, New York, 1993, p 503.
125. Bruno, E, et al: Perilymphatic fistula following trans-tympanic trauma: A clinical case presentation and review of the literature. An Otorrinolaringol Ibero Am 29(4):359, 2002.
126. Dobie, TG, and May, JG: Cognitive-behavioral management of motion sickness. Aviat Space Environ Med 65(Suppl 10):C1, 1994.
127. Rine, RM, et al: Visual-vestibular habituation and balance training for motion sickness. Phys Ther 79:949, 1999.
128. Reason, JT: Motion sickness adaptation: A neural mismatch model. J R Soc Med 71:819, 1978.
129. Bagshaw, M, and Stott, JR: The desensitization of chronically motion sick aircrew in the Royal Air Force. Aviat Space Environ Med 56:1144, 1985.
130. Golding, JF, and Stott, JR: Objective and subjective time courses of recovery from motion sickness assessed by repeated motion challenges. J Vestib Res 7:421, 1997.
131. Banks, RD, et al: The Canadian forces airsickness rehabilitation program, 1981–1991. Aviat Space Environ Med 63:1098, 1992.
132. MacGregor, EA, et al: Migraine prevalence and treatment patterns: The global Migraine and Zolmitriptan Evaluation survey. Headache 43(1):19, 2003.
133. Wang SR, and Young, YI: Multiple system atrophy manifested as dizziness and imbalance: A report of two cases. EurArch Otorhinolayrngol 260:404, 2003.
134. Hikosaka, O, and Maeda, M: Cervical effects on abducens motor neurons and their interaction with vestibulo-ocular reflex. Exp Brain Res 18:512, 1973.
135. Wrisley, DM, et al: Cervicogenic dizziness: A review of diagnosis and treatment. J Orthop Sports Phys Ther 30(12):755, 2000.

Supplemental Readings

Baloh, RW, and Honrubia, V: Clinical Neurophysiology of the Vestibular System. Oxford University Press, New York, 2001.

Epley, JM: The canalith repositioning procedure: For treatment of benign paroxysmal positional vertigo. Otolaryngol Head Neck Surg 107:399, 1992.

Fetter, M, and Dichgans, J: Adaptive mechanisms of VOR compensation after unilateral peripheral vestibular lesions in humans. J Vestib Res 1:9, 1990.

Herdman, SJ: Vestibular Rehabilitation, ed 2. FA Davis, Philadelphia, 2000.

Herdman, SJ, et al: Recovery of dynamic visual acuity in unilateral vestibular hypofunction. Arch Otolaryngol Head Neck Surg 129:819, 2003.

Herdman, SJ, Blatt, PJ, and Schubert, MC: Vestibular rehabilitation of patients with vestibular hypofunction or with benign paroxysmal positional vertigo. Curr Opin Neurol 13:39, 2000.

Johnson, RT, Griffin, JW, and MacAuthour, JC: Current Therapy in Neurologic Disease, ed 6. Mosby Year-Book, St. Louis, 2005.

CHAPTER

25

LEARNING OBJECTIVES

1. Describe the major etiological factors leading to amputation surgery.
2. Describe the major concepts involved in amputation surgery.
3. Describe the major components of post-operative management.
4. Effectively examine a patient following lower extremity amputation.
5. Teach patient and family appropriate post-operative positioning.
6. Describe and demonstrate proper residual limb bandaging.
7. Develop an exercise program to prepare the patient for eventual prosthetic fitting.
8. Respond to patient/family from an awareness of the psychological impact of lower extremity amputation.
9. Analyze and interpret patient data, formulate realistic anticipated goals and expected outcomes, and develop a plan of care when presented with a clinical case study.

Amputation

Bella J. May, PT, EdD, FAPTA

OUTLINE

As you enter the physical therapy department this Monday morning, you note several new referrals coming out of the computer printer. You reflect that it is almost a year since you graduated from school. The time has gone by so fast and you have learned so much. You are pleased you took this position in a large regional hospital because you have had the opportunity to rotate through various services. You are currently working with general medical and surgical patients including those who have had vascular surgery.

You reach for the printout of new referrals and see one for a 72-year-old woman with diabetes and atherosclerosis. You treated her several months ago for an ulcer on the plantar surface of her right first metatarsal and know she had some problems with diabetic control. The patient had a right transtibial (below knee) amputation Sunday afternoon and is now referred for therapy. You are a little sad. The patient is a widow and lives alone although she has three grown children and six grandchildren in town. You remember how she talked about her garden and her other activities and wonder what her prognosis will be for rehabilitation.

The major cause of lower extremity (LE) amputation today continues to be **peripheral vascular disease (PVD)**, particularly when associated with smoking and diabetes.[1–3] Major improvements in noninvasive diagnosis, revascularization, and wound healing techniques have lowered the overall incidence of amputations for vascular disease.[4–6] However, it has been reported that between 2 and 5 percent of individuals with PVD without diabetes and 6 to 25 percent of those with PVD and diabetes come to amputation.[6–11] Perioperative mortality has been variously reported between 7 and 13 percent and is usually associated with other medical problems such as cardiac disease and strokes.[12–14] Over the years, the incidence of amputations for vascular disease has decreased probably as a result of improved revascularization techniques, although total numbers of amputations have increased secondary to increased longevity.[15] Recent studies also indicated that the rate of amputation for vascular disease among African-Americans is considerably higher than that for other ethnic groups and seems to be increasing.[16]

The second leading cause of amputation is trauma, usually from motor vehicle accidents or gunshots. Individuals with traumatic amputations are usually young adults and more frequently men.[14,17] Improved imaging techniques, more effective chemotherapy, and better limb salvage procedures have reduced the incidence of amputation from osteogenic sarcoma. Amputation may be necessary if the tumor is large and cannot be resected without major removal of bone and tissue. However, the surgeon may choose to remove the tumor and incorporate one of several limb salvage procedures. There are many factors that go into this decision including the age of the patient, the size of the tumor, and if the patient is young, the potential for future growth.[18] Tumor excision does not affect 5-year survival rates, which have increased from about 20 percent in the 1970s to 60 to 70 percent in more recent years.[19–23] Regardless of the cause of amputation, physical therapists have a major role in the rehabilitation program. Early onset of appropriate treatment influences the eventual outcome of rehabilitation.

Levels of Amputation

Traditionally, levels of amputation have been identified by anatomical considerations such as below knee and above knee. In 1974, the Task Force on Standardization of Prosthetic-Orthotic Terminology developed an international classification system to define amputation levels. Table 25.1 describes the major terms in common use today.

Traumatic amputations may be performed at any level; the surgeon tries to maintain the greatest bone length and save all possible joints. A variety of surgical techniques may be necessary to create a functional residual limb. Guillotine amputations may precede secondary closure with skin flaps; occasionally, free tissue flaps, taken from some other area of the body, may be used to cover deformities. Amputations for vascular diseases are generally performed at partial foot, transtibial, or transfemoral levels. The limited vascular supply mitigates against effective residual limb healing at the Symes level in most instances.

Patients with unilateral transtibial amputations regardless of age are quite likely to become functional prosthetic users; many individuals with bilateral transtibial amputations can be successfully rehabilitated. Older adults with unilateral transfemoral amputations have more difficulty becoming prosthetically independent and most patients with bilateral transfemoral amputations do not become functional prosthetic users.[24,25] Generally, hip disarticulation, hemipelvectomies, and hemicorporectomies are performed either for tumors or for severe trauma and represent a small percentage of the population of individuals with amputations.

As you prepare to go see the patient, you mentally review what you know about amputation surgery and the healing process. You are pleased that her amputation was at a transtibial level but are concerned about the potential for primary healing. You think about the effects of surgery and the factors that will influence healing.

Table 25.1 Levels of Amputation

Partial toe	Excision of any part of one or more toes
Toe disarticulation	Disarticulation at the metatarsal phalangeal joint
Partial foot/ray resection	Resection of the 3rd, 4th, 5th metatarsals and digits
Transmetatarsal	Amputation through the midsection of all metatarsals
Syme's	Ankle disarticulation with attachment of heel pad to distal end of tibia. May include removal of malleoli and distal tibial/fibular flares
Long transtibial (below knee)	More than 50% tibial length
Transtibial (below knee)	Between 20 and 50% of tibial length
Short transtibial (below knee)	Less than 20% tibial length
Knee disarticulation	Amputation through the knee joint; femur intact
Long transfemoral (above knee)	More than 60% femoral length
Transfemoral (above knee)	Between 35 and 60% femoral length
Short transfemoral (above knee)	Less than 35% femoral length
Hip disarticulation	Amputation through hip joint; pelvis intact
Hemipelvectomy	Resection of lower half of the pelvis
Hemicorporectomy	Amputation both lower limbs and pelvis below L4–L5 level

Surgical Process

The specific type of surgery is determined by the surgeon, whose decision depends on the status of the extremity at the time of amputation. The surgeon must remove the part of the limb that must be eliminated, allow for primary or secondary wound healing, and construct a residual limb for optimal prosthetic fitting and function. Numerous factors affect the selection of level of amputation. Conservation of residual limb length and uncomplicated wound healing, for example, are both important. Although a description of each type of surgical procedure is beyond the scope of this chapter, an understanding of the basic principles of amputation surgery is important.

Skin flaps are as broad as possible and the scar should be pliable, painless, and nonadherent. For most transfemoral and nondysvascular transtibial amputations, equal length anterior and posterior flaps are used, placing the scar at the distal end of the bone (Figs. 25.1 and 25.2).

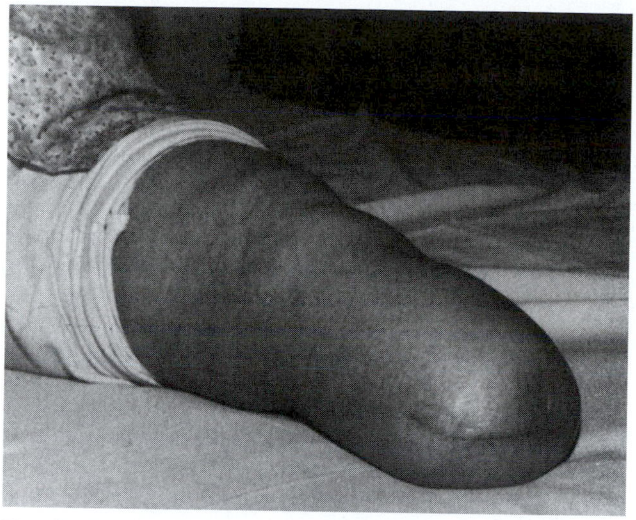

Figure 25.1 Transtibial residual limb with incision from equal length flaps.

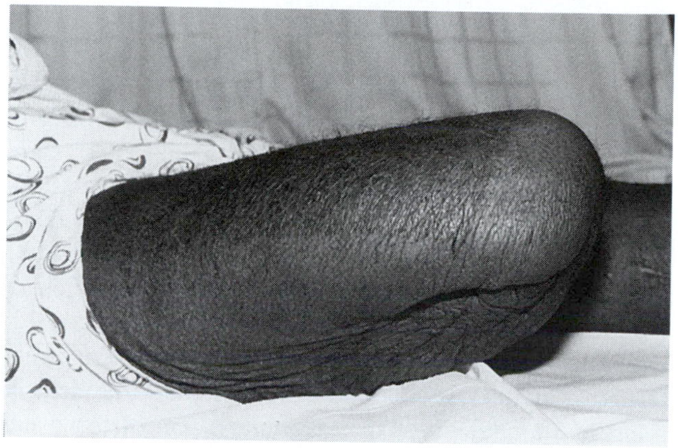

Figure 25.2 Transfemoral residual limb with incision from equal length flaps.

Long posterior flaps are often used in dysvascular transtibial amputations because the posterior tissues have a better blood supply than anterior skin. This places the scar anteriorly over the distal end of the tibia; care must be taken to ensure that the scar does not become adherent to the bone (Fig. 25.3A and B). In recent years, the routine use of the long posterior flap has come into question.[26] The skew flap, developed in England, is believed by some surgeons to be a better approach for individuals with severely compromised distal circulation. The skew flap is an angular medial–lateral incision that places the scar away from bony prominences, a problem with the long posterior flap. Reported research on the use of different skin flaps does not clearly delineate the most advantageous approach and all indicate similar results in terms of rehabilitation.[27–29]

Stabilization of major muscles allows for maximum retention of function. Muscle stabilization may be achieved by *myofascial closure, myoplasty, myodesis,* or *tenodesis*. In most transtibial and transfemoral amputations, a combination of myoplasty (muscle to muscle closure) and myofascial closure is used to ensure that the muscles are properly stabilized and do not slide over the end of the bone.

In some centers, myodesis (muscle attached to periosteum or bone) is employed particularly in transtibial amputations. More rarely, a tenodesis (tendon attached to bone) may be used for muscle stabilization. Whatever the technique, muscle stabilization under some tension is desirable at all levels where muscles must be transected.

Severed peripheral nerves form *neuromas* (a collection of nerve ends) in the residual limb. The neuroma must be well surrounded by soft tissue so as not to cause pain and interfere with prosthetic wear. Surgeons identify the major nerves, pull them down under some tension then cut them cleanly and sharply and allow them to retract into the soft

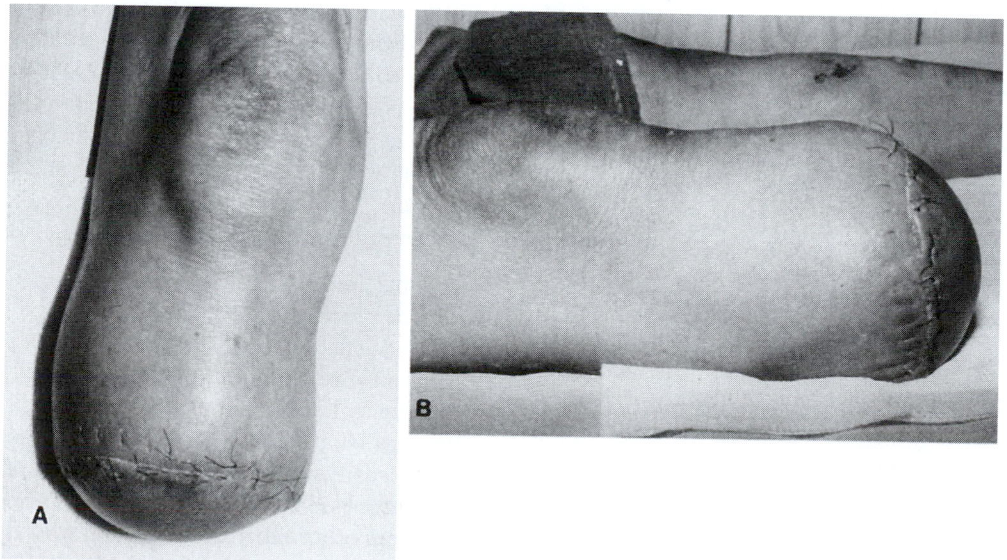

Figure 25.3 (*A*) Anterior and lateral (*B*) view of a transtibial residual limb with anterior incision from a long posterior flap.

tissue of the residual limb. Neuromas that form close to scar tissue or bone generally cause pain and may require later resection or revision.

Hemostasis is achieved by ligating major veins and arteries; *cauterization* is used only for small bleeders. Care is taken not to compromise circulation to distal tissues, particularly the skin flaps, which are important to uncomplicated wound healing.

Bones are sectioned at a length to allow wound closure without excessive redundant tissue at the end of the residual limb and without placing the incision under great tension. Sharp bone ends are smoothed and rounded; in transtibial amputations, the anterior portion of the distal tibia is *beveled* to reduce the pressure between the end of the bone and the prosthetic socket. Care is taken to ensure that the bone is physiologically prepared for the pressures of prosthetic wear.

Tissue layers are approximated under normal physiological tension and the incision is closed, usually with regular sutures. A drainage tube may be inserted as necessary.

In a traumatic amputation, the surgeon attempts to save as much bone length and viable skin as possible and preserve proximal joints while providing for appropriate healing of tissues without secondary complications such as infection. In potentially "dirty" (involving foreign substances) amputations, the incision may be left open with the proximal joint immobilized in a functional position for 5 to 9 days to prevent invasive infection. *Secondary closure* also allows the surgeon to shape the residual limb appropriately for prosthetic rehabilitation.

Amputation for vascular disease is generally considered an elective procedure; the surgeon determines the level of amputation by examining tissue viability through a variety of measures. Segmental limb blood pressures can be determined by Doppler systolic blood pressure measurement. Transcutaneous oxygen measurement, and skin blood flow by radioisotope or plethysmography are also determined. Doppler systolic blood pressure measures have been reported to be quite accurate in predicting viable level of amputation, but have not been as accurate in predicting amputations that do not heal.[30] Improvements in noninvasive examination techniques have greatly reduced the use of **arteriography** to determine amputation level.

Healing Process

The surgeon's goal is to amputate only as much tissue as required to ensure successful healing.[31–33] Numerous factors influence the course of the healing process in each patient. One of the greatest postoperative concerns is infection, whether from external or internal sources. Individuals with contaminated wounds from injury, infected foot ulcers, or other causes are at greater risk of infection. Research indicates that smoking is a major deterrent to wound healing; one study reported that cigarette smokers had a 2.5 percent higher rate of infection and reamputation than nonsmokers.[34] There is some indication that failed attempts at limb revascularization may negatively influence healing at transtibial levels.[35–36] Other factors affecting wound healing are the severity of the vascular problems, diabetes, renal disease, and other physiological problems such as cardiac disease.[36–37]

Expected Outcomes

What will be the most appropriate outcomes for the patient at this time, you ask yourself. You wish you had seen her just before the amputation so you could have begun preparing her for the rehabilitation program. You know you will have only a few days before she is discharged to go home and need to develop outcomes that are as functional as possible. You also wonder if a home health referral will be possible after she leaves the hospital.

The earlier the onset of rehabilitation, the greater the potential for success. The longer the delay, the more likely the development of complications such as joint contractures, general debilitation, and a depressed psychological state. The postoperative program can be arbitrarily divided into two phases: (1) the postsurgical phase is the time between surgery and fitting with a definitive prosthesis or until a decision is made not to fit the patient and (2) the prosthetic phase starts with delivery of a permanent replacement limb. The desired expected outcome of the episode of care is to help the patient regain the presurgical level of function. For some, it will mean return to gainful employment with an active recreational life. For others, it will mean independence in the home and community. For still others, it may mean living in the sheltered environment of a retirement center or nursing home. If the amputation resulted from long-standing chronic disease, the rehabilitation approach may be to help the person function at a higher level than immediately before surgery.[38] Primary aims of the postsurgical period are for the patient to achieve as high a level of independent function as possible and to begin to develop the necessary physical skills and emotional adjustment for eventual prosthetic rehabilitation. Another aim is to determine the feasibility of prosthetic fitting. Examples of general goals for the postsurgical period include:

- The patient will be independent in bed mobility and basic transfers within 1 week.
- The patient will be independent in wheelchair mobility and self-care within 1 week.
- The patient will demonstrate proper residual limb positioning, bandaging, and care within 1 week.
- The patient will demonstrate modified dependence with minimal assistance of one person in ambulation using crutches or a walker within 1 week.

If the cause of amputation was PVD, an additional aim of the postsurgical period would be to ensure that the patient demonstrates proper care of the remaining extremity and adequately understands the disease process. The development of specific anticipated goals and expected outcomes for the individual patient with an amputation is based on the following general goals:

1. Reduce (or prevent) postoperative edema and promote healing of the residual limb
2. Prevent joint contractures, general debility, and integumentary disturbances
3. Maintain or regain strength in the affected LE
4. Maintain or increase strength in the remaining extremities
5. Adjust to the loss of a body part
6. Demonstrate the ability to correctly perform a home exercise program
7. Learn proper care of the remaining extremity.

The success of the rehabilitation program is determined to some extent by the individual's psychological and physiological status and the physical characteristics of the residual limb. The longer the residual limb, the better potential for successful prosthetic ambulation regardless of level of amputation. A well-healed, well-shaped limb with a nonadherent scar is easier to fit than one that is poorly-shaped or has redundant tissue distally or laterally. The vascular status of the remaining extremity will affect the rehabilitation program as will the physiological (but not chronological) age of the individual. The presence of conditions such as diabetes, cardiovascular disease, renal disease, visual impairment, limitation of joint motion, and muscle weakness may affect the eventual level of function. In the final analysis, a cooperative patient who takes an active part in the rehabilitation program is necessary for achievement of rehabilitation goals. If the patient appears passive or depressed, it behooves the therapist to try to understand what is driving the patient's motivation and to make sure the patient understands the relationship between the postsurgical program and eventual prosthetic rehabilitation.

The Clinic Team

The majority of amputations today are performed by vascular surgeons who may or may not be knowledgeable about prosthetic rehabilitation. Referral to an amputation clinic or to physical therapy may be delayed for many weeks as the surgeon waits until the residual limb heals completely and the postoperative edema has been absorbed. Such delays are undesirable and may limit the eventual level of function. Ideally, the clinic team should become involved before surgery, or at least immediately after. Unfortunately, many amputations are performed in hospitals without the services of an amputation clinic or a well-trained team that can develop and supervise the program. The physical therapist may be the only person with competence in prosthetic rehabilitation. Close communication between the vascular surgeon and the physical therapist may serve to increase the likelihood of early referrals.

The clinic team plans and implements comprehensive rehabilitation programs designed to meet the physical, psychological, and economic needs of the patient. Most clinic teams are located in rehabilitation facilities or university health centers. The team generally includes a physician, physical therapist, occupational therapist, prosthetist, and social worker. Other health professionals who often contribute to the team are the nurse, vocational counselor, dietitian, psychologist, and, possibly, administrative coordinator. Table 25.2 outlines the major functions of team members. The clinic team may meet monthly, bimonthly, or weekly depending on the caseload; patients are seen regularly and decisions are made using input from all team members. An initial screening by the physical and occupational therapists prior to the actual clinic visit will guide the examination of each person to be seen and improves the effectiveness of the clinic function.[39] Most patients are seen in environments without amputation clinics. Patients with vascular diseases are treated by vascular specialists and usually come to amputation after many attempts at revascularization. The

Table 25.2 Amputation Clinic Team Functions

Physician	Clinic chief; coordinates team decision making; supervises patient's general medical condition.
Physical therapist	Evaluates and treats patients through postsurgical and prosthetic phases; makes recommendations for prosthetic components and whether or not to fit the patient. May be clinic coordinator.
Prosthetist	Fabricates and modifies prosthesis; recommends prosthetic components; shares data on new prosthetic developments.
Occupational therapist	Evaluates and treats patients with amputations of the upper extremities; makes recommendation for components.
Social worker	Financial counselor and coordinator, liaison with third-party payers and community agencies; helps family cope with social and financial issues.
Dietician	Consultant for patients with diabetes or those needing diet and nutritional guidance.
Vocational counselor	Determines patient's employment potential; provides education and training; assists with placement.

patient may briefly see a physical therapist while in the hospital and may then be discharged without follow-up treatment. Months later, the patient may show up at a prosthetist's office with a prescription for a prosthesis. These individuals may have contractures, the residual limb may be edematous and the person may not have been out of the wheelchair during most of that period.

It is important for the physical therapist in the acute care center to take responsibility for ensuring that some form of follow-up care will be provided, either through outpatient therapy, home care, or referral to a rehabilitation center. It is also important for physical therapists to establish close relationships with regional prosthetic providers. The prosthetist may be knowledgeable about referral resources for postsurgical care as well as for prosthetic training within the patient's community.[40]

Postoperative Dressings

Reading the chart before going to see the patient, you note that the surgeon did not use a rigid postoperative dressing but rather applied a soft dressing covered with an elastic wrap. This information raises your concerns about edema control. Reviewing the chart, you note that the surgery went well, that the patient is afebrile, that vital signs are within normal limits, that she is not spilling sugar, and that she is voiding appropriately. The incision is reported to look clean and the drain is to be removed tomorrow morning. The nursing staff had her out of bed twice yesterday. You also check the patient's medications and find that she is on medication for diabetes, hypertension, and pain as needed. She had pain medication about an hour ago.

Surgeons have several options regarding the postoperative dressing including (1) immediate postoperative fitting or *rigid dressing,* (2) semirigid dressing, or (3) soft dressing. It is important for some sort of edema control to be used because excessive edema in the residual limb can compromise healing and cause pain.

Rigid Dressings

In the early 1960s, orthopedic surgeons in the United States started experimenting with a technique developed in Europe that consisted of fitting the person with a plaster of Paris socket made in the configuration of the definitive prosthesis. An attachment incorporated at the distal end of the dressing allows the later addition of a foot and pylon allowing limited weightbearing ambulation within a few days or a week of surgery *(immediate postoperative prosthesis or IPOP).*[41–43] The IPOP may be handmade from plaster of Paris by the surgeon or a prosthetist. These are not adjustable or removable. The socket must be cut like a cast for removal and a new one applied as the residual limb heals, sutures are removed, and the limb changes shape.

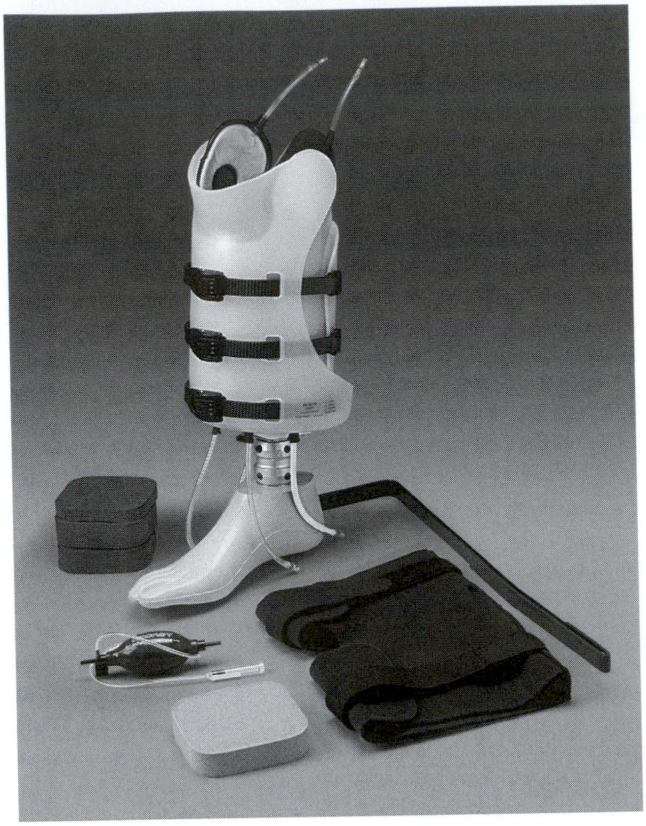

Figure 25.4 AirLimb® (Courtesy of Aircast, Inc, Summit, NJ 07901.).

There are also *removable rigid dressings* (RRD) that may be handmade from plaster or prefabricated from plastic materials and come in different sizes. Prefabricated RRDs are adjustable as the limb changes and may be removed as needed for wound inspection. The commercially available AirLimb® (Aircast Inc, Summit, NJ, 07901) is a plastic socket with inflatable bladders that help maintain proper fit as the residual limb shrinks (Fig. 25.4). The addition of a pylon and foot allows for early, limited, weightbearing ambulation. Like other RRDs, AirLimb® is removable for wound inspection and care but is said to be easier to fit and use.[44]

Use of immediate postoperative rigid dressings vary greatly and are more prevalent in some areas of the country than others. Generally, orthopedic surgeons use the technique more than vascular surgeons. Rigid postsurgical dressing, whether used immediately after surgery or in the early postoperative period, have been found successful in reducing postoperative edema, pain, and enhancing healing even in cases of delayed healing.[45–47] The advantages of the techniques are:

- It greatly limits the development of postoperative edema in the residual limb, thereby reducing postoperative pain and enhancing wound healing.
- It allows for earlier ambulation with the attachment of a pylon and foot.

- It allows for earlier fitting of the permanent prosthesis by reducing the length of time needed for shrinking the residual limb.

The major disadvantages are:

- Prefabricated components can be expensive and their use must be learned.
- Techniques for fabrication of a handmade prosthesis require special training or the involvement of a prosthetist.
- It requires close supervision during the early healing stage.

Semirigid Dressings

There are a number of **semirigid dressings** that have been reported in the literature and may or may not be used in a particular center. All provide better control of edema than the soft dressing but each has some disadvantage that limits its use. **Unna's dressing**, gauze impregnated with a compound of zinc oxide, gelatin, glycerin, and calamine, may be applied in the operating room. Its major disadvantage is that it may loosen easily and is not as rigid as the plaster of Paris dressing. However, it has been shown to be superior to the soft dressing in enhancing healing and reducing edema.[48]

Soft Dressings

The *soft dressing* is the oldest method of postsurgical management of the residual limb. Currently there are two forms of soft dressings: the elastic wrap and the elastic *shrinker.* The major advantages of soft dressings include that:

- They are relatively inexpensive.
- They are lightweight and readily available.
- They can be easily laundered.

The major disadvantages are:

- They provide relatively poor control of edema.
- They can slip and form a tourniquet.
- The elastic wrap requires skill in proper application.
- The elastic wrap needs frequent reapplication.
- New shrinkers must be purchased as the residual limb gets markedly smaller.
- Shrinkers cannot be used until the sutures have been removed and primary healing has occurred.

Elastic Wraps

The elastic wrap may be applied over the postsurgical dressing if care is taken to ensure proper compression. A dressing is applied to the incision followed by some form of gauze pad, then the compression wrap. The soft dressing is indicated in cases of local infection, but is not the treatment of choice for the majority of individuals. The patient or a family member should learn to apply the wrap as soon as possible after wound care is no longer necessary. Many older individuals with transfemoral amputations do not have the necessary balance and coordination to wrap effectively.

Some surgeons prefer delaying elastic wrap until the incision has healed and the sutures have been removed. Leaving the residual limb without any pressure wrap allows for full development of postoperative edema, which may be quite uncomfortable and interfere with circulation in the many small vessels in the skin and soft tissue, thereby potentially compromising healing. The therapist can discuss the benefits of early wrapping if no other form of rigid dressing is used. There is strong evidence in the literature on the benefits of residual limb wrapping and the advantages of early compression.[38,42–47]

One of the major drawbacks of the elastic wrap is that it needs frequent rewrapping. Movement of the residual limb against the bedclothes, bending and extending the proximal joints, and general body movements will cause slippage and changes in pressure. Covering the finished wrap with stockinet helps to reduce some of the wrinkling. However, careful and frequent rewrapping is the only effective way to prevent complications. Nursing staff, family members, and the patient as well as the physical therapist or physical therapist assistant need to assume responsibility for frequent inspection and rewrapping of the residual limb. Residual limb wrapping is described in detail later in this chapter. Evidence Summary Box 25.1 presents data from recent studies examining several types of postsurgical amputation dressings.

Shrinkers

Shrinkers are socklike garments knitted of heavy, rubber-reinforced cotton; they are conical in shape and come in a variety of sizes (Fig. 25.5). As shrinkers come in different sizes, it is not economical to purchase a shrinker while the residual limb is still covered with gauze dressings. Elastic wrap and shrinkers will be discussed in greater detail later in this chapter.

Examination

As you enter the patient's room you find her lying in bed, alert and awake. An incentive spirometer is on the bedside table. The patient looks tired and you realize you will not be able to gather all the information you need during this one visit. You think through the data that must be collected and begin to set priorities, deciding what needs to be done today and what can be put off for another time. Because the patient will probably not be in the hospital long, information regarding the status of the residual limb, her postsurgical cardiopulmonary and general physiological function, her ability to be mobile, the condition of the remaining LE, her feelings about the amputation and discharge plans may be the most important data to obtain. The physical

Evidence Summary Box 25.1

Postsurgical Amputation Dressings

Reference	Subjects	Design/ Intervention	Duration	Results	Comments
Wong,CK, and Edelstein, JE[48] 2000	21 Ss with recent lower limb amputations	Experimental design; 12 Ss treated with semirigid Unna dressings; 9 Ss treated with elastic bandage	Until discharged from inpatient rehabilitation setting	Subjects treated with semirigid dressing healed faster, were ready for fitting sooner and more likely to be discharged ambulating with prosthesis	Semirigid dressings more effective in preparing for prosthetic fitting, less expensive, and less time consuming to apply
Woodburn, KR, et al[a] 2004	Patients requiring transtibial amputation; 46 Ss in the E; 50 Ss in the C	Multicenter randomized controlled trial; E received a rigid dressing; C received nonrigid dressings	Rigid dressings removed at 7 day intervals for inspection	Rigid dressing produced a reduction in time to first casting for prosthesis; however this difference failed to reach statistical significance	Cited advantages of rigid dressing: wound protection, reduced frequency of dressing changes, decreased incidence of contractures, early mobilization. Disadvantages: inability to visualize wound and increased weight
Vigier, S, et al[45] 1999	All Ss with recent transtibial amputation (not yet healed); 28 Ss in the E; 28 Ss in the C	Randomized controlled trial; E rigid plaster cast; C elastic compression bandage	Ss were gradually trained to wear cast up to 5 hours/day	Rigid dressing: accelerated healing, faster limb shrinkage, reduced length of hospitalization	Rigid dressing produced improved reepithelialization and reduced formation of myofibroblasts; deemed safe for limbs with no ischemia

[a]Woodburn, KR, et al.: A randomized trail of rigid stump dressing following trans-tibial amputation for peripheral arterial insufficiency. Prosthet Orthot Int 28(1):22, 2004.

C = Control group; E = experimental group; Ss = subjects.

therapist needs to be involved in early discharge planning to insure continuity of postsurgical care.

Careful examination of each individual is an integral part of physical therapy management. Examination data are obtained continuously throughout this period as the incision heals and the person's tolerance improves. Box 25.2 outlines the typical data needed during a complete postsurgical examination. Some of the data cannot be obtained until some healing has taken place and collecting other data must await complete healing. The availability of some of these data will also depend in part on the treatment of the residual limb by the surgeon. At all times throughout the postsurgical period, the physical therapist must prioritize data collection and integrate it with interventions, always considering immediate patient, family, and caregiver needs.

Range of Motion

Gross range of motion (ROM) estimations are generally adequate for examination of the uninvolved extremity but specific goniometric measurements are necessary for the amputated side and for the ankle motion of the unamputated side. Hip flexion, extension, abduction, and adduction measurements are taken early in the postoperative phase following transtibial amputation. Measurement of knee flexion and extension are taken, if the dressing allows, after some incisional healing has occurred. Hip flexion, extension, abduction, and adduction ROM measurements are taken several days after surgery when the dressing allows, following transfemoral amputation. Measurement of internal and external hip rotation is difficult to obtain and unnecessary if no gross abnormality or pathology is evident. Joint ROM is monitored throughout the postsurgical period.

Muscle Strength

Gross manual muscle testing (MMT) of the upper extremities and uninvolved LE is performed early in the postoperative period. MMT of the involved LE must usually wait

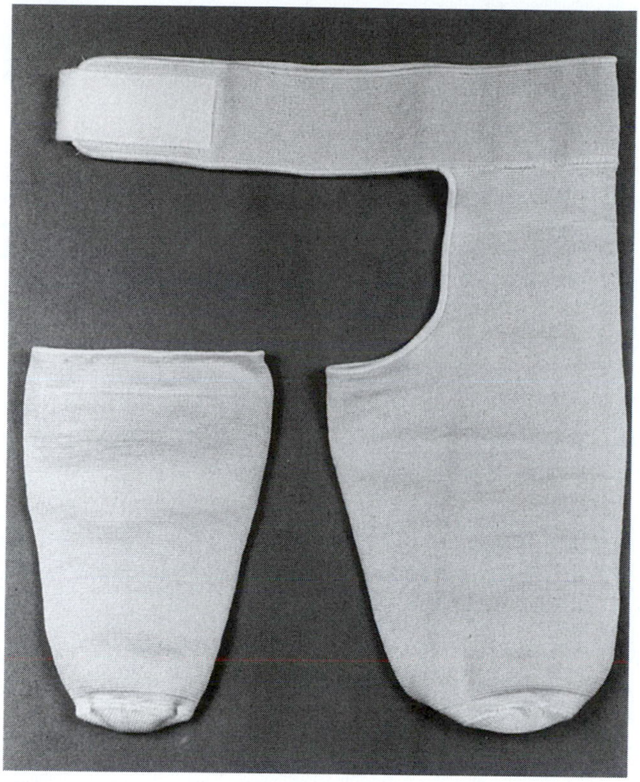

Figure 25.5 (*Left*) Transtibial shrinker. (*Right*) Transfemoral shrinker.

until most healing has occurred. With a transtibial amputation, good strength in the hip extensors and abductors as well as the knee extensors and flexors are needed for satisfactory prosthetic ambulation. For the patient with a transfemoral amputation, good strength of the hip extensors and abductors is a requirement. The strength of these muscles should be monitored throughout the postsurgical program.

Status of the Residual Limb

Residual limb measurements are generally taken and reported in centimeters for uniformity with others involved in the care of individuals who have had an amputation. Circumferential measurements of the residual limb are taken as soon as the dressing will allow, then regularly throughout the postsurgical period. Measurements are made at regular intervals over the length of the residual limb. Circumferential measurements of the transtibial or Symes residual limb are started at the medial tibial plateau and taken every 5 to 8 cm depending on the length of the limb. Length of the residual limb is measured from the medial tibial plateau to the end of the bone.

Circumferential measurements of the transfemoral or through knee residual limb are started at the ischial tuberosity or the greater trochanter, whichever is most palpable, and taken every 8 to 10 cm. Length is measured from the ischial tuberosity or the greater trochanter to the end of the bone. If there is considerable excess tissue distal to the end of the bone, then length measurements are taken to both the end of the bone and the incision line. For accuracy of repeat measurements, exact landmarks are carefully noted. If the ischial tuberosity is used in transfemoral measurements, hip joint position is noted as well.

Other information gathered about the residual limb includes its shape (conical, bulbous, cylindrical redundant tissue), skin condition, sensation, and joint proprioception.

The Phantom Limb

The majority of individuals will encounter **phantom limb sensations** following amputation. In its simplest form, the phantom is the sensation of the limb that is no longer there. The phantom, which usually occurs initially immediately after surgery, is often described as a tingling, burning, itching or pressure sensation, sometimes a numbness. The distal part of the extremity is most frequently felt although, on occasion, the person will feel the whole extremity. The sensation is responsive to external stimuli such as bandaging or rigid dressing; it may dissipate over time or the person may have the sensation throughout life. Phantom sensation may be painless although most people find it uncomfortable and often report it as pain; it usually does not interfere with prosthetic rehabilitation. It is important for the patient to understand that the feeling is quite normal.[49]

Phantom limb pain often follows amputation, occurring in up to 80 percent of individuals undergoing amputation from any cause. It is important to differentiate phantom pain from nonpainful phantom sensation, residual limb pain, and nonpainful residual limb phenomena.[50] Phantom pain is usually characterized as either a cramping or squeezing sensation, or a shooting or a burning pain. Some individuals report all three. The pain may be localized or diffuse; it may be continuous or intermittent and triggered by some external stimuli. It may diminish over time or may become a permanent and often disabling condition. The cause of phantom limb pain has never been well defined, although today there is some agreement that the pain is related to reorganization in the somatosensory cortex. There has been some research on the relationship of cortical reorganization and chronic pain and there is some evidence that individuals who experienced intense preoperative pain were more likely to have phantom limb pain.[50,51]

The residual limb should be carefully examined to differentiate phantom pain from residual limb pain or other conditions such as a neuroma. Sometimes, wearing a prosthesis will ease the phantom pain. On occasion, in the presence of trigger points, injection with steroids or local anesthetic has reduced the pain temporarily. Although the literature is replete with information and studies on phantom sensation and residual limb pain, there is little agreement about the best approach to treatment of these phenomena. In some studies, particularly of individuals who experienced considerable preoperative pain, intrathecal or epidural anesthetic drips

Box 25.2 **Postsurgical Examination Guide**

History
- Patient demographics
- Family and social data
- Preamputation status (work, activity level, independence)
- Financial status
- Other as appropriate

Systems Review
- Cause of amputation (disease, tumor, trauma, congenital)
- Associated diseases/symptoms (neuropathy, visual disturbances, cardiopulmonary disease, renal failure, congenital anomalies)
- Current physiological state (postsurgical cardiopulmonary status, vital signs, shortness of breath, pain)
- Medications

Skin
- Scar (healed, adherent, invaginated, flat)
- Other lesions (size, shape, open, scar tissue)
- Moisture (moist, dry, scaly)
- Sensation (absent, diminished, hyperesthesia)
- Grafts (location, type, healing)
- Dermatological lesions (psoriasis, eczema, cysts)

Residual Limb Length
- Bone length (transtibial limbs measured from medial tibial plateau; transfemoral limbs measured from ischial tuberosity or greater trochanter)
- Soft tissue length (note redundant tissue)

Residual Limb Shape
- Cylindrical, conical, bulbous end, and so forth
- Abnormalities ("dog ears," adductor roll)

Emotional Status
- Acceptance
- Body image

Vascularity (both limbs if amputation cause is vascular)
- Pulses (femoral, popliteal, dorsalis pedis, posterior tibial)
- Color (red, cyanotic)
- Temperature
- Edema (circumference measurement, water displacement measurement, caliper measures)
- Pain (type, location, duration, intensity)
- Trophic changes

Range of Motion
- Residual limb (specific for remaining joints)
- Other lower extremity (gross for major joints)

Muscle Strength
- Residual limb (specific for major muscle groups)
- Other extremities (gross for necessary function)

Neurological
- Pain (phantom [differentiate *sensation* or *pain*], neuroma, incisional, from other causes)
- Neuropathy
- Cognitive status (alert, oriented, confused)

Functional Status
- Transfers (bed-to-chair, to toilet, to car)
- Mobility (ancillary support, supervision)
- Home/family situation (caregiver, architectural barriers, hazards)
- Activities of daily living (bathing, dressing)
- Instrumental activities of daily living (cooking, cleaning)

with opioids were used both pre- and postoperatively with success. However, others have reported no success with such treatments. Noninvasive treatments such as ultrasound, icing, TENS, or massage have been used with varying success. Mild non-narcotic analgesics have been of limited value; biofeedback, guided imagery, psychotherapy, nerve blocks, and dorsal rhyzotomies have all been used with inconsistent results. The treatment of phantom pain can be very frustrating for the clinic team as well as the patient.[49–58]

Status of the Uninvolved Limb

The vascular status of the uninvolved LE is determined and its condition noted. Data gathered include condition of the skin, presence of pulses, sensation, temperature, edema, pain on exercise or at rest, presence of wounds, ulceration, or other abnormalities.

Functional Status

Activities of daily living (ADL) and functional mobility skills including transfer and ambulatory status are examined and documented. Balance both sitting and standing on the remaining extremity is very important and should be examined as long as the person's condition permits. Information on the patient's home situation, including any constraints or special needs, is valuable in establishing an individually relevant treatment program. Data regarding presurgical activity level and the person's own expected outcomes are obtained through interview and will be indicative of potential functional prosthetic use. An individual who had an active lifestyle prior to the amputation is more likely to be able to learn to use a prosthesis well. Individuals with a long history of a sedentary life style may encounter more difficulty, particularly if the amputation is at the transfemoral level.

The person's apparent emotional status and degree of adjustment are noted. Exploration of the patient's suitability and desire for a prosthesis is begun and continues throughout the postsurgical period. Any other problems that may affect the rehabilitation program and outcomes are evaluated and documented.

Emotional Status

As you perform the initial examination of the patient and talk with her about the amputation, you realize that she is quite depressed. Although losing the limb did not come as a shock because she had been struggling with a foot ulcer that would not heal, she verbalizes concern about her ability to return to her own home. She keeps saying, "I don't want to go to one of those places."

Initial reaction to the loss of a limb is usually grief and depression. If the amputation was traumatic, the immediate reaction may include disbelief. The person may experience insomnia, restlessness, and have difficulty concentrating. Some individuals may actually mourn the possible loss of a job or the ability to participate in a favorite sport or other activities rather than the lost limb per se. In the early stages, the person's grief may alternate with feelings of hopelessness, despondency, bitterness, and anger. Socially the patient may feel lonely, isolated, and the object of pity. Concerns about the future, about body image and sexual function, about the responses of family and friends, and about employment all affect the individual's reactions.

Long-term adjustment depends to a great extent on the individual's basic personality structure, sense of accomplishment, and place in the family, community, and world. In general, many individuals with amputations make a satisfactory adjustment to the loss and are reintegrated into a full and active life. In achieving final acceptance, the individual may go through a number of stages including denial, anger, euphoria, and social withdrawal. While it is difficult to predict long range adjustment initially, there is some evidence that early counseling and the opportunity to explore the feelings associated with amputation and rehabilitation may be beneficial for individuals in all age groups.[59,60]

Some individuals may try to avoid distressing thoughts of the lost limb through conscious self-control or by avoiding situations or people that remind them of the lost limb. Some may display temper tantrums or irrational resentment. Some may revert to childlike states of helplessness and dependence.

Many individuals are not fully aware of the consequences of amputation and may fear other physical limitations as a result of the surgery. Fear of impotence or sterility may lead some men to make grandiose statements or display reckless behavior to mask the fear. Thorough explanations of the amputation process and implications by the surgeon or other health worker may alleviate many of these fears.

Generally, people who have had an amputation may dream about themselves as having an intact limb. This image may be so vivid that they fall as they get up at night and attempt to walk to the bathroom without a prosthesis or crutches. Individuals who have lost their leg through injury may dream about the battle or accident in which they were injured. Such reenactments may lead to insomnia, trembling fits, speech impediments, and difficulty with concentration. In general, individuals with congenital amputations or acquired amputations before the age of 5 do not have some of the problems mentioned above because their amputation is a part of their developed self-image.

Psychological Support

The patient needs to receive reassurance and understanding from the entire rehabilitation team. The staff should create an open and receptive environment and be willing to listen. The patient should know what to expect during the entire process. The surgeon and therapists should carefully explain the steps and expectations of rehabilitation. Audiovisual media, such as films or slides, may be helpful.

Others with amputations who have made satisfactory adjustments in their lives and successfully completed rehabilitation may provide support, information on lifestyle changes, and encouragement in private or group sessions. Professionals skilled in group dynamics and patient education are helpful, especially for medical or technical advice regarding such issues as diabetes, medications, or PVD. Family and friends are often included. A nonthreatening atmosphere helps individuals express their feelings and frustrations.

Patients have various attitudes toward the prosthesis. Some are particularly concerned about its appearance, hoping that it will conceal their disability and give the illusion of an intact body. Others claim to be concerned primarily with the restoration of function. When the artificial limb is fitted, the patient must face the fact that the natural limb has been lost irrevocably. If individuals with amputations have been told that the prosthesis will replace their own limb, they may have unrealistic expectations that appearance and function will be as good as in the nonamputated extremity. Realistic adjustment will be necessary as the person learns to use the artificial substitute. Good predictors for adjustment to the prosthesis are motivation to master the prosthesis and to return to an active lifestyle.

The Older Adult

The older individual with a LE amputation is not content to sit in a wheelchair or limp with a walker, but seeks effective rehabilitation services and a meaningful lifestyle. The immediate reaction to amputation is no different than that of any other individual except that the amputation will usually not come as a surprise. The reaction may depend in part on the severity of preoperative pain and the extent of attempts to save the limb. Individuals who have suffered considerable pain may be grateful that the pain has ended. Patients who underwent extensive medical and surgical procedures to save the limb may have a sense of failure. In general, the reactions of older people resemble the reactions of other adults who have experienced an amputation. Some may feel a sense of hopelessness and despair, and have a preoccupation with impending death. Some may have insomnia, anorexia, and be withdrawn. Some older individuals may experience a loss of self-esteem and be afraid of becoming dependent. In some instances, the person may contemplate or attempt suicide, believing that he or she has nothing left to live for. Older people seldom use denial because the functional and anatomical deficit is obvious. Older persons are more likely to dream that the amputation has taken place as compared to younger individuals. The older person may view the amputation as impending death because the rest of the body is vulnerable.

If preoperative attitudes are unrealistically hopeful, postoperative disturbances may be more severe. The older person should not be led to expect a total cure. Learning to use an artificial limb may be a slow and discouraging ordeal and the patient may not express distress or depression in front of the optimism of others. Sharing and support from other older patients can be quite helpful as can a realistic attitude by rehabilitation team members.

Rehabilitation includes not only preparation of the individual physically and psychologically for the community, but preparation of the community for individuals with amputations. Public education media are a useful means of information, particularly for prospective employers. As with other physically challenged individuals, those with amputations need to be accepted and integrated into the community because of their abilities and not their disabilities.

Treatment Interventions

If the patient is to return to her own home, she will need to be ambulatory and able to take care of her residual limb. If she goes to her own home rather than a rehabilitation center, she will need some homemaking help as well as home health care for continued nursing and physical therapy. On the other hand, transfer to a rehabilitation center might help her reach an adequate level of independence to be able to function at home with minimal support until she can be fitted with a prosthesis. You decide to discuss this further with the physician and social worker. In the meantime, you realize that your treatment program will need to focus on functional mobility skills, residual limb care, and care of the intact leg.

Residual Limb Care

Individuals not fitted with a rigid dressing or a *temporary prosthesis* use elastic wrap or shrinkers to reduce the size of the residual limb. The patient, family member, or professional staff member applies the bandage, which is worn 24 hours a day, except when bathing.

Removable rigid dressings for use with transtibial amputations are available and may be an important alternative to the elastic wrap. Regretfully, there are fewer alternatives for the person with a transfemoral amputation; rigid dressings and inexpensive temporary prostheses are more difficult to fabricate and elastic wraps or shrinkers are only minimally effective. It may be advisable to fit the individual following transfemoral amputation with a definitive prosthesis early and then adjust it for shrinkage by using additional socks or a liner.

Edema in the residual limb is often difficult to control owing to complications of diabetes, cardiovascular disease, or hypertension. An intermittent compression unit can be used to reduce edema on a temporary basis. Transfemoral and transtibial sleeves are commercially available.

Proper hygiene and skin care are important. Once the incision is healed and the sutures removed, the person can bathe normally. The residual limb is treated as any other part of the body; it is kept clean and dry. Individuals with dry skin may use a good skin lotion. Care must be taken to avoid abrasions, cuts, and other skin problems. Friction massage, in which layers of skin, subcutaneous tissue, and muscle are moved over the respective underlying tissue, can be used to prevent or mobilize adherent scar tissue. The massage is done gently, after the wound is healed and when no infection is present. Patients can learn to properly perform a gentle friction massage to mobilize the scar tissue and help decrease hypersensitivity of the residual limb to touch and pressure. Early handling of the residual limb by the patient is an aid to acceptance and is encouraged, particularly for individuals who may be repulsed by the limb.

The patient is taught to inspect the residual limb with a mirror each night to make sure there are no sores or impending problems, especially in areas not readily visible. If the person has diminished sensation, careful inspection is particularly important. Because the residual limb tends to become a bit edematous after bathing as a reaction to the warm water, nightly bathing is recommended, particularly once a prosthesis has been fitted. The elastic bandage, shrinker, or removable rigid dressing is reapplied after bathing. If the person has been fitted with a temporary prosthesis, the residual limb is wrapped at night and any time the prosthesis is not worn. Sometimes, individuals fitted in surgery with a rigid dressing then transferred immediately into a temporary prosthesis do not know how to bandage, and encounter difficulties with edema after they remove the prosthesis at night. Learning proper bandaging is part of the therapy program because most people will need to wrap the limb at one time or another.

Patients have been known to apply a variety of "home and folk remedies" to the residual limb. Historically, it was believed that the skin had to be toughened for prosthetic wear by beating it with a towel-wrapped bottle. Various ointments and lotions have been applied; residual limbs have been immersed in substances such as vinegar, salt water, and gasoline to harden the skin. Although the skin does need to adjust to the pressures of wearing an artificial limb, there is no evidence to indicate that "toughening" techniques are beneficial. Such methods may actually be deleterious; research indicates that soft pliable skin is better able to cope with stress than tough dry skin. Patient education regarding proper skin care can reduce the use of home remedies.

The skin of the residual limb may be affected by a variety of dermatological problems such as eczema, psoriasis, or radiation burns. Some of these conditions may mitigate against fitting or wrapping. Treatment may include ultraviolet irradiation, whirlpool, reflex heating, hyperbaric oxygen, or medication. Care must be taken in using ultraviolet or heat in the presence of *dysvascular* disease. The whirlpool may not be the treatment of choice because it increases circulation and edema in the part under treatment. The advantages of the whirlpool as a cleansing agent for skin problems, infected wounds, or incidence of delayed healing must be balanced against its disadvantages before effectiveness can be determined for any individual person.

Residual Limb Wrapping

There are several effective methods of wrapping the residual limb. Patients tend to wrap their own residual limb in a circular manner, often creating a tourniquet, which may compromise healing and foster the development of a bulbous end. Although the transtibial residual limb can be effectively wrapped in a sitting position, it is difficult to properly wrap and anchor the transfemoral limb while sitting. Older patients often cannot balance themselves in the standing position while wrapping. An effective bandage is smooth and wrinkle free, emphasizes angular turns, provides pressure distally, and encourages proximal joint extension. The ends of bandages are fastened with tape, safety pins, or Velcro® rather than clips, which can cut the skin and do not anchor well. A system of wrapping that uses mostly angular or figure-of-eight turns was developed specifically to meet the needs of the older patient and has been successfully in use for the past 40 years.[61] Figures 25.6 and 25.7 illustrate the techniques.

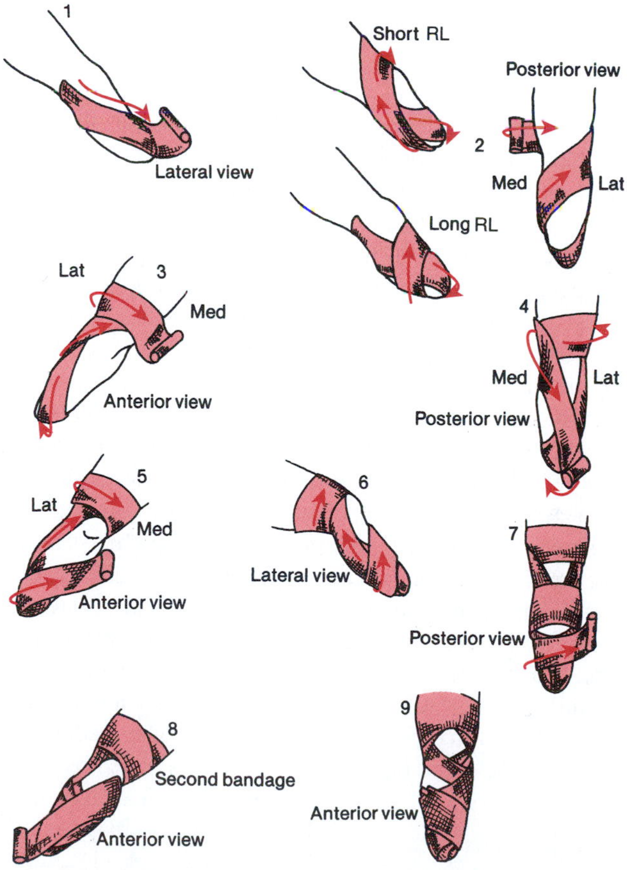

Figure 25.6 Transtibial residual limb wrapping. RL = residual limb.

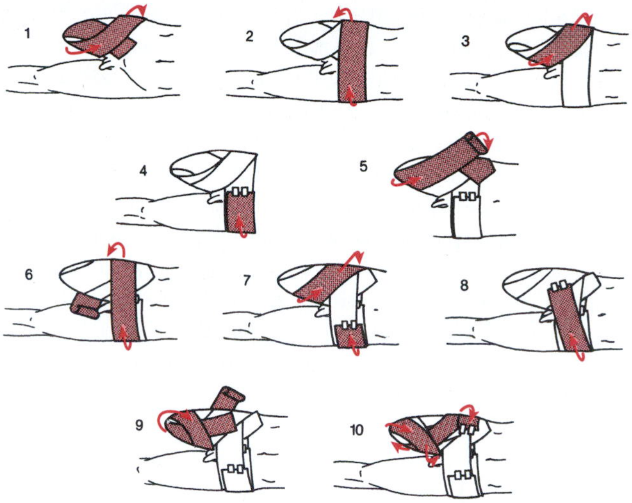

Figure 25.7 Transfemoral residual limb wrapping.

The Transtibial Bandage

Two 4-in. elastic bandages are usually enough to wrap most transtibial residual limbs. Very large residual limbs may require three bandages. The transtibial bandages should not be sewn together so that the weave of each bandage can be brought in contraposition to the other to provide more support. Although an elastic wrap does not provide as much pressure as a rigid dressing, the development of postsurgical edema must be deterred as much as possible; therefore, a firm, even pressure against all soft tissues is desirable. If the incision is placed anteriorly, then an attempt should be made to bring the bandages from posterior to anterior over the distal end.

The first bandage is started at either the medial or lateral tibial condyle and brought diagonally over the anterior surface of the limb to the distal end. One edge of the bandage should just cover the midline of the incision in an anterior-posterior plane. The bandage is continued diagonally over the posterior surface then back over the beginning turn as an anchor. At this point, there is a choice; the bandage may be brought directly over the beginning point as indicated in step 2, or it may be brought across the front of the residual limb in an "X" design. The latter technique is particularly useful with long residual limbs and aids in bandage suspension. An anchoring turn over the distal thigh is made making sure that the wrap is clear of the patella and is not tight around the distal thigh.

After a single anchoring turn above the knee, the bandage is brought back around the opposite tibial condyle and down to the distal end of the limb. One edge of the bandage should overlap the midline of the incision and the other wrap by at least 1/2 in. to ensure adequate distal end support. The figure-of-eight pattern is continued as depicted in steps 4 through 7 until the bandage is used up. Care should be taken to completely cover the residual limb with a firm and even pressure. Semicircular turns are made posteriorly to bring the bandage in line to cross the anterior surface in an angular line. This maneuver provides greater pressure on the posterior soft tissue while distributing pressure anteriorly where the bone is close to the skin. Each turn should partially overlap other turns so the whole residual limb is well covered. The pattern is usually from proximal to distal and back to proximal, starting at the tibial condyles and covering both condyles as well as the patellar tendon. Usually, the patella is left free to aid in knee motion, although with extremely short residual limbs, it may be necessary to cover it for better suspension.

The second bandage is wrapped like the first, except that it is started at the opposite tibial condyle from the first bandage (step 8). Bringing the weave of each bandage in contraposition exerts a more even pressure. With both bandages, an effort is made to bring the angular turns across each other rather than in the same direction.

The Transfemoral Bandage

For most residual limbs, two 6-in. and one 4-in. bandages will adequately cover the limb. The two 6-in. bandages can be sewn together end-to-end taking care not to create a heavy seam; the 4-in. bandage is used by itself. The patient is depicted sidelying in Figure 25.7, which allows a family member or therapist easy access to the residual limb. The patient with good balance on the remaining limb can bandage the residual limb in the standing position, but it is difficult for the patient to self-bandage correctly in the sitting position.

The 6-in. bandages are used first. The first bandage is started in the groin and brought diagonally over the anterior surface to the distal lateral corner, around the end of the residual limb, and diagonally up the posterior side to the iliac crest and around the hips in a spica. The bandage is started medially so that the hip wrap (spica) will encourage extension. After the turn around the hips, the bandage is wrapped around the proximal portion of the residual limb high in the groin, then back around the hips. Although this is a proximal circular turn, it does not create a tourniquet as long as it is continued around the hips. Going around the medial portion of the residual limb high in the groin ensures coverage of the soft tissue in the adductor area and reduces the possibility of an adductor roll, a complication that can seriously interfere with comfortable prosthetic wear. In most instances, the first bandage ends in the second hip spica and is anchored with tape or pin.

The second 6-in. bandage is wrapped like the first but is started a bit more laterally. Any areas not covered with the first bandage must be covered at this time. The second bandage is also anchored in a hip spica after the first figure-of-eight and after the second turn high in the groin. While more of the first two bandages are used to cover the proximal residual limb, care must be taken that no tourniquet is created. Bringing the bandage directly from the proximal medial area into a hip spica helps to keep the adductor tissue covered and prevents rolling of the bandage to some degree.

The 4-in. bandage is used to exert the greatest amount of pressure over middle and distal areas of the residual limb. It is usually not necessary to anchor this bandage around the hips because friction with the already applied bandages and good figure-of-eight turns limit slippage. The 4-in. bandage is generally started laterally to bring the weave across the weave of previous bandages. Regular figure-of-eight turns in varied patterns to cover the entire residual limb are the most effective.

Bandages are applied with firm pressure from the outset. Elastic bandages can be wrapped directly over a soft postsurgical dressing so that bandaging can begin immediately after surgery. The elastic wrap controls edema more effectively if minimal gauze coverage is used over the residual limb. Several gauze pads placed just over the incision are usually adequate protection without compromising the effect of the wrap. Care must be taken to avoid any wrinkles or folds that can cause excessive skin pressure particularly over a soft dressing. It is critically important for the bandage to be rewrapped frequently, especially during the early postoperative period. As has been previously stated, the elastic wrap is not as effective in controlling edema as the rigid or semi rigid dressings.

Shrinkers

The transtibial shrinker is rolled over the residual limb to midthigh and is designed to be self-suspending. Individuals with heavy thighs may need additional suspension with garters or a waist belt. Currently available transfemoral shrinkers incorporate a hip spica, which provides good suspension except with obese individuals (Fig. 25.5). Care must be taken that the patient understands the importance of proper suspension; any rolling of the edges or slipping of the shrinker can create a tourniquet around the proximal part of the residual limb. Shrinkers are easier to apply than elastic bandages and may be a better alternative, particularly for the transfemoral residual limb. Shrinkers are more expensive to use than elastic wrap; the initial cost is greater, and then new shrinkers of smaller sizes must be purchased as the limb volume decreases. However, shrinkers are a viable option for individuals who are not able to properly wrap the residual limb. Shrinkers may not be used until the incision has healed and the sutures have been removed. Sutures can be caught in the shrinker's mesh and the distal distraction forces that accompany donning may cause wound *dehiscence* (splitting open).

Positioning

One of the greatest deterrents to functional prosthetic rehabilitation is contracture of hip or knee. Contractures can develop as a result of muscle imbalance or fascial tightness, from a protective withdrawal reflex into hip and knee flexion, from loss of plantar stimulation in extension, or as a result of faulty positioning such as prolonged sitting or placing the residual limb on a pillow. The patient should understand the importance of proper positioning and regular exercise in preparing for eventual prosthetic fit and ambulation. For all levels of amputation, full ROM in hip extension is critical in allowing the individual to assume a balanced upright posture.

With the transtibial amputation, full ROM in the hips and knee, particularly in extension, is needed. While sitting, the patient can keep the knee extended by using a posterior splint or a board attached to the wheelchair. The patient with a transfemoral amputation needs full ROM in the hip, particularly in extension and adduction. Prolonged sitting is to be avoided. Some time each day should be spent in the prone position. Elevation of the residual limb on a pillow following either transfemoral or transtibial amputation can lead to the development of hip flexion contractures and should be avoided (Figs. 25.8 and 25.9). The early postoperative period is critical in establishing positive patterns of activity that will aid the patient throughout the rehabilitative period. Taking the time to teach the patient to assume responsibility for her or his own care can lead to later benefits.

Management of Contractures

Some individuals will present with hip or knee flexion contractures. Mild contractures may respond to manual mobilization and active exercises but it is almost impossible to reduce moderate to severe contractures by manual stretching, especially hip flexion contractures. Some practitioners advocate holding the extremity in a stretched position with weights for a considerable length of time. There is little evidence that this traditional approach is successful. Facilitated stretching techniques (PNF) are more effective than passive stretching; hold–relax and hold–relax active contraction that utilizes resisted contraction of antagonist muscles may increase ROM, particularly of the knee (see Chapter 13). One of the more effective ways of reducing a knee flexion contracture is to fit the patient with a patellar-tendon-bearing (PTB) prosthesis aligned in a manner that places the hamstrings on stretch with each step. Such prosthetic alignment provides an active stretch that is quite effective. Hip flexion contractures are more frequently found in persons with transfemoral amputations. It is difficult to 'walk out' a hip flexion contracture with the transfemoral prosthesis. In some instances, depending on the severity of the contracture and the length of the residual limb, the contracture can be accommodated in the alignment of the prosthesis. A knee flexion contracture of less than 15° is not usually a problem. Prevention, however, continues to be the best treatment for contractures.

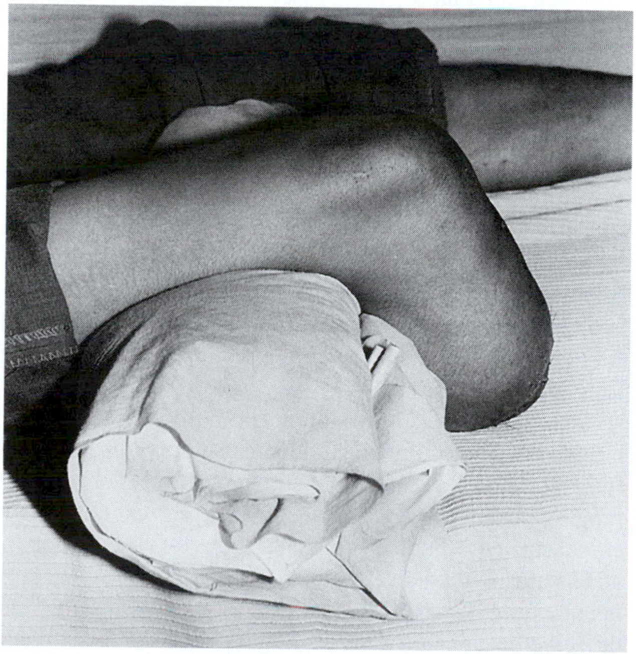

Figure 25.8 Improper positioning of residual limb on a pillow.

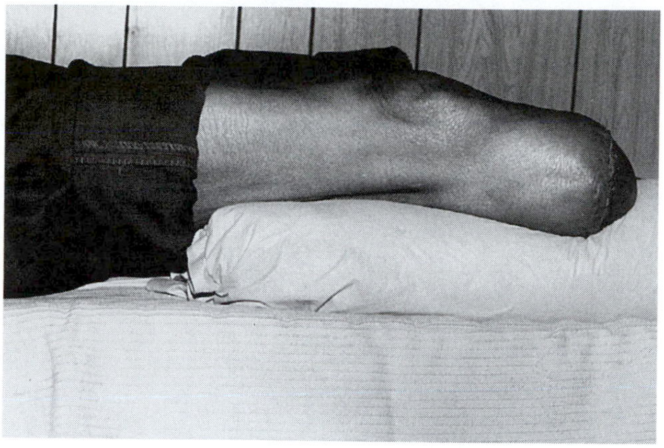

Figure 25.9 Improper positioning of residual limb on a pillow.

Therapeutic Exercise

The exercise program is individually designed and includes strengthening, balance, and coordination activities. The postsurgical dressing, degree of postoperative pain, and healing of the incision will determine when resistive exercises for the involved extremity can be started. The postoperative exercise program can take many forms and a home exercise program (HEP) is necessary. The hip extensors and abductors, and knee extensors and flexors are

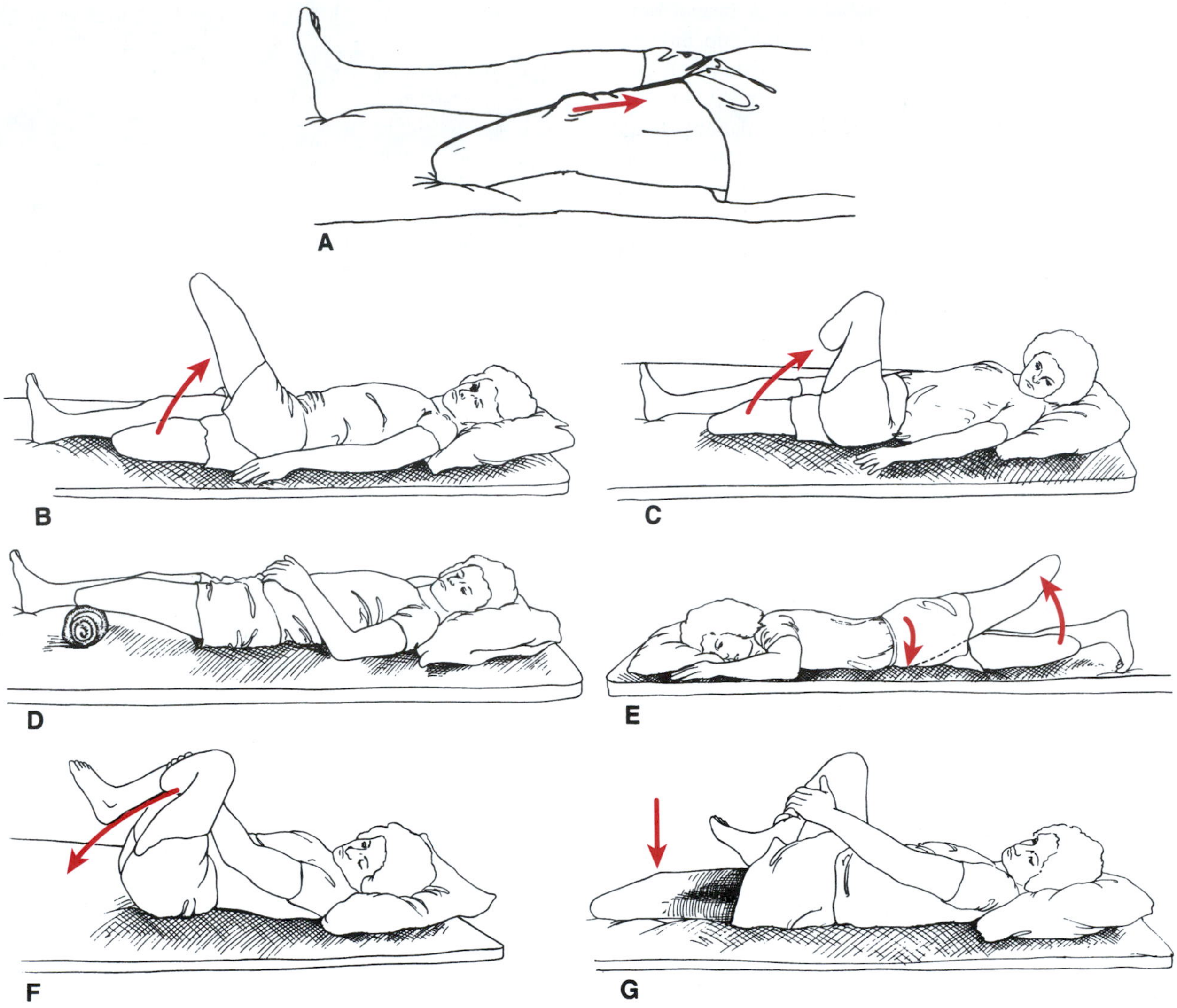

Figure 25.10 (*A–G*) Exercises for individuals with transtibial amputations to maintain or increase muscle strength and flexibility.

particularly important for prosthetic ambulation. Studies have shown a correlation between strength of the key muscle groups and ability to use a prosthesis effectively.[62–64] Figures 25.10 and 25.11 depict a series of exercises particularly well designed to strengthen key muscles around the hip and knee. These exercises can be adapted for a HEP because they are simple to perform and require no special equipment. Exercises need to be graded with increased resistance throughout the postsurgical period.

A general strengthening program that includes the trunk and all extremities is often indicated, particularly for the older person who may have been quite sedentary prior to surgery. Proprioceptive neuromuscular exercise routines are beneficial. The exercise program needs to be individually developed and emphasize those muscles that are most active in prosthetic function. Isometric exercises as depicted in Figures 25.10D and 25.11A may be contraindicated for some individuals with cardiac disease or hypertension. Both exercises can be modified by having the patient actually lift the buttocks off the treatment table in a modified bridging movement.

The younger, more active person with a traumatic amputation does not usually lose a great deal of muscle strength. Many older individuals, however, are relatively sedentary after surgery and need encouragement to develop good strength, coordination, and cardiopulmonary endurance for later ambulation.

Ideally, the exercise program should be sequenced for progressive motor control and increasing coordination and function as well as increased strength. The patient should progress from bed to mat activities using exercises that emphasize coordinated functional mobility. The postoperative status will be determined to a great extent by the preoperative activity level, length of time of disability, and other medical problems as well as the effects of the surgery itself. Because many patients are discharged from the

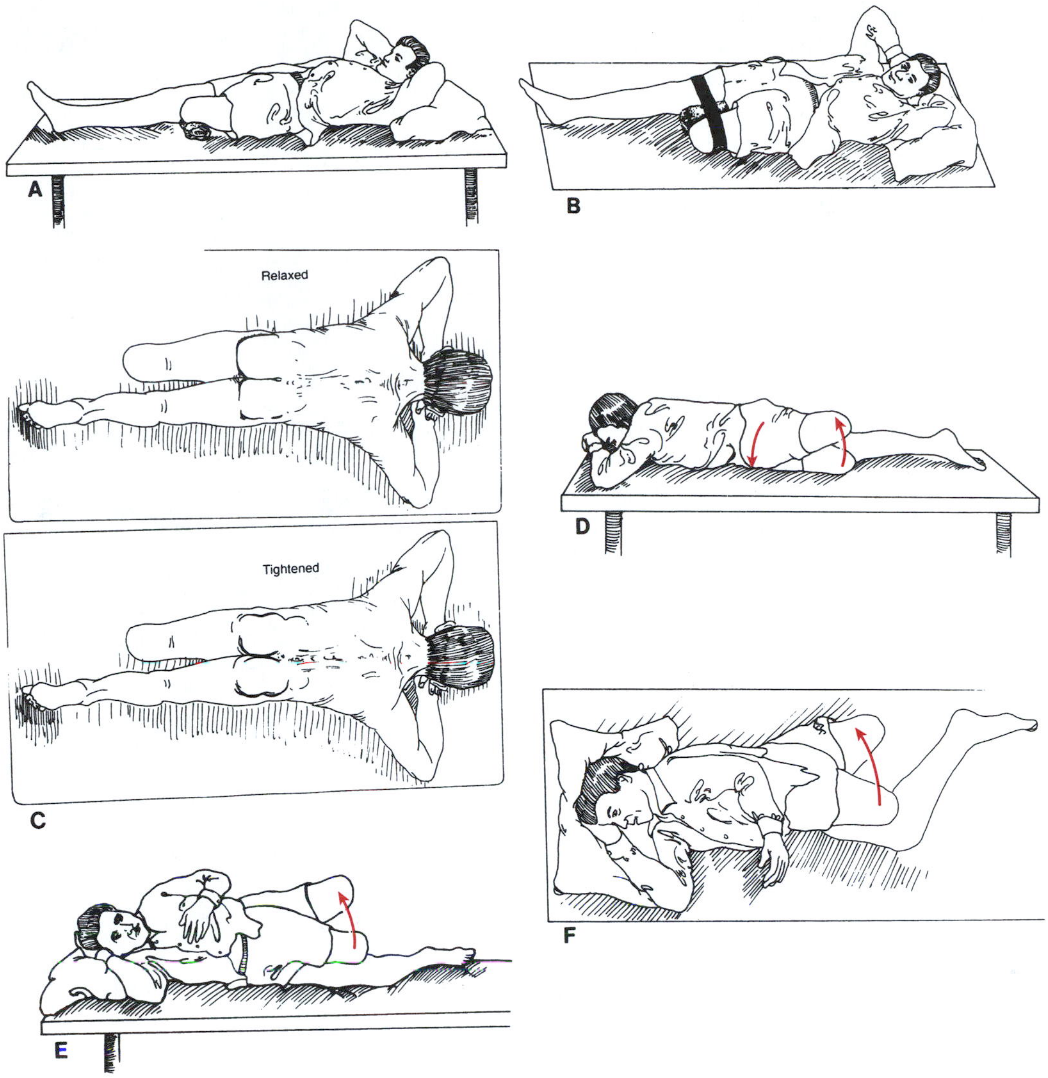

Figure 25.11 (*A–F*) Exercises for individuals with transfemoral amputations to maintain or increase muscle strength and flexibility.

hospital as early as a week after surgery, referral to a rehabilitation center or home health agency is important to provide the necessary continuity of care.

Early mobility is important to total physiological recovery. The patient needs to resume independent activities as soon as possible. Movement transitions (supine-to-sit, sit-to-stand) are preliminary to ambulation activities. Care must be taken during early bed and transfer movements to protect the residual limb from any trauma. The patient must be advised not to push on or slide the residual limb against the bed or chair. The patient also needs to be cautioned against spending too much time in any one position to prevent the development of joint contractures or skin breakdowns.

Most individuals with unilateral amputations have little difficulty adjusting to the change in balance that results from the loss of a limb. Sitting and standing balance activities are a useful part of the postsurgical program, particularly for the older adult who may be afraid of falling. Poor balance and fear of falling have been found to negatively impact successful prosthetic rehabilitation.[65,66] Upper extremity strengthening exercises with weights or elastic bands are important in preparation for crutch walking. Shoulder depression and elbow extension are particularly necessary to improve the ability to lift the body in ambulation. Individuals with bilateral amputations who have one healed residual limb will often use that limb as a prop for bed activities and transfers. Often a debilitated person with bilateral amputations who is unable to lift the body with the arms will be able to transfer when allowed to use the old prosthesis to push on.

Ambulation and Gait Training

Walking is an excellent exercise and necessary for independence in daily life. Gait training can start early in the postoperative phase, and the person with a unilateral LE amputation can become quite independent using a three-point gait pattern on crutches. Many older individuals have difficulty learning to walk on crutches. Some are afraid, some lack the necessary balance and coordination, and others lack endurance. Walking with crutches without a prosthesis requires a greater expenditure of energy than walking with a prosthesis.

Independence in crutch walking is an outcome worthy of considerable therapy time. The individual who can ambulate with crutches will develop a greater degree of general fitness than the person who spends most of the time in a wheelchair. Crutch walking is good preparation for prosthetic ambulation and the person who can learn to use crutches generally will not have difficulty learning to use a prosthesis. However, the individual who cannot learn to walk with crutches independently may still become a very functional prosthetic user. It may take considerable time for an older person to learn to use crutches, but the benefits are worth the efforts. Even if the individual can use crutches only in the sheltered environment of the home, such ambulation should be encouraged. An early graduated mobility program is also important for cardiovascular training and the development of endurance. Cardiovascular endurance is necessary for effective prosthetic ambulation, particularly at the transfemoral level.

There are advantages and disadvantages to using a walker for support during the postsurgical period. Certainly, walking with a walker is physiologically and psychologically more beneficial than sitting in a wheelchair, but it should be used only if the person cannot learn to walk with crutches. A walker is sturdier than crutches but cannot be used on stairs and curbs. It is sometimes difficult for the person who has used a walker during the postsurgical period to switch to crutches or a cane when fitted with a prosthesis, because the gait pattern used with a walker is not appropriate with a prosthesis. A walker encourages a step-to gait pattern whereas efficient prosthetic use requires a step-through gait pattern. A reciprocal walker is not safe during the postsurgical period when the individual is using a three-point gait pattern. All individuals with an amputation need to learn some form of mobility without a prosthesis for use at night or when the prosthesis is not worn for some reason.

Temporary Prostheses

Many individuals are not fitted with any type of prosthetic appliance until the residual limb is free from edema and much of the soft tissue has shrunk, a process that can take many months of conscientious limb wrapping and exercises. During this period, the patient is limited to a wheelchair or to ambulation with crutches or a walker. Most individuals cannot return to work or fully participate in ADL while waiting for the residual limb to mature. Once fitted with a definitive prosthesis, the residual limb continues to change in size and

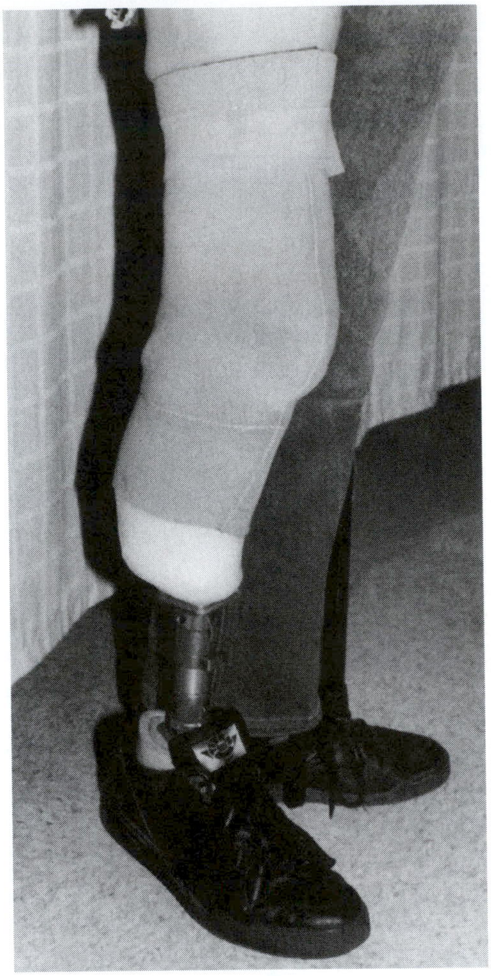

Figure 25.12 Transtibial temporary prosthesis.

a second prosthesis is often required within the first two years. Early fitting with a temporary prosthesis can greatly enhance the postsurgical rehabilitation program. A temporary prosthesis includes a socket designed and constructed according to regular prosthetic principles and attached to some form of pylon, a foot, and some type of suspension. Figures 25.12 and 25.13 depict two different temporary transtibial prostheses, both suspended by a sleeve. Figure 25.13 shows the socket itself with the sleeve removed. (See Chapter 32 for more details on prosthetic components.) Individuals fitted with a temporary prosthesis are taught to use the prosthesis correctly and, depending on physiological status, use little if any external support.

A temporary prosthesis can be fitted as soon as the wound has healed. There are many advantages to using a temporary prosthesis:

- It shrinks the residual limb more effectively than the elastic wrap.
- It allows early bipedal ambulation.
- Many older people can walk safely with a temporary prosthesis and a cane who otherwise would not be ambulatory during the postsurgical period.

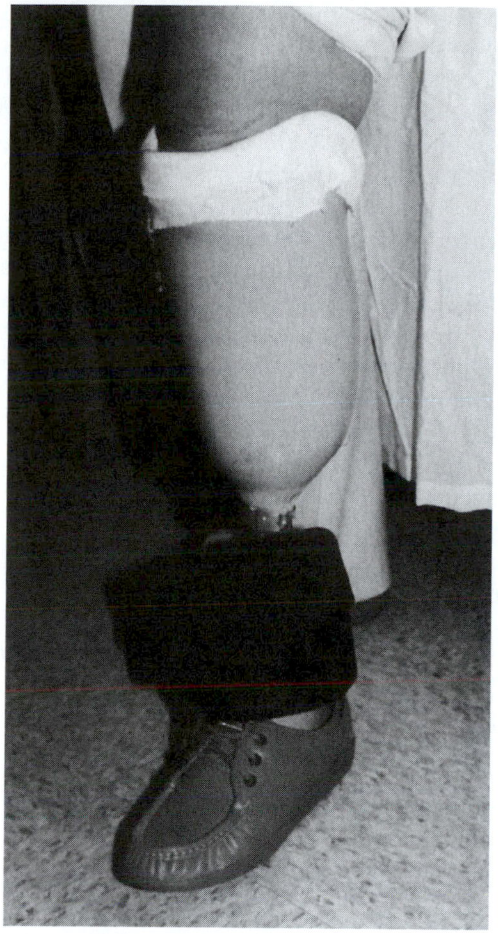

Figure 25.13 Transtibial temporary prosthesis with suspension sleeve lowered to show socket.

- Some individuals can return to work.
- It provides a means of evaluating the rehabilitation potential of individuals with a questionable prognosis.
- It is a positive motivating factor, providing a replacement for the missing part of the body.
- It reduces the need for a complex exercise program because many people can return to full active daily life.
- It can be used by individuals who may have difficulty obtaining payment for a definitive prosthesis.

Many temporary sockets today are made of lightweight thermoplastic materials that can be formed over a positive cast of the residual limb; some are constructed of a fiberglass material that can be formed directly over the residual limb. The prosthesis is usually suspended by a Neoprene sleeve. The prosthesis is worn with a wool sock of appropriate thickness; when the residual limb has shrunk so that three wool socks are needed to maintain socket fit, a new socket needs to be constructed. The temporary prosthesis is usually fabricated by a prosthetist but can be fabricated by a therapist, physician, or any individual who is skilled in the application of prosthetic principles and socket design and who has access to the appropriate materials. Prosthetic components such as feet of various sizes, suspension straps, knee joints, and pylons are now generally available. There are also adjustable temporary prostheses that adjust as the residual limb shrinks. While not fabricated for the individual person, they come in different sizes and the prosthetist can provide necessary adjustments to ensure proper fit. It is easier to fabricate a transtibial socket, but the use of a temporary prosthesis is very important in the rehabilitation of patients with transfemoral amputations.[67] The temporary transfemoral prosthesis should incorporate a well-designed socket, articulated knee joint, foot, and pylon. Suspension may be accomplished with Silesian bandage or pelvic band.

Patient Education

As you work with the patient, you are glad that you started teaching her about PVD and the care of her legs when you were initially treating her. If she is to return home from the hospital, she needs to learn and understand enough to be a partner in the rehabilitation process rather than a passive recipient of information. You know that teaching is not telling and that you have to devise ways to actively involve the patient in learning important concepts and activities. From experience you have learned that the better patients understand the care of their own bodies, the greater the adherence with home programs.

Patient education is an integral and ongoing part of the rehabilitation program. Information on the care of the residual limb, proper care of the uninvolved extremity, positioning, exercises, and diet, if the patient has diabetes, are necessary for the patient to be a full participant in the rehabilitation program.

Many individuals with vascular disease who lose one leg will be concerned about the other leg and receptive to learning proper care. An understanding of the physiological and functional implications of PVD helps the individual assume responsibility for care of the residual limb and remaining extremity. The education program must be individually designed to be relevant and may include:

- A discussion of the disease process, the physiological effects of the symptoms, and lifestyle changes to reduce risk factors
- Information on the benefits of exercises, LE cleanliness, proper foot care, and proper shoe fitting
- Methods of edema control
- The use of exercise to improve circulatory status

Edema, pain, and changes in skin color or temperature may indicate impending problems. If the person is ambulatory on the remaining extremity, the symptoms may reflect too much stress; if the person spends considerable time sitting with the leg in a dependent position, it may be necessary to elevate the extremity. Intermittent claudication (cramping of the calf) during activity indicates the need to stop at least temporarily. The collateral circulation of the remaining extremity is developed slowly through a progressive program of exercises and ambulation. It is important to remember that too much activity may be as harmful as too little.

Care must be taken not to overwhelm the patient with too much information at one time; information overload leads to forgetfulness. It is more effective to prioritize the information and ask the person to remember one new thing each session rather than try to teach a complex program at one time. Written materials are necessary to supplement the teaching and help the patient remember what is required. It is also important for the program to be tailored to the individual's way of life. Involving the patient in establishing priorities enhances adherence. Adherence also improves if the program meets the person's own desired outcomes. The same approach can be used for the HEP. Once the patient is discharged, either weekly clinic visits or home health supervision throughout the postsurgical phase provide a check on home activities, on the condition of the residual limb, and is supportive to the patient, family, and caregiver.

Bilateral Amputation

The postsurgical program for the person with bilateral LE amputations is similar to the program developed for someone with a unilateral amputation except possibly ambulation. If the individual was fitted and ambulated after unilateral amputation, the prosthesis is useful for transfer activities and limited ambulation in the home. Some individuals may be able to use the prosthesis with external support to get around the house more easily, particularly for bathroom activities. Fitting with a temporary prosthesis, as mentioned, is advisable, particularly if the amputations are at transtibial levels. The higher the initial level of amputation, the more difficult ambulation becomes.

All individuals with bilateral amputations need a wheelchair on a permanent basis. The chair should be as narrow as possible with removable desk arms and removable leg rests. Amputee wheelchairs with offset rear wheels and no leg rests are not recommended unless the therapist is sure that the person will never be fitted with prostheses, even cosmetically. It is easier to add anti-tipping devices to the rear of the wheelchair or attach small weights to the front uprights for use when the foot rests are removed.

The postsurgical program includes mat activities designed to help the person regain a sense of body position and balance, upper extremity and residual limb strengthening exercises, and regular ROM exercises. Functional mobility training should stress independence in bed mobility, transfers, and wheelchair use. With bilateral amputations, individuals spend considerable time sitting and are therefore more prone to develop flexion contractures, particularly around the hip joints. The patient should be encouraged to sleep prone if possible, or at least spend some time in the prone position each day. The therapy program also emphasizes ROM of the residual limbs. Some people move about their homes on their knees, or the buttocks. Knee pads made of heavy rubber used by field workers are effective protectors for the residual limbs. Protectors can also be fabricated of foam or felt.

Temporary prostheses are of great value in the rehabilitation of patients with bilateral transtibial amputations. Temporary prostheses are used to evaluate ambulation potential and as an aid to balance and transfer activities. If the individual was initially fitted following the first amputation, the temporary prosthesis will allow resumption of general mobility. The ambulatory potential of patients with bilateral transfemoral amputations is uncertain, particularly among older adults. Some individuals may be fitted with bilateral transfemoral temporary prostheses for use in cardiovascular training but continue to use a wheelchair for functional activities.

The person with bilateral transfemoral amputations can be fitted with shortened prosthesis called "*stubbies*" (Fig. 25.14). Stubby prostheses have regular sockets, no articulated knee joints or shank, and modified rocker bottoms turned backward to prevent the person from falling backward. Because the patient's center of gravity is much lower to the ground and the prostheses are nonarticulated, they are relatively easy to use. Stubbies allow the individual with bilateral transfemoral amputations to acquire erect balance and participate in ambulatory activities quickly and with only moderate expenditures of energy. Stubbies today usually incorporate the ischial containement socket and may be suspended by suction, a locking pin or custom canvas belt.

It is generally recommended that stubbies be only high enough to allow the person to work at a counter. If the center of gravity is raised too high the person will be unstable. Acceptance varies considerably; some people like to use stubbies for ADL in the home but rely on a

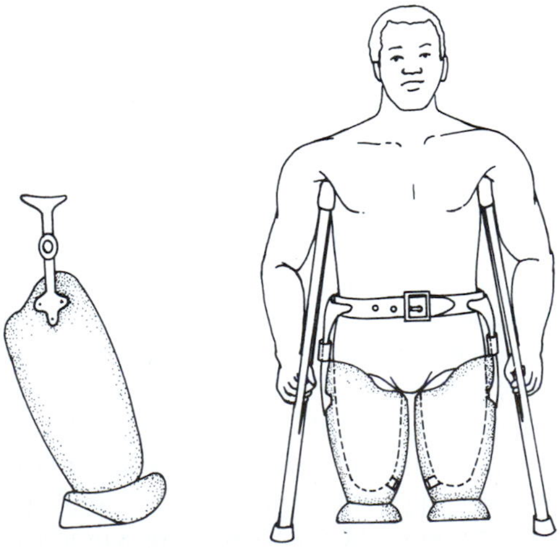

Figure 25.14 Stubbies (bilateral transfemoral amputations).

wheelchair outside the home. Although prescribed rather rarely, they are most effective for individuals with short residual limbs or who will not be able to ambulate with regular prostheses. Temporary prostheses of different heights can be used to determine ambulatory potential, but care must be taken to ensure that the temporary limbs are constructed well enough to tolerate the stresses generated in walking.

Determining Prosthetic Potential

A primary aim of the postsurgical period is to determine the individual's suitability for prosthetic replacement. Not all people with amputations are candidates for a prosthesis, regardless of personal desire. The cost of the prosthesis and the energy demands of prosthetic training require that the clinic team use some judgement in selecting individuals for fitting.

There is no general rule that can safely be applied to all patients in making the decision to fit or not to fit. The patient is part of the decision-making process but the fact that the individual wants a prosthesis is not enough. Many people are not aware of the physiological demands of prosthetic ambulation, particularly at transfemoral levels. The development of lightweight prostheses, stance control knees, hydraulic mechanisms, and energy conserving feet have made it possible to successfully fit many more individuals than in the past; however, some consideration for nonfitting is necessary.

Transtibial Levels

Most individuals amputated at any transtibial level can be successfully fitted with a prosthesis. Flexion contractures, scars, poorly shaped residual limbs, and adherent skin are not contraindications for fitting with today's prosthetic components. Circulatory problems in the nonamputated extremity, unless so severe as to preclude any ambulation, are indications for fitting at the earliest possible time because bipedal ambulation reduces stress on the remaining extremity. In addition, the individual who has learned to ambulate with one prosthesis is more likely to be able to ambulate with two. There are few contraindications to fitting someone with a transtibial amputation other than contraindications to ambulation itself. Individuals who were not ambulatory prior to surgery for reasons other than the problems leading to the amputation will probably not be ambulatory with an amputation. However, individuals who were nonambulatory and debilitated because of infection, lack of diabetic control, and ulcers will probably regain the necessary strength and coordination for ambulation after the diseased limb has been removed. Generally, individuals requiring nursing or custodial care will not be able to use a prosthesis; often equipment sent to a nursing home becomes lost and fitting such individuals may be an inappropriate use of limited resources.

Transfemoral Levels

Many patients can become relatively functional prosthetic users with or without external support. The physiological demands of walking with a transfemoral prosthesis are considerably higher than walking with a transtibial prosthesis and not all individuals have the necessary balance, strength, and energy reserves.[66] Severe hip flexion contractures, obesity, weakness or paralysis of hip musculature, and poor balance and coordination may impede successful ambulation. The person's level of activity and participation in the postsurgical program helps in determining potential for prosthetic ambulation. A temporary prosthesis is a good examination tool.

Most individuals amputated at hip levels are younger and learn to use a prosthesis relatively easily. Although early fitting is physically and psychologically beneficial, active involvement in chemotherapy or radiation therapy may delay fitting. Radiation therapy often burns the skin making fitting impossible until the skin has healed. Patients undergoing chemotherapy may be ill, lose weight, and may not have the energy to participate in a prosthetic training program. The postsurgical program is individually adjusted and supportive until the therapy is complete. If the person has lost considerable weight, fitting may have to be delayed because it is difficult to adjust a prosthesis for increases in weight. Decisions must be individualized and determined by the individual's physical and psychological status.

Bilateral Amputations

Fitting or not fitting someone with bilateral amputations is a difficult decision. Young, agile individuals are generally good candidates for prosthetic fitting regardless of level of amputations. Most patients with bilateral transtibial amputations can become quite functional with prostheses. Most older individuals with bilateral transfemoral amputations have considerable difficulty learning to use two prostheses. Patients with one transfemoral and one transtibial amputation generally can learn to use two prosthesis if the first amputation was at the transfemoral level, and if the person successfully used a transfemoral prosthesis before losing the other leg.

The person who has lost portions of both LEs needs more strength, better coordination, better balance, and greater cardiorespiratory reserves than the person who has lost a portion of one LE. Obesity makes fitting of bilateral prostheses more difficult. The decision to fit or not to fit is made after careful, individual evaluation of the person's total potential and needs. Modern prostheses—lightweight, closer fitting, and with more functional components—have enhanced the rehabilitation potential of individuals with bilateral amputations. The advent of computerized knee components have greatly reduced the energy requirements for ambulation with bilateral transfemoral amputations. However, energy requirements are still quite high and even younger individuals with bilateral transfemoral amputations may need to use a wheelchair some of the time.

Individuals who are not fitted with a prosthesis need to become as independent as possible in a wheelchair. The therapy program includes training in all transfers, wheelchair mobility, and ADL. The program emphasizes sitting balance, moving safely in and out of the wheelchair, and other activities to support as independent a lifestyle as the person's physical and psychological condition allows. Education in the proper care of the residual limb is also important, although wrapping the residual limb may no longer necessary unless the person is more comfortable with the limb covered.

Summary

Most individuals with LE amputations can be helped to return to a full and useful life following the loss of a limb. A program of postoperative care that includes consideration of physical and emotional needs will enable most patients to become functional prosthetic users. Many prosthetic problems can be avoided by properly preparing the individual for prosthetic wear. In this chapter, concepts related to the postoperative management of the individual with a LE amputation have been presented. Through a process of careful evaluation and open communication, a comprehensive program designed to meet the needs of an individual patient can be achieved. The individuality of each person presenting for rehabilitation is one of the challenges of physical therapy practice.

Questions for Review

1. Discuss the advantages and disadvantages of the following methods of postsurgical residual limb management: (a) rigid dressing; (b) AirLimb®; and (c) soft dressing.
2. Discuss the proper method of wrapping the transtibial and the transfemoral residual limb.
3. A 72-year-old man with a history of diabetes, cardiovascular disease, and PVD has been referred for physical therapy 24 hours post right transtibial amputation for gangrene. What examination data are needed to plan an appropriate treatment program? Which are the most critical to obtain on the first visit?
4. Design an exercise program for an 82-year-old individual with a left transfemoral amputation who is referred 2 weeks after amputation.
5. Discuss the advantages and disadvantages of teaching an older person to walk with crutches versus walking with a walker following a unilateral amputation.
6. Which postsurgical activities are more important with bilateral amputations as compared to unilateral amputations? How might you teach these activities?

Case Study

REFERRAL

The patient is a 72-year-old female status post right transtibial amputation yesterday secondary to arteriosclerotic gangrene.

CURRENT MEDICAL HISTORY

Diabetes type 2 since age 48 controlled by insulin 20 units bid. Arteriosclerosis; hypertension controlled by medication; treated for ulcer plantar surface of right first metatarsal area for past 3 months. Ulcer did not heal leading to amputation.

PAST MEDICAL HISTORY

Hysterectomy at age 42, otherwise unremarkable.

SOCIAL HISTORY

Widow who lives alone. Three grown children and six grandchildren in the area.

PHYSICAL THERAPY EXAMINATION (INITIAL)

Chart Review

Patient alert and awake in no apparent distress. Right residual limb wrapped in soft gauze dressing covered with an elastic wrap. Drain in place. Incision clean on dressing change.

BP: 142/70, pulse 66, respiration normal.

Respiratory care practitioner reports patient using spirometer properly, normal cough, no evidence of respiratory problems.

Patient c/o of some pain in residual limb; pain medication given.

Patient has been sitting at the side of the bed twice/day.

Examination Data

Gross muscle strength of left lower extremity and both upper extremities grossly within functional limits (WFL). Muscle strength of right hip flexion, abduction and adduction grossly WFL; hip extension tested sidelying and graded a 3+/5 (Fair +). Demonstrates active motion of right knee flexion and extension with no resistance given at this time.

Residual limb measurements deferred until initial healing has taken place.

Gross range of motion of left lower extremity and both upper extremities WFL. Left hip extension measurements deferred until patient can lie prone or on right side. Gross range of motion of the right hip WFLs except hip extension to 0° measured sidelying. Right knee flexion and extension grossly functional. Specific measurement deferred until dressing can be removed.

Left lower extremity is hairless below the ankle. Skin is warm to touch. Popliteal pulse palpable but not dorsalis pedis pulse. Toes are warm to touch. Proprioceptive sensation intact. Diminished sensation over plantar surface of left foot and dorsum of first metatarsal. No evidence of edema in left lower extremity. Sensation testing of right residual limb deferred secondary to dressing.

FUNCTIONAL STATUS

Bed Mobility

Rolling to left: independent; rolling to right and prone: not tested.

Supine-to-sit and return: modified independent (requires use of "rope ladder" attached to foot of bed).

Transfers

Sit-to-stand with walker: moderate assistance.

Stand-to-sit in chair or bed: moderate assistance.

Locomotion

Ambulation with walker: moderate assistance for 5 feet.

Expected outcomes of physical therapy episode of care (achieved prior to discharge from hospital).

1. The patient will be independent in all transfers.
2. The patient will be independent in ambulation with crutches or walker for 40 feet.
3. The patient will demonstrate knowledge of proper residual limb positioning, bandaging, and care.
4. The patient will demonstrate knowledge of basic residual limb exercises.
5. The patient will demonstrate knowledge of proper care of the left lower extremity.

Upon discharge from the hospital, the patient was referred to home care physical therapy. Examination data obtained following discharge from hospital by home care physical therapist:

Residual limb: Sutures in place, incision healing well, no drainage; length 13.6 cm (5.4 in.) from medial tibial plateau (MTP).

Circumferential measurements from MTP

5 cm (2 in) below MTP = 35 cm (14 in.)
10 cm (4 in.) below MTP = 38 cm (15 in.)
12 cm (5 in.) below MTP = 37 cm (14.5 in.)

Sensation intact.

ROM right knee: WNL.

ROM right hip: extension to 0° (all other motions WNL).

Expected outcomes for physical therapy episode of care during initial postsurgical home care intervention:

1. The patient will be independent in care of residual limb including bandaging or using shrinker.
2. The patient will be independent in crutch (or walker) ambulation within home environment.
3. The patient will be independence in home exercise program (HEP).

GUIDING QUESTIONS

1. The patient's residual limb was wrapped in a soft dressing after amputation. Compare the advantages and disadvantages of the rigid dressing, the semirigid dressing, and soft dressings. What problems might the patient incur with a soft dressing?
2. Review the examination data given for the patient. What data would be important to obtain on the first postoperative visit and what can be deferred? What other data would you obtain and when?
3. Describe your initial treatment program for the patient.
4. What would be the focus of follow-up care after discharge?

References

1. Levy, LA: Smoking and peripheral vascular disease. Clin Podiatr Med Surg 9:165, 1992.
2. Ritz, G, et al: Diabetes and peripheral vascular disease. Clin Podiatr Med Surg 9:125, 1992.
3. McCollum, PT, and Walker, MA: Major limb amputation for end-stage peripheral vascular disease: Level selection and alternative options. In Bowker, JH, and Michael, JW (eds): Atlas of Limb Prosthetics: Surgical, Prosthetic and Rehabilitation Principles, ed 2. Mosby-Year Book, St. Louis, 1992, p 25.
4. Quigley, FG, et al: Impact of femoro-distal bypass on major lower limb amputation rate. Aust N Z J Surg 68:35, 1998.
5. Hallett, JW Jr., et al: Impact of arterial surgery and balloon angioplasty on amputation: A population based study of 1155 procedures between 1973 and 1992. J Vasc Surg 25:29, 1997.
6. Cuson, TM, and Bongiorni, DR: Rehabilitation of the older lower limb amputee: A brief review. J Am Geriatr Soc 44:1388, 1996.
7. Yeager, RA, et al: Surgical management of severe acute lower extremity ischemia. J Vasc Surg 15:385, 1992.
8. Feinglass, J, et al: Peripheral bypass surgery and amputation. Northern Illinois demographics 1993–1997. Arch Surg 135:75, 2000.
9. Edelman, D, et al: Prognostic value of the clinical examination of the diabetic foot ulcer. J Gen Intern Med 12:537, 1997.
10. Moss, SE, et al: The prevalence and incidence of lower extremity amputation in a diabetic population. Arch Intern Med 152:610, 1992.
11. Knighton, DR, et al: Amputation prevention in an independently reviewed at-risk diabetic population using a comprehensive wound care protocol. Am J Surg 160:466, 1990.
12. Krajewski, LP, and Olin, JW: Atherosclerosis of the aorta and lower extremities arteries. In Young, JR, et al (eds): Peripheral Vascular Diseases. Mosby-Year Book, St. Louis, 1991, p 179.
13. Harris, KA, et al: Rehabilitation potential of elderly patients with major amputations. J Cardiovasc Surg (Torino) 32:463, 1991.
14. Ebskov, LB: Relative mortality in lower limb amputees with diabetes mellitus. Prosthet Orthot Int 20:147, 1996.
15. Fletcher, DD, et al: Trends in rehabilitation after amputation for geriatric patients with vascular disease: Implications for future health resource allocation. Arch Phys Med Rehabil 83:1389, 2002.
16. Dillingham, TR, Pezzin, LE, and MacKenzie, EJ: Racial differences in the incidence of limb loss secondary to peripheral vascular disease: A population based study. Arch Phys Med Rehabil 83:1252, 2002.
17. Kay, HW, and Newman, JD: Relative incidence of new amputations: Statistical comparisons of 6,000 new amputees. Prosthet Orthot Int 29:3, 1975.
18. Nagarajan, R, et al: Limb salvage and amputation in survivors of pediatric lower-extremity bone tumors: What are the long-term implications? J Clin Oncol 20:4493, 2002.
19. Stojadinovic, A, et al: Amputation for recurrent soft tissue sarcoma of the extremity: Indications and outcome. Ann Surg Oncol 8:509, 2001.
20. Link, MP, et al: Adjuvant chemotherapy of high-grade osteosarcoma of the extremity. Clin Orthop 270:8, 1991.
21. Simon, M: Limb salvage for osteosarcoma in the 1980s. Clin Orthop 270:264, 1990.
22. Springfield, DS: Introduction to limb-salvage surgery for sarcomas. Orthop Clin North Am 22:1, 1991.
23. Yaw, KM, and Wurtz, LD: Resection and reconstruction for bone tumors in the proximal tibia. Orthop Clin North Am 22:133, 1991.
24. Waters, RL, et al: Energy cost of walking of amputees: The influence of level of amputation. J Bone Joint Surg 58A:42, 1976.
25. Steinberg, FU, et al: Prosthetic rehabilitation of geriatric amputee patients: A follow-up study. Arch Phys Med Rehabil 66:742, 1985.
26. Johnson, WC, et al: Transcutaneous partial oxygen pressure changes following skew flap and Burgess-type below-knee amputation. Arch Surg 132:261, 1997.
27. Allock, PJ, and Jain, AS: Revisiting transtibial amputation with the long posterior flap. Br J Surg, 88:683, 2001.
28. Robinson, KP. Skew-flap below-knee amputation. Ann R Coll Surg Engl 73:155, 1991.
29. Ruckley CV, Stonebridge PA, and Prescott RJ: Skewflap versus long posterior flap in below-knee amputations: Multicenter trial. J Vasc Surg 13:423, 1991.
30. Moore, TJ: Planning for optimal function in amputation surgery. In Bowker, JH, and Michael, JW (eds): Atlas of Limb Prosthetics: Surgical, Prosthetic and Rehabilitation Principles, ed 2. Mosby-Year Book, St. Louis, 1992, p 59.
31. Michaels, JA: The selection of amputation level: An approach using decision analysis. Eur J Vasc Surg 5:451, 1991.
32. Sarin, S, et al: Selection of amputation levels: A review. Eur J Vasc Surg 5:611, 1991.
33. Spence, VA, et al: Assessment of tissue viability in relation to selection of amputation level. Prosth Orthot Int 8:67, 1984.
34. Lind, J, et al: The influence of smoking on complications after primary amputations of the lower extremity. Clin Orthop 267:211, 1991.
35. Evans, WE, et al: Effect of a failed distal reconstruction on the level of amputation. Am J Surg 160:217, 1990.
36. Dormandy, J, et al: Prospective study of 713 below-knee amputations for ischaemia and the effects of a prostacyclin analogue on healing. Br J Surg 81:333, 1994.
37. Dormandy, J, et al: Major amputations: Clinical patterns and predictors (review). Semin Vasc Surg 12:154, 1999.
38. May, BJ: Amputations and Prosthetics: A Case Study Approach, ed 2. FA Davis, Philadelphia, 2002.
39. May, BJ: A statewide amputee rehabilitation programme. Prosthet Orthot Int 2:24, 1978.
40. May, BJ: The prosthetist and the physical therapist: A clinical team. O & P Business News, 11:90, 2002.
41. Burgess, EM: Amputations of the lower extremities. In Nickel, VL (ed): Orthopedic Rehabilitation. Churchill-Livingston, New York, 1982, p 377.
42. Sarmiento, A, et al: Lower-extremity amputation: The impact of immediate postsurgical prosthetic fitting. Clin Orthop 68:22, 1967.
43. Harrington, IJ, et al: A plaster-pylon technique for below-knee amputation. J Bone Joint Surg (Br) 73:76, 1991.
44. Schon, LC, and Short, KW: Benefits of early prosthetic management of transtibial amputees: A prospective clinical study of the Air-Limb™. Journal of Proceedings: AOPA Scientific Sessions, 2000.
45. Vigier, S, et al: Healing of open stump wounds after vascular below-knee amputation: Plaster cast socket with silicone sleeve versus elastic compression. Arch Phys Med Rehabil 80(10):1327, 1999.
46. Goldberg, T, Goldberg, S, and Pollak, J: Postoperative management of lower extremity amputation. Phys Med Rehabil Clin North Am 11:559, 2000.
47. Gendron, B, and Andrews, KL: The use of rigid removable dressings for juvenile amputees: A case report. JACPOC 26(1):4, 1991.
48. Wong, CK, and Edelstein, JE: Unna and elastic post operative dressings: Comparisons of their effect on function of adults with amputations and vascular disease. Arch Phys Med Rehabil 81:1191, 2000.
49. Ehde, DM, et al: Chronic phantom sensations, phantom pain, residual limb pain and other regional pain after lower limb amputation. Arch Phys Med Rehabil 81:1039, 2000.
50. Flor, H: Phantom-limb pain: Characteristics, causes and treatments. Neurology 1:182, 2002.
51. Melzack, R, et al: Central neuroplasticity and pathological pain. Ann NY Acad Sci 933:157, 2001.
52. Oakley, DA, Whitman, LG, and Halligan, PW: Hypnotic imagery as a treatment for phantom limb pain: Two case reports and a review. Clin Rehabil 16:368, 2002.
53. Halbert, J, Crotty, M, and Cameron, ID: Evidence for the optimal management of acute and chronic phantom pain: A systematic review. Clin J Pain 18:84, 2002.
54. Bloomquist, T: Amputation and phantom limb pain: A pain-prevention model. AANA J 69:211, 2001.
55. Belleggia, G, and Birbaumer, N: Treatment of phantom limb pain with combined EMG and thermal biofeedback: A case report. Appl Psychophysiol Biofeedback 26:141, 2001.
56. Flor, H, et al: Effect of sensory discrimination training on cortical reorganisation and phantom limb pain. Lancet 357:1763, 2001.
57. Danshaw, CB: An anesthetic approach to amputation and pain syndromes. Phys Med Rehabil Clin North Am 11:553, 2000.

58. Halbert, J, Crotty, M, and Cameron, ID: Evidence for the optimal management of acute and chronic phantom pain: A systematic review. Clin J Pain 18(2):84, 2002.
59. Price, EM, and Fisher, K: How does counseling help people with amputation? JPO 14:102, 2002.
60. Fisher, K, and Price, EM: The use of a standard measure of emotional distress to evaluate early counseling intervention in patients with amputations. JPO 15:31, 2003.
61. May, BJ: Stump bandaging of the lower extremity amputee. Phys Ther 44:808, 1964.
62. Nadollek, H, Brauer, S, and Isles, R: Outcomes after trans-tibial amputation: The relationship between quiet stance ability, strength of hip abductor muscles and gait. Physiother Res Int 7:203, 2002.
63. Moirenfeld, I, et al: Isokinetic strength and endurance of the knee extensors and flexors in trans-tibial amputees. Prosthet Orthot Int 24:221, 2000.
64. Powers, CM, et al: The influence of lower-extremity muscle force on gait characteristics in individuals with below-knee amputations secondary to vascular disease. Phys Ther 76:369, 1996.
65. Miller, WC, Speechley, M, and Deathe, AB: Balance confidence among people with lower-limb amputations. Phys Ther 82:856, 2002.
66. Miller, WC, et al: The influence of falling, fear of falling, and balance confidence on prosthetic mobility and social activity among individuals with a lower extremity amputation. Arch Phys Med Rehabil 82:1238, 2001.
67. Parry, M, and Morrison, JD: Use of the Femurett adjustable prosthesis in the assessment and walking training of new above-knee amputees. Prosthet Orthot Int 13:36, 1989.
68. Perry, J: Gait analysis: Normal and pathological function. Slack, Thorofare, NJ, 1992.

Supplemental Readings

Aronow, WS: Management of peripheral arterial disease of the lower extremities in elderly patients. J Gerontol A Biol Sci Med Sci. 59:172, 2004.

Bruins, M, et al: Vocational reintegration after a lower limb amputation: A qualitative study. Prosthet Orthot Int 27:4, 2003.

Bussmann, JB, Grootscholten, EA, and Stam, HJ: Daily physical activity and heart rate response in people with a unilateral transtibial amputation for vascular disease. Arch Phys Med Rehabil. 85:240, 2004.

Callaghan, BG, and Condie, ME: A post-discharge quality of life outcome measure for lower limb amputees: Test-retest reliability and construct validity. Clin Rehabil 17:858, 2003.

Condie, E, et al: Slow rehabilitation of a traumatic lower limb amputee. Physiother Res Int 3:233, 1998.

Davis, BL, et al: Lower-extremity amputations in patients with diabetes: Pre- and post-surgical decisions related to successful rehabilitation. Diabetes Metab Res Rev 20 (Suppl 1):S45–50, 2004.

Dillingham, TR, Pezzin, LE, and Mackenzie, EJ: Discharge destination after dysvascular lower-limb amputations. Arch Phys Med Rehabil 84:1662, 2003.

Eskelinen, E, et al: Lower limb amputations in Southern Finland in 2000 and trends up to 2001. Eur J Vasc Endovasc Surg 27:193, 2004.

Gallagher, P, and Maclachlan, M: The trinity amputation and prosthesis experience scales and quality of life in people with lower-limb amputation. Arch Phys Med Rehabil. 85:730, 2004.

Kennedy, MJ: Am I better off with out it? A case study of a patient having a trans-tibial amputation after 52 years of chronic lower limb ulceration and pain. Prosthet Orthot Int 21:187, 1997.

Kern, U, et al: Effects of botulinum toxin type B on stump pain and involuntary movements of the stump. Am J Phys Med Rehabil. 83:396, 2004.

Lin, CC, et al: Effects of liner stiffness for trans-tibial prosthesis: A finite element contact model. Med Eng Phys 26:1, 2004.

Middleton, C. The causes and treatments of phantom limb pain. Nurs Times 99:30, 2003.

Nehler, MR, et al:: Functional outcome in a contemporary series of major lower extremity amputations. J Vasc Surg 38:7, 2003.

Payne MW, and Marks MB. Transtibial amputation management. J Rehabil Res Dev 40:xvi–xvii, 2003.

Paysant, J, et al: Transcranial magnetic stimulation for diagnosis of residual limb neuromas. Arch Phys Med Rehabil 85:737, 2004.

Pinzur, MS, and Angelico, J: A feasibility trial of a prefabricated immediate postoperative prosthetic limb system. Foot Ankle Int 24:861, 2003.

Pinzur, MS, et al: Functional outcome of below-knee amputation in peripheral vascular insufficiency. A multicenter review. Clin Orthop 286:247, 2003.

Sathishkumar, S, et al: A cost-effective, adjustable, femoral socket, temporary prosthesis for immediate rehabilitation of above-knee amputation. Int J Rehabil Res. 27:71, 2004.

Schoppen, T, et al: Physical, mental, and social predictors of functional outcome in unilateral lower-limb amputees. Arch Phys Med Rehabil 84:803, 2003.

Smith, DG, et al: Postoperative dressing and management strategies for transtibial amputations: A critical review. J Rehabil Res Dev 40:213, 2003.

Stapanavatr, W, Ungkittpaiboon, W, and Karnjanabatr, B: Conservative regimen for chronic critical limb ischemia. J Med Assoc Thai 87:310, 2004.

Tuel, SM, et al: Interdisciplinary management of hemicorporectomy after spinal cord injury. Arch Phys Med Rehabil 73:669, 1992.

Whyte, A, and Carroll, LJ: The relationship between catastrophizing and disability in amputees experiencing phantom pain. Disabil Rehabil. 26:649, 2004.

Woodburn, KR, et al; Scottish Vascular Audit Group; and Scottish Physiotherapy Amputee Research Group: A randomised trial of rigid stump dressing following trans-tibial amputation for peripheral arterial insufficiency. Prosthet Orthot Int 28:22, 2004.

Yetzer, EA. Incorporating foot care education into diabetic foot screening. Rehabil Nurs 29:80, 2004.

CHAPTER

26

LEARNING OBJECTIVES

1. Describe the epidemiology, pathology, pathogenesis, disease course, and common clinical manifestations of arthritis.
2. Identify the medical diagnostic procedures commonly used in the examination of patients with arthritis, including laboratory tests and radiography.
3. Describe the medical management of the individual with arthritis.
4. Differentiate between rheumatoid arthritis and osteoarthritis.
5. Identify the tests and measures commonly used in examining the individual with rheumatoid arthritis or osteoarthritis.
6. Discuss the rehabilitation management of the individual with arthritis.
7. Describe responses to psychosocial factors associated with arthritis that affect achievement of anticipated goals and expected outcomes.
8. Explain the importance of a team approach for the individual with arthritis.
9. Analyze and interpret patient data, formulate realistic goals and outcomes, and develop a plan of care when presented with a clinical case study.

Arthritis

Andrew A. Guccione, DPT, PhD, FAPTA
Marian A. Minor, PT, PhD

OUTLINE

The terms "arthritis," "rheumatism," and "rheumatoid disease" are generic references to an array of more than 100 diseases that are divided into 10 classification categories. Two major forms of arthritis are considered in this chapter. **Rheumatoid arthritis (RA)**, a systemic inflammatory disease, is considered in detail; **osteoarthritis (OA)**, a localized process that has been known in the past as **degenerative joint disease (DJD)**, is also discussed. Taken together, these two forms of arthritis account for most of the cases of arthritis that a physical therapist is likely to encounter in clinical practice.

Rheumatoid Arthritis

RA is a major subclassification within the category of diffuse connective tissue diseases that also includes juvenile arthritis, systemic lupus erythematosus (SLE), progressive systemic sclerosis or scleroderma, polymyositis, and dermatomyositis. The first clinical description of the disease is attributed to A.J. Landre-Beauvais in 1800, although analysis of pictorial art of the late Renaissance has provided some evidence for the existence of RA in earlier times. Early descriptive comparisons of patient symptomatology were complicated by the lack of uniform agreement about the distinguishing characteristics of the disease, a difficulty that persists even today given the wide spectrum of clinical presentations associated with this disease. Although the term "rheumatoid arthritis" was first used by Garrod in 1858, it was not accepted by the American Rheumatism Association (ARA) as the official terminology until 1941. The American College of Rheumatology (ACR), formerly the ARA, has revised the diagnostic terminology and criteria for RA several times in the last 45 years and continues to monitor them for accuracy and validity.[1]

Classification Criteria

Clinically, the differential diagnosis of RA is predicated upon the patient's signs and symptoms and careful exclusion of other disorders. When conducting epidemiological and other kinds of research studies, it is often necessary to identify homogeneous groups of individuals with relatively similar signs and symptoms of RA given the wide spectrum of clinical presentations seen in this disease. Although other sets of criteria have existed for this purpose, the ACR classification criteria are most often used to determine whether an individual's clinical presentation should be counted as a case of RA. For most of the 20th century, criteria had allowed four classifications of RA: classical, definite, probable, and possible. The latter two designations were eventually judged to be problematic because many patients with probable or possible RA often were discovered to have a different disease when reexamined at a later time. Therefore, new criteria were tested and established in 1987 based on a combination of signs, symptoms, and laboratory findings that have persisted for a specified period of time (Table 26.1).[2] A diagnosis of RA is now established upon the presentation of four of the seven listed criteria. The joint signs and symptoms described in criteria one through four must have lasted for at least 6 weeks.[1,2]

Epidemiology

The "type" of RA a person had at the time the epidemiological survey was conducted, as well as the criteria used, can complicate the calculation of prevalence rates. It has been estimated that the prevalence rate of definite RA among adults in the United States is approximately 10 cases per 1000 people, or approximately 2.1 million persons.[3] RA affects women two to four times more often than men at all ages.[4] There is a general increase in prevalence for both sexes with increasing age. Although RA is found around the world, there are some differences in the prevalence of RA in certain subpopulations, which suggests a possible role for genetic or environmental factors in the etiology of the disease. For example, black Americans may have a lower prevalence of RA than whites, whereas several Native American groups demonstrate higher prevalence rates. There also is a lower prevalence of RA in native Japanese and native Chinese peoples compared to whites.[1,3,5]

Etiology

Like many other chronic diseases, the etiology of RA is unknown. Current research into the causes of RA is based on a complex, but as yet incomplete, appreciation of the functions of the immune system. Briefly, an **antigen** is a substance, usually foreign to the host, which provokes the immune system into action. The immune system may respond to the antigen directly (cellular immunity) or by the production of **antibodies** that circulate in the serum (humoral immunity). These responses involve two general kinds of lymphocytes: T cells, which are responsible for cellular immunity, and B cells, which produce circulating antibodies specific to the antigen. Antibodies are immunoglobulins, a type of serum protein.[1]

Based on the fact that individuals with RA produce antibodies to their own immunoglobulins, there is some reason to

Table 26.1 The 1987 Revised Criteria For the Classification of Rheumatoid Arthritis[a]

Criterion	Definition
1. Morning stiffness	Morning stiffness in and around the joints, lasting at least one hour before maximal improvement.
2. Arthritis of three or more joint areas	At least three joint areas simultaneously have had soft tissue swelling or fluid (not bony overgrowth alone) observed by a physician. The 14 possible areas are right or left PIP, MCP, wrist, elbow, knee, ankle, and MTP joints.
3. Arthritis of hand joints	At least one area swollen (as defined above) in a wrist, MCP, or PIP joint.
4. Symmetric arthritis	Simultaneous involvement of the same joint areas (as defined in 2) on both sides of the body (bilateral involvement of PIPs, MCPs, or MTPs is acceptable without absolute symmetry).
5. Rheumatoid nodules	Subcutaneous nodules, over bony prominences, or extensor surfaces, or in juxtaarticular regions, observed by a physician.
6. Serum rheumatoid factor	Demonstration of abnormal amounts of serum rheumatoid factor by any method for which the result has been positive in <5% of normal control subjects.
7. Radiographic changes	Radiographic changes typical of rheumatoid arthritis on posteroanterior hand and wrist radiographs, which must include erosions or unequivocal bony decalcification localized in or most marked adjacent to the involved joints (osteoarthritis changes alone do not qualify).

From Arnett, FC,[2] p 319 with permission.

[a]For classification purposes, a patient shall be said to have rheumatoid arthritis if he or she has satisfied at least four of these seven criteria. Criteria 1 through 4 must have been present for at least 6 weeks. Patients with two clinical diagnoses are not excluded. Designation as classic, definite, or probable rheumatoid arthritis is *not* to be made.

believe that RA is an *autoimmune* disorder. It is not clear, however, whether this antibody production is a primary event or results as a response to a specific antigen from an external stimulus. Current theory and research on the cellular basis of autoimmunity suggest that aberrant functioning of cell-mediated immunity and defective T lymphocytes may trigger the autoimmune response that underlies RA.[6,7] A specific etiological agent for RA has not been identified, even though investigators have been able to identify that specific external etiological agents may produce an inflammatory arthritis, for example, **Lyme disease**. The disease that is finally manifested may be more dependent on the host's manner of response than on the agent or the mechanism involved.

Evidence suggests that a variety of agents may initiate arthritis through a number of different mechanisms. A number of bacterial organisms have been suggested, including streptococcus, clostridia, diphtheroids, and mycoplasmas, but no connections have been definitively proven. There has also been discussion of a viral etiology for RA. As with other investigations that seek to identify an etiology for RA, research in this area remains speculative.[1]

Rheumatoid factors (RF) have received considerable attention in the search for a causative agent in RA because they are found in the sera of approximately 70 percent of all patients with RA. RF are antibodies specific to IgG. Current theory suggests that RF arise as antibodies to "altered" autologous (the patient's own) IgG. Some modification of IgG changes its configuration and renders it an autoimmunogen, stimulating the production of RF. IgM is the first class of immunoglobulins formed after contact with an antigen and most RF are of this class, although RF may be of any immunoglobulin class.[1] The exact biological role of RF is unknown and given less weight in current theories on the pathogenesis of RA.[7] RA occurs in the absence of RF in a substantial number of individuals. Individuals with RA, however, who do have RF, or seropositive disease, have increased frequency of subcutaneous nodules, vasculitis, and polyarticular involvement.[1]

Recent studies have also sought to establish a genetic predisposition to the development of RA.[8] Human leukocyte antigens (HLA) are found on the cell surface of most human cells, and are capable of generating an **immune response** when genetically incompatible tissues are grafted to each other, for example, during organ transplants. Genes controlling these HLA are found on the sixth chromosome. Four loci have been described: HLA-A, HLA-B, HLA-C, and HLA-D. RA has been associated with increased HLA-D and HLA-DR (D related) antigens, suggesting that certain genes determine whether a host is more or less at risk for an immunological response that leads to RA.[5] A "rheumatoid epitope" has been identified through DNA typing of HLA-DR4 as a particular sequence of amino acids common among patients with rheumatoid arthritis.[7] Further studies of genomic organization of the HLA-D region specifically implicate a short sequence on the HLA-DRB1 gene and suggest that HLA-DRB1 alleles modify disease expression and progression.[1] Various studies of different ethnic groups have also shown that particular variations of the HLA-DRB1 allele are over-represented in people with RA.[1]

Pathology

Long-standing RA is characterized by the grossly edematous appearance of the **synovium** with slender villous or hair-like projections into the joint cavity. There are distinctive vascular changes, including venous distention, capillary obstruction, neutrophilic infiltration of the arterial walls, and areas of thrombosis and hemorrhage. Synovial proliferation of vascular granulation tissue, known as **pannus**, dissolves collagen as it extends over the joint cartilage. Eventually, if RA continues, the granulation tissue will result in adhesions, **fibrosis** or bony **ankylosis** of the joint. Chronic inflammation can also weaken the joint capsule and its supporting ligamentous structures, altering joint structure and function. Tendon rupture and fraying tendon sheaths may produce imbalanced muscle pull on these pathologically altered joints resulting in the characteristic musculoskeletal deformities seen in advanced RA.[1,9]

Pathogenesis

The key features that differentiate synovial joints from other kinds of joints are exactly those features that make them susceptible to persistent inflammation. Rapid changes in the cellular content and volume of the synovial fluid following alterations in blood flow are possible owing to low pressure in the joint space and the lack of a limiting membrane between the joint space and the synovial blood vessels. High molecular weight substances such as macroglobulins and fibrinogens can pass through the synovial capillaries during periods of inflammation and are not easily cleared.[1] Because the cartilage is avascular, antigen-antibody complexes may be sequestered within the joint cavity and may facilitate a process of phagocytosis and further development of pannus. Although it is accepted that sustained **synovitis** requires the proliferation of new blood vessels, the exact mechanism of capillary growth is not currently understood. One attractive hypothesis is that activated macrophages, responding to antigen-antibody complexes, may stimulate this development.

In established synovitis, polymorphonuclear (PMN) leukocytes are chemotactically drawn into the joint cavity and contribute to the inflammatory destruction of the synovium, although the exact mechanism of this destruction is unknown. It is known that the lysosomal enzymes, which are released from these leukocytes, can directly injure synovial tissues.[1,10]

Clinical Diagnostic Criteria

The clinical diagnosis of RA is based on careful consideration of three factors: the clinical presentation of the patient, which is elucidated through history-taking and physical examination; the corroborating evidence gathered through laboratory tests and radiography; and the exclusion of other possible diagnoses.[1,9]

Signs and Symptoms

Systemic Manifestations

Morning stiffness lasting more than 3 minutes is a hallmark symptom of RA. Difficulty in moving upon awakening and generalized stiffness despite morning activity help to differentiate this sign from the stiffness of a particular joint seen in osteoarthritis following inactivity.[2] Morning stiffness can be qualified in terms of its severity and duration, both of which are directly related to the degree of disease activity. As with other systemic diseases, anorexia, weight loss, and fatigue also may be present.[1,2,11]

Joint Involvement

RA is marked by a bilateral and symmetrical pattern of joint involvement. Clinically, the patient presents with immobility and the cardinal signs of inflammation: pain, redness, swelling, and heat.[1] The term **arthralgia** is used to refer to pain in a joint. The joint examination also may reveal **crepitus**, which is audible or palpable grating or crunching as the joint is moved through its range of motion (ROM). Crepitus is the result of uneven degeneration of the joint surface.

Cervical Spine

The cervical spine is often involved in RA.[12,13] The atlantoaxial joint and the midcervical region are the most common sites of inflammation, which leads to decreased ROM, particularly in rotation, 50 percent of which takes place at the C1 to C2. Involvement of these two vertebrae may produce life-threatening situations if the transverse ligament of the atlas should rupture or if the odontoid process should fracture or herniate through the foramen magnum. Magnetic resonance imaging (MRI) is particularly useful for visualizing both the spinal column and the cord.[1,14]

Ankylosing spondylitis is an inflammation of one or more vertebrae of the spine that may accompany rheumatoid disease. It primarily affects the sacroiliac, spinal facet, and costovertebral joints, and progresses to eventual fusion (ankylosis) of the involved joints.

Temporomandibular Joint

Involvement of this synovial joint results in an inability to open the mouth fully (approximately 2 in.) with normal side-to-side gliding and protrusion. In resting position, the normal approximation of the upper and lower teeth may be altered following persistent inflammation.[9,15]

Shoulders

Shoulder involvement may be seen in the glenohumeral, sternoclavicular, or acromioclavicular joints. These joints may demonstrate degeneration, pain, and loss of ROM. The scapulothoracic articulation may secondarily exhibit a loss of ROM as well. Chronic inflammation of the shoulders causes the capsule and the ligaments to become distended and thinned. Joint surfaces may be eroded until the shoulder eventually becomes unstable. In addition, **tendinitis** and **bursitis** may complicate management.[1,15–17]

Elbows

Inflammation, capsular and ligamentous distension, and joint surface erosion may lead to elbow instability and irregular or catching movements. Flexion contractures frequently develop, the outcome of persistent spasm secondary to pain.[1,16]

Wrists

Early synovitis between the eight carpal bones and the ulna leads to a fairly rapid development of a flexion contracture, which ultimately diminishes the individual's ability to execute power grasp. Chronic inflammation of the proximal row of carpals can lead to a volar **subluxation** of the wrist and hand on the radius, accentuating the normal 10 to 15° of volar inclination of the carpus on the distal radius (Fig. 26.1). Chronic inflammation leads to the loss of radial ligamentous support and destruction of the extensor carpi ulnaris and the fibrocartilage on the distal side of the ulna. The attenuation of these restraining structures allows the proximal carpals to slide down the distal radius toward the ulna, creating a radial deviation of the distal row of carpals in the wrist relative to the two bones of the forearm, where normally there are 5 to 10° of ulnar deviation (Fig. 26.2).[16] Stenosing tenosynovitis of the first dorsal compartment of the wrist (*deQuervain's disease*) may also occur.

Hand Joints

Metacarpophalangeal. Soft-tissue swelling around the metacarpophalangeal (MCP) joints is very common. The volar subluxation and ulnar drift of the MCPs frequently seen in RA are thought to result from accentuation of the normal structural shapes of these joints that tilt the proximal phalanges in an ulnar direction. The anatomical placement and length of the collateral ligaments, which are most stretched during MCP flexion, and the insertions of the intrinsics, which also pull from an ulnar direction, also contribute to ulnar drift at the MCPs during hand motion.

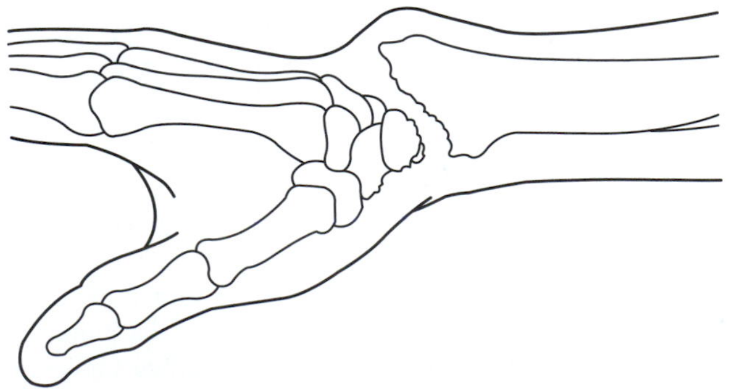

Figure 26.1 Volar subluxation of the carpus on the radius as a result of erosive synovitis of the radiocarpal joint. (From Melvin, J,[16] p 280, with permission.)

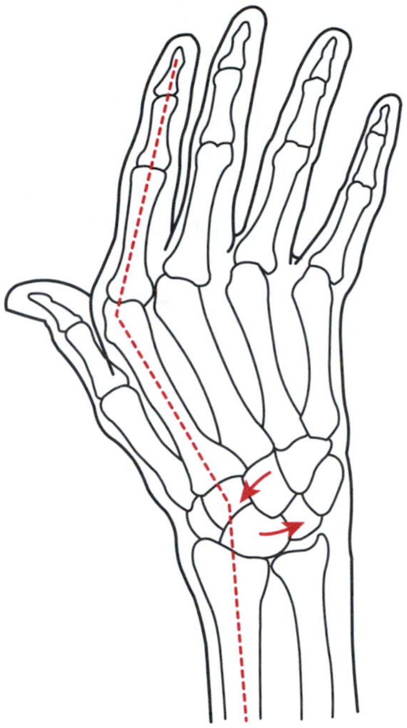

Figure 26.2 Relationship between wrist and metacarpophalangeal joint deformity. (Adapted from Melvin, J,[16] p 281, with permission.)

Weakened ligaments cannot resist a pull toward volar subluxation during power pinch or grasp when flexor tendons "bowstring" across MCPs through frayed tendon sheaths damaged by long-term synovitis.[16] The bowstring effect results from moving the fulcrum of the flexor tendons distally which places an ulnar and volar pull on the proximal phalanges (Fig. 26.3). Radial deviation of the carpals will further enhance MCP ulnar drift as the phalanges try to compensate for the loss of normal ulnar deviation at the wrist. This is known as the *zigzag effect,* where forces in the

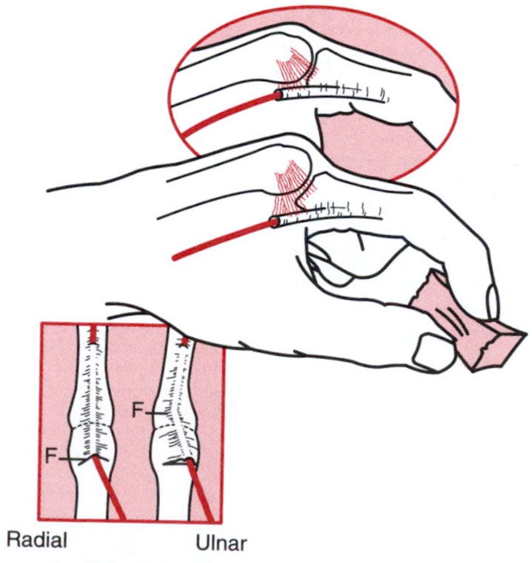

Figure 26.3 Influence of the long flexors in metacarpophalangeal drift deformity. (Adapted from Melvin, J,[16] p 283, with permission.)

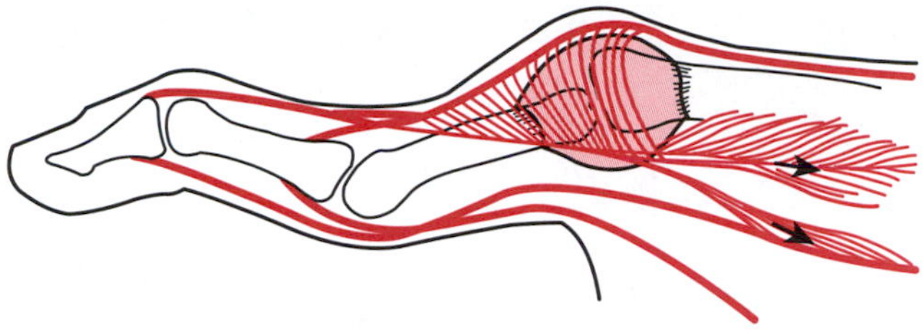

Figure 26.4 Swan neck deformity with initial synovitis at the metacarpophalangeal joint. (Adapted from Melvin, J,[16] p 285, with permission.)

hand try to move the index finger back into its normal functional position in line with the radius (see Fig. 26.2).[16,18–22]

Proximal Interphalangeal. Swelling of the proximal interphalangeal (PIP) joints produces a fusiform or "sausage"-like appearance in the fingers. There are two characteristic deformities seen at the PIP in individuals with RA. The first of these is known as **swan neck deformity** and consists of PIP hyperextension and distal interphalangeal (DIP) flexion. Swan neck deformities arise in three distinct ways, depending on the site of initial involvement.[16,22] Most commonly, swan neck deformity follows from initial synovitis of the MCP, where the pain of chronic synovitis leads to reflex muscle spasm of the intrinsics (Fig. 26.4). The biomechanical force of the intrinsics then combines with the hypermobility found in the chronically inflamed and structurally changed PIP, resulting in volar subluxation and PIP hyperextension. Swan neck deformity may also result when the volar capsule of the PIP is stretched, the lateral bands move dorsally, and tension placed on the flexor digitorum profundis by the PIP flexes the DIP (Fig. 26.5). In these instances, a rupture of the flexor digitorum sublimus further predisposes an individual to swan neck deformity. A third mechanism for developing swan neck deformity involves a rupture of the extensor digitorum communis at its insertion on the DIP resulting in DIP flexion and PIP hyperextension owing to unrestrained pull by the flexor digitorum profundis (Fig. 26.6).[16]

The other characteristic deformity of the PIP is known as a *boutonniere deformity* and consists of DIP extension with PIP flexion (Fig. 26.7). As a result of chronic synovitis, the insertion of extensor digitorum communis into the middle phalanx (known as the central slip) lengthens, and the lateral bands slide volarly to force the PIP into flexion. Bony formation or outgrowths around the end of a joint are

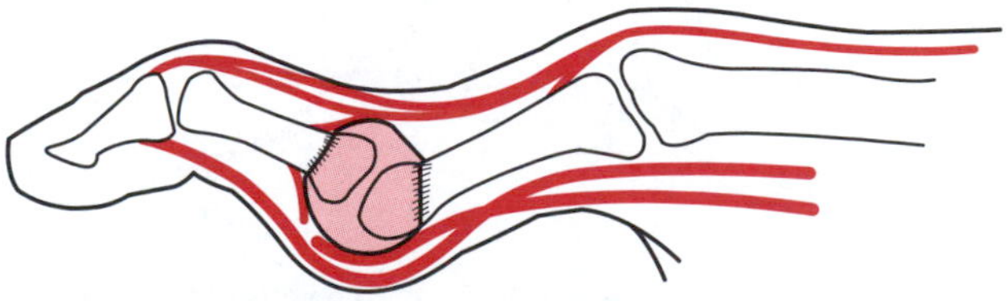

Figure 26.5 Swan neck deformity with initial synovitis at the proximal interphalangeal joint. (Adapted from Melvin, J,[16] p 286, with permission.)

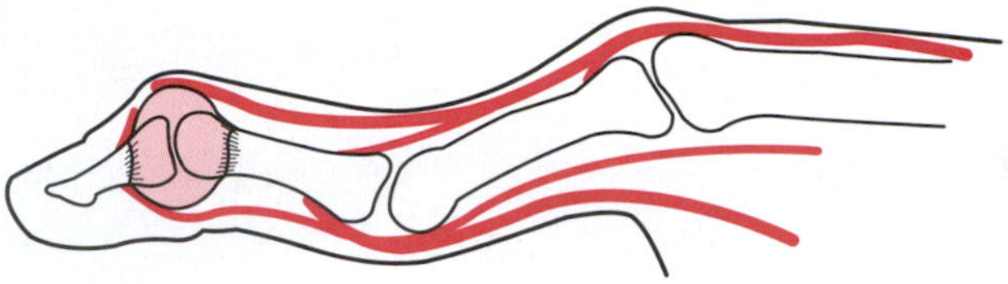

Figure 26.6 Swan neck deformity with initial synovitis at the distal interphalangeal joint. (Adapted from Melvin, J,[16] p 287, with permission.)

termed *osteophytes*. Those found at the PIP are known as *Bouchard's nodes*, and may be seen in OA. They are unrelated to RA, although an individual may have both kinds of arthritis at the same time.[16]

Distal Interphalangeal. The distal interphalangeal (DIP) joints are most often uninvolved in RA. Osteophytes are, however, common in OA and are called *Heberden's nodes*. Occasionally, the tendon of the extensor digitorum communis will rupture, and the unopposed pull of the flexor digitorum profundis will pull the DIP into flexion. This condition is known as *mallet finger* deformity.[16]

Thumb. As in the other digital joints, the primary cause of deformity in the thumb is synovial swelling. The fibers of the dorsal hood mechanism over the MCP, the joint capsule and the collateral ligaments, and the tendons of extensor pollicis brevis and extensor pollicis longus are particularly affected. The exact mechanism of thumb deformities depends on the particular combination of affected structures and may be classified according to the criteria elaborated by Nalebuff.[23] Similar to other hand deformities, the actual presentation depends on the site of initial synovitis, the direction of imbalanced muscle forces, and the integrity of the surrounding joint structures. A *type I deformity*, consisting of MCP flexion with interphalangeal (IP) hyperextension without involvement of the carpometacarpal (CMC) joint, is most commonly seen. *Type II deformity* is assigned when the CMC is subluxed and the IP is held in hyperextension. CMC subluxation and MCP hyperextension is classified as a *type III deformity*, and is more commonly found in RA than a type II deformity.[16,23]

Mutilans Deformity (Opera-Glass Hand). Grossly unstable thumbs and severely deformed phalanges are indicative of *mutilans-type deformity.* Also known as opera glass hand, the transverse folds of the skin of the thumb and fingers resemble a folded telescope. Radiographic study of the bones of the hand reveal severe bone resorption, erosion, and shortening of the MCP, PIP, radiocarpal, and radioulnar joints especially. The negative impact of this deformity on hand function and activities of daily living (ADL) is significant.[16]

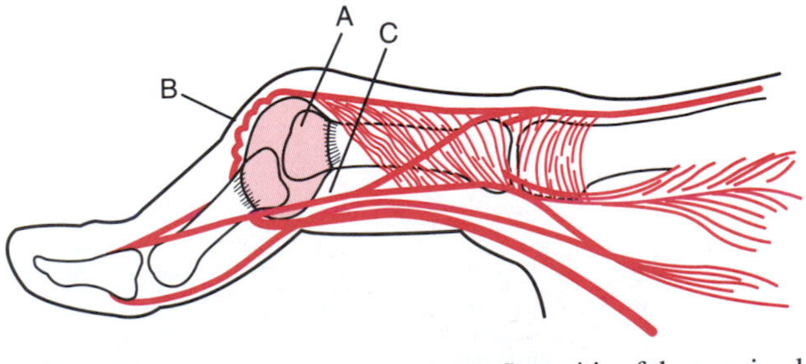

Figure 26.7 Boutonniere deformity. *A*. Synovitis of the proximal interphalangeal joint; *B*. Osteophytes at the end of the joint (Bouchard's nodes); *C*. Rupture of the central tendinous slip of the extensor hood. (Adapted from Melvin, J,[16] p 287, with permission.)

Hip

Although patients may present with complaints of pain in the groin, often owing to trochanteric bursitis, the hip is less commonly involved in RA than in other kinds of arthritis. Radiographic hip disease is seen in about half of all patients with RA. Severe inflammatory destruction of the femoral head and the acetabulum may push the acetabulum into the pelvic cavity, a condition known as *protrusio acetabuli*.[1,15,16]

Knees

Because of the relatively large amount of synovium in the knee, it is one of the most frequently affected joints in RA. Chronic synovitis results in distension of the joint capsule, attenuation of the collateral and cruciate ligaments, and destruction of the joint surfaces. Painful knees may be held in slightly flexed positions, ultimately resulting in flexion contractures.[1,15,16]

Ankles and Feet

Chronic synovitis accentuates the natural tendency of the talus to glide medially and plantarward, resulting in pressure on the calcaneus and leading to hindfoot pronation. The spring ligament is also stretched by these occurrences, flattening the medial longitudinal arch (Fig. 26.8). The calcaneus may erode or develop bony **exostoses** known as spurs. As synovitis weakens the transverse arch, the metatarsals spread

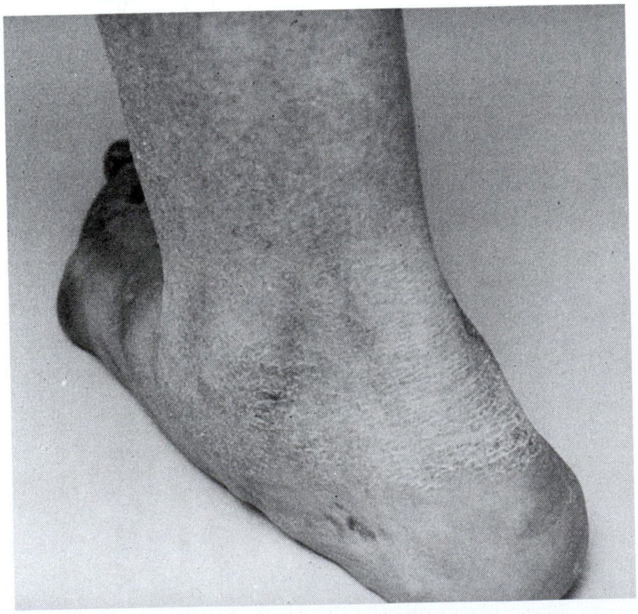

Figure 26.8 Posterior–medial view of the foot and ankle showing calcaneal valgus, pes planus (flatfoot) and hallux valgus. (Used by permission of the Arthritis Foundation.)

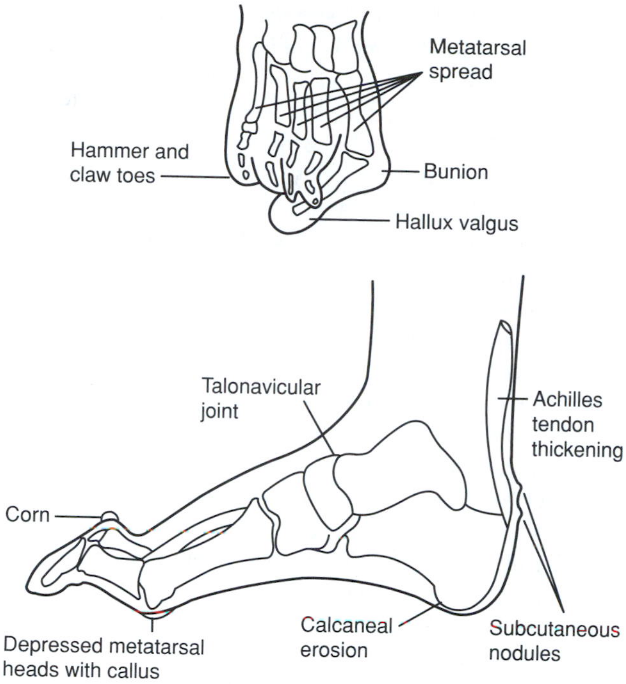

Figure 26.9 Major foot and ankle deformities seen in rheumatoid arthritis. (From Dimonte, P, and Light, H,[81] p 1149, with permission.)

and a splayed forefoot (*splayfoot*) may develop (Fig. 26.9). Synovitis of the metatarsophalangeal (MTP) joints is extremely common and *metatarsalgia* (pain over the metatarsal heads) may develop. A *hallux valgus* and *bunion* (a painful bursitis over the medial aspect of the first MTP joint) may also be present. When volar subluxation of the MTP combines with flexion of the PIP and hyperextension of the DIP joints, this condition is commonly referred to as **hammer toes** (Fig. 26.10). The MTPs may also exhibit volar

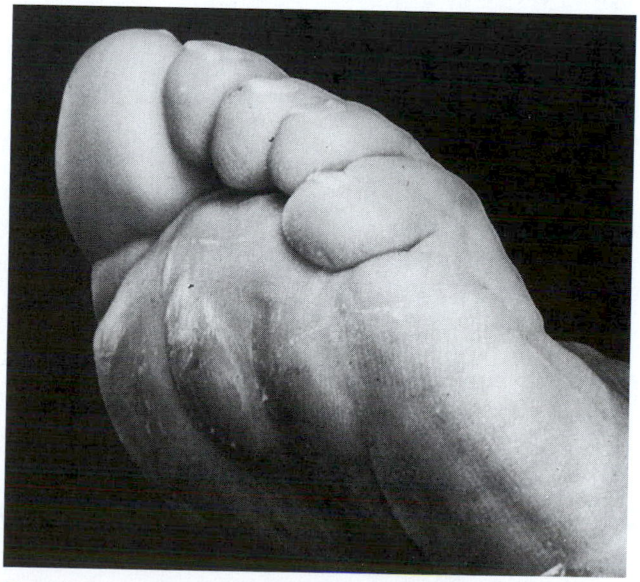

Figure 26.10 Metatarsophalangeal subluxation. (Used by permission of the American College of Rheumatology.)

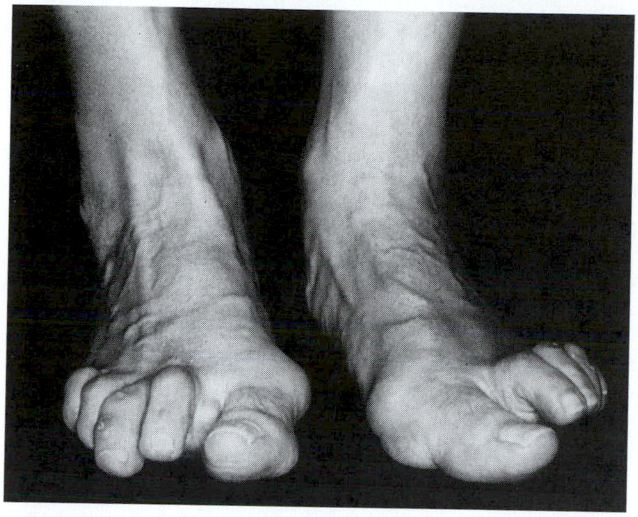

Figure 26.11 Common deformities of the rheumatoid foot. (Used by permission of the American College of Rheumatology.)

subluxation of the metatarsal head with flexion of the PIP and DIP joints, known as *cock-up* or *claw toes* (Fig. 26.11). As the capsule and intertarsal ligaments are weakened and stretched, the proximal phalanges move dorsally on the metatarsal head (Fig. 26.12). Similar to conditions observed in the hand, the long toe extensors "bowstring" over the PIP joints while the flexors are displaced into the intertarsal spaces.[1,15,16,24,25]

Muscle Involvement

Muscle atrophy around affected joints may be present early. It is not definitively known, however, whether this atrophy is the result simply of disuse or selective attrition of muscles owing to some unknown mechanism specifically related to the disease itself. Atrophy in the intrinsic muscles of the hand and the quadriceps are particularly evident in long-standing disease, although the mechanisms for these changes may not be the same. It appears that individuals with RA experience selective attrition of type II (phasic) muscle fibers through some unknown mechanism.[26,27] There is also some evidence that type I (tonic) muscle fibers of the quadriceps will undergo selective atrophy following anterior cruciate damage.[28] Loss of muscle bulk may also be

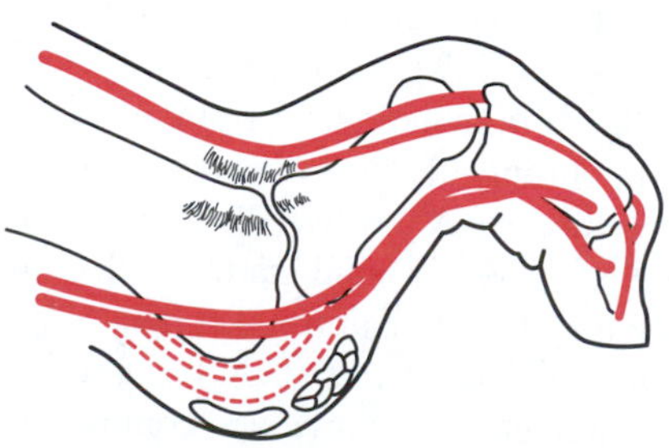

Figure 26.12 Relationship of structures to the metatarsal heads in metatarsalgia. (From Moncur, C, and Shields, M,[24] p 10, with permission.)

the result of a peripheral neuropathy, **myositis**, or steroid-induced myopathy. Muscle weakness may be due to either reflex inhibition secondary to pain or atrophy.[26–28]

Tendons

Inflammation of the synovial lining of the tendon sheaths results in a tenosynovitis that interferes with the smooth gliding of the tendon through the sheath. This may directly damage the tendon itself, and may eventually lead to a tendon rupture. A patient with tendon damage or muscle weakness may exhibit a *lag phenomenon,* which refers to a substantial difference in passive versus active ROM. This is a nonspecific finding that therapists need to examine carefully to determine its cause and design appropriate treatment.[16]

Laboratory Tests

Two concepts are essential to a full understanding of the use of laboratory tests in the detection of RA. The first is the concept of the *sensitivity* of a test, which indicates the proportion of truly diseased individuals who have a positive test. The clinical value of sensitive tests is particularly evident in those instances when a negative misdiagnosis would be deleterious to the health of the patient. In research terms, sensitivity is equivalent to the laboratory test's ability to avoid a false negative result. The concept of *specificity,* on the other hand, refers to the proportion of truly nondiseased individuals who have a negative test. In other words, the specificity of a laboratory test is a measure of its ability to avoid false positives. The clinical diagnostician will usually choose a combination of both sensitive and specific tests to confirm clinical impressions during the diagnostic process.

Elevated erythrocyte sedimentation rate (ESR) or *C reactive protein (CRP),* acute phase reactants, indicate the presence of active inflammation. Although it is characteristic that patients with RA have active inflammation, up to 40 percent of patients with RA have normal values for these tests despite marked clinical evidence of inflammation. Normal ESR and CRP values do not exclude a diagnosis of RA, nor do elevated levels signify a diagnosis of RA. Rheumatoid factor (RF) is the result of the binding of two immunoglobulins. The presence or absence of RF neither confirms nor rules out a diagnosis of RA. Up to 25 percent of people with RA do not have a positive RF (seronegative RA), whereas a positive RF is seen in a number of other diseases with an immunological component (e.g., leprosy, tuberculosis, chronic hepatitis) and occasionally in individuals with no disease. A positive RF cannot confirm a diagnosis of RA; however, in combination with clinical criteria, positive RF may help to confirm a clinical impression.

A *complete blood count (CBC)* is routinely ordered because a number of findings are commonly associated with RA. Red blood cell counts are often decreased, indicating the anemia of chronic disease found in approximately 20 percent of individuals with RA. By comparison, the white blood cell count is generally normal. *Thrombocytosis,* a high platelet count, is not uncommon in active RA.

A synovial fluid analysis can greatly enhance the process of differential diagnosis. Normal synovial fluid is transparent, yellowish, viscous, and without clots. Synovial fluid from inflamed joints is cloudy, less viscous owing to a change in hyaluronate proteins, and will clot. Significant inflammation will also increase the number of proteins in the fluid. A culture can be done to identify potential bacterial agents as the cause of the joint inflammation. If the joint is inflamed, there will be an elevation of white blood cells in the fluid. The presence of crystals may confirm the diagnosis of **gout** (urate crystals) or *pseudogout* (calcium pyrophosphate crystals). A mucin clot is formed in synovial fluid by mixing it with acetic acid. If the synovial fluid is normal, a ropelike mass will form in a clear solution after mixing. Shredding indicates fair mucin clotting, and the formation of small masses with shreds is indicative of a poor mucin clot. Poor clotting accompanies acute infectious arthritis. Inflammatory arthritis, such as RA, produces fair mucin clotting. Good mucin clotting of the synovial fluid is found in a joint that presents with a noninflammatory arthritis.[1]

Radiography

Radiographic study is an essential component of the diagnostic workup for RA. Physical therapists practicing in rheumatology should be avid consumers of the radiographic information available in a patient's record. They should also develop a basic proficiency in identifying abnormalities in joint structure and the surrounding soft tissues that influence the course and outcome of rehabilitation. The ability to identify abnormalities assumes the therapist has a firm notion of how a normal joint appears on a radiograph. Therapists can orient themselves to a radiograph by considering three parameters: alignment, bone density and surface, and cartilaginous spacing (Figs. 26.13

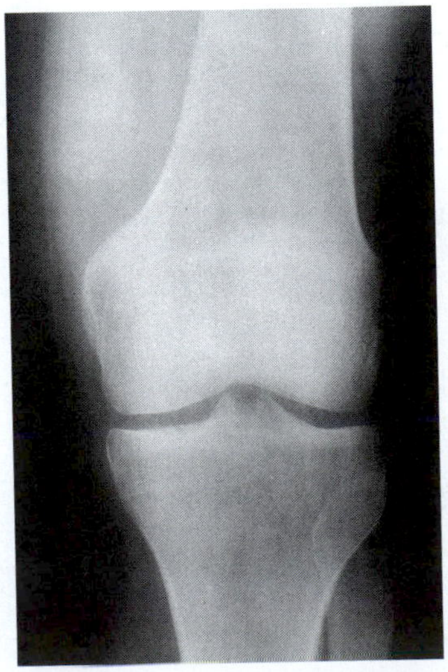

Figure 26.13 Frontal view of the normal knee. (Used by permission of the American College of Rheumatology.)

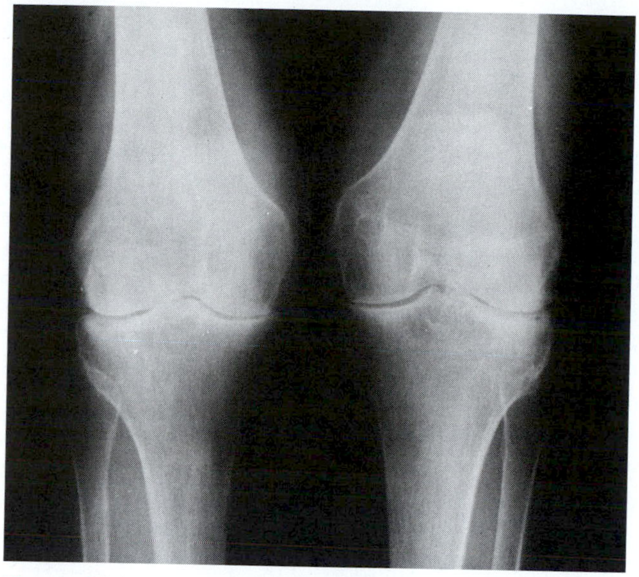

Figure 26.14 Frontal view of the knee with characteristics of rheumatoid arthritis. (Used by permission of the American College of Rheumatology.)

and 26.14). In determining alignment, the therapist should note whether the long axes of the proximal and distal bones of the joint are in their normal spatial relationships and whether the convex surface of one fits well with the concavity of the other. Bone density, in the absence of **osteoporosis**, should be somewhat opaque and milky and appear evenly distributed throughout. The cortices of each bone should be distinct, appropriately thick, and well defined. The soft tissues surrounding the joints should conform to known anatomical shape. The therapist should note any soft tissue swelling evident on the radiograph that might limit function. Finally, the therapist should note whether there is even spacing between the joint surfaces. Uneven, reduced, or absent spacing suggests loss of cartilage or erosion of the joint surfaces. Overall, the joint surface should be smooth and conform to known anatomical shape without osteophytes. The progression of the disease can be characterized along four stages following periodic radiographic examination (Box 26.1). The radiographic changes seen early in the disease are nonspecific, and usually limited to swelling in the surrounding soft tissues, joint effusion, and periarticular demineralization. Diagnostic confirmation is available only later in the disease process when the typical joint space narrowing and erosions in the hands and feet are seen in the characteristic bilateral distribution.[1,29]

Box 26.1 Classification of Progression of Rheumatoid Arthritis

Stage I, Early
1. No destructive changes on radiographic examination.[a]
2. Radiographic evidence of osteoporosis may be present.

Stage II, Moderate
1. Radiographic evidence of osteoporosis, with or without slight subchondral bone destruction; slight cartilage destruction may be present.[a]
2. No joint deformities, although limitation of joint mobility may be present.[a]
3. Adjacent muscle atrophy.
4. Extra-articular soft tissue lesions, such as nodules and tenosynovitis may be present.

Stage III, Severe
1. Radiographic evidence of cartilage and bone destruction, in addition to osteoporosis.[a]
2. Joint deformity, such as subluxation, ulnar deviation, or hyperextension, without fibrous or bony ankylosis.[a]
3. Extensive muscle atrophy.
4. Extra-articular soft tissue lesions, such as nodules and tenosynovitis may be present.

Stage IV, Terminal
1. Fibrous or bony ankylosis[a]
2. Criteria of stage III

From Schumacher, Klippel, and Robinson (eds.): Primer on Rheumatic Diseases, ed 9, Arthritis Foundation, Atlanta, 1988, p 318, with permission.

[a]These criteria must be present to permit classification of a patient in any particular stage or grade.

Impairments and Complications

Deconditioning

People with RA are less physically fit (cardiorespiratory status, muscular strength and endurance, flexibility, and body composition) than their peers without arthritis. Rheumatologic research in conditioning exercise has demonstrated that this situation is not entirely due to the disease process, but is compounded by inadequate levels of regular physical activity.[30,31] In addition to the deconditioning of inactivity, studies of body composition in individuals with RA have shown a marked degree of *cachexia* (wasting of lean body mass) and elevated resting energy expenditure. It appears that immune system activity and inflammation even in individuals with ostensibly well-controlled disease, create an increased metabolism with subsequent loss of lean body tissue.[32]

Rheumatoid Nodules

Rheumatoid nodules are the most common extra-articular manifestations of RA and occur in approximately 25 percent of patients. They are most commonly found in the subcutaneous or deeper connective tissues in areas subjected to repeated mechanical pressure such as the olecranon bursae, the extensor surfaces of the forearms, and the Achilles tendons. Nodules are usually asymptomatic, although they can be tender and may cause skin breakdown or become infected.[1]

Vascular Complications

Most forms of vascular lesions associated with RA are silent, although the fulminant form of rheumatoid arteritis can be life threatening, and accompanied by malnutrition, infection, congestive heart failure, and gastrointestinal bleeding. Foot or wrist drop may occur as a result of vasculitis of the vasa arteriosum to the nerve supply of the radial or superficial peroneal nerves.[1]

Neurological Manifestations

Mild peripheral neuropathies are often seen in RA, particularly in elderly patients, and are unrelated to vasculitis. Most neuropathies result from nerve compression or entrapment, such as *carpal tunnel* or *tarsal tunnel syndromes.*[1]

Cardiopulmonary Complications

Pericarditis can be demonstrated at autopsy in about 4 percent of patients, but clinically detectable heart disease from RA is rare. Similarly, pleuropulmonary manifestations are most commonly asymptomatic, although pleuritis is commonly found on autopsy.[1,9]

Ocular Manifestations

Ocular lesions are usually associated with the dry eyes of *Sjögren's syndrome,* which is an inflammatory disorder of the lacrimal and salivary glands. Scleritis and the relatively more benign episcleritis can also be present, and require careful medical treatment.[1,9,33]

Disease Onset and Course

Disease onset in RA is most usually accompanied by complaints of generalized joint pain and stiffness, most often lasting weeks to months. Disease progression is highly variable. High titers of RF can indicate a more severe disease course. Spontaneous remissions can occur, although it often remains unclear if the individual had an accurately diagnosed case of RA or some other disease. Some patients experience an intermittent course, characterized by partial to complete remissions longer than the periods of exacerbations. A third group of patients experience the full unremitting destructive process of progressive RA.[1,15] Comparisons of elderly-onset RA with early-onset RA have revealed that abrupt onset and large joint involvement, particularly of the shoulder girdle, were more common in the older group. The elderly-onset group also more commonly had features of *polymyalgia rheumatica,* a distinct disease affecting the shoulder and pelvic girdles, with which elderly-onset RA can be confused.[34]

Prognosis

The question of mortality associated with RA is controversial. Previously, it was widely believed that RA itself was not usually a cause of death, although conditions such as systemic vasculitis and atlantoaxial subluxation could be fatal. Now there is a growing body of evidence that individuals with RA may not live as long as their counterparts without disease, especially if the early years of RA were marked by aggressive disease and poor functional status.

Table 26.2 American College of Rheumatology Revised Criteria for Classification of Functional Status in Rheumatoid Arthritis[a]

Class I	Completely able to perform usual activities of daily living (self-care, vocational, and avocational)
Class II	Able to perform usual self-care and vocational activities, but limited in avocational activities
Class III	Able to perform usual self-care activities, but limited in vocational and avocational activities
Class IV	Limited in ability to perform usual self-care, vocational, and avocational activities

From Hochberg, MC, et al: The American College of Rheumatology 1991 revised criteria for the classification of global functional status in rheumatoid arthritis. Arthritis Rheum 35:498, 1992, with permission.

[a]Usual self-care activities include dressing, feeding, bathing, grooming, and toileting. Avocational (recreational and/or leisure) and vocational (work, school, homemaking) activities are patient-desired and age- and sex-specific.

Causes of death occurring more frequently in patients with RA as compared to the general population are infections and renal, respiratory, and gastrointestinal disease.[35,36] Even in patients with milder forms of RA, long-term inflammation ultimately results in joint destruction and significant functional loss. Almost 50 percent of individuals with RA will eventually have marked restrictions in ADL or will be incapacitated.[1] Individuals with late-onset RA appear to have a better functional outcome than those with early onset, but it is unclear whether this finding is the result of having the disease for a shorter period of time or of having a different form of the disease itself.[34] A broad classification of functional disability has been developed by the ARA to characterize the progressive impacts of the disease (Table 26.2). Loss of income is the most severe loss and is directly attributable to work disability secondary to loss of physical function.[37–41]

Osteoarthritis

OA is marked by two localized, pathological features: the progressive destruction of articular cartilage and the formation of bone at the margins of the joint.[1] The disease process of OA confines itself to the affected joint. However, the impairment, functional limitation, and disability related to OA can reach far beyond the perimeters of articular cartilage and subchondral bone. Research documenting the personal and socioeconomic impact of OA increasingly recognizes its importance in both personal and socioeconomic terms.

Classification

Although joint inflammation is implied by the "it is" in osteoarthritis, inflammation is typically found only after there has been substantial articular degeneration. The synovium of an osteoarthritic joint, however, can demonstrate marked changes, similar to those seen in RA in some joints. In epidemiological studies, OA is often graded on radiographs according to the criteria of Kellgren and Lawrence,[42] using an ordinal scale of five levels:

- Grade 0: normal radiograph
- Grade 1: doubtful narrowing of the joint space and possible osteophytes
- Grade 2: definite osteophytes and absent or questionable narrowing of the joint space
- Grade 3: moderate osteophytes and joint space narrowing, some sclerosis, and possible deformity
- Grade 4: large osteophytes, marked narrowing of joint space, severe sclerosis, and definite deformity

Most studies have used grade 2 (the presence of definite osteophytes) as the criterion for defining disease, although a few others have required evidence of joint space narrowing (grade 3), corresponding to clinically identified disease, to designate OA.[42] Although radiographic evidence of joint space narrowing and osteophytes may help confirm the diagnosis and classify the stage of OA, the clinical criteria for hip and knee OA are described in terms of pain and limitation of motion (Box 26.2).[43,44] Radiography adds little to the accuracy of the clinical diagnosis, and there is no clear association between radiographic findings and function or pain. In OA of the knee, muscle strength and pain are more explanatory of functional loss than radiographic findings.[45]

Box 26.2 Clinical Classification Criteria for Knee and Hip Osteoarthritis

Knee osteoarthritis[a]
- Knee pain
- Joint stiffness ≤30 minutes
- Crepitus
- Bony enlargement
- Bony tenderness
- No palpable warmth

Hip osteoarthritis[b]
- Hip internal rotation ≥15° with pain; morning stiffness ≤60 minutes; and age >50 years, and pain on internal rotation, *or*
- Hip pain and hip internal rotation <15°, and hip flexion <115°

[a]95% sensitivity, 69% specificity.
[b]86% sensitivity, 75% specificity.
From Altman, R, et al,[43] and Altman, R, et al.[44]

Patients with OA can be further differentiated in two ways. Some cases of OA are classified as *idiopathic,* when the etiology of the disease is unknown. Idiopathic OA may be localized to a specific joint, or generalized, affecting three or more joints. OA is classified as *secondary,* when the etiology (e.g., trauma, congenital malformation, or other musculoskeletal disease) can be identified.

Epidemiology

OA is an extremely common condition after 40 years of age, although it may not always be symptomatic when present. It is widespread in adults older than 65, and affects men more than women before the age of 50, but reverses after age 50.[1] More than 20 million people in the United states are affected by OA.[46] Studies concerning racial predisposition to OA have yielded conflicting data, depending on the joint studied.

Etiology

Similar to RA, no single factor that predisposes an individual to OA has been identified. Although aging is indeed strongly associated with OA, it must be emphasized that aging in itself does not cause OA, nor should OA be considered synonymous with the "normal" aging process.[1,47] Several factors related to aging may, however, contribute to its development. Trauma prior to adulthood may initiate a remodeling of bone that alters joint mechanics and nutrition in a way that becomes problematic only later in life. The role of repetitive "microtrauma" in the etiology of OA has also received attention.[1] Specifically, occupational tasks, such as repetitive knee bending, have been linked to the development of OA.[48,49] Finally, obesity has been shown to be a risk factor for the development of OA in later life.[1,48,50]

Pathology

Animal models involving knee trauma have provided much of the basis for what we now know about the earliest changes associated with OA in humans. Thus, it is possible that subtle, crucial, and as yet undiscovered differences in humans may alter our understanding of OA in the future. The first osteoarthritic change in articular cartilage, which has been confirmed in humans, is an increase in water content. This increase suggests that the proteoglycans have been allowed to swell with water far beyond normal, although the mechanism by which this occurs is unknown.[1] In addition, there are changes in the composition of newly synthesized proteoglycan. In later stages of disease progression, proteoglycans are lost, which diminishes the water content of cartilage. As proteoglycans are lost, articular cartilage loses its compressive stiffness and elasticity, which in turn, results in the transmission of compressive forces to underlying bone. Changes in cartilage proteoglycans will also negatively affect the ability of the cartilage to form a squeeze film over its surface during joint loading. Collagen synthesis is increased initially, although there is a shift from type II collagen fibers to a larger proportion of type I collagen, the kind found in skin and fibrous tissue. As the articular cartilage is destroyed, the joint space narrows.[51]

One of the first noticeable changes in cartilage is the mild fraying or "flaking" of superficial collagen fibers. Deeper fraying, or "fibrillation," of the upper third of the cartilage follows in areas of greater weightbearing. The cartilage may degenerate to the point that subchondral bone is exposed. Subchondral bone in turn can then become sclerotic and stiffer than normal bone.[51] These changes in cartilage and bone result in increased friction, decreased shock absorption, and greater impact loading of the joint. The traditional view of OA is that the disease process starts with an unrepaired injury to articular cartilage; however, there is also evidence that reduced compliance in bone and periarticular structures may initiate the degenerative processes.[52,53]

The process of osteophyte formation in OA is not well understood. Current hypotheses have implicated increased vascularity in degenerated cartilage, venous congestion from subchondral cysts and thickened subchondral trabeculae, and the continued sloughing of articular cartilage. Each of these hypotheses may explain how this bony growth contributes to the pain and loss of motion that accompany OA.

Pathogenesis

Unlike the synovium in RA, the major pathological changes of OA are found in the articular cartilage, particularly the concentration of proteoglycan, which diminishes according to the severity of the disease. Furthermore, there are metabolic changes in the rate of enzyme production that facilitate the destruction of cartilage. Even though proteoglycan concentration decreases with OA, it is also true that proteoglycan and collagen synthesis increases until the later stages of the disease. This seeming paradox has given rise to several hypotheses concerning the pathogenesis of OA, which have yet to be proven. Given that proteoglycan synthesis increases with OA, it is possible that the quality of this newly synthesized product may not be equal to meeting the biomechanical load normally placed on an adult joint.[1]

Clinical Diagnostic Criteria

Signs and Symptoms

Clinically, a diagnosis is often made on the basis of symptoms and signs (e.g., pain and swelling, loss of ROM, and bony deformity). Not all joints are equally affected by OA. In the upper extremity (UE), the DIPs, PIPs, and CMC of the thumb are commonly involved. The cervical and lumbar spine, hips, knees, and first MTP are also sites for OA. The MCPs, wrists, elbows, and shoulders are usually spared in primary OA.[54] Unlike RA, OA does not have a bilateral, symmetrical presentation. A single joint or any combination of joints on one individual may be affected. OA is not a systemic disease, and is therefore not associated with systemic complaints such as generalized morning stiffness, fever, or loss of appetite. Individuals with OA may experience some stiffness in particular joints upon awakening that is similar to the stiffness felt when mobilizing the same joints after inactivity during the day, but this stiffness does not last nearly as long as in individuals with RA nor is it generalized to the entire body.[54] Crepitus is a common clinical finding in OA as well as in RA.[54]

Although cartilage degeneration is the primary manifestation of OA, cartilage is aneural, and therefore not the cause of a person's pain. Pain in OA may be attributed to incongruent articulations of joint surfaces, periosteal elevation secondary to bone proliferation at the joint margin, abnormal pressures on subchondral bone, trabecular microfractures, and distention of the joint capsule. Many patients will also experience a secondary synovitis, especially when the knee is involved.[54]

Symptoms do not always match the severity of the disease on radiographs. Some patients may magnify the pain they experience. More importantly, unlike individuals with RA who report pain on motion and at rest, the pain associated with OA is likely to occur or worsen only with motion, except in the later stages of the disease.[54]

OA of the hip commonly results in decreased ROM with a tendency for the hip to be held in a somewhat flexed, abducted, and externally rotated position and the knee in flexion. Decreased hip ROM is clearly associated with decreased walking speed, decreased stride length, and increased energy expenditure. Maximum walking speed of 1.8 miles per hour is not uncommon in older persons with hip OA and decreased hip motion.[55] Overall, OA of the knee can impose functional limitations to a degree equivalent to heart disease, congestive heart failure, and chronic obstructive pulmonary disease and accounts for a substantial proportion of the burden of disability among community-living elders.[56]

Patients with the most severe disease may not move their joints as often or in the ways that exacerbate their symptoms. Therefore, pain and disease severity in individuals with OA are potentially related to functional loss, although not in the same way. Among elders, it has been shown, for example, that the functional loss associated with severe radiographic OA without symptoms is more likely than the loss associated with the presence of symptoms but milder disease.[57] One explanation of this finding is that individuals with OA limit their functional activities to avoid movements that are painful. In the clinical examination of the patient with OA one might assume that pain is a primary factor in limiting function as is the case in patients with RA. A clinical examination predicated on this assumption could lead to the hasty conclusion that the patient's functional status is normal if pain is absent. Given that individuals with OA may reduce or eliminate their symptoms by avoiding certain activities, clinicians should explore functional limitations in patients with OA separately from the evaluation of symptoms.

Medical Management

Pharmacological Therapy in Rheumatoid Arthritis

In RA, joint destruction and irreversible damage are most pronounced in the first years after disease onset. Therefore, medical management includes an aggressive approach to stop or retard the disease process as well as to control pain and inflammation. It is currently believed that adequate pharmacological therapy initiated in the early stages of the disease results in less joint damage and functional loss. There are two major classifications of drugs used in RA management: nonsteroidal anti-inflammatory drugs (NSAIDs) and disease-modifying antirheumatic drugs (DMARDs), which includes the biologic response modifiers (BRMs), and corticosteroids.[58]

Nonsteroidal Anti-inflammatory Drugs

Nonsteroidal anti-inflammatory drugs (NSAIDs) are a basic element in long-term treatment of RA, having both *analgesic* and *anti-inflammatory* actions. At lower doses, the NSAID effect is analgesic, through the peripheral inhibition of pro-inflammatory prostaglandin synthesis. At higher doses, the effect is anti-inflammatory probably through both prostaglandin inhibition and alteration in macrophage and neutrophil function. Although NSAIDs provide symptomatic relief, they do not alter the underlying disease process. The major serious and most common side effects are gastrointestinal complaints ranging from nausea to gastrointestinal bleeding and ulcers. There are a great many NSAIDs available over the counter and by prescription.

The two major categories are the traditional NSAIDs, many of which are now available over the counter, and the newer, selective, COX-2 inhibitors. Traditional NSAIDs block both COX-2 and COX-1 enzymes. The COX-1 enzyme is important for the health of the stomach lining and kidneys. Individuals at increased risk for gastrointestinal complications are the elderly, smokers, those taking corticosteroids, and those with severe arthritis, comorbidities, and history of gastrointestinal symptoms. The COX-2 inhibitors were designed to reduce the risk of gastrointestinal toxicity by blocking only the COX-2 enzyme, which is responsible for the pain and swelling associated with inflammation. Early evidence from short term trials supported the decreased risk of gastrointestinal side effects and increased tolerability of COX-2 inhibitors.[59] However, longer term trials identified that patients who had been prescribed COX-2 inhibitors experienced serious and sometimes fatal adverse events compared to patients on traditional NSAIDs. While once thought to be the "wave of the future," the clinical use of these particular drugs is uncertain at best. Concurrent prophylactic therapy to decrease gastrointestinal damage also is an option. Other possible side effects of continuing NSAID use include dizziness, headache, drowsiness or tinnitus, kidney dysfunction, and elevation of liver enzymes. Patients taking NSAIDs should be monitored every 3 to 4 months with CBC and biochemical profiles, as well as stool guaiac analysis for occult blood.

The original NSAID was aspirin, which is still comparable in effectiveness, but requires up to 35 tablets a day to achieve an anti-inflammatory effect. The decision of which NSAID to prescribe is based on risk factors, known toxicities, dosing preferences, and cost. Individual response to an NSAID is extremely variable in terms of both effectiveness and tolerance. Therefore, it often requires several month-long trials to find the best product. Taking more than one NSAID increases the risk of toxicity with no increase in benefit. NSAIDs are prescribed for patients with RA at the onset of symptoms to provide rapid pain relief and control of inflammation while waiting for the slower-acting DMARD to become effective. Table 26.3 lists the NSAIDs currently available.

Disease-Modifying Antirheumatic Drugs

Disease-modifying antirheumatic drugs (DMARDs) are a heterogeneous group of drugs exhibiting a wide range of chemical structures, modes of actions, clinical indications, and toxicities. To be classified as a DMARD, a drug must show evidence of changing the course of RA for at least 1 year (improved function, reduced inflammation, and slowing or prevention of structural damage). DMARDs are slow acting, requiring from 3 weeks to 3 months to become effective. These drugs once were known as "second-line agents," denoting their late introduction in treatment for fear of serious toxicity. However, evidence shows that these drugs are no more toxic than NSAIDs, and current philosophy is to initiate DMARDs early and attempt to maintain treatment for at least 2 to 5 years. Individuals taking DMARDs should be monitored regularly for the toxicities accompanying the specific drug. Some DMARDs were developed specifically for RA; others were first used to treat cancer, malaria, or to prevent rejection of transplanted organs. DMARDs are most often used to treat RA; however, some are used to treat juvenile RA, ankylosing spondylitis, psoriatic arthritis, and systemic lupus erythematosus.

A new group of DMARDs has been developed that inhibit inflammatory cytokine activity, by blocking either tumor necrosis factor-alpha or interleukin-1. They represent a significant advance in the treatment of systemic, inflammatory rheumatic diseases. These so called "biologics," or *biologic response modifying (BRM) agents*, have

Table 26.3 Drugs in the Management of Osteoarthritis and Rheumatoid Arthritis

Drug	Common Brand Names	Adverse Effects	Cautions and Contraindications
Analgesics Acetaminophen	Tylenol, Excedrin caplets, Panadol, Anacin-3	Potential for renal and liver toxicity	Not recommended with high alcohol consumption
NSAIDs Traditional	**OTC:** Advil, Motrin IB, Nuprin, Actron, Orudis KT, Aleve **Prescription:** Voltaren, Lodine, Nalfon, Ansaid, Indocin, Motrin, Orudis, Meclomen, Relafen, Naprosyn, Anaprox, Daypro, Feldene, Clinoril, Tolectin	Gastrointestinal bleeding, ulcers, nausea, diarrhea, indigestion, rash, dizziness, drowsiness, slowed blood clotting, tinnitus, fluid retention	Sensitivity or allergy to similar drugs; kidney, liver or heart disease; hypertension; asthma; ulcers; anticoagulant therapy
COX-2 Inhibitors	celecoxib (Celebrex), meloxicam (Mobic), nabumetone (Relafen)	May result in serious adverse events including cardiac complications and less serious GI side effects than traditional NSAIDS; allergic reactions; elevated blood pressure	Same as above; allergy to sulfa-containing drugs for celecoxib
Corticosteroids Systemic: oral or intravenous	Prednisone, prednisolone, methylprednisolone, triamcinolone, cortisone, hydrocortisone, dexamethasone	With long-term/high-dose: Cushing syndrome, osteoporosis, cataracts, insomnia, hypertension, immune suppression, elevated blood sugar, mood changes, restlessness, increased appetite	Diabetes, infection, hypothyroidism, hypertension, osteoporosis, gastric ulcer
Injection	Triamcinolone, prednisolone, methylprednisolone, dexamethasone, hydrocortisone, betamethasone	Post-injection flare (4–24 hours), transient systemic reaction, increased diabetic symptoms, soft tissue disruption from direct injection	Presence of infection, previous failure to respond
DMARDs Methotrexate	Rheumatrex	Common adverse effects: decreased appetite, abdominal discomfort, nausea, diarrhea, skin rash, itching, oral ulcers, photosensitivity, infection, unusual bleeding/bruising, bone marrow suppression Individual drugs may also have other specific toxicities and increase risk for other conditions	Liver or lung disease, alcoholism, immune system or bone marrow suppression, infection, pregnancy
Injectable gold	Myochrysine, Solganal		Kidney disease, bone marrow suppression, colitis
Oral gold—Auranofin	Ridaura		Previous adverse reaction to gold compound, kidney, liver or inflammatory bowel disease
Azathioprine	Imuran		Kidney or liver disease, pregnancy
Cyclophosphamide	Cytoxan		Kidney or liver disease, pregnancy, infection
Cyclosporin	Sandimmune Neoral		Kidney or liver disease, pregnancy, infection

Table 26.3 Drugs in the Management of Osteoarthritis and Rheumatoid Arthritis (continued)

Drug	Common Brand Names	Adverse Effects	Cautions and Contraindications
Hydroxychloroquine	Plaquenil		Antimalarial drug allergy, retinal abnormality, pregnancy
Penicillamine	Cuprimine Depen		Penicillin allergy, blood disease, kidney disease
Sulfasalazine	Azulfidine		Sulfa or aspirin allergy, kidney or liver disease, blood disease, bronchial asthma
Leflunomide	Arava		Liver disease
Minocycline	Minocin		Tetracycline or sun sensitivity
Biologic Response Modifiers	Etanercept (Enbrel), adalimumab (Humira), anakinra (Kineret), infliximab (Remicade)		Require subcutaneous injection or intravenous infusion (infliximab); increased risk for lymphoma

proved to be effective and offer the possibility of controlling rheumatic diseases to an extent not previously possible. Evidence demonstrates both inhibition of the progression of structural damage and improvement of physical function in RA.[60] The number of diseases in which these agents are useful continues to expand as do the number and types of agents available. Table 26.3 lists the most common DMARDs and the BRMs.

Corticosteroids

Corticosteroids are analogues of the naturally occurring hormone cortisone and are the most powerful anti-inflammatory drugs available. Corticosteroids may be given systemically via oral or intravenous routes, or locally via intra-articular or periarticular injection. After the discovery of cortisone in the 1940s and until the serious, life threatening side effects of long-term use were recognized in the late 1950s, cortisone was thought to be a "wonder drug." Side effects of long-term, high-dose systemic corticosteroids are now known to include osteoporosis, muscle wasting, adrenal suppression, increased susceptibility to infections, impaired wound healing, cataracts, glaucoma, hyperlipidemia, and aseptic bone necrosis. The use of systemic corticosteroids to halt inflammation is still indicated in cases where there is unremitting disease and severe extra-articular inflammation. However, the drug is administered in as low a dose as possible for as short a period of time as possible to maximize benefit and minimize adverse effects. Monitoring should include blood counts, serum potassium and glucose levels, and observation for side effects.

Local injection into a joint, bursa, tendon, or tendon sheath may be used when inflammation is localized. It is generally agreed that intra-articular injections provide benefit for local inflammation with minimal systemic effect, but should be limited to no more than two to four per year to reduce the risk of osteonecrosis and soft tissue damage.

Pharmacological Therapy in Osteoarthritis

Drug therapy in OA has no effect on disease progression and is ancillary to the more general measures of pain control, which include patient-related instruction, joint protection, and exercise.[46] The goals of drug therapy in patients with OA are to relieve pain and decrease inflammation when it is present. Oral analgesics, NSAIDs, and corticosteroid injections are the primary medications used in OA management.[58]

Acetaminophen, an oral analgesic, is usually the drug of first choice. Acetaminophen-containing compounds (Tylenol, Panadol, Anacin-3) have almost no toxicity in recommended doses and do not cause GI bleeding. However, there is no anti-inflammatory effect; acetaminophen cannot be substituted for NSAIDs in this regard. Clinical studies in OA demonstrate that acetaminophen (3 to 4 g/day) provides similar symptom relief to NSAIDs. Acetaminophen may be taken episodically as needed for pain or regularly when symptoms are more severe and long lasting.[46] Liver and kidney toxicity can occur with acetaminophen use. Hepatoxicity most often occurs after a drug overdose, but also may appear with therapeutic use, especially in individuals who drink excessive amounts of alcohol. Kidney toxicity is less common.

NSAIDs have a place in the management of persons with OA who do not respond to acetaminophen and nonpharmacological measures. NSAIDs may be used in combination with acetaminophen, and should be kept to the lowest effective dose to minimize GI toxicity. The COX-2 NSAIDs, described for RA management, had been prescribed for people who are at increased risk until longer-term trials called their safety into question. Common analgesics and NSAIDs are listed in Table 26.3.

Intra-articular corticosteroid injections are often used for acute episodes with an expected modest response. The knee is the most common site; however, soft tissue injections for subacromial, anserine, and trochanteric bursitis also may be effective.

Viscosupplementation or intra-articular injections of the knee with a form of hyaluronic acid (HA) is sometimes used. There are a number of synthetic forms available (Synvisc, Hyalgan, Artzal). HA is a naturally occurring polysaccharide that contributes to the thickness and viscosity of joint fluid in the healthy joint. In the OA knee, the levels of HA are lower and the joint fluid is thinner and less dense, reducing the ability of the fluid to lubricate and attenuate shock. Viscosupplementation therapy consists of a series of weekly injections. The reported effects of treatment are reduced pain and improved function in people with mild to moderate knee OA, which may last for several months. It is not clear if HA injections are more effective than corticosteroid injections, NSAIDs, or placebo injections.[61] The injected HA does not replace normal joint fluid to achieve its effect as most is absorbed and cleared from the joint within a week. The risk of side effects is low. The most serious reported adverse event is an allergic reaction and less serious effects are injection site reactions and joint swelling. There is no evidence that supports increased efficacy of one product over another.

Topical analgesics may be either rubifacients, which contain methyl salicylate, chemical compounds that produce a counterirritant effect, or capsaicin compounds, which reduce pain through depletion of the neurotransmitter substance P in peripheral nerves. To date, the only topical analgesic to show consistent efficacy in controlled clinical trials is capsaicin.[62] Capsaicin is an alkaloid derived from red chili peppers and is available in topical analgesic creams in varying concentrations (Zostrix, Capsaicin-P, Dolorac). It has been shown to decrease pain approximately 40 percent when applied to specific joints four times daily. The initial stinging or burning sensation disappears after several days of use; however, the need for frequent daily applications may limit the acceptability of this therapy for some patients.[46]

Surgical Management

Surgery represents one of the greatest advances in the management of arthritis in the last 40 years. Surgery is not appropriate, however, for every individual with either RA or OA, and the careful selection of the patient and the timing of the procedure are critical. The primary indications for surgery are pain, loss of function, and progression of deformity, although the last two are not always correlated. Surgical outcomes are greatly affected by the personal characteristics of the individual patient, such as motivation and the quality of postoperative rehabilitation. Postoperative rehabilitation goals are to restore mobility to the affected joint, promote stability within the joint, and regain active control of joint motion.

In general, there are three procedures that may be performed on soft tissues: **synovectomy**, soft tissue release, and tendon transfers. Similarly, there are three general bone and joint procedures: **osteotomy**, prosthetic **arthroplasty**, and **arthrodesis**. The choice of specific postoperative physical therapy procedures will depend on the particular surgical intervention, the extent of joint involvement prior to surgery, individual characteristics of the patient, and manifestations of the disease. It is particularly important to remember that a patient with RA, compared to a peer with OA, will have multiple joint involvement, which will ultimately affect the functional outcome of the procedure. A patient with RA is also likely to be a surgical candidate at a much younger age than a patient with OA.[1]

More than 500,000 *total joint arthroplasty (TJA)* surgeries of the hip or knee are performed annually, the majority of which are for patients with OA.[63] These highly successful procedures have revolutionized the management of disabling arthritis in the lower extremity (LE).[64] While studies reporting improved function and quality of life following TJA are not randomized controlled trials, a meta-analysis performed on more than 70 studies of outcomes found significant and lasting benefit.[65] The physical therapist is an important member of an interdisciplinary team involved in preoperative education, postoperative management, and rehabilitation. The primary goals following TJA are to restore function, decrease pain, and gain muscle control to enable the individual to return to previous, or improved, levels of functioning. Immediate postoperative and rehabilitation management is shaped by a variety of factors, including the type of prosthesis, as well as surgical technique and approach. Initial treatment includes therapeutic exercise, transfer and gait training, and instruction in ADL.[63] Once the individual has achieved an adequate level of function and is released from surgical precautions, instruction in establishing a routine of regular exercise and physical activity to support musculoskeletal and cardiovascular fitness is crucial to long-term outcomes and quality of life. A study investigating knee joint motion, strength, and gait in older persons who had undergone unilateral TJA at the knee 1 year previously and were considered to be "rehabilitation successes," found significant differences between the OA subjects and control subjects without arthritis in LE range of motion, muscle performance, and gait. During walking, active knee ROM was less than expected, ROM and angular velocity of knee and hip were less on the side with the arthroplasty and greater on the unaffected side, and joint loading was less at heel strike on the side with the arthroplasty and greater and more rapid on the unaffected side. Push off was diminished bilaterally, as were gait velocity and stride length.[66]

Rehabilitative Management

Because arthritis is a chronic, often progressive disease, care providers must always concern themselves with the long-range trajectory of the illness beyond the particular point in time that the care is provided. RA is a systemic disease with multiple impacts on all facets of the individual's life. OA can significantly alter a person's function and quality of life. Although each professional regards the individual as a whole person, the expertise of each professional addresses only certain aspects of the complex and interconnected problems faced by that individual. Without a broad range of expertise, none of these problems can be adequately solved. Therefore, the rehabilitation of the individual with arthritis requires the intense and coordinated efforts of a variety of health professionals, including physical therapists. Although a therapist may provide services to assist a person in adjusting to the effects of a medical condition, it is the individual who must live within the constraints imposed by the illness each day and who is the ultimate authority on the goals of therapy in whatever setting services are provided. The patient's ability to self-manage successfully is a major predictor of better health outcomes.[67] The physical therapist can play an important role in helping the patient with minimal disability gain confidence and experience in using self-management skills to deal with the condition. The objectives of treatment of OA and RA are similar: to manage pain, maximize function and impede or remediate musculoskeletal impairment, and teach self-management skills. The remainder of this chapter will discuss physical therapist examination and interventions for people with RA and OA of the hip and knee. Although OA also presents at other joints, these two are the most common and disabling sites for OA and are most frequently seen by a physical therapist.

Physical Therapy Examination

An extensive and careful examination of the musculoskeletal system as it contributes to the overall functional ability of the patient is imperative. Because quality care of the individual with RA involves an entire team of professionals, the physical therapist must carefully review the chart, if one is available in the setting in which the services will be provided, and consult with all other caregivers to ascertain their proposed plans and goals of intervention.

The physical therapist should begin an examination by taking a patient history that will orient the therapist to the nature and extent of the current problem and relate that problem to the patient's past medical history. During the interview, the therapist should elicit from the patient that individual's understanding of the disease and what is personally seen as the major problem at hand. In particular, the therapist should be concerned with identifying "red flag" signs and symptoms that indicate the need for immediate medical follow up (Table 26.4).[68] Pain should be examined in terms of its location, duration, and intensity along with the other signs of inflammation (heat, erythema, and swelling). Specific information on joint symptoms, morning stiffness, previous level of activity, pattern and degree of fatigue, and current medication regimen should also be gathered. Although the majority of tests and measures used in examining the individual with RA and OA are generic to the practice of physical therapy, many of these procedures require particular adaptations owing to the nature of joint involvement. Following the history, a review of the cardiopulmonary, integumentary, and neuromuscular systems should be undertaken before performing more definitive examination of the musculoskeletal system.

Range of Motion

Goniometric measurement of passive range of motion (PROM) is indicated at all affected joints following a gross ROM screening. Common wisdom suggests that a complete goniometric baseline is useful for documenting the progression of a chronic disease. The method of measurement for each joint must be standardized in the clinical setting and used in every application. Specific training and periodic review of technique by all clinic staff should be conducted to ensure the long-term value of the data, especially with individuals with a chronic disease. Otherwise, the potential variations in intrarater and interrater reliability of goniometry will weaken the opportunity to compare data throughout the course of the disease.[69] Although such a database may be useful in terms of a particular physical therapy episode of care, it is of questionable value when compared to data collected by another therapist using a different instrument and method of measurement. If joint pain or poor activity tolerance prohibit measurement of PROM, the therapist may consider substituting a functional ROM test by asking the patient to touch various body parts (e.g., the top of the head and small of the back) to determine the ROM available for performing self-care activities. During the ROM examination, the therapist should note any tenderness, crepitus, or pain on movement.

A number of studies demonstrate that arthritis in "only one joint" is more typically a multi-joint problem. A consistent finding regarding LE ROM in the presence of OA of the knee is decreased ROM in the hip, knee, and ankle of the involved side, as well as significantly limited motion in all three joints of the uninvolved limb. When older persons with knee OA are compared to nonarthritic controls, ROM in both limbs and at all joints is diminished.[70]

Table 26.4 "Red Flags" Suggesting The Need for Urgent Evaluation and Management

Flag	Differential Diagnosis
History of significant trauma	Soft tissue injury, internal derangement, or fracture
Hot, swollen joint	Infection, systemic rheumatic disease, gout, pseudogout
Constitutional signs (e.g., fever, weight loss, malaise)	Infection, sepsis, systemic rheumatic disease
Weakness	
Focal	Focal nerve lesion (compartment syndrome, entrapment neuropathy, mononeuritis multiplex, motor neuron disease, radiculopathy[a])
Diffuse	Myositis, metabolic myopathy, paraneoplastic syndrome, degenerative neuromuscular disorder, toxin, myelopathy,[a] transverse myelitis
Neurogenic pain (burning, numbness, parathesia)	
Asymmetric	Radiculopathy,[a] reflex sympathetic dystrophy, entrapment neuropathy
Symmetric	Myelopathy,[a] peripheral neuropathy
History of significant trauma	Soft tissue injury, internal derangement, or fracture
Claudication pain pattern	Peripheral vascular disease, giant cell arteritis (jaw pain), lumbar spinal stenosis

[a] Radiculopathy and myelopathy may be due to infectious, neoplastic, or mechanical processes.

When there is OA in a hip or knee, active motion in functional positions should be examined in all joints of both LEs. It is important to observe motion for symmetry and smoothness during gait, stair climbing, and arising from a chair. Ascending stairs requires the greatest amount and velocity of knee flexion and may be one of the best activities for determination of knee function.[66] Decreased ROM at the hip and knee increases the risk for injury and falls. Nearly 50° hip flexion and 90° knee flexion are required to recover balance from a stumble during walking.[71]

Strength

Application of standard manual muscle tests to determine strength may be limited because of pain at various points in the range. A patient may be strong in the pain-free portion of range but weak secondary to reflex inhibition in the very portion of the range that is essential to a functional activity. Joint effusions also inhibit muscle contraction.[72] Individuals with severe deformity and deranged joints are inappropriate candidates for traditional tests of strength. A functional test of strength, therefore, is more indicative of rehabilitation needs and will help identify the anticipated goals of strengthening programs prior to initiating treatment. An additional complicating factor in the application of conventional muscle tests is the frequent display of the lag phenomenon. Because the patient is able to move only partway through the available range, traditional grading systems are not sensitive to recording changes, because the gap between active and passive ROM narrows as a result of treatment. A therapist may want to comment specifically on the degrees of active motion and the grade of strength exhibited in that arc of motion. If a traditional testing method is used, therapists should also document the particular approach to testing used (e.g., break testing, isometric holding at the end of range, or resistance throughout the ROM), which will clarify the meaning of the grade assigned. Break testing generally yields higher grades than would be received if full range testing were done. It is also important to record whether the patient was receiving any medications that might alter performance or exercise tolerance. The therapist also may wish to document the time of day to account for the effects of morning stiffness.

The functional threshold for LE strength has yet to be determined. However, reports from studies that have examined knee strength as a percentage of body weight suggest that isokinetic strength measured at velocities between 60° and 180° per second should be 20 and 30 percent body weight for knee extension and 20 to 25 percent for knee flexion.[66,70] Isometric knee extension below 10 kg of force (measured with the hip at neutral and knee at 90°) corresponded to marked disability in a study of persons with OA of the knee.[45]

Joint Stability

The ligamentous laxity of any affected joint should be fully investigated. Ligamentous instability of UE and LE joints may be a significant deterrent to ADL and ambulation. Improper loading of an unstable joint may also further contribute to joint damage and pain.

Endurance

Fatigue is one of the systemic manifestations of RA and a symptom frequently reported by individuals with OA. Fatigue should be carefully examined both during the course of a single day and over several days to obtain a full understanding of its pattern. The decreased cardiovascular fitness of individuals with RA demands specific attention.[30] Heart rate, respiratory rate, blood pressure and ratings of perceived exertion should all be measured during a functional activity that is reasonably stressful for the patient's current level of fitness. Excessive increases may indicate the presence of inflammation or impairment of pulmonary and cardiac function and require more extensive and sophisticated tests and measures. Because the costosternal and costovertebral articulations are synovial joints, chest expansion, breathing, and coughing may be compromised in the patient with RA and should be examined. It is also important to determine cardiovascular fitness in individuals with OA, as cardiovascular deficits are clearly associated with long standing or severe disease.[73]

Functional Examination

As with any long-term disease process, a number of different functional tests may be indicated. Functional measures may include ADL, work, and leisure activities (see Chapter 11). The choice of a functional instrument is influenced by several factors including the characteristics and needs of the individual patient, the level and depth of information required, and its predictive value in gauging the efficacy of treatment.[74–76] As with goniometric measurement, the reliability and validity of the instrument should be known if the data are to be used for comparative purposes. The *Functional Status Index,* which was designed expressly to be used in outpatient rheumatologic settings, is an instrument known to be reliable and valid, as well as provide enough baseline data to be an effective screen of patient performance (see Appendix A).[77,78] This instrument is used to establish an individual's function in a representative sample of typical ADL along the parameters of pain, difficulty, and dependence experienced by the individual in performing these activities. Another arthritis specific instrument, the revised *Arthritis Impact Measurement Scales (AIMS2),* expands the concept of function to include performance in psychological and social domains as well as physical function. The AIMS2 also measures the patient's satisfaction with current functional status and individual preferences for outcome.[79] The *Western Ontario MacMasters Osteoarthritis Index (WOMAC)* is a widely used, valid and reliable self-report instrument of 24-items in three categories specific to OA of the hip and/or knee (pain, stiffness, function). The WOMAC takes about 10 minutes to administer and is easily scored by hand. It is available in either Likert form (0–4) or visual analog scales.[80] Both the AIMS2 and the WOMAC are sensitive to clinical intervention and provide excellent clinically feasible, standardized measures in the domains of function and disability to monitor change over time.

Mobility and Gait

A complete and detailed gait examination is one of the most important contributions of the physical therapist to the rehabilitation team's understanding of the individual's functional abilities and serves to identify additional areas for examination and intervention (Table 26.5)[81] (see Chapter 10 for a complete discussion). Substantial differences in knee ROM and gait velocity between patients with either OA or RA and their peers without arthritis have been demonstrated.[82]

Sensory Integrity

Any indication of peripheral neuropathy or nerve involvement should be investigated using standard examination procedures (see Chapter 5). Sensory changes that are concomitant with other conditions such as diabetes or the normal aging process should be considered when appropriate.

Psychological Status

There is no personality type specific to individuals with RA or any other kind of arthritis that has been demonstrated in any scientifically acceptable way. Individuals with chronic arthritis experience years of functional and social loss that would stress any person's ability to cope and adapt.[83] Reports of pain, however, are significantly correlated with self-reports of depression, but not correlated with functional level.[84] The overall psychological status of the individual with RA is generally similar to those individuals with other chronic diseases that threaten a severe change in body image and disruption of social integration (see Chapter 2). Individuals respond to these threats with various coping strategies to maintain psychological equilibrium. No single strategy is better than another, although some strategies ultimately facilitate the achievement of positive outcomes, whereas others hinder an individual's progress toward self-chosen goals. Exploration of the patient's attitude toward rehabilitation, as well as that of family members, can assist the therapist in achieving goals and instill a realistic, yet positive, orientation to future functional ability. The individual with RA is requested to implement a series of changes in daily life with respect to medications, exercise, and self-care. Failure to comply with professional recommendations is often interpreted as a rejection of the care provider's assistance or psychologically maladaptive behavior. The physical therapist must avoid using one's professional authority as a reason to exert control over another person. Allowing the individual to set the

Table 26.5 Analysis of Gait Deviations, Physical Examination Findings, and Treatment Goals

Gait Deviations	Physical Examination Findings	Treatment Goals
Pronated foot Shuffled progression Decreased step length Initial contact with medial border of foot Decreased single-limb balance Prolonged double-support phase Late heel rise Plantarflexion of ipsilateral ankle in swing Genu valgus with weightbearing	Tenderness over subtalar midtarsal area Limited inversion range Weak and painful posterior tibialis muscle Pronated weightbearing posture of foot Lax medial collateral ligament of knee	Relieve subtalar and midtarsal joint stresses Increase ankle inversion Strengthen posterior tibialis muscle Stabilize hypermobile joints with rigid orthosis Maintain neutral alignment in stance by foot positioning
Hallux valgus Lateral and posterior weight shift Late heel rise Decreased single-limb balance	Lateral deviation of great toe Swelling of first MTP joint Shortening of flexor hallucis brevis muscle Tenderness of great toe Weakness of great toe abduction	Accommodate foot with wide toe box shoe Increase extension of great toe Relieve weightbearing stresses
Metatarsophalangeal joint subluxation Diminished roll off Decreased single-limb stance Apropulsive progression Decreased single-limb balance	Painful MTP heads with weightbearing Callus formation over MTP heads Ulcerations over MTP heads Limited MTP flexion Prominent MTP heads	Redistribute pressure with metatarsal bar Relieve pressure with soft cutout shoe insert Increase flexion mobility of MTP joints Accommodate foot with extra-depth shoe
Hammer or claw toes Diminished roll off Decreased single-limb stance Apropulsive progression Decreased single-limb balance	Posture of MTP joint hyperextension with proximal and distal interphalangeal joint flexion Posture of MTP and distal interphalangeal joint hyperextension with proximal interphalangeal flexion Callus formation at plantar tips and dorsum of proximal interphalangeal joint Limited MTP flexion	Improve toe alignment with metatarsal bar Accommodate foot with extra-depth shoe Diminish pressure with soft insert Increase toe mobility
Painful heel Toe-heel pattern No heel contact in stance Decreased stride length Decreased velocity Plantarflexion of ankle in swing Increased hip flexion in swing Decreased step length of contralateral limb	Painful active plantarflexion Painful passive and active dorsiflexion Swelling and pain at Achilles insertion Tenderness over spur Decreased ankle dorsiflexion range	Decrease inflammation with steroid injection or modalities Relieve weightbearing stress Decrease pressure over spur with soft shoe insert Maintain ankle mobility

From Dimonte and Light,[81] with permission.
MTP = metatarsal-phalangeal.

direction of treatment and to use the expertise of the care provider to attain these self-chosen goals offers the greatest opportunity for responsible and humane care.

Environmental Barriers

The therapist should be aware of physical barriers in the home and work environments that might require specific examination and recommendations for change (see Chapter 12). A discussion about the home and work environments may reveal conditions that impede regaining complete independence and make the individual aware of the possibilities for altering these environments. The costs of such changes may be a limiting factor for implementing these recommendations. The work environment affects employment and disability in more ways than the physical setting and task requirements. Acceptance and understanding by supervisors and co-workers of the disease and self-management requirements of the worker with arthritis are important determinants of maintaining employment and income.

Physical Therapy Intervention

The development of specific anticipated goals and expected outcomes for the individual with arthritis is based on the following general goals:

- Decrease pain.
- Increase or maintain the ROM of all joints sufficient for functional activities.
- Increase or maintain muscle strength sufficient for functional activities.
- Increase joint stability and decrease biomechanical stress on all affected joints.
- Increase endurance for all functional activities.
- Promote independence in all ADL, including bed mobility and transfers.
- Improve efficiency and safety of gait pattern.
- Establish patterns of adequate physical activity or exercise to maintain or improve musculoskeletal and cardiovascular fitness and general health.
- Educate the patient, family, and other personnel to promote the individual's capacity for self-management.

The specific goals and outcomes identified for each patient will depend on the type of arthritis, the clinical presentation, and individual circumstances. Goal-setting is best done cooperatively with the patient to ensure ongoing and open communication during the course of treatment. It is the physical therapist's responsibility to determine the plan of care (POC), implement that plan safely and effectively, and delegate responsibility appropriately to ensure that the patient's goals can be reached. Another component of professional accountability is clear and precise documentation that allows an outside party to determine the purposes of intervention and the degree to which the therapist realized these objectives. The therapist should also be able to ensure that these objectives are attained in the most expedient manner. Goals and outcomes should be specifically tailored to meet the needs of the patient and should be stated clearly in terms of measurable criteria and the time period proposed for achievement (e.g., increase ROM of the left shoulder in 3 weeks, and independent ambulation with platform crutches for at least 250 ft without fatigue within 1 month). Stating time frames for achievement of goals and outcomes serves as a check for the therapist. Failure to achieve a certain goal in a proposed period of time suggests that the therapist needs to reevaluate the nature of the problem or reformulate the POC along different lines to produce the desired effect. Goals and outcomes should be revised to reflect changes owing to other factors that may affect progress or alter the proposed time frames.

Modalities for Pain Relief

Therapists may choose from a variety of physical agents that provide heat or cold to affected areas. The primary purpose of these modalities is to manage pain and facilitate more comfortable exercise and physical activity. Superficial heat is used to produce localized analgesia and increase local circulation in the area to which it is applied. It penetrates only a few millimeters and does not enter the depth of the synovial cavity. Superficial heat can be delivered through a number of means: moist hot pack, dry heating pads and lamps, paraffin, and hydrotherapy. There is no conclusive evidence that any method of application achieves a significantly better therapeutic effect, but patients often report a greater tolerance for and comfort derived from moist heat. Paraffin is particularly useful in delivering superficial heat to irregularly shaped joints or to individuals who cannot tolerate the weight of a moist hot pack. Although paraffin mixtures can be concocted at home by the patient, instructions for their use should be provided cautiously because of the high flammability of the wax. Although hydrotherapy is one of the most expensive and time-consuming methods for delivering superficial heat, it does have the added advantage that the therapist can combine heat with exercise. It may also orient the patient to the value of a therapeutic aquatic program that can be undertaken in conjunction with or following treatment.

Deep heating modalities may affect the viscoelastic properties of collagen and increase the plastic stretch of ligaments, however their efficacy in arthritis is not demonstrated. Their use in treating individuals with RA during the acute stage of inflammation is contraindicated, as they may stimulate collagenase activity within the joint furthering its destruction.[85–87] Furthermore, modalities that do not readily translate to home use foster a dependency on clinical care and do not promote self-management.

Local applications of cold will also produce local analgesia and increase superficial circulation at the site of application following an initial period of vasoconstriction. Cold is particularly useful around joints that are swollen, a condition that usually worsens with the application of superficial heat modalities. Therapists may use either wet or dry application techniques. Superficial cold is contradicted in patients with **Raynaud's phenomenon** or *cryoglobulinemia,* linked to an abnormal protein (cryoglobulins) in the blood that gels at low temperatures. Both may be associated with RA.

Therapists may also wish to consider using other modalities for pain relief in treating the individual with RA, including transcutaneous electrical nerve stimulation (TENS), although the value of TENS as reported in the literature is inconsistent. A meta-analysis of studies investigating TENS for knee OA pain concluded that the mode of TENS applied did affect results, repeated use was more effective than a single application, and use for at least 4 weeks was the most effective.[88]

In RA, hand and wrist orthoses may be used to immobilize specific joints and help reduce pain and swelling by providing local rest and support. Splints may be functional splints, corrective splints, resting splints that are worn at night or periodically during the day, or soft compression devices. The use of functional wrist splints to decrease pain and increase function in RA appears to have merit. Reduced pain and improved grip and pinch strength are reported. There is some evidence that strength and dexterity may be impaired initially when a splint is applied. A study that investigated the effect of functional wrist splint wear on task performance reported that wearing a commercially available elastic wrist orthosis resulted in some decrement in performance speed on a number of common tasks, though pain was significantly reduced for all tasks.[89]

Orthoses also may be used to alleviate pain through biomechanical support or correction for individuals with knee OA. Foot orthoses designed to reduce calcaneal valgus or foot pronation and reduce mechanical stress at the knee appear to reduce pain in some individuals with knee OA.[90] Other methods that show promise in treating knee OA pain are patellofemoral taping[90] and load shifting knee braces.[91] All orthotic interventions require professional evaluation, selection, education, and monitoring of use.

Complete bed rest is rarely recommended. Adequate quality and quantity of sleep at night and short rests during the day are preferred. Inactivity is a common problem for people with arthritis. Inadequate physical activity results in deconditioning, depression, lower pain thresholds, diminished bone and soft tissue health, and increased risk for a number of serious conditions. Thus, a major goal of care is to assist the person to maintain or regain adequate levels of physical activity and avoid the unnecessary consequences of inactivity.

Joint Mobility

A major factor affecting joint mobility in individuals with RA is the level of inflammation and position in which they are kept when not in motion. Patients should be taught proper positioning when resting and should be encouraged to perform self-ROM to the extent possible to maintain motion. Therapists may apply neurophysiological principles of therapeutic exercise to lengthen shortened muscles.[92] Patients should be given the opportunity to rest frequently when performing these exercises. Pain should be respected at all times and should be minimal after exercise. Common wisdom recommends that *exercise-induced pain should subside within 1 hour*. If the patient reports discomfort in excess of 1 hour, it is a potential indicator that either the intensity or the duration of the exercise was too great and should be reduced at the next exercise session. Patients should be encouraged to exercise on their own during those times of the day when they feel best. Local pain relief modalities prior to or following treatment are important considerations and should be used as indicated.

In hip and knee OA, manual therapy may offer some benefit within a comprehensive treatment program that includes exercise.[93] Manual therapy is not generally recommended for individuals with RA who have joint inflammation or resultant laxity.

Strengthening

Decreased muscle function (strength, endurance, power) in persons with arthritis arises from a number of sources: intra-articular and extra-articular inflammatory disease processes, side effects of medication, disuse, reflex inhibition in response to pain and joint effusion, impaired proprioception, and loss of mechanical integrity around the joint. A variety of conditioning programs can be effective for improving strength, endurance, and function without exacerbation of pain or disease activity.

Initially, isometric exercise may be indicated to improve muscle tone, static endurance, and strength and to prepare joints for more vigorous activity. Although isometric exercise does avoid the concern of joint motion and mechanical irritation, it can produce other unwanted effects. Isometric exercise at more than 40 percent maximal voluntary contraction constricts blood flow through the exercising muscle. Restricted circulation in the muscle can produce unnecessary postexercise muscle soreness, and the increased peripheral vascular resistance produces increased blood pressure. In the knee and hip, high-intensity isometric contraction has been shown to significantly increase intra-articular pressure and reduce synovial circulation.[94,95]

Instructions to a patient for isometric exercise should include the cautions to: (1) maintain the contraction for no more than 6 seconds; (2) avoid maximal effort because it is neither necessary nor desirable; (3) exhale during the contraction and inhale during a similar time period of relaxation; and (4) not contract more than two muscle groups at a time.

Dynamic exercise includes both shortening (concentric) and lengthening (eccentric) contractions. Strength and endurance may be improved through resistance (physiological overload) supplied by weight of the body part or external resistance in the form of free weights, elastic bands, or a variety of resistive exercise equipment. A cautious approach to resistance training is recommended to protect unstable or

Table 26.6 **Purposes, Parameters, and Precautions for Isometric and Dynamic Exercises for Strengthening**

Isometric	Dynamic
Purpose	
• Minimize atrophy • Improve function and weightbearing activity • Improve muscle tone • Maintain/increase static strength and endurance	• Increase muscle power • Improve function • Promote strength of bone and cartilage • Maintain/increase dynamic strength and endurance • Enhance synovial blood flow
Parameters	
• Perform at functional joint angles • Intensity: ≤ 70% one MVC • Duration: 6 second contraction • Frequency: 5–10 repetitions daily	• Perform in pain-free range • Use functional activities/movement patterns • Intensity: Progress to ≤70% one RM • Capable of 8–10 repetitions of motion against gravity before additional resistance • Duration: Progress to 8–10 exercises, 8–10 repetitions • Frequency: 2–3 times/week on alternate days
Precautions	
• May increase blood pressure • Exhale during contraction; avoid Valsalva maneuver • May increase intra-articular pressure • Decreased muscle blood flow	• May increase biomechanical stress on unstable or malaligned joints • Avoid forces on involved hands and wrists • May increase intra-articular pressure

MVC = maximal voluntary contraction; RM = repetition maximum.

inflamed joints from damage. Strengthening exercise should be performed within the pain-free range. Maximum benefit and maintenance can be achieved by incorporating functional movements and body positions in the recommended exercise routine. The patient should learn to perform exercises rhythmically with well-controlled movement toward the end part of the range and to modify resistance, repetitions, or frequency as needed. Gradual progression of resistance and repetition is recommended. Reduction in intensity, frequency, or motion should be made if increased joint swelling or pain occurs. Table 26.6 summarizes major considerations in selecting isometric or dynamic strengthening.

Individuals with RA benefit from maintaining or restoring muscular fitness. A number of well-controlled studies have reported results of strengthening regimes that provide overload and result in positive adaptations in muscle and functional performance with no exacerbation of disease symptoms.[96] Loads of up to 70 percent one repetition maximum (1RM) used in a circuit resistance training program of persons with controlled RA demonstrated no exacerbation in joint symptoms and significant improvements in strength and function.[32]

In persons with knee osteoarthritis, the evidence is strong and consistent that LE exercise that includes neuromuscular and functional training reduces pain and improves function. Interventions have included isometric, isotonic, and functional exercise, as well as proprioceptive and balance training. Interventions have been tested in both clinically supervised and self-directed settings with positive results and acceptable adherence.[97] Evidence supporting the use of exercise in the management of knee OA is presented in Evidence Summary Box 26.3.[98–101]

Joint Protection

Therapists should target functional activities that require specific techniques of joint protection.[102] A randomized controlled trial that compared the effects of an education-behavioral joint protection program to standard education (each consisting of 4 two-hour sessions), demonstrated that patients in the joint protection group adhered to joint protection strategies and had significantly less pain, morning stiffness, disease flares, visits to the doctor, and difficulties with ADL at 6 and 12 months following the intervention.[98] Patients should be encouraged to incorporate joint care into all ADL to minimize pain and conserve energy (see Appendix B).

In addition to reducing pain and improving function, orthoses also may provide support and protection for vulnerable and painful joints. Foot orthotics or specially designed shoes can serve the dual purpose of relieving biomechanical stresses and enhancing function for the person with RA foot involvement.[24,103,104] The cost of special shoes may not be reimbursable under many insurance programs. A good shoe will provide support and eliminate unnecessary joint motion in the talocalcaneal joint with a firm and wide heel counter. It should also help to maintain normal bony alignment and accommodate all existing foot deformities within a toe box of adequate dimensions. Pressure should be evenly distributed along the plantar surface of the

Evidence Summary Box 26.3

Therapeutic Exercise in the Management of Knee Osteoarthritis (OA)

Reference	Subjects	Methods	Duration	Results
Baker, KR, et al[98] 2001	46 Ss Mean age 69 ± 6 Knee pain and radiographic OA	RCT; 2 groups Lower extremity strength training HEP: 3×/week, with home visits	4 months	Significant improvements in pain, strength and function. Strength gains correlated with functional gains
Thomas, RS, et al[99] 2002	786 Ss Mean age 62 ± 9 self-reported knee pain	RCT Strength training HEP daily	24 months; evaluations every 6 months	Significant improvements in pain, stiffness, function, and isometric strength
Huang, MH, et al[100] 2003	132 Ss mean age 62 ± 5 radiographic OA	RCT Compared isotonic, isokinetic, isometric strength training 3×/week	8 weeks with 1 year follow-up	Significant improvements in pain, and disability walking speed in all exercise groups; isotonic group had more pain reduction and better retention.
Fransen, M, et al[101] 2002	1 RCTs 1633 Ss	Systematic review		Moderate improvements in pain and small improvements for function

HEP = home exercise program; RCT = randomized clinical trial; Ss = subjects.

foot during weightbearing. To achieve this goal may require the fabrication of orthoses. A *rocker sole* (shoe sole that is curved at the toe) can be used to facilitate toe off with limited ankle motion. A controlled trial was conducted of the effect of off-the-shelf extra-depth orthopedic footwear for people with RA and at least one year of foot pain. Outcomes were pain, gait, and physical function after 2 months of wearing the extra-depth shoes. The footwear group improved significantly on self-reported disability, weightbearing and non-weightbearing pain, and gait. In addition to extra depth in the shoe toe box, the shoes provided greater rear foot stability, an arch support, a stiff shank, and a padded heel collar above the heel counter for improved fit. This study reported that walking pain accounted for 75 percent of the variability in physical function level of the subjects.[105]

Endurance Training

The cardiovascular fitness of individuals with RA or OA may be compromised. A number of well-controlled trials have reported the ability to improve this impairment through regular cardiovascular conditioning without aggravating joints. Programs similar to those designed for deconditioned individuals can be instituted for individuals with arthritis. If weightbearing is a barrier to exercise, a non-weightbearing apparatus such as a cycle ergometry or aquatic program may be used. For most people, walking and stationary bicycles are a safe and effective means of aerobic exercise.[96] Furthermore, patients who have engaged in such a program often report an increase in self-esteem and improved emotional status.[106–113] Medical screening as appropriate for age and medical condition should occur prior to beginning an exercise program that entails marked increase in physical activity levels.

Functional Training

Functional training for the individual with arthritis proceeds in the same fashion as for other individuals with similar deficits. Therapists may choose to reduce the functional demands of an activity either temporarily, such as under conditions of acute inflammation, or permanently by incorporating a variety of aids into ADL that substitute for lost ROM and strength. These modifications can include long-handled appliances and devices with built-up handles for easier grasp. There are aids for dressing and grooming as well as personal hygiene.

UE involvement in RA, particularly of the wrist and hands, may complicate the choice of an ambulation aid by precluding any weightbearing on these affected joints. In these instances, platform attachments can be used to transform the forearm into a weightbearing surface. Rearranging the home or work environment also can improve a person's functional abilities. Raising beds or chairs can reduce the effort needed to stand up. Railings placed around the bed, bath, and along stairways also can help increase an individual's independence.

Gait Training

Specific deviations will be evident throughout the gait cycle. These may include gait asymmetries, decreased velocity, cadence and stride length, prolonged period of double support, inadequate heel strike and toe-off, and diminished joint excursion through both swing and stance. Gait deviations in the patient with RA, specifically owing to foot pain or deformities, may also be evident (see Table 26.5).[81] Therapists should address the underlying joint and muscle impairments that contribute to these deviations in the gait training program with persons with any type of arthritis.

The degree to which the gait of an individual with arthritis should, or can, approximate normal is one of the most difficult questions in designing a therapeutic program. Some "abnormalities" such as antalgic limping may in fact reduce joint loading. Joint destruction may necessitate the introduction of ambulation aids as cumbersome as platform crutches or rolling walkers with platform attachments. The gait of the individual with RA or OA should be safe, functional, and cosmetically acceptable to the patient rather than an unattainable idealized version of the norm.

Decreased walking speed in arthritis is common, and there is general agreement that increased speed is a meaningful measure of functional improvement. For example, a person's ability to walk fast enough to cross the street with the timing of the traffic light is important for functional community locomotion. However, increased walking speed without attention to joint biomechanics may be undesirable. In a clinical trial of a nonsteroidal drug for persons with knee OA, all with a varus deformity, gait variables were included as outcome measures. The researchers found that self-reported pain diminished and walking speed increased in the active therapy group. At the same time, kinetic analysis of joint forces showed the increased speed was accompanied by increased adductor moment at the knee and greater loading of the medial compartment.[114] This additional loading of the joint and increased stress on lateral supporting tissue may not be worth the gains of increased speed. Attention to biomechanical factors thus should be considered in comprehensive management, even when drug therapy decreases pain and improves gait speed.

Education

Patient education in the rheumatic diseases has been shown to result in positive changes in knowledge, health behaviors, beliefs, and attitudes that affect health status, quality of life, and health care utilization.[115] As in any chronic illness, education should include information needed to deal with the condition (taking medications, exercise), self-management skills necessary to carry out important social and vocational roles, and resources needed to deal with the emotional consequences of chronic illness such as depression, fear, and frustration. The evidence is overwhelming that education designed to teach self-management skills and increase client self-efficacy for these tasks is the most effective.[116] The *Arthritis Foundation* (1330 West Peachtree Street, Atlanta, GA 30309, 404/872-7100; http://www.arthritis.org), can supply the clinician or the individual with a variety of educational materials, pamphlets, and self-help courses that will increase cognitive understanding of the disease process and self-management skills. Many local chapters of the Foundation hold individual and family support groups to increase psychosocial adaptation as well as run aquatic and land exercise programs in public facilities. The *Association of Rheumatology Health Professionals,* a division of the American College of Rheumatology (http://www.rheumatology.org), can provide the therapist with scientific and clinical enrichment for enhanced practice, as well as a network of professional colleagues who work in rheumatology.

Summary

RA and OA are the two kinds of arthritis that a physical therapist is likely to see in clinical practice. The primary functional limitations of the individual with RA or OA result from musculoskeletal impairments. Irregularities on the bone surface, loss of joint mobility, muscle weakness, and atrophy contribute directly to limitations in ADL and the ability to work. Pain secondary to changes in normal joint structure and function often limits function as well. Musculoskeletal impairments related to arthritis may also lead to impairments of other systems, such as decreased cardiovascular endurance for functional activities. The physical therapist is well suited to evaluate and treat these impairments, remediate the functional limitations, and educate the patient in self-management skills to avoid unnecessary disability. Rehabilitation of the individual with arthritis is most often directed toward restoring or maintaining joint mobility and strength and emphasizes functional retraining and health promotion.

Questions for Review

1. What epidemiological factors are related to RA?
2. What are the major pathological changes seen in RA?
3. State two hypotheses concerning the pathogenesis of RA.
4. Describe three factors that may predispose an individual to osteoarthritis.
5. Describe two changes in articular cartilage associated with OA.
6. Name at least two laboratory tests used in the diagnosis of RA and state their purposes.
7. Explain three parameters for orienting to radiographs.
8. Describe the typical joint changes seen with RA for the following joints: atlantoaxial, temporomandibular, carpals, knees, and talocalcaneal.
9. Define the following deformities: ulnar drift, swan neck, boutonniere, hammer toes, claw toes, and hallux valgus.

10. Describe the overall goals of medical management for RA and OA.
11. What are the primary indications for surgery in RA?
12. Describe the key points in taking a history for the individual with arthritis.
13. What adaptations of standard tests and measures should be made in examining the individual with RA?
14. What are the general goals of physical therapy in treating individuals with RA or OA?
15. Explain the goals and progression of a strengthening program.
16. Discuss treatment alternatives for increasing ROM.
17. Design a cardiovascular conditioning program for an individual with LE joint involvement.
18. State at least four principles of joint protection and give a practical application of each.
19. What criteria guide the selection of shoes for the individual with RA?
20. What are the purposes of splints?
21. Describe gait deviations commonly associated with RA.
22. Describe what kinds of assistive devices and ambulation aids are most often needed by the individual with.

Case Study

Two case studies are presented: Case 1 presents a patient with rheumatoid arthritis and Case 2 considers a patient with osteoarthritis.

CASE 1: RHEUMATOID ARTHRITIS

History

The patient is a 35-year-old married woman who has two children in elementary school and is a tax accountant. At this time, she works about 20 hours a week. She has been referred to physical therapy by her rheumatologist whom she has just seen for the third time. Her history indicates a 2-year period since her initial complaints of joint swelling and pain, fatigue, and increasing weakness. She had been diagnosed over this time with carpal tunnel syndrome, knee osteoarthritis, fibromyalgia, and Lyme disease; however, her symptoms continued to worsen on NSAIDs and antidepressants, and she was referred to the rheumatologist 3 months ago. History, physical examination, laboratory, and radiographic evidence have confirmed a diagnosis of seronegative RA. She began a course of methotrexate and NSAIDs 1 month ago.

Physical Therapy Examination

At the initial examination by a physical therapist, she reports that her morning stiffness is now less than 30 minutes (previous high of 3 hours), pain and swelling in hands, feet, and elbows is markedly less, and she is feeling more energetic. Systems review of the integumentary system is unremarkable except for a slight edema and redness of the distal joints of the UE. Her blood pressure and respiratory rate are within normal limits. Her resting heart rate is 72 but increases to 96 with modest exertion.

ROM is limited at the shoulder, elbows, wrists, and MCPs. She lacks 10° of knee extension and has no ankle dorsiflexion or hip extension beyond neutral. Strength is good minus to fair. She exhibits a forward head, rounded shoulder posture, with the beginning of a marked kyphosis. She complains of the most pain in wrists, elbows, and ankles, and general weakness. She is relieved that at last she has been diagnosed with a condition for which there is effective treatment and she trusts her rheumatologist. Her immediate goals are to regain comfortable motion, strength, and stamina and to avoid deformity. Eventually she expects to be able to return to full time employment.

GUIDING QUESTIONS

1. What are the anticipated goals and expected outcomes of intervention in this case?
2. Formulate a physical therapy plan of care.
3. What resources are available to her in the community as part of her program of patient-related instruction?
4. What supportive devices might be used to decrease symptoms and increase function?
5. How would her physical therapist optimally schedule her return visits to clinic?

CASE 2: OSTEOARTHRITIS

History

The patient is a 68-year-old African-American woman whose bilateral knee pain has increased over the past 6 months. She is 5 ft 2 in. tall and weighs 180 lbs. She has type 2 diabetes, hypertension, and hypercholesterolemia for which she takes prescribed medication. She lives with her daughter's family, takes care of the two elementary school-age grandchildren, and helps with housework during the day while the parents are at work. She is having trouble getting up and down from sitting, using stairs, getting in and out of the car, bathing the children, and walking for more than 10 minutes at a time. She has had intermittent knee pain and stiffness for the past 5 years and has treated symptoms with over-the-counter medications including aspirin, acetaminophen, and NSAIDs. She also has used topical agents and a number of alternative therapies.

She recently visited her primary care physician because the increased knee pain and stiffness has made it extremely difficult for her to continue her work in the home. Radiographs show bilateral joint space narrowing, more in the medial compartments, and greater on the right. There is evidence of bony sclerosis and osteophytes. Joint alignment is good on the left, but there is slight genu varum on the right. Her physician has suggested a course of conservative measures at this time and a consult with a physical therapist. The patient and her doctor have agreed to discuss surgical options if she is not satisfied with her condition in 3 to 6 months.

Physical Therapy Examination

Beginning with a history and systems review at the initial examination by the physical therapist, the patient reports that she no longer goes out to shop, visit, or eat out with the family because she is so slow, tires quickly, and requires help to get in and out of the car and up curbs and steps without rails. She admits to feeling low and blue much of the time. Her pain is usually relieved by rest, and wakes her up only occasionally at night. Her concerns are being able to stay active and to continue her role in the family. She has heard about glucosamine and chondroitin sulfate and asks about their effectiveness and safety. Her heart rate is 84, her blood pressure is 140/80, and her respiratory rate is 16. There is no appreciable increase of her vital signs with increased activity owing to the slow pace at which she moves. The integumentary integrity of all four extremities is unremarkable. Sensory integrity of the distal extremities is intact.

Selected tests and measures reveal weakness and loss of motion in hips, knees, and ankles bilaterally, an antalgic and slow gait, left knee pain of 7 out of 10 while walking and 9 out of 10 while climbing stairs, and right knee pain at 6 out of 10 for all activities on a visual analog scale (VAS). She is wearing house slippers and shows marked ankle pronation on the right. Weightbearing calcaneal valgus is 10° on the right; 5° on the left.

GUIDING QUESTIONS

1. What kinds of goals should the physical therapist discuss with the patient as the anticipated goals of intervention?
2. Formulate a home exercise program for this patient and determine an optimal schedule for follow-up by the physical therapist.
3. What kind of orthotic device would reduce this patient's impairments and increase her function?
4. What should be included in patient-related instruction to maximize this patient's function?
5. What strategies would maximize this patient's adherence to her home program?

References

1. Klippel, JH (ed): Primer on the Rheumatic Diseases, ed 9. Arthritis Foundation, Atlanta, 1997.
2. Arnett, FC, et al: The American Rheumatism Association 1987 revised criteria for the classification of rheumatoid arthritis. Arthritis Rheum 31:315, 1988.
3. Lawrence, RC, et al: Estimates of the prevalence of arthritis and selected musculoskeletal disorders in the United States. Arthritis Rheum 41:778, 1998.
4. Hannan, MT: Epidemiology of rheumatic diseases. In Robbins L (ed): Clinical Care in the Rheumatic Diseases. Association of Rheumatology Health Professionals, Atlanta, 2001, p 9.
5. Spector, TD: Rheumatoid arthritis. Rheum Dis Clin North Am 16:513, 1990.
6. Crow, MK, and Friedman, SM: Microbial superantigens and autoimmune response. Bull Rheum Dis 41:1, 1992.
7. Carpenter, AB: Immunology and inflammation. In Robbins, L, et al (eds): Clinical Care in the Rheumatic Diseases, ed 2. American College of Rheumatology, Atlanta, 2001, p 15.
8. Reveille, JD: The genetic contribution to the pathogenesis of rheumatoid arthritis. Curr Opin Rheumatol 10:187, 1998.
9. Gornisiewicz, M, and Moreland, LW: Rheumatoid arthritis. In Robbins, L, et al (eds): Clinical Care in the Rheumatic Diseases, ed 2. American College of Rheumatology, Atlanta, 2001, p 89.
10. Firestein, GS, and Zvaifler, NJ: The pathogenesis of rheumatoid arthritis. Rheum Dis Clin North Am 13:447, 1987.
11. Nichols, LA: History and physical assessment. In Robbins, L, et al (eds): Clinical Care in the Rheumatic Diseases, ed 2. American College of Rheumatology, Atlanta, 2001, p 31.
12. Moncur, C, and Williams, HJ: Cervical spine management in patients with rheumatoid arthritis. Phys Ther 68:509, 1988.
13. Kramer, J, et al: Rheumatoid arthritis of the cervical spine. Rheum Dis Clin North Am 17:757, 1991.
14. Hardin, J: Pain and the cervical spine. Bull Rheum Dis 50(10):1, 2001.
15. Jones, JV, and Covert, A: Diagnosis and management of arthritic conditions. In Walker JM, and Helewa A (eds): Physical Therapy in Arthritis. WB Saunders, Philadelphia, 1996, p 47.
16. Melvin, JL: Rheumatic Disease: Occupational Therapy and Rehabilitation, ed 3. FA Davis, Philadelphia, 1989.
17. Gibson, KR: Rheumatoid arthritis of the shoulder. Phys Ther 66:1920, 1986.
18. Hakstian, RW, and Tubiana, R: Ulnar deviation of the fingers. J Bone Joint Surg 49:299, 1967.
19. Pahle, JA, and Raunio, P: The influence of wrist position on finger deviation in the rheumatoid hand. J Bone Joint Surg 51:664, 1969.
20. Swezey, RL, and Fiegenberg, DS: Inappropriate intrinsic muscle action in the rheumatoid hand. Ann Rheum Dis 30:619, 1971.
21. Smith, EM, et al: Role of the finger flexors in rheumatoid deformities of the metacarpophalangeal joints. Arthritis Rheum 7:467, 1964.
22. English, CB, and Nalebuff, EA: Understanding the arthritic hand. Am J Occup Ther 7:352, 1971.
23. Nalebuff, EA: Diagnosis, classification and management of rheumatoid thumb deformities. Bull Hosp Joint Dis 24:119, 1968.
24. Moncur, C, and Shields, M: Clinical management of metatarsalgia in the patient with arthritis. Clin Manage Phys Ther 3:7, 1983.
25. Kirkup, JR, et al: The hallux and rheumatoid arthritis. Acta Orthop Scand 48:527, 1977.
26. Edstrom, L, and Nordemar, R: Differential changes in type I and type II muscle fibers in rheumatoid arthritis. Scand J Rheum 3:155, 1974.
27. Nordemar, R, et al: Changes in muscle fiber size and physical performance in patients with rheumatoid arthritis after 7 months physical training. Scand J Rheum 5:233, 1976.
28. Edstrom, L: Selective atrophy of red muscle fibers in the quadriceps in longstanding knee-joint dysfunction. J Neurol Sci 11:551, 1970.
29. Forrester, DM, and Brown, JC: The radiographic assessment of arthritis: The plain film. Clin Rheum Dis 9:291, 1983.
30. Ekblom, B, et al: Physical performance in patients with rheumatoid arthritis. Scand J Rheum 3:121, 1974.
31. Minor, MA, et al: Exercise tolerance and disease related measures in patients with rheumatoid arthritis and osteoarthritis. J Rheumatol 15:905, 1988.

32. Rall, LC, and Roubenoff, R: Body composition, metabolism, and resistance exercise in patients with rheumatoid arthritis. Arthritis Care Res 9:151, 1996.
33. Tessler, HH: The eye in rheumatic disease. Bull Rheum Dis 35:1, 1985.
34. Deal, CL, et al: The clinical features of elderly-onset rheumatoid arthritis. Arthritis Rheum 28:987, 1985.
35. Pincus, T, and Callahan, LF: Early mortality in RA predicted by poor clinical status. Bull Rheum Dis 41:1, 1992.
36. Callahan, LF, and Pincus, T: Mortality in the rheumatic diseases. Arthritis Care Res 8:229, 1995.
37. Yelin, EH, et al: The work dynamics of the person with rheumatoid arthritis. Arthritis Rheum 30:507, 1987.
38. Yelin, E, and Felts, WR: A summary of the impact of musculoskeletal conditions in the United States. Arthritis Rheum 33:750, 1990.
39. Lubeck, DP: The economic impact of arthritis. Arthritis Care Res 8:304, 1995.
40. Yelin, EH: Musculoskeletal conditions and employment. Arthritis Care Res 8:311, 1995.
41. Allaire, SH, et al: Reducing work disability associated with rheumatoid arthritis: Identification of additional risk factors and persons likely to benefit from intervention. Arthritis Care Res 9:349, 1996.
42. Kellgren, JH, and Lawrence, JS: Atlas of Standard Radiographs: The Epidemiology of Chronic Rheumatism, vol. 2. Blackwell Scientific, Oxford, 1963.
43. Altman, R, et al: Development of criteria for the classification and reporting of osteoarthritis: Classification of osteoarthritis of the knee. Arthritis Rheum 29:1039, 1986.
44. Altman, R, et al: The American College of Rheumatology criteria for the classification and reporting of osteoarthritis of the hip. Arthritis Rheum 34:505, 1991.
45. McAlindon, TE, et al: Determinants of disability in osteoarthritis of the knee. Ann Rheum Dis 52:258, 1993.
46. Lozada, CJ, and Altman, RD: Osteoarthritis. In Robbins L et al. (eds): Clinical Care in the Rheumatic Diseases, ed 2. American College of Rheumatology, Atlanta, 2001, p 113.
47. Brandt, KD, and Fife, RS: Ageing in relation to the pathogenesis of osteoarthritis. Clin Rheum Dis 12:117, 1986.
48. Anderson, JJ, and Felson, DT: Factors associated with knee osteoarthritis (OA) in the HANES I survey: Evidence for an association with overweight, race and physical demands of work. Am J Epidemiol 128:179, 1988.
49. Coggon, D, et al: Occupational physical activities and osteoarthritis of the knee. Arthritis Rheum 43:1443, 2000.
50. Felson, DT, et al: Obesity and knee osteoarthritis: The Framingham Study. Ann Intern Med 109:18, 1988.
51. Threlkeld, AJ, and Currier, DP: Osteoarthritis: Effects on synovial joint tissues. Phys Ther 68:364, 1988.
52. Radin, EL, and Paul, IL: Does cartilage compliance reduce skeletal impact loads? The relative force-attenuating properties of articular cartilage, synovial fluid, periarticular soft tissues and bone. Arthritis Rheum 13:139, 1970.
53. Radin, EL, and Paul, IL: Response of joints to impact loading. I. In vitro wear. Arthritis Rheum 14:356, 1971.
54. Moscowitz, RW: Osteoarthritis—signs and symptoms. In Moskowitz, RW, et al (eds): Osteoarthritis: Diagnosis and Medical/Surgical Management, ed 2. Philadelphia, WB Saunders, 1992, p 255.
55. Gussoni, M, et al: Energy cost of walking with hip joint impairment. Phys Ther 70:295, 1990.
56. Guccione, AA, et al: The effects of specific medical conditions on the functional limitations of elders in the Framingham Study. Am J Publ Health 84:351, 1994.
57. Guccione, AA, et al: Defining arthritis and measuring functional status in elders: Methodological issues in the study of disease and disability. Am J Publ Health 80:945, 1990.
58. Miller, DR: Pharmacologic interventions in the 21st century. In Robbins, L, et al (eds): Clinical Care in the Rheumatic Diseases ed 2. American College of Rheumatology. Atlanta, 2001, p 169.
59. Watson, DJ, et al: Gastrointestinal tolerability of the selective cyclooxygenase-2 (COX-2) inhibitor rofecoxib compared with nonselective COX-1 and COX-2 inhibitors in osteoarthritis. Arch Intern Med 160:2998, 2000.
60. Furst, DE, et al: Updated consensus statement on biological agents for the treatment of rheumatoid arthritis and other immune mediated inflammatory diseases. Ann Rheum Dis 62 Suppl 2:ii2, 2003.
61. Lo, GH, et al: Intra-articular hyaluronic acid in the treatment of knee osteoarthritis: A meta-analysis. JAMA 290: 3115, 2003.
62. Zhang, WY, and Li Wan Po, A: The effectiveness of topically applied capsaicin: A meta-analysis. Eur J Clin Pharmacol 46:517, 1994.
63. Ganz, SB, and Viellion, G: Pre- and post-surgical management of the hip and knee. In Robbins L, et al (eds): Clinical Care in the Rheumatic Diseases, ed 2. American College of Rheumatology, Atlanta, 2001, p 221
64. The Orthopaedic Forum: NIH Consensus Statement on Total Knee Replacement December 8–10, 2003. J Bone Joint Surg Am 86:1328, 2004.
65. Ethgen, O, et al: Health-related quality of life in total hip and total knee arthroplasty. A qualitative and systematic review of the literature. J Bone Joint Surg 86:963, 2004.
66. Jesevar, DS, et al: Knee kinematics and kinetics during locomotor activities of daily living in subjects with knee arthroplasty and in healthy controls. Phys Ther 73:229, 1993.
67. Superio-Cabuslay, E, et al: Patient education intervention in osteoarthritis and rheumatoid arthritis: A meta-analytic comparison with nonsteroidal drug treatment. Arthritis Care Res 9:292, 1996.
68. American College of Rheumatology Ad Hoc Committee on Clinical Guidelines: Guidelines for the initial evaluation of the adult patient with acute musculoskeletal symptoms. Arthritis Rheum 39:1, 1996.
69. Norkin, CC, and White, DJ: Measurement of Joint Motion: A Guide to Goniometry, ed 3. FA Davis, Philadelphia, 2003, p 39.
70. Messier, SP, et al: Osteoarthritis of the knee: Effects on gait, strength, and flexibility. Arch Phys Med Rehabil 73:29, 1992.
71. Grabiner, MD, et al: Kinematics of recovery from a stumble. J Gerontol 48:M97, 1993.
72. Geborek, P, et al: Joint capsular stiffness in knee arthritis. Relationship to intraarticular volume, hydrostatic pressures, and extensor muscle function. J Rheumatol 16:1351, 1989.
73. Philbin, EF, et al: Cardiovascular fitness and health in patients with end-stage osteoarthritis. Arthritis Rheum 38:799, 1995.
74. Liang, MH, et al: Comparative measurement efficiency and sensitivity of five health status instruments for arthritis research. Arthritis Rheum 28:542, 1985.
75. Guccione, AA, and Jette, AM: Assessing limitations in physical function in patients with arthritis. Arthritis Care Res 1:120, 1988.
76. Guccione, AA, and Jette, AM: Multidimensional assessment of functional limitations in patients with arthritis. Arthritis Care Res 3:44, 1990.
77. Jette, AM: Functional capacity evaluation: An empirical approach. Arch Phys Med Rehabil 61:85, 1980.
78. Jette, AM: Functional Status Index: Reliability of a chronic disease evaluation instrument. Arch Phys Med Rehabil 61:395, 1980.
79. Meenan, RF, et al: AIMS2: The content and properties of a revised and expanded Arthritis Impact Measurement Scales health status questionnaire. Arthritis Rheum 35:1, 1992.
80. Katz, PP (ed): Health outcome measures. Arthritis Care Res 49(5 Suppl) S1–232, 2003.
81. Dimonte, P, and Light, H: Pathomechanics, gait deviations, and treatment of the rheumatoid foot. Phys Ther 62:1148, 1982.
82. Brinkmann, JR, and Perry, J: Rate and range of knee motion during ambulation in healthy and arthritic subjects. Phys Ther 65:1055, 1985.
83. Parker, JC, Wright, GE, and Smarr, KL: Psychological assessment. In Robbins L, et al (eds): Clinical Care in the Rheumatic Diseases, ed 2. American College of Rheumatology, Atlanta, 2001, p 69
84. Bradley, LA: Psychological aspects of arthritis. Bull Rheum Dis 35:1, 1985.
85. Harris, ED, Jr, and McCroskery, PA: The influence of temperature and fibril stability on degradation of cartilage collagen by rheumatoid synovial collagenase. New Engl J Med 290:1, 1974.
86. Feibel, A, and Fast, A: Deep heating of joints: A reconsideration. Arch Phys Med Rehabil 57:513, 1976.
87. Oosterveld, FGJ, et al: The effect of local heat and cold therapy on the intraarticular and skin surface temperature of the knee. Arthritis Rheum 35:146, 1992.

88. Osiri, M, et al: Transcutaneous electrical nerve stimulation for knee osteoarthritis. The Cochrane Database of Systematic Reviews 2003 (1). Retrieved September 25, 2004 from htttp://www.chochrane.org.
89. Pagnotta, A, et al: The effect of a static wrist orthoses on hand function in individuals with rheumatoid arthritis. J Rheumatol 25:879, 1998.
90. Fitzgerald, GK, and Oatis, C: Role of physical therapy in management of knee osteoarthritis. Curr Opin Rheumatol 16:143, 2004.
91. Giori, NJ: Load-shifting brace treatment for osteoarthritis of the knee: A minimum 11/2-year follow-up study. J Rehab Res Dev 41:187, 2004.
92. Kisner, C, and Colby, LA: Therapeutic Exercise. Foundations and Techniques, ed 4. FA Davis, Philadelphia, 2002.
93. Deyle, G, et al: Effectiveness of manual physical therapy and exercise in osteoarthritis of the knee: A randomized, controlled trial. Ann Intern Med 132:173, 2000.
94. James, MJ, et al: Effect of exercise on 99mTc-DPTA clearance from knees with effusions. J Rheumatol 21:501, 1994.
95. Krebs, DE, et al: Exercise and gait effects on in vivo hip contact pressures. Phys Ther 71:301, 1990.
96. Stenstrom, CH, and Minor, MA: Evidence of the benefit of aerobic and strengthening exercise in rheumatoid arthritis. Arthritis Care Res 49:428, 2003.
97. Minor, MA: Impact of exercise on osteoarthritis outcomes. J Rheumatol 31 (Suppl 70): 81, 2004.
98. Baker, KR, et al: The efficacy of home based progressive strength training in older adults with knee osteoarthritis: A randomized controlled trial. J Rheumatol 28:1655, 2001.
99. Thomas, RS, et al: Home-based exercise program for knee pain and knee osteoarthritis: Randomized controlled trial. BMJ 325:752, 2002.
100. Huang, MH, et al: A comparison of various therapeutic exercises on the functional status of patients with knee osteoarthritis. Semin Arthritis Rheum 32:398, 2003.
101. Fransen, M, et al: Therapeutic exercise for people with osteoarthritis of the hip or knee. A systematic review. J Rheumatol 29:1737, 2002.
102. Cordery, JC: Joint protection, a responsibility of the occupational therapist. Am J Occup Ther 19:285, 1965.
103. Locke, M, et al: Ankle and subtalar motion during gait in arthritic patients. Phys Ther 64:504, 1984.
104. Marks, RM, and Myerson, MS: Foot and ankle issues in rheumatoid arthritis. Bull Rheum Dis 46:1, 1997.
105. Fransen, M, and Edmonds, J: Off-the-shelf footwear for people with rheumatoid arthritis. Arthritis Care Res 10:250, 1997.
106. Harkcom, TM, et al: Therapeutic value of graded aerobic exercise training in rheumatoid arthritis. Arthritis Rheum 28:32, 1985.
107. Ekblom, B, et al: Effect of short-term physical training on patients with rheumatoid arthritis I. Scand J Rheum 4:80, 1975.
108. Ekblom, B, et al: Effect of short-term physical training on patients with rheumatoid arthritis II. Scand J Rheum 4:87, 1975.
109. Nordemar, R, et al: Physical training in rheumatoid arthritis: A controlled long-term study. I. Scand J Rheum 10:17, 1981.
110. Nordemar, R: Physical training in rheumatoid arthritis: A controlled long-term study. II. Functional capacity and general attitudes. Scand J Rheum 10:25, 1981.
111. Minor, MA, et al: Efficacy of physical conditioning exercise in patients with rheumatoid arthritis and osteoarthritis. Arthritis Rheum 32:1396, 1989.
112. Kovar, PA, et al: Supervised fitness walking in patients with osteoarthritis of the knee. Ann Intern Med 116:529, 1992.
113. Melton-Rogers, S, et al: Cardiorespiratory responses of patients with rheumatoid arthritis during bicycle riding and running in water. Phys Ther 76:1058, 1996.
114. Schnitzer, TJ, et al: Effect of piroxicam on gait in patients with osteoarthritis of the knee. Arthritis Rheum 36:1207, 1993.
115. Boutaugh, ML, and Brady, TJ: Patient education. In Robbins, et al (eds): Clinical Care in the Rheumatic Diseases, ed 2. American College of Rheumatology, Atlanta, 2001, p 155.
116. Lorig, K, and Gonzalez, V: The integration of theory and practice: A 12-year case study. Health Educ Q 19:355, 1992.

Supplemental Reading

Ottawa Panel Evidence-Based Clinical Practice Guidelines for Therapeutic Exercises in the Management of Rheumatoid Arthritis in Adults. Phys Ther 84:934, 2004.

Ottawa Panel Evidence-Based Clinical Practice Guidelines for Electrotherapy and Thermotherapy in the Management of Rheumatoid Arthritis in Adults. Phys Ther 84:1016, 2004.

Appendix A: Functional Status Index

Activity	Assistance (1–5)	Pain (1–4)	Difficulty (1–4)	Comments
Mobility				
Walking inside	______	______	______	______
Climbing up stairs	______	______	______	______
Rising from a chair	______	______	______	______
Personal Care	______	______	______	______
Putting on pants	______	______	______	______
Buttoning a shirt/blouse	______	______	______	______
Washing all parts of the body	______	______	______	______
Putting on a shirt/blouse	______	______	______	______
Home Chores				
Vacuuming a rug	______	______	______	______
Reaching into low cupboards	______	______	______	______
Doing laundry	______	______	______	______
Doing yardwork	______	______	______	______
Hand Activities				
Writing	______	______	______	______
Opening container	______	______	______	______
Dialing a phone	______	______	______	______
Social Activities				
Performing your job	______	______	______	______
Driving a car	______	______	______	______
Attending meetings/appointments	______	______	______	______
Visiting with friends and relatives	______	______	______	______

Used by permission of Alan M. Jette.

KEY:

ASSISTANCE: 1 = independent; 2 = uses devices; 3 = uses human assistance; 4 = uses devices and human assistance; 5 = unable or unsafe to do the activity

PAIN: 1 = no pain; 2 = mild pain; 3 = moderate pain; 4 = severe pain

DIFFICULTY: 1 = no difficulty; 2 = mild difficulty; 3 = moderate difficulty; 4 = severe difficulty

TIME FRAME: On average during the past 7 days

Appendix B: Joint Protection, Rest, and Energy Conservation

Joint Protection

Why Is Joint Protection Important?
Overuse and abuse of arthritic joints may lead to progressive deterioration of the joint and its surrounding tissues. Positive action is necessary to protect joints, conserve energy, and preserve function.

During activity, a normal joint is protected by the muscles around it that absorb the forces on the joint, preventing undue strain on the tendons, ligaments, and cartilage. A diseased joint is mechanically weak and poorly stabilized, which can contribute to the overstretching of the tendons and ligaments and damage to the cartilage. This increased stress can increase the destruction of the joint and cause increased pain.

How Can Joints Be Protected?
The main idea in joint protection is to minimize the strain on joints in daily activities. Joint protection techniques try to reduce the force on the joint, to slow down the joint damage. Good posture and positioning, changing the method of an activity, and pacing all help to protect the joint.

Which Joints Need Protection?
People with a local type of arthritis, like osteoarthritis, need to pay close attention to the joints that are involved with the arthritis. People with a systemic or whole-body type of arthritis, like rheumatoid arthritis, need to reduce the stress on all their joints. In addition to the joint protection principles and examples listed below, people with rheumatoid arthritis should look at the section below entitled Additional Reminders for Protection of the Rheumatoid Hand.

In planning your joint protection, start by concentrating on the joints that are currently giving you the most trouble. Check off the principles that apply most strongly to you, and list several examples of how you can apply that principle to your problem joints.

JOINT PROTECTION PRINCIPLES — Your Examples

☐ 1. *Respect Pain.*
- a. It is important to distinguish between discomfort and pain. __________
- b. Pain that lasts for more than 1 to 2 hours after an activity indicates that the activity is too stressful and needs to be modified. __________
- c. If there is a sharp increase in pain during activity, stop and rest, then modify the activity. __________
- d. If there is unusual pain or stiffness the next day, look back at the previous day's activities to see if they were too strenuous. __________

☐ 2. *Avoid Positions of Deformity.*
The foremost position of deformity for most joints is flexion, bending of the joint. Maintaining a bent position increases the possibility of deformity.
- a. Stand erect, with weight evenly divided on both feet. __________
- b. Lay as flat as possible in bed; do not curl up or prop yourself up on several pillows. __________
- c. Work with your hands flat. __________
- d. Avoid tight grip or squeezing. __________

☐ 3. *Avoid Awkward Positions.*
Use each joint in its most stable and functional position. Extra strain is placed on a joint when it is twisted or rotated.
- a. Rise straight up from sitting, rather than leaning to one side for support. __________
- b. Reposition feet rather than twisting trunk or knees. __________
- c. Stand on a stool to reach overhead. __________
- d. Reposition yourself closer to object rather than stretch your reach. __________
- e. Sit to clean or garden, rather than squatting or kneeling down. __________
- f. Use good posture when you stand, sit, and lie down. __________

☐ 4. *Use Strongest Joints or Distribute the Force over Several Joints.*
The stress on each individual joint is less if it is divided over several joints. The larger joints have greater muscles surrounding them to absorb the stress.
- a. Use two hands whenever possible. __________
- b. Carry packages in both arms rather than in one. __________
- c. Carry a shoulder purse, or purse handle over forearm rather than in fingers. __________
- d. Use knapsack to carry packages on back. __________
- e. Lift objects from underneath, using wrist and elbow, rather than pinch gripping the sides. __________
- f. Lift objects with your knees bent, your back straight. __________

g. Move large objects with body weight behind it, the push coming from the legs. __________
h. Push with open palm or forearm rather than fingers. __________

☐ 5. *Use Adapted Equipment.*
Find equipment that will reduce the stress on the joint or make the job easier.
The Self-Help Manual for People with Arthritis is a catalog of adapted equipment available from the local Arthritis Foundation. __________

a. Equipment can be modified by:
   1. Building up the handle so it is easier to grasp. __________
   2. Extending the handle so it is easier to reach. __________

b. Equipment available:
Walking aids
Self-care aids
Bathroom safety
Homemaking equipment
Job modification equipment

Joints that need protection: ____
____

Activities to be modified: ____
____
____

ADDITIONAL REMINDERS FOR THE PROTECTION OF THE RHEUMATOID HAND

1. Through exercise, maintain wrist extension (ability to pick hand up off table) to ensure power grip.
2. Through exercise, maintain supination (ability to turn palm up) to ensure ability to hold and to carry objects.
3. Avoid positions of deformity.
   a. Finger flexion
      1. Avoid making fist or tight grip—use built-up handles.
      2. Work with hand flat—use dust mitts, sponges.
      3. Avoid prolonged holding of objects: pen, book, pan, needle.
      4. Avoid putting any pressure on bent knuckles.
   b. Ulnar deviation (tendency of fingers to slide to little finger side)
      1. Avoid pressure toward little finger side of hand.
      2. Any twisting of hand, open door knobs, jars, etc., should be turned toward thumb.
      3. Grip objects parallel across palm, not diagonal; for example, hold utensil like dagger to cut food, stir with wooden spoon.
4. Avoid stress on small joints of hand.
   a. Use two hands whenever possible.
   b. Substitute larger stronger joints: for example, lift or carry with palms or forearm, not small finger joints; carry bag over elbow or shoulder, not in fingertips.
   c. Avoid activities involving pinching motions.
   d. Avoid twisting and squeezing motions with hands.

GETTING ADDITIONAL REST

Rest is important because it reduces the pain and fatigue that accompany arthritis. In addition, it aids the body's healing process and helps control the inflammation. Rest also may reduce the stress on joints and protect them from further damage. All of these benefits are important in managing arthritis.

Each day you need to make sure you get enough whole body rest, local joint rest, and emotional rest. There are many options: Mark off the options that may be possible for you.

☐ 1. *Plenty of Nightly Rest*
Get the usual 8 to 10 hours of nightly rest. It is not as important that you sleep for that length of time, but make sure you stretch out with your joints supported, so that your body can rest.

☐ 2. *Daily Rest Periods*
Ideally, several times a day you can stretch out for 15 to 60 minutes with your joints supported. Again, it is the body rest, not sleep, that is most important.

☐ 3. *Five-Minute "Breathers"*
Partway through a task, sit back and take it easy for a few minutes. This will allow you to finish the task almost as quickly but more comfortably and with less fatigue.

☐ 4. *Local Joint Rest*
When a joint hurts, stop and rest. If your hip or knee hurts while walking, sit down for a few minutes with your legs supported; if your hand hurts while writing, stop and lay it flat for a few minutes. Splints can be used to rest painful wrists or fingers. If your neck hurts, lay down with just a small pillow supporting the curve of your neck. Any painful joint can be given extra rest.

☐ 5. *Take Time for Relaxing Activities*
Listening to music, reading, playing cards, or other light leisure activites all can be a pleasant change of pace and can be restful and refreshing for you.

There are unlimited options for getting additional rest. It takes creativity to find ways to fit extra rest into your schedule; then it takes self-discipline to make sure you follow through, incorporating the additional rest in your activities. Making the effort to get more rest can pay off in a reduction of pain and fatigue.

Ways to get more rest:
Systemic, whole body rest ____________________
Local joint rest ____________________
Emotional rest ____________________

ENERGY CONSERVATION TO REDUCE FATIGUE

Why is Energy Conservation Important?

One of the major symptoms of arthritis may be fatigue—getting tired very easily. In the inflammatory types of arthritis, fatigue may be part of the disease process. In all types of arthritis, pain and difficult movement may use up energy, so you tire more easily.

It is important to avoid getting overtired. Fatigue may increase the possibility of a flare-up in inflammatory types of arthritis like rheumatoid arthritis. In all types of arthritis, fatigue may make the pain and stiffness seem worse, and it will make activities more difficult. We hope to reduce this fatigue by conserving energy and using it carefully.

How Can You Reduce Fatigue?

Some people try to conserve energy and reduce fatigue by staying in bed all day. Others stop doing anything that is not absolutely necessary each day. Unfortunately, the activities that are usually cut out are the leisure activities—the enjoyable things people do for themselves or for fun. These are not good ideas.

You can conserve energy and reduce fatigue by modifying and simplifying your activities, pacing yourself, getting additional rest, and using adapted equipment.

Energy Conservation

By conserving your energy, you may be able to do as much or more activity with less pain and fatigue. We are trying to avoid both overactivity and underactivity. Conserving your energy and simplifying your work is *not* being lazy. It is not sensible to overtire yourself. Overwork will not keep your joints mobile, but it may damage your joints further.

It is not so much *what* you do, but *how* you do it that can help control your fatigue. An attempt should be made to modify any activities that leave you overly tired or cause pain that continues for more than 1 to 2 hours.

You will need to identify ways that your own daily activities can be simplified. As you read through the energy conservation strategies, check off strategies that may work for you, and list several of your own examples.

☐ 1. *Plan the Task.*

Your Examples

a. Think the task through. ____________
b. Decide when and where the job is best done. ____________
c. Plan out the simplest approach to the job. ____________
d. Gather all supplies before you begin. ____________
e. Arrange step sequence so that it moves in one direction (usually left to right). ____________
f. Use fewer, more efficient movements to complete task. ____________

☐ 2. *Eliminate Extra Trips.*

a. Organize your shopping list according to how the store is laid out. ____________
b. Stay in the laundry room until your laundry is finished. ____________
c. Clean one area at a time. ____________

☐ 3. *Use Good Posture and Body Mechanics.*

a. Sit to work; you will be more stable and use your strength more efficiently. ____________
b. Use large strong muscle groups, rather than straining individual muscles and joints. ____________
c. Lift with your knees bent, your back straight. ____________
d. Carry objects close to your body. ____________
e. Push objects, with body weight behind it, rather than pulling or carrying. ____________
f. Avoid awakward bending, reaching, and twisting. ____________

☐ 4. *Don't Fight Gravity.*

a. Slide, rather than lift objects. ____________
b. Use wheeled cart. ____________
c. Use lightweight equipment. ____________
d. Stabilize pitcher on surface and tilt to pour, rather than picking it up. ____________

☐ 5. *Pace Yourself.*

a. Get plenty of nightly rest. ____________
b. Plan several rest periods during the day. ____________
c. Rest before you get tired. ____________
d. Avoid a rush. ____________
e. Work at a steady rate with rest period. ____________
f. Develop a rhythm to your movements. ____________

☐ 6. *Use Energy-Saving Devices.*

a. Convenience foods. ____________
b. Adapted equipment. ____________

Strategies to be tried: ____________________

Activities to be modified: ____________________

Excerpted from Brady, TJ: Home Management of Arthritis: Developing Your Own Plan. Arthritis Foundation, Minnesota Chapter, Minneapolis, 1983. Used by permission of the author.

CHAPTER

27

LEARNING OBJECTIVES

1. Describe the anatomy and physiology of the skin as an organ in the healthy state and damaged condition that occurs with a burn injury.
2. Describe the pathology, symptoms, and sequela of burn injuries.
3. Explain the treatment for a patient with various depths and extent of burn injury in relation to medical, surgical, and physical therapy management.
4. Identify the consequences of contracture formation after burn injury and the treatment of this condition.
5. Identify approaches to management of hypertrophic scars.
6. Provide a rationale for the type of skin care necessary after burn wound healing.
7. Analyze and interpret patient data, formulate anticipated goals and expected outcomes, and develop a plan of care when presented with a clinical case study.

Burns

Reginald L. Richard, PT, MS
R. Scott Ward, PT, PhD

OUTLINE

Burn injuries are one of the major health problems of the industrial world. In the United States, more than 1 million persons are burned each year (4.2/10,000) with approximately 4500 to 5000 related deaths.[1–3] In addition, it has been estimated that burn injuries account for 45,000 hospitalizations per year, with half being admitted to specialized burn treatment centers and half to other types of medical facilities.[1]

Although these data report the extent of the health care problem caused by burn injury, recent medical advances have significantly reduced the number of deaths from burn injuries and have improved the prognosis and functional abilities of surviving patients.[4,5] The survival rate has improved annually owing to improved resuscitation techniques, the acute medical and surgical care that are now available, and continued research into the management and care of the patient with burns. As a result of improvement in care, treatment, and survival of burned patients, more physical therapists will become responsible for treating these patients for a significant portion of their rehabilitation in settings other than a hospital burn center (e.g., outpatient clinics, community hospitals).

This chapter introduces the problems that occur with the different depths of burn injury and the complications that can result from thermal destruction of the skin. Current techniques used in the medical, surgical, and rehabilitative management of the patient who has been burned will be described. For more in-depth information regarding the examination and treatment of the patient with a burn injury, the reader is referred to additional sources.[6–9]

Epidemiology of Burn Injuries

Although the morbidity and mortality of patients with burns has dramatically decreased in recent years, the epidemiology of burns remains basically the same. There is a peak incidence of burn injury in children 1 to 5 years of age, primarily from scalds from hot liquids.[2,3] The primary cause of burn injury in adolescents and adults is accidents with flammable liquids. Men between the ages of 16 and 40 have the highest incidence of injury.[2] Fires that occur in homes and other structural dwellings are responsible for less than 5 percent of the hospital admissions for burn injuries, but account for nearly 12 percent of the burn-related deaths in this country.[2] Most of these deaths are due to inhalation injury. The number of burn-related accidents has decreased presumably because of better preventative measures, such as smoke detectors, education, and more stringent fire codes.[10]

A major reason for the improved prognosis and survival of patients with severe burn injury is the availability of specialized burn centers.[4] The advent of the burn center and the concentrated team care and focused research that has been generated by these facilities has improved the prognosis and survival of the most severely burned patient, as well as reduced the average hospital stay in most cases.

The American Burn Association[11] has established criteria for admission to a designated burn center as follows:

1. Partial-thickness burns greater than 10 percent of total body surface area (TBSA).
2. Full-thickness burns in any age group.
3. Burns that involve the hands, feet, face, perineum, genitalia, or skin overlying major joints.
4. Electrical burns including lightning injury.
5. Chemical burns.
6. Inhalation injury.
7. Burn injury in patients with preexisting illness that could complicate management.
8. Patient with a burn and coexistent trauma (e.g., fractures).
9. Patients who require special social, emotional, or long-term rehabilitation, including cases involving suspected child abuse.
10. Children with burns in hospital settings without qualified burn management personnel or equipment.

Twenty-five years ago, there were only 12 specialized burn centers. Today there are approximately 135 specialized centers for the care of patients with burn injuries and other skin disorders. This accounts for approximately 1700 beds in the United States.[12] Furthermore, burn centers now have begun to undergo the process of verification (voluntary quality assurance review) through the American Burn Association.[13]

A burn center is staffed by specialists—physicians, nurses, physical therapists, occupational therapists, dieticians, psychiatrists, psychologists, social workers, child life therapists, chaplains, pharmacists, vocational rehabilitation specialists, and other support personnel—who direct all their expertise toward the care, treatment, and rehabilitation of the patient with a burn injury. Each member is an integral part of the team, and the most effective burn centers are successful because of their team approach to the care of each patient.[4] It is historically noteworthy to mention that the interdisciplinary "team" approach to patient care was initiated by burn personnel with the founding and establishment of the American Burn Association in 1967.

Skin Anatomy and Burn Wound Pathology

The skin is the largest organ of the body, comprising approximately 15 percent of a person's total body weight. Anatomically, the skin consists of two distinct layers of tissue: the *epidermis*, which is the outermost layer exposed to the environment, and the deeper layer, termed the *dermis*.[14] Although not part of the skin per se, a third layer involved in the anatomical consideration of the skin is the subcutaneous fat cell layer directly under the dermis and above muscle fascial layers. These layers are illustrated in Figure 27.1. The epidermis is avascular, but it performs several vital functions. The stratum corneum gives the skin its waterproof characteristic and serves the role of protection from infection. The stratum granulosum is the layer responsible for water retention and heat regulation. The stratum spinosum adds a layer of protection to the underlying stratum basale layer. Cells in the basal layer enable the epidermis to regenerate. This layer also contains melanocytes, the cells that determine skin pigmentation. The interface between the epidermis and the dermis is termed the *rete peg region*. This area consists of an extensive series of epidermal–dermal ridges and valleys that serve to increase the surface area between the epidermis and the dermis. These ridges act as a reservoir of skin and are needed to overcome frictional forces that skin is exposed to in daily activity. Lack of these ridges in the healed burn wound will result in blisters from abrasion and poor adherence of the new epidermal tissue when it comes in contact with clothing or other surfaces.

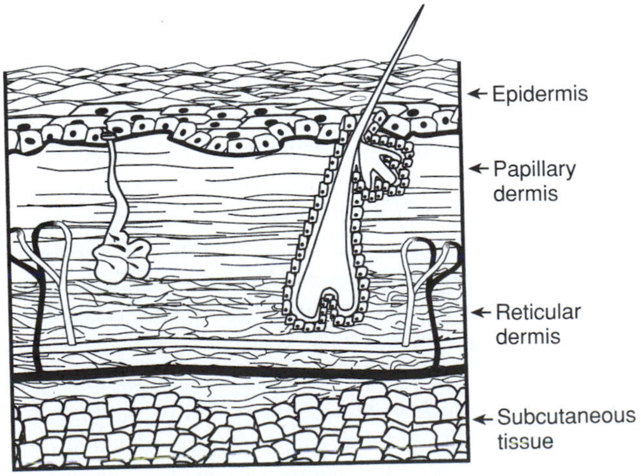

Figure 27.1 Cross-section of skin.

The dermis is considered the "true skin," because it contains blood vessels, lymphatics, nerves, collagen and elastic fibers. It also encloses the epidermal appendages (sweat ducts and sebaceous glands, and hair follicles), which provide a deep source of epidermal cells. The dermis is 20 to 30 times thicker than the epidermis. It is comprised primarily of interwoven collagen and elastic fibers, which provide the skin with its tensile strength and elasticity to resist deformation. The predominantly parallel orientation of normal collagen in the dermis is different than the whorls of collagen typically seen in scar tissue that result from burn injury.[15] The hierarchical location of sensory receptors in the skin is an important consideration for determining depth of burn injury (Table 27.1). The dermis can be subdivided into two layers: the superficial papillary layer and the deep reticular layer.[14] The papillae of the papillary layer project upward and interdigitate with the epidermis. The papillae contain vascular plexuses that serve, in part, to nourish the epidermis through osmosis. Morphologically, this layer is composed of a loose basket-weave network of collagen fibers. The reticular dermis lies below the papillary dermis and is composed of densely interwoven collagen fibers. The reticular dermis attaches to the subcutaneous tissue by an irregular interlacing network of fibrous connective tissue.

In addition to the functions mentioned already, the skin is important in temperature regulation through the excretion of sweat and electrolytes, secretion of oils that lubricate the skin, vitamin D synthesis, sensation, and cosmetic appearance and identity. As the result of a burn injury, some or all of these functions may be impaired and/or lost, and the patient's defense mechanisms will be compromised.

One basic pathophysiological consideration in a burn injury is the alteration of vascular integrity, which results in the formation of edema in the interstitial spaces. Edema formation occurs in the area of burn as well as in adjacent tissues. An initial concern of the physical therapist on the burn team is a decrease in joint range of motion (ROM) due to swelling.

The amount of skin destruction is based on temperature and length of time the tissue is exposed to heat.[16] The type of insult (i.e., flame, liquid, chemical, or electrical) also will affect the amount of tissue destruction. A tremendous amount of heat is not required to cause damage. At temperatures below 111°F (44°C), local tissue damage will not occur unless the exposure is for prolonged periods. In the temperature range between 111°F and 124°F (44°C to 51°C), the rate of cellular death doubles with each degree rise in temperature, and short exposures will lead to cell destruction.[16,17] At temperatures in excess of 124°F (51°C), exposure time needed to damage tissue is extremely brief.

Table 27.1 Location of Sensory Receptors in the Layers of the Skin

Structure	Location	Function
Free nerve ending	Epidermis	Pain, itch
Free nerve ending	Dermis	Pain
Merkel's disks	Stratum spinosum	Touch
Meissner's corpuscle	Papillary dermis	Touch
Ruffini's corpuscle	Papillary dermis	Warm
Krause's end bulb	Papillary dermis	Cold
Pacinian corpuscle	Reticular dermis	Pressure, vibration

Classifications of Burn Injury

Until recently, burn injuries were classified according to their severity as first, second, and third degree. Although the lay public may still use these classifications, most medical literature now classifies burn injuries by the depth of skin tissue destroyed.[17] The Guide to Physical Therapist Practice also describes impairments of the integument in relation to the depth of the tissue injury.[18] The degree to which a burn causes skin damage depends on many factors, including the duration and intensity of heat, skin thickness and area exposed, vascularity, and age.

The different classifications of burn wounds will present different clinical pictures, and each can change dramatically during the course of treatment. In addition to the amount of direct tissue damage from a burn, a patient's metabolic, physiological, and psychological condition can greatly affect the patient's clinical status. This section will present general clinical signs and symptoms seen in each of the burn wound classifications (Table 27.2).

Superficial Burn

A superficial, sometimes also referred to as an epidermal burn, causes cell damage only to the epidermis (Fig. 27.2). This depth of burn correlates to practice pattern 7B, Impaired Integumentary Integrity Associated with Superficial Skin Involvement, in the *Guide to Physical Therapist Practice*.[18] The classic "sunburn" is the best example of a superficial burn. Clinically, the skin appears red or erythematous.[19] The erythema is a result of epidermal damage and dermal irritation, but there is no injury to the dermal tissue. There is diffusion of inflammatory mediators from sites of epidermal damage and release of vasoactive substances from mast cells. The surface of a superficial burn is dry. Blisters will be absent, but slight edema may be apparent. After a superficial burn, there is usually a delay in the development of pain, at which point the area becomes tender to the touch.

The inflammatory reaction will cease, and the injured epidermis will peel off or desquamate in 2 to 3 days. Healing is spontaneous; that is, the skin will heal on its own, and no scar will be present.

Table 27.2 Burn Wound Classifications: Differential Diagnosis

Depth of Burn	Color/ Vascularity	Surface Appearance/ Pain	Swelling/Healing/ Scarring
Superficial	Erythematous, pink or red; irritated dermis	No blisters, dry surface; delayed pain, tender	Minimal edema; spontaneous healing; no scars
Superficial partial-thickness	Bright pink or red, mottled red; inflamed dermis; erythematous with blanching and capillary refill	Intact blisters, moist surface, weeping or glistening; painful; sensitive to changes in temperature, exposure to air currents, light touch	Moderate edema; spontaneous healing; minimal scarring; discoloration
Deep partial-thickness	Mixed red, waxy white; blanching with slow capillary refill	Broken blisters, wet surface; sensitive to pressure but insensitive to light touch or soft pin prick	Marked edema; slow healing; excessive scarring
Full-thickness	White (ischemic), charred, tan, fawn, mahogany, black, red; hemoglobin fixation; no blanching; thrombosed vessels; poor distal circulation	Parchment-like, leathery, rigid, dry; anesthetic; body hairs pull out easily	Area depressed; heals with skin grafting; scarring
Subdermal	Charred	Subcutaneous tissue evident; anesthetic; muscle damage; neurological involvement	Tissue defects; heals with skin grafting; scarring

Superficial Partial-Thickness Burn

With a superficial **partial-thickness burn** (Fig. 27.3) damage occurs through the epidermis and into the papillary layer of the dermis. The epidermal layer is destroyed completely, but the dermal layer sustains only mild to moderate damage. This depth of burn corresponds to practice pattern 7C, Impaired Integumentary Integrity Associated with Partial-Thickness Skin Involvement and Scar Formation, in the *Guide to Physical Therapist Practice*.[18] The most common sign of a superficial partial-thickness burn is the presence of intact blisters over the area that has been injured.

Although the internal environment of a blister is felt to be sterile, it has been shown that blister fluid contains substances that increase the inflammatory response and retard the healing process, and it is recommended that blisters be evacuated.[20–24] Healing will occur more rapidly if the skin is removed and an appropriate wound dressing applied.

Once blisters have been removed, the surface appearance of the burn area will be moist. The wound will be

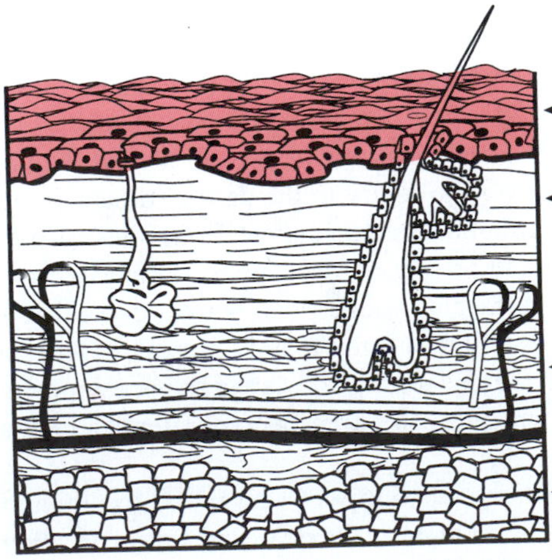

Figure 27.2 Shading represents depth of skin involved in a superficial burn.

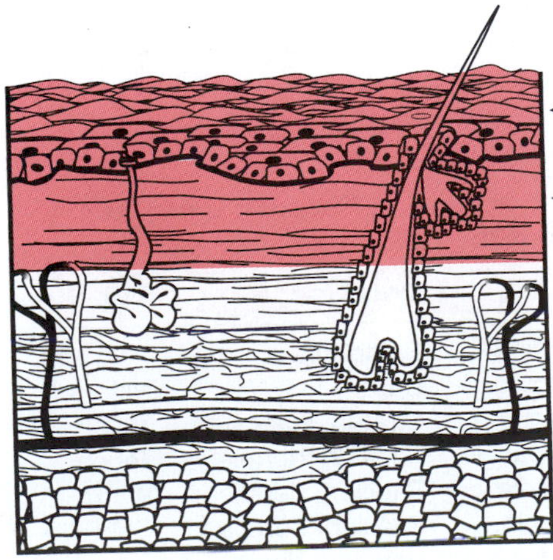

Figure 27.3 Shading represents depth of skin involved in a superficial partial-thickness burn.

bright red because the dermis is inflamed. The wound will **blanch**, which means that if pressure is exerted against the tissue with a finger, a white spot appears as a result of displacement of blood in the capillaries under pressure. On release of pressure, the white area will demonstrate brisk capillary refill. Edema can be moderate.

This type of burn is extremely painful secondary to irritation of the nerve endings contained in the dermis. When the wound is open, the patient will be highly sensitive to temperature changes, exposure to air, and light touch. In addition to pain, fever may be present if areas become infected.

Some topical antimicrobial creams will cause the wound to develop a gelatin-like film that eventually will peel off, similar to the **desquamation** that occurs with sunburn. This exudate is a coagulum of the topical antibiotic used to prevent infection and serum that seeps from the wound as a result of the insult to capillary integrity.

Superficial partial-thickness burns heal without surgical intervention, by means of epithelial cell production and migration from the wound's periphery and surviving skin appendages. Coverage by new epithelium resumes the barrier function of the skin, and complete healing should occur in 7 to 10 days. There may be some residual skin color change owing to destruction of melanocytes, but scarring is minimal.

Deep Partial-Thickness Burn

A deep partial-thickness burn injury (Fig. 27.4) involves destruction of the epidermis with damage of the dermis down into the reticular layer. As this burn nears the deepest dermis it begins to resemble a full-thickness burn. The depth best matches practice pattern 7C, Impaired Integumentary Integrity Associated with Partial-Thickness Skin Involvement and Scar Formation, in the *Guide to Physical Therapist Practice.*[18] Most of the nerve endings, hair follicles, and sweat ducts will be injured because most of the dermis is destroyed.

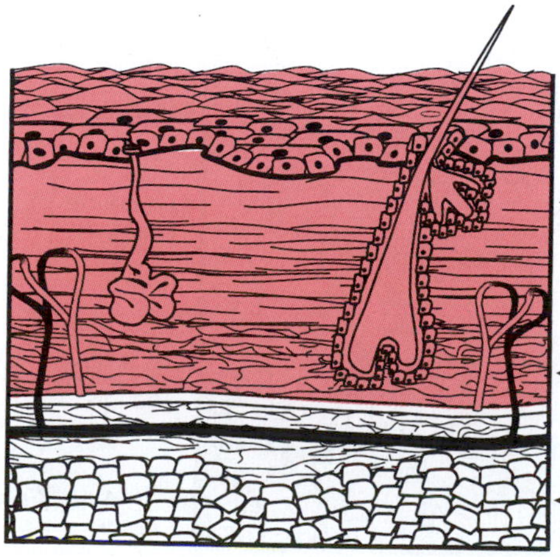

Figure 27.4 Shading represents depth of skin involved in a deep partial-thickness burn.

Deep partial-thickness burns appear as a mixed red or waxy white color. The deeper the injury, the more white it will appear. Capillary refill will be sluggish after the application of pressure on the wound.

The surface usually is wet from broken blisters and alteration of the dermal vascular network, which leaks plasma fluid. Marked edema is a hallmark sign of this burn depth. There is a large amount of evaporative water loss (15 to 20 times normal) because of tissue and vascular destruction.[16,25] An area of deep partial-thickness burn has diminished sensation to light touch or soft pin-prick, but retains the sense of deep pressure due to the location of the Pacinian corpuscles deep in the reticular dermis. Healing occurs through scar formation and re-epithelialization. By definition, the dermis is only partially destroyed; therefore, some viable epidermal cells may remain within the surviving epidermal appendages and serve as a source for new skin growth.

The depth of a deep partial-thickness injury is difficult to determine, so allowing the wound to demarcate during the first few days is necessary. Demarcation becomes evident after several days as the dead tissue begins to slough. Hair follicles that penetrate into the deeper dermal regions below the burn level remain viable. Preservation of hair follicles and new hair growth will indicate a deep partial-thickness burn rather than a full-thickness injury, and there is a corresponding greater potential for spontaneous healing. Factors that determine which epidermal structures survive and which die include the thickness of the skin in a particular location and/or the distance of the area from the source of heat.

Deep partial-thickness burns that are allowed to heal spontaneously will have a thin epithelium and may lack the usual number of sebaceous glands to keep the skin lubricated. New tissue usually appears dry and scaly, is itchy, and is easily abraded. Creams are necessary to artificially lubricate the new surface. Sensation and the number of active sweat ducts will be diminished.

A deep partial-thickness burn generally will heal in 3 to 5 weeks if it does not become infected. It is critical to keep the wound free of infection, because infection can convert a deep partial-thickness burn into a deeper injury. The development of **hypertrophic** and *keloid scars* are a frequent consequence of a deep partial-thickness burn.

Full-Thickness Burn

In a **full-thickness burn** (Fig. 27.5) all of the epidermal and dermal layers are destroyed completely. In addition, the subcutaneous fat layer may be damaged to some extent. This burn depth is consistent with practice pattern 7D, Impaired Integumentary Integrity Associated with Full-Thickness Skin Involvement and Scar Formation, in the *Guide to Physical Therapist Practice.*[18]

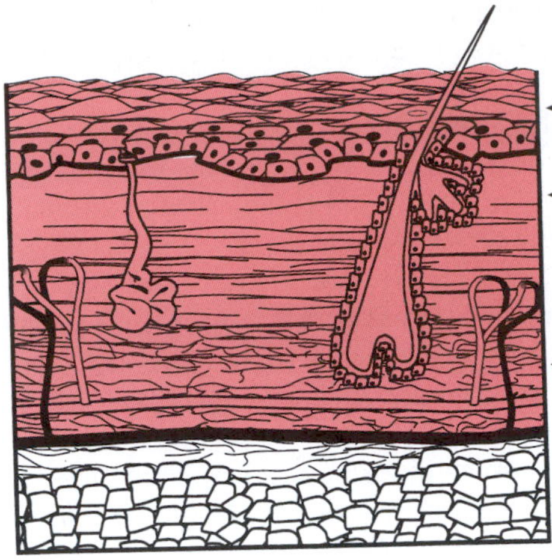

Figure 27.5 Shading represents depth of skin involved in a full-thickness burn.

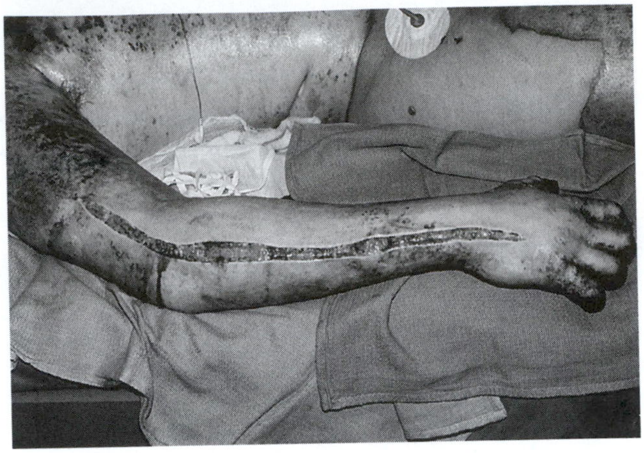

Figure 27.6 Escharotomy of the right upper extremity. (From Richard and Staley,[6] p 113, with permission.)

A full-thickness burn is characterized by a hard, parchment-like eschar covering the area. **Eschar** is devitalized tissue consisting of desiccated coagulum of plasma and necrotic cells. Eschar feels dry, leathery, and rigid. The color of eschar can vary from black to deep red to white; the latter indicates total ischemia of the area. Frequently, thrombosis of superficial blood vessels is apparent and no blanching of the tissue is observed. The deep red color of the tissue is due to hemoglobin fixation liberated from destroyed red blood cells.

Hair follicles are completely destroyed, so bodily hair will pull out easily. All nerve endings in the dermal tissue are destroyed, and the wound will be *insensate* (without feeling); however, a patient may experience a significant amount of pain due to adjacent areas of partial-thickness burn that usually surround a full-thickness injury.

A major problem that arises from deep burns is the damage to the peripheral vascular system. Because large amounts of fluid leak into the interstitial space beneath unyielding eschar, the pressure in the extravascular space increases, potentially constricting the deep circulation to the point of occlusion of blood flow. Because eschar does not have the elastic quality of normal skin, edema that forms in an area of circumferential burn can cause compression of the underlying vasculature. If this compression is not relieved, it may lead to eventual occlusion with possible necrosis of tissue distal to the site of injury. To maintain vascular flow, an **escharotomy** may be necessary. An escharotomy is a midlateral incision of the eschar.[26,27] Figure 27.6 shows an escharotomy and the result of pressure that forces the incision to gape. Following an escharotomy, pulses are monitored frequently. If the escharotomy is successful, there will be an immediate improvement in the peripheral blood flow, demonstrated by normal pulses distal to the wound, and by return of normal temperature, and capillary refill of the distal extremity.

Although it may be difficult to differentiate a deep-partial from a full-thickness burn in the early postburn period, the differences will become evident after several days. With a full-thickness burn, there are no sites available for re-epithelialization of the wound. All epithelial cells have been destroyed, and skin grafting of tissue over the wound will be necessary. Grafting will be discussed in detail in the section on surgical intervention in the treatment of burns.

Subdermal Burn

An additional category of burn, the *subdermal burn,* involves complete destruction of all tissue from the epidermis down to and through the subcutaneous tissue (Fig. 27.7). This depth of injury correlates with practice pattern 7E, Impaired Integumentary Integrity Associated with Skin Involvement Extending into Fascia, Muscle, or Bone and Scar Formation, in the *Guide to Physical Therapist Practice.*[18] Muscle and bone are subject to necrosis when burned. This type of burn occurs with prolonged contact

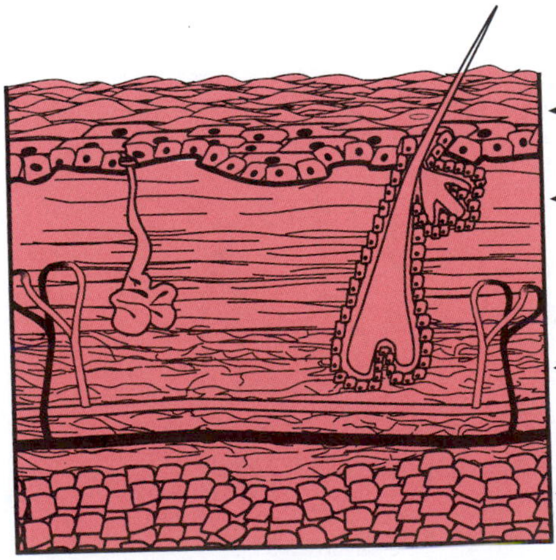

Figure 27.7 Shading represents depth of skin involved in a subdermal burn.

with a flame or hot liquid and routinely occurs as a result of contact with electricity. Extensive surgical and therapeutic management is necessary to return a patient to some degree of function.

Electrical Burn

The signs and symptoms of an **electrical burn** may vary according to the type of current, intensity of the current, and the area of the body the electric current passes through.[28] A burn results from the passage of an electric current through the body after the skin has made contact with an electrical source. Electric current follows the course of least resistance offered by various tissue. Nerves, followed by blood vessels, offer the least resistance. Bone offers the most resistance.

Typically, contact sites will exist where the patient first came into contact with the electricity and a second site where the patient was grounded. The wound where initial contact was made (may be referred to as the entrance wound) will appear charred and depressed, and many times, is smaller than the ground site. The skin appears yellow and ischemic. The ground site (may be referred to as the exit wound) sometimes appears as though there was an explosion out of the tissue at the site. It is dry in appearance. Tissues along the pathway of the current may be damaged as a result of the heat that developed. An extremity or area that appears viable after an injury may become necrotic and gangrenous in a few days. Arteries may undergo spasm, and there may be necrosis of the vascular wall. The blood supply to the surrounding tissues, including muscle, may be altered. Damaged muscle will feel soft. Because the course of tissue destruction is unpredictable, there may be unequal and uneven muscle damage. Time will be required to determine which tissues will remain viable and which will not.

There are other consequences of electricity passing through the body. One of the cardiac effects is arrhythmias, and possible causes of death from electrical burns are ventricular fibrillation or respiratory arrest. There also may be renal consequences leading to renal failure as a result of excessive protein breakdown and the shock to the kidney that follows a major trauma. One of the most severe complications of electric current damage is acute spinal cord damage or vertebral fracture. Clinically, these patients will have spastic paresis but may or may not have any sensory pathway changes over concomitant areas of spasticity.

Burn Wound Zones

The burn wound consists of three zones (Fig. 27.8).[17] In the *zone of coagulation* cells are irreversibly damaged and skin death occurs. This area is equivalent to a full-thickness burn and will require a skin graft to heal. Because of the lack of viable tissue and the amount of eschar, the risk of infection is increased. This potential complication emphasizes the need for careful monitoring, the use of antibiotics, and the treatment of a burned patient in a specialized burn center. The *zone of stasis* contains injured cells that may die within 24 to 48 hours without diligent treatment. It is in the zone of stasis that infection, drying, and/or inadequate perfusion of the wound will result in conversion of potentially salvageable tissue to completely necrotic tissue and enlargement of the zone of coagulation. Splints or compression bandages, if applied too tightly, can compromise this area. Finally, the *zone of hyperemia* is the site of minimal cell damage, and the tissue should recover within several days with no lasting effects.[29]

Extent of Burned Area

In addition to depth of burn injury, another major factor to consider when determining the severity of a burn is the extent of body burn. To calculate rapidly an estimate of the percentage of total body surface area burned, Polaski and Tennison[30] developed the **Rule of Nines**. The rule of nines divides the body surface into areas that are 9 percent, or multiples of 9 percent, of the total body surface. Figure 27.9 shows the percentages using the rule of nines for adults and children. Lund and Browder[31] modified the percentages of body surface area to account for a continuum of age and to accommodate for growth of the different body segments. This method is the more accurate means of the two methods to determine the extent of burn injury. Figure 27.10 shows the relative percentages of burned area for children and adults according to the Lund and Browder formula.

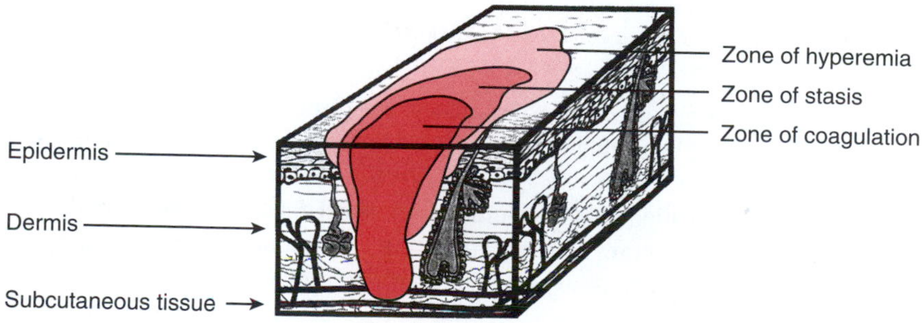

Figure 27.8 Zones of tissue damage as the result of a burn injury.

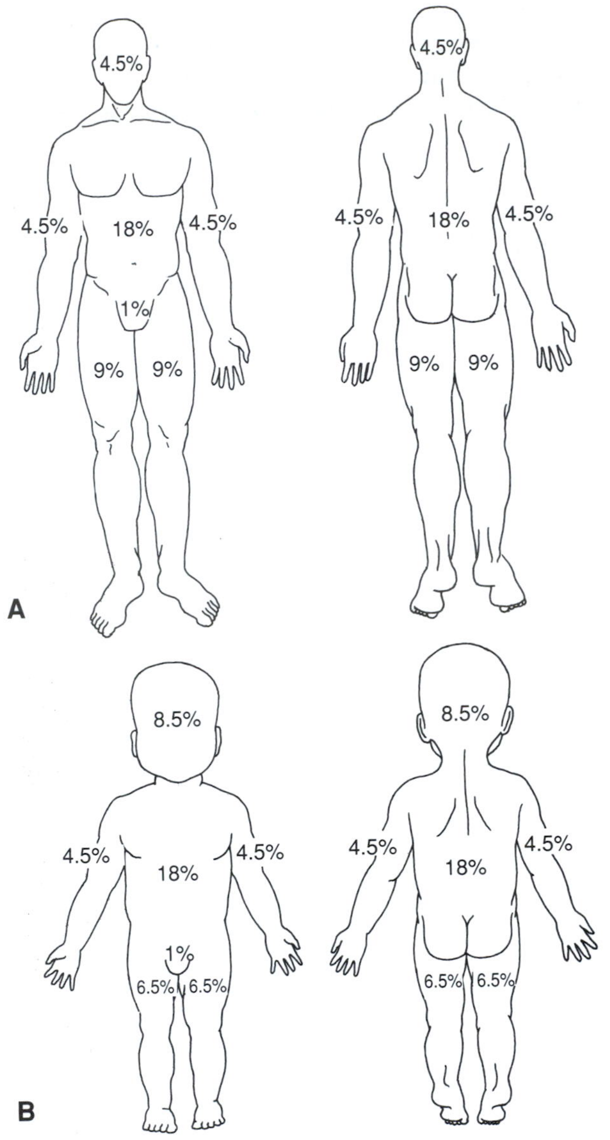

Figure 27.9 Rule of Nines to determine percentage of body surface area burn in adults (*A*) and children (*B*).

Although this formula provides an accurate examination of TBSA, the use of the rule of nines is more practical in the emergent triage of a patient with a burn injury.

Complications of Burn Injury

Depending on the extent of burn injury, the depth of the burn, and the type of burn, there may be secondary systemic complications.[32] In addition, the health, age, and psychological status of a patient who is burned will affect these complications. This section will highlight some systemic complications a patient may experience after a significant burn injury.

Infection

Infection, in conjunction with organ system failure, is a leading cause of mortality from burns.[33] Some virulent strains of *pseudomonas aeruginosa* and *staphylococcus aureus* are resistant to antibiotics and have been responsible for epidemic infections in burn centers.[1,33] Systemic antibiotics are used to treat both burn and general system infections once they have been documented.[33,34] A bacterial count in excess of 10^5 per gram of tissue constitutes burn wound infection and levels of 10^7 to 10^9 are usually associated with lethal burns. Most wounds are treated with topical antibiotics, and these will be discussed in the section on medical care of burns.

Pulmonary Complications

Any patient who has been burned in a closed space should be suspected of having an **inhalation injury**.[35] Among patients with burns, the incidence of smoke inhalation may be in excess of 33 percent,[36] and this rises to 66 percent in patients with facial burns.[37] Several studies have indicated that the incidence of pulmonary complications is extremely high after severe burns, and that death due to pneumonia alone is attributed to a majority of the deaths following burn injury.[38]

Signs of an inhalation injury include facial burns, singed nasal hairs, harsh cough, hoarseness, abnormal breath sounds, respiratory distress, and carbonaceous sputum and/or hypoxemia.[38]

The primary complications associated with this injury are carbon monoxide poisoning, tracheal damage, upper airway obstruction, pulmonary edema, and pneumonia. Lung damage from inhaling noxious gases and smoke may be lethal. To determine the extent of inhalation injury, several diagnostic procedures can be performed. The most helpful diagnostic procedure is bronchoscopy.[38]

Metabolic Complications

Thermal injury poses a great metabolic and catabolic challenge to the body. Most of the recent advances in burn treatment and rehabilitation have come directly from the increased understanding of the metabolic demands of a burn injury and from the ability to improve the patient's nutritional status to meet these demands.[39] The consequences of increased metabolic and catabolic activity following a burn are a rapid decrease in body weight, negative nitrogen balance, and a decrease in energy stores that are vital to the healing process.[40]

As a result of the increased metabolic activity, there will be an increase of 1.8°F to 2.6°F (1°C to 2°C) in core temperature that seems to be due to a resetting of the hypothalamic temperature centers in the brain.[1] Wilmore et al[41] hypothesized that there is a significant relationship between the increased evaporative heat loss from the impaired skin

**Burn Estimate and Diagram
Age vs Area**

Initial Examination

Cause of Burn_____

Date of Burn_____

Time of Burn_____

Age _____

Gender_____

Weight _____

Date of Admission_____

Signature _____

Date_____

Burn Diagram

Color Code

**Red – FT
Blue – PT**

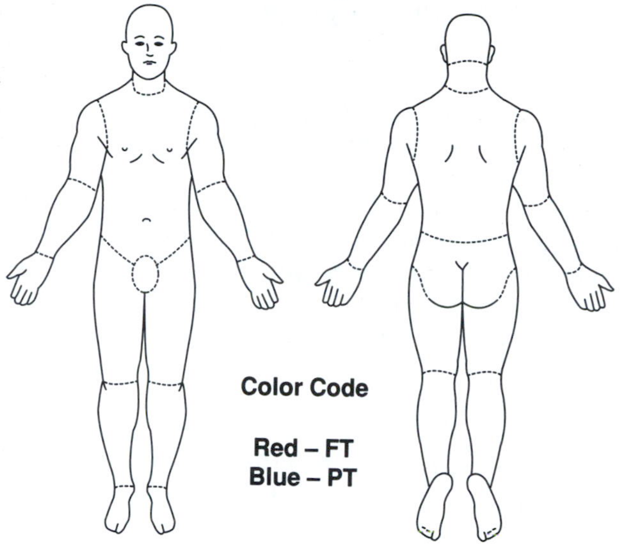

Area	Birth yr.	1–4 yrs.	5–9 yrs.	10–14 yrs.	15 yrs.	Adult	PT	FT	Total	Donor Areas
Head	19	17	13	11	9	7				
Neck	2	2	2	2	2	2				
Anterior Trunk	13	13	13	13	13	13				
Posterior Trunk	13	13	13	13	13	13				
Right Buttock	2$\frac{1}{2}$	2$\frac{1}{2}$	2$\frac{1}{2}$	2$\frac{1}{2}$	2$\frac{1}{2}$	2$\frac{1}{2}$				
Left Buttock	2$\frac{1}{2}$	2$\frac{1}{2}$	2$\frac{1}{2}$	2$\frac{1}{2}$	2$\frac{1}{2}$	2$\frac{1}{2}$				
Genitalia	1	1	1	1	1	1				
Right Upper Arm	4	4	4	4	4	4				
Left Upper Arm	4	4	4	4	4	4				
Right Lower Arm	3	3	3	3	3	3				
Left Lower Arm	3	3	3	3	3	3				
Right Hand	2$\frac{1}{2}$	2$\frac{1}{2}$	2$\frac{1}{2}$	2$\frac{1}{2}$	2$\frac{1}{2}$	2$\frac{1}{2}$				
Left Hand	2$\frac{1}{2}$	2$\frac{1}{2}$	2$\frac{1}{2}$	2$\frac{1}{2}$	2$\frac{1}{2}$	2$\frac{1}{2}$				
Right Thigh	5$\frac{1}{2}$	6$\frac{1}{2}$	8	8$\frac{1}{2}$	9	9$\frac{1}{2}$				
Left Thigh	5$\frac{1}{2}$	6$\frac{1}{2}$	8	8$\frac{1}{2}$	9	9$\frac{1}{2}$				
Right Leg	5	5	5$\frac{1}{2}$	6	6$\frac{1}{2}$	7				
Left Leg	5	5	5$\frac{1}{2}$	6	6$\frac{1}{2}$	7				
Right Foot	3$\frac{1}{2}$	3$\frac{1}{2}$	3$\frac{1}{2}$	3$\frac{1}{2}$	3$\frac{1}{2}$	3$\frac{1}{2}$				
Left Foot	3$\frac{1}{2}$	3$\frac{1}{2}$	3$\frac{1}{2}$	3$\frac{1}{2}$	3$\frac{1}{2}$	3$\frac{1}{2}$				
						Total				

Key: FT – Full Thickness
PT – Part Thickness

Figure 27.10 Modified Lund and Browder chart for determination of percentage of body surface area burn for various ages. (Courtesy Shriners Burns Hospital, Cincinnati, OH.)

barrier over a burn and the hypermetabolic state. In any event, if individuals with burns are placed in a room with normal ambient temperature, excessive heat loss will be exhibited, and this will further exaggerate the stress response seen in these patients.[1,41] Therefore, it is recommended that room temperature be kept at 86°F (30°C), which will significantly reduce the metabolic rate.

As part of the patient's altered metabolism, protein from muscle tissue is preferentially used as a source of energy. This situation, coupled with the effects of bed rest, causes muscles to atrophy and renders patients weak from both their burn injury and hospitalization.

Much of the improved management of burns has been attributed to the greater focus of research on the nutritional needs of patients. It is beyond the scope of this chapter to detail nutritional supplementation, and the interested reader is referred to several excellent reviews of advances in burn nutrition.[42–44]

Cardiovascular Complications

Hemodynamic changes result from a shift in fluid to the interstitium, which subsequently reduces plasma and intravascular fluid volume. Following these changes, there will be a tremendous initial decrease in cardiac output, which may reach 15 percent within the first hour after injury.[45,46]

Hematological and circulatory changes also occur after a severe burn injury. These changes include alterations in platelet concentration and function, clotting factors, and white blood cell components; red blood cell dysfunction; and decreases in hemoglobin and hematocrit.[47] These physiological alterations, coupled with cardiac changes and injured vascular beds, will significantly impact initial resuscitation efforts and, if the patient survives, how rapidly he or she will recover. In addition, patients will exhibit decompensation from an endurance standpoint.

Heterotopic Ossification

Patients with burns are highly susceptible to the development of *heterotopic ossification (HO),* as shown by prospective studies demonstrating a very high reported incidence.[48–51] However, the actual number of cases that progress on to becoming clinically problematic is relatively low.[50,51] Why HO occurs in patients with burn injuries is uncertain. Suspected etiologies include greater than 20 percent TBSA burn, immobilization, microtrauma, high protein intake, and sepsis. The most common areas affected are the elbows, followed by the hips and shoulders; however, HO can appear anywhere throughout the body.[50,51] Usually HO occurs in areas of full-thickness injury or sites that remain unhealed for prolonged periods of time. Symptoms appear late in a patient's course of recovery and include decreased ROM, point-specific pain, and a quality of reported pain that differs from that experienced by patients with a generalized burn injury.

Neuropathy

Peripheral neuropathy in patients with burns can take two forms: **polyneuropathy** or local neuropathy.[52] The cause of polyneuropathy is unknown. As with patients with HO, patients with peripheral neuropathy generally have a large TBSA burn, and the condition may be associated with sepsis. Fortunately, most neuropathies resolve over time.

Local neuropathies can be caused by a number of factors, most of which center on burn treatment issues, such as compression bandages applied too tightly, poorly fitted splints, or prolonged and inappropriate positioning of a patient.[52] The most common sites of involvement are the brachial plexus, ulnar nerve, and common peroneal nerve.

Pathological Scars

Burn scars occur in areas of deep partial-thickness burn that are allowed to heal spontaneously and in full-thickness burns that have been skin grafted, but where graft coverage is incomplete. Scars become pathological when they take on the form of hypertrophy, contracture or both. Each of these scar conditions is unique and should not be viewed as synonymous. A patient can have a hypertrophic scar that does not interfere with movement or a scar contracture band that is not hypertrophied. However, both conditions can exist simultaneously, and specific treatment for each is discussed later in this chapter.

Burn Wound Healing

The burn wound has been described and the causes and complications of burn injury have been reviewed. The remaining sections of this chapter will concentrate on the various types of medical and surgical therapeutic interventions and physical rehabilitation of the patient with a burn. First, however, it is necessary to outline the healing process of a burn wound.[53]

The two layers of the skin—the epidermis and dermis—differ morphologically, and they heal by separate mechanisms. In the following sections, the physiology of each component is described, and the clinical implications of burns to these areas are addressed.

Epidermal Healing

When a burn injures just the epidermis, or if there are viable cells lining the skin appendages, **epithelial healing** can occur on the surface of a wound. The stimulus for epithelial growth is the presence of an open wound exposing subepithelial tissue of the body to the environment. The intact epithelium attempts to cover an exposed wound through mitosis and the ameboid movement of cells from the basal layer of the surrounding epidermis into the wound. The epithelial cells stop migration when they are completely in contact with other epithelial cells. After this *contact inhibition,* cells can begin to differentiate to form the various layers of the epithelium. While epithelial cells move about the wound site, they maintain a connection with the normal epithelium at the wound margin. To continue migration and proliferation, a suitable base for the epithelial cells must be provided by adequate nutrition and blood supply, or else the new cells will die.

The process of epithelialization is most evident clinically in the partial-thickness wound that has intact hair follicles and glands. The epithelial cells from the skin appendages provide a source from which the wound may heal. The cells migrate outwardly from the appendages and appear as epidermal islands from which they spread peripherally into the wound. Skin growth and coverage actually can be seen over time from these epithelial islands.

Damage to sebaceous glands may cause dryness and itching of a healing wound. Lubrication can be a problem, and the new skin is characteristically dry and may split. Dryness may continue for a long time, because many of the sebaceous glands do not return to their normal function after a wound is epithelialized. Therapists need to educate patients about the type, frequency, and techniques of moisturizing cream application to lubricate newly healed tissue.

Dermal Healing

When an injury involves tissue deeper than the epidermis, **dermal healing**, or scar formation occurs. Scar formation can be divided into three phases: inflammatory, proliferative, and maturation. Although these phases will be described separately, they occur on a continuum and one phase often overlaps another.

Inflammatory Phase

The primary reaction of viable tissue to a burn wound is inflammation, which prepares the wound for healing through hemostatic, vascular, and cellular events. Inflammation begins at the time of injury, ends in about 3 to 5 days, and is characterized by redness, edema, warmth, pain, and decreased ROM. Initially, when a blood vessel is ruptured, the wall of the vessel contracts to decrease blood flow. Platelets aggregate, and fibrin is deposited to form a clot over the area. Fibrin serves a threefold function: (1) to partially retain body fluids, (2) protect the underlying cells from desiccation, and (3) to provide a firm coagulum substance from which cells can infiltrate. Therefore, fibrin can be thought of as forming a lattice network, from which cells can climb and work themselves into the healing structure.

After a transient vasoconstriction of the vasculature, which lasts about 5 to 10 minutes, vessels vasodilate to increase blood flow to the area. There is increased permeability of the blood vessels, with leaking of plasma into the interstitial space and subsequent edema formation. Leukocytes infiltrate the area and begin to rid the site of contamination. Of particular importance is the presence of the macrophage, which is responsible for attracting fibroblasts into the area.

Proliferative Phase

During this phase, re-epithelialization is occurring at the surface of the wound, while deep within the wound, fibroblasts are migrating and proliferating. **Fibroblasts** are the cells that synthesize scar tissue, which is composed of collagen and protein polysaccharides. In addition, the fibroblasts produce a viscous ground substance that surrounds the collagen strands. The collagen is deposited with a random alignment and no true architectural arrangement of fibers. Stress (e.g., a force intended to elongate the scar) applied to the developing tissue during this time causes the fibers to align along the direction of force.[54] During this period of fibroplasia, the tensile strength of the wound increases at a rate proportional to the rate of collagen synthesis.

In conjunction with collagen deposition, granulation tissue is formed during this phase. Granulation tissue consists of macrophages, fibroblasts, collagen, and blood vessels.[53] These newly formed blood vessels bring a rich blood supply to the area and encourage further wound healing. However, granulation tissue formation is not necessary for skin graft adherence, and excess granulation tissue may lead to increased hypertrophic scarring.

During the proliferative phase, **wound contraction** occurs. Wound contraction is an active process in which the body attempts to close a wound where a loss of tissue has occurred. The amount of contraction is determined by the amount of available mobile skin around the defect. It involves movement of existing tissue at the wound edge toward the center, not formation of new tissue. Wound contraction is stopped when (1) the edges of the wound meet, or (2) tension in the surrounding skin equals or exceeds the force of contraction. Skin grafting may decrease contraction, with thick grafts causing less contraction.

Maturation Phase

A wound is considered closed at the time epithelium covers the surface; however, wound healing involves remodeling of the scar tissue. During the maturation phase, there is a reduction in the number of fibroblasts, a decrease in vascularity due to a lesser metabolic demand, and remodeling of collagen, which becomes more parallel in arrangement and forms stronger bonds. The ratio of collagen breakdown to production determines the type of scar that forms. If the rate of breakdown equals or slightly exceeds the rate of production, maturation results in a pale, flat, and pliable scar. If the rate of collagen production exceeds breakdown, then a hypertrophic scar may result. This scar is characterized by being red and raised in appearance, and rigid in texture; it stays within the boundary of the original wound. A keloid is a large, firm scar that overflows the boundaries of the original wound; it is more common in darkly pigmented individuals. Both of these scars take a prolonged period of time to mature and can lead to both functional and cosmetic deformities.

Medical Management of Burns

Advances in the medical management of burns have resulted in the survival of thousands of patients who 15 or 20 years ago would have died of their injuries.[55] The research base and techniques available today at modern burn centers have enabled patients to receive better care through the use of more sophisticated techniques for the treatment of major burn injuries. This section will discuss the initial treatment of burn injuries and the surgical procedures associated with excision and grafting of new skin onto a burn wound.

Initial Management and Wound Care

The goals in the initial management of a patient with a burn are to address the major life-threatening problems and stabilize the patient through procedures designed to:

1. Establish and maintain an airway.
2. Prevent cyanosis, shock, and hemorrhage.
3. Establish baseline data on the patient, such as extent and depth of burn injury.

4. Prevent or reduce fluid losses.
5. Clean the patient and wounds.
6. Examine injuries.
7. Prevent pulmonary and cardiac complications.

Triage using these procedures applies to major burn trauma.

Initially, a patient must be transported from the site of injury to a treatment facility. If possible, transportation will be directly to a burn center, rather than to a hospital emergency room. The goals of treatment in transit are to stabilize the patient and maintain an airway. During the initial transportation phase, patient history and personal data are gathered when possible. The type of agent causing the burn is noted, and initial examination of the burn injury takes place. Emergency medical personnel may use the rule of nines to estimate the percent of burn injury. Furthermore, they will prepare the individual for triage at the burn center by removing all burned clothing and jewelry and initiating the administration of fluid through an intravenous line.

One of the major advances in burn care has been in fluid volume replacement initially and throughout a patient's treatment. Research has led to an improved understanding of the physiological changes that occur in a patient after a burn injury and of the fluid volumes necessary to improve the chance for survival.[44,46] Information about the physiological changes responsible for the shifts in body fluids and protein has led to the use of intravenous solutions in an amount necessary to replace vital fluid and electrolytes.[56]

After a patient arrives at a burn center and adequate fluid resuscitation has been initiated, the burn team determines the extent and depth of injury, and begins initial wound cleansing. Wound cleansing may be performed using a variety of approaches, although the majority of burn centers still incorporate hydrotherapy.[57-59] The initial wound care session allows the team to establish body weight, examine a patient fully, remove hair where necessary, and start the **débridement** process by removing any loose skin. The goals of wound cleansing and debridement are to remove dead tissue, prevent infection, and promote revascularization and/or epithelialization of the area. Depending on the facility, physical therapists may be involved in the wound cleaning procedure.[58,60,61]

A large hydrotherapy tank or whirlpool tub usually will have some form of disinfectant in the water to assist in infection control.[57,62,63] Water temperature should be between 98.6°F and 104°F (37°C to 40°C). While a patient is in the water, adherent dressings (if present) are removed. Care must be taken when removing the dressings to ensure minimal or no bleeding. The removal of dressings in the water is less painful than dry removal. Some burn units have converted to the use of showers, spraying, or "bed baths" for the removal of dressings and daily cleaning of wounds.[64] Regardless of the wound cleansing approach, most patients require pain medication prior to wound care.

After dressings are removed, the wound should be inspected carefully. The appearance, depth, size, exudate, and odor are noted. *Infection* is characterized by thick purulent drainage, odor, fever, a brownish-black discoloration, rapid separation of eschar, boils in adjacent tissue, or conversion of a deep partial-thickness burn to a full-thickness injury.

Wound care is carried out using clean technique and sterile instruments. If **sharp débridement** (the use of surgical scissors or scalpel and forceps to remove eschar) is performed, sloughed epidermis and loose eschar are removed and pockets of pus are drained. The procedure needs to be performed carefully so that bleeding is minimal.

After the wounds have been cleaned, the patient should be kept warm to reduce any further metabolic demands due to additional heat loss. Topical medications and/or dressings are then reapplied. Table 27.3 presents common topical medications used in the treatment of burns. The technique of applying a topical cream or ointment without dressings is called the **open technique** and allows for ongoing inspection of the wound and monitoring of the healing process. With this technique, the topical medication must be reapplied throughout the day.

The **closed technique** consists of applying dressings over a topical agent. Dressings serve several purposes: (1) they hold topical antimicrobial agents on the wound, (2) they reduce fluid loss from the wound, and (3) they protect the wound. Dressings are changed once or twice a day, depending on the size and type of wound, and the type of topical antimicrobial used.

Dressings consist of several layers. The first layer is nonadherent to protect the fragile healing surface from disruption. This may be followed by cotton padding to absorb wound drainage. The final layer consists of roll gauze or elastic bandages, which hold the other layers in place but allow movement.

Surgical Management of the Burn Wound

Primary excision is surgical removal of eschar. Much of the increased survival rate of patients with extensive burns has been due to the early primary excision of burn wounds.[65] Normally, a patient is taken to surgery after successful resuscitation, usually within 1 week of injury. As much of the eschar is removed at one time as possible. Proponents of early primary excision believe that this approach is easier on a patient than repeated débridements, and that it promotes more rapid healing, reduces infection and scarring, and is more economical in terms of staff and hospital time.[65]

In many burn centers, a burn wound is closed with a graft at the time of primary excision. There are many types of grafts that can be used to close a wound. An **autograft** is a patient's own skin, taken from an unburned area and transplanted to cover a burned area. Autografts are desirable because they provide permanent coverage of the wound. An **allograft (homograft)** is skin taken from an individual of the same species, usually cadaver skin. The skin can be kept

Table 27.3 Common Topical Medications Used in Treatment of Burns

Medication	Description	Method of Application
Silver sulfadiazine	Most commonly used topical antibacterial agent; effective against *pseudomonas* infections.	White cream applied with sterile glove 2–4 mm thick directly to wound or impregnated into fine mesh gauze.
Mafenide acetate (Sulfamylon)	Topical antibacterial agent; effective against gram-negative or gram-positive organisms; diffuses easily through eschar.	White cream applied directly to wound with thin 1–2 mm layer twice daily; may be left undressed or covered with thin layer of gauze.
Mafenide acetate solution (Sulfamylon 5% solution)	Topical solution with antimicrobial function against gram-negative and gram-positive organisms. Maintains moist environment.	50 gram packet of white powder mixed with either 1000 mL of sterile water or 0.9% sodium chloride soaked gauze.
Silver nitrate	Antiseptic germicide and astringent; will penetrate only 1–2 mm of eschar; useful for surface bacteria; stains black.	Dressings or soaks used every 2 hours; also available as small sticks to cauterize small open areas.
Bacitracin/Polysporin	Bland ointment; effective against gram-positive organisms.	Thin layer of ointment applied directly to wound and left open.
Collagenase, Accuzyme	Enzymatic débriding agent selectively débrides necrotic tissue; no antibacterial action.	Ointment applied to eschar and covered with moist occlusive dressing with or without an antimicrobial agent.

frozen in skin banks for prolonged periods. Allografts are temporary grafts used to cover large burns when there is insufficient autograft available. **Xenograft (heterograft)**, is skin from another species, usually a pig. Allografts or xenografts are used until there is sufficient normal skin available for an autograft.

Perhaps the most progressive advancement in the care of patients with burns in recent years is the use of **skin substitutes** for coverage of an excised wound.[66-71] Skin substitutes consist of cultured autologous skin, which is grown in a laboratory from a biopsy of a patient's own tissue, the use of altered cadaver skin, or other biologically engineered tissues. Skin substitutes are used when large areas of burn exist and coverage is necessary for a patient's survival. Cultured autologous skin takes several weeks to grow and is highly susceptible to infection. Other biologically engineered tissues are more readily available and have demonstrated more reliable adherence than in the past. With the use of most skin substitutes, ROM exercises may be delayed and shearing forces must be avoided. Although skin substitutes are an expensive intervention for wound coverage, they are useful and have proved effective in managing patients with large burn wounds. A few types of skin substitutes include:

1. *Cultured epidermal autografts (CEA)*: A skin biopsy is obtained from a patient, and only the epidermal cells are cultured.[66,67]
2. *Cultured autologous composite grafts*: A skin biopsy is obtained from a patient, and both epidermal and dermal cells are cultured. This forms a bilayer structure.
3. *Allogenic skin substitute*: The epidermal layer of skin and all immune cells are removed from cadaver skin. This tissue is applied to the graft bed and once adhered, a thin epidermal autograft or CEA is applied.[68]
4. *Cultured dermis (temporary)*: Cultured dermal matrix is seeded with human neonatal fibroblasts and used as a temporary covering in place of cadaver skin. This substitute eventually is removed and replaced with an autograft.[69,70]
5. *Cultured dermis (definitive)*: This skin substitute is composed of cultured bovine collagen with a silicone outer layer. Pores in the material allow for controlled growth of a neodermis. After approximately 14 days, the silicone layer is removed and a very thin skin graft or CEA is applied.[71]

Skin Grafting Procedure

The removal of skin to graft onto a burn wound is done surgically under anesthesia. The skin used for a graft usually is removed with a *dermatome*. This instrument not only allows the surgeon to obtain a large amount of skin, but a more consistent thickness of skin can be obtained. The dermatome is adjusted to remove a predetermined thickness of skin for a **split-thickness skin graft**. A split-thickness skin graft contains epidermis and only the superficial layers of the dermis, as opposed to a **full-thickness skin graft**, which consists of the full dermal thickness.

The site from which a skin graft is taken is called a **donor site**. Common donor sites include the thighs, buttocks, and

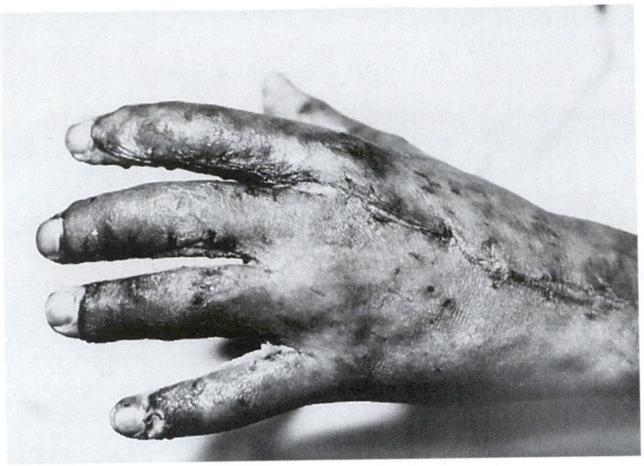

Figure 27.11 Sheet graft on dorsum of left hand, postoperative day 7. (From Richard and Staley,[6] p 183, with permission.)

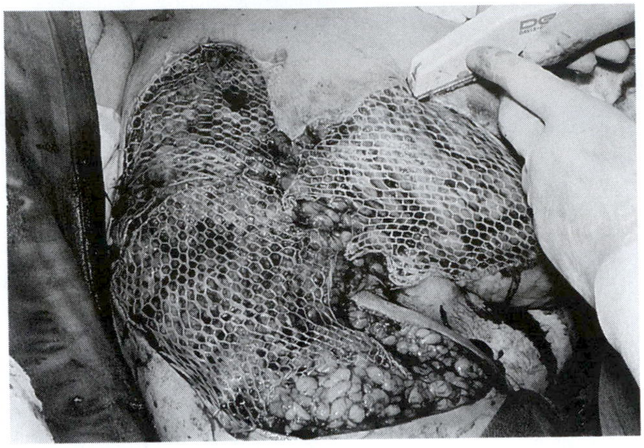

Figure 27.12 Meshed split-thickness skin graft applied to freshly excised wound and secured with staples.

back. These wounds heal by re-epithelialization, like a partial-thickness burn, and require appropriate care to prevent additional dermal damage with resultant scar formation. A full-thickness skin graft has the disadvantage of leaving a full-thickness wound that will require either primary closure or grafting with a split-thickness skin graft.

Generally, the thinner the skin graft, the better the adherence, and the thicker the graft, the better the cosmetic result. In addition, a thin graft will contract more than a thick skin graft once it has adhered to the wound bed. Selection of depth depends on many factors, including whether or not the donor site needs to be used again for another skin graft. Taking a thicker graft adversely affects the possibility of taking another graft from the same site for a prolonged period of time. Harvesting from split-thickness skin graft sites may be repeated in 10 to 14 days, depending on the amount of time the donor site takes to heal.

A **sheet graft** is a skin graft applied to a recipient bed without alteration following harvesting from a donor site (Fig. 27.11). The face, neck, and hands are covered with this type of graft for optimal cosmesis and function. When limited donor skin is available, most areas are covered with a **mesh graft** (Fig. 27.12). The meshing of a graft consists of processing the sheet graft through a device that makes tiny parallel incisions in a linear arrangement. This process permits the skin graft to be expanded before it is applied to the wound bed.[72] This technique allows coverage of a larger area, and once the graft adheres, the interstices heal through re-epithelialization.

A skin graft usually is held in place with sutures, staples, or Steri-Strips® (elastic skin closures). Once a graft is fixed in position, any blood or serum that might have become located between the graft and the recipient site should be removed. Application of a pressure dressing facilitates contact between the graft and recipient site.

One of the basic necessities for successful adherence of a graft is sufficient vascularity within the wound bed. Grafts will not adhere to poorly vascularized areas, such as tendon. Once a skin graft has been applied, separation of a graft from its bed must be prevented. Separation may result from shear force, mechanical trauma, or hematoma formation. Initially, an area is immobilized with a dressing that provides firm, even compression on the wound. Other reasons for graft failure include inadequate excision of necrotic tissue and infection.

Survival of a skin graft depends on several factors: (1) circulation, which provides a nutritive supply to the graft; (2) inosculation, or the process by which a direct connection is established between a graft and the host vessels; and (3) penetration of the host vessels into a graft site. Except in darkly pigmented persons, grafts are white in color at the time of transplantation and begin to show a pinkish hue within a matter of hours after their placement on an adequate vascular bed.

The re-establishment of circulation in a skin graft will take place through the formation of direct anastomosis between respective vessels, invasion from the host bed forming new channels, or both. Twenty-four hours after grafting, numerous host vessels will have penetrated the graft.[53] The invasion of new capillaries seems to be the most important consideration in vascularization. Normally, within 72 hours, inosculation has proceeded to the point where the skin graft is secure. Initially, structural connections are fibrous. Collagen is then laid down to secure the attachment of the graft.

Surgical Correction of Scar Contracture

If physical therapy interventions are unsuccessful in averting scar contracture formation, and limitations are noted in ROM and function, surgery may be required. In the past, reconstructive surgery usually was postponed while a burn wound was in the active, immature phase of scar formation.[73] More recently, however, successful release of scar contractures before scar maturation has

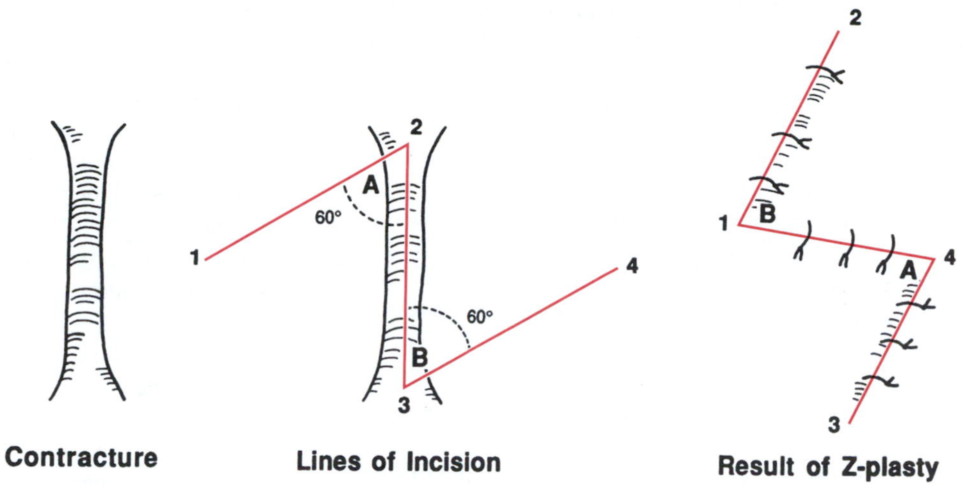

Figure 27.13 Schematic diagram of Z-plasty procedure. Lengthening of scar tissue introduce normal tissue on each side of the elongated scar band. (From Richard and Staley,[6] p 192, with permission.)

been documented.[74] Each patient's scar will require an individualized evaluation and treatment. Surgical treatment options are beyond the scope of this chapter, but common procedures to eliminate scar contractures are skin grafts and Z-plasties. A **Z-plasty** is shown in Figure 27.13. The Z-plasty serves to lengthen a scar by interposing normal tissue in the line of the scar. Skin grafts are used for more severe contractures.

Physical Therapy Management

Treatment of a patient with burns begins the moment he or she arrives at the hospital and is an evolving process that may need to be modified daily.[7–9,75] The previous sections of this chapter have discussed the pathophysiological changes and alterations of the skin that occur in the burn wound and the closure of that wound, including various types of skin graft materials. While the skin is healing, it is imperative that physical therapy intervention occurs concurrently. Treatment is directed toward prevention of scar contracture, preservation of normal ROM, prevention or minimization of hypertrophic scar formation and deformity, maintenance or improvement in muscular strength and cardiovascular endurance, return to preburn function, and performance of activities of daily living (ADL).[6] The physical therapist interacts with other members of the burn team to assist patients in obtaining these outcomes. For many patients, the most difficult phase of rehabilitation occurs after the wounds have healed and the scar tissue begins to contract. Early physical therapy intervention to establish a program of exercise and functional movement in conjunction with the wound healing process, will facilitate rehabilitation efforts once healing is complete. The remainder of this chapter will address the physical therapist's role in the rehabilitation program of a patient who has sustained a burn injury.

Examination

After the initial examination of the depth of burn and amount of TBSA involved, the physical therapist then examines the patient to determine the presence of impairments and functional limitations. The therapist must also consider the potential for development of indirect impairments as the burn wounds heal and mature. For example, active or passive ROM may be limited as a result of edema, restrictive eschar, or pain, and an initial baseline measure should be obtained. In addition, the therapist needs to obtain an accurate history from the patient and family members regarding any preexisting limitations or previous injuries that may affect rehabilitation potential.

Other tests and measures discussed in this text can be included in the initial examination and reexamination of a patient following burn injury (e.g., gait, functional status). Because healing of a burn wound is a dynamic process and changes may occur daily, the physical therapist must examine and monitor patients routinely for changes in skin integrity, ROM, and mobility. Frequent evaluation will keep the physical therapist and other members of the burn care team abreast of potential problems so that intervention can occur before a potential problem becomes a real one.

In addition to the physical damage a burn has on a patient, there also may be an enormous psychological impact.[76,77] The physical therapist should be cognizant of a potential problem during ongoing evaluations, because psychological trauma may affect the patient's progress and outlook toward his or her future and rehabilitation. Referral to an appropriate professional for intervention may be necessary.

Anticipated Goals and Expected Outcomes

Based on the evaluation, the extent and depth of burn, and the patient's current health status, age, and physical and mental condition, the patient's prognosis can be estimated by the burn care team. Goals and outcomes of physical therapy must be carefully individualized and are contingent on the patient's prognosis and current medical status. The development of specific anticipated goals and expected outcomes is based on the following general goals from the *Guide to Physical Therapist Practice*[18] and include:

1. Wound and soft tissue healing is enhanced.
2. Risk of infection and complications is reduced.
3. Risk of secondary impairments is reduced.
4. Maximal ROM is achieved.
5. Pre-injury level of cardiovascular endurance is restored.
6. Good to normal strength is achieved.
7. Independent ambulation is achieved.
8. Independent function in BADL and IADL is increased.
9. Scar formation is minimized.[10]
10. Patient, family, and caregivers understanding of expectations and goals and outcomes is increased.[11]
11. Aerobic capacity is increased.[12]
12. Self-management of symptoms is improved.

The optimal outcome of rehabilitation is the return of a patient to preinjury function and lifestyle.

Intervention

Patients with burns usually will begin physical therapy on the day of admission. The initial examination of a patient will determine which areas need to be addressed first. Control and resolution of edema and preserving ROM usually are first priorities. Elevation of the extremities and active movement, especially of the hands and ankles, help to minimize edema formation. Prevention of scar contractures can be accomplished through positioning, splinting, and exercise. Exercise and ambulation also will help to minimize the deleterious effects of bed rest. Following wound closure, massage and compression will assist with minimizing contracture formation and management of burn scars.

The scar that forms across a joint skin crease while healing is composed of immature collagen. A scar will shorten as a result of the contractile or pulling forces in scar tissue and limit ROM and function unless interventions are taken against this process. Although measures to prevent a contracture are undertaken in expectation of the best result, there will be patients who develop scar contractures. There are several interventions available to the physical therapist to aid in the prevention and/or treatment of scar contracture.

As stated, positioning, splinting, and exercise are three interventions effective in opposing the scar contracture process. Active exercise and patient participation in functional activities are the best treatments to prevent or minimize contractures. However, owing to the relentless forces of scar tissue formation and pain associated with

Table 27.4 Positioning Strategies for Common Deformities

Joint	Common Deformity	Motions to Be Stressed	Suggested Approaches
Anterior neck	Flexion	Hyperextension	Use double mattress; position neck in extension (Fig. 27.14); with healing use rigid cervical orthosis
Shoulder and axilla	Adduction and internal rotation	Abduction, flexion and external rotation	Position with shoulder flexed and abducted (airplane splint)
Elbow	Flexion and pronation	Extension and supination	Splint in extension
Hand	Claw hand (also called intrinsic minus position)	Wrist extension; metacarpophalangeal flexion, proximal interphalangeal and distal interphalangeal extension; thumb abduction	Wrap fingers separately. Elevate to decrease edema. Position in *intrinsic plus* position: wrist in extension, metacarpophalangeal in flexion, proximal interphalangeal and distal interphalangeal in extension, thumb in abduction with large web space
Hip and groin	Flexion and adduction	All motions, especially hip extension and abduction	Hip neutral with slight abduction
Knee	Flexion	Extension	Posterior knee splint
Ankle	Plantarflexion	All motions especially dorsiflexion	Plastic ankle-foot orthosis with cutout at Achilles tendon and ankle positioned in neutral.

exercising a burned area, additional interventions may be necessary. Early and ongoing patient and/or family education is needed to help these individuals understand the necessity of the burn rehabilitation process.

Positioning and Splinting

A patient's positioning program should begin on the day of admission.[8,9,60,78] Outcomes of a positioning program are to (1) minimize edema; (2) prevent tissue destruction; and (3) maintain soft tissues in an elongated state. General guidelines and examples of proper positioning are provided in Table 27.4 and Figures 27.14 through 27.17. Burned areas should be positioned in an elongated state or neutral position of function.

Splinting can be viewed as an extension of the positioning program. There are certain "antideformity" positions in which patients generally are splinted; however, the therapist needs to examine the location of the burn and which movements are difficult for the patient to achieve. With the exception of immobilizing a skin graft after surgery, splints should be fabricated for patients only if ROM or function would be lost without them. General indications for the use of splints include (1) prevention of contractures, (2) maintenance of ROM achieved during an exercise session or surgical release, (3) correction of contractures, and (4) protection of a joint or tendon.[79] Splint design should be kept simple so that a splint is easy to apply, remove, and clean. Splints usually are worn at night, when a patient is resting, or continuously for several days following skin grafting. Splints should conform to the body part, and care must be taken to ensure that there are no pressure points that may cause a breakdown in healing or normal skin. Splints should be checked routinely for proper fit and revised if necessary. Active motion is important, and splints and positioning are intended to serve as adjuncts to the therapy program until full active motion can be achieved.

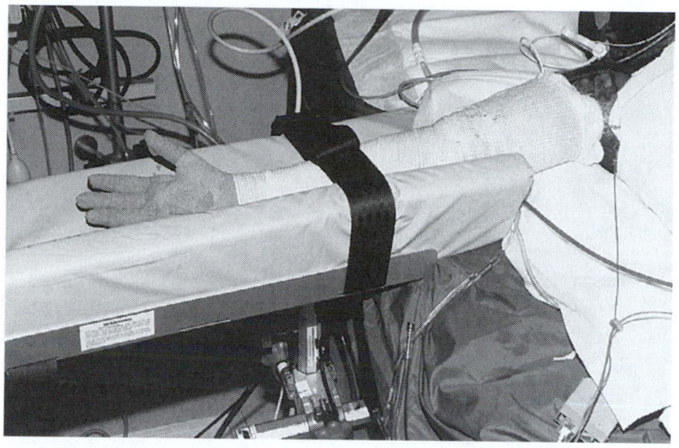

Figure 27.15 Positioning in bed of patient with burns of the axilla. (From Richard and Staley,[6] p 228, with permission.)

Most splints used for burn injuries are static. This type of splint has no moveable parts, and maintains a position or immobilizes an area following skin grafting (Fig. 27.18). Dynamic splints also have been used successfully in the care of patients with a burn injury (Fig. 27.19).[80-82] These splints have moveable parts that allow joint movement. Dynamic splints apply a low-load, prolonged stress that can be adjusted to a patient's tolerance. They offer great potential for correcting a developing contracture and the early return of active function in areas of extensive burn and grafting.[83] The use of continuous passive motion devices also is appropriate for certain patients with burn injuries.[84–88]

Active and Passive Exercise

Active exercise begins on the day of admission.[7–9,60,89] Any patient who is alert and able to follow commands is encouraged to perform active exercises of involved body parts frequently throughout the day. A patient should perform active exercise of all extremities and trunk, including unburned

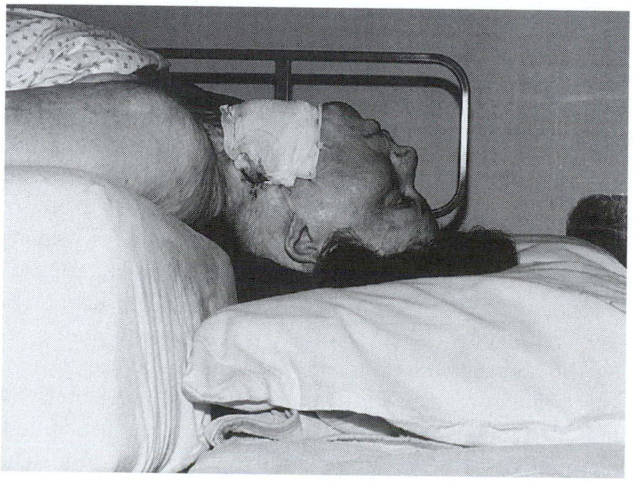

Figure 27.14 Positioning in bed of patient with burns of the anterior neck. (From Richard and Staley,[6] p 225, with permission.)

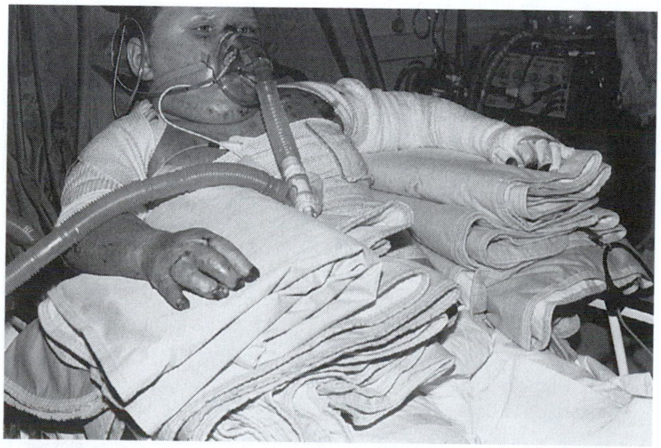

Figure 27.16 Positioning of upper extremities to reduce edema while seated. (From Richard and Staley,[6] p 231, with permission.)

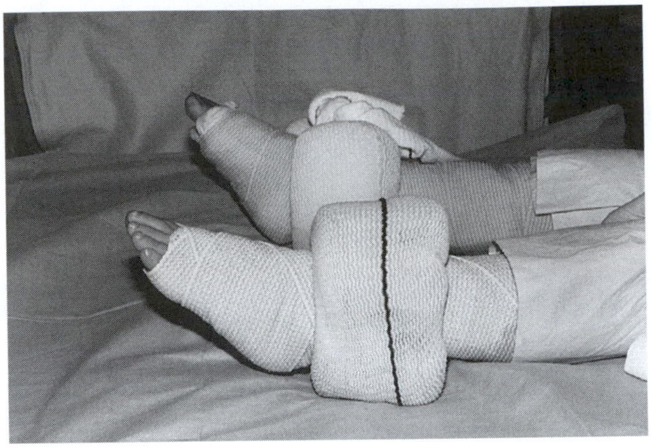

Figure 27.17 Elevation of heels off bed, with use of foam rolls encased in elastic netting. Note: this technique would not be used with burns to Achilles tendon area.

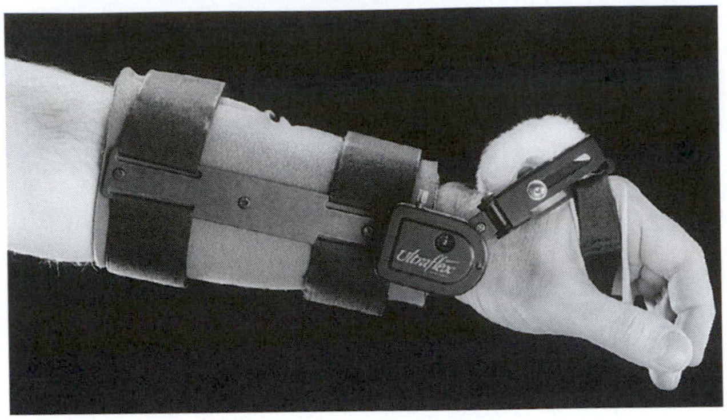

Figure 27.19 Dynamic splint used to provide a low-load, prolonged stress to scar tissue.

areas. Dressing changes are an opportune time for an exercise session because the burn wound is visible, and the therapist can monitor the wound during the session. If a patient has just received a skin graft, active and passive exercise of the area may be discontinued for 3 to 5 days to allow the graft to adhere.[75,90,91] After the surgeon determines it is safe to begin exercise again, gentle ROM—first active and then passive, if needed—is reinstituted.

Active-assistive and passive exercise should be initiated if a patient cannot fully achieve active ROM (see Evidence Summary Box 27.1). To keep the healed burned area moist, it should be lubricated before exercise is initiated. Care should be taken around areas of skin grafts, and stress should be applied in a gentle, prolonged, and gradual fashion. If the burn wounds are well healed, heating modalities (e.g., paraffin, ultrasound) may be used to increase the pliability of the tissue before exercise therapy.[94,95]

ROM in the area of unhealed burns can be extremely painful, and many patients will indicate they would rather lose their motion than be subjected to the additional pain that occurs with movement. It usually is difficult and mentally draining on the physical therapist to push patients to exercise in and through pain, but it is critical that the therapist be persistent. Coordinating an exercise session with the administration of pain medication will lessen the painful experience for the patient.[74,89] Physical therapists should elicit the assistance of the family in keeping the patient motivated and mobile as much as possible.

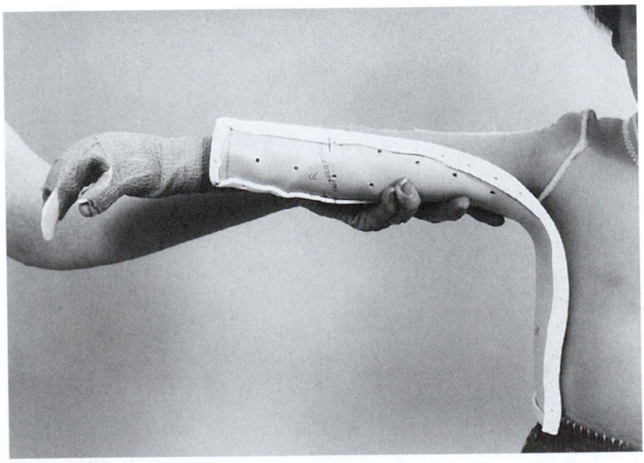

Figure 27.18 Static splint that immobilizes the shoulder in abduction and the elbow in extension.

Resistive and Conditioning Exercise

As a patient continues to recover, the rehabilitation program can be progressed to include strengthening exercises.[7,60,89] Patients with major burns may lose body weight, and lean muscle mass can decrease rapidly. Exercise may consist of isokinetic, isotonic, or other resistive training devices. General principles of exercise training and strength improvement should be followed, but they may need to be modified on the basis of a patient's condition and stage of wound healing. Resistive devices such as free weights and pulleys can be used to prevent loss of strength in areas not burned.

When a patient initially begins strengthening or endurance exercises, the physical therapist should monitor vital signs to examine cardiovascular and respiratory responses to treatment.[96] Overexertion may occur. Monitoring of pulse, blood pressure, and respiratory rate before, during, and after exercise, particularly in the recovery period after exercise, will yield valuable information as to the status of the cardiovascular and pulmonary systems.

Patients should be encouraged to participate in exercises that will stress the cardiovascular system, such as walking from the burn unit to the physical therapy department. Cycling or rowing ergometry, treadmill walking, stair climbing, and other forms of aerobic exercise should be encouraged. These activities will not only work to increase cardiovascular endurance, but can have the added benefit of improving strength and ROM of the extremities. In addition, they introduce variety into the rehabilitation program. The physical therapist needs to be creative and innovative to motivate patients to increase their exercise capacity.

Evidence Summary Box 27.1

Passive Range-of-Motion Exercises Following Burns

Reference	Subjects	Methods	Duration	Results	Comments
Richard, RL, et al[92] 1987	6 Ss S/P full and partial-thickness hand burns; mean age 35.5 years	Pretest, posttest design; alternating treatment/control; T1: PROM by therapist T2: Static wrap of digits	1 treatment session	Significant increase in finger joint flexion, mainly MCP, measured in all digits following PROM versus static wrapping ($p < .001$); increases in motion noted with static wrapping in PIP joints	Overall import of the study demonstrates varying passive stretch methods to increase joint ROM
Covey, MH, et al[87] 1988	10 Ss Bilateral deep hand burns; mean age 45 years	Pretest, posttest design; one hand of each subject randomly assigned; C: Conventional hand therapy E: Continuous passive motion; both groups carried out active motion exercises and self-care when not being passively exercised	C: 30 min 2×day; E: 2-8 hours daily; Tests were discontinued when a subject would reach a ROM goal	80% of fingers in both groups achieved the goal ROM within the same period of time (9 days); neither group reported more pain than the other during treatment; no complications from the motion were reported	Authors recommend regular passive stretch for joints with burn wound or scar contraction
Edstrom, LE, et al[93] 1979	222 hand burns (deep hand burns not healed within 14 days postburn)	Pretest, posttest design; hands were randomly assigned to a group at postburn day 10; C: Hand burns allowed to heal spontaneously; E: Hand burns grafted after 214 days of postburn nonhealing; Both groups participated in the same program of splinting and ROM exercises	Followed for at least 35 days; appears that long term follow-up may have occurred in many cases, although not specifically reported	Eventual outcome listed as "perfect function" in hands of both groups	Although it was reported that measurement of ROM was taken—the numbers were not reported or analyzed; therefore, only increases in ROM can be assumed
Ward, RS, et al[95] 1994	9 Ss 14 joints examined; mean age 36 years	Pretest, posttest design; 14 UE joints were randomly assigned to a group C: Placebo ultrasound E: Ultrasound Both groups received passive stretching to the test joint between outcome measures; each joint treated and examined 6 times during the study, for a total of 84 joint examinations	Measurements taken prior to and following each session; a total of 6 sessions were held for each patient during the study period	The majority (87%) of joints in both the treatment and control groups demonstrated an increase in ROM with passive stretch; 12% of the joints showed no increase in range and 1% exhibited a loss of range	Although the aim of this study was to examine the effect of ultrasound on ROM and pain, the results are applicable because passive ROM exercise was the primary intervention to gain range
Richard, R, et al[83] 2000	52 cases of burn scar contracture; mean age 22 years	Retrospective review of patients with burn scar contractures; T1: Treated with multiple interventions including exercise, massage, passive stretch T2: Included either dynamic splints, and serial casts or splints	Reports of the types of treatments initiated and the outcome of scar contracture	The scar contractures treated with splinting, which stretched the scar as passive ROM exercise might, improved in less than half the time of the contractures of patients treated with varying interventions	This study examined existing contractures related to scar formation and may not be applicable to burn wound contraction or to scar contraction that has not achieved the level of contracture

C = Control; E = experimental; MCP = metacarpophalangeal; PIP = proximal interphalangeal; PROM = passive range of motion; ROM = range of motion; S/P = status post; Ss = subjects; T1 = treatment group 1; T2 = treatment group 2; UE = upper extremity.

Ambulation

Ambulation should be initiated at the earliest appropriate time. If the lower extremities are skin grafted, ambulation may be discontinued until it is safe to resume.[97-100] When ambulation is initiated after a skin graft, the lower extremities should be wrapped in elastic bandages in a figure-of-eight pattern to support the new grafts and promote venous return. If a patient cannot tolerate the upright position because of orthostatic intolerance or pain from the lower extremities in a dependent position, gradual increases in tilt-table treatment time will assist in preparing the patient for standing.[101-103] Initially, a patient may require an assistive device to ambulate. However, independent ambulation without an assistive device should be achieved as soon as possible.

The physical therapist will spend a great deal of time with an individual patient during each exercise session. The rewards of a successful treatment program are tremendous when a patient who has suffered a life-threatening burn is able to walk out of the hospital and return to productive community involvement.

Scar Management

Following wound closure, a skin graft or healed burn wound is vascular, flat, and soft. During the following 3 to 6 months, dramatic changes may occur. The newly healed areas may become raised and firm. Pressure has been used successfully to hasten scar maturation and minimize hypertrophic scar formation.[104] However, no one study validates the mechanism by which pressure alters scar tissue. Pressure may exert control over hypertrophic scarring by (1) thinning the dermis, (2) altering the biochemical structure of scar tissue, (3) decreasing blood flow to the area, (4) reorganizing collagen bundles, or (5) decreasing tissue water content. Constant pressure dressings or garments exerting pressure exceeding 25 mm Hg will decrease the vascularity, decrease the amount of mucopolysaccharides, decrease collagen deposition, and significantly lessen localized edema.[7,104,105] The early hypertrophic scar is readily influenced by compressive forces and thus will respond to pressure therapy. The earlier the scar tissue is exposed to pressure, the better the result.[106,107] Usually, if the scar is less than 6 months old, it will respond to pressure therapy by conforming to the pressure, remaining flat on the surface, and not developing into a hypertrophic scar.[107] However, if the scar is still active or shows evidence of vascularity (red color), pressure therapy may be successful, even if the scar is 1 year old.

In general, if a patient's wounds heal in less than 10 to 14 days, which would be indicative of a superficial partial-thickness burn, pressure may not be needed. If wound healing takes longer than 10 to 14 days (as in a deep partial-thickness burn) or is skin grafted, pressure usually is indicated.[108]

Pressure Dressings

Elastic wraps can be used to provide vascular support of skin grafts and donor sites as well as to control edema and scarring. Elastic wraps should be used until a patient's skin or scars can tolerate the shearing force of pressure garment application, and open areas are minimal. Elastic wraps are applied in a figure-of-eight pattern on the lower extremities. A spiral wrap can be used on the upper extremities and a circular wrap on the trunk.[104]

A self-adherent elastic bandage can be used for the hand and toes.[104,109,110] This bandage adheres only to itself and can be used over dressings before the wounds have healed. It helps to minimize edema and control scar formation. It may be used before application of a glove or as definitive pressure on an infant's hand.

Tubular support bandages come in various circumferences and garment styles. They provide a moderate amount of compression and may be used as interim garments before a custom-made garment is fit.[104,111] The tubular support bandage is especially useful for small children who grow rapidly and require frequent alterations in garment size.

Several companies manufacture pressure garments. Some are ready made and come in several sizes to fit most patients; others are custom made for the individual patient. For the custom-made garments, a physical therapist uses a tape measure to determine the circumference of each limb every 1.5 in. (38 mm) of its length to fit the garment exactly to the limb with the proper pressure. Garments are measured when a patient has only a few remaining open areas. The garments are very tight, and difficult to apply, but the pressure is necessary to prevent scar hypertrophy. Garments can be ordered for any or all body parts, including the face and head, and they come in many styles, options, and colors (Fig. 27.20).[104] Garments can be worn when the skin or scars can tolerate the shearing force of application. Pantyhose may be used under waist-height pressure garments to assist with donning. Garments usually are worn 23 hours a day (removed for bathing) for as long as 12 to 18 months to assist with scar remodeling. Garments should be washed daily to prevent buildup of perspiration and moisturizing cream, which may lead to scar maceration. The patient usually receives two sets of garments, one to wear and one to wash.

Adequate pressure may not be obtained with elastic wraps or pressure garments over concave surfaces, such as the sternum or axilla, and an insert may be necessary.[112,113] Inserts can be made of many materials including foam, silicone elastomer, elastomer putty, and gel pads.[104,111,114–116] These items need to be removed and cleaned regularly to prevent maceration of the underlying tissue.

Early, consistent use of pressure will result in flat, pliable scars, desensitization and protection of scars, and relief of itching. Pressure is necessary until scar maturation, when the scars are pale, flat, and soft.

Massage

Massage is useful to assist with ROM exercise by making the tissue more pliable. Deep friction massage is thought to loosen scar tissue by mobilizing cutaneous tissue from

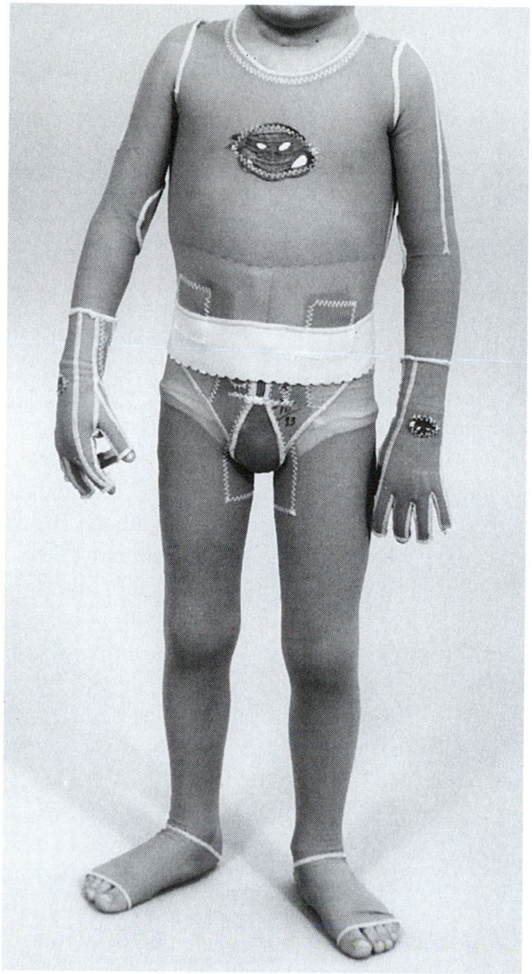

Figure 27.20 Pressure garments such as gloves, vest, and waist-height pants are worn to minimize hypertrophic scar formation.

underlying tissue and act to break up adhesions.[7,117] When massage is used in conjunction with ROM exercise, the immature scar can be elongated more easily, and contracture can be corrected. Although no study has validated the use of massage for patients with burn injuries,[118] in the long term, skin pliability and texture appear improved by the use of massage. Firm scars that are routinely massaged tend to soften. Edges or seams of grafts or any area that is raised and firm may benefit from massage. Scars should be massaged in a slow, firm manner for 5 to 10 minutes, three to six times daily.

Camouflage Makeup

For scars of the face, neck, and hands, camouflage makeup can be used.[9,104] This type of makeup may be useful when a person has either hyperpigmentation or hypopigmentation of the skin due to the burn injury. In addition, makeup can be used before scar maturation, when the scar is still red, and a patient wants to go out in public without his or her pressure garments or devices for short periods of time. The cosmetics are opaque, color correct burn scars, and are available in multiple shades to accommodate various skin colors. They also are waterproof and can be worn during all activities. These products can be purchased in larger department stores or where theatrical products are sold.

Follow-Up Care

Before patients are discharged from the hospital, the therapist should provide information regarding a home exercise program (HEP), splinting and positioning program, and skin care.

A HEP should continue to stress frequent ROM exercises in combination with massage. In addition, patients should be encouraged to perform as many ADL skills as possible independently. Therapists can videotape the patient's exercise program to provide the patient, family, and outpatient therapist with the actual ROM and movement pattern used in each exercise. A video facilitates education of those involved in the patient's rehabilitation program and helps to ensure consistency of treatment after discharge.[119]

The splinting schedule and pressure program that was followed in the hospital just before the patient's discharge should be continued at home. Before discharge, the patient family members, and/or caregivers should be able to apply and remove all splints and pressure appliances independently.

Proper skin care requires specifying the type of soap and cream a patient is to use. In general, soap should be mild without perfumes or other irritants. A moisturizing soap can be used after all open areas are healed. Moisturizing creams should be applied two to three times daily and should not contain perfumes or have a significant alcohol content. Patients should be instructed to massage the cream completely into their skin to avoid buildup on the surface. If a patient will be exposed to the sun, a sunscreen with a skin protection factor of at least 15 should be used and reapplied frequently.[120] Patients should be cautioned to avoid the sun if at all possible and to use hats or clothing to help protect their skin against the sun's rays.

Small, superficial open areas may plague a patient for many months after wound closure because of the fragility of a healed burn wound. The patient should be instructed to wash these areas twice daily, apply a small amount of antibiotic ointment, and cover the areas with a nonadherent dressing. Further irritation or maceration can be prevented by avoiding shearing forces, improper fit of clothing, brisk cleansing, and soaking in water too long, or application of too much cream.

Itching may intensify when wounds have healed. A patient should be instructed to pat, rather than scratch, the irritated areas. Application of cream may help decrease itching; however, some patients may require oral medication to help control this problem.

Some patients with burn injury may require outpatient therapy to supplement the HEP and monitor and adjust their splinting and pressure program. Frequency of outpatient therapy is based on individual patient need. Regardless of whether or not a patient receives outpatient therapy, he or she should be monitored at regular intervals through an outpatient clinic. This will allow burn team members to monitor the patient's adjustment back into society and alter the rehabilitation program according to the patient's physical abilities and extent of scar maturation. When an adult patient's burns have matured and full ROM is achieved, further follow-up care is unnecessary. However, a child will need to be monitored until he or she is fully grown, because burn scars may not keep pace with a child's growth; surgical release of scar tissue may be necessary.[121]

Community Programs

There are various community programs available to individuals who have survived a burn injury. The therapist should be aware of those in the patient's home community so that an appropriate referral can be made. If programs are not available, someone in the hospital or community may want to initiate a program. Programs may include:

1. Burn Prevention Programs: The American Burn Association, 625 N. Michigan Ave., Chicago, IL 60611; (800) 548-2876, has a Burn Prevention Committee with a myriad of printed materials.
2. School Re-entry Programs: Provided by the hospital personnel for the students and staff in the child's school.[9,121]
3. Burn Camps: Weekend- to week-long camps provide an opportunity for children to interact in a controlled, outdoor environment with peers who have sustained a similar injury.[9,121] The American Burn Association has a Burn Camp Special Interest Group with readily available information about camps throughout the United States and Canada.
4. Adult Support Groups: Provide an opportunity for individuals with or without their families to share experiences and gain support from others who have had similar injuries.[121]

Summary

Burn injuries represent a major health problem in terms of management and care of surviving patients. Specific impairments and complications vary according to the extent and depth of thermal destruction of the skin. The classification of burn injuries is based on the depth of tissue destroyed and includes superficial burn, superficial partial-thickness burn, deep partial-thickness burn, full-thickness burn, and subdermal burn. The rule of nines[30] and the Lund and Browder [31] formula were developed to assist with the initial determination of the extent of burn injury. The specific clinical signs and symptoms that result from a burn injury vary according to the different classifications. Indirect impairments can include infection, and pulmonary, metabolic, skeletal, muscular, neurological, and cardiovascular and pulmonary complications. Medical management addresses life-threatening problems and stabilization of the patient. Dressings with topical medications, débridement, surgical excision, and skin grafting are primary treatment measures. Skin substitutes are slowly becoming a practical alternative to skin grafting. Physical therapy management focuses on the prevention of scar contracture, maintenance of normal ROM, development of muscular strength and endurance, improvement of cardiovascular conditioning, independence in functional activities, and prevention of hypertrophic scarring. Although burn trauma and subsequent recovery can be a devastating life occurrence, there are treatment facilities and medical professionals to assist patients with burn injuries and their families return to as normal a lifestyle as possible.

Questions for Review

1. Identify the two primary layers of skin and list two functions of each.
2. Describe the differences between superficial, partial-thickness, and full-thickness burns.
3. Explain how a deep partial-thickness burn can convert to a full-thickness burn.
4. Compare the treatments for deep partial-thickness and full-thickness burns.
5. Describe the primary complications of the pulmonary system due to extensive burns.
6. What are the major metabolic complications associated with burns, and how are they treated?
7. List the three phases that occur in the healing of a burn wound.
8. What are the goals of the initial medical management and resuscitation of a patient with an acute burn injury?
9. Describe the various types of skin grafts.
10. Differentiate between a split-thickness and full-thickness skin graft.
11. List three essential factors for successful skin graft adherence.
12. Discuss the types of exercise that are useful in a burn rehabilitation program.
13. What interventions can be used to prevent burn scar contractures?
14. What interventions can be used to prevent hypertrophic scar formation?
15. What information should be included in patient, family, and caregiver education before discharge from the hospital?

Case Study

Patient History

A 29-year-old man sustained a 30% TBSA burn 6 weeks before this outpatient examination and evaluation. The patient was burned at home while he was refueling a lawnmower with gasoline, which ignited. Areas of the body affected by the burn included the right upper extremity (UE), portions of the posterior and anterior trunk, lateral neck, right side of face, and thigh. Areas skin grafted included the right dorsal hand, forearm, and arm up to the axillary crease. The remaining burn wounds healed secondarily. The neck, face, and thigh burns were superficial. The patient was initially treated at a regional burn center and now is referred to the local hospital for follow-up outpatient physical therapy due to decreased right elbow extension, decreased shoulder flexion, and inability to reach overhead.

Physical Therapy Examination Findings

The right UE lacks 15° degrees elbow extension (i.e., 15° to 120°) and flexion of the shoulder is limited to 0° to 155°. Scar contracture bands are noted at both locations at the end of available range with movement. The patient states he has some difficulty donning shirts and his jacket. All other movements are within functional limits (WFL). The patient's strength overall is considered WFL, as are other physical parameters. His wounds are all closed. The patient lives with his girlfriend and has medical benefits through his employer.

One week after his discharge from the hospital, the patient presented for his initial outpatient examination wearing interim pressure garments, as instructed. He also brought the static elbow splint that had been issued to him during his acute hospitalization, but which "doesn't fit right anymore." The expected outcome for this patient is to regain full right UE ROM and function.

GUIDING QUESTIONS

1. Describe how you would approach the clinical problems presented. Your answer should address positioning, splinting, exercise, and scar-management interventions.
2. What patient education would you provide? Would this differ if the patient is adherent versus nonadherent with the therapy program?
3. What is the anticipated rehabilitation potential for this patient? Your decision making should consider time from burn injury and stage of healing.

References

1. American Burn Association: Burn Incidence and Treatment in the US: 2000 Fact Sheet. American Burn Association, Chicago, IL, 60611 Retrieved October 14, 2004, from http://www.ameriburn.org.
2. Pruitt, BA, Jr, and Mason, AD, Jr: Epidemiological, demographic and outcomes characteristics of burn injury. In Herndon, DN (ed): Total Burn Care. WB Saunders, Philadelphia, 1996, p 5.
3. Baker, SP, et al: Fire, burns and lightning. In Baker, SP, et al (eds): The Injury Fact Book. Oxford University Press, New York, 1992, p 161.
4. Herndon, DN, et al: Teamwork for total burn care: Achievements, directions and hopes. In Herndon, DN (ed): Total Burn Care. WB Saunders, Philadelphia, 1996, p 1.
5. Saffle, JR, et al: Recent outcomes in the treatment of burn injury in the United States: A report from the American Burn Association patient registry. J Burn Care Rehabil 16:219, 1995.
6. Richard, RL, and Staley, MJ (eds): Burn Care and Rehabilitation: Principles and Practice. FA Davis, Philadelphia, 1994.
7. Ward, RS: Physical rehabilitation. In Carrougher, GJ (ed): Burn Care and Therapy. CV Mosby, St. Louis, 1998, p 293.
8. Moore, M: The burn unit. In Campbell, SK, et al (eds): Physical Therapy for Children. WB Saunders, Philadelphia, 1994, p 763.
9. Grigsby de Linde, L: Rehabilitation of the child with burns. In Tecklin, JS (ed): Pediatric Physical Therapy, ed 3. Lippincott, Philadelphia, 1999, p 468.
10. Shani, E, and Rosenberg, L: Are we making an impact? A review of a burn prevention program in Israeli schools. J Burn Care Rehabil 19:82, 1998.
11. Committee on Trauma: Guidelines for Operation of Burn Units. In Resources for Optimal Care of the Injured Patient. American College of Surgeons, Chicago, 1999, p 55.
12. Burn Care Resources in North America 1996-1997. American College of Surgeons, Chicago, 1996.
13. Supple, KG, Fiala, SM, and Gamelli, RL: Preparation for burn center verification. J Burn Care Rehabil 18:58, 1997.
14. Holbrook, KA, and Wolff, K: The structure and development of skin. In Fitzpatrick, TB, et al (eds): Dermatology In General Medicine. McGraw-Hill, New York, 1993, p 97.
15. Lanir, Y: The fibrous structure of the skin and its relation to mechanical behavior. In Marks, R, and Payne, PA (eds): Bioengineering and the Skin. MIT Press, Cambridge, MA, 1981, p 93.
16. Moncrief, JA: The body's response to heat. In Artz, CP, et al (eds): Burns: A Team Approach. WB Saunders, Philadelphia, 1979, p 24.
17. Johnson, C: Pathologic manifestations of burn injury. In Richard, RL, and Staley, MJ (eds): Burn Care and Rehabilitation: Principles and Practice. FA Davis, Philadelphia, 1994, p 31.
18. Guide to Physical Therapist Practice, ed 2. American Physical Therapy Association, Alexandria, VA, 2001.
19 Norris, PG, et al: Acute effects of ultraviolet radiation on the skin. In Fitzpatrick, TB, et al (eds): Dermatology in General Medicine. McGraw-Hill, New York, 1993, p 1651.
20. Heggers, JP, et al: Evaluation of burn blister fluid. Plast Reconst Surg 65:798, 1980.
21. Rockwell, WB, and Ehrlich, HP: Fibrinolysis inhibition in human burn blister fluid. J Burn Care Rehabil 11:1, 1990.
22. Garner, WL, et al: The effects of burn blister fluid on keratinocyte replication and differentiation. J Burn Care Rehabil 14:127, 1993.
23. Ono, I, et al: A study of cytokines in burn blister fluid related to wound healing. Burns 21:352, 1995.
24. Richard, R, and Johnson, RM: Managing superficial burn wounds. Adv Skin Wound Care 15:246, 2002.
25. Lund, T, et al: Pathogenesis of edema formation in burn injuries. World J Surg 16:2, 1992.
26. Mozingo, DW: Surgical management. In Carrougher, GJ (ed): Burn Care and Therapy. CV Mosby, St. Louis, 1998, p 233.
27. Miller, SF, et al: Triage and Resuscitation of the Burn Patient. In Richard, RL, and Staley, MJ (eds): Burn Care and Rehabilitation: Principles and Practice. FA Davis, Philadelphia, 1994, p 107.

28. Wittman, MI: Electrical and chemical burns. In Richard, RL, and Staley, MJ (eds): Burn Care and Rehabilitation: Principles and Practice. FA Davis, Philadelphia, 1994, p 603.
29. Williams, WG, and Phillips, LG: Pathophysiology of the burn wound. In Herndon, DN (ed): Total Burn Care. WB Saunders, Philadelphia, 1996, p 65.
30. Polaski, GR, and Tennison, AC: Estimation of the amount of burned surface area. JAMA 103:34, 1948.
31. Lund, CC, and Browder, NC: Estimation of area of burns. Surg Gynecol Obstet 79:352, 1955.
32. Sheridan, RL, and Tompkins, RG: Etiology and prevention of multisystem organ failure. In Herndon, DN (ed): Total Burn Care.WB Saunders, Philadelphia, 1996, p 302.
33. Heggers, J, et al: Treatment of infections in burns. In Herndon, DN (ed): Total Burn Care. Philadelphia, WB Saunders, 1996, p 98.
34. Weber, JM: Epidemiology of infections and strategies for control. In Carrougher, GJ (ed): Burn Care and Therapy. CV Mosby, St. Louis, 1998, p 185.
35. Moylan, JA: Smoke inhalation and burn injury. Surg Clin North Am 60:1530, 1980.
36. Greenberg, MI, and Walter, J: Axioms on smoke inhalation. Hosp Med 19:13, 1983.
37. Chu, CS: New concepts of pulmonary burn injury. J Trauma 21:958, 1981.
38. Cioffi, WG, Jr: Inhalation injury. In Carrougher, GJ (ed): Burn Care and Therapy. CV Mosby, St. Louis, 1998, p 35.
39. Mancusi-Ungaro, HR, et al: Caloric and nitrogen balances as predictors of nutritional outcome in patients with burns. J Burn Care Rehabil 13:695, 1992.
40. Demling, RH, and DeSanti, L: Increased protein intake during the recovery phase after severe burns increases body weight gain and muscle function. J Burn Care Rehabil 19:161, 1998.
41. Wilmore, DW, et al: Effect of ambient temperature on heat production and heat loss in burn patients. J Appl Physiol 38:593, 1975.
42. Prelack, K, et al: Energy and protein provisions for thermally injured children revisited: An outcome-based approach for determining requirements. J Burn Care Rehabil 18:177, 1997.
43. Dominioni, L, et al: Enteral feeding in burn hypermetabolism: Nutritional and metabolic effects on different levels of calorie and protein intake. J Parenter Enteral Nutr 9:269, 1985.
44. Matsuda, T, et al: The importance of burn wound size in determining the optimal calorie:nitrogen ratio. Surgery 94:562, 1983.
45. Demling, RH, et al: The study of burn wound edema using dichromatic absorptiometry. J Trauma 18:124, 1978.
46. Kramer, GC, and Nguyen, TT: Pathophysiology of burn shock and burn edema. In Herndon, DN: Total Burn Care. WB Saunders, Philadelphia, 1996, p 44.
47. Gordon, MD, and Winfree, JH: Fluid resuscitation after a major burn. In Carrougher, GJ (ed): Burn Care and Therapy. CV Mosby, St. Louis, 1998, p 107.
48. Munster, AM, et al: Heterotopic calcification following burns: A prospective study. J Trauma 12:1071, 1972.
49. Schiele, HP, et al: Radiographic changes in burns of the upper extremity. Diagnostic Radiology 104:13, 1971.
50. Rubin, MM, and Cozzi, GM: Heterotopic ossification of the temporomandibular joint in a burn patient. J Oral Maxillofac Surg 44:897, 1986.
51. Edlich, RF, et al: Heterotopic calcification and ossification in the burn patient. J Burn Care Rehabil 6:363, 1985.
52. Dutcher, K, and Johnson, C: Neuromuscular and musculoskeletal complications. In Richard, RL, and Staley, MJ (eds): Burn Care and Rehabilitation: Principles and Practice. FA Davis, Philadelphia, 1994, p 576.
53. Greenhalgh, DG, and Staley, MJ: Burn wound healing. In Richard, RL, and Staley, MJ (eds): Burn Care and Rehabilitation: Principles and Practice. FA Davis, Philadelphia, 1994, p 70.
54. Arem, AJ, and Madden, JW: Is there a Wolff's law for connective tissue? Surg Forum 25:512, 1974.
55. Saffle, JR, et al: Recent outcomes in the treatment of burn injury in the United States: A report from the American Burn Association patient registry. J Burn Care Rehabil 16:219, 1995.
56. Warden, GD: Fluid resuscitation and early management. In Herdon, DN (ed): Total Burn Care. WB Saunders, Philadelphia, 1996, p 53.
57. Thomson, PD, et al: A survey of burn hydrotherapy in the United States. J Burn Care Rehabil 11:151, 1990.
58. Saffle, JR, and Schnebly, WA: Burn wound care. In Richard, RL, and Staley, MJ (eds): Burn Care and Rehabilitation: Principles and Practice. FA Davis, Philadelphia, 1994, p 119.
59. Shankowsky, HA, et al: North American survey of hydrotherapy in modern burn care. J Burn Care Rehabil 15:143, 1994.
60. Ward, RS: The rehabilitation of burn patients. Crit Rev Phys Rehab Med 2:121, 1991.
61. Neville, C, and Dimick, AR: The trauma table as an alternative to the Hubbard tank in burn care. J Burn Care Rehabil 8:574, 1987.
62. Heggers, JP, et al: Bactericidal and wound-healing properties of sodium hypochlorite solutions. J Burn Care Rehabil 12:420, 1991.
63. Richard, RL: The use of chlorine bleach as a disinfectant and antiseptic in whirlpools. Phys Ther Forum 7:7, 1988.
64. Carrougher, GJ: Burn wound assessment and topical treatment. In Carrougher, GJ (ed): Burn Care and Therapy, CV Mosby, St. Louis, 1998, p 142.
65. Miller, SF, et al: Surgical management of the burn patient. In Richard, RL, and Staley, MJ (eds): Burn Care and Rehabilitation: Principles and Practice. FA Davis, Philadelphia, 1994, p 180.
66. Cuono, C, et al: Use of cultured epidermal autografts and dermal allografts as skin replacement after burn injury. Lancet 8490:1123, 1986.
67. Munster, AM: Cultured epidermal autographs in the management of burn patients. J Burn Care Rehabil 13:121, 1992.
68. Lattari, V, et al: The use of a permanent dermal allograft in full-thickness burns of the hand and foot: A report of three cases. J Burn Care Rehabil 18:147, 1997.
69. Hansbrough, J, et al: Clinical trials of a biosynthetic temporary skin replacement, Dermagraft-Transitional Covering, compared with cryopreserved human cadaver skin for temporary coverage of excised burn wounds. J Burn Care Rehabil 18:43, 1997.
70. Purdue, G, et al: A multicenter clinical trial of a biosynthetic skin replacement, Dermagraft-TC, compared with cryopreserved human cadaver skin for temporary coverage of excised burn wounds. J Burn Care Rehabil 18:52, 1997.
71. Heimbach, D, et al: Artificial dermis for major burns: A multicenter, randomized clinical trial. Ann Surg 208:313, 1988.
72. Richard, R, et al: A comparison of the Tanner and Bioplasty skin mesher systems for maximal skin graft expansion. J Burn Care Rehabil 14:690, 1993.
73. Larson, D, et al: Prevention and treatment of burn scar contracture. In Artz, CP, et al (eds): Burns: A Team Approach. WB Saunders, Philadelphia, 1979, p 466.
74. Greenhalgh, DG, et al: The early release of axillary contractures in pediatric patients with burns. J Burn Care Rehabil 14:39, 1993.
75. Richard, RL, and Staley, MJ: Burn patient evaluation and treatment planning. In Richard, RL, and Staley, MJ (eds): Burn Care and Rehabilitation: Principles and Practice. FA Davis, Philadelphia, 1994, p 201.
76. Moss, BF, et al: Psychologic support and pain management of the burn patient. In Richard, RL, and Staley, MJ (eds): Burn Care and Rehabilitation: Principles and Practice. FA Davis, Philadelphia, 1994, p 475.
77. Adcock, RJ, et al: Psychologic and emotional recovery. In Carrougher, GJ (ed): Burn Care and Therapy. CV Mosby, St. Louis, 1998, p 329.
78. Apfel, L, et al: Approaches to positioning the burn patient. In Richard, RL, and Staley, MJ (eds): Burn Care and Rehabilitation: Principles and Practice. FA Davis, Philadelphia, 1994, p 221.
79. Daugherty, M, and Carr-Collins, J: Splinting techniques for the burn patient. In Richard, RL, and Staley, MJ (eds): Burn Care and Rehabilitation: Principles and Practice. FA Davis, Philadelphia, 1994, p 242.
80. Richard, RL: Use of Dynasplint to correct elbow flexion burn contracture: A case report. J Burn Care Rehabil 7:151, 1986.
81. Richard, R, and Staley, M: Dynamic splinting: Basic science + modern technology. Physical Therapy Forum 11:21, 1992.
82. Richard, RL, et al: Dynamic versus static splints: A prospective case for sustained stress. J Burn Care Rehabil 16:284, 1995.
83. Richard, R, et al: Multimodal versus progressive treatment techniques to correct burn scar contractures. J Burn Care Rehabil 21:506, 2000.

84. Covey, MH, et al: Efficacy of continuous passive motion (CPM) devices with hand burns. J Burn Care Rehabil 9:397, 1988.
85. McAllister, LP, and Salazar, CA: Case report on the use of CPM on an electrical burn. J Burn Care Rehabil 9:401, 1988.
86. McGough, CE: Introduction to CPM. J Burn Care Rehabil 9:494, 1988.
87. Covey, MH: Application of CPM devices with burn patients. J Burn Care Rehabil 9:496, 1988.
88. Richard, RL, et al: The physiologic response of a patient with critical burns to continuous passive motion. J Burn Care Rehabil 11:554, 1990.
89. Humphrey, C, et al: Soft tissue management and exercise. In Richard, RL, and Staley, MJ (eds): Burn Care and Rehabilitation: Principles and Practice. FA Davis, Philadelphia, 1994, p 324.
90. Herndon, DN, et al: Management of the pediatric patient with burns. J Burn Care Rehabil 14:3, 1993.
91. Schwanholt, C, et al: A comparison of full-thickness versus split-thickness autografts for the coverage of deep palm burns in the very young pediatric patient. J Burn Care Rehabil 14:29, 1993.
92. Richard, RL, et al: Comparison of the effect of passive exercise v static wrapping on finger range of motion in the burned hand. J Burn Care Rehabil 8:576, 1987.
93. Edstrom, LE, et al: Prospective randomized treatments for burned hands: Nonoperative vs. operative. Preliminary report. Scand J Plast Reconstr Surg 13:131, 1979.
94. Ward, RS: The use of physical agents in burn care. In Richard, RL, and Staley, MJ (eds): Burn Care and Rehabilitation: Principles and Practice. FA Davis, Philadelphia, 1994, p 419.
95. Ward, RS, et al: Evaluation of therapeutic ultrasound to improve response to physical therapy and lessen scar contracture after burn injury. J Burn Care Rehabil 15:74, 1994.
96. Black, S, et al: Oxygen consumption for lower extremity exercises in normal subjects and burn patients. Phys Ther 60:1255, 1980.
97. Schmitt, P, et al: Lower Extremity Burns and Ambulation. In Richard, RL, and Staley, MJ (eds): Burn Care and Rehabilitation: Principles and Practice. FA Davis, Philadelphia, 1994, p 361.
98. Schmitt, MA, et al: How soon is safe? Ambulation of the patient with burns after lower extremity skin grafting. J Burn Care Rehabil 12:33, 1991.
99. Burnsworth, B, et al: Immediate ambulation of patients with lower-extremity grafts. J Burn Care Rehabil 13:89, 1992.
100. Grube, BJ, et al: Early ambulation and discharge in 100 patients with burns of the foot treated by grafts. J Trauma 33:662, 1992.
101. Temmen, HJ, et al: Tilt table exercise guidelines for burn patients: Are cardiac exercise parameters appropriate? Proc Am Burn Assoc 30:221, 1998.
102. Boyea, BL, et al: Use of the tilt table for postural reconditioning of burn patients prior to ambulation. Proc Am Burn Assoc 30:233, 1998.
103. Trees, DW, Ketelsen, CA, and Hobbs, JA: Use of a modified tilt table for preambulation strength training as an adjunct to burn rehabilitation: A case series. J Burn Care Rehabil 24:97, 2003.
104. Staley, MJ, and Richard, RL: Scar management. In Richard, RL, and Staley, MJ (eds): Burn Care and Rehabilitation: Principles and Practice. FA Davis, Philadelphia, 1994, p 380.
105. Johnson, CL: Physical therapists as scar modifiers. Phys Ther 64:1381, 1984.
106. Kischer, CW, and Shetlar, MR: Microvasculature in hypertrophic scars and the effects of pressure. J Trauma 19:757, 1979.
107. Leung, PC, and Ng, M: Pressure treatment for hypertrophic scars. Burns 6:224, 1980.
108. Deitch, EA, et al: Hypertrophic burn scars: Analysis of variables. J Trauma 23:895, 1983.
109. Ward, RS, et al: Use of Coban self-adherent wrap in management of postburn hand grafts: Case reports. J Burn Care Rehabil 15:364, 1994.
110. Lowell, M, et al: Effect of 3M™ Coban™ self-adherent wraps on edema and function of the burned hand: A case study. J Burn Care Rehabil 24:253, 2003.
111. Kealey, GP, et al: Prospective randomized comparison of two types of pressure therapy garments. J Burn Care Rehabil 11:334, 1990.
112. Cheng, JCY, et al: Pressure therapy in the treatment of post-burn hypertrophic scar: A critical look into its usefulness and fallacies by pressure monitoring. Burns 10:154, 1984.
113. Mann, R, et al: Do custom-fitted pressure garments provide adequate pressure. J Burn Care Rehabil 18:247, 1997.
114. Alston, DW, et al: Materials for pressure inserts in the control of hypertrophic scar tissue. J Burn Care Rehabil 2:40, 1981.
115. Moore, ML, et al: Effectiveness of custom pressure garments in wound management: A prospective trial within wounds and with verified pressure. J Burn Care Rehabil 21:S177, 2000.
116. Perkins, K, et al: Current materials and techniques used in a burn scar management programme. Burns 13:406, 1987.
117. Miles, WK, and Grigsby, L: Remodeling of scar tissue in the burned hand. In Hunter, JM, et al (eds): Rehabilitation of the Hand. CV Mosby, St. Louis, 1984, p 841.
118. Patino, O, and Novick, C: Massage on hypertrophic scars. J Burn Care Rehabil 20:268, 1999.
119. Gallagher, J, et al: Discharge videotaping: A means of augmenting occupational and physical therapy. J Burn Care Rehabil 11:470, 1990.
120. Braddom, RL, et al: The physical treatment and rehabilitation of burn patients. In Hummel, RP (ed): Clinical Burn Therapy. John Wright PSG, Boston, 1982, p 297.
121. Leman, CJ, and Ricks, N: Discharge planning and follow-up burn care. In Richard, RL, and Staley, MJ (eds): Burn Care and Rehabilitation: Principles and Practice. FA Davis, Philadelphia, 1994, p 447.

Supplemental Readings

Allison, K and Porter, K: Consensus on the pre-hospital approach to burns patient management. Injury 35(8):734, 2004.
Brown, TP, et al: Survival benefit conferred by topical antimicrobial preparations in burn patients: A historical perspective. J Trauma 56(4):863, 2004.
Caruso, DM, et al: Randomized clinical study of hydrofiber dressing with silver or silver sulfadiazine in the management of partial-thickness burns. J Burn Care Res 27(3):298, 2006.
Clayman, MA, Clayman, SM, and Mozingo, DW: The use of collagen-glycosaminoglycan copolymer (integra) for the repair of hypertrophic scars and keloids. J Burn Care Res 27(3):404, 2006.
Dauber, A, et al: Chronic persistent pain after severe burns: A survey of 358 burn survivors. Pain Med 3(1):6, 2002.
Herndon, DN (ed): Total Burn Care, ed 2. WB Saunders, Philadelphia, 2002.
Herndon, DN, and Tompkins, RG: Support of the metabolic response to burn injury. Lancet 363(9424):1895, 2004.
Mustoe, TA, et al: International clinical recommendations on scar management. Plast Reconst Surg 110:560, 2002.
Prakash, S, Fatima, T, and Pawar, M: Patient controlled analgesia with fentanyl for burn dressing changes. Anesth Analg 99(2):552, 2004.
See, P, et al: Our clinical experience using cryopreserved cadaveric allograft for the management of severe burns. Cell Tissue Bank 2(2):113, 2001.
Sheridan, RL, and Tompkins, RG: What's new in burns and metabolism. J Am Coll Surg 198:243, 2004.
Simons, M, Ziviani, J, and Tyack, ZF: Measuring functional outcome in pediatric patients with burns: Methodological considerations. Burns 30(5):411, 2004.
Ward, RS: Physical rehabilitation. In: Carrougher, GJ (ed): Burn Care and Therapy. CV Mosby, St. Louis, 1998, p 293.
Weinstock-Zlotnick, G, Torres-Gray, D, and Segal, R: Effect of partial pressure garment work gloves on hand function in patients with hand burns: A pilot study. J Hand Ther 17(3):368, 2004.

CHAPTER

28

Chronic Pain

Lisa Janice Cohen, PT, MS, OCS

LEARNING OBJECTIVES

1. Understand the usefulness and limitations of modern pain theories in explaining the clinical variance of patients with chronic pain.
2. Explain the physiology of pain and the anatomical mechanisms that contribute to chronic pain.
3. Analyze and classify pain based on signs, symptoms, function, and subjective data.
4. Describe common clinical presentations of chronic pain.
5. Discuss advantages and disadvantages of pain measurement tools.
6. Distinguish between open and closed ended questions and generate examples of both types of questions.
7. Distinguish between anxiety/fear-avoidance and nonadherence.
8. Identify appropriate techniques to build and/or repair rapport in the clinical relationship.
9. Develop appropriate goals when presented with a case study of a patient with chronic pain.
10. Generate an appropriate plan of care based on objective and subjective examination data.
11. Describe the contributions of the members of an interdisciplinary pain management team.

OUTLINE

Patients who present with chronic pain pose significant challenges to the physical therapist. The clinical picture is complicated by functional limitations that do not seem supported by physical impairments and physical impairments that do not seem related to the disease process or mechanism of injury. Psychological distress, distorted self image, and fear often accompany the impairments and confound the examination and treatment process.

Management of chronic pain is a significant health care concern. Treatment for back pain alone accounted for 2.5 percent of the country's total health care outlay, with 75 percent of the costs driven by 25 percent of patients. Chronic symptoms accounted for much of the difference.[1]

Although it is likely that the practicing physical therapist will encounter patients with chronic pain, pain management is not a recognized as a specialty within the profession.[2] Physical therapy practice is broadly organized under four categories: musculoskeletal, neurological, cardiovascular/pulmonary, and integumentary. Since pain and chronic pain can accompany diagnoses associated with *any* of these areas, understanding the multidimensional aspects of pain is crucial to a physical therapist practicing in any setting.

History of Pain

The history of pain is as old as the history of mankind. In ancient cultures, pain and illness were inseparable from spiritual beliefs. Many of these cultures believed that suffering was caused by the malicious influence of spirits of the dead or the gods (Ancient Egyptians, Ancient Greeks) or punishment for misdeeds (Mesopotamians). In ancient India, the universality of the pain experience was attributed to unfulfilled desires. The ancient Chinese held that pain was a result of an imbalance of yin and yang, resulting in either excess or blocked chi. Rebalancing the chi, or the flow of energy throughout the body, was believed necessary to restore physiological balance and health. Medicinals, derivatives of many plant extracts, were also used by many ancient cultures. The Ancient Greeks and Romans devoted much study to the course of illness and recovery, and there is strong evidence that both Greek and Roman civilizations used opium derivatives for pain relief.[3] In Europe during the Dark and Middle Ages, the church became the focus of culture and learning. Pain, illness, and recovery were left to the will of God. Much of the Greek and Roman medicinal knowledge was banned as heretical. In fact, although Galen described the rudiments of our current nervous system early in the 2nd century, his teachings were banned by the church and were largely forgotten.[3]

Plato deduced that pain and pleasure, though opposite sensations, were linked together on a continuum, originating from the heart and representing passions of the soul. Aristotle taught that pain arose from an imbalance of hot influences from the heart and cool influences from the brain. Because Aristotle's views were supported by the church, they remained to profoundly influence the development of science in the Western world. Despite descriptions of pain related to inflammation by Celsus and Galens, the concept described by Aristotle prevailed for 23 centuries, attributing pain to a "passion of the soul."[3] The link between pain and physiology was not re-forged until well after the Renaissance in the 17th and 18th centuries.

In 1628, Harvey discovered the circulation of blood. Dissection of human bodies was still largely forbidden because of the strong religious convictions that had predominated for centuries. As long as the heart was considered the center of the soul and mind, the church forbade the study of the human body. To remove such strong prohibition by the church, Descartes conceptualized the separation of the mind and body. He described the pineal body as the connecting point, the center of the brain. Descartes proposed that for a person to be conscious of something, the experience had to go through this center. The pineal body then was believed to be the point at which the physical transmission of information along the nervous system became transformed into conscious thoughts, feelings, and emotions. Descartes placed the brain as the center of perception and described the nerves as tubes containing delicate threads that connected sensation in the periphery with awareness (Fig. 28.1).[4] Despite huge advances in science, this simplistic view of the nervous system continued to dominate medical understanding of pain for several centuries.

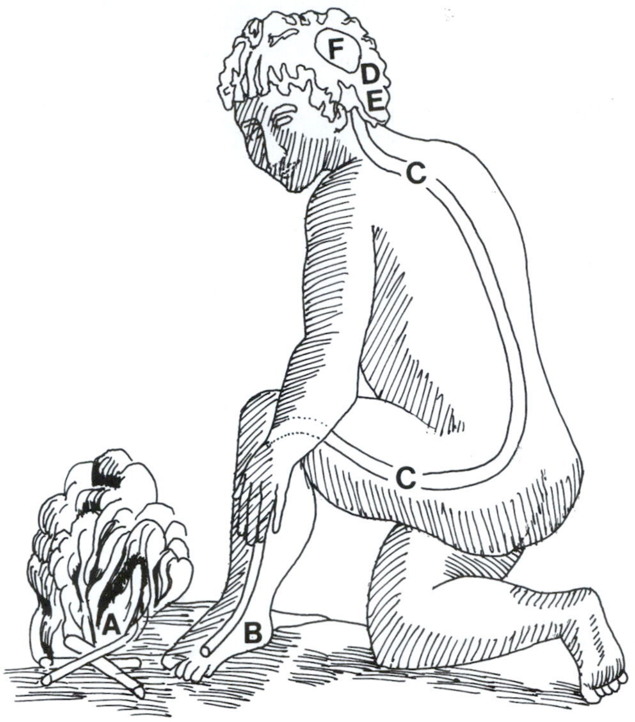

Figure 28.1 Descartes' "delicate thread." Descartes (1664) considered nerves to be tubes that contain a large number of fine threads, connecting the brain with the skin and other tissues. (From Melzack and Wall,[4] p 72, with permission.)

Pain Theories

Early Medical Models

In modern western medicine until the mid-20th century, pain was assumed to be a symptom of an underlying physiological cause. To stop the pain, the underlying problem needed to be corrected. This view is fairly mechanistic and is consistent with Descartes' belief of the duality between mind and body. Medical models work well in pain that arises as a result of acute tissue damage or acute illness. However, they cannot account for pain that persists after healing is presumed to have taken place. Pain in complex situations, such as in phantom limb pain, also cannot be easily fit into this theory. Medical models are not robust enough to explain the variability of pain experience seen in clinical practice.[5,6]

However, these theories (summarized in Table 28.1) and their evolution are instructive in understanding historical influences on how pain has been managed. For example, the *Specificity Theory,* which describes pain as a specific physical sensation, led to medical practice that "cut out" the pain, or the tissue from which the pain was believed to originate. Other theories, such as the *Fourth Theory of Pain,* suggest the intensity of the stimulus and the reaction to it create the pain experience. Such a theory suggests that two individuals experiencing the same problem (i.e., a fractured leg) would vary in their responses to that pain. Current scientific understanding of pain experience has incorporated the influence of cultural, environmental, and personality factors. However, when we examine two patients who we believe to have the same pain problem, we may still consider one patient's response as being what we would expect from that experience

Table 28.1 Historical Theories of Pain

Theory	Author	Summary
Intensive (summation) Theory	Erb 1874	This theory, built on Aristotle's concept that pain resulted from excessive stimulation of the sense of touch, was described by several authors in the 1840s. Erb maintained that every stimulus was capable of producing pain if it reached sufficient intensity. The theory was further developed by Goldscheider in 1894, who described both stimulus intensity and central summation as critical determinants of pain. It was implied that the summation occurred in the dorsal horn cells.
Specificity Theory	VonFrey 1895	This theory is based on the assumption that the free nerve endings are pain receptors, and that the other three types of receptors are also specific to a sensory experience. Pain perception was viewed as a function of the amount of physical damage alone.
Strong's Theory	Strong 1895	Strong believed that pain was an experience based on both the noxious stimulus and the psychic reaction or displeasure provoked by the sensation.
Pattern Theories	Nafe 1934	Early pattern theories suggested that all cutaneous qualities are produced by spatial and temporal patterns of nerve impulses rather than by separate, modality-specific transmission routes.
Central Summation Theory	Livingston 1943	This theory proposed that the intense stimulation resulting from nerve and tissue damage activated fibers that projected to internuncial neuron pools within the spinal cord. Abnormal reverberating circuits were created, with self-activating neurons. Prolonged abnormal activity bombarded cells in the spinal cord, and information was projected to the brain for pain perception.
The Fourth Theory of Pain	Hardy, Wolff, and Goodell 1940s	This theory expanded on Strong's theory and stated that pain was composed of two components: the perception of pain and the reaction one has to it. The reaction was described as a complex physiopsychological process involving cognitive functions of the individual, and influenced by past experiences, culture, and various psychological factors that produce great variation in the "reaction pain threshold."
Sensory Interaction Theory	Noordenbos 1959	This is a description of two systems involving transmission of pain and other sensory information with a fast and slow system. The slow system, composed of unmyelinated small diameter fibers, was presumed to conduct somatic and visceral afferents. The fast system, composed of large fibers, was said to inhibit transmission of the small fibers.
Gate Control Theory	Melzack and Wall 1965	This theory proposed that the neural mechanisms in the dorsal horns of the spinal cord act like a gate that can increase or decrease the flow of nerve impulses from peripheral fibers to the spinal cord cells that project to the brain. The somatic input is therefore subjected to the modulating influence of the gate before it evokes pain perception and response. It is suggested that large-fiber inputs tend to close the gate, whereas small-fiber inputs generally open it. Descending controls from the brain also influence what is experienced.

whereas another individual's response falls outside these expectations. Livingston's theory of a *Central Summation of Impulses* has been expanded by many of the current theorists. Livingston proposed a "vicious cycle of reflexes" involving a chronic irritation of a peripheral sensory nerve with increased afferent impulses. This irritation resulted in abnormal activity in an internuncial pool of neurons in the lateral and anterior horn of the spinal cord, and in turn increased sympathetic reflex efferent activity, including increased heart rate, vasoconstriction, and muscle spasm. This heightened sympathetic activity was thought to produce further abnormal input, thereby creating a feedback loop that perpetuated the experience. The prolonged excitability of the internuncial pool is further maintained by fear and anxiety. Such pain was thought to no longer be triggering an alarm of imminent danger, but to have become itself the pathology, residing within the nervous system. The pain pathways were thought to fire although no noxious stimuli were present.

The transmission of the signal was thought to be faulty, so that when a very minor, non-noxious stimulus was present, the information was garbled and distorted, causing the pain pathways to fire inappropriately.[7,8]

The Gate Control Theory

In the 1960s, Melzack and Wall's research showed that the experience of pain could be modulated through alternative input to the nervous system. Their theory, modified in the 1980s, identified the substantia gelatinosa (SG) in the spinal cord as a structure that acts as a "gate" to control access to the pain pathways. A schematic diagram of the theory is shown in Figure 28.2. In this model, noxious stimuli can be modified both by activity within the spinal cord and by descending influences from the brain. They were able to demonstrate that pain perception is an individualized and complex response of our nervous system that integrates purely physiologic processes with more subjective beliefs and interpretation. The **Gate Control Theory** helps to account for some of the variance in pain expression and treatment outcomes with its intricate feedforward and feedback loops between the central and peripheral nervous systems.[4]

Many common physical therapy interventions are thought to be effective based on this model. For example, **transcutaneous electrical nerve stimulation (TENS)** and ice massage may act as counterirritant stimuli to close the gate to other noxious impulses at the spinal cord level.

Biopsychosocial Models

The work of Melzack and Wall led to the development of cognitive/behavioral or **biopsychosocial models** of pain and the widespread acceptance of the interdisciplinary pain management program. The biopsychosocial approach seeks

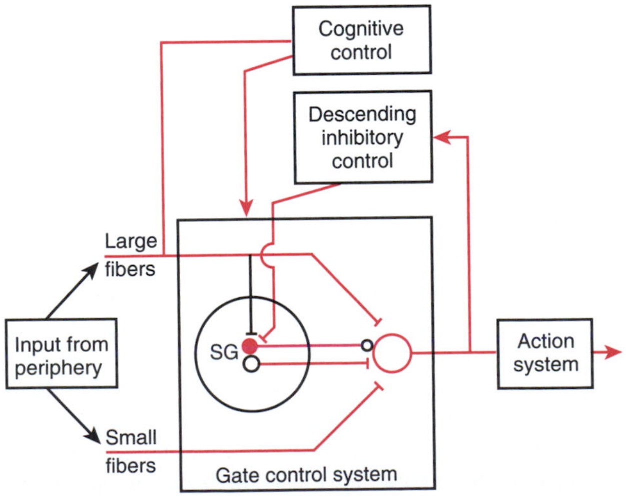

Figure 28.2 Melzack and Wall's 1983 Revised Gate Control Theory. (From Bonica,[3] p 10, with permission.)

to explain pain as a complex interaction of a person's physiology, thoughts, feelings, and social milieu. A new lexicon was developed to explore the complexity of this theory including *nociception, pain, suffering,* and *pain behavior.*[9] **Nociception** refers to the stimulation of peripheral pain sensitive nerve endings by mechanical, thermal, or chemical energy that activates A-delta and C fibers which transmit a signal to the central nervous system. **Pain** is the perception or identification of stimuli as painful. **Suffering** is a subjective valuation placed on the experience of pain. It is the feeling associated with anticipation of or an actual threat to our well being. **Pain behavior** is the observable actions of an individual in response to his or her experience of pain and/or suffering.

In this paradigm, mind and body are inseparable; indeed perception and physiology interact in highly complex ways that science is just beginning to understand. Further, there is no one-to-one correspondence between nociception and pain, pain and suffering, or suffering and pain behavior. Pain, suffering, and pain behavior can all occur *without actual stimulation of pain structures*. The degree to which nociception is expressed as pain is often contextually determined. Examples of this phenomenon include soldiers wounded on the battlefield who do not report pain and young children who glance at their caregivers before reacting to a playground fall. The brain does not discriminate between actual tissue damage and the threat of or perceived tissue damage. Suffering, too, can be based on perception rather than nociceptive input.

Pain Behavior

Pain behavior is one of the most puzzling and challenging aspects of pain management. It lends itself to misinterpretation and observer bias and complicates the pattern of objective findings. Pilowski[10] defines *abnormal illness behavior* in terms of the interaction between health provider and patient. In essence, it is a value judgment *on the part of the practitioner* in determining what proportion of the symptoms the patient is "entitled" to express. Pain behavior is a type of illness behavior and includes elements of what an observer interprets as suggesting pain. These elements include postural asymmetry, antalgic movements, facial expression, pain verbalization, and seeking medical assistance.[9] Interpreting pain behavior as purely negative behavior to be extinguished negates its importance as a communication tool.[11,12] All behavior has a purpose. It is estimated that most communication occurs on a nonverbal level. Humans are quite skilled from birth in decoding the nonverbal portion of communication. We employ these techniques unconsciously both expressively and receptively.[13] In the vast majority of cases, pain behaviors are unconscious rather than deliberate and are used to convey distress rather than to manipulate interactions. Figure 28.3 presents components of the complex psychophysiological dimensions of chronic pain.

One of the dangers in overinterpreting pain behavior is in assuming all behaviors to be pain behaviors. For example, a

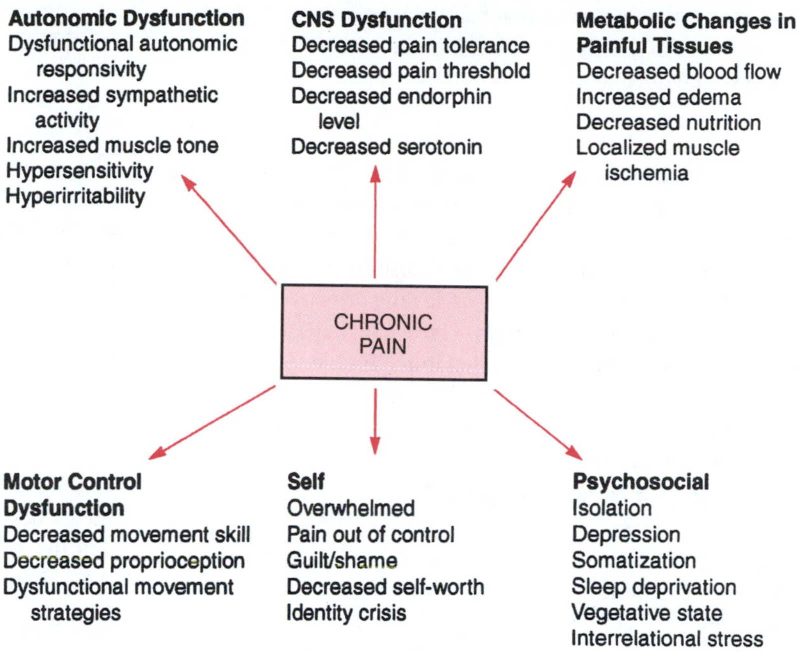

Figure 28.3 Components of the complex psychophysiological dimensions of chronic pain.

patient who limps into the treatment room may be limping from back pain, but he may also be limping from a preexisting leg length discrepancy. Making value judgments on the basis of observed behavior is not compatible with a therapeutic relationship.

Neuroplasticity, Wind-Up, and Learning

Novel imaging techniques and advances in neuroscience have led to an increased understanding of the role that perception, anticipation, and past experience has on the human central nervous system (CNS). Neuroplasticity is the concept that our CNS reorganizes in response to peripheral input. We know that these changes occur and that some of these changes predispose individuals to experience chronic pain.[14] Coghill et al describe structural differences in the brain and brain activation using functional magnetic resonance imaging (fMRI) data from volunteers who described themselves as more or less sensitive to pain.[15]

There is compelling animal model and human evidence of changes in the somatosensory cortex[16–20] and spinal cord[21,22] with exposure to painful stimuli. Melzack et al[23] present an excellent review of our current knowledge in this area.

Wind-up is a specific type of neuroplasticity in which the receptive fields of CNS neurons expand, sensitizing the individual's nervous system and effectively lowering the threshold to the transmission of nociceptive impulses.[23] Studies of induced chronic pain in animal models suggest that wind-up can be effectively blocked with *preemptive analgesia.* Preemptive analgesia is the administration of pain relieving medication, most often to a specific tissue, prior to a medical or surgical intervention that is likely to give rise to nociceptive input in that tissue. Data from human investigation of preemptive analgesia in the reduction of postsurgical pain has been mixed. Several controlled studies have found no difference in amount of anaesthesia required for surgery or self-report of pain after surgery with use of preemptive analgesia.[24–26] Other studies have found significant differences in postsurgical pain with preemptive analgesia.[27–29]

Pain is a complex phenomenon that involves more than biology, physiology, and pharmacology. Any theory of pain must take into account the compelling problem of individuals with comparable illness or injury who fail to respond to comparable interventions. Biopsychosocial models of pain are currently the best fit to explain this complexity and guide optimum practice and research.

The Biology of Pain

A working knowledge of pain physiology is essential to navigate the literature in pain management, as well as rationally examine and select appropriate pain management tools in patient care.

Nociceptors

Nociceptors are the pain specific nerve endings in the periphery. They fire in response to potential tissue damage. They are abundant in the skin and musculoskeletal system. Nociceptors consist of free nerve endings: *A-delta,* and *C fibers.* The A-delta fibers respond to mechanical and thermal stimulation and elicit the first, localized sharp pain. They are thought to produce the *withdrawal reflex* and are of short duration. C fibers are polymodal receptors. They respond to chemical, thermal, and mechanical stimuli and produce the secondary aching or burning pain and are of long duration.

Pain modulation can occur in the periphery by the stimulation of *A-beta* afferents. These are large diameter, non-nociceptive neurons that can "close the gate" via activation of the SG. This activation inhibits ascending response at the spinal cord level.[30]

Ascending Pathways

The *spinothalamic tract* carries the information for pain discrimination ("what, where") from spinal level to thalamus. This pathway serves to localize the nociceptive input and primarily travels to the somatosensory cortex. The *spinoreticulothalamic system* carries the affective (feeling/interpretive) component of pain. These pathways travel from spinal level to thalamus, hypothalamus, limbic system, and sensory cortex. The spinoreticulothalamic system connects nociception with the older centers of our brain that mediate memory and emotion. Chronic pain is neurologically hard wired to link pain and affect.[30]

Descending Pathways

The brain is able to modulate the intensity and frequency of ascending tract cell firing through the action of descending pathways.[30] The descending pathways can inhibit the ascending pathways via interneurons in the dorsal horn of the spinal cord. Descending impulses travel from the periaqueductal gray (PAG) to the raphe nuclei in the upper medulla and to the dorsal horn via reticulospinal fibers. Other pain-suppressing impulses pass from the PAG to the dorsal horn via the locus coeruleus. Communication between pathways occurs via neurotransmitters. Cognitive and emotional factors either enhance or inhibit activity in the descending pathways to alter pain perception. Treatment techniques like relaxation, meditation, imagery, and distraction are thought to enhance the activity of the descending pathways to inhibit pain. Release of *endorphins* (endogenous morphine) and *enkephalins* via exercise or relaxation response can inhibit pain.[31] These substances are located in the periaquaductal gray (PAG) matter, thalamus, SG, and the limbic system.

Neurotransmitters

Neurotransmitters are used for communication between neurons. They are synthesized in the neuron that stores it and are stored in the vesicles of the neuron. They are released with nerve impulses and bind/activate a specific receptor. Neurotransmitters are able to be inactivated by other neurotransmitters. Examples of neurotransmitters include dopamine, serotonin, norepinephrine, acetylcholine, glutamate, gamma-aminobutyric acid (GABA), and glycine.

Neurons receive a constant barrage of synaptic signals, some inhibitory, some excitatory. Impulses are summed at the level of the nerve cell, and if the balance favors excitation, the nerve will fire. If the balance favors inhibition, the nerve cell will not fire. Many of the current drugs used in chronic pain are thought to act on neurotransmitters that may be relevant in pain modulation. For example, some of the antidepressant medication (SSRIs, or selective serotonin reuptake inhibitors) can be effective in pain management. Research has shown their pain modulation effect to be independent of their effect on depression. In addition, endorphins and enkephalins act to inhibit transmission of substance P.[31]

Peripheral Mechanisms

The Inflammatory Response

The inflammatory response has been identified as a crucial peripheral modulator of pain.[32–35] Inflammatory mediators—prostaglandins and leukotrienes increase peripheral nociception. Also in local edema, there is local formation of bradykinin, another irritant. Degranulation of inflammatory cells releases histamine and serotonin, which can act locally to drive increased nociception. Small-caliber nerves release substance P and calcitonin-gene-related peptide (CGRP), which are also implicated in driving nociception. Medications such as corticosteroids and nonsteroidal anti-inflammatory drugs (NSAIDs) are thought to act on these inflammatory mediators. Local application of heat and/or cold, as well as soft tissue mobilization and exercise can all act to modulate the inflammatory response to decrease pain.

The Sensitization of Nociceptors

Repeated noxious stimuli to the polymodal nociceptors lower their threshold to stimulation. This is thought to "open the gate" at the spinal cord level, which increases the barrage of pain impulses on the CNS. This also can help explain the phenomena of **allodynia**, in which non-painful stimuli such as light touch or air moving across the skin can be perceived as painful.[4]

Peripheral Nerve Injury

If injured, peripheral nerves regenerate at a slow rate of approximately 1 mm/day. If the path for nerve regeneration is blocked, **neuromas** form. Sprouts within neuroma are sensitive to mechanical stimulation. In addition, excitation of the neuroma may occur and be sustained by electrical "crosstalk" between bare axons. This can be a source of **neuropathic pain**.

Medical Management of Pain

Medical management of chronic pain may include pharmacological interventions, interventional (minimally invasive) pain management, and surgical pain management. Treatment may be provided by primary care physicians or tertiary pain specialists. Chronic pain is best addressed by collaborative team management; interventions provided within this framework are more likely to be successful than those provided on a unimodal basis.

Pharmacological Intervention

Analgesics are the most common class of medications used for pain management. These include nonsteroidal NSAIDs, acetaminophen, and narcotic (opioid) medications. Other classes of drugs used in pain treatment include antidepressant and anticonvulsant medication. Topical preparations are also used, ranging from transdermal delivery of opioids to

Table 28.2 Common Classes of Medications Used in Chronic Pain Management

Medication Class/ Generic Name	Examples	Clinical Indication	Adverse Effects
Paraaminophenols	Acetaminophen	Mild to moderate pain, no anti-inflammatory effect	Liver toxicity
NSAIDs	Aspirin Ibuprofen Roxicob	Mild to moderate pain, antiinflammatory effect Antiinflammatory effect, GI symptom sparing	GI bleeding, nausea
Opioids	Morphine Fentanyl Oxycodone	Moderate to severe pain	Tolerance, addiction, sedation, constipation, immune suppression
Antidepressants	Amitriptyline Nortriptyline	Chronic pain	Anticholinergic effects (dry mouth, constipation, blurred vision), sedation, insomnia,
Antiepileptics	Gabapentin Carbamazepine	Neuropathic pain	Dizziness, fatigue, ataxia, liver damage

over-the-counter creams for temporary pain relief. Examples of each of these classes of drugs are presented in Table 28.2. The use of analgesics for acute pain management is common. The function of these medications is to minimize tissue damage and to maximize tissue healing. Reducing patient anxiety and fear also reduces the sympathetic arousal level, allowing for increased blood flow and changes in pain perception. Prolonged use of any medication can be problematic, because adverse side effects may develop over time. Generally, nonaddictive medications may be taken for a longer time if side effects do not become a problem.

NSAIDs are available as both over-the-counter medications and prescription medications. Some of the newest classes of NSAIDs are the COX-2 inhibitors. These drugs provide powerful and effective antiinflammatory action with less gastrointestinal side effects. Several studies have shown the effectiveness of COX-2 inhibitors in chronic pain.[36,37]

Narcotic analgesics are often both physiologically and psychologically addicting, but research evidence shows that when the medication is properly adjusted to the pain level, psychological addiction is less likely.[38] The use of narcotic analgesics in chronic non-cancer pain is controversial. Nedeljkovic et al provide two thorough reviews of the literature and issues associated with the prescription of narcotic medication in patients with chronic pain.[39,40] Some of the major concerns include issues of physiological tolerance, addiction, opioid-induced pain sensitivity, and immune function effects. More minor side effects include nausea and constipation. In addition, there are certain types of pain in which narcotics are not effective, most notably neuropathic pain. Patients on narcotic pain medications must be carefully screened and monitored. Some may stay on these medications for years, enabling them to reach a level of activity with significantly higher function.[41,42] Patients using properly managed narcotics sometimes report they perceive the nociceptive component of their pain, but "it no longer bothers them," (i.e., there is less suffering associated with the pain experience). The use of narcotics designed to fill the same receptor sites as the endorphins made within the body results in a decreased production of endorphins. Endorphin depletion can occur with prolonged use of narcotics and, with such depletion, the need for the drug increases. New advances in pharmacology are enabling narcotic medication dosages to remain stable for long periods of time. The use of pumps to continuously infuse narcotic medication locally or systemically has been developed for immediate postoperative use as well as long-term pain management.

Antidepressant medications are thought to have analgesic properties separate from their effect on depression. This may include both central and peripheral mechanisms. Antidepressants have been shown to block reuptake of noradrenaline and 5-hydroxytryptamine. They also have direct and indirect actions on opioid receptors. Some antidepressants also potentiate the activity of systemic morphine.[43] Anticonvulsive medications are used primarily in neuropathic pain. There is strong support for their use in animal models of neuropathic pain.[44] Gabapentin has been shown to be effective in animal models of allodynia[45] and in human treatment of trigeminal neuralgia.[46]

As pain becomes chronic, adjustments must be made to the medication regimen. Medications that were helpful in the acute phase are often no longer helpful in chronic pain. Data from pain clinics, often the last stop for patients seeking help within the medical model, indicate that the most important factor in increasing level of function and successfully managing the pain is the reduction of excessive use of multiple addictive medications.[8] Patients with chronic pain often end up on a wide array of drugs, including pain medications, muscle relaxants, anti-anxiety medication, and tranquilizers. Chronic use of such medication may contribute to the withdrawn, depressed appearance of some patients with pain.

Interventional Pain Management

Anesthetic blocks, injections, or other procedures may be performed for several reasons:

- To determine the anatomical source of the pain
- To ascertain specific nociceptive pathways
- To differentiate between local and referred somatic pain
- To determine the role of the sympathetic nervous system in the pain experience
- To differentiate local pathology from reflex muscle spasm in such disorders as torticollis and the piriformis syndrome

These procedures also may be used to block pain to determine the patient's response to the elimination of pain. By blocking afferent (nociceptive) or efferent (sympathetic) fibers for several hours, abnormal activity may not return when the blockade wears off. In addition, during that time rehabilitation is facilitated and more aggressive therapy can be performed that otherwise might not be tolerated. The restoration of normal movement patterns may enhance the perpetuation of relief after the block wears off. These procedures, which may be diagnostic and/or therapeutic in nature, are listed in Table 28.3.

Table 28.3 Interventional Pain Management

Procedure	Diagnostic	Therapeutic
Facet block	Identify location of pain in facets rather than disks.	Not repeated routinely but may be used if long-term relief (months) obtained by interrupting reflex cycle.
Epidural injection done with fluroscope	Considered best intervention when pain is one sided (e.g., lateral foraminal disk herniation); 1–3 steroid injections done when nerve root is pain generator to decrease swelling.	In some patients, may be repeated every 1–2 years if symptoms relieved for several months.
SI injection	Identify SI as source of pain; steroid injections to determine duration of pain relief.	If SI is primary pain generator steroid injection may be repeated only when severe irritation/inflammation limits function up to maximum of 3 per year.
Diskogram	Used prior to surgery when fusion considered; several disks are injected, including one normal to identify disks causing symptoms.	New techniques include intradiscal steroid for annular tear or internal disk derangement.
Nerve block	Identify nerve as pain generator; may include steroid use to decrease inflammation.	May be repeated in some patients if significant relief is followed by return of significant pain.
Piriformis/other muscle block	Identify pain generator; steroid injected to decrease muscle tone and decrease inflammation of nerve.	Allows aggressive rehabilitation efforts to stretch muscle, decrease nerve entrapment, relieve pain; may need to be repeated for full therapeutic effect.
Sympathetic blocks	Determine role of complex regional pain syndrome in pain complaint.	May be repeated 4–10 times to reverse complex regional pain syndrome cycle; done in conjunction with aggressive therapy and prior to sympathectomy.
Dorsal column stimulator	Determine if pain can be controlled after all other conservative attempts have failed.	Considered for neuropathic pain; implanted for long-term pain control.
Indwelling pain pump	N/A	Indicated for nociceptive pain; may be used for long term pain control if surgery is not an option and pain cannot be altered. Provides better pain management than oral medications, or injections.

N/A = not applicable; SI = sacroiliac joint.

When pathology cannot be corrected surgically and tissue health restored, occasional treatment using blocks or injections may improve function as well as quality of life. Stimulators can be implanted along the spinal cord (Gait Control Theory) to block pain impulses from traveling to the brain where perception of pain occurs. This procedure, most commonly used for failed low back syndrome, requires careful patient selection. It may be more successful than alternatives such as additional surgery for segmental stabilization, rhizotomies, and ganglionectomies.[47] The development of scar tissue, altered nociceptive feedback loops, and permanent tissue compromise from either the injury or surgery may be indications for pain management provided by the anesthesiologist. These interventions are generally accompanied by patient instruction in self-management, pain medication (in some cases), and rehabilitation efforts.

Blocks may be used after surgery to reduce postoperative pain or in the early stages of **chronic regional pain syndrome (CRPS)** to reduce progression to full CRPS. Therapeutic blocks for CRPS interrupt the cycle of continuous pain transmission and allow treatment to mobilize and restore function. The effect of a block may extend beyond the duration of the drugs, allow for normalization of sensory feedback loops, and provide some relief from physical pain. Patients often are more able to work and function at a higher level with an increased sense of control over the pain. Patients may also be more willing to work on the psychosocial aspects of their lives that impact the pain experience.[48]

Surgical Pain Management

Techniques such as rhizotomies and cordotomies had previously been considered last-resort techniques. In many cases, the short-term results were excellent, but the long-term results were found to be poor; the pain found other tracts or neurons on which to travel, and the pain returned after variable time periods of several months to years.[49–51]

Permanent sympathectomy for any of the CRPS may be very successful. Usually, multiple sympathetic nerve blocks are performed first to determine the effectiveness of the blockade. If the block relieves pain but the duration of the relief does not increase with several blocks, a permanent sympathectomy might be very beneficial. This technique is more successful in the earlier stages of the disorder as compared to the later stages.

Clinical Presentation of Pain

Pain is not a single entity; nor can it be clearly categorized by its pathophysiology. Rather, pain, its evaluation, and its treatment are multifaceted. To accurately evaluate and manage pain, the clinician must attempt to categorize the pain experience on the basis of signs, symptoms, and patient self-report. Pain management techniques vary widely in their success. Research studies, in some part, fail to find efficacy in pain treatment because many studies do not adequately differentiate patients or treatments. Many studies, in fact, compare medications or interventional pain treatments to physical therapy as if "physical therapy" were a single intervention. It is hardly surprising that such studies fail to find "physical therapy" treatment successful in the management of pain. Far more research needs to be done that matches the appropriate treatments to the appropriate patients in the study of pain management.

Acuity

Pain can be understood as a function of its acuity. Many definitions simply relate acuity to a rigid time frame of, for example, 6 months. Pain of less than 6 months duration is "acute," while pain lasting longer than 6 months is "chronic." This is a simplistic definition and is not ultimately helpful in describing the kind of problems seen in clinical practice. A better definition of **acute pain** links an unpleasant sensory, perceptual, emotional, and mental experience provoked by acute disease or injury with autonomic, psychological, and behavioral responses.[52]

Chronic pain can be defined as persistent pain that lasts beyond the expected time frame for tissue healing. Chronic pain lends itself to behavioral and/or emotional interpretations and is a multifaceted problem. Its effective treatment must address the wide range of issues involved: biological, psychological, and social. Researchers also define **chronic pain syndrome** as a subset of chronic pain in which secondary impairments from disuse, depression, and loss of self-efficacy lead to significant dysfunction that may be out of proportion to physiologic findings.

Subacute pain is somewhat of a puzzle. It does not have a structured definition, but exists to explain the spectrum of pain experience between the acute and the chronic. Subacute pain is a useful category for patients who have pain somewhat longer than healing time would account for, but whose pain is not so long standing that it has caused significant behavioral and or physiological alterations.

It is also clinically useful to distinguish between chronic pain and ongoing or intermittent acute pain. For example, pain from sickle cell crisis or spinal tumors may last longer than 6 months, but may not have other features of chronic pain. Also, an acute pain episode can occur superimposed on a patient with a history of chronic pain or chronic pain syndrome. The presentation of the acute pain process in such individuals will be significantly different than in patients with pain-naïve nervous systems. There are both psychological/behavioral and physiological/neurological changes in the person with chronic pain. Science is just beginning to acquire the tools to investigate those differences. Table 28.4 outlines the major differences between acute and chronic pain presentations.

Table 28.4 Differentiating Acute from Chronic Pain

Acute Pain	Chronic Pain
Pain is a symptom.	Pain is a disease.
Onset is well defined.	Onset is ill defined.
Pathology is identifiable.	Pathology is often unidentifiable.
Signs of autonomic activity.	None or adapted autonomic response.
Response to tissue injury.	Response to change in nervous system.
Has biological function.	Unknown biological function.
Responds to pain treatment.	Less responsive to pain treatment.
Responds to medication.	Less responsive to medication.
Associated with anxiety.	Associated with depression.
Affects the individual.	Involves social network.
Fits the medical model.	Poor fit to medical model.

Adapted from Wittink H, and Michel T (eds): Pain Management for Physical Therapists, ed 2. Heinemann, Boston, 2002, p 5.

Tissue of Origin

Pain can be categorized as originating from one of three major structures: musculoskeletal, neuropathic, and visceral. Musculoskeletal pain arises from injury or irritation of fascia, muscle, bone, and/or joint structures. It is easily localized and the most easily understood by patient and clinician. Ligamentous strains, muscle tears, and arthritic pain are all examples of musculoskeletal pain problems.

Neuropathic pain is pain from injury to or irritation of the nervous system. The pain is described as more diffuse, and often characterized as "burning" and "aching" pain. Trigeminal neuropathy and diabetic neuropathy are common examples of this type of pain.

CRPS can be categorized as a type of neuropathic pain. CRPS is recent terminology applied to what was previously called *"causalgia"* and *reflex sympathetic dystrophy (RSD)*. A recent consensus statement issued by The National Institutes of Health (NIH) calls CRPS a disease of the CNS. Patients with CRPS exhibit changes in somatosensory, sympathetic, and motor systems that are likely related to changes in the CNS. There are widespread effects of CRPS including allodynia, sudomotor changes, poor motor control, and problems with muscle recruitment. CRPS often occurs as a result of peripheral trauma. The mechanisms underlying CRPS and its expression are not yet known. It is likely that alterations occur in the immune system, the CNS (spinal cord and higher brain structures), and the integration of multiple nervous system inputs.[53] This complex disorder has been recognized for more than a century. Dr. Weir Mitchell, a physician during the American Civil War, documented his observations of soldiers suffering from what we now call CRPS:

> *Its intensity varies from the most trivial burning to a state of torment. . . . Exposure to the air is avoided by the patient with a care which seems absurd, and most of the bad cases keep the hand constantly wet, finding relief in the moisture rather than in the coolness of the application. . . . As the pain increases, the general sympathy becomes more marked. The temper changes and grows irritable, and the face becomes anxious, and has a look of weariness and suffering . . . the rattling of a newspaper, a breath of air, the step of another across the ward, the vibrations caused by a military band, or the shock of the feet in walking, gives rise to an increase of pain.*[54, p 221]

Visceral pain arises from injury or irritation of internal organs. This pain is often quite distant from the site of tissue irritation (*referred pain*), and, as a consequence, it is often least understood by patients. Pain from interstitial cystitis and irritable bowel syndrome are examples of visceral pain. Visceral pain patterns often mimic musculoskeletal pain. For example, kidney disease often manifests as lower back pain. Gall bladder disease can manifest as scapular pain. It is important for the clinician to be familiar with these visceral referral pain patterns in order to rule in or rule out non-musculoskeletal contributors to pain.[55] In general, visceral pain will not change in response to provocation tests of the musculoskeletal area it refers to. Visceral pain must be ruled out, for example, in a patient whose low back pain does not change in response to palpation, segment testing, or physiological movement. Referral to a physician for diagnostic testing in cases like these is essential.

Mind–Body Dualism

Stratifying patients by acuity and/or by tissue of origin is only part of the diagnostic process. In practice, it is rare for patients to present with absolutely clear-cut patterns of signs and symptoms that match specific categories. In some cases, rigidly applying diagnostic criteria will lead to a less than optimal plan of care (POC). Taken to an extreme, patients with confusing pain patterns can be dismissed by health care providers as malingerers, crazy, or hysterical. All suffering is real, regardless of whether it has a specific physiologic cause. The physical therapist treating the chronic pain population must temper his or her tendency to use strict hierarchical diagnostic criteria for identifying tissue pathology, such as herniated disc or spinal stenosis, and look more broadly at suffering and dysfunction.

In acute pain of musculoskeletal origin (e.g., an ankle sprain), signs (swelling, ROM limitations, joint capsule tightness) will closely mirror symptoms (pain, stiffness, difficulty walking) and observed physical function. The more chronic a problem is, the less concordance there is between signs, symptoms, and function. There are both physiological and sociological reasons for this. The fact that the spinoreticulothalamic tract is active in chronic pain and has rich connections with the limbic system leads to the affective component of pain. Social and cultural factors in pain behavior and reinforcement lead to changes in self-image and the perception or meaning of pain. Biopsychosocial models do a better job of accounting for a full range of responses to pain than do the medical models.[56,57]

In treatment of pain, it may be useful for the clinician to look at degree of concordance vs divergence among signs, symptoms, and function. In cases where there is high concordance, impairment-based treatments will likely be more successful. In cases where there is high divergence, a functionally based approach may be more appropriate (Fig. 28.4).

Table 28.5 presents a comparison of the physical therapy examination findings from two patients with ankle injuries. The findings vary greatly depending on whether the patient presents with acute versus chronic injury.

In the acute pain example, there is high concordance among symptoms (patient complaints), signs (examination findings), and function. Treatment aimed toward ameliorating the physical findings has a high probability of success with the patient's eventual return to function. In the chronic pain example, there is a high divergence among symptoms, signs, and function, with the patient's report of function and complaints apparently out of proportion to

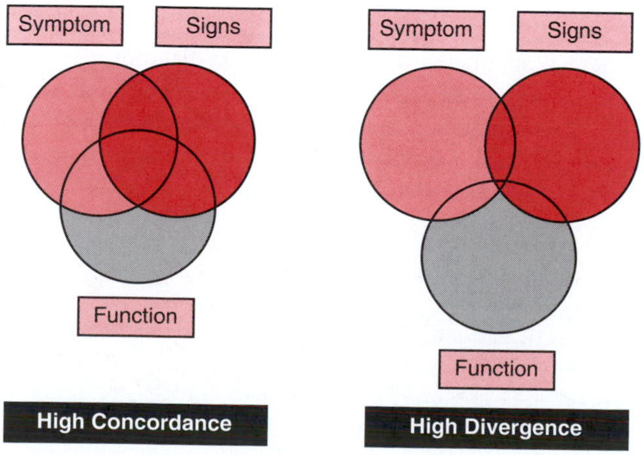

Figure 28.4 Relationship among signs, symptoms, and function in chronic pain.

physical findings. There appears to be significant disability in this case. Physical therapy treatment focused only on impairments is unlikely to lead to resolution of symptoms and return to function.

Pain Measurement

Pain is a purely subjective phenomenon. Unlike ROM, strength, or tissue extensibility, pain has no accurate or specific measurement tool. However, the measurement of pain has become a vital part of patient examination. The Joint Commission on Accreditation of Healthcare Organizations (JCAHO)[58] has emphasized the importance of pain and pain treatment by suggesting that pain be recognized as "the fifth vital sign" in health care settings.

Pain measurement allows the therapist to establish the baseline level of a patient's pain and determine if the interventions have altered the pain in a significant way. There are multiple tools in use to examine pain. Some of the commonly used tools include the *Visual Analogue Scale (VAS), body diagrams, pain questionnaires,* and *functional impairment/health-related quality of life measures.* There are advantages and disadvantages of each type of tool. Choosing a tool depends, in part, on the type of setting in which the clinician is practicing and the amount of time available for pain measurement.[59]

Visual Analogue Scale

The VAS is one of the most basic pain measurement tools. It consists of a 10 centimeter line, bounded by terminal anchors. Beneath the anchors are written cues (e.g., pain as bad as it could be, no pain at all). Research on the VAS has shown it to be a more reliable tool when the line does not have numeral markings on it and the patient is allowed to mark the line relative to the intensity of the pain. The clinician can measure the place on the line and convert it into a score between 0 and 10, where 0 is no pain at all and 10 is pain as bad as it could be. The VAS is widely used because it is easily administered and requires little to no training or equipment. However, it has several limitations in clinical use. Because pain is subjective, the difference between a score of 1 and 3 is not necessarily the same as the difference between a score of 8 and 10, even though the interval between the numbers is the same. Therefore, it is not a valid use of the scale to say that a particular patient whose VAS scored dropped from 10 to 5 has experienced a 50 percent reduction in his or her pain. It is likely that this represents a *significant reduction* of pain, but we cannot determine the percentile using VAS scores.[60] A sample VAS is presented in Appendix A. The FACES scale (Fig. 28.5) is an adaptation of a visual analogue scale for children.

Table 28.5 Brief Case Example: Acute vs. Chronic Pain

Selected Examination Data	Acute Pain	Chronic Pain
Social history	38-year-old married man, manager at a major corporation.	38-year-old married man, last worked 1 year ago as manager at a major corporation.
History of present illness	3 weeks status postsurgical repair of right Achilles tendon complete rupture, sustained playing softball on the company team	1 year ago, history of R Achilles complete rupture at company softball game; successful surgical repair 1 day post-injury; patient reports cast was fabricated too tightly and caused "nerve damage;" he has active litigation against the community hospital where he was treated; he reports that physical therapy (exercise and gait training) in the past made him worse; referring physician has cleared him for full weightbearing.
Chief complaint	R LE pain at rest, difficulty walking	Severe pain, unable to walk, unable to work, spends most of the day on the sofa at home.
Patient's goals	Full function without ankle pain, independent ambulation without crutches, return to softball	"Get rid of this pain." "Have a normal life."
Pain measured on a 10 cm VAS	At rest: 2/10; when ambulating: 7/10	At rest: 8/10; when ambulating 10+/10
Range of motion (ROM)	Significant limitations of AROM R ankle PF: 5°–45°; INV: 0–5°; EV: 0–5°	Patient is unwilling to move ankle owing to pain.
Joint mobility	Limited calcaneal mobility	Unable to test due to pain.
Observation/palpation	Adherent surgical scar, moderate swelling R ankle	Well-healed scar; smooth, hairless limb; significant atrophy throughout R LE; mild swelling R ankle/calf; unable to palpate R LE due to complaints of pain.
Gait	Independent PWB w/axillary crutches, cast boot	Independent NWB w/axillary crutches, cast boot; patient unwilling to attempt weightbearing RLE due to pain

AROM = active range of motion; EV = eversion; INV = inversion; LE = lower extremity; NWB = non-weightbearing; PF = plantarflexion; PWB = partial weightbearing; R = right; VAS = visual analogue scale.

Body Diagrams

Body diagrams (Fig. 28.6) consist of a line drawing of the human figure, generally front, back, and side views, with a key consisting of symbols for different kinds of pain. The patient is instructed to mark the body diagram using the symbols to represent the location of his or her pain. These are somewhat more time consuming to administer, and requires patient instruction in how to complete the diagram. The data obtained from body diagrams is more difficult to

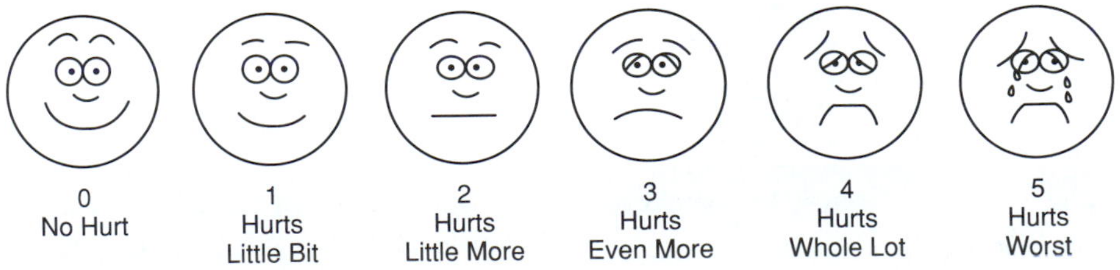

Figure 28.5 FACES. (From Wong, DL, et al: Wong's Essentials of Pediatric Nursing, ed 6. Mosby, St. Louis, 2001, p 1301, with permission.)

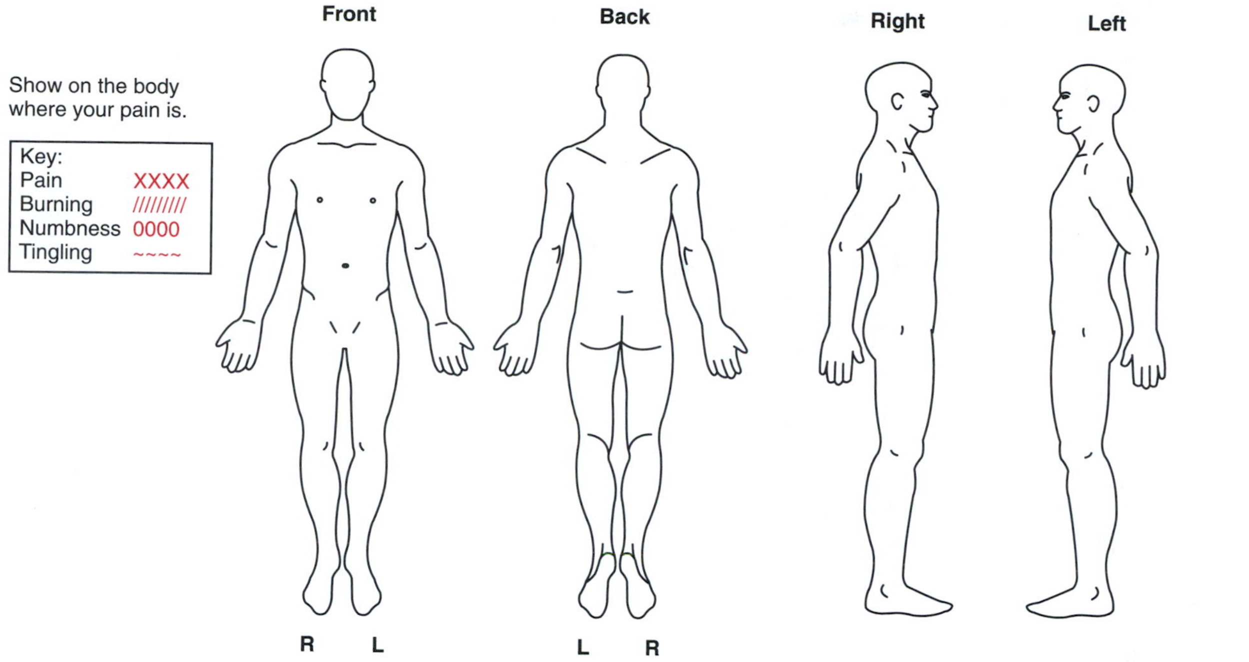

Figure 28.6 Body diagram tool.

objectively analyze than that obtained from VAS or other pain tools. Observer bias has been shown to influence analysis of body diagram data.[61]

Body diagrams have been shown to have good reliability in patients with pain.[62,63] Margolis et al measured test–retest reliability in 51 patients with chronic pain. Body diagrams were scored for percentage of body area in pain in addition to pain location. The interval between body diagram testing averaged 71 days. The authors found a test–retest reliability coefficient of 0.85.[63]

The diagrams can be "scored" as *organic* (in concordance with anatomical patterns of pain) or *nonorganic* (not in accordance with anatomical patterns of pain) (see Figs. 28.7 and 28.8). There is some evidence of a correlation between nonorganic body diagrams with psychological distress and poor outcome.[64] However, other studies have shown little predictive value between organic and nonorganic body

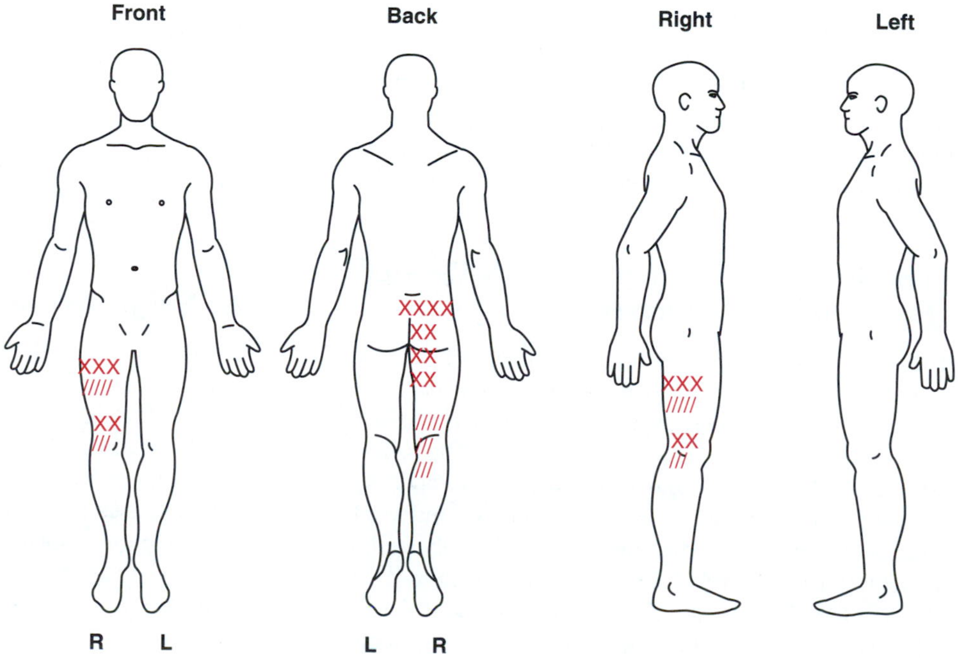

Figure 28.7 Dermatomal pain pattern. Example of a dermatomal/organic pattern of self-reported radicular low back pain. The pattern and distribution of pain follows the anatomical distribution of nerves to the periphery.

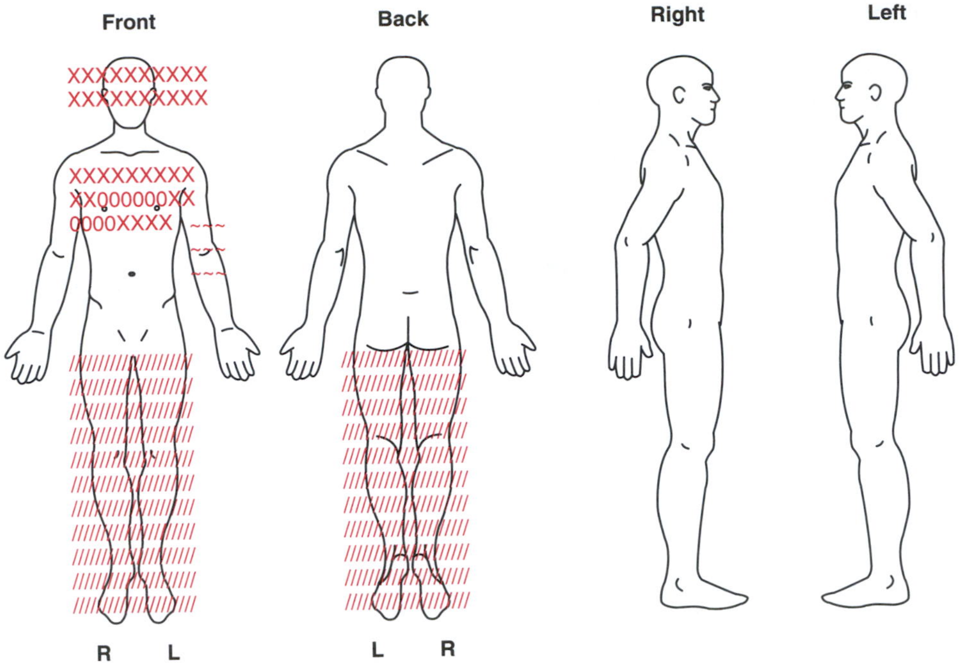

Figure 28.8 Nondermatomal pain pattern. Example of a nonanatomic/nondermatomal pattern of self-reported chronic pain. The pattern and distribution of pain does not follow the anatomical distribution of nerves to the periphery. Pain is indicated outside the confines of the body.

diagrams, physical findings, and treatment outcomes in chronic back pain.[65–67]

Pain Questionnaires

Pain questionnaires seek to examine pain through the language a patient uses to describe pain. The most well researched tool of this type is the *McGill Pain Questionnaire (MPQ)*. It consists of three portions: a body diagram, a pain intensity rating, and a list of words a patient is asked to choose from in describing his or her pain. It is lengthier than either the VAS or a body diagram alone, and it may be culturally inappropriate for patients who may not understand all or some of the vocabulary used to describe the pain. The MPQ has been used extensively in the pain literature, with diverse populations and diagnoses[68–71] and refinements of the tool are ongoing.[72,73] Appendix B presents the word choices the patient is asked to use in describing his or her pain.

Functional Impairment/Health-Related Quality of Life Measures

These measures attempt to examine impact of pain on a patient's daily life rather than measuring the pain itself. They are self-report tools; the patient is shown a list of activities along with a corresponding Likert Scale. The patient is asked to mark the degree to which pain interferes or does not interfere with the particular activity. There are many other functional impairment measures used clinically and for research purposes. The *Dallas Pain Questionnaire,*[74,75] the *SF-36,*[76] the *Glasgow Pain Questionnaire,*[77] and the *Pain Disability Index*[78] are all examples of these types of tools.

Like the MPQ, these measures can also be culturally inappropriate, particularly if they ask a patient to rate his or her ability to perform tasks that would not be culturally appropriate, regardless of pain. These types of measures can also be time consuming to administer and to score as compared with the VAS.

Physical Therapy Examination

The physical therapy examination provides an opportunity to obtain objective signs and to administer appropriate tests and measures. It also provides an opportunity to build rapport essential for a positive therapeutic relationship. There are several factors that make the examination of chronic pain more challenging than acute pain. Secondary dysfunction due to disuse, fear/avoidance, dual diagnosis, and/or past treatment failures can "muddy the waters" in interpreting the results of an examination.

The Subjective Interview

The subjective interview offers an opportunity to begin to develop a positive therapeutic relationship with the patient. Patients with chronic pain often present with histories of multiple treatment failures and attendant anxiety and the potential for expression of anger or mistrust. The language a therapist uses to address the patient can help make this first interaction a positive one. Components of the subjective interview are identified in Table 28.6.

An effective interview will incorporate a combination of open-ended and closed-ended questions. Open-ended

Table 28.6 Components of the Subjective Interview

Interview Component	Guiding Question(s)
Chief complaint	*Tell me about your problem*
Mode and time of onset	*When did the pain problem start?* *How did it start?*
History of treatment since onset	*When did you first seek treatment for your problem?* *Who did you see? What happened then?*
History of progression since onset	*Over the past 6 months, has your problem gotten better, worse, or stayed the same?*
Pain	
• Location	*Where is your pain?*
• Intensity	*How strong is your pain?* *Can you rate it on this pain scale? [instruct patient in use of VAS or other pain measurement device]*
• Pattern	*What makes the pain better? What makes the pain worse?*
• Description	*Show me where your pain is.*
Patient's general health	*Have you gained or lost weight recently?* *Has your appetite changed?* *How are you sleeping?*
Current medication list	*What medications or supplements do you take?* *Do you take any medications or supplements not related to your pain?*
Current functional limitations	*What can't you do because of the pain?*
Opportunity to add information	*Is there anything we haven't discussed that might be important to your problem?*
Establish goals and ways to measure improvement	*How will you know you're better?* *What will you be able to do when you're better?* *What do you want to be able to do better a month from now that you're unable to do now?*

VAS = visual analogue scale.

questions are questions that cannot be answered with a "yes" or "no" response, but require narrative explanations. For example, "*What happened on the day of your accident?*" or "*Why are you here?*" Open-ended questions encourage disclosure. They can be used to clarify responses or have the patient elaborate on a previous answer. They are a good starting place for any interview.

Closed-ended questions are used when the desired response is succinct, such as "yes," "no," "always," "sometimes," or "never." For example, "*How many surgeries have you had?*" or "*Did you have a fusion?*" are examples of closed-ended questions. The closed-ended questions allow the therapist to control the flow of information. They are used to narrow down or clarify a narrative response. They are also helpful in focusing and redirecting an anxious or overly talkative patient.

The talkative patient will require more structure (closed-ended questions) in an interview. The reticent patient will need to be drawn out with the use of open-ended questions. Alternating between these types of questions will help ensure a thorough, organized, and accurate interview. A partial example of a subjective interview can be found in Table 28.7.

There is no substitute for a thorough patient interview. During a face-to-face conversation, the therapist can ask follow-up questions, take the interview in a different direction, observe pain behavior and affect, and establish the partnership that is essential to the therapeutic process. An interview takes time, particularly for the patient with chronic pain whose history may include decades of treatments.

Tests and Measurements

The information obtained during the subjective interview and the physical therapist's initial observation of the patient will guide the therapist in the selection of the most appropriate tests and measures. The tests and measures used for patients with chronic pain are not different than those used in any physical therapy examination. Certain elements of the physical examination will be appropriate in nearly all patients with chronic pain: vital signs, reflex integrity, sensory integrity, posture, ROM, muscle performance,

Table 28.7 A Partial Example of a Subjective Interview

Physical Therapist (open- and closed-ended questions)	Patient Response
Tell me why you are here (*open*)	*I have neck pain and headaches.*
How did the pain start? (*open*)	*I was rear ended at a stop light by a newspaper truck 4 years ago.*
Were you able to walk away from the accident on your own? (*closed*)	*Yes, but I was dizzy and my neck hurt right away.*
So what happened after that? (*open*)	*They took me to the hospital and took x-rays. They said nothing was broken so they sent me home with pain killers.*
What tests did you have? (*open*)	*More X-rays and an MRI.*
Were you able to go back to work? (*closed*)	*No, are you kidding?! I couldn't even sit 5 minutes and when I try to use a computer, my head just throbs and my arms go numb.*
What do you hope to achieve working with me? (*open*)	*The pain pills don't really work and I don't know what else to try. My doctor told me to try physical therapy again.*
Starting with the time you wake up, what do you do in a typical day? (*open*)	*I get up before 5 and can't get back to sleep. I usually get out of bed so I don't wake my husband. I take a hot bath. Then I lie down on the sofa in the living room.*
Are there things that you are unable to do because of pain that you would like to be able to do? (*open*)	*I wish I could use a computer or go out to dinner and a movie with my husband.*
How will you know you are better? (*open*)	*I don't know, maybe I could sit through a movie without pain.*

Note: Questions are abstracted from a thorough interview and are presented here primarily to illustrate the differences between open and closed ended questions with sample responses.

and gait. Other elements of the physical examination will be diagnosis specific or specific to particular patient complaints. Some of these include (but are not limited to) examination of aerobic capacity, functional skills, circulation, body mechanics, joint mobility and motor control, orthotic devices, and work/functional integration. These examinations will give the therapist a baseline measure of signs, symptoms, and functional ability, as well as a determination of the need for orthotic or assistive devices and the ability to return to work (work place evaluation). Table 28.8 illustrates examples of selected examination techniques and their relationship to chronic pain findings.

Examination findings may be normal, or the patterns of signs and symptoms may be contradictory. Some impairments are direct and related to the initial injury or diagnosis. Others are indirect, owing to disuse or compensatory motor patterns that have developed due to pain. Postural asymmetries are common in patients with chronic pain. These asymmetries often develop immediately after an injury, as the body seeks to protect the injured area. Tissue lengths adapt over time, and become part of the established, or habituated, movement pattern. The movement patterns of patients with chronic pain are frequently rigid and guarded to compensate first for the pain and later for balance disturbances that may arise from the postural asymmetries. Joints distant from the original injury eventually may be limited in ROM as these asymmetries become chronic.[79] Movement dysfunction becomes a perpetuating factor and may persist long after the initial pathology is resolved. With extensive postural and movement dysfunction, the patient may report virtually all movements to be painful. Movements also may be limited by fear as the patient experiences pain in areas distant from the initial injury. Testing ROM in standing and then in a prone position may result in marked differences in joint excursion. Testing the same task in two different positions can assist in determining the influence of shortening of muscles or other soft tissue involved in the test movement. Discrepancies in findings have been seen by some as support for the patient attempting to "fake" limitations. In reality, they represent differences in selection of movement strategies. This phenomenon of apparent changes in ROM and movement strategies can be demonstrated in normal, healthy subjects as well. Cardiovascular fitness often is poor in these

Table 28.8 Components of the Physical Therapy Examination and Common Findings in Patients with Chronic Pain

Components of Examination	Common Findings with Chronic Pain
Reflex integrity	Often inhibited owing to muscle holding.
Sensory integrity	May be inconsistent, impairments nondermatomal, hypersensitivity to cutaneous stimulation common.
Posture	Muscle dysfunction, poor sense of body position, and disuse often contribute to postural asymmetries.
ROM	Changes in ROM may be inconsistent and related to both primary and secondary symptom complaints.
Muscle performance	Adaptive changes in muscle length and tension, and myofascial trigger points are often prevalent; strength may be inconsistent; trigger points and pain may inhibit muscles during break testing (MMT) as a reflex protective mechanism.
Gait	Postural asymmetries and poor self-awareness may lead to antalgic gait.
Aerobic capacity	Patients may have long-standing habit of self-limiting activity; aerobic exercise without pain is not possible, so they avoid.
Ergonomics and body mechanics	Often impaired, awareness of these impairments is often poor.
Joint mobility	Limitations are more commonly a result of muscle holding, muscle shortening, pain related inhibition as opposed to actual joint restrictions.
Motor control	Often impaired as a result of long-term disuse and pain related changes in kinesthetic awareness and movement.

MMT = manual muscle test; ROM = range of motion.

patients, and low endurance combined with rapid muscle fatigue may result in inconsistent testing.

Evaluation and Treatment Planning

Clinical decision making must take into account both the physical and psychological changes associated with pain. The overall goal of treatment is to decrease pain-related disability. This can be accomplished with a coordinated treatment plan that focuses on improved function along with resolution of treatable direct and indirect impairments. Functional goals must be measurable, specific, and attainable and mutually agreed upon by the physical therapist and patient.

Specific treatments matter less than the matching the treatment to the specific functional problems and goals presented by each patient. In addition, the therapist must understand the philosophical difference between pain treatment and pain management as that difference applies to chronic pain.

Chronic pain is more likely to produce diffuse and unrelated impairments and functional problems than is acute pain. In acute pain, it is appropriate to identify a specific tissue impairment that is responsible for the majority of symptoms involved. In the case of acute knee pain resulting from a recent skiing injury, it would be reasonable to assume that the pain arises from small tears of knee ligaments if confirmed by the physical exam. It would also be reasonable to develop a POC based on the goals of decreasing inflammation, instability, and pain using a variety of passive modalities and active exercise.

The patient who presents with knee and lower leg pain that is diffuse, long standing, and not consistent with a specific impairment typically demonstrates significant functional limitations. It is not logical to look to identify a single specific tissue as the root cause of the problem. A better fit here is treatment geared toward improving function and managing pain. This type of pain rehabilitation is consistent with the philosophies of functional restoration, work hardening, cognitive–behavioral therapy, and pain rehabilitation.[80–84]

Psychosocial Factors

There may be little concordance among signs, symptoms, and function in the patient with chronic pain. This can lead to difficulty in the interpretation of findings and the development of a logical and coherent POC. Indeed, the skills of matching subjective complaints to examination findings that work so well in patients with more straightforward acute pain can be misleading and must be carefully evaluated. Pain-related disability is inextricably linked to problems of fear-avoidance, ineffective coping, depression, trauma, and inappropriate social reinforcement. These psychosocial issues may confuse the pattern of findings that clinicians rely on in treatment planning.

Fear-Avoidance

Chronic pain involves the limbic system and evokes an emotional response along with CNS recognition of pain intensity and localization. Patients with chronic pain often have histories of treatment failures and pain flares as a result of functional activity. These past experiences lead to anticipatory anxiety and pain. Thus, a patient may be locked into a cycle in which activity causes pain that increases fear and decreases physical activity.[85] Along with this constraining of activity come secondary impairments of disuse that can include, but are not limited to, ROM limitations, joint stiffness, muscle atrophy, deconditioning, and coordination impairments. *Fear-avoidance* can often be misinterpreted as nonadherence.[86–88]

Fear-avoidance can be addressed by patient education and close monitoring of home exercise and activity programs. Exercise prescription must be carefully planned and monitored so that the patient will experience success from the beginning. In addition, the program and its progression must be matched with the individual. Exercise prescription is fully addressed later in this chapter.

Coping, Catastrophizing, and Acceptance

In the case of chronic pain, there is little direct correspondence among impairments, experience of pain, and function. Clinicians and researchers have investigated psychosocial measures to identify critical risk factors in chronicity. One of the measures extensively studied is **coping**, or the individual's ability to manage his or her distress. It has been theorized that preexisting poor coping styles may place an individual at higher risk for developing chronic pain from an injury that a more effective coper would recover from. Research with the *Multidimensional Pain Inventory (MPI)* has shown it to be a reliable and valid tool in examining coping styles in a chronic pain population.[89] Patterns of answers on the MPI questionnaire group patients on the basis of coping into one of three subsets: *dysfunctional*, *interpersonally distressed*, and *adaptive coper*. Studies using this classification have shown that dysfunctional and interpersonally distressed profiles negatively correlate with function.[90,91] Other studies have shown no correlation in outcomes among the patients subgrouped into the different coping styles.[91–93] This may indicate that biopsychosocial-based rehabilitation can be effective no matter the coping profile of the patient or that other variables in addition to coping may be crucial.

Another variable is *catastrophizing*, or the perception of pain as terrible, incapacitating, and unbearable. Catastrophizing has been correlated with increased pain perception in experimental[94] and clinical pain in patients with fibromyalgia[95] and with depression and pain severity in chronic pain.[96]

The concept of *acceptance* may also be useful in pain rehabilitation. Acceptance represents a patient's shift away from a search for a cure for pain toward a focus on non-pain-related life tasks. Acceptance has been related to subjective report of well-being, psychological functioning, and physical functioning in patients with chronic pain.[97,98]

Depression

The relationship between depression and pain is a complex one. Recent studies confirm depression as a significant and independent risk factor for development of back pain[99,100] and neck pain.[100] Back pain is also a significant risk factor for development of major depression.[101] This relationship appears to be a linear one, with increased pain intensity associated with higher risk of depression. Furthermore, pain appears to adversely affect the outcome of treatment for depression in a significant majority of patients presenting with depression in primary care.[102] The combination of pain and depression is associated with higher rates of perceived disability than pain or depression alone.[101] While no specific causative relationship between pain and depression has been found, the covariance of pain and depression is a significant and confounding variable in the effective treatment of chronic pain.

Pain and Trauma

There has been a long standing anecdotal linking of chronic pain with abuse and trauma. History of physical and or sexual abuse has been shown to interfere with pain management in patients with chronic pain.[103] There is evidence for a high correlation between sexual abuse and chronic pelvic pain in women,[104] childhood abuse or neglect and fibromyalgia,[105] childhood abuse or neglect and chronic low back pain,[106] and childhood psychological trauma and poor outcome in lower back pain (LBP) surgery.[107] It is likely that a physical therapist working with pain problems will encounter patients who are survivors of childhood physical and/or sexual abuse, trauma, and neglect. It is vital for the clinician to develop the sensitivity and skills required to work with trauma survivors. An excellent resource for clinicians is a study by Schachter et al[108] that employed semistructured interviews with adult survivors of childhood trauma and their experiences with physical therapy treatment.

Social Reinforcement

Patients with chronic pain often call pain the invisible disability. Pain is a subjective construct and communication of distress occurs within a social milieu that can include family, friends, co-workers, and health care workers.[108] Social reinforcement can be a powerful tool in shaping pain behavior. Negative spousal response to pain has been associated with increased anxiety and depression[109] and decreased physical activity[110] in patients with chronic pain. In clinical practice, the physical therapist can actively support and reinforce appropriate well behaviors rather than inadvertently reinforce inappropriate pain behavior by avoiding pain language and focusing on function.

Rapport, Relationship, and Compliance

There is a perception among clinicians that patients with chronic pain are difficult patients. Although there are patients who may be difficult to work with, use of the label "difficult patient" is at best unhelpful and at worst destructive to the therapeutic process. In the majority of cases, the difficulty stems from mismatches between patient and therapist expectations. The effective clinician develops strategies for identifying and dealing with difficult behavior to enhance patient adherence and reduce the chance of frustration and burnout. Strategies to diffuse anger, anxiety, eliminate ambiguity, and maintain appropriate professional boundaries are as important to clinical practice as the skillful application of any treatment technique.[111–114]

Problematic Behaviors

There are many types of problematic behavior. They can include intense emotions expressed verbally, demands expressed verbally, nonadherence, manipulation, and disruptive conduct. Any of these behaviors can interfere with the therapeutic process.

There are several distinct behaviors and response patterns that may emerge within the treatment process that can affect both the clinician and patient. These include:

- Passive–Dependent response
- Overanxious response
- Hostile response
- Passive–Aggressive response
- Help Rejecting response

The patient in a *passive–dependent* mode may continuously demand reassurance, defer to the clinician, or act powerless. The clinician may be overly solicitous, fail to follow through on plans, or avoid making decisions. The *overanxious* patient may appear to be magnifying symptoms, express high anxiety, or internalize blame for the condition. The overanxious clinician may be overly cautions, feel anxious, unprepared, or take responsibility for the patient's status. The patient who acts with *hostility* may be suspicious of clinician's motives, feel mistreated and/or persecuted, or reject all or part of the POC. The clinician who responds with hostility may be suspicious of the patient's motives, feel taken advantage of, or ignore the patient's input. In a *passive–aggressive* response style, the patient may use a "yes, but . . ." response pattern, appear to be helpless, or blame others for his or her condition. The clinician who responds in a passive–aggressive manner may be help rejecting, complain about lack of support, or blame the patient for lack of progress. The patient in the *help rejecting* pattern may have difficulty asking for help, act belligerently, or minimize symptoms/disability. The clinician may feel threatened by supervision, act overconfidently, or minimize problems.

In clinical situations, responses are often mixed. A patient may present in a way that is both passive aggressive and help rejecting. The clinician may react to this patient with features of hostility and anxiety. It is important for the clinician to be able to identify emerging behavior/response patterns so that he or she may employ techniques to enhance rapport.[111–114]

Managing Problematic Behaviors

Two of the main techniques for managing problematic behavior in the clinic are relationship building and good communication. These techniques are closely related. The specific components of relationship building include (1) setting clear expectations,(2) mutual goal setting, and (3) the treatment contract.

Relationship Building

If there is a mismatch in the overall expectations of the therapy process between the clinician and the patient, it is likely that treatment will fail. In the arena of chronic pain, a common mismatch is that of pain management versus pain elimination. The philosophy of pain rehabilitation for chronic pain is similar to the philosophy of treatment of any chronic illness: patient education and self-management. In the case of type 1 diabetes, treatment goals might include patient self-monitoring of diet and blood sugars and independence in administering insulin. In the biopsychosocial model of pain rehabilitation, treatment goals include self-monitoring of activity and body mechanics, pacing and home exercise, and self-application of independent pain control modalities such as heat, cold, and self-massage. If the patient expects the clinician to "take away the pain" using passive treatment modalities, then the stage is set for significant conflict and poor outcomes.

The skilled clinician will use the initial examination and the goal setting process as an opportunity to share and shape expectations of the treatment process. Questions such as: *How will you know when you are better?* or *What will you be able to do at the end of treatment that you have difficulty doing now?* help set up expectations that highlight enhanced function as the ultimate goal of therapy. Treatment goals are not determined by the therapist. Rather, the process of goal setting emerges from the dialogue between therapist and patient in which the therapist helps the patient articulate his or her hopes for future functioning.

The concept of the *treatment contract* comes from the psychodynamic arena. It is useful in pain rehabilitation because it objectifies the roles of each participant in the healing partnership. At its most basic, the treatment contract specifies that the clinician will bring his or her skills to work with the patient in a professional manner. The patient agrees to work to his or her capacity on the shared goals developed with the clinician. In many cases, this contract emerges as a verbal agreement from the communication and goal setting process. In other cases, the contract can be written, with agreed upon responsibilities and rights that is signed and held by both parties. In a team setting, a contract can help all parties stay focused on the goals and help to moderate treatment disputes that may arise. It is important to remember that the contract binds both parties—the clinician as well as the patient.

Communication Skills

Difficulties with communication often underlie stressful professional and/or patient interactions. There are specific communication skills that the effective clinician can employ to decrease ambiguity and conflict.[113] They include:

- "I" statements
- Reference to standards/rules
- Active listening
- Reflecting emotion
- Use of "we" or teambuilding
- Limit setting

"I" Statements. Beginning a sentence with "you" at best widens the gap in the relationship between patient and clinician, and at worst can set up an expectation of hostility and blame. "You didn't do your home exercises last week," and "You always make me worse when I come to therapy" are examples of accusatory statements that increase friction and stress in a working relationship. Statements that begin with "I" help to diffuse an emotionally laden interchange and do not confer blame. "I am concerned about your home exercise program" and "I keep getting pain flares after physical therapy."

Reference to Standards and Rules. Referring to standards can help to remove personal conflict from a stressful situation. Rather than argue or persuade an individual that a course of action is "right" because the clinician believes it is, he or she can reference the standard of care, the research literature, or the rules of the institution. For example, "According to physical therapy research, active exercise is more helpful than hot packs and ultrasound for your condition." This is an extremely useful tool when objective confrontation of behavior is necessary.

Active Listening. Listening skills are just as important to communication as are speaking skills. The active listener is empathic, nonjudgmental, does not interpret, and encourages appropriate disclosure. The active listener is willing to suspend disbelief and listen completely and objectively without jumping to conclusions or drawing hasty assumptions.

Reflecting Emotion. Techniques of mirroring emotions can diffuse difficult situations. Two specific techniques for reflecting emotion include acknowledging and restating. In acknowledging, the clinician verbally labels the emotion in a way that the patient feels heard and validated. For example, "it sounds like you are very frustrated, Mr. Jones." That simple statement can allow the patient to move beyond the emotion and back into healthy rapport. Restating can be a very powerful tool to handle misunderstandings and intense emotion. Restating is an error checking device—it allows for further clarification in a problematic situation. An example of restating is: "Let me make sure I understand what you are saying. It sounds as if you believe your doctor doesn't want to prescribe your medications anymore. Is that what you are telling me?" Both techniques (reflecting and restating) can be used together to great effect.

Use of "We" or Teambuilding. The language we use helps set up expectations. Using the words "we" and "us" rather than "'I" and "you" can help reinforce the treatment contract concept in which both parties (therapist and patient) have rights and together are responsible for the outcome of treatment. Some examples of teambuilding include: "How can we solve this problem?" or "Let's look at this with your doctor's input," and "Where should we go from here?"

Limit Setting. Difficult behavior not only makes the job of rehabilitation harder, it also creates an unsafe working environment for all the patients and staff in the area. Using clear and nonaggressive language can help to set appropriate limits and increase safety and adherence. For example, "Shouting disrupts the exercise class," or "It is not appropriate to raise your voice in the clinic," or "I can only help you when you attend scheduled sessions," are all good examples of limit setting. The clinician can use a combination of the above techniques to curb disruptive behavior.

Physical Therapy Interventions

Because impairments and functional limitations in chronic pain can arise from and can affect the musculoskeletal, neuromuscular, cardiopulmonary, or integumentary systems, therapists can employ a wide variety of treatment techniques. These techniques run the gamut from modalities to patient education, mobilization and massage, therapeutic exercise, and gait training and conditioning. Interventions that are not diagnosis and impairment specific include pain control modalities, therapeutic exercise, and patient education.

Pain Control Modalities

Passive modalities such as heat (moist hot pack, diathermy, ultrasound), cold, manual therapy (massage, mobilization) and electro therapy (electrical stimulation, interferential, high-voltage galvanic stimulation [HVGS]) are for the most part useful in addressing specific tissue level impairments. Although these impairments (e.g., inflammation, tissue restriction, joint stiffness) can coexist with chronic pain, treatment limited to addressing impairments will not significantly change pain-related disability. Furthermore, application of treatment techniques that require the patient be a passive recipient encourages disability[115] by reinforcing that the patient has no power to effect change in his or her life. There is a body of literature on the concept of locus of control and evidence that an external locus of control is consistent with a higher degree of perceived disability.[116–118] Pain rehabilitation consistent with the biopsychosocial model aims to increase self-efficacy, increase internal locus of control, and reduce pain-related disability.

There can be a role in chronic pain management for passive modalities. However, that role is small and must be explained well to the patient. For example, ultrasound can be a useful tool for providing deep heat to a tight muscle or joint, allowing the structure to move more normally, thus enabling the patient to be successful with a home exercise program. In this case, the ultrasound is used only as a bridge until the patient can actively participate in the prescribed exercises. The cornerstones of physical therapy management of chronic pain are therapeutic exercise and patient education.

Therapeutic Exercise

The Cochrane Collaborative group was unable to perform a meta-analysis of the available studies on pain and exercise because of significant heterogeneity of study populations, exercise protocols, and outcome measures. They conclude there is little evidence supporting a positive effect of exercise on acute pain and only moderate evidence of exercise's positive effect on function in patients with chronic low back pain.[119] However, a review by Liddle et al identified 16 randomized controlled trials of exercise and chronic pain in which positive effects of exercise on chronic back pain were demonstrated. Two common features in these successful trials were adequate supervision for exercise and patient adherence with the program.[120] One significant limitation of these studies is that their outcome measures did not adequately focus on function and focused instead on impairments. Staal et al reported a significant decrease in absence from work using a structured activity and exercise program. However, there was no statistically significant difference between the nonstructured group and the structured group on measures of pain perception and functional status (measured by patient questionnaire).[121] Despite conflicting levels of evidence, there is a consensus, however, that exercise can decrease chronic pain and disability.[122,123]

It is common for patients to be frightened of exercise and experience difficulty in physical therapy. Fear/avoidance has a large part to play in this difficulty. The physical therapist must employ techniques to minimize fear/avoidance and gain the patient's trust. In order for any exercise program to be effective, it needs to be: (1) individualized to the patient's goals, (2) matched to the patient's current physical abilities, and (3) progressed at a rate that will build function without increasing distress. This requires a high level of skill on the part of the physical therapist. Exercise programs need to be carefully developed and implemented and monitored closely. Patients with chronic pain who have experienced long-term disability often have poor abilities to self-assess and self-regulate activity. In fact, some research has shown a link between pain and kinesthetic impairments and motor learning difficulties.[128–130] This difficulty with motor planning and motor learning can account for many of the inconsistencies seen in task performance of patients with chronic pain. Patients with chronic pain are prone to cycles of overdoing and underdoing and need to be taught the skills of pacing and self-management.

Exercise prescription starts with those activities the patient says he or she wants to do but has difficulty doing because of pain. The therapist then breaks down those activities into functional components that relate to a specific exercise goal. Exercises are then chosen to support the specific goals (Table 28.9).

Instruction and implementation depend on the patient's current functional and physical status. Exercise must be done consistently with proper pacing and body mechanics if it is to be effective and help the patient reach his or her expected outcome.

Setting Initial Exercise Baselines

Because of difficulties with fear/avoidance and poor self-assessment/self-regulation, the physical therapist must carefully set the beginning level of exercise in order to allow the patient to experience success. This can be done by prescribing several exercises, which the patient is instructed to do over the course of several days, while monitoring *how many the patient is able to do before pain or fatigue interferes*. The

Table 28.9 Exercise Analysis and Prescription

Expected Outcome	Functional Limitation	Anticipated Goals	Exercise(s)
Go to the movies.	Patient is currently limited by poor sitting, standing, and walking tolerance; stiffness of the lumbar spine and loss of balance when walking.	Sitting >2 hours Walking >2 city blocks Standing >15 minutes	• Aerobic training: stationary bicycle, treadmill • Lumbar mobility exercises • Functional strengthening exercises: standing • Standing balance and coordination exercises

Table 28.10 Setting the Exercise Baseline

Exercise	Day 1	Day 2	Day 3	Day 4	Average	Baseline
Pelvic tilt	12	2	6	8	7	**7**
Bridging	12	0	2	2	4	**3**
Hamstring stretch	10	3	0	3	4	**3**

therapist then evaluates the pattern, determines the average of all the trials, and sets an appropriate baseline (Table 28.10).

In setting the baseline, the therapist should aim for a submaximal level of exercise that will allow the patient to be consistently successful in the early stages of the exercise program. In the case of large differences in exercise trials, that baseline is set at a percentage of the average. The percentage is based on the patient's age, fitness level, degree of fluctuation, amount of fear/avoidance, among other factors. Where the trials are relatively stable over time, the baseline can be safely set to the average.

Once the baseline is set, it is important to establish a rate of increase along with a target goal. The more specific a POC is, the less difficulty the patient will have in following it safely with less pain-related disability. Ambiguity increases the experience of pain. Even in the treatment of patients with acute pain, ambiguous instructions have been shown to increase perception of disability.[115] Table 28.11 presents an example of an exercise flow sheet, with space for current quota, patient's current level, and goal.

The therapist can use the quota sheet as a tool for patient education, pacing, exercise modification, and patient motivation and adherence.[131] There is little in the literature that addresses specificity of exercise prescription and behavioral management of exercise programs for patients with chronic pain. This is an area in which additional research is warranted.

Postural retraining, pacing, and instruction in proper body mechanics are also crucial elements of the pain rehabilitation program. Long standing poor postural body habits can sustain musculoskeletal pain after the original injury has healed. Physical therapy interventions aimed at improving kinesthetic awareness and efficient muscle recruitment can be very effective for these faulty postural habits. Surface electromyography (sEMG) can be a valuable tool because it can identify abnormal muscle firing patterns and help the patient learn better movement strategies.[132–135]

Patient Education

Patient education is not a separate component of pain management. Rather, it is the primary element of the self-management paradigm. Like any chronic condition, management of chronic pain is enhanced through increased patient *self-advocacy, self-management,* and *self-efficacy.* From the initial contact with the patient, through the examination, goal setting, and POC the therapist must use skills and techniques to foster patient self-reliance. Effective management of chronic pain employs an appropriate home exercise program (HEP) and targeted patient education.

Pain control modalities can be used as part of a HEP to independently manage pain symptoms. These include use of heat, cold, and self-massage. There are a variety of commercially available hot packs, providing both dry and most heat. Some of the most useful of these are easily heated in the microwave. Some are dual use and can also be placed in the freezer for use as a cold pack. Cold can be applied via a commercial cold pack, cubed or crushed ice in a plastic bag, and direct application of ice to the skin in an ice massage. Ice massage can be applied either to the site of pain or to the web space of the thumb. There is some evidence that this engages gating mechanisms at the spinal

Table 28.11 Sample Quota Sheet for Exercise Prescription

Exercise	Goal	Mon	Tues	Wed	Thurs	Fri	Sat	Sun
Exercise 1	25	Quota						
		Actual						
Exercise 2								
Exercise 3								
Exercise 4								

cord for pain relief.[136,137] Appendix C contains patient directions for performing an ice massage.

Patients can be taught to use a variety of simple tools for self-massage. One of the most useful of these tools is a tennis ball. A single tennis ball can be used for shiatsu-like pressure point massage on nearly any muscle belly. The patient simply places the ball between his or her body and a firm surface and the weight of the body part on the ball provides the needed force. Larger balls can be used for larger muscle groups. Suboccipital release is a useful tool for patients with neck pain and/or headaches. Two tennis balls are tethered together in a sock or examination glove. The patient is instructed to lie supine and place the balls beneath his or her neck in the suboccipital area. The apex of each ball provides counter pressure against the suboccipital muscles and the spinous processes of the cervical spine fit in the space between the balls. Appendix D provides sample patient instructions for cervical self-massage. A variety of commercial devices are available for patient self-massage.

Patients with chronic pain often harbor many misconceptions about their pain, its prognosis, and their functional ability. Often these misconceptions emerge from fear. One of the first components of an education program is for the therapist to teach the difference between *hurt* and *harm.* Acute pain functions as a signaling device that something is wrong with the body and needs to be addressed. Chronic pain is often self-sustaining and not directly linked to acute tissue damage; the patient needs to understand that pain itself does not mean danger. It is particularly important that the patient understand that delayed onset muscle soreness (DOMS) is likely to accompany any change in his or her activity. Patients with chronic pain have difficulty differentiating between types of discomfort owing to the central neurological changes that accompany chronic pain.

The Interdisciplinary Team

Chronic pain is not generally amenable to unimodal treatment—whether medical, surgical, rehabilitative, or psychological.[139,140] Physical therapy is likely to be most effective for long term functional improvement of individuals with chronic pain when it is integrated with medical and psychological treatments in an interdisciplinary team-based program. The composition of the team in pain rehabilitation may vary, but at its core are specialists in medical care (e.g., neurology, orthopaedics, physiatry, anesthesia, nursing), rehabilitation care (e.g., physical therapy, occupational therapy, vocational rehabilitation), and psychosocial care (e.g., psychiatry, psychology, social work). The *functional restoration approach*, popularized by Mayer et al[139] consists of intensive physical rehabilitation in a behavioral management milieu. Most team-based rehabilitation programs incorporate elements of functional restoration.

There is a wealth of literature in support of interdisciplinary rehabilitation of chronic pain. In a Cochrane Collaborative Review, 10 randomized trials of nearly 2000 patients were analyzed. The researchers concluded there is:

> *(1) ". . . strong evidence that intensive multidisciplinary biopsychosocial rehabilitation with functional restoration improves function when compared with inpatient or outpatient non-multidisciplinary rehabilitation," and (2) ". . . moderate evidence that intensive multidisciplinary biopsychosocial rehabilitation with functional restoration reduces pain when compared with outpatient non-multidisciplinary rehabilitation or usual care."*[140, p 1514]

Summary

Chronic pain is a distinct diagnostic entity and differs from acute pain in its pathology, physiology, and psychological meaning. It also differs in its emotional, behavioral, and functional sequelae. Pain behavior, difficulties in motor planning/motor learning, and fear/avoidance can complicate the clinical picture of individuals with chronic pain. Effective management of chronic pain addresses biological, psychological, and social realms and is best provided in an intensive rehabilitation setting by an interdisciplinary team.

The physical therapist is an essential member of the chronic pain management team. Physical therapists need to employ strong communication and rapport building skills in order to foster a healthy therapeutic relationship and patient self-reliance. Specific physical therapy interventions do not differ significantly in chronic pain versus acute pain; the major focus is on active rather than passive intervention with the expected outcome of improving function rather than the primary elimination of specific impairments.

Acknowledgment

Acknowledgment is extended to Barbara J. Headley, whose earlier version of this chapter provided the foundation for the current work.

Questions for Review

1. Name three ways in which psychological distress might be manifested in a patient with chronic pain.
2. Differentiate between open and closed ended questions for gathering patient data. Describe the benefit of each.
3. Your patient had not done his home exercise program (HEP) for 2 weeks. The first week, he lost the quota sheet. The second week, he complained of increased pain after physical therapy. How will you determine if

your patient has a high fear/avoidance or is being nonadherent?

4. A patient was referred by her nurse case manager from workman's compensation. The case manager has provided you with a thorough job description. The patient is a computer assembly worker injured 2 years ago on the job. During the examination, the patient is anxious and verbalizes hostility about her employer. She states emphatically that she will not go back to that job. Which of the following is the most appropriate strategy for goal setting:
   A. Compare the job description with the patient's current functional status and set goals that will allow the patient to function at the level needed for the job.
   B. Do not discuss the job description with the patient and focus on the patient's current status and impairments only in the goal setting process.
   C. Ascertain the patient's expected outcomes of physical therapy intervention. Discuss the job description in terms of generic skills that will translate into any job and set goals that are mutually agreeable.

Case Study

The patient is a 53-year-old right-hand dominant, single woman, currently not working, who presents to physical therapy with chief complaint of left knee pain and stiffness 2 months status post left total knee arthroplasty.

PATIENT HISTORY

The patient reports a multiyear history of left knee pain with episodes of patellar dislocation while ambulating in the community. She underwent left (L) total knee arthroplasty 2 months ago and reports medication complications during her hospital stay that delayed the start of inpatient physical therapy. Postoperative care included use of a constant passive motion (CPM) machine and referral to outpatient physical therapy following discharge.

The patient reports significant difficulty participating in physical therapy with anxiety and panic attacks during sessions. Patient reports experiencing flashbacks of childhood abuse during therapy. This was particularly problematic when her knee ROM was being measured with a goniometer and the therapist would forcefully hold her knee into flexion.

The patient has been told by her surgeon that if she does not gain sufficient range of knee motion, she will need to undergo manipulation under anesthesia.

FUNCTIONAL LIMITATIONS

The patient is limited in ambulation to household distances using a straight cane. She demonstrates significant gait deviations and is unable to bend L knee to allow for ease of sitting, using stairs, and activities of daily living (ADL) such as dressing and bathing.

PAST MEDICAL HISTORY

Multijoint osteoarthritis, chondromalacia patella, epilepsy, bipolar disorder

PSYCHOSOCIAL HISTORY

The patient lives alone. She is on medical disability. She has a history of severe childhood abuse and trauma.

MEDICATIONS

Depakote, Tegretol, Paxil, Lithium, Tylenol prn

PHYSICAL THERAPY EXAMINATION FINDINGS

Palpation/observation

Marked swelling of the L knee, with marked tightness of the L knee arthroplasty scar as well as restrictions in the fascia throughout the L thigh, L knee, and L lower leg. Significant anxiety when L knee is touched.

Strength, ROM, and Sensation

ROM of L knee limited by pain; not measured owing to anxiety. By observation, AROM appeared to be quite limited (approximately 5–75°). Strength of adjacent muscles (L hip, ankle) 4/5; R LE strength WNL.

Gait

Antalgic, with slow, lateral whip of L LE during swing phase. Patient unable to ascend or descend stairs step over step. She uses a straight cane in the R UE.

Pain

Reported as 0/10 in sitting, 7–8/10 during walking, and 9–10/10 during exercises (VAS).

GUIDING QUESTIONS/ACTIVITIES

1. Provide an example of one closed-ended and one open-ended question that might be used in this patient's interview. Describe the differences and benefits of each type of question.
2. Formulate a problem list for this patient including impairments, functional limitations, and disability.
3. Formulate a POC for this patient.
4. Name three ways in which psychological distress might manifest in this patient.
5. This patient demonstrates a complex psychosocial history as well as an atypical postsurgical course with difficulties in her early rehabilitation. How will you modify her POC in order to minimize patient anxiety and maximize patient

compliance? Specifically, how will you monitor her ROM if she has a panic reaction to the goniometer?

6. The patient has not done her home exercise program (HEP) for 2 weeks. The first week, she reports having lost the quota sheet. The second week, she complained of increased pain during and after exercises. How will you determine if this patient has high fear/avoidance or is being noncompliant?

7. The *Difficult Behavior Worksheet* below provides examples of potential patient verbal responses.
   A. Match the verbal response to the response type (see list on bottom of worksheet)
   B. List a specific strategy you might employ to increase rapport and decrease difficult behavior.

Difficult Behavior Worksheet

Response Type	Examples of Patient Verbal Responses	Strategy to Increase Rapport and Decrease Difficult Behavior
	Are you sure this is safe? My doctor says I have brittle bones, you know. Well, you know best, dear.	
	The exercises are no problem. I'm fine. I'll do it myself.	
	I tried to do my exercises, but I just had too much pain. You worked me so hard last session!	
	It's no use. I'll never be able to sit at a computer again. I'll just end up right back where I started.	
	My last physical therapist put me in bed for 2 weeks. If you ask me to lift those weights, I'm out of here.	

Response Type: Passive–Dependent, Overanxious, Hostile, Passive–Aggressive, Help Rejecting

References

1. Luo, X, et al: Estimates and patterns of direct health care expenditures among individuals with back pain in the United States. Spine 29(1):79, 2004.
2. American Physical Therapy Association: Guide to Physical Therapist Practice, ed 2. Phys Ther 81(1):1, 2001.
3. Bonica, JJ: History of pain concepts and therapies. In Bonica, JJ (ed): The Management of Pain. Lea & Febiger, Philadelphia, 1990, p 2.
4. Melzack, R, and Wall, PD: Pain mechanisms: A new theory. Science 150:971, 1965.
5. Talo, S, et al: An empirical investigation of the Biopsychosocial Disease Consequence Model: Psychological impairment, disability, and handicap in chronic pain patients. Disabil Rehabil 17(6):281, 1995.
6. Fordyce, WE: On the nature of illness and disability: An editorial. Clin Orthop (336):47, 1997.
7. Bonica, JJ: General considerations of chronic pain. In Bonica, JJ (ed): The Management of Pain. Lea & Febiger, Philadelphia, 1990, p 180.
8. Gildenberg, PL, and DeVaul, RA: The chronic pain patient: Evaluation and management. In Gildenberg, PL (ed): Pain and Headache. Karger, New York, 1985.
9. Fordyce, WE: Pain and suffering: A reappraisal. Am Psychol 43(4):276, 1988.
10. Pilowski, I: A general classification of abnormal illness behavior. Br J Med Psychol 51:131, 1978.
11. Turk, DC, and Flor, H: Pain greater than pain behaviors: The utility and limitations of the pain behavior construct. Pain 31(3):277, 1987.
12. Keefe, FJ: Pain behavior observation: Current status and future directions. Curr Rev Pain 4(1):12, 2000.
13. Mehrabian, A: Silent messages: Implicit communication of emotions and attitudes, ed 2. Wadsworth, Belmont, CA, 1981.
14. Petersen-Felixa, S, and Curatolob, M: Neuroplasticity—an important factor in acute and chronic pain. Swiss Med Wkly 132:273, 2002.
15. Coghill, R, McHaffie, J, and Yen, Y: Neural correlates of interindividual differences in the subjective experience of pain. PNAS 100(14):8538, 2003.
16. Druschky, K, et al: Alteration of the somatosensory cortical map in peripheral mononeuropathy due to carpal tunnel syndrome. NeuroReport 11:3925, 2000.
17. Byl, NN, Merzenich, MM, and Jenkins, WM: A primate genesis model of focal dystonia and repetitive strain injury: Learning-induced dedifferentiation of the representation of the hand in the primary somatosensory cortex in adult monkeys. Neurology 47(2):508, 1996.
18. Tinazzi, M, et al: Neuroplastic changes related to pain occurring at multiple levels of the human somatosensory system: A somatosensory-evoked potentials study in patients with cervical radicular pain. J Neurosci 20(24):9277, 2000.
19. Schwoebel, J, et al: Pain and the body schema, evidence for peripheral effects on mental representations of movement. Brain 124:2098, 2001.
20. Karl, A, et al: Reorganization of motor and somatosensory cortex in upper extremity amputees with phantom limb pain. Neuroscience 21(10):3609, 2001.
21. Luo, D, et al: Upregulation of dorsal root ganglion a2d (alpha 2 delta) calcium channel subunit and its correlation with allodynia in spinal nerve-injured rats. Neuroscience 21(6):1868, 2001.
22. Goff, JR, et al: Reorganization of the spinal dorsal horn in models of chronic pain: Correlation with behavior. Neuroscience 82(2):559, 1998.

23. Melzack, R, et al: Central neuroplasticity and pathological pain. Ann NY Acad Sci 933:157, 2001.
24. Fagan, DJ, Martin, W, and Smith, A: A randomized, double-blind trial of pre-emptive local anesthesia in day-case knee arthroscopy. Arthroscopy 19(1):50, 2003.
25. Campbell, WI, Kendrick, RW, and Fee, JP: Balanced pre-emptive analgesia: Does it work? A double-blind, controlled study in bilaterally symmetrical oral surgery. Br J Anaesth 81(5):727, 1998.
26. Millar, AY, Mansfield, MD, and Kinsella, J: Influence of timing of morphine administration on postoperative pain and analgesic consumption. Br J Anaesth 81(3):373, 1998.
27. Priya, V, et al: Efficacy of intravenous ketoprofen for pre-emptive analgesia. J Postgrad Med 48(2):109, 2002.
28. Akural, EI, et al: Pre-emptive effect of epidural sufentanil in abdominal hysterectomy. Br J Anaesth 88(6):803, 2002.
29. Katz, J, et al: Pre-emptive lumbar epidural anaesthesia reduces postoperative pain and patient-controlled morphine consumption after lower abdominal surgery. Pain 59(3):395, 1994.
30. Bonica, JJ: Anatomic and physiologic basis of nociception and pain. In Bonica, JJ (ed): The Management of Pain. Lea &Febiger, Philadelphia, 1990, p 28.
31. Bonica, JJ: Biochemistry and modulation of nociception and pain. In Bonica, JJ (ed): The Management of Pain. Lea & Febiger, Philadelphia, 1990, p 95.
32. Takeuchi, Y, et al: Effects of experimentally induced inflammation on temporomandibular joint nociceptors in rats. Neurosci Lett 354(2):172, 2004.
33. Hou, SX, et al: Chronic inflammation and compression of the dorsal root contribute to sciatica induced by the intervertebral disc herniation in rats. Pain 105(1–2):255, 2003.
34. Leis, S, et al: Substance-P-induced protein extravasation is bilaterally increased in complex regional pain syndrome. Exp Neurol 183(1):197, 2003.
35. Song, XJ, et al: Somata of nerve-injured sensory neurons exhibit enhanced responses to inflammatory mediators. Pain 104(3):701, 2003.
36. Fine, P: The role of rofecoxib, a cyclooxygenase-2-specific inhibitor, for the treatment of non-cancer pain: A review. J Pain 3(4):272, 2002.
37. Birbara, C, Puopolo, A, and Munoz, D: Treatment of chronic low back pain with etoricoxib, a new cyclo-oxygenase-2 selective inhibitor: Improvement in pain and disability—a randomized, placebo-controlled, 3-month trial. J Pain 4(6):307, 2003.
38. Block, AR: Presurgical Psychological Screening in Chronic Pain Syndromes. Erlbaum, Mahwah, NJ, 1996.
39. Nedeljkovic, S, Wasan, A, and Jamison, R: Assessment of efficacy of long-term opioid therapy in pain patients with substance abuse potential. Clin J Pain 18(4 Suppl):S39, 2002.
40. Ballantyne, J, and Mao, J: Opioid therapy for chronic pain. N Engl J Med 349(20):1943, 2003.
41. Wen-hsien, W: Pain Management: Assessment and Treatment of Chronic and Acute Syndromes. Human Sciences Press, New York, 1987.
42. Benedetti, C, and Butler, SH: Systemic analgesics. In Bonica, JJ (ed): The Management of Pain. Lea & Febiger, Philadelphia, 1990, p 1640.
43. Sawynok, J, Esser, M, and Reid, A: Antidepressants as analgesics: An overview of central and peripheral mechanisms of action. J Psychiatry Neurosci 26(1):21, 2001.
44. Fox, A, Gentry, C, and Patel, S: Comparative activity of the anticonvulsants oxcarbazepine, carbamazepine, lamotrigine, and gabapentin in a model of neuropathic pain in the rat and guinea-pig. Pain 105(1–2):355, 2003.
45. Pan, HL, Eisenach, JC, and Chen, SR: Gabapentin suppresses ectopic nerve discharges and reverses allodynia in neuropathic rats. J Pharmacol Exp Ther 288(3):1026, 1999.
46. Cheshire, WP: Defining the role for gabapentin in the treatment of trigeminal neuralgia: A retrospective study. J Pain 3(2):137, 2002.
47. North, RB, et al: A prospective, randomized study of spinal cord stimulation versus reoperation for failed back surgery syndrome: Initial results. In Proceedings of the 11th Meeting of the World Society for Stereotactic and Functional Neurosurgery, Ixtapa, Mexico, 1993.
48. Bonica, JJ, and Buckley, FP: Regional analgesia with local anesthetics. In Bonica, JJ (ed): The Management of Pain. Lea & Febiger, Philadelphia, 1990, p 1883.
49. Hurt, R, and Ballantine, H: Stereotactic anterior cingulate lesions for persistent pain: A report on 68 cases. Clin Neurosurg 21:334, 1973.
50. Nashold, BJ: Current status of the DREZ operation. Neurosurgery 15:942, 1984.
51. Spiegel, E, and Wycis, H: Present status of stereoencephalotomies for pain relief. Confin Neurol 27:7, 1966.
52. Vasudevan, SV, and Lynch, TN: Pain centers—organization and outcome. West J Med 154(5):532, 1991.
53. Baron, R, et al: National Institutes of Health Workshop: Reflex sympathetic dystrophy/complex regional pain syndromes—state of the science. Anesth Analg 95(6):1812, 2002.
54. Bonica, JJ: Causalgia and other reflex sympathetic dystrophies. In Bonica, JJ (ed): The Management of Pain. Lea & Febiger, Philadelphia, 1990, p 220.
55. Goodman, C, and Snyder, T: Differential Diagnosis in Physical Therapy. WB Saunders, Philadelphia, 1990.
56. Martelli, MF, et al: Psychological, neuropsychological, and medical considerations in assessment and management of pain. J Head Trauma Rehabil 19(1):10, 2004.
57. Grace, VM: Mind/body dualism in medicine: The case of chronic pelvic pain without organic pathology: A critical review of the literature. Int J Health Serv 28(1):127, 1998.
58. Joint Commission of Accreditation of Healthcare Organizations (JCAH)) Improving the Quality of Pain Management Through Measurement and Action, Joint Commission Resources, Inc, One Renaissance Blvd, Oakbrook Terrace, IL, 2003 Retrieved March 11, 2005 from http://www.jcaho.org/news+room/health+care+issues/pain+mono_jc.pdf.
59. Ong, KS, and Seymour, RA: Pain measurement in humans. J R Coll Surg Edinb Irel 2:15, 2004.
60. Wewers, ME, and Lowe, NK: A critical review of visual analogue scales in the measurement of clinical phenomena. Res Nurs Health 13(4):227, 1990.
61. Reigo, T, Tropp, H, and Timpka, T: Pain drawing evaluation—the problem with the clinically biased surgeon. Intra-and interobserver agreement in 50 cases related to clinical bias. Acta Orthop Scand 69(4):408, 1998.
62. Ohnmeiss, DD: Repeatability of pain drawings in a low back pain population. Spine 25(8):980, 2000.
63. Margolis, RB, Chibnall, JT, and Tait, RC: Test-retest reliability of the pain drawing instrument. Pain 33(1):49, 198.
64. Dahl, B, et al: Nonorganic pain drawings are associated with low psychological scores on the preoperative SF-36 questionnaire in patients with chronic low back pain. Eur Spine J 10(3):211, 2001.
65. Von Baeyer, CL, et al: Invalid use of pain drawings in psychological screening of back pain patients. Pain 16(1):103, 1983.
66. Brismar, H, Vucetic, N, and Svensson, O: Pain patterns in lumbar disc hernia drawings compared to surgical findings in 159 patients. Acta Orthop Scand 67(5):470, 1996.
67. Hagg, O, et al: Pain-drawing does not predict the outcome of fusion surgery for chronic low-back pain: A report from the Swedish Lumbar Spine Study. Eur Spine J 12(1):2, 2003.
68. Turk, DC, Rudy, TE, and Salovey, P: The McGill Pain Questionnaire reconsidered: Confirming the factor structure and examining appropriate uses. Pain 21(4):385, 1985.
69. Melzack, R, et al: Trigeminal neuralgia and atypical facial pain: Use of the McGill Pain Questionnaire for discrimination and diagnosis. Pain 27(3):297, 1986.
70. Melzack, R: The short-form McGill Pain Questionnaire. Pain 30(2):191, 1987.
71. Mongini, F, et al: Confirmation of the distinction between chronic migraine and chronic tension-type headache by the McGill Pain Questionnaire. Headache 43(8), 867, 2003.
72. Towery, S, and Fernandez, E: Reclassification and rescaling of McGill Pain Questionnaire verbal descriptors of pain sensation: a replication. Clin J Pain 12(4):270, 1996.
73. Fernandez, E, and Boyle, GJ: Affective and evaluative descriptors of pain in the McGill Pain Questionnaire: Reduction and reorganization. J Pain 3(1):70, 2002.

74. Lawlis, GF, et al: The development of the Dallas Pain Questionnaire: An assessment of the impact of spinal pain on behavior. Spine 14(5):511, 1989.
75. Ozguler, A, et al: Using the Dallas Pain Questionnaire to classify individuals with low back pain in a working population. Spine 27(16):1783, 2002.
76. Meyer-Rosberg, K, et al: A comparison of the SF-36 and Nottingham Health Profile in patients with chronic neuropathic pain. Eur J Pain 5(4):391, 2001.
77. Thomas, RJ, McEwen, J, and Asbury, AJ: The Glasgow Pain Questionnaire: A new generic measure of pain, development, and testing. Int J Epidemiol 25(5):1060, 1996.
78. Jerome, A, and Gross, RT: Pain disability index: Construct and discriminant validity. Arch Phys Med Rehabil 72(11):920, 1991.
79. Riegger-Krugh, C, and Keysor, JJ: Skeletal malalignments of the lower quarter: Correlated and compensatory motions and postures. JOSPT 23:164, 1996.
80. Fordyce, W, Roberts, A, and Sternbach, R: The behavioral management of chronic pain: A response to critics. Pain 22:113, 1985.
81. Gatchel, RJ: Occupational low back disability: Why function needs to "drive" the rehabilitation process. Am Pain Soc J 3:107, 1994.
82. Hazard, R, et al: Functional restoration with behavioral support: A one year prospective study of patients with chronic low back pain. Spine 14:157, 1989.
83. Mayer, T, et al: A prospective two-year study of functional restoration in industrial low back injury. JAMA 258:1763, 1987.
84. Mayer, T, and Gatchel, R: Functional Restoration for Spinal Disorders: The Sports Medicine Approach. Lea & Febiger, Philadelphia, 1988.
85. Al-Obaidi, SM, et al: The role of anticipation and fear of pain in the persistence of avoidance behavior in patients with chronic low back pain. Spine 25(9):1126, 2000.
86. Fritz, JM, and George, SZ: Identifying psychosocial variables in patients with acute work-related low back pain: The importance of fear-avoidance beliefs. Phys Ther 82(10):973, 2002.
87. Buer, N, and Linton, SJ: Fear-avoidance beliefs and catastrophizing: Occurrence and risk factor in back pain and ADL in the general population. Pain 99(3):485, 2002.
88. Vlaeyen, JW, et al. The treatment of fear of movement/(re)injury in chronic low back pain: Further evidence on the effectiveness of exposure in vivo. Clin J Pain 18(4):251, 2002.
89. Jamison, RN, et al: Cognitive behavioral classifications of chronic pain: Replication and extension of empirically derived patient profiles. Pain 57:277, 1994.
90. Epker, J, and Gatchel, RJ: Coping profile differences in the biopsychosocial functioning of patients with temporomandibular disorder. Psychosom Med 62:69, 2000.
91. Bergstrom, G, et al: The impact of psychologically different patient groups on outcome after a vocational rehabilitation program for long-term spinal pain patients. Pain 93(3):229, 2001.
92. Gatchel, RJ, et al: A preliminary study of multidimensional pain inventory profile differences in predicting treatment outcome in a heterogeneous cohort of patients with chronic pain. Clin J Pain 18(3):139, 2002.
93. Davis, PJ, et al: Multidimensional subgroups in migraine: Differential treatment outcome to a pain medicine program. Pain Med 4(3):215, 2003.
94. Gracely, RH, et al: Pain catastrophizing and neural responses to pain among persons with fibromyalgia. Brain 127(4):835, 2004.
95. Hassett, AL, et al: The role of catastrophizing in the pain and depression of women with fibromyalgia syndrome. Arthritis Rheum 43(11):2493, 2000.
96. Tan, G, et al: Coping with chronic pain: A comparison of two measures. Pain 90(1-2):127, 2001.
97. Viane, I, et al: Acceptance of pain is an independent predictor of mental well being in patients with chronic pain: Empirical evidence and reappraisal. Pain 106(1-2):65, 2003.
98. McCracken, LM, and Eccleston, C: Coping or acceptance: What to do about chronic pain? Pain 105(1-2):197, 2003.
99. Larson, SL, Clark, MR, and Eaton, WW: Depressive disorder as a long-term antecedent risk factor for incident back pain: A 13-year follow-up study from the Baltimore Epidemiological Catchment Area sample. Psychol Med 34(2):211, 2004.
100. Carroll, LJ, Cassidy, JD, and Cote, P: Depression as a risk factor for onset of an episode of troublesome neck and low back pain. Pain 107(1-2):134, 2004.
101. Currie, SR, and Wang, J: Chronic back pain and major depression in the general Canadian population. Pain 107(1-2):54, 2004.
102. Bair, MJ, et al: Impact of pain on depression treatment response in primary care. Psychosom Med 66(1):17, 2004.
103. Spertus, IL, et al: Gender differences in associations between trauma history and adjustment among chronic pain patients. Pain 82(1):97, 1999.
104. Walker, EA, et al: Psychiatric diagnoses and sexual victimization in women with chronic pelvic pain. Psychosomatics 36(6):531, 1995.
105. Walker, EA, et al: Psychosocial factors in fibromyalgia compared with rheumatoid arthritis: II. Sexual, physical, and emotional abuse and neglect. Psychosom Med 59(6):572, 1997.
106. Schofferman, J, et al: Childhood psychological trauma and chronic refractory low-back pain. Clin J Pain 9(4):260, 1993.
107. Schofferman, J, et al: Childhood psychological trauma correlates with unsuccessful lumbar spine surgery. Spine 17(6 Suppl):S138, 1992.
108. Schachter, CL, Stalker, CA, and Teram, E: Toward sensitive practice: Issues for physical therapists working with survivors of childhood sexual abuse. Phys Ther 79(3):248, 1999.
109. Cano, A, et al: Marital functioning, chronic pain, and psychological distress. Pain 107(1-2):99, 2004.
110. Flor, H, Kerns, RD, and Turk, DC: The role of spouse reinforcement, perceived pain, and activity levels of chronic pain patients. J Psychosom Res 31(2):251, 1987.
111. Hahn, SR, et al: The difficult doctor-patient relationship: Somatization, personality, and psychopathology. J Clin Epidemiol 47:647, 1994.
112. Kahana, R, and Bibring, GL: Personality types. In Zinberg, NE (ed): Medical Management in Psychiatry and Medical Practice in a General Hospital. International Universities Press, Guilford, CT, 1965, p 108.
113. Purtilo, R, and Haddad, A: Health Professional and Patient Interaction, ed 6. WB Saunders, Philadelphia, 2002.
114. Smith, S: Dealing with the difficult patient. Postgrad Med J 71:653, 1995.
115. Fordyce, WE, et al: Acute back pain: A control-group comparison of behavioral vs traditional management methods. J Behav Med 9(2):127, 1986.
116. Harkapaa, K, et al: Health locus of control beliefs and psychological distress as predictors for treatment outcome in low-back pain patients: Results of a 3-month follow-up of a controlled intervention study. J Pain 46(1):35, 1991.
117. French, DJ, et al: Perceived self-efficacy and headache-related disability. Headache 40(8):647, 2000.
118. Coughlin, AM, et al: Multidisciplinary treatment of chronic pain patients: Its efficacy in changing patient locus of control. Arch Phys Med Rehabil 81(6):739, 2000.
119. van Tulder, M, et al: Exercise therapy for low back pain: A systematic review within the framework of the cochrane collaboration back review group. Spine 25(21):2784, 2000.
120. Liddle, SD, Baxter, GD, and Gracey, JH: Exercise and chronic low back pain: What works? Pain 107(1-2):176, 2004.
121. Staal, JB, et al: Graded activity for low back pain in occupational health care: A randomized, controlled trial. Ann Intern Med 140(2):77, 2004.
122. Rainville, J, et al: The influence of intense exercise-based physical therapy program on back pain anticipated before and induced by physical activities. Spine 4(2):176, 2004.
123. Rainville, J, et al: Exercise as a treatment for chronic low back pain. Spine 4(1):106, 2004.
124. Chok, B, et al: Endurance training of the trunk extensor muscles in people with subacute low back pain. Phys Ther 79(11):1032, 1999.
125. Moffat, JK, et al: Randomised controlled trial of exercise for low back pain: Clinical outcomes, costs, and preferences. BMJ 319:279, 1999.
126. Viljanen, M, et al: Effectiveness of dynamic muscle training, relaxation training, or ordinary activity on chronic neck pain: Randomized controlled trial relaxation training. BMJ 327:475, 2003.

127. Schachter, C, et al: Effects of short versus long bouts of aerobic exercise in sedentary women with fibromyalgia: A randomized controlled trial. Phys Ther 83(4):340, 2003.
128. Jull, GA, and Richardson, CA: Motor control problems in patients with spinal pain: A new direction for therapeutic exercise. J Manipulative Physiol Ther 23(2):115, 2000.
129. Luoto, S, et al: Mechanisms explaining the association between low back trouble and deficits in information processing: A controlled study with follow-up. Spine 24(3):255, 1999.
130. Gill, KP, and Callaghan, MJ: The measurement of lumbar proprioception in individuals with and without low back pain. Spine 23(3):371, 1998.
131. Dolce, JJ, et al: Exercise quotas, anticipatory concern and self-efficacy expectancies in chronic pain: A preliminary report. Pain 24(3):365, 1986.
132. Kasman, G: Use of integrated electromyography for the assessment and treatment of musculoskeletal pain: Guidelines for physical medicine practitioners. In Cram, J (ed): Clinical EMG for Surface Recordings, vol 2. Clinical Resources, Nevada City, 1990, p 255.
133. Khalil, T, et al: Electromyographic symmetry in patients with chronic low back pain and comparison to controls. Advances in Industrial Ergonomics and Safety 3:483, 1991.
134. Seidel, H, et al: Electromyographic evaluation of back muscle fatigue with repeated sustained contractions of different strengths. Eur J Appl Physiol 56:592, 1987.
135. Sihvonen, T, et al: Electric behavior of low back muscles during lumbar pelvic rhythm in low back pain patients and healthy controls. Arch Phys Med Rehabil 72:1080, 1991.
136. Melzack, R, et al: Ice massage and transcutaneous electrical stimulation: Comparison of treatment for low-back pain. Pain 9(2):209, 1980.
137. Melzack, R, Guite, S, and Gonshor, A: Relief of dental pain by ice massage of the hand. Can Med Assoc J 122(2):189, 1980.
138. Bogduk, N: Management of chronic low back pain. Med J Aust 180(2):79, 2004.
139. Mayer, TG, et al: A prospective two-year study of functional restoration in industrial low back injury: An objective assessment procedure. JAMA 258(13):1763, 1987.
140. Guzmán, J, et al: Multidisciplinary Bio-Psycho-Social Rehabilitation for Chronic Low Back Pain. BMJ 322(7301):1511, 2001.

Supplemental Readings

Joint Commission on Accreditation of Healthcare Organizations: Pain: Current Understanding of Assessment, Management, and Treatments (JCAHO Pain Management Monograph) Retrieved October 28, 2005 from http://www.jcaho.org/news+room/health+care+issues/pain_mono_npc.pdf (www.jcaho.org)

Joint Commission on Accreditation of Healthcare Organizations: Improving the Quality of Pain Management Through Measurement and Action, (JCAHO Pain Management Monograph) Retrieved October 28, 2005 from http://www.jcaho.org/news+room/health+care+issues/pain_mono_jc.pdf (www.jcaho.org)

Main, CJ, and Spanswick, CC: Pain Management: An Interdisciplinary Approach. Churchill Livingstone (Elsevier), New York, 2000.

Monga, T, and Grabois, M: Pain Management in Rehabilitation. Demos Medical Publishing, New York, 2002.

Wittink H, and Michel T. (eds). Pain Management for Physical Therapists, ed 2. Heinemann, Boston, 2002.

Appendix A: Visual Analogue Scale

Visual Pain Scale

Name: ______________________________ Date: ____________________

Instructions: Numerical scores can be obtained by measuring the placement of the mark along a 10 cm line. Scores may be compared with repeat administration of the scale.

Please mark an "X" along the line to show how your pain has effected your level of function.

1. At what level do you perceive your pain?
   No pain ____ Worst possible
2. At what level do you experience pain at night?
   No pain ____ Worst possible
3. Has the pain effected your level of activity?
   No problem ____ Total change
4. How well does medication relieve your pain?
   Complete relief ____ No relief
5. How stiff is your back/neck?
   No stiffness ____ Totally stiff
6. Does your pain interfere with sitting?
   No problem ____ Cannot sit
7. Is it painful for you to walk?
   No pain ____ Cannot walk
8. Does your pain keep you from standing/sitting still?
   No problem ____ Cannot do it
9. Does your pain interfere with your normal household chores?
   No problem ____ Cannot do them
10. Does your pain effect your driving time in a car?
    No problem ____ Cannot do it
11. Do you get relief from your pain by lying down?
    Complete relief ____ No relief at all
12. How much have you had to change your job responsibilities?
    No change ____ So much I can't work
13. How much control do you feel you have over the pain?
    Total control ____ No control
14. How much control have you lost over other areas of your life due to the pain?
    No control lost ____ Total loss of control

Developed by Barbara Headley, PT, MS.

Appendix B: The McGill Pain Questionnaire

What does your pain feel like?

Some of the words below describe your present pain. Circle ONLY those words that best describe it. Leave out any word-group that is not suitable. Use only a single word in each appropriate group—the one that applies best.

1	2	3	4
Flickering	Jumping	Pricking	Sharp
Quivering	Flashing	Boring	Cutting
Pulsing	Shooting	Drilling	Lacerating
Throbbing		Stabbing	
Beating		Lancinating	
Pounding			
5	**6**	**7**	**8**
Pinching	Tugging	Hot	Tingling
Pressing	Pulling	Burning	Itchy
Gnawing	Wrenching	Scalding	Smarting
Cramping		Searing	Stinging
Crushing			
9	**10**	**11**	**12**
Dull	Tender	Tiring	Sickening
Sore	Taut	Exhausting	Suffocating
Hurting	Rasping		
Aching	Splitting		
Heavy			
13	**14**	**15**	**16**
Fearful	Punishing	Wretched	Annoying
Frightful	Gruelling	Blinding	Troublesome
Terrifying	Cruel		Miserable
	Vicious		Intense
	Killing		Unbearable
17	**18**	**19**	**20**
Spreading	Tight	Cool	Nagging
Radiating	Numb	Cold	Nauseating
Penetrating	Drawing	Freezing	Agonizing
Piercing	Squeezing		Dreadful
	Tearing		Torturing

Includes 20 categories of word descriptors covering 3 main classes: sensory (1–10), affective (11–15), evaluative (16); miscellaneous properties of pain are included in 17–20. Scoring can include: (1) number of words chosen (NWC), and (2) pain intensity (the first word in each category implies the least pain and is scored as a 1, the next word indicates higher intensity and is assigned a value of 2, and so forth); a score can be obtained for each category and a total score for all categories.

Reprinted from Melzack, R: The McGill Pain Questionnaire (MPQ): Major Properties and Scoring Methods. Pain 1:277, 1975, p 281, with permission from the International Association for the Study of Pain.

Appendix C: Patient Instructions for Ice Massage

Ice massage can be a powerful tool for pain relief. Ice massage is also effective in reducing swelling.

You will need:

- A paper or Styrofoam cup of completely frozen water; peel away the top portion of the cup so about an inch or more of the ice is exposed; an ice cube can also be used
- A towel

Directions:

1. Apply the ice to the primary place of pain or to the web-space of the thumb (*or as indicated by your therapist*).
2. Apply the ice to bare skin. *If you are using an ice cube, use an insulating cloth between the ice and the hand holding the ice.*
3. Move the ice in slow circles (two or three circles per second), lightly on the surface of your skin.
4. Continue icing for 3–5 minutes, or until the part iced becomes numb.
5. You may feel four distinct stages of icing: cold, burning, pain/ache, and numbing.
6. Stop icing when the part feels numb. You may dry off any water that remains on the skin.
7. You may repeat the icing every 2 hours as needed for pain relief.

Appendix D: Patient Instructions for Cervical Self-Massage

Releasing tension behind the neck can be a powerful tool for relaxation, pain relief, and range of motion.

You will need:

- Two tennis balls
- A sock or latex-type glove
- A small rolled towel (you may need to place the towel underneath your neck if the balls roll or slide down your neck [optional])

Directions

1. Place the tennis balls inside the sock or glove so they are close together.
2. Tie a knot in sock/glove so the tennis balls are tethered together.
3. Lay on a firm, flat surface (not a bed). You may place a pillow under your knees, or bend your knees if desired.
4. Place the tethered tennis balls horizontally behind your neck, pressing on the muscles at the juncture of the head and neck. This is your *suboccipital* area. Your spine should rest in the space between the two tennis balls, so there is no pressure on the bones of your spine.

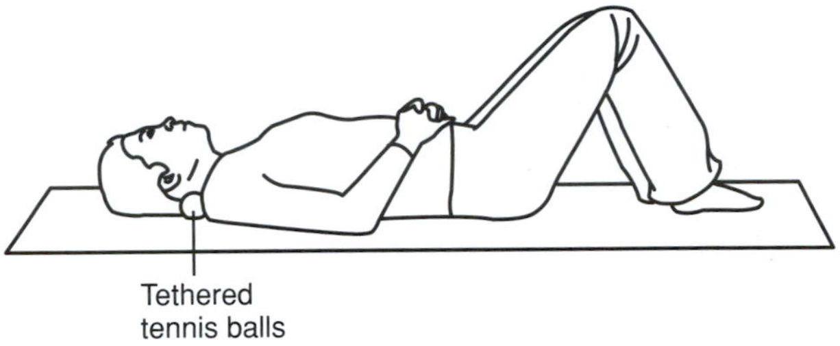

5. Lie on the tennis balls for *2–4 minutes*.

CHAPTER

29

LEARNING OBJECTIVES

1. Recognize the signs of cognitive and perceptual deficits.
2. Describe how cognitive and perceptual deficits affect the ability of the patient to participate in rehabilitation.
3. Explain how a patient can be assisted to compensate for body scheme and/or body image disorders.
4. Describe how spatial relations impairments can affect the patient's ability to follow directions.
5. Explain the effect of the various agnosias on the patient's ability to recognize stimuli in the environment.
6. Differentiate between ideomotor and ideational apraxia. Describe how a patient with apraxia might behave in response to different instructional sets commonly employed in rehabilitation.
7. Describe how the psychological and emotional status of a patient with cognitive and perceptual deficits may affect participation in rehabilitation.
8. Analyze and interpret patient data, formulate realistic anticipated goals and expected outcomes, and identify appropriate interventions when presented with a clinical case study.

Cognitive and Perceptual Dysfunction

Carolyn A. Unsworth, OTR, PhD

OUTLINE

Cognitive and perceptual deficits are among the chief causes of confusion about and lack of progress in patients who have sustained brain damage, even among those whose motor skills have returned. Cognitive and perceptual deficits are some of the most puzzling and disabling difficulties that a person can experience. Thinking, remembering, reasoning, and making sense of the world around us is fundamental to carrying out daily living activities. When individuals experience problems with these capacities, it can have a devastating effect on their lives and the lives of their family. These people may not be able to live alone, fulfill the responsibilities of paid employment, or sustain a family life and relationships.[1] Thus, effective treatment of many patients with brain damage depends on understanding perception and cognition.

The brain may be damaged through several mechanisms including infections such as encephalitis; anoxia as may occur following near drowning; cardiopulmonary arrest, or carbon monoxide poisoning; tumors that are benign or malignant; trauma resulting from motor vehicle accidents, falls, or violent incidents (e.g., traumatic sports-related injury, gunshot wound); toxins such as alcohol or substance abuse; and vascular disease, which may produce an infarct or hemorrhagic stroke. The largest two groups of people who acquire cognitive and perceptual impairments following brain damage are persons who experienced stroke and traumatic brain injury.[1] The physical aspects of rehabilitation of these patient groups are addressed in Chapters 18 and 22, respectively.

The patient who has sustained an initial cerebral vascular accident (CVA) is thought to have focal or localized damage to discrete areas of the brain, often resulting in discrete cognitive or perceptual deficits. In contrast, patients who have sustained a traumatic brain injury are presumed to have generalized brain damage resulting in cognitive impairment with generalized deficits in attention, memory, learning, and so forth, rather than specific difficulties in discrete cognitive or perceptual functions. However, elements of both perceptual and cognitive dysfunction may occur in brain damage owing to either CVA or trauma. The distinctions between the two groups of patients become particularly blurred when one considers the patient who has suffered multiple strokes; this patient may in fact present with combined elements of both focal and generalized brain damage. Throughout this chapter, the patient with hemiplegia in whom brain damage has occurred as a result of a stroke will be the focus. The primary objective of this chapter is to introduce the reader to concepts relating to cognitive and perceptual dysfunction following brain damage.

An important focus for the physical therapist should be an understanding of how a particular cognitive or perceptual impairment might be manifested clinically, and how examination and treatment of movement disorders might be adjusted to capitalize on the abilities and minimize the cognitive or perceptual limitations of the patient. Deficits in the cognitive or perceptual domain must be considered to accurately determine the patient's true residual abilities. Using sets of directions that would confuse a patient with apraxia during a specific examination procedure may paint a picture of a greater or different motor disability than that which actually exists. Often the first clue to a cognitive or perceptual problem appears during initial sensorimotor testing. Awareness of the possibility and nature of cognitive or perceptual deficits will signal the therapist to redirect the method of testing, particularly the instructional sets and cues.

Cognition and Perception

The perceptual–motor process is a chain of events through which the individual selects, integrates, and interprets stimuli from the body and the surrounding environment. Cognition can be conceived of as the method used by the central nervous system (CNS) to process information. Cognitive processes include knowing, understanding, awareness, judgement, and decision making.[2] The difficulty of separating perceptual and cognitive deficits is readily apparent, both in patient behavior and in contradictory conceptualizations of these two domains of function. For example, according to some authors, cognition is conceived of as a general term that includes perception, attention, thinking, and memory.[3] According to other authors, perception is an umbrella term that encompasses both cognition and visual perception as subcomponents.[3] At this time, there is insufficient research evidence to suggest which approach most accurately reflects the way we think about and perceive information. What is clear is that normally functioning perceptual and cognitive systems are a necessary key to successful interaction with the environment. Because the majority of work in this field does distinguish between cognition and perception[1] and because it is probably easier to learn about these processes individually, they are defined separately for the purposes of this chapter.

Cognitive and perceptual capacities are clearly prerequisites for learning[4] and rehabilitation is largely a learning process.[2] Thus, it is not surprising that patients with cognitive and perceptual disorders are limited in their ability to learn self-care and activities of daily living (ADL) skills; hence, as a group, they are more limited in their potential for achieving independence.[5] In any rehabilitation program geared toward achievement of maximum independence, there is a compelling need for therapists to learn to recognize behavior related to perceptual deficits. The therapist's modification of examination and treatment approaches in light of these deficits will ensure that patients receive the full benefit of these services.

Cognition and Higher-Order Cognition

Cognition is the act or process of knowing, including awareness, reasoning, judgment, intuition and memory. **Executive functions** are sometimes discussed under this heading as well. Executive functions include the capacity to plan, manipulate information, initiate and terminate activities, recognize errors, problem solve, and think abstractly. Commonly, executive functions are categorized as *higher order cognitive functions*[6] or *metacognitive functions*.[7,8]

Perception

Lezak[4] defines **perception** as the integration of sensory impressions into information that is psychologically meaningful. Thus, perception is the ability to select those stimuli that require attention and action, to integrate those stimuli with each other and with prior information, and finally to interpret them. The resulting awareness of objects and experiences within the environment enables the individual to make sense out of a complex and constantly changing internal and external sensory environment.[9]

The terms perception and **sensation** are often confused with each other. Sensation may be defined as the appreciation of stimuli through the organs of special sense (e.g., eyes, ears, nose, and so forth), the peripheral cutaneous sensory system (e.g., temperature, taste, touch, and so forth), or internal receptors (e.g., deep receptors in muscles and joints).[9] Perception cannot be viewed as independent of sensation. However, the quality of perception is far more complex than the recognition of the individual sensation.[9] Perceptual deficits do not lie in the sensory ability itself, but rather with the individual's ability to interpret the sensation accurately, and therefore respond appropriately.[1]

Responsibilities of the Physical Therapist and the Occupational Therapist

Occupational therapists are the members of the rehabilitation team who are specially trained to examine and treat cognitive and perceptual deficits in relation to functional adaptation. They are responsible for the selection and administration of an appropriate constellation of tests and measures, accurate interpretation of results, and formulation of an overall plan of care (POC) for cognitive and perceptual rehabilitation. If appropriate, the occupational therapist may refer a patient to a neuropsychologist for specific intellectual testing.

In the hospital setting, the physical therapist is often the first member of the rehabilitation team to see a patient with brain injury. The physical therapist must understand the nature of cognitive and perceptual dysfunction and recognize that individuals in certain diagnostic categories, such as those with stroke or traumatic head injury, are likely to behave in ways that indicate the presence of particular cognitive or perceptual deficits.[10] When this occurs, the physical therapist should be aware that it is appropriate to refer the patient to occupational therapy for evaluation and treatment.

The tests and measures described in this chapter are included to assist the reader in understanding the nature of the different cognitive and perceptual disabilities. They are not meant to be used as a substitute for an intensive evaluation by a trained occupational therapist when it is deemed necessary.

An understanding of cognitive and perceptual dysfunction may go a long way toward alleviating much of the potential frustration that often accompanies treatment of a patient with brain damage, most of which is the result of inappropriate expectations on the part of the therapist, the patient, and the family. By collaborating with the occupational therapist, other members of the rehabilitation team, and the family, consistent treatment strategies may be developed and carried out, with obvious benefits to the patient.

Clinical Indicators

Cognitive and perceptual deficits ought to be ruled out as a cause of diminished functioning in all patients who have experienced brain damage. Such problems are particularly likely culprits in cases in which the patient seems unable to participate fully in self-care tasks and has difficulty participating in physical therapy for reasons that cannot be accounted for by lack of motor ability, sensation, comprehension, or motivation. Cognitive and perceptual dysfunction resulting from acquired brain damage must be differentiated from premorbid cognitive perceptual deficits (from previous trauma, illness, congenital abnormality, or dementing process) and from the general confusion and emotional sequelae that often accompany stroke and brain injury.[4]

Often, patients with cognitive and perceptual difficulties may display the following characteristics: inability to do simple tasks independently or safely, difficulty in initiating or completing a task, difficulty in switching from one task to the next, and a diminished capacity to locate visually or to identify objects that seem obviously necessary for task completion. In addition, they may be unable to follow simple one-step instructions, despite apparently good comprehension. They may make the same mistakes over and over. Activities may take an inordinately long time to complete, or they may be done impulsively. Patients may hesitate many times, appear distracted and frustrated, and exhibit poor planning. They are frequently inattentive to one side of the body and extrapersonal space, and may deny the presence or extent of their disability. These characteristics, all or some of which may be present, often make participation in daily living activities and therapy seem an insurmountable problem. These clinical features are explained and expanded upon throughout the remainder of this chapter.

Two typical scenarios are presented to give the reader an idea of when to suspect perceptual dysfunction. The first case involves a patient with a right hemisphere stroke who presents clinically with a left hemiparesis and good speech. Upon observation in the nursing unit, the patient appears to have functional strength in the unaffected right extremities and fair return on the affected left side. Yet the patient seems to have difficulty with simple range of motion (ROM) activities, even in the intact extremities, appearing confused and unable to move the arm up or down on command. The patient cannot seem to follow instructions for walking with a quad cane, constantly confuses the proper step sequence, and is unable to maneuver a wheelchair around the corner without crashing into the wall.

This patient should not be dismissed as uncooperative, intellectually inferior, or confused. In this instance, the patient is likely experiencing difficulty in spatial relations, right–left discrimination, and vertical disorientation, or perhaps left-sided neglect and apraxia. Further observation and examination should reveal the precise cause of the difficulties.

The second case involves a patient with left hemisphere damage and a resulting right hemiparesis and mild **aphasia**. The patient can respond reliably to "yes/no" questions and is able to follow simple one-stage commands such as, "Put the pencil on the table," or "Give me the cup." However, if asked to point to the arm, or asked to imitate the therapist's movements during an active ROM test even with the unaffected limbs, the patient does not respond and appears totally uncooperative. During therapy, the same patient is on a mat table. The therapist explains and then demonstrates the proper techniques for rolling to one side. The patient does not move. However, a moment later when his wife arrives, the patient quickly initiates rolling in an attempt to sit up to greet his wife. The astute therapist will realize that this patient may not be confused, stubborn, or uncooperative, as indeed he may appear. Rather, he may be suffering from a lack of awareness of body structure and relationship of body parts (somatagnosia), as evidenced by the ROM test incident, and an inability to perform a task on command or to imitate gestures **(ideomotor apraxia)**, as demonstrated in the rolling episode.

Hospitalization Following Brain Damage

The brain that has been damaged functions as a whole, just as it does in individuals without brain damage. When one part is damaged, the behavior observed is not merely the result of the brain operating precisely as in the intact individual minus the function of the area that was subject to anoxia. Rather, it is an outward manifestation of the reorganization of the entire CNS, at multiple levels, working to compensate for the loss.[11]

Because of the brain damage, the patient must cope with a nervous system operating without normal sensory input at all levels, both cortical and subcortical.[11] Normal responses to environmental stimuli are difficult to obtain when the input on which they have to act is deranged or incomplete. Recovery of function can be attributed to structural reorganization of the CNS into a new dynamic system widely dispersed within the cerebral cortex and lower segments.[12,13]

A significant contributor to the clinical picture of a patient after a CVA is the response to hospitalization. From a cognitive and perceptual perspective, when a patient is hospitalized (with or without brain damage), the inputs imposed on that patient's nervous system are radically different from the ones normally received. On the one hand, the environment is sensorially impoverished. There is no variation in temperature and lighting, and familiar background noises (e.g., telephones, airplanes, dogs, and buses) are missing. On the other hand, an enormous array of unfamiliar noises are present: nurses talking, loudspeakers, and the whir of machines. Strange and different smells, and unfamiliar, unavoidable, and unpleasant sights abound. Often, because of motor impairment, the patient cannot move around to seek or to escape inputs; therefore, a multiplicity of sensory inputs bombards the nervous system. Even if orienting responses are preserved, there is a profound sense of loss of control. This sensory derangement compounds the problems faced by the patient with brain damage, because those very abilities that enable the individual to select, filter out, and integrate incoming sensations to organize the self for appropriate action often fail in this sensorially bizarre environment.

To gain insight into the experience of the patient under such circumstances, it is enlightening to browse through the biographical and autographical reports of some noted neurologists and neuropsychologists, themselves victims or relatives of victims of CVAs. Particularly instructive are the reports of Bach-y-Rita,[14] Brodal,[15] and Gardner.[16]

Theoretical Frameworks

The theoretical bases of five approaches to therapy are examined in this section. The therapist will be guided in the selection of examination and treatment approaches consistent with the theoretical model. It is important to note that these approaches are not mutually exclusive. Many therapists use a combination of approaches, guiding selection by their clinical expertise and the patient's response to the techniques. Specific applications of these approaches will be presented following the description of individual cognitive and perceptual deficits in the final section of this chapter. Further information on a variety of theoretical approaches used by occupational therapists when working with patients who have cognitive and perceptual problems can be found in Averbuch and Katz[17] and Unsworth.[1]

The Retraining Approach

This approach was described by Averbuch and Katz[17] and focuses on the remediation of underlying skills the patient has lost. Sometimes this approach is referred to as the *transfer-of-training approach*. The approach is based on the assumption that a disruption in one brain region can have a negative impact on brain functioning as a whole. An underlying assumption of this approach is that skills learned for one task can generalize to others. In other words, transfer-of-training is assumed. The premise underlying transfer-of-training is that practice in one task with particular cognitive or perceptual requirements will enhance performance in other tasks with similar perceptual demands.[1,18,19] Thus, doing specifically selected perceptual exercises, such as pegboard activities, or parquetry blocks and puzzles will result in improving the perceptual skills required to perform those functional tasks. For example, Young et al[20] demonstrated that training patients with left hemiplegia in block design, in addition to *visual scanning* and *visual cancellation tasks,* resulted in improvements in reading and writing, although no specific training in these areas was offered. Because all tasks require the use of multiple perceptual skills, it is difficult to ascertain precisely which perceptual skills are being trained during any one session.[21]

Research to date has not unequivocally demonstrated a generalization from perceptual–motor training to functional skills.[18,21] Neistadt[19] suggests that the patient's capacity to learn must be evaluated and that learning capacity is the key to a patient's ability to generalize material learned in one situation to others. If transfer of training does occur, then strategies to enhance this can be incorporated into other components of the treatment program such as those aimed at maintaining sitting or standing balance, weight-bearing exercises, or functional use of the affected extremities.

The Sensory Integrative Approach

Ayres developed the theory of **sensory integration (SI)** in an effort to explain the relationship between neural functioning and the behavior of children with sensorimotor or learning problems.[22] The theory, strongly influenced by the neurobehavioral literature, describes normal sensory integrative development and functioning, defines patterns of sensory integrative dysfunction, and suggests treatment techniques.[22] Sensory integration can be defined as the organization of sensation for use.[23,24]

Integration of basic sensorimotor functions (tactile, proprioceptive, and vestibular) proceeds in a developmental sequence in the normal child within the context of goal-directed, meaningful activity. It is assumed that the production of an adaptive response facilitates sensory integration, which in turn enhances the ability to produce higher-level adaptive behaviors. Sensory integration is thought to occur at all levels of the nervous system.

The underlying assumption for treatment is that, by offering opportunities for controlled sensory input, the therapist can effect normal CNS processing of sensory information and thus elicit specific desired motor responses.[25] The performance of these adaptive responses, in turn, influences the way in which the brain organizes and processes sensation, thus enhancing the ability to learn.

Some of the treatment modalities employed include rubbing or icing to provide sensory input, resistance, and weightbearing to impart proprioceptive input, and the use of spinning to provide vestibular input. Following the controlled sensory input, an adaptive motor response is required by the patient to integrate the sensations provided by the therapist. In young children, the use of compensatory or **splinter skills** (skills acquired in a manner inconsistent with, or incapable of being integrated with, those already present) is avoided in favor of remediating underlying deficits. For more detailed information the reader is referred to the work of Ayres.[23,24]

Zoltan[2] argues that elderly patients, who comprise the majority of the stroke population, experience sensory integrative dysfunction similar to that of children with learning disabilities, and that this is because of the physiological changes associated with aging, along with environmentally induced sensory deprivation. The limitations in mobility caused by a stroke further prevent the patient from receiving and thus processing adequate sensory input.

The application of this theory to the adult post-stroke population, however, is open to serious debate. Bundy et al[22] argue that the theory explains mild to moderate learning and behavioral problems that are the result of a central deficit in processing sensations that are specifically not associated with frank brain damage. Further, there are a number of problems with the application of this approach to adult populations, even if it is theoretically tenable.

The treatment process is ordinarily quite lengthy. In addition, specific tests and measures and treatment approaches have been developed for and standardized on children, who presumably have sufficiently plastic nervous systems to be influenced by this form of therapy. The neurophysiological literature is replete with examples of ability that would be completely lost in mature individuals with similar lesions.[26–28] Furthermore, a mature adult with diffuse cerebral damage may have other complicating medical concerns and deficits in mobility that actually contraindicate the use of the equipment that is essential to the treatment process.[22] It is likely that many of the treatment regimes described as sensory integration are best described as a *sensorimotor approach*, which utilizes handling or directed sensory stimulation to elicit a specific motor response.[22]

The Neurofunctional Approach

The *neurofunctional approach* was first described by Giles and Wilson in 1992[29] and is based on learning theory. In contrast to the *retraining approach,* which assumes that transfer-of-training can occur, the authors of the neurofunctional approach assume that patients with acquired brain injury must practice every activity in its true context in order to recover function. Hence, the focus of this approach is on retraining real world skills rather than on retraining specific cognitive and perceptual processes.[30] Giles[30] argues that remediation approaches are largely unproven and thus may result in little functional improvement for the patient. He also suggests that compensatory skills or techniques are taught to a patient without considering if the gains made in terms of quality of life justify the considerable effort required.

The Rehabilitative/Compensatory (Functional) Approach

Probably the most widely used approach in treating perceptual deficits is the *rehabilitative/compensatory approach*[31–33] (also referred to as the *functional approach*), which offers a great deal of practical support for the physical therapist. The basic assumptions underlying this approach are that adults with brain trauma will have difficulty generalizing and learning from dissimilar tasks.[34] Direct repetitive practice of specific functional skills that are impaired is an efficient means of enhancing the patient's independence in those specific tasks. More recently, Fisher[35] extended the work of Trombly by (1) articulating more explicitly assumptions made about people within the rehabilitative/compensatory model; (2) generalizing this model beyond persons with physical disabilities to those with developmental, cognitive, or psychosocial disabilities; and (3) adding collaborative consultation to education and adaptation as strategies used to effect change.

The proponents of this approach favor addressing the functional problem over and above the treatment of its underlying cause when working with an adult post-stroke population. For example, a patient with difficulty in depth and distance perception, who is therefore unable to navigate a flight of stairs, would be made aware of the deficit, provided with external cues to compensate for the perceptual disorder, and would repetitively practice adapted techniques for safe stair climbing. The more closely the therapeutic practice situation resembles the home situation in terms of stair depth and height, amount of traffic, lighting, and so forth, the less generalizing is required and the more success the patient is likely to have when he or she returns home. However, problems might still be displayed in depth and distance perception in other areas of daily function.

In this functional approach, therapy is viewed as a learning process that takes into consideration the unique strengths and limitations of the individual patient. It is composed of two complementary components: compensation and adaptation.[1] *Compensation* refers to the changes that need to be made in the patient's approach to tasks. *Adaptation* refers to the alterations that need to be made in the human/social and physical environment in order to facilitate relearning of skills. In relation to the human/social environment, the therapist is concerned with altering the actions of others' functioning in the environment to enhance the patient's performance.

To compensate for the disability, the patient first has to be made aware of deficiencies (*cognitive awareness*) and must then be taught how to circumvent them using intact sensations and perceptual skills. The patient should be instructed in specific techniques and assisted in developing successful functional habits. The patient will need to be taught to attend to cues from the environment to enhance skill performance. The therapist helps the patient identify and then call upon these new cues. For example, if the patient has a visual field cut, the therapist should explain that because of a visual problem, the patient is seeing only one half of the environment. The patient should then be shown how to turn the head to compensate for the deficit. Environmental scanning could be incorporated into general therapy sessions as well.

A few general suggestions when teaching compensatory techniques are: (1) use simple directions; (2) establish and carry out a routine; (3) do each activity in a consistent manner; and (4) employ repetition as much as necessary.

Adaptation refers to the alteration not of the patient's strategy, but of the environment. For example, if the patient cannot differentiate between right and left, or tends to neglect the left side of the body, a piece of red tape on the left shoe during gait training will allow the patient to attend more easily to the left side and thus to follow the therapist's instructions more accurately. The therapist can use this functional approach to assist patients in improving specific motor skills related to treatment goals.

There are several inherent benefits to the rehabilitation/compensatory (functional) approach. First, in the current managed care environment there is a limited amount of time for inpatient rehabilitation.[36] Therefore, therapists need to concentrate on outcome-directed real-life functional activities because independent performance of these activities at home is the ultimate goal of therapeutic intervention. Interventions directed toward specific functional outcomes are typically reimbursable.[31] In addition, the activities are age appropriate, specific, and clearly relevant to the patient's concerns. For this reason, they tend to be the most motivating. The tasks can also be incorporated into a daily hospital routine. Dressing can be reinforced at bedside by the nursing staff, and eating skills can be reinforced at each mealtime.

The major limitation of this approach is that the methods learned in one task are not typically generalized to the performance of another task. The functional approach has been criticized as the teaching of splinter skills, in which the causes of the dysfunction are not addressed.

Cognitive Rehabilitation and the Quadraphonic Approach

Cognitive rehabilitation focuses on training individuals with brain injury to structure and organize information.[37] It addresses memory, high language disorders, and perceptual dysfunction under one umbrella.[38] Information processing, problem solving, awareness, judgement, and decision making are among the areas included. The therapist using a cognitive remediation approach might be concerned with the patient's perceptual style, including perceptual strategy, response to different types of cues, and rate and consistency of task performance.[39] Diller and Gordon[40] provide a review of the literature pertaining to intervention strategies for cognitive deficits.

Research has demonstrated that even in a non-brain-injured population, skills learned in one task do not automatically transfer to other tasks.[41] Hence, cognitive strategies can be used to facilitate the carryover of skills learned in therapy to functional activities. In her multicontext treatment approach to cognition, Toglia[41] proposes that learning can be conceptualized as a dynamic interplay between characteristics of the patient, characteristics of the task, and the environment in which it is performed. This has also been termed a *dynamic interactional approach*.[42] Characteristics of the individual patient that might affect learning include information processing strategies, metacognition (including awareness of one's own performance) and prior experience, attitudes, and emotions. Task-related variables that are proposed to affect learning include the nature of the task itself (familiarity with the task, spatial arrangements, instruction set, and movement and postural requirements), and the criteria that are used to determine the learner's abilities. Environmental variables include the social and cultural environment in which treatment occurs, as well as the physical context.

The *cognitive treatment approach* proposes a number of treatment strategies that may be relevant to the practice of physical therapy. These treatment strategies include[41]:

- Using multiple environments in which to carry out the training activity to enhance transfer of learning.
- Analyzing the characteristics of the task to establish criteria to determine if transfer of learning in fact took place.
- Providing training to make the patient aware of abilities, the level of difficulty of the task, and promote self-examination of performance.
- Relating new information or skills to previously learned ones.

Although these treatment strategies are well known within the field of cognitive–perceptual rehabilitation, the efficacy of the techniques remains to be established with the post-stroke population. For a comprehensive understanding and practical guidelines to the evaluation and treatment of patients with cognitive impairments from a dynamic perspective the reader is referred to Toglia[42] and Abreu.[43]

Abreu[44] has developed these treatment strategies as the *quadraphonic approach*. The quadraphonic approach is an interactive rehabilitation approach that provides a holistic perspective for the management of stroke, traumatic brain injury, brain tumors, cerebral palsy, and other neurologic conditions. The quadraphonic approach uses both a micro and a macro perspective for evaluation and treatment. The macro perspective provides guidelines for the management of functional performance and real life occupations. Evaluation and treatment is accomplished through the use of narrative analysis and synthesis of real life occupations to explain and predict the behavior of an individual based on four characteristics: *lifestyle*, *lifestage*, *health*, and *disadvantage status*. Real life occupations include shopping, cooking, meal preparation, money management, and mobility. The use of this dual perspective provides a holistic basis for the quadraphonic approach. The micro perspective provides guidelines for the management of performance components or subskills that include attention, visual perception, memory, motor planning, postural control, and problem solving. Evaluation and treatment of these performance components is based on a frame of reference that incorporates four theories: (1) information processing; (2) teaching/learning; (3) neurodevelopmental; and (4) biomechanical. Diagrammatic presentations of the components of the micro and macro perspectives are provided in Figures 29.1 and 29.2. An example of a therapist using this approach when working with a patient who has memory and learning problems may be found in Abreu.[43]

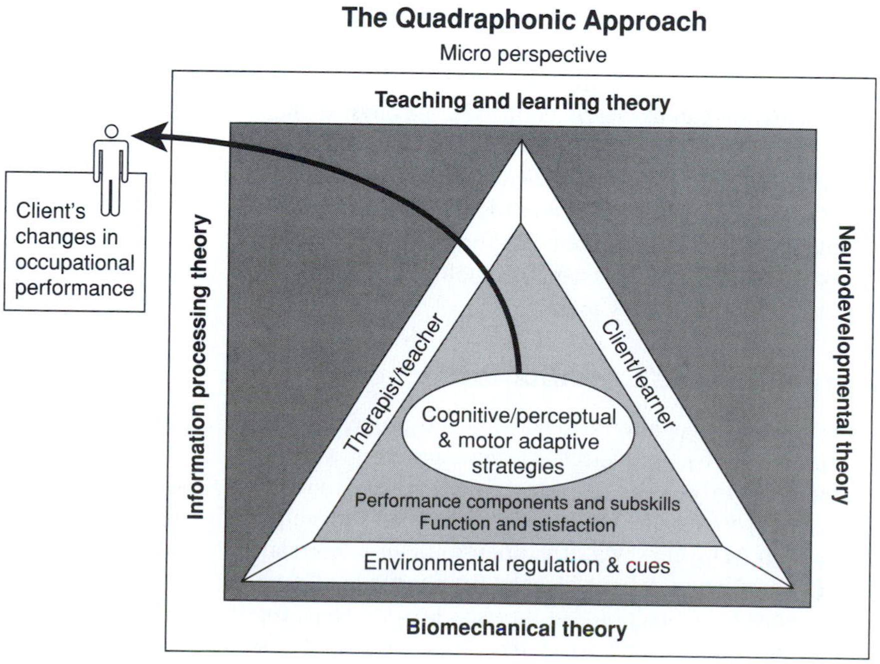

Figure 29.1 The quadraphonic approach—micro perspective. (From Abreu,[43] p 185, with permission.)

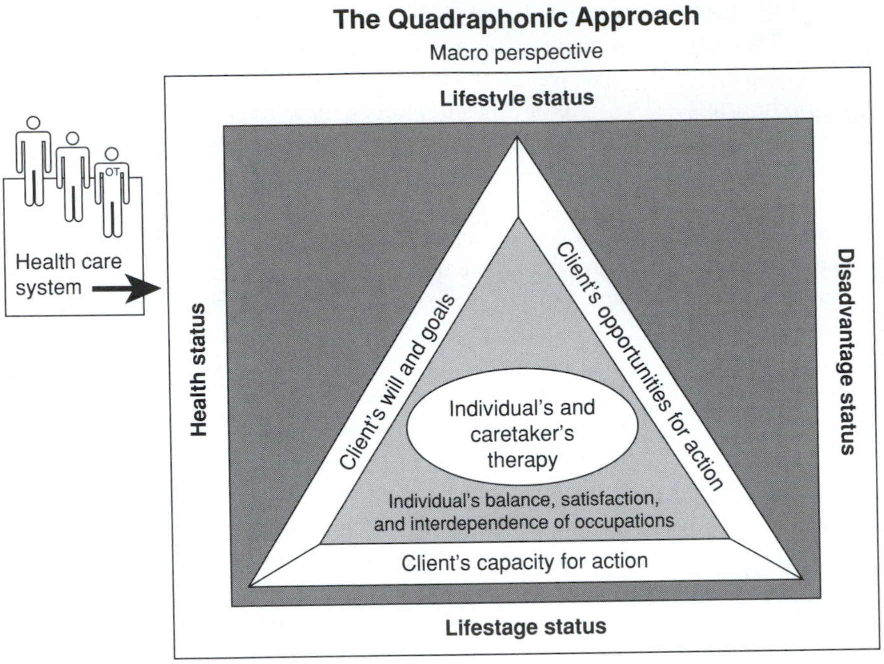

Figure 29.2 The quadraphonic approach—macro perspective. (From Abreu,[43] p 187, with permission.)

Examination of Cognitive and Perceptual Deficits

The use of systematic data collection provides the scientific basis for guiding intervention. Its importance cannot be overemphasized with respect to all facets of therapeutic intervention, including remediation of cognitive and perceptual dysfunction. **Task analysis** is the breakdown of an activity or task into its component parts together with a delineation of the specific motor, perceptual, and cognitive abilities necessary to perform each component. Task analysis is another tool critical to appropriate therapeutic intervention. For example, the strength, ROM, and balance abilities necessary to accomplish bed mobility and ambulation activities can be clearly defined by the physical therapist. However, the specific perceptual and cognitive requirements of each step needed to perform these two tasks may not be known. Without knowledge of the perceptual and cognitive requirements for successful completion of a task, the therapist cannot simplify the task for the patient and progressively upgrade it.

Purpose of the Examination

The presence of cognitive and perceptual dysfunction must be confirmed if it is suspected to be interfering with the patient's ability to carry out functional activities.[1] Perceptual performance is positively correlated with ability to perform ADL; however, it is often difficult to correlate specific perceptual deficits gleaned from testing with specific elements of functional ability and loss.[1,45] Thus, formal testing is indicated when there is a functional loss unexplained by motor deficit, sensory deficit, or deficient comprehension. It should be noted that not all areas of functional loss are typically detected within the hospital setting. It is not uncommon for the patient to perform adequately in self-care skills after therapy in the hospital but to fail on the same tasks in other environmental contexts, such as the home. Higher-level tasks, such as driving, banking, or planning a meal may only emerge as areas of difficulty once the patient is discharged home. When appropriate, the patient's competence in these areas should be considered within the context of an instrumental activities of daily living (IADL) examination with the occupational therapist while the patient is still hospitalized.

The purpose of patient examination is to determine which cognitive and perceptual abilities are intact and which are limited. Understanding the manner in which a particular deficit influences task performance will foster the application of a therapeutic strategy in which intact capabilities may be used to compensate for or to overcome deficits.[1]

Failure in the performance of a task may result from any number of processes underlying cognition and perception. For example, a patient's inability to complete a jigsaw puzzle may result from an inability to organize the pieces or problem solve where they go (disorder of executive function) or difficulty in attending to one half of the picture (unilateral neglect). The patient may be incapable of concentrating on the instructions (attention deficit), unable to know what the pieces are for (ideational apraxia), or unable to manipulate them (ideomotor apraxia). Although it is often difficult to implicate reliably one or another of these problem areas, the therapist must be aware of the different deficits that may produce similar patterns of behavior.[1,5]

A fascinating study conducted by Galski et al[46] concerning the prediction of driving ability following brain injury (including stroke) in 35 patients underscores the critical nature of carefully selected perceptual and cognitive tests. In this study, 64 percent of actual behind-the-wheel driving performances were predicted by performance on a selected battery of neuropsychological tests that measured visual perception. Examination of individual test results uncovered the reasons for unsafe driving, enabling instructors to focus on remediating the specific deficits in preparation for safe driving.

Patient examination is not an end in itself. Careful examination paves the way for realistic and cost-effective intervention.[47] Continuous monitoring of the patient's cognitive and perceptual status will ensure the use of appropriate treatment regimens and their modification when necessary.

Factors Influencing Patient Examination

Psychological and emotional status plays an important role in the patient's ability to cope with disability and with the testing situation. The therapist needs to be aware of behaviors that reflect a patient's psychological response to illness rather than particular cognitive or perceptual abilities. Psychological adjustment to disability depends on many factors, including age, vocational status, education, economic situation, attitude toward the reactions of others, family support, and feelings of competence prior to the onset of disease (see Chapter 2).[45,48,49]

When examining psychological and emotional status the following should be noted: whether the patient is confused; the level of comprehension for verbal instructions (written and spoken); whether communication is enhanced through the use of visual cues and demonstration; the ability to recognize errors; the level of cooperation and initiative (whether the patient is realistic about capabilities and goals); and emotional stability.[50] Disturbances of emotional response are evidenced by rapid and frequent mood changes and low frustration tolerance. Difficult tasks may cause a catastrophic reaction.[45]

The patient's ability to detect relevant cues from the environment or to discriminate between relevant and irrelevant stimuli (necessary for cognitive and perceptual competence) may be adversely influenced by poor judgement, fatigue, and prior expectations. Poor judgment is a major contributor to accidents in patients with hemiplegia. This is related in part to the diminished awareness by these patients as to their altered capabilities. The ambiguity of having one set of limbs that works normally and one set that is not functional may lead the patient to rely on solutions to the problems of daily living that are familiar but now inappropriate.[45]

Anxiety over capabilities may inhibit optimal performance during examination and treatment. The patient's capacity to perform optimally on testing and to learn is enhanced if anxiety can be reduced.[45] Motivation is influenced by many factors, among them premorbid personality. It is of utmost importance for the therapist to structure the therapeutic environment so that the patient will be positively motivated to learn to his or her maximum ability.[45] To this end, therapeutic tasks should be structured to ensure success, thereby diminishing frustration.

Other factors that may limit a patient's performance on cognitive and perceptual tests include reduced receptive and expressive communication skills, depression, and fatigue. Prior to a formal examination, the therapist should consider the patient's language skills, and confirm these observations with the speech–language pathologist. The therapist should also be aware of any medications the patient is taking and how these may affect performance. For example, many medications produce drowsiness as a side effect that would affect patient performance during testing.[1] Following stroke, 30 to 50 percent[12] of people are said to experience depression, the symptoms of which can easily be mistaken for cognitive or perceptual problems. Finally, a determination should be made of the patient's level of fatigue prior to any examination procedure.

The patient's behavior should not be misinterpreted because of a cultural bias, such as a lack of experience in taking tests. Premorbid intellectual ability should be ascertained from an interview with family or friends, because intellectual abilities may affect performance on some of the tests and measurements as well as affecting behavior in general. Premorbid memory should also be determined.

Finally, it is very important to conduct a sensory examination prior to cognitive or perceptual testing to establish whether the patient has sufficient sensory abilities to proceed with testing (this includes visual screening as well). Distinguishing between sensory and cognitive or perceptual problems is explored in more detail in the next section of this chapter. Each of these problems may adversely influence performance and may also reduce the patient's performance in treatment and capacity to learn from treatment. The therapist should be aware of the potential for these problems arising, and seek to minimize their impact.

Distinguishing Between Sensory and Cognitive and Perceptual Deficits

Cognitive and perceptual dysfunction must be differentiated from sensory loss, language impairment, hearing loss, motor loss (weakness, spasticity, incoordination), visual disturbances (poor eyesight, **homonymous hemianopsia**), disorientation, and lack of comprehension. The therapist must rule out pure sensory impairments prior to testing for cognitive and perceptual deficits, otherwise the therapist may incorrectly attribute poor performance to perceptual problems and design treatment accordingly when in fact the problem has a sensory base and should be treated quite differently. The therapist should conduct tests of deep (proprioceptive) sensations (kinesthesia, position sense, vibration), superficial sensations (pain, temperature, light touch, and pressure), and combined cortical sensations (stereognosis, tactile localization two-point discrimination, barognosis, graphesthesia, and recognition of texture) using methods described in Chapter 5. The patient's hearing also requires testing. For example, if the patient does not seem to understand what the therapist is saying, hearing problems should be ruled out before more extensive language and cognitive tests are conducted. The therapist may need to confirm with the family if the patient wears a hearing aid and ensure its availability during therapy. If in doubt, the therapist may need to request testing by the speech–language pathologist or audiologist.

The therapist must also determine if the patient has any visual impairments because they can easily be mistaken for perceptual problems. Given the prevalence of sensory-based visual problems, the following section focuses on identification of these impairments and the importance of distinguishing between visual and perceptual origins for treatment purposes.

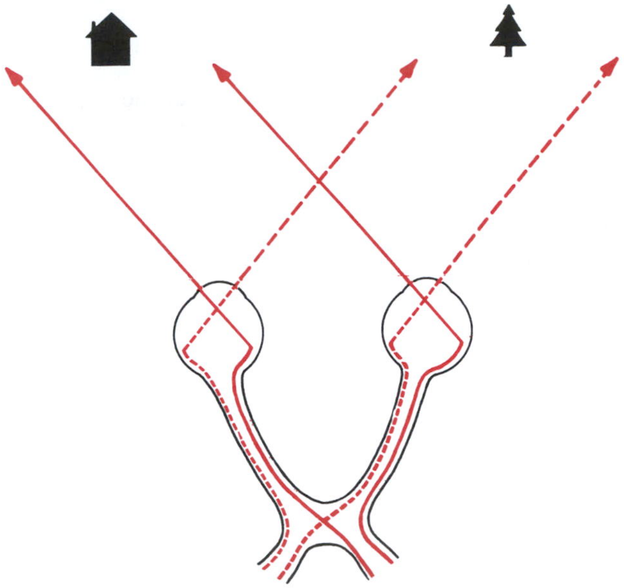

Figure 29.3 Normally functioning visual system; right and left visual fields. See text for explanation. (From Sharpless,[9] p 247, with permission.)

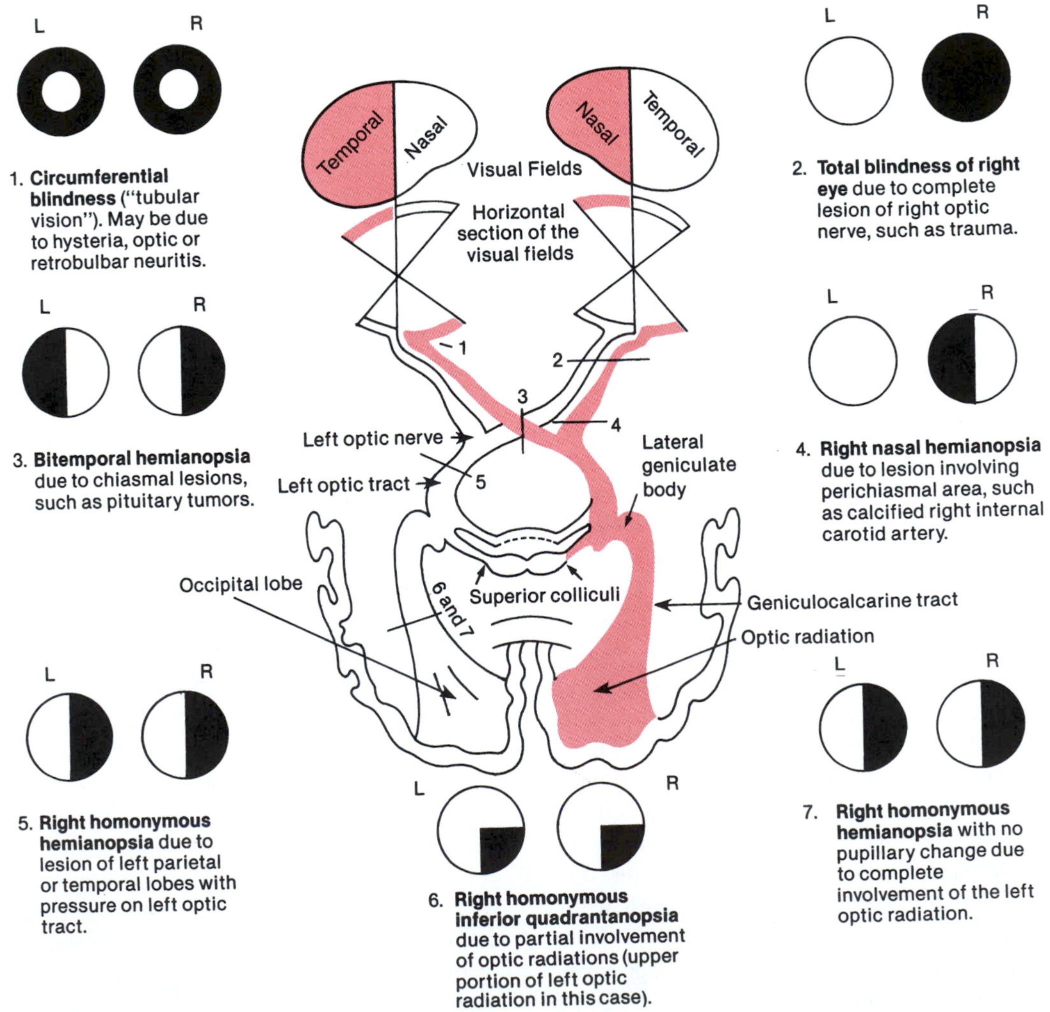

Figure 29.4 Visual field deficits and associated lesions sites. (From Chusid,[59] p 114, with permission.)

Visual Impairments

Visual impairments are one of the most common forms of sensory loss affecting the patient with hemiplegia.[51,52] The lesion resulting from a stroke may affect the eye, optic radiation, or visual cortex and subsequently the reception, transmission, and appreciation of any visual array. Visual impairments commonly encountered by patients with hemiplegia include poor eyesight, diplopia, homonymous hemianopsia, damage to the visual cortex, and retinal damage. Awareness of the presence of these deficits is important so as not to confuse them with visual perceptual deficiencies, and to ensure their consideration during treatment planning and therapeutic intervention.

The critical nature of the basic visual skills (i.e., acuity, oculomotor control, and intact visual fields) in forming a basis for higher level visual perception is highlighted by Warren[53,54] in a hierarchical model for the evaluation and treatment of visual perceptual dysfunction. In this developmental model, the basic visual skills enumerated above form the foundation for the next level of visual skills, which include visual attention, visual scanning, and pattern recognition. These skills, along with memory, are required to facilitate the highest level visual skill termed visual cognition.[53,54] This model has implications for the evaluation and treatment of visual perceptual disorders in a bottom-up sequence[54] (i.e., working from the "bottom" initially focusing on underlying skills that will then promote recovery of the next level of skills).

Impairments of oculomotor control (control of eye movements) are a common occurrence following a CVA. Poor visual acuity is another frequent finding following stroke or brain injury, even in the absence of other visual problems.[55] Therefore, it is recommended that the patient receive a comprehensive eye examination and have his or her eyeglass prescription checked.

Diplopia, or double vision, is often present following brain damage. The patient sees two of the entire environment. Diplopia is usually the result of defective function of extraocular muscles in which both eyes are used but not in focus. Treatment usually consists of exercises for the eye muscles. In addition, the patient usually is instructed to wear a patch on alternate eyes until the condition clears. If the condition does not clear, the optometrist may recommend prisms.

Visual field deficit is probably the most common visual deficit affecting patients with hemiplegia[56] and occurs most frequently following damage to the middle cerebral artery near the internal capsule.[9] The diagnostic term for this deficit is homonymous hemianopsia. Studies indicate that the frequency of hemianopsia following a right-hemisphere stroke is around 17 percent.[12] In addition, there is a significant correlation between the presence of visual field deficits and visual neglect.[57] Most important, the presence of a visual field deficit is a significant prognostic sign, predicting both a higher death rate following stroke and poorer performance in ADL, even following rehabilitation.[12,58]

Figure 29.3 demonstrates the normal functioning of the visual fields, in which the left side of the environment (the house) is perceived by the nasal retina of the left eye and the temporal retina of the right eye, and the right side of the environment (the tree) is perceived by the nasal retina of the right eye and the temporal retina of the left eye.[9]

The lesion producing homonymous hemianopsia interrupts inflow to the optic pathways on one side of the brain. This produces a loss of the outer half of the visual field from one eye and the inner half of the visual field of the other eye. The result is a loss of incoming information from half of the visual environment (left or right) contralateral to the side of the lesion. Thus, the loss of the left half of the visual field accompanies left hemiplegia and loss of the right visual field accompanies right hemiplegia. Figure 29.4 illustrates visual field deficits associated with a number of lesions to the visual system.[59]

The presence of a visual field cut may inhibit performance in many daily activities. The patient is usually unaware of the condition and does not automatically compensate by turning the head unless specifically instructed. One of the dangers in this condition is street crossing (Fig. 29.5).[60] Another example of the effects of a visual field cut is illustrated in Figure 29.6.[9] When presented with a tray of food, a patient with right homonymous hemianopsia may attend to the plate and fork on the left side and fail to see the knife, spoon, and cup on the right side of the plate. The patient might read only one half of the newspaper page, either to or from the midline.

Because of its prevalence, it is essential for the therapist to determine whether hemianopsia is present or not. A number of testing procedures are currently employed. In the confrontation method, the patient sits opposite the therapist and is instructed to maintain his or her gaze on the therapist's nose (Fig. 29.7).[61] The therapist slowly brings a target, such as a pen, into the patient's field of view simultaneously or alternately from the right or left. The patient is instructed to indicate when and where he or she sees the targets.

To help the patient compensate for the visual field deficit, the patient can first be made aware of the deficit and then be instructed to turn the head to the affected side. Patients usually require constant reminders at first, which may be tapered off with time and practice. Early in therapy, items (e.g., eating utensils, writing implements) should be placed where the patient is most apt to see them (on the intact side). They can be moved progressively to the midline and then to the affected side, when appropriate. The nursing staff should be made aware of the condition and be requested to place the patient's essential bedside needs such as telephone, tissues, and so forth within the intact visual field. The therapist initially should sit on the patient's intact side when instructing or giving demonstrations and should alternate this with the affected side so that the patient receives maximum stimulation. Of course, the patient will have to be reminded to turn the head at first. External cues can be employed as well. For reading, a red line can be drawn on the side of the page that is not seen.

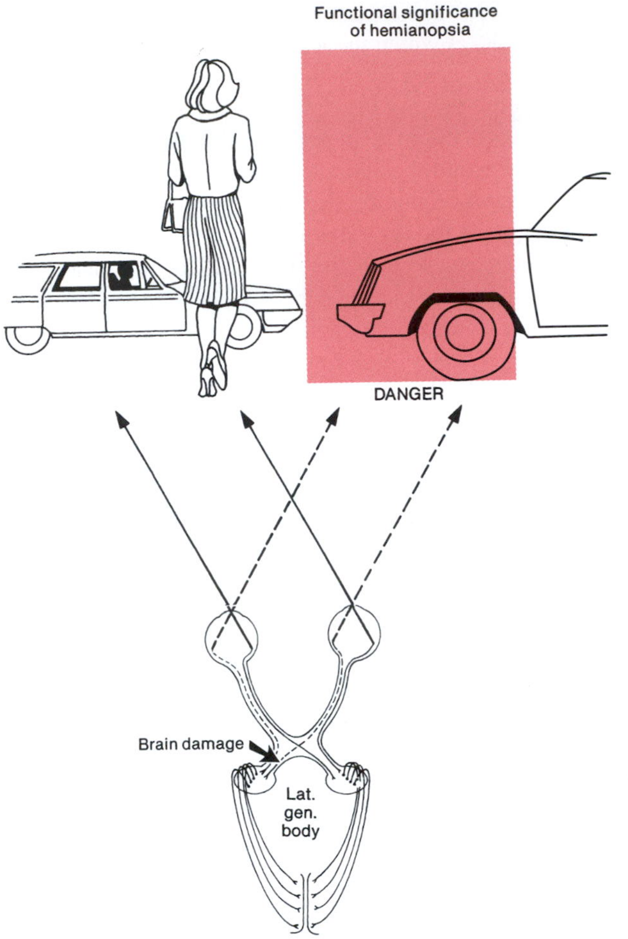

Figure 29.5 The functional significance of hemianopsia—it may lead to accidents. (From Tobis and Lowenthal,[60] p 78, with permission.)

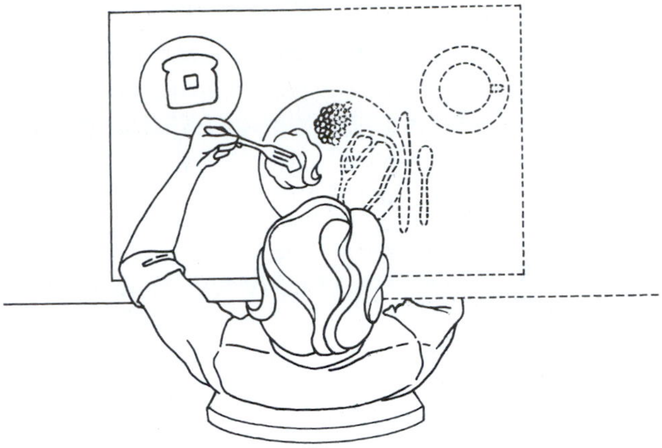

Figure 29.6 A table setting as it might appear to a patient with right homonymous hemianopsia following a stroke. The dotted lines indicate that she may be unable to locate her knife, spoon, cup, and so forth. (From Sharpless,[9] p 248, with permission.)

Red tape can be placed on the floor, mat, or parallel bars to attract the patient to scan to the side of the environment that is not seen. The patient should be taught to look for these cues. These external cues can be slowly tapered off over time. Patients can be instructed that they can devise their own cues to clue them into the unseen side of the environment in situations that have not been addressed per se in therapy. Exercises that require motor crossing of the midline can be used to reinforce visual crossing of the midline and turning of the head.[61,62]

Oculomotor impairment is the third potential area of deficit in basic visual skills that is common in patients who have had a stroke. Eye movements, which are controlled by the extraocular muscles, are used to detect, identify, and derive meaning from objects and the environment. They allow a person to become oriented to and explore the critical visual aspects of the environment.[11] Two types of eye movements are important to examine: (1) **visual fixation**, which allows the patient to maintain focus on an object as it is brought nearer or farther away; and (2) **ocular pursuits**, which enable the eyes to follow a moving object and visually scan the environment. Often the eyes will not follow a moving object visually, although the patient seems aware of the presence of that object and can locate it if asked. The patient is visually hypoactive. Oculomotor dysfunction often accompanies visual–perceptual dysfunction[63] and is frequently related to attention deficits.[64]

Visual scanning can be tested as follows. Sit opposite the patient. Hold up a pencil with a colorful pencil topper 18 in. in front of the patient's eyes. Slowly move the pencil horizontally, then vertically, then diagonally. Repeat each direction two to three times. Note the smoothness of eye movements, the presence of a midline jerk or jump, and whether the eyes move together.[2,63]

Aside from the visual sensory impairments outlined above, many patients suffer from visual–perceptual impairment. Damage to areas of the cortex upon which visual information converges with information from other senses may interfere with the recognition and interpretation of visual information, even though the visual stimuli may have arrived at the visual cortex uninterrupted. A total failure to appreciate incoming visual sensory information

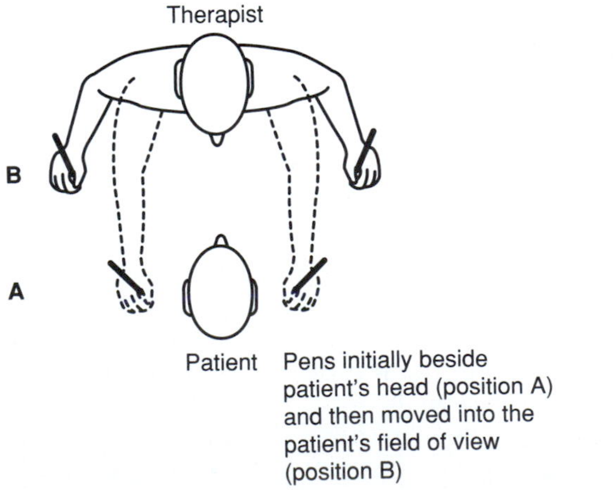

Figure 29.7 Method for testing hemianopsia. (Modified from Predretti,[61] p 99, with permission.)

owing to a lesion in the cortex is referred to as **cortical blindness**.[63] There is no statistical correspondence between the presence of visual field cuts and the presence of visual–perceptual disorders.[65] Similarly, there is no correspondence between aphasia, age, and time since infarct, and measures of visual–perceptual dysfunction.[65] However, within the realm of visual–perceptual impairments, there is a significant difference between the performances of patients with right hemiplegia and those with left hemiplegia. Patients with left hemiplegia have frequently been found to perform more poorly on measures of visual–perceptual dysfunction than patients with right hemiplegia. Thus, therapists should be aware of the possibility of visual–perceptual deficits, particularly in the population with left hemiplegia.

Standardized Cognitive and Perceptual Tests

A standardized test is one that has a uniform procedure to administer and score, provides operational definitions for all terms, is norm-referenced,[66] and information is available concerning its reliability and validity, which is essential for correct interpretation of results.[67] Results from standardized tests of cognition and perception can be communicated to other therapists who will share an understanding of the patient's capacities or abilities. Standardized tests can be administered both at admission and at discharge to provide the therapist with a reliable and valid measure of the outcome of therapy.

When conducting a standardized test, the patient should be sitting comfortably and wearing glasses and/or a hearing aid if needed. Ideally, the room should be quiet and free of distraction. The therapist should be positioned opposite or next to the patient. Age, gender, and hand dominance should be noted.[1] In addition, the performance of a patient who has had a stroke may vary from day to day; a single testing session is, therefore, usually unreliable.[68] A number of short sessions scheduled on successive days are preferable. To enhance its practical value, perceptual testing must be done in conjunction with observation in self-care and ADL skills, where the patient's judgement and discriminative abilities with regard to real-life tasks can be determined. It is not uncommon for patients to test poorly for visual–perceptual skills but to perform adequately in ADL with minimal effort or assistance.[64]

The quality of the patient's response to the test media (e.g., how the task is approached, how and why the error is made) is as important to note as the success or failure in completing the selected task. Some aspects of response in the testing situation or during ADL can be referred to as the patient's individual *perceptual style*. Included under this rubric are the patient's perceptual strategy, response to various cues (such as auditory, visual, and tactile), rate of performance, and consistency of performance.[37]

Occupational therapists use a variety of standardized tests to determine the presence of cognitive and perceptual impairments and resulting disabilities. When selecting a standardized test the therapist must consider many factors. The selection depends on what the therapist wants to learn about the patient, and what the test can potentially reveal.[1] In many cases a single test will not provide all the information required by a therapist to plan treatment, so several tests may be administered (Table 29.1).[69–83] In addition to those presented in Table 29.1, other more global instruments used to measure the outcome of rehabilitation are the *Medical Outcomes Study (MOS), Short Form Health Survey (SF-36),*[84] *Therapy Outcome Measure (TOM),*[85] the *Canadian Occupational Performance Measure (COPM),*[86] *Rivermead Rehabilitation Centre Life Goals Questionnaire,*[87] *Reintegration to Normal Living Index (RNL),*[88] and the *Functional Independence Measure (FIM$_{MR}$^{SM}).*[89] Some of these instruments also incorporate items that measure cognition and perception. For example, the FIM$_{MR}$^{SM} includes three cognition-related items (memory, problem solving, and social interaction). The tests described in the section on specific cognitive and perceptual deficits are used widely in the clinic. Although some of the instruments presented are not standardized, they are still useful, particularly for examining the quality of response to the test stimuli.

Intervention

Treatment Approaches

Five major approaches to cognitive and perceptual rehabilitation are commonly employed by occupational therapists. They are the *retraining approach,* the *sensory integrative approach,* the *neurofunctional approach,* the *rehabilitation/compensatory approach,* and the *cognitive rehabilitation/quadraphonic approach.* These approaches were described earlier in the chapter. Although research directly comparing the efficacy of the various approaches has been sparse, attempts have been made recently to empirically define and test the methodologies.[21,25,34,90] Issues to consider in examining the approaches are the availability of standardized measures of change in functional status and ADL, length and frequency of feedback, group versus individual treatment, specific stimulus properties, format and frequency of feedback, and individual information processing styles.[21]

Neistadt[25,34] described these treatments dichotomously as either remedial or adaptive/compensatory. The remedial approach encompasses the retraining approach, the sensory integrative approach, and the cognitive approach.[1] The neurofunctional approach and the rehabilitation/compensatory approach are described as adaptive or compensatory. The quadraphonic approach brings together aspects of both the remedial and compensatory approaches. A description of

Table 29.1 Summary of Standardized Tests

Test	Description
Arnadottir OT-ADL Neurobehavioral Evaluation (A-ONE)[5]	This test was developed to measure a patient's neurobehavior through daily living tasks (dressing, grooming, hygiene, transfer and mobility, feeding, and communication). Occupational therapists must undertake a 5-day training and certification course to qualify to administer this test. A wide variety of cognitive and perceptual impairments can be detected with this instrument.
Structured Observational Test of Function (SOTOF)[69]	The SOTOF was designed to examine older persons' level of occupational performance and neuropsychological functioning following neurological damage of cortical origin.[70] The instrument consists of a screening test, neuropsychological checklist, and four ADL scales (eating from a bowl, pouring a drink and drinking, putting on an upper body garment, and washing and drying hands). After analyzing observational data, a wide variety of neuropsychological deficits are extrapolated.[69]
Allen Cognitive Level Test (ACL)[71,72]	The ACL is used as a screening tool to estimate a person's cognitive level. Although originally developed for use with clients who have psychiatric problems, this test is also used with people who have acquired brain damage, or experience a dementing illness such as Alzheimer's disease. Following an interview to gain information concerning the client's educational and work background, the client is observed performing the visuomotor task of leather lacing. It is assumed that the client's cognitive functioning is reflected through his or her motor actions.[1]
Chessington Occupational Therapy Neurological Assessment Battery (COTNAB)[73]	The COTNAB was designed to examine cognitive and perceptual deficits in patients 16 years of age and older following stroke or head injury. The battery consists of 12 tests divided into four sections examining visual perception, constructional ability, sensory-motor ability, and ability to follow instructions. Further information about this instrument may be found in Stanley et al[74] and Sloan et al.[75]
Loewenstein Occupational Therapy Cognitive Assessment (LOTCA)[76]	The LOTCA is a battery-style test lasting 35 to 40 minutes and composed of 20 subtests that examine four areas: orientation, visual and spatial perception, visuomotor organization, and thinking operations. The instrument was developed for use with people who have experienced stroke, traumatic brain injury, or tumor. Further information about this test is contained in Katz et al.[77]
The Behavioural Inattention Test (BIT)[78]	The BIT was developed to examine clients for the presence of unilateral visual neglect and to provide the therapist with information concerning how the neglect impacts the client's ability to perform everyday occupations.[79] The BIT consists of nine activity-based subtests and six pen-and-paper subtests. Many of these test items have been used in the past in a nonstandardized way to examine for the presence of neglect.
Rivermead Perceptual Assessment Battery (RPAB)[80]	This instrument was designed to examine visual perceptual impairments in patients following head injury or stroke. The RPAB is a battery consisting of 16 performance tests that examine form discrimination, color constancy, sequencing, object completion, figure-ground discrimination, body image, inattention, and spatial awareness. The test can be completed in approximately 1 hour. For further information on the RPAB, the reader is referred to Jesshope et al.[81]
Rivermead Behavioural Memory Test (RBMT)[82]	This battery was designed to examine everyday memory abilities. It offers the therapist an initial determination of the client's memory function, an indication of appropriate areas for treatment, and enables the therapist to monitor memory skills throughout the treatment program. The RBMT can be administered in approximately 30 minutes by occupational therapists, speech–language pathologists, and psychologists. For further information on the RBMT, the reader is referred to Wilson et al[82,83]

the key components of these two main approaches is outlined below. A discussion on education is also provided because no intervention program would be complete without the provision of education to both the patient and the caregivers. Finally, a discussion is provided on integrating these three elements within a rehabilitation program.

The Remedial Approach

Remedial approaches focus on the patient's deficits and attempt to improve functional ability by retraining specific perceptual components of behavior.[25] The assumption uniting this set of tactics is that facilitation of, or training in, underlying skills will enhance the recovery or reorganization of deficient CNS functioning.[21,25] This, in turn, will automatically translate into improvement in functional skills. Remedial approaches are also referred to as bottom-up approaches. These approaches work from the bottom, which is the recovery of underlying skills, and assume that the patient will be able to generalize skills to occupational performance, which is at a higher level.[1,47]

The Adaptive/Compensatory Approach

The adaptive or compensatory approach mandates direct training in the functional skills that are deficient. It does not assume automatic carryover from tasks that are not obviously similar to the functional task to be learned, and thus minimizes the need for generalization. In an adaptive or "top-down" approach, the therapist works with the patient on specific tasks that are required, or those that the patient wants to achieve. In other words, the therapist starts at the top, which is the desired functional outcome, rather than working with the patient on the underlying performance components.[35] Table 29.2 presents a comparison of the assumptions underlying the remedial and adaptive approaches.

Patient, Family, and Caregiver Education

Education for the patient, family, and caregivers is essential for continuity of care. The patient and caregivers should understand why it is inadvisable or impossible for the patient to do some things safely or independently, and why other things must be done in a specific way. Explaining the reasons why the patient behaves in a particular way reduces the likelihood of inappropriate expectations from those without the background to know that brain damage affects not only how the patient moves but how he or she experiences and thus responds to the world.

Feedback is essential to the patient's learning. The patient's own feedback may be inaccurate owing to perceptual and cognitive dysfunctions. Thus, the individual may be unaware that a task has not been accomplished or that it has not been performed in the safest or most efficient manner. Feedback should be provided in the form of **knowledge of results (*KR*)**, and **knowledge of performance (KP)**. Knowledge of results is information regarding whether or not the patient attained the correct outcome. Knowledge of performance is information regarding the manner in which the task was accomplished.[91]

The form in which this feedback is delivered depends on the specific limitations and strengths of the patient. For example, the physical therapy goal for a patient with left hemiplegia and visual perceptual involvement might be to walk to the end of the parallel bars. KR would consist of a verbal confirmation by the therapist as to whether or not the patient reached the end of the parallel bars. KP might include comments by the therapist concerning the adequacy of the patient's visual scanning, positioning of the lower extremities, correct posture, and appropriate use of the upper limbs. For the patient with communication impairments, the feedback would have to be visual. Tactile input also can be used effectively to cue patients with either right or left hemiplegia. A combination of inputs, using a number of sensory modalities, often facilitates patient success at a given task.

When involving the patient in education sessions, the patient must be addressed as a competent adult, and not patronized. He or she must be regarded as the principal participant in the rehabilitation process. In situations in which the perceptual deficit does not interfere with

Table 29.2 Common Assumptions of Adaptive and Remedial Approaches

Adaptive Approach	Remedial Approach
The adult brain has limited potential to repair and reorganize itself after injury.	The adult brain can repair and reorganize itself after injury.
Intact behaviors can be used to compensate for ones that are impaired.	This repair and reorganization is influenced by environmental stimuli.
Adaptive retraining can facilitate the substitution of intact behaviors for impaired ones.	Cognitive, perceptual, and sensorimotor exercises can promote brain recovery and reorganization.
Adaptive ADL provide training in functional behaviors.	Cognitive, perceptual, and sensorimotor exercises provide training in the cognitive and perceptual skills needed for those exercises.
Training in specific, essential activities of daily living tasks is necessary because adults with brain injury have difficulty generalizing learning.	Remedial training in cognitive and perceptual skills will be generalized across all activities requiring those skills.
Functional activities require cognitive and perceptual skills.	Functional activities require cognitive and perceptual skills.
Adaptation and compensation will lead to improved functional performance.	Cognitive and perceptual remediation will lead to improved functional performance.

assimilation of information, the patient should have the major role in the decision making process regarding the goals of therapy.

Refocusing Intervention

Many clinicians begin an intervention program by adopting remedial strategies. In these circumstances, therapists are aiming to maximize recovery of function and educate their patients about the problems experienced and ways that can improve their function. However, some patients may not make much progress. In some cases, the patient may have inadequate language skills to be able to work with the therapist, or may have limited insight to his or her problems and therefore will not work with the therapist. In other cases still, improvements simply do not seem to occur for a variety of reasons that the therapist may not be able to pinpoint. Finally, in the current climate of managed care, the therapist may not have very much time allocated to work with the patient using remedial techniques. The patient's discharge may be imminent, and yet he or she may not be independent or safe enough to be discharged. In such cases, the therapist may switch from a remedial approach to a compensatory one.

When using an adaptive compensatory approach, the therapist will address education of the caregivers as well as the patient. Intervention strategies will focus on changing the environment or the strategy for task completion so that the patient can be safe and independent as quickly as possible. In many instances, therapists use a three-point approach to intervention where they educate patients and caregivers, begin the program using remedial techniques, and then switch to compensation techniques when the patient's improvements have plateaued and/or discharge is imminent.

The Impact of Managed Care

The introduction of managed care in the U.S. health care system has many implications for treatment of patients with cognitive and perceptual deficits. The most striking of these is the reduction in time allocated for inpatient evaluation and treatment.[36] Cognitive and perceptual problems are not readily visible and are therefore more easily overlooked than physical problems. Hence, pressure to discharge patients quickly, possibly before the full extent of cognitive and perceptual deficits has been revealed means that patients may be discharged to potentially hazardous situations at home. Therapists need to do an initial screening of all patients with brain damage to determine potential problems as early as possible, and ensure that patients are discharged to a safe environment. Although inpatient rehabilitation time is reduced, there is more opportunity for outpatient services conducted in the clinic or in the patient's home.[92] The advantage of home care is that therapists have an opportunity to work with the patient in his or her own environment, and tailor therapy to the patient's current circumstances. Patients with cognitive and perceptual deficits often perform better in their own familiar environments.

The major disadvantage of reduced inpatient treatment time for many patients, including those with cognitive and perceptual deficits, is that a home discharge may not be safe after only limited inpatient rehabilitation. The situation is complicated by having to discharge a patient who does not have family support to another type of institutional care (possibly a nursing home or skilled nursing facility) when in the long term this level of care may not be necessary. It is distressing for patients who are confused owing to cognitive and perceptual problems to be moved, particularly when they may believe the move is permanent.

Discharge Planning

Discharge planning begins as soon as the patient is admitted for rehabilitation.[93] The most important question to be answered during this stage is where the patient will live upon discharge. There are two major types of housing available to persons with disabilities: community-based accommodation and supported accommodation. Community-based accommodation includes private homes, retirement villages, and hotels or rooming houses. Supported accommodation may be defined as any accommodation that provides personal care and medical services on a consistent, continual, or per need basis, and includes nursing homes, skilled nursing facilities, assisted living centers, and sheltered or group housing.[94,95]

The key to discharge planning is to consider the match between the patient's skills and the demands of the environment, and then factor in the support systems available from a spouse, friends, or family to assist with tasks that the patient cannot manage.[95,96] This approach works well when patients and their families have insight and an understanding of the patient's problems. However, cognitive and perceptual deficits are often not very visible and it may be difficult for the family and the patient to understand the functional impact of these deficits. For example, a patient may regain full motor function following a stroke, but experience ongoing difficulties with unilateral neglect. This problem is not readily apparent to the untrained onlooker. However, this patient cannot drive and may be in danger when simply crossing the road. These problems have major lifestyle implications for the patient.

Interventions that facilitate a patient's return to community-based housing usually center on enabling the patient to carry out ADL skills in an acceptable and safe manner. If this cannot be achieved and the patient does not have a live-in caregiver, then supported housing such as a nursing home may be the only alternative. Research examining the discharge process for a sample of 62 patients following stroke revealed that the majority were reluctant to consider alternatives to returning home despite having significant self-care deficits.[96] Our housing is central to who we are as individuals and it is very difficult for patients, particularly those with limited insight, to understand and accept that they can no longer live in the community.

Review of Cognitive and Perceptual Deficits

This section is divided into seven parts: attention deficits, memory impairments, impairments of executive function, body scheme and body image impairments, spatial relations impairments, agnosia, and apraxia (Table 29.3). Each category encompasses a constellation of deficits, which are grouped together for ease of understanding. Information pertaining to each deficit will be organized identically as follows:

1. Definition(s)
2. Clinical Examples
3. Lesion Area
4. Testing
5. Treatment Suggestions

The value of dwelling on probable areas of cortical damage is controversial. The indication of cortical loci is an attempt to relate the study of neuroanatomy to actual patient behavior involving cognitive and perceptual dysfunction. An examination of cortical loci will give the reader a sense of which cognitive and perceptual deficits are likely to be seen together.

As therapists, we are required to assist the patient to bridge the gap between maladaptive behavior and independent function in ADL skills. Whether or not the area of the brain purported to produce a particular dysfunction appears damaged on a computed tomography (CT) scan or other neurological or radiological test is not a key determinant of the rehabilitative approach to therapy. The patient's approach to task performance and the relative strengths or weaknesses of the patient (motor, cognitive, and perceptual), which the therapist ascertains through thorough observation and testing, are much more pertinent to the selection of appropriate therapeutic strategies than the locus of the lesion.

Testing tools are described for each cognitive or perceptual deficit to enhance the reader's awareness of the complexity of behavior ascribed to perceptual deficiencies. Familiarity with the tools used to examine cognitive or perceptual deficits can serve as an aid in communication between physical and occupational therapists engaged in the treatment of the same patient.

The following section also includes specific treatment suggestions from the sensorimotor, transfer of training, and functional approaches described. The treatment techniques most relevant are those dealing with the functional approach and adaptation of the environment. In these sections, examples are given of how to facilitate the patient's success within a treatment session. Information is provided on how the therapist might gear language, demonstrations, feedback, and the use of media and the environment to the individual needs of the cognitively or perceptually impaired patient. The evidence base for treatment is not strong for many of these treatment techniques, and further research is required to support their efficacy.

Table 29.3 Summary of Cognitive and Perceptual Impairments

Area of Deficit	Specific Impairments

Cognition	Attention disorders
	  Sustained attention
	  Selective attention
	  Divided attention
	  Alternating attention
	Memory disorders
	  Immediate recall
	  Short-term memory
	  Long-term memory

Higher-order cognition	Executive functions
	  Volition
	  Planning
	  Purposive action
	  Effective performance

Perception	Body scheme/body image disorders
	  Unilateral neglect
	  Anosognosia
	  Somatoagnosia
	  Right–left discrimination
	  Finger agnosia
	Spatial relation disorders (complex perception)
	  Figure–ground discrimination
	  Form discrimination
	  Spatial relations
	  Position in space
	  Topographic disorientation
	  Depth and distance perception
	  Vertical disorientation
	Agnosias
	  Visual object agnosia
	  Auditory agnosia
	  Tactile agnosia
	Apraxia
	  Ideomotor apraxia
	  Ideational apraxia
	  Buccofacial apraxia

Attention Deficits

1. *Definitions.* The inability of many patients with hemiplegia to maintain attention during therapy is a frequent

complaint of therapists. **Attention** is the ability to select and attend to a specific stimulus while simultaneously suppressing extraneous stimuli.[97] A patient who is inattentive or distractible will have difficulty in processing and assimilating new information or techniques.[98] Often, patients who have suffered a CVA will have low arousal levels, and require a great deal of sensory input to be alerted to the environment. Low arousal thus must be considered as a cause for seeming inattention.

Four different kinds of attention are generally discussed in the literature. These are sustained attention, focused or selective attention, alternating attention, and divided attention. **Sustained attention** is a capacity to attend to relevant information during activity. Sustained attention implies that a person can maintain a consistent response during a continuous activity. **Focused** or **selective attention** is the capacity to attend to a task despite environmental visual or auditory stimuli. **Alternating attention** is the capacity to move flexibly between tasks and respond appropriately to the demands of each task. **Divided attention** is the capacity to respond simultaneously to two or more tasks or stimuli when all stimuli are relevant.[1]

2. *Clinical Examples.* Clinically, the patient with a disorder of sustained attention may report that he or she starts to watch a TV program and then "just drifts off." A patient who has to stop a dressing activity to talk to the therapist may be demonstrating difficulties with focused attention. Patients who are easily disturbed by music or other forms of background noise may also be experiencing problems with focused attention.

   Hence, a problem with focused attention is often referred to as distractibility. Divided attention is required when more than one response is needed or more than one stimuli needs to be monitored.[99] Selective attention is required when certain stimuli need to be ignored.[100] Patients who have difficulty with divided and alternating attention may have great difficulties with more complex daily living activities such as cooking a meal or driving.
3. *Lesion Areas.* Multiple brain regions are thought to be responsible for producing attention. These include the reticular formation (which regulates arousal), the various sensory systems that deliver and code relevant sensory information, and the limbic and frontal regions that underlie the drive and affective components of concentration.[100]
4. *Testing.* General screening tests such as the *Loewenstein Occupational Therapy Cognitive Assessment*[76] or *Chessington Occupational Therapy Neurological Assessment Battery (COTNAB)*[73] include subtests that examine attentional abilities. To investigate problems of attention, neuropsychologists generally administer the *Stroop Test*,[101] the *Paced Auditory Serial Attention Test (PASAT)*,[102] and the *Trail Making Test*.[103]
5. *Treatment Suggestions.* The purpose of therapy is to increase the patient's attention to appropriate stimuli, and disregard inappropriate stimuli.
   a. *Remedial Approach.* Clinically, the ability to attend to a task has implications for the therapeutic process. Patients should be trained to scan the visual environment in a slow and systematic manner. In the presence of right hemiplegia, the patient should be spoken to more slowly to afford an opportunity to process verbal information. In addition, patients with left hemiplegia should be encouraged to use verbalization to improve performance in visual tasks, and patients with right hemiplegia should be taught to use visualization techniques to facilitate attendance to verbal tasks.

      Some additional tools that may be used for the remediation of attentional deficits and distractibility are setting time or speed limits, amplification of critical stimuli, and making the crucial stimuli salient (noticeable) to the patient.[64] The environment can be graded by having the patient initially perform some aspects of therapy in a nondistracting setting (closed environment) and then slowly increasing potentially distracting elements, both visual and auditory, as patient tolerance improves.[1]
   b. *Compensatory Approach.* For many patients, the inability to attend to significant stimuli is compounded by distraction due to extraneous stimuli in the environment. Often noise is the most distracting stimulus, causing irritability and diminished concentration. Ponsford, Sloan, and Snow[104] provide further ideas for working with patients who have limited attention.

      A Cochrane Review entitled "Cognitive rehabilitation for attention deficits following stroke" was conducted in 2002.[105] This review revealed only two controlled trials of attention training in stroke. The results of these studies suggested that training improved alertness and sustained attention on measures of these capacities, but there was no evidence to support or refute the use of cognitive rehabilitation for attention deficits to improve functional independence.

Memory Impairments

Memory can be defined as a "mental process that allows the individual to store experiences and perceptions for recall at a later time."[98, p 78] All memory is not localized in one particular place in the nervous system; rather, many and perhaps all regions of the brain may contain neurons with adequate plasticity for memory storage.[106] Memory comprises acquisition or learning, storage or retention, and retrieval or recall.[107] Learning is a crucial element of rehabilitation. If the patient is unable to learn then time in rehabilitation may not be well spent. Hence, it is very important for the therapist to take steps to evaluate the patient's memory before beginning physical retraining programs. Three levels of memory will be examined: immediate recall, short-term memory, and long-term memory.

Immediate Recall and Short-Term Memory

1. *Definitions.* **Immediate recall** involves retention of information that has been stored for a few seconds. **Short-term memory** mediates retention of events or learning that has taken place within a few minutes, hours, or days.[4]
2. *Clinical Examples.* A patient with immediate recall difficulties may not be able to remember the instructions given only seconds before by the therapist for what the patient is to do. A patient with a short-term memory problem may not come back to the physical therapy department, even though the therapist asked him or her to return in an hour. Alternatively, the therapist may teach the patient a new transfer technique, and on the following day find that the patient has not retained any of the steps involved. Patients with severe short-term memory problems may not even be able to hold a simple conversation.[1]
3. *Lesion Areas.* Memory is a complex capacity involving many brain regions including four of the major structures of the cerebral cortex (the frontal, parietal, temporal, and occipital lobes) and the limbic system.[4]
4. *Testing.* The *Rivermead Behavioural Memory Test (RBMT)*[82] can be used to examine memory function. Alternatively the adequacy of memory functions can be ascertained by having the patient recall lists or collections of objects that have just been presented (immediate recall) or by teaching the patient a new verbal or visual task and asking him or her to recall it a few hours or a day later (short-term memory). Frequently there is a loss of short-term memory following stroke, and this particularly interferes with the patient's ability to benefit from rehabilitation, especially from those activities involving the use of new and heretofore unfamiliar techniques.[45]
5. *Treatment Suggestions.* The purpose of memory retraining is to enable the patient to effectively encode and recall information so that learning can occur.
   a. *Remedial Approach.* As good attention skills are vital for memory, the therapist must ensure that attention problems are addressed and improvements are noted before initiating work on memory retraining.[1,43] A primary focus of this approach is working with the patient to effectively encode information so it can be more easily retrieved when appropriate. This may include organizing material to be remembered, and making logical associations. A determination should be made of how the patient used to remember information and build on these past strategies. There is very little evidence to suggest that drills, computer games, or memory tests such as recalling a list of items that have been covered over have any effect on retraining memory. However, if the therapist assists the patient to develop memory strategies when playing these games, then these strategies can be generalized to everyday activities.
   b. *Compensatory Approach.* The use of a diary or notebook system (memory log) can help many patients to manage their daily living activities. However, the patient needs to have sufficient memory to use this system. Environmental prompts such as a beeper or a wall calendar can be useful to assist patients to remember their routine, or to look at their diary. When external aids are used, the patient needs to be taught how to use them. Guidelines for the use of such devices may be found in Sohlberg and Mateer.[108]

Long-Term Memory

1. *Definition.* **Long-term memory** consists of early experiences and information acquired over a period of years. Patients who do not have long-term memory are often described as having amnesia.[45]
2. *Clinical Examples.* Patients who experience long-term memory problems may have difficulty recalling events from many years ago such as a child's birth, or work experiences. Long-term memory problems are common following brain injury and in Alzheimer's disease, but are not commonly seen following stroke.[45]
3. *Lesion Areas.* As described, memory is a complex capacity involving many brain regions. For a detailed discussion, the reader is referred to Fuster[109] and Lezak.[4]
4. *Testing.* The adequacy of memory functions can be determined by having the patient recall personal historical events. The *Rivermead Behavioural Memory Test (RBMT)*[82] can be used to test memory in a standardized way. It is advisable to question the patient's family as to premorbid memory, because many patients in the stroke-prone age group have already begun to experience declining memory as part of the aging process.
5. *Treatment Suggestions.* Treatments for assisting patients overcome long-term memory impairments are similar to those outlined above for immediate recall and short-term memory impairments. Further information on the management of memory impairments may be found in Wilson and Moffat.[110]

Although the literature contains many studies exploring a variety of memory treatments, few of these were designed as randomized controlled trials. A recent Cochrane Review[111] found only one controlled trail in which at least 75 percent of participants had a stroke. The study reviewed was conducted by Doornheim and De Haan,[112] and showed that memory training had no significant effect on memory impairment or subjective memory complaints. The Cochrane reviewers concluded that there is currently insufficient evidence at this time to support or refute the effectiveness of cognitive rehabilitation for memory problems after stroke.

Impairments of Executive Functions

1. *Definition.* As defined by Lezak, "executive functions consist of those capacities that enable a person to engage successfully in independent, purposive, self-serving behavior."[4, p 42] Lezak goes on to describe executive

functions as consisting of four overlapping components: volition, planning, purposive action, and effective performance.

Volition is the capacity to determine what one needs and wants to do. It also encompasses a future realization of one's needs and wants. Volition encompasses goal planning and task initiation, self-awareness, awareness of the environment, and social awareness. *Planning* is ". . . the identification and organization of the steps and elements (e.g., skills, material, other persons) needed to carry out an intention or achieve a goal."[4, p 653] Planning involves weighing alternatives and making choices. *Purposive action* includes productivity and self-regulation, which encompasses the ability to initiate, maintain, switch, and stop complex action sequences in an orderly manner to realize a goal. *Effective performance* is the capacity for quality control, including the ability to self-monitor and self-correct one's behavior. Because ineffective self-monitoring and difficulty with self-correction are the primary features of the performance of persons with problems with effective performance, patients may not even perceive their mistakes, whereas others may identify them but take no action to correct them.[113]

2. *Clinical Examples.* Although some patients with executive function disorders are unable to formulate realistic goals or intentions (volition) or plan, others may be able to formulate goals and initiate goal-directed task performance, but owing to defective planning are not able to realize their goals. Patients with planning problems may say or intend one thing, but do another.[4] Patients who have difficulty with effective performance may not even perceive their mistakes, whereas others may identify them but do not take corrective action. Family and hospital staff may complain of the patient's apparent apathy, poor or unreliable judgment, inappropriate behavior, difficulty adapting to new situations, and/or lack of attention to the needs and feelings of others.[113]
3. *Lesion Area.* Executive functions have traditionally been associated with the frontal and prefrontal cortex,[6] but the current view is that these capacities are mediated by reciprocal connections with other cortical and subcortical regions via the dorsolateral prefrontal–subcortical circuit.[114]
4. *Testing.* Tests of executive functions include the *Behavioural Assessment of the Dysexecutive Syndrome (BADS),*[115] the *Executive Functions Assessment,*[116] and the *Good Samaritan Hospital for Cognitive Rehabilitation's Executive Functions Behavioural Rating Scale.*[117]
5. *Treatment Suggestions.* The combination of impulsiveness, poor judgment, poor planning ability, and lack of foresight, which is particularly problematic in patients with left hemiplegia, does not bode well for independent functioning. The severity of these impairments may diminish somewhat over time.[9] Although some general remedial and adaptive treatment suggestions are described here, for more specific details refer to Ponsford, Sloan, and Snow[104] and Duran and Fisher.[113]
   a. *Remedial Approach.* By providing structure, feedback, and routine, a person's performance can be enhanced (e.g., providing structure by giving the patient steps to follow, assisting the task to become routine by repeated practice, or providing immediate feedback about the patient's behavior and the effect it has on others). The therapist initially acts as the patient's frontal lobes, and gradually transfers these responsibilities to the patient. Unless the patient has some awareness of the problems, a remedial approach will not be particularly successful.[104] Honda[118] recently reported a study with three patients over a 6-month period who were provided with self-instructional training, a problem-solving procedure, and physical-set changing exercises described as moving the four extremities and trunk in time to a metronome. In this study, "Patients were instructed to follow a videotape for 20 minutes. In the tape, a physical therapist moves four extremities and his trunk in time to a metronome. He changes activities every 2 or 3 minutes. The patients were trained with these methods for a total of 6 months. In the self-instructional procedure and problem-solving training phase, psychologists guided and trained patients 1 hour per day twice a week. In the physical set changing exercise phase, patients were advised to practice twice a day watching the instruction video tape. Each training phase lasted 6 weeks."[118, p 18] While two of the subjects revealed improvements on the neuropsychological test used as an outcome measure, all subjects improved in personal and instrumental activities of daily living. Of course, a limitation of this study is the small sample size and lack of control subjects, since it could be expected that these patients would make spontaneous recovery over the 6-month study period.
   b. *Compensatory Approach.* The therapist can assist the patient to compensate for poor abilities by utilizing other intact cognitive functions and/or modifying the environment. For example, the therapist might ask the patient to perform a task in a room with minimal distractions, or change the demands of the patient's work, home, or community to diminish the need to employ executive functions. A beeper or alarm clock may be used to assist a patient overcome poor initiation.

Body Scheme and Body Image Impairments

Body image is defined as a visual and mental image of one's body that includes feelings about one's body, especially in relation to health and disease.[119] The term **body scheme** refers to a postural model of the body, including the relationship of body parts to each other and the relationship of the body to the environment. Body awareness is derived from the integration of tactile, proprioceptive, and interoceptive sensations, in addition to the individual's subjective feelings about the body.[119] An awareness of body scheme is considered one of the essential foundations for the performance of all purposeful motor behavior.[119] According to Van Duesen, body image is "a dynamic synthesis of the body schema and those environmental inputs providing relevant emotional and conceptual components."[119, p 118] The two terms, body image and body scheme, are often used interchangeably; therefore, when researching this topic, close attention should be paid to the particular definition put forth by each individual author. Specific impairments of body image and body scheme are unilateral neglect, somatoagnosia, right–left discrimination, finger agnosia, and anosognosia.

Unilateral Neglect

1. *Definition.* **Unilateral neglect** is the inability to register and integrate stimuli and perceptions from one side of the body (body neglect) and the environment or **hemispace** (spatial neglect of the area surrounding one side of the body), which is not due to a sensory loss. Unilateral neglect is also referred to as unilateral spatial neglect, hemi-inattention, hemineglect, and unilateral visual inattention.[120] It is important for the therapist to be familiar with this disorder because it is a frequent clinical finding. Neglect following right cerebral infarction has been reported in between 12 and 95 percent of patients.[121] The reporting rates vary enormously due to differences in time selected for reporting and techniques used to detect the neglect. Unilateral neglect usually, although not always, affects the left side of the body or hemispace, and for purposes of this discussion, we will assume that it is the left. If a patient has unilateral neglect, he or she seems to ignore the left side of the body and stimuli occurring in the left personal space. This may occur despite intact visual fields, or concomitantly with right or left homonymous hemianopsia; however, it is not caused by homonymous hemianopsia.[122]

When working with a patient who has unilateral neglect, the therapist should also determine which sensory modalities are affected including visual, tactile, and auditory. One or all of these modalities may be neglected. Neglect can also be understood in terms of the area of space that is neglected. For example, unilateral neglect may express itself as a disorder of attention and goal directed behavior in:

- Contralesional personal space (defined as pertaining to the body) such as shaving only the right half of the face, or failing to wash the left side of the body, or
- Contralesional peripersonal space (that area of space within arm distance), for example failing to use objects on the contralesional side of the meal tray, or
- Contralesional extrapersonal space (that area of space beyond arm length) such as failing to negotiate obstacles, doorways and so forth during locomotion.[50,120]

Unilateral neglect is also demonstrated by an impaired ability to attend to either the object or the environment as a whole. It is possible that while some patients may neglect half of the environment, others may neglect half of objects in the total environment. In the first case, the patient may neglect the left side of the entire visual scene (Fig. 29.8). In the second case, a patient may neglect the left side of an object, regardless of its absolute position in the visual display. For example, the patient may neglect the left side of a cup even though it is on his or her right side or omit the left side of objects when drawing items such as a flower, house, or tree as depicted in Figure 29.9.

Frequently, a patient with unilateral neglect has sensory loss on the affected side, which compounds the problem. Although a patient with left-sided hemianopsia has actual loss of vision from the left visual field of both eyes, he or she may be aware of the problem and compensate automatically or learn to compensate by turning the head. A patient with visual neglect has intact vision but seems unaware of the problem and does not attempt to compensate spontaneously by turning the

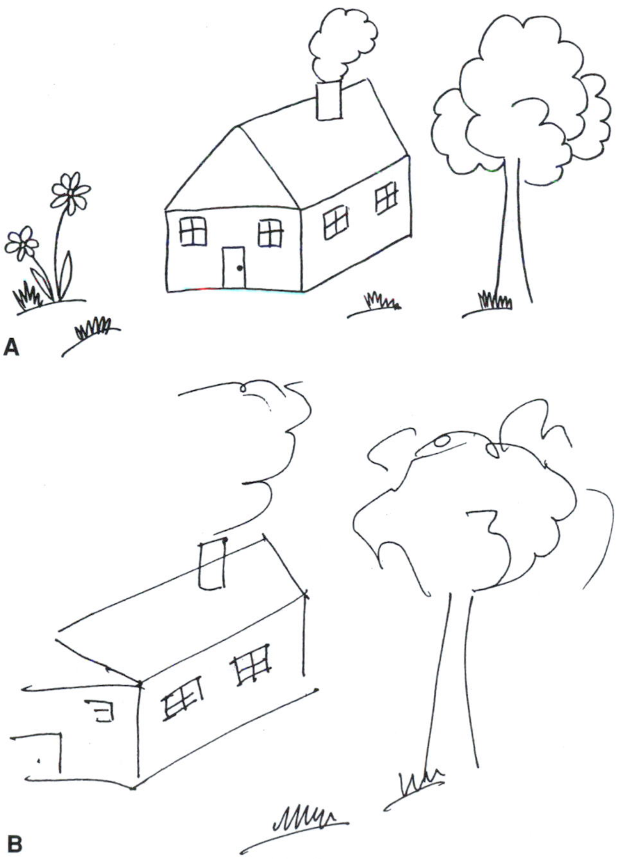

A

B

Figure 29.8 Example of a drawing by a patient with unilateral neglect. Therapist's drawing of a house and yard (A). Impaired copying by a patient with unilateral neglect—environment neglect following a stroke (B). (From Corben and Unsworth,[120] p 360, with permission.)

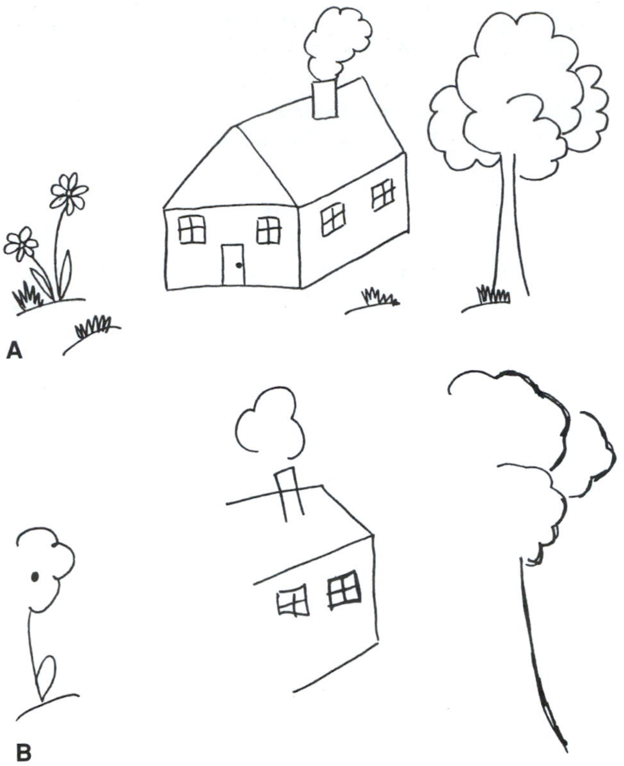

Figure 29.9 Example of a drawing by a patient with unilateral neglect. Therapist's drawing of a house and yard (A). Impaired copying by a patient with unilateral neglect—object neglect following a stroke (B). (From Corben and Unsworth,[120] p 363, with permission.)

head. In extreme cases the patient appears totally indifferent to the left side of the body and environment, and may deny that the left extremities belong to him or her.[123] More time seems to be required to learn to compensate for this impairment than for hemianopsia. There is great difficulty in integrating all stimuli from the left half of the body and personal space for use in ADL skills. As with hemianopsia, the patient with visual unilateral neglect often avoids crossing the midline visually or motorically.[62]

2. *Clinical Examples.* The patient may ignore the left half of the body when dressing and forget to put on the left sleeve or left pants leg. Often a male patient will forget to shave the left half of his face. A woman may neglect to put makeup on the left side of her face.[124] The patient may neglect to eat from the left half of a plate and will start reading a newspaper from the middle of the line. Typically, the patient bumps into objects on the left side or tends to veer toward the right when walking or propelling a wheelchair.
3. *Lesion Area.* It has been suggested that lesions involving the inferior–posterior regions of the right parietal lobe are significant determinants of neglect.[122,125]
4. *Testing.* A variety of techniques are useful. No single test is adequate to identify unilateral neglect in all patients because the impairment may be manifested differently in each patient.
   a. The *Behavioural Inattention Test (BIT)*[78] can be used to examine unilateral neglect (Table 29.1). The patient may also be observed during ADL such as dressing, or an IADL such as preparing a meal. The therapist observes performance, and observes changes in the patient's behavior in response to cueing.
   b. The purpose of therapy is to increase awareness of the left side of the body and space. Current beliefs concerning the mechanisms underlying unilateral neglect guide the majority of treatment approaches. Rizzolatti and Berti[126] combine the popular attentional and representational models in their premotor theory of neglect. The basis of this theory is that spatial attention is dependent on several independent neural circuits. Attention, and therefore perception of stimuli, is enhanced as a direct result of activation of motor circuits, as occurs when a person moves. Hence, activating motor circuits of the ipsilesional hemisphere (via voluntary movements of the left upper or lower limbs) may facilitate associated sensory circuits. Such movement may in turn lead to improvements in the processing of stimuli from the contralesional (left) side.[120]
5. *Treatment Suggestions.*
   a. *Remedial Approach.* Capitalizing on the rationale of the premotor theory of neglect, the following suggestions are proposed. Stimuli that are specialized for the right side of the brain, such as shapes and blocks, should be used to enhance right brain activation. At the same time, the presence of stimuli that are known to activate the left side of the brain, such as letters and numbers, should be minimized. Use of verbal instructions should be minimized. Simple verbal instructions should be used to encourage the patient to turn the head to the left to anchor his or her attention to that side of space.[123] In addition, research suggests that conducting motor activities with the left body side, such as simply clenching and unclenching the fist, can improve attention to the left body side and hemispace. Robertson et al[127] conducted a study with six individuals with hemiplegia who were asked to walk through a doorway. Each of the subject's walking trajectory (pathway) was measured, and it was found that all trajectories were significantly deviated to the right of center. The subjects were then asked to clench and unclench their left hands prior to, and during, walking through the doorway. The researchers found that this procedure significantly assisted subjects to center their walking trajectories. Other techniques that have been used to treat patients with unilateral neglect include eye-patching and prism glasses. These techniques are not common in therapy and a review of their effectiveness is included in Evidence Summary Box 29.1.
   b. *Compensatory Approach.* The patient is initially educated about the condition, and then strategies to assist

Evidence Summary Box 29.1

Evidence Addressing the Use of Cognitive Rehabilitation Techniques to Increase Activity in Patients with Unilateral Neglect Following Stroke[129]

Reference	Subjects	Design/ Intervention	Duration	Results	Comments
Fanthome et al[130] 1995	Patients with recent RH stroke E = 9; C = 9 Gender (M/F): E = 6/3 C = 6/3 Time post-onset (months): E = 1.0; C = 0.6 IC: <80 years age, no history of dementia or psychiatric problems, not unwell, right-handed, score > 6 on Abbreviated Mental Test, score <130 on BIT	RCT Blinded examiner E: Ss wear specially modified glasses which provide a reminder beep if patient fails to move eyes to the left in a 15-second interval C: No treatment for visual inattention	4 weeks E = Treatment 2 hours 40 minutes per week C = No treatment	After the 4 weeks, no significant difference between groups in either eye movements or BIT scores	E and C groups appeared adequately matched on demographic and clinical data although control group slightly older than experimental; no baseline BIT data
Kalra et al[131] 1997	Patients 2–14 days post-stroke with VN E = 24; C = 23 Mean age (SD): E = 78 (9); C = 76 (10) Median time post-onset: 6 days (2–14 range) EC: TIAs, reversible neurological deficits, hemianopsia or severe dysphasia	RCT (blinded examiner) E = Spatiomotor cueing based on *attentional–motor integration* model; early emphasis on restoration of function; C = Conventional therapy focusing on restoration of tone, movement pattern, and motor activity before addressing skilled functional activity	12 weeks Initial baseline measures and following the 12 weeks; mean therapy time = 47.7 hours	6 types of outcome data collected: (1) mortality; (2) BI; (3) discharge destination; (4) length of hospital stay; (5) duration of therapy input; and (6) RPAB (cancellation subtest and discharge home) Patients with VN have similar discharge destination despite lower BI scores (compared to patients without VN); spatiomotor cueing improves ($p < .05$) outcome in patients with VN	Principle behind approach: Movements of affected limb in the deficit hemispace led to summation of activation of affected receptive fields of 2 distinct but linked spatial systems for personal and extrapersonal space; this resulted in improvements in attentional skills and appreciation of spatial relationships on the affected side
Robertson et al[132] 1990	30 patients with left visual field neglect on BIT; E = 17; C = 13 Mean age: E = 64.2(12.6); C = 63.1 (9.6) Gender (M/F) E = 9/11; C = 10/6; Onset of neglect in weeks: E = 19.2 (21.1); C = 10.8 (6.3) IC: presence of neglect (failure on at least 3/9 behavioral tests); oriented to time and place;	RCT Random blinded allocation of patients to conditions with blocks of severe versus mild neglect patients; E = computerized scanning and attentional training (intensive briefing about nature of subjects problems, feedback on L and R latencies, trainer reinforcement and encouragement)	7 weeks E = 15.5 hours (14 sessions of 75 minutes each; 2 per week) C = 11.4 hours of recreational computing	6 types of outcome data collected: (1) BIT (principal outcome measure); (2) WAIS-R subtests (Picture Completion and Block Design); (3) Neale Reading Test; (4) Letter cancellation; (5) Observer's report of neglect; and (6) ReyCFT (copy only); blind follow-up at the end of training and 6 months after revealed no statistically	Findings suggest this type of computerized training may not be useful on a routine basis; further study is warranted to establish the type, frequency, and duration of training that could produce clinically significant changes in unilateral visual neglect

(*continued*)

Evidence Summary Box 29.1

Evidence Addressing the Use of Cognitive Rehabilitation Techniques to Increase Activity in Patients with Unilateral Neglect Following Stroke[129] (continued)

Reference	Subjects	Design/ Intervention	Duration	Results	Comments
	ability to consent; ability to concentrate sufficiently to sit at computer-based task for 15 minutes	C = recreational computing (such as games, quizzes and simple logical games)		or clinically significant results between groups	
Rossi et al[133] 1990	39 patients following stroke with HHA or VN E = 18; C = 21 Mean age: E = 72.6; C= 63.3; Gender (M/F): E = 10/8; C = 9/12; Mean weeks post-stroke: E = 4.4; C = 4.7; Side of stroke (R/L): E = 16/2; C = 13/8; IC: Presence of HHA or VN (HHA/VN): E = 12/6 C = 15/6; EC: best-corrected visual acuity less than 20/200; inability to comprehend and cooperate with testing	RCT E = 15 diopter plastic press-on Fresnel prisms (to fit on inside of spectacle lenses for all daytime activities); C = no prism treatment; Eight types of outcomes data collected: (1) Modified MMSE; (2) MVPT; (3) Line Bisection; (4) Line Cancellation; (5) HFVS; (6) Tangent Screen Examination (7) BI; and (8) Frequency of falls	4 weeks; outcomes examined at baseline, 2 weeks, and 4 weeks	Prism-treated group performed significantly better than controls on the following: (1) MVPT; (2) Line Bisection Task; (3) Line Cancellation Task; (4) HFVS; and (5) Tangent Screen Examination; there was no significant difference in BI scores at 4 weeks	C group younger but otherwise groups were similar on demographic and clinical background factors including BI; while treatment using the prisms improves visual perception test scores, it does not seem to lead to improvements in ADL function in patients with stroke with HHA or unilateral VN, thus limiting its use
Wiart et al[134] 1997	22 patients post-stroke with severe left lateral neglect (positive findings for neglect on 3 tests); E = 11; C = 11; Mean age: E = 66; C = 72; Gender (M/F): E 6/5, C 6/5; Time post-onset (mean days): E = 35; C = 30; EC: history of stroke; alteration of general status; cognitive difficulties incompatible with rehabilitation	RCT E = experimental treatment is Bon Saint Come (one of the author's) method; thoracolumbar vest worn with attached metal pointer above head; patient points to target on mobile panel; audible and luminous signals provide biofeedback when targets are touched; therapist participates actively during the session, stimulating, guiding, and correcting; C = 3–4 hours traditional rehabilitation per day	E = 1 hour/day (20 days) of experimental treatment followed by traditional rehabilitation (physical therapy for 1–2 hours and 1 hour of occupational therapy) C = 3–4 hours traditional rehabilitation per day	Two types of outcome data collected: (1) quantitative scoring of neglect (line bisection, line cancellation, bell cancellation); (2) autonomy (FIM); Data collected: day 0, day 30 (after therapy) and day 60. All quantitative and FIM scores improved significantly more in the E group than in the C group	E group was younger and had a higher initial FIM score (66) than the C group (54); C group had more, but not significantly so, omissions on line cancellation (C = 16; E = 14) and right deviations on line bisection (C = 53%; E = 50%) at baseline compared with E group; the Bon Saint Come method shows promise and should be further tested.

BI = Barthel Index; BIT = Behavioural Inattention Test; C = control group; E = experimental group; EC = exclusion criteria; FIM = Functional Independence Measure; HFVS = Harrington Flocks Visual Field Screener; HHA = homonymous hemianopia; IC = inclusion criteria; MMSE = Mini-Mental Status Examination; MVPT = Motor-Free Visual Perceptual Test; RCT = randomized controlled trial; ReyCFT = Rey Complex Figure Test; RH = right hemisphere; RPAB = Rivermead Perceptual Assessment Battery; S, Ss = subject, subjects; TIA = transient ischemic attack; UK = United Kingdom; VN = visual neglect; WAIS-R = Wechsler Adult Intelligence Scale-Revised.

managing everyday activities are devised. For example, when reading a book or newspaper, a red ribbon may be placed on the left margin and the patient is taught to scan back to this point after completing each line. The environment may also be adapted within this approach. The patient is addressed and given demonstrations from the unaffected side. The nursing staff should place the patient's call button, telephone, and other essential items on the unaffected side. A bold red line may be drawn on the side of the page that is neglected.[119] A mirror may be placed in front of the patient while he or she is dressing or ambulating to draw attention to the neglected side.

c. Several Cochrane Reviews have been conducted concerning the effectiveness of cognitive and perceptual rehabilitation. An overview of findings from small Cochrane Reviews in the areas of attention and memory rehabilitation were presented earlier. A more extensive Cochrane Review[129] was conducted concerning the effectiveness of therapy for unilateral neglect as there has been an abundance of studies and trials conducted on this puzzling disorder over the past 20 years. Evidence Summary Box 29.1 contains a summary of selected controlled trails included in the Cochrane Review.[129] Cochrane Reviews only include controlled trails and each trial is rated (A, B, or C) on the quality of its randomization process. "A" studies are considered adequate, "B" unclear, and "C" inadequate. Of the 15 studies included in the Cochrane review, The Evidence Summary Box contains all the studies with an A classification (Fanthome et al,[130] Kalra et al,[131] and Robertson et al[132]) and two randomly selected studies rated as B (Rossi et al[133] and Wiart et al[134]). As a result of conducting this review, Bowen, Lincoln, and Dewey[129] concluded that there is some evidence that cognitive rehabilitation for patients with unilateral neglect improves performance on some impairment-based tests. However, the effects of cognitive rehabilitation on reducing activity limitations are unclear. Additional well-designed randomized controlled trials (RCTs) and more basic research are required to develop outcome measures in the field.

Anosognosia

1. *Definition.* **Anosognosia** is a severe condition including denial and lack of awareness of the presence or severity of one's paralysis.[50] Anosognosia is defined as a lack of awareness, or denial, of a paretic extremity as belonging to the person, or a lack of insight concerning, or denial of, paralysis.[50] Presence of this disability may compromise rehabilitation potential greatly, because it limits the patient's ability to recognize the need for, and thus to use, compensatory techniques.
2. *Clinical Examples.* Typically, the patient maintains that there is nothing wrong and may disown the paralyzed limbs and refuse to accept responsibility for them. The patient may claim that the limb has a mind of its own or that it was left at home, or in a closet.
3. *Lesion Area.* The pathogenesis of anosognosia remains unclear,[50] although the region of the supramarginal gyrus has been proposed.[59]
4. *Testing.* Anosognosia is identified by talking to the patient. The patient is asked what happened to the arm or leg, whether he or she is paralyzed, how the limb feels, and why it cannot be moved. A patient with anosognosia may deny the paralysis, say that it is of no concern, and fabricate reasons why a limb does not move the way it should.
5. *Treatment Suggestions.* Anosognosia often resolves spontaneously in the first 3 months following stroke.[135] Maeshima et al[135] also noted that until the condition resolves, it seriously hampers rehabilitation. If the condition persists long term, is extremely difficult to compensate for. Safety is of paramount importance in the treatment and discharge planning for patients suffering from anosognosia, because they typically do not acknowledge their disability and will therefore refuse to be careful.[9]

Somatoagnosia

1. *Definition.* **Somatoagnosia**, or impairment in body scheme, is a lack of awareness of the body structure and the relationship of body parts to oneself or to others. Somatoagnosia is also referred to as *autopagnosia* or simply *body agnosia.*[136] Patients with this deficit may display difficulty following instructions that require distinguishing body parts and may be unable to imitate movements of the therapist.[68] Often patients report that the affected arm or leg feels unduly heavy. Lack of proprioception may underlie or compound this disorder.[137]
2. *Clinical Examples.* The patient may have difficulty performing transfer activities because he or she does not perceive the meaning of terms related to body parts; for example, "Pivot on your leg and reach for the armrest with your hand." In addition, a patient with a body scheme disorder will have difficulty dressing. Patients may have a hard time participating in exercises that require some body parts to be moved in relation to other body parts; for example, "Bring your arm across your chest and touch your shoulder."
3. *Lesion Area.* The lesion site is often the dominant parietal lobe.[59] Therefore, this disorder is seen primarily with right hemiplegia. However, impairment in body scheme may also occur with left hemiplegia.
4. *Testing.*
   a. The patient is requested to point to body parts named by the therapist, on him- or herself, on the therapist, and on a picture or puzzle of a human figure. Zoltan[2] provides details of these testing procedures. An example of verbal directives from these tests is, "Show me your feet. Show me your chin. Point to your back." The words "right" and "left" should not be used because they may lead to an inaccurate diagnosis in patients who

have difficulty with right–left discrimination. Aphasia should be ruled out as a cause of poor performance.

b. The patient is asked to imitate movements of the therapist. For example, the therapist touches his or her cheek, arm, leg, and so forth. A mirror-image response is acceptable.[2]

c. The patient is requested to answer questions about the relationship of body parts. For example, "Are your knees below your head? Which is on top of your head, your hair or your feet?" For patients with aphasia, questions should be phrased to require a yes or no, or true or false response. Patients with intact function in this area should respond correctly most of the time and within a reasonable period of time. Those patients with receptive aphasia are particularly likely to do poorly on tests for somatagnosia.[136]

5. *Treatment Suggestions.* Using a remedial approach, the therapist aims for the patient to associate sensory input with an adaptive motor response.[2] Facilitation of body awareness is accomplished through sensory stimulation to the body part affected. For example, the patient is asked to rub the appropriate body part with a rough cloth as the therapist names it or points to it.[22] Alternatively, the patient verbally identifies body parts, or points to pictures of them as the therapist touches them.

Right–Left Discrimination

1. *Definition.* A **right–left discrimination disorder** is the inability to identify the right and left sides of one's own body or of that of the examiner.[122] This includes the inability to execute movements in response to verbal commands that include the terms "right" and "left." Patients are often unable to imitate movements.[122]
2. *Clinical Examples.* The patient cannot tell the therapist which is the right arm and which is the left. The right shoe cannot be discerned from the left shoe, and the patient is unable to follow instructions using the concept of right–left, such as "turn right at the corner." The patient cannot distinguish the right from the left side of the therapist.
3. *Lesion Area.* The lesion site is the parietal lobe of either hemisphere.[122] A close relationship between aphasia (usually owing to left hemisphere damage) and deficits in right–left discrimination has been reported. In patients without aphasia (usually those with right hemisphere damage), a relationship has been reported between general mental impairment and right–left discrimination disorder.[136]
4. *Testing.* The patient is asked to point to body parts on command, such as: right ear, left foot, right arm, and so forth. Six responses should be elicited on the patient's own body, on that of the therapist, and on a model or picture of the human body.[136] To rule out somatoagnosia, the patient should be tested first without using the words "right" and "left."
5. *Treatment Suggestions.* If using a compensatory approach, when giving instructions to the patient, the words "right" and "left" should be avoided. Instead, pointing or providing cues using distinguishing features of the limb may be more effective (e.g., "the arm with the watch"). These guidelines are particularly salient for the therapist teaching locomotion or transfers, where confusing instructions may have dangerous consequences. The right side of all common objects such as shoes and clothing should be marked with red tape or seam binding.

Finger Agnosia

1. *Definition.* **Finger agnosia** can be defined as the inability to identify the fingers of one's own hands or of the hands of the examiner.[122]
2. *Clinical Examples.* The disorder is characterized by difficulty in naming the fingers on command, identifying which finger was touched, and, by some definitions, mimicking finger movements. This deficit usually occurs bilaterally and is more common in the middle three fingers.[138] Finger agnosia correlates highly with poor dexterity in tasks that require movements of individual fingers in relation to each other,[1] such as buttoning, tying laces, and typing.
3. *Lesion Area.* Finger agnosia may be the result of a lesion located in either parietal lobe,[139] often in the region of the angular gyrus of the left hemisphere. It is often found in conjunction with an aphasic disorder,[136] or with general mental impairment.[122,136] Bilateral finger agnosia along with right–left discrimination problems, **agraphia**, and *acalculia* is termed *Gerstmann's syndrome.*[122] Gerstmann's syndrome usually is associated with a focal lesion of the dominant hemisphere in the region of the angular gyrus.[59]
4. *Testing.* A portion of *Sauguet's test*[2,136] is recommended. Sauguet's test includes asking the patient to move or point to his or her finger when named by the therapist to determine if finger agnosia is present. Between five and ten commands from the therapist is adequate. The test is not standardized.
   a. The patient is asked to name the fingers touched by the therapist, with the eyes open (five times) and if successful, with vision occluded (five times).
   b. The patient is asked to point to the fingers named by the therapist on the patient's own hands (10 times), on the therapist's hands (10 times), and on a schematic model (10 times).
   c. The patient is asked to point to the equivalent finger on a life-sized picture when each finger is touched by the therapist.
   d. The patient is asked to imitate finger movements; for example, curl the index finger, touch the thumb to the middle finger.
5. *Treatment Suggestions.* There is very limited evidence to support treatment techniques for patients with finger

agnosia. When using a remedial approach, the patient's discriminative tactile systems (touch and pressure) are stimulated. A rough cloth can be used to rub the dorsal surface of the affected arm, hand, and fingers, and the ventral surface of the affected fingers. Pressure can be applied to the ventral surface of the hand. For additional details the reader is referred to Zoltan.[2]

Spatial Relations Disorders (Complex Perception)

Spatial relations disorders encompass a constellation of impairments that have in common a difficulty in perceiving the relationship between the self and two or more objects.[140] Research suggests that the right parietal lobe plays a primary role in space perception. Thus, a spatial relations impairment most frequently occurs in patients with right-sided lesions with resulting left hemiparesis.[140]

Spatial relations disorders include impairments of figure–ground discrimination, form discrimination, spatial relations, position in space, and topographical disorientation. Additional visuospatial impairments, such as depth and distance perception and vertical disorientation will also be discussed in this section. In a study comparing the effectiveness of the cognitive remediation (sometimes referred to as the *transfer of training technique*) versus the functional approach, Edmans, Webster, and Lincoln[141] found that both approaches were equally successful in treating perceptual impairments. However, since this study did not control for the effects of spontaneous recovery in both groups, further research is required.

Figure–Ground Discrimination

1. *Definition.* An impairment in visual figure–ground discrimination is the inability to visually distinguish a figure from the background in which it is embedded.[5] Functionally, it interferes with the patient's ability to locate important objects that are not prominent in a visual array. The patient has difficulty ignoring irrelevant visual stimuli and cannot select the appropriate cue to which to respond.[5] This may lead to distractibility, resulting in a shortened attention span,[142] frustration, and decreased independent and safe functioning.[68]
2. *Clinical Examples.* The patient cannot locate items in a pocketbook or drawer, locate buttons on a shirt, or distinguish the armhole from the remainder of a solid-colored shirt. The patient may not be able to tell when one step ends and another begins on a flight of stairs, especially when descending.
3. *Lesion Area.* Parieto-occipital lesions of the right hemisphere and less frequently the left hemisphere commonly produce this disorder.[143]
4. *Testing.*
   a. The *Ayres Figure–Ground Test* (subtest of the *Southern California Sensory Integration Tests*)[144] requires the subject to distinguish the three objects in an embedded test picture, from a possible selection of six items (Fig. 29.10). This test was standardized on children but may be useful as a clinical tool in identifying perceptual disorders in adults with brain damage.[4] Normative data have been generated for normal adult males.[145]
   b. *Functional Tests.* A white towel can be placed on a white sheet, and the patient is asked to find the towel. The patient can be asked to point out the sleeve, buttons, and collar of a white shirt, or to pick out a spoon from an unsorted array of eating utensils. It is necessary to rule out poor eyesight, hemianopsia, visual agnosia, and poor comprehension to improve the validity of these testing techniques.
5. *Treatment Suggestions.*
   a. *Remedial Approach.* The therapist should arrange for practice in visually locating objects in a simple array (such as three very different objects), and progress to more difficult ones (four or five dissimilar objects and three similar ones).
   b. *Compensatory Approach.* The patient is taught to become aware of the existence and nature of the deficit. The patient should be cautioned to examine groups of objects slowly and systematically and should be instructed to use other, intact senses (e.g., touch) when searching for items such as clothing or silverware. When learning to lock a wheelchair, the patient should be advised to locate the brake levers by touch rather than by searching for them visually. Red tape may be placed over the Velcro strap of the shoe

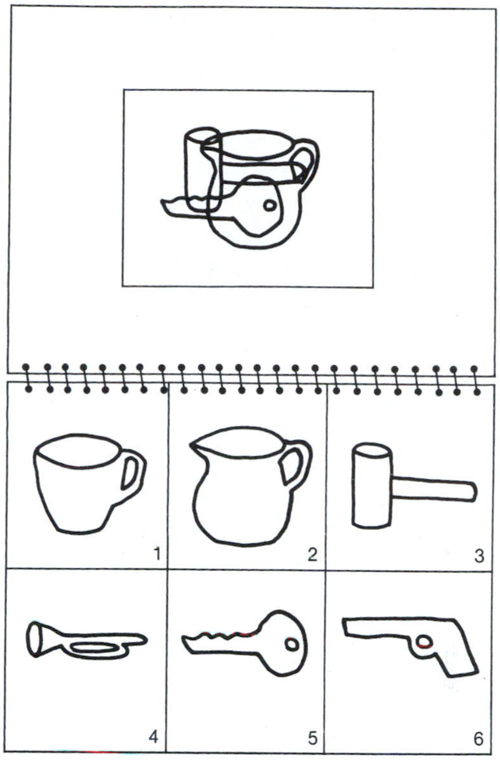

Figure 29.10 An example of the figure–ground perception test. (From Ayres,[144] Plate 2A, with permission.)

or orthosis to aid the patient in locating it. Few items should be placed in the patient's drawers or nightstand, and they should be replaced in the same location each time. Brightly colored tape can be used to mark the edges on stairs. Repetition is a key element of this approach and repeated practice is used in each specific area of difficulty. The same procedure should be employed during each practice session, incorporating verbal cues and touch as adjuncts to vision.

Form Discrimination

1. *Definition.* Impairment in **form discrimination** is the inability to perceive or attend to subtle differences in form and shape. The patient is likely to confuse objects of similar shape or not to recognize an object placed in an unusual position.
2. *Clinical Examples.* The patient may confuse a pen with a toothbrush, a vase with a water pitcher, a cane with a crutch, and so forth.
3. *Lesion Area.* The lesion site is the parieto-temporo-occipital region (posterior association areas) of the nondominant lobe.[4]
4. *Testing.* A number of items similar in shape and different in size are gathered. The patient is asked to identify them. One set of items might be a pencil, pen, straw, toothbrush, watch, and the other might be a key, paper clip, coins, and a ring. Each object is presented several times in different positions (e.g., upside down). Visual object agnosia must be ruled out as a cause for poor performance by first presenting objects separately and asking the patient to identify them or to demonstrate how they are used.
5. *Treatment Suggestions.*
   a. *Remedial Approach.* The patient should practice describing, identifying, and demonstrating the use of similarly shaped and sized objects. The patient should sort like objects and should be assisted to focus on differentiating cues.
   b. *Compensatory Approach.* The patient must be made aware of the specific deficit. If the patient can read, frequently used and confused objects can be labeled. The patient should be encouraged to use vision, touch, and self-verbalization in combination when objects are confused.

Spatial Relations

1. *Definition.* A **spatial relations disorder**, or spatial disorientation, is the inability to perceive the relationship of one object in space to another object, or to oneself. This may lead to, or compound, problems in constructional tasks and dressing.[5] Crossing the midline may be a problem for patients with spatial relations deficits.[140] Spatial relations skills are required to manage most activities of daily living.
2. *Clinical Examples.* The patient might find it difficult to place the cutlery, plate, and spoon in the proper position when setting the table. The patient may be unable to tell the time from a clock because of difficulty in perceiving the relative positions of the hands.[2,29] The patient may have difficulty learning to position his or her arms, legs, and trunk in relation to the wheelchair to prepare for transferring.
3. *Lesion Area.* The lesion site is predominantly the inferior parietal lobe or parieto-occipital-temporal junction, usually of the right side.[5] Arnadottir [140] explains how a patient with perceptual deficits may have difficulty putting on a shirt. This is illustrated in Figure 29.11. Since the CNS works in a holistic way, the task of putting on a shirt requires visual, tactile, and auditory information as well as attentional and memory capacities and motor output. Figure 29.11 suggests that while damage in a variety of brain areas may affect visuospatial processing, the most common lesion site is the right inferior parietal lobe.
4. *Testing.* Recommended tests include the *Rivermead Perceptual Assessment Battery (RPAB)*[80] and the *Arnadottir OT-ADL Neurobehavioural Evaluation (A-ONE)*.[5] To improve the validity of these tests, unilateral neglect and hemianopsia should be ruled out as the causes of poor performance. If these impairments are present, the stimulus array should be positioned appropriately.
5. *Treatment Suggestions.* When using a remedial approach, patient ability to orient to other objects can be improved by giving the patient instructions to position himself or herself in relation to the therapist or another object. The therapist might say, "Sit next to me," "Go behind the table," *or* "Step over the line." In addition, the therapist can set up a maze of furniture. Having the patient copy block or matchstick designs of increasing difficulty will increase awareness of the relationship between one object (block or matchstick) and the next. If the patient avoids crossing the midline, activities that require crossing the midline both motorically and visually can be incorporated into other therapeutic activities. One specific activity is to have the patient hold a dowel with both hands. The therapist guides it from the uninvolved side to the involved side. Later, the patient can progress to manipulating the dowel with only verbal or visual cues, and finally to guiding it independently.[146]

Position in Space

1. *Definition.* **Position in space impairment** is the inability to perceive and to interpret spatial concepts such as up, down, under, over, in, out, in front of, and behind.
2. *Clinical Examples.* If a patient is asked to raise the arm "above" the head during ROM activities or is asked to place the feet "on" the footrests, the patient may behave as if he or she does not know what to do.
3. *Lesion Area.* The lesion is usually located in the nondominant parietal lobe.[143]

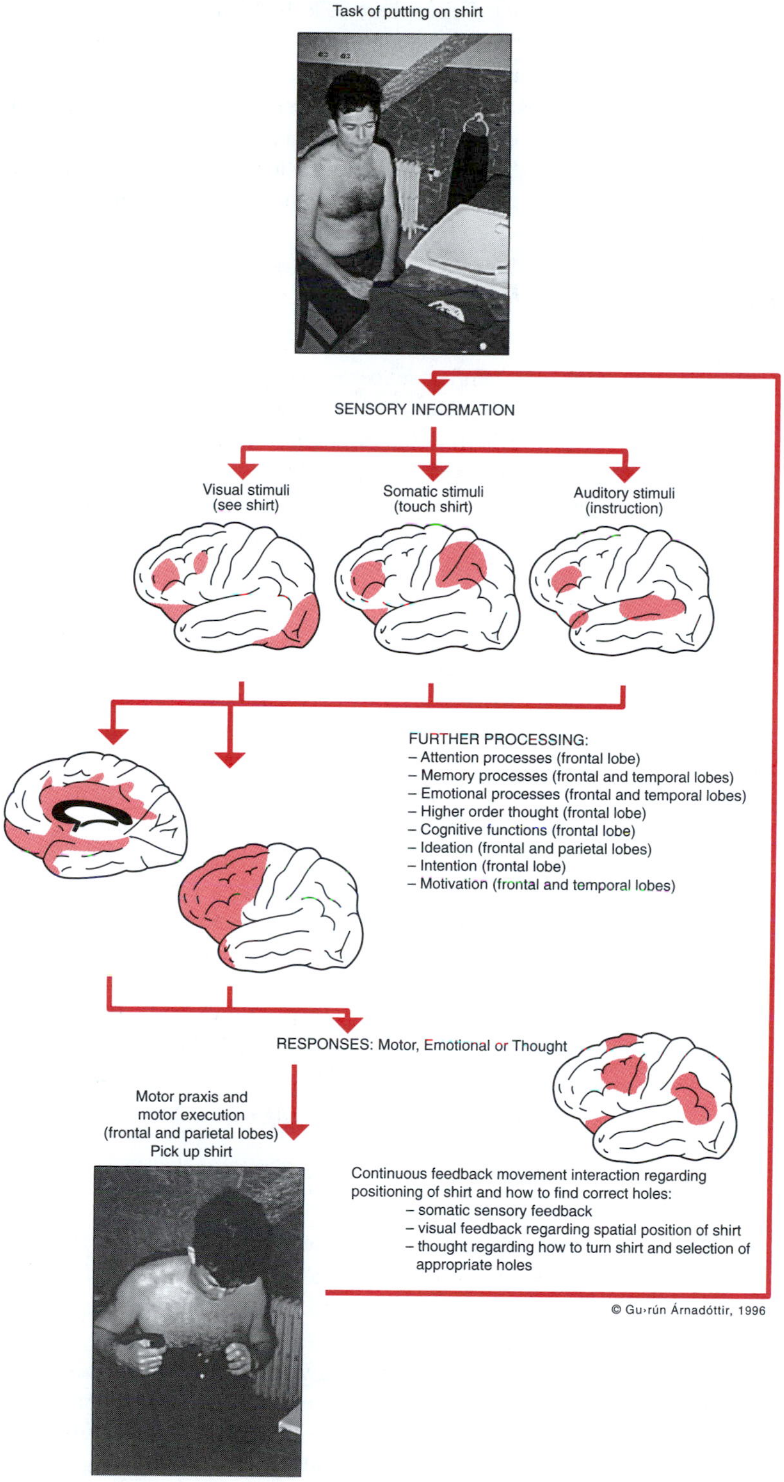

Figure 29.11 Spatial relation processing as a man puts on a shirt. (From Arnadottir,[140] p 405, with permission.)

4. *Testing.* To test function, two objects are used, such as a shoe and a shoebox. The patient is asked to place the shoe in different positions in relation to the shoebox; for example, in the box, on top of the box, or next to the box. Alternatively, the patient is presented with two objects and asked to describe their relationship. For example, a toothbrush can be placed in a cup, under a cup, and so forth, and the patient is then asked to indicate the location of the toothbrush.

Another mode of testing is to have the patient copy the therapist's manipulations with an identical set of objects. For example, the therapist hands the patient a comb and a brush. The therapist then takes an identical set and places them in a particular relationship to each other, such as the comb on top of the brush. The patient is requested to arrange his or her comb and brush in the same way. Success in this task may represent sufficient ability to use position in space functionally.

Figure–ground difficulty, apraxia, incoordination, and lack of comprehension should be ruled out when performing these tests. Objects should be positioned to avoid compounding of results with hemianopsia and unilateral spatial neglect.

5. *Treatment Suggestions.* If using a retraining approach, three or four identical objects are placed in the same orientation (wrist weights, combs, mugs, and so forth). An additional object is placed in a different orientation. The patient is asked to identify the odd one, and then to place it in the same orientation as the other objects.

Topographic Disorientation

1. *Definition.* Topographic disorientation refers to difficulty in understanding and remembering the relationship of one location to another.[147] As a result, the patient is unable to get from one place to another, with or without a map. This disorder is frequently seen in conjunction with other difficulties in spatial relations.[45]
2. *Clinical Examples.* The patient cannot find the way from his or her room to the physical therapy clinic, despite being shown repeatedly. The patient cannot describe the spatial characteristics of familiar surroundings, such as the layout of his or her bedroom at home.[143]
3. *Lesion Areas.* The majority of cases involve damage to the right retrosplenial cortex, with Brodmann's area 30 compromised in most patients.[147] Bilateral parietal lesions, and more rarely, left-side parietal lesions, can produce this problem.[143]
4. *Testing.* The patient is asked to describe or to draw a familiar route, such as the block on which he or she lives, the layout of his or her house, or a major neighborhood intersection.[137] An impaired patient will be unable to succeed in this task. However, the therapist must differentiate between memory problems and topographical orientation difficulties.
5. *Treatment Suggestions.* This deficit usually resolves 8 weeks post-onset.[147] However, several treatment techniques can be used to hasten recovery, or to assist long term if the condition persists.
   a. *Remedial Approach.* The patient practices going from one place to another, following verbal instructions. Initially, simple routes should be used, and then more complicated ones.[2]
   b. *Compensatory Approach.* Frequently traveled routes can be marked with colored dots. The spaces between the dots are gradually increased and eventually eliminated as improvement takes place.[2] This is an example of taking a normally right-hemisphere task and (because there is right-sided damage) converting it into a left-hemisphere task. In this instance we take the spatial task of remembering routes (right-hemisphere task) and substitute sequential landmarks (sequencing is typically a left-hemisphere strength) to accomplish the goal of getting from place to place. The patient should be reminded not to leave the clinic, room, or home unattended, because he or she may get lost.

Depth and Distance Perception

1. *Definition.* The patient with a disorder of depth and distance perception experiences inaccurate judgment of direction, distance, and depth. Spatial disorientation may be a contributing factor in faulty distance perception.
2. *Clinical Examples.* The patient may have difficulty navigating stairs, may miss the chair when attempting to sit, or may continue pouring juice once a glass is filled.[142]
3. *Lesion Areas.* This impairment may occur with a lesion in the posterior right hemisphere in the superior visual association cortices; may be evident with right-sided or bilateral lesions.[143]
4. *Testing.*
   a. For a functional test of distance perception, the patient is asked to take or to grasp an object that has been placed on a table. The object may also be held in front of the patient, in the air, and the patient is again asked to grasp it. The impaired patient will overshoot or undershoot.[2]
   b. To determine depth perception functionally, the patient can be asked to fill a glass of water.[2] A patient with a depth perception deficit may continue pouring once the glass is filled.
5. *Treatment Suggestions.* The patient should be assisted in becoming aware of the deficit (education to increase cognitive awareness). Emphasis should be placed on the importance of walking carefully on uneven surfaces, particularly the stairs.
   a. *Remedial Approach.* The patient is requested to place the feet on designated spots during gait training.[55] Also, blocks can be arranged in piles 2 to 8 in. high. The patient is asked to touch the top of the piles with the foot. This is done to reestablish a sense of depth and distance.[146]
   b. *Compensatory Approach.* Practice in compensating for disturbances in depth and distance perception occurs intrinsically in many ADL skills, both those involving moving through space and those that involve manipulation.

Vertical Disorientation

1. *Definition.* **Vertical disorientation** refers to a distorted perception of what is vertical. Displacement of the vertical position can contribute to disturbance of motor performance, both in posture and in gait. Early in recovery most patients post-CVA demonstrate some impairment in the sense of verticality.[148] This is not influenced by the

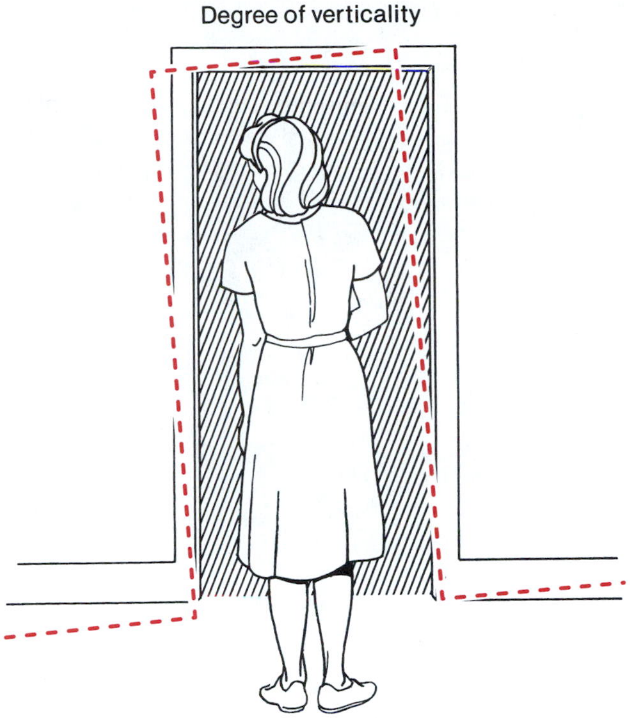

Figure 29.12 Vertical disorientation may contribute to disturbances of posture and gait. (From Tobis and Lowenthal,[60] p 37, with permission.)

presence of homonymous hemianopsia.[68] Scores on one test for visual perception of the vertical position were found to correlate with differences in walking ability.[68]

2. *Clinical Examples.* An example of the way in which a person with distorted verticality views the world and the way this may affect posture is depicted in Figure 29.12.
3. *Lesion Area.* The lesion site is in the nondominant parietal lobe.
4. *Testing.* The therapist holds a cane vertically and then turns it sideways to a horizontal plane. Researchers use a luminous rod with patients seated in a darkened room.[148] The patient is handed the cane and asked to turn it back to the original position. If the patient's perception of the vertical position is distorted, the cane will most likely be placed at an angle, representing the patient's conception of the world around him- or herself.
5. *Treatment Suggestions.* The patient must be made aware of the deficit. The patient should be instructed to compensate by using touch for proper self-orientation, especially when going through doorways, in and out of elevators, and on the stairs.

Agnosias (Simple Perception)

Agnosia is the inability to recognize or make sense of incoming information despite intact sensory capacities. Although this condition is relatively rare, it can affect any sensory modality (e.g., vision, audition, touch, taste) and anything (e.g., faces, sounds, colors, familiar or less familiar objects). Although there is an inability to recognize familiar objects using one or two of the sensory modalities, the ability to recognize the same object using other sensory modalities is usually present.[59,149]

Visual Agnosias

1. *Definitions* and 2. *Clinical Examples.* **Visual object agnosia** is the most common form of agnosia.[4] It is defined as the inability to recognize familiar objects despite normal function of the eyes and optic tracts.[149] One remarkable aspect of this disorder is the readiness with which the patient can identify an object once it is handled (i.e., information is received from another sensory modality).[150] The patient may not recognize people, possessions, and common objects. Specific types of visual agnosia and some clinical presentations are described below.

   Simultanagnosia, also known as Balint's syndrome,[4] is the inability to perceive a visual stimulus as a whole. The patient perceives an entire array one part at a time. The lesion is usually in the dominant occipital lobe.

   Prosopagnosia was traditionally considered to be the inability to recognize familiar faces. This phenomenon is now thought to be related to any visually ambiguous stimulus, the recognition of which depends on evoking a memory context, such as different species of birds or different makes of cars. Prosopagnosia is usually accompanied by visual field impairments. Bilaterally symmetric occipital lesions are thought to be responsible for this impairment.[50,151]

   Color agnosia is the inability to recognize colors; it is not color blindness. The patient is unable to identify or name colors on command, although color chips can be correctly paired.[50] However, the meaning of color is lost so that the patient no longer associates a duckling as yellow or the sea as blue.[149] Color agnosia is frequently associated with facial or other visual object agnosias.[4,143] It is usually the result of a dominant hemisphere lesion.[4] The simultaneous occurrence of left-sided hemianopsia, alexia, and color agnosia is a classic occipital lobe syndrome.[4]
3. *Lesion Area.* The lesions associated with visual object agnosias are thought to occur in the occipito-temporo-parietal association areas of either hemisphere. These areas are responsible for the integration of visual stimuli with respect to memory.[59]
4. *Testing.* To test for this deficit, several common objects are placed in front of the patient. The patient is asked to name the objects, to point to an object named by the therapist, or to demonstrate its use. It is important to rule out aphasia and apraxia, although this is not easily done. Details of other nonstandardized and standardized testing procedures are provided in Laver and Unsworth.[149]

5. *Treatment Suggestions.*
   a. *Remedial Approach.* Drills can be used to practice discrimination between faces that are important to the patient (using photographs), in discrimination between colors, and common objects. The therapist should assist the patient in picking out salient visual cues for relating names to faces.

   As with many cognitive and perceptual deficits, a therapist may treat a patient with visual agnosia in an Easy Street Environment®. These environments have been incorporated into rehabilitation centers in the United States for almost 20 years. The Easy Street Environment® is a modular "world" of life size streets (with a variety of ambulation surfaces, stairs, curbs, and so forth), vehicles, shops, and offices which are constructed in a dedicated area within the rehabilitation setting. The Easy Street Environment® has many advantages since it allows occupational therapists, physical therapists, and speech–language professionals to work with a patient in a safe, private, and comfortable environment where the patient can try out relearned or new skills. The therapist can also save considerable time by taking the patient down the corridor to the Easy Street Environment® rather than to their own local community, although ultimately such an outing to the local community may be undertaken. Figure 29.13 shows a patient with a visual object agnosia learning to use the Easy Street Environment® Automatic Teller Machine (ATM). This patient may also learn new strategies to identify groceries and therefore be able to practice shopping in the Easy Street Environment® Market Place (Fig. 29.14).

   b. *Compensatory Approach.* The patient is instructed to use intact sensory modalities, such as touch or audition, to distinguish people and objects.

Auditory Agnosia

1. *Definition.* **Auditory agnosia** refers to the inability to recognize nonspeech sounds or to discriminate between them. This rarely occurs in the absence of other communication disorders.[4]
2. *Clinical Examples.* The patient with auditory agnosia cannot tell, for example, the difference between the ring of a doorbell and that of a telephone, or between a dog barking and thunder.
3. *Lesion Area.* The lesion is located in the dominant temporal lobe.[4]
4. *Testing.* Testing is usually carried out by a speech–language pathologist. The patient is asked to close the eyes and to identify the source of various sounds. The therapist rings a bell, honks a horn, rings a telephone, and so forth, and asks the patient to identify the sound (verbally or by pointing to a picture).
5. *Treatment Suggestions.* Treatment generally consists of drilling the patient on sounds, but this has not been found to be particularly effective.[1,2]

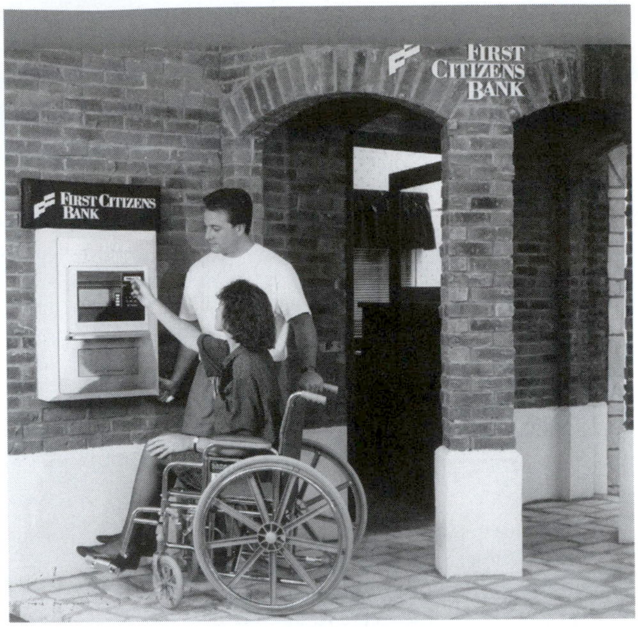

Figure 29.13 A client with an agnosia learns to use an ATM with help from a therapist in the Easy Street Environment®. (Courtesy of Easy Street Environments,® Scottsdale, AZ 85260.)

Tactile Agnosia or Astereognosis

1. *Definition.* Tactile agnosia, or *astereognosis,* is the inability to recognize forms by handling them, although tactile, proprioceptive, and thermal sensations may be intact. This impairment commonly causes difficulties in ADL skills, inasmuch as many self-care activities that are normally done in the absence of constant visual monitoring require the manipulation of objects. If tactile

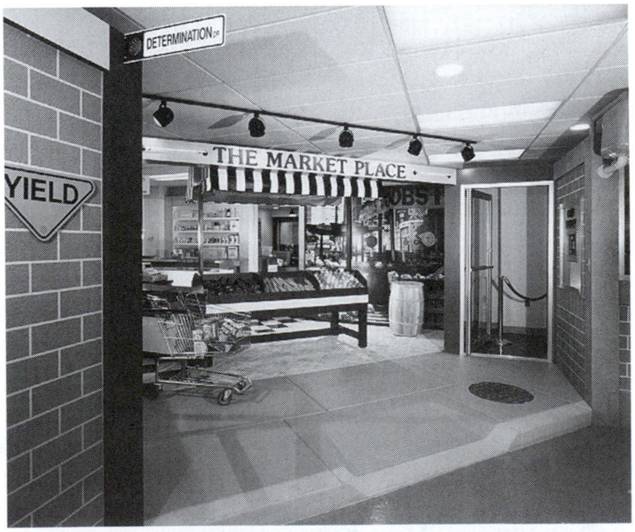

Figure 29.14 Clients with agnosias and many other cognitive and perceptual deficits can practice daily living skills in the controlled Easy Street Environment® such as provided in the market store. (Courtesy of Easy Street Environments,® Scottsdale, AZ 85260.)

agnosia is present in combination with unilateral neglect or sensory loss, performance in ADL skills may be severely hampered.[68]

2. *Clinical Examples.* If a patient is handed an object (key, comb, safety pin) with vision occluded, the patient will fail to recognize it.
3. *Lesion Area.* The lesion is in the parieto-temporo-occipital lobe (posterior association areas) of either hemisphere.[4]
4. *Testing.* The patient is asked to identify objects placed in the hand by examining them manually without visual cues.
5. *Treatment Suggestions.*
   a. *Remedial Approach.* The patient practices feeling various common objects, shapes, and textures with vision occluded. The patient is instructed to immediately look at the object for visual feedback and note special characteristics of the object.
   b. *Compensatory Approach.* To improve cognitive awareness, the patient is educated concerning the nature of the deficit and is instructed in visual compensation.

Apraxia

Apraxia is an impairment of voluntary skilled learned movement. It is characterized by an inability to perform purposeful movements, which cannot be accounted for by inadequate strength, loss of coordination, impaired sensation, attentional difficulties, abnormal tone, movement disorders, intellectual deterioration, poor comprehension, or uncooperativeness.[152–154] Many patients with apraxia also present with aphasia, and the two deficits are sometimes difficult to distinguish.[4] Donkervoot et al[155] report the prevalence of apraxia among patients with first left hemisphere stroke in rehabilitation as around 28 percent. The two main forms of apraxia discussed in the literature are *ideomotor* and *ideational apraxia*. Ideomotor and ideational apraxias are generally thought to be the result of dominant hemisphere lesions and may be particularly difficult to test in the patient with aphasia. Although aphasia and apraxia often occur together, there is not a strong correlation between the severity of the aphasia and the severity of the apraxia. A third form of apraxia, *buccofacial apraxia,* is actually a type of ideomotor apraxia and is characterized by difficulties with performing the purposeful movements that involve facial muscles related to the mouth. This may include responding to the command "pretend to blow out a candle," or producing an orderly sequence of phonemes to produce speech. Hence, apraxia is a disorder of skilled movement and not a language disorder.[50] Some rehabilitation texts also describe constructional and dressing apraxias. However, it is generally believed that these are not true apraxias, but rather are difficulties in the application of cognitive and perceptual skill to these tasks. In other words, they are terms used to describe specific difficulties with a construction or drawing task or dressing. Both these problems are more frequently associated with right hemisphere lesions.[156]

Ideomotor Apraxia

1. *Definition.* Ideomotor apraxia refers to a breakdown between concept and performance. There is a disconnection between the idea of a movement and its motor execution. It appears that the information cannot be transferred from the areas of the brain that conceptualize to the centers for motor execution. Thus the patient with ideomotor apraxia is able to carry out habitual tasks automatically and describe how they are done but is unable to imitate gestures or perform on command.[157,158] Patients with this form of apraxia often **perseverate**[59]; that is, they repeat an activity or a segment of a task over and over, even if it is no longer necessary or appropriate. This makes it difficult for them to finish one task and go on to the next. Patients with ideomotor apraxia appear most impaired when requested to perform tasks that require use of many implements and that have many steps. This form of apraxia can be demonstrated separately in the facial areas, upper extremity, lower extremity, and for total body movements.[159] Patients with apraxia are often observed to be clumsy in their actual handling of objects. Impairment is often suspected when observing the patient during ADL or during a routine motor examination.
2. *Clinical Examples.* Several examples of ideomotor apraxia follow. The patient is unable to "blow" on command. However, if presented with a bubble wand, the patient will spontaneously blow bubbles. The patient may fail to walk if requested to in a traditional manner. However, if a cup of coffee is placed on a table at the other end of the room and the patient is told, "Please have coffee," the patient is likely to traverse the room to get it.[137] A male patient is asked to comb his hair. He may be able to identify the comb and even tell you what it is used for; however, he will not actually use the comb appropriately when it is handed to him. Despite this observation in the clinic, his wife reports that he combs his hair spontaneously every morning. A female patient is asked to squeeze a dynamometer. She appears not to know what to do with it, although her comprehension is adequate, the task has just been demonstrated, and it is clear that she has adequate strength.
3. *Lesion Area.* Apraxia results most frequently from lesions in the left, dominant hemisphere. There is evidence that both frontal lesions and posterior parietal lesions can result in apraxia.[160]
4. *Testing.* The *Goodglass and Kaplan*[159] test for apraxia is composed of universally known movements, such as blowing, brushing teeth, hammering, shaving, and

so forth. It is based on what the authors consider a hierarchy of difficulty for patients with apraxia. First the patient is asked, "Show me how you would bang a nail with a hammer." If the patient fails to do this or uses his or her fist as if it were a hammer, the patient is told, "Pretend to hold the hammer." If the patient fails following this instruction, the therapist demonstrates the act and asks the patient to imitate it. The patient with apraxia typically will not improve after demonstration but will improve with use of the actual implements.[4] The ability to correct oneself on following verbal cueing is considered not indicative of apraxia. Additional apraxia tests may be found in Butler,[156] or the work of van Heugten et al,[161] who have adapted the Arnadottir OT-ADL Neurobehavioural Evaluation (A-ONE)[5] as an observational method of testing for apraxia.

5. *Treatment Suggestions.*
   a. *Remedial Approach.* In the remediation of apraxias, it is advised that the therapist speak slowly and use the shortest possible sentences. One command should be given at a time, and the second command should not be given until the first task is completed. When teaching a new task, it should be broken down into its component parts. One component is taught at a time, physically guiding the patient through the task if necessary. It should be completed in precisely the same manner each time.[156] When all the individual units are mastered, an attempt to combine them should be made. A great deal of repetition may be necessary.[68] Family members must be advised to use the exact approach found to be successful in the clinic. Performing activities in as normal an environment as possible is also helpful. A case example of a young woman relearning how to drink from a cup using this technique is provided by Butler.[156] Using the sensorimotor approach, multiple sensory inputs are used on the affected body parts to enhance the production of appropriate motor responses. The reader is referred to the work of Okoye[162] for additional details on this approach.
   b. *Compensatory Approach.* Donkervoot et al[163] report a randomized controlled trial that showed the effectiveness of an occupational therapy treatment program including "strategy training" over regular occupational therapy. Strategy training involves teaching the patient compensatory techniques to overcome the apraxia such as use of pictures in the correct sequence to support ADL skills.

Ideational Apraxia

1. *Definition.* Ideational apraxia is a failure in the conceptualization of the task. It is an inability to perform a purposeful motor act, either automatically or on command, because the patient no longer understands the overall concept of the act, cannot retain the idea of the task, or cannot formulate the motor patterns required. Often the patient can perform isolated components of a task but cannot combine them into a complete act. Furthermore, the patient cannot verbally describe the process of performing an activity, describe the function of objects, or use them appropriately.[164,165]
2. *Clinical Examples.* When presented in the clinic with a toothbrush and toothpaste and told to brush the teeth, the patient may put the tube of toothpaste in the mouth, or try to put toothpaste on the toothbrush without removing the cap. Further, the patient may be unable to describe verbally how tooth-brushing is done. Similar phenomena may be evident in all aspects of ADL (washing, meal preparation, and so forth) and so may limit the safety and potential independence of the patient.[5] It has been shown that patients with ideational apraxia who test poorly in the clinical situation appear more able to perform ADL skills at the appropriate time and in a familiar setting.[162]
3. *Lesion Area.* The lesion causing ideational apraxia is thought to be in the dominant parietal lobe. This deficit also may be seen in conjunction with diffuse brain damage, such as cerebral arteriosclerosis.[59]
4. *Testing.* The tests for ideational apraxia are similar to those for ideomotor apraxia. The major expected response difference is that the patient with ideomotor apraxia can perform a motor act spontaneously and automatically at the appropriate time, but the patient with ideational apraxia is unable to do so. Refer to Butler[156] for full testing protocols.
5. *Treatment Suggestions.* The treatment techniques are the same as those for ideomotor apraxia.

Buccofacial Apraxia

1. *Definition.* Buccofacial or oral apraxia involves difficulties with performing purposeful movements with the lips, tongue, cheeks, larynx, and pharynx on command. An unusual condition, Pederson et al[166] report the prevalence rate in rehabilitation patients as around 6 percent.
2. *Clinical Examples.* A patient may have difficulty responding to the command "pretend to blow out a candle" or "blow a kiss." However, in a normal context where the patient may perform these actions automatically, performance is not impaired. In addition, while patients may be able to produce the individual phonemes required for speech, the patient may have difficulty in producing an orderly sequence of phonemes. Formulaic speech, or automatic expressions such as "have a nice day" may be preserved.[167]
3. *Lesion Area.* Difficulties with buccofacial apraxia seem associated with lesions in the frontal and central oper-

cula, anterior insula, and a small area of the first temporal gyrus (adjacent to the frontal and central opercula). While buccofacial apraxia often coexists with Broca's aphasia, the two may be seen independently.[167]

4. *Testing*. The patient should be examined by a speech–language pathologist.
5. *Treatment Suggestions*. The speech–language pathologist can advise the health care team on strategies to communicate with patients who have buccofacial apraxia.

Summary

Cognition and perception, the processes by which an individual thinks and selects, integrates, and interprets stimuli from the body and surrounding environment, are critical to the normal functioning of each human being. The patient with brain damage may be lacking in those abilities that allow one to make sense of and to respond appropriately to the outside world. It is essential for the physical therapist to be able to recognize when a patient is experiencing some type of perceptual dysfunction and to have the requisite tools to understand the causes of the behavior.

This chapter provided an overview of cognitive and perceptual deficits that may occur following brain damage, particularly those resulting from a stroke, and how such deficits can affect the functioning of the patient, especially within the context of the rehabilitation setting. The importance of differentiating cognitive and perceptual deficits from problems related to lack of motor ability, inadequate sensation, poor language skills, and simple uncooperativeness has been emphasized. Although alluded to in a very abbreviated fashion, activity analysis and systematic data collection remain two of the most powerful tools at the disposal of the therapist attempting to develop a firm rationale for, and to empirically justify the efficacy of any treatment selected. Treatment in the form of adaptation of the physical environment and instructional sets and the teaching of compensatory techniques has been singled out as the most effective avenue for intervention.

Acknowledgment

Gratitude is extended to Chaye Lamm Warburg, whose earlier version of this chapter provided the foundation for the current work.

Questions for Review

1. What general characteristics are displayed by patients with cognitive and perceptual deficits during execution of a task?
2. Identify the underlying premise of the *transfer-of-training approach* to treatment.
3. What is the underlying assumption of the *sensory integrative approach* to treatment? Provide examples of the treatment modalities employed with this approach.
4. How is the performance of specific functional skills enhanced using the *functional approach* to treatment? What are the inherent benefits of using the functional approach?
5. Describe general suggestions for optimizing teaching/learning strategies when using compensatory techniques.
6. Identify the four treatment strategies included in the *cognitive approach* to treatment.
7. What potential influencing factors must be considered when examining a patient with cognitive and perceptual disabilities?
8. What examination procedures will assist the therapist in distinguishing between sensory and cognitive or perceptual problems?
9. Distinguish the difference between feedback provided in the form of knowledge of results (KR) versus knowledge of performance (KP).
10. Identify and define the four different types of attention.
11. What is the purpose of memory retraining? Compare and contrast the focus of the *remedial approach* and the *compensatory approach* to memory retraining.
12. Define the following terms: unilateral neglect, somatoagnosia, right–left discrimination, finger agnosia, and anosognosia.
13. Identify four spatial relations deficits. What general clinical manifestation do these disorders have in common? Define each of the four deficits identified and provide an example of how each would influence patient performance of a task.
14. Provide examples of the functional implications of a *visual figure–ground discrimination* deficit. What is the most common lesion site producing this disorder?
15. What is the characteristic feature of apraxia? Define the three types of apraxias. Provide examples of task performance characteristics associated with each type of apraxia.

Case Study

The patient is a 72-year-old woman who has just been admitted to a rehabilitation facility following a stroke. The patient experienced a right parietal hemorrhagic stroke. A CT scan revealed a 1.5 in. (4 cm) hemorrhage that was subsequently drained. She will be able to stay in the rehabilitation facility for 20 days. Although the patient has some physical problems, the emphasis of this case study is on cognitive and perceptual tests and interventions. The occupational therapist and the physical therapist are collaboratively using a combination of cognitive retraining and the functional approach in therapy.

PAST MEDICAL HISTORY

The patient's past medical history includes insulin-dependent diabetes and mild rheumatoid arthritis in her right shoulder and both hands.

SOCIAL

The patient lives alone in her own home. Supportive friends and family, her two children and their families live nearby. She is insured by a local HMO. She is retired from the police force and enjoys gardening, reading, and watching television. She previously drove an automobile with an automatic transmission.

PHYSICAL THERAPY EXAMINATION

When the patient was approached from the left, she seemed to ignore the physical therapist and did not respond to greetings. However, when the therapist sat in the chair on the patient's right side, she seemed to have no problems talking to the therapist.

Range of Motion, Muscle Tone, and Balance

Examination revealed full ROM, reduced strength in the left arm and hand and some reduced dynamic standing balance reactions.

Sensation

The physical therapist tested sensation and noted normal sensation in all areas (sharp/dull, light touch, temperature, proprioceptive sensations, cortical sensations) on the right side. However, the patient seemed to have difficulties on the left side and her performance in detecting stimuli seemed inconsistent. Because the physical therapist suspected cognitive and perceptual deficits, a complete sensory test was deferred until the occupational therapist could fully examine the patient.

Functional Status

The physical therapist examined the patient's transfers and instructed her in a safer way to get in and out of bed. The therapist scored the patient on the *Functional Independence Measure (FIM)*[89] and found:

Self-Care

Eating: FIM level = 4
Grooming: FIM level = 5
Bathing: FIM level = 3
Dressing—upper body: FIM level = 5
Dressing—lower body: FIM level = 4
Toileting: FIM level = 6

Transfers

Bed, chair, wheelchair: FIM level = 5
Toilet: FIM level = 5
Tub: FIM level = 4

Locomotion

Walk: FIM level = 5

The physical therapist asked about her family and she was able to provide many details. However, she seemed puzzled about where she was and was concerned that she was not looking her best and needed to do her hair. The therapist suggested that she might like to brush her hair. The brush was on the table on the patient's left side, and she said she did not have one. The physical therapist cued her to check her bedside table, but on checking she maintained she did not have a brush. At the end of the session (which lasted about 40 minutes) the therapist asked her to demonstrate the bed transfer technique again that she had been taught at the beginning of the session. She seemed confused and could not do what the physical therapist had taught her.

OCCUPATIONAL THERAPY COGNITION AND PERCEPTION EXAMINATION

The occupational therapist conducted two standardized tests: the *Rivermead Behavioural Memory Test (RBMT)*[82] because the patient demonstrates memory impairments, and the *Arnadottir OT-ADL Neurobehavioral Evaluation (A-ONE)*[5] to examine the impact of the patient's problems on her daily living activities. The occupational therapist also reasoned that further tests of the patient's IADLs including home and driving abilities would need to be conducted closer to her discharge. The patient's FIM scores for the Social Cognition Items were:

Social Cognition FIM

Social interaction: FIM level = 6
Problem solving: FIM level = 6
Memory: FIM level = 3

GUIDING QUESTIONS

1. What are some of the functional difficulties the patient is having and what cognitive and perceptual deficits might be causing these? Please note that there may be more than one possible impairment for the functional problems noted.
2. Develop a clinical asset and problem list.
3. Identify anticipated goals and expected outcomes appropriate for this patient.
4. Identify two treatment strategies to improve spontaneous use of left upper extremity and decrease unilateral neglect.
5. Identify two treatment strategies to improve the patient's memory.
6. How can the success of the patient's rehabilitation program be measured?

References

1. Unsworth, C: Cognitive and Perceptual Dysfunction: A Clinical Reasoning Approach to Evaluation and Intervention. FA Davis, Philadelphia, 1999.
2. Zoltan, B: Vision, Perception and Cognition: A Manual for Evaluation and Treatment of the Neurologically Impaired Adult, ed 3 rev. Charles B. Slack, Thorofare, NJ, 1996.
3. Katz, N, et al: Lowenstein Occupational Therapy Cognitive Assessment (LOTCA) battery for brain injured patients: reliability and validity. Am J Occup Ther 43:184, 1989.
4. Lezak, MD: Neuropsychological Assessment, ed 3. Oxford University Press, New York, 1995.
5. Arnadottir, G: The Brain and Behavior: Assessing Cortical Dysfunction Through Activities of Daily Living. CV Mosby, St. Louis, 1990.
6. Glosser, G, and Goodglass, H: Disorders of executive control functions among aphasic and other brain-damaged patients. J Clin Exp Neuropsychol 12:485, 1990.
7. Katz, N, and Hartman-Maeir, A: Occupational performance and metacognition. Can J Occup Ther 64:53, 1997.
8. Winegardner, J: Executive functions. In Cohen, H (ed): Neuroscience for Rehabilitation. Lippincott, Philadelphia, 1993, p 346.
9. Sharpless, JW: Mossman's A Problem Oriented Approach to Stroke Rehabilitation, ed 2. Charles C Thomas, Springfield, IL, 1982.
10. Edwards, S: Neurological Physiotherapy: A Problem Solving Approach. Churchill Livingstone, New York, 1996.
11. Luria, AR: Higher Cortical Functions in Man. Basic Books, New York, 1966.
12. Pak, R, and Dombrovy, ML: Stroke. In Good, DC, and Couch, JR (eds): Handbook of Neurorehabilitation. Marcel Dekker, New York, 1994, p 461.
13. Meir, M, et al: Individual differences in neuropsychological recovery: An overview. In Meier, M, et al (eds). Neuropsychological Rehabilitation. Churchill Livingstone, London, 1987, p 71.
14. Bach-y-Rita, P: Brain plasticity as a basis for therapeutic procedures. In Bach-y-Rita, P (ed): Recovery of Function: Theoretical Considerations for Brain Injury Rehabilitation. University Park Press, Baltimore, 1980, p 225.
15. Brodal, A: Self-observations and neuro-anatomical considerations after a stroke. Brain 76:675, 1973.
16. Gardner, H: The Shattered Mind: The Person After Brain Damage. Alfred A Knopf, New York, 1975.
17. Averbuch, S, and Katz, N: Cognitive rehabilitation: A retraining approach for brain-injured adults. In Katz, N (ed): Cognitive Rehabilitation: Models for Intervention in Occupational Therapy. Andover Medical, Boston, 1992, p 219.
18. Neistadt, ME: The neurobiology of learning: Implications for treatment of adults with brain injury. Am J Occup Ther 48:421, 1994.
19. Neistadt, ME: Assessing learning capabilities during cognitive and perceptual evaluations for adults with traumatic brain injury. Occup Ther Health Care 9:3, 1995.
20. Young, GC, Collins, D, and Hren, M: Effect of pairing scanning training with block design training in the remediation of perceptual problems in left hemiplegics. J Clin Neuropsychol 42:312, 1983.
21. Neistadt, ME: Occupational therapy for adults with perceptual deficits. Am J Occup Ther 42:434, 1988.
22. Bundy, AC, Lane, SJ, and Murray, EA (eds): Sensory Integration: Theory and Practice, ed 2. FA Davis, Philadelphia, 2002.
23. Ayres, JA: Sensory Integration and Learning Disorders. Western Psychological Service, Los Angeles, 1972.
24. Ayres, JA: Sensory Integration and the Child. Western Psychological Services, Los Angeles, 1980.
25. Neistadt, ME: A critical analysis of occupational therapy approaches for perceptual deficits in adults with brain injury. Am J Occup Ther 44:299, 1990.
26. Moore, J: Neuronanatomical considerations relating to recovery of function following brain injury. In Bach-y-Rita, P (ed): Recovery of Function: Theoretical Consideration for Brain Injury Rehabilitation. University Park Press, Baltimore, 1980, p 9.
27. Finger, S, and Stein, DG: Brain Damage and Recovery: Research and Clinical Perspectives. Academic Press, New York, 1982.
28. Braziz, PW, Masdeu, J, and Biller, J: Localization in Clinical Neurology, ed 3. Little, Brown, Boston, 1996.
29. Giles, GM, and Wilson, JC: Occupational Therapy for the Brain Injured Adult: A Neurofunctional Approach. Chapman & Hall, London, 1992.
30. Giles, GM: A neurofunctional approach to rehabilitation following severe brain injury. In Katz, N (ed): Cognitive Rehabilitation: Models for Intervention in Occupational Therapy. Andover Medical, Boston, 1992, p 195.
31. Trombly, CA (ed): Occupational Therapy for Physical Dysfunction, ed 5. Williams &Wilkins, Baltimore, 2002.
32. Trombly, CA: Conceptual foundations for practice. In Trombly, CA (ed): Occupational Therapy for Physical Dysfunction, ed 5. Lippincott Williams & Wilkins, Baltimore, 2002, p 1.
33. Trombly, CA: Restoring the role of independent person. In Trombly, CA (ed): Occupational Therapy for Physical Dysfunction, ed 5. Lippincott Williams & Wilkins, Baltimore, 2002, p 629.
34. Neistadt, ME: Occupational therapy treatment for constructional deficits. Am J Occup Ther 46:141, 1992.
35. Fisher, AG: An expanded rehabilitative model of practice. In Fisher, AG (ed): Assessment of Motor and Process Skills, ed 2. Three Star Press, Fort Collins, CO, 1997, p 73.
36. Ellek, D: Managed competition: Maintaining health care within the private sector. Am J Occup Ther 49:468, 1995.
37. Toglia, J, and Abreu, BC: Cognitive Rehabilitation Supplement to Workshop: Management of Cognitive–Perceptual Dysfunction in the Brain-Damaged Adult. Sponsored by Braintree Hospital, Braintree, MA and Cognitive Rehabilitation Associates, New York, May, 1987.
38. Giantusos, R: What is cognitive rehabilitation? J Rehabil 46:36, 1980.
39. Abreu, BC, and Toglia, JP: Cognitive rehabilitation: A model for occupational therapy. Am J Occup Ther 41:439, 1987.
40. Diller, L, and Gordon, WA: Intervention strategies for cognitive deficits in brain-injured adults. J Consult Clin Psychol 49:822, 1981.
41. Toglia, JP: Generalization of treatment: A multicontext approach to cognitive perceptual impairment in adults with brain injury. Am J Occup Ther 45:505, 1991.
42. Toglia, JP: A dynamic interactional model to cognitive rehabilitation. In Katz, N (ed): Cognition and Occupational in Rehabilitation: Cognitive Models for Intervention in Occupational Therapy. The American Occupational Therapy Association, Inc, Bethesda, 1998, p 5.
43. Abreu, BC: Evaluation and intervention with memory and learning impairment. In Unsworth, CA (ed): Cognitive and Perceptual Dysfunction: A Clinical Reasoning Approach to Evaluation and Intervention. FA Davis, Philadelphia, 1999, p 163.

44. Abreu, BC: The quadraphonic approach: Holistic rehabilitation for brain injury. In Katz, N (ed): Cognition and Occupation in Rehabilitation: Cognitive Models for Intervention in Occupational Therapy. The American Occupational Therapy Association, Inc, Bethesda, 1998, p 51.
45. Wilcock, AA: Occupational Therapy Approaches to Stroke. Churchill Livingstone, Melbourne, 1986.
46. Galski, T, Beuno, RL, and Ehle, HT: Driving after cerebral damage: A model with implications for evaluation. Am J Occup Ther 46:324, 1992.
47. Vining Radomski, M, and Schold David, E: Optimizing cognitive abilities. In Trombly, CA (ed): Occupational Therapy for Physical Dysfunction, ed 5. Lippincott, Williams & Wilkins, Baltimore, 2002, p 609.
48. Gainotti, G: Emotional and psychosocial problems after brain injury. Neuropsychol Rehab 3:259, 1993.
49. Bronstein, KS, Popovich, JM, and Stewart-Amidei, C: Promoting Stroke Recovery. CV Mosby, St. Louis, 1991.
50. Bradshaw, JL, and Mattingley, JB: Clinical Neuropsychology: Behavioral and Brain Science. Academic Press, San Diego, 1995.
51. Cate, Y, and Richards, L: Relationship between performance on tests of basic visual functions and visual-perceptual processing in persons after brain injury. Am J Occup Ther 54:326, 2000.
52. Dirette, DK, and Hinojosa, J: The effects of a compensatory intervention on processing deficits in adults with acquired brain damage. Occup Ther J Res 19:223, 1999.
53. Warren, M: A hierarchical model for evaluation and treatment of visual perceptual dysfunction in adult acquired brain injury, I. Am J Occup Ther 47:42, 1993.
54. Warren, M: A hierarchical model for evaluation and treatment of visual perceptual dysfunction in adult acquired brain injury, II. Am J Occup Ther 47:55, 1993.
55. Sandin, KJ, and Mason, KD: Manual of Stroke Rehabilitation. Butterworth-Heinemann, Boston, 1996.
56. Gresham, GE, et al: Post-Stroke Rehabilitation: Clinical Practice Guidelines. Aspen, Gaithersburg, MD, 1995.
57. Hier, DB, Mondlock, J, and Caplan, LR: Recovery of behavioral abnormalities after right hemisphere stroke. Neurology 33:345, 1983.
58. Haerer, AF: Visual field defects and the prognosis of stroke patients. Stroke 4:163, 1977.
59. Chusid, JG: Correlative Neuroanatomy and Functional Neurology, ed 19. Lange Medical Publications, Los Altos, CA, 1985.
60. Tobis, JS, and Lowenthal, M: Evaluation and Management of the Brain-Damaged Patient. Charles C Thomas, Springfield, IL, 1960.
61. Pedretti, LW: Evaluation of sensation, perception and cognition. In Pedretti, LW (ed): Occupational Therapy: Practice Skills for Physical Dysfunction, ed 2. CV Mosby, St. Louis, 1985, p 99.
62. Stilwell, JM: The meaning of manual midline crossing. Sens Integr Q 21:1, 1994.
63. Chaikin, LE: Disorders of vision and visual perceptual dysfunction. In Umphred, DA (ed): Neurological Rehabilitation, ed 4. CV Mosby, St. Louis, 2001, p 821.
64. Diller, L, and Weinberg, J: Differential aspects of attention in brain-damaged persons. Percept Motor Skills 35:71, 1972.
65. Van Ravensberg, CD, et al: Visual perception in hemiplegic patients. Arch Phys Med Rehabil 65:304, 1984.
66. Anastasi, A: Psychological Testing, ed 6. Macmillan, New York, 1988.
67. de Clive-Lowe, S: Outcome measurement, cost-effectiveness and clinical audit: The importance of standardised assessment to occupational therapists in meeting these new demands. Br J Occup Ther 59:357, 1996.
68. Wall, N: Stroke rehabilitation. In Logigian, MK (ed): Adult Rehabilitation: A Team Approach for Therapists. Little, Brown, Boston, 1982, p 225.
69. Laver, AJ, and Powell, GE: The Structured Observational Test of Function (SOTOF). NFER-NELSON, Windsor, England, 1995.
70. Laver, AJ: The structured observational test of function. Gerontol Spec Int Sect Newsl 17:1, 1994.
71. Allen, CK: Allen cognitive level test manual. S & S/ Worldwide, Colchester, 1990.
72. Allen, CK, Earhart, CA, and Blue, T: Occupational therapy treatment goals for the physically and cognitively disabled. American Occupational Therapy Association, Rockville, MD, 1992.
73. Tyerman, R, et al: COTNAB-Chessington Occupational Therapy Neurological Assessment Battery Introductory Manual. Nottingham Rehab Limited, Nottingham, 1986.
74. Stanley, M, et al: Chessington Occupational Therapy Neurological Assessment Battery: Comparison of performance of people aged 50–65 years with people aged 66 and over. Austral Occup Ther J 42:55, 1995.
75. Sloan, RL, et al: Routine screening of brain damaged patients: A comparison of the Rivermead Perceptual Assessment Battery and the Chessington Occupational Therapy Neurological Assessment Battery. Clin Rehab 5:265, 1991.
76. Itzkovich, M, et al: The Loewenstein Occupational Therapy Assessment (LOTCA) manual. Maddak, Inc, Pequanock, NJ, 1990.
77. Cooke, DM, McKenna, K, and Fleming, J: Development of a standardized occupational therapy screening tool for visual perception in adults. Scand J Occup Ther 12(2): 59, 2005.
78. Wilson, B, et al: Behavioural Inattention Test. Thames Valley Test Company, Bury St Edmunds, 1987.
79. Wilson, B, Cockburn, J, and Halligan, P: Development of a behavioural test of visuospatial neglect. Arch Phys Med Rehabil 68:98, 1987.
80. Whiting, S, et al: RPAB-Rivermead Perceptual Assessment Battery. NFER-NELSON, Windsor, 1985.
81. Jesshope, HJ, Clark, MS, and Smith, DS: The RPAB: Its application to stroke-patients and relationship with function. Clin Rehab 5:115, 1991.
82. Wilson, B, et al: RBMT-The Rivermead Behavioural Memory Test. Thames Valley Test Company, Bury St. Edmunds, 1991.
83. Wilson, B, et al: Development and validation of a test battery for detecting and monitoring everyday memory problems. J Clin Exp Neuropsychol 11:885, 1989.
84. Ware, JJ, and Sherbourne, CD: The MOS 36-item short-form health survey (SF-36): I. Conceptual framework and item selection. Med Care 30:473, 1992.
85. Enderby, P: Therapy Outcome Measures. Singular Publishing Group, San Diego, CA, 1997.
86. Law, M, et al: Canadian Occupational Performance Measure. Canadian Association of Occupational Therapists, Toronto, Ontario, 1991.
87. Davis, A, et al: First steps towards an interdisciplinary approach to rehabilitation. Clin Rehab 6:237, 1992.
88. Wood-Dauphinee, SL, et al: Assessment of global function: The Reintegration to Normal Living Index. Arch Phys Med 69:583, 1988.
89. Guide for the Uniform Data Set for Medical Rehabilitation (Adult FIM SM): Version 5.0. State University of New York at Buffalo, Buffalo, 1999.
90. Jongbloed, L, et al: Stroke rehabilitation: Sensory integrative treatment versus functional treatment. Am J Occup Ther 43:391, 1989.
91. Gentile, AM: A working model of skill acquisition with special reference to teaching. Quest Monograph 17:61, 1972.
92. Evanofski, M: Occupational therapy reimbursement, regulation, and the evolving scope of practice. In Crepeau, EB, Cohn, ES, and Schell, BAB (eds): Willard and Spackman's Occupational Therapy, ed 10. Lippincott Williams & Wilkins. Philadelphia, 2003, p 887.
93. McKeehan, KM: Conceptual framework for discharge planning. In McKeehan, KM (ed): Continuing Care: A Multidisciplinary Approach to Discharge Planning. CV Mosby, Toronto, 1981, p 3.
94. Unsworth, CA, and Thomas, SA: Information use in discharge accommodation recommendations for stroke patients. Clin Rehabil 7:181, 1993.
95. Unsworth, CA, Thomas, SA, and Greenwood, KM: Rehabilitation team decisions concerning discharge housing for stroke patients. Arch Phys Med Rehabil 76:331, 1995.
96. Unsworth, CA: Clients' perceptions of discharge housing decisions following stroke rehabilitation. Am J Occup Ther 50:207, 1996.
97. Stringer, AY: A Guide to Adult Neurological Diagnosis. FA Davis, Philadelphia, 1996.
98. Strub, RL, and Black, FW: The Mental Status Examination in Neurology, ed 2. FA Davis, Philadelphia, 1985.
99. Mateer, CA, Kerns, KA, and Eso, KL: Management of attention and memory disorders following traumatic brain injury. J Learn Disabil 29:618, 1996.

100. van Zomeren, AH, and Brouwer, WH: The Clinical Neuropsychology of Attention. Oxford University Press, New York, 1994.
101. Stroop, JR: Studies of inference in serial verbal reactions. J Exp Psychol 18:643, 1935.
102. Gronwall, D: Paced auditory serial addition task: A measure of recovery from concussion. Percept Motor Skills 44:367, 1977.
103. US Army: Army Individual Test Battery. Manual of directions and scoring. Adjutant General's Office, 1944.
104. Ponsford, J, Sloan, S, and Snow, P: Traumatic brain injury: Rehabilitation for everyday adaptive living. Lawrence Erlbaum, Hove, 1995
105. Lincoln, NB, et al: Cognitive rehabilitation for attention deficits following stroke (Cochrane review). In The Cochrane Library, Issue 3, Update Software, Oxford, 2002.
106. Kepferman, I: Learning and memory. In Kandel, ER, Schwartz, JH, and Jessell, TM (eds): Principles of Neuroscience, ed 3. Elsevier, New York, 1991, p 996.
107. Wickelgren, WA: Learning and Memory. Prentice-Hall, Englewood Cliffs, NJ, 1977.
108. Sohlberg, MM, and Mateer, CA: Introduction to cognitive rehabilitation: Theory and practice. The Guilford Press, New York, 1989.
109. Fuster, JM: Memory in the Cerebral Cortex: An Empirical Approach to Neural Networks in the Human and Nonhuman Primate. MIT Press, Cambridge, MA, 1995.
110. Wilson, BA, and Moffat, N: Clinical Management of Memory Problems. Chapman & Hall, London, 1992.
111. Majid, M.J, et al: Cognitive rehabilitation for memory deficits following stroke (Cochrane Review). In: The Cochrane Library, Issue 3. Update Software, Oxford, 2002.
112. Doornheim, K, and De Haan, EHF: Cognitive training for memory deficits in stroke patients. Neuropsychol Rehabil 8:393, 1998.
113. Duran, L, and Fisher, AG: Evaluation and intervention with executive functions impairment. In Unsworth, CA: Cognitive and Perceptual Dysfunction: A Clinical Reasoning Approach to Evaluation and Intervention. FA Davis, Philadelphia, 1999, p 209.
114. Cummins, JL: Anatomic and behavioral aspects of frontal-subcortical circuits. In Grafman, J, et al (eds): Annals of the New York Academy of Sciences: Structure and Function of the Human Prefrontal Cortex, vol. 769. New York Academy of Sciences, New York, 1995, p 1.
115. Wilson, BA, et al: Behavioural Assessment of the Dysexecutive Syndrome. Thames Valley Test Company, Bury St. Edmunds, UK, 1996.
116. Pollens, R, et al: Beyond cognition: Executive functions in closed head injury. Cogn Rehabil 65:23, 1988.
117. Sohlberg, MM, Mateer, CA, and Stuss, DT: Contemporary approaches to the management of executive control dysfunction. J Head Trauma Rehab 8:45, 1993.
118. Honda, T: Rehabilitation of executive function impairment after stroke. Top Stroke Rehabil 6(1):15, 1999.
119. Van Deusen, J: Body Image and Perceptual Dysfunction in Adults. WB Saunders, Philadelphia, 1993.
120. Corben, L, and Unsworth, CA: Evaluation and intervention with unilateral neglect. In Unsworth, CA (ed): Cognitive and Perceptual Dysfunction: A Clinical Reasoning Approach to Evaluation and Intervention. FA Davis, Philadelphia, 1999, p 357.
121. Robertson, IH, and Halligan, PW: Spatial Neglect: A Clinical Handbook for Diagnosis and Treatment. Psychology Press, Hove, 1999.
122. Benton, A, and Sivan, AB: Disturbances of the body schema. In Heilman, KM, and Valenstein, E (eds): Clinical Neuropsychology, ed 3. Oxford University Press, New York, 1993, p 123.
123. Herman, EWM: Spatial neglect: New issues and their implications for occupational therapy practice. Am J Occup Ther 46:207, 1992.
124. Gordon, WA, et al: Perceptual remediation in patients with right brain damage: A comprehensive program. Arch Phys Med Rehabil 66:353, 1985.
125. Vallar, G: The anatomical basis of spatial hemineglect in humans. In Robertson, IH, and Marshall, JC (eds): Unilateral Neglect: Clinical and Experimental Studies. Lawrence Erlbaum, Hove, 1993, p 27.
126. Rizzolatti, G and Berti, A: Neural mechanisms of spatial neglect. In Robertson, IH and Marshall, JC (eds): Unilateral Neglect: Clinical and Experimental Studies. Lawrence Erlbaum, Hove, 1993, p 87.
127. Robertson, IH, et al: Walking trajectory and hand movements in unilateral left neglect: A vestibular hypothesis. Neuropsychologia 32:1495, 1994.
128. Stanton, KM, et al: Wheelchair transfer training for right cerebral dysfunctions: An interdisciplinary approach. Arch Phys Med Rehabil 64:276, 1983.
129. Bowen, A, et al: Cognitive rehabilitation for spatial neglect following stroke (Cochrane Review). In The Cochrane Library, Issue 3. Update Software, Oxford, 2002.
130. Fanthome, Y, et al: The treatment of visual neglect using feedback of eye movements: A pilot study. Disabil Rehabil 17:413, 1995.
131. Kalra, L, et al: The influence of visual neglect on stroke rehabilitation. Stroke 28: 1386, 1997.
132. Robertson, I, et al: Microcomputer-based rehabilitation for unilateral left visual neglect: A randomised controlled trial. Arch Phys Med Rehabil 71:663, 1990.
133. Rossi, P, Kheyfets, S, and Reding, MJ: Fresnel prisms improve visual perception in stroke patients with homonymous hemianopia or unilateral visual neglect. Neurol 40:1597, 1990.
134. Wiart, L, et al: Unilateral neglect syndrome rehabilitation by trunk rotation and scanning training. Arch Phys Med Rehabil 78:424, 1997.
135. Maeshima, S, et al: Rehabilitation of patients with anosognosia for hemiplegia due to intracerebral haemorrhage. Brain Injury 11: 691, 1997.
136. Sauguet, J, et al: Disturbances of the body scheme in relation to language impairment and hemispheric locus of lesion. J Neurol Neurosurg Psychiatry 34:496, 1971.
137. Johnstone, M: Restoration of Motor Function in the Stroke Patient, ed 2. Churchill Livingstone, New York, 1983.
138. Hecaen, H, et al: The syndrome of apractagnosia due to lesions of the minor vertebral hemisphere. Arch Neurol Psychiatry 75:400, 1956.
139. Gainotti, G: Emotional behaviour and hemispheric side of the lesion. Cortex 8:41, 1972.
140. Arnadottir, G, and Gudrun, A: Evaluation and intervention with complex perceptual disorder. In Unsworth, CA (ed): Cognitive and Perceptual Dysfunction: A Clinical Reasoning Approach to Evaluation and Intervention. FA Davis, Philadelphia, 1999, p 393.
141. Edmans, JA, Webster, J, and Lincoln, NB: A comparison of two approaches in the treatment of perceptual problems after stroke. Clin Rehabil 14:230, 2000.
142. Halperin, E, and Cohen, BS: Perceptual-motor dysfunction. Stumbling block to rehabilitation. Md Med J 20:139, 1971.
143. Benton, A, and Tranel, D: Visuoperceptual, visuospatial, and visuoconstructive disorders. In Heilman, KM, and Valenstein, E (eds): Clinical Neuropsychology, ed 3. Oxford University Press, New York, 1993, p 165.
144. Ayres, JA: Southern California Sensory Integration Tests. Western Psychological Services, Los Angeles, 1972.
145. Peterson, P, and Wikoff, RL: The performance of adult males on the Southern California figure–ground visual perception test. Am J Occup Ther 37:554, 1983.
146. Anderson, E, and Choy, E: Parietal lobe syndromes in hemiplegia: A program for treatment. Am J Occup Ther 24:13, 1970.
147. Maguire, EA: The retrosplenial contribution to human navigation: A review of lesion and neuroimaging findings. Scand J Psychol 42:225, 2001.
148. Yelnik, AP, et al: Perception of verticality after recent cerebral hemispheric stroke. Stroke 33:2247, 2002.
149. Laver, AJ, and Unsworth, CA: Evaluation and intervention with simple perceptual impairment (agnosias). In Unsworth, CA (ed): Cognitive and Perceptual Dysfunction: A Clincial Reasoning Approach to Evaluation and Intervention. FA Davis, Philadelphia, 1999, p 299.
150. Wade, DT, et al: Stroke: A Critical Approach to Diagnosis. Treatment, and Management. Yearbook, Chicago, 1986.
151. Damasio, AR, Damasio, H, and van Hoesen, GW: Prosopagnosia: Anatomical basis and behavioral mechanism. Neurology 32:331, 1982.
152. Croce, R: A review of the neural basis of apractic disorders with implications for remediation. Adapt Phys Act Q 10:173, 1993.

153. Tate, R, and McDonald, S: What is apraxia? The clinician's dilemma. Neuropsychol Rehab 5:273, 1995.
154. Kirshner, H: The Apraxias. In Bradley, W, et al (eds): Neurology in Clinical Practice: Principles of Diagnosis and Management, vol 1. Butterworth-Heinmann, London, 1991, p 117.
155. Donkervoot, M, et al: Prevalence of apraxia among patients with a first left hemisphere stroke in rehabilitation centres and nursing homes. Clin Rehabil 14:130, 2000.
156. Butler, J: Evaluation and intervention with apraxia. In Unsworth, CA (ed): Cognitive and Perceptual Dysfunction: A Clincial Reasoning Approach to Evaluation and Intervention. FA Davis, Philadelphia, 1999, p 257.
157. Raade, AS, Roth, LJ, and Heilman, KM: The relationship between buccofacial and limb apraxia. Brain Cognition 16:130, 1991.
158. Mozaz, M, et al: Apraxia in a patient with lesion located in right sub-cortical area: Analysis of errors. Cortex 26:651, 1990.
159. Goodglass, H, and Kaplan, E: The Assessment of Aphasia and Related Disorders, ed 2. Lea & Febiger, Philadelphia, 1983.
160. Halsband, U, et al: The role of the pre-motor and the supplementary motor area in the temporal control of movement in man. Brain 116:243, 1993.
161. Van Heugten, CM: Assessment of disabilities in stroke patients with apraxia: Internal consistency and inter-observer reliability. Occup Ther J Res 19:55, 1999.
162. Okoye, R: The apraxias. In Abreu, BC (ed): Physical Disabilities Manual. Raven Press, New York, 1981, p 241.
163. Donkervoot, M, et al: Efficacy of strategy training in left hemisphere stroke patients with apraxia: A randomized clinical trial. Neuropsychol Rehabil 11:549, 2001.
164. De Renzi, E, and Lucchelli, F: Ideational apraxia. Brain 111:1173, 1988.
165. Mayer, NH, et al: Buttering a hot cup of coffee: An approach to the study of errors of action in patients with brain damage. In Tupper, DE, and Cicerone, KD (eds): The Neuropsychology of Everyday Life: Assessment and Basic Competencies. Kluwer, London, 1990, p 259.
166. Pedersen, PM, et al: Manual and oral apraxia in acute stroke, frequency and influence on functional outcome. Am J Phys Med Rehabil 80:685, 2001.
167. Heilman, KM, and Valenstein, E (eds): Clinical Neuropsychology, ed 4. Oxford University Press, New York, 2003.

Supplemental Readings

Banich, MT: Cognitive Neuroscience and Neuropsychology, ed 2. Houghton Mifflin, Boston, 2004.
Cohen, H (ed): Neuroscience for Rehabilitation, ed 2. Lippincott, Philadelphia, 1999.
Gravell, R, and Johnson, R (eds): Head Injury Rehabilitation: A Community Team Perspective. Whurr Publishers, London, 2002.
Ponsford, J (ed): Cognitive and Behavioral Rehabilitation: From Neurobiology to Clinical Practice. The Guilford Press, New York, 2004.
Sacks, O: The Man who Mistook his Wife for a Hat. Harper & Row, New York, 1985.
Strub, RL, and Black, FW: The Mental Status Examination in Neurology, ed 4. FA Davis, Philadelphia, 2000.
Stuss, DT, Winocur, G, and Robertson, IH (eds): Cognitive Neurorehabilitation. Cambridge University Press, Cambridge, UK, 1999.
Unsworth, C (ed): Cognitive and Perceptual Dysfunction: A Clinical Reasoning Approach to Evaluation and Intervention. FA Davis, Philadelphia, 1999.

CHAPTER

30

LEARNING OBJECTIVES

1. Explain the organization of language with respect to the role of phonological, lexical, syntactic, and semantic systems.
2. Gain an understanding of the role of the motor speech system in the speech production process.
3. Explain and characterize the classic aphasic syndromes.
4. Identify and explain the critical factors in the evaluation of the recovery and rehabilitation of aphasia.
5. Identify and describe general approaches to aphasia rehabilitation and some specific treatment methods.
6. Describe the primary types of dysarthria and rationales for dysarthria treatment.
7. Describe speech apraxia and its treatment.
8. Gain an understanding of neurogenic swallowing disorder.
9. Describe the goals and rationales for the use of augmentative communication systems.

Neurogenic Disorders of Speech and Language

Martha Taylor Sarno, MA, MD (hon)

OUTLINE

Most people take the ability to produce and understand speech for granted and pay little attention to the nature and function of the processes involved in communication. Yet speech, like tool making, sets us apart from animals and is one of our most human behaviors. Even in primitive societies, humans have used the oral–motor speech code to share experiences, ideas, and feelings. Not all communities have developed writing and reading systems.

The use of speech for communication contributes to our identity as human beings and to the perception of "self." As a result, disruptions in the ability to communicate, whether caused by structural abnormalities (e.g., cleft palate), neurological conditions (e.g., stroke, Parkinson's disease), or nonorganic conditions (e.g., nonorganic articulatory disorders) may impact on a person's daily life in important ways. For some, the acquisition of a communication disorder may have sufficient impact to cause an individual to withdraw from the workforce. For those whose communication disorders have persisted since childhood, the disorder may represent a significant vocational handicap. In other cases, a disorder that does not impede an individual's vocational life nonetheless interferes with everyday socialization. Communication disorders are complex, multifaceted behavioral impairments often associated so closely with a person's self-image as to threaten the quality of his or her life.

The term **communication** encompasses all of the behaviors, including speech, that human beings use to transmit information and interact with others. Speech comprises a delicate and rapid sequence of sensory and motor events requiring the coordinated activity of several parts of the body. The use of speech for communication involves many levels of human activity, ranging from the fine motor coordination of components of the oral–motor system to the subtle shades of meaning that occur at the cognitive/semantic level. Gestures, pantomime, and other nonverbal *pragmatic language* behaviors, such as turn taking, are also essential elements of communication.

Among unimpaired speakers, speech behavior varies greatly, yet the oral–motor system is efficient for the exchange of even complicated information. The range of variability is so wide that individuals generally produce different sound waves with different characteristics even when producing the same word. But listeners do not rely solely on information derived from speech waves. We also depend on cues, which are components of what is referred to as *context*. Context includes aspects of a communicative exchange such as the purpose of the activity, the location of the exchange, the knowledge of the participants, the roles of each participant, and the level of formality required by the situation.

This chapter addresses the neurogenic disorders of communication, a category of communication disorders represented by the majority of patients receiving speech–language pathology services in rehabilitation medicine programs. The most common of these disorders are **aphasia**, a language disorder, and **dysarthria**, a motor–speech disorder.

The field of speech–language pathology, which came into being in 1925 with the establishment of the American Speech–Language–Hearing Association (ASHA), is dedicated to the diagnosis and treatment of individuals with congenital or acquired disorders of speech and language. Communication disorders exact a large economic toll, costing the United States economy an estimated $30 billion a year in lost productivity, special education costs, and medical costs. The National Institute on Deafness and Other Communication Disorders (NIDCD) estimated the number of individuals in the United States with a speech, voice, or language disorder at 14 million.[1] Approximately 28 million Americans have a hearing loss. Fifty-five percent of those with hearing impairments are older than 65 years of age and 12 out of every 1000 children younger than 18 has a hearing impairment.[2,3]

In the population older than the age of 65, 10.8 percent have speech and language disorders, whereas among those younger than 45 years of age, 9.9 percent have speech and language disorders. The largest population of communication impaired are children with language disorders (43.7 percent) and *articulation disorders* (32.1 percent).[1] Aphasia affects approximately 15 percent of the adult speech–language impaired population.[4]

The speech–language pathology profession has grown rapidly. Affiliates (members and certificate holders) in the American Speech–Language–Hearing Association increased from 1623 to 35,000 between 1950 and 1980. Speech–language pathology is a master's degree entry field and more than 85 percent of all states require a license to practice. The ASHA awards the Certificate of Clinical Competence (CCC) to speech–language pathologists who meet specified academic and clinical experience requirements, which includes a Clinical Fellowship Year (CFY). Today, there are over 100,000 speech–language pathologists certified by ASHA, of whom more than 95.6 percent are female. Health care facilities account for about 35.5 percent of the settings in which certified speech–language pathologists are employed with 14.1 percent working in hospital settings.[5] The term *speech–language pathologist* is the official designation of professionals in the field who hold the CCC. The term *speech therapist,* although no longer considered professionally appropriate, is a term that is often used informally.

In order that the presence and degree of speech or language pathology manifested by a given person can be identified and measured, his or her performance must be compared with a standard of "normal." One may choose as the standard (1) the language common to the cultural community of unimpaired persons in which the patient lives, in which case an individual's verbal function would be compared with that of others in the same community of similar age, gender, education, and achievement, or (2) the patient's verbal behavior prior to the onset of illness or trauma. The latter will vary from individual to individual and is based on premorbid educational achievement, specific cultural characteristics, personality, and other factors. A patient is verbally impaired when he or she deviates in any parameter of language and/or speech processing from the "normal" communication behavior of the community in which he or she functioned premorbidly.

A "normal" standard is implied in the terms *impairment, disability,* and *handicap*. In 1980, the World Health Organization (WHO) presented a classification schema that distinguished among the terms: *impairment* is the pathology itself (its location, measured size, and so forth); *disability* is the consequence of an impairment and its impact on everyday personal, social, and vocational life; and *handicap* is the value the individual, family, and community place on the disability and the degree to which the individual is disadvantaged.[6] In 2001, the classification was revised. The term disability was replaced by *activities,* defined as the nature and extent of functioning; and handicap was replaced by *participation,* defined as a person's involvement in life situations.[7]

The Organization of Language

When an individual generates an idea that he or she wants to express, it is transformed into words and sentences by calling into play certain physiological and acoustic events. The message is converted into linguistic form at the listener's end. The listener, in turn, fits the auditory information into a sequence of words and sentences that are ultimately understood.

We refer to the system of symbols that are strung together into sentences expressing our thoughts and the understanding of those messages as *language*. In the first few years of life, infants and children gain a great deal of practice and experience in the use of language, until it becomes habitual and is used without conscious awareness.

Phonology refers to the study of the sound system of language. Words are made up of speech sounds or *phonemes,* which are generally classified as either *vowels* or *consonants*. Phonemes in and of themselves do not symbolize ideas or objects, but when put together they are the basic linguistic units that make words. Words comprise the *lexicon,* or vocabulary, of a language. In English, there are 16 vowels and 22 consonants, which are combined into larger units called *syllables*.

There are between 1000 and 2000 syllables in English, which usually consist of a vowel as a central phoneme surrounded by one or more consonants. Most languages have their own rules about how phonemes may be combined into larger units. For example, in English, syllables never start with the *ng* phoneme. The most frequently used words in English are sequences of from two to five phonemes. Some have as many as 10 phonemes or as few as 1. Generally, however, the most frequently used words have few phonemes. New words are added to the English language every day, even though only a small number of phoneme combinations are possible. Although there are several hundred thousand English words, we use a repertoire of only about 5000 to 10,000 words 95 percent of the time.

The grammar, or *syntax,* of a language determines the sequence of words that are acceptable in the formation of sentences. In English, for example, it is possible to say "The black box is on the table," but the sequence "Box black table on the" is unacceptable. Another example is "The old radio played well," is syntactically correct but "Old the well played radio" is not. The sentence, "The boy walked to the store" is meaningful, but the sentence, "The book walked to the store" is not. The language system that refers to the meanings of words is called *semantics.*

In addition to the phonological (sounds), lexical (vocabulary), syntactical (grammar), and semantic (meaning) systems of a language, we also utilize *prosody* (stress and intonation) to help make distinctions between questions, statements, expressions of emotional feelings, shock, exclamations, and so forth.

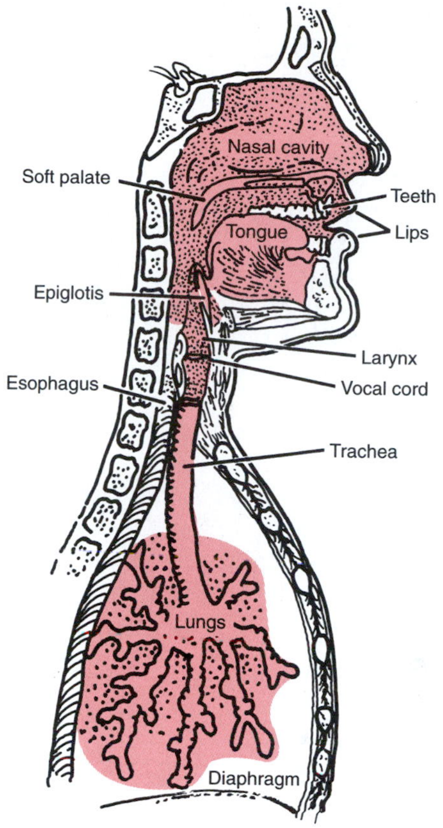

Figure 30.1 The human vocal organ.

Speech Production

The speech organs consist of the lungs, trachea, larynx (which contains the vocal cords), pharynx, nose, and mouth. When considered together, these organs comprise a "tube" referred to as the *vocal tract,* which extends from the lungs to the lips. Vocal tract shape is varied by moving the tongue, lips, and any other parts of the tract. Changes in the configuration of the vocal tract act to modify the aerodynamic qualities of the air stream during speech (Fig. 30.1)

The primary function of the vocal organs relates to basic life-sustaining functions such as breathing and swallowing. These organs not only take on different roles for speech, but function differently when engaged in speech production. For example, breathing for life-sustaining purposes is far more rapid than for speech production. A full cycle inhalation/exhalation takes approximately 5 seconds, whereas during speech we control the breathing rate according to the demands of the words and sentences we are producing, sometimes reducing the rate of breathing to as little as 15 percent devoted to inhalation. This is dictated in part by the fact that, when speaking, we generally take in enough air to vocalize a complete thought and we exhale the air gradually during the articulation of the thought.

The steady stream of air exhaled from the lungs is the source of energy for speech production, which is made audible by the rapid vibration of the vocal cords. During speech, we continuously alter the shape of the vocal tract by moving the tongue, lips, and other parts of the system. By moving parts of the vocal tract, thereby modifying its acoustic properties, we are able to produce the different sounds. That is, by altering the shape of the vocal tract upon *phonation,* we transform the air stream into a resonance chamber (Figs. 30.2 and 30.3).

The *larynx* acts as a barrier to prevent food from entering the trachea and lungs by closing automatically during the act of swallowing, which is also helped by the action of the epiglottis. By opening and closing the flow of air from the lungs, the larynx acts as a valve between the lungs and the mouth. The laryngeal valve also acts to lock air into the lungs, which we do automatically when we perform heavy work with our upper extremities. The larynx is not a fixed, rigid organ but, because of its cartilaginous construction and corresponding connecting muscles and ligaments moves up and down during both swallowing and speaking.

The *vocal cords* extend on either side of the larynx from the Adam's apple at the front to the arytenoid cartilages at

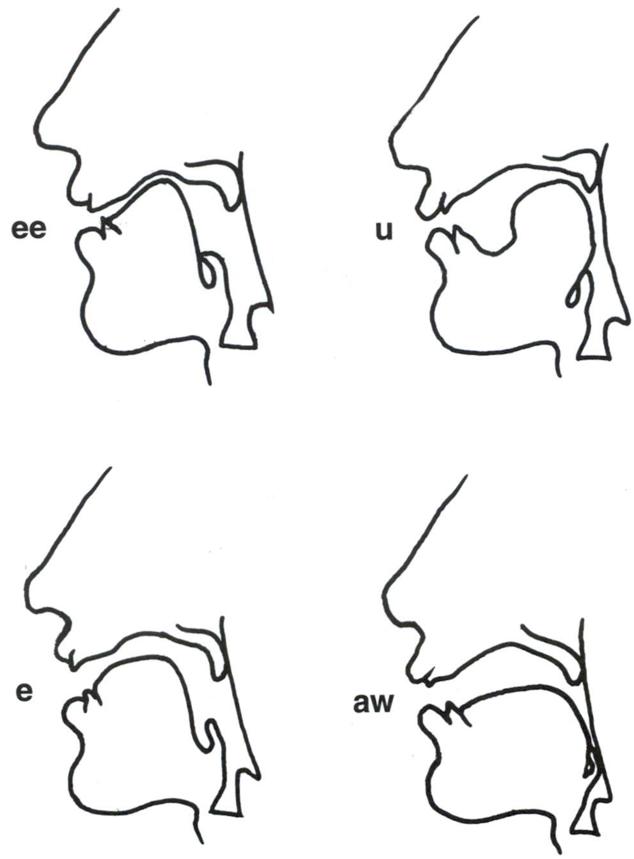

Figure 30.2 Outlines of the vocal tract during articulation of various vowels.

the back. We refer to the space between the vocal cords as the *glottis*. When the cords are pressed together, the passage of air is sealed off and the valve is shut. Because the cords are held together at the front where they articulate with the Adam's apple, the open glottis is V-shaped, opening only at the back. When we speak, we vibrate the vocal cords in a rhythmic fashion, opening and closing the air passage from the lungs to the oral/nasal cavities.

The frequency of sound produced by the vocal cords is directly related to their mass, tension, and length. We alter the tension and length of the vocal cords continuously while speaking. In normal speech, the range of vocal cord frequencies is from about 60 to 350 cycles per second (cps). Most people use a vocal cord frequency range that covers about one and a half octaves.

The *pharynx* is the area of the vocal tract connecting the larynx with the nose and mouth. We isolate the nasal cavity from the pharynx and back of the mouth by raising the soft palate. The most adjustable component of the vocal tract is the mouth, whose shape and size can be modified more than any other organ of the oral–motor system by changing the relative position of the palate, tongue, lips, and teeth. The lips are rounded, spread, or closed to alter the shape and length of the vocal tract or to stop airflow. The teeth and their relationship to the lips or tongue tip change the airflow. An important component of the teeth ridge is the *alveolus*, which is the area covered by the gums.

The term *articulation* refers to the articulating, or "meeting," of the various organs of the oral-pharyngeal cavity to produce the sounds of speech. Speech *intelligibility* refers to how a person "sounds" when speaking. A number of factors can influence judgments of intelligibility such as the presence or absence of visual cues or of extraneous movements (i.e., tremor). The precision of the production of consonant sounds is one of the primary factors that contributes to speech intelligibility. Consonants are described by specifying their place and manner of articulation and whether they are voiced or unvoiced (Table 30.1). The "places" of articulation are the lips (labial), teeth, gums (alveolar), palate, and glottis. The *manner of articulation* refers to the plosive, fricative, nasal, liquid, and semivowel categories.

Plosive sounds, sometimes referred to as "stop" sounds, are those produced by building up air pressure in the oral cavity and suddenly releasing it (e.g., *p, t*). The blockage can occur by pressing the lips together or by pressing the tongue against either the gums or soft palate. There are plosive consonants that are labial, alveolar, or velar.

Fricatives are produced by making the air turbulent (e.g., *f, v*). Most consonants are produced with the soft

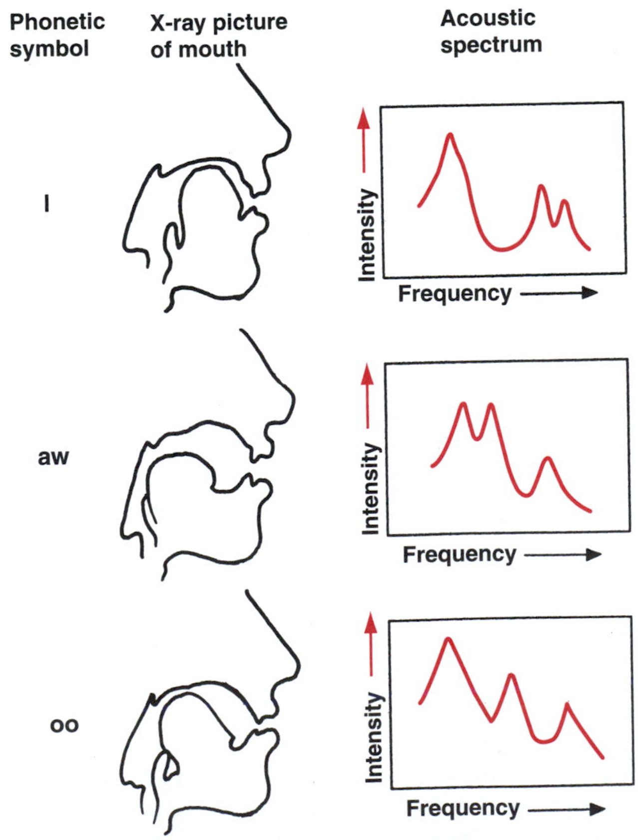

Figure 30.3 Vocal tract configuration and corresponding spectra for three different vowels. The peaks of the spectra represent vocal tract resonances. The vertical lines for individual harmonics are not shown.

Table 30.1 Classification of English Consonants by Place and Manner of Articulation

Place of Articulation	Manner of Articulation				
	Plosive	Fricative	Semivowel	Liquids (including laterals)	Nasal
Labial	p b	—	w	—	m
Labiodental	—	f v	—	—	—
Dental	—	θ th	—	—	—
Alveolar	t d	s z	y	l r	n
Palatal	—	sh zh	—	—	—
Velar	kg	—	—	—	ng
Glottal	—	h	—	—	—

palate raised, thereby closing off the flow of air to the nasal cavity, except for the *nasals* (e.g., *m, n, ng*), which are made by lowering the soft palate and blocking the oral cavity somewhere along its length. *Liquids* are sounds made with the soft palate raised: /r/, /l/.

Semivowels refer to those sounds produced by maintaining the vocal tract in a vowel-like position, then changing the position rapidly for the vowel that follows (e.g., *w, y*).

Speech sounds are affected by their *context,* that is, the sounds that immediately precede or follow. A speech sound wave is a continuous event rather than a sequence of discrete segments. The identification of a speech sound depends on relating acoustic features of the sound wave at different points in time.

A standard reference for the quality of vowels is the eight cardinal vowels (Fig. 30.4). This schema of the positions of the tongue for the production of the vowels of the language help us to visualize the tongue's movements during speech. It is, in a sense, a map of the tongue positions for vowel production. Tongue placement is described by specifying the location of the main body of the tongue at its highest point. For example, for the sound /ee/ as in the word *beat,* the tongue tip is pointed in a high frontal configuration, whereas for the sound /ah/ as in the word *father,* the highest point of the tongue is low and posterior in the oral cavity.

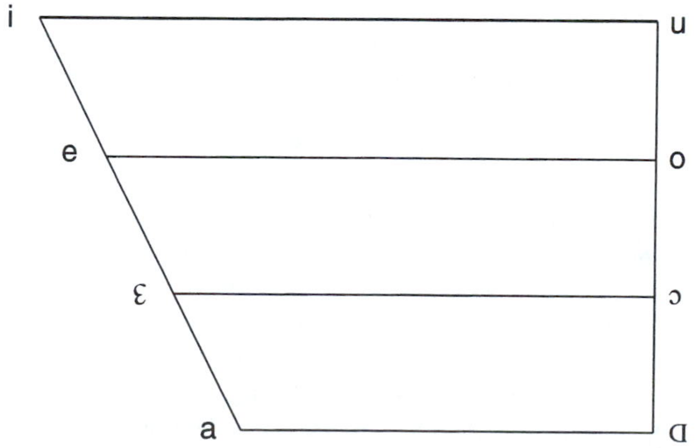

Figure 30.4 The cardinal vowels represented as a vowel quadrilateral. The cardinal vowels are extremely placed reference points for vowel articulation. Vowels on the same horizontal line are believed to have an equally high tongue height while vowels in the left–right position are assumed to be equally backed and fronted. (Adapted from Ladefoged, P: A Course in Phonetics. Harcourt Brace Jovanovich, New York, 1975, with permission.)

All vowel sounds and some consonant sounds are *voiced.* That is, the vocal cords vibrate during their production. When a sound is produced without vocal cord vibration, we say that it is *unvoiced* (e.g., *p, s*). Table 30.1 shows that many consonant sounds are articulated in the same manner, and differ only with respect to voicing (e.g., *p-b; s-z; f-v; k-g*).

Speech behavior comprises a complex motor event that goes well beyond the skilled movements required of the oral–motor system. Yet we produce speech without thinking about it, even while simultaneously involved in other activities. However, to transform thought into speech takes some voluntary, conscious behavior that allows us to take information stored in memory and translate it into a coherent production of words and utterances that follow certain grammatical rules.

In addition to its linguistic aspects, neurogenic communication disorders often involve coexisting mild to severe cognitive deficits that may not only aggravate the communication disorder but also make it difficult to differentiate cognitive from communication deficits. Although the communication disorder manifests in patients with right brain damage will not be addressed in this chapter, it is an example of a disorder in which the cognitive component is a major issue.

The importance of the communication process and its underlying systems becomes apparent when we consider the two most common neurogenic communication disorders: *aphasia* and *dysarthria.* This chapter focuses primarily on aphasia and dysarthria and will also consider verbal apraxia, dysphagia, and the use of augmentative/alternate systems of communication.

Aphasia

The proportion of persons older than 65 years of age is projected to reach 21 to 22 percent of the total population by the year 2050.[8] It is estimated that there are more than 1 million individuals with aphasia in the United States alone[9,10] and that there are approximately 84,000 new patients with aphasia in the United States each year, most of whom desire treatment.[11] The majority are older than 65 years of age and acquired aphasia as a result of a stroke. A smaller number are the consequence of head trauma and neoplasms. Aphasia is also frequently present in the early stages of Alzheimer's disease. It was estimated that the cost of speech–language aphasia in the 1969 calendar year was $13.2 million.[12] This number has probably tripled in the intervening years.

Classification and Nomenclature

In this chapter, the term **aphasia** refers to the acquired communication disorder that is manifest in individuals who were previously capable of using language appropriately. It does not refer to those developmental language disorders that may be present in individuals who never developed normal language and for whom the ability to use language may never reach age-appropriate performance levels.

In acquired aphasia, central nervous system disease or trauma compromises certain structures in a focal rather than generalized fashion. The study of the neuroanatomical correlates of the aphasias has engaged neurologists since the late nineteenth century, and the correlation between aphasic syndromes and cerebral localization is relatively consistent. However, recent advances in neuroradiological technology have made aphasia localization a subject of increased research.

Aphasiologists generally agree that there are distinct major aphasic syndromes that adhere to specific profiles of impairment. This is not surprising, because the lesions that produce aphasia, particularly in the patient with cerebrovascular disease, tend to be located in brain loci that are especially vulnerable. It is not always possible, however, to classify patients according to these syndromes. Estimates of the proportion of cases that can be unambiguously classified range from 30 to 80 percent.[13]

The characteristics of an individual's speech production are used to determine aphasia classification. Speech output that is characterized as hesitant, awkward, interrupted, and produced with effort is referred to as *nonfluent aphasia* in contrast to speech output that is facile in articulation, produced at a normal rate, with preserved flow and melody, and is referred to as *fluent aphasia*. Fluency judgments are made during extended conversation with a patient and are defined as follows.

Fluent aphasia is characterized by impaired auditory comprehension and fluent speech that is of normal rate and melody. Fluent aphasia is usually associated with a lesion in the vicinity of the posterior portion of the first temporal gyrus of the left hemisphere. When fluent aphasia is severe, word and sound substitutions may be of such magnitude and frequency that speech may be rendered meaningless. Patients with fluent aphasia tend to have greatest difficulty in retrieving those words that are substantive (nouns and verbs). They also tend to have some degree of impaired awareness and are rarely physically disabled, because their lesions are located in the posterior portion of the brain, distant from motor areas. There are several types of syndromes subsumed under the fluent aphasia classification (Table 30.2).

Nonfluent aphasia is characterized by limited vocabulary, slow, hesitant speech, some awkward articulation, and restricted use of grammar in the presence of relatively preserved auditory comprehension. Nonfluent aphasia is associated with anterior lesions usually involving the third frontal convolution of the left hemisphere. Patients with nonfluent aphasia tend to express themselves in vocabulary that is substantive (nouns, verbs) and lack the ability to retrieve less substantive parts of speech (prepositions, conjunctions, pronouns). Patients with nonfluent aphasia tend to have good awareness of their deficit and usually have impaired motor function on the right side (right hemiplegia–paresis).

A severe aphasia with marked dysfunction across all language modalities and with severely limited residual use of all communication modes for oral–aural interactions is referred to as *global aphasia*. Global aphasia is not a type of aphasia but rather a designation of severity. The patient with global aphasia generally has extensive damage, which may be anywhere in the left hemisphere, and is sometimes bilateral.[14] Global aphasia has been cited as among the most common type of aphasia in patients referred for speech rehabilitation services.[15,16]

The most common category of fluent aphasia is *Wernicke's aphasia* (also referred to as sensory aphasia and/or receptive aphasia). Wernicke's aphasia is usually the result of a lesion in the posterior portion of the first temporal gyrus of the left hemisphere. It is characterized by impaired auditory comprehension and fluently articulated speech marked by word substitutions. Reading and writing are usually severely impaired as well. Although patients with Wernicke's aphasia may produce what seem like complete utterances and use complex verb tenses, they often add a word or phrase and "augment" speech production. They may also speak at a rate greater than normal. Although the production of speech sounds is generally precise, patients with Wernicke's aphasia may reverse phonemes and/or syllables (hopspipal/trevilision) and may produce *neologisms* (nonsense words).

Table 30.2 Classification by Aphasia Syndromes

	Wernicke's Aphasia	Broca's Aphasia	Global Aphasia	Conduction Aphasia	Anomic Aphasia	Transcortical Motor Aphasia	Pure Word Deafness
Area of infarction	Posterior portion of temporal gyrus	Third frontal convolution	Third frontal convolution and posterior portion of superior temporal gyrus	Parietal operculum or posterior superior temporal gyrus	Angular gyrus	Supplementary motor areas	Both Heschl's gyri or connection between Heschl's gyrus and posterior superior temporal gyrus
Spontaneous speech	Fluent	Nonfluent	Nonfluent	Fluent or nonfluent	Fluent	Nonfluent	Fluent
Comprehension	Poor	Good	Poor	Good	Good	Good	Poor
Repetition	Poor	Poor (but may be better than spontaneous speech)	Poor	Very poor	Good	Excellent	Poor
Naming	Poor	Poor (but may be better than spontaneous speech)	Poor	Poor	Very poor	Poor	Good
Reading comprehension	Poor	Good	Poor	Good to poor	Good to poor	Good	Good
Writing	Poor	Poor	Poor	Poor	Good to poor	Poor	Good

Wernicke's aphasia may evolve into anomic aphasia in the course of recovery. *Anomic aphasia* is characterized by a significant word finding difficulty in the context of fluent, grammatically well-formed speech. Auditory comprehension is relatively preserved for most speaking situations. Speech output may be somewhat vague and the patient may be proficient in producing *circumlocutions* to skirt the lack of specificity of language use.

Broca's aphasia is a nonfluent type of aphasia also referred to as expressive aphasia, motor aphasia, and/or verbal aphasia. Broca's aphasia is the result of a lesion involving the third frontal convolution of the left hemisphere, the subcortical white matter, and extending posteriorly to the inferior portion of the motor strip (precentral gyrus). It is characterized by awkward articulation, restricted vocabulary, and restriction to simple grammatical forms in the presence of a relative preservation of auditory comprehension. Writing skills generally mirror the pattern of speech. Reading may be less impaired than speech and writing. The patient may be limited to one and two word productions for expression and find it impossible to combine words into sentences. Articulation may be awkward and effortful (see the section on Verbal Apraxia). Nonfluent Broca's aphasia is rarely found in aphasia after traumatic brain injury (TBI). Anomic disturbances predominate in aphasia secondary to TBI. In children, aphasia after TBI is generally characterized by a reduction of output with hesitancy, difficulty initiating speech, and sometimes mutism.[17]

Many measures of aphasia and related disorders have been developed for use in both clinical and research settings. In an inpatient setting, patients with aphasia are generally screened at bedside. The purpose of a bedside screening is to obtain a general idea of a patient's profile of deficits and preserved areas of language function as a basis for recommendations for more comprehensive testing and possible rehabilitation. Obviously, screening tests have limited value because they offer few details about the type and severity of aphasic deficits that lead to a syndrome classification. An important purpose of a comprehensive examination is to provide a baseline measure against which to gauge progress in the course of rehabilitation.

Aphasia Measures

Comprehensive language tests designed to measure aphasic impairment generally contain specific domains of performance. In addition to the general requirements for the construction of tests, such as reliability, standardization, and demonstrated validity, certain factors are considered important in the design of tests intended to identify and measure aphasia. These include range of item difficulty, use in measuring recovery, and ability to contribute to diagnostic classification. [18,19] Aphasia tests are generally based on examinations of linguistic task performance and at a minimum include tasks of visual confrontation *naming;* a spontaneous or conversational *speech sample* that is analyzed for fluency of output, effort, articulation, phrase length, prosody, word substitutions, and omissions; *repetition* of digits, single words, multisyllable words, and sentences of increasing length and complexity; *comprehension of spoken language* of single words, of sentences that require only yes–no responses, and pointing on command; *word retrieval* (word finding) measuring the ability to generate words beginning with a particular letter of the alphabet or in a particular semantic category (animals); *reading;* and *writing* from dictation and spontaneously. Some widely used aphasia measures include the *Boston Diagnostic Aphasia Examination (BDAE)*,[13] the *Neurosensory Center Comprehensive Examination for Aphasia (NCCEA)*,[20] and the *Western Aphasia Battery*.[21]

In addition to the measurement of performance on specific linguistic tasks, an aphasia examination also requires supplementary measures of *functional communication*. This is necessary because an individual's actual use of language in everyday life may not correspond to the degree of pathology measured by specific language task performance.[22,23] Functional communication measures are usually produced in the form of rating scales with high interrater reliability. The *Functional Communication Profile (FCP)*.[24,25] *Communicative Activities of Daily Living (CADL)*,[26] and ASHA's *Functional Assessment of Communication Skills (ASHA FACS)*,[27] which have high interrater reliability, are widely used for this purpose.

Historical Perspective

Language disturbances were recorded as early as 3500 BC and attempts to "retrain" individuals with aphasia have been recorded throughout history.[28] Some of the first documented cases of both natural recovery and intervention were the patients of Nicolo Massa and Francisco Arceo in 1558.[29]

In a landmark paper in the late nineteenth century, "Du siège de la faculté du langage articulé," Paul Broca was one of the first to discuss the possibility of retraining in aphasia.[30] Dr. Charles K. Mills was the first to address recovery and rehabilitation in aphasia in an English-language publication. He reported the training of a patient with post-stroke aphasia whom he and Donald Broadbent treated, using methods largely determined by the patient, who began by systematically repeating letters, words, and phrases.[31,32] Mills's observations and approach to aphasia rehabilitation, published over a century ago, are remarkably similar to much present-day practice and thought. Mills noted that not all patients benefit from retraining to the same degree and acknowledged that spontaneous recovery might have an influence on the course and extent of recovery.

World War I and its brain-injured combat survivors led to the establishment of treatment centers where patients with posttraumatic aphasia were treated, especially in Europe. Reports of aphasia rehabilitation experiences during and after the war in England and the United States were also published.[33,34] One of the most comprehensive descriptions of the systematic treatment of a large number of patients with brain injuries, of whom 90 to 100 were followed for a 10-year period, was provided by Kurt Goldstein in Frankfurt during the Second World War.[35]

Until World War II, reports of retraining civilians with post-stroke aphasia were rare. The aphasia literature was based almost exclusively on posttraumatic aphasia. In 1933, Singer and Low reported the case of a 39-year-old woman who suffered an apparent vascular infarct after a full-term delivery and showed continuous language improvement with consistent training over a 10-year period.[36]

In a landmark 5-year study supported by the Commonwealth Fund, Weisenburg and McBride addressed the general topic of aphasia and commented on the effectiveness of reeducation.[37] The study concerned 60 patients who were younger than 60 years of age, a majority of whom had suffered strokes, and concluded that reeducation increased the rate of recovery, assisted in facilitating the use of compensatory means of communication, and improved morale. Their work also documented the psychotherapeutic benefits of treatment.

Aphasia and its concomitant neurological deficits in the patient with stroke were generally viewed as natural and necessary components of the aging process in the period before World War II. The treatment of aphasia in the civilian population was not considered an option.

Many variables had an influence on making the treatment of aphasia the common practice that it is today. The advent of speech pathology as a health profession, the emergence of rehabilitation medicine as a medical specialty, the mass media explosion, a larger and more affluent middle class, an increase in the life span, the number of stroke and brain injury survivors, and public expectations of medicine in the age of technology are among them. The last has been particularly true in the industrialized world, where it is widely believed that there is a treatment for every human ill.[38]

Journals devoted to brain/language issues have become indispensable information sources for aphasiologists (e.g., *Aphasiology, Brain and Language,* and *Cortex*). The Academy of Aphasia, a scholarly society dedicated to the study of aphasia, was established in 1962. The National Aphasia Association (NAA) was founded in the United States in 1987 for the purpose of providing information to the public about aphasia, advocating for the aphasic community, and encouraging the establishment of support groups called Aphasia Community Groups (ACGs).[39]

Several informational publications designed for use by the families and friends of patients with aphasia also appeared in the period following World War II.[40–45] One of these, "Understanding Aphasia," is still widely read and has been published in 12 languages.[45]

Evaluation of Recovery

If complete recovery from aphasia is to occur, it usually happens within a matter of hours or days following onset. Once aphasia has persisted for several weeks or months, a complete return to a premorbid state is usually the exception.

Most patients do not consider themselves recovered unless they have fully recovered to previous levels of language performance.[38,46] When unrecovered patients are satisfied with their level of competence and consider themselves recovered, this is a psychological perception and should not be confused with an objective evaluation of communication abilities. The true test of aphasia rehabilitation outcome is the patients' perception of the quality of their lives. Measures of life function that include activity levels, socialization, mobility, and community reintegration can be used for this purpose.[47,48]

It is useful to distinguish between two separate recovery dimensions in aphasia: one that is objective and attempts to quantify the extent to which the patient has regained language abilities; and a second, which in humanistic terms may be more important, that measures the recovery of functional communication.

The concept of a functional dimension of communication behavior emerged logically from the experience of treating patients with aphasia in the rehabilitation medicine setting. Historically, rehabilitation medicine has acknowledged that the ability of patients to function in their daily lives (activities of daily living [ADL]), does not necessarily correlate with the extent of physical disability. Improvement in quantitative measures of language performance does not necessarily correlate with improvement in functional communication.[38]

Efficacy of Treatment in Post-Stroke Aphasia

Many methodological problems have limited the number of studies that examine the efficacy of aphasia rehabilitation.[49–55] Nevertheless, treatment accountability issues are compelling and a focus of professional concern.

Studies that investigate treatment effects, specific techniques, and approaches have been reported since the late 1950s.[56] Vignolo,[57] Hagen,[58] and Basso et al[59,60] have utilized untreated control and treated groups and shown a treatment effect. The work of Shewan and Kertesz[61] and Poeck et al[62] with treated and untreated groups has also yielded positive treatment effects. Variables such as spontaneous recovery,[63–65] age,[66,67] duration and treatment intensity,[52] and specific treatment techniques[68,69] have been studied.

Although studies have varied methodologically and by research focus, the results provide strong indication for positive treatment effects. Some have maintained that single case studies rather than randomized, controlled trials are the most appropriate method for addressing treatment efficacy.[70,71] A single case approach to the study of aphasia treatment efficacy has not escaped criticism but is far less frequent than criticism of studies based on groups of people with aphasia.[55] Negative views of the group study model are based primarily on the view that individuals are unique especially with respect to communication behavior.

Recently the Academy of Neurologic Communication Disorders and Sciences (ANCDS) has been engaged in an effort to develop evidence based practice guidelines for neurogenic communication disorders.[72,73] At this writing the ANCDS initiative is still in progress and the speech–language pathology profession continues to depend on meta-analyses of efficacy studies reported for 45 studies published between 1946 and 1988 and for 55 studies that support better clinical outcome for patients who received early, intensive treatment.[74,75]

Recovery

Aphasia is most often of sudden onset as the result of a stroke or head trauma. Generally some degree of natural recovery takes place in the majority of patients with or without intervention in the period immediately following onset. However, there is a lack of consensus about the duration of the *spontaneous recovery* period.[76–78] Culton reported rapid spontaneous language recovery in the first month following the onset of aphasia.[79] A number of studies have concluded that the greatest improvement occurs in the first 2 to 3 months post-onset.[57,59,63,79,81] Butfield and Zangwill,[82] Sands et al,[83] and Vignolo[57] found that the recovery rate dropped significantly after 6 months. Others have reported that spontaneous recovery does not occur after 6 months[55] or 1 year.[59,79] Sarno and Levita[84] reported that the greater change took place within a 3-month than a 6-month post-onset period in a sample of patients with severe aphasia seen up to 6 months after strokes.

In a survey of 850 patients following acute stroke (within the past month), aphasia was present in 177 patients during the acute phase. In the four to twelve weeks following the stroke, aphasia improved in 74 percent of the patients and cleared in 44 percent.[11]

An exception to the possible occurrence of spontaneous recovery exists in the case of *primary progressive aphasia (PPA),* a condition first described in 1982 which has become a diagnostic category.[85] PPA is a slowly progressive isolated aphasia which has been described sufficiently to be considered a distinct clinical–behavioral entity. It can exist in the absence or relative absence of generalized cognitive impairment.[86,87] It generally begins as a difficulty with a particular language function (e.g., naming) which gradually worsens over a period of at least 2 years before cognitive deficits begin to become evident.

Investigators who have addressed prognostic factors in aphasia recovery have generally concluded that factors such as age, gender, and handedness do not affect recovery from aphasia.[88,89]

In the healthy aged, language performance declines significantly between the seventh and eighth decades. Comprehension performance begins to decline in the sixth decade and continues through the eighth decade.[90–92] Although age has been reported as a significant prognostic factor[57,90,93,94] many do not support this view.[59,67,88,95–98] The wide discrepancy regarding the influence of age in the aphasia recovery literature may relate to differences in sampling and methodology. Gender does not appear to have an important influence on outcome[88,99,103] while handedness may have an effect.[100]

It is generally agreed that posttraumatic aphasia has a better prognosis than aphasia secondary to vascular lesions.[57,82] In fact, some cases of aphasia secondary to TBI have been reported to recover completely.[63,101] The finding that traumatic aphasia carries a better prognosis than vascular aphasia may be influenced by the fact that patients involved in traumatic events are generally neurologically healthy whereas patients who have had strokes may have widespread vascular involvement.[88]

Both type and severity of aphasia appear to carry predictive value, with global aphasia having the poorest prognosis.[60,102–104] Basso reported that when patients with fluent and nonfluent aphasia of the same severity were compared, there were no differences in degree of recovery. In 881 consecutive acute stroke admissions to a community-based hospital, it was possible to make valid prognoses within one to four weeks after stroke depending on the initial severity of aphasia.[88]

The majority of investigators report that patients with severe aphasia do not recover as well as those with mild aphasia.[52,63,83,102,104] Sarno and Levita found that people with fluent aphasia reached the highest level of functional communication, whereas patients with nonfluent and global aphasia made smaller gains in the 8- to 52-week post-stroke period.[103] Global aphasia sometimes evolves to severe Broca's aphasia when there is significantly improved comprehension. Broca's aphasia may become *anomic aphasia,* and Wernicke's aphasia may evolve to anomic or *conduction aphasia.*[63,102–106] When patients with aphasia recover a great deal of language function they are usually left with residual *anomia.*

Patients whose computed tomography (CT) scans show large dominant hemisphere lesions, many small lesions, or bilateral lesions are less likely to recover than those with smaller or fewer lesions.[46,102] Lesions in Wernicke's area or those that extend more posteriorly tend to lead to severe and persistent aphasia. The neuroradiological correlates of aphasia recovery have been addressed by some investigators.[81,107] Yarnell et al reported little prognostic value in angiographic and radioscintigram findings.[46] Similarly, CT scans did not help in predicting who might profit from language retraining in a Norwegian study.[77]

Comprehension tends to recover to a greater degree than expression.[16,57,80,108–110] Educational level or occupational status before illness does not always correlate with recovery; however, Sarno and Levita reported that aphasic individuals who were employed at the time of stroke recovered more than those who were unemployed.[84]

The presence of depression, anxiety, and paranoia have been cited as negative factors in recovery.[111–113] Premorbid personality traits have been identified as important prognostic factors. Eisenson and Herrmann felt that patients with outgoing personalities had a better prognosis than those with introverted, dependent, or rigid personalities.[114–116]

It is the general consensus that language gains in aphasia take place earlier rather than later, and that time since onset is an important recovery variable.[103,117–121]

Psychological and Related Factors

Psychological factors such as depression, anxiety, premorbid personality, fatigue, and paranoia are often cited as deterrents to recovery and communication. The social isolation experienced by people with aphasia and their families has a profound impact on their quality of life.[54] The effect of aphasia on the individual's sense of "self" is often extremely negative, leading to a loss of self-esteem and feelings of helplessness. The opportunity for "healing conversation," so essential to individuals who have suffered losses, is often unavailable to those with aphasia. Deep depression is frequently the result of this combination. The influence of these psychosocial variables is usually negative and is believed to be considerable.

Treatment of Aphasia

Literally hundreds of specific treatment techniques are cited in the aphasia literature. Aphasia treatment is rarely the same in any two settings. The lack of therapeutic uniformity has undoubtedly impeded carefully controlled studies on the effects of language retraining. Most methods derive essentially from traditional pedagogic practices, relying heavily on repetition.[121]

The primary assumption in treatment of aphasia is that language in the brain is not "erased," but that retrieval of its individual units has been impaired. Approaches to aphasia therapy have generally followed one of two models: a *substitute skill model* or a *direct treatment model,* both of which are based on the assumption that the processes that subserve normal performance need to be understood if treatment is to succeed.[122] An example of the *substitute skill model* can be found in deaf individuals, some of whom use speech reading, a visual input rather than an auditory input, as an aid to comprehend spoken language. If a *direct treatment model* is followed, specific exercises individually designed to ameliorate specific linguistic deficits are the basis of treatment.

In general, treatment methods can be categorized as those that are largely indirect stimulation-facilitation and those that are essentially direct structured-pedagogic.[101,111,118,120,123,124] The two principles that underlie most treatment methods reflect contrasting views of aphasia as either impaired access to language or a "loss" of language. The stimulation methods generally follow an impaired access theory and pedagogic approaches are based on a theory of aphasia as a language loss.

In practice, however, much of aphasia treatment addresses the *performance* aspect of language in which repeated practice and "teaching" strategies are assumed to help restore impaired skills through a "task-oriented" approach (i.e., naming practice). One of the commonly used techniques involves self-cueing and repetition exercises that manipulate components of grammar and vocabulary. Another approach involves "stimulating" the patient to use residual language by encouraging conversation in a permissive setting where a patient's responses are unconditionally accepted and topics are of personal interest.[124]

Visual communication therapy (VIC) is an experimental technique designed for global aphasia.[125–129] VIC employs an index card system of arbitrary symbols representing syntactic and lexical components that patients learn to manipulate so as to (1) respond to a command and (2) express needs, wishes, or other emotions. The system attempts to circumvent the use of natural oral language, which is severely impaired and often unavailable to the patient with global aphasia. An adaptation and application of the VIC system called *Computer-Aided Visual Communication system (C-VIC)* was developed by Steele et al.[127,128] Weinrich et al demonstrated that C-VIC training can lead to improved spoken language.[130]

Investigators conclude that the evidence supports the view that some patients who have severe aphasia can master the basics of an artificial language and that some of the cognitive operations entailed in natural language are preserved despite severity of involvement.

Visual Action Therapy (VAT) developed at the Boston Veterans Administration Medical Center by Helm-Estabrooks et al is designed to train people with global aphasia to use symbolic gestures representing visually absent objects.[131–132] The tasks leading to this goal include associating pictured forms with specific objects, manipulating real objects appropriately, and finally producing symbolic gestures that represent the objects used (e.g., cup, hammer, razor).

In an attempt to utilize systematized gestural language to facilitate oral production, American Indian sign language has been modified in a method that combines common gestural sign with oral speech production (Amerind) for selected cases.[133–135]

In the *functional communication treatment (FCT)* method developed by Aten et al, emphasis is placed on restoration of communication in the broadest sense.[134] Treatment is designed to improve information processing in the activities necessary to conducting ADL, social interactions, and self-expression of both physical and psychological needs.[136,137]

Promoting Aphasics' Communicative Effectiveness (PACE), is a technique intended to reshape structured interaction between clinicians and patients into more natural communicative exchanges, includes several pragmatic components common to natural conversation.[138]

In addition to these approaches, some investigators have reported the use of drawing as a potential means of communication.[139–142] Others describe interactive approaches to treatment of aphasia. These approaches include: the *communication partners* approach of Lyon,[139–141] a treatment plan designed to enhance communication and well-being in settings where the person with aphasia and the caregiver live; the *supported conversation* approach introduced by Kagan,[143,144] in which volunteers are trained as conversation partners to facilitate conversation in the person with aphasia by using all available modalities, thereby revealing the individual's competence and permitting a communicative interaction; and the *social model of aphasia* approach introduced by Simmons-Mackie[145] and Simmons-Mackie and Damico[146,147] which focuses on the fulfillment of social needs and the encouragement of a greater conversational burden on the part of communication partners. Partners are trained to facilitate interaction by modifying some of their interactive behavior.

The unfortunate reality is that once the condition of aphasia has stabilized, very few patients recover normal communication function, with or without speech therapy. Accordingly, aphasia rehabilitation should be viewed as a process of patient management in the broadest sense of the term. That is, the task is primarily one of helping the patient and his or her intimates adjust to the alterations and limitations imposed by the disability. Effective aphasia rehabilitation management requires the participation of a variety of disciplines, including medicine, psychology, physical therapy, occupational therapy, social work, vocational counseling, and, most critically, aphasia therapy.

The Patient with Aphasia

It has been observed that the variability of patients' psychological reactions is rarely determined by the type or location of their lesions but is an expression of the whole life experience of the person who has had a stroke.[47,88,113,148]

In a study of patients with aphasia participating in a group psychotherapy program, Friedman investigated the nature of psychological regression with impaired reality testing in aphasia.[149] Beyond the communication difficulties posed by aphasia, he observed that patients remained psychologically isolated. They did not maintain a consistent level of group participation and expressed intense feelings that they were very different from other people. Both withdrawal and projection were apparent as each patient acted in isolation and yet complained of this characteristic in others.

The selective and discriminating use of speech therapy to stimulate and support the patient through the various stages of recovery is an effective management tool.[78,150,151] Experienced aphasia therapists recognize that while working on aphasic deficits, they are simultaneously dealing psychotherapeutically with a readjusting personality.[113] Speech therapy, therefore, serves different purposes at different points along the way. Sometimes it allows patients to "borrow time," as Baretz and Stephenson have aptly stated.[152] Occasionally depression lifts after speech therapy has been initiated, reflecting the supportive and nurturing nature of the therapeutic relationship rather than an objective improvement in recovery of speech–language.[148]

Aphasia rehabilitation can be viewed as a dynamic process consisting of a series of stages like the stages of mourning described by Kübler-Ross, through which the majority of patients evolve.[153] Some, of course, never emerge from a state of severe depression.[154] Kübler-Ross and other authors have suggested that the stages through which someone with aphasia passes—including denial, rage, bargaining, and acceptance—could be characterized as attempts to overcome the sense of loss.[153]

By directly addressing a patient's linguistic deficits and channeling attention and energies toward constructive ends, speech therapy may produce a noticeable reduction in depression. Therapy tasks in this instance act as an equivalent for work, which has long been recognized as an antidote for depression.

There is a great tendency to overestimate the capacity of individuals with aphasia to return to work, particularly if the verbal deficits are mild. Premature attempts to return to work can have a negative psychological impact. Professional rehabilitation counselors are best equipped to explore and evaluate a patient's vocational potential and carry out the long and arduous process of evaluating work performance and job requirements.

Experienced aphasia clinicians stress the importance of the patient's family in the rehabilitation process. Some of the potentially negative reactions of the family include overprotectiveness, hostility, anger, unrealistic expectations, overzealousness, lack of knowledge of the dimensions of the disorder, and inability to cope with practical difficulties. The apparently natural tendency of family members to minimize the patient's communication impairment, particularly in the early stages of recovery, requires understanding and tactful management.[113]

The quality of premorbid relationships generally tends to be intensified after a catastrophic event; those that were problematic may deteriorate further, whereas the bond between a loving couple may become stronger. The reversal of roles, changes in levels of dependency, and a changed economic situation, so often a consequence of chronic disability, can have a critical negative impact on the patient and his or her family.

In a positive family milieu, patients are encouraged to develop regular daily routines as close to premorbid patterns as possible and are treated as contributing members of the family. Patients need to be allowed some sense of control. Including the patient in rehabilitation planning promotes restoration of feelings of self-worth. In this regard, the emphasis on function rather than complete recovery, pointing out success rather than performance failure, adds to a patient's sense of self. It is essential to listen to patients, particularly to their expressions of loss. Commiseration is often more comforting than optimistic prognostic statements.

Group speech therapy, stroke clubs, and other social groups are frequently used resources that can be effective tools in the management of some patients with chronic aphasia. The National Aphasia Association (NAA) was founded in the United States in 1987, following the lead of existing organizations established in Finland in 1971, Germany in 1978, the United Kingdom in 1980, and Sweden in 1981. An extensive array of educational and resource information appropriate for patients, families, and professionals is available on the NAA Web site (http://www.aphasia.org). Knowledge that one is not alone often helps to reduce depression and loneliness.[77,111]

Group therapy with peers also provides a comfortable atmosphere in which patients can meet new friends and share feelings, although not all individuals with aphasia find it beneficial. A positive effect seems related to level of comprehension, time since onset, and personality factors. Although group therapy generally plays an important role in aphasia rehabilitation, it should be noted that much of its effectiveness depends on the skill and experience of the group leader.[155,156]

In our present state of knowledge, aphasia rehabilitation remains eclectic and specifically tailored to the individual patient. Fundamental to this therapeutic philosophy is the acknowledgement and appreciation of the uniqueness of the individual. No two persons with aphasia are exactly alike in pathology, personality, linguistic deficits, reactions to catastrophic illness, life experience, spiritual values, or a host of other factors. The influence of these factors carries different weight and strength at different stages of recovery and they are all related to recovery outcome.

Experience suggests that, except for severely depressed individuals with aphasia, patients generally participate as fully as possible during rehabilitation. Therapists must not allow their expectations to contaminate the therapeutic interaction; this is not uncommon and is usually motivated by laudatory aspirations—therapists want to see their patients improve—but is nonetheless counterproductive. Patients with involvement of subcortical areas may have low levels of activation, a purely physiological process independent of psychological motivation. The distinction between these two processes must be understood.

Many ethical–moral dilemmas face those who manage the rehabilitation of patients with aphasia. One of the principal issues is a result of the necessity to select those individuals who will receive treatment. Rehabilitation medicine services are not only scarce in many situations, but they are also not considered to be a right or entitlement. Services are usually provided on a selective basis to those individuals believed to have the potential to benefit. This process assumes that we know who can benefit.[9,157–160] Many who are experienced in aphasia rehabilitation management hold the view that all people should be given a trial treatment period to determine their candidacy for further treatment and that trials should be provided at different points in the recovery course. Goal setting, the patient's right to self-determination, and the criteria appropriate in determining the termination of therapy are also important ethical issues.[113,160]

Dysarthria

The term **dysarthria** refers to an impairment of speech production resulting from damage to the central or peripheral nervous system, which causes weakness, paralysis, or incoordination of the motor–speech system. Any one or all of the components of the motor–speech system (respiration, phonation, articulation, resonance, and prosody) may by compromised by neural damage. The type and degree of dysarthria depends on the underlying etiology, degree of neuropathology, coexistence of other disabilities, and the individual response of the patient to the condition. It is not unusual for dysarthria to coexist with aphasia in patients who have suffered cerebrovascular accidents or TBI. The severity of dysarthria may range from the production of occasional imprecisely articulated consonant sounds to speech that is rendered totally unintelligible by the degree of impairment to the underlying systems. When patients are totally unintelligible as the result of severe motor–speech system impairment, they exhibit **anarthria**.

The incidence of dysarthria in the population of individuals with neurogenic disorders is approximately 46 percent, representing a significant proportion of the patients with communication impairments seen in medical settings.[86]

Dysarthria is generally reflected in deficits occurring in multiple motor–speech systems, but may sometimes occur in a single system (i.e., an impairment of soft palate movement resulting in hypernasality). It is most notably prevalent in cerebral palsy, TBI, cerebrovascular accidents, demyelinating diseases (e.g., multiple sclerosis) Parkinson's disease, amyotrophic lateral sclerosis, and neoplasm.

There are five primary types of dysarthria: *spastic, flaccid, ataxic, hypokinetic,* and *hyperkinetic.* When two or more types coexist, the term *mixed dysarthria* is used. Coexisting physical disabilities are present in a majority of patients who manifest dysarthria.

Classification and Nomenclature

Spastic dysarthria is characterized by imprecise articulation, slow labored articulation, hypernasality, harsh to strained phonation, and monotonous pitch. Syllables may be given equal stress and inflection. There is often reduced control of exhalation, with shallow inhalations and slow breaths. Spastic dysarthria is the result of bilateral pyramidal system damage involving the corticobulbar tracts (upper motor neurons). The pathology may cause weakness and paresis of the face and tongue musculature on the side opposite to the lesion. There is a high incidence of spastic dysarthria among those with cerebral palsy.[86]

Flaccid dysarthria is characterized by slow/labored articulation, hypernasality, and hoarse, breathy phonation. Phrases may be short, inhalation is shallow, and the control of exhalation may be reduced. There is often a reduction in the variation of pitch and loudness with audible inspirations. Most of these deviant speech characteristics are related to muscular weakness and reduced muscle tone, which affect the speech, accuracy, and range of speech movements.

Ataxic dysarthria is characterized by disturbances of timing, movement, range, and control and coordination of the muscles of speech and respiration. Speech is imprecise, slow, and irregular. There may be intermittent periods of explosive inflection, syllable stress, and loudness patterns. Phonemes may be prolonged; pitch and loudness are monotonous. The lesions producing ataxic dysarthria are bilateral, generalized lesions involving the deep midline nuclei and pathways of the cerebellum. Patients with multiple sclerosis often manifest ataxic dysarthria.

Hypokinetic dysarthria is characterized by variable articulatory precision, slow rate of speech, harsh, hoarse voice quality, excessive and overly long pauses, prolonged syllables and reduced phonation. Patients with Parkinson's or parkinsonian-like symptoms often manifest hypokinetic dysarthria, which is caused by lesions of the substantia nigra.

Hyperkinetic dysarthria is characterized by variable articulatory precision, vocal harshness, prolonged sounds and intervals between words, monotonous pitch, and loudness. Patients with Huntington's disease manifest hyperkinetic dysarthria, which is caused by lesions of the basal ganglia and/or their extrapyramidal projections.

Treatment of Dysarthria

Dysarthria treatment must be individually designed and account for the profile of impairment as well as the variability of its disabling effects. The performance of components of the motor–speech system does not necessarily result in changes in the disabling effects of the dysarthria; that is, the intelligibility of speech.[157] Goals that relate to the level of disability rather than normal speech are generally more realistic because they do not focus on normalcy, which is usually an unachievable goal, or improvement in the performance of a single component of the motor speech system, which may not, in the overall picture, be functionally important. There is relatively little data-based information available on the long-term prognosis for patients with dysarthria.

The focus of dysarthria treatment is sometimes based on an approach that stresses compensatory skills. These techniques tend to encourage the patient to minimize the overall disability by using strategies that may actually deviate from normal (i.e., slowing down the rate of speech production to increase intelligibility of consonant production).

The primary objective of dysarthria treatment is to improve the intelligibility of speech, which can be negatively affected if the speaker is in a dark, noisy place. Patients and communication partners must be trained to seek the most optimal situations for communication interactions. Exercises are generally administered to increase the precision, strength, and coordination of movements of the motor-speech system and the coordinated action of various components of the system. However, the general focus of dysarthria treatment is phonetic, because it is articulatory precision that contributes most to overall intelligibility. Clearly, as a patient's overall physical coordination and precision of movement increase, corresponding improvements occur in the control of the motor–speech system, and hence in speech intelligibility.

Verbal Apraxia

Some patients with nonfluent (Broca's) aphasia present with articulatory difficulty that manifests as imprecise and awkward articulation, distortion of phoneme production, and some literal *paraphasic* (sound substitution) errors in the absence of impaired strength or coordination of the motor speech system. This characteristic, which may be so severe that the patient is barely intelligible, can appear to be independent of difficulty in language processing and is referred to as **verbal apraxia** (or speech dyspraxia, apraxia of speech, cortical dysarthria, phonetic disintegration). Unlike dysarthric speakers, apraxic speakers do not generally have deficits in performing nonspeech movements of the oral musculature. The possible independence of this deficit from the language disorder of Broca's aphasia remains controversial.

Treatment of Dyspraxia

The disorder of articulation referred to as speech dyspraxia seldom, if ever, is manifest in the absence of a coexisting Broca's aphasia, however mild. The speech dyspraxia component of this multifaceted communication disorder appears to be especially amenable to direct therapeutic intervention using approaches adapted primarily from traditional articulation therapy techniques, including stress and intonation drills. These approaches, designed to improve phonetic placement accuracy, typically depend on imitation, stress, and progressive approximation, which are drilled using kinesthetic, visual, and auditory cues. Generally, the stimuli used as the bases for these exercises are selected in a presumed order of difficulty, beginning with nonoral imitation, followed by sounds, words, phrases, and finally utterances.

Treatment techniques for speech dyspraxia have been described by many clinicians.[162–170] Dworkin et al reported an effective treatment approach in a study of a single subject.[171] Various rhythmic techniques in which the patient generates the rhythm have also been reported as facilitory methods to increase articulation accuracy.[172] In contrast, Shane and Darley found that articulation precision tended to deteriorate under externally imposed rhythmic stimulation.[173] *Melodic intonation therapy* has also been employed as a facilitory technique in the treatment of patients with speech dyspraxia.

The long-term nature of recovery of phonemic production in patients with verbal apraxia was confirmed in a study of a patient with Broca's aphasia who received speech therapy for 10 years. The errors that prevailed in the first poststroke year were compared with performance at 10 years. The features of place and manner of production had improved; although voicing and addition errors (the addition of sounds) persisted, omission errors (the omission of sounds) were virtually eliminated.[174]

Dysphagia

The swallowing process is composed of a number of complex neuromuscular events. Normal swallowing requires that an individual be able to move food or liquid from the mouth (*oral phase of swallowing*), through the pharynx (*pharyngeal phase of swallowing*), and into the esophagus. In the oral swallow phase food is collected in the oral cavity in a single mass, or bolus, which is then propelled into the pharynx and further propelled under pressure into the esophagus. During the oral phase of swallowing, the bolus is first held between the tongue and palate and then propelled by the tongue from the front to the back of the oral cavity. The bolus moves over the back of the tongue into the pharynx, triggering the pharyngeal swallow and the neuromuscular events that propel the bolus into the esophagus. Velopharyngeal closure, tongue base posterior motion, pharyngeal contraction, laryngeal elevation and closure, and upper esophageal opening occur to allow bolus passage into the esophagus. Airway protection involves closure of the airway entrance and airway. Closure occurs by the vocal folds to the epiglottis moving downward to prevent food from entering the trachea during this process.

Dysphagia is defined as a condition in which an individual has had an interruption in either eating function or the maintenance of nutrition and hydration.[175] Many patients with neurogenic communication disorders also manifest deficits in swallowing (dysphagia). From 30 to 40 percent of individuals who have suffered strokes may have swallowing deficits ranging from mild to severe.[176–179] In some cases dysphagia is only present in the acute phase with rapid recovery of swallowing function taking place in the first 3 weeks post-stroke.[180] Swallowing deficits in poststroke patients are often due to a combination of weakness and incoordination of the oral, pharyngeal, and laryngeal musculature, resulting in inefficient propulsion of a food bolus or liquid through the oral cavity, pharynx, and into the esophagus. Delayed triggering of swallowing is common after stroke.[175] Oral or pharyngeal transit times may be slow. Reduced elevation or closure of the larynx may result in material being misdirected into the airway (aspiration). Dysphagia is also often present in patients with Parkinson's disease, Huntington's disease, the dystonias and dyskinesias, amyotrophic lateral sclerosis, multiple sclerosis, neoplasm, dementia, Alzheimer's disease, and other degenerative neurological conditions, as well as cerebral palsy. In addition, dysphagia is often seen in traumatically brain injured individuals.[177]

A dysphagia examination usually begins at bedside and is followed by more objective, instrumental techniques if a pharyngeal phase swallowing disorder is suspected. The most frequently used instrumental technique to view swallowing physiology in a dysphagia examination is the modified barium swallow because it provides a radiographic view of the entire oropharyngeal swallow, including structural movement and bolus flow. Precise physiological swallowing disorders can be identified. In addition, the effects of therapeutic strategies on swallow physiology, safety, and efficiency can be examined. Another useful examination procedure is videoendoscopy. In most settings, the swallowing evaluation is carried out by the speech–language pathologist.[180]

Treatment of Dysphagia

Dysphagia treatment is designed to improve swallowing efficiency for nutritional purposes and to increase swallowing safety. This can be accomplished by compensatory strategies and/or techniques designed to change swallowing physiology and reduce the risk of aspiration. Compensatory strategies include postural changes that affect the way food passes through the mouth and pharynx, dietary management, and placing food in the mouth in optimal positions. Postural techniques may also be introduced to reduce the possibility of aspiration.[179] Specific exercises (and maneuvers) are used to increase the coordination, range of motion, strength, and sensory input of the muscles and structures involved in the oral and pharyngeal phases of swallowing. These exercises are designed to improve lingual initiation, lingual propulsion, laryngeal elevation, closure and tongue base approximation to the posterior pharyngeal wall.[181]

The physical therapist can play an important role in positioning the patient for optimum swallowing, and providing treatment to reduce muscle spasticity, improve muscle strength and coordination, and prevent primitive reflex patterns from interfering with swallowing.[182–187]

Alternative/Augmentative Communication Systems and Devices

New technology, especially synthetic speech and microcomputers, has been adapted for use as augmentative communication devices. These devices provide a compensatory means of communication and are used as a facilitory technique to enhance or substitute for impaired speech (aphasia, dysarthria). Since the advent of microcomputers, they have been adapted for use in the treatment of aphasia.

Microcomputers were the basis for an approach that Seron et al found effective in treating patients with writing disorders associated with aphasia.[188] With continued exposure to training, improvement in accuracy and recognition time in reading commonly used words,[189] and improvement in auditory comprehension were noted in a patient with aphasia who, when followed up at a later date, showed additional gains.[190,191] Computer-generated phonemic cues were effective in improving naming in five patients with Broca's aphasia.[192] An augmentative system was developed for a patient with Broca's aphasia[193]; a word retrieval facilitation program was developed for individuals with aphasia[194]; and Steele et al[128] and Weinrich et al[195] replicated and extended the findings of Gardner et al[125] and Baker et al[196] by training those with aphasia to use a computerized version of the VIC system.

If an individual who is unable to make him- or herself understood still has residual writing and spelling skills, aids that utilize the alphabet can provide a means of communication (e.g., an alphabet board). A communication book may consist of pictures or words arranged according to topics (e.g., foods, family members) in a notebook for easy access. The same type of material has also been adapted for computerized access in the form of portable or table-top devices. Augmentative and alternative communication aids can be divided into high-tech and low-tech categories. Typewriters, telephones, communication books, and other similar devices are in the low-tech category, requiring only batteries or electricity. The high-tech category includes specially adapted computers and switching systems.

Thus far, only a small proportion of the aphasia population has benefited from alternative and augmentative communication devices. A larger number of persons with motor–speech impairments (e.g., those with cerebral palsy) have been able to increase their communicative effectiveness with technical aids. The complex interaction of the language, motor–speech system, and cognition in aphasia pose a challenge to current and future technology.[192]

Implications for the Physical Therapist

Physical therapists often work in settings where they may be the first to become aware of a patient's communication disorder, and should refer such patients to a speech–language pathologist for evaluation. The physical therapist can contribute to the patient's improvement in communication function in two important ways: by providing physiological support for speech functions, and by stimulating and facilitating communication through successful, fulfilling interaction with the patient. In either case, the physical therapist will want to work closely with the speech–language pathologist to ensure that their treatment goals and interventions are compatible.

The provision of physiological support for speech functions is especially relevant to the patient with pathology of the oral-motor system (e.g., dysarthria). The physical therapist will want to explore the influence of physiological support on the patient's speech in determining a comprehensive plan of care. Proper posture, for example, can help to inhibit reflexes that may trigger primitive movements. When a patient's speech function is influenced by overflow movements, stabilization techniques may be indicated.

Control of respiration is essential to the improvement of vocalization and the phrasing of speech. The muscles of respiration can be strengthened along with exercises designed to increase head control, stability, and sitting balance. Proper posture and eye contact enhance the possibility that speech will be audible and clear.

When a patient with a communication impairment is prescribed a communication board, the physical therapist contributes by determining a patient's sitting balance and tolerance, upper extremity motor control, and the best method for responding (e.g., pointing).

Strengthening exercises to increase the speech and range of motion of the tongue, lips, and general facial musculature and to improve coordination of the oral–motor system also increase the probability of intelligible speech and help the patient with dysarthria and dysphagia. Postural techniques are especially important for patients with dysphagia, who require individually tailored treatment programs designed to facilitate swallowing and prevent aspiration.

Because communication is a social activity, the physical therapy setting is a natural context for social interaction. The setting can be supportive by providing an atmosphere that is conducive to conversation and allows the patient to engage in a successful verbal interaction.

Patients who are neurologically compromised often have difficulty processing information in a distracting setting. Excessive noise, competing voices, and the presence of other stimuli can make communication particularly difficult. When possible, the physical therapist should strive to work with patients who are communicatively impaired in a closed environment that is free of these distractions. Patients with communication impairments do best when they are positioned in such a way that face-to-face communication is possible, including the visualization of gestures and facial expressions. For this reason, room lighting needs to be sufficient.

Patients who manifest neurogenic speech-language disorders, especially those with aphasia pose a considerable challenge to effective communication. The individual nature of each manifestation of aphasia argues for a close working relationship with the speech-language pathologist. This will ensure that the most effective communication strategies are used with an individual patient.

One of the greatest difficulties in addressing the needs of patients with acquired aphasia has to do with determining and accounting for the patient's level of auditory comprehension. Virtually all patients with aphasia have some degree of difficulty in comprehending spoken language. Physical therapists need to become skilled at recognizing and dealing with auditory comprehension deficits because they can be a major deterrent to successful rehabilitation.

Misconceptions of the auditory comprehension level of a patient with aphasia can range from the assumption that a patient understands everything to the assumption that the patient comprehends nothing and must be excluded from conversation. A guiding principle to keep in mind is that auditory comprehension can vary greatly, depending on the context and complexity of the task at hand. Switching topics quickly, speaking too quickly, background noises, talking while a patient is engaged in physical activity, and conversing with more than one person at a time can impede the individual's ability to process auditory information. Sentences should be short and simple and the patient should be given sufficient time to process the information and formulate a response. Questions that require elaborate answers, such as "Tell me about your vacation" or "What do you think about the latest news?" are generally difficult for patients with aphasia to answer. It is best to ask questions that can be answered with "yes," "no," or another single word. Physical cues to comprehension such as gestures, facial expression, and voice inflection can facilitate and enhance a patient's understanding. It is important for the physical therapist to know that patients with aphasia often find it easier to respond to whole body or axial commands ("stand up," "sit down") than distal commands ("point," "pick up").

It can be tempting to try to remedy a laborious communication situation by "talking down" to a patient with aphasia as if speaking to a child, or raising one's voice as if speaking to someone with impaired hearing. The best strategy is to speak a little more slowly, using language that is not too complex, and remaining consistent in giving instructions. This can be particularly important in the physical therapy setting, where verbal commands are a fundamental element in the patient–therapist interaction. At times, it may be necessary to repeat a sentence to be understood.

Rehabilitation team members almost universally overestimate the degree to which a person with aphasia understands spoken language. Physical therapists, when possible, should turn to the speech–language pathologist for an indication of the patient's preserved auditory comprehension. It may be necessary to rephrase questions and supplement with body language to ensure comprehension.

The use of accompanying visual cues, such as gestures and facial expressions, can be extremely helpful for some patients. Others may understand best if a message is supplemented by written cues. Sometimes one can assist by asking questions that can be answered by *yes* or *no* in a "20 questions" format. When someone with aphasia is having trouble expressing him- or herself, it usually helps to allow them extra time to speak. If the patient becomes visibly frustrated, it is desirable to remain calm and suggest that the patient wait and try again later.

During physical therapy interventions, patients with aphasia can be encouraged to produce single-word, repetitive speech that coincides with physical movements as a means of providing supplemental speech practice. Activities such as counting movements in series one to ten, and using words like up, down, left, and right while performing physical movements are examples of such techniques. The physical therapist, however, should always remain sensitive to the possibility of making speech demands that are beyond a patient's level of preserved communicative skill.

Summary

Ever since World War II, speech–language pathologists have played an important role on the rehabilitation team in the management of patients with neurogenic speech–language disorders, especially aphasia and dysarthria. For the physical therapist, an understanding of normal and pathological communication behaviors can not only make this population of patients more interesting to work with, but can also enhance the quality of treatment he or she provides.

Communication using speech is a complex, species-specific behavior that consists of the coordinated interaction of cognitive, motor, sensory, psychological, and social skills. The neurogenic disorders of speech and language, specifically aphasia and dysarthria, dominate the population of communication impaired patients in the rehabilitation setting. Viewed as a group, patients with neurogenic communication disorders comprise a relatively severely impaired segment of the disabled population.

The impact of neurogenic speech–language disorders on the self, family, community life, and vocational options makes these disorders especially challenging. The close relationship of one's verbal characteristics to personality and identity may cause even the mildest neurogenic communication disorder to affect the psychosocial domain. Current research is investigating the interaction of linguistic, cognitive, and psychosocial variables and their influence on the outcome of recovery and rehabilitation.

Questions for Review

1. Define aphasia.
2. Describe the differences that distinguish nonfluent from fluent aphasic syndromes and give clinical examples.
3. Discuss the components of a comprehensive language test designed to measure aphasic impairment.
4. Describe some critical factors that influence recovery from aphasia.
5. Describe the psychological sequelae that may have a negative effect on the outcome of aphasia rehabilitation.
6. Define dysarthria.
7. What neurological conditions are generally associated with dysphagia?
8. Describe augmentative communication systems and some specific techniques/devices that may enhance the treatment of aphasia.
9. How can the physical therapist contribute to the physiological support for speech?

Case Study

The patient is a 62-year-old man who teaches high school. He sustained a right hemiplegia and difficulty communicating as the result of a hemorrhagic stroke, which occurred 8 months ago. At this time, except for dressing, he is ADL independent and ambulates with a cane.

At one month post-stroke, the patient was limited to yes or no responses and a vocabulary ranging from 30 to 50 nouns and verbs as well as everyday greetings (hello, goodbye). In the course of a communicative interaction, he often resorted to writing a letter or word or gesturing to help in his communication efforts. He appeared to understand most of what was said especially when the topic was familiar. He received rehabilitation services during the acute poststroke phase while hospitalized and received 20 sessions of speech–language pathology services as an outpatient.

At 8 months post-stroke, the patient's communication disorder is marked by a slow, hesitant production of one- and two-word utterances; easily produced automatic speech (i.e., everyday greetings); difficulty expressing complex information; awkward and labored articulation, which causes occasional articulatory imprecision; impaired writing; and some difficulty reading lengthy or complex material. Although the majority of his speaking vocabulary consists of nouns and verbs, adverbs and adjectives are now used with greater frequency. There is a persistent lack of conjunctions, articles, and prepositions in speech, which causes him to have impaired grammar. The patient has no apparent difficulty understanding spoken language except when it is rapid, complex, and/or unfamiliar.

Both the patient and his caregiver report that the frequency of social interactions in his current life has been curtailed dramatically. He continues to see close family members on a regular basis but he rarely sees friends or work companions. The family reports that he is frustrated and depressed over this and feels isolated from the community much of the time. They also indicate that there has been a gradual but noticeable increase in his speaking vocabulary, ability to write, and reading skill. He has recently joined a local stroke group where he hopes to meet others with similar communication difficulties.

GUIDING QUESTIONS

1. A team conference is scheduled the day after you assume treatment responsibilities for the patient. What types of information would you obtain in consultation with the speech–language pathologist?
2. What communication strategies are generally useful with patients who have sustained a stroke?
3. What approach might you use if the patient became frustrated trying to express himself during a physical therapy treatment?
4. As a physical therapist, what might you do to decrease the patient's sense of isolation and enhance his emotional well-being?
5. In what ways can physical therapy treatment sessions serve to reinforce communication behavior?

References

1. National Institute on Deafness and Other Communication Disorders (NIDCD): Research in Human Communication. NIH Publication No. 92-3317. Bethesda, MD, 1995.
2. NIDCD: National Strategic Research Plan for Hearing and Hearing Impairments. Bethesda, MD, 1996.
3. Adams, PF, Hendershot, GE, and Marano, MA: Current estimates from the National Health Interview Survey, 1996. Centers for Disease Control and Prevention/National Center for Health Statistics. Vital Health Stat (200):1, 1999.
4. Slater, SC: Portrait of the Professions: 1992 Omnibus Survey. ASHA 34:61, 1992.
5. ASHA: Highlights and Trends: ASHA Member Counts. Rockville, MD, 2006. Retrieved May 18, 2006 from http://www.asha.org/about/membership-certification/member-counts.htm.
6. World Health Organization (WHO) ICIDH-2: International classification of impairment, disabilities and handicap. World Health Organization, Geneva, Switzerland, 1980.

7. WHO: International classification of functioning, disability and health. World Health Organization, Geneva, Switzerland, 2001. Retrieved October 25, 2004, from www3.who.int/icf/icf.
8. U.S. Census Bureau: U.S. Interim Projections by Age, Sex, Race and Hispanic Origin. Retrieved May 18, 2006 from http://www.census.gov/ipc/www/usinterimproj/, 2004.
9. National Institutes of Health (NIH): Aphasia: Hope through research. NIH Publication No. 80-391. Bethesda, MD, 1979.
10. National Institute on Deafness and Other Communication Disorders: NIDCD Fact Sheet: Aphasia. NIH Publication No. 97-4257. Bethesda, MD, 1997.
11. Brust, JC, et al: Aphasia in acute stroke. Stroke 7:167, 1976.
12. NIH: Decade of research: Answers through scientific research. The National Advisory Neurological and Communicative Disorders and Stroke Council. The National Institutes of Health, Bethesda, MD, 1989.
13. Goodglass, H, et al: The Assessment of Aphasia and Related Disorders, ed 3. Lippincott Williams & Wilkins, Philadelphia, 2001.
14. Damasio, A: Signs of aphasia. In Sarno, MT (ed): Acquired Aphasia, ed 3. Academic Press, New York, 1998, p 25.
15. Sarno, MT: A survey of 100 aphasic Medicare patients in a speech pathology program. J Am Geriatr Soc 18:471, 1970.
16. Prins, R, et al: Recovery from aphasia: Spontaneous speech versus language comprehension. Brain Lang 6:192, 1978.
17. Levin, HS: Linguistic recovery aphasia closed head-injury. Brain Lang 12:360, 1981.
18. Spreen, O, and Risser, A: Assessment of aphasia. In Sarno, MT (ed): Acquired Aphasia, ed 3. Academic Press, New York, 1998, p 71.
19. Spreen, O, and Risser, AH: Assessment of Aphasia. Oxford University Press, New York, 2000.
20. Spreen, O, and Benton, AL: Neurosensory Center Comprehensive Examination for Aphasia, ed 2. University of Victoria, Department of Psychology, Neuropsychology Laboratory, Victoria, BC, 1977.
21. Kertesz, A: Western Aphasia Battery. Grune & Stratton, New York, 1982.
22. Sarno, MT: The functional assessment of verbal impairment. In G. Grimby (ed) Recent advances in rehabilitation medicine. Almquist & Wiksell, Stockholm, 1983, p 75.
23. Worrall, LE: A conceptual framework for a functional approach to acquired neurogenic disorders of communication. In Worrall, LE and Frattali, CM (eds): Neurogenic Communication Disorders: A Functional Approach. Thieme, New York, 2000, p 3.
24. Sarno, MT: A measurement of functional communication in aphasia. Arch Phys Med Rehabil 46:107, 1965.
25. Sarno, MT: The Functional Communication Profile: Manual of Directions (Rehabilitation Monograph No. 42). New York University Medical Center, Rusk Institute of Rehabilitation Medicine, New York, 1969.
26. Holland, AL: Communicative Abilities in Daily Living. University Park Press, Baltimore, 1980.
27. Frattali, CM, et al: Functional Assessment of Communication Skills for Adults: Administration and Scoring Manual. American Speech & Hearing Association, Rockville, MD, 1995.
28. Benton, AL: Contributions to aphasia before Broca. Cortex 1:314, 1964.
29. Benton, AL, and Joynt, RJ: Early descriptions of aphasia. Arch Neurol 3:109, 1960.
30. Broca, P: Du siège de la faculté du language articulé. Bull Soc Anthropol 6:377, 1885.
31. Broadbent, D: A case of peculiar affection of speech, with commentary. Brain 1:484, 1879.
32. Mills, CK: Treatment of aphasia by training. JAMA 43:1940, 1904.
33. Head, H: Aphasia and Kindred Disorders of Speech, vols. 1 and 2. Cambridge University Press, Cambridge, UK, 1926.
34. Nielsen, J: Agnosia, Apraxia, Aphasia: Their Value in Cerebral Localization. Hoeber, New York, 1946.
35. Goldstein, K: After Effects of Brain Injuries in War: Their Evaluation and Treatment. Grune & Stratton, New York, 1942.
36. Singer, H, and Low, A: The brain in a case of motor aphasia in which improvement occurred with training. Arch Neurol Psychiatry 29:162, 1933.
37. Weisenburg, T, and McBride, K: Aphasia: A Clinical and Psychological Study. Commonwealth Fund, New York, 1935.
38. Sarno, MT: Recovery and rehabilitation in aphasia. In Sarno, M.T. (ed) Acquired Aphasia, ed 3. Academic Press, San Diego, 1998, p 595.
39. Klein, K: Community-based resources for persons with aphasia and their families. Top Stroke Rehabil 2:18, 1996.
40. American Heart Association: Aphasia and the family. Publication EM 359, Dallas, 1969.
41. Backus, O, et al: Aphasia in Adults. University of Michigan Press, Ann Arbor, 1947.
42. Boone, D: An Adult Has Aphasia: For the Family, ed 2. Interstate Printers and Publishers, Danville, IL, 1984.
43. Sarno, JE, and Sarno, MT: Stroke: A Guide for Patients and Their Families, ed 3. McGraw-Hill, New York, 1991.
44. Simonson, J: According to the aphasic adult. University of Texas (Southwestern) Medical School, Dallas, 1971.
45. Sarno, MT: Understanding Aphasia: A Guide for Family and Friends. Monograph No. 2, ed 4. Rusk Institute of Rehabilitation Medicine, New York University Medical Center, New York, 2004.
46. Yarnell, P, et al: Aphasia outcome in stroke: A clinical neuroradiological correlation. Stroke 7:514, 1976.
47. Sarno, MT: Quality of life in aphasia in the first poststroke year. Aphasiology 11:665, 1997.
48. Sorin-Peters, R: Viewing couples with aphasia as adult learners: Implications for promoting quality of life. Aphasiology 17(4): 405, 2003.
49. Darley, F: The efficacy of language rehabilitation in aphasia. J Speech Hear Disord 37:3, 1972.
50. Prins, R, et al: Efficacy of two different types of speech therapy for aphasic stroke patients. Appl Psycholing 10:85, 1989.
51. Wertz, RT, et al: VA cooperative study on aphasia: A comparison of individual and group treatment. J Speech Hear Disord 24:580, 1981.
52. Wertz, RT, et al: Comparison of clinic, home, and deferred language treatment for aphasia: A VA cooperative study. Arch Neurol 43:653, 1986.
53. Wertz, RT: Language treatment for aphasia is efficacious, but for whom? Top Lang Disord 8:1, 1987.
54. Sarno, MT: Recovery and rehabilitation in aphasia. In Sarno, MT (ed): Acquired Aphasia, ed 3. Academic Press, San Diego, 1998, p 595.
55. Basso, A: Aphasia and Its Therapy. Oxford University Press, New York, 2003.
56. Marks, M, et al: Rehabilitation of the aphasic patient: A survey of three years experience in a rehabilitation setting. Neurology 7:837, 1957.
57. Vignolo, LA: Evolution of aphasia and language rehabilitation: A retrospective exploratory study. Cortex 1:344, 1964.
58. Hagen, C: Communication abilities in hemiplegia: Effect of speech therapy. Arch Phys Med Rehabil 54:545, 1973.
59. Basso, A, et al: Etude controlée de la reéducation du language dans l'aphasie: Comparaison entre aphasiques traites et non-traites. Rev Neurol (Paris) 131:607, 1975.
60. Basso, A, et al: Influence of rehabilitation on language skills in aphasic patients. Arch Neurol 36:190, 1979.
61. Shewan, C, and Kertesz, A: Effects of speech and language treatment on recovery from aphasia. Brain Lang 23:272, 1984.
62. Poeck, K, et al: Outcome of intensive language treatment in aphasia. J Speech Hear Disord 54:471, 1989.
63. Kertesz, A, and McCabe, P: Recovery patterns and prognosis in aphasia. Brain Lang 100:1, 1977.
64. Levita, E: Effects of speech therapy on aphasics' responses to the Functional Communication Profile. Percept Motor Skills 47:151, 1978.
65. Shewan, CM: Expressive language recovery in aphasia using the Shewan Spontaneous Language Analysis (SSLA) System. J Commun Disord 17:175, 1988.
66. Wertz, RT, and Dronkers, N: Effects of age on aphasia. Paper presented at the American Speech-Language-Hearing Association Research Symposium on Communication Sciences and Disorders and Aging, Washington, DC, 1988.
67. Sarno, MT: Final Report. Age, linguistic evolution, and quality of life in aphasia. DHHS Grant No. CMS 5 R01 DC 00432-04. NIDCD, 1997.
68. Helm-Estabrooks, N, and Ramsberger, G: Treatment of agrammatism in long-term Broca's aphasia. Br J Disord Commun 21:39, 1986.

69. Glindemann, R, et al: The efficacy of modeling in PACE-therapy. Aphasiology 5:425, 1991.
70. Howard D: Beyond randomized controlled trials: The case for effective studies of the effects of treatment in aphasia. Br J Dis Commun 21:89, 1986.
71. Byng, S: Hypothesis testing and aphasia therapy. In Holland, AL, and Forbes, M (eds): Aphasia treatment. World Perspectives. San Diego, 1993, p 115.
72. Golper, L, et al: Evidence-based practice guidelines for the management of communication disorders in neurologically impaired individuals: Project Introduction. Academy of Neurologic Communication Disorders and Sciences, Minneapolis, MN, 2001. Retrieved October 23, 2004 from http://www.ancds.duq.edu/guidelines.html.
73. Frattali, C, et al:Development of evidence-based practice guidelines: Committee update. J Med Speech-Lang Pathol 11(3):ix, 2003.
74. Whurr, R, et al: A meta-analysis of studies carried out between 1946 and 1988 concerned with the efficacy of speech and language therapy treatment for aphasic patients. Eur J Commun 27:1, 1992.
75. Robey, RR: The efficacy of treatment for aphasic persons: A meta-analysis. Brain Lang 47:172, 1998.
76. Darley, F: Language rehabilitation: Presentation 8. In Benton, A (ed): Behavioral Change in Cerebrovascular Disease. Harper, New York, 1970, p 51.
77. Reinvang, I, and Engvik, E: Language recovery in aphasia from 3–6 months after stroke. In Sarno, MT, and Hook, O (eds): Aphasia: Assessment and Treatment. Almquist & Wiksell, Stockholm, Sweden, 1980, p 79.
78. Sarno, MT: Review of research in aphasia: Recovery and rehabilitation. In Sarno, MT, and Hook, O (eds): Aphasia: Assessment and Treatment. Almquist & Wiksell, Stockholm, Sweden, 1980, p 15.
79. Culton, G: Spontaneous recovery from aphasia. J Speech Hear Res 12:825, 1969.
80. Lomas, A, and Kertesz, A: Patterns of spontaneous recovery in aphasic groups: A study of adult stroke patients. Brain Lang 5:388, 1978.
81. Demeurisse, G, et al: Quantitative study of the rate of recovery from aphasia due to ischemic stroke. Stroke 11:455, 1980.
82. Butfield, E, and Zangwill, O: Re-education in aphasia: A review of 70 cases. J Neurol Neurosurg Psychiatry 9:75, 1946.
83. Sands, E, et al: Long term assessment of language function in aphasia due to stroke. Arch Phys Med Rehabil 50:203, 1969.
84. Sarno, MT, and Levita, E: Natural course of recovery in severe aphasia. Arch Phys Med Rehabil 52:175, 1971.
85. Mesulam, MM: Slowly progressive aphasia without generalized dementia. Ann Neurol 11:592, 1982.
86. Duffy, JR: Motor Speech Disorders. CV Mosby, St. Louis, 1995.
87. Davis, G. Aphasiology: Disorders and Clinical Practice. Allyn and Bacon, Needham Heights, MA, 2000.
88. Basso, A: Prognostic factors in aphasia. Aphasiology 6:337, 1992.
89. Cappa, S: Spontaneous recovery from aphasia. In Stemmer, B, and Whitaker, HA (eds.): Handbook of Neurolinguistics. Academic Press, San Diego, 1998, p 535.
90. Nicholas, M, et al: Empty speech in Alzheimer's disease and fluent aphasia. J Speech Hear Res 28:405, 1985.
91. Bayles, KA, and Kaszniak, AW: Communication and Cognition in Normal Aging and Dementia. Little, Brown, Boston, 1987.
92. Obler, LK, et al: On comprehension across the adult life span. Cortex 21:273, 1985.
93. Nicholas, M, et al: Aging, language, and language disorders. In Sarno, MT (ed): Acquired Aphasia, ed 3. Academic Press, San Diego, 1998, p 413.
94. Holland, AL, et al: Predictors of language restriction following stroke: A multivariate analyses. J Speech Hearing Res 31:232, 1989.
95. Kertesz, A: Recovery from aphasia. Adv Neurol 42:23, 1984.
96. Wertz, RT, and Dronkers, NF: Effects of age on aphasia. Paper presented at the American Speech-Language-Hearing Association Research Symposium on Communication Disorders and Aging, Washington, DC, 1988.
97. Pedersen, M, et al: Aphasia in acute stroke: Incidence, determinants, and recovery. Ann Recov 38:659, 1995.
98. Sarno, MT: Preliminary findings: Age, linguistic evolution and quality of life in recovery from aphasia. Scand J Rehabil Med Suppl 26:43, 1992.
99. Sarno, MT, et al: Gender and recovery from aphasia after stroke. J Nerv Ment Dis 173:605, 1985.
100. Borod, J, et al: Long term language recovery in left handed aphasic patients. Aphasiology 78:301, 1990.
101. Kertesz, A: Aphasia and Associated Disorders: Taxonomy, Localization and Recovery. Grune & Stratton, New York, 1979.
102. Schuell, H, et al: Aphasia in Adults. Harper, New York, 1964.
103. Sarno, MT, and Levita, E: Recovery in treated aphasia in the first year post-stroke. Stroke 10:663, 1979.
104. Selnes, OA, et al: Recovery of single-word comprehension CT scan correlates. Brain Lang 21:72, 1984.
105. Pashek, GV, and Holland, AL: Evolution of aphasia in the first year post onset. Cortex 24:411, 1988.
106. Kertesz, A: Evolution of aphasic syndromes. Top Lang Disord 1:15, 1981.
107. Goldenberg, G, and Scott, J: Influence of size and site of cerebral lesions on spontaneous recovery of aphasia and success of language therapy. Brain Lang 47:684, 1994.
108. Kenin, M, and Swisher, L: A study of pattern of recovery in aphasia. Cortex 8:56, 1972.
109. Lebrun, Y: Recovery in polyglot aphasics. In Lebrun, Y, and Hoops, R (eds): Recovery in Aphasics. Neurolinguistics, vol. 4. Swets and Zeitlinger BV, Amsterdam, 1976, p 96.
110. Basso, A, et al: Sex differences in recovery from aphasia. Cortex 18:469, 1982.
111. Benson, DF: Aphasia, Alexia, and Agraphia. Churchill Livingston, New York, 1979.
112. Damasio, AR: Aphasia. N Engl J Med 336:531, 1992.
113. Sarno, MT: Aphasia rehabilitation: Psychosocial and ethical considerations. Aphasiology 7:321, 1993.
114. Eisenson, J: Adult Aphasia: Assessment and Treatment. Prentice-Hall, Englewood Cliffs, NJ, 1973.
115. Herrmann, M, et al: The impact of aphasia on the patient and family in the first year post-stroke. Top Stroke Rehabil 2:5, 1995.
116. Eisenson, J: Aphasia: A point of view as to the nature of the disorder and factors that determine prognosis and recovery. Int JNeurol 4:287, 1964.
117. Marshall, RC, and Phillipps, DS: Prognosis for improved verbal communication in aphasic stroke patients. Arch Phys Med Rehabil 4:597, 1983.
118. Darley, FL, et al: Motor Speech Disorders. WB Saunders, Philadelphia, 1975.
119. Sarno, MT: Aphasia rehabilitation. In Dickson, S (ed): Communication Disorders: Remedial Principles and Practices. Scott, Foresman, Glenview, IL, 1974, p 404.
120. Sarno, MT: Disorders of communication in stroke. In Licht, S (ed): Stroke and Its Rehabilitation. Williams & Wilkins, Baltimore, 1975, p 380.
121. Sarno, MT: Language rehabilitation outcome in the elderly aphasic patient. In Obler, LK, and Albert, ML (eds): Language and Communication in the Elderly: Clinical, Therapeutic and Experimental Issues. DC Heath, Lexington, MA, 1980, p 191.
122. Goodglass, H: Neurolinguistic principles and aphasia therapy. In Meier, M, et al (ed): Neuropsychological Rehabilitation. The Guilford Press, New York, 1987.
123. Burns, MS, and Halper, AS: Speech/Language Treatment of the Aphasias: An Integrated Clinical Approach. Aspen, Rockville, MD, 1988.
124. Sarno, MT: Management of aphasia. In Bornstein, RA, and Brown, GG (eds): Neurobehavioral Aspects of Cerebrovascular Disease. Oxford University Press, New York, 1990, p 314.
125. Gardner, H, et al: Visual communication in aphasia. Neuropsychologia 14:275, 1976.
126. Weinrich, MP, et al: Implementation of a visual communicative system for aphasic patients on a microcomputer. Ann Neurol 18:148, 1985.
127. Steele, RD, et al: Evaluating performance of severely aphasic patients on a computer-aided visual communication system. In Brookshire, RH (ed): Clinical Aphasiology: Conference Proceedings. BRK Publications, Minneapolis, 1987, p 46.
128. Steele, RD et al: Computer-based visual communication in aphasia. Neuropsychologia 27:409, 1999.
129. Weinrich, MP: Computerized visual communication (C-VIC) therapy. Paper presented at the Academy of Aphasia, Phoenix, AZ, 1987.

130. Weinrich, M, et al: Training on an iconic communication system for severe aphasia can improve natural language production. Aphasiology 9:343, 1995.
131. Helm, N, and Benson, DF: Visual action therapy for global aphasia. Presentation at the 16th Annual Meeting of the Academy of Aphasia, Chicago, 1978.
132. Helm-Estabrooks, N, et al: Visual action therapy for aphasia. J Speech Hear Disord 47:385, 1982.
133. Skelly, M, et al: American Indian sign (AMERIND) as a facilitator of verbalization for the oral verbal apraxic. J Speech Hear Disord 39:445, 1974.
134. Rao, P, and Horner, J: Gesture as a deblocking modality in a severe aphasic patient. In Brookshire, RH (ed): Clinical Aphasiology: Conference Proceedings. BRK Publications, Minneapolis, 1978, p 180.
135. Rao, P, et al: The use of American-Indian Code by severe aphasic adults. In Chapey, R (ed): Language Intervention Strategies in Aphasia and Related Neurogenic Communication Disorders, ed 4. Lippincott Williams & Wilkins, Baltimore, 2001, p 688.
136. Aten, JL, et al: The efficacy of functional communication therapy for chronic aphasic patients. J Speech Hear Disord 47:93, 1982.
137. Aten, JL: Function communication treatment. In Chapey, R (ed): Language Intervention Strategies in Adult Aphasia, ed 2. Williams & Wilkins, Baltimore, 1986, p 266.
138. Wilcox, M, and Davis, G: Promoting aphasics' communicative effectiveness. Paper presented to the American Speech-Language-Hearing Association, San Francisco, 1978.
139. Lyon, JG: Drawing: Its value as a communication aid for adults with aphasia. Aphasiology 9:33, 1995.
140. Lyon, JG: Coping with Aphasia. Singular Publishing Group, San Diego, CA, 1997.
141. Lyon, JG: Communication use and participation in life for adults with aphasia in natural settings: The scope of the problem. Am J Speech Lang Pathol 1:7, 1992.
142. Rao, PR: Drawing and gesture as communication options in a person with severe aphasia. Top Stroke Rehabil 2:49, 1995.
143. Kagan, A, and Gailey, GF: Functional is not enough: Training conversation partners for aphasic adults. In Holland, A, and Forbes, MM (eds): Aphasia Treatment: World Perspectives. Singular Publishing Group, San Diego, 1993, p 199.
144. Kagan, A: Revealing the competence of aphasic adults through conversation: A challenge to health professionals. Top Stroke Rehabil 2:15, 1995.
145. Simmons-Mackie, N: An Ethnographic Investigation of Compensatory Strategies in Aphasia. Unpublished doctoral dissertation. Louisiana State University, Baton Rouge, 1993.
146. Simmons-Mackie, N, and Damico, J: Communication competence in aphasia: Evidence from compensatory strategies. In Lemme, ML (ed): Clinical Aphasiology, vol. 23. Pro-Ed, Austin, TX, 1995, p 3.
147. Simmons-Mackie, N, and Damico, J: Reformulating the definition of compensatory strategies in aphasia. Aphasiology 11:761, 1997.
148. Ullman, M: Behavioral Changes in Patients Following Strokes. Charles C Thomas, Springfield, IL, 1962.
149. Friedman, M: On the nature of regression. Arch Gen Psychiatry 3:17, 1961.
150. Brumfitt, S, and Clarke, P: An application of psychotherapeutic techniques to the management of aphasia. Paper presented at Summer Conference: Aphasia Therapy. Cardiff, England, July 19, 1980.
151. Tanner, D: Loss and grief: Implications for the speech-language pathologist and audiologist. J Am Speech Hear Assoc 22:916, 1980.
152. Baretz, R, and Stephenson, G: Unrealistic patient. NYS J Med 76:54, 1976.
153. Kübler-Ross, E: On Death and Dying. Macmillan, New York, 1969.
154. Espmark, S: Stroke before fifty: A follow-up study of vocational and psychological adjustment. Scand J Rehab Med (Suppl) 2:1, 1973.
155. Kearns, KJ: Group therapy for aphasia: Theoretical and practical considerations. In Chapey, R (ed): Language Intervention Strategies in Adult Aphasia, ed 2. Baltimore, Williams & Wilkins, 1986, p 304.
156. Bollinger, R, et al: A study of group communication intervention with chronic aphasic persons. Aphasiology 7:301, 1993.
157. Caplan, AL, et al: Ethical and policy issues in rehabilitation medicine. A Hastings Center Report, Briarcliff Manor, NY. Special Supplement, 1987.
158. Hass, J, et al: Case studies in ethics and rehabilitation. The Hastings Center, Briarcliff Manor, NY, 1988.
159. Sarno, MT: The case of Mr. M: The selection and treatment of aphasic patients. Case studies in ethics and rehabilitation medicine. The Hastings Center, Briarcliff Manor, NY, 1988, p 24.
160. Sarno, MT: The silent minority: The patient with aphasia. Hemphill Lecture. Rehabilitation Institute of Chicago, Chicago, 1986.
161. Yorkston, KM, et al (eds): Clinical Management of Dysarthric Speakers. Little, Brown, Boston, 1988.
162. Deal, J, and Florance, C: Modification of the eight-step continuum for treatment of apraxia of speech in adults. J Speech Hear Disord 43:89, 1978.
163. Halpern, H: Therapy for agnosia, apraxia, and dysarthria. In Chapey, R (ed): Language Intervention Strategies in Adult Aphasia. Williams & Wilkins, Baltimore, 1981, p 420.
164. Rosenbek, JC: Treating apraxia of speech. In Johns, DF (ed): Clinical Management of Neurogenic Communication Disorders. Little, Brown, Boston, 1978, p 191.
165. Rosenbek, JC, et al: A treatment for apraxia of speech in adults. J Speech Hear Disord 38:462, 1973.
166. Houston Wiedl, IM: The basic foundation approach for decreasing aphasia and verbal apraxia in adults (BFA). In Brookshire, RH (ed): Clinical Aphasiology: Conference Proceedings. BRK Publications, Minneapolis, 1976, p 209.
167. Rosenbek, JC: Advances in the evaluation and treatment of speech apraxia. In Rose, FC (ed): Advances in Neurology. Progress in Aphasiology, vol. 42. Raven, New York, 1984, p 327.
168. Wertz, RT, et al: Apraxia of Speech in Adults: The Disorder and Its Management. Grune & Stratton, New York, 1984.
169. Wertz, RT: Language disorders in adults: State of the clinical art. In Holland, AL (ed): Language Disorders in Adults. College Hill, San Diego, 1984, p 1.
170. Rubow, R, et al: Vibrotactile stimulation for intersystemic reorganization in the treatment of apraxia of speech. Arch Phys Med Rehabil 63:97, 1982.
171. Dworkin, JP, et al: Dyspraxia of speech: The effectiveness of a treatment regimen. J Speech Hear Disord 53:289, 1988.
172. Rosenbek, JC, et al: Treatment of developmental apraxia of speech: A case study. Lang Speech Hear Serv Sch 5:13, 1974.
173. Shane, H, and Darley, FL: The effect of auditory rhythmic stimulation on articulatory accuracy in apraxia of speech. Cortex 14:444, 1978.
174. Sands, E, et al: Progressive changes in articulatory patterns in verbal apraxia: A longitudinal case study. Brain Lang 6:97, 1978.
175. Buchholz, D: Editorial: What is dysphagia? Dysphagia 11:23, 1996.
176. Groher, MD, and Bukulman, R: The presence of swallowing disorders in two teaching hospitals. Dysphagia 1:3-6, 1986.
177. Veis, S, and Logemann, J: The nature of swallowing disorders in CVA patients. Arch Phys Med Rehabil 66:372, 1985.
178. Wade, DT, and Hewer, RL: Motor loss and swallowing difficulty after stroke: Frequency, recovery, and prognosis. Acta Neurol Scand 76:50, 1987.
179. Cherney, LR: Dysphagia in adults with neurologic disorders: An Overview. In LR Cherney (ed): Clinical Management of Dysphagia in Adults and Children. Aspen Publishers, Gaithersburg, MD, 1994, p 1.
180. Logemann, JA: Evaluation and Treatment of Swallowing Disorders, 2nd ed. Pro-Ed, Austin, TX, 1998.
181. Logemann, JA, and Kahrilas, P: Relearning to swallow post CVA: Application of maneuvers and indirect biofeedback: A case study. Neurology 40:1136, 1990.
182. Lazarus, C., and Logemann, J: Swallowing disorders in closed head trauma patients. Arch Phys Med Rehabil 68: 79, 1987.
183. Lazarus, CL, et al: Effects of bolus volume, viscosity, and repeated swallows in nonstroke subjects and stroke patients. Arch Phys Med Rehabil 74:1066, 1993.
184. Lazzara, G, Lazarus, C, and Logemann, JA: Impact of thermal stimulation on the triggering of swallowing reflex. Dysphagia 1, 73, 1986.
185. Logemann, JA, et al: Closure mechanisms of laryngeal vestibule during swallowing. Am J Physiol 262(2 Pt 1):G338, 1992.
186. Martin, BJW, et al: Normal laryngeal valving patterns during three breath-hold maneuvers: A pilot investigation. Dysphagia, 8:11, 1993.

187. Kahrilas, PJ, et al: Volitional augmentation of upper esophageal sphincter opening during swallowing. Am J Physiol 260(3 Pt 1): G45, 1991.
188. Seron, X, et al: A computer-based therapy for the treatment of aphasic subjects with writing disorders. J Speech Hear Disord 45:45, 1980.
189. Katz, RC, and Nagy, V: A computerized approach for improving word recognition in chronic aphasic patients. In Brookshire, RH (ed): Clinical Aphasiology: Conference proceedings. BRK Publishers, Minneapolis, 1983.
190. Mills, RH: Microcomputerized auditory comprehension training. In Brookshire, RH (ed): Clinical Aphasiology: Conference Proceedings. BRK Publications, Minneapolis, 1982, p 147.
191. Mills, RH, and Hoffer, P: Computers and caring: An integrative approach to the treatment of aphasia and head injury. In Marshall, RC (ed): Case Studies in Aphasia Rehabilitation. University Park Press, Baltimore, 1985.
192. Bruce, C, and Howard, D: Computer-generated phonemic cues: An effective aid for naming in aphasia. Br J Disord Commun 22:191, 1987.
193. Garrett, K, et al: A comprehensive augmentative communication system for an adult with Broca's aphasia. Augment Altern Commun 5:55, 1989.
194. Hunnicutt, S: Access: A lexical access program. Proceedings of RESNA 12th Annual Conference, New Orleans, LA, 1989, p 284.
195. Weinrich, MP, et al: Processing of visual syntax in a globally aphasic patient. Brain Lang 36:391, 1989.
196. Baker, E, et al: Can linguistic competence be dissociated from natural language functions? Nature 254:609, 1975.

Supplemental Readings

Avent, JR: Manual of Cooperative Group Treatment for Aphasia. Butterworth-Heinemann, Boston, 1997.

Bhatnager, S: Neuroscience for the Study of Communicative Disorders. Lippincott Williams & Wilkins, Philadelphia, 2001.

Chapey, R (ed): Language Intervention Strategies in Aphasia and Related Neurogenic Communication Disorders. Lippincott Williams & Wilkins, Baltimore, 2001.

Code, C (ed): The Characteristics of Aphasia. Taylor & Francis, London, 1989.

Connor, LT, and Obler, LK (eds): Neurobehavior of Language and Cognition Studies of Normal Aging and Brain Damage. Kluwer Academic, New York, 2000.

Duffy, JR: Motor Speech Disorders. CV Mosby, St. Louis, 1995.

Elman, RJ (ed): Group Treatment of Neurogenic Communication Disorders: The Expert Clinician's Approach. Butterworth-Heinemann, Boston, 1999.

Hegde, MN: A Coursebook on Aphasia and Other Neurogenic Language Disorders. Singular Publishing Group, San Diego, 1998.

Helm-Estabrooks, N, and Albert, ML: Manual of Aphasia and Aphasa Therapy. Pro-Ed, Austin, TX, 2003.

Helm-Estabrooks, N, and Holland, AL (eds): Approaches to the Treatment of Aphasia. San Diego: Singular Publishing Group, San Diego, 1998.

Lapointe, II (ed): Aphasia and Related Neurogenic Language Disorders, ed 2. Thieme, New York, 1997.

Murdoch, B, and Theodoros, D: Traumatic brain injury: Associated speech, language, and swallowing disorders. Singular Publishing Group, San Diego, 2001.

Myers, P: Right Hemisphere Damage: Disorders of Communication and Cognition. Singular Publishing Group, San Diego, 1999.

Owens, R, Metz, D, and Haas, A: Introduction to Communication Disorders: A Life Span Perspective. Allyn & Bacon, Needham Heights, MA, 2003.

Pound, C, et al: Beyond Aphasia: Therapies for Living With Communication Disability. Winslow Press Ltd, UK, 2000.

Sarno, MT (ed): Acquired Aphasia, ed 3. Academic Press, New York, 1998.

Sarno, MT: Quality of life in aphasia in the first poststroke year. Aphasiology 11:665, 1997.

Simmons-Mackie, N, Damico, J, and Damico, H: A qualitative study of feedback in aphasia treatment. Am J Speech Lang Pathol J Clin Pract 8:218, 1999.

SECTION FOUR

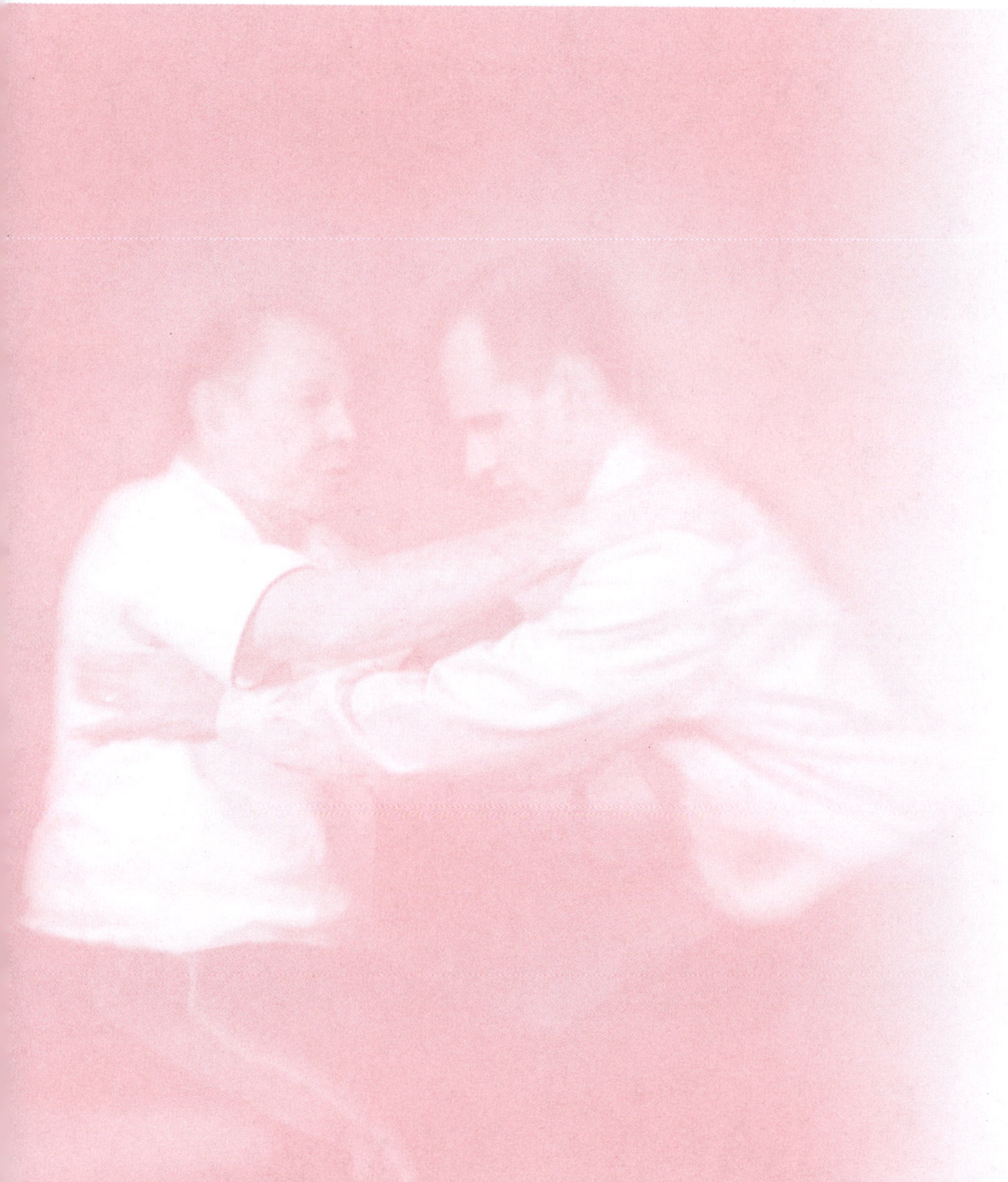

Orthotics, Prosthetics, and the Prescriptive Wheelchair

CHAPTER

31

LEARNING OBJECTIVES

1. Relate the major parts of the shoe to the requirements of individuals fitted with lower-limb orthoses.
2. Compare the characteristics, advantages, and disadvantages of plastics, metals, and other materials used in orthoses.
3. Describe the components of contemporary foot, ankle–foot, knee–ankle–foot, hip–knee–ankle–foot, trunk–hip–knee–ankle–foot, and trunk orthoses.
4. Explain the orthotic options available for patients with paraplegia.
5. Identify the features of lower-limb and trunk orthoses that are considered during the examination process.
6. Outline the physical therapist's role in management of patients fitted with lower-limb and trunk orthoses.
7. Analyze and interpret patient data, formulate realistic goals and outcomes, and develop a plan of care when presented with a clinical case study.

Orthotics

Joan E. Edelstein, PT, MA, FISPO

OUTLINE

An **orthosis** is an external appliance worn to restrict or assist motion or to transfer load from one area to another. The older term, *brace,* is a synonym. A splint connotes an orthosis intended for temporary use. An orthotist is the health care professional who designs, fabricates, and fits orthoses for the limbs and trunk, while a pedorthist is the health care professional who designs, fabricates, and fits only shoes and foot orthoses. *Orthotic* is an adjective, although some use the word as a noun. Archaeological evidence indicates that orthoses have been used at least since the fifth Egyptian dynasty (2750 to 2625 BC). The term orthosis appears to have been coined in the mid-twentieth century.

This chapter presents the most frequently prescribed orthoses for the lower limb and the trunk, as well as new developments in the field. Key elements in training patients to use orthoses are discussed. The focus is on orthotic design characteristics, their biomechanical rationale, merits of specific materials, and criteria for judging the adequacy of orthotic fit, function, and construction.

Terminology and Types of Orthoses

Generic terminology is superseding the traditional use of eponyms. Naming orthoses by the joints they encompass and the type of motion control facilitates communication among clinicians and consumers. Thus, *foot orthoses (FOs)* are appliances applied to the foot and placed inside or outside the shoe, such as metatarsal pads and heel lifts. *Ankle–foot orthoses (AFOs)* encompass the shoe and terminate below the knee. The *knee–ankle–foot orthosis (KAFO)* extends from the shoe to the thigh. A *hip–knee–ankle–foot orthosis (HKAFO)* is a KAFO with a pelvic band that surrounds the lower trunk. A *trunk–hip–knee–ankle–foot orthosis (THKAFO)* covers part of the thorax as well as the lower limbs. A *knee orthosis (KO)* and a *hip orthosis (HO)* are other applications of the same system of nomenclature.

Lower-Limb Orthoses

Lower-limb orthoses range from shoes used for clinical purposes to THKAFOs. Characteristics and functions of the principal FOs, AFOs, KAFOs, HKAFOs, and THKAFOs, and trunk orthoses, together with the clinically important attributes of shoes, will be described. Although physical therapists also encounter KOs, HOs, and orthoses for special purposes, such as management of Legg Calve Perthes' disease, these orthoses are not included because they are used less frequently than the appliances that do appear in this chapter. Similarly, orthoses for the upper limb are omitted from this chapter because they are less commonly prescribed and in most instances are used only for a brief duration.

Shoes

The shoe is the foundation for most lower-limb orthoses. Each part of the shoe contributes to the efficacy of orthotic management and offers many options for selection.[1] Shoes transfer body weight to the ground and protect the wearer from the terrain and the weather. The ideal shoe should distribute bearing forces so as to provide optimum comfort, function, and appearance of the foot. For the individual with an orthopedic disorder, footwear can serve two additional purposes: (1) it reduces pressure on sensitive deformed structures by redistributing force toward pain-free areas; and (2) it serves as the foundation for AFOs and more extensive bracing. Unless the shoe is correctly fitted and appropriately modified, the alignment of the orthosis will not provide the designed pattern of weightbearing. The major parts of the shoe are the upper, sole, heel, and reinforcements (Fig. 31.1). These features are found in both the traditional leather shoe and the athletic sneaker.

Upper

The portion of the shoe over the dorsum of the foot is the *upper*. It consists of an anterior component called the *vamp* and the posterior part, the *quarter*. If the shoe is to be used with an AFO having an insert as its distal attachment, then the vamp should extend to the proximal portion of the dorsum to secure the shoe and thereby the rest of the orthosis

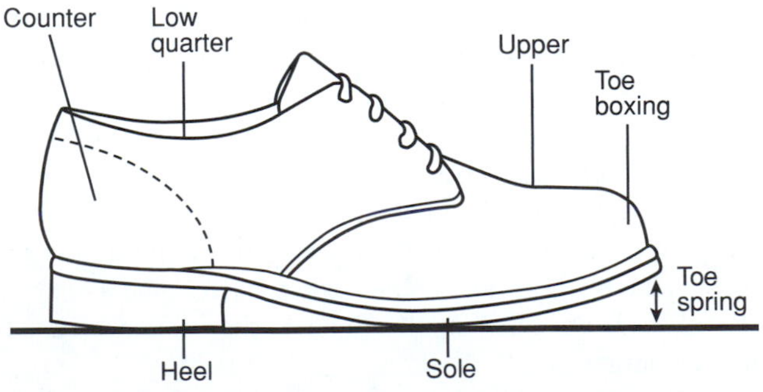

Figure 31.1 Parts of a low quarter shoe with a Blucher lace stay. Note that the counter and toe boxing are internal reinforcing structures of the shoe.

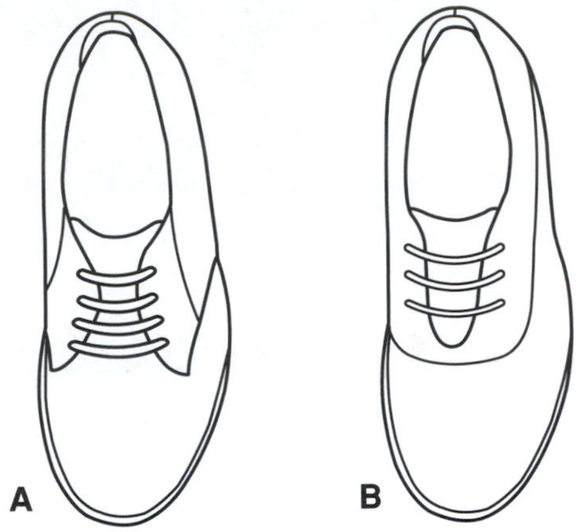

Figure 31.2 Low quarter shoes: (*A*) Blucher and (*B*) Bal (Balmoral). The Blucher lace stay is generally preferred for orthotic use owing to ease in donning and adjustability.

high onto the foot. In a laced shoe, the vamp contains the lace stays, which have eyelets for shoelaces (Fig. 31.2). Laces provide more precise adjustment over the entire opening than do strap closures. The latter, however, enable some individuals with limited manual dexterity to manage the shoe more easily. For most orthotic purposes, a *Blucher* lace stay is preferable; it is distinguished by the separation between the anterior margin of the lace stay and the vamp. The alternate design is the *Bal,* or *Balmoral,* lace stay, in which the lace stay is continuous with the vamp. The Blucher opening permits substantial adjustability, an important feature for the patient with edema. It also offers a large inlet into the shoe, so that one can determine whether paralyzed toes lie flat within the shoe. An extra depth shoe is one having an upper contoured with additional vertical space. The shoe is manufactured with a second inner sole that can be removed to accommodate an insert or thick surgical dressing.

Quarter height is another consideration in shoe prescription. The low-quarter terminates below the malleoli and is satisfactory for most clinical purposes. This style does not restrict foot or ankle motion. If the patient will be wearing a plastic orthosis molded about the ankle, it is not necessary to go to the additional expense of providing a high-quarter shoe for ankle support. A high-quarter shoe, covering the malleoli, is indicated to cover the foot having rigid pes equinus. It is also appropriate to augment foot stability in the absence of an AFO. The high-quarter shoe, however, is more difficult to don and more expensive than a comparable low-quarter one.

Sole

The *sole* is the bottom portion of the shoe. For use with a riveted metal attachment between shoe and orthosis, the sole should have two parts, the outer and the inner sole, both made of leather. Between the two lies a metal reinforcement that receives the rivets. This type of shoe, however, is heavier than an athletic shoe with a single sole. Leather soles absorb little impact shock and provide minimal traction as compared to rubber soles. To absorb shock, the shoe may have a resilient outer sole, inner sole, or insert.[2]

Regardless of material, the outer sole should not contact the floor at the distal end; the slight rise of the sole is known as *toe spring* (see Fig. 31.1), which allows a rocker effect at late stance. If a lift is added to the sole to compensate for leg length discrepancy, the lift should be beveled to achieve toe spring.

Heel

The *heel* is the portion of the shoe adjacent to the outer sole, under the anatomical heel. A broad, low heel provides greatest stability and distributes force between the back and front of the foot. For adults, a 1 in. (2.5 cm) heel tilts the center of gravity slightly forward to aid transition through stance phase, but does not disturb normal knee and hip alignment significantly. A higher heel places the ankle in its extreme plantarflexion range and forces the tibia forward. The wearer compensates either by retaining slight knee and hip flexion or by extending the knee and exaggerating lumbar lordosis. The high heel transmits more stress to the metatarsals. Nevertheless, transferring load anteriorly may be desirable if the patient has heel pain. The higher heel also reduces tension on the Achilles tendon and other posterior structures and accommodates rigid **pes equinus**. Although most heels are made of firm material with a rubber plantar surface, a low resilient heel is indicated to permit slight plantarflexion if the ankle cannot move because of orthotic or anatomical limitation.

Reinforcements

Reinforcements located at strategic points preserve the shape of the shoe. *Toe boxing* in the vamp protects the toes from stubbing and vertical trauma; it should be high enough to accommodate hammer toes or similar deformity. The *shank* piece is a longitudinal plate that reinforces the sole between the anterior border of the heel and the widest part of the sole at the metatarsal heads. A corrugated steel shank is necessary if an orthotic attachment is to be riveted to the shoe. The *counter* stiffens the quarter and generally terminates at the anterior border of the heel. The patient with **pes valgus**, however, should have a shoe with a long medial counter that provides reinforcement along the medial border of the foot to the head of the first metatarsal, thus resisting the tendency of the foot to collapse medially.

Last

The *last* is the model over which the shoe is made. The last, whether of traditional wood, custom-made plaster, or computer-generated design, remains with the manufacturer; the shoe shape duplicates the last's contour. A given shoe size may be achieved with many lasts, each transmitting different forces to the foot. Consequently, the physical therapist should ascertain that the shoe shape fits the foot satisfactorily, rather than relying on a particular shoe size. The patient with a markedly deformed foot requires a shoe made over a special last, either factory- or custom-made.

Foot Orthoses

Foot orthoses are appliances that apply forces to the foot. These may be an *insert* placed in the shoe, an internal modification affixed inside the shoe, or an external modification attached to the sole or heel of the shoe. They can enhance function by relieving pain. This may be accomplished by transferring weightbearing stresses to pressure-tolerant sites, protecting painful areas from contact with the shoe, correcting alignment of a flexible segment, or accommodating a fixed deformity. Inserts can also improve the wearer's transition during stance phase, by altering the rollover point in late stance and by equalizing foot and leg lengths on both limbs. In many instances, a particular therapeutic aim can be achieved by a variety of devices.

Internal Modifications

Generally, the closer the modification is to the foot, the more effective it is. Consequently, inserts and internal modifications are widely used. The insert permits the patient to transfer the orthosis from shoe to shoe, if the shoes have the same heel height; otherwise, a rigid insert may rock in the shoe. Most inserts terminate just behind the metatarsal heads; thus, they may slip forward, particularly if the shoe has a relatively high heel. Some inserts extend the full length of the sole, preventing slippage, but occupying the often limited space in the anterior portion of the shoe. Internal modifications are fixed to the shoe's interior, guaranteeing the desired placement, but limiting the patient to the single pair of modified shoes. Both inserts and internal modifications reduce shoe volume, so proper shoe fit must be judged with these components in place.

Inserts made of soft materials, such as the *viscoelastic* plastics (e.g., Sorbothane and Viscolas), reduce shear and impact shock, thus protecting painful or insensitive feet.[3] Inserts are also constructed of semirigid or rigid plastics, rubber, or metal, often with a resilient overlay. A heel-spur insert orthosis (Fig. 31.3), for example, may be made of

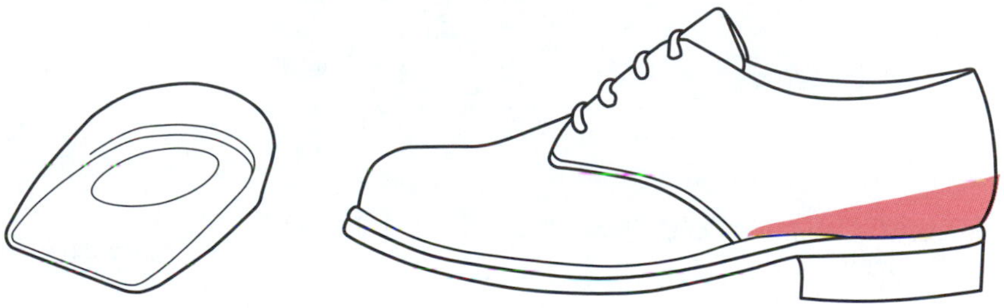

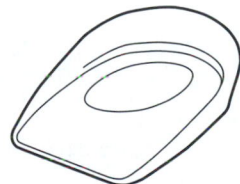

Figure 31.3 Plastic tapered heel spur cushion with concave relief to reduce pressure. The shaded area of the shoe on the far right indicates the relative position of the heel spur when placed in a shoe.

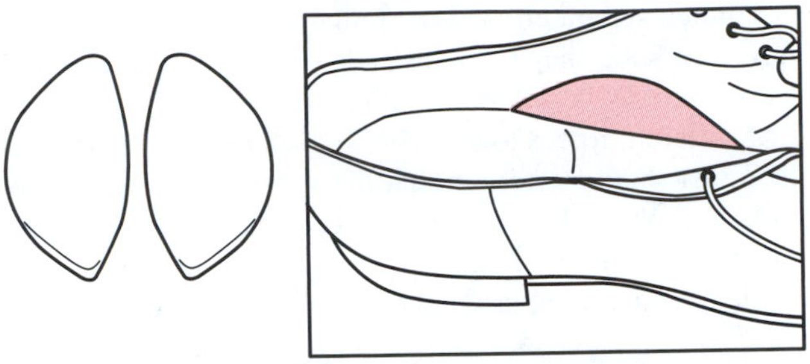

Figure 31.4 Scaphoid pads (*left*) are available with self-adhesive backing; scaphoid pad (*right*) glued to the inside of the shoe.

viscoelastic plastic or rubber.[4] The orthosis slopes anteriorly to reduce load on the painful heel. In addition, the orthosis has a concave relief to minimize pressure on the tender area.

Longitudinal arch supports are intended to prevent depression of the subtalar joint and flattening of the arch **(pes planus)**. The orthosis may include a wedge (post) to alter foot alignment. The minimum support is a rubber *scaphoid pad* (Fig. 31.4) positioned at the medial border of the insole with the apex between the sustentaculum tali and the navicular tuberosity.[5–7] Flexible flat foot can be realigned with a semirigid plastic *University of California Biomechanics Laboratory (UCBL) insert* (Fig. 31.5).[8] It is molded over a plaster model of the foot, taken with the foot in maximum correction. It encompasses the heel and midfoot, applying medialward force to the calcaneus, and lateral and upward force to the medial portion of the midfoot. Inserts appear to have minimal effect on metatarsophalangeal function.[9] With regard to the effect of inserts on proximal joints, the evidence is equivocal; some investigations show that orthoses alter the onset of erector spinae and gluteus medius activity[10] and support the positive effect of FOs on reducing patellofemoral pain,[11,12] while others show little or no effect.[13] Inserts appear not to change the strike pattern used by runners[14] and evidence suggests improved foot alignment.[15]

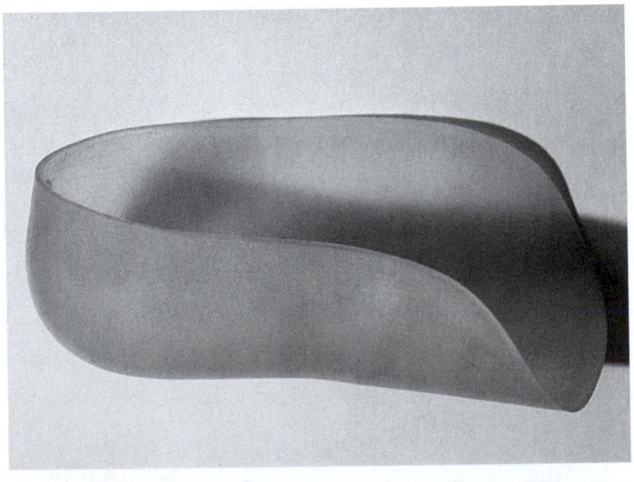

Figure 31.5 University of California Biomechanics Laboratory (UCBL) insert.

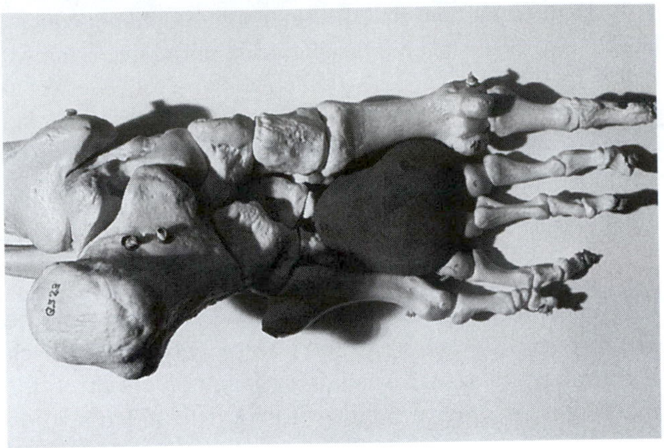

Figure 31.6 Rubber metatarsal pab. Whether used as an internal modification or as part of an insert, the pad should be oriented as shown on the skeletal model.

The *metatarsal pad* (Fig. 31.6) is a convexity that may be incorporated in an insert or may be a resilient domed component glued to the inner sole so that its apex is under the metatarsal shafts. The pad transfers stress from the metatarsal heads to the metatarsal shafts.[16] Occasionally, modifications are sandwiched between the inner and outer soles; for example, the patient with marked arthritic changes in the front of the foot probably will be more comfortable if the shoe has a long steel spring between the soles to eliminate motion at the painful joints. The same effect can be achieved with a rigid insert.

External Modifications

An external modification ensures that the patient wears the appropriate shoes and does not reduce shoe volume, but will erode as the patient walks and is somewhat conspicuous. In addition, the client is limited to wearing the modified shoe, rather than being able to choose from a wide selection of shoes.

A *heel wedge* (Fig. 31.7) is a frequently prescribed external modification. It alters alignment of the calcaneus. A

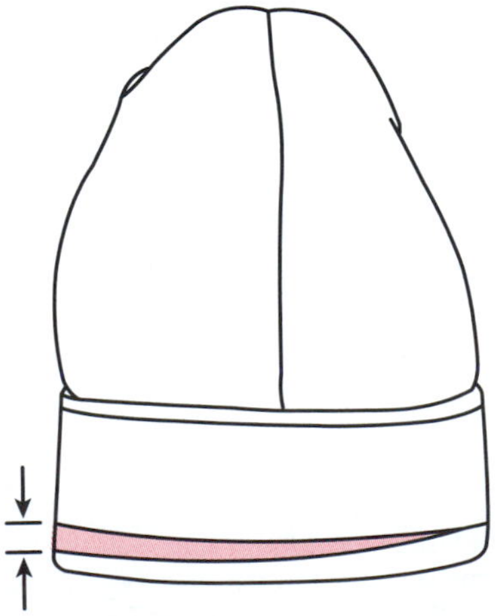

Figure 31.7 Medial heel wedge.

medial heel wedge, by applying laterally directed force, can aid in realigning flexible **pes valgus** or can accommodate rigid **pes varus** by filling the void between the sole and the floor on the medial side. A medial wedge is incorporated in a *Thomas heel,* intended for flexible pes valgus (Fig. 31.8). The anterior border of the Thomas heel extends forward on the medial side to augment the effect of the medial wedge in supporting the longitudinal arch. A cushion heel is made of resilient material to absorb shock at heel contact. Because it provides slight plantarflexion, the cushion heel is indicated when the patient wears an orthosis with a rigid ankle. Sole wedges alter medial–lateral metatarsal alignment. A lateral wedge shifts weight bearing to the medial side of the front of the foot. It compensates for fixed forefoot valgus, allowing the entire front of the foot to contact the floor.

A *metatarsal bar* (see Fig. 31.8) is a flat strip of leather or other firm material placed posterior to the metatarsal heads. At late stance, the bar transfers stress from the metatarsophalangeal joints to the metatarsal shafts. A *rocker bar* (see Fig. 31.8) is a convex strip affixed to the sole proximal to the metatarsal heads. It reduces the distance the wearer must travel during stance phase, improving late stance,[17] as well as shifting load from the metatarsophalangeal joints to the metatarsal shafts.

The patient with leg length discrepancy of more than 1/2 in. (1 cm) will walk better with a shoe lift made of cork or lightweight plastic. Approximately 3/8 in. (0.8 cm) of the elevation can be accommodated inside a low-quarter shoe at the heel.

Ankle–Foot Orthoses

The AFO is composed of a foundation, ankle control, foot control, and a superstructure.

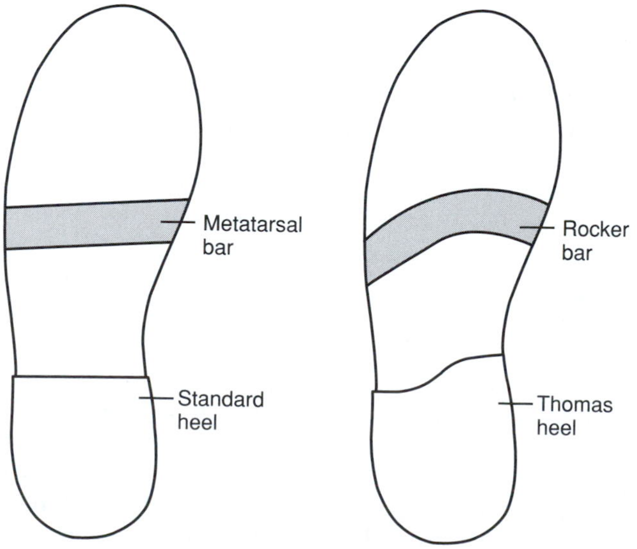

Figure 31.8 Illustrated here are (*left*) a metatarsal bar and standard heel and (*right*) a rocker bar with a Thomas heel.

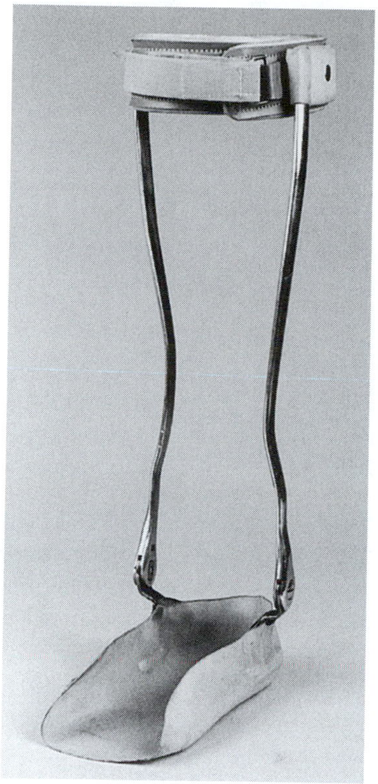

Figure 31.9 AFO with plastic shoe insert.

Foundation

The foundation of the orthosis consists of the shoe and a plastic or metal component.

Insert

A plastic or metal insert or foot plate foundation (Fig. 31.9) has several advantages. Because internal modifications can be incorporated in it, the insert provides good control of the foot. It must be worn with a shoe that closes high on the dorsum of the foot to retain the orthosis. The insert facilitates donning the orthosis because the shoe can be separated from the rest of the brace. The insert also permits interchanging shoes, assuming that all shoes have been made on the same last. Less expensive shoes, such as sneakers, can also be worn, because the foundation does not need to be riveted to the shoe. The orthosis with an insert is relatively lightweight; the insert is usually made of a thermoplastic material, such as polyethylene or polypropylene. These materials are heated, then molded over a plaster model of the patient's limb. The orthotist modifies the model, removing some plaster in areas where the orthosis is to apply substantial pressure, and adding plaster where pressure relief is required.

An insert foundation is inappropriate if the patient cannot be relied on to wear the orthosis with a shoe of proper heel height. If the orthosis is placed in a shoe with too low a heel, the uprights would incline posteriorly, increasing the tendency of the wearer's knee to extend. Conversely, if the orthosis is worn with a higher heeled shoe,

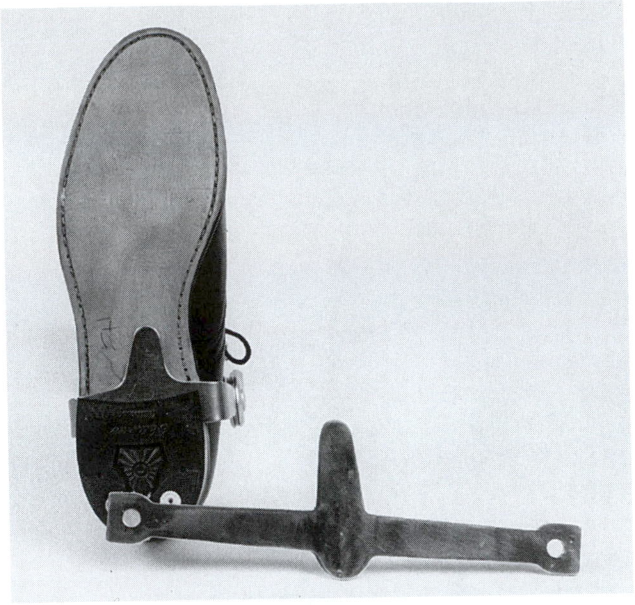

Figure 31.10 Solid stirrup. Note that the stirrup in the foreground is as it appears from the manufacturer before it is fitted to the shoe.

the patient might experience knee instability. The insert reduces interior shoe volume, and thus must be used with suitably spacious shoes. Custom-molded foot plates may be more expensive than other types of foundations. If the orthosis is to be used by a very obese or exceptionally active individual, a plastic foot plate may not provide adequate support.

Stirrup

The traditional foundation for the AFO is a steel *stirrup,* a U-shaped fixture, the center portion of which is riveted to the shoe through the shank. The arms of the stirrup join the brace uprights at the level of the anatomical ankle, providing congruency between orthotic and anatomical joints. The *solid stirrup* (Fig. 31.10) is a one-piece attachment that provides maximum stability of the orthosis on the shoe. The *split stirrup* (Fig. 31.11) has three segments. The central portion has a transverse rectangular opening on each side. Medial and lateral angled side pieces fit into the openings. The split stirrup simplifies donning the orthosis because the wearer can detach the uprights from the shoe. If a central piece is riveted to other shoes, then shoes can be interchanged. The extremely active client may dislodge a side piece from its receptacle unintentionally. The split stirrup is bulkier and heavier than a solid stirrup or foot plate.

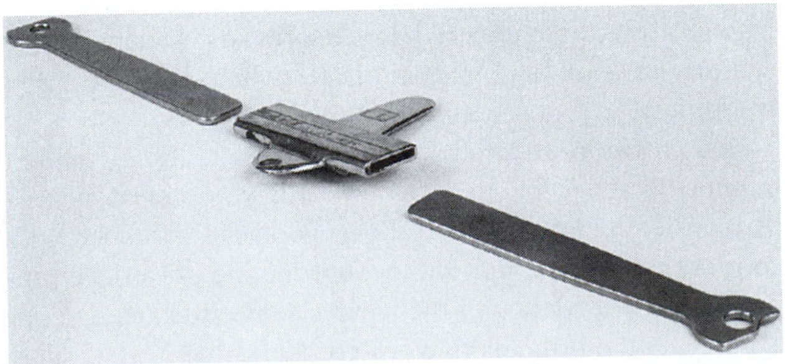

Figure 31.11 Split stirrup.

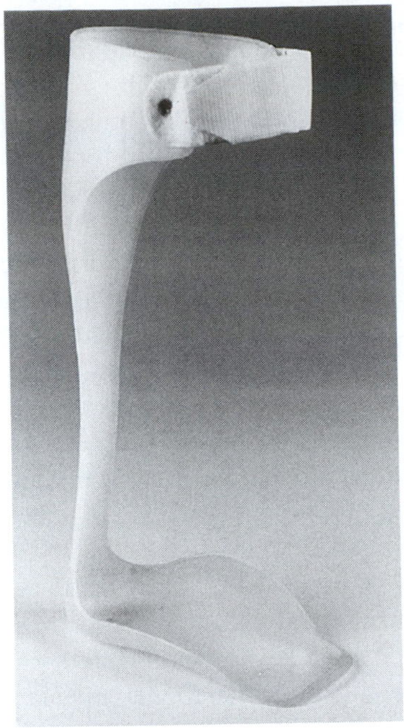

Figure 31.12 Plastic foot plate on posterior leaf spring AFO.

Ankle Control

Most AFOs are prescribed to control ankle motion by limiting plantarflexion and/or dorsiflexion, or by assisting motion. The patient with dorsiflexor weakness or paralysis risks dragging the toe during swing phase. Dorsiflexion assistance can be provided by a *posterior leaf spring* that arises from a plastic insert (Fig. 31.12). During early stance, as the patient applies force to the braced foot, the upright bends backward slightly. When the patient progresses into swing phase, the plastic recoils forward to lift the foot. Thinner, narrower plastic permits relatively greater motion. Motion assistance can also be achieved with a steel dorsiflexion spring assist (Klenzak joint) (Fig. 31.13) incorporated into each stirrup. The coil spring compresses in stance and rebounds during swing. The tightness of the coil can be adjusted. An orthosis with a dorsiflexion spring assist is noticeably bulkier than the posterior leaf spring model. Both types of spring assists yield slightly into plantarflexion at heel contact, affording the wearer protection against inadvertent knee flexion. Other AFO designs are presented in Figures 31.14 and 31.15.

The alternate approach to prevent toe drag is plantarflexion resistance, which prevents the foot from plantarflexing so that the patient with drop foot will not catch the toe and stumble during swing phase. Adults with hemiplegia who wore AFOs demonstrated increased cadence, walking speed, step length, and ankle dorsiflexion.[18] A joint placed in a plastic hinged solid ankle AFO (Fig. 31.16) or a metal posterior stop (Fig. 31.17) can be incorporated in the stirrup. The posterior stop tends to impose a flexion force at the knee during early stance and prevents the lax knee from hyperextending.

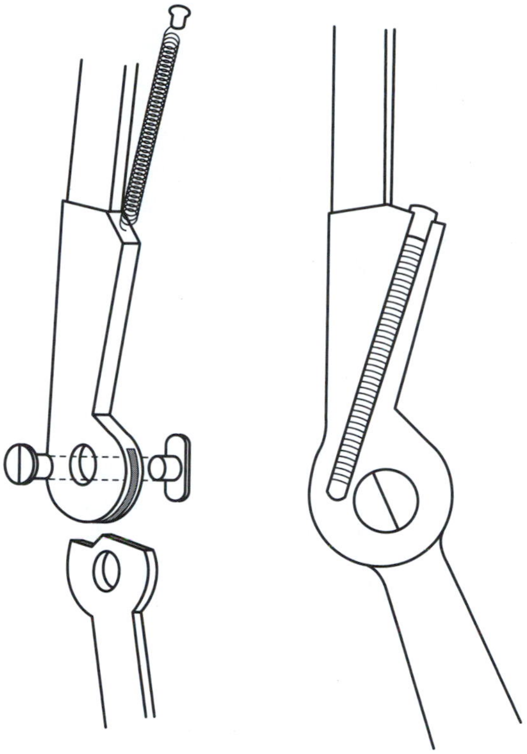

Figure 31.13 Steel dorsiflexion assist.

An anterior stop limits dorsiflexion, aiding the individual with paralysis of the triceps surae to achieve late stance.[19]

Limiting all foot and ankle motion can be achieved with a plastic *solid ankle–foot orthosis* (Fig. 31.18); its trimline is anterior to the malleoli. The solid ankle orthosis may be divided transversely at the ankle, with the two sections hinged, creating the *hinged solid ankle–foot orthosis* (see Fig. 31.16). It provides slight sagittal motion, fostering achievement of the foot-flat position in early stance and enabling some patients with hemiplegia to walk with increased stride length and cadence.[20] Children with spastic diplegia preferred the hinged AFO, rather than the solid AFO, although gait velocity, cadence, and stride length were unaffected.[21] The joint at the hinge may be a plastic overlap or a plastic rod. A versatile option is a pair of metal hinges that can be adjusted to alter the excursion of ankle motion. An alternative to the plastic solid ankle AFO is a metal joint that resists both plantarflexion and dorsiflexion, known as a limited motion joint. One type of limited motion joint is a pair of *bichannel adjustable ankle locks (BiCAALs)* (Fig. 31.19) which consist of a pair of joints, each of which has an anterior and a posterior spring. Ordinarily, the springs are replaced by metal pins, the lengths of which determine the amount of motion provided by the orthosis. To compensate for lack of plantarflexion in early stance, the shoe used with the solid AFO or the orthosis with a limited motion stop should have a resilient heel. Similarly, to facilitate early rollover in late stance, the shoe sole should have a rocker bar.

Foot Control

Medial–lateral motion can be controlled with a solid ankle AFO. The rigidity of the orthosis can be increased by using thicker or stiffer plastic, corrugating the plastic, forming the edges with a rolled contour, or embedding carbon fiber reinforcements. A solid ankle AFO (see Fig. 31.18) or a hinged

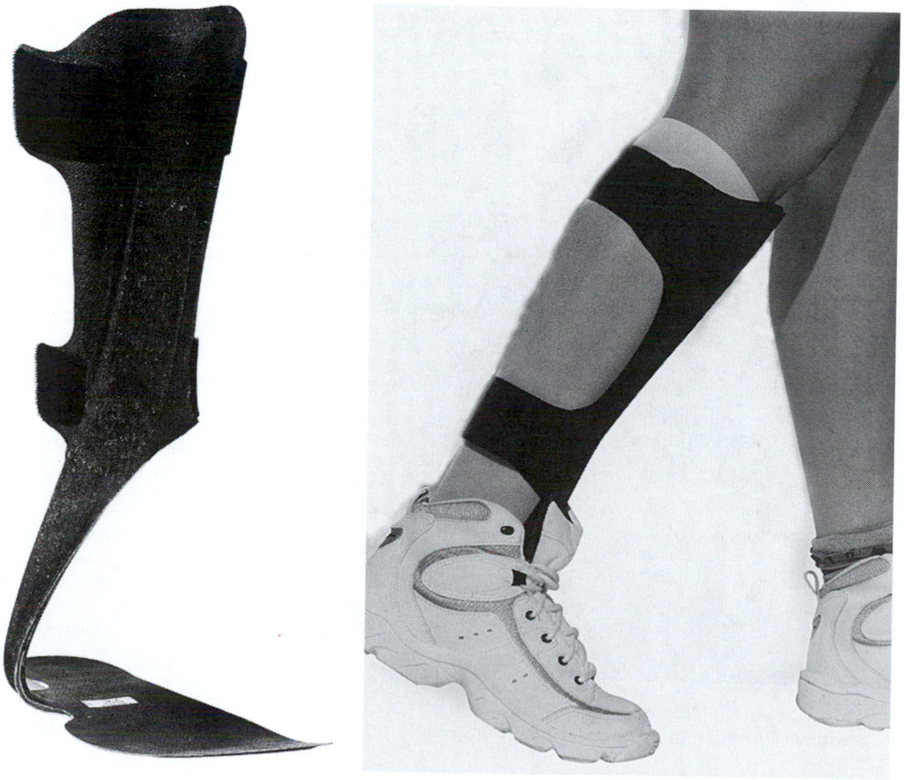

Figure 31.14 ToeOFF® ankle foot orthosis. This orthosis is designed to provide dorsiflexion assistance in the presence of mild to severe footdrop accompanied by mild to moderate ankle instability. It is fabricated from fiber glass, carbon fiber, and Kevlar. Note: This orthosis would not be indicated in the presence of moderate to severe spasticity or edema. (Courtesy of CAMP Scandinavia AB. SE 254 67 Helsingborg, Sweden.)

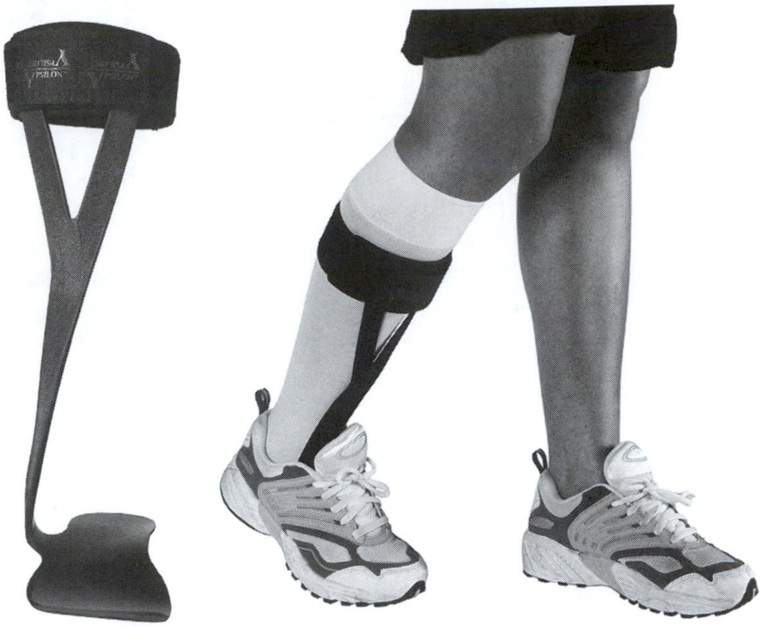

Figure 31.15 Ypsilon™ ankle foot orthosis. This carbon composite AFO is designed to provide dorsiflexion assistance in the presence of mild to moderate isolated drop foot. It promotes free ankle movements (medial, lateral, and rotational movement). The proximal Y-shape provides tibia crest clearance. Note: This orthosis would not be indicated for an unstable ankle joint or in the presence of moderate to severe spasticity or edema. (Courtesy of CAMP Scandinavia AB. SE 254 67 Helsingborg, Sweden.)

solid ankle AFO (see Fig. 31.16) also controls frontal and transverse plane foot motion. Less effective is a metal and leather orthosis to which a leather valgus (varus) correction strap is attached. The valgus correction strap (Fig. 31.20) is sewn to the medial portion of the shoe upper near the sole, and buckles around the lateral upright, exerting a laterally directed force to restrain pronation. The varus correction strap has opposite attachments and force application. Either strap, although adjustable, complicates donning.

Superstructure

The proximal portion of the orthosis, the superstructure, consists of uprights, and a shell, band, or brim. Plastic AFOs usually have a single upright or shell. Both the solid ankle and the hinged solid ankle AFOs have a posterior shell extending from the medial to the lateral midline of the

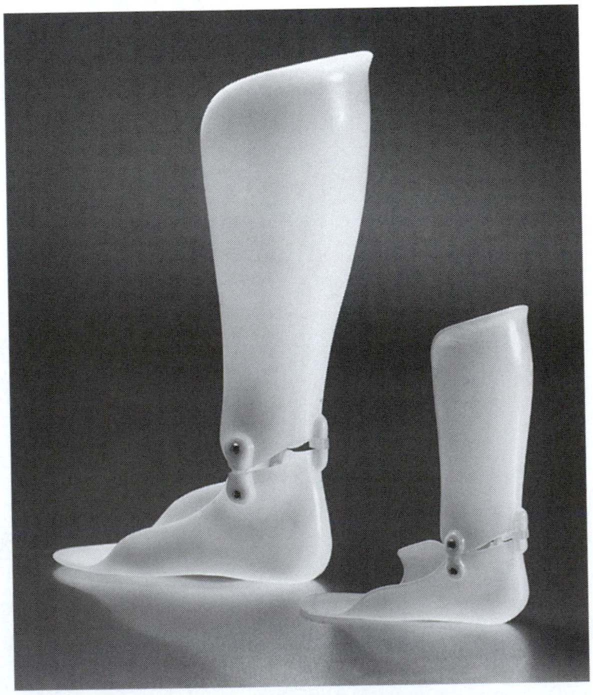

Figure 31.16 Plastic hinged solid ankle foot orthoses. (Courtesy of Otto Bock, Minneapolis, MN 55447.)

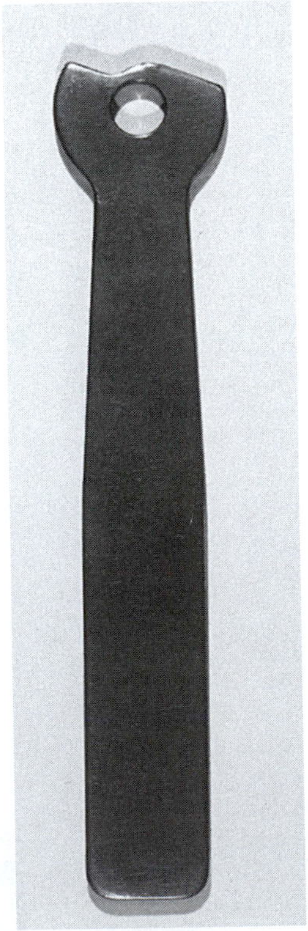

Figure 31.17 Steel stirrup with posterior stop at its proximal end. Stop is to the left.

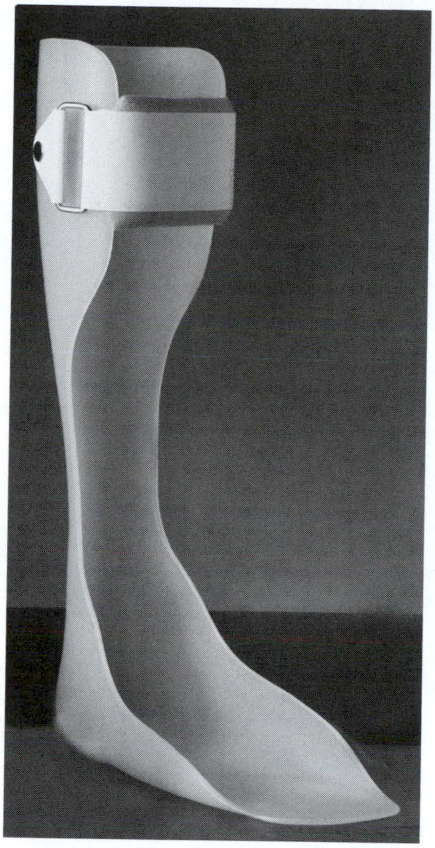

Figure 31.18 Plastic solid AFO. (Courtesy of Otto Bock, Minneapolis, MN 55447).

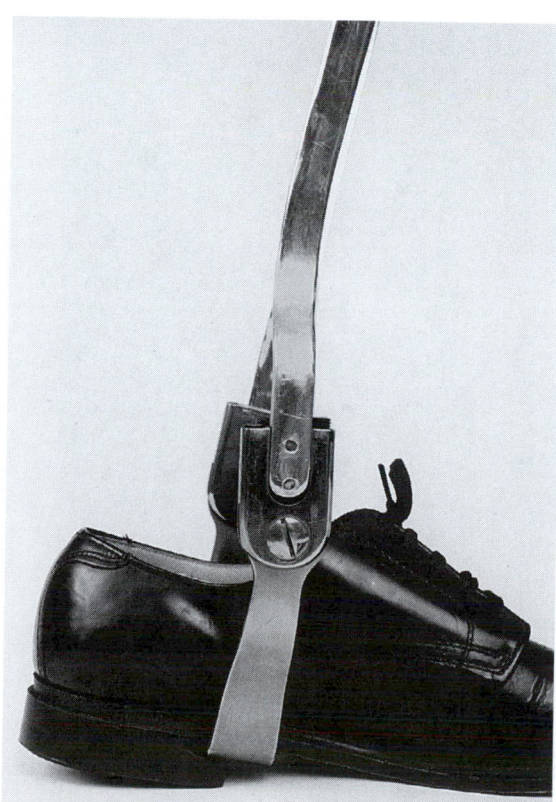

Figure 31.19 Bichannel adjustable ankle locks (BiCAALs).

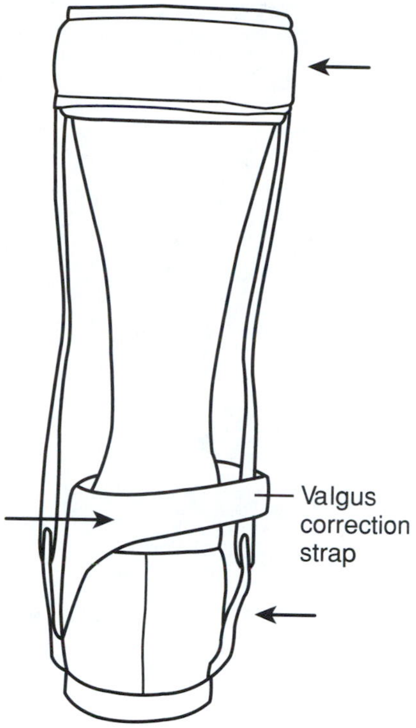

Figure 31.20 Valgus correction strap (also called a "T-strap"). The arrows denoted the three-point pressure system created by the correction forces (right lower extremity).

leg, thus providing excellent medial-lateral control and a broad surface to minimize pressure. The posterior leaf spring AFO (see Fig. 31.12) has a single posterior upright that does not contribute to frontal or transverse plane control.

The spiral AFO (Fig. 31.21) is a design in which a single upright spirals from the foot plate around the leg, terminating in a proximal band. It may be made of polypropylene, nylon acrylic, or carbon fiber. The spiral orthosis controls, but does not eliminate, motion in all planes.[22] Orthoses with plastic shells or uprights are molded over a cast of the patient's leg and are designed to fit snugly for maximal control and minimal conspicuousness. Such AFOs are contraindicated for the individual whose ankle and leg volume fluctuates markedly, because the orthoses cannot be adjusted readily.

Metal and leather orthoses usually have medial and lateral uprights to maximize structural stability. Occasionally, a single side upright will suffice when the patient insists on a less conspicuous orthosis and the person is not expected to exert undue force. Aluminum uprights are lighter in weight than steel. Carbon graphite and titanium uprights weigh appreciably less than aluminum and rival the strength of steel; however, orthoses made of the newer materials are more expensive.

Most orthoses have a posterior calf band made of plastic or leather-upholstered metal. The band has an anterior buckled or pressure closure strap (Fig. 31.22). The farther the band is from the ankle joint, the more effective the leverage of the orthosis; however, the band must not impinge on

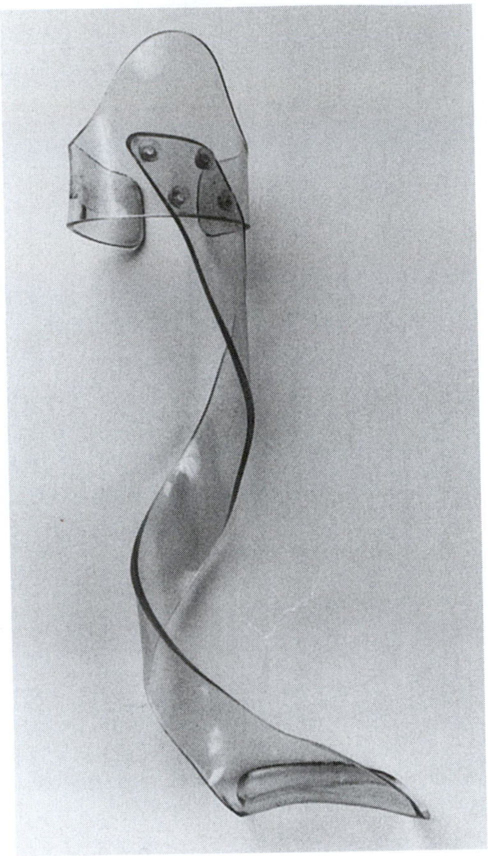

Figure 31.21 Spiral AFO.

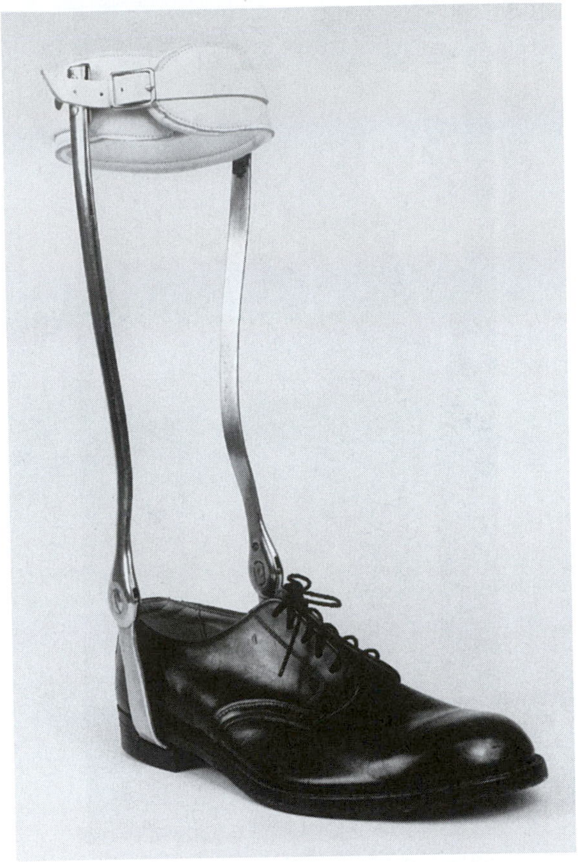

Figure 31.22 AFO with stirrup attachment, limited motion ankle joints, bilateral uprights, and upholstered metal calf band.

the peroneal nerve. An anterior band that is part of a solid ankle AFO imposes posteriorly directed force near the knee, enabling the AFO to resist knee flexion. Such an orthosis is sometimes known as a *floor reaction orthosis* (Fig. 31.23). In fact, all lower-limb orthoses are influenced by the floor reaction when the wearer stands or is in the stance phase of gait. If the AFO is to reduce the amount of weight transmitted through the foot, it may have a *patellar-tendon-bearing brim* (Fig. 31.24), resembling a transtibial (below-knee) prosthetic socket. The plastic brim has a slight indentation over the patellar tendon, and is hinged to facilitate donning. The brim must be used with a plastic solid ankle or a steel limited-motion ankle joint.

Tone-reducing orthoses are plastic AFOs designed for children with spastic cerebral palsy and adults with spastic hemiplegia. The foot plate and broad upright are designed to modify reflex hypertonicity by applying constant pressure to the plantarflexors and invertors. They are particularly useful for individuals who have moderate spasticity with varus instability, but do not have fixed deformity. They control the tendency of the foot to assume an equinovarus posture; in addition, some versions have a foot plate that maintains the toes in an extended or hyperextended position, thus assisting children with spasticity to walk with better foot and knee control.[23–26] Similar versions have proved successful with adults who have sustained cerebral vascular accidents.[27,28] The *supramalleolar orthosis,*

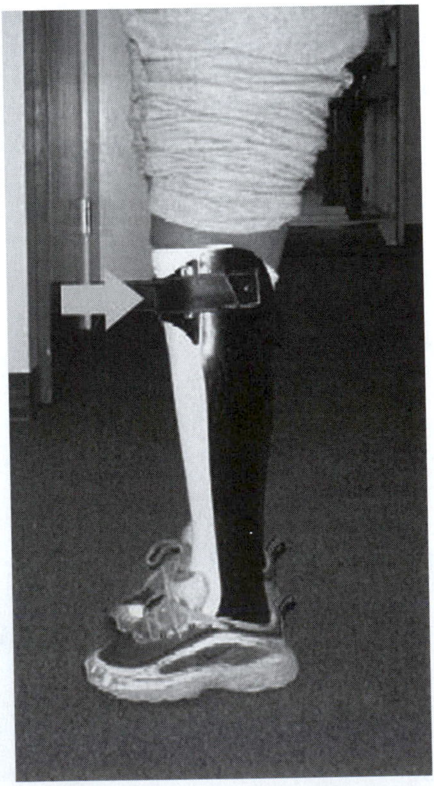

Figure 31.23 Floor reaction force orthoses provide a knee extension moment to control knee flexion in stance. (Courtesy of Ortho-Bionics Laboratory, Inc. South Ozone Park, NY 11420.)

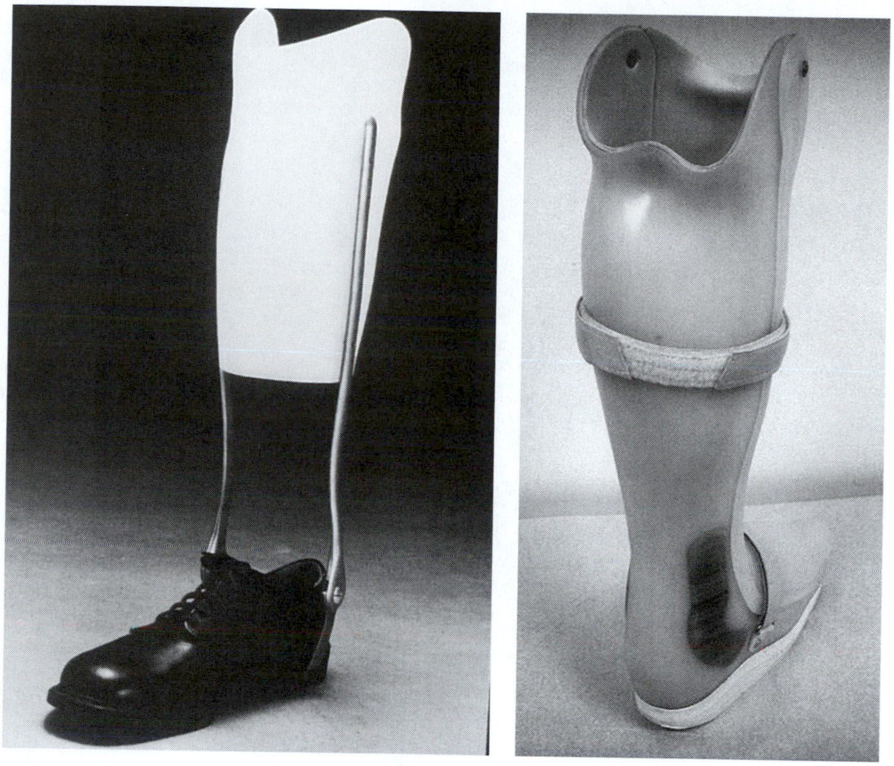

Figure 31.24 (*Left*) AFO with stirrup, hinged ankle joint, steel uprights, and plastic patellar-tendon-bearing brim. (*Right*) Plastic AFO with patellar tendon bearing brim to reduce weightbearing on foot. (Courtesy of Ortho-Bionics Laboratory, Inc, South Ozone Park, NY 11420.)

sometimes prescribed for children with spastic diplegia, offers less restriction of ankle motion than a solid ankle AFO.[28]

Knee–Ankle–Foot Orthoses

Individuals with more extensive paralysis or limb deformity may benefit from KAFOs, which consist of a shoe, foundation, ankle control, knee control, and superstructure. KAFOs often include foot control. The shoe, foundation, ankle control, and foot control of the KAFO may be selected from the components already described. Donning a plastic and metal KAFO is appreciably faster than putting on a metal and leather orthosis.

Knee Control

The simplest knee joint is a hinge. Because most KAFOs include a pair of uprights, the orthosis has a pair of knee hinges that provide medial–lateral and hyperextension restriction while permitting knee flexion.

The *offset joint* (Fig. 31.25) is a hinge placed posterior to the midline of the leg. The patient's weight line falls anterior to the offset joint, stabilizing the knee in extension during the early stance phase of gait when the wearer is on a level surface. The offset joint does not hamper knee flexion during swing or sitting. The joint may, however, flex inadvertently when the wearer walks on ramps.

The most common knee control is the drop ring lock (Fig. 31.26). When the client stands with the knee fully extended, the ring drops, preventing the uprights from bending. Although both medial and lateral joints should be

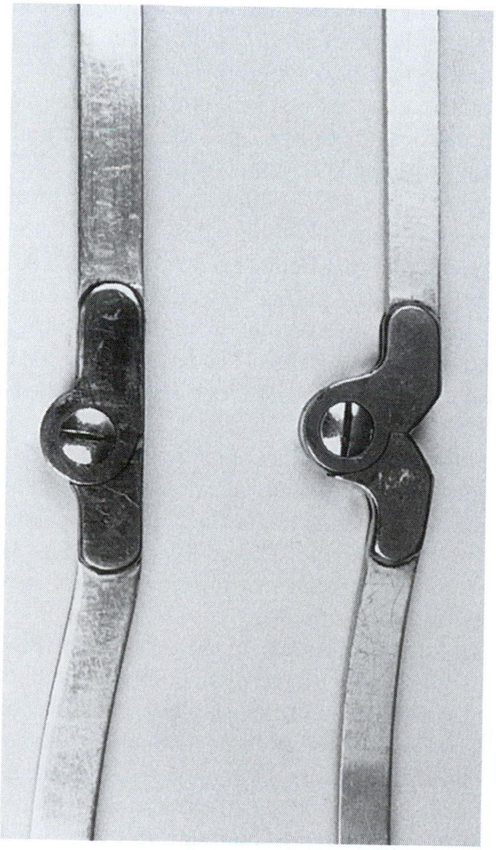

Figure 31.25 Knee joint-offset hinge.

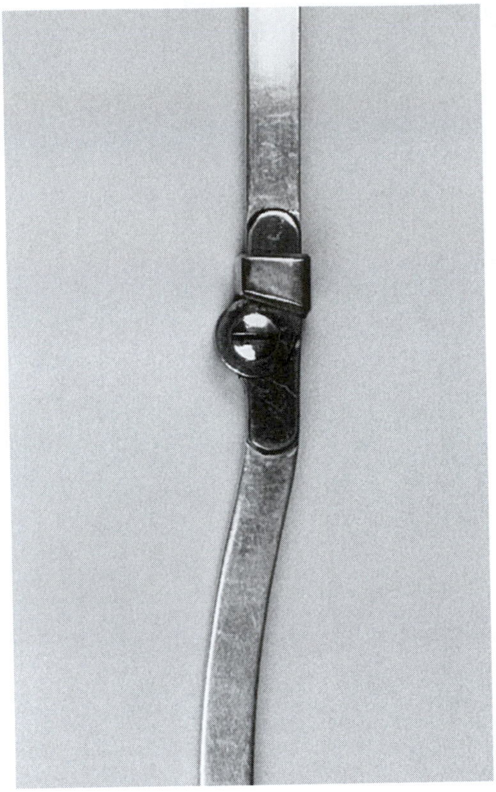

Figure 31.26 Hinge with drop ring lock.

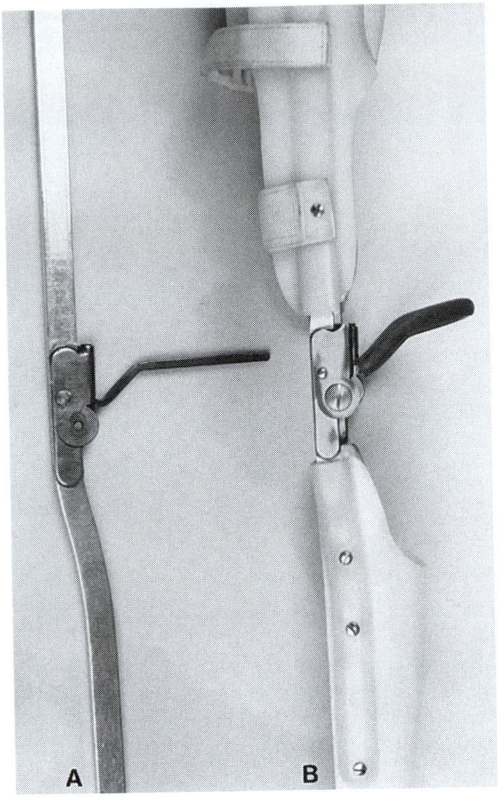

Figure 31.27 Pawl lock: basic component (*A*) and pawl lock installed in KAFO with bail shaped to curve posteriorly (*B*).

locked for maximum stability, manipulating a pair of drop ring locks is inconvenient, unless each upright is equipped with a spring-loaded *retention button*. The button permits the wearer to unlock one upright, then attend to the other one without having the first lock drop. The buttons also enable the physical therapist to give the patient a trial period of walking with the knee joints unlocked.

The *pawl lock with bail release* (Fig. 31.27) provides simultaneous locking of both uprights. The pawl is a spring-loaded projection that fits into a notched disk. The patient unlocks the brace by pulling upward on the posterior bail. Some people are agile enough to be able to nudge the bail by pressing it against a chair. The bail is bulky and may release the locks unexpectedly if the wearer is jostled against a rigid object.

The offset joint and knee joints with basic drop ring or pawl locks are contraindicated in the presence of knee flexion contracture. If one cannot achieve full passive knee extension, an adjustable serrated knee joint (Fig. 31.28) is required. Such joints have a drop ring lock for stability in the partially flexed attitude.

Sagittal stability is augmented by a kneecap (Fig. 31.29) or an anterior band or strap that completes the three-point pressure system necessary for stability. The cap or band applies a posteriorly directed force to complement the anteriorly directed forces from the back of the shoe and the thigh band. The leather kneecap is the traditional component. It has four straps buckled to both uprights above and below the knee and applies a posteriorly directed force to oppose any tendency of the knee to flex. The kneecap requires the patient to buckle two straps when donning the orthosis. When the straps are tight enough to stabilize the knee, the

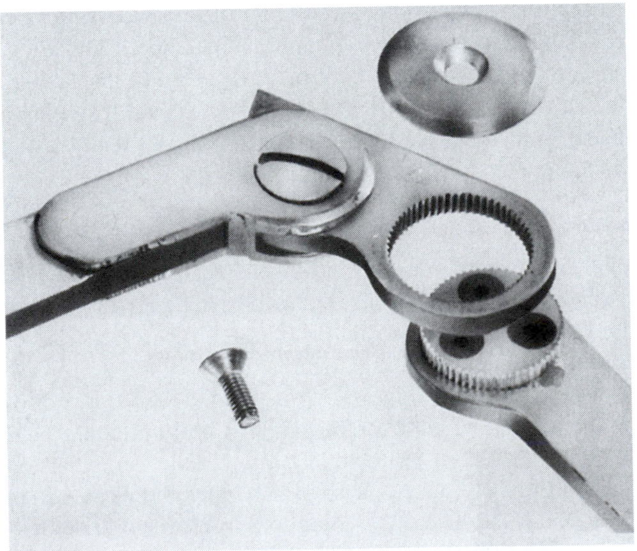

Figure 31.28 Serrated knee lock. Note the location of the knee hinge and the serrated disk. (From Fishman, S, et al: Lower-limb orthoses. In American Academy of Orthopaedic Surgeons: Atlas of Orthotics, ed 2. Mosby, St. Louis, 1985, p 213, with permission.)

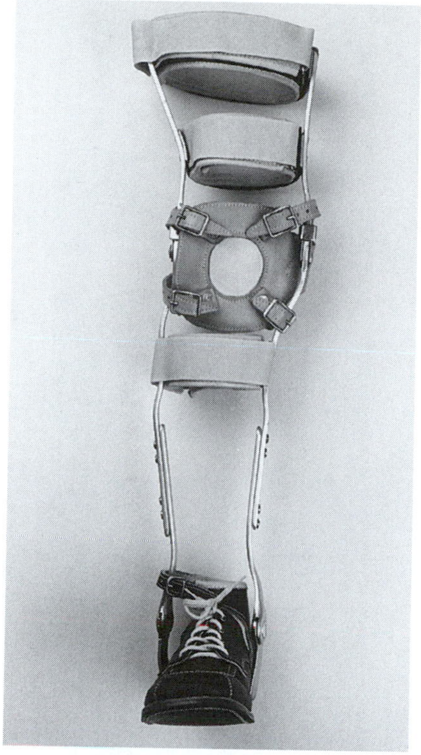

Figure 31.29 KAFO with knee cap.

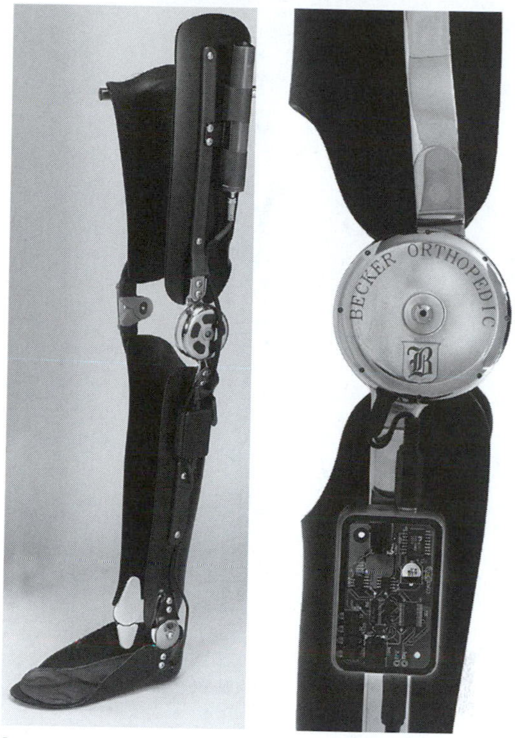

A B

Figure 31.30 KAFO with computer-controlled knee joint. (Becker E-Knee, Becker Orthopedic, Troy, MI 48083.)

pad is likely to restrict flexion when the wearer sits. A more practical alternative is a rigid anterior band, either a pretibial band or a suprapatellar band, both of which apply posteriorly directed force,[29] but do not interfere with sitting and are easier to don. The bands generally are molded of plastic and thus not readily adjustable. The prepatellar band rests over the bony proximal portion of the leg and requires careful contouring to be comfortable. The suprapatellar band fits over the fleshy anterodistal thigh.

A newer means of obtaining sagittal stability involves a KAFO with electronic stance control mechanisms that prevent knee flexion during stance phase, without interfering with knee extension, and permit knee flexion during swing phase. By moving a lever on the side of the joint, the patient can select the mode of action: (1) stance control which is disengaged during swing phase, (2) no stance control, and (3) lock in full extension. Preliminary investigation indicates that adults with lower-limb paralysis walked faster, with increased cadence and step length, and fewer compensatory trunk movements, as compared with use of a locked KAFO.[30] KAFOs with computer-controlled knee joints are also available (Fig. 31.30).

Frontal plane control may be achieved with plastic calf shells shaped to apply corrective force for **genu valgum** or **genu varum**. To reduce genu valgum, the medial portion of the shell extends proximally in order to apply laterally directed force at the knee. The semirigid shell is more effective than a valgum correction strap, which is a kneecap with a fifth strap designed to be buckled around the lateral upright. The opposite force application is indicated for the patient who has genu varum. The shell does not require time in donning and applies force over a broad area without impinging on the popliteal fossa.

Superstructure

Thigh bands provide structural stability to the orthosis. If the distal portion of the limb cannot tolerate full weightbearing, then the proximal thigh band may be shaped to form a weightbearing brim. Either the quadrilateral or the ischial containment design can be used. To eliminate all weightbearing through the entire leg, the orthosis must include a weightbearing brim, a locked knee joint, and a *patten* bottom. The patten is a distal extension that keeps the shoe on the braced side off the floor. To maintain a level pelvis, the patient must also wear a lift on the opposite shoe; the height of the lift should equal the height of the patten.

Hip–Knee–Ankle–Foot Orthoses

Addition of a pelvic band and hip joints converts the KAFO to an HKAFO.

Hip Joint

The usual hip joint is a metal hinge (Fig. 31.31) that connects the lateral upright of the KAFO to a pelvic band. The joint prevents abduction and adduction, as well as hip

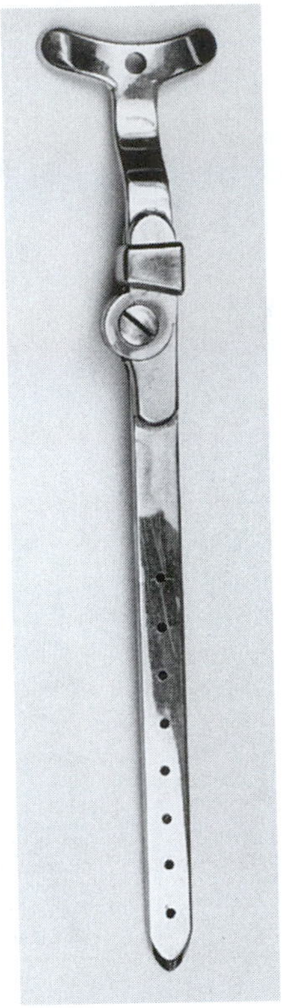

Figure 31.31 Hip joint with drop ring lock.

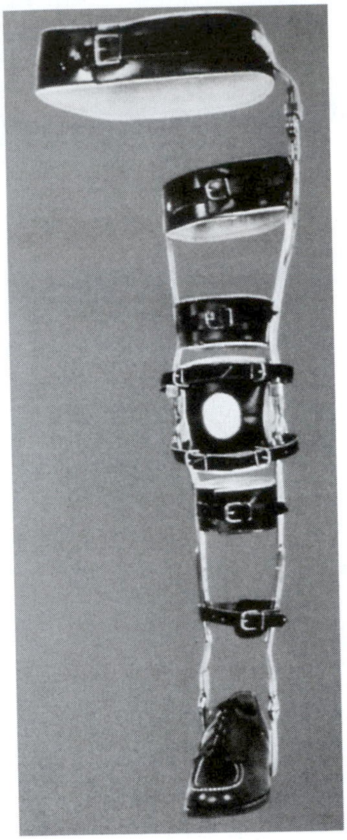

Figure 31.32 HKAFO with stirrup; steel uprights; hinged ankle, knee, and hip-joints; drop ring locks at the knee and hip; and pelvic band.

rotation. If the patient requires only control of hip rotation, a simpler alternative to the hip joint and pelvic band is a webbing strap. To reduce internal rotation, the strap resembles a prosthetic Silesian bandage. To reduce external rotation, the strap joins the lateral uprights of the KAFOs and passes anteriorly at the level of the groin. If flexion control is required, a drop ring lock is added to the hip joint. A two-position lock stabilizes the patient in hip extension for standing and walking, and at 90 of hip flexion for sitting.

Pelvic Band

An upholstered metal band (Fig. 31.32) will anchor the HKAFO to the trunk. The band is designed to lodge between the greater trochanter and the iliac crest on each side. HKAFOs are not used very often because they are much more awkward to don than KAFOs, and, if the hip joints are locked, they restrict gait to the swing-to or swing-through pattern. The pelvic band is likely to be uncomfortable when the wearer sits.

Trunk–Hip–Knee–Ankle–Foot Orthoses

Patients who require more stability than provided by HKAFOs may be fitted with THKAFOs (Fig. 31.33), which incorporate a lumbosacral orthosis attached to KAFOs. The pelvic band of the trunk orthosis serves as the pelvic band used on HKAFOs. Because the THKAFO is very difficult to don and is heavy and cumbersome, it is seldom worn

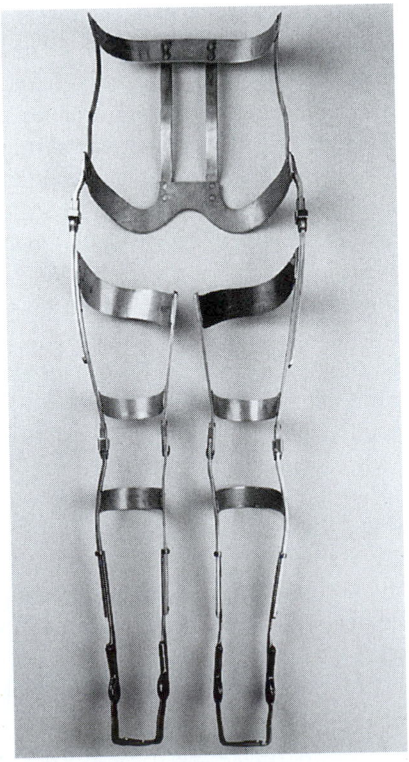

Figure 31.33 THKAFO without upholstery.

after the client is discharged from the rehabilitation program. Alternative orthoses providing standing stability, with or without provision for walking, are available for individuals with paraplegia.

Orthotic Options for Patients with Paraplegia

Orthoses are often prescribed for patients with spina bifida, spinal cord injury, or other disorders that result in paraplegia. The functional goals for such people include standing to maintain skeletal, renal, respiratory, circulatory, and gastrointestinal function and some form of ambulation.[31] Upright posture also affords the individual important psychological benefits.

Mass-Produced Orthoses

Several appliances are readily available for children with spina bifida or other disorders resulting in paraplegia. The mass-produced orthoses provide the youngster with considerable function and are less expensive and easier to don than many custom-made devices.

Standing Frame and Swivel Walker

Designed for children, the *standing frame* (Fig. 31.34) consists of a broad base, posterior nonarticulated uprights extending from a flat base to a midtorso chest band, and a posterior thoracolumbar band. Anterior leg bands contribute to stability. The child wears ordinary shoes without any special attachments. The shoes are strapped to the base of the frame. A similar orthosis is the *swivel walker,* which is made in both child and adult sizes.[32,33] The major difference is the base, which has two distal plates that rock slightly to enable a swiveling gait. A variety of standing frames are also available for adults (Fig. 31.35)

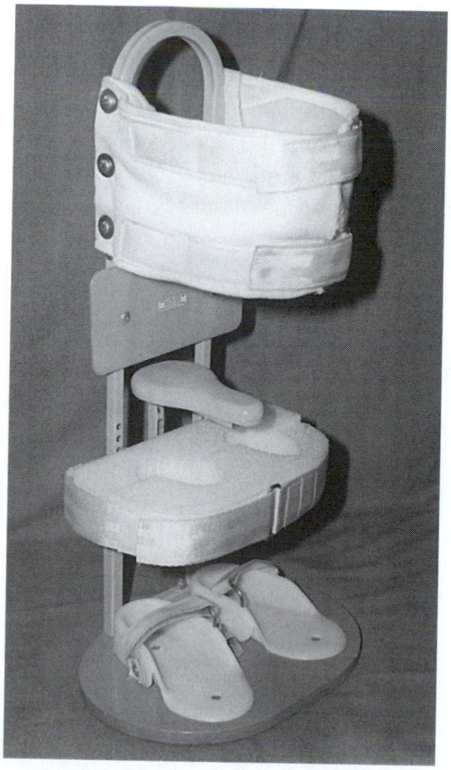

Figure 31.34 Standing frame. (Courtesy of Variety Village, Electro Limb Production Centre, Scarborough [Toronto], Ontario, Canada.)

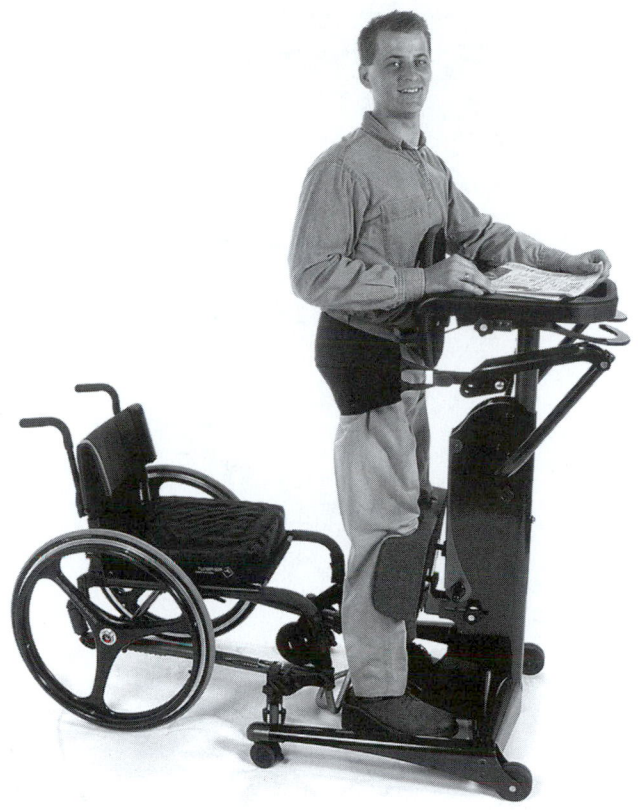

Figure 31.35 Adult standing frame. (Courtesy of Altimate Medical, Inc, Morton, MN 56270.)

Parapodium

The *parapodium* (Fig. 31.36) differs from the standing frame by virtue of joints that permit the wearer to sit. The base is flat. The stabilizing points on the standing frame, swivel walker, and the parapodium are the same. One version of parapodium has a provision for keeping the knees locked while the child unlocks the hips for leaning forward to pick up objects from the floor. The mass-produced standing frame, walker, and parapodium are less expensive than custom-made orthoses. They permit the wearer to stand without crutch support, freeing the hands for play or vocational activities. With some of these devices, the child can move from place to place by rotating the upper torso to shift weight, causing the frame to rock and rotate alternately on one edge then the other. For walking longer distances, the youngster uses crutches or a walker in the

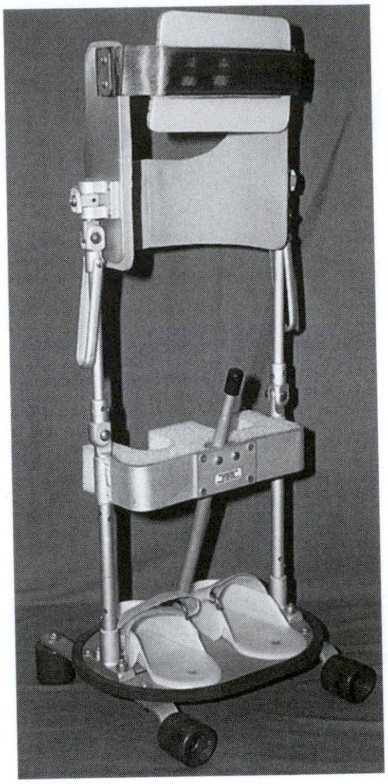

Figure 31.36 Parapodium. (Courtesy of Variety Village, Electro Limb Production Centre, Scarborough [Toronto], Ontario, Canada.)

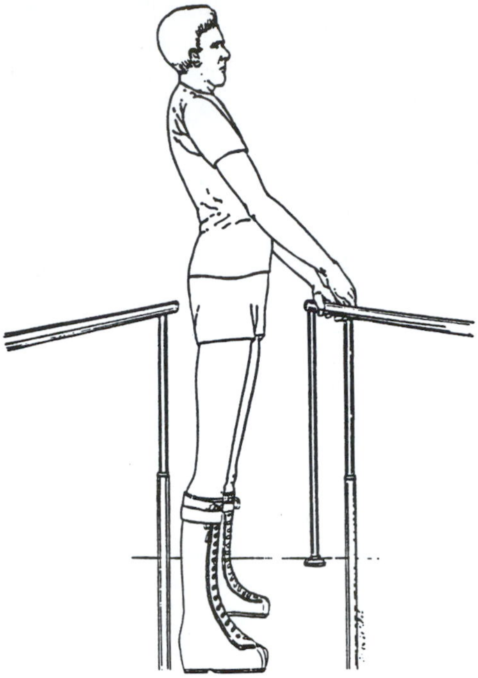

Figure 31.37 Standing balance with lumbar lordosis using stabilizing boots set in approximately 15 degrees of plantarflexion. (From Kent,[34] p 304, with permission.)

swing-to or swing-through pattern. The appliances are worn on the outside of trousers, which school-age children eventually find cosmetically objectionable.

Custom-Made Orthoses

Whereas the mass-produced devices afford considerable function to their users, many individuals seek more streamlined orthoses. Custom-made AFOs, KAFOs, and THKAFOs provide sufficient rigidity, either by metal joints or orthotic alignment, to enable selected individuals to stand. Ambulation requires crutches or similar aids, together with well-coordinated use of the upper trunk and upper limbs. Some patients may not realize the extent of the physical conditioning program required to prepare them for ambulation. Consequently, a trial period is advisable using mass-produced, adjustable, temporary orthoses.

Stabilizing Boots

AFOs designed for adults with paraplegia include a pair of plastic orthoses molded to conform to the patient's legs and feet (Fig. 31.37). The foot plate is angled at approximately 15° plantarflexion to shift the wearer's center of gravity anterior to the ankles.[34,35] The plastic component is inserted into leather boots with flat soles. The legs are thus inclined posteriorly to keep the knees extended. The patient maintains standing stability by leaning backward, with the iliofemoral ligaments resisting a backward fall. Crutches, a walker, or a pair of canes are needed for two- or four-point gait. Ambulation requires shifting the upper torso diagonally forward to allow one leg to swing ahead. The orthoses are easy to don and do not restrict sitting. The candidate must not have any hip or knee flexion contractures, and must be able to extend the hips and lumbar trunk fully.

Craig-Scott KAFOS

A pair of *Craig-Scott KAFOs* (Fig. 31.38) may be prescribed for adults with paraplegia. Each orthosis includes either a shoe reinforced with transverse and longitudinal plates and BiCAAL ankle joints set in slight dorsiflexion or a plastic solid ankle section, as well as a pretibial band, a pawl lock with bail release, and a single thigh band. The orthoses enable the patient to stand with sufficient backward lean so as to prevent untoward hip or trunk flexion. The gait pattern usually is swing-to or swing-through, with the aid of crutches or a walker. Although the orthoses do not restrict hip motion, the patient with thoracic spinal injury cannot flex the hips voluntarily, and the orthosis has no mechanism to aid single-leg progression. Some individuals perform a two- or four-point gait by shifting the trunk enough to allow the leg to swing forward in a pendular manner.

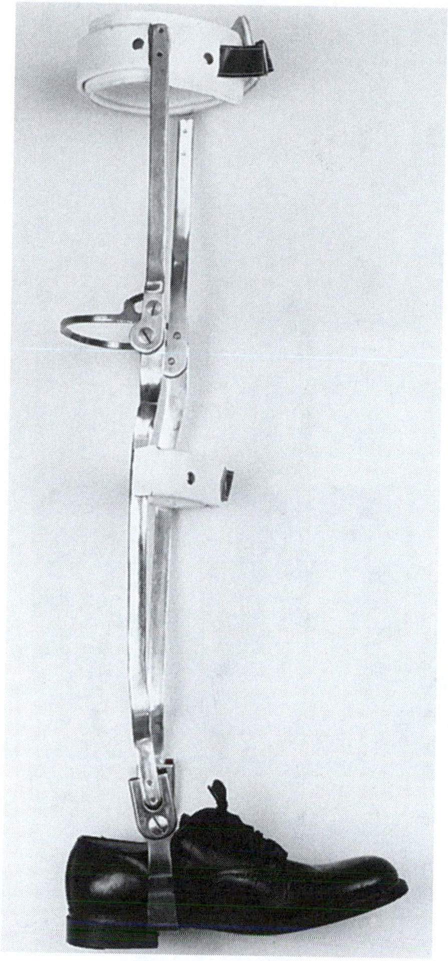

Figure 31.38 Craig-Scott KAFO.

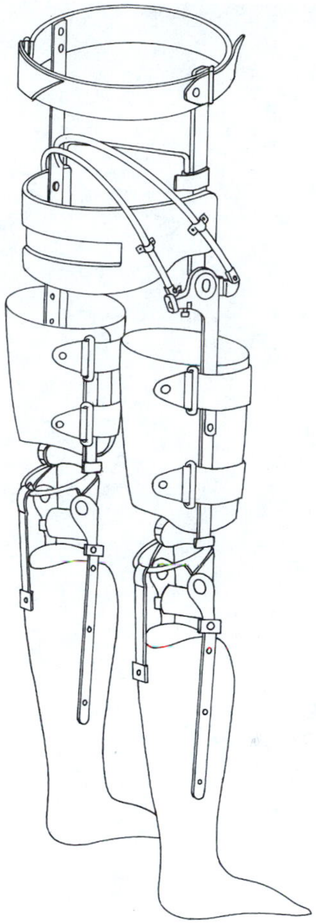

Figure 31.39 Reciprocating gait orthosis. (Courtesy of Fillauer Companies, Inc, Chattanooga, TN 37406.)

The *Walkabout orthosis* consists of a pair of KAFOs with a hinge mechanism joining the medial uprights of the two orthoses. The mechanism permits hip flexion and extension, but restricts abduction, adduction, and rotation.[36,37] A pair of KAFOs with a medial hip joint that is linked to the ankle joints enables patients to walk with greater cadence and velocity.[38]

Reciprocating Gait Orthoses

Both children and adults can be fitted with a *reciprocating gait orthosis (RGO)* (Figs. 31.39 and 31.40), a THKAFO in which the hips are joined by one or two metal cables or rods.[39–45] The knees are stabilized with knee locks, offset knee joints, or pretibial bands, and the feet are encased in solid ankle orthoses. To walk, the wearer uses a four-stage procedure: (1) shift weight to the right leg, (2) tuck the pelvis by extending the upper thorax, (3) press on the crutches, and (4) allow the left leg to swing through. The procedure is reversed for the next step. The steel cable(s) or rods prevent inadvertent hip flexion on the supporting leg. Reciprocal four- or two-point gait is stable, because one foot is always on the floor, but the pace is slow. For sitting, the wearer releases the cable(s) to enable the hips to flex.

Externally Powered Orthoses

Orthoses may be combined with *pneumatic foot control*[46,47] or *functional electrical stimulation (FES)* to enable selected patients to achieve household, or in rare cases, community ambulation.[48] This technique involves the use of electrical current to produce muscular contractions. Typically, stimulation is provided to the quadriceps and gluteus maximus. If the ankles are not supported by AFOs, then the system also includes surface electrodes over the peroneal nerves to initiate dorsiflexion, as well as reflex hip flexion. The candidate should have full passive mobility in all joints and should be able to use a control system that regulates the timing and amount of current needed to transfer from the chair to the standing position and to walk in various directions. FES is occasionally used to foster lower-limb exercise, thereby maintaining muscle bulk and reducing the risk of pressure ulcers. Nevertheless, the metabolic cost of orthotically assisted ambulation is very high.[49,50]

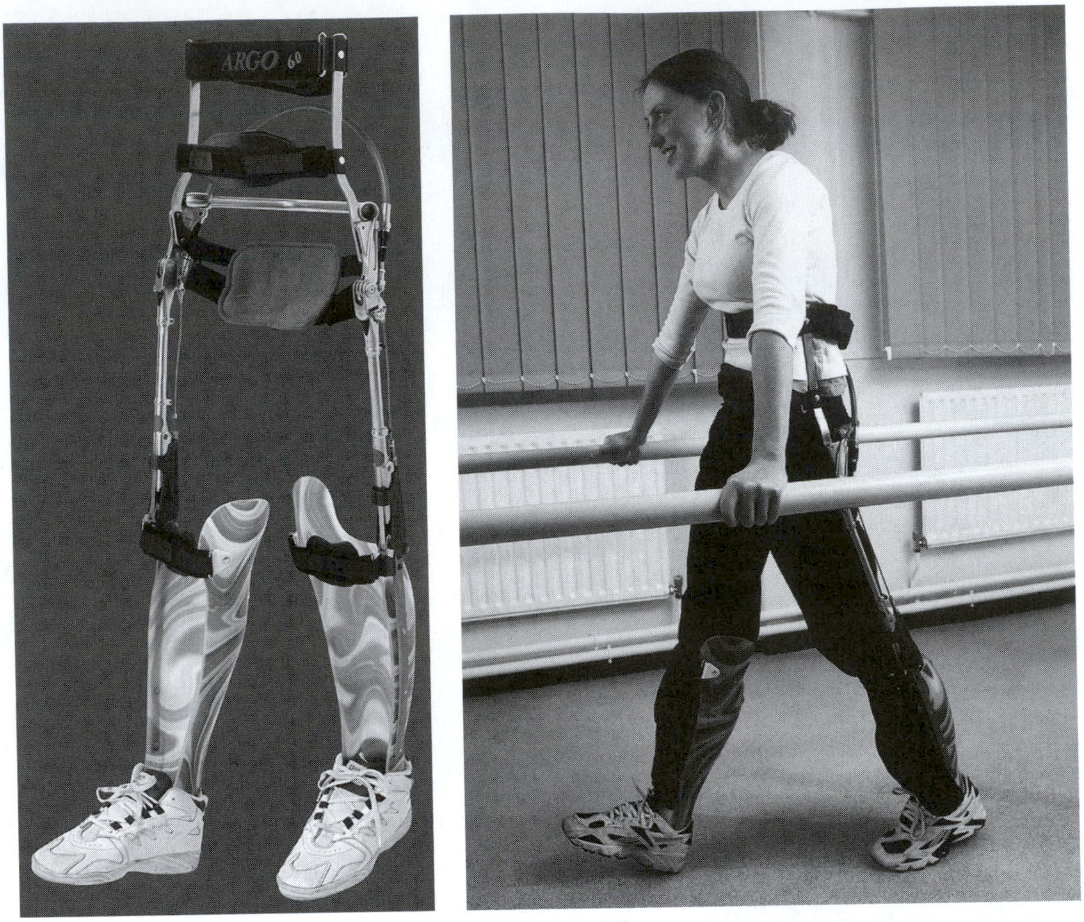

A B

Figure 31.40 The ARGO 60 Reciprocating gait orthosis. This system includes pneumatic struts at the knee which extend the knees and ensure locks are engaged on standing. (Courtesy of RSL Steeper, Rochester Kent ME2 4DP, United Kingdom.)

Trunk Orthoses

Trunk orthoses may be used in association with lower-limb orthoses or may be worn to reduce the disability caused by low-back pain, neck sprain, scoliosis, or other skeletal or neuromuscular disorders. By supporting the trunk, the orthosis assists in controlling spinal motion; however, forces that the orthosis exerts are modified by the skin, subcutaneous tissue, and musculature that surround the vertebral column, and, in the case of higher orthoses, by the thoracic cage. Patients with spinal cord injury benefit from trunk orthoses in two ways: (1) the orthoses impart control of motion of the lumbar region, with or without thoracic control, and (2) they compress the abdomen to improve respiration. Individuals with cervical lesions may need to wear an orthosis that restrains neck motion until stability is achieved by surgery or other means. A special group of trunk orthoses are intended for children and adolescents with scoliosis.

Corset

If abdominal compression is the sole goal, a *corset* (Fig. 31.41) will suffice. It is a fabric orthosis that has no horizontal rigid structures, although some have vertical rigid reinforcements. The corset may cover only the lumbar and sacral regions, or may extend superiorly as a thoracolumbosacral corset. The primary effect of a corset

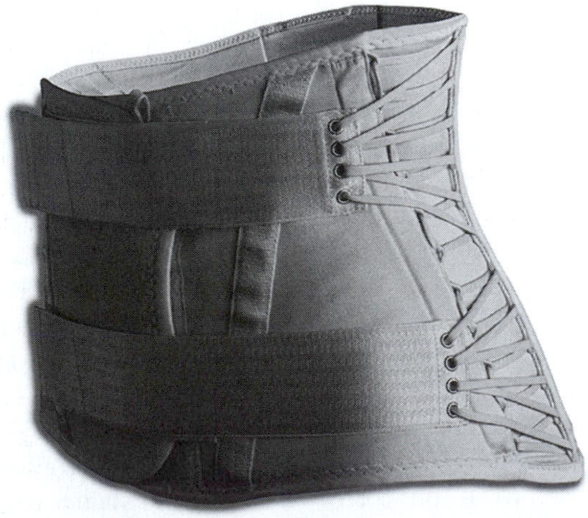

Figure 31.41 Narrow lumbosacral corset (cotton/elastic polymer) with front Velcro® closure. (Courtesy of Camp Healthcare Corporation, Jackson, MI 49204.)

is to increase intra-abdominal pressure, although the orthosis does reduce frontal movement.[51]

Some individuals with low back disorders find that corsets relieve pain.[52] The increase in intra-abdominal pressure reduces stress on posterior spinal musculature, thus diminishing the load on the lumbar intervertebral disks. Although temporary reduction of abdominal and erector spinae muscular activity is therapeutic, long-term reliance on a corset can promote muscular atrophy and contracture, as well as psychological dependence on the appliance.

Rigid Orthoses

Most lumbosacral and thoracolumbosacral orthoses include a corset or a fabric abdominal front to compress the abdomen. Rigid orthoses are distinguished by the presence of horizontal, as well as vertical, rigid plastic or metal components. Motion limitation is accomplished by a series of three-point pressure systems, in which force in one direction is counteracted by two forces in the opposite direction.

Lumbosacral Flexion, Extension, Lateral Control Orthoses

A typical example of a rigid trunk orthosis is the *lumbosacral flexion, extension, lateral control (LS FEL)* orthosis (Fig. 31.42), also known as a *Knight spinal orthosis.* This appliance includes a pelvic band, which should provide firm anchorage over the midsection of the buttocks, and a thoracic band, intended to lie horizontally over the lower thorax without impinging on the scapulae. The bands, which may be foam-lined rigid plastic or leather-upholstered metal, are joined by a pair of posterior uprights, which lie on either side of the vertebral spines, and a pair of lateral uprights placed at the lateral midline of the torso. A corset or abdominal front completes the LS FEL orthosis. The orthosis restrains flexion by a three-point system consisting of posteriorly directed force from the top and bottom of the abdominal front or corset and an anteriorly directed force from the midportion of the posterior uprights. Extension is controlled by posteriorly directed force from the midsection of the abdominal front or corset and anteriorly directed force from the thoracic and pelvic bands. The lateral uprights resist lateral flexion.[52] Other rigid lumbosacral (LS) orthosis are made entirely of polyethylene with removable replaceable liners (Fig. 31.43).

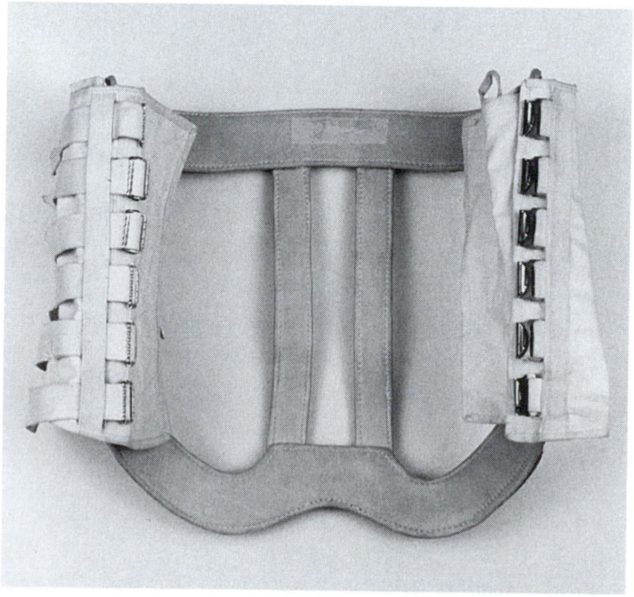

Figure 31.42 Lumbosacral flexion-extension-lateral control orthosis.

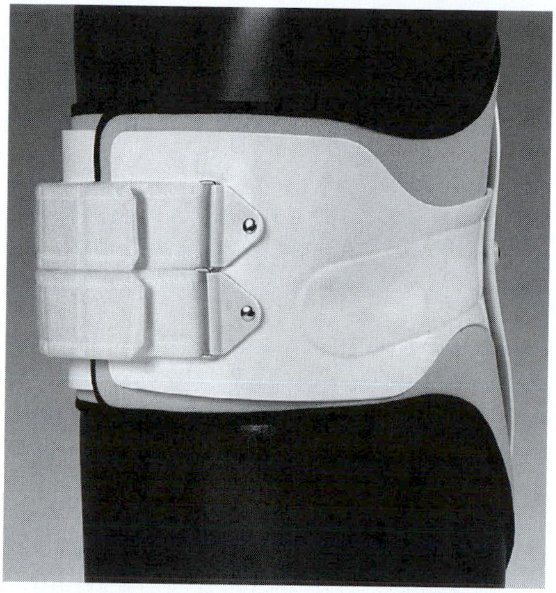

Figure 31.43 Polyethylene lumbosacral flexion-extension-lateral control orthosis. (Courtesy of Boston Brace International, Inc, Avon, MA 02322.)

A plastic lumbosacral jacket restricts motion in all directions. An alternate version combining the jacket with the LS FEL has been shown to be effective at controlling spondylolisthesis.[53] The efficacy of orthotic intervention to reduce[54,55] or prevent low back pain remains controversial.[56]

Thoracolumbosacral Flexion, Extension Control Orthoses

Also called a *Taylor brace,* the *thoracolumbosacral flexion, extension control (TLS FE)* orthosis consists of a pelvic band, posterior uprights terminating at midscapular level, an abdominal front or corset, and axillary straps attached to an interscapular band. This orthosis reduces flexion by a three-point system consisting of posteriorly directed force from the axillary straps and the bottom of the abdominal front or corset, and anteriorly directed force from the midportion of the posterior uprights. Extension resistance is provided by posteriorly directed force from the midsection of the abdominal front or corset and anteriorly directed force from the pelvic and interscapular bands.[57] Addition of lateral uprights converts the orthosis

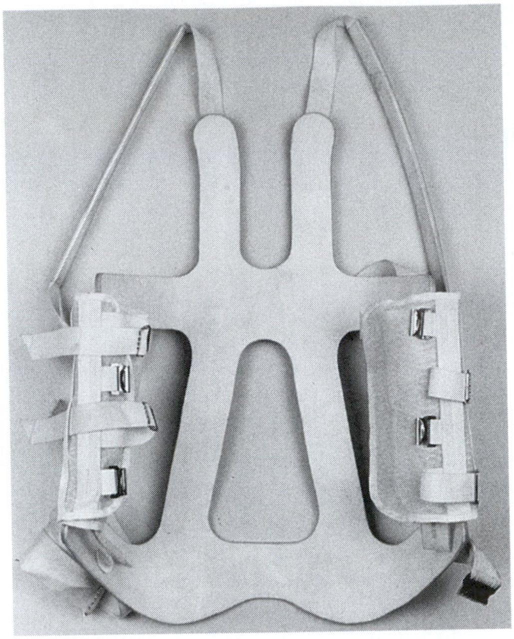

Figure 31.44 Thoracolumbosacral flexion–extension–lateral control orthosis.

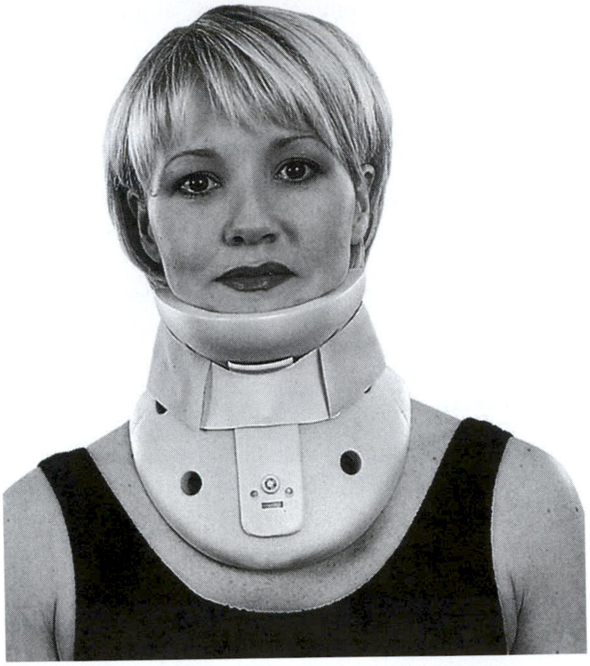

Figure 31.46 Philadelphia collar. (Courtesy of Camp Healthcare Corporation, Jackson, MI 49204.)

to a TLS FEL orthosis (Fig. 31.44). Although TLSOs reduce segmental and gross spinal movements, the amount of movement reduction varies greatly from one person to another.[58] A plastic thoracolumbosacral jacket limits trunk motion in the frontal, sagittal, and transverse planes, and provides maximum support.

Cervical Orthoses

Cervical orthoses are classified according to design characteristics.[59] Minimal motion control is provided by collars (Fig. 31.45) that encircle the neck with fabric, resilient foam, or rigid plastic. The *Philadelphia collar* (Fig. 31.46) has mandibular and occipital extensions and a rigid anterior strut; it is sometimes used for upper cervical injuries.[60] For moderate control, a *four-post orthosis* (Fig. 31.47) is used. Usually it has two anterior adjustable posts joining a

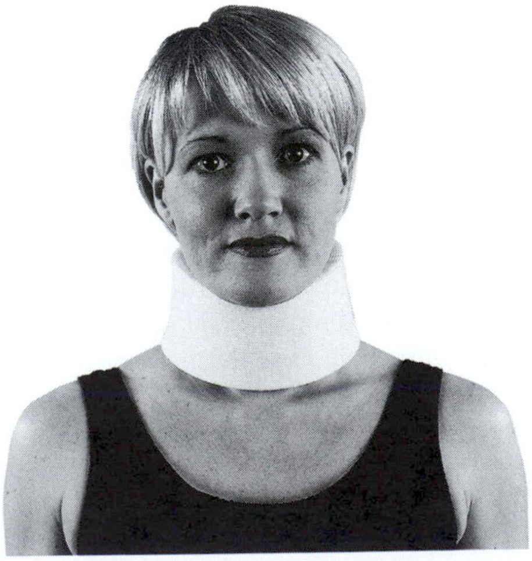

Figure 31.45 Soft foam rubber collar. (Courtesy of Camp Healthcare Corporation, Jackson, MI 49204.)

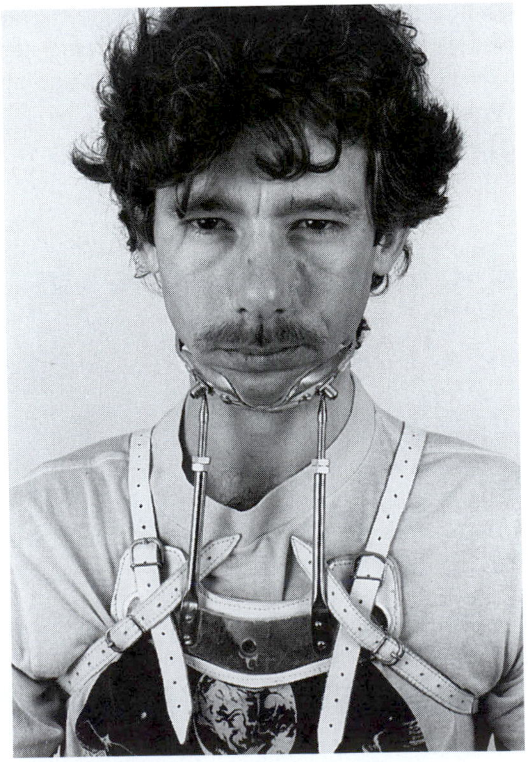

Figure 31.47 Four-post cervical orthosis.

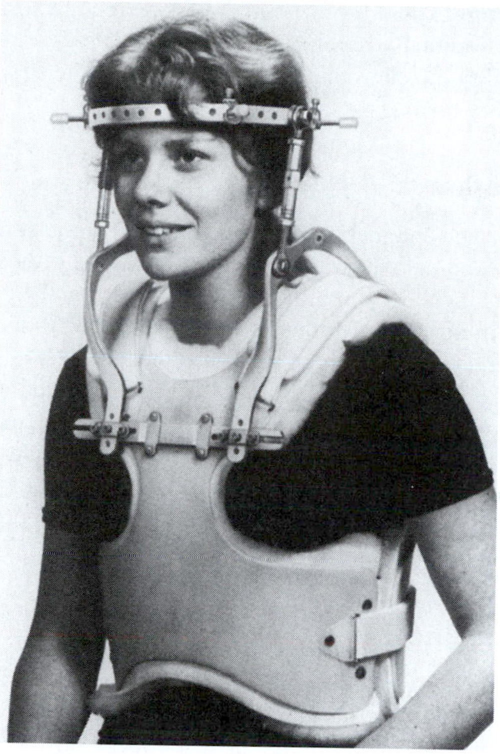

Figure 31.48 Halo-vest orthosis. (Fillauer Companies, Inc, Chattanooga, TN 37406.)

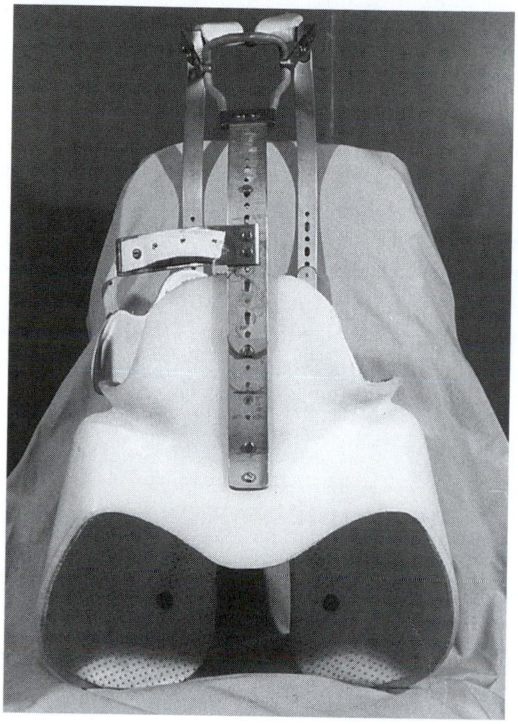

Figure 31.49 Anterior view of the plastic and metal Milwaukee orthosis.

sternal plate to a mandibular plate and two posterior uprights connecting a thoracic plate to an occipital plate. The sternal plate is strapped to the thoracic plate and the occipital plate is strapped to the mandibular plate.[61–63]

Maximum orthotic control of the neck may be achieved either with a *Minerva* or a *halo* orthosis[64–66] (Fig. 31.48). The Minerva orthosis is a noninvasive appliance that has a rigid plastic posterior section extending from the head to the midtrunk; the superior portion is held in place by a forehead band. The halo orthosis has a circular band of metal that is fixed to the skull by four tiny screws. Uprights connect the halo to a thoracic orthosis.

Scoliosis Orthoses

Children and adolescents with kyphoses or thoracic, thoracolumbar, or lumbar scolioses may be fitted with a TLSO that applies forces to realign the vertebral column and thoracic cage. Although substantial improvement is evident when the orthosis is worn, long-term follow up indicates that the major achievement is that the orthosis prevents the curve from increasing beyond its original contour.[67–69] The *Milwaukee orthosis*[70,71] (Fig. 31.49), the oldest of contemporary scoliosis orthoses, is still prescribed. It consists of a frame composed of a pelvic girdle, two posterior uprights, an anterior upright, and a superior ring that lies on the upper chest and can be hidden by most clothing. Various pads are strapped to the frame to apply corrective forces. The *Boston orthosis*[72,73] (Fig. 31.50) usually does not extend as high as the Milwaukee orthosis; its foundation is a mass-produced plastic module that the orthotist alters to meet the needs of the individual patient. The *Wilmington orthosis*[74] is another option; it is a custom-made thoracolumbosacral jacket intended to guide the trunk to

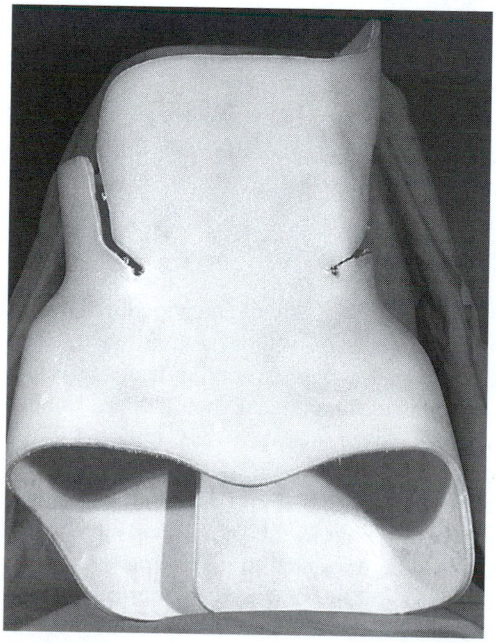

Figure 31.50 Plastic Boston orthosis.

straighter alignment. These and most other scoliosis orthoses are most effective on patients who have immature spines and moderate vertebral curves in the midthoracic or more inferior portions of the trunk. Although part-time wearing is better tolerated by adolescents, the classic protocol, which requires the youngster to wear the orthosis snugly 23 hours each day is associated with more favorable results.[75–77]

Another approach to scoliosis management requires the patient to wear an orthosis only at night when the effects of gravity are minimized. Both the *Charleston bending brace*,[78,79] and the *Providence brace*[80] provide overcorrection of the spinal curve.

Orthotic Maintenance

To obtain the best service from orthoses, the patient should observe basic routine inspection and care procedures. Written instructions help reinforce the recommendations of the orthotist and therapist.

Shoes

Whether or not the shoe is attached directly to the orthosis, it is important that footwear be kept in good condition, with replacement of the sole and heel as soon as moderate wear is evident. The replacements should include whatever wedges, bars, or elevations were originally prescribed. The patient who tends to strike on the toe may need metal toe plates to preserve the sole. Shoes that are outgrown or distorted will not afford the wearer optimal function from the orthosis. If a stirrup is attached to the shoe, the patient should inspect the rivets to make certain that none have separated; if they have, the shoe should be returned to the orthotist for repair.

Clean hose without holes or repairs should be worn. In addition, long hosiery or cotton leggings shield the leg from pressure at the edges of the brace uprights, bands, and shells.

Shells, Bands, and Straps

Plastic bands and shells should be wiped with a damp cloth to remove any surface soil. It is inadvisable to try to hasten drying by using a hair dryer or other heat source that might soften the plastic. The patient should check the plastic periodically for any cracking; if any is noted, the orthosis should be brought to the orthotist for immediate repair. Pressure straps eventually become infiltrated with lint, which interferes with the hook and loop closing action; the straps should be inspected to determine when they should be replaced. Leather bands require periodic cleaning and can be washed with mild saddle soap. If the original leather deteriorates to the point that portions of the underlying metal are exposed, new leatherwork is required. Leather straps eventually become brittle and may break. A loss of flexibility indicates that it is time to replace the straps, before they break.

Uprights

In a plastic and metal KAFO for a child, the metal upright is screwed or riveted to the plastic shell. The orthosis can be lengthened by removing the fasteners and inserting them in new holes drilled farther up on the calf shell and farther down on the thigh shell. In a metal and leather AFO or KAFO for a child, the uprights are overlapped and secured with screws. The screws tend to work loose, reducing the stability of the orthosis. This problem should be reported to the orthotist. The orthosis is lengthened by removing all screws, setting the uprights at the appropriate distance, and reinserting the screws.

Joints and Locks

Metal components should be kept away from sand, liquids, and other foreign substances. If the joints do not articulate smoothly or become noisy or if the locks do not engage properly, then cleaning and lubrication may remedy the problem. Otherwise, professional attention is required.

Physical Therapy Management

Physical therapists participate in management of the wearer of an orthosis (1) prior to orthotic prescription, (2) at orthotic prescription, (3) upon delivery of the orthosis, and (4) during training to facilitate proper use and care of the orthosis. In the ideal situation, the therapist is a member of an orthotic clinic team, working directly with the physician and orthotist to develop the orthotic prescription and examine the patient and orthosis before and after training. The physical therapist is also responsible for training the patient. Whether or not the hospital or rehabilitation center has a clinic team, the physical therapist is expected to accomplish the following:

Preorthotic Examination

- Contribute to the orthotic prescription (analyze potential of orthotic components to remediate impairment, functional limitation, or disability).[59]
- Examine the prescribed orthosis through analysis of (1) effects and benefits in terms of improved function, (2) movement while patient wears the device, (3) practicality and ease of use, (4) alignment and fit, and (5) safety during use of device.[59]
- Facilitate orthotic acceptance.
- Train the patient to don, use, and maintain the orthosis.

Matching the patient's biomechanical requirements to the appropriate orthosis requires careful examination.

Joint Mobility

A thorough goniometric examination, including both active and passive range of motion, is a prerequisite to orthotic prescription. If the patient has a fixed foot deformity, either the shoe will have to be modified to accommodate the foot, or an insert will have to be fabricated. In either instance, the goal is to achieve comfortable contact of the entire plantar surface of the foot on the inner sole of the shoe. Knee flexion contracture necessitates prescription of accommodative joints, because the regular drop ring and pawl locks can be used only with a knee that can be brought to the fully extended position. Hip flexion contracture precludes the prescription of orthoses that depend on alignment for stability, such as the offset knee joint, stabilizing boots, or Craig-Scott KAFOs.

Limb Length

The therapist should ascertain whether there is a discrepancy in leg length. If the patient can stand, one can check the pelvis to determine if it is level. For the recumbent individual, one can measure each lower extremity (LE) from the anterior superior iliac spine to the medial malleolus. With a difference of more than 1/2 in. (1 cm) there should be compensation by a shoe elevation. For the patient with weakness in one limb, a 1/2-in. (1-cm) lift on the contralateral shoe will aid clearance of the involved LE during swing phase.

Muscle Function

The manual muscle test (MMT) should be augmented by an examination of functional activities to determine what substitutions the patient is able to make to accomplish standing and walking. Although the muscle test may reveal marked weakness, if the patient can manage without an orthosis, it is unlikely that it will be accepted. For example, the person with dorsiflexor weakness who can ambulate by exaggerating hip flexion during swing phase may not agree to an AFO with a posterior stop. An important consideration in examination of muscle function is that traditional MMTs may be inappropriate in the presence of marked spasticity. In such instances, functional tests of motor performance are essential.

Sensation

The clinician should record the extent of any sensory loss. Intimately fitted plastic orthoses are satisfactory for individuals with sensory loss if the edges of the orthosis are smooth and the orthosis does not pinch the patient's flesh. Proprioceptive loss may indicate the need for orthotic stabilization, such as a solid ankle AFO to control a Charcot neuropathic ankle. Patients should be taught to regularly inspect the skin (including presence of volume changes) and instructed to bring any changes to the attention of the physical therapist.

Upper Limbs

Although the patient is being considered as a candidate for LE or trunk orthoses, the therapist must determine the mobility and muscle power of the upper extremities (UEs). Significant weakness, stiffness, or deformity will interfere with donning the orthosis. Substitution of pressure closures for leather buckles may suffice. If the individual cannot ambulate without canes or crutches, the therapist should determine whether standard aids will be satisfactory or whether modification of the hand pieces is required. If the upper limbs are very weak, the patient will not be able to use the LE orthoses for walking. Alternate standing arrangements may be preferable, such as the use of a standing frame, standing table, or standing wheelchair to provide weightbearing stress.

Psychological Status

Realistic orthotic prescription requires ascertaining that the patient is willing to wear the orthotic device. The patient with a recent spinal cord injury may still deny the permanence of paralysis and thus be against wearing orthoses that are visible reminders of disability. The adolescent with spina bifida may prefer to sit unbraced in a wheelchair rather than struggle with donning orthoses and walking slowly, in a manner very different from the individual's peers. The patient with spinal cord injury must be prepared to work vigorously to increase upper limb and trunk strength and aerobic capacity. The person who has sustained a cerebral vascular accident resulting in severe perceptual deficits may not be able to walk, even with orthotic assistance, because the environment now seems unfamiliar. An orthosis for prevention of deformity may be prescribed, rather than one that is designed to aid gait.

The therapist should determine the extent to which the patient is likely to comply with instructions pertaining to orthotic use and care. For example, if it is doubtful that the individual will wear appropriate shoes with an insert orthosis, then the prescription should specify stirrup attachment to suitable shoes.

Orthotic Prescription

Lower-limb orthoses benefit individuals with a wide variety of musculoskeletal and neurological disorders. The particular diagnosis is less important in formulating the prescription than consideration of the patient's impairments and functional limitations. Prognosis also influences prescription. The person who is likely to recover partial or full function should have an orthosis that can be adjusted to accommodate the changing status. An individual with recent hemiplegia, for example, may exhibit marked spasticity, indicating a need for a limitation in motion at the ankle. As the person regains voluntary control and spasticity decreases, the ankle can be adjusted to permit more movement.

Lifestyle has a bearing on orthotic selection. A very active patient requires an orthosis made of exceptionally sturdy materials. Split stirrups, for example, may not be appropriate because they can spring loose from the receptacle on the shoe if excessive medial–lateral stress is applied. The patient's concern with appearance is another practical consideration; it may dictate use of a shoe insert so that reasonably fashionable shoes may be worn. Similarly, plastic shells are less bulky than metal uprights and calf bands, and do not present a shiny metal appearance. Although most people want the orthosis to be as inconspicuous as possible, some children and adults opt for bright colors, which can be achieved with various plastics.

Ankle–Foot Orthoses

The primary candidates for AFOs are those with peripheral neuropathy, especially peroneal lesions, and hemiplegia. Those with foot drag can be fitted with an AFO with a posterior stop; this design, however, tends to cause the knee to flex excessively in early stance when controlled plantarflexion is normally achieved. In the absence of plantarflexion, the patient may flex the knee to effect a foot-flat position. The alternative is a resilient shoe heel, or an AFO with a plastic posterior leaf spring or a metal dorsiflexion spring assist, both of which permit controlled plantarflexion early in stance to prevent knee stress.

Orthotic management of a patient with hemiplegia depends on the extent of spasticity and paralysis. If the motor loss is confined to poor dorsiflexion, the posterior leaf spring AFO suffices. An even simpler and less expensive option is a 1/2 in. (1 cm) lift on the heel and sole of the contralateral shoe to provide clearance for the weak limb during swing phase. Those with medial–lateral and sagittal plane instability require an AFO with limited-motion ankle joints or a plastic spiral AFO. With pain or severe instability, a solid ankle AFO is required. In the presence of severe spasticity, a spring assist for joint motion is contraindicated because the spring action may serve to increase spasticity.

Knee–Ankle–Foot and Other Lower-Limb Orthoses

A KAFO may be used to compensate for paralysis of the entire LE. The physical therapist should allow the patient the use a temporary orthosis in order to proceed more confidently with prescription of an expensive, custom-made orthosis. Several versions of temporary orthoses are manufactured and prove exceedingly useful in demonstrating whether the patient is likely to benefit from orthotic knee control.

Stabilizing AFOs, Craig-Scott KAFOs, HKAFOs, the reciprocating gait orthosis, are some options for patients with paraplegia. For the child, the orthotic program should start with a simple standing frame and progress to the parapodium before involving the child in the greater expense and donning difficulty of form-fitting bracing. Children and adults may begin with a swivel walker or lightweight modular frames.

Trunk Orthoses

A corset may be adequate to increase intra-abdominal pressure and thereby may reduce the discomfort of low back pain. Where greater motion restriction is indicated, such as for the individual with trunk paralysis, the LS FEL, TLS FE, or TLS FEL orthosis will provide substantial support. Plastic lumbosacral or thoracolumbosacral jackets offer maximum support. Cervical orthoses, whether collars or post devices, restrain motion and remind the wearer not to move the head in an abrupt manner. Collars also retain body heat, which may prove therapeutic. For maximum neck control, a Minerva or halo orthosis is required.

An array of orthoses is available for management of patients with scoliosis. These include the Milwaukee orthosis, which is the most extensive, as well as the Boston and Wilmington orthoses, which do not terminate quite so high on the trunk. The Providence and Charleston braces are designed for nighttime use only.

Orthotic Examination

Examination is an essential element of orthotic management. The physical therapist should be certain that the orthosis fits and functions properly before attempting to train the patient to use it. Analysis may be conducted under the aegis of a formal orthotic clinic team. If so, when the orthosis is delivered, the team should determine the adequacy of the orthosis as pass, provisional pass, or fail. *Pass* indicates that the orthosis is altogether satisfactory and the patient is ready for training. *Provisional pass* means that minor faults exist, generally having to do with the cosmetic finishing of the appliance; the patient can wear the orthosis in the training program without harmful effect. *Failure* signifies that the orthosis has a major defect that would interfere with training; for example, shoes that are too tight for the patient. The problem must be resolved before training can begin. If the orthosis is not prescribed by a clinic team, then the physical therapist should use the examination procedure to assure that the orthosis meets the patient's needs. Final examination is performed at the conclusion of training to judge the fit and function of the orthosis and the patient's skill in using it.

Lower-Limb Orthotic Static Examination

Examination involves *static examination* of the orthosis on the patient while standing and sitting, as well as examination of the device off the individual. *Dynamic examination* refers to analysis of the wearer's gait.

The orthosis is inspected as the wearer stands and sits. The patient's skin and the construction of the orthosis are checked with the orthosis off the patient. The orthosis should be compared with the prescription. Departures from the original specifications must be approved by the individual(s) who developed the prescription.

The patient should stand in parallel bars, or other secure environment, and should attempt to bear equal weight on both feet. The shoe should fit satisfactorily, particularly in length, width, and snugness of the counters. Whether or not wedges or lifts have been added to the shoe, the sole and heel should rest flat on the floor, except for the distal portion, which should curve upward slightly to aid in late stance. The ankle joint should be at the distal tip of the medial malleolus to be congruent with the anatomical ankle and avoid vertical motion of the orthosis on the leg during gait.

The calf band should terminate below the fibular head to avoid impingement on the peroneal nerve. If a patellar-tendon-bearing brim is used, it should have a concave relief to limit pressure on the fibular head. This component does not eliminate distal weightbearing; however, one should judge to see that the shoe heel is somewhat unloaded. This can be estimated by placing a ribbon in the shoe before the patient dons the shoe. One end of the ribbon hangs out the back of the shoe. When the patient stands with the shoe and orthosis on, the therapist should be able to pull the ribbon out of the shoe. The calf shell, band, or patellar-tendon-bearing brim should not intrude on the popliteal fossa so that the patient has difficulty flexing the knee when sitting. Donning ease is affected by the type of closure of both the shoe and band.

The mechanical knee joints should be congruent with the anatomical knee; for the adult, the usual placement is approximately 3/4 in. (2 cm) above the medial tibial plateau. The knee lock should function properly, because use of a lock is often the major reason for wearing a KAFO. The medial upright should terminate approximately 1.5 in. (4 cm) below the perineum. The calf and distal thigh shells or bands should be equidistant so that when the orthosis is flexed, as in sitting, the plastic or metal parts will contact one another, rather than pinch the back of the wearer's leg.

If the KAFO has a quadrilateral brim to reduce weightbearing through the bony skeleton, the brim should have adequate provision for the sensitive adductor longus tendon and should provide a sufficient seat for the ischial tuberosity.

The pelvic joint is set slightly above and anterior to the greater trochanter to compensate for the usual angulation of the femoral neck; setting the joint anterior to the trochanter takes into account the medial rotation of the femur. The pelvic band should conform to the contours of the wearer's torso, without edge pressure.

When the brace is off, the therapist should inspect the patient's skin to detect any irritations attributable to the orthosis. One should move the joints slowly to check range of motion. *Binding* refers to tilting of the distal portion of the joint in relation to the proximal member so as to interfere with movement. If the medial and lateral stops do not contact their respective stops at the same time, the stop that contacts first will erode rapidly and may contribute to twisting of the orthosis.

Dynamic Examination

The gait pattern exhibited by the person who wears an orthosis reflects both the contribution of the wearer's general health status and the orthotic motion control and assistance. Table 31.1 relates orthotic and anatomical causes of the most commonly observed gait deviations. Sagittal plane deviations are easier to judge than are those that occur in the frontal or transverse plane.

During early stance, the patient may exhibit foot slap, striking with toes first, or flat-foot contact, indicating inability to restrain plantarflexion or failure of the orthosis to support the foot and ankle. Excessive medial or lateral contact may indicate that the orthosis does not track the way the patient's limb does. Knee hyperextension or excessive flexion indicates that the orthosis is not applying adequate control. A posterior stop on the AFO should prevent the lax knee from hyperextending. If the patient wears a KAFO and has knee hyperextension, the stops in the knee joint are set improperly or have eroded, or the calf and thigh shells or bands are too deep. Anterior and posterior trunk bending are seen at early stance when the patient attempts to control a weak knee or hip. If the quadriceps are weak, the patient will bend forward. The person who fears that the knee may collapse may benefit from an AFO with a solid ankle and an anterior band, or a KAFO with a knee lock. If the gluteus maximus is weak, the individual is apt to lean backward. Lordosis indicates hip flexion contracture or a KAFO that does not fit properly. Lateral trunk bending in early stance phase may result from hip abductor weakness or hip instability; however, uncompensated shortness of the limb will also give rise to this problem, as will a medial upright on a KAFO that is too high, or an abducted pelvic joint on an HKAFO. A wide walking base may be the patient's compensation for a medial upright or shell that impinges into the perineum.

The client may have difficulty during late stance either delaying weight transfer or being unable to transfer weight over the affected foot. The problem can be mitigated with an anterior stop and a rocker bar. One should be certain that the trimlines of the solid ankle AFO or the stops on the stirrup function properly.

During swing phase, the patient must be able to clear the floor with the braced leg. Hip hiking occurs when the hip flexors are weak, as well as when the limb is functionally longer than the contralateral limb. Increased length may be produced by a faulty posterior stop that no longer limits plantarflexion, or by a locked knee joint. The problem should be anticipated and, for the unilateral KAFO wearer, can be prevented by adding a 1/2 in. (1 cm) lift to the contralateral shoe. Internal or external hip rotation may be caused by motor imbalance between medial and lateral musculature; the orthotic causes relate to malalignment of the brace. Similarly, excessive medial or lateral foot contact may indicate that the orthosis does not track the way the patient's limb does. A walking base that is abnormally wide can be caused by a limb that is longer than that on the opposite side. Vaulting refers to exaggerated plantarflexion on the contralateral limb during swing phase of the affected side. Vaulting occurs because the braced leg is functionally

Table 31.1 Orthotic Gait Analysis

Deviation	Orthotic Causes	Anatomical Causes
Early Stance		
1. Foot slap: forefoot slaps the ground	Inadequate dorsiflexion assist Inadequate plantarflexion stop	Weak dorsiflexors
2. Toes first: tiptoe posture may or may not be maintained throughout stance	Inadequate heel lift Inadequate dorsiflexion assist Inadequate plantarflexion stop Inadequate relief of heel pain	Short LE Pes equinus Extensor spasticity Heel pain
3. Flat foot contact: entire foot contacts ground initially	Inadequate traction from sole Requires walking aid (e.g., cane) Inadequate dorsiflexion stop	Poor balance Pes calcaneus
4. Excessive medial (or lateral) foot contact: medial (or lateral) border contacts floor	Transverse plane malalignment	Weak invertors (evertors) Pes valgus (varus) Genu valgum (varum)
5. Excessive knee flexion: knee collapses when foot contacts ground	Inadequate knee lock Inadequate dorsiflexion stop Plantarflexion restriction (stop) Inadequate contralateral shoe lift	Weak quadriceps Short contralateral LE Knee pain Knee and/or hip flexion contracture Flexor synergy Pes calcaneus
6. Hyperextended knee: knee hyperextends as weight is transferred to LE	Genu recurvatum inadequately controlled by plantarflexion stop Excessively concave (deep) calf band Pes equinus uncompensated by contralateral shoe lift Inadequate knee lock	Weak quadriceps Lax knee ligaments Extensor synergy Pes equinus Short contralateral LE Contralateral knee and/or hip flexion contracture
7. Anterior trunk bending: patient leans forward as weight is transferred to LE	Inadequate knee lock	Weak quadriceps Hip flexion contracture Knee flexion contracture
8. Posterior trunk bending: patient leans backward as weight is transferred to LE	Inadequate hip lock Knee lock	Weak gluteus maximus Knee ankylosis
9. Lateral trunk bending: patient leans toward stance leg as weight is transferred to LE	Excessive height of medial upright of KAFO Excessive abduction of hip joint of HKAFO Requires walking aid (e.g., cane) Insufficient shoe lift	Weak gluteus medius Abduction contracture Dislocated hip Hip pain Poor balance Short leg

10. Wide walking base: heel centers more than 4 in. (10 cm) apart	Excessive height of medial upright of KAFO Excessive abduction of hip joint of HKAFO Insufficient lift on contralateral shoe Knee lock Requires walking aid (e.g., cane)	Abduction contracture Poor balance Short contralateral LE
11. Internal (or external) rotation: LE internally (or externally) rotated	Uprights incorrectly aligned in transverse plane Requires orthotic control (e.g., rotation control straps, pelvic band)	Internal (or external) hip rotators spastic External (or internal) hip rotators weak Anteversion (retroversion) Weak quadriceps: external rotation
Late Stance		
1. Inadequate transition: delayed or absent transfer of weight over the forefoot	Plantarflexion stop Inadequate dorsiflexion stop	Weak plantarflexors Achilles tendon sprain or rupture Pes calcaneus Forefoot pain
Swing		
1. Toe drag: toes maintain contact with ground	Inadequate dorsiflexion assist Inadequate plantarflexion stop	Weak dorsiflexors Plantarflexor spasticity Pes equinus Weak hip flexors
2. Circumduction: LE swings outward in a semicircular arc	Knee lock Inadequate dorsiflexion assist Inadequate plantarflexion stop	Weak hip flexors Extensor synergy Knee and/or ankle ankylosis Weak dorsiflexors Pes equinus
3. Hip hiking: LE elevated at pelvis to enable the limb to swing forward	Knee lock Inadequate dorsiflexion assist Inadequate plantarflexion stop	Short contralateral LE Contralateral knee and/or hip flexion contracture Weak hip flexors Extensor synergy Knee and/or ankle ankylosis Weak dorsiflexors Pes equinus
4. Vaulting: exaggerated plantarflexion of contralateral LE to enable the limb to swing forward	Knee lock Inadequate dorsiflexion assist Inadequate plantarflexion stop	Weak hip flexors Extensor spasticity Pes equinus Short contralateral LE Contralateral knee and/or hip flexion contracture Knee and/or ankle ankylosis Weak dorsiflexors

LE = Lower extremity.

too long, possibly because the posterior ankle stop has eroded or a knee lock is used. The less agile patient may obtain foot clearance by hip hiking, that is, elevating the pelvis on the swing side.

Trunk Orthosis Static Examination

Lumbosacral and thoracolumbosacral orthoses usually include thoracic and pelvic bands, which should fit flat against the trunk without edge pressure. Uprights should not press against bony prominences, particularly when the patient sits. The abdominal front should extend from just below the xiphoid process to just above the pubic symphysis. The cervical orthosis should hold the head in the best tolerated position. Rigid components, such as a mandibular plate, occipital plate, sternal plate, or thoracic plate should be shaped to apply maximum area to the body segment.

Facilitating Orthotic Acceptance

Clinic team management is valuable in fostering acceptance of the orthosis by the patient. The team also enables clinicians to join efforts to help the client achieve the maximum benefit from orthotic rehabilitation. Bringing the new wearer of an orthosis in contact with other users in the physical therapy department can help the new patient recognize that orthotic use is not a strange occurrence. Peer support groups for patients and their families are helpful for sharing concerns and anxieties, and reaching workable solutions to common problems. Support groups usually are organized for people having particular disabilities, such as paraplegia or hemiplegia; many clients will have orthoses as part of their rehabilitation. The physical therapist can guide some meetings of the group. The therapist works most closely with the patient, usually on a daily basis, and thus is able to identify those individuals whose response to disability is sufficiently aberrant as to require psychological attention.

Orthotic Training

Orthoses are designed to provide the individual with a maximum of function with a minimum of discomfort and effort. No single training program suits every orthosis wearer because of the wide range of disorders for which orthotic management is indicated. To the extent possible, however, the physical therapist should instruct the patient in the correct manner of donning the orthosis, developing standing balance, walking safely, and performing other ambulatory activities.

Optimal performance depends on the favorable interaction of many factors. Foremost is the extent of skeletal and neuromuscular involvement. The mobility, strength, and coordination of all body segments, especially in the LEs and trunk, are important, as are the individual's muscle tone, cardiovascular and pulmonary health, body weight, psychological status, and chronological age. The quality of the orthosis also influences the client's achievements.

Most orthosis wearers have chronic conditions, such as rheumatoid arthritis, or permanent sequelae from trauma, such as paraplegia following spinal cord injury. Orthotic management enhances function without necessarily influencing the underlying pathology. Training prepares the patient for lifelong activity with an orthosis. Persons with reversible disorders, such as peroneal nerve injury, often benefit from temporary use of an orthosis. Such individuals should learn proper use of the orthosis to prevent secondary disorders and should receive reexamination so that the orthosis may be altered as the condition changes. Patients with progressive disorders, such as muscular dystrophy and multiple sclerosis, require vigilant reexamination so that the extent of physical deterioration may be reflected in orthotic changes, as well as continual training to cope with altered functional abilities. For all situations, a carefully devised exercise and activity program should enable the patient to manage efficiently for maximum independence.

Donning Orthoses

Regardless of type of LE orthosis, the patient should wear clean, properly fitting hose. The AFO with shoe insert is most easily donned by applying the orthosis to the foot and leg, prior to placing the braced limb in the shoe. If the AFO has a split stirrup, the shoe should be donned first; then the orthosis should be fitted into the box caliper on the shoe. If the AFO has a solid stirrup, the patient will have to insert the foot into the shoe, then fasten the calf band.

The same general procedures are useful with KAFOs. The patient may find donning easier if the brace is applied while lying on a bed or a mat table. If the KAFO is donned while the patient sits, the therapist should check the tightness of the kneecap, if this component is part of the orthosis. A kneecap that is comfortable for sitting will probably be too loose for effective knee control when the wearer stands. Donning HKAFOs and THKAFOs is much more arduous. The beginner should lie on a mat table alongside the orthosis. By rolling to one side, the patient should be able to pull the brace under the legs so as to permit lying in it. Then the patient dons the shoes and fastens the various straps.

Lumbosacral and thoracolumbosacral corsets and rigid orthoses should be donned while the patient is supine to achieve maximum compression of the abdomen. The orthosis should be fastened from the bottom upward.

Standing Balance

The problem of standing safely is most difficult for the individual who wears a pair of KAFOs or more extensive bracing. In ordinary standing, all weight passes through the feet, whereas when standing and walking with orthoses and crutches, the patient must learn to distribute weight partly on the hands and partly on the feet. The line of gravity falls within a tripod bounded by the hands and feet. The tripod is a compromise between leaning too far forward on the hands, to increase stability at the price of fatiguing the arms, and leaning too far backward, which reduces arm strain but makes balance precarious. As balance improves, the patient uses the hands only for balance, rather than for substantial weightbearing.

The person who wears bilateral KAFOs will need crutches or other aids for independent gait. A prerequisite for crutch ambulation is the ability to shift weight. Shifting weight to the heels takes pressure off the hands so they can be moved. Using parallel bars, the beginner shifts all weight to the feet and raises and lowers one hand, then the other hand. The goal is to be able to lift both hands simultaneously, as may be done with crutches when performing a drag-to or similar gait. Once the patient is able to shift weight from the feet to the hands and back to the feet confidently, the same exercise should be done with crutches. Advanced skills, such as moving the hands and eventually the crutches, behind the body, should be practiced. Those who will walk in reciprocal fashion, alternating footsteps, need to practice diagonal weight shifting.

Gait Training

The various crutch gaits differ in the sequence of crutch and footsteps. Patterns vary in speed, safety, and amount of energy required. The patient should learn as many gaits as possible, so as to modify walking in crowds, over long distances, and in situations in which speed is desired. In addition to walking forward, the client needs to be able to walk sideward, turn corners, and maneuver on different surfaces, such as rugs, gravel, grass, and through doors. A repertoire of gaits permits the client to adjust to environmental requirements. Gait selection depends on the individual's functional ability, including:

- *Step ability*: Can the patient take steps with either or both LEs?
- *Weightbearing and balance ability*: Can the patient bear weight and remain balanced on one or both LEs?
- *Upper-limb power*: Can the patient push the body off the floor by pressing down on the hands?

Reciprocal Gaits

The four- and two-point gaits require that one move the LEs alternately by hip flexion or pelvic elevation. The patient shifts weight as each LE is moved. The four-point sequence is (1) right hand, (2) left foot, (3) left hand, and (4) right foot. The two-point sequence requires greater balance and coordination, but is a faster mode of walking: (1) right hand and left leg; (2) left hand and right leg. The patterns also are useful when one is confronted with crowds or slippery surfaces. These gaits are suited to persons who lack the coordination and balance needed for simultaneous gaits.

Simultaneous Gaits

If both LEs are moved simultaneously, the patient places considerable stress on the upper limbs. The series includes the drag-to, swing-to, and swing-through patterns. Although the swing-through gait can be performed rapidly, simultaneous gaits generally are slow and very fatiguing, because the upper limbs are poorly adapted for ambulatory function; a sizable amount of nonfunctioning bodily structure must be controlled by a smaller muscular apparatus. The weight of the orthoses and, in the case of a patient with spinal cord lesion, absence of peripheral sensation, aggravate the problem of using a simultaneous gait pattern.

The drag-to gait is the most elementary of the group, but it is very slow. The sequence is (1) advance both hands, then (2) push on the crutches enough to drag the feet forward. The feet do not pass ahead of the hands. The swing-to pattern is more rapid, because the patient swings rather than drags the LEs. Swinging is accomplished by extending the elbows and depressing the shoulder girdle to elevate the trunk and LEs. The swing-through gait is the most advanced pattern, requiring much balance, strength, and coordination of the upper limbs, because the patient swings the LEs beyond the hands, or crutch tips. The sequence is (1) advance both hands, (2) swing both LEs to a point in front of the hands to reverse the basic tripod position, and (3) advance both hands to the starting position. The swing-through gait requires extensive preliminary training, including push-ups to strengthen the arms. The gait is rapid but requires more floor space than the other patterns, to permit alternate swinging of LEs and crutches. Detailed instructions in gait training are provided in Chapter 14.

The ultimate test of walking proficiency is the ability to conduct a conversation while ambulating, an activity pattern that indicates some degree of automatic functioning. Practice in the clinical setting should be extended to walking on varied terrain, indoors and outdoors.

Related Activities

The patient should learn as many activities as physical condition permits. Daily life often involves negotiating stairs, curbs, and ramps, as well as transferring from the chair to the upright position, and into an automobile. Instruction in driving a suitably equipped automobile is an important part of rehabilitation. Not all individuals who wear orthoses achieve the full range of ambulatory activities, yet they benefit from partial independence in accomplishing tasks, at least from the psychological and physiological values attendant to ambulation.

Final Examination and Follow-Up Care

Prior to discharge, the orthosis wearer and the brace should be examined to make certain that fit, function, appearance, and use are acceptable. The patient should return to the hospital or rehabilitation center at regular intervals so that the clinic team can monitor the individual's function and the orthosis, and can spot incipient abrasions or other signs of misfit or disrepair. The follow-up visit also enables the physical therapist to reinforce skills taught in the intensive program and address any new problems the patient may present.

Functional Capacities

The patient's ambulatory ability and capacity for other physical activities reflect both orthotic and anatomical factors. Energy measurement is a valuable guide to functional capacity. Energy cost is calculated from the amount of oxygen consumed as the subject performs. Consumption may be determined either per unit of distance traversed or per unit of time. One tends to select a walking speed that requires the least energy per unit of distance. If the energy cost is too high, the patient will realize that ambulation is not a practical mode of locomotion. Sometimes, high energy cost is tolerable for short distances, as in household ambulation. Community ambulation, however, demands sustained effort for longer distances, plus the ability to maneuver over curbs and other irregularities in the walking surface. Many energy studies have been conducted with the two largest groups of individuals who wear orthoses, namely those with paraplegia and those with hemiplegia.

Paraplegia

The level of spinal cord damage is a critical determinant of functional capacity. Investigators generally conclude that functional ambulation is not feasible for those with lesions above the T11 segment of the spinal cord. Children wearing the reciprocating gait orthosis while performing the swing-through crutch gait have approximately the same energy expenditure as when propelling a wheelchair.[61] Adults with thoracic injuries consume nine times the energy expended by nondisabled individuals per meter, while those with lumbar lesions require triple the normal amount of oxygen, when walking at self-selected speeds. Those with high-level paraplegia use three times their own basal oxygen rate ambulating with Craig-Scott KAFOs; they choose a very slow walking pace. Subjects with lesions between T11 and L2 wearing bilateral KAFOs select walking speeds less than half that of nondisabled persons, with oxygen uptake six times normal. Wheelchair propulsion by the same group increases oxygen uptake less than 10 percent more than normal, at a considerably faster speed.[81,82] The very high-energy cost may be accounted for by the fact that the LE paralysis requires that the individual move by upper limb and thoracic action, usually in a swing-to or swing-through gait. This pattern is extremely strenuous, taxing nondisabled adults by at least 75 percent more energy than normal walking.

Of less significance in determining functional capacity is the type of orthosis. Restraining both plantarflexion and dorsiflexion, as provided by Craig-Scott KAFOs, reduces energy demand very slightly. Ankle restraint, however, makes no appreciable difference in the energy required to negotiate stairs and ramps. Performance is somewhat more efficient with molded plastic KAFOs, which weigh slightly less than traditional metal and leather braces. Most subjects fitted with a reciprocating gait orthosis preferred it primarily because of its appearance and perception of stability.

One should not lose sight of the principal purpose of ambulation, namely to get from one place to another, rather than to execute an exhausting physical stunt. The near universal abandonment of orthoses by individuals with thoracic spinal cord injury upon discharge from the rehabilitation center attests to the fact that most decide that accomplishing vocational and recreational tasks is more important than struggling with brace donning and energy costly ambulation.

Hemiplegia

Although the increased energy demand occasioned by hemiplegic ambulation is not nearly as dramatic as that for paraplegic gait, the cost should be considered in planning reasonable goals. Energy cost rises in proportion to the amount of spasticity. The increase ranges from no appreciable difference for persons with hemiplegia to a 100 percent increase for relatively inexperienced walkers. On average, comfortable gait is approximately half the speed of that for nondisabled individuals.[82]

The type of orthosis does not appear to make much difference in functional capacity, although patients with hemiplegia perform more efficiently with some form of AFO than without any bracing. Investigation of the factors that influence energy expenditure, especially physical status, help the clinician plan the most appropriate rehabilitation program and forecast long-term performance.

Summary

This chapter has focused on lower-limb and trunk orthoses. The most frequently prescribed orthoses and orthotic components have been presented. In addition, the responsibilities of the physical therapist in orthotic management have been emphasized.

Ideally, an orthosis is prescribed by an orthotic clinic team composed of a physician, physical therapist, and orthotist. The prescription should be based on a thorough examination, with particular attention to the specific factors discussed in this chapter. Input from the patient and all team members during the decision making process is critical. This approach will ensure an optimum match between the patient's biomechanical and psychological requirements and an appropriate orthosis capable of performing its intended function. Once the orthosis has been prescribed, it should be evaluated to ensure satisfactory fit, function, and construction, and the patient should have the benefit of a suitable training program for donning the orthosis and using it effectively.

Questions for Review

1. Describe the major parts of the shoe. What is the advantage of the Blucher opening? A low quarter?
2. Specify the purpose and placement of a metatarsal bar.
3. What are the advantages and disadvantages of the shoe insert as compared with the solid stirrup?
4. Indicate the clinical use of a posterior leg band, an anterior leg band, and a patellar-tendon-bearing brim.
5. How do tone-inhibiting AFOs improve the patient's function?
6. What orthotic knee joint is indicated for the patient with knee flexion contracture?
7. How do stabilizing AFOs or Craig-Scott KAFOs support a client with paraplegia?
8. What orthoses permit the child with paraplegia to stand without the aid of crutches?
9. Describe the three-point system in a lumbosacral, flexion, extension control orthosis.
10. Outline a maintenance program for a plastic and metal KAFO with solid ankle and pawl lock.
11. What data should be gathered prior to formulating an orthotic prescription?
12. What features of the AFO are considered in static examination?
13. Delineate the training program for a person with paraplegia who has been fitted with bilateral KAFOs.
14. Compare and contrast the orthotic options for a patient with hemiplegia.
15. What are the anatomical and orthotic causes of vaulting?

Case Study

PATIENT HISTORY AND CURRENT PROBLEM

The patient is a 55-year-old woman who had poliomyelitis at the age of 3. She sustained complete paralysis of the right LE and left foot and ankle. During childhood she wore bilateral knee–ankle–foot (KAFO) orthoses and ambulated with a four-point gait with the aid of a pair of axillary crutches. When she was 18, she had a left ankle and subtalar fusion. She was fitted with a right KAFO, which included a stirrup foundation, posterior ankle stop, drop ring knee lock, knee pad, and leather-covered calf and thigh bands. For the next 30 years, she wore the same brace, and had the leather and shoe replaced whenever they became worn. She used a cane in the left hand when she walked outdoors. She returned to the rehabilitation department today complaining of pain in the knee and fatigue. She also said that her brace tears her stockings at the knee. She is curious about new orthotic developments.

PAST MEDICAL HISTORY

Except for the poliomyelitis, she enjoyed good health although her endurance was always less than that of her friends.

SOCIAL HISTORY

The patient is a reference librarian who lives with her husband. She enjoys visiting her grandchildren, attending the theater, and participating in political campaigns.

PHYSICAL THERAPY EXAMINATION FINDINGS

Review of Systems

Cognitive status: Alert, oriented, memory intact

Endurance: Limited, primarily restricted by discomfort in her right knee. She can walk for three city blocks before having to rest.

Vision: Intact with corrective lens

Blood pressure: 136/74
Respiratory rate: WFL

Range of Motion Examination

		Right	Left
Hip	Flexion	WFL	WFL
	Extension	WFL	WFL
	Abduction	WFL	WFL
	Adduction	WFL	WFL
	External rotation	WFL	WFL
	Internal rotation	WFL	WFL
Knee		25-0-120°*	WFL
Ankle	Dorsiflexion	0–5°	0° (no motion)
	Plantarflexion	0–40°	0° (no motion)
	Inversion	0–10°	0° (no motion)
	Eversion	0–5°	0° (no motion)

*Right knee exhibits 25° of hyperextension.

Sensation

- All modalities WFL bilaterally in both limbs
- Sensation in both upper limbs WFL

Strength: Manual Muscle Test (MMT) Grades

		Right	Left
Hip	Flexion	2−/5	4/5
	Extension	0	4/5
	Abduction	0	4/5
	Adduction	0	4/5
	Internal rotation	0	4/5
	External rotation	0	3+/5
Knee	Flexion	0	4−/5
	Extension	0	3+/5
Ankle	Dorsiflexion	0	N/A
	Plantarflexion	0	N/A
	Inversion	0	N/A
	Eversion	0	N/A
	Upper limb strength	WFL	WFL

N/A = not applicable owing to fusion; WFL = within functional limits.

Orthotic Examination

Uprights malaligned permitting 20° knee hyperextension. Posterior ankle stop worn, permitting 10° plantarflexion. Leather on calf and thigh bands is worn.

Balance

Standing
- Static: Good; able to maintain static position for unlimited period
- Dynamic: Good on level surface. Not tested on ramp; patient reports that balance on ramps is precarious
- Sitting: WFL

Gait

Patient walks slowly with a right KAFO with considerable lateral trunk bending to the right. Trunk bending reduces when she uses a cane in the left hand. She reports that she has great difficulty ascending and descending ramps. Additional findings include:

- Overall decrease in speed of movement
- Broad walking base
- Circumducts right leg
- Right knee hyperextends within the orthosis
- Right ankle plantarflexion limited by orthosis
- Left foot and ankle fused in neutral position

Functional Status

- Independent in transfers: sit-to-stand; floor-to-stand transfer
- Independent in all BADL
- Independent in approximately 85 percent of IADL (limitations imposed by pain, fatigue, and low ambulatory tolerance)

PATIENT-DESIRED OUTCOME AND GOALS

- Walk without knee pain.
- Improve endurance.
- Improve appearance.
- Reduce frequency of torn stockings in the vicinity of the knee.

GUIDING QUESTIONS

1. Formulate a clinical problem list.
2. Formulate a patient asset list.
3. Establish anticipated goals and expected outcomes of physical therapy.
4. Formulate a physical therapy plan of care.

References

1. Janisse, DJ: The shoe in rehabilitation of the foot and ankle. In Sammarco, GJ (ed): Rehabilitation of the Foot and Ankle. Mosby Yearbook, St. Louis, 1995.
2. Shiba, N, et al: Shock-absorbing effect of shoe insert materials commonly used in management of lower extremity disorders. Clin Orthop 310:130, 1995.
3. Mohamed, O, et al: The effects of Plastazote and Aliplast/Plastazote orthoses on plantar pressures in elderly persons with diabetic neuropathy. J Prosthet Orthot 16:55, 2004.
4. Seligman, DA, and Dawson, DR: Customized heel pads and soft orthotics to treat heel pain and plantar fasciitis. Arch Phys Med Rehabil 84:1564, 2003.
5. Bennett, P, et al: Analysis of the effects of custom moulded foot orthotics. Gait Posture 3:183, 1994.
6. Kogler, GF, Solomonidis, SE, and Paul, JP: Biomechanics of longitudinal arch support mechanisms in foot orthoses and their effect on plantar aponeurosis strain. Clin Biomech 11:243, 1996.
7. McCulloch, MU, Brunt, D, and Vander Linden, D: The effect of foot orthotics and gait velocity on lower limb kinematics and temporal events of stance. J Orthop Sports Phys Ther 17:69, 1993.
8. Leung, AKL, et al: Biomechanical gait evaluation of the immediate effect of orthotic treatment for flexible flat foot. Prosthet Orthot Int 22:25, 1998.
9. Nawoczenski, DA, and Ludewig, PM: The effect of forefoot and arch posting orthotic designs on first metatarsophalangeal joint kinematics during gait. J Orthop Sports Phys Ther 34:317, 2004.
10. Bird, AR, Bendrups, AP, and Payne, CB: The effect of foot wedging on electromyographic activity in the erector spinae and gluteus medius muscles during walking. Gait Posture 18:81, 2003.
11. Gross, MT, and Foxworth, JL: The role of foot orthoses as an intervention for patellofemoral pain. J Orthop Sports Phys Ther 33:661, 2003.
12. Saxena, A., and Haddad, J: The effect of foot orthoses on patellofemoral pain syndrome. J Am Podiatr Med Assoc 93:264, 2003.
13. Nester, CJ, van der Linden, ML, and Bowker, P: Effect of foot orthoses on the kinematics and kinetics of normal walking gait. Gait Posture 17:180, 2003.
14. Stackhouse, CL, Davis, IM, and Hamill, J: Orthotic intervention in forefoot and rearfoot strike running patterns. Clin Biomech 19:64, 2004.
15. Gross, ML, et al: Effectiveness of orthotic shoe inserts in the long-distance runner. Am J Sports Med 19:409, 1991.
16. Postema, K, et al: Primary metatarsalgia: The influence of a custom moulded insole and a rocker bar on plantar pressure. Prosthet Orthot Int 22:35, 1998.
17. Richardson, JK: Rocker-soled shoes and walking distance in patients with calf claudication. Arch Phys Med Rehabil 72:554, 1991.
18. Gok, H, et al: Effects of ankle-foot orthoses on hemiparetic gait. Clin Rehabil 17:137, 2003.
19. Lehmann, JF: Push-off and propulsion of the body in normal and abnormal gait: Correction by ankle-foot orthoses. Clin Orthop 288:97, 1993.
20. Tyson, SF, and Thornton, HA: The effect of a hinged ankle foot orthosis on hemiplegic gait: Objective measures and users' opinions. Clin Rehabil 15:53, 2001.
21. Smiley, SJ, et al: A comparison of the effects of solid, articulated, and posterior leaf-spring ankle-foot orthoses and shoes alone on gait and energy expenditure in children with spastic diplegic cerebral palsy. Orthopedics 25:411, 2002.
22. Armesto, DG, et al: Orthotics design with advanced materials and methods: A pilot study. Rehabilitation Research and Development Reports, Department of Veterans Affairs, Baltimore, 1997, p 215.
23. Shamp, JK: Neurophysiologic orthotic designs in the treatment of central nervous system disorders. J Prosthet Orthot 2:14, 2000.
24. Crenshaw, S, et al: The efficacy of tone-reducing features in orthotics on the gait of children with spastic diplegic cerebral palsy. J Pediatr Orthop 20:210, 2000.
25. Lin, SS, and Bibbo, C: Orthotic and bracing principles in neuromuscular foot and ankle problems. Foot Ankle Clin 5:235, 2000.
26. Lohman, M, and Goldstein, H: Alternative strategies in tone-reducing AFO design. J Prosthet Orthot 5:1, 1993.
27. Dieli, J, et al: Effect of dynamic AFOs on hemiplegic adults. J Prosthet Orthot 9:82, 1997.
28. Carlson, WE, et al: Orthotic management of gait in spastic diplegia. Am J Phys Med Rehabil 76:219, 1997.
29. Lehmann, JF, et al: Knee-ankle-foot orthoses for paresis and paralysis. Phys Med Rehabil Clin N Am 3:161, 1992.
30. McMillan, AG, et al: Preliminary evidence for effectiveness of a stance control orthosis. J Prosthet Orthot 16:6, 2004.
31. Ogilvie, C, Bowker, P, and Rowley, DI: The physiological benefits of paraplegic orthotically aided walking. Paraplegia 31:111, 1993.
32. Stallard, J, et al: The ORLAU VCG (variable center of gravity) swivel walker for muscular dystrophy patients. Prosthet Orthot Int 16:46, 1992.
33. May, CS, et al: Comparison of rocking edge spacing for two common designs of swivel walkers. Prosthet Orthot Int 28:75, 2004.
34. Kent, HO: Vannini-Rizzoli stabilizing orthosis (boot): Preliminary report on a new ambulatory aid for spinal cord injury. Arch Phys Med Rehabil 73:302, 1992.
35. Lyles, M, and Munday, J: Report on the evaluation of the Vannini-Rizzoli stabilizing limb orthosis. J Rehabil Res Dev 29:77, 1992.
36. Saitoh, E, et al: Clinical experience with a new hip-knee-foot orthotic system using a medial single hip joint for paraplegic standing and walking. Am J Phys Med Rehabil 75:198, 1996.
37. Harvey, LA, et al: Functional outcomes attained by T9-T12 paraplegic patients with the walkabout and the isocentric reciprocal gait orthoses. Arch Phys Med Rehabil 78:706, 1997.
38. Genda, E, et al: A new walking orthosis for paraplegics: Hip and ankle linkage system. Prosthet Orthot Int 28:69, 2004.
39. Guidera, KJ, et al: Use of the reciprocating gait orthosis in myelodysplasia. J Pediatr Orthop 6:341, 1993.
40. Bernardi, M, et al: The efficiency of walking of paraplegic patients using a reciprocating gait orthosis. Paraplegia 33:409, 1995.
41. Sykes, L, et al: The reciprocating gait orthosis: Long-term usage patterns. Arch Phys Med Rehabil 76:779, 1995.
42. Franceschini, M, et al: Reciprocating gait orthoses: A multicenter study of their use by spinal cord injured patients. Arch Phys Med Rehabil 78:582, 1997.
43. Baardman, G, et al: The influence of the reciprocal hip joint link in the Advanced Reciprocating Gait Orthosis on standing performance in paraplegia. Prosthet Orthot Int 21:210, 1997.
44. Massucci, M, et al: Walking with the Advanced Reciprocating Gait Orthosis (ARGO) in thoracic paraplegic patients: Energy expenditure and cardiorespiratory performance. Spinal Cord 36:223, 1998.
45. Roussos, N, et al: A long-term review of severely disabled spina bifida patients using a reciprocal walking system. Disabil Rehabil 23:239, 2001.
46. Yano, et al: A new concept of dynamic orthosis for paraplegia: The weight bearing control (WBC) orthosis. Prosthet Orthot Int 21:222, 1997.
47. Kawashima, N, et al: Energy expenditure during walking with weight-bearing control (WBC) orthosis in thoracic level of paraplegic patients. Spinal Cord 41:506, 2003.
48. Solomonow, M, et al: Reciprocating gait orthosis powered with electrical muscle stimulation (RGO II): Performance evaluation of 70 paraplegics. Part I: Orthopedics 20:315, 1997, and Part II: 20:411, 1997.
49. Spadone, R., et al: Energy consumption of locomotion with orthosis versus Parastep-assisted gait: A single case study. Spinal Cord 41:97, 2003.
50. Merati, G, et al: Paraplegic adaptation to assisted-walking: Energy expenditure during wheelchair versus orthosis use. Spinal Cord 38:37, 2000.
51. Vogt, L, et al. Lumbar corsets: Their effect on three-dimensional kinematics of the pelvis. J Rehabil Res Dev 37:495, 2000.
52. Tuong, NH, et al: Three-dimensional evaluation of lumbar orthosis effects on spinal behavior. J Rehabil Res Dev 35:34, 1998.
53. Smith, KM: A preliminary report on a new design of a spinal orthosis for spondylolytic patients: Review of the literature and initiation for future study of a new design. J Prosthet Orthot 10:45, 1998.
54. Van Tulder, MW, et al: Lumbar supports for prevention and treatment of low back pain. Cochrane Database Syst Rev CD001823, 2000.
55. Jellema, P, et al: Lumbar supports for prevention and treatment of low back pain: A systematic review within the framework of the Cochrane Back Review Group. Spine 26:377, 2001.

56. van Poppel, MN, et al: Lumbar supports and education for the prevention of low back pain in industry. JAMA 279:1789, 1998.
57. Spratt, KF, et al: Efficacy of flexion and extension treatments incorporating braces for lower-back pain patients with retrodisplacement, spondylolisthesis, or normal sagittal translation. Spine 18:1839, 1993.
58. van Leeuwen, PJ, et al: Assessment of spinal movement reduction by thoraco-lumbar-sacral orthoses. J Rehabil Res Dev 37:395, 2000.
59. Fisher, SV: Cervical orthotics. Phys Med Rehabil Clin North Am 3:29, 1992.
60. Cosan, TE, et al: Indications of Philadelphia collar in the treatment of upper cervical injuries. Eur J Emerg Med 8:33, 2001.
61. Gavin, TM, et al: Biomechanical analysis of cervical orthoses in flexion and extension: A comparison of cervical collars and cervical thoracic orthoses. J Rehabil Res Dev 40:527, 2003.
62. Sandler, AJ, et al: The effectiveness of several cervical orthoses: An in vivo comparison of the mechanical stability provided by several widely used models. Spine 21:1624, 1996.
63. Lunsford, T, et al: The effectiveness of four contemporary cervical orthoses in restricting cervical motion. J Prosthet Orthot 6:93, 1994.
64. Sharpe, KP, Rao, S, and Ziogas, A: Evaluation of the effectiveness of the Minerva cervicothoracic orthosis. Spine 20:1475, 1995.
65. Vieweg, U, and Schultheiss, R: A review of halo vest treatment of upper cervical spine injuries. Arch Orthop Trauma Surg 121:50, 2001.
66. Pringle, RG: Review article: Halo versus Minerva: Which orthosis? Paraplegia 28:281, 1990.
67. Nachemson, AL, and Peterson, LE: Effectiveness of treatment with a brace in girls who had adolescent idiopathic scoliosis: A prospective, controlled study based on data from the brace study of the Scoliosis Research Society. J Bone Joint Surg 77-A:815, 1995.
68. Rowe, DE, et al: A meta-analysis of the efficacy of non-operative treatments for idiopathic scoliosis. J Bone Joint Surg 79-A:664, 1997.
69. van Rhijn, LW, Veraart BE, and Plasmans, CM: Application of a lumbar brace for thoracic and double thoracic lumbar scoliosis: A comparative study. J Pediatr Orthop 12:178, 2003.
70. Lonstein, JE, and Winter, RB: The Milwaukee brace for the treatment of idiopathic scoliosis: A review of 1020 patients. J Bone Joint Surg 76-A:1207, 1994.
71. Patwardhan, AG, et al: Biomechanical comparison of the Milwaukee brace and the TLSO for treatment of idiopathic scoliosis. J Prosthet Orthot 8:115, 1996.
72. Olafsson, Y, et al: Boston brace in the treatment of idiopathic scoliosis. J Pediatr Orthop 15:524, 1995.
73. Mac-Thiong, JM, et al: Biomechanical evaluation of the Boston brace system for the treatment of adolescent idiopathic scoliosis: Relationship between strap tension and brace interface forces. Spine 29:26, 2004.
74. Lou, E., et al: Correlation between quantity and quality of orthosis wear and treatment outcomes in adolescent idiopathic scoliosis. Prosthet Orthot Int 28:49, 2004.
75. Katz, DE, and Durani, AA: Factors that influence outcome in bracing large curves in patients with adolescent idiopathic scoliosis. Spine 26:2354, 2001.
76. Wong, MS, et al: Effectiveness and biomechanics of spinal orthoses in the treatment of adolescent idiopathic scoliosis (AIS). Prosthet Orthot Int 24:148, 2000.
77. Allington, NJ, and Bowen, JR: Adolescent idiopathic scoliosis: Treatment with the Wilmington brace: A comparison of full-time and part-time use. J Bone Joint Surg 78-A:1056, 1996.
78. Katz, DE, et al: A comparison between the Boston brace and the Charleston bending brace in adolescent idiopathic scoliosis. Spine 22:1302, 1997.
79. Gepstein, R, et al: Effectiveness of the Charleston bending brace in the treatment of single-curve idiopathic scoliosis. J Pediatr Orthop 22:84, 2002.
80. D'Amato, CR, Griggs, S, and McCoy, B: Nighttime bracing with the Providence brace in adolescent girls with idiopathic scoliosis. Spine 26:2006, 2001.
81. Bowker, P, et al: Energetics of paraplegic walking. J Biomed Eng 14:34, 1992.
82. Gonzalez, E and Edelstein, J. Energy expenditure in ambulation: In Gonzalez, et al (eds): Downey and Darling's Physiological Basis of Rehabilitation Medicine. ed. 3. Butterworth-Heinemann, Boston, 2001, p 417.

Supplemental Readings

Aisen, ML: Orthotics in Neurologic Rehabilitation. Demos Medical Publishing, New York, 1992.
Bowker, P, et al (eds): Biomechanical Basis of Orthotic Management. Butterworth-Heinemann, Oxford, 1993.
Edelstein, JE, and Bruckner, J: Orthotics: A Comprehensive Clinical Approach. Slack, Thorofare, NJ, 2002.
Goldberg, B, and Hsu, J: Atlas of Orthoses: Rehabilitation Principles and Application of Orthotic and Assistive Devices, ed 3. CV Mosby, St. Louis, 1996.
Lusardi, MM, and Nielsen, CC: Orthotics and Prosthetics in Rehabilitation. Butterworth Heinemann, Boston, 2000.
McKee, P, and Morgan, L: Orthotics in Rehabilitation: Splinting the Hand and Body. FA Davis, Philadelphia, 1998.
Nawoczenski, DA, and Epler, ME: Orthotics in Functional Rehabilitation of the Lower Limb. WB Saunders, Philadelphia, 1997.
Redford, JB, et al: Orthotics: Clinical Practice and Rehabilitation Technology. Churchill Livingstone, New York, 1995.
Seymour, R: Prosthetics and Orthotics: Lower Limb and Spinal. Lippincott Williams & Wilkins, Philadelphia, 2002.
Smidt, GL (ed): Gait in Rehabilitation. Churchill Livingstone, New York, 1990.
Wu, KK: Foot Orthoses: Principles and Clinical Applications. Williams & Wilkins, Baltimore, 1990.

Appendix A: Lower-Limb Orthotic Examination

1. Is the orthosis as prescribed?
2. Can the client don the orthosis easily?

Standing

3. Is the shoe satisfactory and does it fit properly?
4. Are the sole and heel of the shoe flat on the floor?
5. If a shoe insert is used, is there minimal rocking between insert and shoe?

Ankle

6. Do the mechanical ankle joints coincide with the anatomical ankle (anatomic ankle joint axis is approximated by a horizontal line between the malleoli at level of the distal tip of the medial malleolus)?
7. Is there adequate clearance between the anatomical ankle and the mechanical ankle joints?
8. Does the valgus or varus correction strap control the foot position?

Knee

9. Does the mechanical knee joint(s) coincide with the anatomical knee (.5–.75 in. [1.2–1.9 cm]) above medial tibial plateau)?
10. Is there adequate clearance between the anatomical knee and the mechanical knee joint?
11. Is the knee lock secure and easy to operate?

Shells, Bands, Cuffs, and Uprights

12. Do the shells, bands, cuffs, and uprights conform to the contours of the leg and thigh?
13. Is there adequate clearance between the top of the calf shell or band and the head of the fibula?
14. Is there adequate clearance between the orthosis and the perineum?
15. Is the orthosis below the greater trochanter but at least 1 in. (2.5 cm) higher than the medial shell or upright?
16. Are the uprights at the midline of the leg and thigh?
17. Do the shells, bands, and cuffs conform to the contours of the leg and thigh?
18. Is any flesh roll above the shell or band minimal?
19. Are the bottom of the thigh shell or distal thigh band and the top of the calf shell or band equidistant from the knee?
20. In a child's orthosis, is there adequate provision for lengthening the orthosis?

Weight-Relieving Components

21. In a patellar-tendon-bearing brim, is there adequate relief for the head of the fibula?
22. With a quadrilateral brim, is the client free from excessive pressure in the anteromedial and medial aspect of the brim?
23. With a quadrilateral brim, does the ischial tuberosity rest on the ischial seat?
24. With a patellar-tendon-bearing brim, is there adequate reduction in weightbearing through the orthosis?

Hip

25. Is the center of the pelvic joint slightly above and ahead of greater trochanter?
26. Is the hip lock secure and easy to operate?
27. Does the pelvic band fit the torso accurately?

Stability

28. Does the orthosis provide adequate stability to the client?

Sitting

29. Can the patient sit comfortably with hips and knees flexed 90°?
30. Can the patient lean forward to touch the shoes?

Walking

31. Is the patient's performance in level walking satisfactory?
32. Is the patient's performance on stairs and ramps satisfactory?

33. Is the orthosis sufficiently rigid?
34. Does the varus or valgus correction strap provide adequate support?
35. Does the orthosis operate quietly?
36. Does the patient consider the orthosis satisfactory as to comfort, function, and appearance?

Orthosis Off the Patient

37. Is the skin free of abrasions or other discolorations attributable to the orthosis?
38. Is the construction satisfactory?
39. Do all components function satisfactorily?

Appendix B: Trunk Orthotic Examination

1. Is the orthosis as prescribed?
2. Can the client don the orthosis easily?

Standing

Pelvic Band

3. Does the pelvic band lie flat on the trunk below the posterior superior iliac spines?
4. Does the pelvic band pass between the trochanters and iliac crests?

Thoracic Band

5. Does the thoracic band lie flat on the trunk below the scapulae?
6. Does the thoracic band lie horizontally on the trunk?

Uprights

7. Do the posterior uprights avoid pressure on bony prominences, such as the vertebral spines or scapulae?
8. Do the lateral uprights extend along the lateral midlines of the trunk?

Abdominal Front

9. Is the abdominal front of adequate size?

Cervical Orthosis

10. Is the head in the prescribed position?
11. Do all rigid components fit properly?

Sitting

12. Can the patient sit comfortably with the hips and knees flexed 90°?
13. Does the patient consider the orthosis satisfactory as to comfort, function, and appearance?

Orthosis Off the Patient

14. Is the skin free of abrasions or other discolorations attributable to the orthosis?
15. Is the construction satisfactory?
16. Do all components function satisfactorily?

CHAPTER

32

Prosthetics

Joan E. Edelstein, PT, MA, FISPO

LEARNING OBJECTIVES

1. Describe the major components of transtibial and transfemoral prostheses, including advantages and disadvantages of alternative components and materials.
2. Explain the distinctive features of partial foot, Syme's, and knee and hip disarticulation prostheses.
3. Outline the maintenance program for prosthetic components.
4. Conduct static and dynamic examination of transtibial and transfemoral prostheses.
5. Summarize the physical therapist's role in management of individuals with lower-limb amputation.
6. Analyze and interpret patient data, formulate realistic goals and outcomes, and develop a plan of care when presented with a clinical case study.

OUTLINE

Physical therapists are concerned with the care of individuals with lower- and upper-limb amputations. Such individuals are often fitted with a *prosthesis,* a replacement of all or part of the leg or arm. A *prosthetist* is a health care professional who designs, fabricates, and fits limb prostheses. In the broadest sense, however, prostheses include dentures, titanium femoral heads, and plastic heart valves.

The major causes of amputation are peripheral vascular disease, trauma, malignancy, and congenital deficiency. Vascular disease accounts for most leg amputations, particularly among patients with diabetes. Individuals older than 60 constitute the largest group of people with amputation.[1] Trauma is responsible for the majority of amputations in younger adults and adolescents. Trauma and vascular disease are more common among men. Bone and soft tissue tumors are sometimes treated by removal of the limb, and adolescence is the period of peak incidence. Congenital deficiency refers to the absence or abnormality of a limb evident at birth.

This chapter focuses on the lower extremity (LE) because many more people have lost a portion of the LE, as compared with the upper extremity (UE). Physical therapists are key members of the rehabilitation team, working with prosthetists, physicians, occupational therapists and others to foster the patient's welfare. For patients with LE amputation, physical therapists have the major role in assisting the patient to regain function. For those with UE amputation, physical therapists may play a lesser role, cooperating with occupational therapists, depending on the administrative organization of the health care facility. Lower-limb prostheses will be described, together with a program for training patients in their use.

Historic records confirm that the concept of replacing a missing limb is very old. A forked stick formed a peg leg to support a **transtibial** (below-knee) amputation limb was known in antiquity. Museums display artificial hands, resembling the glove of a suit of armor. Today, most individuals with LE amputation are provided with a prosthesis because function with one LE is very different from maneuvering with two. In contrast, most daily activities and vocational tasks can be performed with a single upper limb.

The principal lower-limb prostheses are partial foot, Syme's, transtibial, and transfemoral (above-knee), as well as knee and hip disarticulation. The physical therapist should be familiar with their characteristics and maintenance, as well as the rehabilitation of patients fitted with these devices.

Partial Foot Prostheses

The purposes of partial foot prostheses are to (1) restore, as much as possible, foot function, particularly in walking and (2) simulate the shape of the missing foot segment. The patient who has lost one or more toes may simply pad the toe section of the shoe to improve the appearance of the upper portion of the shoe. Standing will not be affected, assuming the metatarsal heads remain. When the individual walks, late stance will be less forceful, particularly if the phalanges of the great toe are absent. An arch support helps to maintain alignment of the amputated foot.[2]

Transmetatarsal amputation disturbs foot appearance more noticeably. A prosthesis prevents the shoe from developing an unnatural crease in the forefoot area. The patient bears most weight on the heel and reduces the amount of time spent on the affected foot during walking. A particularly useful prosthesis consists of a plastic socket for the remainder of the foot. The socket is affixed to a rigid plate that extends the full length of the inner sole of the shoe. The plate has a cosmetic toe filler. The socket protects the amputated ends of the metatarsals, while the rigid plate restores foot length so that the person can spend more time during the stance phase of gait on the affected side than would otherwise be the case. To aid late stance, the bottom of the prosthesis or the sole of the shoe may have a convex rocker bar.[3]

Amputation or disarticulation through the tarsals poses the additional problem of retaining the small foot segment in the shoe during swing phase. Foot length is apt to be diminished further by an equinus deformity of the amputated limb, resulting from unbalanced contraction of the triceps surae. Consequently, the prosthesis described for the transmetatarsal amputation may be augmented with a plastic calf shell, which is strapped around the leg.

Transtibial Prostheses

The transtibial level refers to an amputation in which the tibia and fibula are transected. The patient retains the anatomical knee and its motor and sensory functions. This is the predominant site of amputation, particularly for individuals with vascular disease. From a functional and prosthetic viewpoint, the **Syme's amputation** is similar; amputation is just above the malleoli, with all foot bones removed and the calcaneal fat pad retained. The Syme's amputation limb is longer than the transtibial amputation limb, improving prosthetic control; in addition, the individual with a Syme's amputation may be able to tolerate significant weight through the end of the limb. Prostheses for both the Syme's and transtibial levels include a foot–ankle assembly and socket; the transtibial prosthesis also has a shank and a suspension component.

Foot–Ankle Assembly

The prosthetic foot restores the general contour of the patient's foot, absorbs shock at heel contact, plantarflexes in early stance, and simulates metatarsophalangeal hyperextension (toe-break action) in the latter part of stance phase (Fig. 32.1). The foot is in the neutral position during swing phase. Many assemblies also provide slight motion in the frontal and transverse planes.[4–9]

Nonarticulated Feet

In the United States, the most popular foot type is nonarticulated, without a cleft between the foot and lower portion of the shank. As compared with articulated feet, nonarticulated components are lighter in weight, more durable, and more attractive; some versions are made to suit high-heeled shoes.

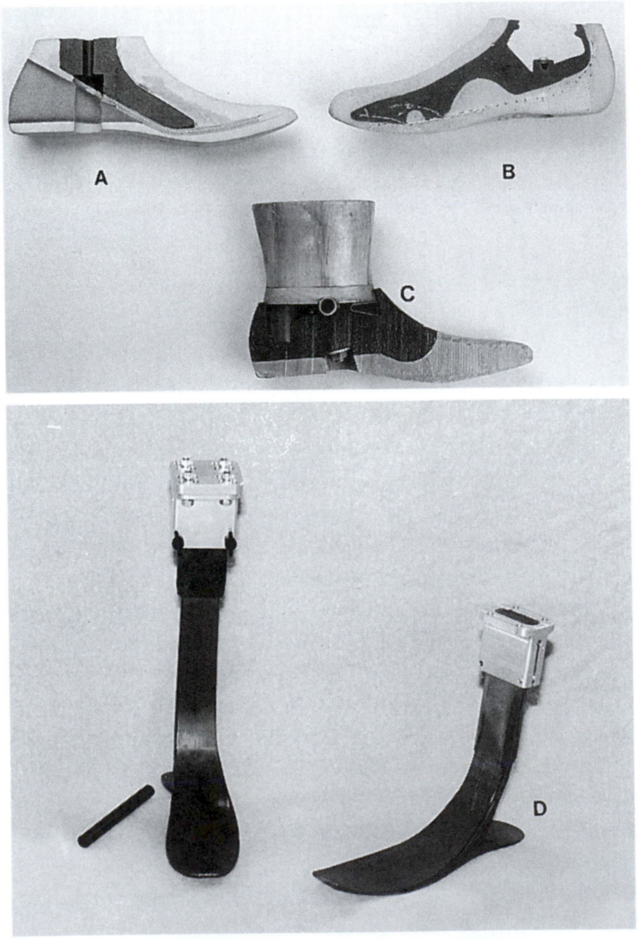

Figure 32.1 Cross section of foot-ankle assemblies. (*A*) SACH. (*B*) SAFE. (*C*) Single-axis. (*D*) Two models of the Springlite with adjustment rod.

SACH Foot

The nonarticulated *solid ankle cushion heel (SACH)* assembly is the most commonly prescribed foot in current practice (see Fig. 32.1A). It consists of a wooden or metal *keel*, which terminates at a point corresponding to the metatarsophalangeal joints. The keel is covered with rubber; the posterior portion is resilient, to absorb shock and permit plantarflexion in early stance. Anteriorly, the junction of the keel and the rubber toe sections allows the foot to hyperextend in late stance. The SACH foot is manufactured in a wide range of sizes to accommodate infants, adolescents, and adults. It is available with heel cushions of varying degrees of compressibility for those who strike the heel with different amounts of force, as well as in several plantarflexion angles to fit shoes with diverse heel heights. The heel cushion allows a very small amount of medial–lateral and transverse motion.

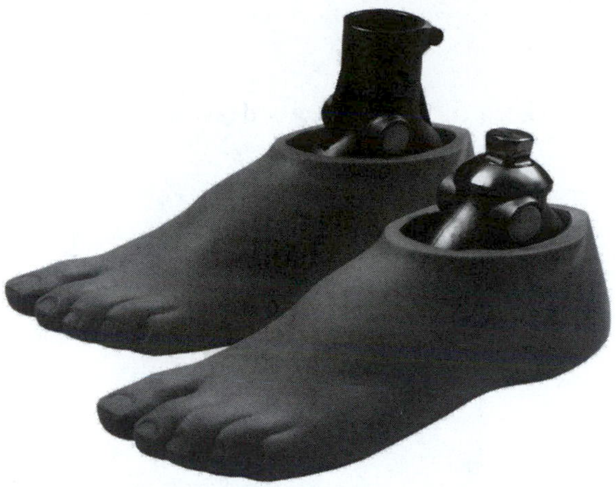

Figure 32.2 Cosmetic foot covers (Courtesy of Ossur, Aliso Viejo, CA 92656)

Other Nonarticulated Feet

A version of the SACH foot is the *stationary attachment flexible endoskeleton (SAFE)* foot (see Fig. 32.1B). It has a rigid ankle block joined to the posterior portion of the keel at a 45° angle, which is comparable to that of the anatomical subtalar joint. The junction permits the wearer to maintain contact with moderately uneven terrain, because of the greater range of medial–lateral motion permitted in the rear foot. The SAFE foot, however, is somewhat heavier and more expensive than the SACH foot. Feet that have a springy sole store energy in early and midstance as the wearer moves over the foot, bending it slightly. In late stance, as the wearer transfers loading to the opposite foot, the spring in the prosthetic foot recoils, returning some of the stored energy. Such feet are described as energy storing/energy releasing, or dynamic.[10–14] For example, the *Carbon Copy II* foot has two carbon fiber longitudinal flexible plates. When the wearer walks at regular speed, the distal plate bends, then springs back to its resting shape. When the wearer runs, both plates bend, then straighten.[15] The *Seattle foot* incorporates a slightly flexible plastic keel, which bends somewhat at heel contact, storing energy.[16] At late stance, the keel recoils as the wearer unloads the foot, releasing energy for a springy termination to stance. Both the *Flex-Foot* and the *Springlite foot* (see Fig. 32.1D) include a long band of carbon fiber material, which extends from the toe to the proximal shank, as well as a posterior heel section. The long band acts as a leaf spring, enabling the foot to store considerable energy in early and midstance, and then to release energy at the end of stance phase. Active wearers, such as those who play basketball or run, utilize the energy-storing and energy-releasing capacity of these feet.[17–19] Many of these feet are available with cosmetic covers (Fig. 32.2) and tend to be more expensive than alternative assemblies.

A large variety of prosthetic feet are currently available (Fig. 32.3). Selection of the appropriate foot is based on the needs of the individual with consideration to the wearer's activity level, weight, level of amputation as well as the length and shape of the residual limb.

Articulated Feet

Manufactured with separate foot and lower shank sections, articulated feet have the sections joined by a metal bolt or cable. The ease of foot motion is controlled by rubber bumpers. In the rear is a resilient bumper to absorb shock and control plantarflexion excursion; it is easy for the prosthetist to substitute a firmer or softer bumper, depending on the force which the patient applies in early stance. A heavy or very active client requires a firm bumper, whereas a frail individual needs a bumper that is soft enough to permit the foot to plantarflex with minimal loading. At early stance, weightbearing on the heel causes the foot to plantarflex, ensuring that the wearer achieves the stable foot-flat position. Anterior to the ankle bolt is firmer rubber or similar material, the dorsiflexion stop, which resists dorsiflexion as the wearer transfers weight forward over the foot. Articulated feet are subject to eventual loosening, which may be signaled by a squeaking noise.

Single-Axis Feet

The most common example of an articulated foot is the *single-axis foot* (see Fig. 32.1C). It permits plantarflexion and dorsiflexion, as well as toe-break action, but does not allow medial–lateral or transverse motion. Some people prefer this simplicity of control.

Multiple-Axis Feet

These components move slightly in all planes to aid the wearer in maintaining maximum contact with the walking surface, even if the surface slopes or has slight irregularities. *Multiple-axis feet* are heavier and less durable than single-axis or nonarticulated feet.

The clinician can select from a wide array of foot–ankle assemblies, in addition to the representative components described here.

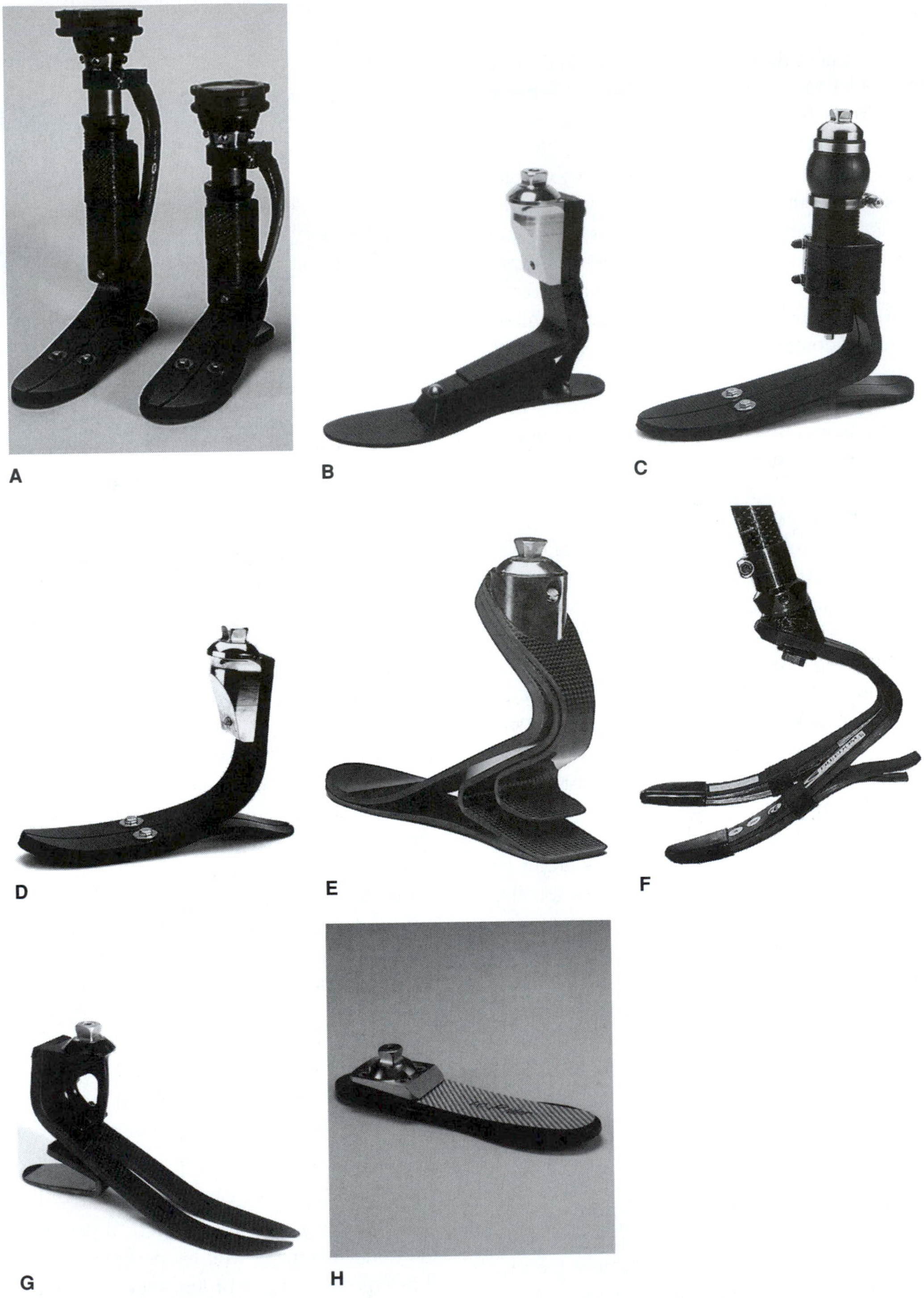

Figure 32.3 Examples of prosthetic feet. (*A*) Re-Flex VSP® and Re-Flex VSP Low Profile®, (*B*) Talux®, (*C*) Ceterus®, (*D*) Vari-Flex® (Courtesy of Ossur, Aliso Viejo, CA, 92656), (*E*) The Renegade, (*F*) Toe Split (Courtesy of Freedom Innovations, Fayette, UT 84630), (*G*) the ELITE® (Courtesy of Endolite, Centerville, OH 45459), and (*H*) Lo Rider (Courtesy of Otto Bock, Minneapolis, MN 55447-4467).

Rotators

A rotator is a component placed above the prosthetic foot to absorb shock in the transverse plane. This action protects the user from skin chafing, which would otherwise occur if the socket were permitted to rotate against the skin. Rotators are most often used with single-axis feet and by very active individuals, especially those with transfemoral amputations.

Shank

The shank is the substitute for the human leg, restoring leg length and shape. The shank is located above the foot–ankle assembly (or rotator) and below the socket in a transtibial prosthesis. The Syme's prosthesis does not have a shank because the socket encasing the amputated limb extends to the foot–ankle assembly. Two types of shank are used: *exoskeletal* and *endoskeletal*.

Exoskeletal Shank

The *exoskeletal shank* (Fig. 32.4), sometimes called *crustacean,* is made of wood or rigid plastic. The rigid exterior is shaped to simulate the contour of the anatomic leg. Although the shank is usually finished with plastic tinted to match the wearer's skin color; some individuals opt for a multicolored or patterned shank. The exoskeletal shank is very durable and, with the plastic finish, impervious to liquids and most abrasives. Because they are less lifelike and do not permit changes in angulation of the prosthesis, they are less frequently prescribed.

Endoskeletal Shank

The *endoskeletal* (Fig. 32.5, see also Fig. 32.4), or *modular shank* consists of a central aluminum or rigid plastic pylon covered with foam rubber and a sturdy stocking or similar finish. With its cover, the endoskeletal shank is more natural in appearance than the shiny exoskeletal shank. In addition, the pylon has a mechanism that permits making slight adjustment of the angulation of the prosthesis; this may contribute to comfort and ease of walking. A variety of prosthetic foot–ankle assemblies, such as the Flex Foot, incorporate an endoskeletal shank. Sometimes a mechanism is incorporated in the shank to absorb vertical shock,[20] thereby reducing stress on the amputation limb and adjacent joints.

Socket

The amputated limb fits into a plastic receptacle called the socket (Fig. 32.6). Although the original name for the modern transtibial socket was the *patellar-tendon-bearing (PTB)* socket, the socket is designed to contact all portions of the amputated limb for maximum distribution of load, as well as to assist venous blood circulation and provide tactile feedback. The PTB socket features a prominent indentation over the patellar tendon. Newer socket variations are the hypobaric, in which soft tissues are drawn inferiorly to increase distal cushioning, and total surface bearing, which has less anterior indentation. Sockets are custom made of plastic molded over a model of the patient's amputation limb. The model may be produced from a plaster cast of the amputation limb or by *computer-aided design/computer-aided manufacture (CAD–CAM).* The latter involves an electronic sensor, which transmits a detailed map of the limb to a computerized program consisting of socket-shape variations; the prosthetist selects the appropriate shape, which is transmitted to an electronic carver that creates the model over which the plastic is shaped. Whether the model is made by hand or by computer, it provides *reliefs;* these are concavities in the socket over areas contacting sensitive structures, such as bony prominences;

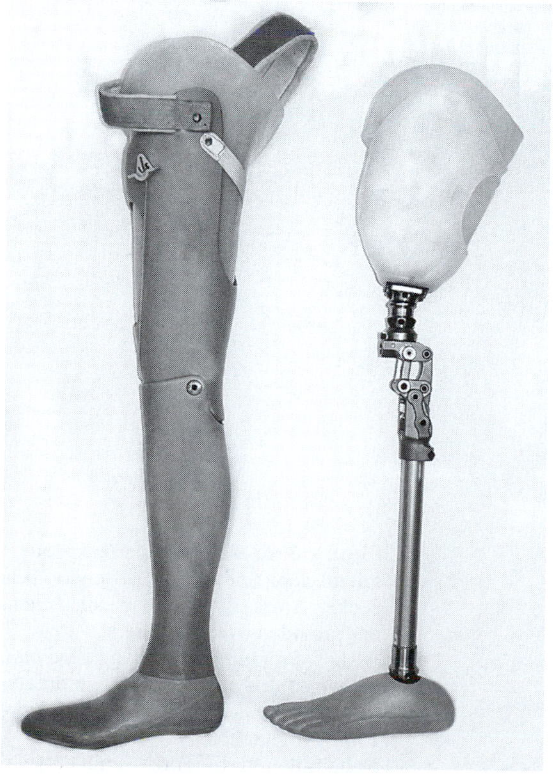

Figure 32.4 (*Left*) Exoskeletal transfemoral prosthesis. (*Right*) Endoskeletal transfemoral prosthesis with cosmetic cover removed.

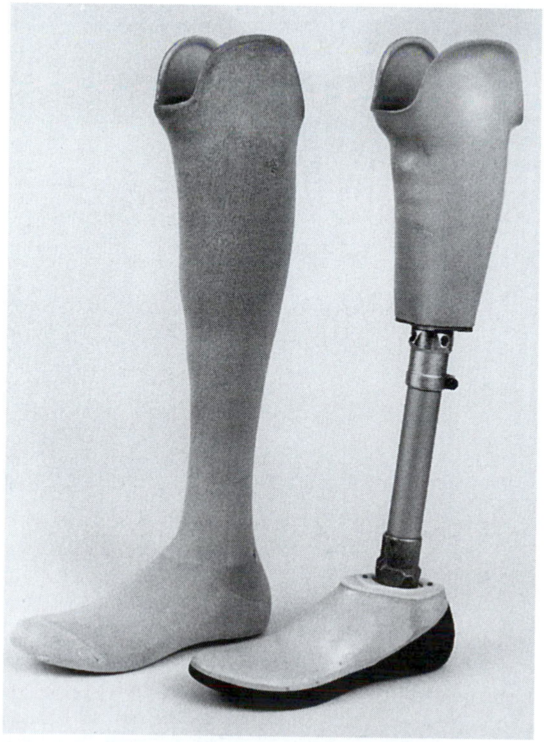

Figure 32.5 Transtibial prosthesis with SACH foot, endoskeletal shank, patellar-tendon-bearing socket, and supracondylar suspension with and without foam rubber covering.

reliefs are located over the fibular head, tibial crest, tibial condyles, and anterior–distal tibia. The posterior brim is trimmed to provide adequate room for the medial and lateral hamstring tendons, so that the patient is comfortable when sitting. *Buildups* are convexities in the socket over areas contacting pressure-tolerant tissues, such as the belly of the gastrocnemius; the patellar tendon; proximomedial tibia, corresponding to the pes anserinus; and the tibial and fibular shafts.

When viewed from above, the socket resembles a triangle, the apex of which is formed by the relief for the tibial tubercle and crest, and the base angles of which are the hamstring reliefs. The anterior wall terminates at the mid patella, or above. The medial and lateral walls extend at least to the femoral epicondyles. The posterior wall lies across the popliteal fossa.

The socket is aligned on the shank in slight flexion to enhance loading on the patellar tendon, prevent genu recurvatum, and resist the tendency of the amputated limb to slide too deeply into the socket. Flexion also facilitates contraction of the quadriceps muscle. The socket is also aligned with a slight lateral tilt to reduce loading on the fibular head.

Lined Socket

The transtibial socket generally includes a resilient *polyethylene foam liner*. In addition to cushioning the amputated limb, the removable liner facilitates alteration of socket size; the prosthetist can add material to the outside of the liner, reducing the volume of the socket while preserving smooth interior contours. The liner, however, adds to the bulk of the prosthesis and is a heat insulator, which the wearer may find uncomfortable in the summer. The Syme's prosthesis has a liner that assists entry of the bulbous distal end of the amputated limb, enabling the wearer to don the prosthesis easily. Individuals with Syme's and transtibial amputations usually wear cotton, wool, or synthetic fabric socks to ensure a snug socket fit. An alternative to the polyethylene liner is a sheath made of silicone or similar material, which fits so snugly that the wearer has little risk of abrasion between the socket and skin.[21–24]

Unlined Socket

Although the unlined socket is sometimes referred to as a hard socket, that term is a misnomer, because the wearer has a soft interface provided by socks or a sheath worn

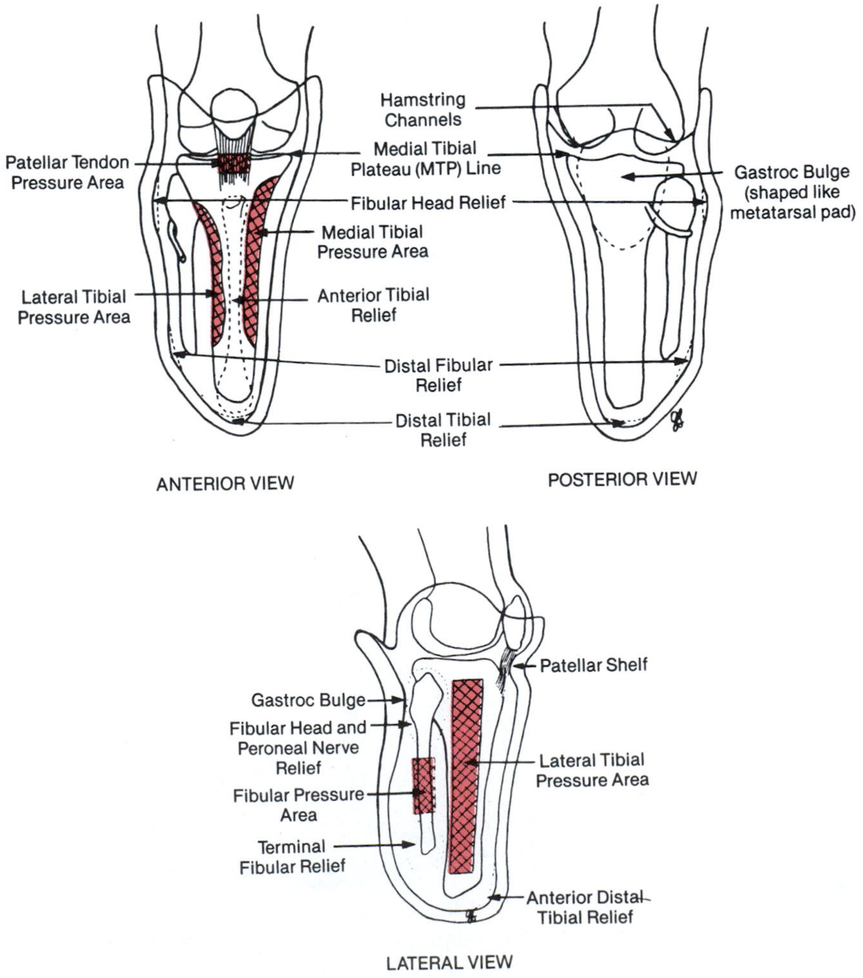

Figure 32.6 Anterior, posterior, and lateral depiction of patellar-tendon-bearing socket. Areas of relief (also called *channels*) are provided over pressure sensitive tissues. Pressure areas (also called *buildups* or *bulges*) indicate contact with pressure-tolerant tissues. (From Sanders, GT: Lower Limb Amputations: A Guide to Rehabilitation. FA Davis, Philadelphia, 1986, p 176, with permission.)

with the unlined socket. Occasionally, a resilient pad is placed in the bottom of the unlined socket to cushion the distal end of the amputated limb. The unlined socket is a more satisfactory choice for the person whose limb has stabilized in volume, because it is easier to clean; however, it is more difficult to alter the shape of the unlined socket in comparison to the lined socket.

A newer type of unlined socket is made of thin thermoplastic in a rigid frame. The plastic can be spot-heated to facilitate alteration of socket fit. It adheres to the skin better than does rigid plastic, thereby improving suspension. It contributes to comfort by dissipating body heat more effectively and responds to changes in amputation limb shape as the patient contracts and relaxes various muscles.

Syme's Socket

The patient with a Syme's amputation can usually bear significant weight through the distal end of the amputated limb. Consequently, the Syme's socket (Fig. 32.7) does not need to provide proximal loading. The socket trimlines (edges) are slightly lower, and the frontal and sagittal plane alignment less tilted, as compared to the transtibial socket. Relief for the tibial crest remains an important feature of the socket. If the distal end of the Syme's limb is markedly bulbous, the lower part of the medial wall can be made removable; the patient dons the socket, and then fastens the wall section in place.

Suspension

During the swing phase of walking, or whenever the wearer is not standing on the prosthesis, such as when climbing stairs or jumping, the prosthesis requires some form of suspension to hold it in place.

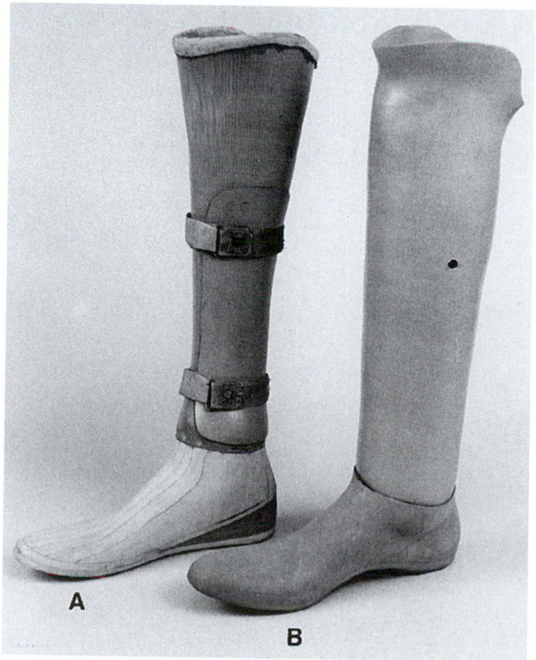

Figure 32.7 Syme's prostheses. (*A*) Socket with medial opening. (*B*) Socket with continuous walls and flexible liner.

Cuff Variants

The modern transtibial prosthesis originated with a supracondylar cuff (Fig. 32.8), which is still widely used. The cuff, a leather strap encircling the thigh immediately above the femoral epicondyles, permits the user to adjust the snugness of suspension easily. Some individuals, however, object to the profile of the distal thigh created by the cuff. Others who have severely arthritic hands or limited vision have difficulty engaging the buckle or pressure loop closure on the cuff.

The cuff may be augmented by a *fork strap* and *waist belt*. The elastic fork strap extends from the outside of the anterior portion of the socket to a waist belt. The fork strap and waist belt may be indicated for individuals who climb ladders or engage in other activities during which the prosthesis is unsupported by the ground for long periods. An alternative to the cuff is a rubber sleeve, a tubular component that covers the proximal socket and the distal thigh (Fig. 32.9). The sleeve provides excellent suspension and a streamlined silhouette when the wearer sits. Donning the sleeve, however, requires two strong hands and a thigh that does not have excessive subcutaneous tissue.

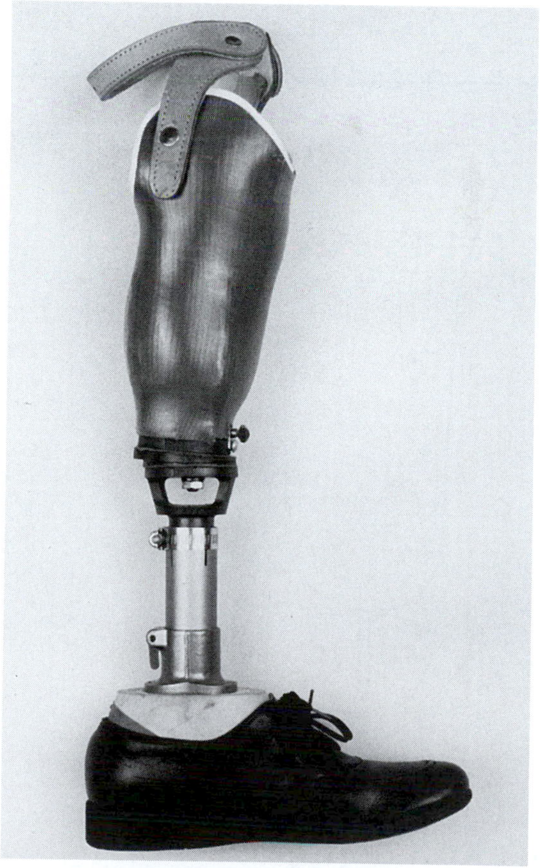

Figure 32.8 Transtibial temporary prosthesis with supracondylar cuff suspension. Socket is mounted on an adjustable pylon shank with SACH foot.

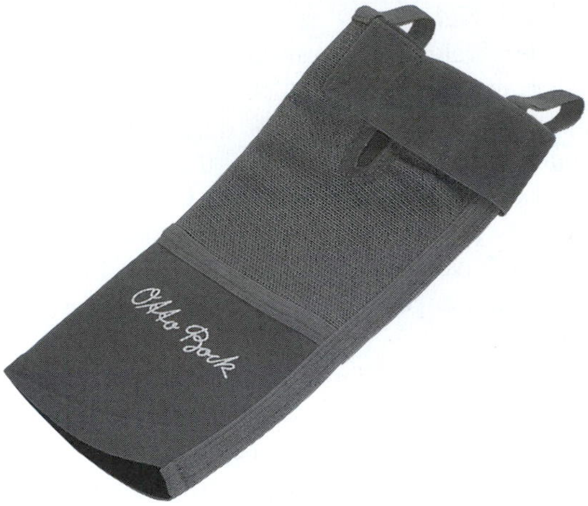

Figure 32.9 Transtibial Suspension Sleeve. (Courtesy of Otto Bock, Minneapolis, MN 55447-4467.)

Distal Attachment

Very secure suspension is achieved with the use of a silicone sheath with a distal metal pin (Fig. 32.10). The sheath clings to the skin. The user inserts the sheathed limb into the prosthesis, guiding the attached pin into a receptacle in the socket. During swing phase, the pin mechanism prevents the prosthesis from slipping.

A surgical approach to distal attachment is known as *osseointegration*.[25] The surgeon implants metal posts in the distal bone. The posts protrude through the skin and lock into a mechanism in the prosthesis. Osseointegration eliminates the need for other suspension apparatus; however, fluid drainage and infection at the skin/post interface are sometimes troublesome. The procedure was developed in Europe and is not yet readily available in North America.

Brim Variants

The prosthesis may be suspended by its socket walls extended proximally. With *supracondylar (SC) suspension* (Fig. 32.11), the medial and lateral walls extend above the femoral epicondyles. The medial wall has a plastic wedge. When donning the prosthesis, the client removes the wedge, places the amputation limb in the socket, then places the wedge between the socket and the medial epicondyle to retain the prosthesis on the limb. Alternatively, the wedge can be incorporated in a liner; for donning, the patient applies the liner, and then inserts the limb, with liner, into the socket. Supracondylar suspension increases medial–lateral stability of the prosthesis, presents a pleasing contour at the knee, and eliminates the need to engage a buckle or hook and pile loop on a cuff. It is more difficult to fabricate (and, hence, more expensive), and it is not readily adjustable.

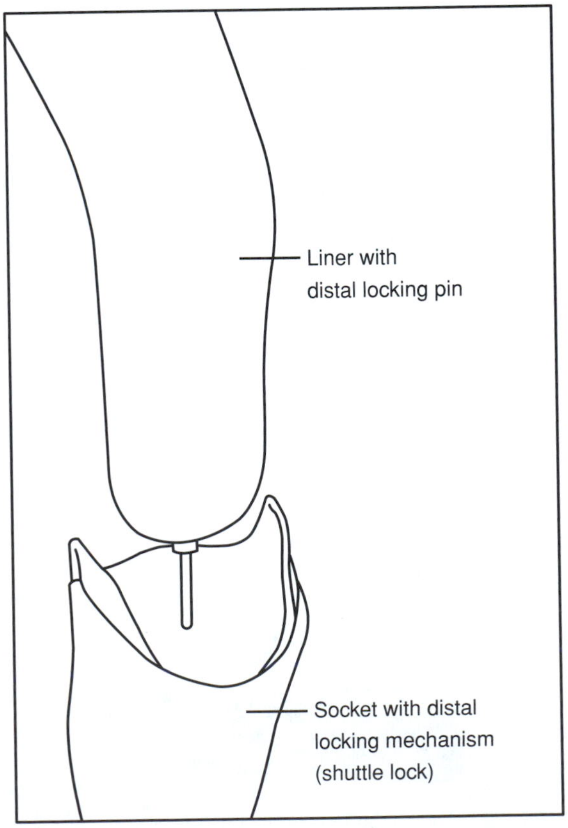

Figure 32.10 Transtibial distal pin attachment (sometimes referred to as a *shuttle lock*).

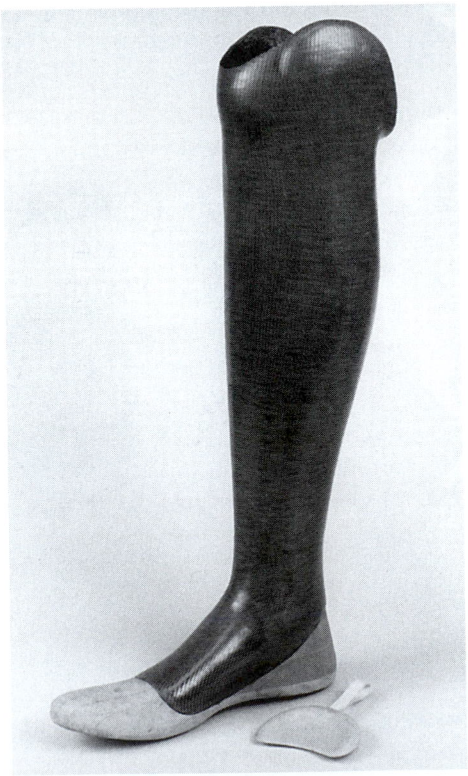

Figure 32.11 Transtibial prosthesis with SACH foot, exoskeletal shank, patellar-tendon-bearing socket, and supracondylar wedge suspension.

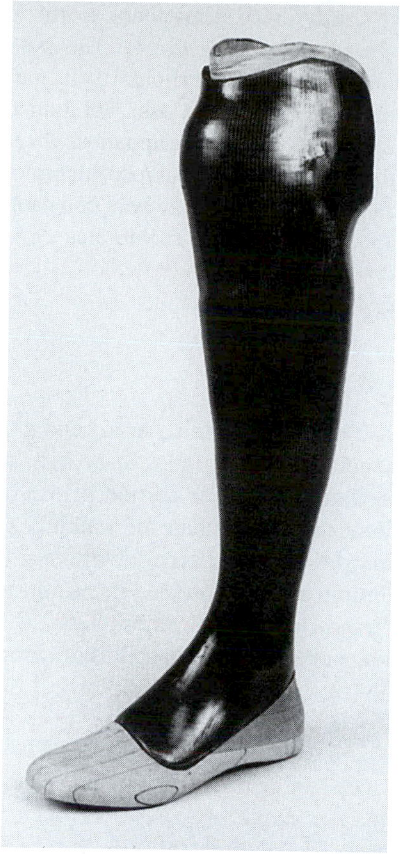

Figure 32.12 Transtibial prosthesis with supracondylar/suprapatellar (SC/SP) suspension.

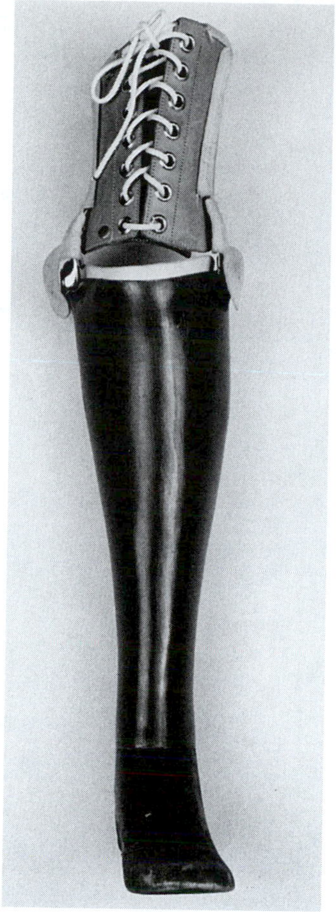

Figure 32.13 Transtibial prosthesis with leather thigh corset suspension.

Presenting a contour of medial and lateral walls similar to the supracondylar suspension, the **supracondylar/suprapatellar (SC/SP) suspension** (Fig. 32.12) also features an anterior wall, which terminates above the patella. The short amputated limb is well accommodated by SC/SP suspension. The high anterior wall may interfere with kneeling and presents a conspicuous appearance when the wearer sits.

Thigh Corset

Some individuals with very sensitive skin may benefit from thigh corset suspension (Fig. 32.13). Metal hinges attach distally to the medial and lateral aspects of the socket and proximally to a leather or flexible plastic corset. Corset heights vary and may reach the ischial tuberosity for maximum weight relief on the amputated limb. The hinges increase frontal plane stability, and the corset increases area for weightbearing load distribution. The resulting prosthesis, however, is heavier and apt to foster **piston action** because the hinges have a single pivot joint that does not articulate collinearly with the anatomical knee. Prolonged use of a thigh corset produces pressure atrophy of the thigh. A prosthesis with corset suspension is more difficult to don because the wearer must fasten laces or series of pressure-loop straps.

Syme's Suspension

The Syme's prosthesis is suspended by the contour of its brims and socket walls, without a cuff or other suspension mechanism.

Vacuum-Assisted Socket System

Used less frequently with transtibial amputations owing to reduced surface area of the residual limb, vacuum assisted suspension may be another alternative for some patients. The *Harmony® Volume Management System* (Fig. 32.14) uniquely combines use of a pump, liner, and sleeve to achieve elevated vacuum in an airtight environment. The vacuum is believed to promote fluid exchange, reduce moisture buildup, regulate volume fluctuations, and increase proprioceptive awareness of where the limb is in space.

Transfemoral (Above-Knee) Prostheses

Individuals with amputation between the femoral epicondyles and greater trochanter are fitted with **transfemoral**

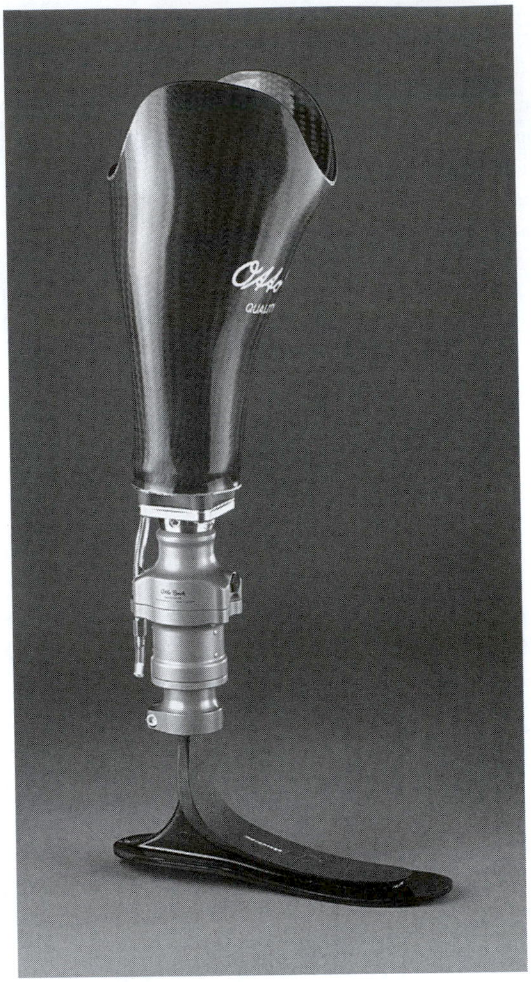

Figure 32.14 The Harmony® Volume Management System. (Courtesy of Otto Bock, Minneapolis, MN 55447.)

prostheses. Those whose limbs retain the distal part of the femur can wear a knee disarticulation prosthesis, which differs from the transfemoral prosthesis in the type of knee unit and socket. If the amputation is proximal to the greater trochanter, the patient cannot retain or control a transfemoral prosthesis and is therefore a candidate for a hip disarticulation prosthesis. The transfemoral prosthesis consists of (1) foot–ankle assembly; (2) shank; (3) knee unit; (4) socket; and (5) suspension device.

Although the SACH foot is most commonly used for transfemoral prostheses, the single-axis foot is somewhat more frequently prescribed for transfemoral than for transtibial prostheses. The single-axis foot reaches the foot-flat position with minimal application of weightbearing load. Nevertheless, any foot, including the energy storing/releasing designs, can be incorporated in a transfemoral prosthesis. As compared with wearers of transtibial prostheses, however, most wearers of transfemoral prostheses do not load the prosthesis as vigorously. Consequently, less energy would be stored and released in a dynamic response foot.

Either the sturdy exoskeletal shank or the endoskeletal shank may be used (see Fig. 32.4). The latter creates a more pleasing appearance, particularly in the knee area, and is adjustable; in addition, it is lighter than an exoskeletal shank. Limited research is inconclusive regarding the merit of light prosthetic weight.[26] Problems of durability remain, particularly at the knee, where constant bending of the joint, especially kneeling, accelerates deterioration of the rubber cover. A rotator with or without a shock absorber may be incorporated in the shank.[27]

Knee Unit

The prosthetic knee enables the user to bend the knee when sitting or kneeling and, in most instances, also permits knee flexion during the latter portion of the stance phase and throughout the swing phase of walking. Commercial knee units may be described according to four features: (1) **axis**; (2) **friction mechanism**; (3) **extension aid**; and (4) *mechanical stabilizer*. Many combinations of features are available; not every knee unit has all four components.

Axis System

The thigh piece can be connected to the shank either by a simple *single-axis hinge* (Fig. 32.15), which is the usual arrangement, or by *polycentric linkage* (see Fig. 32.15). Polycentric systems (Fig. 32.16) have four or more pivoting bars and provide greater stability to the knee, inasmuch as the momentary center of knee rotation is posterior to the wearer's weight line during most of stance phase.[28] This style is less common because of its greater complexity and because other means are available to stabilize the knee.

Friction Mechanisms

In the simplest sense, the leg of the transfemoral prosthesis is a pendulum swinging about the knee. For the elderly individual who walks slowly for short distances, a basic pendulum is adequate. More energetic walkers, however, benefit from adjustable friction mechanisms that modify the pendular action of the knee to reduce the asymmetry

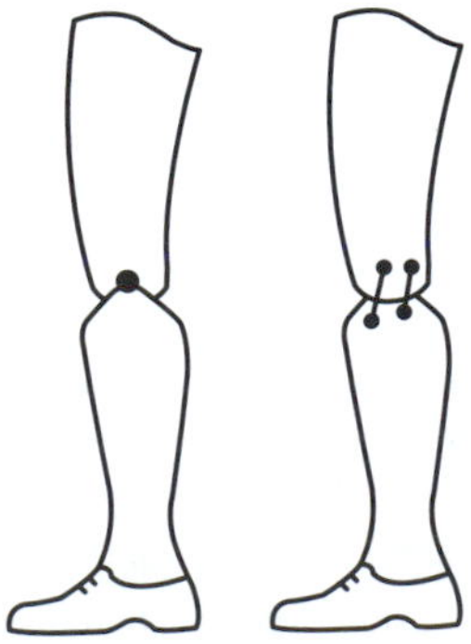

Figure 32.15 Single-axis knee (*left*), polycentric knee (*right*).

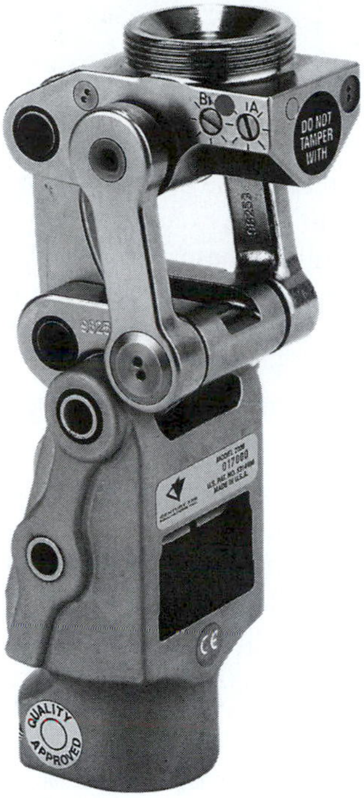

Figure 32.16 Polycentric knee unit designed to provide stability during stance (Courtesy of Ossur, Aliso Viejo, CA 92656.)

between the motions of the sound and prosthetic legs. If the knee does not have sufficient friction to retard its natural pendular action, the individual who walks rapidly experiences excessive knee flexion at the beginning of swing phase and abrupt, often noisy, knee extension at the end of swing phase. Friction mechanisms change the knee swing by modifying the speed of knee motion during various parts of swing phase and by affecting knee swing according to walking speed. Two interrelated issues involved in friction mechanism are the time during swing phase when friction affects the knee unit and the medium through which the mechanism operates.

Constant and Variable

The most popular knee unit has **constant friction** (Fig. 32.17), generally a clamp that grasps the knee bolt. Throughout a given swing phase, the amount of friction is unvarying. The clamp is easy to loosen or tighten to change the ease of knee motion. A more sophisticated device applies **variable friction**, in which the amount of friction changes during a given swing phase. At early swing, high friction is applied to retard excessive knee flexion; during midswing, friction diminishes to permit the knee to swing easily; at late swing, friction increases to dampen impact.

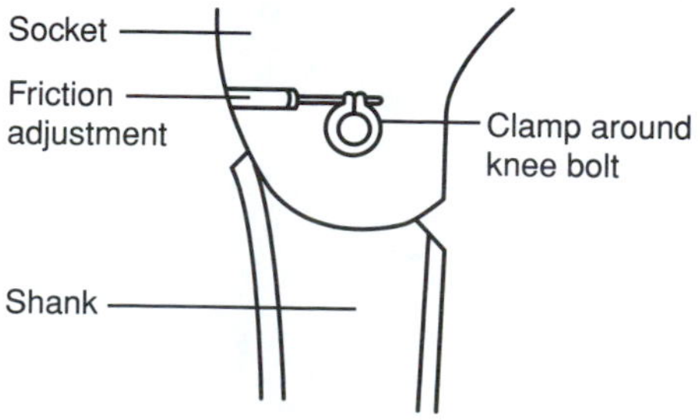

Figure 32.17 Constant friction is achieved by a clamp that encircles the knee bolt and provides the same amount of resistance throughout swing phase.

Medium

The medium through which friction is applied influences performance. The usual medium is *sliding friction,* contact of one solid structure on another. A clamp sliding about the knee bolt is simple and inexpensive, but it does not accommodate automatically to changes in walking speed. A more complex approach is *fluid friction,* either oil (*hydraulic friction*) (Fig. 32.18) or air (*pneumatic friction*). Unlike sliding friction, fluid friction varies directly with velocity. Thus with a hydraulic or pneumatic unit, if the wearer suddenly walks faster, the knee increases friction instantly to prevent excessive knee flexion and abrupt extension. Consequently, the movements of the prosthetic and sound limbs are more symmetrical than would be the case with sliding friction. Oil or air is contained in a cylinder in the knee unit. A piston descends in the cylinder during early swing, causing the knee to flex. The speed of piston descent depends on the type of fluid and the walking speed. Later, the piston ascends, extending the knee. Hydraulic units provide more friction than do pneumatic devices. Both types are more expensive than the simpler sliding friction designs. Various combinations of friction

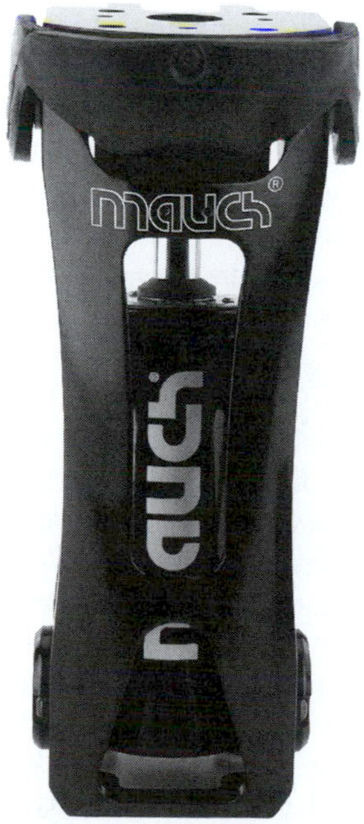

Figure 32.18 Mauch® single-axis hydraulic knee unit swing control or swing and stance control (SNS®); the stance control feature allows foot-over-foot stair descent. (Courtesy of Ossur, Aliso Viejo, CA 92656.)

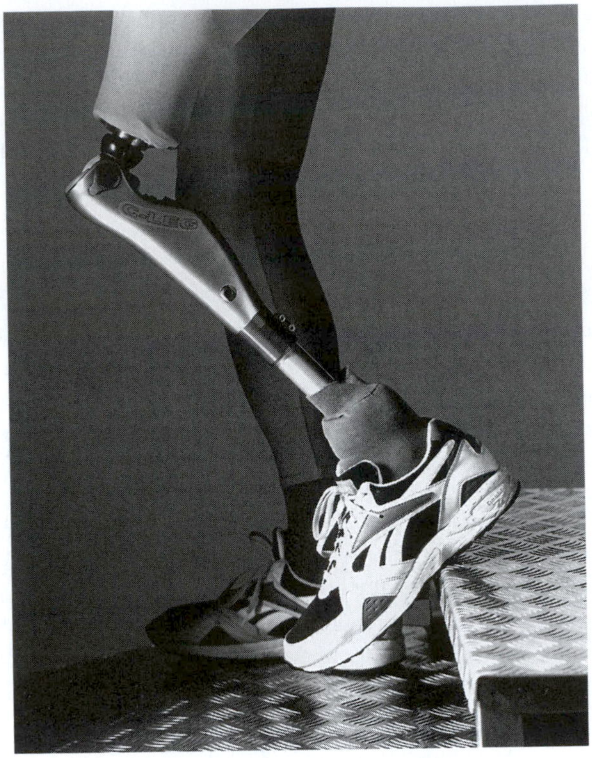

Figure 32.19 Otto Bock C-Leg® is a microprocessor-controlled knee with force sensors that detect loading of the foot and ankle and the precise angle of the knee joint. (Courtesy of Otto Bock, Minneapolis, MN 55447.)

designs are manufactured, such as constant sliding friction, variable sliding friction, and variable fluid friction.

Microprocessor control (Fig. 32.19) utilizes electronic sensors, which detects the rate and range of shank movement 50 or more times per second, providing almost instant friction adjustment to changes in the gait pattern.[29] Units are programmed with a computer, and may provide stumble recovery, accommodation to walking on various terrain and bicycle riding, while others have a locking option.

Extension Aid

A mechanism to assist knee extension during the latter part of swing phase is common. The simplest type is an external aid, consisting of *elastic webbing* in front of the knee axis. The elastic stretches when the knee flexes in early swing and recoils to extend the knee in late swing. Webbing tension is easily adjusted, but tends to pull the knee into extension when the wearer sits. The *internal extension aid* is an elastic strap or coiled spring within the knee unit. It functions identically to the external aid during walking, but unlike the external aid, the internal type keeps the knee flexed when the individual sits. Acute knee flexion causes the strap or spring to pass behind the knee axis, maintaining the flexed attitude. Fluid-controlled knee units incorporate an internal extension aid.

Stabilizers

Most knee units do not have a special device to increase stability. The patient controls knee action by hip motion, aided by the alignment of the knee in relation to other components of the prosthesis. The prosthetic knee joint is usually aligned posterior to a line extending from the trochanter to the ankle (TKA line). The patient who has excellent balance and muscular control may have the knee bolt placed on the line, thus creating TKA alignment. Elderly or debilitated patients may benefit from a stabilizing mechanism, as do some people who walk on very rough terrain, such as hunters.

Manual Lock

The simplest mechanical stabilizer is a manual lock (Fig. 32.20), in which a pin lodges in a receptacle and is released only when the wearer manipulates an unlocking lever. When engaged, the manual lock prevents knee flexion. The user is secure not only during early stance, but throughout the entire gait cycle. To compensate for difficulty in advancing the locked prosthesis, the shank should be shortened approximately 1/2 in. (1 cm). Another problem inherent with the manual lock is the need to disengage it when the wearer sits. Nevertheless, some older adults prefer the stability of the locked knee.[30]

Friction Brake

A more elaborate stabilizing system, the *friction brake* (Fig. 32.21), provides very high friction during early stance, resisting any tendency of the knee to flex. One design, incorporated in a sliding friction unit, involves the mating of a wedge and groove upon loading, assuming the

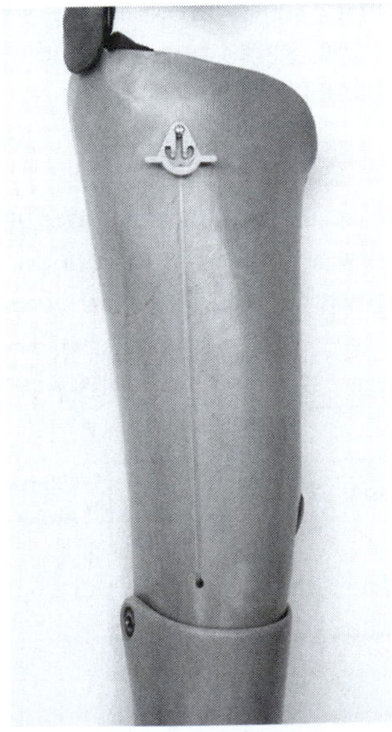

Figure 32.20 Manual knee lock on a single axis knee unit. Note that this configuration has a proximal release attached by a high-density plastic wire to the knee.

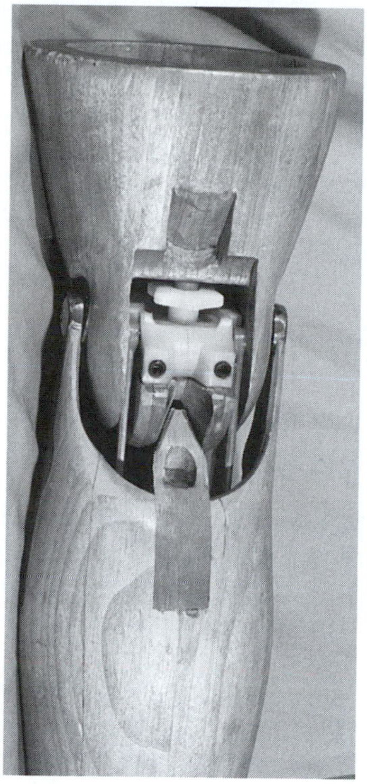

Figure 32.21 Single-axis knee unit with constant friction and weight-activated friction brake. The wedge-shaped surfaces in the knee unit and upper shank are forced together during weightbearing to lock the knee.

knee is flexed less than 25°. Another version of friction brake is found in several hydraulic units; during early stance, additional fluid resistance markedly retards piston descent within the fluid cylinder and thus stabilizes the knee.

From midstance through heel contact, friction brakes do not interfere with knee motion. In addition, they do not impede the patient who transfers from standing to sitting. Such devices add to the cost of the prosthesis and, if improperly used, may not protect the patient from falling.

Socket

As with all prosthetic sockets, the transfemoral one should be a total-contact receptacle to distribute load over the maximum area, thereby reducing pressure. Total-contact fitting also provides counterpressure to assist venous return and prevent distal edema, and enhances sensory feedback to foster better control of the prosthesis.

Most transfemoral sockets are made of a flexible plastic socket (Fig. 32.22) encased in a rigid frame so that the wearer may transmit weight through the distal components of the prosthesis to the ground. The flexible plastic provides sensory input from external objects, such as chairs.

Transfemoral sockets are designed to emphasize loading on pressure-tolerant structures, such as the gluteal musculature, sides of the thigh, and, to a lesser extent, distal end of the amputated limb. The socket must avoid excessive pressure on the pubic symphysis and perineum.

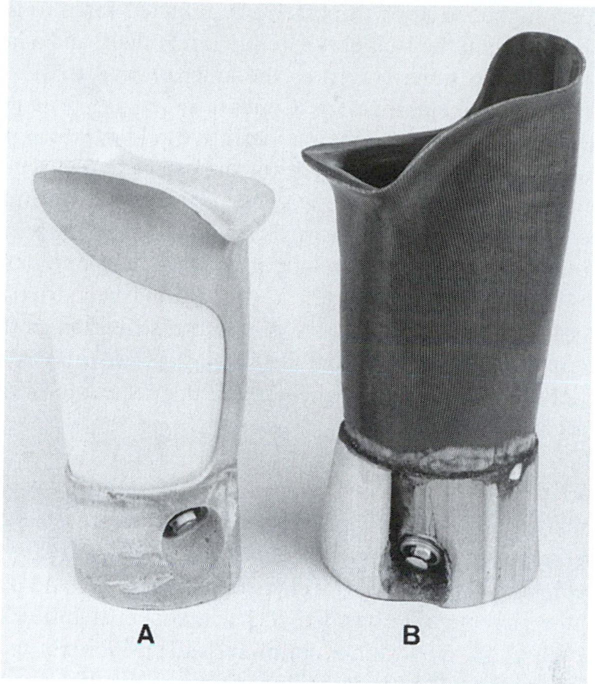

Figure 32.22 Quadrilateral sockets. (*A*) Flexible socket in rigid frame. (*B*) Rigid polyester laminate socket.

Quadrilateral Socket

The traditional transfemoral socket shape is quadrilateral when viewed from above (Fig. 32.23). The socket features a horizontal posterior shelf for the ischial tuberosity and gluteal musculature, a medial brim at the same level as the posterior shelf, an anterior wall 2.5 to 3 in. (6 to

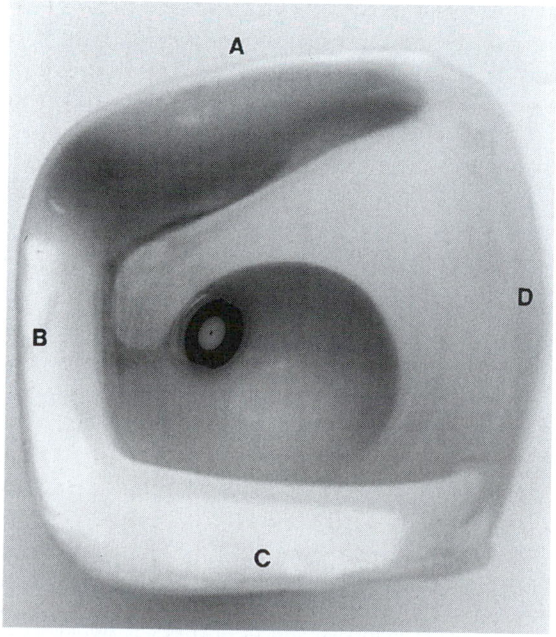

Figure 32.23 Quadrilateral flexible socket in rigid frame viewed from above. (*A*) Anterior wall. (*B*) Medial wall. (*C*) Posterior wall. (*D*) Lateral wall.

8 cm) higher to apply a posteriorly directed force to the thigh to retain the ischial tuberosity on its shelf, and a lateral wall the same height as the anterior wall to aid in medial–lateral stabilization. Concave reliefs are (1) anterior–medial, for the pressure-sensitive adductor longus tendon; (2) posterior–medial, for the sensitive hamstring tendons and sciatic nerve; (3) posterior–lateral, to permit the gluteus maximus to contract and bulge without being crowded; and (4) anterior–lateral, to allow adequate room for the rectus femoris. The anterior wall has a convexity, Scarpa's bulge, to maximize pressure distribution in the vicinity of the femoral triangle. The lateral wall may have reliefs for the greater trochanter and the distal end of the femur.

Ischial Containment Socket

An alternate design (Fig. 32.24) type is sometimes called the *contoured adducted trochanter-controlled alignment method*.[31,32] Its walls cover the ischial tuberosity and part of the ischiopubic ramus to augment socket stability. To increase frontal plane stability and minimize bulk between the thighs, the medial–lateral width of the socket is narrower than that of the quadrilateral socket. The anterior wall is lower than in the quadrilateral socket, whereas the lateral wall covers the greater trochanter. Weightbearing occurs on the sides and bottom of the amputated limb.

Fit and Alignment

Regardless of shape and materials, the socket should fit snugly to minimize the risk of chafing and maximize the wearer's control of the prosthesis. Slight socket flexion is desirable for several reasons: (1) to facilitate contraction of the hip extensors; (2) to reduce lumbar lordosis; and (3) to provide a zone through which the thigh may be extended to permit the wearer to take steps of approximately equal length. For wearers of quadrilateral sockets, socket flexion also enhances positioning of the ischial tuberosity on the posterior brim.[33]

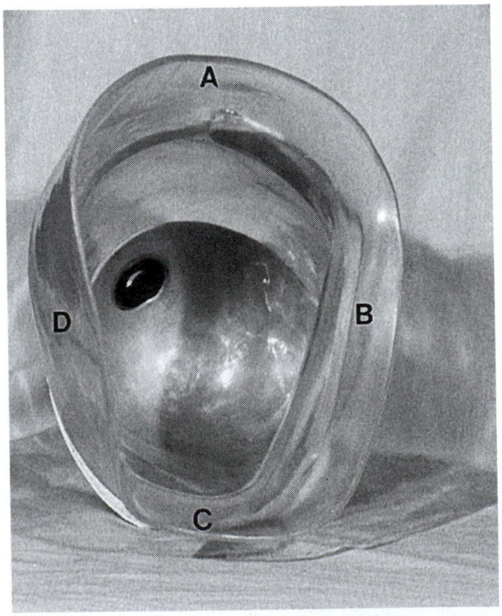

Figure 32.24 Ischial containment flexible transfemoral socket. Note the relatively narrow medial–lateral dimension. (*A*) Anterior brim. (*B*) Medial brim. (*C*) Posterior brim. (*D*) Lateral brim.

Suspension

Three means are used to suspend the transfemoral prosthesis: (1) total suction, (2) partial suction, and (3) no suction.

Suction Suspension

Suction refers to the pressure difference inside and outside the socket. With suction suspension, internal socket pressure is less than external pressure; consequently, atmospheric pressure causes the socket to remain on the thigh. The socket brim must fit snugly; a one-way air-release valve located at the bottom of the socket enables residual air to be expelled.

Total Suction

Maximum control of the prosthesis, without any encumbering auxiliary suspension, can be achieved only if the socket fits very snugly to give total suction (Fig. 32.25). If the patient experiences changes in amputated limb volume, suction will be lost and an auxiliary suspension will be required.

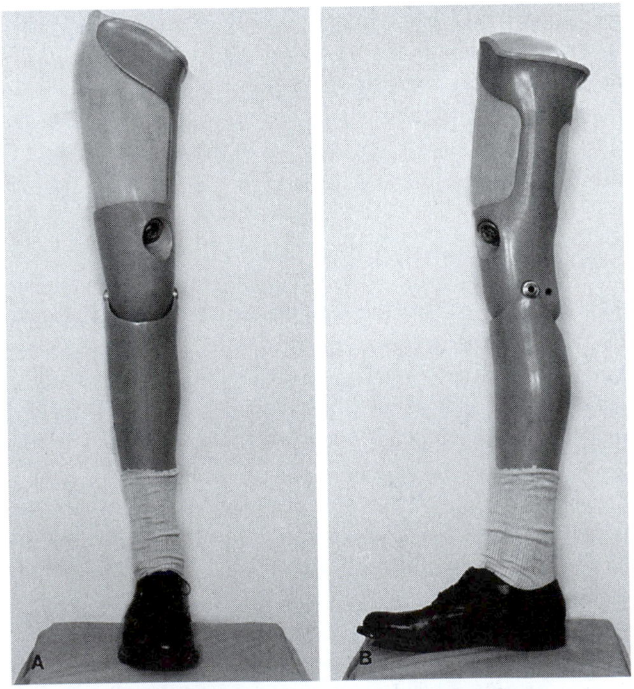

Figure 32.25 Transfemoral prosthesis with SACH foot, exoskeletal shank, single-axis constant friction knee unit, and quadrilateral flexible socket with suction suspension. (*A*) Anterior view. (*B*) Medial view.

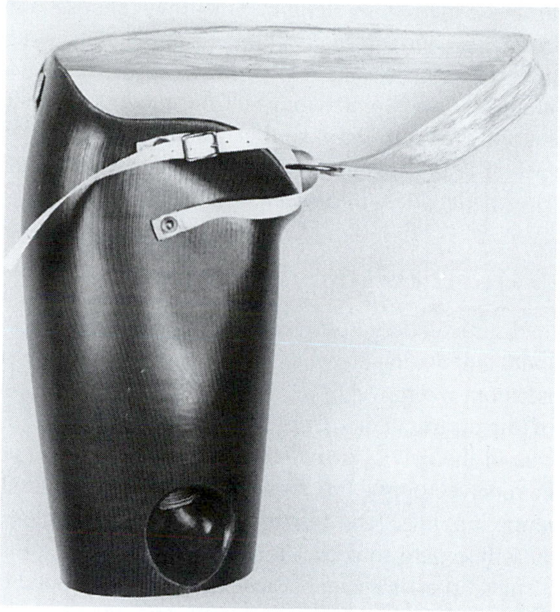

Figure 32.26 Quadrilateral partial suction socket with Silesian bandage.

Partial Suction

A socket that is slightly loose may enable partial suction suspension. The patient wears one or more socks, or a liner made of silicone or other synthetic material. Because socket fit is looser, an auxiliary suspension aid is needed, either a fabric Silesian bandage (Fig. 32.26), or a rigid plastic or metal hip joint and pelvic band (Fig. 32.27). These aids encircle the pelvis. The Silesian bandage also controls the transverse plane orientation of the prosthesis on the thigh, while the hip joint restricts transverse and frontal motion at the hip. The pelvic band adds weight to the prosthesis and may impose uncomfortable pressure against the torso when the wearer sits.

No Suction

If the socket has a distal hole but no valve, then there is no pressure difference between inside and outside the socket. The client wears one or more socks and requires a pelvic band. The relatively loose socket makes donning easy, but hinders control of the prosthesis and sitting comfort. Another alternative is the addition of a transfemoral suspension sleeve (Fig. 32.28).

Osseointegration is the newest alternative to suction. One or more metal posts implanted in the femur lock into a fixture embedded in the distal portion of the socket.[34]

Disarticulation Prostheses

Individuals with knee or hip disarticulation wear prostheses that include the same distal components as prostheses for

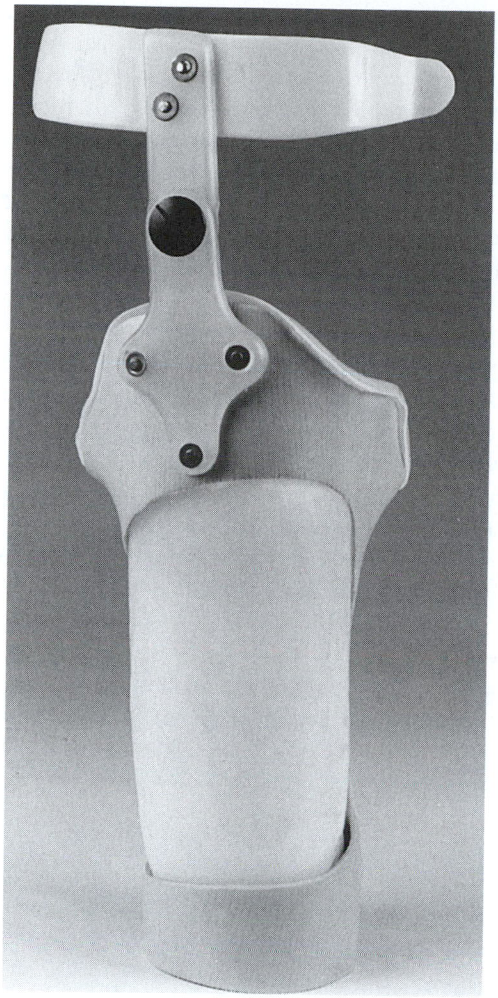

Figure 32.27 Quadrilateral partial suction socket with rigid plastic pelvic band attachment (to which a leather or fabric belt is secured that wraps around the pelvis).

lower levels. Any prosthetic foot can be used with either an endoskeletal or exoskeletal shank. The major distinction, therefore, is in the proximal portion of the prostheses.

Knee Disarticulation Prostheses

When amputation is at or distal to the femoral epicondyles, the patient should have excellent prosthetic control

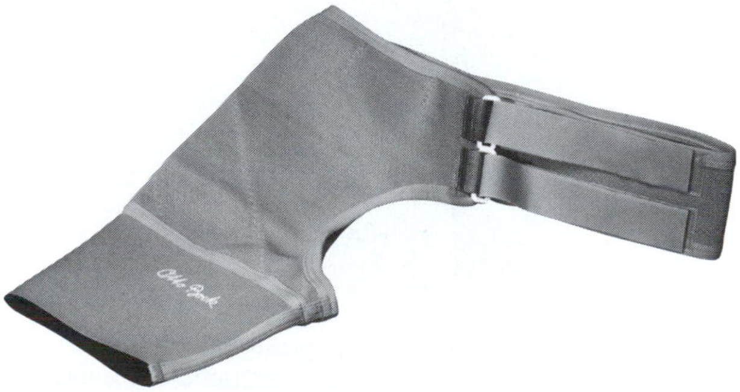

Figure 32.28 Transfemoral suspension sleeve. (Courtesy of Otto Bock, Minneapolis, MN 55447.)

because (1) thigh leverage is at a maximum; (2) most of the body weight can be borne through the distal end of the femur; and (3) the broad epicondyles provide rotational stability. The problem presented by knee disarticulation is primarily cosmetic; when the individual sits, the thigh on the amputated side may protrude slightly. The knee disarticulation prosthesis (Fig. 32.29) has a streamlined knee that minimizes protrusion, as well as a specially designed socket.

Socket

Two types of sockets are currently in use. Both are made of plastic and usually terminate below the ischial tuberosity. Generally, no additional suspension aids are needed. One version features an anterior opening to accommodate a bulbous amputated limb. After the limb is inserted, the wearer closes the socket with lacing or pressure-loop tapes. The other design has no anterior opening and is suitable for limbs that are not bulbous.

Knee Unit

Several units are specifically manufactured for knee disarticulation. All have a thin proximal attachment plate to minimize added thigh length. One may choose among hydraulic, pneumatic, and sliding friction units, with or without polycentric linkage. Even with a special knee unit, the thigh will be slightly longer. Consequently, the shank is shortened equivalently, so that when the person stands, the pelvis is level. When the individual sits, the thigh on the prosthetic side will project slightly.

Hip Disarticulation Prostheses

A hip disarticulation prosthesis (Fig. 32.30) is fitted to a person with amputation above the greater trochanter (very short transfemoral), removal of the femoral head from the acetabulum (hip disarticulation), or removal of the femur and some portion of the pelvis (**transpelvic amputation**, also known as hemipelvectomy). Prostheses for proximal levels share common hip, knee, and foot assemblies and alignment, but differ with regard to socket design. The endoskeletal thigh and shank predominate because they afford appreciable weight saving in these massive prostheses.

Socket

The basic socket is plastic molded to provide weightbearing on the ipsilateral ischial tuberosity and buttock (gluteal

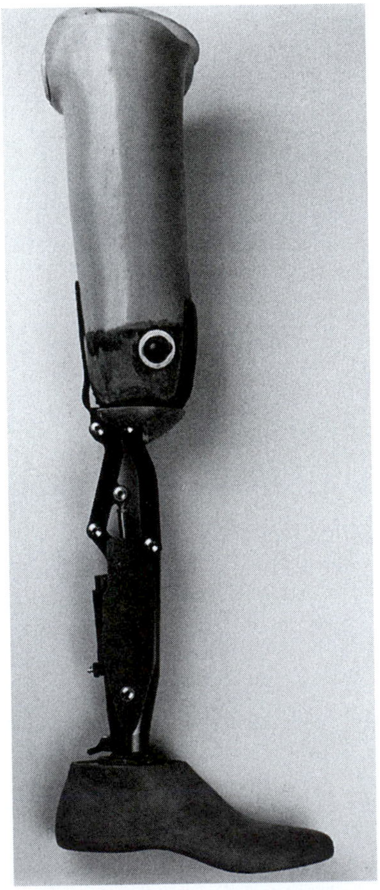

Figure 32.29 Knee disarticulation prosthesis with SACH foot, endoskeletal shank, polycentric hydraulic friction knee unit, and quadrilateral socket with suction suspension.

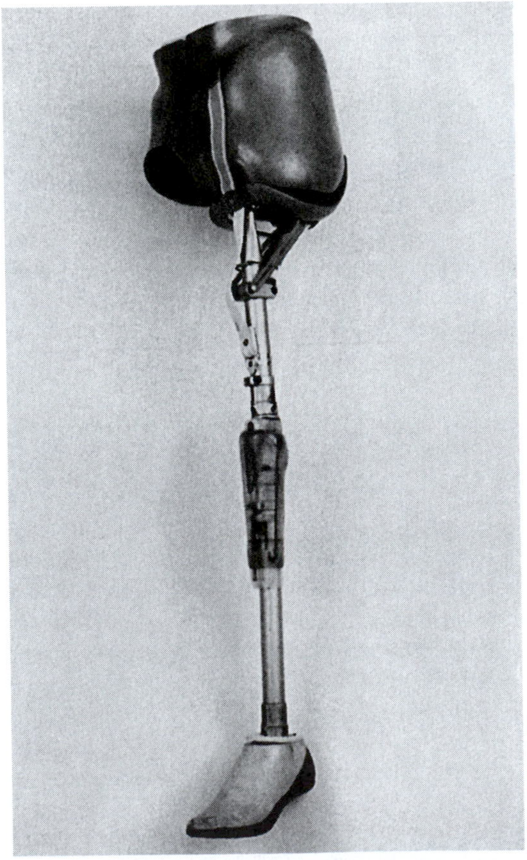

Figure 32.30 Hip disarticulation prosthesis with SACH foot, endoskeletal shank, single-axis knee and extension aid, single-axis hip with extension aid, and rigid socket.

musculature). The person with transpelvic amputation who does not retain the ipsilateral tuberosity or iliac crest has a socket with a higher proximal trimline, sometimes encompassing the lower thorax. This individual supports weight on the remainder of the pelvis, on the abdomen, and perhaps on the lower ribs.

Hip Unit

Various joints provide hip flexion. The joints have an extension aid to bias the prosthesis toward the stable neutral position. Positioning the mechanical hip anterior to a point corresponding to the anatomical hip also contributes to hip stability. The joint is set below the normal hip, so that with sitting, the prosthetic thigh will not protrude unattractively.

Stability

Several attributes combine to make the hip disarticulation prosthesis very stable, namely the hip extension aid, anterior placement of the hip joint, posterior placement of the knee unit, and a knee extension aid. The prosthesis may be shortened slightly, primarily to aid clearance during swing phase, but also to encourage the wearer to apply maximum weight to the prosthesis and to increase stability.

Socks, Sheaths, and Liners

All individuals with LE amputations, except those wearing transfemoral prostheses suspended by total suction or those using a sheath, require a supply of clean socks of appropriate material, size, and shape. It is expeditious to order at least a dozen socks at the time the prosthesis is prescribed, so that third-party payment may cover this relatively inexpensive but important accessory.

Fabric socks are woven in various thicknesses, referred to as *ply,* designating the number of threads knitted together. Cotton socks absorb perspiration readily and are the least allergenic; they are made in two-, three-, and five-ply, the last being the thickest. Wool socks provide good cushioning, woven in three-, five-, and six-ply; they are expensive and must be laundered carefully. Orlon/Lycra socks are manufactured in two- and three-ply thicknesses. They can be washed easily without shrinking. This synthetic fabric combination affords considerable resilience, but does not absorb much perspiration.

A nylon sheath creates a smooth surface over the skin, thereby reducing the risk of chafing, especially in hot weather and among those with much scarring. Some transtibial prosthesis wearers are able to use a woman's knee-high nylon stocking if the amputated limb is slender. Because nylon does not absorb perspiration, liquid passes through the weave to be absorbed by an outer sock of cotton or wool. Silicone, urethane, and other synthetic sheaths provide excellent shock absorption and abrasion resistance; they also can aid in suspending the socket on the patient's limb, and are designed to be worn next to the skin. They are, however, more expensive than fabric socks or sheaths.

Figure 32.31 The Iceross® Dermo is an example of a locking silicone gel liner that provides a cushioned residual limb environment as well as suspends the prosthesis. (Courtesy of Ossur, Aliso Viejo, CA 92656.)

It is common practice to add more socks as the amputated limb shrinks. Nevertheless, when the patient requires a total of 15-ply of socks to achieve snug fit, the socket should be altered or replaced by the prosthetist. Excessive sock padding distorts the weightbearing characteristics of the socket, losing the effect of strategically placed buildups and reliefs.

Regardless of material, the shape of the sock or sheath is important for comfort. An interface of proper size fits smoothly without wrinkling or undue stretching. The sock or sheath should be long enough to terminate above the most proximal part of the socket.

Silicone gel suspension liners are another form of socket-residual limb interface. These liners provide cushioning and added comfort to the residual limb as well as function as a primary or secondary suspension system. Some include a nylon outer cover, with liner thickness tapering distally and may be indicated for particularly active users and those with fragile or sensitive residual limbs. They are available in both locking (Fig. 32.31) and seal-in designs.

Prosthetic Maintenance

Optimal function depends on proper care of socks or sheaths, prosthesis, amputated limb, and intact limb, as well as general health maintenance. Guidelines for personal hygiene are presented in Chapter 25. In addition to ensuring cleanliness, the individual should wear a well-fitting sock and shoe on the sound foot. It must be the mate to the shoe on the prosthesis. Both shoes should be in excellent condition.

As with any appliance, the prosthesis benefits from simple regular maintenance, which generally avoids costly, time-consuming repairs. Printed instructions pertaining to the prosthesis and socks or sheath are helpful for patient education.

Socket and Suspension

Plastic sockets should be washed with a cloth dampened in warm water that has a very small amount of mild soap dissolved in it. The socket is then wiped with a damp, soap-free cloth, and dried with a fresh towel. In warm climates, the socket should be washed every evening so that it will be completely dry when the patient dresses the following morning.

The transfemoral suction valve should be brushed daily to remove talcum and lint, which might clog the tiny aperture. The valve should be inserted and removed only with one's fingers, because tools are apt to damage the internal mechanism or outer threads.

Leather corsets should be kept dry. Use of saddle soap will keep leather clean. If the patient is incontinent, the thigh corset should be made of flexible *polyester laminate* or polypropylene, which are impervious to urine.

Socket liners made of polyethylene foam can be washed by hand in tepid water with mild soap, rinsed, and air-dried overnight. They should not be subjected to direct sunlight when removed from the prosthesis.

Knee Unit

Sliding friction mechanisms tend to loosen with walking and thus require periodic tightening to retain the original adjustment. The frequency of tightening depends on how much the wearer walks. Most units have a pair of screws in front or in the rear of the knee unit that can be turned clockwise with an Allen wrench or common screwdriver. After turning each screw a quarter turn, the client should walk for at least 5 minutes to ascertain the effectiveness of the adjustment.

Squeaking at the knee or articulated ankle indicates the need for oil. The rubber or felt extension bumper in the knee unit will erode after prolonged vigorous use, and the wearer will then notice that the knee begins to hyperextend. The bumper, visible when the knee is flexed, must be replaced by the prosthetist.

The external kick strap extension aid gradually loses its elasticity. The user will then experience high heel rise in early swing and slow knee extension at the end of swing phase. The simplest approach is to tighten the strap through its buckle. Eventually, the prosthetist will need to replace the elastic webbing. Internal elastic extension aids are not subject to rubbing from the trouser leg or skirt and thus do not lose elasticity as readily. Steel spring internal aids retain their effectiveness for the life of the prosthesis.

Pneumatic and hydraulic units must be protected against tears of the rubber shield protecting the piston. The piston must not be scratched, because this would allow air and debris to enter the cylinder. Air bubbles in the unit will cause a spongy feeling, and possibly noise with walking. At night, the prosthesis should be stored upright, with the knee extended to exclude air from the cylinder.

Foot–Ankle Assembly

One should avoid getting the prosthetic foot wet, especially if the foot is an articulated model. If this happens, the shoe and sock should be removed to allow the foot to dry completely, away from direct heat. The wearer should also avoid stepping into sand and similar materials that might enter the cleft between the foot and shank section and restrict the excursion of the foot. The prosthetist would have to disassemble the foot to clean it.

The client should inspect the foot periodically to spot cracking at the toe-break or tip of the keel; such a crack will curl the toes and prevent smooth transition during late stance. A deteriorated heel cushion or plantar bumper will cause one to appear to be walking in a hole. Although most feet are now molded to simulate toes, the patient should not walk without a shoe because the sole of the prosthetic foot is not intended to resist much abrasion.

Foot socks wear much more quickly on the prosthetic side, because the hard foot-ankle assembly and shank rub against the fabric. Stair risers also scuff the sock. Some people find that wearing two socks helps cushion the outer one against premature formation of holes.

The individual must be instructed regarding wearing shoes of the same heel height as was the case when the prosthesis was aligned. Too low a heel interrupts late stance; an unduly high heel makes the knee less stable. If the prosthesis has the usual foot designed for low-heeled shoes, and the wearer wishes to wear flat-heeled shoes, a 1/2 in. (1 cm) shim should be placed inside both shoes at the heel. High-heeled shoes require that the foot be changed, either by unbolting it and replacing it with a foot with an appropriate plantarflexion angle, or by adjusting a heel-height screw found in certain models of feet. Boots and other footwear with stiff upper sections restrict the action of any foot assembly that is designed to provide substantial dorsiflexion and plantarflexion.

Removing the shoe is easier if the prosthesis is not worn. With the shoe unlaced completely, one grasps the counter, then pulls the heel of the shoe off the back of the foot. Finally, the shoe is moved upward off the forefoot.

The shoe should be put on the prosthetic foot with the aid of a shoehorn.

Exterior Finish

The usual finish of exoskeletal shanks is polyester laminate, which is impervious to most liquids. It needs to be wiped only periodically with a cloth dampened with dilute detergent to remove surface soil. Marks can be scoured gently with kitchen cleanser; excessive abrasion will dull the finish.

The soft foam cover of the endoskeletal prosthesis requires reasonable caution against exposure to direct heat, penetrating objects, and solvents. The outer covering will need replacement whenever it becomes unacceptably soiled or torn. The transfemoral version tends to deteriorate at the knee, especially if the wearer kneels a great deal.

Physical Therapy Management

Physical therapists participate in the management of patients with amputation at several key stages: (1) preoperative; (2) postoperative–preprosthetic; (3) prosthetic prescription; (4) prosthetic examination; and (5) prosthetic training.

The first two stages are described in Chapter 25. The following discussion emphasizes the responsibilities of the physical therapist with regard to the patient and prosthesis. Ideally, the therapist works as a member of a **clinic team**, together with the physician and prosthetist. Others, such as a social worker, vocational counselor, and psychologist may participate in the team on a regular basis or as needed. The clinic team provides the best environment for exchange of information and viewpoints regarding the patient and fosters efficient treatment. The team meets to formulate the prospective prescription, examine the newly delivered prosthesis, and reexamine the patient and prosthesis upon completion of prosthetic training. The therapist, therefore, has an integral part to play in these critical points in rehabilitation, as well as conducting prosthetic training. If a formal clinic team is not established in the therapist's work setting, then one must coordinate the recommendations of the physician and prosthetist.

With either administrative situation, the physical therapist:

- Addresses preprescription considerations.
- Contributes to prosthetic prescription.
- Examines the prosthesis.
- Facilitates prosthetic acceptance.
- Trains the patient to don, use, and maintain the prosthesis.

Preprescription Considerations

Successful prosthetic rehabilitation depends on matching the individual's physical and psychosocial characteristics to a prosthesis composed of carefully selected components. Although everyone who wears a prosthesis has an amputation or comparable limb deficiency, the reverse is not true. That is, some people with amputations are not candidates for prostheses or prefer not to use prostheses.[35] Prostheses are contraindicated for patients with severe dementia or depression, or advanced cardiopulmonary disease. If the person displays significant changes associated with organic brain syndrome, then prosthetic fitting is contraindicated. Individuals with bilateral amputations who are unable to transfer independently or don underwear by themselves are unlikely to benefit from a definitive prostheses. Similarly, a patient with bilateral amputations who had sustained unilateral amputation previously and was unable to don and walk with a prosthesis is not a candidate for prostheses. Some people with high amputations, especially hip disarticulation, find that a prosthesis is unduly cumbersome; they prefer to ambulate with a pair of crutches or depend on a wheelchair. Several sports, particularly swimming, are easier to perform without a prosthesis.

Physical Examination

The physical therapist should examine joint mobility and active and passive range of motion of all joints on both LEs. Knee and hip flexion contractures compromise prosthetic alignment and appearance. A knee lock may be needed in a transfemoral prosthesis, and an alternative socket design for a transtibial prosthesis. Severe contractures preclude fitting with conventional components, or may contraindicate provision of any prosthesis. The deleterious effects of contractures are especially serious with bilateral amputations.

The length of the amputated limb should be measured. The individual with a short transtibial amputation may require SC/SP suspension. Every attempt should be made to fit the patient with a short transfemoral amputation with suction or partial-suction suspension to retain the prosthesis on the thigh.

Strength of all limb and trunk muscles should be examined. Frequently, the elderly patient with vascular disease experiences reduced physical activity as LE pains and foot ulceration develop. Such an individual may present with marked debility, which would interfere with prosthetic use or necessitate use of a unit with a knee lock.

The therapist should inspect the skin, noting the status of the incision and any lesions. The patient may require a nylon or silicone sheath to provide a smooth interface between socket and skin to avoid irritating tender or grafted skin.

An examination of sensory function should be performed. For example, an individual with impaired proprioception at the knee will need extra prosthetic stability in the form of higher medial and lateral walls, or side joints attached to a thigh corset, on the transtibial prosthesis. Blindness does not preclude fitting, but it does pose problems with regard to selecting components that are easy to don, as well as altering the training program. If the patient complains of a neuroma, the problem must be addressed surgically or conservatively before fitting can proceed.

The therapist should examine the patient's ability to learn and retain new information including both short- and long-term memory. Neurological conditions such as cerebrovascular accident, complicate fitting and training. Ipsilateral hemiplegia is not as detrimental to prosthetic rehabilitation as contralateral paralysis. In both instances, the prosthesis should be designed for maximum stability. Patients with mild neurological impairments often respond favorably to altered training strategies, which the therapist designs on an individualized basis.

The circulation and anthropometric dimensions of the amputated and sound limbs require careful scrutiny. The physical therapist should teach the patient to inspect the intact foot, using a hand mirror to visualize the plantar surface. Inspection aims to identify skin lesions and incipient areas of abrasion so that corrective measures may be instituted before ulceration or infection ensues. In addition, the patient should be taught to keep the sound foot clean and should wear clean hose and a well-fitting shoe (see Chapter 17 for additional guidelines for managing the patient with peripheral vascular disease). Sequential measurements of amputated limb circumference as well as palpation will indicate whether the patient has edema. Measures should be instituted to stabilize limb volume so that the patient can retain the fit of the prosthetic socket. The patient with vascular impairment may benefit from prosthetic fitting, which transfers some stress from the contralateral limb. In addition, should the person come to bilateral amputation, previous experience with donning and controlling a unilateral prosthesis is invaluable in adjusting to a pair of prostheses.

Prosthetic prescription is also based on the patient's aerobic capacity and endurance. The clinic team must formulate realistic goals based on the individual's physical capacity, particularly related to exercise tolerance and level of deconditioning. The person who is not expected to walk rapidly is an unlikely candidate for an energy-storing/releasing foot or a fluid-controlled knee unit. Nevertheless, a fluid-controlled knee unit that incorporates a braking mechanism is appropriate for selected patients with generalized weakness.

Obesity is another factor to be considered in the preprescription examination. The obese individual is more apt to fluctuate in body weight, necessitating provision of socket liners and several socks to compensate for changing limb circumference. Similarly, those who have renal disease, especially if requiring dialysis, experience volume changes that need prosthetic accommodation.

Arthritis affects prosthesis prescription. Diminished LE mobility or deformity compromises prosthetic alignment. Patients with hip or knee arthroplasty, however, function quite well with a prosthesis. Hand and wrist function or malalignment affect the mode of donning; a laced corset should be avoided. Canes and crutches may require modification.

One of the most useful examination procedures involves observing the patient's ability to transfer from bed to wheelchair. To accomplish this maneuver, the individual must have reasonable strength, balance, and coordination, as well as adequate comprehension. Functional examination is an essential component of physical therapy management (see Chapter 11).

Psychosocial Considerations

Ordinarily, the physical therapist treats the patient more frequently than any other member of the clinic team and thus is more likely to be attuned to changes in the individual's psychosocial status. The patient who is excessively fearful will be served best by prosthetic rehabilitation beginning with a *temporary (provisional) prosthesis.* Motivation is a cardinal determinant of prosthetic outcome. Again, strong motivation demonstrated through use of a temporary prosthesis and adherence with other elements of the rehabilitation program is a reliable predictor of prosthetic success. One should guard against unrealistic expectations. Involving the patient and family in group situations with other persons with amputation, in the physical therapy department, and in social environments fosters constructive attitudes. The therapist should also weigh the likelihood that the individual will be able to care for complex prosthetic mechanisms and have the financial resources to obtain prosthetic servicing, especially of components, such as the foam rubber covering of the endoskeletal shank, which is less durable.

Prosthetic Prescription

Because no prosthetic component is ideal for all clients, it is necessary to select components that are most apt to meet the individual's needs. Alternatives to every element of the prosthesis have advantages and disadvantages. The task of the physical therapist, in conjunction with other team members, is to judge the relative merits of various feet, shanks, and other components in light of objective and subjective information pertaining to the prosthetic candidate.

Some people can be expected to function best with a sophisticated prosthesis that enhances the wearer's ability to engage in vigorous walking and athletics. Others are best served by a simple, inexpensive device. The most accurate predictor of future function is the patient's performance with a previous prosthesis. For the wearer who seeks a replacement prosthesis, the clinic team should consider the extent of use of the previous limb, together with any changes in the patient's health status and lifestyle. For example, if the person fitted with one prosthesis now returns with bilateral amputation, never having used the original prosthesis, that patient is a very poor candidate for bilateral prosthetic fitting. In contrast, another person who had been fitted with a simple transfemoral prosthesis expresses the wish to participate in sports. By demonstrating good use of the original prosthesis, that individual is likely to derive considerable benefit from a new prosthesis with a fluid-controlled knee unit and an energy-storing/releasing foot.

Prescription for the new patient is more difficult. Depending on the interval between amputation surgery and prescription, the amputated limb may not have stabilized in volume; the patient may not have achieved the maximum benefit from the preprosthetic program. The best criterion for prosthetic prescription in such an instance is performance with a temporary (provisional) prosthesis. This appliance includes a well-fitting socket, suitable suspension, pylon, and foot; with the transfemoral model, it usually has a knee unit. The temporary prosthesis allows preliminary gait and activities training. The major difference between the temporary and definitive (permanent) prosthesis is appearance. The temporary socket is designed for easy alteration to accommodate change in amputated limb volume. Ordinarily, little attention is paid to the color and exterior shape of the temporary prosthesis.

Temporary Prostheses

Transtibial (Below-Knee) Temporary Prosthesis

Most transtibial temporary prostheses have sockets made of thermoplastic material that becomes malleable at temperatures low enough to permit forming directly on the patient. One can also obtain mass-produced adjustable sockets; it may be necessary to pad the socket bottom so that the amputated limb does not develop distal edema. Some temporary prostheses have a plaster socket molded to the amputated limb. Plaster is inexpensive, readily available, and easy to use. The resulting socket, however, is rather heavy and bulky. Suspension is usually by a cuff or thigh corset. The pylon can be an aluminum component manufactured for this purpose; such a pylon has a proximal fixture that permits small changes in prosthetic alignment. A simpler pylon can be made with polyvinylchloride piping, such as used for plumbing. The pipe is lightweight and can be spot-heated to enable slight alteration in alignment. A SACH foot is customarily used on temporary prostheses.

Transfemoral (Above-Knee) Temporary Prosthesis

The easiest approach is to use a polypropylene socket (Fig. 32.32), which is manufactured in several sizes and has straps for circumferential adjustment. The socket can be suspended with a Silesian bandage or pelvic band, and is mounted on a knee unit, which may include a manual lock. Alternatively, a custom-fabricated socket of plaster or low-temperature thermoplastic can be used. Some individuals with bilateral transfemoral amputations use a pair of stubbies (Chapter 25, Fig. 19-25). These are nonarticulated prostheses; the sockets are mounted on short platforms, drastically reducing the wearer's height in order to increase balance stability. The platforms each have a rearward projection to protect the patient from a backward fall.

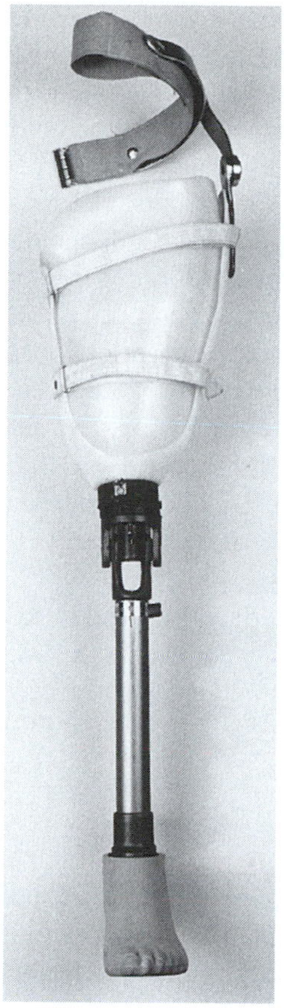

Figure 32.32 Transfemoral temporary prosthesis with adjustable polypropylene socket, pelvic band, knee unit with manual lock, and adjustable pylon shank with SACH foot.

Prosthetic Examination

The prosthesis should be examined before the patient engages in prosthetic training and should be reexamined at the conclusion of training. The procedure is intended to determine the adequacy of prosthetic fit and function, as well as the wearer's opinion of appearance and overall satisfaction. This process typically follows a sequence of examining the prosthesis while the patient stands (static analysis), examining the patient's gait (dynamic analysis), and finally examining the prosthesis off the patient (additional static analysis). In many institutions, the physical therapist examines the prosthesis and presents a summary of findings to the clinic team. The team makes the final determination regarding the acceptability of the prosthesis. At initial examination, the team has three options: (1) pass, (2) provisional pass, or (3) fail. Pass indicates that no changes are needed in the prosthesis and the patient can proceed to training. Provisional pass signals that one or more minor problems require correction, none of which would interfere with training. Failure is the team's judgment that the prosthesis has a major fault that should be corrected to the team's satisfaction before commencement of prosthetic training. For example, poor finishing of the prosthetic foot merits a provisional pass, whereas a socket that abrades the amputated limb should be graded as fail. If the therapist intends to train a patient who is not managed by a formal clinic team, it is especially critical that one examine the prosthesis prior to initiating training to discover any problems that would negate the future program. At the final examination, two ratings are available: pass indicates that no problems exist and the patient uses the prosthesis in a manner commensurate with that individual's physical capacity; fail means that major or minor problems remain.

No special materials are needed to examine the prosthesis, except for a checklist and a straight chair. For final examination, stairs and a ramp are needed. Appendices A and B contain the checklists referred to in the following sections.

Transtibial (Below-Knee) Examination

Most items on the checklist in Appendix A are self-explanatory. Each contributes to forming an accurate judgment of the adequacy of the prosthesis.

Static Analysis

The prosthesis is examined while the wearer stands and sits. In addition, the amputated limb and details of the prosthesis are examined. The prosthesis should be compared with the prescription. Departures from the original specifications must be approved by the individual who authorized the prescription.

The new wearer should stand in the parallel bars or other secure environment, attempting to bear equal weight on both feet. The therapist should solicit subjective comments about comfort. Estimates of anterior–posterior and medial–lateral alignment are aided by slipping a sheet of paper under various parts of the shoe. Ideally, the patient should stand with both heels and soles flat on the floor. Malalignment, indicated by excessive weightbearing on one portion of the shoe, may be confirmed by subsequent analysis of gait.

Most prostheses are constructed so that when the individual stands, the pelvis is level.[36] If the pelvis tilts, the therapist should place lifts under the foot on the shorter side to restore a level pelvis. If the total lift measures 1/2 in. (1 cm) or less, no attention is needed. For greater discrepancy, one should seek causative factors. An amputated limb that sinks too far into the socket will make the prosthetic side appear short, and the wearer will probably complain of discomfort.

Piston action refers to vertical motion of the socket when the patient elevates the pelvis. Socket slippage is caused by looseness, inadequate suspension, or both. Socket walls should fit snugly, as should the thigh corset if it is part of the prosthesis.

Comfortable sitting is a primary need for all people. The posterior brim should not impinge into the popliteal fossa, and hamstring reliefs should be adequate, especially on the medial side where the semitendinosus and semimembranosus insert relatively distally. Placement of the tabs of the cuff or the joints of the corset also influences sitting comfort.

Dynamic Analysis

Analysis of the gait pattern and performance of other ambulatory activities is an essential part of rehabilitation. For most patients, a major reason for being fitted with a prosthesis is to resume walking. Nevertheless, no prosthesis eradicates entirely the anatomical and physiological changes produced by amputation. When walking, the person who wears a prosthesis compensates for anatomical and prosthetic deficiencies. Some are inherent to amputation; others are abnormalities of the body or the prosthesis. Because virtually all people walk with a prosthesis in a manner different from the nondisabled walking pattern, prosthetic gait represents compensation for the patient's altered locomotor apparatus. The term "gait compensation" may be a more accurate descriptor than the more commonly used "gait deviation" inasmuch as the patient with amputation is most unlikely ever to walk exactly like a nondisabled person.

No prosthesis restores sensation, skeletal continuity, muscle integrity, and full body weight. Anatomical deficiencies are aggravated in the presence of pain, contracture, weakness, instability, or incoordination. Similarly, prosthetic components do not replace every function of the missing limb. For example, most prosthetic feet do not move through the full excursion of the human counterpart. Inadequacies in the prosthesis compel the wearer to adopt gait compensations. Such problems include a poorly fitted socket, prosthetic malalignment, malfunctioning components, and improper height of the prosthesis. Compounding the problem are incorrect donning of the prosthesis and wearing inappropriate shoes. The physical therapist must determine when gait compensation exists and what its cause is likely to be so that remedial action may be taken. Otherwise, the patient is compelled to expend more energy walking and to exhibit a more conspicuously abnormal gait. The new wearer will have had brief experience walking in the prosthesis during the course of prosthetic fabrication. Although a smooth gait is unlikely on the day of the initial examination, gross departure from the usual gait exhibited by others with similar prostheses should be noted and causes sought.

Transtibial analysis focuses on action of the knee on the amputated side during stance phase. Both knees should flex in a controlled manner during their respective early and late stance phases. Excessive flexion indicates that the socket is aligned too far anterior in relation to the foot, or is excessively flexed; this deviation may cause the patient to fall. If the knee flexes too much only during early stance, the cause may be a heel cushion that is too firm for

Table 32.1 Transtibial Prosthetic Gait Analysis

Compensation/Deviation	Prosthetic Causes	Anatomical Causes
Early Stance		
1. Excessive knee flexion	High shoe heel Insufficient plantarflexion Stiff heel cushion Socket too far anterior Socket excessively flexed Cuff tabs too posterior	Flexion contracture Weak quadriceps
2. Insufficient knee flexion	Low shoe heel Excessive plantarflexion Soft heel cushion Socket too far posterior Socket insufficiently flexed	Extensor spasticity Weak quadriceps Anterior-distal pain Arthritis
Midstance		
1. Lateral thrust	Excessive foot inset	
2. Medial thrust	Excessive foot outset	
Late Stance		
1. Early knee flexion: also referred to as "drop off"	High shoe heel Insufficient plantarflexion Keel too short Dorsiflexion stop too soft Socket too far anterior Socket excessively flexed Cuff tabs too posterior	Flexion contracture
2. Delayed knee flexion: perception of walking uphill	Low shoe heel Excessive plantarflexion Keel too long Dorsiflexion stop too stiff Socket too far posterior Socket insufficiently flexed	Extensor spasticity

that wearer. Conversely, insufficient knee flexion results from posterior displacement of the socket or inadequate socket tilting. When viewed in the frontal plane, the socket brim should maintain reasonable contact with the leg; excessive lateral thrust of the prosthetic brim suggests that the prosthetic foot has been positioned too far medially. Table 32.1 summarizes the prosthetic and anatomical causes of gait compensations/deviations.[37–41]

At the initial examination, performance on stairs and inclines may be omitted because the patient has not had training in these activities.

Inspection of the Prosthesis Off the Patient

After conducting the dynamic analysis, the therapist should examine the amputated limb for signs of proper loading. The posterior wall should be at the same level as the build-up for the patellar ligament when the patient stands. Because one cannot ascertain this relationship when the prosthesis is being worn, a substitute check is performed. Stand the prosthesis on a table; place the end of a long pencil or ruler on the anterior socket bulge and rest the ruler on the posterior brim. In a well-constructed prosthesis, the ruler will slant upward toward the rear, indicating that when the individual stands in the prosthesis and compresses the heel cushion, the wall will be at the proper height.

Any straps or cuff should provide reasonable adjustability. Construction is a guide to future durability, as well as contributing to acceptable appearance of the prosthesis.

Transfemoral (Above-Knee) Examination

A similar checklist is used to examine the transfemoral prosthesis (Appendix B). It is important to recognize that seldom is one item of major significance. The therapist and entire team should look for patterns that might herald future difficulty. For example, malalignment detected in static analysis should be confirmed during gait.

Static Analysis

The patient who has a flesh roll above the socket either did not don the socket properly or has a thigh that is larger than that for which the socket was made. Perineal pressure results from sharpness of the medial brim or insufficiency of the adductor longus relief in a quadrilateral socket.

The knee unit should be stable enough to withstand a blow delivered by the therapist to the posterior aspect of the unit. Stability is influenced by the *alignment* of the knee in relation to the hip and prosthetic ankle. The farther posterior the knee bolt, the more stable the knee will be. Polycentric linkage and mechanical stabilizers also contribute to stability. If the socket is opaque, the only way to judge its snugness is by palpating tissue protruding through the valve hole when the valve is removed.

The checklist is designed to help the clinician determine the fit of the socket, regardless of shape or material. If the prosthesis has a quadrilateral socket, proper location of the adductor longus tendon and ischial tuberosity ensures that the patient has donned the socket correctly. A horizontal posterior brim allows weight to be borne on the gluteal musculature as well as the ischial tuberosity. The ischial containment socket is intended to cover the ischial tuberosity, yet allow the client to move the hip in all directions comfortably, without socket gapping.

The lateral attachment of the Silesian bandage should be superior and posterior to the greater trochanter for best control of prosthetic rotation. Anteriorly, the attachment should be at the level of the ischial seat, or slightly below, to aid in adducting the prosthesis.

The pelvic joint and band should fit the torso snugly for optimum control of the prosthesis and to minimize bulkiness.

The patient should be able to sit comfortably with the prosthesis. Posterior discomfort may indicate inadequate hamstring relief, or a sharp or thick posterior brim.

Dynamic Analysis

Gait analysis gives the clinic team members the opportunity to determine the adequacy of socket fit, and of prosthesis alignment and adjustment. The patient also influences the walking pattern by the timing and force of muscular contraction and the presence or absence of contractures. The goal of walking with a transfemoral prosthesis is a comfortable, safe, efficient gait, rather than duplicating the gait of someone wearing a transtibial prosthesis or one who does not have amputation. Table 32.2 summarizes transfemoral prosthetic gait compensations/deviations.

Compensations/Deviations Best Viewed from Behind. Many individuals with transfemoral amputation abduct the prosthesis to improve frontal plane balance. Hip abduction contracture predisposes patients to this deviation, which is seen in stance phase. Inadequate socket adduction, socket looseness, or medial discomfort causes the fault. Circumduction is a displacement exhibited in swing phase if the prosthesis is too long or if the patient is reluctant to allow the knee to bend. Socket looseness also may result in circumduction. The patient may shift the trunk excessively. Lateral trunk bending toward the prosthetic side during stance phase generally accompanies abducted gait. It should be noted, however, that all individuals with transfemoral amputation have an incomplete abductor mechanism, and tend to compensate by bending toward the prosthetic side. Although the hip joint and gluteus medius are usually in good condition, lack of skeletal continuity to the ground compromises the effectiveness of abductor contraction. If the prosthesis is too long, the patient will abduct; if it is too short, the patient will bend laterally without abducting.

Whips refer to rotation of the heel at late stance. If the socket does not fit well, contraction with bulging of the thigh musculature will cause the prosthesis to rotate abruptly as it is being unloaded at the end of stance phase. Although less likely, malrotation of the knee unit or foot-ankle assembly may contribute to whipping. Rotation of the foot on heel contact is a much more serious deviation. It indicates inadequate compression of the heel cushion or plantar bumper and can result in a fall.

Compensations/Deviations Best Viewed from the Side. Forward trunk shifting in stance phase is a compensation that some patients use to cope with knee instability. If the walker or crutches are too short, the individual will lean forward. Lumbar lordosis results from inadequate socket flexion and is aggravated by a hip flexion contracture.

Improper adjustment of the knee unit gives rise to *uneven heel rise* (excessive knee flexion) and *terminal swing impact* (abrupt knee extension). If both deviations are present, the probable cause is insufficient friction. If the knee exhibits impact without undue heel rise, it is more likely that the extension aid is too tight.

To compensate for reduced knee motion, the vigorous walker may *vault*, excessively plantarflexing the sound ankle to afford extra room to clear the prosthesis during prosthetic swing phase. A less strenuous compensation for actual or functional prosthesis length is *hip hiking*, when the patient elevates the pelvis on the prosthetic side.

Step lengths will be unequal if the patient has a hip flexion contracture or inadequate balance; a longer step is taken with the prosthesis. The longer prosthetic step gives the person more time on the sound limb. A flexion contracture prevents the sound limb from passing the prosthetic side during swing phase on the sound side.

Inspection of the Prosthesis Off the Patient

Following the static examination, the therapist should examine the prosthesis and amputated limb as indicated on the checklist. A resilient back pad enables the patient to sit quietly without undue trouser or skirt abrasion. The pad is unnecessary with a flexible socket.

Facilitating Prosthetic Acceptance

Amputation generally is regarded as a grievous occurrence, with its visibility a constant reminder of the individual's abnormality.[42–48] The physical therapist can help

Table 32.2 Transfemoral (Above-Knee) Prosthetic Gait Analysis

Compensation/Deviation	Prosthetic Causes	Anatomical Causes
Lateral Displacements		
1. Abduction: stance	Long prosthesis Abducted hip joint Inadequate lateral wall adduction Sharp or high medial wall	Abduction contracture Weak abductors Lateral/distal pain Adductor redundancy instability
2. Circumduction: swing	Long prosthesis Locked knee unit Loose friction Inadequate suspension Small socket Loose socket Foot plantarflexed	Abduction contracture Poor knee control
Trunk Shifts		
1. Lateral bend: stance	Short prosthesis Inadequate lateral wall adduction Sharp or high medial wall	Abduction contracture Weak abductors Hip pain Instability Short amputation limb
2. Forward flexion: stance	Unstable knee unit Short walker or crutches	Instability
3. Lordosis: stance	Inadequate socket flexion	Hip flexion contracture Weak extensors
Rotations		
1. Medial (or lateral) whip: heel off	Faulty socket contour Knee bolt externally (or internally) rotated Foot malrotated Prosthesis donned in malrotation	With sliding friction unit, fast pace
2. Foot rotation at heel contact	Stiff heel cushion Malrotated foot	
Excessive Knee Motion		
1. High heel rise: early swing	Inadequate friction Slack extension aid	
2. Terminal impact: late swing	Inadequate friction Taut extension aid	Forceful hip flexion
Reduced Knee Motion		
1. Vault: swing	See above: circumduction	With sliding friction unit, fast pace
2. Hip hike: swing	See above: circumduction	Weak dorsiflexors Plantarflexor spasticity Pes equinus Weak hip flexors
Uneven Step Length	Uncomfortable socket Insufficient socket flexion	Hip flexion contracture Instability

the patient and family accept the reality of amputation and the prosthesis by verbal and nonverbal communication. One's calm respect for the patient as a worthy human being, regardless of limb condition, should set a model for the attitudes of others. Clinic team management accords not only the benefits of better prosthetic provision but also brings the individual in contact with clinicians who convey experience and confidence in dealing with problems that the person may have considered unique.

As soon as possible, the hospitalized patient should be treated in the physical therapy department, rather than at bedside. The bustle of the department should help dispel despondency. Although postoperative mourning is expected, prolonged depression is not constructive. Peer support groups are often very effective in aiding acceptance of the prosthesis and in learning special procedures for accomplishing activities. Observation and eventual participation in specially designed sports programs is another way people learn to cope and gain the most from rehabilitation. The physical therapist, by virtue of close daily contact with the patient, is also in a position to recommend to the clinic those who might profit from psychological counseling and psychiatric services.

Prosthetic Training

Learning to use a prosthesis effectively involves being able to don it correctly, develop good balance and coordination, walk in a safe and reasonably symmetrical manner, and perform other ambulatory and self-care activities. Anticipated goals and expected outcomes depend on the patient's physical and psychological status, preprosthetic experience, and quality of prosthesis. Using the prosthesis only to assist in transferring from the wheelchair to the toilet may be an appropriate outcome for an elderly person with multiple disabilities, whereas the program for the youngster with traumatic amputation might extend to a full range of sports.

Donning

Correct application of the prosthesis and frequent inspection of the amputated limb are very important, especially for the beginner and those with poor circulation. Patients with partial foot, Syme's, and transtibial amputations can don the prosthesis while seated, after having applied the correct number and sequence of socks or sheath. Then, in most instances, the individual simply inserts the amputated limb into the socket. With SC/SP suspension, one applies the liner to the amputated limb, then inserts the limb and liner into the socket. The initial entry into the socket with corset suspension may be made while sitting; however, final tightening of laces or straps should be done in the standing position to ensure that the limb is lodged suitably in the socket.

Those with transfemoral amputation also can begin the donning process while seated. Total suction wearers may use either a pulling or pushing method. To pull oneself into the socket, the patient applies a light dusting of talcum powder to the thigh to reduce friction. Then one applies a pulling sock, a tubular cotton stockinet approximately 30 in. (76 cm) long, a roll of elastic bandage wound around the thigh, or a nylon stocking. Whatever the donning aid, it should be placed high in the groin to pull in proximal tissues. After placing the sock-encased thigh into the socket, one draws the distal end of the aid through the valve hole. Although it is possible to complete the donning process while seated, most people prefer to stand while pulling the sock or other aid out through the valve hole. By leaning forward, the body's weight line will prevent the prosthetic knee from flexing inadvertently. The patient alternately flexes and extends the sound hip and knee while tugging downward on the donning aid until it slips out from the prosthesis. Finally, one inserts the valve.

Another approach to donning is to coat the thigh with a lubricating lotion, push it into the socket, then install the valve. Patients who use partial suction apply a sock, making certain the proximal margin of the sock extends to the inguinal ligament. The patient then introduces the amputated limb into the socket, taking care that the thigh is correctly oriented; pulls the distal end of the sock down through the valve hole enough to ensure that the skin is smooth; tucks the sock back into the socket; and inserts the valve. Finally, one secures the pelvic band or Silesian bandage. If suction is not used, donning is similar to the method used with partial suction, except that there is no valve.

Balance and Coordination

Exercises are similar for all patients with LE amputations, although the individual with a transfemoral or hip disarticulation prosthesis may be expected to encounter more difficulty controlling the mechanical knee, as compared to those with two anatomical knees. All must learn to balance on the amputated side. A graduated program for increasing prosthetic tolerance minimizes the danger of skin abrasion, particularly if the amputated limb presents skin grafts, poor circulation, or diminished sensation. The patient should alternately exercise and rest, with cardiopulmonary monitoring a routine part of the program, especially for high-risk individuals.

Some clinicians eschew parallel bars because the fearful patient pulls on them, which will be fruitless when progressing to a cane. When bars are used, the therapist should encourage the patient to rest the open hand on the bar for support, rather than using a viselike grip. A plinth or sturdy table offers the dual advantages of providing good support on only one side, ordinarily the contralateral side, and unidirectional control, because the patient can only push, never pull, for balance.

Static erect balance reintroduces the novice to bipedal posture. The patient should strive for level pelvis and shoulders, vertical trunk without excessive lordosis, and equal weightbearing. The therapist should guard and assist the patient as necessary. When the physical therapist stands near the prosthesis, this encourages the patient to shift his or her weight onto it. To suggest symmetrical performance, refer to the limbs as "right" and "left," or "sound" and "prosthetic," rather than discouraging the patient with "good" and "bad." The client must learn to utilize proximal sensory receptors to maintain balance and perceive the position of the prosthesis without looking at the floor. Some patients respond well to increased use of visual feedback (e.g., using a mirror).

Dynamic exercises improve medial–lateral, sagittal, and rotary control. The patient learns that hip flexion causes the knee to bend, and hip extension stabilizes the knee during stance phase. Placing the sound foot ahead of the prosthesis makes the prosthetic knee more stable. Patients should be instructed in weight shifting in both symmetrical and stride positions and in stepping movements. Stepping on a low stool or step platform with the sound leg obliges the patient to shift weight onto the prosthesis and increases stance phase duration on the prosthesis. Symmetrical performance is fostered by having all exercises performed rhythmically with both the right and left LEs.

Gait Training

Walking is a natural progression from dynamic balance exercises as the patient takes successive steps. Some people respond well to proprioceptive neuromuscular facilitation.[44] Rhythmic counting and walking in time with music in 2/4 time also improves gait symmetry and speed. In the physical therapy department, an apparatus that includes a suspension harness provides a protected environment for the patient to learn gradual weightbearing on the prosthesis.[45] A balance apparatus providing electronic feedback[46] with or without emphasis on psychological awareness of bodily position[47] is another training option.

Either a cane or pair of forearm crutches is an appropriate aid for the client who is unable to achieve a safe gait without undue fatigue. Sometimes the cane is used only outdoors to aid in negotiating curbs and other ground irregularities and to signal oncoming traffic. Ordinarily the cane is used on the contralateral side to enhance frontal plane balance. If bilateral assistance is required, a pair of forearm crutches is preferable to two canes. The crutches remain clasped around the forearms when the user opens a door. Axillary crutches tempt the patient to lean on the axillary bars, risking impingement of the radial nerves; they are also inconvenient when climbing stairs. An aluminum walker provides maximum stability, which is particularly useful for patients with generalized weakness. The walker should be adjusted so that the user does not lean too far forward. Patients with transtibial amputation walked faster with a two-wheeled walker as compared with a four-footed walker.[48]

Fear of falling can undermine walking and social activity participation. Improving the patient's balance confidence is essential to lessen this concern.[49]

Functional Training

The prosthesis wearer who is learning to walk also should gain experience in performing a wide variety of functional mobility skills. Activities such as transferring to various chairs add interest to the program and, for some patients, may be more important than long-distance ambulation. The training program for vigorous individuals includes stair climbing, negotiating ramps, retrieving objects from the floor, kneeling, sitting on the floor, running, driving a car, and engaging in sports. The fundamental difference between these activities and walking is the way each LE is used. Walking implies symmetrical usage, but the other activities are done asymmetrically, with greater reliance on the strength, agility, and sensory control of the sound limb.

Generally, the patient should have the opportunity to analyze each new situation and arrive at a solution to the problem, rather than depending on directions from the therapist. Most tasks can be accomplished safely in several ways. The learner profits from observing other prosthesis wearers as well as from professional instruction.

Transfers

Rising from different chairs, the toilet, and car are primary skills even for people who are elderly or debilitated. Most patients enter the physical therapy department in a wheelchair. Initially, the patient can park the chair at the parallel bars or at a plinth. After locking the wheelchair and raising the footrests, the patient should sit forward and transfer weight to the intact leg, then push down on the chair armrests. The individual will find that placing the sound foot close to the chair enables rising by extending the knee and hip on the sound side. Sitting is accomplished by placing the sound foot close to the chair and lowering oneself by controlled hip and knee flexion on the sound side.

For both standing and sitting, the beginner should have the advantage of a chair with armrests that enable use of the hands to control and assist trunk movement. Later the person should practice sitting in deep upholstered sofas and low chairs, as well as benches, the toilet, and other seats that do not have armrests. Transfer into an automobile should be an integral part of the training activities; otherwise, the patient faces a gloomy future, confined to home or dependent on special transportation systems. To enter the right (passenger) side of an automobile, the prosthetic wearer faces toward the front of the car. The person with a right prosthesis puts the right hand on the door post and the left hand on the back of the front seat, then swings the left leg into the car, slides onto the car seat, and finally places the prosthesis in the car. The individual with a left prosthesis may find that sitting sideways with both feet out the car door is easiest. One then pivots on the seat while swinging the prosthesis into the car, then puts the intact right foot inside the car.

Climbing Stairs, Ramps, and Curbs

Patients with Syme's and transtibial amputations generally ascend and descend stairs and inclines with steps of equal length in step-over-step progression.[50] Those with unilateral transfemoral amputation, in contrast, ascend by leading with the sound foot and learn to descend by first placing the prosthesis on the lower step. A few individuals with transfemoral amputation subsequently learn to control prosthetic knee flexion in order to descend step-over-step. Curbs present a slightly different problem, because there is no handrail. The techniques are basically the same, however. If the stairs, ramp, or curb are too steep, the individual may climb diagonally or sidestep with the prosthesis kept on the downhill side.

Final Examination and Follow-Up Care

Economic strictures may compel the therapist to conclude the training program after the patient is able to walk and to negotiate basic transfers and stair climbing but before the full range of training activities is completed. Before discharge, the patient and prosthesis should be reexamined to make certain that socket fit, prosthetic appearance, and function are acceptable. The checklist used for initial examination can be used. The physical therapist should instruct the patient with regard to the patient's responsibility for reporting skin redness and any loose or missing parts from the prosthesis.

The new prosthesis wearer should return to the training site at regular intervals so that the clinic team may examine socket fit. Most will require major socket revision or replacement during the first year to accommodate shrinkage. Follow-up visits are good opportunities to augment training and to encourage the individual to engage in the widest possible range of activities.

Functional Capacities

Functional capacities refer to the individual's ability to walk, transfer from chairs, climb stairs, and perform other ambulatory activities, including recreational endeavors. A primary responsibility of the clinic team is to predict the probable function of the person with a new amputation, to determine whether the individual would benefit from a prosthesis, and what degree of activity is likely.[51–54] Because many people with LE amputation are elderly with several medical problems, the need for accurate forecasting and ongoing monitoring is especially critical.[55–61]

Walking with a prosthesis increases energy cost.[62–66] Compared with those people with two sound limbs, the individual with a unilateral transtibial prosthesis requires slightly more oxygen when walking at a comfortable speed; the person wearing a transfemoral prosthesis consumes nearly 50% more oxygen than normal. The prosthesis wearer chooses a comfortable pace, because at a speed that is natural for the individual, the energy cost per minute is similar to that of the person who does not require a prosthesis, although speed is slower.[67,68] The lower the amputation level, the less the metabolic disadvantage. Among persons with transtibial amputations older than 40, those with long amputated limbs average minimal increase in energy, but persons with shorter limbs work harder. Those with bilateral transtibial amputations expend less energy than those with unilateral transfemoral amputations. Individuals whose amputation was traumatic perform more efficiently than those whose amputation was caused by vascular disease at every amputation level. People who sustained trauma walk faster and use less oxygen than their dysvascular counterparts.

The increased metabolic expenditure results in part from the socket, which surrounds semifluid tissue, giving imperfect anchorage. The resulting pseudoarthrosis is more difficult to control than in an intact limb. The foot–ankle assembly transmits no plantar tactile or proprioceptive sensation, does not move through as large an excursion as the normal foot, and does not initiate the dynamic propulsion characteristic of normal gait. The transfemoral prosthesis also incorporates a knee unit that provides no proprioception to the wearer. The problem is aggravated by the fact that a prosthesis is operated by remotely located muscles that contract longer and more forcefully than in normal gait. With transfemoral amputation, for example, the prosthetic foot is placed by hip motion. The resulting alteration of motion is reflected in asymmetry of timing, further disturbing gait smoothness. Individuals with prostheses walk with greater vertical movement, inasmuch as the knee, whether prosthetic for the transfemoral prosthesis wearer or anatomical in the transtibial wearer, does not flex as much as the contralateral knee during stance phase.

With the exception of patients on beta-blockers, heart rate response is an important indication of the metabolic cost of prosthetic use for most individuals. Response from those wearing a unilateral transtibial prosthesis is not appreciably different from that of people of comparable age who did not have amputation, although the latter group were more active.[69]

Sports participation (Fig. 32.33) is an excellent extension of rehabilitation for patients of all ages. Older adults may enjoy fishing, golfing, dancing, Tai Chi Chuan, and shuffleboard, and younger people may add basketball, tennis, archery, and track events to their range of activities. Most sports do not require any adaptation to the prosthesis. Horseback riding is a superb activity that fosters trunk control and seated balance. The hiker should pack extra amputated limb socks or a sheath to protect the skin; a well-fitting, comfortable hiking boot is essential. Bowling and participating in shot put are facilitated by emphasizing balance on the intact LE. For sports that involve running, an energy storing/releasing foot is most suitable. The socket should fit snugly with very secure suspension to minimize abrasion of the amputated limb. Clients with Syme's or transtibial amputations usually run with reasonably symmetrical step lengths, although they will favor the sound

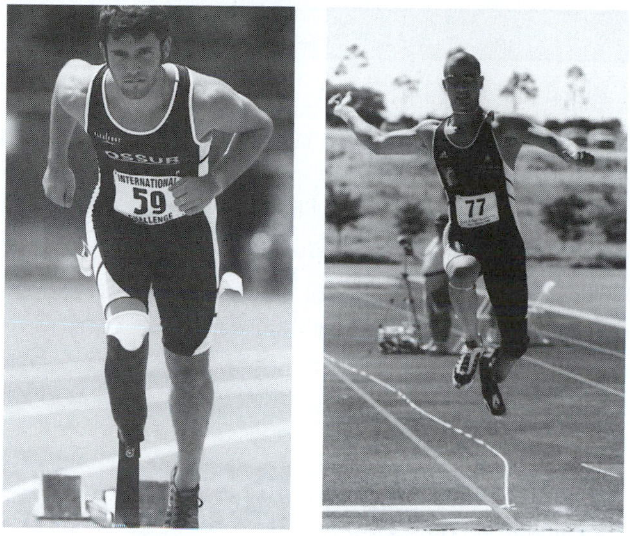

Figure 32.33 Participants in a distance run (*left*) and long jump (*right*) event. (Courtesy of Ossur, Aliso Viejo, CA 92656.)

limb, which has greater propulsive ability.[70,71] Those with a knee disarticulation or transfemoral amputation will derive most of the propulsive force from the sound leg and use the prosthesis as a momentary prop. Many marathon competitions have a category for people with disabilities. Jumping, as in basketball, requires the athlete to generate a substantial upward force with the sound leg; landing is more comfortable on the sound leg, particularly for those who wear transfemoral prostheses. Some activities are facilitated by minor modification of the equipment, such as a toe loop on a bicycle pedal or an adapted prosthesis.[72,73] Other activities are generally performed without a prosthesis, such as swimming and skiing. The skier will probably use ski poles equipped with small rudders, in a "three-track" manner. Soccer is usually played without a prosthesis, with the player using a pair of crutches. Some individuals enjoy playing tennis and field events in a wheelchair. Equipment and techniques developed for individuals with paraplegia usually can be adapted for people with amputations. Recreational programs designed for children and adults with amputations help the participants to return to active lifestyles.[74] The physical therapist should be able to refer patients to convenient recreational clubs, camps, and sporting events. The desired outcome is to maximize each person's functional capacity and quality of life.

Overall satisfaction with prosthetic rehabilitation depends on many factors. Difficulty with wound healing and prosthetic fit delay return to work,[75] while women and adults with higher educational level are more likely to express satisfaction with rehabilitation. Neither amputation etiology nor level make a significant impact on the patients' perceptions.[76]

Summary

This chapter has focused on management of people with lower-limb amputations. Characteristics and function of the principal lower-limb prostheses and prosthetic components have been discussed. In addition, the responsibilities of the physical therapist in prosthetic management have been emphasized. Successful prosthetic rehabilitation depends on close collaboration among the patient, physical therapist, physician, prosthetist, and other team members. This will provide an environment for information exchange and foster coordinated management. The result will be an optimum match between the patient's physical and psychosocial characteristics and a prosthesis capable of fulfilling its intended purposes.

Questions for Review

1. What are the principal causes of amputation in the elderly? In the young?
2. Describe appropriate prostheses for individuals with various partial foot amputations.
3. Distinguish between the Syme's and the transtibial amputation limbs and prostheses.
4. What prosthetic feet are especially suitable for geriatric patients? Why?
5. Name the reliefs and buildups in the transtibial socket.
6. Contrast the modes of suspension for the transtibial prosthesis. Which suspension is indicated for an individual with a short amputated limb?
7. Classify knee units according to friction mechanisms.
8. Compare the quadrilateral and the ischial containment transfemoral sockets.
9. Describe the modes of suspension of the transfemoral prosthesis. In which type(s) does the client wear a sock?
10. How is the wearer of a hip disarticulation prosthesis prevented from inadvertently flexing the hip and knee?
11. Outline a maintenance program for a transfemoral prosthesis with hydraulic knee unit and endoskeletal shank.
12. What factors should be considered prior to formulating a prosthetic prescription?
13. How can the physical therapist determine and improve the patient's psychological status?
14. What features of the transtibial prosthesis are considered in static examination? In dynamic examination?
15. Delineate the training program for a patient with a transfemoral prosthesis.

Case Study

The patient is a 67-year-old man with diabetic arteriosclerosis. He sustained a right transtibial amputation 5 months ago. He was treated in the inpatient physical therapy department for 3 weeks. The wound healed satisfactorily. His physical therapist taught him to transfer independently and ambulate using a temporary prosthesis and a walker. He was discharged with a home program consisting of exercises to promote strength, joint mobility, and endurance. He was also told to keep an elastic shrinker on his amputated limb whenever he was not wearing the temporary prosthesis. In addition, the physical therapist instructed the patient in care of the left foot, including thorough foot washing every evening; inspecting all surfaces of the foot, using a mirror; wearing a clean sock and well-fitting shoe each day; and careful nail trimming. He was fitted with a permanent prosthesis 3 months after surgery. The prosthesis consisted of a SACH foot, endoskeletal shank, total contact socket, and cuff suspension. He returned to the rehabilitation department today complaining of difficulty keeping his balance on the irregular terrain on the golf course where he had gone for the first time since his surgery. He also mentioned that his golf score was poorer than it had ever been.

PAST MEDICAL HISTORY

The patient was in fairly good health until 6 months ago, when he went on a long-awaited trip to Europe. On the trip he did much more walking than usual, even though he had to stop every 50 ft because of cramping pain in his legs. His wife noticed that the hallux and second toe on his right foot were discolored. The discolored area became painful. Upon his return home, he was examined by his primary care physician and was diagnosed with gangrene and adult-onset diabetes. Despite aggressive wound care, the gangrene progressed to involve the entire foot. An amputation was required. His diabetes is now stabilized with diet.

SOCIAL HISTORY

The patient is a retired accountant who lives with his wife. For years, he played golf on vacations. Upon retirement last year, he had looked forward to more frequent golfing.

PHYSICAL THERAPY EXAMINATION FINDINGS

Review of Systems

- Cognitive status: Alert, oriented, memory intact.
- Endurance: Fair, tolerance to activity is approximately 30 minutes (with some fluctuation); occasional rest periods required.
- Vision: Intact with corrective lens
- Blood pressure: 140/86
- Respiratory rate: WFL

Range of Motion

Goniometric examination of both lower limbs: WNL

Observational Gait Analysis (general findings)

- Overall decrease in speed of movement
- Diminished, awkward weight transfer.

Hip/Pelvis (Bilateral)

- Decreased pelvic rotation
- Diminished hip flexion

Knee

- Diminished right knee flexion

Foot/Ankle

- Minimal medial–lateral motion of the right foot

Gait

The patient is a functional ambulator using a transtibial prosthesis. Gait is slow, with longer steps on the right side; without the cane he leans to the right side. When outdoors he uses a cane in the left hand. He can climb stairs slowly, using the handrail. On uneven surfaces, he widens his walking base and walks slowly.

Sensation

- Lower limbs: sharp/dull, light touch, temperature, proprioception: WFL bilaterally.
- Sensation in both upper limbs: WFL

Strength

Manual Muscle Test (MMT) Grades

		Right	Left
Hip	Flexion	4/5	4/5
	Extension	4/5	4/5
	Abduction	4/5	4/5
	Adduction	4/5	4/5
	Internal rotation	4−/5	4−/5
	External rotation	4−/5	4−/5
Knee	Flexion	4−/5	4/5
	Extension	3+/5	4−/5
Foot/Ankle	Dorsiflexion	N/A	4/5
	Plantarflexion	N/A	4/5
	Inversion	N/A	4/5
	Eversion	N/A	4/5
Upper limb	WFL	WFL	WFL

N/A = not applicable owing to amputation; WFL = within functional limits.

Prosthetic Examination

Socket is loose, as indicated by piston action

Balance

- Standing
  - Static: Good; able to maintain static position for unlimited period
  - Dynamic: Fair +; difficulty maintaining balance on uneven terrain
- Sitting: WFL

Examination of Function

- Patient independent in all transfers: bed, chair (FIM level = 7); requires minimal assistance in floor-to-stand transfers.
- Patient is independent in all BADL.
- Patient is independent in approximately 80% of IADL (limitations imposed by fatigue and low ambulatory tolerance).

PATIENT DESIRED OUTCOME (GOALS)

- Play golf at previous level of proficiency
- Walk without depending on cane when outdoors
- Improve endurance

GUIDING QUESTIONS

1. Formulate a clinical problem list.
2. Formulate a patient asset list.
3. Establish anticipated goals and expected outcomes.
4. Formulate a plan of care.

References

1. Epidemiology of lower extremity amputation in centres in Europe, North America and East Asia: The global lower extremity amputation study group. Br J Surg 87:328, 2000.
2. Mueller, MJ, and Strube, MJ: Therapeutic footwear: Enhanced function in people with diabetes and transmetatarsal amputation. Arch Phys Med Rehabil 78:952, 1997.
3. Boyd, LA, et al: Forefoot rocker mechanics in individuals with partial foot amputation. Gait Posture 9:144, 1999.
4. Doyle, W, et al: The Syme prosthesis revisited. J Prosthet Orthot 5:95, 1993.
5. Edelstein, JE: Current choices in prosthetic feet. Clin Rev Phys Rehab Med 2:213, 1991.
6. Barth, DG, et al: Gait analysis and energy cost of below-knee amputees wearing six different prosthetic feet. J Prosthet Orthot 4:63, 1992.
7. Huang, GF, Chou, YL, and Su, FC: Gait analysis and energy consumption of below-knee amputees wearing three different prosthetic feet. Gait Posture 12:162, 2000.
8. Czerniecki, JM, and Gitter, AJ: Prosthetic feet: A scientific and clinical review of current components. State Art Rev PM&R 8:109, 1994.
9. Powers, CM, et al: Influence of prosthetic foot design on sound limb loading in adults with unilateral below-knee amputations. Arch Phys Med Rehabil 75:825, 1994.
10. Menard, MR, et al: Comparative biomechanical analysis of energy-storing prosthetic feet. Arch Phys Med Rehabil 73:451, 1992.
11. Perry, J, and Shanfield, S: Efficiency of dynamic elastic response prosthetic feet. J Rehabil Res Dev 30:137, 1993.
12. Alaranta, H, et al: Subjective benefits of energy-storing prostheses. Prosthet Orthot Int 18:92, 1994.
13. Snyder, RD, et al: The effect of five prosthetic feet on the gait and loading of the sound limb in dysvascular below-knee amputees. J Rehabil Res Dev 32:309, 1995.
14. Torburn, L, et al: Energy expenditure during ambulation in dysvascular and traumatic below-knee amputees: A comparison of five prosthetic feet. J Rehabil Res Dev 32:111, 1995.
15. Barr, AE, et al: Biomechanical comparison of the energy-storing capabilities of SACH and Carbon Copy II prosthetic feet during the stance phase of gait in a person with below-knee amputation. Phys Ther 72:344, 1992.
16. Arya, AP, et al: A biomechanical comparison of the SACH, Seattle and Jaipur feet using ground reaction forces. Prosthet Orthot Int 19:37, 1995.
17. Lehmann, JF, et al: Comprehensive analysis of energy storing prosthetic feet: Flex Foot and Seattle foot versus standard SACH foot. Arch Phys Med Rehabil 74:1225, 1993.
18. Macfarlane, PA, et al: Transfemoral amputee physiological requirements: Comparisons between SACH foot walking and Flex-Foot walking. J Prosthet Orthot 9:138, 1997.
19. Ehara, Y, et al: Energy storing property of so-called energy-storing prosthetic feet. Arch Phys Med Rehabil 74:68, 1993.
20. Ross, J, et al: Study of telescopic pylon on lower limb amputees. Orthopad Technik 3:1, 2003.
21. Kristinsson, O: The ICEROSS concept: A discussion of philosophy. Prosthet Orthot Int 17:49, 1993.
22. Datta, D, et al: Outcome of fitting an ICEROSS prosthesis: Views of transtibial amputees. Prosthet Orthot Int 20:111, 1996.
23. Sewell, P, et al: Developments in trans-tibial prosthetic socket fitting process: A review of past and present research. Prosthet Orthot Int 24:97, 2000.
24. Astrom, I, and Stenstrom, A: Effect on gait and socket comfort in unilateral trans-tibial amputees after exchange to a polyurethane concept. Prosthet Orthot Int 28:28, 2004.
25. Branemark, R, et al: Osseointegration in skeletal reconstruction and rehabilitation. J Rehabil Res Dev 38:175, 2001.
26. Meikle, B, et al: Does increased prosthetic weight affect gait speed and patient preference in dysvascular transfemoral amputees? Arch Phys Med Rehabil 84:1657, 2003.
27. Van der Linden, ML, Twiste, N, and Rithalia, SV: The biomechanical effects of the inclusion of a torque absorber on trans-femoral amputee gait. Prosthet Orthot Int 26:35, 2002.
28. Radcliffe, CW: Four-bar linkage prosthetic knee mechanisms: Kinematics, alignment and prescription criteria. Prosthet Orthot Int 18:159, 1994.
29. Chin, T, et al: Effect of an Intelligent Prosthesis (IP) on the walking ability of young transfemoral amputees: Comparison of IP users with able bodied people. Am J Phys Med Rehabil 82:447, 2001.
30. Devlin, M, et al: Patient preference and gait efficiency in a geriatric population with transfemoral amputation using a free-swinging versus a locked prosthetic knee joint. Arch Phys Med Rehabil 83:246, 2002.
31. Pritham, CH: Biomechanics and shape of the above-knee socket considered in light of the ischial containment concept. Prosthet Orthot Int 14:9, 1990.
32. Gailey, RS, et al: The CAT-CAM socket and quadrilateral socket: A comparison of energy cost during ambulation. Prosthet Orthot Int 17:95, 1993.

33. Gottschalk, FA, and Stills, M: The biomechanics of trans-femoral amputation. Prosthet Orthot Int 8:12, 1994.
34. Sullivan, J, et al: Rehabilitation of the trans-femoral amputee with an osseointegrated prosthesis: The United Kingdom experience. Prosthet Orthot Int 27:114, 2003.
35. Lilja, M, and Oberg, T: Proper time for definitive transtibial prosthetic fitting. J Prosthet Orthot 9:90, 1997.
36. Isakov, E, et al: Influence of prosthesis alignment on the standing balance of below-knee amputees. Clin Biomech 9:258, 1994.
37. Edelstein, JE: Prosthetic and orthotic gait. In Smidt, GL (ed): Gait in Rehabilitation. Churchill Livingstone, New York, 1990, p. 281.
38. Lemaire, ED, et al: Gait patterns of elderly men with transtibial amputations. Prosthet Orthot Int 17:27, 1993.
39. Isakov, E, et al: Double-limb support and step-length asymmetry in below-knee amputees. Scand J Rehabil Med 29:75, 1996.
40. Powers, CM, et al: The influence of extremity muscle force on gait characteristics in individuals with below-knee amputations secondary to vascular disease. Phys Ther 76:369, 1996.
41. Sanderson, DJ, and Martin, PE: Lower extremity kinematic and kinetic adaptation in unilateral below-knee amputees during walking. Gait Posture 6:126, 1997.
42. Ryarczyk, BD, et al: Social discomfort and depression in a sample of adults with leg amputations. Arch Phys Med Rehabil 73:1169, 1992.
43. Breakey, JW: Body image: The lower-limb amputee. J Prosthet Orthot 9:58, 1997.
44. Yigiter, K, et al: A comparison of traditional prosthetic training versus proprioceptive neuromuscular facilitation resistive gait training with trans-femoral amputees. Prosthet Orthot Int 26:213, 2002.
45. Hunter, D, and Smith-Cole, E: Energy expenditure of below-knee amputees during harness-supported treadmill ambulation. J Orthop Sports Phys Ther 21:268, 1995.
46. Matjacic, Z, and Burger, H: Dynamic balance training during standing in people with trans-tibial amputation: A pilot study. Prosthet Orthot Int 27:214, 2003.
47. Sjodahl, C, et al: Gait improvement in unilateral transfemoral amputees by a combined psychological and physiotherapeutic treatment. J Rehabil Med. 33:114, 2001.
48. Tsai, HA, et al: Aided gait of people with lower-limb amputations: Comparison of 4-footed and 2-wheeled walkers. Arch Phys Med Rehabil 84:584, 2003.
49. Miller, WC, et al: The influence of falling, fear of falling, and balance confidence on prosthetic mobility and social activity among individuals with lower extremity amputation. Arch Phys Med Rehabil 82:1238, 2001.
50. Powers, CM, et al: Stair ambulation in persons with transtibial amputation: An analysis of the Seattle LightFoot. J Rehabil Res Dev 34:9, 1997.
51. Heinemann, AW, Bode, RK, and O'Reilly, C: Development and measurement properties of the Orthotics and Prosthetics Users' Survey (OPUS): A comprehensive set of clinical outcome instruments. Prosthet Orthot Int 27:191, 2003.
52. Rommers, GM, et al: Mobility of people with lower limb amputations: Scales and questionnaires. Clin Rehabil 15:92, 2001.
53. Franchignoni, F, et al: Reliability, validity, and responsiveness of the Locomotor Capabilities Index in adults with lower-limb amputation undergoing prosthetic training. Arch Phys Med Rehabil 85:743, 2004.
54. Gallagher, P, and MacLachlan, M: The Trinity Amputation and Prosthesis Experience Scales and quality of life in people with lower-limb amputation. Arch Phys Med Rehabil 85:730, 2004.
55. Hagberg, K, and Branemark, R: Consequences of non-vascular transfemoral amputation: A survey of quality of life, prosthetic use and problems. Prosthet Orthot Int 25:186, 2001.
56. Siriwardena, GA, and Bertrand, PV: Factors influencing rehabilitation of arteriosclerotic lower limb amputees. J Rehabil Res Dev 28:35, 1991.
57. Bilodeau, S, et al: Lower limb prosthetics utilization by elderly amputees. Prosthet Orthot Int 24:124, 2000.
58. Fletcher, DD, et al: Rehabilitation of the geriatric vascular amputee patient: A population-based study. Arch Phys Med Rehabil 82:776, 2001.
59. Davies, B, and Datta, D: Mobility outcome following unilateral lower limb amputation. Prosthet Orthot Int 27:186, 2003.
60. Dillingham, TR, Pezzin, LE, and Mackenzie, EJ: Discharge destination after dysvascular lower-limb amputations. Arch Phys Med Rehabil 84:1662, 2003.
61. Johannesson, A, Larsson, GU, and Oberg, T: From major amputation to prosthetic outcome: A prospective study of 190 patients in a defined population. Prosthet Orthot Int 28:9, 2004.
62. Gonzalez, E, and Edelstein, J: Energy expenditure in ambulation. In Gonzalez, E, et al (eds).Downey and Darling's Physiological Basis of Rehabilitation Medicine. ed 3. Butterworth-Heinemann, Boston, 2001, p 417.
63. Gailey, RS, et al: Energy expenditure of trans-tibial amputees during ambulation at self-selected pace. Prosthet Orthot Int 18:84, 1994.
64. Boonstra, AM, et al: Energy cost during ambulation in trans-femoral amputees: A knee joint with a mechanical swing-phase control vs. a knee joint with a pneumatic swing-phase control. Scand J Rehabil Med 27:77, 1995.
65. Schmalz T, Blumentritt, S, and Jarasch, R: Energy expenditure and biomechanical characteristics of lower limb amputee gait: The influence of prosthetic alignment and different prosthetic components. Gait Posture 16:255, 2002.
66. Jaegers, SM, et al: The relationships between comfortable and most metabolically efficient walking speed in persons with unilateral above-knee amputation. Arch Phys Med Rehabil 74:521, 1993.
67. Hermodsson, et al: Gait in transtibial amputees: A comparative study with healthy subjects in relation to walking speed. Prosthet Orthot Int 18:68, 1994.
68. Jones, ME, et al: Weight-bearing and velocity in transtibial and transfemoral amputees. Prosthet Orthot Int 21:183, 1997.
69. Bussmann, JB, et al: Daily physical activity and heart rate response in people with a unilateral transtibial amputation for vascular disease. Arch Phys Med Rehabil 85:240, 2004.
70. Czerniecki, JM, and Gitter, A: Insights into amputee running: A muscle work analysis. Am J Phys Med Rehabil 71:209, 1992.
71. Prince, F, et al: Running gait impulse asymmetries in below-knee amputees. Prosthet Orthot Int 16:19, 1992.
72. Farley, R, Mitchell, F, and Griffiths, M: Custom skiing and trekking adaptations for a trans-tibial and trans-radial quadrilateral amputee. Prosthet Orthot Int 28:60, 2004.
73. Fergason, JR, and Boone, DA: Custom design in lower limb prosthetics for athletic activity. Phys Med Rehabil Clin North Am. 11:681, 2000.
74. Legro, MW, et al: Recreational activities of lower-limb amputees with prostheses. J Rehabil Res Dev 38:319, 2001.
75. Bruins, M, et al: Vocational reintegration after a lower limb amputation: A qualitative study. Prosthet Orthot Int 27:4, 2003.
76. Pezzin, LE, et al: Use and satisfaction with prosthetic limb devices and related services. Arch Phys Med Rehabil 85:723, 2004.

Supplemental Reading

Burgess, EM, and Rappoport, A: Physical Fitness: A Guide for Individuals with Lower Limb Loss. Department of Veterans Affairs, Washington, DC, 1992.

Engstrom, B, and Van de Van, C: Physiotherapy for Amputees, ed 2. Churchill Livingstone, Edinburgh, 1993.

Fitzlaff, G, and Heim, S: Lower Limb Prosthetic Components: Design, Function and Biomechanical Properties. Verlag Orthopadie Technik, Dortmund, Germany, 2002.

Ham, R, and Cotton, L: Limb Amputation: From Aetiology to Rehabilitation. Chapman & Hall, London, 1991.

Lusardi, MM, and Nielsen, CC: Orthotics and Prosthetics in Rehabilitation. Butterworth Heinemann, Boston, 2000.
May, BJ: Amputations and Prosthetics: A Case Study Approach, ed 2. FA Davis, Philadelphia, 2002.
Mensch, G, and Ellis, PM: Physical Therapy Management of Lower Extremity Amputations. Aspen, Gaithersburg, MD, 1986.
Murdoch, G, et al (eds): Amputation: Surgical Practice and Patient Management. Butterworth Heinemann, Oxford, 1996.
Parker, JN, and Parker, PM (eds): Amputation: A Medical Dictionary, Bibliography & Annotated Research Guide to Internet References. ICON Health Publications, San Diego, CA, 2003.
Rehabilitation Institute of Chicago. Lower Extremity Amputation: A Guide to Functional Outcomes in Physical Therapy Management. Pro-Ed, Austin, TX, 2005.
Seymour, R: Prosthetics and Orthotics: Lower Limb and Spinal. Lippincott Williams & Wilkins, Philadelphia, 2002.
Smith, DG, et al (eds): Atlas of Amputations and Limb Deficiencies, ed 3. American Academy of Orthopaedic Surgeons, Chicago, 2004.

Appendix A: Transtibial (Below-Knee) Prosthetic Examination

1. Is the prosthesis as prescribed?
2. Can the client don the prosthesis easily?

Standing

3. Is the client comfortable when standing with the heel midlines 6 in. (15 cm) apart?
4. Is the anterior–posterior alignment satisfactory?
5. Is the medial–lateral alignment satisfactory?
6. Do the contours and color of the prosthesis match the opposite limb?
7. Is the prosthesis the correct length?
8. Is piston action minimal?
9. Does the socket contact the amputation limb without pinching or gapping?

Suspension

10. Does the suspension component fit the amputation limb properly?
11. Does the cuff, fork strap, or thigh corset have adequate provision for adjustment?

Sitting

12. Can the client sit comfortably with hips and knees flexed 90°?

Walking

13. Is the client's performance in level walking satisfactory?
14. Is the client's performance on stairs and ramps satisfactory?
15. Can the client kneel satisfactorily?
16. Does the suspension function properly?
17. Does the prosthesis operate quietly?
18. Does the client consider the prosthesis satisfactory as to comfort, function, and appearance?

Prosthesis Off the Client

19. Is the skin free of abrasions or other discolorations attributable to this prosthesis?
20. Is the socket interior smooth?
21. Is the posterior wall of the socket of adequate height?
22. Is the construction satisfactory?
23. Do all components function satisfactorily?

Appendix B: Transfemoral (Above-Knee) Prosthetic Examination

1. Is the prosthesis as prescribed?
2. Can the client don the prosthesis easily?

Standing

3. Is the client comfortable when standing with the heel midlines 6 in. (15 cm) apart?
4. Is any flesh roll above the socket minimal?
5. Is the client free from vertical pressure in the perineum?
6. Do the contours and color of the prosthesis match the opposite limb?
7. Is the prosthesis the correct length?
8. Is the knee stable?
9. When the socket valve is removed, is the distal tissue firm?

Quadrilateral Socket

10. Does the ischial tuberosity rest on the posterior brim?
11. Is the posterior brim approximately parallel to the floor?
12. Is the adductor longus tendon located in the anterior–medial corner?

Ischial Containment Socket

13. Does the posterior–medial corner of the socket cover the ischial tuberosity?
14. Can the client hyperextend the hip on the amputated side comfortably?
15. Can the client flex the hip 90° comfortably, without socket gapping?
16. Can the client abduct the hip on the amputated side comfortably, without socket gapping?

Suspension

17. Does the Silesian bandage control prosthetic rotation and adduction adequately?
18. Does the pelvic band conform to the torso?

Sitting

19. Can the client sit comfortably with hips and knees flexed 90°?
20. Does the socket remain securely on the thigh, without gapping or rotating?
21. Are both thighs approximately the same length and height from the floor?
22. Can the client lean forward to touch the shoes?

Walking

23. Is the client's performance in level walking satisfactory?
24. Is the client's performance on stairs and ramps satisfactory?
25. Does the suspension function properly?
26. Does the prosthesis operate quietly?
27. Does the client consider the prosthesis satisfactory as to comfort, function, and appearance?

Prosthesis Off the Client

28. Is the skin free of abrasions or other discolorations attributable to this prosthesis?
29. Is the socket interior smooth?
30. With the prosthesis fully flexed on a table, can the thigh piece be brought to at least the vertical position?
31. If the socket is totally rigid, is a back pad attached?
32. Is the construction satisfactory?
33. Do all components function satisfactorily?

CHAPTER

33

LEARNING OBJECTIVES

1. Identify the postural support components of a wheelchair seating system.
2. Identify the components that make up a wheeled mobility base.
3. Describe the components of the patient examination process.
4. Describe the measurements required for correct fitting of a prescriptive wheelchair.
5. Understand the function and indications for common wheelchair features and postural support components.
6. Recognize the functional implications of a properly prescribed wheelchair for environmental access.
7. Analyze and interpret patient data and identify appropriate prescriptive elements when presented with a clinical case study.

The Prescriptive Wheelchair

Adrienne Falk Bergen, PT, ATP

OUTLINE

Physical therapists are often called on to prescribe a wheelchair.[1,2] A properly prescribed wheelchair can be a useful device in reintegrating a person with a disability into the community, whereas a poorly prescribed one can actually exacerbate the problems associated with functional limitations and disability. This chapter presents a systematic approach to determining the appropriate components of a prescriptive wheelchair, beginning with a thorough examination and culminating with a plan of care (POC) that includes the proper seating system and wheeled mobility base. The seating system and mobility base combine to create a prescriptive wheelchair, a seated environment from which the patient can achieve maximum function.

A wheelchair is truly a mobility orthosis. An *orthosis* is a device used to provide support or to straighten or to correct a deformity. It is typically a brace made of metal or plastic that increases or maintains a person's level of function. If properly prescribed, a wheelchair will provide sufficient support to help deter the effect of deforming forces or weakened structures on function of the system. In simpler terms, it should support the user as needed to allow maximum function. Inasmuch as it is on wheels, the system can be called a *mobility orthosis,* providing appropriate support to allow maximum functional mobility.

Like a well-made orthosis, the wheelchair should fit correctly. It should be reasonably cosmetic to the user. It should also be as lightweight and yet as strong as possible. It can be obtained from a stock supply when appropriate, but most often individual modifications for the patient's special needs are required.

Like a well-made orthosis, the wheelchair should be prescribed by qualified professionals. The entire team should make the decision concerning a prescriptive wheelchair. It is important that all those concerned with the person's present and future function be a part of this team. This includes the wheelchair user, therapists, family members, caregivers, nurses, physicians, educators, vocational counselors, and a qualified rehabilitation technology supplier. To ensure that the most suitable device is obtained, the team must have a clear idea of who will be using it, what functional level is expected, and where the chair will be used. All the members should contribute to the examination reports and letter of medical necessity, which must be prepared to secure funding. Once the chair is supplied, the team is responsible for adjusting and fitting the final device, as well as teaching the patient and any caregivers how to use and maintain the device to ensure optimal long-term performance.

A prescriptive wheelchair is a combination of a postural support system and a mobility base that are joined to create a dynamic seated environment (Fig. 33.1). The *postural support system* is made up of the surfaces that contact the user's body directly. This includes the seat, back, and foot supports as well as any additional components needed to maintain postural alignment. Maintenance of postural alignment may require such additions as a head support; lateral supports for the trunk, hips, and knees; medial support for the knees; and upper extremity (UE) support surfaces, as well as straps or bands (e.g., anterior chest or pelvis) needed to keep the user interfaced with the support surfaces. The *mobility base* consists of the tubular frame, armrests, foot supports, and wheels. Once the decisions are made about the type of support system needed, the team must then decide what type of mobility base best suits the user's functional level and environmental needs. For some patients, caregiver needs are of paramount importance. Clear information will be needed to ensure that the postural support system and the mobility base interface properly. For users who utilize more than one mobility base (e.g., power and manual), the most cost-effective approach is to have one support system interface with all the mobility bases. This is not always practical, and sometimes it is best to have the full-support system on the chair used most frequently, and forgo optimal postural support in the backup system to facilitate transport for short trips.

Creating a dynamic seating system involves three steps: (1) examining the patient/client and evaluating the data; (2) determining the diagnosis and prognosis, anticipated goals and expected outcomes; and (3) planning the intervention. This process will allow appropriate recommendations and product choices. As noted, the overall desired outcome is to create a dynamic seating system that is a comfortable base from which the user can attain a maximal functional level. Before the physical examination is begun, information must be gathered from the entire team regarding their expectations. A great deal can be learned at this point about what the various team members hope the system will be able to do for the patient. It is extremely important to bring all the obvious and hidden issues out into full view before the process is begun. Patients, family members, or caregivers may assume that the wheelchair and seating system can achieve unrealistic goals (normalize posture, provide total pain relief, facilitate independent transfers). When these hidden goals are not met, these individuals are often so disappointed that they cannot see the other benefits of the system. Open discussion is absolutely necessary.

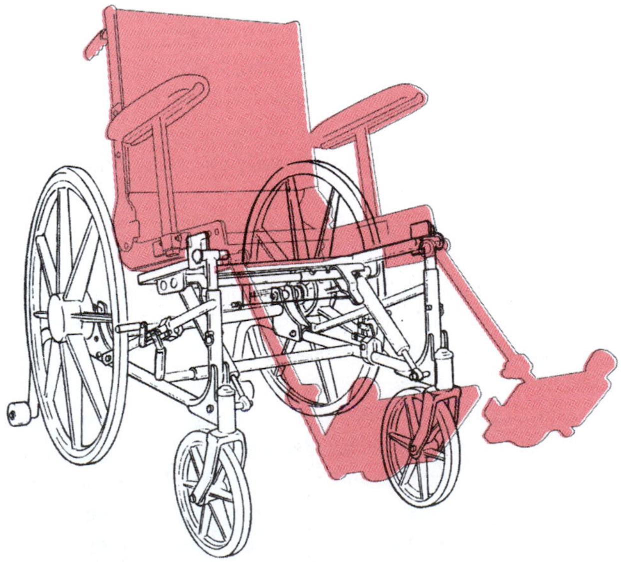

Figure 33.1 A prescriptive wheelchair consists of the postural support system and a mobility base.

The Examination Process

It is important to take time at the beginning of the examination process to explain to the patient and caregivers what will be happening, what information will be gathered, and why the information is important. Everyone should be made to feel that his or her input is necessary and valuable. Time should be allocated during data collection for comments or questions from the patient, caregivers, and other team members. Prior to each stage of the process, the patient should be asked if it is acceptable to proceed. For example, "I would like to put my hands on your pelvis, is that okay?" It is important to move slowly and speak calmly, because quick movements or loud speech may increase anxiety. In some patients, this may increase muscle tone, interfering with data collection. It is important to explain what is being observed or measured so that patients and caregivers can understand information exchanged between team members, and so they can fully comprehend the team's findings and the subsequent recommendations.

Information must be gathered from the entire team to determine the person's present level of function and the targeted goals and outcomes. The tests and measures should be completed by the appropriate professionals and submitted to the wheelchair team for review. The team must be totally informed about the patient's medical and surgical history and plans, neurological status, postural control, musculoskeletal status, sensory status, functional skill level, cognitive-perceptual–behavioral status, and communication level. Accurate information about the patient's home, work, educational, and recreational environments must be considered, along with the method the patient will use to transport the wheelchair. Funding sources should be identified so that the team is aware of any possible problems and advanced planning can begin.

Physical Examination

Although time consuming, it is absolutely critical that the physical examination be complete and accurate because changes may be difficult to make later. Accurate recording provides a permanent record of why certain decisions were made. During the ordering or manufacturing process, additional decisions concerning modifications may be needed. If accurate measurements are on file, decisions can often be made without recalling the person to the clinic.

The purpose of the physical examination is to learn as much as possible about the person's strength and range of available movement and about how movement of one body part affects tone, comfort, position, control, and performance in other body segments. The goal is to preserve spinal alignment whenever possible, maintaining the natural lumbar curve whenever it can be produced. The person should be examined in a gravity-minimized position (supine or sidelying), as well as a gravity-dependent position (sitting), whenever possible. To create a properly fitted system, range of motion (ROM) measurements are required. Accurate measurements are also needed of under thigh length; leg length; distance from the seat to the lower scapula, midscapula, and shoulder; distance from hanging elbow-to-seat surface; and width across the hips, shoulders, and from outside the knee to outside the opposite knee. Linear measurements must be taken in a corrected sitting position, accommodating for any limitations found in the supine or sidelying position.

Examination of Function Using Existing Equipment

A great deal can be learned by observing the patient in his or her existing wheelchair. The patient should be in the best or most commonly assumed position, with supports and straps in place. Questions should include how the patient and or caregiver feels the device is working, has it always worked like this, or has its function decreased over time. If it worked well initially, but does not work well now, is this because of patient change (weight gain or loss, growth, functional gain or loss) or equipment change (broken or missing parts, decreased reliability)? Information can be gathered during this portion of the examination about the patient's and caregiver's attitudes and technology savvy, as well as their physical use of the equipment. Throughout the initial visit, team members should continuously observe the existing equipment, the patient, the caregivers, and their physical and psychosocial interactions.

The team should gather data about the patient's postural alignment at the head, shoulders, trunk, pelvis, and lower extremities (LEs) using both visual observation and hands-on palpation. Pelvic alignment is examined by palpation along the pelvis crests, and on the anterior superior iliac spines (ASIS). The position of the pelvis (e.g., rotation, posterior or anterior tilt) should be carefully documented.

With the patient's shirt removed or at least lifted to nipple level, trunk posture can be observed directly. A combination of visual observation and palpation will allow determination of alignment (for example, abdominal wrinkles usually mean a rounded spine). In the presence of abnormal alignment, the therapist should determine (1) if alignment can be corrected using gentle pressure; and (2) what factors may be interfering with good postural alignment.

The patient should transfer onto a mat table. Observation of the specific transfer method used and level of assistance required will avoid creating a new system that interferes with this function.

Supine Examination

The physical examination usually requires more than one examiner. The patient should be positioned supine on a firm surface (a mat or carpeted floor works well; a bed may not be firm enough). The range of available pelvic and hip movements as they relate to spinal and pelvic alignment should be determined. The purpose is to determine the maximum ROM available before spinal alignment is disturbed. The LEs must be well supported by the examiner, with the knees flexed 95° to 100° or as much as is needed to eliminate the influence of the hamstring muscle group (Fig. 33.2). Care should be taken to neutralize pelvic tilt if at all possible. This may require tone reduction techniques in the presence of spasticity. The examiner palpates the ASIS of the pelvis and monitors position of the lumbar spine to ensure that the available degree of curvature is maintained. If gross ROM limitations such as abduction and/or adduction contractures are present, the LEs should be allowed to assume whatever posture is needed to achieve optimal pelvic alignment.

With the LEs positioned as needed, both hips can then be flexed at the same time to obtain a gross estimate of ROM. This can be followed by more detailed examination of each limb individually. ROM measurements should include hip flexion, abduction, adduction, and internal and external rotation; their affect on pelvic position and general body alignment should be noted as well. If the pelvis is asymmetric when the knees are aligned, this may

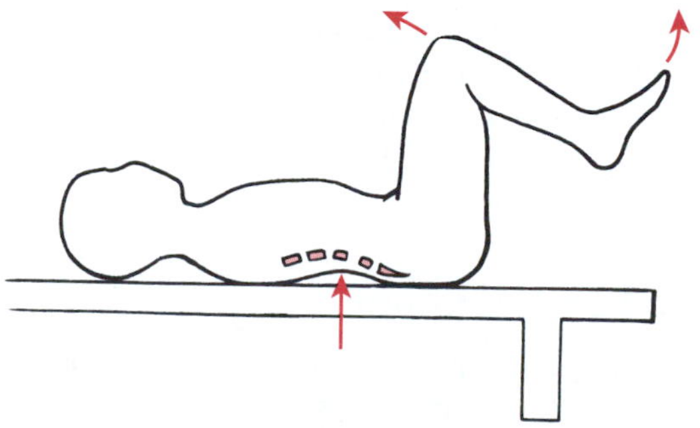

Figure 33.2 The examiner must monitor the lumbar curve as the hips are flexed and the knees extended.

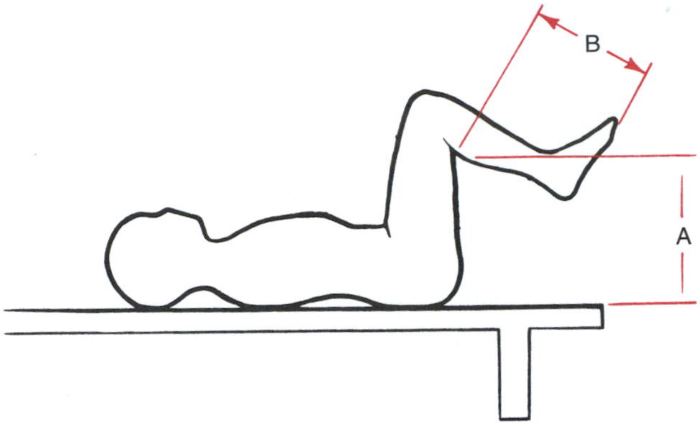

Figure 33.3 In the supine position with the hips and knees flexed the examiner can measure the undersurface of the thigh from the popliteal fossa to a firm support surface (*A*). Note that this position can also be used to measure leg length from the popliteal fossa to the heel (*B*).

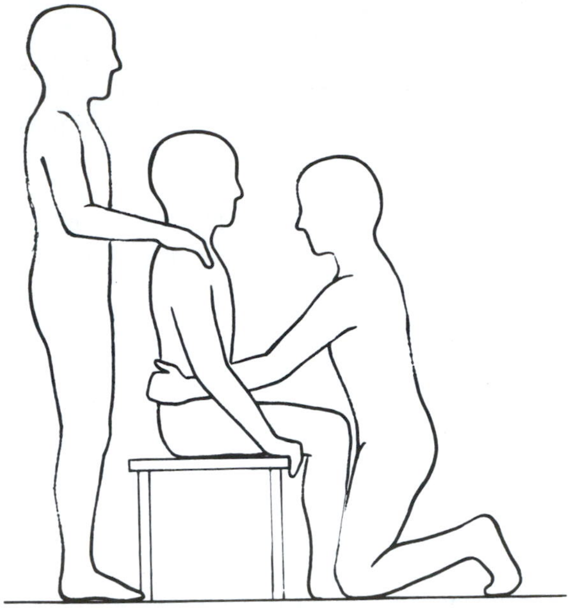

Figure 33.4 It is recommended that sitting measurements be taken with the patient on a thin seating surface to ensure adequate room for knee flexion as needed.

indicate limited range of hip abduction or adduction. In some cases, it will be necessary to allow the LEs to rotate off to one side (*windblown position*), be widely abducted, and/or internally or externally rotated, to achieve good pelvic alignment and minimize any negative effect on spinal alignment. If movement through hip ROM and/or opening of the knee angle (introducing hamstring influence) in one or both LEs negatively impacts pelvic alignment and the lumbar curve, decisions must be made about eliminating this influence in the seating unit. If spasticity is problematic, the team may consider recommending therapeutic interventions such as chemical blocks, medications, or surgery.

This period on the mat also presents a unique opportunity to discuss skin integrity history, examine present skin condition, and identify any problem areas. Bony prominences may change location once the patient is sitting again, so this information should be reconfirmed during the seated examination.

Once ROM is documented, a linear measurement of seat depth should be determined. From a supine position, the examiner should support the LEs in an optimal position and neutralize the pelvis. A second person measures the undersurface of the thigh from the popliteal fossa directly down to the support surface. This should be done for each LE individually, obtaining a left and right measurement of seat depth (Fig. 33.3). If the LEs are abducted or in a windblown position, the examiner must use caution to measure a line perpendicular to the support surface, not along the line the limbs assume.

Seated Examination

Once examination in the supine position is completed, the patient should be placed in a supported sitting position with the knees flexed to 100° or more to eliminate the influence of the hamstring muscle group. Accommodation must be made for any limitations documented in the supine position. Ideally, seated examination should be done on a simulator, a chair specifically designed for planar seated examinations. If a simulator is not available, this can be done on a mat table with a thin front edge to allow 100° of knee flexion. If support is needed, one examiner can be positioned in front of the person and another behind, offering support (Fig. 33.4). The examiner in front should now determine pelvic position and mobility with the hips in the amount of flexion available as previously determined in the supine position. Pressure is used at the front of the knees and counterbalanced by manipulation of the pelvis to achieve a neutral posture with good lumbar and trunk alignment. The examiner determines the degree of flexibility and the influence of gravity on posture. Initial ideas can be formulated about where control may be needed to achieve postural goals.

In the supported sitting position, the examiner should remeasure the sitting depth from behind the buttocks to the popliteal fossa (Fig. 33.5A). This may differ from the supine measurement, and careful examination should reveal whether the difference is secondary to correctable postural difficulties or simply variable flesh distribution in sitting versus supine. Leg measurement (Fig. 33.5B), from the popliteal fossa to the heel with customary footwear in place, will be needed to determine footrest length on the wheelchair. The sitting knee flexion angle should also be documented (Fig. 33.5C). Measurement of back height should be taken from the sitting surface to the posterior superior iliac crests (Fig. 33.5D), lower scapula (Fig. 33.5E), top of the shoulder (Fig. 33.5F), occiput (Fig. 33.5G), and crown of the head (Fig. 33.5H). These measurements will provide a detailed record should

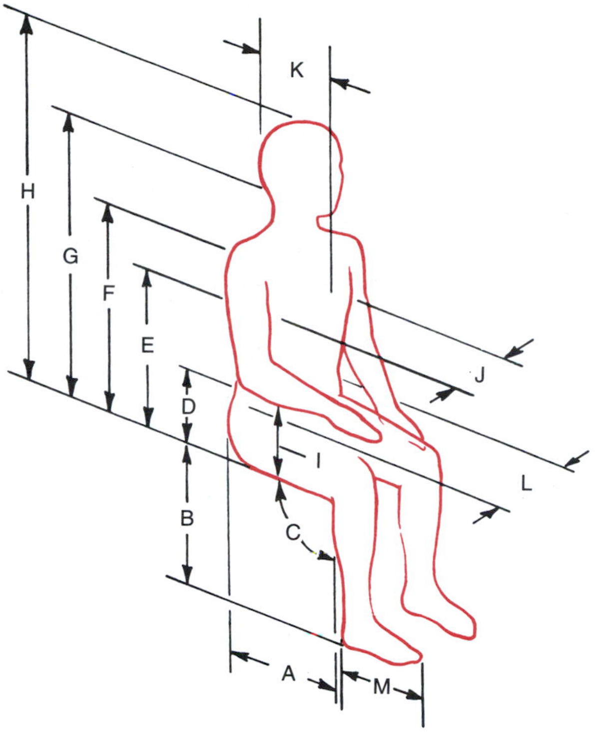

Figure 33.5 The following measurements are added to those taken in the supine position. (*A*) Sitting depth from behind the buttocks to popliteal fossa (right and left side); (*B*) leg measured from popliteal fossa to heel (right and left side); (*C*) knee flexion angle; (*D*) back height from sitting surface to posterior superior iliac crest, (*E*) from sitting surface to lower scapula, (*F*) from sitting surface to top of shoulder, (*G*) from sitting surface to occiput, and (*H*) from sitting surface to crown of head; (*I*) hanging elbow from sitting surface to the elbow or forearm; (*J*) width and (*K*) depth of trunk; (*L*) width of hips; and (*M*) measurement of foot length.

decisions regarding wheelchair back height be needed once the examination is completed. Measurement of the *hanging elbow* (Fig. 33.5I) is needed to determine proper armrest height. With the person in a corrected sitting position, the UE is positioned at the side of the body with 90° of elbow flexion and the shoulder in a neutral position. A measurement is taken from the bottom of the elbow or forearm to the sitting surface.

During the seated examination, measurements should be taken of width (Fig. 33.5J) and depth (Fig. 33.5K) of the trunk and width (Fig. 33.5L) of the hips for decisions regarding support accessories and width of the seating system and the mobility base. If the patient is seated asymmetrically, it will be necessary to measure across the widest span of the patient's seated body (e.g., outside hip on the adducted side to outside knee of the abducted leg). A measurement of foot length (Fig. 33.5M) should also be taken. To ensure accurate recommendations it is important to consider orthoses, clothing, and recent weight loss or gain, as well as the patient's potential for growth when recording these measurements. If it takes more than a few months to secure funding it may be necessary to remeasure the client before placing the order.

Anticipated Goals and Expected Outcomes

Data from the entire team is compiled and evaluated to determine the patient's present level of function, establish goals and outcomes, and create a seating technology POC. It is important that all goals and outcomes be thoroughly discussed to avoid system failure owing to poor planning, poor communication and/or unrealistic expectations from any of the team members. It may be necessary to set priorities if all of the goals cannot be met.

A well-planned seating system may be able to normalize tone, decrease pathological reflex activity, improve postural symmetry, enhance range of movement, maintain and/or improve skin condition, increase comfort and sitting tolerance, decrease fatigue, and improve function of the autonomic nervous system.[3] In addition, the base of the seating system can allow for changes in orientation in space (recline and tilt). A properly prescribed mobility base will improve access to the physical environment (both manual and power-activated), whether alone or with a caregiver. It should be effective for accomplishing all home, school, work, and recreational activities and, where necessary, assist the caregiver with patient management.

When setting priorities, it is important that clinical team members do not overload the patient with their professional opinions. Clinical teams may not be fully aware of the barriers facing the individual using a wheelchair in his or her physical environment. Clinicians may observe a patient ambulating in the clinic and feel that with added practice he or she could ambulate full time. This clinician may consider recommending crutches and a simple manual wheelchair. In the patient's real environment, however, long distances may need to be traversed to independently shop, attend community activities, and function at school or work. Walking to these activities would require extraordinary effort, and propelling a standard manual wheelchair may not offer much additional assistance. A motorized scooter or wheelchair may be more effective as a supplement for environmental mobility.

Intervention

Once all of the information is evaluated, the team creates a POC. The general, over-all *postural goal* is to achieve optimal trunk position because all function, both central (control, alignment, internal organ function) and distal (gross and fine motor control in the head and UEs), is based on the position and control of the trunk and limb girdles. The *mobility goal* is to provide efficient ease of movement from the user's and caregiver's perspectives. The *system outcome* is to provide comfort and maximal functional independence. The intervention consists of prescription of the seating system and the mobility base.

The data gathered during the examination can now be used to determine whether the patient is functioning at his or her highest potential, or whether additional support would be helpful to improve function of distal body parts.[4,5] The impact of positioning on skin condition, respiratory function, speech, and general functioning should also be considered. It is usually helpful at this point to simulate various interventions. This can be accomplished using a simulator chair that has various adjustments for surface dimensions (e.g., seat depth, back height, calf length), angles between seat and back, seat and calf, and calf and foot, as well as tilt-in-space and postural support features.[6] If a simulator chair is not available, it is important to establish an alternative approach to simulate the type of seating environment under consideration. This gives the team an opportunity to observe the patient with the proposed intervention components in place. If the patient has any pressure problems, the pressure mapping should occur in this corrected and supported position to determine how to approach the intervention.

If the patient is capable of self-propulsion in a manual wheelchair, or if he or she is being considered for powered mobility, product trials may be necessary. The patient should have an opportunity to try various pieces of equipment prior to product selection. The mode of propulsion, method of transfer, and interaction with the environment can be observed during each trial. Performance will be influenced by the individual's strength, posture, and tone, and can be modified by support system intervention. Proper intervention may enhance function (e.g., respiratory, motor), whereas improper intervention (e.g., insufficient support, poorly placed wheels, excessive chair width) may interfere with function.

In choosing chair properties, careful attention must be given to possible secondary problems that may be created. For example, if the intervention includes a high seat cushion for pressure relief, will the user be able to get under tables and desks, transfer, or reach the wheels for self-propulsion? If the recommendation includes a custom support system, will the weight preclude easy self-propulsion or caregiver management? Will the bulk make automobile transport difficult or impossible? Attention to these issues can produce modifications that will create workable systems; inattention can produce impaired function and disability. Simulation and trials give the team an opportunity to make informed decisions prior to final product selection.

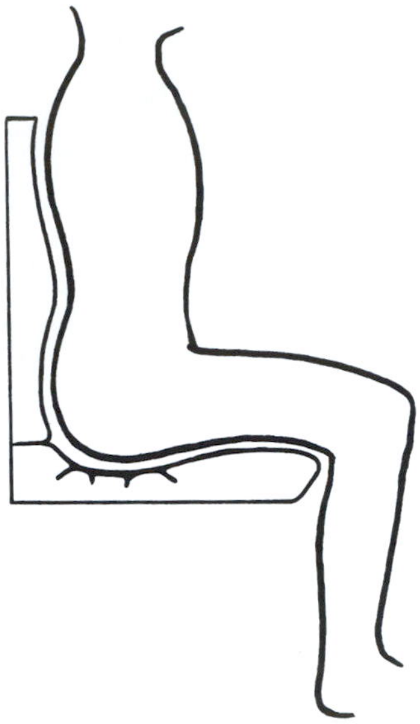

Figure 33.7 Some types of foam will contour as a response to body weight.

Postural Support System

The components of the system that will directly affect comfort and maintenance of posture are the seat surface,

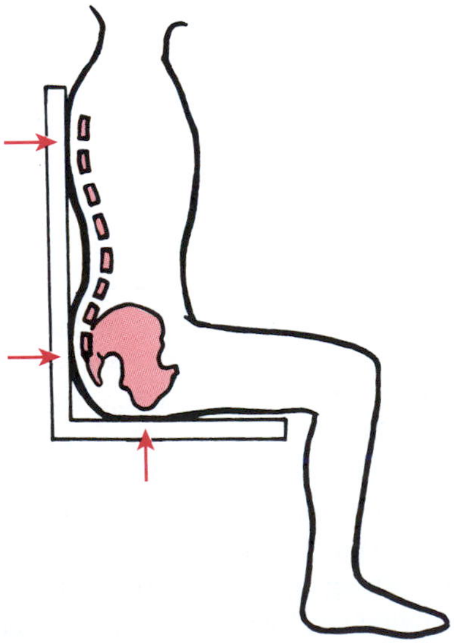

Figure 33.6 Patients seated on planar surfaces may show increased pressure over bony prominences.

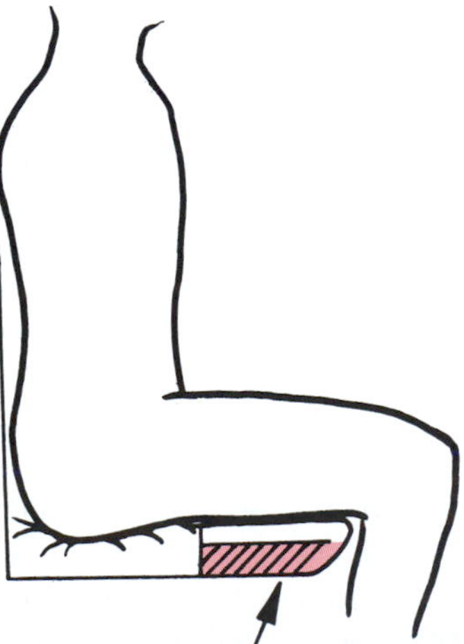

Figure 33.8 An option for creating contoured seats is use of varying density (firmness) of foam.

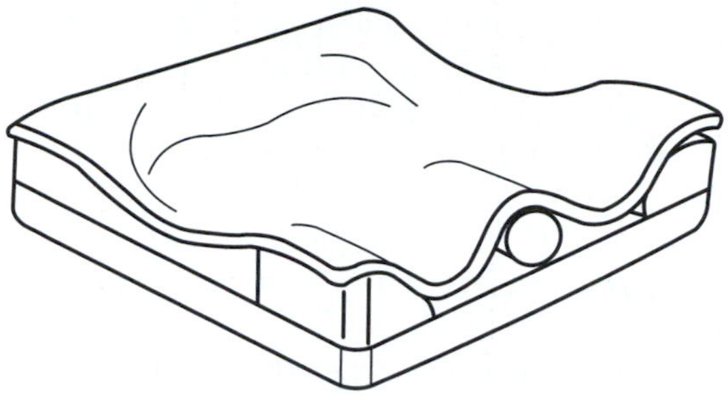

Figure 33.9 Firmer foam shapes can be placed under a more flexible foam to create a contoured cushion.

back surface, pelvic belt, and UE and LE supports. These areas should be addressed together as the postural support system. Increased contact between the user and the support surfaces increases comfort and control and decreases pressure over bony prominences.[7–10] The continuum of available support surfaces runs from firm *planar surfaces* (wood, firm foam) (Fig. 33.6), through deformable surfaces (knit-covered foam) (Figs. 33.7 and 33.8), and *contoured surfaces* (Fig. 33.9), up to and including *custom-molded surfaces* (Fig. 33.10).

Angular relationships between the surfaces at the hip and knee joints (seat and back surfaces, seat and calf surfaces) must be determined based on the ROM measures obtained during the physical examination. This information will allow the planned intervention to accommodate limitations in ROM, assure proper alignment of body segments, and minimize pressure distal to the joint. Changes of orientation in space (fixed or dynamic) affect the user's comfort level, pressure over skin surfaces, fatigue, and ability to work in gravity-minimized and gravity-influenced positions. Attention to these features will help ensure the success of the seating intervention. Appendix A provides an overview of features of the wheelchair postural support system.

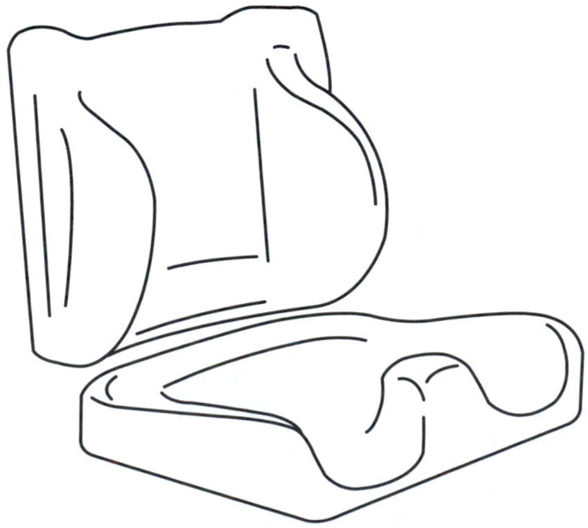

Figure 33.10 Custom-molded cushions match the patient's body contours.

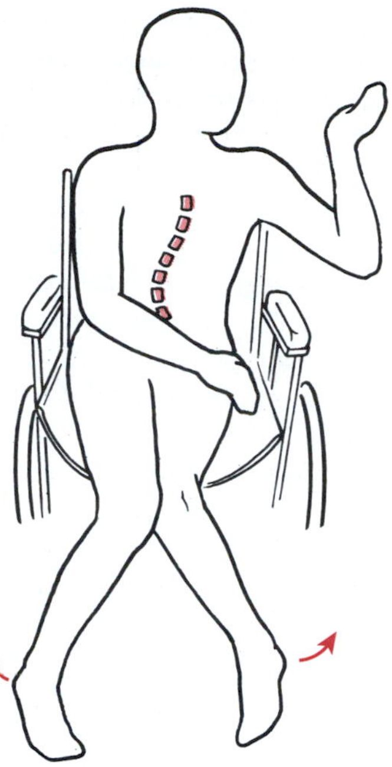

Figure 33.11 Overall poor sitting posture and asymmetries created by a sling seat.

Seat Surface

Many wheelchairs come with a fabric or *sling seat*. This type of surface reinforces a poor pelvic position because the hips tend to slide forward, creating a posterior pelvic tilt. The thighs typically move toward adduction and internal rotation, and the patient tends to sit asymmetrically (Fig. 33.11). Most wheelchair users can benefit from a firm sitting surface (Fig. 33.12). Total contact between the

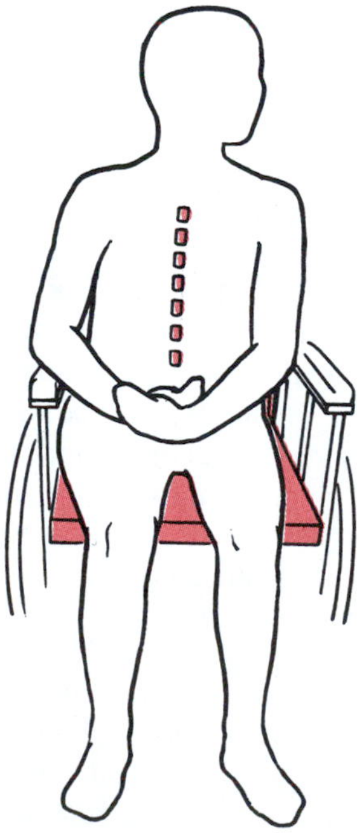

Figure 33.12 A firm sitting surface enhances sitting posture and provides a stable base of support.

undersurface of the thigh and the seating surface will enhance sitting ability by providing a stable base of support on which to mount upper body function.[7–10] In most cases, the front of the seat should actually extend into the popliteal fossa. It is imperative that the front edge is well padded and contoured to provide relief for hamstring tendons, calf bulk, and/or bracing. This surface many require specialized foam in one or varying firmnesses, or a specific contour. The patient also may require a special cushion for comfort, control, and/or pressure relief. Cushions are generally made of foam, gel, liquid, pockets of air, or a combination of these elements.

The depth of the seat should be measured carefully, because an overly deep seat will create pressure behind the knee and encourage a posterior pelvic tilt and a resultant tendency toward *kyphotic posturing*. A seat that is too shallow will not provide enough support, making maintenance of LE alignment more difficult.

For persons with neuromuscular problems (e.g., multiple sclerosis, muscular dystrophy, cerebral palsy, traumatic brain injury), the seat may require *lateral hip*, or *medial* or *lateral knee positioners* to maintain alignment of the LE.[11] The seating system must be prepared for these additions before being upholstered. The seat also may require a change in orientation, or increased contour, to affect tone at the hips. This can be done with varying foam firmnesses, contouring, hardware changes, or properties built into the chosen mobility base.

Back Surface

Individuals using a wheelchair who have fair to good trunk control usually require only back support to the mid-scapula. Many prefer it lower. Some sit well with just the upholstery in place while others require additional support in front of or instead of the upholstery.

Although some low wheelchair backs work well in the short run, they may cause problems over longer periods of use, with users experiencing fatigue and back pain. In these cases, a higher back is more appropriate. In most cases, the standard fabric back that comes with a wheelchair does not provide sufficient support for long periods of sitting. Some wheelchairs are available with back upholstery that has reinforcing straps that can be adjusted to provide contoured support. This type of support may be sufficient for some patients. It provides moderate support, only slightly increases overall chair weight, and does not interfere with folding.

Most full time wheelchair users require some additional back support for comfort and/or postural control such as an insert or cushion placed in front of the wheelchair's back upholstery, a panel placed into a custom sewn pocket behind the back upholstery, or, in many cases, a back installed instead of the back upholstery. These supports add some amount of weight to the chair and must be removed for folding. This type of support can be whatever height the patient requires for support and/or comfort. For patients with good trunk control, the back can be below the scapula. For persons who have poor trunk control and those who tend to push into extension, the back height should be to the shoulders (approximately to the level of the acromion process). This is especially critical if any type of anterior shoulder support is to be used.

A higher back may make it more difficult for caregivers to adjust posture, but the added control offered will decrease the need for frequent postural adjustments. It is very important to create the correct seat/back angle for comfortable postural alignment of the head over the shoulders and pelvis. With a high back, this may require customized foam additions or angulation at the seat/back junction or at the superior pelvis (a biangular back). In some cases, it may also be necessary to make the back dynamic by providing spring loaded mounting hardware to allow maximum support with accommodation for patient tone and comfort level.

The back insert is fabricated from a firm base such as very firm foam, wood, plastic, or metal padded with foam or a layer of air filled cells. The padding can vary in thickness and firmness allowing more or less control at the pelvis or across the scapular and shoulder areas. The team must observe the patient's response to a back insert and vary the surface consistency, shape, and/or angle to the seat surface according to postural needs, function, and comfort level. A very firm foam may work well for individuals with low central tone by encouraging more extension, but those with prominent bony protuberances may not tolerate this type of surface. Others may achieve good extension following alignment but lose lateral stability, thus requiring additional lateral contour and/or lateral supports.

As with the back insert, persons with neuromuscular problems (e.g., multiple sclerosis, muscular dystrophy, cerebral palsy, traumatic brain injury), may require *lateral trunk* and *lateral hip positioners* to maintain alignment of the hips and trunk.[11] The back must be prepared for these additions before being upholstered. When interfacing the seating to the mobility base it is critical to make sure that none of the components interfere with UE mobility and/or good wheel approach for pushing.

Pelvic Positioner

A belt or more rigid pelvic positioner may be needed for safety and for assistance with postural control.[12] Padding is recommended if the belt is pulled tightly to influence or maintain pelvic alignment. The direction, angle of pull, and number of anchor points of the belt is important.[13] For example, if one hip tends to pull forward consistently, it may be useful to have the belt tighten by pulling it down toward that hip. The angle of pull to the seating surface should normally be 45 to 60° (Fig. 33.13).[12] Some

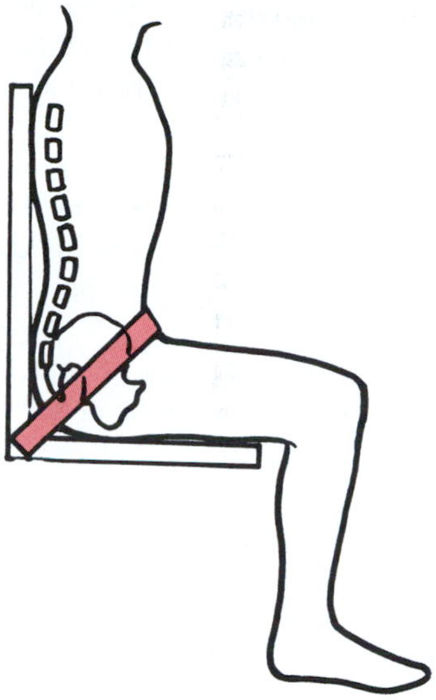

Figure 33.13 The pelvic belt should cross the pelvic-femoral junction at approximately a 45° to 60° angle to the seating surface.

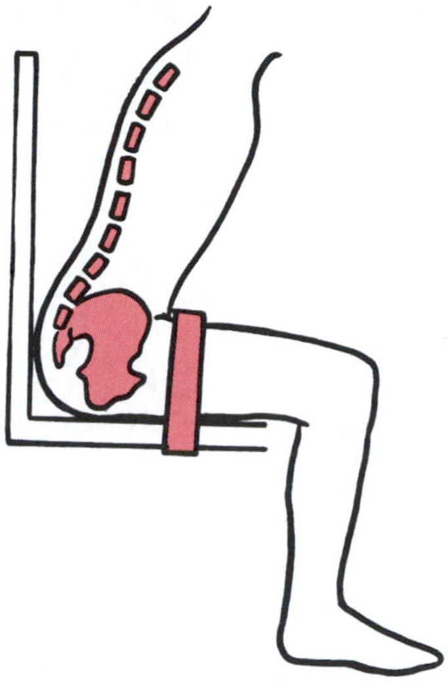

Figure 33.14 A belt placed over the upper thigh (at a 90° angle to the sitting surface) will free the pelvis for natural anterior tilting.

patients respond well to belts that form a 90° angle with the sitting surface. This pull discourages patients who tend to extend in their wheelchairs as a result of increases in tone. This 90° placement also leaves the pelvis free for anterior tilting, an assist for those patients who can use this mobility for added function (Fig. 33.14). Some patients can benefit from multiple angles of pull. For these clients, a four-point belt might be most appropriate.

Upper Extremity Supports

Wheelchair armrests have many important functions. They provide assistance for pushing up to standing, a support surface for arms and UE support surfaces such as lap boards, a mechanism for relief of ischial pressure (sitting pushups), and some small amount of lateral stability. Attention should be directed to the height of the armrests, and the length and size of the support surface. It may be necessary for the patient to use the armrests to support the UE and thus decrease pull on the shoulders and trunk, which may also affect head position. This approach is often used for individuals with significant weakness, such as those with high-level spinal cord injuries or muscular dystrophy. Individuals who lean on their armrests for postural assistance will have decreased functional use of the UE.

For some individuals, the armrests will be used to mount an *upper extremity support surface (UESS)* such as a tray or trough. These surfaces provide several important functions. They can be used to achieve symmetric positioning of the UEs, maintain corrected alignment of the glenohumeral joint and scapula, and serve as a work or communication surface. They also can act as an adjunct to the postural control system by supporting the weight of the upper limbs and decreasing pull on the shoulders and trunk. In addition, in special cases, high (elevated) UESSs can be used to inhibit tone around the shoulders and neck. In extreme cases, the UEs of individuals with athetosis may be purposely anchored beneath the UESS to decrease interference from involuntary movement when using a head pointer or when eating. Some individuals with involuntary movements find that stabilizing their UEs under the UESS, or with a combination of side walls and straps on the top of the UESS, allows them to isolate head and oral movements for eating, switch access, and so forth.

Lower Extremity Supports

Style and position are important considerations when selecting foot support systems. Placement of the foot support system will directly affect the position of the entire lower body, affecting tone and posture in the trunk, head, and arms. Adequate hip flexion will help keep the pelvis well positioned on the sitting surface. Good foot support height and style are required for maintenance of this position. Foot supports that are too low will result in lower knees, placing the hips in a more open angle and encouraging forward sliding of the pelvis. Foot supports that are too high may unload the thighs, placing increased weight on the ischial tuberosities. Elevating leg rests even in their lowered position may place excessive stretch on tight hamstrings, pulling the pelvis into a posterior tilt (Fig. 33.15). Any limitation of motion imposed by the hamstrings will directly influence the choice of foot positioners. To achieve maximum comfortable hip flexion, it may be necessary to flex the knees more than 90°, requiring special intervention on the foot supports. Decisions regarding

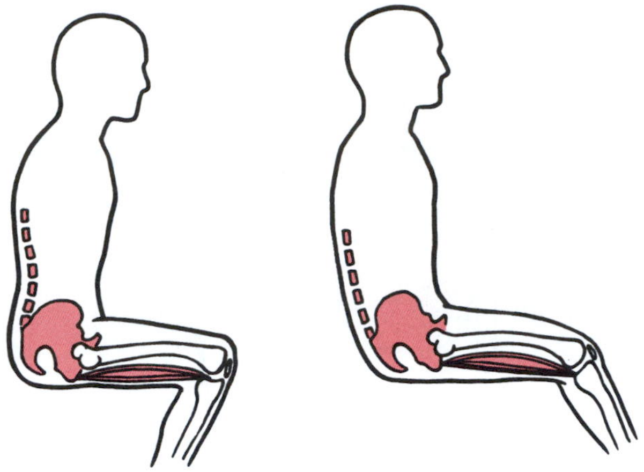

Figure 33.15 Sitting alignment with the hamstrings on slack and the knees flexed (*left*) and positioning assumed with feet resting on elevating foot rests (*right*) causing tension on the hamstring that pulls the pelvis into a posterior tilt.

straps and foot positioners must be made early, based on available ROM, to ensure clearance for placement on the final unit.

The Wheeled Mobility Base

The wheeled base forms the mobility structure for the seating system. Mobility bases include dependent systems, independent systems activated manually, and independent systems activated under battery power.

Dependent systems include strollers, pushchairs, and many of the elaborate postural support systems used by individuals with severe disability and mental impairments. These systems may have small wheels that are not intended for self-propulsion. When considering a dependent mobility system, it is important to determine the function of the unit. Is this a primary mobility system, or a backup for the person who has a powered mobility unit? If the ability to use any independent movement system exists (i.e., using one UE, one LE, or even an eye blink, breath, or tongue movement), the person should be considered for either a manual or powered wheelchair as the primary mobility system. Sophisticated technology allows even those with the most severe disability to achieve independent mobility. If at all possible, even very young children (12 to 18 months or older) and the elderly should be provided with a means of independent mobility that allows them to extend beyond the boundary of their functional limitation or disability. Research supports the beneficial impact of independent functioning on all aspects of cognitive and psychosocial well-being.[14–17]

When considering a *manual self-propelled mobility base*, it is critical to consider the possible implications for long term function of the shoulder girdle. Research indicates that patients that use manual wheelchairs, especially if they are not properly fitted to their bodies and functional level, are in danger of UE damage from repetitive strain injuries (RSI). RSI can result in damage to soft tissue (tendons, ligaments, nerves) or bony structures secondary to frequent repeated motions such as wheelchair push strokes. The damage can include inflammation, compression, and/or tears in the shoulder joint and surrounding structures, resulting in pain and decreased function.[18,19]

RSI have been identified in the shoulders, wrists, and hands of wheelchair users. Even patients without documented RSI report increased pain in these joints with prolonged wheelchair use.[20,21] Small muscles are required to produce large forces repeatedly to move the chair through space. These same muscles are typically required for a variety of activities of daily living (ADL) tasks, thus increasing the trauma. Muscles are used in atypical positions, and become overstretched and overused. Stress on the muscles and joints increases with increased wheelchair weight, increased user weight, and environmental factors. Many symptoms are not felt until the condition is well advanced. Rotator cuff injuries and instability of the glenohumeral joint are common at the shoulder. Since a number of muscles cross the wrist and elbow, problems occurring at the wrist often create pain at the elbow. Medial epicondylitis and carpal tunnel syndrome are common. See Evidence Summary Box 33.1 for a summary of studies addressing UE pain associated with wheelchair propulsion.

When prescribing wheelchairs and features for patients who are able to self-propel, consideration must be given to preventing RSI whenever possible. An important prevention strategy is careful positioning of the UE to allow the most efficient stroke during propulsion, reducing the amount of force needed per stroke and reducing the number of strokes required to move the chair. It is also critical to observe wrist alignment in order to minimize trauma and the chance of impingement leading to carpal tunnel syndrome (CTS).[22–24] Other criteria that should be considered in prescribing a self-propelled wheelchair include selecting a chair that:

- Has the lightest weight possible.
- Has a stable frame for most efficient movement.
- Is well-manufactured, with high-quality bearings (increased ease of motion for moving parts) for less roll resistance when push forces are applied, and secure non-moving parts.
- Has optimal wheel size and type for individual patient function.
- Provides the best possible combination of ease of propulsion and stability.

Careful attention should be directed toward the patient's position in the chair. The pelvis should be in a neutral position with the trunk upright. The spine should be extended slightly over the pelvis into a ready posture for pushing. It

(text continues on page 1300)

Evidence Summary Box 33.1

Studies Addressing Pain Associated with Wheelchair Propulsion

Reference	Purpose	Subjects/Design	Results	Conclusions/Comments
Sie, IH, et al[18] 1992	To document the prevalence of UE pain according to specific UE regions, and the relationship of UE pain to time since injury in Ss with SCI.	Nonrandomized cohort study; Questionnaire sent to 239 Ss > 1-year post SCI; mean age 37.4 years. Ss interviewed for presence of UE pain (shoulders, upper arms, elbows, lower arms, wrists, and hands), screened for CTS.	55% of Ss with tetraplegia (quadriplegia) reported pain in at least one region of UE, 40% in more than one region. 64% of Ss with paraplegia reported UE pain, 32% in more than one region. 59% of all Ss reported some UE pain, 30% reported pain requiring medication, limiting function, or causing pain with ADL. Ss with paraplegia reported less significant pain than those with tetraplegia. 41% of all Ss reported shoulder pain.	Shoulder region was the most common painful area in Ss with tetraplegia, and second most common in Ss with paraplegia. There was a general trend indicating that UE pain increased with time past since injury, up to 20 years. There was a steady increase in frequency of CTS-related complaints with time since injury up to 19 years, in Ss with paraplegia.
Fullerton, HD, et al 2003[a]	To directly compare the onset and prevalence of shoulder pain in the athletic and non-athletic W/C user populations.	Cohort study; 20-item questionnaire, mailed to a randomized group of 500 individuals through the Virginia SCI Registry, 257 Ss were obtained, 86% had SCI. Patients were considered athletic if: 1) trained at least 3 hours/week, 2) involved in at least 3 competitions per year, 3) had a W/C modified for sports. 172 of the Ss were identified as athletes.	48% of all Ss reported shoulder pain, 70% of these Ss sought treatment for pain, and 92% had pain with ADL. 66% of non-athletes reported pain, only 39% of athletes reported pain. Pain and athletic status were not significantly related to onset on shoulder pain. There was no significant difference between Ss with tetraplegia and Ss with paraplegia. Age had a strong effect for both pain and athletic status. Non-athletic Ss were found to be more than twice as susceptible to shoulder pain as athletes independent of age, SCI level, and number of years in W/C.	A limitation of this study is that one question remains unanswered: do non-athletes have more pain because they are not athletic, or are they not athletic because of shoulder pain? There is a possibility of sampling bias because many of the questionnaires were hand-distributed.

(continued)

Evidence Summary Box 33.1

Studies Addressing Pain Associated with Wheelchair Propulsion (continued)

Reference	Purpose	Subjects/Design	Results	Conclusions/Comments
Curtis, KA, et al 1999[b]	To compare the prevalence and intensity of shoulder pain experienced during daily functional activities in wheelchair users with tetraplegia and paraplegia.	Nonrandomized cohort study; Self-report survey; 55 women and 140 men; 92 Ss with tetraplegia (mean age 32.9 years) and 103 Ss with paraplegia (mean age 34.4 years). Ss used manual wheelchair for 3 hours per week and had at least 1 year since onset of SCI. Groups were partitioned according to age, level of daily activity, and years of W/C use.	There was no significant difference between Ss with tetraplegia and with paraplegia in terms of age, years of wheelchair use, and weekly hours of activity. Ss with paraplegia performed more transfers per week and spent more hours per week driving (both significant). Less than 15% of all Ss experienced shoulder pain before becoming W/C users, 78% with tetraplegia and 59% with paraplegia had felt shoulder pain since they started using the W/C. There was significantly higher prevalence of previous, bilateral, and current shoulder pain in Ss with tetraplegia than those with paraplegia. Both groups had most severe shoulder pain when pushing the W/C up an incline, pushing for more than 10 minutes, and while sleeping.	This study documents a strong influence of shoulder pain on the performance of functional activities after SCI. Ss with tetraplegia, increased age and duration of W/C use were associated with avoiding strenuous functional activities.
Veeger, HEJ, et al 2002[c]	To examine the mechanical load on the glenohumeral joint and on the shoulder muscles during W/C propulsion at everyday intensities.	Nonrandomized cohort study; Three experienced male W/C users, ages 22, 27, and 38. Weight 180, 176, and 209 lbs (81.5, 80 and 95 Kg) respectively. All participated in W/C sports on weekly bases. Each underwent four, 4 minute W/C exercise tests at two target resistances (10 and 20 N), and target speeds (0.83 and 1.39 m.s[−1]), during which data were collected for construction of a musculoskeletal model of the UE. Antropometric parameters of the model based on data from two cadaver studies. Individual muscle performance estimated based on this model.	Push time shortened significantly when velocity increased, while recovery time was reduced considerably with an increase power output. The muscle that produced the largest force during the push phase was the subscapularis. Supraspinatus and infraspinatus were also highly active. Pectoralis major produced a moderate internal rotational force. Biceps produced more force than triceps during push phase. During recovery phase, the scapular part of the deltoid produced more force than all other muscles. The supraspinatus was by far the most taxed muscle when force output is considered relative to maximal force. Also highly active were the forearms (pronators and the supinating effect of the biceps).	Peak glenohumeral contact forces varied between 800 and 1400 N. The supraspinatus and infraspinatus may be responsible for an external rotation compensatory moment for the deltoid (excessive internal rotation may cause the greater tubercle to move directly under the acromion, thus increasing probability for impingement). Despite the relatively low contact forces, the peak forces and peak stresses in the rotator cuff muscles, (particularly supraspinatus) appear high. These high peak stresses might cause overuse injuries.

Boninger, ML, et al 2004[d]	To investigate MRI and radiographic abnormalities in individuals with paraplegia who were W/C users.	Nonrandomized cohort study; 28 Ss with paraplegia, 19 male and 9 female (mean age 35 yrs), with a traumatic SCI at the 4th thoracic level or below, occurring more than 1-year before the start of the study. Ss used manual W/C full-time for mobility. Each subject completed a standardized questionnaire, had a uniform physical examination focusing on the shoulder, and underwent imaging studies (radiographic and MRI). BMI was calculated.	5 Ss displayed osteolysis of the distal clavicle, 11 displayed subacromial spur, and 8 displayed AC DJD. Only nine Ss had radiographs that were read as entirely normal. One subject was found to have a rotator cuff tear. Distal clavicular edema was the most common abnormality found in MRI (20 subjects), 18 Ss displayed AC DJD, CA ligament problems were common as well. Ss with a high BMI had a greater degree of abnormality.	It is hypothesized that shoulder injuries are due to the repetitive loading that occurs during transfers and W/C propulsion. BMI alone was not related to abnormalities, which may suggest that taller subjects have musculoskeletal systems that are better able to handle increased stresses.
Samuelsson, KAM, et al 2004[e]	To describe the consequences of shoulder pain on activity and participation in Ss with paraplegia who use a W/C, and describe the prevalence and type of shoulder pain.	Nonrandomized cohort study; 56 potential Ss with paraplegia due to SCI (12 women, 44 men, mean age 49 years), more than 1-year prior to study were screened for participation via questionnaire, 21 (37.5%) of those responding had shoulder pain. 13 of these Ss were used to delineate the type and consequence of shoulder pain. The CMS, WUSPI, KBADLI and COPM were used to describe the impact of shoulder pain on activity.	The highest pain intensity was found for loading a wheelchair into a car, followed by pushing up inclines outdoors and usual ADL at work and school. 54% of Ss presented with problems related to self-care activities; 23% productivity; 23% leisure activities. The most common problem was transferring in and out of a car (62%) and W/C propulsion 46%.	Sitting posture may be related to shoulder pain in this population. W/C users with SCI tend to adopt a kyphotic posture, which causes an abnormal rotation of the scapula. This could contribute to entrapment of the greater tubercle beneath the acromion. The most defined problems related to shoulder pain were related to W/C use.

Evidence Summary Box prepared by Stephen A. Caronia.

[a]Fullerton, HD, et al: Shoulder pain: A comparison of wheelchair athletes and nonathletic wheelchair users. Med Sci Sports Exerc 35(12):1958, 2003.

[b]Curtis, KA, et al: Shoulder pain in wheelchair users with tetraplegia and paraplegia. Arch Phys Med Rehabil 80(4):453, 1999.

[c]Veeger, HEJ, et al: Load on the shoulder in low intensity wheelchair propulsion. Clin Biomech 17(3):211, 2002.

[d]Boninger, ML, et al: Shoulder imaging abnormalities in individuals with paraplegia. J Rehabil Res Dev 38(4):401, 2001.

[e]Samuelsson, KAM, Tropp, H, and Gerdle, B: Shoulder pain and its consequences in paraplegic spinal cord-injured, wheelchair users. Spinal Cord 42(1):41, 2004.

~ Approximately; > more than; AC = acromio-clavicular (joint); ADL = activities of daily living; BMI = body mass index; CA = coraco-acromial (ligament); CMS = Constant Murley Scale; COPM = Canadian Occupational Performance Measure; CTS = carpal tunnel syndrome; DJD = degenerative joint disease; KBADLI = Klien and Bell ADL Index; NI = not indicated; RCI = rotator cuff injury; SCI = spinal cord injury; Sh = shoulder; Ss = subjects; UE = upper extremity; WUSPI = Wheelchair Users Shoulder Pain Index; W/C = wheelchair.

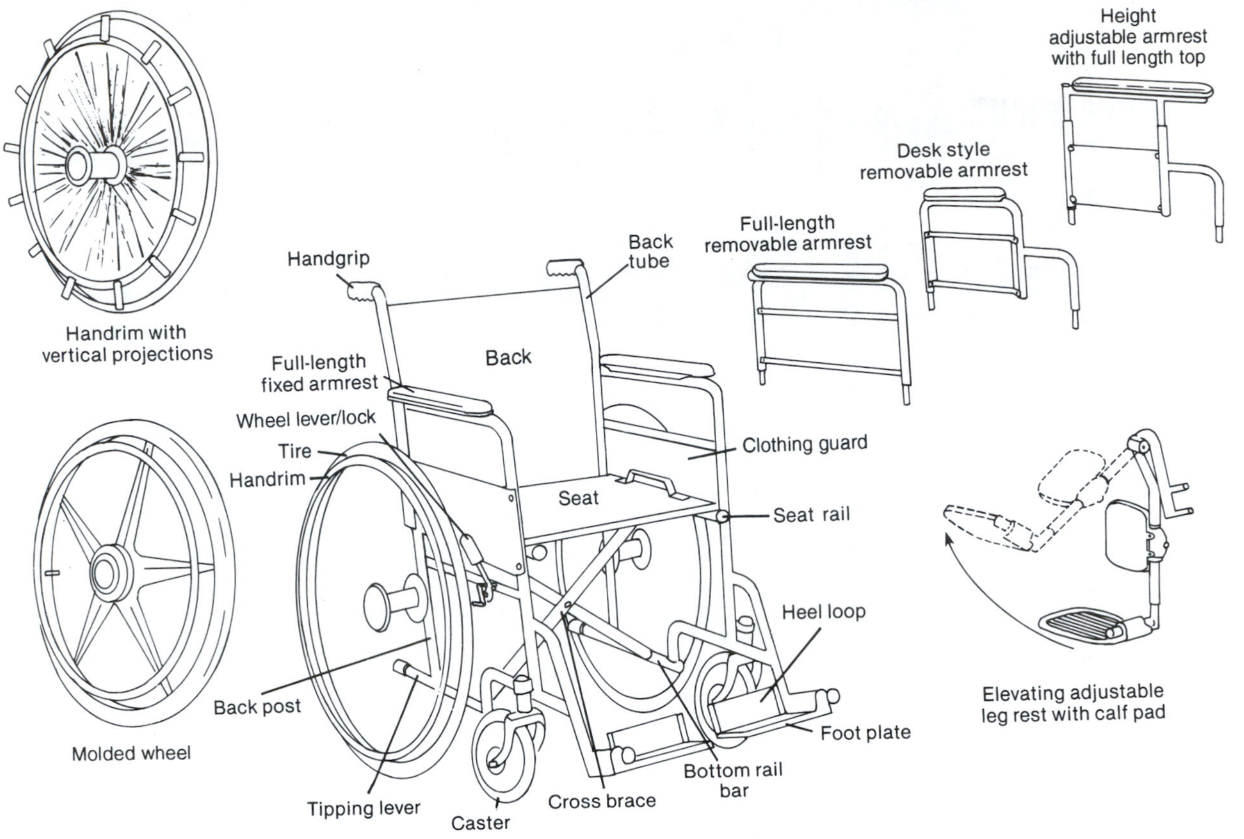

Figure 33.16 Foundation components of a prescriptive wheelchair.

may be necessary to open the seat/back angle to achieve this for some patients. The trunk and hips should be stable to allow full release of the UE for wheel approach and push. If the patient does not have trunk stability, it may be necessary to provide additional external support.

When preparing the specifications for a wheeled mobility base, many features must be carefully considered. There are dozens of bases available, each with subtly different features. The team will be challenged in their effort to make the correct match between user and product. Figure 33.16 presents an overview of the foundational components of a prescriptive wheelchair.

The Wheelchair Seat

Seat Depth

Correct seat depth is particularly important to achieve maximum postural support and control. Wheelchairs are readily available from manufacturers in various seat depths. Manufacturers' seat depth listings usually correspond to the depth of the upholstery or seat itself from the back to the front edge. Depending on the manufacturer, the upholstery or seat depth may be equal to, less than, or greater than that of the metal seat rail. The team must be aware of different manufacturers' features. If the patient does not fit a listed size, modifications can be made by use of a back insert, by frame construction, or by upholstery/seat modifications. Most seat depth modifications can be made on a new or existing wheelchair.

Back Insert/Support: Impact on Seat Depth

A back insert/support can be used to alter the overall depth of the sitting surface. This back insert/support, or cushion, can be ordered with any specified overall thickness, and usually consists of a piece of wood or dense plastic with foam padding. Inserts can be placed in front of the wheelchair's upholstery, or the upholstery can be removed and the back insert can be mounted with specialized hardware (Fig. 33.17). When ordering back inserts, it is imperative to know the manufacturer's standard thickness and type of foam. Through selection or specification one can choose whether the insert or replacement back is to be narrow (positioned between the back tubes) or full width (positioned in front of the back tubes). The choice will affect overall available sitting surface, as well as impact shoulder mobility for wheel approach. If the upholstery is to remain in place, it is important to note whether it is mounted in front of the back tubes, between the back tubes, or half and half, inasmuch as this will directly affect the placement of the back insert. It is also critical to note whether the back tube has a bend, which will affect the vertical orientation of the back insert. Putting the insert in front of the back tubes

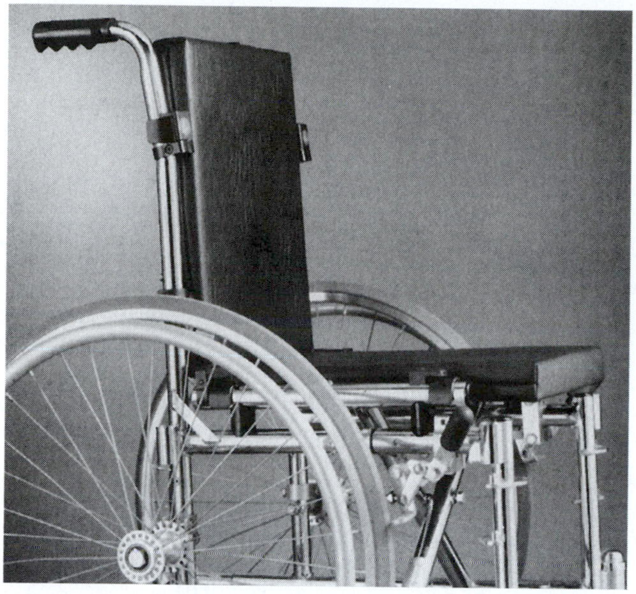

Figure 33.17 Wheelchair seat upholstery can be replaced with firm inserts held to the frame by specialized hardware. Usually the seat, or a cushion with a seat board inside, can safely extend approximately 2 in. (5 cm) beyond the end of the seat rail.

will position the user forward, and this factor plus the full width support across the shoulders may affect the ability to reach the wheels for self-propulsion. It is sometimes useful to position the back insert forward to create a system with an adjustable seat depth if growth or weight gain is anticipated. If this is needed, the back may need custom foam and/or profile (shape) to allow free movement of the shoulders and arms.

Frame Construction

Frame Construction: Impact on Seat Depth

Seat depth also can be modified (increased or decreased) by frame construction. Modifications by construction should be considered with short and wide individuals, very tall persons, or long-legged individuals who have slowed or completed their growth cycle. An important factor to consider is that lengthening the chair frame will increase the turning radius and may prevent the user from maneuvering the chair in small spaces. A few manufacturers supply seat extension kits or special frame designs that extend the seat rail a few inches without changing the overall length of the frame. Seat rail extension kits work well on many frames, but on others they may extend over the top of the legrest attachment and prevent removal of the legrest when the wheelchair is in the open position.

Upholstery Modifications: Impact on Seat Depth

Wheelchair seat depth may also be altered by upholstery changes. This can be achieved symmetrically if leg length is equal, or asymmetrically if leg length is unequal. Seat depth can be increased or decreased within specific dimensions set by the manufacturer. Generally, a seat insert or a seat cushion with a board inside its cover can be extended 1 to 2 in. (2.54 to 5.08 cm) beyond the front end of the seat rail without creating an unstable sitting surface (see Fig. 33.17). The seat upholstery, insert, or cushion can also be cut back several inches to shorten the seat surface. Inserts can be fabricated with *growth tails* that fit between the back tubes as unused sitting surface; more seat depth can be exposed by pulling the seat forward along the seat rail as needed. The effects on foot placement of any of these modifications must be determined. Subsequent foot plate adjustments may be required.

Decisions about the chair upholstery require detailed knowledge of what each manufacturer considers standard. For instance, is upholstery depth as listed the same as seat rail length, 1 in. (2.54 cm) shorter, or 1 in. (2.54 cm) longer? If the chair is offered with a seating system, are the measurements supplied taken from the seating system or the wheelchair frame? Are standard foot plates a large or small size, and how close are they to the front end of the frame? Can they be ordered closer to the frame to minimize effect on overall length, so that the seat can be deepened without affecting turning radius? Careful scrutiny of various wheelchairs will reveal differences in available parts and interfaces depending on wheelchair style and manufacturer.

Seat Width

The width of the seat, as well as the overall width of the wheelchair, is important to functional use. Special considerations will be needed for individuals who wear orthoses, require *control blocks* at the hip or lateral thigh/knee, wear bulky clothing, or experience weight fluctuations. The natural tendency is to increase the width of the seat. Such a solution must be approached cautiously, however, inasmuch as this will also increase the overall width of the chair and may create difficulty for those needing to reach the wheels for self-propulsion or for those who must maneuver in tight places. The overall outside width of the chair should be as narrow as possible for optimal function. Excessive width makes the chair difficult to maneuver through doorways and in small areas. It is also more difficult to propel the chair if the user must widely abduct his or her arms to reach the wheels. This wide abduction requires the patient to use available muscular strength around the shoulder girdle for stability and posture, leaving less to use for functional push (Figs. 33.18 and 33.19). The goal is to create a chair that fits as close to the user's body as possible. This will make the chair easy to wheel and maneuver. It also will make the chair seem, visually, more congruent with the user's body lines.

Available seat width can be changed in several ways. Widening can be accomplished by: (1) use of fixed offset or removable arms; (2) use of attachable armrest receivers that space one or both arms out further (can only be done with small rear wheels); (3) construction design of a new chair; and (4) changing or in some cases adjusting the bottom cross braces on an existing chair. Seat narrowing can be achieved by upholstery or by construction modifications.

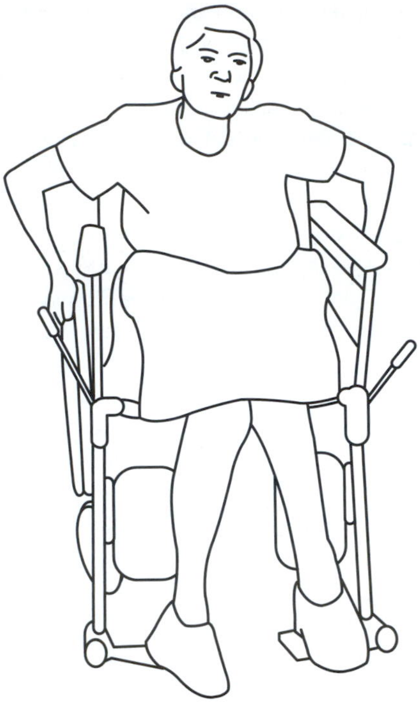

Figure 33.18 A wheelchair that is too wide will make wheel access and propulsion more difficult for the patient.

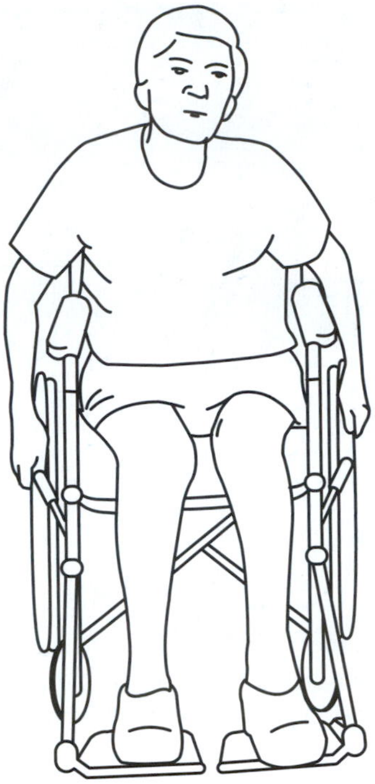

Figure 33.19 A narrower wheelchair allows easier wheel access and propulsion.

Narrowing a chair by upholstery essentially creates a "growing" chair out of any size chair. The chair is simply folded a bit. A limiter strap and/or narrower upholstery is mounted, preventing full-width opening. This will raise the seat height. This should not be done on chairs where the top seat rail must clip to the bottom rail for stability. Other width modifications include various hand rim and armrest options, internal mounting of the wheel axle plate on some ultralight wheelchairs, and wheelchair narrowing devices (which can be used to move the chair through a narrow space for a short distance). Narrowing devices are useful only for individuals who have sufficient coordination to rock the chair from side-to-side while turning the crank handle of the device. The device will not work with solid seat inserts, or with reclining wheelchairs that have spreader bars to reinforce the back. If there is enough room to use the wheelchair-narrowing device comfortably, perhaps the wheelchair should have been narrower in the first place.

Seat Height

The wheelchair's seat height is measured from the seat rail to the floor with the chair fully opened. It is more important to think about the finished height of the wheelchair seat (including any cushion or seating insert); this is important for optimal independent functioning in foot-assisted self-propulsion, transfers (especially reentering the chair using a sliding or stand pivot approach), ground clearance under the footplates on various terrains, approaching working surfaces, interacting with peers, and transferring into a van via lift or ramp. Finished seat height must be examined with respect to the entire chair, inasmuch as it may alter the user's position relative to the armrests, back height, wheel locks, wheels,[25] and footrests. Seat height can be altered by one or more methods, including: (1) altering the frame construction when ordering the chair; (2) changing the wheel size; (3) altering the rear axle and front caster placement on frames that allow this; (4) altering the thickness of the seat inserts or cushions; and (5) removing the seat upholstery and using solid hook-out seat boards with adjustable hardware to raise or drop the seat on the frame.

Seat Surface

A firm sitting surface will provide a more symmetric sitting base. The firm surface will provide a more stable base of support for the upper body, usually resulting in improved function. A firm sitting surface can be achieved in a variety of ways, with or without specialized cushions (see Appendix A).

Prior to deciding on a nonstandard seat surface, the team should inspect what the manufacturer considers a standard seat. Some manufacturers use extremely taut fabric for their seat slings (notably some of the ultralight wheelchairs). In combination with a firm cushion, no other support may be needed. Others use a fabric design that allows the sling component to be adjusted. This works adequately for some users, allowing them to adjust the tension as the sling becomes slack with extended use. Some manufacturers of nonfolding manual wheelchairs and powered wheelchairs replace the seat upholstery with a solid metal or plastic base, allowing a cushion to be attached to the surface with Velcro®.

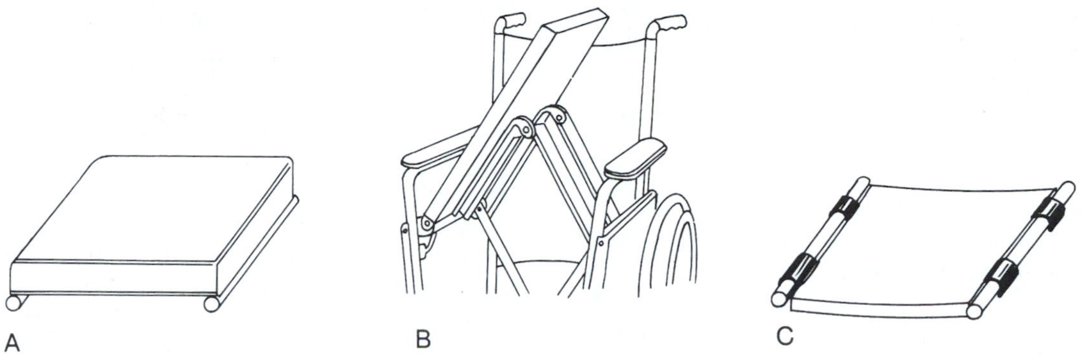

Figure 33.20 Firm seat options. A solid seat insert (*A*), a solid folding seat (*B*), or a solid hook-on seat (*C*).

If a firmer seat is needed, there are several ways this can be achieved (Fig. 33.20). The simplest is to incorporate a homemade or commercially fabricated board into the cushion that comes with the chair. An off-the-chair cushion that comes with a removable cover can be purchased separately from the chair. It is possible, however, that these lightweight units may slide about in the chair, producing an asymmetric sitting surface. Many cushions have special nonslip fabric or Velcro® strips on the underside that discourages slippage. It may be helpful for some patients to have extra Velcro® attached to the seat upholstery and to the bottom of a zip-on cushion cover to avoid cushion shift during transfers. Some manufacturers offer cushion *rigidizers*. This is usually a plastic panel attached by Velcro® between the seat upholstery and the underside of the cushion. These work well with many patients, but may also slip out of place and provide asymmetrical seating.

A second option for a firm seat is to order the wheelchair with a standard hammock seat and a solid seat insert on top (Fig. 33.20A). This type of insert adds slight additional weight to the wheelchair system. The insert is usually made of foam and wood, and is covered with vinyl to match the chair. The standard thickness and firmness of the foam varies with each manufacturer. The individual rehabilitation technology supplier will provide information on standard foam characteristics. Custom thicknesses and firmnesses are available if requested, either directly from the primary manufacturer or from a manufacturer of wheelchair component parts. The solid seat insert has several drawbacks. The insert may slip about in the seat, especially when the armrests are spaced away from the seat, creating an asymmetric sitting surface with one side on the seat rail and the other on the upholstery only. The insert must be removed to fold the chair.

Another option for firm seating is a solid folding seat (Fig. 33.20B). This type of seat is an integral part of the frame. It is permanently hinged to one seat rail, folding up when the chair is folded and dropping down into place as it is opened. When the chair is folded, this style of seat alters the shape of the chair. It is important to determine whether this shape will fit into the patient's car. When the seat is in the opened position, it rests between the seat rails, leaving the rails exposed. If it is 1 in. (2.54 cm) thick overall, its top surface will be level with the seat rails. If it is fabricated with thicker foam, the solid folding seat surface will be above the seat rails. In a 16-in. (40.64 cm) wide wheelchair, for instance, there will be 14 in. (35.56 cm) of upholstered and padded seating surface and 1 in. (2.54 cm) of rail exposed on each side. Some users find this uncomfortable if they are using the full seat width as a sitting surface. The advantage of a solid folding seat is that it cannot get lost, or be eliminated from the seating system for convenience. Some manufacturers use hardware for solid folding seats that adds strength to the frame but will also add 7 to 10 pounds to the weight of the chair. Other manufacturer's use a simpler mechanism, adding neither weight nor additional strength to the frame of the chair.

A fourth option for providing a solid seating surface is the solid hook-on seat (Fig. 33.20C). This is a separate seat board that has hook-type hardware along both sides. These hooks clip onto the seat rail, securing the seat in the chair. The seat can hook on at the level of the seat rails, or below or above them. With this variability, and with the different thicknesses of foam available for the insert and/or separate seat cushions, it is possible to change the height and/or pitch of the sitting surface without altering the frame. When the seat is removed to fold the chair, there is no sitting surface on the chair frame and there is no extra hardware. The hook-on seat does not add weight to the folded frame, but will add weight to the open frame. Care should be taken in providing this alternative to users who drive, because the wheelchair's seat upholstery is frequently used as a handle for pulling the chair into the car. In addition to the standard bent hooks, the solid hook-on seat can be equipped with specialized hardware that allows the seat surface to be angled. Many styles of hardware are available from different manufacturers. Several wheelchair manufacturers include angle-adjustable seats in their product options.

The Wheelchair Back

To determine the height of the back, the degree of back support needed to achieve optimal function must be ascertained.

The wheelchair back can be ordered to specification. Until the person's medical status is stable, consideration should be given to ordering add-on or removable parts, such as a headrest extension, a sectional-height back that can be removed and replaced later with lower upholstery and back tubes, or an adjustable-height back. The additional back height may make the folded chair too large to fit into a car, or may not allow adequate clearance for entering a van. In such cases, or in cases in which a custom chair is not possible or an existing chair is in good condition, a removable back insert or replacement back in a custom height might suffice.

When increasing or decreasing the back height, attention should be directed to the level of the push handles. On many chairs, these can be mounted at a height most useful for the caregivers. Some manufacturers even offer plug-in or adjustable-angle push handles to provide the correct push handle heights for multiple caregivers. An extra reinforcement cap of upholstery may provide additional strength to the upper edge of the upholstery. A few wheelchairs are upholstered with the top edge of the back upholstery wrapped around the top of the back tubes while, on other chairs, the upholstery forms a sleeve around the back tubes. Most manufacturers offer an optional style of back upholstery that features straps that can be adjusted to create a more custom contour for the seated user. Tightening the straps in the posterior pelvic area and loosening the straps in the upper trunk area is a common technique to help balance the upper trunk while providing proper support for a neutral pelvic tilt.

On standard wheelchairs, the back tubes rise straight to midback level and then angle backward. When a user leans on these for support, they tend to facilitate shoulder retraction and back extension. Patients often need this leeway to feel comfortable. If a strapped on solid back insert is used, the user may push the top edge until it rests on the tubes, forcing the bottom edge to push the pelvis forward on the wheelchair seat. If this problem is anticipated, it is possible to order the chair with straight tubes instead of the standard angled ones. It is also possible to brace the insert to maintain the designated angle for good posture. For active individuals who require full UE clearance to access the wheels efficiently, it may be necessary to use a special back support with a rounded upper contour, or a scapula cut-out. This type of back will provide good support along the spine while freeing scapula, shoulder, and humerus for wheel access and push.

In addition to back height, many wheelchairs offer angle adjustable back tubes, allowing the chair to be set up with a more open or closed seat/back angle. This adjustment point is either at the back tube/seat rail junction or at a point closer to the pelvic crest. Again, this can be achieved with a back insert on angle adjustable hardware, or a biangular back, if only a small amount of adjustment range is required. It should be noted that back inserts add extra weight to the chair for pushing and must be removed for folding.

The Pelvic Positioner

The pelvic belt is one of the simplest features on a prescription wheelchair. Most clinicians know that the pelvic belt should cross the pelvis at a 45 to 60° angle to the sitting surface, and many understand that the closure style is often critical. There is more than this involved, however, in deciding on a proper pelvic belt. The style of closure is important in facilitating independent use. Many patients can manage only Velcro®, whereas others can manage only buckles. If the user is not able to use the belt independently, and/or significant postural control is required, the style of belt is limited. Some Velcro® closure belts are not strong enough for use by persons with severe extensor spasms. For these, and for others who require a great deal of control, a Velcro® and D-ring style closure belt, or a belt with a cinching-style buckle arrangement, is the most suitable. Cinching-style buckles similar to those on automobile seat belts are available in push-button, airline, and side release styles. Side release buckles are difficult to release, making them a good choice for patients who might try to open a belt at an inappropriate time. However, they are made of plastic and should be monitored continuously for cracks and breaks. The critical feature desired on all styles is that, once the initial contact has been made with the fastener, the belt can be adjusted further to increase tightness.

Mounting the belt to the wheelchair's seat rail is common. Caution should be used with patients who push into excessive extension. This type of belt placement may cause the wheelchair to fold as the rider pushes upward on the belt. In such situations, a custom-made piece of hardware may be needed to mount the belt at a specific point on the frame rail directly below the seat rail (Fig. 33.21). Mounting the belt to the seating insert is not recommended since seat hardware failure or the improper installation of the seat when reassembling the chair after folding could result in injury.

The width of the belt and size of the buckle will affect the level of control offered. The belt and buckle must be correctly proportioned to the user's body. Small children should have belts 1 in. (2.54 cm) wide; larger children and small adults, belts 1.5 in. (3.81 cm) wide; and adults, belts 2 in. (5.08 cm) wide. The buckles should be comfortable. Plastic buckles may be more comfortable for some users. Padding may increase comfort and allow for tighter control.

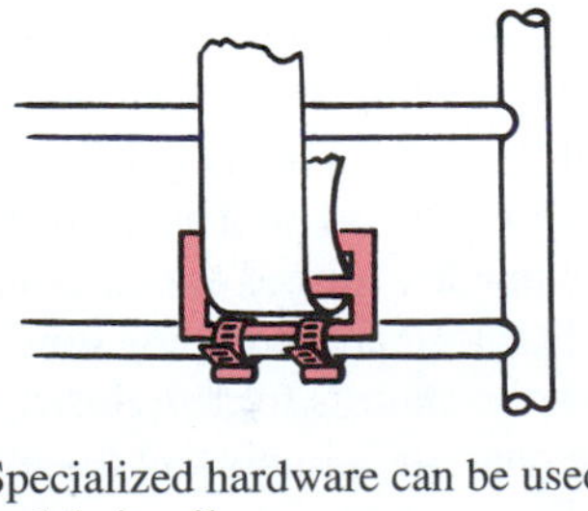

Figure 33.21 Specialized hardware can be used to clamp a lapbelt to the wheelchair rail.

Footrests and Legrests

The footrest (swing-away) and legrest (elevating and swing-away) lengths are determined by measuring the leg length from the popliteal fossa to the heel and subtracting 1 inch. The corresponding measurement on the wheelchair is called the *minimum footboard extension (MinFBX)*. This measurement is the distance from the seat rail to the foot plate. If separate cushions or an insert with or without special foam thickness has been added, or if the seat itself must be angled, the MinFBX measurement must be modified accordingly when the chair is ordered from the manufacturer. For example, if the distance from the popliteal fossa to the heel is 16 in. (40.64 cm), and the patient is to sit on a cushion 2 in. (5.08 cm) thick, a MinFBX of approximately 13 in. (33 cm) will be needed if the seat is firm, or 14 in. (36 cm) if the seat is of soft foam.

Optimal foot placement may be difficult to achieve in the presence of postural control problems, limited ROM, and/or abnormal tone. Proper sitting posture for maximum control may call for a 90° knee flexion angle with a neutral ankle position. Many times, this knee-foot alignment is imperative for maintaining total body alignment, especially for people with tightness in the hamstring muscle group. For small individuals this is rather simple, since the footplate will be above the caster fork and not interfere with caster rotation during movement. When dealing with larger patients, it may be necessary to (1) raise them on cushions if only an additional 1–3 in. (2.5–7.6 cm) is needed; (2) order special, smaller casters (with or without special-length stem bolts or forks); (3) use a special extended, or flared wheelchair frame; or (4) order a chair with the large fixed wheels in the front (or mid-frame on a power base) to allow the knees to be flexed to 90° or more without the feet interfering with caster movement. Positioning the patient forward on the wheelchair frame by using custom back supports can put too much weight on the front casters. On some manual wheelchair frames, this anterior weight shift can make the chair unbalanced. On rear-wheel-drive power chairs, this reduces the weight on the drive wheels and may result in motor and tire problems.

The style of hardware the particular manufacturer uses to mount footrests (called *hangers*) will change the orientation of the foot support to the frame of the chair and to the user's body. Swing-away hangers, for example, may place the foot plates parallel to the floor, or at an angle, and may locate them close to the chair frame or as much as 3 to 4 in. (7.6–10 cm) anterior to the front upright. Many manufacturers offer hangers as standard options at various angles (90, 80, 70, 75, 60, and 65° being the most common), and still others will make custom hangers on request. Angle adjustable hangers that allow seat/calf board adjustment from 60° to 180° are also available. Rotational hangers (also called spica clamps) can be adjusted to properly support LEs that are abducted or adducted when the patient is properly seated. These can be ordered on the original wheelchair, or as a later addition on some frames.

The mounting style should be chosen for function as well as posture. For individuals with edema, detachable elevating legrests may be required. For patients with increased hamstring tone or tightness (e.g., cerebral palsy, multiple sclerosis, muscular dystrophy), elevating legrests are usually not recommended because opening the knee angle will stretch the hamstrings and may pull the pelvis out of alignment. Detachable swing-away footrests do not elevate, but do swing away (in and/or out) to allow clearance for transfers and a better approach to the front of the wheelchair. Lift-off footrests are usually the strongest and can withstand the extra force exerted by patients with high tone, excessive thrusting, or those who "stand" on their footplates to change position. Lift-off footrests usually require removal for transfers. On a chair with a fixed front end, the footrest "hanger" is not a separate part but a continuous part of the wheelchair's side frame. These are extremely strong and can be angled very close to the front of the wheelchair allowing for tighter knee angles. When ordering front-rigging styles, consideration must be given to both present and future function so that the user will be able to continue to improve within the chair and not have a chair that actually exacerbates problems of management.

There are several styles of foot support: a one-piece solid or tubular footboard, or two individual foot plates (solid or open tubular). Some offer angle adjustability in two or four directions. The size of the foot plate surface can vary. Some manufacturers offer several different sizes; others offer only one or two. Several of the manufacturers that produce seating systems also offer foot support systems that mount to the wheelchair's hangers or directly to the seating system. The ultralight wheelchairs are often available with open or filled-in foot plates. The foot plate should accommodate the length of the foot, as well as the width of orthoses or oversized shoes. Narrowing a chair for a better fit around the hips and better hand placement on the rims also decreases the available space between the front tubes for the foot plates. Some of the flip-up style foot plates have additional hardware, which further limits the available space in this area. If the area for foot placement is too narrow, LE position can be compromised.

Calf straps, pads or a calf panel can be used to help keep the feet on the foot plates. Several options are available for actually positioning the foot on the foot plate. Heel loops will stop the foot from sliding off the back of the foot plate and can be mounted as needed to keep the heel positioned correctly. They can be made of webbing, heavy vinyl or plastic in various heights. Ankle straps will keep the foot interfaced with the heel loop. The straps should make a 45° angle with the foot plate surface, causing weight to be placed into the heel. These straps can have varying closure styles: simple Velcro®, Velcro® with D rings, or buckles. Care should be taken to avoid having hard portions of the straps pressing on bony prominences. Some manufactures offer curved buckles and pads to increase comfort and avoid pressure. Crossed ankle straps or figure-of-eight strapping also can be effective. Rigid shoe holders with ankle straps, toe straps, and/or crossed straps provide posterior and lateral control for patients who need more assistance maintaining proper alignment on the foot plate. Ankle cuffs can be used to help maintain the foot on the foot plate while allowing some degree of movement. The straps that attach the cuff to the foot plate are adjustable to provide the correct amount of movement restriction for each patient. Rigid supports such as plastic heel loops or shoe holders will prevent the footplates from flipping up for transfers.

Armrests

Nonremovable armrests offer no specific benefits for an individual using a wheelchair unless it is likely that removable armrests will be lost. They are often ordered in an attempt to reduce the overall width of the chair. This can be achieved with wraparound or space saver armrests that are removable and allow for transfers, sitting without armrests, use of special adapted inserts, changing from fixed-height to adjustable-height armrests, and so forth. Although adjustable and wraparound armrest styles may be more costly on the initial frame, they provide for a more flexible system that can be altered as the patient's functional needs change.

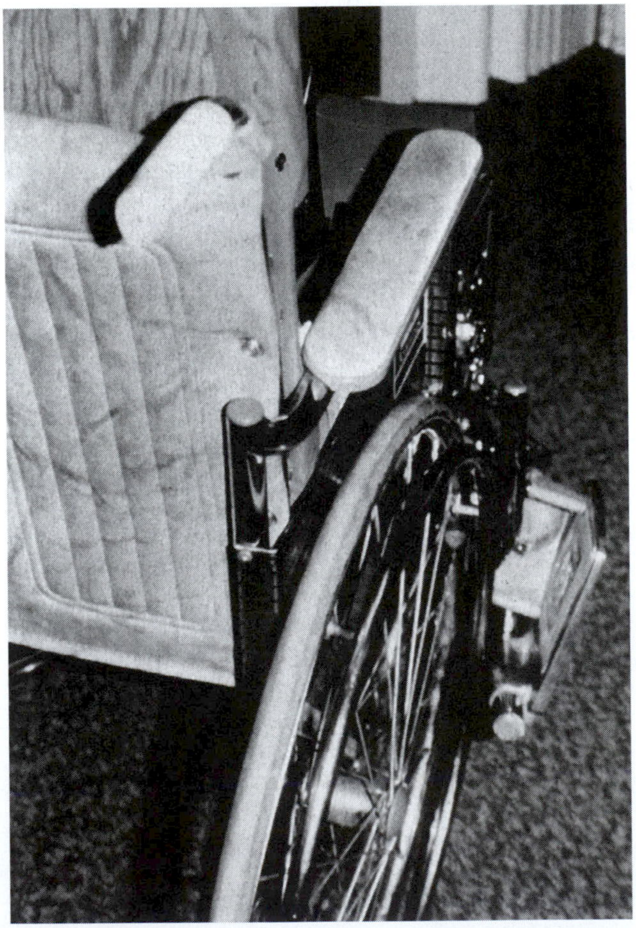

Figure 33.22 Wraparound or space-saver armrests insert behind the wheelchair's back tube.

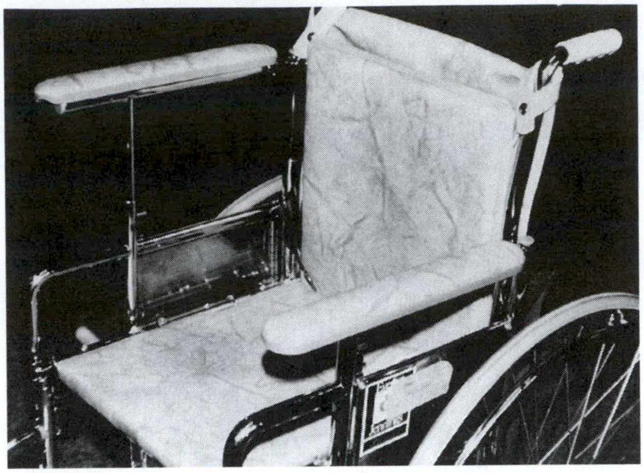

Figure 33.23 Height adjustable arms are available in desk or full length. They allow variable arm heights with a simple adjustment.

Wraparound armrests reduce the overall outside width of the chair by 1.5 in. (3.81 cm) because they allow the wheels to be mounted closer to the side frame. This is accomplished by structural placement of the posterior upright of the armrest behind (wrapped around) the back tube (Fig. 33.22). This narrows the chair for easier maneuverability and places the wheels closer for better hand approach. Removal and repositioning of this style armrest may be difficult for some individuals.

Height-adjustable armrests (Fig. 33.23) are important for children, especially those whose chair frames have been ordered with built-in growth allowance. This type of adjustability is also useful for users who need more or less support depending on the time of day or activity. For example, the arms can be raised to assist in sit-to-stand transfers and lowered for everyday wheelchair use. They also permit placement of a UESS without extensive custom modifications.

Full-length armrests give more room for an UESS to be secured. They also afford the user a larger surface to grasp for push-ups and transfers. Standard full-length armrests, however, may prevent the user from getting close to tables or work surfaces. Shorter-length, desk arms can be ordered to allow for this function. Alternately, full-length height-adjustable armrests allow the user to remove the armrest top or to raise it above the table or work surface for closer access, while providing the longer top surface of a full-length pad.

Some armrests are tubular, with rounded tops rather than flat armrest pads. Several of these styles have only one point of mounting on the chair (Fig. 33.24). Although they may appear unstable, most of these work well for weight-bearing (e.g., pressure relief, depression transfers). Some styles flip up but do not remove, and others swing out to the side. Some have clothing guards, and others do not. Knowledge of all available options, in combination with patient examination data, will inform selection of armrest style to maximize function.

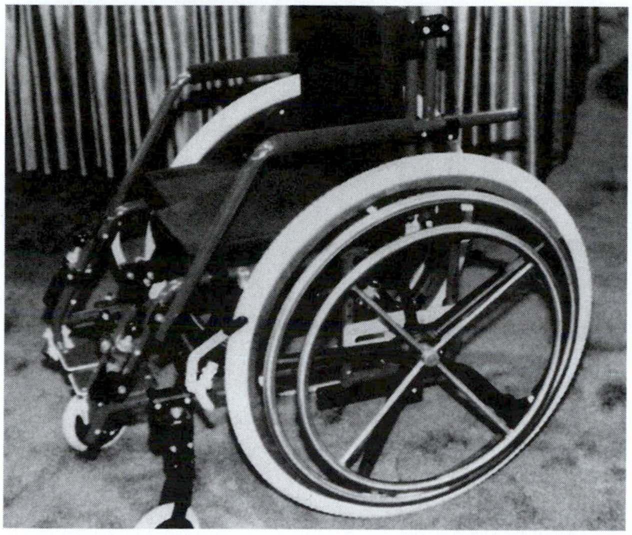

Figure 33.24 Tubular arm rests with single point of mounting on chair. As pictured here, traditional wheelchairs have the large wheel in the rear and a smaller wheel, or caster, in the front. This chair has a single post arm, swing away footrests, and spoked wheels. (Courtesy of Sunrise Medical, Carlsbad, CA 92008.)

When ordering a specific armrest style, the height of the armrest from the finished seat surface should be checked. After comparing this to the measurement obtained for the hanging elbow (see Fig. 33.5), a custom-ordered armrest height may be required. Wheelchair armrest height is determined by adding 1 in. (2.54 cm) to the hanging elbow measure. Armrests that are too high will cause shoulder elevation, and those that are too short may encourage leaning. Those spaced too far apart may interfere with ability to wheel the chair.

Wheels, Hand Rims, and Tires

Wheel choice and placement are critical. The size of the wheel will affect the ability to get the wheel into the correct anterior/posterior and vertical position on chairs which have adjustability. Movement of the rear wheel forward or backward affects overall stability as well as wheel approach for pushing. Up and down adjustment affects seat height in the rear, seat tilt, wheel approach for pushing, as well as overall stability. Wheels that are too low or too small are difficult for seated riders to reach, especially if they are using any type of pressure relieving cushion that has not been dropped between the seat rails.[25] Wheels that are too large or too high result in shoulder elevation when the patient begins his or her stroke, forcing the humerus into the acromion.

When the wheels are too small, or the ratio between the seated rider and the wheels makes the wheels functionally "too small," riders will use short inefficient strokes. Seeking more force to move the chair, some patients who have weak UEs or who are placed too far from the wheels will often bend forward to push. Some can be seen "pumping" in their chairs, actually coming up off the seat to add pushing force to the wheels. Children are often provided with smaller wheels to achieve lower seat heights for transfers and peer approach, but these small wheels require more effort when actively moving the chair. These patients have the smallest, shortest UE muscles and are very vulnerable to RSI. Careful consideration should be given to the size of the wheel if the child will be pushing the chair actively immediately or in the future.

Proper center of mass adjustment is important for safety as well as ease of mobility for caregivers and independent wheelchair riders. It is critical for any patient at risk for RSI. Moving the rear wheel backward along the frame moves the patient's center of mass more forward, away from the "drive" wheels. Patients will then require more energy to keep the casters tracking correctly, especially in turns and on slopes. The rider must reach further back to grab the wheel, a poor lever arm position resulting in decreased efficiency in the stroke and increased stress on muscles and joints. The overall length of the chair frame is increased, making the turning radius larger and decreasing general maneuverability.

Moving the rear wheels more forward moves the rider's center of mass over the "drive" wheels, and decreases the weight on the casters and therefore decreases the amount of power needed to keep the chair tracking well during turns and on slopes. This results in less stress on the UE muscle groups.[26] The chair will be more maneuverable but it will also have more tendency to tip.

For patients of varying age groups and body size, the issue of wheel placement is extremely critical if RSI and CTS is to be minimized and function maximized.[18–28] The goal is to make the chair as responsive as possible while maintaining stability. Children are often positioned in chairs with an eye toward growth adjustability for the future. The seating surface is moved forward on the seat frame and there is limited ability to move the rear wheel forward because of interference by frame parts. Children have short muscles because of their body size, and yet they are often asked to push chairs that weigh as much or more than adult systems, with the rear wheels in the poorest position. Extra attention must be paid to wheelchair set up for this age group.

Older patients are usually given the least adjustable wheelchairs. The wheels are set far back along the side frame. The seated rider is often kyphotic, placing the shoulder girdle more forward in the wheelchair. Elders often have decreased strength and decreased ROM. Use of these standard configuration wheelchairs places the individual at risk for RSI when asked to use the UEs for functional self propulsion.

Users who fall in or near the obesity categories (body mass index [BMI] of 30 kg/m^2 or above[29]) must be placed in wheelchairs that are rated for this population (a bariatric chair). Most of these riders have excessive tissue mass in the hip and buttock area. If this is not accommodated, the person will balance his or her trunk several inches anterior to the center of mass. This results in the shoulders being far anterior to the rear wheel. In addition, these patients have increased body weight. They are asked to push a heavier wheelchair, as well as their heavy body weight, using a wheel that is posterior to the shoulder line, resulting in excessive stress on shoulder and arm musculature.

The ideal UE position for wheelchair propulsion is with the hands posterior to the shoulder girdle and the elbows flexed between 100° and 120°.[28]

The wheel and tire choice also affects energy expenditure required to move the chair. The goal is to decrease the amplitude and frequency of the force needed to push the chair by decreasing the weight of the wheel, decreasing compression in the wheel, and decreasing rolling resistance. Historically, spoked wheels were not often used as they were more difficult to maintain. However, new technology has made them stronger and more suitable for everyday use. Spoked wheels are lighter and more durable than spokeless wheels making them the wheel of choice for wheelchair riders who are pushing their chairs.

It is important to consider the patient's lifestyle as well as wheelchair performance when choosing tires. Can the rider or caregiver maintain the tires and repair them if needed? What type of terrain does the chair regularly traverse? Solid tires have little or no tread, and therefore have decreased traction on uneven surfaces. They are less shock absorbing but maintenance free. Pneumatic tires have increased rolling resistance, increased traction, and absorb road shocks. However, pneumatics carry the risk of a flat tire, and if the proper inflation is not maintained the patient will need more force to push the chair. Adding no flat inserts to pneumatic tires will decrease maintenance, but they are heavy and have almost no shock absorbing factor. In addition, no flats usually force wheel locks out of adjustment quickly, requiring that the wheel locks be adjusted frequently. Patients with limited strength may find applying wheel locks to tires with no flat inserts requires more strength than they have. Kevlar® tires or "tuff" strips may be a better choice so that pneumatic tires can be used.

Some patients cannot reach and push both wheels even if the chair is set up perfectly. Some of these patients may be able to use a one-arm drive system. In this type of system, chair movement is controlled by two handrims placed on one wheel and a cross linkage that spans the frame to the other wheel (Fig. 33.25). The user must push one or the other or both rims together. This type of system adds 5 to 10 pounds to the weight of the chair and the wheels have a limited range of adjustability. All of this makes pushing more taxing. Use of this type of system requires careful consideration.

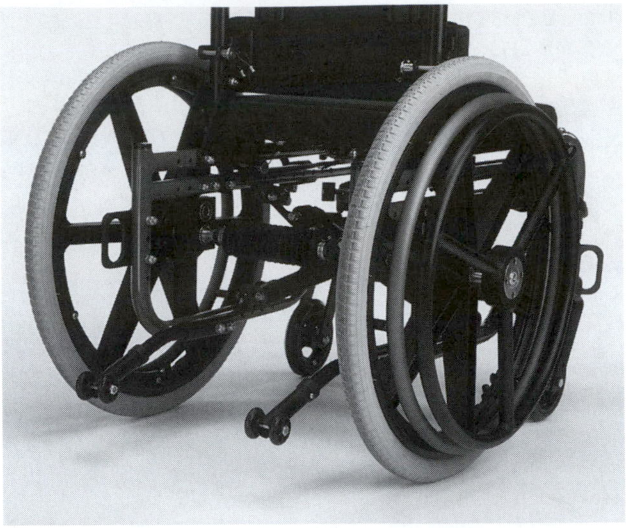

Figure 33.25 A double hand rim on one side allows the user to drive a one-arm drive wheelchair with one hand. (Courtesy of Sunrise Medical, Carlsbad, CA 92008.)

The Frame

Most people who use manual wheelchairs utilize outdoor frames (see Fig. 33.24). This means that the large wheels are in the back and the casters are in the front. Chairs with large wheels in the front (Fig. 33.26) are sometimes ordered for individuals with severe knee flexion contractures, for those whose UE ROM is limited, and for children who do better if they see the wheels. Although access to the wheels may be easier with the indoor model, overall maneuverability may be more difficult, and transfers may present a problem. Use of these chairs outdoors is difficult because it is almost impossible to pull them up curbs or steps. Front-wheel and mid-wheel drive power wheelchairs have their larger wheel in the front or center of the frame.

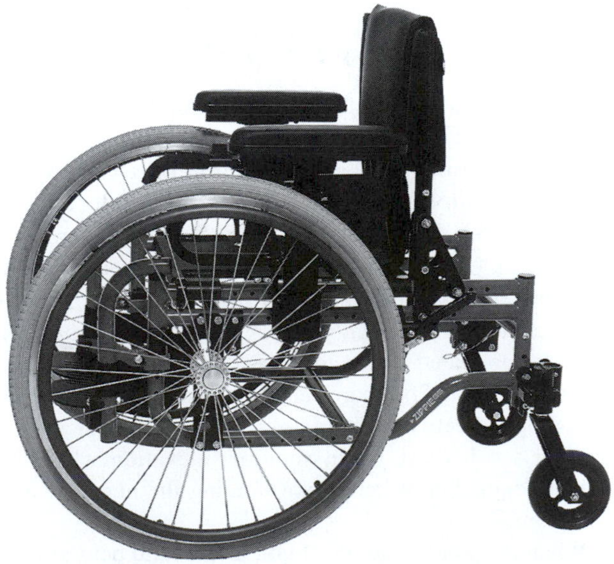

Figure 33.26 Wheelchairs with large front wheels and small rear casters may be easier for some patients to push, but are more difficult to use outdoors. (Courtesy of Sunrise Medical, Carlsbad, CA 92008.)

They are usually powerful enough to climb small curbs, but the wheel configuration precludes a caregiver's pulling them up larger curbs and steps.

Chair frames are available in rigid or folding styles. Most rigid frames offer fold-down backs and removable wheels to allow some breakdown for stowage in vehicles. Rigid frames allow each of the user's pushes to translate more efficiently into chair motion. However, on uneven terrain the user of a rigid frame may be uncomfortable, because the frame transfers rather than absorbs shock. Some specialty chairs have shock absorbers built into the frame to smooth out the ride for patients who have a problem with road shock which may increase spasms or result in severe discomfort. Rigid frames are the lightest available, with some weighing 20 pounds or less with the wheels in place (Fig. 33.27). Folding styles provide a slightly more comfortable ride, as the frame provides some shock absorption. They are easier to store when traveling (e.g., in the trunk of a car) but tend to be heavier compared to rigid frames.

Chair frames are available in heavy-duty, standard, lightweight, active-duty lightweight, and ultra-lightweight construction. Patients and their caregivers who are functioning in the community should be offered the lightest, strongest possible frame feasible. The lighter frames are easier for the user to propel and easier for caregivers to manage. For chairs used exclusively indoors, or when caregivers do not have to lift and carry the unit, the issue of weight may be secondary to the issue of price. To justify the added expense of an active-duty lightweight or ultra-lightweight chair, explanation for its necessity must be provided to the third-party payer as a medical need.

Accessories

Many accessories are available to personalize the chair for functional and aesthetic reasons. Crutch holders, antitippers, utility bags, and UESS all serve a functional purpose. A choice of frame and upholstery color, usually at no extra cost, will help to personalize the chair. Making the perfect match between consumer and product will require a careful determination of the user's needs and a matching of these to the product features. Something as simple as the style of a lock or the type of push handle may have important long-term functional or care-giving implications.

Specialized Wheelchairs

Positioning

Patients with poor postural control, abnormal tone, muscle shortening, or skeletal deformities often require wheelchairs that offer varied positioning possibilities. A frame may be needed that offers a fixed or adjustable posterior *tilt-in-space* orientation (Fig. 33.28). This frame may need to be combined with a reclinable back or an angle-adjustable seating surface or both. Some chairs allow caregivers to change the seat position, whereas others afford the rider this control. Some offer components for positioning, such as head and torso supports. Several

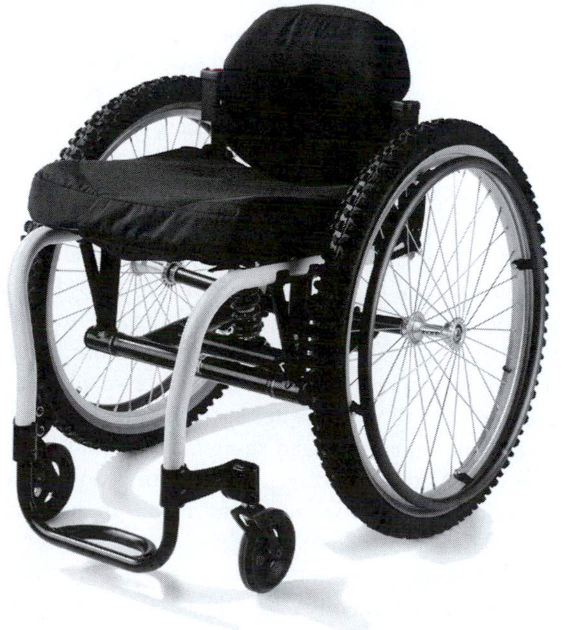

Figure 33.27 Lightweight rigid frame chair with adjustable suspension system, seat back angle, wheel base, and footrest lengths. The chair has knobby tires on spoked wheels (Courtesy of Sunrise Medical, Carlsbad, CA 92008.)

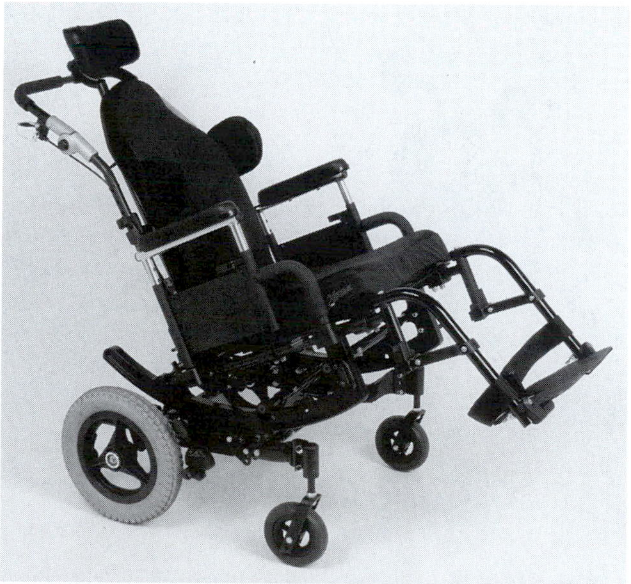

Figure 33.28 Wheelchairs that tilt through space with all their angles preset are called tilt-in-space wheelchairs. They are available in manual and motorized models. (Courtesy of Sunrise Medical, Carlsbad, CA 92008.)

manufacturers offer systems that include positioning components on a mobility base. Others do not offer the components and it becomes necessary to interface more than one manufacturer's products to have a complete chair (see Appendix A).

Power

A *powered mobility system* (Fig. 33.29) consists of a base or frame, a seat, and electronics (batteries, motors, control module, and driver control). A powered mobility system should be considered when a person cannot independently access his or her environment via ambulation or a manual wheelchair. Some wheelchair riders are marginal self-propellers in manual wheelchairs. They may be able to move around indoors, and on level surfaces outdoors, but cannot move around in the community environment without unduly stressing muscles and joints, creating postural problems, and/or imposing cardiovascular strain. The long-term overuse injury of muscles and joints and the possibility of skeletal deformity must be discussed with the patient and caregiver as part of the examination process. Patients must face the possibility that they may create problems significant enough to impede function in critical areas such as transfers and ADL.[18–28,30]

An examination of the patient's full environment must be made to determine if powered mobility will be helpful and usable. Architectural barriers such as steps might preclude the use of powered mobility or require that the patient have both a powered and manual system for use at different times. In addition, attention should be given to how the chair will be transported, and the level of technology tolerance of both the consumer and caregiver. For patients whose condition is changing, a long-term plan must be established to guide decision making when choosing products. When considering powered mobility for individuals that may have cognitive impairments, the rule of thumb is that the driver is aware of safety for themselves and others. In most cases, the ability to stop and to judge when to stop is more difficult to teach than driving itself. Awareness, reliable movement, and good response time are all important factors in wheelchair use. Some patients who can drive using a joystick cannot release it quickly enough, and might be safer using a different control site and/or a different type of control mechanism.

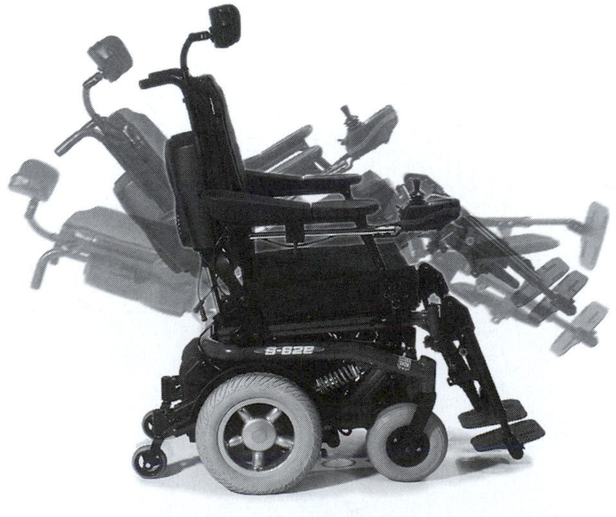

Figure 33.29 Motorized wheelchairs offer patients with poor coordination, weakness or paralysis, an opportunity to move around in their environment. This chair also has a power operated seating system. (Courtesy of Sunrise Medical, Carlsbad, CA 92008.)

The base or frame of the powered chair and the seat portion are the mechanical parts of the chair. As in all other areas, there are advantages and disadvantages to the various systems available. Frame-style wheelchairs were the norm in previous years, but are not as popular any more. In this type of chair the seat and base are one continuous structure. Many of these can be folded like a traditional manual wheelchair once the batteries (and their support frame if necessary) are removed. This type of system may offer a more shock-absorbing ride and more room underneath the seat for positioning of a ventilator and extra batteries if needed. However, because there are more moving parts, they may require higher maintenance.

A base style frame is usually a one-size-fits-all wheeled component that accepts different seating units. This allows positioning of wider seating units without affecting the base width proportionally as with frame-style chairs. Most manufacturers use the same base even with extra-wide seats, but may require the use of wider tires and casters. Therefore, for most adult users a base style chair will be narrower. This type of chair usually has a lower seat height, accepts larger batteries, and more easily accepts power seat components. They are usually extremely stable, making it more difficult for caregivers to assist with tilting the chair to mount curbs.

Belt-driven chairs are rare. These chairs perform best over firm surfaces, but some of the energy produced by the motors is lost in the belt and to slippage before going to the wheel. Direct drive systems allow all of the energy to pass directly from the motor into the wheel. They are quieter, can have more torque when needed, and can use smaller, wider wheels for stability and an overall narrower footprint. Direct drive wheels can have rear, middle, or front placement. Although rear-wheel placement is more common, mid- and front-wheel drive chairs have a smaller turning radius and may allow for better knee positioning to accommodate tight hamstrings and shorten the overall length of the systems. Mid-wheel drive chairs perform well outdoors, but may produce a "rocking chair" effect on acceleration and deceleration, which may be problematic for users with postural instability, or startle responses. Having the drive wheels positioned directly under the seated user may make steering more intuitive for some patients.

Power seat and positioning functions (e.g., power recline, power tilt, power elevating legrests, power seat elevator, and power stand-up) are extremely important for individuals using a powered wheelchair who are prone to pressure ulcers or orthostatic hypotension, those with poor endurance for upright sitting, as well as those with painful conditions that require frequent change of position.[31] They are available in many combinations, with a few chairs offering all of the features in one system. Addition of these features makes the chair heavier and more costly.

Motorized three-, and four-wheeled power operated vehicles and wheelchairs are available in many styles with varying degrees of portability, power, and electronic sophistication. In all cases it would be ideal if a proportional drive system could be used. *Proportional drives* respond to pressure like an automobile accelerator; the more pressure, the more speed. Because the speed and degree of acceleration are controlled by the rider's movement of the joystick, this type of system gives the user the greatest degree of control.

With the advent of microprocessor-controlled wheelchairs, the performance parameters of the joystick can be altered to adapt to the user's ability. Such systems allow individuals with severe spasticity and those who are extremely weak to achieve wheelchair mobility with a proportional system. Alternate access spots for users who cannot use their hands should be considered. This might include the head, foot, chin, tongue, or extensions of body parts, such as using pointers or similar adapted accessors.

For patients who cannot use a proportional controller the team may want to consider using a microswitching system. A *microswitching system* is an all-or-none drive system. The speed is preset. Some systems have only one speed while others have two or three speeds. The operator applies any degree of pressure, and as soon as the switch (mechanical or electrical) is activated, the system runs at the preset speed. Individual switches are provided for the four directions (forward, reverse, right, left), and a series of individual movements are required to maneuver in tight spaces. Individual switches can be operated through a puff-n-sip tube placed in the mouth, or by pressing a surface or interrupting a beam. They can be arranged around a joystick in a control box, or they can be placed anywhere around the body to allow the user to drive the chair. For example, there might be two switches on an UESS for gross pressing with the hand, and additional switches at the head, knees, or feet to allow mobility in all four directions. For patients with less than four or five movements, chairs with dual- and single-switch accessing systems are available; however, such systems make the chair progressively more tedious to operate. Voice operated technology is available on a limited basis for driving and for operating power seat functions.

Sports and Recreation

Many users are active in recreational and competitive sports, some of which are done from the wheelchair. These patients may need more than one wheelchair: a *street* or *everyday* chair, and a finely tuned *competition chair* or *recreational chair* (Figs. 33.30 to 33.36). For

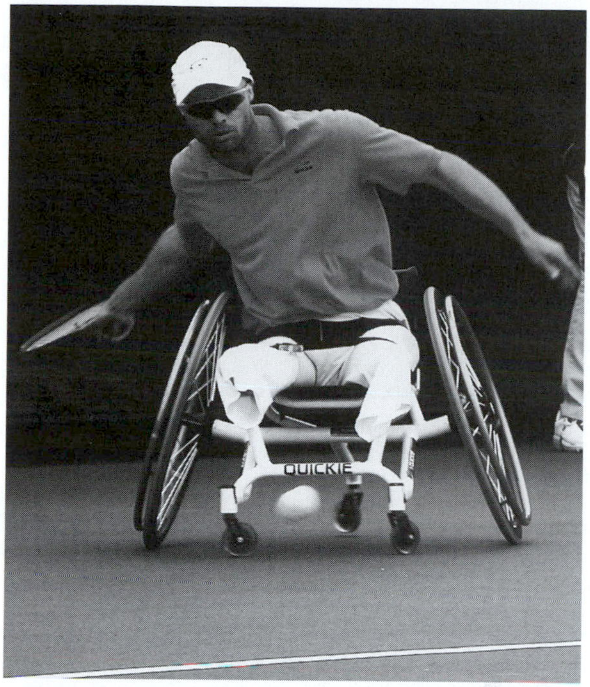

Figure 33.30 This court chair is shown being used for tennis play. It can also be used for basketball. The back is very low to allow free trunk and arm movement. The wheels are radically cambered for stability. (Courtesy of Sunrise Medical, Carlsbad, CA 92008.)

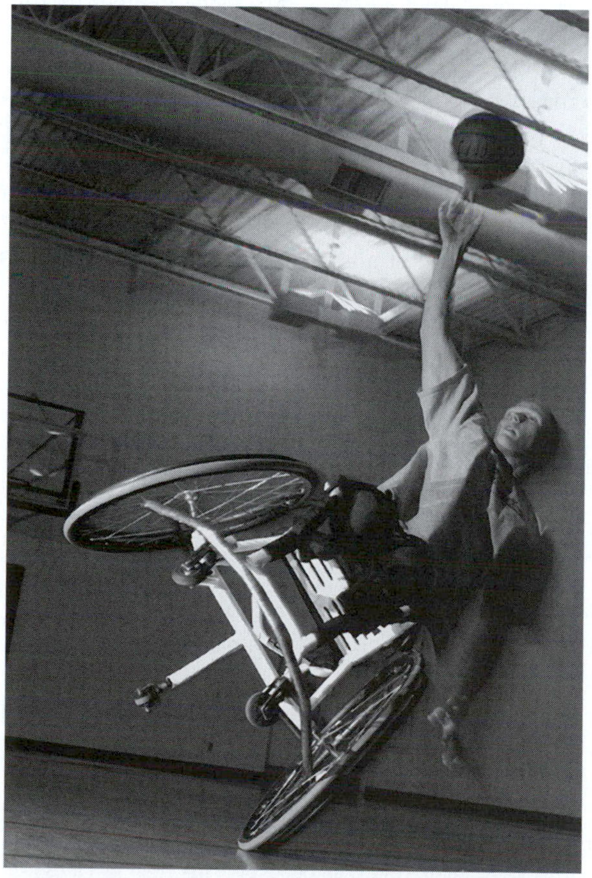

Figure 33.31 This court chair is being used for basketball. (Courtesy of Sunrise Medical, Carlsbad, CA 92008.)

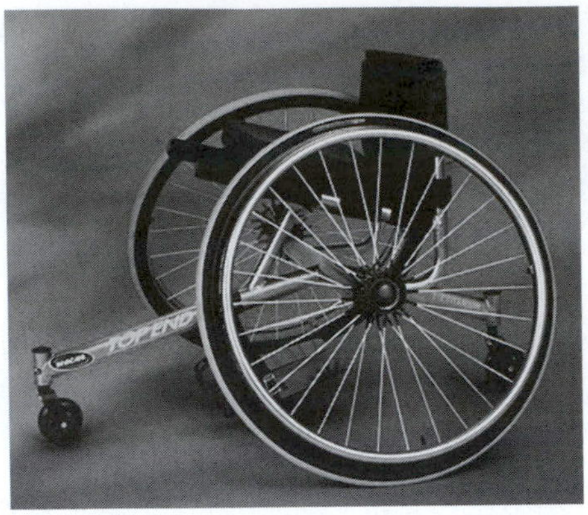

Figure 33.32 This tennis chair has a single front caster and a very low back. (Courtesy of Invacare Corporation, Elyria, OH 44035.)

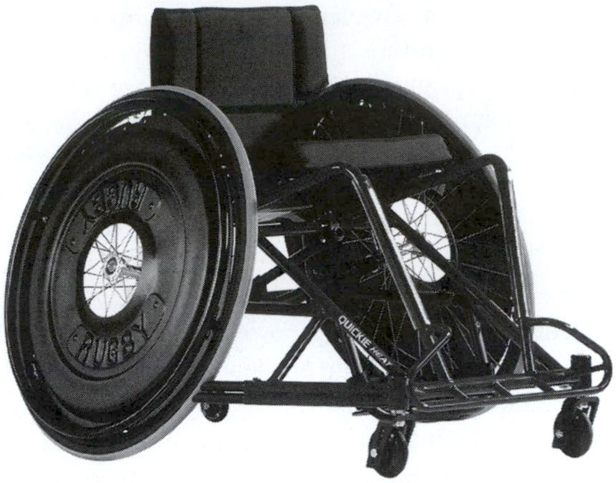

Figure 33.34 This wheelchair has been designed for use in Quad Rugby which is a high contact sport. (Courtesy of Sunrise Medical, Carlsbad, CA 92008.)

some sports such as archery, discus, shot put, and precision javelin, a more stable chair is an advantage. A wide wheel camber can achieve this even on a lightweight frame. For basketball, tennis, and dancing the chair's responsiveness is critical. Competition chairs are usually of rigid construction, and made of very strong lightweight materials. Wheel and caster placement, tires, axles, and bearings can make a radical difference in chair performance when matched with the user's body weight and configuration. Users who participate in more than one activity may want a chair with a great deal of adjustability to allow parameter changes for various activities or multiple chairs, if possible.

Individuals who use their wheelchairs on off-road, challenging trails will require knobby tires (see Fig. 33.27), because the tread of normal wheelchair tires will tend to get stuck in softer ground. Those who compete in road racing will need competition chairs that have taken many of their design features from racing bicycles: narrow, hard tires; frames made of lightweight alloys, titanium or carbon; low seats for minimum air resistance; and small push rims for higher gearing. Racers usually sit in a tucked position, with approximately 120° of hip flexion and knees and legs strapped together to present a very sleek line and minimal wind resistance as the unit (wheelchair and user) moves quickly along the track. For tennis and dance, the chair is trimmed down to its sleekest configuration with all accessories, even wheel locks, removed. Wheel hubs and spoke configurations are designed to hold a tennis ball during competition. The backs are as low as possible to leave the user's upper body free for movement (see Fig. 33.30).

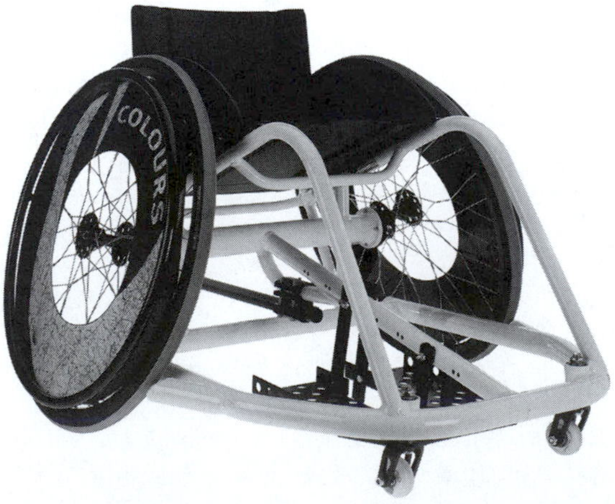

Figure 33.33 Some sports chairs are designed for high contact sports like football, rugby, and hockey. This chair has a rigid frame with larger than standard tubing and a very wide front end. (Courtesy of Colours in Motion, Anaheim, CA 92806.)

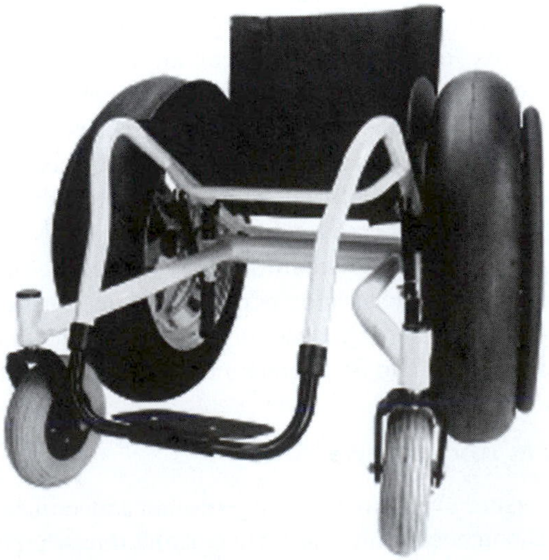

Figure 33.35 This wheelchair and its tires and casters have been designed for use on sand and in the water. (Courtesy of Colours in Motion, Anaheim, CA 92806.)

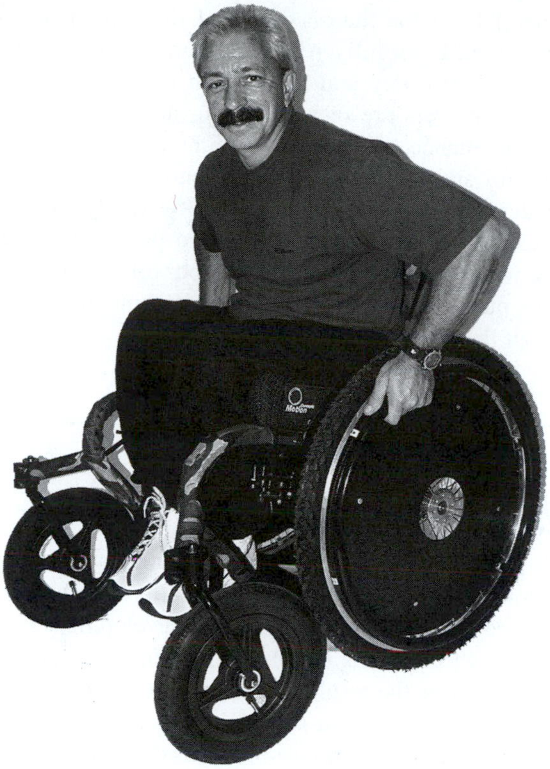

Figure 33.36 This wheelchair is designed for all terrain use. (Courtesy of Motion Concepts, Concord, Ontario, Canada, L4K 3C1.)

Wheelchair Training Strategies

Many individuals using a wheelchair for the first time will require a training period. During this time the patient will learn how to propel the chair in all directions (i.e., using both arms, one or two arms in combination with one or two legs, or one arm using a dual-wheel drive system). He or she must also learn how to operate the wheel locks, foot supports, and armrests, and to use the mechanisms safely without tipping forward or sideways out of the chair seat. He or she will learn how to transfer in and out of the chair with the least possible assistance. Some users will always require maximal assistance for transfer activities, but others will be able to achieve functional independence. Chair features such as removable or swing-away arm and foot supports, and lowered seat heights may be important features for independence. For patients who perform standing transfers (independent or assisted), special attention should be given to the user's ability to get out of or back into the chair, because the seat height may prove problematic. Most chairs with a cushion allow a user to slide forward and come to standing. Some patients (e.g., the patient with bilateral transfemoral amputation) may benefit from adjustable height armrests. The armrests are raised during sit-to-stand transfers.

Although sidewalk cutouts are now mandated in many areas, patients who are capable of independent community mobility benefit from learning to do *wheelies* to negotiate existing curbs. The chair is balanced on the rear wheels while the front casters are elevated and then propelled forward to mount the curb.

Patients who drive need to practice transfers from the wheelchair to the car seat. The wheelchair is then pulled into the vehicle either behind the seat, or across his or her body into the passenger seat. Either method is very dependent on the chair's folded size and weight, the user's upper body skill and strength, and the internal configuration of the car. Active patients also need to practice controlled falls out of the wheelchair and floor-to-wheelchair transfers that can be utilized in the event of falls.

Power chair training is slightly different, and usually concentrates primarily on driving skill and safety. The initial challenge is to locate a reliable access control site and method (e.g., hand control with a joystick, head control with individual switches). Training then involves working with the user on consistent responses (especially to "stop" commands, or the recognized need to stop based on the user's awareness), and accurate maneuverability. Although switch activation can be judged using a computer program, actual road time is necessary for training and ensuring the driver knows how to respond to a variety of situations, distractions, and obstacles.

It is also important for wheelchair users to learn how to ask for help and how to direct helpers who might be touching them or the wheelchair. Some rehabilitation facilities have large fleets of sample chairs that can be used with patients for examination and training. If this option is not available, a qualified supplier or manufacturer's representative in the area should be located.

The Role of the Certified Rehabilitation Technology Supplier

Traditional home care and/or durable medical equipment companies are well qualified to accept prescriptive wheelchair information over the phone. They keep standard-sized items in stock, and can get them to the user quickly, often within 24 hours. More specialized equipment usually requires input to the team from an *Assistive Technology Supplier (ATS)* who has passed the RESNA national certification exam or a *Certified Rehabilitation Technology Supplier (CRTS)* who is a member of the National Registry of Rehabilitation Technology Suppliers who is also an ATS. He or she is a specialist and can work with the team to design a system that fits the patient's unique needs. Once the team's goals are explained to the supplier, he or she will be able to provide a list of available products that match the user's needs. It is critical that the team hear about all of the options, not just the products available from one manufacturer. The CRTS or ATS will be able to explain the pros and cons, as well as the prices of various products and options to everyone involved. It may be advisable for the user to actually try several products before a decision is made. The supplier can work with the team to arrange this opportunity.

Once a system has been selected, the clinical team's recommendations (including physical, psychosocial, and cognitive factors if applicable) are compiled into a *letter of medical necessity*. The letter of medical necessity (with physician and clinic team member signatures), a physician's prescription, and price estimate are then forwarded to the third-party payer(s). The justification package should explain the medical need for each feature requested, along with an expected outcome from the intervention. Providing measurable functional outcomes is essential to help the payer make an informed decision.

The CRTS or ATS should keep all of the team members apprised as the process moves along from submission through approval, ordering, and receipt of the chair and its components. Once the system is complete, the supplier must deliver it as instructed by the prescriber (to the clinic, school, or home of the user). At delivery, those involved with formulating the prescription should have an opportunity to inspect the system and be sure that it meets the specifications, as well as to observe and assist as the supplier makes final adjustments. The process may require more than one or two visits for complex systems that require interim fittings.

On final delivery, the CRTS or ATS explains to the user and/or caregivers how to use the chair, including use of all safety features (straps, wheel locks, anttippers), assembly and disassembly for folding, and normal maintenance (including battery maintenance on power wheelchairs and scooters). Once the chair is delivered, the user and/or caregivers should carefully read any manuals provided and mail in all warranty and registration materials. The user and/or caregivers are responsible for all normal cleaning and maintenance. The supplier and the company he or she works for should be located close enough to the user to provide emergency repairs as needed. Warranty repairs are the responsibility of the supplier who provided the chair (most warranties cover the cost of labor for 12 months following purchase and then labor costs become the responsibility of the owner).

Summary

A systematic approach to prescribing a wheelchair has been presented. The individual components of both the postural support and the wheeled mobility base have been described. The primary outcome in developing any prescriptive wheelchair is maximum function and independence. It must be the result of a thorough evaluation using a patient centered problem-solving approach, with attention to the specific factors discussed in this chapter. Input from the user and all team members during the decision making phase is critical. This process will result in an optimally designed chair capable of achieving its intended purpose. Using a patient-centered approach, with open communication among team members, rehabilitation technology supplier, and manufacturer will ensure that each prescriptive wheelchair will meet the needs of the individual.

Questions for Review

1. Explain what information or data is gathered during each of the following portions of the examination process.
   a. Physical examination
   b. Examination of function using existing equipment
   c. Examination in the supine position
   d. Examination in the seated position
2. Describe the following seating components and provide two indications for their use.
   a. Firm seat
   b. Firm back
   c. Lapboard/UESS
   d. Lapbelt
3. Describe the following wheelchair components; compare and contrast their functional benefits.
   a. Detachable swing-away footrests/elevating legrests
   b. Fixed-height armrests/adjustable-height armrests
   c. Single-axle placement/multiple-axle placement
   d. Proportional drive/microswitching system
4. When measuring for seat depth, what two positions would you place the patient in and why?
5. Identify landmarks and measurements needed to help determine the size of the following parts of a wheeled mobility system:
   a. Seat width
   b. Seat depth
   c. Seat back height
   d. Armrest height
   e. Minimum footboard extension (MinFBX).
6. Compare and contrast the characteristic features, postural control provided, as well as the advantages and disadvantages of:
   a. Wheelchair seats: (1) solid insert and (2) solid hook-on seat
   b. Wheelchair seat cushions: (1) comfort cushion (planar/contoured), (2) pressure relieving foam (contoured, custom contoured), (3) pressure-relieving fluid or fluid/foam combination, and (4) pressure-relieving air
   c. Back supports: (1) adjustable strap upholstery, (2) solid insert, and (3) solid hook-on back

Case Study

The patient is a 24-year-old man who suffered a traumatic brain injury when he was 15 years old. He presents in a tilt-in-space manual wheelchair with a high back, back insert, planar seat with a loose gel pad covering, anterior chest support and padded lap belt. He sits poorly in the chair and caregivers report he consistently slips down on the seat, curves his trunk to the side and keeps his head flexed forward and to the side. He is dependent in eating and transfers. He makes eye contact occasionally and can indicate yes/no with a hand movement. The immediate goal of his team and caregivers is to improve postural alignment and then, in the future, determine a site where he can consistently access a switch that will allow use of a computer for communication, learning, and recreational activities.

Physical Therapy Examination Findings

When seated in the chair his head is down and laterally flexed to the left. His trunk is shortened on the left with the shoulder depressed; the pelvis is in an oblique position with the left side raised. The pelvis is tilted posteriorly with both LEs abducted. His hips are shifted toward the left. The seat/back angle of the chair is set at 90°. The knees are positioned at 90° and the feet do not remain in position on the foot plates. The UEs rest on an UESS.

A supine examination reveals that the patient's head, trunk, and pelvis can be neutrally aligned. There is some pelvic mobility, and the hips can be flexed to 75° before the pelvis begins to rotate posteriorly. There is limited hip adduction and internal rotation, but both LEs can achieve neutral position. The hamstrings are moderately tight, but should not interfere with sitting. There are no red or scarred areas over bony prominences despite a marked pelvic obliquity in sitting.

Using a simulator chair, the patient sat with a seat/back angle of 105°. Lateral trunk, hip, and knee supports were placed to help keep him centered on the sitting surface. The lateral knee supports were very effective in preventing the abduction pattern typically assumed. A head/neck support was used posteriorly and laterally. An additional support pad was placed at the left temple to address the lateral flexion. A forehead strap was suggested to assist with upright head positioning, but was uncomfortable and rejected by the patient. The patient answered yes/no questions while postural response to the support and angle changes were observed. He was able to remain symmetrically seated with the pelvis well positioned on the seat surface for approximately 45 minutes, with the chair in 10° of posterior tilt.

GUIDING QUESTIONS

1. What adjustments should be made and what components would you recommend be added to the patient's tilt-in-space wheelchair to improve postural alignment for each of the following areas? Identify the *degree of accommodation*, *postural control*, and *functional assistance* that will be provided by each of your recommendations for the following areas:
   a. Head and neck
   b. Trunk
   c. Hip
   d. Knee
2. The patient already has an anterior chest support. What function does this component provide?
3. What recommendations would you make to address the problem of foot positioning on the foot plates?
4. What type of seat cushion would you recommend for this patient? Provide a rationale for your selection.

References

1. Bolin, I, Bodin, P, and Kreuter, M: Sitting position—posture and performance in C5-C6 tetraplegia. Spinal Cord 38(7):425, 2000.
2. Kennedy , P, et al: The effect of a specialist seating assessment clinic on the skin management of individuals with spinal cord injury. J Tissue Viability 13(3):122, 2003.
3. Troy, BS, et al: An analysis of work postures of manual wheelchair users in the office environment. J Rehabil Res Dev 34(2):151, 1997.
4. Curtis, KA, et al: Functional reach in wheelchair users: The effects of trunk and lower extremity stabilization. Arch Phys Med Rehabil 76(4):360, 1995.
5. Aissaoui, R, et al: Effect of seat cushion on dynamic stability in sitting during a reaching task in wheelchair users with paraplegia. Arch Phys Med Rehabil 82(2):274, 2001.
6. Saftler, F, et al: Use of a positioning chair in conjunction with proper seating principles for a seating evaluation. Proceedings from ICCART, 1988.
7. Sprigle S, Chung KC, and Brubaker CE: Reduction of sitting pressures with custom contoured cushions. J Rehabil Res Dev 27(2):135, 1990.
8. Sprigle, S, Chung, KC, and Brubaker, CE: Factors affecting seat contour characteristics. J Rehabil Res Dev 27(2):127, 1990.
9. Hobson, DA: Comparative effects of posture and pressure distribution at the body-seat interface. J Rehabil Res Dev 29(4):21, 1992.
10. Sprigle, S, and Chung, K: The use of contoured foam to reduce seat interface pressures. Proceedings of the 12th Annual Conference of the Rehabilitation Engineering Society of North America (RESNA), New Orleans, LA, June 25–30, 1989. RESNA Press, Washington, DC, 1989.
11. Holmes, KJ, et al: Management of scoliosis with special seating for the non-ambulant spastic cerebral palsy population—a biomechanical study. Clin Biomech (Bristol, Avon). 18(6):480, 2003.
12. Bergen, AF: A seat belt is a seat belt is a. . . . Assist Technol 1:7, 1989.
13. Margolis, S, et al: The sub-ASIS bar: An effective approach to pelvic stabilization in seated position. Proceedings of the 8th Annual Conference of RESNA, Memphis, TN, June 24–28, 1985. RESNA Press, Washington, DC, 1985.
14. Butler, C: Effects of powered mobility on self-initiated behaviors of very young children with locomotor disability. Dev Med Child Neurol 28:325, 1986.
15. Butler, C, Okamoto, GA, and McKay, TM: Powered mobility for very young disabled children. Dev Med Child Neurol 25:472, 1983.
16. Lotto, W, and Milner, M: Evaluations and Development of Powered Mobility Aids for 2–5 Year Olds with Neuromuscular Disorders. Ontario Crippled Child Centre, Toronto, Ontario, 1983.

17. Trefler, E, et al: Selected Readings on Powered Mobility for Children and Adults with Severe Physical Disabilities. RESNA Press, Washington, DC, 1986.
18. Sie, IH, et al: Upper extremity pain in the postrehabilitation spinal cord injured patient. Arch Phys Med Rehabil 73:44, 1992.
19. Boninger, ML, et al: Shoulder imaging abnormalities in individuals with paraplegia. J Rehabil Res Dev 38(4):401, 2001.
20. Boninger, ML, et al: Wheelchair pushrim kinetics: Body weight and median nerve function. Arch Phys Med Rehabil 80(8):910, 1999.
21 Boninger, ML, et al: Shoulder magnetic resonance imaging abnormalities, wheelchair propulsion, and gender. Arch Phys Med Rehabil 84(11):1615, 2003.
22. Brubaker, CE: Wheelchair prescription: An analysis of factors that affect mobility and performance. J Rehabil Res Dev 23(4):19, 1986.
23. Highes, CJ, et al: Biomechanics of wheelchair propulsion as a function of seat position and user-to-chair interface. Arch Phys Med Rehabil 73(3):263, 1992.
24. Masse, LC, Lamontagne, M, and O'Riain, MD: Biomechanical analysis of wheelchair propulsion for various seating positions. J Rehabil Res Dev 29(3):12, 1992.
25. Wei, SH, et al: Wrist kinematic characterization of wheelchair propulsion in various seating positions: Implication to wrist pain. Clin Biomech (Bristol, Avon). 18(6):S46, 2003.
26. Boninger, ML, et al: Manual wheelchair push rim biomechanics and axle position. Arch Phys Med Rehabil 81(5):608, 2000.
27. Lal, S: Premature degenerative shoulder changes in spinal cord injury patients. Spinal Cord 36(3):186, 1998.
28. van der Woude, LH, et al: Seat height in handrim wheelchair propulsion. J Rehabil Res Dev 26(4):31, 1989.
29. World Health Organization: Obesity: Preventing and Managing the Global Epidemic. Report of a WHO Consultation. World Health Organ Tech Rep Ser 894, Geneva, Switzerland, 2000.
30 Beaumont-White, S, and Ham, RO: Powered wheelchairs: Are we enabling or disabling? Prosthet Orthot Int 21(1):62, 1997.
31. Lacoste, M, et al: Powered tilt/recline systems: Why and how are they used? Assist Technol 15(1):58, 2003.

Supplemental Readings

Algood, SD, et al: Effect of a pushrim-activated power-assist wheelchair on the functional capabilities of persons with tetraplegia. Arch Phys Med Rehabil 86(3):380, 2005.

Axelson, P, et al: The Manual Wheelchair Training Guide. PAX Press, Santa Cruz, CA, 1998.

Bain, B, and Leger, D: Assistive Technology: An Interdisciplinary Approach. Churchill Livingstone, New York, 1997.

Centers for Medicare & Medicaid Services (CMS), HHS, Medicare program: Conditions for payment of power mobility devices, including power wheelchairs and power-operated vehicles: Interim final rule with comment period. Fed Regist 70(165):50939, 2005.

Clarke, P, and Colantonio, A: Wheelchair use among community-dwelling older adults: Prevalence and risk factors in a national sample. Can J Aging 24(2):191, 2005.

Cook, AM, and Hussey, SM: Assistive Technologies: Principles and Practice. CV Mosby, St. Louis, 2002.

Cooper, RA, et al: Braking electric-powered wheelchairs: Effect of braking method, seatbelt, and legrests. Arch Phys Med Rehabil 79(10):1244, 1998.

Cooper, RA, et al: Evaluation of a pushrim-activated, power-assisted wheelchair. Arch Phys Med Rehabil 82(5):702, 2001.

Cooper, RA, et al: Performance of selected lightweight wheelchairs on ANSI/RESNA tests. Arch Phys Med Rehabil 78(10):1138, 1997.

De Groot, S, et al: Course of gross mechanical efficiency in handrim wheelchair propulsion during rehabilitation of people with spinal cord injury: A prospective cohort study. Arch Phys Med Rehabil 86(7):1452, 2005.

Dutta, T, and Fernie, GR: Utilization of ultrasound sensors for anti-collision systems of powered wheelchairs. IEEE Trans Neural Syst Rehabil Eng 13(1):24, 2005.

Engstrom, B: Ergonomic Seating: A True Challenge When Using Wheelchairs. Posturalis Books, Hasselby, Sweden, 2002.

Ferguson-Pell, M, et al: The role of wheelchair seating standards in determining clinical practices and funding policy. Assist Technol 17(1):1, 2005.

Gaal, RP, et al: Wheelchair rider injuries: Causes and consequences for wheelchair design and selection. J Rehabil Res Dev 34(1):58, 1997.

Gavin-Dreschnack, D, et al: Wheelchair-related falls: Current evidence and directions for improved quality care. J Nurs Care Qual 20(2):119, 2005.

Gibson, J, and Frank, A: Pain experienced by electric-powered chair users: A pilot exploration using pain drawings. Physiother Res Int 10(2):110, 2005.

Gutierres, DD, et al: Effect of fore-aft seat position on shoulder demands during wheelchair propulsion, part 2: An electromyographic analysis. J Spinal Cord Med 28(3):222, 2005.

Hall, K, et al: Power mobility driving training for seniors: A pilot study. Assist Technol 17(1):47, 2005.

Hoenig, H, et al: A clinical trial of a rehabilitation expert clinician versus usual care for providing manual wheelchairs. J Am Geriatr Soc 53(10):1712, 2005.

Holliday, PJ, et al: Understanding and measuring powered wheelchair mobility and manoeuvrability, part I: Reach in confined spaces. Disabil Rehabil 19;27(16):939, 2005.

Kernozek, TW, and Lewin, JE: Seat interface pressures of individuals with paraplegia: Influence of dynamic wheelchair locomotion compared with static seated measurements. Arch Phys Med Rehabil 79(3):313, 1998.

Kirby, RL, DiPersio, M, and MacLeod, D: Wheelchair safety: Effect of locking or grasping the rear wheels during a rear tip. Arch Phys Med Rehabil 77(12):1266, 1996.

Kotajarvi, BR, et al: The effect of seat position on wheelchair propulsion biomechanics. J Rehabil Res Dev 41(3B):403, 2004.

Levy, CE, and Chow, JW: Pushrim-activated power-assist wheelchairs: Elegance in motion. Am J Phys Med Rehabil 83(2):166, 2004.

Levy, CE, et al: Variable ratio power assist wheelchair eases wheeling over a variety of terrains for elders. Arch Phys Med Rehabil 85(1):104, 2004.

Minkel, JL: Seating and mobility considerations for people with spinal cord injury. Phys Ther 80(7):701, 2000.

Mortenson, WB, et al: Perceptions of power mobility use and safety within residential facilities. Can J Occup Ther 72(3):142, 2005.

Mulroy, SJ, et al: Effect of fore-aft seat position on shoulder demands during wheelchair propulsion, part 1: A kinetic analysis. J Spinal Cord Med 28(3):214, 2005.

Postma, K, et al: Validity of the detection of wheelchair propulsion as measured with an Activity Monitor in patients with spinal cord injury. Spinal Cord 43(9):550, 2005.

Reed, MP, and van Roosmalen, L: A pilot study of a method for assessing the reach capability of wheelchair users for safety belt design. Appl Ergon 36(5):523, 2005.

Richter, WM, and Axelson, PW: Low-impact wheelchair propulsion: Achievable and acceptable. J Rehabil Res Dev 42(3 Suppl 1):21, 2005.

Sawatzky, BJ, et al: Prevalence of shoulder pain in adult-versus childhood-onset wheelchair users: A pilot study. J Rehabil Res Dev 42(3 Suppl 1):1, 2005.

Simpson, R, et al: A prototype power assist wheelchair that provides for obstacle detection and avoidance for those with visual impairments. J Neuroeng Rehabil 3(2):30, 2005.

Souza, AL, et al: Upper limb strength in individuals with spinal cord injury who use manual wheelchairs. J Spinal Cord Med 28(1):26, 2005.

Van Drongelen, S, et al: Mechanical load on the upper extremity during wheelchair activities. Arch Phys Med Rehabil 86(6):1214, 2005.

Van Drongelen, S, et al: Glenohumeral contact forces and muscle forces evaluated in wheelchair-related activities of daily living in able-bodied subjects versus subjects with paraplegia and tetraplegia. Arch Phys Med Rehabil 86(7):1434, 2005.

Zollars, JA: Special Seating: An Illustrated Guide. Otto Bock, Minneapolis, MN, 1996.

Appendix A: Features of the Wheelchair Postural Support System

	Characteristics	Postural Control Provided (at impairment level)	Functional Assistance Provided (at the functional limitation/ disability level)	Advantages	Disadvantages
Seat Supports					
Solid insert	• Padded insert board; reinforcement board inside cushion cover; contoured or flat insert board between cushion and wheelchair upholstery. • Can be used with any cushion, custom or pre-made, for comfort or pressure relief. • Velcro® interface to upholstery. • Spans seat rails or mounts to upholstery between seat rails. • Works best with cushions that have zip-off cover to allow use of wide strips of Velcro® interfacing to hold cushion securely. • Addition of extra Velcro® sewn to upholstery and underside or cover will hold better during sliding transfers.	• Creates stable, level base of support. • Decreases tendency toward adduction and internal rotation of LEs, posterior pelvic tilt, and slipping forward in the seat. • Improves pelvic position. • Encourages level pelvis, neutral pelvic tilt, symmetrical spinal alignment.	• Good base on which to promote trunk extension and upper body stability. • Enhances distal function (head and UEs).	• Low cost. • Adds minimal weight to frame. • Removes easily for chair folding. • Wheelchair can still be used if solid insert is lost or forgotten.	• Increases seat height. • Can shift on seat and produce asymmetrical sitting surface.
Solid hook-on seat	• Seat upholstery is removed and solid seat is installed using hardware to hook to seat rails. • Hardware can be fixed level with seat rails or dropped lower than seat rails. • Angle and height adjustable; allows changing position of seat surface on frame of new or existing frame.	• Improves pelvic position. • Creates stable, level base of support. • Decreases tendency toward adduction and internal rotation of LEs, posterior pelvic tilt, and slipping forward on the seat. • Encourages level pelvis, neutral pelvic tilt, symmetrical spinal alignment.	• Good base on which to promote trunk extension and upper body stability. • Enhances distal function (head and UEs). • With forward slope, allows increased ROM in UE for reach and wheel approach.	• Can change slope of seat without tilt-in-space chair. • Wheelchair cannot be used if seat support is missing; ensures use at all times. • Dropped style can reduce effect of thick seat cushion on seat height. • Does not shift during transfers.	• More difficult to remove for folding than Velcro® interface. • Adds weight to frame.

(*continued*)

Appendix A: Features of the Wheelchair Postural Support System (continued)

	Characteristics	Postural Control Provided (at impairment level)	Functional Assistance Provided (at the functional limitation/ disability level)	Advantages	Disadvantages
		• Raising anterior portion of seat can help keep patient back on wheelchair seat. • Raising posterior aspect of seat can facilitate trunk cocontraction.		• Seat angles can be changed to accommodate limited ROM.	
Seat Cushions					
Comfort cushion (planar/contoured)	• Usually planar, but may have slight generic contour. • Varying degrees of firmness available for different comfort levels. • Can be made of layered foam to mix firmness for postural control and to accommodate limited ROM (e.g., more flexion in one hip as compared to the other can be accommodated by different firmnesses, or by actually cutting the foam into different shapes).	• Increases comfort; facilitates level pelvis; promotes a neutral pelvic position. • Provides surface to create stable base of support.	• Appropriate for patients with minimal seating needs. • Does not interfere with sliding transfers.	• Inexpensive. • Lightweight. • Patient can sit anywhere on cushion without discomfort. • Totally flat cushions with one firmness throughout can be rotated to decrease spot wear.	• No pressure relief. • Minimal support. • Minimal postural control.
Pressure-relieving foam (contoured, custom contoured)	• Based on principle that increased surface contact results in improved pressure distribution/relief. • Custom or pre-made contour depends on need to accommodate individual postural asymmetries. • Varying degrees of firmness available. • Can be made of layered foam to mix firmness for postural control and to accommodate limited ROM. • Generic shapes work best with symmetrical individuals.	• Shaped to control postural alignment. • Increases comfort; facilitates level pelvis; promotes a neutral pelvic position. • Provides surface to create stable base of support. • Custom-made contour more effective when accommodating asymmetries.	• Appropriate for patients with moderate to significant seating needs. • Assists with controlling posture and/or accommodating pelvic asymmetries to allow level shoulders and more erect head position. • Increases sitting time; decreases problems with pressure over bony prominences; improves postural stability that results in increased upper body function.	• Increased surface contact, creating improved pressure distribution. • Accommodates moderate to severe postural asymmetry. • Easier for caregivers to position and reposition the patient. • Low maintenance.	• More expensive. • May interfere with sliding transfers. • Patient may feel "locked in" because movement on cushion surface is restricted.

Pressure-relieving fluid or fluid/foam combination	• Based on the principle that increased surface contact results in improved pressure distribution/relief; generic contour or planar surface with fluid filled sack. • Bony prominences are "immersed" in the fluid, increasing surface contact. • Some types have positioning components to accommodate for postural asymmetries and provide improved postural control. • Combination units allow the foam base to be cut to accommodate limited ROM. • Generic contoured shapes work best with symmetrical individuals. • Firm under base provides stable support for proper seating alignment.	• Provides surface to create stable base of support. • Some have add-on pieces to control postural alignment. • Increases comfort; facilitates level pelvis; promotes a neutral pelvic position. • Increases sitting tolerance for patients who sit with oblique pelvis. • Provides appropriate support for pelvis to promote level shoulders and erect head.	• Appropriate for patients with moderate to significant seating needs. • Assists with controlling posture and/or accommodating pelvic asymmetries to allow level shoulders and more erect head position. • Results in increased sitting time; decreased problems with pressure over bony prominences; improved postural stability; and increased upper body function. • Gel medium usually increases stability at the pelvis; the pelvis sinks in and is "held" by the foam, essentially broadening the base of support area.	• Increases surface area, contact creates improved pressure distribution. • Accommodates moderate to severe postural asymmetry. • Increases stability at the pelvis. • Easier for caregivers to position and reposition patient.	• More expensive. • Some maintenance required. • Heavier than foam or air. • Patient may feel "locked in" because movement on cushion surface is restricted.
Pressure-relieving air	• Appears planar, but responds to patient weight. • Patient is "immersed" in the cushion based on regulation of the amount of air. • Based on principle that increased surface contact results in improved pressure distribution/relief; bony prominences are "floating."	• Does not provide a very stable base of support; some users find it too unstable. • Individuals with decreased trunk stability tend to keep arms closer to the body for stability, decreasing UE reach distance.	• Imperative for patients with moderate to significant pressure-relieving needs. • Results in increased sitting time; decreased problems with pressure over bony prominences.	• Very lightweight. • Accommodates moderates to severe postural asymmetry. • Increases surface contact for improved pressure distribution.	• More expensive. • Base provided may be too unstable for some user; unstable base may make transfers difficult. • Air pressure must be monitored carefully. • Continuous maintenance required.

(*continued*)

Appendix A: Features of the Wheelchair Postural Support System (continued)

	Characteristics	Postural Control Provided (at impairment level)	Functional Assistance Provided (at the functional limitation/ disability level)	Advantages	Disadvantages
		• Some air cushions are segmented to allow more air into selected segments to improve postural control (it should be noted that segmented cushions are less pressure relieving because the air cannot flow from one segment of the cushion to another). • Additional postural accommodation can be provided by placing foam pieces under the cushion.			
Back Supports					
Pita back	• Solid board (padded or unpadded) that slips in to a pocket in the back upholstery. • Provides mild to moderate level of support. • Useful for patients who need a slight reminder to sit upright.	• Assists patients who need a reminder to sit with trunk extension. • Assists with maintaining a neutral pelvis and an upright sitting posture.	• Provides enough support to encourage trunk extension.	• Lightweight. • Slips in and out easily for folding.	• Only provides slight degree of support. • Wheelchair can be used without this back support. • It can be lost or left behind when the chair is folded.

Solid insert	• Maintains pelvic alignment when correctly interfaced with seat surface (based on ROM examination to determine available hip flexion). • If attached to the upholstery by Velcro®, or hung between the back canes, it provides moderate support and will not decrease seat surface depth on the chair. • If hung or belted in front of the back canes, will decrease seat surface depth. • Will assume the angle of the back canes unless braced across the top. • Special foaming can be used to accommodate back contour or provide some postural control.	• Maintains pelvic alignment when interfaced with seat surface. • Enhances upright sitting, trunk and head alignment. • Provides some lateral control if shaped foaming is used.	• Enhances trunk control to allow improved distal function.	• Removes easily for folding. • Assists with postural control. • Adds minimal weight to chair.	• May not be stable in chair. • Wheelchair can be used without this back support. • It can be lost or left behind when the chair is folded.
Solid hook-on back	• Very stable back support that can be aligned and angled as needed to create appropriate seat/back angle; accommodates for limited ROM. • Can hold planar, contoured, or molded back, or air flotation cushion for pressure relief. • Can be manufactured or custom-made. • Allows for provision of maximum support when needed. • Mounts using permanent or removable hardware; with use of permanent hardware, can actually strengthen frame.	• Enhances upright sitting; accommodates for limited ROM; accommodates for any degree of deformity; provides support as needed. • Maintains client in position deemed appropriate based on examination findings.	• Provides support to enhance movement control of the UE and the head. • Increases surface area, contact provides improved comfort and pressure relief. • Maintains trunk alignment to enhance pelvic positioning.	• Solid support structure. • Resists extensor thrusting. • Accepts planar, contoured, or molded surfaces. • Wheelchair cannot be used without this back support in place. • Allows attachment of additional supports such as headrests which work best when back structure is solid and stable.	• Increases weight of wheelchair. • Requires manipulation of hardware to remove and fold wheelchair.

(continued)

Appendix A: Features of the Wheelchair Postural Support System (continued)

	Characteristics	Postural Control Provided (at impairment level)	Functional Assistance Provided (at the functional limitation/ disability level)	Advantages	Disadvantages
Specialized Support Components					
Head/neck supports	• Provides support for patients with fair, poor, or absent head control. • Mounting hardware can be fixed, removable, and/or flip back; hardware can be adjusted in one, two, or multiple planes.	• Posterior, lateral, and anterior head or neck controllers available. • Promotes maintenance of a neutral cervical spine and head position. • Eliminates lateral flexion and rotation, which, when not controlled, can disturb trunk and pelvic alignment.	• Supports the head to assist with respiration, visual interaction with environment, feeding, and swallowing. • Improves safety during transport on level surfaces and when patient is transported seated in wheelchair placed a motor vehicle.	• Provides support and improves alignment. • Improves safety during transport.	• May interfere with head movement. • May trigger extensor thrust. • May cause skin problems in areas of high pressure.
Lateral trunk supports	• Indicated in the presence of weak or spastic trunk muscles. • Can be straight or contoured for more control. • Mounting hardware can be fixed or swing away for transfers.	• Improves trunk stability and alignment (within available range); improves pelvic alignment. • Controls lateral trunk flexion.	• Improves trunk control; facilitates UE movement and distal control. • Improves respiration, feeding, and swallowing.	• Improves stability and alignment. • Improves head alignment and control. • Enhances safety during movement through space.	• May interfere with trunk movement. • Increases weight of the system. • May interfere with attempts to self-propel with UE.
Anterior chest support	• Assists with maintenance of upright trunk posture and control of shoulder position. • Can be minimally supportive or maximally supportive depending on configuration of features (e.g., straps, padded straps, butterfly, and bib).	• Supports trunk along anterior surface of trunk and shoulders, eliminates forward lean. • May influence and discourage shoulder protraction.	• Trunk support may improve respiration, eating, and swallowing. • Stabilizes trunk to allow improved UE function and head control. • Shoulder control promotes better head posture.	• Supports trunk in upright position. • Stabilizes trunk to free arms and head for movement. • Improves head position for respiration, eating, swallowing, and visual interaction with environment.	• Restricts trunk movement. • Overuse limits patient's opportunity to improve trunk control.

Lateral hip guides	• Improves pelvic alignment on seat. • Assists with maintaining pelvic position on contoured seat.	• Improves weight distribution on pelvis. • Improves pelvic positioning; enhances alignment of upper and lower body segments; contributes to alignment of entire body. • Assists with maintenance of pelvic alignment, which reduces asymmetries in trunk and LEs.	• Allows patient to achieve or tolerate better alignment. • Increases sitting time.	• Improves and maintains alignment. • Improves symmetrical weightbearing through pelvis.	• May interfere with transfers if not removable. • Patient may feel "locked in" on seat. • Increases weight of the system.
Lateral knee guides	• May be built into the cushion contours, or fabricated from separate pieces of padded wood or plastic attached to the seat or armrest of the wheelchair; • Should extend to the end of the knee if maximal control is required.	• Helps to maintain LE alignment; reduces excessive abduction and external rotation (e.g., patients who tend to fall into abduction, push into abduction, or whose legs do not come into neutral). • Improves neutral alignment of LEs; assists with maintenance of pelvic position. • Maintains LE alignment in combination with anterior knee block.	• Improves pelvic position. • Promotes improved trunk position and UE function. • Maintains neutral alignment of LEs. • Reduces forward sliding of pelvis on seat.	• Maintains LE alignment. • Assists with maintenance of pelvic position on seat.	• If high enough to provide control, may interfere with transfers unless removable. • Adds weight to the seating system.

(*continued*)

Appendix A: Features of the Wheelchair Postural Support System (continued)

	Characteristics	Postural Control Provided (at impairment level)	Functional Assistance Provided (at the functional limitation/disability level)	Advantages	Disadvantages
Medial knee block	• May be built into the cushion contours, or be a separate or removable flip-down block. • For maximal control, the medial knee block should be positioned at the distal portion of the limb, between the condyles. • The support should never be used to stabilize the pelvis on the seat by pressing into the groin; it also should not be used to stop the user from sliding off the front of the seat.	• Prevents LEs from moving into adduction. • If wide enough, may decrease spasticity. • Maintains LE alignment. • When used with windblown position,[a] medial knee block can prevent pelvis from continuing to rotate forward. • Use of wider blocks will keep the greater trochanter properly seated in the hip joint.	• Helps to maintain a broad, stable base of support; this base improves alignment of the upper body.	• Maintains LE alignment. • Reduces extensor tone. • May help to elongate adductors. • Provides broad base of support.	• May interfere with transfers. • Increases weight of seat.
Anterior knee block	• Increases pelvic stability; most effective way to maintain proper pelvic position on the seat. Note: if hips are subluxed, dislocated, or not properly formed, approval from an orthopedist should be obtained.	• Maintains pelvic alignment; maintains pelvis in neutral tilt; prevents pelvis form moving forward on seat surface. • Assists with maintenance of LE alignment when used with medial and lateral knee controls.	• Helps to maintain a broad, stable base of support with neutral pelvic alignment; this base will promote improved alignment and functional use of upper body. • When used in conjunction with forward sloped seat, may facilitate trunk cocontraction, extension, and improved UE ROM.	• Maintains LE alignment. • Reduces extensor tone. • Provides broad base of support. • Increases stability.	• May impose too much pressure at the hips and over the patellas. • Patient may feel restricted.

[a]Windblown position: Both LEs oriented to one side with one LE adducted and the other abducted.

Glossary

Abarognosis: Inability to recognize weight.

Acalculia: Inability to perform simple arithmetic operations; inability to calculate.

Acceleration: The rate of change of velocity with respect to time.

Accelerometer: A device used to measure the vertical, anterior–posterior, and medial–lateral accelerations of the body.

Accessibility: The degree to which an environment affords use of its resources with respect to an individual's level of function.

Accessible design: The structural plan of buildings or dwellings that meet prescribed standards for accessibility.

Accessory (joint play) motions: Motions between adjacent joint surfaces that occur when a bone moves through a range of motion; includes slides (glides), distractions, compressions, rolls, and spins.

Acoustic neuroma: Benign tumor of the vestibulocochlear cranial nerve.

Activation: The production of a movement response once critical threshold for neuronal firing is reached.

Active coping strategies: Techniques used to deal actively with stressful situations, such as assertiveness.

Active range of motion (AROM): The amount of joint motion obtained with unassisted voluntary joint motion.

Activities of daily living (ADL): Daily living skills necessary for an adult to manage life. *Basic ADL* (BADL) include grooming skills such as oral hygiene, showering or bathing, dressing, feeding, toilet hygiene, and personal device care (e.g., a splint). *Instrumental ADL* (IADL) include money management, functional communication and socialization, functional and community mobility, and health maintenance. Often included in ADL are sexual expression, medication routine, and emergency response.

Activity: The nature and extent of functioning at the level of the person. Activities may be limited in nature, duration, and quality.

Activity pacing: The balancing of activity with rest periods interspersed throughout the day.

Acute stress disorder (ASD): A diagnostic subset of stress disorders generally indicating a sudden onset of relatively short duration.

Adaptation: Alteration of the environment to compensate for dysfunction.

Adaptive equipment: Devices or equipment designed and fabricated to improve performance in activities of daily living.

Adaptive motor performance: The ability of the central nervous system to modify sensory and motor systems in response to changing demands (task, environment, injury); modification is based on feedback and experience (practice).

Adventitious breath sounds: Crackles or wheezes; heard during auscultation, in addition to the overall quality of the breath sound.

Aerobic exercise: Any sustained exercise in which the required energy is supplied by the available oxygen within the system.

Affect management: Controlling emotions by actively using various techniques or strategies.

Affective function: Mental and emotional skills and coping strategies needed to manage everyday tasks and stresses as well as the more traumatic events each person encounters over the course of a lifetime.

Agenesis: The failure of an organ or part of an organ to develop or grow.

Agnosia: The inability to recognize familiar objects with one sensory modality, while retaining the ability to recognize the same object with other sensory modalities.

Agraphia: Disorders of writing not due to motor difficulties in letter formation.

Akathisia: Extreme motor restlessness.

Akinesia: Inability to initiate or execute movement.

Allesthesia: Sensation experienced at a site remote from point of stimulation.

Allodynia: Pain produced by non-noxious stimulus (e.g., light touch).

Allograft (or homograft): Skin used for temporary coverage of a burn wound; the skin is taken from the same species (usually cadaver skin).

Alternating attention: The capacity to move between tasks and respond appropriately to the demands of each task.

Amnesia: A loss of memory.

Amyotrophic lateral sclerosis (ALS): A degenerative disease of the nervous system of unknown cause, affecting both upper and lower motor neurons; commonly known as Lou Gehrig's disease.

Analgesia: Complete loss of pain sensibility.

Analgesic: Medication or modality used to relieve pain.

Anarthria: Unintelligible speech resulting from a brain lesion, particularly in the brainstem, causing severe impairment of the motor–speech system. See also *Dysarthria*.

Anesthesia: Loss of sensation.

Aneurysm: Localized arterial wall weakness with abnormal dilatation of a blood vessel due to congenital defect.

Angina (angina pectoris): An oppressive pain or pressure in the chest caused by inadequate blood flow and oxygenation of heart muscle.

Angle of Louis: Anatomical landmark on the chest wall for the right atrium; the bony demarcation of the manubrium from the body of the sternum.

Angular velocity: The rate of motion in rotation of a body segment around an axis.

Ankylosing spondylitis: Chronic bone and joint disease in which the inflammatory process affects primarily the sacroiliac, spinal facet, and costovertebral joints.

Ankylosis: Immobility or fixation of a joint.

Anorexia: Loss of appetite.

Anosognosia: A perceptual impairment including denial, neglect, and lack of awareness of the presence or severity of one's paralysis.

Anoxia: Absence of oxygen.

Anterior cord syndrome: An incomplete spinal cord lesion with primary damage in the anterior cord; there is loss of motor function and sense of pain and temperature, with preservation of proprioception, kinesthesia, and vibration below the level of the lesion.

Antibody: A protein developed in response to an antigen, belonging to one of the immunoglobulin classes.

Anticipatory postural control: The ability of the CNS to modify sensory and motor systems in advance of movement; pretuning is based on previous learning and feedforward mechanisms.

Antidromic conduction: Propagation of an action potential in a direction opposite the normal (orthodromic) direction for that fiber (i.e., conduction along motor fibers toward the spinal cord, and conduction along sensory fibers away from the spinal cord).

Antigen: Any substance that induces the formation of antibodies that will react specifically to that antigen.

Anxiety: An emotional state consisting of uneasy feelings of anticipation or dread of real or imagined danger; associated with an autonomic response.

Aphasia: Communication disorder caused by brain damage and characterized by an impairment of language comprehension, formulation, and use; excludes disorders associated with primary sensory deficits, general mental deterioration, or psychiatric disorders. Partial impairment is often referred to as *dysphasia*.

Apnea: Absence of respirations, usually temporary in duration.

Apoptosis: A mode of cell death in which the cell actively participates in its own destruction by activating preprogrammed intracellular mechanisms.

Apraxia: An impairment of voluntary learned movement that is characterized by an inability to perform purposeful movements not accounted for by inadequate strength, loss of coordination, impaired sensation, attentional deficits, or lack of comprehension.

Arousal: Alertness; the state of being prepared to act.

Arteriography: Radiographic visualization of an artery following insertion of a radiopaque material.

Arteriole: The smallest subunit of the arterial system.

Arteriosclerosis obliterans: Arteriosclerosis in which the lumen of the artery is completely occluded.

Arteriovenous malformation (AVM): An abnormality in embryonic development leading to a skein of tangled arteries and veins, usually without an intervening capillary bed; its rupture produces hemorrhage.

Arthralgia: Pain in a joint.

Arthrodesis: Surgical procedure designed to produce fusion of a joint.

Arthrokinematics: The motion of adjacent joint surfaces that occurs when a bone moves through a range of motion.

Arthroplasty: Any surgical reconstruction of a joint; may or may not involve prosthetic replacement.

Artifacts (EMG or ECG): Voltage signals generated by a source other than the one of interest.

Aspiration: Penetration of food, liquid, saliva, or gastric reflux into the airway; common in patients with dysphagia.

Asset: An individual's strengths and abilities that can be used for reinforcement and emphasis during therapy; also includes supportive social structure and environment.

Associated reactions: Automatic responses of the limbs that occur as a result of action occurring in some other part of the body, either by voluntary or reflex stimulation. In hemiplegia, associated reactions are stereotyped and abnormal.

Association: Strong feelings of identification with another person.

Associative stage (motor learning): The second or middle stage of learning (Fitts-Posner) in which the skill strategy has been selected and the skill is refined through continued practice.

Astereognosis (tactile agnosia): Inability to recognize the form and shape of objects by touch.

Asthenia: Generalized muscle weakness, especially in muscular or cerebellar disease.

Asthma: A clinical syndrome characterized by increased reactivity of the tracheobronchial tree to various stimuli.

Asynergia: Loss of ability to associate muscles together for complex movements.

Ataxia: Uncoordinated movement that manifests when voluntary movements are attempted; may influence gait, posture, and patterns of movements.

Atelectasis: Alveolar collapse involving part or all of the lung due to obstruction of a bronchus or the inability of the alveoli to expand.

Atherosclerosis: A form of arteriosclerosis in which yellowish plaques (atheromas) form within the vessel walls; plaques consist of lipids and other blood-borne substances.

Athetosis: A condition in which slow, involuntary, writhing, twisting, "wormlike" movements occur.

Atopognosia: Inability to localize a sensation.

Atrophy: Loss of muscle bulk (wasting); origin can be primary neurogenic (lower motor neuron disease or injury) or disuse (inactivity).

Attention: Capacity of the brain to process information from the environment or from long-term memory.

Augmentative communication device: A device used by a person impaired by a communication disorder that provides a compensatory means of communication or enhances the individual's residual communication skills (e.g., manual and electronic communication boards).

Autograft: Skin taken from an unburned area of a patient, which is then transplanted to cover a wound.

Autoimmune disease: A disease produced when the body's normal tolerance of the antigens of its own cells (i.e., self-antigens or autoantigens [Aag]) is disrupted.

Autolytic débridement: Use of the body's endogenous enzymes to digest devitalized tissue and promote granulation tissue formation.

Automatic postural synergies: Discrete patterns of extremity and trunk muscle contractions characterized by consistency in muscle combinations, timing, and intensity (e.g., to preserve standing balance).

Automaticity: The process by which skills, or certain aspects of skills, can be performed with minimum conscious effort and attention.

Autonomic dysreflexia (hyperreflexia): A pathological autonomic reflex seen in patients with high-level spinal cord injuries. It is precipitated by a noxious stimulus below the level of the lesion and produces an acute onset of autonomic activity. It is considered an emergency situation characterized by hypertension, bradycardia, headache, and sweating.

Autonomous stage (motor learning): The third stage of learning (Fitts-Posner) in which the spatial and temporal aspects of movement become highly organized through continued practice; skills are characterized by automaticity and a low degree of attention.

Autonomy: A quality or state of self-governance or independence. The patient's right to choose for his or her life, and to voice that choice for as long as possible.

Avascular necrosis: Necrosis of part of a bone secondary to ischemia; most commonly seen in the femoral or humeral head.

Babinski sign: Dorsiflexion of the great toe with fanning of the other toes on stimulation of the lateral sole of the foot.

Balance (postural stability): The condition in which all the forces acting on the body are balanced such that the center of mass (COM) is within the limits of stability, the boundaries of the base of support (BOS).

Bandwidth feedback (bandwidth KR): Augmented feedback given when performance exceeds a predetermined range of errors.

Barognosis: Ability to recognize weight.

Behavioral shaping techniques: Techniques that involve the modification of behavior through the use of reinforcement and rewards given for correct performance (e.g., praise); a program of self-monitoring training is also an important component.

Beneficence: Doing what is best for the patient.

Benevolence: Being kind and good hearted.

Benign paroxysmal positional vertigo (BPPV): Vertigo and nystagmus that occurs as a result of otoconia in the semicircular canals, displaced from the utricle.

Beveled (surface): Smooth, slanted angle between two surfaces; for example, a slant or inclination between two uneven surfaces to allow easier passage of a wheelchair.

Bilateral transfer: Transfer of learning that occurs between limbs.

Biopsychosocial model: A model of illness that uses a combined approach, incorporating biological/physiological, psychological, and social realms.

Blanch: A white spot seen on the skin when pressure is applied; an indication of the presence of viable capillary beds.

Blocked practice: A practice schedule in which one skill is practiced repeatedly before progressing to practice of another skill during the practice session.

Blood pressure: The amount of pressure within the arteries throughout the cardiac cycle; a product of CO_2 and peripheral vascular resistance.

Body image: A visual and mental image of one's body that includes feelings about one's body, especially in relation to health and disease.

Body mass index (BMI): An index used to control for both height and weight; determined by dividing body weight by standing height.

Body scheme: A postural model of one's body, including the relationship of the body parts to each other and the relationship of the body to the environment.

Bouchard's nodes: Osteophyte formation around the proximal interphalangeal joint.

Boutonniere deformity: Contracture of hand musculature marked by proximal interphalangeal joint flexion and distal interphalangeal joint extension.

Bradycardia: Abnormally slow (low) pulse rate, below approximately 50 beats per minute.

Bradykinesia: Extreme slowness and difficulty maintaining movement.

Bradyphrenia: A disorder of intellectual function characterized by a slowing of thought processes with lack of concentration and attention.

Bradypnea: Abnormally slow respiratory rate; 10 or fewer breaths per minute.

Brain attack: See *Stroke*.

Brainstem herniation: Secondary brain damage and neurological deterioration resulting from significant edema, elevated intracranial pressures, with resulting contralateral and caudal shifts of brain structures.

Break test: A method of applying resistance during manual muscle testing or hand-held dynamometry in which the patient holds a joint position until the therapist gradually overpowers the patient and an eccentric contraction begins to occur.

Brown-Sequard syndrome: Incomplete spinal cord lesion caused by hemisection of the cord; characterized by loss of motor function, proprioception, and kinesthesia on the side of the lesion with loss of sense of pain and temperature on the opposite side.

Bulbocavernosus reflex (positive): Pressure on the glans penis or glans clitoris that elicits a contraction of the external anal sphincter.

Bunion: Hallux valgus with a painful bursitis over the medial aspect of the first metatarsophalangeal joint.

Bursitis: Inflammation of a bursa that can be due to frictional forces, trauma, or rheumatoid diseases.

Cachexia: State of ill health with an appearance of malnutrition and wasting; associated with many chronic diseases.

Cadence: Number of steps per unit of time.

Calculation ability: Competence in foundational mathematical abilities such as addition, subtraction, multiplication, and division.

Capsular pattern: A characteristic pattern of restricted passive osteokinematic motion, usually involving more than one motion at a joint; indicates intra-articular joint inflammation or capsular fibrosis.

Cardiac index (CI): Cardiac output expressed in relation to body surface area.

Cardiac output (CO): The volume of blood that leaves the left ventricle per minute; it is a product of heart rate (HR) and stroke volume (SV); expressed in L/min.

Cardiogenic shock: Inadequate cardiac output and arterial blood pressure to perfuse the major organs; a life-threatening event.

Cardiomyopathies: Any disease that affects heart muscle and diminishes cardiac performance.

Caregivers: Individuals who are responsible for the patient's/client's care, including home health aides, day-care providers, teachers, or educational aides.

Carpal tunnel syndrome: Compression of the median nerve in the carpal flexor space; commonly seen in patients with flexor tenosynovitis.

Catecholamine: One of many biologically active amines, including dopamine, norepinephrine, epinephrine, and metanephrine. They have a marked effect on the nervous and cardiovascular systems, metabolic rate, temperature, and smooth muscle.

Cauda equina lesion: A spinal injury with damage to peripheral nerve roots below the first lumbar vertebra; some regeneration is possible.

Center of mass (COM): The midpoint of the body; in the erect standing posture, the CoM is located at the level of the second sacral segment.

Center of pressure (COP): The point of application of the ground reaction forces located between the feet in bilateral stance.

Central cord syndrome: Incomplete spinal cord lesion characterized by greater neurological involvement in upper extremities (cervical tracts more centrally located) than in the lower extremities (lumbar and sacral tracts more peripheral).

Central post-stroke (thalamic) pain: Central pain that occurs after infarction involving the spinothalamic system, the ventral posterolateral thalamus, or subcortical parietal lobe; pain is described as constant, burning pain with intermittent sharp pains; aggravated by noxious stimuli.

Cerebral embolus (CE): Bits of matter (blood clot, plaque, and less commonly air, fat) formed elsewhere are released into the bloodstream and travel to the cerebral arteries where they lodge in a vessel, producing occlusion and infarction.

Cerebral infarction (CI): Ischemia and necrosis of an area of the brain following a reduction of blood flow that falls below the critical level necessary for cell survival.

Cerebral shock: Transient hypotonia following injury to the brain.

Cerebral thrombosis: The formation or development of a blood clot within the cerebral arteries or their branches; also includes extracranial vessels (carotid or vertebral arteries).

Cerebrovascular accident (CVA): See *Stroke*.

Cervical vertigo: Symptoms of dizziness, imbalance, lightheadedness occurring as a result cervical pathology.

Charcot's triad: Cardinal symptoms of multiple sclerosis including intention tremor, scanning speech, and nystagmus.

Checklist: Functional instrument in which a description of various tasks is scored using a nominal measure (e.g., present/absent; completed/not completed).

Chorea: A movement disorder characterized by involuntary, rapid, irregular, jerky movements; seen in Huntington's disease (also called *choreiform movements*).

Choreoathetosis: Movement disorder with features of both chorea and athetosis; seen in some forms of cerebral palsy.

Chronic obstructive pulmonary disease (COPD): A disease process characterized by nonreversible airflow limitation. Clinical symptoms include cough, sputum production, and dyspnea.

Chronic venous insufficiency (CVI): Venous insufficiency that persists over a long period of time.

Chronotropic incompetence: Inability to increase heart rate appropriately in response to an increase in oxygen demand.

Circadian rhythm: Variations in vital sign values that occur on a regular and predictable 24-hour cycle.

Circle of Willis: Union of the anterior, middle, and posterior cerebral arteries (branches of the carotid and vertebrobasilar arteries), forming an anastomosis at the base of the brain.

Clasp-knife response: A sudden relaxation or letting go of a spastic muscle in response to a stretch stimulus.

Clients: Individuals who engage the services of a physical therapist and who can benefit from the physical therapist's consultation, interventions, professional advice, health promotion, fitness, wellness, or prevention services. Clients also are businesses, school systems, and others to whom physical therapists provide services.

Clinical decision making (clinical reasoning): A multidimensional process that involves a wide range of cognitive skills individuals use to process information, reach decisions, and determine actions.

Clonus: Cyclical, spasmodic alteration of muscular contraction and relaxation in response to a sustained stretch of a spastic muscle.

Closed motor skill: A movement skill performed in a stable, nonchanging environment.

Closed technique: The wound-care technique of covering a wound from the outside environment with an appropriate dressing.

Closed-loop control system: A motor control system that employs feedback and a reference for correctness to compute error and initiate subsequent corrections.

Clubbing: Bulbous swelling of the distal fingers and toes accompanied by a loss of the normal angle between the nailbed and the skin; associated with diagnoses imposing long-standing hypoxia and cyanosis such as congenital heart defects and pulmonary disorders.

Cock-up (claw) toe: Deformity with hyperextension of the metatarsophalangeal joint and flexion of the proximal and distal interphalangeal joints.

Code of Ethics: A set of moral norms adopted by a professional group to direct value-laden choices in a way consistent with professional responsibility.

Cognition: The act or process of knowing, including awareness, reasoning, judgment, intuition, and memory.

Cognitive deficits: Impaired functioning in memory, judgment, construction, attention, sequencing, planning, recognition, or sorting.

Cognitive rehabilitation: An approach to the remediation of cognitive–perceptual skills that focuses on how the individual acquires and uses knowledge, and seeks overall strategies for the brain-damaged patient to approach task performance.

Cognitive restructuring: The cognitive–behavioral therapy technique of reshaping a person's thoughts/beliefs.

Cognitive stage (motor learning): The initial stage of learning (Fitts-Posner) in which the cognitive plan for the skill is developed; the learner develops an understanding of the task, develops initial strategies, and determines how to evaluate the task.

Cognitive therapy: A psychosocial intervention that changes negative maladaptive thoughts and beliefs into positive, more adaptive ones.

Cogwheel rigidity: A hypertonic state of rigidity with superimposed rachet-like jerkiness; characterized by and alternate giving way and then increased resistance to movement.

Collateral sprouting (regenerative synaptogenesis): A form of function-induced plasticity in which growth of surviving nerve fibers is stimulated following injury.

Coma: A state of unconsciousness from which one cannot be aroused; the patient is unresponsive to stimulations.

Coma stimulation (early recovery management program): An organized program of sensory and environmental stimulation designed to improve the overall level of alertness and arousal of patients with brain injury who are emerging from coma and vegetative states.

Communication: Any means by which an individual relates experiences, ideas, knowledge, and feelings to another; includes speech, sign language, body language, gestures, writing; the process by which meanings are exchanged between individuals through a system of symbols.

Community integration: Introducing or reintroducing a person into a community.

Compassion: Sympathetic consciousness of another's situation and the desire to alleviate pain or suffering.

Compensated heart failure: Left ventricular dysfunction in which the compensatory mechanisms have provided an adequate cardiac output and blood pressure response; there are no systemic signs of congestion.

Compensation: Behavioral substitution of alternate strategies to accomplish a task.

Compensatory training: Intervention that is aimed at modifying the task, activity, or environment in order to allow the patient to maintain or regain function; behavioral substitution of alternate patterns of movement to accomplish the task.

Complete lesion (SCI): A spinal cord injury characterized by no sensory or motor function below the neurological level of lesion and no sensory or motor function in the lowest sacral segments (S4 and S5).

Complex Regional Pain Syndrome (CRPS): A complex disorder or group of syndromes that include causalgia and reflex sympathetic dystrophy (RSD); symptoms include pain and related sensory abnormalities, abnormal blood flow and sweating, abnormal motor function, and trophic changes.

Compression: The approximation of joint surfaces.

Conduction distance: Distance measured (in centimeters) between two points of stimulation along a nerve in a nerve conduction velocity test.

Conduction time (NCV): Time difference (in milliseconds) between the distal and proximal points of stimulation along a nerve trunk in a nerve conduction velocity test.

Conduction velocity (CV): Speed of propagation of an action potential along a nerve or muscle fiber; calculated in meters per second by dividing the conduction distance by the conduction time.

Confabulation: The patient fills in memory gaps with inappropriate words or fabricates stories.

Confidentiality: Keeping another person's trust private and secret, whether requested or not.

Congestive heart failure (CHF): The presence of pulmonary and/or peripheral congestion due to heart failure, most commonly left ventricular dysfunction.

Consciousness: A state of awareness; implies orientation to person, place, and time.

Context: Includes the features, aspects, attributes of, or objects, structures, human-made organization, service provision, and agencies in, the physical, social, and attitudinal environment in which people live and conduct their lives.

Contextual interference: The interference that results from practicing one task within the context of other tasks; e.g., high contextual interference occurs with practice of multiple skills in a random practice order.

Continuous motor skill: A motor skill with arbitrary beginning and end points.

Conversion disorder: A psychological disorder expressed by symptoms or deficits in sensory or motor systems that mimic a neurological or general medical disease.

Coordination: The ability to execute smooth, accurate, and controlled motor responses.

Cor Pulmonale: Hypertrophy or failure of the right ventricle from a primary pulmonary cause.

Coronary artery bypass graft (CABG): Surgical revascularization procedure to restore coronary blood flow through new blood vessel grafts.

Coronary artery disease (CAD): Heart disease resulting from a narrowing of the coronary arteries as a result of atherosclerosis.

Coronary spasm: Transient occlusion of a coronary artery due to spasm of the arterial smooth muscle.

Cortical blindness: A total failure to appreciate incoming visual sensory information owing to a lesion in the cortex, rather than injury to the eyes.

Costal breathing: A breathing pattern characterized by use of accessory muscles of respiration; also called *thoracic breathing*.

Coup-contrecoup injury: Injury caused by back-and-forth movement of the brain in the skull; coup contusions occur at the site of impact while contrecoup contusions occur in the brain opposite the initial point of impact.

Crackles (rales): An abnormal auscultatory finding within the lungs characterized by rattling or bubbling sounds that occur owing to secretions in the air passages of the respiratory tract; the sound is often compared to that of rustling a cellophane bag.

Credé maneuver: Technique for emptying urine from a flaccid bladder; repeated pressure is placed between the umbilicus and symphysis pubis in a downward direction; manual pressure is also placed directly over the bladder to further facilitate removal of urine.

Crepitus: A grating, crunching, or popping sensation (or sound) that occurs during joint or tendon motion.

Cumulative trauma disorder (CTD): Direct and indirect impairments with concomitant dysfunction and disability related to, but not solely caused by repetitive work tasks.

Cyanosis: Dusky, bluish, gray, or dark purple color changes in the mucous membranes or skin caused by deoxygenated or reduced hemoglobin in the blood.

Cystic fibrosis: A genetic disorder characterized by an exocrine gland dysfunction that results in abnormally viscid secretions.

Débridement: The removal of foreign material and necrotic or damaged tissue.

Decerebrate rigidity: Sustained contraction and posturing of the trunk and limbs in a position of full extension; seen in the unconscious patient with severe brain injury and a lesion in the brainstem between the superior colliculi and vestibular nucleus.

Declarative learning: Cognitive learning that occurs through processes of conscious recall, awareness, attention, and reflection.

Declarative memory: Memory of facts that can be consciously recalled.

Decorticate rigidity: Sustained contraction and posturing of the trunk and lower limbs in extension, and the upper limbs in flexion; seen in the unconscious patient with severe brain injury and a lesion at the level of the diencephalon (above the superior colliculus).

Deep brain stimulation (DBS): The implantation of electrodes in the brain (ventral intermediate nucleus of the thalamus) where they block nerve signals that cause symptoms; the pacemaker is implanted within the chest; used in the treatment of Parkinson's disease.

Deep tendon reflex (DTR): Muscle contraction resulting from brisk tapping and stimulation of the stretch-sensitive IA afferents of the neuromuscular spindle via a monosynaptic pathway.

Deep vein thrombosis (DVT): Formation of a blood clot in the deep venous system; occurring most frequently in the lower extremities; clinical manifestations include warmth, pain, and swelling in the affected extremity.

Defense mechanism: A psychological means of coping with conflict or anxiety; examples include denial, sublimation, repression, rationalization, conversion, and dissociation.

Degenerative joint disease (DJD): See *Osteoarthritis*.

Degrees of freedom: The number of separate independent dimensions of movement that must be controlled by engaging cooperative units of muscle action.

Delirium (acute confusional state): A clouding of consciousness with dulling of cognitive processes and general impairment of alertness; patients may demonstrate confusion, agitation, disorientation, and illusions or hallucinations.

Dementia: A broad base of cognitive deficits caused by a progressive organic mental disorder; characterized by confusion, disorientation, memory loss, personality disintegration, and deterioration of intellectual capacity and function.

Demyelination: Destruction or removal of the myelin sheath of nerve tissue by a disease process.

Denial: Refusal to acknowledge the truth or reality of a situation; a defense mechanism used to alleviate the anxiety and pain associated with functional limitation or disability; removes realities from conscious awareness.

Depersonalization: Detraction from an individual's dignity or worth; failure to honor a person's uniqueness.

Depression: A mental state characterized by feelings of despair, hopelessness, and loss of interest or pleasure in living.

Depth perception: Judgment of the distance between objects and self.

de Quervain's disease: Stenosing tenosynovitis of the first dorsal compartment of the wrist involving the abductor pollicis longus and the extensor pollicis brevis.

Dermal healing: The process whereby the dermis is repaired via scar formation.

Dermatome: A band or region of skin supplied by a single sensory nerve.

Desquamation: Peeling of the outer layers of the epidermis.

Developmental motor skills: Functional skills acquired during early motor development; used as landmarks or "milestones" of patient progression or change.

Diagnosis: The diagnostic process includes integrating and evaluating data obtained during the examination to describe the patient/client condition in terms that will guide the prognosis, the plan of care, and intervention strategies. Physical therapists use diagnostic labels that identify the impact of a condition on function at the level of the system (especially the movement system) and at the level of the whole person.

Diaschisis: The recovery of brain activity after the resolution of temporary blocking factors (e.g., shock, edema, decreased blood flow, decreased glucose utilization).

Diastole: Period of relaxation of the ventricles of the heart; the muscle fibers lengthen and the heart dilates.

Diastolic pressure: The pressure of the blood during relaxation (diastole) of the ventricles.

Diffuse axonal injury (DAI): Widely scattered shearing of axons that can occur during traumatic brain injury; although not intense in any one location, it can cause dramatic disability as a result of its cumulative effects.

Dignity: The quality of being worthy, honored, esteemed; to have distinction as a person.

Diplopia: Double vision.

Disability: The inability to perform or a limitation in the performance of actions, tasks, and activities usually expected in specific social roles that are customary for the individual or expected for the person's status or role in a specific sociocultural context and physical environment. Categories of required roles are self-care, home management, work (job/school/play), and community/leisure.

Disablement: An interaction/complex relationship between health condition and contextual factors (i.e., environmental and personal factors).

Discrete motor skill: A motor skill with clearly defined beginning and end points.

Disease: A pathological condition of the body or abnormal entity with a characteristic group of signs and symptoms affecting the body; with known or unknown etiology.

Dislocation: Displacement of a bone or vertebral body from its normal position.

Distraction: A traction force; separation of joint surfaces.

Distress: A term denoting a negative perception or response to a stressor; the stressor becomes immobilizing and overwhelming; initiates a sympathetic physiological stress response in the individual. See also *Stress reaction, Eustress.*

Distributed practice: An alternating sequence of practice and rest periods in which practice time is equal to or less than rest time.

Disuse atrophy: Lack of muscle activity following injury; results in wasting due to decreased protein synthesis; associated with length changes in muscle, changes in connective tissue, and loss of fast twitch fibers.

Divided attention: The capacity to respond simultaneously to two or more tasks or stimuli when all stimuli are relevant.

Dizziness: Sensation of lightheadedness, unsteadiness, loss of spatial orientation, or loss of balance.

Donor site: Site from which a skin graft is taken.

Dual-task training: Training that utilizes performance of simultaneous tasks, with a degree of interference caused by one task on the other (e.g., walking and talking).

Dynamic postural control (dynamic balance, controlled mobility): The ability to maintain postural stability and orientation with the center of mass over the base of support while parts of the body are in motion.

Dysarthria: A category of motor speech disorders caused by impairment in parts of the central or peripheral nervous system that mediate speech production. Respiration, articulation, phonation, resonance, and/or prosody may be affected; volitional and automatic actions (e.g., chewing and swallowing) and movement of the jaw and tongue may also be deviant. It excludes apraxia of speech and functional or central language disorders.

Dyscalculia: Impaired ability to perform simple arithmetic operations; difficulty in accomplishing calculations.

Dysdiadochokinesia: Impaired ability to perform rapid alternating movements.

Dysequilibrium: Impaired balance ability.

Dysesthesia: An abnormal and unpleasant sensation, such as a sense of burning, numbness, pins and needles, or tingling sensation.

Dyskinesia: Impaired ability to perform voluntary movement. *Tardive dyskinesia* is characterized by slow, rhythmic, involuntary movements that occur as an undesired effect of drug therapy, e.g., phenothiazine medications.

Dysmetria: Impaired ability to judge the distance or range of a movement.

Dysphagia: Inability to swallow or difficulty in swallowing.

Dysphasia: See *Aphasia.*

Dysphonia: Impaired volume, quality, or pitch of the voice.

Dysphoria: Psychological distress marked by anxiety and dissatisfaction.

Dyspnea: The feeling of breathlessness that occurs when there is a higher demand for ventilation than can be met by comfortable breathing; air hunger; normally accompanies vigorous exercise.

Dyssynergia: Impaired ability to associate muscles together for complex movement; decomposition of movement.

Dysthymic disorder: Variability in dysphoric mood or atypical depression characterized by intermittent episodes of severe anxiety.

Dystonia: A hyperkinetic movement disorder characterized by disordered tone and involuntary movements involving large portions of the body, typically twisting or writhing motions.

Edema: A local or generalized condition characterized by excessive accumulation of fluid in the tissues.

Effusion: Excess fluid in the joint indicating irritation or inflammation of the synovium; escape of fluid into a body cavity.

Ejection fraction (EF): The percent of left ventricular end diastolic volume (LVEDV) that was ejected from the left ventricle during systole; expressed as the ratio of stroke volume (SV) to LVEDV (SV divided by LVEDV).

Electrical burn: Injury sustained from the passage of electric current through the tissues of the body.

Electrical silence: The absence of measurable EMG activity, typically recorded at rest in normal muscles.

Electrode: A device capable of recording electrical potentials or conducting electricity to provide a stimulus.

Electromyography: The recording and study of the electrical activity of muscle; provides a graphic record of resting and voluntary muscle activity as well as activity resulting from electrical stimulation (e.g., nerve conduction studies).

Elevation activities: A general term used in gait training to describe an ambulatory activity requiring movement from one level surface to another (e.g., negotiating curbs, climbing stairs or ramps).

Empathy: A three-stage process that includes (1) identification with another's experience or situation,
(2) a shared experience with another person, and
(3) a reclaiming of one's individuality separate from the shared moment.

Endarterectomy: A surgical opening of the carotid arteries to remove plaque and reduce stenosis.

End-feel: The tissue resistance experienced by the therapist when overpressure is applied at the end of a range of motion or accessory motion.

End-of-dose deterioration (wearing off): A worsening of symptoms during the expected time frame of medication effectiveness; seen with long-term use of L-dopa therapy.

Endorphins: A group of neurotransmitters that activate opiate receptors and have pain-relieving properties similar to morphine. There are three types of endorphins: beta-endorphins, found primarily in the pituitary gland, and enkephalins and dynorphin, distributed throughout the nervous system.

Energy conservation: The adoption of strategies that reduce overall energy requirements of the task and overall level of fatigue.

Environmental accessibility: Absence or removal of physical barriers from the entrance and within a building or dwelling to allow use by individuals with disabilities.

Environmental barrier: Physical impediments that prevent individuals from functioning optimally in their surroundings and include safety hazards, access problems, and home or workplace design difficulties (e.g., revolving doors, stairways, narrow doorways).

Environmental control unit (ECU): An electrical interface that allows the user to control a variety of electrical appliances and devices; operation is accomplished by use of a central control panel.

Epidural hematoma: Extravascular blood mass located between the dura and the skull.

Epithelial healing: The process of regeneration of the epidermis through epithelial cell migration, proliferation, and differentiation.

Epithelial islands: Surviving tissue from which new epithelial cell growth will originate.

Ergonomic examination: Data collection concerned with fitting a job to a person's anatomical and physiological characteristics in a way that enhances human efficiency and performance; identifies potential risks of injury for an individual worker.

Erythema: Reddening of the skin.

Eschar: The dead, necrotic tissue cast off from the skin, especially after a burn wound.

Escharotomy: Midlateral incision of the burned eschar used to relieve pressure in an extremity or on the trunk.

Ethical dilemma: A conflict of values where each value action is seen to be equally bad or good, and to act on one value cancels out the other so that you can't have it "both ways."

Ethical distress: A conflict of duties when one knows the best or right thing to do, but is prohibited from doing it by some structure or process, for example, organizational policy.

Euphoria: An exaggerated feeling of well-being, a sense of optimism incongruent with the patient's incapacitating disability.

Eupnea: Normal respiration.

Eustress: A positive perception or response to a stressor whereby the stressor is seen as, or becomes, enervating or motivating, rather than overwhelming or negative. See also *Stress reaction, Distress.*

Euthymic mood: A normal mood, neither manic nor dysthymic.

Evoked potential (EMG): Waveform elicited by a stimulus.

Exacerbation (relapse): Acute worsening or flare-up of neurological signs and symptoms; usually associated with multiple sclerosis and inflammation and demyelination in the brain and spinal cord.

Executive functions (higher order cognitive functions): Includes the capacity to plan, manipulate information, initiate and terminate activities, recognize errors, problem solve, and think abstractly.

Exercise prescription (FITT equation): An individualized exercise program specifying the frequency, intensity, time (duration), and type (mode) of therapeutic intervention.

Exercise tolerance test (ETT, graded exercise or stress test): A measure of the efficiency of the cardiorespiratory system; the subject's ability to tolerate increasing intensities of exercise is monitored using electrocardiographic, hemodynamic, and symptomatic responses. Manifestations of myocardial ischemia, electrical instability, and other exertional intolerance abnormalities are determined.

Exhaustion: The limit of endurance beyond which no further performance is possible.

Exostoses: Ossifications of muscular or ligamentous attachments.

Expected outcomes: The intended results of patient/client management; the changes in impairment, functional limitations, and disabilities and the changes in health, wellness, and fitness needs that are expected as a result of implementing the plan of care.

Exteroceptors: Sensory receptors that provide information from the external environment.

Extrinsic feedback (augmented feedback): Feedback that supplements feedback normally received during a movement task and comes from an external source (auditory or visual).

Facilitated stretching: The application of techniques that promote reflex relaxation of the muscle to be elongated prior to or during the stretching maneuver (e.g., contract-relax, hold-relax techniques).

Facilitation: Increased capacity to initiate a movement response through increased neuronal activity and altered synaptic potential.

Fading feedback (fading knowledge of results [KR]): The frequency of augmented feedback is systematically reduced during the course of practice.

Fasciculation potentials (EMG): Electrical activity during electromyography characterized by random, spontaneous twitching of a group of muscle fibers that may be visible through the skin. The amplitude, configuration, duration, and frequency are variable.

Fatigue: The failure to generate the required or expected force during sustained or repeated contractions.

Fear/avoidance: Fear of reinjury that prevents an individual from believing he or she is able to exercise or be functionally active.

Febrile: Pertaining to a fever; state of elevated body temperature.

Feedback: Response-produced information received during or after a movement; used to monitor output for corrective actions.

Feedforward: The sending of signals in advance of movement to ready the sensorimotor systems for incoming sensory feedback or for a future motor command.

Fibroblasts: A connective tissue cell that forms the fibrous tissues in the body.

Fibrosis: Abnormal formation of fibrous tissue.

Fidelity: Being faithful (steadfast, respectful) to one's patients, to one's colleagues, and to one's profession, even when one disagrees.

Fight or flight response (alarm or stress response): Defensive responses initiated by the sympathetic nervous system (mass discharge) to protect the individual under varying circumstances.

Figure–ground discrimination: The ability to distinguish a figure from the background in which it is embedded.

Finger agnosia: The inability to identify the fingers on one's own hands or on the hands of the examiner, including difficulty in naming the fingers on command, identifying which finger was touched, and mimicking finger movements.

Flaccid bulbar palsy: Degeneration of the lower motor neurons of the bulbar muscles.

Flaccidity: Absence of muscle tone.

Flat affect: Displaying little or no emotion.

Focused attention: See *Selective attention.*

Force plates: Load transducers that are capable of measuring ground reaction forces and the center of pressure.

Forced gaze deviation: Deviation of the eyes secondary to unopposed action of eye muscles.

Forced-use training (constraint induced movement training): A training strategy in which patients are required to use their affected extremity while the intact extremity is restrained (e.g., post-stroke).

Form discrimination: The ability to perceive or to attend to subtle differences in form and shape.

Free-floating anxiety: A psychodynamic construct denoting generalized feelings of anxiety whereby the individual is unable to state or locate the source, cause, or reason for such feelings; the anxiety is not attached to a source or event.

Freezing: A sudden episode of immobility or block in movement, seen in Parkinson's disease.

Full-thickness burn: Burn involving the entire dermis.

Full-thickness skin graft: Graft containing epidermis and full dermal thickness.

Functional activities: Activities identified by an individual as essential to support physical and psychological well-being as well as to create a personal sense of meaningful living.

Functional capacities: The ability to execute performance components of essential activities, including cognitive and social interactions, activities of daily living, mobility skills, and life roles.

Functional limitation: The restriction of the ability to perform, at the level of the whole person, a physical action, task, or activity, in an efficient, typically expected, or competent manner.

Functional maintenance program: A rehabilitation program designed to manage the effects of progressive disease; includes strategies to prevent or slow decline of function, and promote regular exercise, good health, and self-management skills.

Functional mobility skills (FMS): Mobility skills required for daily function, such as bed mobility (rolling, turning, supine-to-sit, and sit-to-supine), sit-to-stand and stand-to-sit, transfers, locomotion and walking, and stair climbing.

Functional/task-oriented training: A therapeutic approach to retraining the patient with movement disorders; practice is task- and context-specific with an overall goal of functional independence.

Function-induced plasticity: Neural reorganization following brain injury that occurs as a result of experience (practice) and training.

Fund of knowledge: Mental status screening test utilizing questions related to the patient's learning history and life experiences.

Gate control theory: A theory of pain, developed by Melzack and Wall, that suggests pain can be blocked at various gate locations in the spinal cord.

General adaptation syndrome (GAS): The sum total of an organism's response to stress originally described by Hans Seyle, who divided the body's chemical and structural response to stress into three stages: (1) alarm, (2) resistance or adaption, and (3) exhaustion.

Generalizability: The extent to which practice on one task contributes to the performance of other, related skills.

Generalized anxiety disorder: Excessive worry, apprehension, and concern persisting for at least 6 months; may be accompanied by irritability, fatigue, and disturbed sleep patterns.

Genu valgum: A deformity in which the lower extremities curve inward with knees close together; knock knees.

Giant motor units: Motor unit potentials with a peak-to-peak amplitude and duration much greater than normal ranges; often seen after collateral sprouting with regeneration of peripheral nerves.

Glasgow Coma Scale: A scale that documents level of consciousness and severity of brain injury; based on best motor response, verbal response, and eye opening.

Glide (slide): Translatory (linear) joint motion of one bony surface sliding over another surface; the same point on one surface comes into contact with new points on the other surface.

Gliosis: Proliferation of neuroglial tissue within the central nervous system that results in glial scars (plaques).

Goals: The intended results of patient/client management. Anticipated goals indicate changes in impairment, functional limitations, and disabilities and changes in health, wellness, and fitness needs that are expected as a result of implementing the plan of care.

Gold standard: Accepted, accurate measure of a particular phenomenon that can serve as the normative standard for other measures.

Gout: Disease characterized by acute episodes of arthritis with the presence of sodium urate crystals in the synovial fluid or deposits of urate crystals in or about the joints and other tissues.

Granulation tissue: A matrix of collagen, hyaluronic acid, and fibronectin in a newly formed vascular network.

Graphesthesia (traced figure identification): Recognition of numbers, letters, or symbols traced on the skin.

Grief: A psychological state of distress or sadness associated with a significant loss.

Ground (floor) reaction force (GRF): Vertical, anterior–posterior, and medial–lateral forces created as a result of foot contact with the supporting surface; forces are equal in magnitude and opposite in direction to the force applied by the foot to the ground.

Guided movement: A training strategy in which the movements of the learner are assisted or controlled by various means to prevent errors; manual guidance assists movement (passive or active assisted movement) or restricts (constrains) segments.

Habituation: A decrease in responsiveness of sensory receptors from repeated exposure.

Hallpike-Dix maneuver: A positional test used to reproduce vertigo and nystagmus and diagnose benign positional vertigo; the patient is moved from sitting to supine with the head tilted over the end of the table and turned to either side.

Hallucination: Sensing things that are not tangibly real and believing that they are; may be visual, auditory, tactile, gustatory, or olfactory.

Hallux valgus: Valgus deformity at the first metatarsophalangeal joint of the great toe.

Hammer toe: Deformity with hyperextension of the metatarsophalangeal joint, flexion of the proximal interphalangeal, and hyperextension of the distal interphalangeal joints.

Hand-held dynamometer: A portable testing device placed between the patient's body part and the therapist's hand that measures mechanical force.

Handicap: The value that an individual, family, and community place on a disability and the degree to which an individual is disadvantaged because of it.

Health: A state of complete physical, mental, and social well-being, and not merely the absence of disease and infirmity.

Health-related quality of life (HRQOL): The total effect of individual and environmental factors on function and health status; includes three major dimensions: *physical function* (BADL, IADL), *psychological function*, and *social function*.

Heart rate reserve (Karvonen) formula: Resting heart rate (HR_{rest}) is subtracted from maximal heart rate (HR_{max}) to obtain the heart rate reserve. The conditioning intensity, 40 to 85 percent of heart rate reserve, is calculated. These values are added to HR_{rest} to obtain the target heart rate range (THRR).

Heart sounds: The auscultatory sounds of the cardiac cycle. S_1: The normal first heart sound, produced by the closure of the mitral and tricuspid valves; marks the beginning of systole. S_2: The normal second heart sound, produced by the closure of the aortic and pulmonic valves; marks the end of systole and the beginning of diastole. S_3: Ventricular gallop, an abnormal heart sound associated with the presence of congestive heart failure. S_4: Atrial gallop, an abnormal heart sound associated with a myocardial infarction.

Heberden's nodes: Bony enlargement of the distal interphalangeal joint; characteristic of osteoarthritis.

Hemianopia (hemianopsia): Inability to see in one half of the visual field.

Hemiballismus: Sudden, jerky, forceful, flailing motions of one side of the body.

Hemispace: One half of the spatial field around the body.

Hemorrhagic stroke: Abnormal bleeding into the extravascular areas of the brain secondary to aneurysm and rupture or bleeding from an arteriovenous malformation; associated with long-standing hypertension or may be the result of trauma.

Hemosiderin staining: A brownish discoloration of the skin due to a pigment released from hemoglobin following red blood cell lysis.

Heterotopic ossification (HO): Abnormal bone growth in muscle or other connective tissue; can restrict range of motion and lead to impaired function; also known as *ectopic bone formation*.

Holistic: An approach that values the multifaceted dimensions of a patient's life, including social roles, culture, religion, gender, age, community, ethnicity, personality, and social support.

Hostility (externalized): Anger or hostility toward others or inanimate objects in situations when reaction is unwarranted; often associated with depression; may occur as a reactive response to functional limitations or disability.

Hypalgesia: Decreased sensitivity to pain.

Hyperalgesia: Increased sensitivity to pain.

Hypercapnia: An increase in the amount of carbon dioxide within the arterial blood.

Hyperesthesia: Increased sensitivity to sensory stimuli.

Hyperkinesia: A general term used to describe abnormally increased muscle activity or movement; restlessness.

Hypermetria: Excessive distance or range of a movement; an overestimation of the required motion needed to reach a target object.

Hypermobility: Excessive joint motion.

Hyperpyrexia: Extremely high fever; temperature reading of 106°F (41.1°C) or greater.

Hypertension: Higher than normal blood pressure.

Hyperthermia: Extremely high fever; temperature reading of 106°F (41.1°C) or greater.

Hypertonia: Increased muscle tone above normal resting levels.

Hypertrophic scar: Raised scar that stays within the boundaries of a wound and is characteristically red, raised, and firm.

Hypertrophy: Increased size or bulk of muscle.

Hyperventilation: Abnormally fast rate and depth of respiration.

Hypesthesia: Decreased sensitivity to sensory stimuli.

Hypokinesia: A general term used to describe decreased motor responses (especially to a specific stimulus); sluggishness, listlessness.

Hypokinetic dysarthria: Difficult and defective speech characterized by decreased voice volume, monotone/monopitch speech, imprecise or distorted articulation, and uncontrolled speech rate.

Hypometria: Shortened distance or range of a movement; an underestimation of the required motion needed to reach a target object.

Hypomobility: Restricted joint motion.

Hypotension: Lower than normal blood pressure.

Hypothermia: Body temperature below average normal range.

Hypotonia: Muscle tone reduced below normal resting levels.

Hypoventilation: Decrease in the rate and depth of respiration.

Hypovolemia: Abnormally low volume of circulating blood in the body.

Hypovolemic shock: Shock caused by substantial fluid loss from intravascular space (e.g., blood or electrolyte solution loss).

Hypoxemia: Decrease in the amount of oxygen within the arterial blood.

Hypoxia: Oxygen deficiency in body tissues.

Hypoxic-ischemic injury: Brain damage from arterial hypotension and hypoxemia; complicated by raised intracranial pressure, cerebral vasospasm, edema, and combinations of these, as well as an impaired ability of the vessels of the brain to autoregulate.

Ideational apraxia: An inability to perform a purposeful motor act, either automatically or upon command; an inability to retain the idea of the task and to formulate the necessary motor patterns; the patient no longer understands the overall concept of the act.

Ideomotor apraxia: The inability to perform a task on command and to imitate gestures, even though the patient understands the concept of the task and is able to carry out habitual tasks automatically.

Illness: Encompasses the personal behaviors that emerge when the reality of having a disease is internalized and experienced by an individual.

Imagery: Visualizing a scene or rehearsing a script for a specific purpose such as relaxation.

Immune: Protected from or resistant to a disease or infection as a result of the development of antibodies or cell-mediated immunity.

Impairment (direct): A loss or abnormality of anatomical, physiological, mental, or psychological structure or function; the natural consequence of pathology or disease.

Inclinometer: A device that uses gravity's effect on pointers or fluid levels to measure joint position and motion.

Incomplete lesion (SCI): Motor and/or sensory function below the neurological level including sensory and/or motor function at S4 and S5; some preservation of sensory or motor function below the level of the lesion.

Indifference: Lack of concern or interest; aloofness; detachment.

Inhalation injury: Injury to the lungs due to breathing hot and/or toxic gases; usually occurs when individual is burned in a closed space.

Inhibition: Decreased neuronal activity and synaptic output leading to decreased capacity to initiate a movement response.

Input impedance: A form of resistance to current flow in an alternating current circuit. Skin, electrodes, and amplifier input terminals provide sources of impedance to electromyography potentials.

Insertion activity (EMG): Electrical activity caused by insertion or movement of a needle electrode in a muscle during electromyography; can be normal, reduced, increased, or prolonged.

Inspiratory capacity: The total amount of air that can be inspired after a tidal exhalation; inspiratory reserve volume plus residual volume equals inspiratory capacity.

Inspiratory reserve volume (IRV): The amount of air that can be inspired after a tidal inspiration.

Instrumental activities of daily living (IADL): See *Activities of daily living.*

Intention (kinetic) tremor: Oscillatory movements that occur during voluntary motion.

Interference pattern: Electrical activity, recorded from a muscle during electromyography involving maximal voluntary effort, in which identification of each of the contributing motor unit potentials is not possible.

Interoceptor: Sensory receptors that provide information about the body's internal environment (such as oxygen levels and blood pressure).

Intertask transfer: Transfer of learning between tasks or skills.

Intervention: The purposeful interaction of the physical therapist with the patient/client and, when appropriate, with other individuals involved in the care of the patient/client, using various physical therapy procedures and techniques to produce changes in the condition.

Intracerebral hematoma: Extravascular blood mass located within the brain tissue.

Intracerebral hemorrhage: Rupture of a cerebral vessel with subsequent bleeding into the cerebral hemispheres.

Intracranial pressure (ICP): Measure of pressure inside the cranium; normal ICP is 5 to 10 mm Hg.

Intrathecal injection: A central (within the spinal canal) chemical injection that interrupts the reflex arc; used to decrease severe spasticity.

Intrinsic feedback: The feedback normally received during the execution of movement from the various sensory systems (e.g., visual, somatosensory, vestibular).

Inverted-U theory (Yerkes-Dodson law): A description of the relationship between arousal and performance; too much or too little arousal can cause marked deterioration in performance.

Ipsilateral pushing (contraversive pushing, Pusher syndrome): An unusual motor behavior following stroke characterized by active pushing with the stronger extremities toward the hemiparetic side, leading to a lateral postural imbalance and a tendency to fall toward the hemiparetic side.

Ischemia: A temporary deficiency in oxygenated blood supply to an organ or tissue.

Ischemic cascade (secondary injury): Brain cell injury and death that progresses rapidly within the core infarction area and over time within the ischemic penumbra (the transitional area surrounding the ischemic core); results from loss of brain cells' ability to produce energy, particularly adenosine triphosphate (ATP), with elevation of intracellular calcium, and release of excessive excitatory neurotransmitter, proteases, lipases, and free radicals.

Ischemic stroke: Loss of cerebral circulation resulting in anoxia and infarction; includes embolic and thrombotic stroke.

Isokinetic dynamometer: A testing and exercise device that controls the velocity of a limb movement, keeping it at a constant rate while offering accommodating resistance throughout the range of motion.

Job analysis: Identification of the specific components of work tasks and features of the environment in which they must be accomplished.

Joint mobilization: Passive therapeutic techniques applied specifically to joint structures that utilize arthrokinematic motions; used to increase or maintain joint play and range of motion or to treat pain.

Joint play (accessory) motions: Motions that occur between joint surfaces that accompany osteokinematic motions, but are not under voluntary control; includes slides (glides), distractions, compressions, rolls, and spins; also refers to the distensibility of the joint capsule and ligaments that allow joint motion to occur.

Joint reaction forces: The forces between articular surfaces created by muscle, gravity, and inertial forces; measured in Newtons.

Justice: The quality of impartiality or fairness.

Key muscles: Muscles that add significantly to a patient's functional capacity at each successive level of lesion following spinal cord injury.

Kinematic analysis: A description of the type, amount, and direction of motion; does not include the forces producing the motion.

Kinesthesia: Sensation and awareness of active or passive movement; awareness of movement.

Kinetic analysis: The study of the forces that cause motion.

Knowledge of performance (KP): A type of augmented feedback that provides information about the nature of the movement pattern produced.

Knowledge of results (KR): A type of augmented feedback that provides information about the outcome of the movement or skill performance in terms of overall goal.

Korotkoff's sounds: Sounds heard in auscultation of blood pressure.

Kyphosis: An exaggeration or angulation of the posterior curve of the spine; usually found in the dorsal spine.

Lacunar infarction (lacunar syndrome): Blood flow is blocked in very small arterial vessels deep within the cerebral white matter with involvement of the internal capsule; characterized by contralateral pure motor or sensory deficits without visual field, cognitive, or speech deficits.

Lag phenomenon: Difference between active and passive range of motion.

Leadpipe rigidity: A constant, uniform resistance to passive movement, with no fluctuations.

Learned nonuse: A learned pattern of disuse that follows sensory or motor loss affecting involved segments of the body; usually accompanied by overcompensation with intact segments.

Lethargy: A state of general slowing of motor responses, including speech and movement.

Level of cognitive function (LOCF) (Rancho Los Amigos Scale): A descriptive scale that outlines a predictable sequence of cognitive and behavioral recovery seen in individuals with traumatic brain injury.

Lhermitte's sign: A sign of posterior column damage in the spinal cord; flexion of the neck produces an electric shock-like sensation running down the spine and into the lower extremities.

Ligamentous instability test (ligament stress test): A test in which a patient's joint is passively maneuvered to determine the integrity of ligaments and other joint structures.

Limits of stability (LOS): The maximum distance an individual is able or willing to lean in any direction without loss of balance or changing the base of support (BOS); the midpoint of limits of stability is centered alignment (center of mass [COM] alignment).

Linear velocity: The rate at which a body moves in a straight line.

Linear work: Force multiplied by distance.

Locked-in syndrome (LIS): Tetraplegia and lower bulbar palsy (anarthria) with preserved consciousness following stroke involving bilateral infarction of the ventral pons.

Lordosis: Abnormally increased anterior curvature of the lumbar spine.

Lower motor neuron (LMN) syndrome: Lesions affecting the anterior horn cell or peripheral nerve produce decreased or absent tone along with associated symptoms of paralysis, muscle fasciculations and fibrillations with denervation, and neurogenic atrophy.

Lyme disease: Systemic inflammatory disorder characterized by recurrent episodes of polyarthritis, skin lesions, and involvement of the cardiac and nervous systems following a tick bite.

Lymphedema: A chronic disorder characterized by an abnormal accumulation of lymph fluid in the tissues of one or more body regions.

Maceration: Softening of a solid by exposure to water or other fluid; usually pertains to the skin.

Maintenance therapy: A series of occasional clinical, educational, and/or administrative services designed to maintain the patient's current level of function.

Make test (active resistance test): A method of applying resistance during manual muscle testing in which the patient moves through an arc of motion against the therapist's resistance. In hand-held dynamometry, the term has also been used to indicate a patient's performance of a maximal isometric contraction against the therapist's resistance.

Malingering: A legal term referring to the faking of injury or illness symptoms for secondary gain.

Mallet finger deformity: Deformity involving only flexion of the distal interphalangeal joint; secondary to disruption of the insertion of the extensor tendon into the base of the distal phalanx.

Manual Muscle Testing (MMT): A formal examination and grading system that uses arc of motion, gravity, and manually applied resistance to quantify muscle strength on an ordinal scale.

Marcus Gunn pupil: Paradoxical dilation of pupil in response to ophthalmologic examination using a light test; indicative of unilateral pupillary defect (normal response is constriction as light is shone into the eye).

Masked face: Lack of facial expression with infrequent blinking; commonly seen in Parkinson's disease.

Massed practice: A prolonged period of practice in which the practice time is much greater than rest time.

Mechanical insufflation–exsufflation (MI–E) device: A device designed to inflate the lung with positive pressure and assist cough with negative pressure through the flip of a switch.

Memory: The mental registration, retention, and recall of past experience, knowledge, and ideas.

Ménière's disease: A syndrome characterized by recurrent symptoms of vertigo, tinnitus, sensation of fullness in the ear, and hearing loss, often resulting in gradual progressive deafness.

Mental function: See *Cognition.*

Mental practice: A practice strategy in which performance of the task is imagined or visualized without overt physical practice.

Mesh graft: Process whereby the donor skin is placed through a device that increases the surface area of the graft.

Metabolic equivalent (MET): A rating of energy expenditure for a given activity based on oxygen consumption; one MET equals 3.5 mL of oxygen used per kilogram of body weight per minute.

Metatarsalgia: Pain over the metatarsal heads on the plantar aspect of the foot.

Micrographia: An abnormally small handwriting that is difficult to read; commonly seen in Parkinson's disease.

Micturition: Voiding of urine; urination.

Mind–body techniques: Methods in which patients use mental processes to promote healing.

Minimally conscious state: Severely altered consciousness with definite, but minimal behavioral evidence of self or environmental awareness.

Mobility: The ability to move from one place to another independently and safely.

Moral values: Values that dictate how one interacts with or treats another human being; reflects a person's basic uniqueness, dignity, and worth.

Morning stiffness: Prolonged generalized stiffness upon awakening that is associated with inflammatory arthritis; indicative of systemic involvement.

Motivation: The internal state that tends to affect or stimulate behavior and direct an individual toward a goal.

Motor capacity: The inborn, hereditary potential for general motor performance.

Motor control: An area of study dealing with the understanding of the neural, physical, and behavioral aspects of movement.

Motor function (motor control and motor learning): The ability to learn or perform the skillful and efficient assumption, maintenance, modification, and control of voluntary movement patterns and postures.

Motor impersistence: An inability to sustain a movement or a posture.

Motor learning: A set of internal processes associated with practice or experience leading to relatively permanent changes in the capability for skilled behavior.

Motor level (SCI): Following spinal cord injury, the most caudal segment of the spinal cord with normal motor function bilaterally.

Motor memory (procedural or implicit memory): The recall of movements or motor information; involves storage of motor programs, subroutines, or schema.

Motor neuron disease: A heterogeneous spectrum of inherited or acquired clinical disorders of the upper motor neurons, lower motor neurons, or both.

Motor plan (complex motor program): An idea or plan for purposeful movement that is made up of several component motor programs.

Motor program: A set of commands that, when initiated, results in the production of a coordinated movement sequence.

Motor skill: The ability to consistently perform coordinated movement sequences for the purposes of investigation and interaction with the physical and social environment; a learned skill that is dependent on practice and experience.

Motor unit: The anatomical unit consisting of an anterior horn cell, its axon, the neuromuscular junctions, and all the muscle fibers innervated by that axon.

Motor unit action potential: Action potential reflecting the electrical activity of a single motor unit capable of being recorded by an electrode; characterized by its amplitude, configuration, duration, frequency, and sound.

Movement decomposition: See *Dyssynergia.*

Movement time (MT): The interval of time between the initiation of movement and the completion of movement.

Multi-infarct dementia: Deteriorative mental state characterized by reduction in intellectual faculties; the result of multiple small strokes.

Muscle endurance: The ability of a muscle to contract repeatedly over time.

Muscle performance: The capacity of a muscle to do work; the product of force and distance.

Muscle power: Work produced per unit of time; the product of strength and speed.

Muscle strength: The measurable force exerted by a muscle or group of muscles to overcome a resistance.

Mutilans-type deformity (opera-glass hand): Severe bony destruction and resorption in a synovial joint; telescopic shortening in the fingers.

Mutism: Condition of being unable to speak or speaking only in whispers.

Myelin: The phospholipid–protein of the cell membranes of Schwann cells and oligodendrocytes (CNS) that forms the myelin sheath of neurons; acts as an electrical insulator and increases the velocity of impulse transmission.

Myelotomy: Severance of nerve fibers of the spinal cord; used to reduce severe spasticity.

Myocardial infarction (MI): Death of myocardial cells as a result of coronary artery occlusion.

Myocardial oxygen demand ($M\dot{V}O_2$): The amount of oxygen required for the metabolic needs of the myocardium.

Myositis: Inflammatory disease of striated muscle.

Myotomy: Surgical sectioning or release of a muscle; used to reduce spasticity.

Myotonic discharge (EMG): A high-frequency discharge, characterized by repetitive firing (2080 Hz) of biphasic or monophasic potentials recorded on electromyography after needle insertion or after voluntary muscle contraction, with a waxing and waning amplitude and frequency and a sound likened to a "dive-bomber."

Nerve conduction velocity (NCV): The speed with which a peripheral motor or sensory nerve conducts an impulse.

Neurectomy: Partial or total excision or resection of a nerve; used to reduce severe spasticity.

Neurological level (SCI): Following spinal cord injury, the most caudal level of the spinal cord with normal motor and sensory function on both the left and right sides of the body.

Neuromas: A tumor or mass growing from a nerve; composed of nerve cells.

Neuromotor development: The acquisition and evolution of movement skills that occurs throughout the life span.

Neuropathy: Any disease of nerves including peripheral nerves, cranial nerves, and/or autonomic nerves.

Neuroplasticity (plasticity): The capacity of brain and nerve cells to repair and change in response to experience or environment; defines recovery of function following injury and disease.

Nociception: The stimulation of peripheral pain sensitive nerve endings (C-fibers, A-delta fibers) and the transmission of impulses along peripheral nerves to the CNS where the stimulus is perceived as pain.

Nociceptor: A receptor for injurious or painful stimuli; a pain sense organ.

Nocturia: Excessive urination during the night.

Nominal measures: Classification scheme based on categories without order or rank, the simplest of which are dichotomous response sets such as "present/absent" and "yes/no;" also have more than two categories.

Noncapsular pattern: A restriction of passive osteokinematic motion; restriction is not proportioned similar to a capsular pattern; indicates a cause other than intra-articular inflammation or capsular fibrosis.

Nonmoral values: Values that do not reflect on how one treats another person but reflects esthetic, political, intellectual, personal, or social choices.

Numbing (psychic numbing or emotional anesthesia): Feelings of being detached or estranged from others; a loss of ability or interest in previously enjoyable activities, or the lack of any emotions or feelings.

Nystagmus: Involuntary back-and-forth or cyclical movements of the eyes; movements may be rotatory, horizontal, or vertical.

Obtundation: Dulled or blunted sensitivity.

Obtunded: A state of altered consciousness in which the patient sleeps often and when aroused exhibits decreased alertness and interest in the environment and delayed reactions.

Ocular pursuit: The ability of the eyes to follow a moving object.

Off-state: Plasma concentrations of medications decline and do not adequately control symptoms.

On–off phenomenon: Abrupt and often unpredictable fluctuations in motor performance and response; common in Parkinson's disease with progression and long-term use of L-dopa therapy.

On-state: Plasma concentrations of medications are therapeutic and optimally control the symptoms.

Open-loop control system: A motor control system that employs motor programs without the influence of peripheral feedback or error detection processes.

Open motor skill: A movement skill performed in a variable, changing environment.

Open wound care technique: Absence of dressings; often used after skin grafting to the face.

Ophthalmoplegia: Complete ocular paralysis.

Opisthotonus: Strong and sustained contraction of the extensor muscles of the neck and trunk; seen in the unconscious patient with severe brain injury.

Ordinal (or rank order) measures: Classification scheme that rates observations in terms of the relationship between items (e.g., less than, equal to, or greater than).

Orientation: The ability to comprehend and to adjust oneself within an unfamiliar environment with respect to awareness of time, person, and place.

Orthodromic conduction: Propagation of an action potential in the same direction as physiological conduction (i.e., motor nerve conduction away from the spinal cord and sensory nerve conduction toward the spinal cord).

Orthostatic (postural) hypotension: A prolonged drop in blood pressure that accompanies a position change from supine to upright; dizziness or loss of consciousness occurs as a result of decreased venous return and cerebral blood flow.

Oscillopsia: Blurring of the visual environment during head motion.

Oscilloscope: A device for displaying electronic signals on a screen.

Osteoarthritis (OA): The most common rheumatic disease, characterized by the progressive loss of articular cartilage and the formation of bone at the joint margin.

Osteokinematics: Gross, angular motions of bones around a joint axis, such as flexion, extension, abduction, adduction, or rotation.

Osteophytes: Bone growths at joint margins.

Osteoporosis: Condition characterized by a loss of bone mass throughout the skeleton, predisposing patients to fractures.

Osteotomy: Surgical cutting of a bone.

Ototoxic: Having a detrimental effect on cranial nerve VIII or the organs of hearing.

Overload principle: To strengthen muscle, the loads must be greater than normally incurred.

Overwork weakness (injury): A prolonged decrease in absolute strength and endurance due to excessive activity of partially denervated muscle.

Oxygen consumption ($\dot{V}o_2$): The volume of oxygen consumed per unit of time; during aerobic exercise, an accurate reflection of energy expenditure.

Pain: The perception or identification of stimuli as painful.

Pain behavior: Observable actions of an individual in response to their experience of pain and/or suffering.

Pallesthesia: Ability to perceive or to recognize vibratory stimuli.

Pallidotomy: A destructive lesion produced in the basal ganglia (the globus pallidus internus [Gpi]); used to lessen the symptoms of Parkinson's disease.

Pallor: Paleness or absence of coloration in the skin.

Panic attack: Sudden onset of intense apprehension, fear, or discomfort; may include feelings of imminent danger or impending doom.

Pannus: Inflamed synovial granulation tissue seen in rheumatoid arthritis.

Paraplegia: Paralysis of all or part of the trunk and both lower extremities from lesions of the thoracic or lumbar spinal cord or sacral roots.

Paresthesia: Abnormal sensation such as numbness, prickling, or tingling, without apparent cause.

Paroxysmal nocturnal dyspnea (PND): Labored or difficult breathing that awakens a person suddenly from sleep.

Partial-thickness burn: Burn involving the epidermis and part of the dermis. Subcategories are superficial partial-thickness and deep partial-thickness burns, depending on the amount of dermis involved.

Participation: The extent of a person's involvement in life situations in relation to impairments, activities, health condition, and contextual factors. Participation may be restricted in type, duration, and quality.

Parts-to-whole practice: Practice of separate component parts occurs in addition to practice of the integrated whole; useful in acquiring skills with highly independent steps (e.g., transfers).

Passive range of motion (PROM): The amount of joint motion available when a therapist moves the joint through the range without assistance from the patient.

Patronizing: To adopt an air of condescension.

Perception: The process of selection, integration, and interpretation of stimuli from one's own body and the surrounding environment.

Percussion: A force rhythmically applied with the therapist's cupped hands to the patient's thorax; used to promote release of secretions from the wall of the airways.

Percutaneous endoscopic gastrostomy (PEG): A type of gastrostomy tube inserted via endoscopy.

Performance: An observable motor behavior, the result of practice or experience.

Performance-based test: Examination of a particular skill based on observation of an actual attempt, as compared to acceptance of a self-report of skill level.

Perilymphatic fistula (PLF): A rupture of the oval or round windows of the ear, causing an opening between the middle and inner ear.

Peripheral nerve block: A local chemical injection used to block transmission of a motor nerve selectively; used to decrease spasticity.

Peripheral neuropathy: Pathological condition of the peripheral nerves; characterized by muscle weakness, paresthesias, impaired reflexes, and autonomic symptoms.

Peripheral vascular disease (PVD): A general term used to describe any disorder that interferes with arterial or venous blood flow of the extremities.

Peripheral vascular resistance (PVR): The resistance to blood flow; a property primarily of the arterial vascular system.

Perseveration: Abnormal compulsive and inappropriate repetition of words or behaviors; observed in patients with diseases of the frontal lobes of the brain or schizophrenia.

Pes equinus: A foot deformity in which the heel is elevated and the foot is maintained in plantarflexion.

Pes planus: A flattening of the longitudinal arch of the foot; flat foot.

Pes valgus (talipes valgus): A foot deformity in which the heel and foot are turned outward.

Pes varus (talipes varus): A foot deformity in which the heel and foot are turned inward.

Phantom limb: The sensation that a part of the body that has become desensitized or has been amputated is still there.

Phantom pain: Pain originating from the desensitized or amputated body part.

Phobia: An unrelenting, irrational, intense fear of a specific object or situation; associated with a persistent desire to avoid the feared (phobic) stimulus; may interfere with social functioning.

Physical signs: Directly observable or measurable changes in an individual's organs or systems as a result of pathology or disease.

Physiologic cost index (PCI): The difference between walking heart rate and resting heart rate divided by the average walking speed and expressed in beats per meter.

Pitting edema: The indentation to the skin when pressure is applied; a measure of the severity of peripheral edema.

Pity: Sympathetic heartfelt sorrow.

Plan of care (POC): Statements that specify anticipated goals and the expected outcomes; predicted level of optimal improvement; specific interventions with proposed duration and frequency; and anticipated discharge plans.

Polycythemia: A greater than usual amount of circulating red blood cells.

Polymyalgia rheumatica: A rheumatologic illness characterized by muscle pain and stiffness, especially of the shoulder and pelvic girdle muscles, fever, malaise, weight loss, and stiffness.

Polyneuropathy: Any disease that affects multiple peripheral nerves.

Position in space impairment: The inability to perceive and interpret spatial concepts such as up, down, under, over, in, out, in front of, and behind.

Positive sharp waves (EMG): Electrical potentials associated with fibrillating muscle fibers, recorded with electromyography as biphasic, positive-negative action potentials initiated by needle movement and recurring in uniform patterns.

Posterior cord syndrome: A rare incomplete spinal cord injury with primary damage to the posterior cord; characterized by preservation of motor function, sense of pain, and light touch, with loss of proprioception and epicritic sensations below the level of the lesion.

Posttraumatic seizure: Seizure disorder that develops following brain injury.

Postural drainage: Positioning a patient such that the bronchus is perpendicular to the ground and the mucociliary transport of secretions is facilitated.

Postural orientation: The control of relative positions of body parts by skeletal muscles, with respect to each other and gravity.

Postural (static) tremor: Oscillation of the body (usually proximal segments) that occurs when maintained against gravity.

Postural stress syndrome: Discomfort and stress associated with lack of movement, muscle rigidity, faulty posture, and/or ligamentous strain.

Practice: Repeated performance trials.

Preferred practice patterns: The generally accepted elements of patient/client management that physical therapists provide for patients/clients who are classified in these patterns; the pattern title reflects the diagnosis made by the physical therapist.

Prejudice: To prejudge or to classify a person as belonging to a larger group and thus to believe things about that person that one believes about the larger group.

Premorbid: Occurring before a patient became ill or injured.

Pressure autoregulation: Autoregulation of arterioles in response to a decrease in blood flow.

Pressure sore (decubitus ulcer): Damage to the skin or underlying structures as a result of tissue compression and inadequate perfusion.

Preventative intervention: Intervention that is aimed at minimizing potential impairments, functional limitations, and disabilities and maintaining health.

Primary excision: Surgical removal of eschar.

Primary lymphedema: Lymphedema caused by a condition that is congenital or hereditary; lymph node or lymph vessel formation is abnormal.

Problem-oriented medical record (POMR): An organized approach to the patient–treatment documentation process characterized by four phases: (1) formation of a database; (2) identification of a specific problem list; (3) identification of a specific treatment plan; and (4) evaluation of the effectiveness of treatment plans.

Procedural learning: Learning that enables a person to know "how to do" a motor skill or procedure; procedural learning is typically not verbalized.

Procedural memory: See *Motor memory*.

Prognosis: The determination of the predicted optimal level of improvement in function and amount of time needed to reach that level.

Proprioception: The awareness of position sense and posture.

Proprioceptors: Sensory receptors that respond to pressure, position, or stretch; found in muscles, tendons, ligaments, joints, and fascia.

Prosopagnosia: An inability to recognize faces or other visual stimuli as being familiar and distinct from one another.

Protrusio acetabuli: Condition in which the head of the femur pushes the acetabulum into the pelvic cavity.

Proximal latency: The time (in milliseconds) for an action potential to travel from the proximal point of stimulation along a nerve to the recording electrode; used in calculating nerve conduction velocity.

Pseudobulbar affect (emotional dysregulation syndrome): Unstable or changeable emotional state characterized by emotional outbursts of uncontrolled or exaggerated laughing or crying that are inconsistent with mood. The patient quickly changes from laughing to crying with only slight provocation.

Psychological function: Ability to use mental and affective resources effectively relative to the requirements of a particular situation.

Psychomotor retardation: Slow movements that result from depression.

Psychosomatic: Pertaining to the relationship of the brain and body; disorders that have a physiological component but are thought to originate in the psychological and emotional state of the patient.

Pulmonary capillary wedge pressure (PCWP): The pressure within a pulmonary capillary determined by a balloon catheter.

Pulmonary edema: Pulmonary congestion; may be due to an increase in capillary hydrostatic pressure (e.g., left ventricular dysfunction), decreased plasma oncotic pressure, lymphatic insufficiency, altered alveolar–capillary membrane permeability, or other less common causes.

Pulse deficit: The difference between the apical and radial pulses.

Pulse oximetry: Noninvasive method of determining arterial blood oxygenation.

Pulse pressure: The difference between the diastolic and systolic pressures.

Pusher syndrome: See *Ipsilateral pushing*.

Pyrexia: Increased body temperature; fever.

Pyrogens: Fever-producing substances.

Quality of life (QOL): A sense of total well-being that encompasses both physical and psychosocial aspects of an individual's life.

Ramp grade: Degree of inclination or slope of a ramp; 1:12, or 1 in. of threshold height for every 12 in. of ramp length.

Random practice: A practice schedule in which there is no specified order for practicing several motor skills.

Rate pressure product (RPP): An estimation of myocardial oxygen demand; the product of heart rate and systolic blood pressure.

Rating of perceived exertion scale (the Borg RPE Scale): A scale that allows an individual to estimate effort and exertion, breathlessness, and fatigue during physical work; a 15-grade interval scale with grades ranging from 6 (no exertion at all) to 20 (maximum exertion); developed by Gunnar Borg.

Rating of perceived shortness of breath (dyspnea scale): A subjective assessment of shortness of breath as it relates to exercise intensity.

Raynaud's disease: A process initiated by exposure to cold or emotional disturbance, resulting in intermittent episodes of pallor followed by cyanosis, then redness of the digits, before a return to normal; known as Raynaud's phenomenon when describing the condition associated with rheumatic and/or autoimmune disorders such as scleroderma or lupus erythematosus.

Reaction: The response of an organism, or part of it, to a stimulus.

Reaction time (RT): The interval of time between the onset of a stimulus and the initiation of a movement response.

Rebound phenomenon: Normally, when resistance to an isometric contraction is suddenly removed, the body segment forcibly moves a short distance in the direction in which effort was focused before "rebounding" in the opposite direction. Absence of this check reflex is associated with cerebellar disease.

Recovery: The re-acquisition of skills lost through injury or insult.

Redundancy: The recovery of function through use of available back-up or fail-safe systems (pathways) within the CNS; e.g., reliance on somatosensory or vestibular inputs for maintenance of balance in the presence of visual deficits.

Reference of correctness (motor learning): Representation of the ideal performance of a task critical to early cognitive stage learning; achieved through demonstration and modeling.

Reflex: An involuntary response to a stimulus; reflexes are specific and predictable.

Regress: To revert to a more primitive state.

Relaxation response: The sense of calm and well-being attained by using stress management techniques.

Remediation/restorative approaches: Neurotherapeutic approaches that have as their primary focus the use of therapeutic exercises and neuromuscular facilitation techniques to reduce sensorimotor impairments underlying disability and promote functional recovery (e.g., neurodevelopmental treatment [NDT], proprioceptive neuromuscular facilitation [PNF]).

Resistance to contextual change: The adaptability required to perform a motor task in altered environmental situations; ability to "resist" environmental factors from impacting performance.

Respect: The act of giving particular attention to a person; worthy of high regard.

Respiration: The exchange of gas within the body. *External respiration* is the exchange of gas between the alveoli and the pulmonary capillaries. *Internal respiration* is the exchange of gas between the capillary and the tissue.

Response time: The time interval that includes both reaction time and movement time, from onset of stimulus to completion of movement.

Resting tremor: Involuntary oscillatory movements that occur when a body segment is at rest; typically disappears or decreases with purposeful movement.

Restorative rehabilitation: Treatment intervention focused on the improvement of impairments, functional limitations, and disabilities.

Restrictive lung disease: A group of pulmonary disorders characterized by difficulty in expanding the lungs and a reduction in total lung volume.

Retention (motor learning): Persistence of the ability to perform a motor skill; an acquired capability as a result of practice or experience with a task.

Retention test: A performance test of a practiced skill given after a period of no practice (retention interval).

Retinal slip: Visual images fall off the fovea of the retina.

Retraining approach: Intervention that focuses on practice of tasks with particular perceptual requirements that will enhance performance in tasks with similar perceptual demands.

Retrograde amnesia: Loss of memory for events that occurred before a brain insult.

Rheumatism: General term for acute and chronic conditions characterized by inflammation, muscle stiffness and soreness, and joint pain.

Rheumatoid arthritis (RA): A systemic disease characterized by a bilateral, symmetrical pattern of joint involvement and chronic inflammation of the synovium.

Rheumatoid factor (RF): An immunoglobulin found in the blood of a high percentage of adults with rheumatoid arthritis; may be seronegative or positive.

Rhizotomy: Surgical severance of a nerve root; used to relieve pain or reduce spasticity.

Rhythmic auditory stimulation (RAS): The use of a device to impart a steady beat to trigger movements (e.g., metronome, musical listening device).

Right–left discrimination disorder: The inability to identify the right and left sides of one's own body or that of the examiner.

Rigidity (leadpipe): A hypertonic state characterized by increased uniform resistance that persists throughout the whole range of motion and is independent of the velocity of movement; seen in disorders of the basal ganglia.

Risk factors: Behaviors, attributes, or environmental influences that increase the chance of developing impairments, functional limitations, or disability.

Roll (joint): An angular motion between two bony surfaces, similar to the bottom of a rocking chair rolling over the floor. New points on one surface come into contact with new points on the other surface.

Roll-gliding (joint): The combination of a roll and glide. As a roll occurs between two surfaces, one surface slides on the other.

Romberg sign: Inability to maintain standing balance when vision is occluded.

Rotational work: Torque multiplied by the arc of movement.

Rule of nines: Estimation used to determine the amount of total body surface area that has been burned. It divides the body into segments that are approximately 9% of the total.

Sacral sparing: An incomplete spinal cord lesion in which some sacral innervation remains intact; complete loss of motor function and sensation in other areas below the level of the lesion.

Scanning speech: A speech pattern that is slow, and may be slurred, hesitant, with prolonged syllables and inappropriate pauses; the melodic quality of speech is altered.

Schema: An abstract representation or set of rules governing movement formed on the basis of experience and stored in memory.

Schizophrenia: A chronic mental illness characterized by hallucinations, delusions, disorganized speech and behavior, flat affect, and social withdrawal; progressive decrease in overall functioning.

Scleroderma: A chronic disease of unknown etiology that causes a sclerosis or hardening of the skin and other internal organs.

Scoliosis: A lateral curvature of the spine.

Secondary (indirect) impairments: Sequelae or complications occurring in systems other than the system affected by the original pathology or insult; the result of preexisting impairments or expanding multisystem dysfunction.

Selective (focused attention): The capacity to attend to a task despite competing environmental visual or auditory stimuli.

Selective stretching: The application of stretching techniques selectively to improve overall function; some muscles and joints are stretched while motion is limited in other muscles or joints (e.g., tenodesis grasp following spinal cord injury).

Self-efficacy: The belief that an individual will be able to deal with particular situations that may contain novel, unpredictable, and stressful elements.

Self-mutilation: The act of causing physical harm to oneself (e.g., cutting one's own skin, pulling out hair).

Self-transposal: The attempt to put oneself cognitively in the place of the other, to "walk in another person's shoes."

Semirigid dressing: Postoperative dressing made of a semirigid material and designed to contain edema. See also *Unna's dressing*.

Sensation: A feeling or awareness that results from stimulation of the body's sensory receptors and transmission of the nerve impulse along an afferent fiber to the brain.

Sensorimotor strategies (sensory stimulation): An organized application of sensory stimuli from visual, somatosensory, and vestibular systems for coordinating posture and movement.

Sensory integration: The ability of the brain to process and organize disparate information from the different senses and to develop meaningful perceptions to guide adaptive responses (cognitive or motor).

Sensory integration treatment: An approach to perceptual remediation that focuses on offering specific sensory stimulation and carefully controlling the subsequent motor output; influences the way in which the brain organizes and processes sensations.

Sensory level (SCI): Following spinal cord injury, the most caudal segment of the spinal cord with normal sensory function bilaterally.

Serial casting: Repeated application and removal of casts for the purpose of progressively increasing passive range of motion and decreasing tone.

Serial motor skill: A skill involving a series of discrete components.

Serial practice: A practice schedule in which several skills are practiced in a specified and repeating order during the practice session.

Shaking (respiratory): A bouncing maneuver applied to the rib cage throughout the expiratory phase of breathing by the hands of the therapist to assist the mucociliary transport system; promotes release of secretions.

Sharp débridement (wound care): Use of sterile scissors and forceps to remove eschar.

Sharp/dull discrimination: Ability to discriminate between pointed and blunt cutaneous stimuli.

Shear: An applied horizontal force or pressure against the surface and layers of the skin; tissues slide in opposite and parallel directions.

Sheet graft: Autograft that is applied in a single sheet without alteration; may be split-thickness or full-thickness in depth.

Shock (psychological): A sudden mental disorder occurring as a consequence of, or reaction to, emotional trauma or sudden physical injury; overwhelming state of mental and physical depression.

Short-term memory (recent memory): The ability to remember current day-to-day events, learn new information, and retrieve information after an interval of minutes, hours, or days.

Sialorrhea: Excessive saliva; drooling.

Sigh (respiration): A deep inspiration followed by a prolonged, audible expiration; occasional sighs are normal and function to expand alveoli; frequent sighs are abnormal and may be indicative of emotional stress.

Simultanagnosia: The inability to perceive a visual stimulus as a whole; also known as *Balint's syndrome*.

Single motor unit pattern (EMG): An interference pattern recorded on electromyography at maximal effort when single motor unit potentials can still be identified.

Situational exposure exercises: The cognitive–behavioral therapy technique of desensitization where the patient is slowly exposed to anxiety-producing activities that were previously avoided; often used in the treatment of anxiety disorders such as posttraumatic stress disorder and phobias.

Sjögren's syndrome: Disease of the lacrimal and parotid glands, resulting in dry eyes and mouth; frequently occurs with rheumatoid arthritis, systemic lupus erythematosus, and systemic sclerosis.

Skin resistance: The opposition to electrical conduction offered by skin cells and other substances on the skin, usually necessitating some form of skin preparation before application of surface electrodes.

Skin substitutes: Tissues engineered in a laboratory that are used to restore the essential functions of the skin, provide a barrier to the environment, and control evaporative water loss.

SOAP format (subjective, objective, assessment, plan): Progress note format utilized in the problem-oriented medical record; delineation is made among subjective findings, objective examination findings, assessment results, and plan of care.

Social function: Ability to interact successfully with others in the performance of social roles and obligations; includes social interactions, roles, and networks.

Somatoagnosia: Impairment in body scheme; a lack of awareness of the body structure and the relationship of body parts of oneself or of others.

Somatosensation: Sensory information received from peripheral cutaneous, muscle (spindles, Golgi tendon organs), and joint receptors.

Spastic bulbar palsy: Degeneration of the upper motor neurons supplying the muscles innervated by the cranial nerves.

Spasticity: A hypertonic motor disorder characterized by velocity-dependent resistance to passive stretch; the result of an upper motor neuron lesion.

Spatial relations disorder: A constellation of deficits that have in common a difficulty in perceiving the relationship between objects in space, or the relationship between the self and two or more objects; included are disorders of figure–ground discrimination, form discrimination, spatial relations, position in space perception, and topographic orientation.

Spatial summation: Summation of sensory inputs from multiple cells synapsing on the same neuron that results in depolarization and propagation of the nerve signal.

Specificity of training principle: Physiological responses to training are specific to the particular type and velocity of exercise utilized (e.g., isometric, isotonic, isokinetic), specific body segments utilized, and the environmental context in which training occurs.

Speed–accuracy tradeoff: A characteristic of motor skill performance in which speed of performing the movement influences the accuracy of the response (e.g., increasing speed decreases movement accuracy and vice versa); especially evident when learning complex skills.

Spin: The rotation of a surface around a stationary axis. The same point on the moving surface creates an arc of a circle as the surface moves.

Spinal shock: Period immediately following injury to the spinal cord, characterized by absence of all reflex activity, flaccidity, and a loss of sensation below the level of the lesion; generally subsides within 24 hours.

Splayfoot: Transverse spreading of the forefoot.

Splinter skill: A trained or learned skill that is acquired in a manner inconsistent with, or incapable of being integrated with, skills the individual already possesses; not easily generalized to other environments or to variations of the same task.

Split-thickness skin graft: Graft containing epidermis and only the superficial layers of the dermis.

Splitting (psychological): Defense mechanism in which the patient represents things or situations as either very good (because they support his or her desires) or as very bad (because they are obstacles to his or her desires).

Spontaneous potentials (EMG): Action potentials recorded from muscle or nerve at rest after insertion activity has subsided and when there is no voluntary contraction or external stimulus.

Stability (static postural control, static balance): The ability to maintain postural stability and orientation with the center of mass (COM) over the base of support (BOS) and the body at rest.

Starling's length–tension relationship: The force of blood ejected by the heart is determined primarily by the length of the fibers of its muscular wall.

Static–dynamic control: The ability to shift weight onto support segments, freeing a limb for dynamic activities.

Stereognosis: The ability to recognize the shape of objects by touch.

Stereotaxic surgery: Surgical lesioning of the brain.

Stertor: A snoring sound owing to secretions in the trachea and large bronchi (*adj.* stertorous).

Stress reaction: The observable consequences of the stressor; accompanied by sympathetic signs and symptoms such as palpitations, cold sweat, faint feelings, dilated pupils, pallor, fear, and a host of other complaints.

Stridor: A harsh, high-pitched crowing sound that occurs with upper airway obstructions caused by narrowing of the glottis or trachea (e.g., tracheal stenosis, presence of a foreign object).

Stroke (brain attack; cerebrovascular accident [CVA]): Acute onset of neurological dysfunction due to an abnormality in cerebral circulation with signs and symptoms that correspond to involvement of focal areas of the brain.

Stroke volume (SV): The volume of blood ejected from the left ventricle (LV) with each contraction, expressed in mL/min; the difference between LV end diastolic volume and LV end systolic volume.

Stupor: A state of semiconsciousness; the patient lacks responsiveness and can be aroused only by intense stimuli.

Subarachnoid hemorrhage: Rupture and bleeding of a cerebral vessel into the subarachnoid space; may occur spontaneously, the result of an aneurysm or arteriovenous malformation or secondary to trauma.

Subclavian steal syndrome: Shunting of blood, which was destined for the brain, away from the cerebral circulation; occurs when the subclavian artery is occluded. Blood then flows from the opposite vertebral artery across to and down the vertebral artery on the side of the occlusion.

Subdural hematoma: Extravascular blood mass located beneath the dura mater of the brain.

Subluxation: Incomplete or partial dislocation.

Subordinate part (subroutine): Element of movement without which the task cannot proceed safely or efficiently.

Suffering: The subjective valuation placed on the experience of pain; the feeling associated with anticipation of or an actual threat to our well being.

Summary (or additive) measure: Approach to grading a specific series of skills by awarding points for each task or activity; totals the score as a percentage of 100 or as a fraction.

Summed feedback (summary KR): Augmented feedback given after a predetermined set of performance trials is completed.

Superficial (epidermal) burn: Burn involving only the epidermal layer (e.g., sunburn).

Sustained attention (vigilance): The ability to attend to relevant information; sustained attention implies the ability to maintain consistent performance during a continuous activity.

Swan neck deformity: Finger deformity involving hyperextension of the proximal interphalangeal joint and flexion of the distal interphalangeal joint.

Sympathy: Feeling at one with another's feelings.

Symptoms: Subjective evidence of physical abnormality; the reactions to the changes experienced by an individual as a result of pathology or disease.

Synergies (obligatory, stereotyped): Stereotyped, mass movement patterns associated with neurological deficit; movements are primitive, automatic, reflexive, and highly stereotyped; characteristic of patients with stroke in the early and middle stages of recovery.

Synergy (normal): Normal association of functionally linked muscles that are constrained by the CNS to act cooperatively to produce an action; coordinative structures.

Synesthesia: A sensation in one area from a stimulus applied in another location; subjective perception of a sense different from the one applied (e.g., an auditory stimulus perceived as a sensation of smell).

Synovectomy: Surgical procedure to remove the synovial lining of joints or tendon sheaths.

Synovitis: Inflammation of the synovium.

Synovium: Tissue lining synovial joints, tendon sheaths, and bursa. In the joint, it produces fluid to lubricate the joint and is the part of the joint that becomes inflamed in inflammatory joint disease.

Systemic: A condition that affects the body as a whole.

Systemic lupus erythematosus (SLE): Systemic inflammatory disease characterized by small vessel vasculitis and a diverse clinical picture.

Systole: Period during which the ventricles of the heart are contracting.

Systolic pressure: The pressure of the blood during contraction (systole) of the ventricles.

Tachycardia: An abnormally rapid (high) pulse rate; greater than 100 beats per minute in adults.

Tachypnea: An abnormally fast respiratory rate; greater than 24 breaths per minute.

Target heart rate (THR): For a specific patient, the most appropriate heart rate within the prescribed heart rate range to ensure endurance training.

Tarsal tunnel syndrome: Neuropathy of the distal portion of the tibial nerve at the ankle caused by chronic pressure on the nerve at the point it passes through the tarsal tunnel.

Task analysis: The breakdown of an activity or task into its component parts and a delineation of the specific motoric, perceptual, and cognitive abilities that are necessary to perform each component.

Team approach: A widely used approach to inpatient rehabilitation in which a group of professionals provide multidisciplinary interventions; participants typically include a physiatrist, physical therapist, occupational therapist, social worker, speech-language therapist, and a nurse.

Telemetry: Transmission of signals (EMG or ECG) via radiofrequency transmitter and receiver.

Temporal dispersion (NCV): Distortion of duration, amplitude, or shape of the M wave potential in a motor nerve conduction velocity test.

Temporal summation: Summation of potentials from a presynaptic neuron arriving close together in time that results in depolarization and propagation of the nerve signal.

Temporary prosthesis: Prosthesis constructed and aligned like the permanent appliance but cosmetically incomplete.

Tendonitis: Inflammation of a tendon.

Tenodesis: Surgical attachment of a tendon to a bone.

Tetraplegia (quadriplegia): Complete paralysis of all four extremities and trunk, including the respiratory muscles from lesions of the cervical spinal cord.

Thalamotomy: A destructive lesion is produced within the thalamus, the ventral intermediate nucleus (VIN).

Thermanalgesia: Inability to perceive heat.

Thermanesthesia: Inability to perceive sensations of heat and cold.

Thermesthesia: Ability to perceive heat and cold sensations; temperature sensibility.

Thermhyperesthesia: Increased sensitivity to temperature.

Thermhypesthesia: Decreased sensitivity to temperature.

Thigmanesthesia: Loss of light touch sensibility.

Thoracic breathing: A breathing pattern characterized by use of accessory muscles of respiration.

Thrombotic stroke (atherothrombotic brain infarction [ABI]): Formation of a blood clot or thrombus within the cerebral arteries or their branches or the internal carotid or vertebral arteries, causing an occlusion and cerebral infarction; large vessel thrombosis is the most common and is associated with long-standing atherosclerosis.

Thrombus: A blood clot that obstructs a blood vessel or a cavity of the heart.

Tidal volume: Volume or amount of air exchanged with a single breath.

Tone (muscle): The resistance of muscle to passive elongation or stretch.

Topographical disorientation: Difficulty understanding and remembering the relationship of one place to another.

Torque: A force that produces rotation; force multiplied by perpendicular distance from the axis of rotation.

Transcutaneous electrical nerve stimulation (TENS): A physical modality in which electrical impulses are transmitted through the skin, thought to inhibit pain according to the gate control theory.

Transfer of learning: The gain (or loss) of performance in a criterion task as a result of practice or experience with some other task.

Transient ischemic attack (TIA or mini-stroke): Temporary interruption of blood supply to the brain; symptoms of neurological deficit may last for only a few minutes or hours but do not last longer than 24 hours. After the attack no evidence of residual brain damage or neurological damage remains.

Tremor: An involuntary oscillatory movement resulting from alternate contractions of opposing muscle groups. Types include *intention* (kinetic), *postural* (static), and *resting*.

Trendelenburg position: An inclined bed position such that the head of the bed is lower than the foot.

Trigger points: Discrete, focal, hyperirritable spots located in a taut band of skeletal muscle that produce pain locally and in a referred pattern; often accompanies chronic musculoskeletal disorders.

Two-point discrimination: Ability to distinguish two blunt points applied to the skin simultaneously.

Unilateral neglect: The inability to register and to integrate visual stimuli and perceptions from one side of the environment (usually the left), not attributable to sensory-based problems. As a result, the patient ignores stimuli occurring in that side of personal space.

Universal design (life-span design): A structural plan for buildings and dwellings that meet the requirements of all people including those with functional limitations and disability; takes into consideration the needs of a wide range of individuals as well as the changing needs of human beings across the life-span.

Universal goniometer: A device with a central protractor (body) and two extensions (arms) used to measure joint position and motion.

Unna's dressing: A semirigid dressing consisting of gauze impregnated with zinc oxide, gelatin, glycerin, and calamine that is wrapped on the foot and lower limb; used in the management of venous ulcers primarily and occasionally with arterial foot ulcers.

Upper motor neuron (UMN) syndrome: Motor dysfunction observed in patients with lesions of the corticospinal or pyramidal tract in the brain or spinal cord. Characterized by spasticity, abnormal reflex behaviors, loss of precise autonomic control, impaired muscle activation, paresis, decreased dexterity, and fatigability.

Uthoff's symptom: An adverse reaction to heat seen in patients with multiple sclerosis; the effect is usually immediate and dramatic in terms of reduced function and increased fatigue.

Validity: The degree to which an instrument or tool measures what it is designed to measure.

Valsalva maneuver: An attempt to exhale forcibly with the glottis, nose, and mouth closed; causes increased intrathoracic pressure, slowing of the pulse, decreased return of blood to the heart, and increased venous pressure.

Value: An inner force that provides the standards by which patterns of choice are made.

Variable practice: Practice of several variations of the same task or within the same category or class of movements.

Ventilation: The act of moving air in and out of the lungs.

Verbal apraxia (speech apraxia): Impairment of volitional articulatory movement secondary to cortical, dominant hemisphere lesion; manifested in imprecise and awkward articulation, distortion of phoneme production without commensurate pathology to the motor–speech system.

Vertebrobasilar insufficiency (VBI): Ischemia in the area of junction for the vertebral and basilar arteries.

Vertical disorientation: A distorted perception of the upright (vertical) position.

Vertigo: An illusion of movement, a sense of spinning.

Vesicular breath sounds: The normal intensity of a breath sound heard during auscultation of the lungs.

Vicariance: The recovery of function through the utilization of different and underutilized areas of the brain.

Visual (linear) analog scale: A measurement scale in which a horizontal or vertical straight line is labeled with descriptive or numeric terms to anchor the extremes of the scale; the individual is asked to bisect the line at a point representing self-reported position on the scale.

Visual fixation: The ability to maintain focus on an object as it is brought closer to and farther away from the eyes.

Visual object agnosia: The inability to recognize familiar objects despite normal function of the eyes and optic tracts.

Visual proprioception: Detection of the relative orientation of the body parts and orientation of the body in space by the visual system; provides a basis for movement control.

Vital capacity (VC): The greatest volume of air that can be exhaled from a full inspiration, or the greatest volume of air that can be inhaled from a full exhalation.

Vital signs (cardinal signs): The signs of life; that is, pulse, body temperature, respiration, and blood pressure.

Volume conduction: Spread of current from a potential source through a conducting medium, such as body tissues.

Walking velocity: The rate of linear forward motion of the body; measured in either centimeters per second or meters per minute. Walking velocity = distance/time.

Wheeze: A musical adventitious sound heard during lung auscultation when expired air is forced through a narrowed airway.

Withdrawal: Symptoms that accompany cessation of alcohol, amphetamines, sedatives, opioids, cocaine, hypnotics, or anxiolytics that have been abused over a period of time; withdrawal symptoms differ with the substance abused and are usually the opposite of the symptoms of intoxication, but may also include perspiration, agitation, and physical pain.

Work: The application of a force through a distance; accomplished whenever a force moves an object through a distance; the product of force and distance.

Wound contraction: Movement of the wound margins toward the center of the defect; thought to be caused by the active movement of the fibroblasts in the wound bed.

Xenograft (or heterograft): Skin used as a temporary wound cover, which is harvested from another species of animal, usually a pig.

Zigzag effect: Ulnar drift at the metacarpophalangeal joints associated with radial deviation of the wrist.

Zone of partial preservation: Following spinal cord injury, areas of intact motor and/or sensory function below the neurological level, but no function at S4 and S5.

Z-plasty: Procedure used to surgically lengthen a burn scar or contracture to allow for greater range of motion.

Some definitions from: American Physical Therapy Association: Guide to Physical Therapist Practice, ed 2. Alexandria, VA, 2001.

Index

Note: Illustrations are indicated by *(f)*; tables by *(t)*; boxes by *(b)*.

A

B

C

D

H

M

S

T

U

V

W

X

Y

Z